SPINE

VOLUME ONE

Second Edition

SURGERY

Techniques, Complication Avoidance, and Management

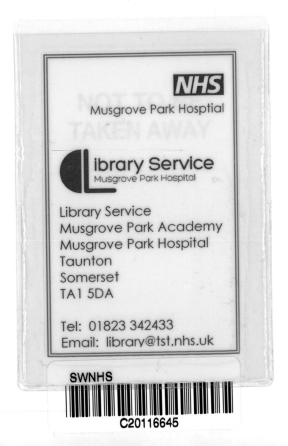

SPINE

VOLUME ONE

Second Edition

SURGERY

Techniques, Complication Avoidance, and Management

EDWARD C. BENZEL, MD

Chairman, Cleveland Clinic Spine Institute
Vice Chairman, Department of Neurosurgery
The Cleveland Clinic Foundation
Cleveland, Ohio

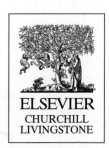

ELSEVIER
CHURCHILL
LIVINGSTONE

ELSEVIER
CHURCHILL
LIVINGSTONE

The Curtis Center
170 S Independence Mall W 300E
Philadelphia, Pennsylvania 19106

SPINE SURGERY: TECHNIQUES, COMPLICATION AVOIDANCE,   ISBN 0-443-06616-7
AND MANAGEMENT
Copyright 2005, Elsevier, Inc. All rights reserved.

First edition 1999.

Library of Congress Cataloging-in-Publication Data

Spine surgery: techniques, complication avoidance, and management / [edited by] Edward
C. Benzel.– 2nd ed.
   p. ; cm.
   Includes bibliographical references and index.
   ISBN 0-443-06616-7
     1. Spine–Surgery. I. Benzel, Edward C.
   [DNLM: 1. Spinal Diseases–surgery. 2. Spinal Diseases–complications.
   3. Spine–surgery. WE 725 S7599 2005]
   RD768.S684 2005
   617.5′6059–dc22   2004045517

Acquisitions Editor: *Rebecca Schmidt Gaertner*
Developmental Editor: *Agnes Hunt Byrne*
Publishing Services Manager: *Joan Sinclair*
Project Manager: *Daniel Clipner*

Printed in the United States of America.

Last digit is the print number: 9 8 7 6 5 4 3 2 1

This book is dedicated to my wife, Mary; my children, Morgan, Jason, Brian, and Matthew; and my mother and father, Anna and Carl, for their past and present encouragement, tolerance, and guidance.

A special thanks to Christine Moore for her energy, diligence, and effort, as well as her continued and perpetual commitment to this project; to all the contributors for their masterful "works" and for the privilege of their friendships, both new and old; and to prior residents and fellows, who have provided energy, encouragement, and guidance.

Contributors

Mark F. Abel, MD
Professor, Department of Orthopedics, University of Virginia School of Medicine, Charlottesville, Virginia

Kuniyoshi Abumi, MD, Dr Med Sci
Professor, Department of Orthopaedic Surgery, Health Administration Center, Hokkaido University, Sapporo, Japan

Mark S. Adams, MD
Saginaw Valley Neurosurgery, Saginaw, Michiga

Cary D. Alberstone, MD
Ventura County Neurosurgery Associates, Oxnard, California

Joseph T. Alexander, MD
Assistant Professor, Department of Neurosurgery, Wake Forest University School of Medicine, Winston-Salem, North Carolina

John A. Anson, MD, FACS
Las Vegas, Nevada

Ronald I. Apfelbaum, MD
Professor of Neurosurgery, Department of Neurosurgery, University of Utah Health Sciences Center, Salt Lake City, Utah

Paul M. Arnold, MD
Professor of Neurosurgery, Department of Surgery, University of Kansas Medical Center, Kansas City, Kansas

L. Brett Babat, MD
Premier Orthopaedics and Sports Medicine, Nashville, Tennessee

Julian E. Bailes, MD
Professor and Chairman, Department of Neurosurgery, West Virginia University, Morgantown, West Virginia

Jamie Baisden, MD
Assistant Professor of Neurosurgery, Medical College of Wisconsin, Milwaukee, Wisconsin

Nevan G. Baldwin, MD, FACS
Clinical Associate Professor, Texas Tech University, Lubbock, Texas

Perry A. Ball, MD
Dartmouth-Hitchcock Medical Center, Lebanon, New Hampshire

Giancarlo Barolat, MD
Thomas Jefferson University Hospital, Philadelphia, Pennsylvania

H. Hunt Batjer, MD
Department of Neurosurgery, Northwestern University Medical School, Chicago, Illinois

Thomas W. Bauer, MD, PhD
Departments of Orthopaedic Surgery and Pathology, The Cleveland Clinic Foundation, Cleveland, Ohio

James R. Bean, MD
Neurosurgical Associates, Lexington, Kentucky

Brion J. Beerle, MD
Chair, Department of Anesthesiology, Alaska Regional Hospital, Anchorage, Alaska

Gordon R. Bell, MD
The Cleveland Clinic Foundation, Cleveland, Ohio
Cleveland Clinic Spine Institute

Gregory J. Bennett, MD
Clinical Director-Neurosurgery, Erie County Medical Center, Buffalo, New York

Edward C. Benzel, MD
Chairman, Cleveland Clinic Spine Institute,
Vice Chairman, Department of Neurosurgery,
The Cleveland Clinic Foundation, Cleveland, Ohio

Darren Bergey, MD
Loma Linda University Medical Center, Loma Linda, California

Marc L. Bertrand, MD
Assistant Professor and Director, Neuroanesthesia, Department of Anesthesiology, Dartmouth-Hitchcock Medical Center, Lebanon, New Hampshire

Mark H. Bilsky, MD
Memorial Sloan Kettering Cancer Center, New York, New York

Barry D. Birch, MD
Department of Neurosurgery, Mayo Clinic Scottsdale, Scottsdale, Arizona

Robert S. Biscup, MS, DO, FAOAO
Cleveland Clinic Florida Spine Center, Weston, Florida

Kevin Blaylock, CPA
CFO, Neuroscience Specialists, CEO, Oklahoma Spine Hospital, LLC, Oklahoma City, Oklahoma

Oheneba Boachie-Adjei, MD
Hospital for Special Surgery, New York, New York

Maxwell Boakye, MD
Assistant Professor of Neurosurgery,
Stanford School of Medicine, Stanford, California

Scott D. Boden, MD
Professor of Orthopaedics, Director, The Emory Spine
Center, Emory University School of Medicine, Atlanta,
Georgia

Henry Bohlman, MD
Professor, Case Western Reserve University and
University Hospitals, Cleveland, Ohio

Michael Bolesta, MD
Associate Professor, Department of Orthopedics,
Southwestern Medical School, Dallas, Texas

Mary B. Bondy, MBA
Cleveland Clinic Spine Institute, The Cleveland Clinic
Foundation, Cleveland, Ohio

Christopher M. Boxell, MD
Oklahoma Spine & Brain Institute, Tulsar, Oklahoma

Keith H. Bridwell, MD
Washington University School of Medicine, St. Louis,
Missouri

Darrell S. Brodke, MD
Associate Professor, Department of Orthopedics,
Director, Spine Service, University of Utah, Salt Lake
City, Utah

James Butler, MD
Resident, Department of Neurosurgery, The Cleveland
Clinic Foundation, Cleveland, Ohio

David W. Cahill, MD (deceased)
Department of Neurosurgery, College of Medicine,
University of South Florida, Tampa, Florida

Robert C. Cantu, MA, MD, FACS, FACSM
Chief, Neurosurgery Service and Director, Service
Sports Medicine, Emerson Hospital, Concord,
Massachusetts; Adjunct Professor, Exercise and Sport
Science, University of North Carolina, Chapel Hill,
North Carolina

Allen L. Carl, MD
Professor, Division of Orthopaedic Surgery, Albany
Medical College, Albany, New York

John A. Carrino, MD, MPH
Assistant Professor of Radiology, Harvard Medical
School, Clinical Director, Magnetic Resonance Therapy
Program, Co-Director, Spine Intervention Service,
Boston, Massachusetts

John R. Caruso, MD
Neurosurgical Specialists, LLC, Hagerstown, Maryland

Andrew G. Chenelle, MD, MS
DuPage Neurosurgery, S.C., Glen Ellyn, Illinois

Joseph S. Cheng, MD
Assistant Professor and Co-Director, Section of Spinal
Surgery, Department of Neurosurgery, Vanderbilt
Medical Center North, Nashville, Tennessee

Yong-Jun Cho, MD
Department of Neurosurgery, Stanford University,
Stanford, California

Tanvir F. Choudhri, MD
Assistant Professor and Director, Neurosurgery Spine
Program, Department of Neurosurgery, Mount Sinai
Medical Center, New York, New York

Frank Conguista, MD
Resident, Division of Orthopaedic Surgery, Albany
Medical College, Albany, New York

Edward S. Connolly, MD
Professor of Neurosurgery, Ochsner Clinic Foundation,
Louisiana State University School of Medicine, New
Orleans, Louisiana

Paul R. Cooper, MD
Professor of Neurosurgery, New York University School
of Medicine, New York, New York

Jean-Valéry C.E. Coumans, MD
Department of Neurosurgery, Massachusetts General
Hospital, Boston, Massachusetts

Albert E. Cram, MD
Professor, Department of Neurosurgery, University of
Iowa Hospitals and Clinics, Iowa City, Iowa

H. Alan Crockard, MD
The National Hospital for Neurology and Neurosurgery,
London, United Kingdom

Richard Crownover, MD
The Cleveland Clinic Foundation, Cleveland,
Ohio

Bryan W. Cunningham, MD
Director, Biomechanics Laboratory, Union Memorial
Hospital, Baltimore, Maryland

William T. Curry, Jr, MD
Department of Neurosurgery, Massachusetts General
Hospital, Boston, Massachusetts

Joseph F. Cusick, MD
Professor, Medical College of Wisconsin, Madison,
Wisconsin

Scott D. Daffner, MD
Thomas Jefferson University, Philadelphia,
Pennsylvania

Mark D. D'Alise, MD, FACS
Neurosurgical Associates, Complex and Reconstructive Spinal Surgery, Lubbock, Texas

Vinay Deshmukh, MD
Carolina Neurosurgery and Spine, Charlotte, North Carolina

Denis DiAngelo, MD
Associate Professor, School of Biomechanical Engineering, University of Tennessee Health Science Center, Memphis, Tennessee

Curtis A. Dickman, MD
Associate Chief, Spine Section, Director, Spinal Research, Division of Neurological Surgery, Barrow Neurosurgical Associates, Phoenix, Arizona

Thomas B. Ducker, MD
Maryland Neurological Institute, Annapolis, Maryland

Scott T. Dull, MD, FACS
Neurosurgical Network, Toledo, Ohio

Stewart B. Dunsker, MD
Emeritus Faculty, Mayfield Clinic and Spine Institute, Cincinnati, Ohio

Michael J. Ebersold, MD
Professor of Neurosurgery, Mayo Clinic College of Medicine, Department of Neurologic Surgery, Luther Middlefort Clinic—Mayo Health System, Eau Claire, Wisconsin

Jason Eckhardt
Spine Research Laboratory, The Cleveland Clinic Foundation, Cleveland, Ohio

Bruce L. Ehni, MD
Neurosurgical Group of Texas; and Clinical Associate Professor, Baylor College of Medicine, Houston, Texas

Matthew Eichenbaum, MD
Spine Research Fellow, Department of Orthopaedic Surgery, Thomas Jefferson University and the Rothman Institute, Philadelphia, Pennsylvania

Kurt M. Eichholz, MD
Resident, Department of Neurosurgery, University of Iowa, Iowa City, Iowa

Marc E. Eichler, MD
Division of Spine Surgery, Department of Neurosurgery, Brigham and Women's Hospital, Boston, Massachusetts

Samer K. Elbabaa, MD
Resident, Division of Neurosurgery, Department of Surgery, University of North Carolina at Chapel Hill, Chapel Hill, North Carolina

Sanford E. Emery, MD, MBA
Professor and Chairman, Department of Orthopaedics, West Virginia University, Morgantown, West Virginia

Nancy E. Epstein, MD
Clinical Professor of Neurological Surgery, The Albert Einstein College of Medicine, Bronx; Attending in Neurosurgery, Winthrop University Hospital, Mineola; and The North Shore-Long Island Jewish Health System, Manhasset, New York

Jennifer Erdos, MD
Resident in Orthopedic Surgery, Allegheny General Hospital, Pittsburgh, Pennsylvania

Thomas J. Errico, MD
Associate Professor of Orthopedic and Neurologic Surgery, New York University School of Medicine, Chief of the Spine Service, Department of Orthopedic Surgery, NYU/Hospital for Joint Diseases, New York, New York

Tom Faciszewski, MD
Chairman, Department of Orthopedic Spine Surgery, Marshfield Clinic, Marshfield, Wisconsin

Michael G. Fehlings, MD, PhD, FRCS(C)
Professor of Neurosurgery, Krembil Chair in Neurological Repair and Regeneration, University of Toronto; Director Krembil Neuroscience Program, Heed Spinal Program, Toronto Western Hospital, University Health Network, Toronto, Ontario, Canada

Lisa A. Ferrara, MS, PhDc
Spine Research Laboratory, The Cleveland Clinic Foundation, Cleveland, Ohio

Richard G. Fessler, MD, PhD
Professor and Chairman, Section of Neurological Surgery, University of Chicago Hospital, Chicago, Illinois

Kevin T. Foley, MD
Associate Professor, Neurosurgery, University of Tennessee, Memphis, Tennessee

Robert M. Galler, DO
Assistant Professor of Neurosurgery, Stony Brook University Medical Center, Stony Brook, New York

John W. German, MD
Albany Medical College, Department of Neurosurgery, Albany, New York

Alexander J. Ghanayem, MD
Associate Professor and Chief, Division of Spine Surgery, Department of Orthpaedic Surgery, Loyola University Medical Center, Maywood, Illinois

Zoher Ghogawala, MD
Assistant Clinical Professor of Neurosurgery, Yale
University School of Medicine, New Haven,
Connecticut

Vijay K. Goel, PhD
Professor and Chair, Department of Bioengineering,
University of Toledo, Director, Spine Research Center,
Department of Orthopedics, Medical College of Ohio,
Toledo, Ohio

Jan Goffin, MD, PhD
Department of Neurosurgery, Catholic University of
Leuven, University Hospital Gasthuisberg, Leuven,
Belgium

Ziya L. Gokaslan, MD
Professor of Neurosurgery, Johns Hopkins University,
Baltimore, Maryland

Sohrab Gollogly
University of Utah, Salt Lake City, Utah

Jorge Gonzalez-Martinez, MD
Resident, Department of Neurosurgery, The Cleveland
Clinic Foundation, Cleveland, Ohio

James E. Greensmith, MD, PhD
Department of Anesthesia, Saint Elizabeth Hospital,
Appleton, Wisconsin

Jeffrey D. Gross, MD
Comprehensive Spine and Wellness Center, Ladera
Ranch, California

Regis W. Haid, Jr, MD
Atlanta Brain and Spine Care, Atlanta, Georgia

Andrea L. Halliday MD, PA
Center for Neurological Disorders, Fort Worth Brain
and Spine Institute, Fort Worth, Texas

Allan J. Hamilton, MD
Head of Surgery, University of Arizona Health Sciences
Center, Tucson, Arizona

Fadi Hanbali, MD
Assistant Professor of Neurosurgery, University of Texas
Medical Branch, Galveston, Texas

Jürgen Harms, MD
Center for Spine Surgery, Department of Orthopedics
and Traumatology, Klinikum Karlsbad-Langensteinbach,
Karlsbad-Langensteinbach, Germany

James S. Harrop, MD
Assistant Professor, Division of Spinal Surgery,
Department of Neurosurgery, Neurosurgical Director,
Delaware Valley Spinal Cord Injury Center, Thomas
Jefferson University, Philadelphia, Pennsylvania

Blaine I. Hart, MD
Professor, Department of Radiology, University of
New Mexico School of Medicine, Albuquerque,
New Mexico

Robert A. Hart, MD, MA
Chief, Spine Section, Assistant Professor, Department
of Orthopaedic Surgery, Oregon Health and Science
University, Portland Shriner's Hospital, Portland, Oregon

Robert F. Heary, MD
Associate Professor of Neurological Surgery, University
of Medicine and Dentistry-New Jersey, New Jersey
Medical School; Director, The Spine Center of New
Jersey, Neurological Institute of New Jersey, Newark,
New Jersey

Fraser C. Henderson, MD
Associate Professor of Neurosurgery, Director of
Neurosurgery of the Spine and Craniocervical Junction,
Georgetown University Medical Center, Washington, D.C.

Patrick W. Hitchon, MD
Professor, Department of Neurosurgery, University of
Iowa Hospitals and Clinics, Iowa City, Iowa

James P. Hollowell, MD
Integrated Spine Care, Milwaukee, Wisconsin

Paul J. Holman, MD
Department of Neurosurgery, Cleveland Clinic
Foundation, Cleveland, Ohio

John K. Houten, MD
Associate Professor, Department of Neurological Surgery,
Montefiore Hospital, Albert Einstein/Jaboni Hospital,
Bronx, New York

Robert E. Isaacs, MD
Head, Section of Minimally Invasive Spine Surgery,
Cleveland Clinic Florida Spine Institute, Weston, Florida

Manabu Ito, MD, Dr Med Sci
Assistant Professor, Department of Orthpaedic Surgery,
Hokkaido University Graduate School of Medicine,
Sapporo, Japan

John A. Jane, Jr, MD
Department of Neurological Surgery, University of
Virginia, Charlottesville, Virginia

J. Patrick Johnson, MD
Co-Director, Cedars-Sinai Institute for Spinal Disorders,
Los Angeles, California

Christopher Kager, MD
Lancaster Neuroscience and Spine Association,
Lancaster, Pennsylvania

Iain H. Kalfas, MD
Head, Section of Spinal Surgery, Department of Neurosurgery, Cleveland Clinic Foundation, Cleveland, Ohio

George J. Kaptain, MD
Loma Linda University Medical Center, Loma Linda, California

Saad Khairi, MD
Spine Fellow, Cedars-Sinai Institute for Spinal Disorders, Los Angeles, California

Daniel H. Kim, MD
Associate Professor and Director, Spinal and Peripheral Nerve Surgery, Depatment of Neurosurgery, Stanford University Medical School, Stanford, California

David H. Kim, MD
Attending Spinal Surgeon, The Boston Spine Group, Boston, Massachusetts

Thomas A. Kopitnik, Jr., MD
University of Texas Southwestern Medical Center at Dallas, Dallas, Texas

Robert J. Kowalski, MD, MS, PE
Resident, Department of Neurosurgery, The Cleveland Clinic Foundation, Cleveland, Ohio

Ajit A. Krishnaney, MD
Department of Neurosurgery, Cleveland Clinic Foundation, Cleveland, Ohio

John A. Lancon, MD
Associate Professor of Neurosurgery and Pediatrics, Blair E. Batson Hospital for Children, The University of Mississippi Medical Center, Jackson, Mississippi

Giuseppe Lanzino, MD
Associate Professor, Department of Neurosurgery, University of Illinois College of Medicine at Peoria, Peoria, Illinois

Sanford J. Larson, MD, PhD
Medical College of Wisconsin, Department of Neurosurgery, Milwaukee, Wisconsin

Jorge Lastra-Power, MD
Assistant Professor, Neurosurgery Section, University of Puerto Rico, San Juan, Puerto Rico

Nathan H. Lebwohl, MD
Voluntary Associate Professor, Clinical Orthopaedics and Rehabilitation University of Miami School of Medicine, Miami, Florida

Isador H. Lieberman, MD, MBA, FRCS(C)
Department of Orthopaedics and The Cleveland Clinic Spine Institute, The Cleveland Clinic Foundation, Cleveland, Ohio

Donlin M. Long, MD
Johns Hopkins University Medical School, Baltimore, Maryland

Mark G. Luciano, MD, PhD
Head, Section of Pediatric and Congenital Neurosurgery, Department of Neurological Surgery, The Cleveland Clinic Foundation, Cleveland, Ohio

Charles A. Luevano, BS
Component Reliability Development, General Motors Corp., Milford, Michigan

Parley M. Madsen III, MD, PhD
Microsurgery and Brain Research Institute, St. Louis, Missouri

Dennis J. Maiman, MD, PhD
Professor of Neurosurgery, Medical College of Wisconsin and Clement J Zablocki VA Medical Center, Milwaukee, Wisconsin

Jacek M. Malik, MD, PhD
Peninsula Neurosurgical Associates, Salisbury, Maryland

David G. Malone, MD
Oklahoma Spine & Brain Institute, Tulsa, Oklahoma

Joseph C. Maroon, MD
Clinical Professor and Vice Chairman, Department of Neurosurgery, University of Pittsburgh Medical Center, Pittsburgh, Pennsylvania

Eric M. Massicotte, MD, MSc, FRCS(C)
Assistant Professor of Neurosurgery, University of Toronto, Toronto, Ontario, Canada

Shunji Matsunaga, MD
Assistant Professor, Department of Orthopedic Surgery, Kagoshima Graduate School of Medical and Dental Sciences, Kagoshima, Japan

Daniel J. Mazanec, MD, FACP
Vice Chairman, Cleveland Clinic Spine Institute, The Cleveland Clinic Foundation; and Associate Professor of Medicine, Cleveland Clinic Lerner College of Medicine, Cleveland, Ohio

Paul C. McAfee, MD
Chief of Spine Surgery, St. Joseph's Hospital, Baltimore, Maryland

Bruce M. McCormack, MD
Clinical Faculty, University of California San Francisco Medical Center, San Francisco, California

Paul C. McCormick, MD, MPH
Professor of Clinical Neurosurgery, Columbia University College of Physicians and Surgeons, New York, New York

William E. McCormick, MD
Schwartzapfel Novick, West Islip, New York

Robert A. McGuire, Jr., MD
University of Mississippi Medical Center, Jackson,
Mississippi

Robert F. McLain, MD
The Cleveland Clinic Spine Institute, The Cleveland
Clinic Foundation, Cleveland, Ohio

Nagy Mekhail, MD, PhD
The Cleveland Clinic Foundation, Cleveland, Ohio

D. Mark Melton, MD
Resident, Department of Neurosurgery, College of
Medicine, University of South Florida, Tampa,
Florida

Carole A. Miller, MD
Ohio State University, Department of Neurological
Surgery, Columbus, Ohio

Jared H. Miller, BA
Case Western Reserve University, Cleveland, Ohio

Sung Min, MD
The Cleveland Clinic Foundation, Cleveland, Ohio

William Mitchell, MD
Attending Neurosurgeon, JFK Medical Center, Edison,
New Jersey

Junichi Mizuno, MD, PhD
Associate Professor, Department of Neurological Surgery,
Aichi Medical University School of Medicine, Aichi,
Japan

Michael T. Modic, MD
The Cleveland Clinic Foundation, Cleveland, Ohio

Howard W. Morgan, Jr, MD
University of Texas, Southwestern Medical School,
Dallas, Texas

Robert J. Morlock, PhD
Pfizer Incorporated, Worldwide Outcomes Research,
Ann Arbor, Michigan

Michael A. Morone, MD, PhD
Deaconess Billings Clinic, Billings, Montana

Wade M. Mueller, MD
Assistant Professor of Neurosurgery, Medical College
of Wisconsin, Madison, Wisconsin

Praveen V. Mummaneni, MD
Assistant Professor, Department of Neurological Surgery,
Emory University School of Medicine, Atlanta, Georgia

John S. Myseros, MD
Assistant Professor, Division of Neurosurgery, Cincinnati
College of Medicine, Staff Pediatric Neurosurgeon,
Cincinnati Children's Hospital

Sait Naderi, MD
Associate Professor, Department of Neurosurgery, Dokuz
Eylul University, Izmir, Turkey

Dileep Nair, MD
The Cleveland Clinic Foundation, Cleveland, Ohio

Hiroshi Nakagawa, MD, PhD
Professor and Chairman, Department of Neurological
Surgery, Aichi Medical University School of Medicine,
Aichi, Japan

Jaime H. Nieto, MD
Divisions of Neurosurgery and Orthopedic Surgery,
Maimonides Medical Center, Brooklyn, New York

Russ P. Nockels, MD
Associate Professor, Neurological Surgery, Orthopaedic
Surgery and Rehabilitation, Loyola University Medical
Center, Maywood, Illinois

Bruce E. Northrup, MD
Professor Emeritus, Department of Neurosurgery,
Thomas Jefferson University, Philadelphia, Pennsylvania

Chima Ohaegbulam, MD
Resident, Department of Neurosurgery, Brigham and
Women's Hospital, Harvard Medical School, Boston,
Massachusetts

Tunc Oktenoglu, MD
VKV Amerikan Hastanesi, Nisantasi, Istanbul, Turkey

Bernardo Jose Ordonez, MD
Neurosurgical Associates, Norfolk, Virginia

Jeffrey H. Owen, PhD
Sentient Medical Systems, Cockeysville, Maryland

A. Fahir Özer, MD
American Hospital, Istanbul, Turkey

Stephen M. Papadopoulos, MD
Director of Surgical Navigation, Barrow Neurosurgical
Institute, Phoenix, Arizona

Christopher G. Paramore, MD
Lake Norman Neurological and Spine Surgery,
Mooresville, North Carolina

Robert S. Pashman, MD
Director, Scoliosis and Spinal Deformity, Cedars-Sinai
Institute for Spinal Disorders, Los Angeles, California

Warwick J. Peacock, MD
Professor Emeritus, Department of Neurosurgery,
University of California, San Francisco, San Francisco,
California

Stanley Pelofsky, MD
Neuroscience Specialists, Oklahoma City, Oklahoma

Noel I. Perin, MD, FRCS, FACS
Clinical Associate Professor, Department of
Neurosurgery, St. Luke's/Roosevelt Hospital Center,
New York, New York

Christopher J. Pham, DO
Department of Neurosurgery, Stanford University
Hospital School, Stanford, California

Rick J. Placide, MD, PT
West End Orthopaedic Clinic, Richmond, Virginia

Branko Prpa, MD
All Saints Healthcare, Racine, Wisconsin

Gregory J. Przybylski, MD
John F. Kennedy Medical Center, Edison, New Jersey

Ashraf A. Ragab, MD
University of Mississippi Medical Center, Jackson,
Mississippi

Y. Raja Rampersaud, MD, FRCS(C)
Assistant Professor, Division Orthopedic Surgery,
University of Toronto; Spinal Program, Krambil
Neuroscience Center, Toronto Western Hospital,
University Health Network, Toronto, Ontario, Canada

Peter A. Rasmussen, MD
Department of Neurosurgery, The Cleveland Clinic
Foundation, Cleveland, Ohio

Richard B. Raynor, MD
Clinical Professor of Neurosurgery, New York University
School of Medicine, New York, New York

Gary L. Rea, MD, PhD
Department of Orthopaedics, Ohio State University
Hospital East, Columbus, Ohio

Glenn R. Rechtine, MD
Dunspaugh-Dalton Professor of Spinal Surgery,
Department of Neurosurgery, University of Florida,
Gainesville, Florida

John Regan, MD
Medical Director, Institute for Spinal Disorders,
Cedars-Sinai Medical Center, Los Angeles, California

Setti S. Rengachary, MD
Associate Chairman and Professor, Department of
Neurological Surgery, Wayne State University, Detroit
Medical Center, Detroit, Michigan

Daniel K. Resnick, MD
Associate Professor, Department of Neurosurgery,
University of Wisconsin Medical School, Madison,
Wisconsin

Laurence D. Rhines, MD
Assistant Professor and Director, Spine Program,
Department of Neurosurgery, University of Texas MD
Anderson Cancer Center, Houston, Texas

Albert J. Rhoton, MD
Chairman Emeritus, Department of Neurosurgery,
University of Florida – Gainesville, Gainesville, Florida

Donna J. Rodriguez, MS, RD, CNSD
Former Visiting Professor/Lecturer, College of
Education, Nutrition/Dietetics Program, University of
New Mexico; Professional Healthcare Writer, Lovelace
Healthcare Innovations, Lovelace Health Systems,
Albuquerque, New Mexico

Gerald E. Rodts, Jr, MD
Associate Professor and Director of Neurosurgery Spine,
Department of Neurological Surgery, Emory University,
Atlanta, Georgia

Michael J. Rosner, MD
Department of Neurosurgery, Walter Reed Army
Medical Center, Washington, DC

Alexander Sah, MD
Resident, Harvard Medical School Combined
Orthopedic Residency Program, Boston, Massachusetts

Jared P. Salinsky, DO
Resident, Department of Orthopedic Surgery,
NSUCOM/Parkway Regional Medical Center, North
Miami Beach, Florida

Paul Santiago, MD
Assistant Professor, Department of Neurological Surgery,
Washington University School of Medicine, St. Louis,
Missouri

Mehdi Sarkarati, MD
Assistant Clinical Professor, Department of Physical
Medicine and Rehabilitation Tufts University School of
Medicine, Healthsouth N.E. Rehabilitation Hospital,
Woburn, Massachusetts

Richard L. Saunders, MD
Professor Emeritus of Surgery, Dartmouth-Hitchcock
Medical Center, Lebanon, New Hampshire

Paul D. Sawin, MD
Orlando Neurosurgery, Orlando, Florida

Edward H. Scheid, MD
Senior Resident, Thomas Jefferson University,
Department of Neurosurgery, Philadelphia,
Pennsylvania

Meic H. Schmidt, MD
Assistant Professor and Director, Spinal Oncology,
Department of Neurosurgery, University of Utah
Medical Center, Salt Lake City, Utah

Michael Schneier, MD
Neurological Surgery, Philadelphia, Pennsylvania

Dilip K. Sengupta, MD, Dr Med
Professor, Department of Orthopaedics, Dartmouth-
Hitchcock Medical Center, Lebanon, New Hampshire

Christopher I. Shaffrey, MD
Professor, Department of Neurological Surgery,
University of Virginia School of Medicine,
Charlottesville, Virginia

Mark E. Shaffrey, MD
Department of Neurosurgery, University of Virginia
Health System, Charlottesville, Virginia

Alok D. Sharan, MD
Albany Medical College, Albany, New York

Ashwini D. Sharan, MD
Assistant Professor, Department of Neurosurgery,
Thomas Jefferson University, Philadelphia, Pennsylvania

Christopher B. Shields, MD, FRCS(C)
Professor and Norton Hospital Chairman, Department
of Neurological Surgery, University of Louisville,
Louisville, Kentucky

Frederick A. Simeone, MD
Department of Neurosurgery, Thomas Jefferson
University, Philadelphia, Pennsylvania

Kern Singh, MD
Department of Orthopedic Surgery, Rush Presbyterian
St. Luke's Medical Center, Chicago, Illinois

Ran Vijai P. Singh, MD
Neurological Associates, Norfolk, Virginia

Donald A. Smith, MD
Associate Professor, Department of Neurosurgery,
College of Medicine, University of South Florida,
Tampa, Florida

Maurice M. Smith, MD
Semmes-Murphey Clinic, Germantown, Tennessee

Volker K.H. Sonntag, MD, FACS
Vice Chairman and Chief, Spine Section, Division of
Neurological Surgery; Barrow Neurosurgical Associates;
and Director, Residency Program, University of Arizona,
Phoenix, Arizona

Ivan J. Sosa, MD
Chief Resident, Neurosurgery Section, University
of Puerto Rico, San Juan, Puerto Rico

Micheal J. Speck, MD
The Cleveland Clinic Spine Institute, The Cleveland
Clinic Foundation, Cleveland, Ohio

Robert F. Spetzler, MD
Director, Department of Neurosurgery, Barrow
Neurological Institute, Phoenix, Arizona

Sudhakar T. Sridharan, MD
Research Director, Department of Rheumatic and
Immunologic Diseases, The Cleveland Clinic
Foundation, Cleveland, Ohio

Loretta A. Staudt, MS, PT
University of California Los Angeles, Los Angeles,
California

Michael P. Steinmetz, MD
Resident, Department of Neurosurgery, The Cleveland
Clinic Foundation, Cleveland, Ohio

Charles B. Stillerman, MD
Clinical Professor of Surgery, University of North Dakota
School of Medicine, Minot, North Dakota

Kota Suda, MD, Dr Med Sci
Spine Surgeon, Center for Spinal Injury and Disorder,
Bibai Rosai Hospital, Bibai, Japan

Sonia Suys, MD
General Surgeon, Virginia Beach, Virginia

George W. Sypert, MD
Southwest Florida Neurosurgical Association, Fort
Myers, Florida

Charles H. Tator, MD, PhD, MA, FRCSC, FACS
Director, Canadian Paraplegic Association Spinal Cord
Injury Research Centre, Toronto Western Hospital,
Toronto, Ontario, Hospital

Nicholas Theodore, MD
Director, Neurotrauma, Division of Neurological
Surgery, Barrow Neurosurgical Associates, Phoenix,
Arizona

Ajith J. Thomas, MD
MeritCare Neuroscience, Fargo, North Dakota

Nicholas W.M. Thomas, MD
Department of Neurosurgery, Kings College Hospital,
London, England

Robert E. Tibbs, Jr., MD
Mercy Health Center, Oklahoma City, Oklahoma

Daisuke Togawa, MD, PhD
Department of Orthopaedics and The Cleveland Clinic
Spine Institute, The Cleveland Clinic Foundation,
Cleveland, Ohio

Frank J. Tomecek, MD
Oklahoma Brain & Spine Institute, Tulsa, Oklahoma

Richard M. Toselli, MD
University of North Carolina at Chapel Hill, Chapel Hill,
North Carolina

Vincent C. Traynelis, MD
Professor, Department of Neurosurgery, The University
of Iowa, Iowa City, Iowa

Gregory R. Trost, MD
Assistant Professor, Departments of Neurosurgery and
Orthopaedic Surgery, University of Wisconsin Medical
School, Madison, Wisconsin

Eeric Truumees, MD
Staff Spine Surgeon, William Beaumont Hospital, Royal Oak, Michigan; Orthopedic Director, Gehring Biomechanics Laboratory; and Adjunct Faculty, Wayne State University Biomechanics Center, Detroit, Michigan

Gary W. Tye, MD
Department of Neurosurgery, Virginia Commonwealth University Health System, Richmond, Virginia

Abm Salah Uddin, MD
John F. Kennedy Medical Center, Edison, New Jersey

Alexander R. Vaccaro, MD
Professor of Orthopaedic Surgery, Co-Chief of Spine Surgery, Jefferson Medical College, Thomas Jefferson University, The Rothman Institute; and Co-Director, Delaware Valley Regional Spinal Cord Injury Center, Philadelphia, Pennsylvania

Ceslovas Vaicys, MD
Division of Neurosurgery, Memorial Healthcare System, Hollywood, Florida

Alex Valadka, MD
Baylor College of Medicine, Texas Medical Center, Houston, Texas

Arnold B. Vardiman, MD
Neurological Associates of San Antonio, San Antonio, Texas

Anthony A. Virella, MD
Chief Resident, Division of Neurosurgery, University of California Los Angeles Medical Center, Los Angeles, California

Elizabeth Vitarbo, MD
University of Miami, Miami, Florida

Todd W. Vitaz, MD
University of Louisville, Louisville, Kentucky

Dennis G. Vollmer, MD
Division of Neurosurgery, University of Texas Health Science Center at San Antonio, San Antonio, Texas

Jean-Marc Voyadzis, MD
Resident, Department of Neurosurgery, Georgetown University Hospital, Washington, D.C.

John D. Ward, MD
Professor and Vice Chairman, Department of Neurosurgery, Chief, Pediatric Neurosurgery, Virginia Commonwealth University Health System, Richmond, Virginia

Joseph Watson, MD
Assistant Professor, University of California Davis School of Medicine, Davis, California

John K. Webb, FRCS
Chairman, Center for Spinal Studies and Surgery, University Hospital, Nottingham, United Kingdom

Philip R. Weinstein, MD
University of California San Francisco School of Medicine, San Francisco, California

Martin W. Weiser, PhD
Technical Product Manager, Johnson Matthey Electronics, Spokane, Washington

William C. Welch, MD, FACS
Associate Professor, Department of Neurological Surgery, University of Pittsburgh Medical Center, Pittsburgh, Pennsylvania

Simcha J. Weller, MD
Director, Neurosurgery Spinal Disorders Program, Beth Israel Deaconess Medical Center, Boston, Massachusetts

L. Erik Westerlund, MD
CORE Orthopaedic Medical Center, P.C., Encinitas, California

Jonathan A. White, MD
University of Texas, Southwestern Medical Center, Dallas, Texas

Melvin D. Whitfield, MD
The Cleveland Clinic Spine Institute, The Cleveland Clinic Foundation, Cleveland, Ohio

Gregory C. Wiggins, MD
David Grant Medical Center, Travis Air Force Base, California

Jack E. Wilberger, MD
Acting Chairman, Department of Neurosurgery, Allegheny General Hospital, Pittsburgh, Pennsylvania

William S. Wilke, MD
Department of Rheumatic and Immunologic Diseases, The Cleveland Clinic Foundation, Cleveland, Ohio

Diana Barrett Wiseman, MD
Department of Neurosurgery, Naval Hospital, Okinawa, Japan

W. Putnam Wolcott, MD
Neurosurgeon, Newport News, Virginia

Eric J. Woodard, MD
Assistant Professor and Chief, Section of Spine Surgery, Department of Neurosurgery, Harvard Medical School, Brookline, Massachusetts

Philip Yazback, MD
Neuroscience Group of NE Wisconsin, Neenah, Wisconsin

Narayan Yoganandan, PhD
Department of Neurosurgery, Medical College of
Wisconsin, Milwaukee, Wisconsin

Kenneth S. Yonemura, MD
Assistant Professor, SUNY-Upstate Medical University,
Syracuse, New York

Kazuo Yonenobu, MD
Department of Orthopaedic Surgery, Osaka University
Medical School, Osaka, Japan

Hansen A. Yuan, MD
Professor, SUNY-Upstate Medical University, Syracuse,
New York

Seth M. Zeidman, MD
University of Rochester Medical Center, Rochester,
New York

Barry M. Zide, MD
Professor, Department of Surgery (Plastic), New York
University Medical Center, New York, New York

Mehmet Zileli, MD
Professor of Neurosurgery, Ege University Faculty of
Medicine, Department of Neurosurgery, Bornova, Izmir,
Turkey

Preface

This, the second edition, is bigger and (I think) better than the first. This preface is as appropriate for the second edition, as I feel it was for the first. Therefore, it is presented again with minimal modification.

The purpose of this book is to assist the spine surgeon with the avoidance, identification, and management of complications. This differs little from a presentation of operative technique and medical management. Therefore, this book in many respects is a *techniques* book. To achieve its purpose, an understanding of history, decision making, medical management, differential diagnosis, ethics, and even discussions of problems associated with related disorders (such as peripheral nerve injury and metabolic bone diseases) is mandatory. This process requires an understanding of the fundamental basic science components of spine surgery (e.g., anatomy, biomechanics, and physiology).

The book's style was created by its authors, as well as their interactions with each other. In most cases, two or more senior authors were assigned to most chapters. These senior authors were not necessarily chosen on the basis of their philosophical compatibility with their coauthor(s). In fact, coauthors with opposing viewpoints were chosen in many circumstances. Authors were also selected on the basis of experience, educational adeptness, and communication and writing skills. The greater-than-usual number of expert authors contributing to each chapter achieves continuity within the text itself that would not be possible otherwise.

Risk Taking

Surgery is a risk-taking process. The patient places himself or herself in the hands of the surgeon, and the ensuing decision-making process involves the resolution (or the attempts at such) of many technical and quality-of-life–related issues and dilemmas. A surgical procedure may be warranted if the sum of the costs (both financial and personal) and risks is less than the sum of the benefits. This risk/benefit analysis should be of paramount concern and should be emphasized by the surgeon and realized by the patient. This book is designed to help surgeons achieve their goals, by minimizing the *risk-taking* component of this "equation."

Opinion and Dogmatism

This book is intended to be used as a textbook, to serve as a reference, and to function as a resource for information. Much information is available in the pages that follow. Perspectives, *pearls,* conventional wisdom, and objective data are presented, as is opinion. Great care has been taken to identify opinion when presented, and to avoid its extreme dogmatism.

It is important to be objective, fair, and nonjudgmental when assessing complications, particularly those of others. There are clearly many ways to effectively and safely accomplish a task. Very infrequently, if ever, does a single method *always* work. What works for one surgeon may not work for another, and vice versa.

Nomenclature

In this book, some standardization of nomenclature was thought to be important. For example, *ventral* (according to Dorland's, pertaining to the belly or to any venter; denoting a position more toward the belly surface than some other object of reference) is used instead of *anterior* (according to Dorland's, situated in front of or in the forward part of an organ toward the head end of the body; a term used in reference to the ventral or belly surface of the body).[1] Similarly, *dorsal* is used instead of *posterior; rostral* instead of *cephalad;* and *caudal* instead of *caudad.* Exceptions to this are situations in which the term designates a structure or concept that is clearly established (e.g., *anterior* longitudinal ligament).

Repetition

We learn most effectively by having data presented in a repetitive manner, often from different perspectives, using differing techniques (e.g., written, mathematical, or visual). Truly understanding a concept involves a *spiral,* which often involves multiple exposures to information, so that a solid data base is acquired. New data (raw data) are then added and assimilated. This "expanded" knowledge base can then be applied to, and enhanced by, additional basic science and clinical applications. This entire process is perpetually refined by new experiences, such as clinical encounters or through reading (Figure 1). Repetition is good.

Standard of Care

Before undertaking the definition of a complication, the issue of standard of care deserves consideration. S. Haines (personal communication) illustrates the discrepancy between the legal definition (the degree of care a reasonable person would take to prevent injury to another) and the evidence-based definition (a generally accepted principle for patient management reflecting a high degree of clinical certainty) of the standard of care. Emphasis on "certainty" by clinicians and its de-emphasis by the legal system are most certainly noteworthy.

What is a Complication?

Peter McL. Black addressed the issue of defining a complication of neurological surgery in the front matter to *Brain Surgery: Complication Avoidance and Management.*[2] Much of what Black addressed is pertinent to spine surgery. The unique nature of spine surgery, however, dictates the examination of complications from a slightly different approach. The nuances and complexities of the spine and spine surgery are associated with unique concerns.

In order to more clearly understand the nature of a spine surgery complication, each author (of the first

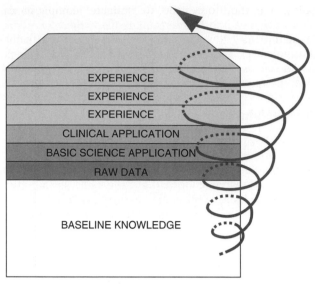

Figure 1 The Learning Spiral.

edition) completed a questionnaire that incorporates some of the concepts and questions used in Black's questionnaire. It was specifically designed to facilitate an understanding of a complication. The results of this questionnaire are reported and discussed for our enlightenment regarding the complications of our "trade." There was a 98% response rate by spine surgeon authors. Fourteen authors, who do not participate significantly in clinical decision making (i.e., engineers, nurses, anesthesiologists, and physiologists), did not complete the questionnaire. What is particularly interesting and revealing is the commentary by the majority (73%) of the respondents.

The first section (Questions 1 and 2) explores surgeon and institutional policy regarding complications. The second section (Questions 3 through 9) concerns the specifics of defining a complication and involves surgeon opinion to a significant degree. Nevertheless, this section provides a baseline for those wishing to derive an "operational definition(s)" of complications. The final question (Question 10) provides a philosophical and speculative slant.

The Responses

Question 1 reveals that spine surgeons do not have an adequate definition of what constitutes a surgical complication. Question 2 implies that in teaching institutions, there is variability regarding what is to be presented at a morbidity and mortality conference. D. Long provides a pertinent response that is worth sharing. He outlines seven rules for morbidity and mortality conferences:

1. All mortality must be discussed. The case must be presented by the residents and the responsible faculty surgeon must be at the meeting to summarize the mortality.
2. All postoperative neurological change, expected or unexpected, must be presented. The responsible surgeon must be present to discuss the case.
3. All postoperative infections are discussed. Those with serious patient implications are discussed in detail.

The others, which are more routine, are listed. For instance, a urinary tract infection is merely listed, but a wound infection or meningitis is discussed.
4. Any surgical or postsurgical event that prolongs the expected hospitalization must be discussed.
5. Any failure of equipment must be discussed. This includes shunts, stimulators, and internal fixators.
6. All serious events involving non-neurosurgical organ systems are discussed.
7. All postanesthetic complications are discussed in anesthesia morbidity and mortality conference but also must be listed at the neurosurgery morbidity and mortality conference.

Excessive cost is treated as a complication. If there is an outlier, when the cost is extreme, that patient case is discussed.

D. Long reported that after the monthly meeting at his institution, chief residents who present the cases produce a written summary that goes into the minutes of the conference. This details the complication that occurred and the discussion that centered on prevention.

Question 3 shows that the majority of respondents thought that a complication was an adverse event that occurred within 1 month of surgery. This has constituted traditional thinking, but without an objective rationale. Question 4 "spreads out" this field even further.

The majority of authors who responded to Question 5 believed that the younger and healthier the patient in whom a pneumonia occurs after routine surgery, the greater the probability that the pneumonia should be considered a complication. Perhaps this should apply to selected other complications as well.

Regarding Question 6, the authors were split on whether a dural tear that was successfully repaired during surgery signifies a complication. Clinical manifestations of this "tear," however, were relatively consistently considered complications by the authors.

Question 7 revealed an interesting response by the authors. Generally, a pedicle screw fracture was not considered to be a complication if asymptomatic and associated with a solid fusion. However, if there was an associated pseudarthrosis, with or without back pain, this same fracture was generally considered to be a complication. Finally, if the back pain persisted but the fusion was solid, no complication was believed to be present. Therefore, in the authors' opinion, the acquisition of fusion was the main determinant regarding definition of a complication in this circumstance.

Similarly, the responses to Question 8 depict a relatively clear demarcation between symptomatic and asymptomatic pseudarthroses after anterior cervical discectomies. The case of a symptomatic patient with a pseudarthrosis was regarded by the majority of respondents to be a complication, whereas those cases in which a pseudarthrosis was asymptomatic, no complication was thought to be present.

Regarding Question 9, a complaint of back pain at the rostral implant insertion site was not believed to be indicative of a complication by the majority of authors, almost regardless of circumstance.

Question 10, although theoretic, elicited consistent responses. The majority of respondents thought that the quality of *our* medical practices and medical reporting would be improved by a more accurate definition of what constitutes a complication. They also believed that quality assurance would be enhanced. They, however, had mixed feelings about whether the medical-legal climate would be improved.

Author Commentary

The majority of authors not only completed the questionnaire but added comments that were of significant relevance. Although most thought that the questionnaire was of some utility, the responses in this regard varied. They ranged from statements such as "Nice try, Ed, but I think this standardization would be difficult to do and really does not matter. . ." (anonymous) to ". . . a very thought-provoking questionnaire that illustrates well the 'gray areas' involved with the definition of complications." (M. Gallagher)

"You touch on a very important point in that standard agreement of what constitutes a complication is highly subjective. We need to develop an analogue of the Glasgow Outcome Scale for spine that can be more universally applied." (E. Woodard) It is in this vein that perhaps the most clear and concise response regarding the definition of a complication was derived. P. McCormick defined a complication as "an untoward unanticipated adverse event." Although this is clear and concise, it is made more specific by J. Lancon. He defined a complication as "any perioperative event which results in persistence or recurrence of symptoms or the development of new symptoms." B. Northrup defined a complication as "a preventable symptomatic maloccurrence that requires additional treatment. . ." This adds specificity to Lancon's definition while broadening McCormick's.

A. Hamilton defines a complication ". . . as any untoward event occurring to a patient while on the neurosurgical service. These are usually subdivided into errors in diagnosis, errors in management, or errors in technique. By this definition, therefore, the development of a urinary tract infection in a patient who had Foley catheter is considered a complication."

J. Bean provided a particularly relevant medical-legal slant to the definition. He stated, "A complication has no generally agreed meaning until it is operationally defined. A medicolegal definition will of necessity vary from a 'scientific' or clinical definition because the responses to and uses of the information will be different. One focuses on culpability, one on the modification of clinical behavior or decision making."

The most pertinent question, perhaps, is not necessarily what constitutes a complication but what constitutes an avoidable versus non-avoidable complication. More importantly, what constitutes negligence? In this vein, R. Apfelbaum responded, "Complication to me doesn't imply failure to provide adequate care—although it can mean that. Most often, it reflects the fact that we work with a biologic system with multiple variables acting concomi-

tantly. We therefore need to evaluate 'complications,' which can be anything short of a perfect result . . ."

In the future, we should perhaps focus on a further breakdown of the term "complication." Perhaps a simple discussion of the concept of "avoidable" and "nonavoidable" complications is the place to start. The use of refined outcome assessment tools will clearly facilitate this process in the future.

The Canadian Thistle

What is a complication? We still have not answered this question. Perhaps we never will. It, indeed, has different meanings and implications, depending on both its definer and the circumstances.

Perhaps an analogy is in order. The *Canadian thistle* is considered a weed on the eastern Washington farm on which I grew up. This weed is a destroyer of wheat crops and the *enemy* of the farmer. Its mere presence in a field, in a sense, is a *complication* of farming; a manifestation, perhaps, of inadequate *control* measures and of less than optimal surveillance, early detection, and eradication techniques. If left unchecked, the Canadian thistle is associated with serious detrimental consequences.

In Albuquerque, New Mexico, where my family had made our home in years gone by, the Canadian thistle is annoying to some, unnoticed by others, and considered a flower by many. Beauty is in the eye of the beholder, and, perhaps more relevant here, *ugly* is clearly a matter of perception and perspective, as is fault and blame.

To the spine surgeon, the patient, and the attorney, a complication has different meanings, and often different consequences. Whereas postoperative pain (as subjective as it may be) may not be considered a complication by the surgeon, and occasionally may be annoying and a source of distress to the patient, it may be a source of revenue, and therefore joy, for the attorney. Beauty is clearly in the eye of the beholder, and without question, *ugly* is indeed a matter of perception and perspective.

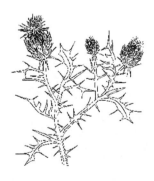

The Components And Factors Involved With The Definition Of A Complication Of Spinal Surgery: A Survey

1. Does your service have an explicit written (or "understood") definition of what constitutes a surgical complication? If so, could you append it to this questionnaire? If not, would you briefly describe your own concept of a complication under comments below?
   Yes 9%   No 88%   No response 3%

2. How do you decide what will be presented at a Morbidity and Mortality conference?
   Residents decide 31%   Faculty decides 24%
   Faculty/residents decide 35%   Other 10%

3. Do you consider a complication as an adverse event occurring (check all that apply):
   a. *Within 48 hours of surgery 45%*
   b. *Within a week of surgery 46%*
   c. *Within a month of surgery 75%*
   d. *While the patient was in the hospital 43%*
   e. *With reasonable assurance as a result of the surgical manipulation 75%*
   f. *None 23%*

4. Do you consider recurrent sciatica, that is identical to the preoperative lumbar laminotomy pain pattern, to be a complication if it occurs (check all that apply):
   a. *Within 48 hours of surgery 35%*
   b. *Within a week of surgery 36%*
   c. *Within a month of surgery 41%*
   d. *Within 2 months of surgery 25%*
   e. *Within 6 months of surgery 35%*
   f. *None 1%*

5. Do you consider the occurrence of pneumonia to be a complication if it occurs (check all that apply):
   a. *In a 25-year-old postoperative ventilated cervical quadriplegic patient 57%*
   b. *In a 65-year-old postoperative lumbar fusion patient with chronic obstructive pulmonary disease 13%*
   c. *In a 25-year-old nonoperated ventilated cervical quadriplegic patient 45%*
   d. *In a 40-year-old healthy nonsmoker on day 2 following a routine lumbar discectomy 96%*

6a. Do you consider a dural tear, that is successfully repaired during surgery and that has no adverse sequelae, to be a complication of surgery?
   Yes 43%   No 57%

6b. Do you consider this same dural tear to be a complication of surgery if (check all that apply):
   a. *It is associated with 2 days of severe positional headaches 74%*
   b. *It is associated with CSF leakage through the wound and that requires lumbar drainage to successfully manage 96%*
   c. *It requires reoperation to manage 96%*

7. Do you consider pedicle screw fracture at 6 months following surgery to be a complication if (check all that apply):
   a. *It is asymptomatic and associated with a solid fusion 24%*
   b. *It is asymptomatic and associated with a pseudarthrosis 65%*
   c. *It is associated with persistent back pain and a solid fusion 38%*
   d. *It is associated with persistent back pain and a pseudarthrosis 86%*
   e. *None of the above 13%*

8. In a patient who has undergone an anterior cervical discectomy with fusion, do you consider a pseudarthrosis (without excessive movement on flexion/extension x-rays) to be a complication if (check all that apply):
   a. *It is asymptomatic 24%*
   b. *It is associated with neck pain 80%*
   c. *It is associated with radicular pain 80%*
   d. *None 15%*

9. One year following a fusion and the placement of a hook-rod system for an unstable L1 fracture in a patient without neurological deficit, the patient complains of back pain at the rostral implant insertion site. Do you consider this a complication if (check all that apply):
   a. *You successfully manage the pain with an exercise program 12%*
   b. *Narcotic analgesics are required to manage the pain 30%*
   c. *The pain is managed successfully by surgical removal of the spinal implant 40%*
   d. *None 52%*

10. If we as surgeons could more accurately define what constitutes a complication (check all that apply):
   a. *Would the quality of our practices be improved?*
      Yes 63%   No 28%   No response 9%
   b. *Would medical reporting in the literature be enhanced?*
      Yes 92%   No 6%   No response 2%
   c. *Would quality assurance be enhanced?*
      Yes 76%   No 14%   No response 10%
   d. *Would the medico-legal climate be:*
      Worsened Improved   No effect No
      29%   38%   29%   response 4%
   e. *And if we could simultaneously standardize which complications were the result of negligence, would the medico-legal climate be:*
      Worsened 20% Improved 50% No effect 23%
      No response 7%

The definition of a complication is not as clear as *outsiders* (e.g., the lay public and the legal system) often believe is the case. With all this in mind, and in the best interest of our patients, we should attain and maintain objectivity. We should not be swayed by uneducated or undeserved accolades from the medically naive, or by *threats* from entrepreneurs. Complications must be defined, avoided, identified, and aggressively managed. Their avoidance, identification, and management should not be charged with emotion and anger but attacked with an armamentarium of logic, thoughtfulness, science, and objectivity.

The avoidance, identification, and management of the complications of spine surgery are addressed in the pages that follow by experts in the field. These experts themselves are not infallible. They address complications with which they have had first-hand experience. We must seize the opportunity to benefit from their wisdom and experience. A wise person can learn from the observations and mistakes of others.

Like a Canadian thistle, a complication means different things to different people. We must put complications in their appropriate perspective by clarifying their definition. Then we should actively avoid them and aggressively identify and manage them when they occur.

Final Comments

Chapter 1 by Robert Grossman, in the sister volume to the first edition of this textbook, is worthy of careful review.[3] His "Maxims Concerning Complications" are repeated here, to emphasize their value.

MAXIMS CONCERNING COMPLICATIONS

Some aphorisms that are useful in guiding one's practice to avoid complications are as follows:

1. There is no such thing as a *simple* neurosurgical (spine surgery) operation.
2. It is easier to stay out of trouble than to get out of trouble.
3. The time expended in avoiding complications will be more than compensated by the time saved in not having to treat them.
4. The patient's well-being is paramount. A neurosurgeon (spine surgeon) should never hesitate to request consultation, or assistance, during surgery.
5. Surgeons should always operate with the meticulousness that they would wish for if they were the patient. It is a salutary exercise for surgeons to think of their own feelings and reactions if they had to undergo the procedures being carried out.

REFERENCES

1. *Dorland's Illustrated Medical Dictionary,* ed 26. Philadelphia, WB Saunders, 1981.
2. Black P McL: What is a complication in neurological surgery? A practical approach. In Apuzzo MLJ (ed): *Brain Surgery: Complication Avoidance and Management. Supratentorial Procedures.* New York, Churchill Livingstone, 1994, pp xxv-xxviii.
3. Grossman RG: Preoperative and surgical planning for avoiding complications. In Apuzzo MLJ (ed): *Brain Surgery: Complication Avoidance and Management. Supratentorial Procedures.* Churchill Livingstone, New York, 1994, p 9.

Contents

Conflict of Interest

In order to minimize bias, the disclosure of potential conflicts of interest is imperative. The following contributors to this book have disclosed financial relationships with industrial partners. These relationships could bias the author's opinion and, therefore, should be considered accordingly.

Author	Industrial Partner
Ronald I. Apfelbaum, MD	Aesculap Instrument Co, Medtronic
Giancarlo Barolat, MD	Advanced Neuromodulation System (ANS), Medtronic
Edward C. Benzel, MD	DePuy Spine, NuVasive, Orthovita, & Spinal Concepts
Scott D. Boden, MD	Medtronic, Centerpulse, Osteotech, & Wright Medical
Joseph S. Cheng, MD	Medtronic Sofamor Danek
Curtis A. Dickman, MD	Johnson and Johnson & Medtronic
Thomas J. Errico, MD	Fastenetix, Medtronic, & Synthes Spine
Jan Goffin, MD, PhD	Spinal Dynamics, Medtronic Sofamor Danek
Regis W. Haid, Jr., MD	MedTronic; Johnson & Johnson;
Allan J. Hamilton, MD	Biogen & Guilford Pharmaceuticals
Robert A. Hart, MD, MA	Stryker Howmedic, MedTronic Sofamor Danek; Depuy Spine; Kyphon; Synthes/AO; Orthovita
Robert F. Heary, MD	DePuy Spine
Patrick W. Hitchon, MD	
Iain H. Kalfas, MD	DePuy Spine, Medtronic Sofamor Danek, Synthes Spine, Spine Tech
Lawrence G. Lenke, MD	Medtronic Sofamor Danek
Alan D. Levi, MD	DePuy Spine & Medtronic
Isador H. Lieberman, MD	Kyphon, DePuy Spine, Orthovita
Paul C. McAfee, MD	DePuy Spine
Nagy Mekhail, MD, PhD	Pfizer, Merck, Medtronic
Hiroshi Nakagawa, MD, PhD	Ammtec (Tokyo, Japan)
Daniel K. Resnick, MD	NuVasiv, Orthovita
Gerald E. Rodts, Jr., MD	Medtronic
Christopher B. Shields, MD, FRCS(C)	Norton Healthcare
Vincent C. Traynelis, MD	Medtronic Sofamor Danek
Kenneth S. Yonemura, MD	Smith & Nephew – Spine

CHAPTER 1

History

Cary D. Alberstone, Sait Naderi, and
Edward C. Benzel

The evolution of spinal surgery has revolved around three basic surgical goals: decompression, surgical stabilization, and deformity correction. To emphasize their importance, these surgical goals form the framework for this chapter. However, other related fundamental arenas, such as anatomy, biomechanics, nonsurgical treatment modalities, contributed to the development of surgical concepts as well.

Although the main advances in spine surgery occurred in the nineteenth and twentieth centuries, their roots date back several thousand years. Without understanding and appreciating the past, it is not possible to understand and appreciate the advancements of the last two centuries. Therefore, before touching upon the last two centuries' spine history, a short history of spine medicine of the antique period, medieval period, and Renaissance is presented.

The Antique Period and Spine Surgery

There is no evidence of surgical decompression and stabilization, nor the surgical correction of deformity, during the antique period except for laminectomy in a trauma case reported by Paulus of Aegina. However, it is known that the antique period's physicians were, to some extent, able to evaluate patients with spinal disorders. They in fact did use frames for reduction of dislocation and gibbus and applied some of the knowledge gained from human and animal dissections.

Srimad Bhagwat Mahapuranam, an ancient Indian epic (3500-1800 BC), depicts the oldest documentation of spinal traction. In a passage from this document, it is described that Lord Krishna applied axial traction to correct a hunchback in one of his devotees.[63]

The Edwin Smith Papyrus (2600-2200 BC) is the most well-known document on Egyptian medicine. This document reports 48 cases. Imhotep (2686-2613 BC), an antique surgeon, authored this papyrus. Six cases of spinal trauma were reported. Hence, nearly 4600 years ago, vertebral subluxation and dislocation and traumatic quadriplegia and paraplegia were described.[12] Recently, it was reported that Egyptian physicians described the "spinal djet column concept."[65]

Antique medicine was also influenced by the Greco-Roman period physicians.[13] *Hippocrates* (460-375 BC) addressed the anatomy and pathology of the spine. He described the normal curvatures of the spine, the structure of the spine, and the tendons attached to the spine. He defined tuberculous spondylitis, posttraumatic kypho-sis, scoliosis, spinal dislocation, and spinous process fracture. He addressed the relationship between spinal tuberculosis and gibbus. According to Hippocrates, spinous process fracture was not dangerous. However, fractures of vertebral body were more important. He described two frames for reduction of the dislocated spine, including the Hippocratic ladder and the Hippocratic board.[2] The details of Hippocratic treatment were recorded by Celsus (25 BC-50 AD).

Aristotle (384-322 BC) focused on kinesiology. His treatises—"parts of animals, movement of animals, and progression of animals—described the actions of the muscles." He analyzed and described walking, in which rotatory motion is transformed into translational motion. Although his studies were not directly related to the spine, they were the first to address human kinesiology and, in fact, biomechanics.

Galen of Pergamon (130-200 AD), another physician of the antique era, worked as a surgeon and anatomist. He studied the anatomy of animals and extrapolated his findings to human anatomy. His anatomic doctrines became the gold standard for more than 1200 years. He used the terms *kyphosis, scoliosis,* and *lordosis,* and he attempted to correct these deformities. He also worked as the official surgeon of gladiators in amphitheaters. Because of this position, he was accepted as "the father of sports medicine." He confirmed the observations of Imhotep and Hippocrates regarding the neurological sequences of cervical spine trauma. Nevertheless, to the best of our knowledge, he did not operate for spinal trauma.[76]

Oribasius (325-400 AD), another antique period physician, added a bar to the Hippocratic reduction device and used it for both spinal trauma and spinal deformity.[113]

One of the most important figures dealing with spinal disorders during the end of this period is *Paulus of Aegina* (625-690 AD). He collected what was known from the previous 1000 years in a seven-volume encyclopedia. Paulus of Aegina not only used the Hippocratic bed, but also worked with a red-hot iron. He is credited with performing the first known laminectomy. This was performed for a case of spinal fracture resulting in spinal cord compression. He emphasized the use of orthoses in spinal trauma cases.[42]

The Medieval Period and Spine Surgery

The studies and reports of Paulus of Aegina are the most important source of information regarding this period of medicine. This age was followed by the dark age in Europe. Whereas Western medicine showed no progress during the dark age, the Eastern world developed the science. The early Islamic civilizations realized the importance of science and scientific investigation. The most important books of the antique age were translated into Syrian, Arabic, and Persian. Therefore, using the Western doctrines, the Islamic civilizations discovered new information and were able to contribute further. In terms of spine medicine, several important contributors, including Avicenna and Abulcasis, added to this movement.

Avicenna (981-1037 AD), a famous physician of this era, worked in all areas of medicine (Figure 1-1). His famous

1

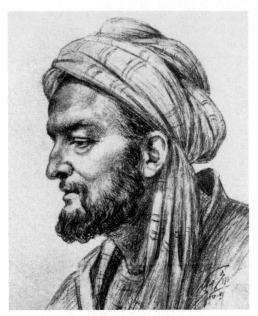

Figure 1.1 Avicenna.

book, the *Canon,* was a seminal textbook until the seventeenth century in Europe. He described the biomechanics-related anatomy of the spine. He also described flexion, extension, lateral bending, and axial rotation of the spine.[86] Avicenna also used a traction system similar to the system described by Hippocrates.

Abulcasis (936-1013 AD), a famous Arabian surgeon of the eleventh century, wrote a surgery treatise, "At-Tasnif." He described several surgical disorders, including low back pain, sciatica, scoliosis, and spinal trauma. He recommended the use of chemical or thermal cauterization for several spinal disorders. He also developed a device to reduce dislocated spine.[99]

Serafeddin Sabuncuoglu (1385-1468 AD), a Turkish physician of the fifteenth century, wrote an illustrated atlas of surgery.[85] He described scoliosis, sciatica, low back pain, and spinal dislocations. He described a technique for reduction of spinal dislocations, using a frame similar to that designed by Abulcasis.

Renaissance and Spine Surgery

The dark age in Europe evolved into the Renassiance. During this period actual academic centers were established in Europe. In addition, centers for the translation of documents, similar to centers established in Islamic regions, were founded. The antique-age classics were translated into Latin from Arabic in such translation centers. This infusion of scientific information contributed to the "character" of the Renaissance. During this time, the Western world spawned disciplines, including art, medicine, physics, and mathematics.

The works of *Leonardo da Vinci* (1452-1519 AD) are of importance in this regard. da Vinci worked on the philosophy of mechanics and on anatomy in *De Figura Humana.* He described spine anatomy, the number of vertebrae, and the joints in detail. By studying anatomy

in the context of mechanics, da Vinci gained some insight into biomechanics. He considered the importance of the muscles for stability of the cervical spine. However, his work was unpublished for centuries, and his brilliant daydreaming had a limited scientific impact on biomechanics.[87]

Andreas Vesalius (1514-1564 AD), an anatomist and physician, wrote his famous anatomy book, *De Humani Corporis Fabrica Liberi Septum*, and changed several doctrines described by Galen. Actually, it took several centuries for the world to accept that Galen had made errors that were corrected by Vesalius. Because he described and defined modern anatomy, he is commonly accepted as the father of anatomy. He described spine, intervertebral disc, and intervertebral foramina. His biomechanical point of view regarding the flexion extension of the head was similar to that of Avicenna.[10]

The early anatomic studies and observations were followed by biomechanical advancements. In this regard *Giovanni Alfonso Borelli* (1608-1679 AD) deserves significant credit. Borelli described the biomechanical aspects of living tissue. He is the founder of the "iatrophysics" concept; a term that subsequently became known as *biomechanics*. He is accepted as the "father of spinal biomechanics." His book, *De Motu Animalium,* describes the movements of animals. He wrote that the intervertebral disc is a viscoelastic material. He reported that the intervertebral disc carries loads. This is so because he observed that muscles could not bear the loads alone. Therefore, he concluded that the intervertebral discs should have function during the load bearing. He was the first scientist to describe the human weight center (center of gravity).[75,82]

The studies and accomplishments of the Renaissance period were not limited to the aforementioned. Many scientists contributed to the body of the literature in this period. The advancements from this period resulted in the formation of early modern surgery, beginning in the nineteenth century.

The Early Modern Period and Spine Surgery
Spinal Decompression and the Early Modern Period

Although an open decompression of the spinal canal for spinal cord compression was recommended by some surgeons between the sixteenth and eighteenth centuries (e.g., Pare, Hildanus), there is no evidence of successful intervention except for two cases reported by Paulus of Aegina and Louis prior to the nineteenth century.

Spinal decompression in the early modern period was primarily via laminectomy. Throughout most of the nineteenth century, laminectomy was developed and its utility debated as the only surgical approach to all spinal pathologies, including tumor, trauma, and infection. At the dawn of the twentieth century, the indications for laminectomy were extended to the decompression of spinal degenerative disease, an understanding of which had eluded nineteenth-century surgeons because they failed to appreciate the connection between its clinical and pathologic manifestations.

During the nineteenth century, spinal surgery was performed almost exclusively for neural element decompression. Numerous nonoperative approaches to deformity correction were attempted over the centuries, but the surgical approach to deformity correction was a twentieth-century development. Nor were the techniques of spinal stabilization a product of the nineteenth century, because both spinal fusion and internal fixation did not appear until after or around the turn of the century. Moreover, a failure to recognize the implications for treatment of degenerative spinal disease, including spondylosis and degenerative disc disease, meant that the solution to these problems had to await the new century.

Thus, during the nineteenth century, the indications for spinal surgery were limited to the treatment of tumor, trauma, and infection. Although each of these conditions posed unique clinical and surgical problems, they shared the need for surgical decompression. Throughout the early modern period, surgical decompression of the spine was the single most common reason to undertake the risks of spinal surgery, and laminectomy was the most commonly used technique to achieve it.

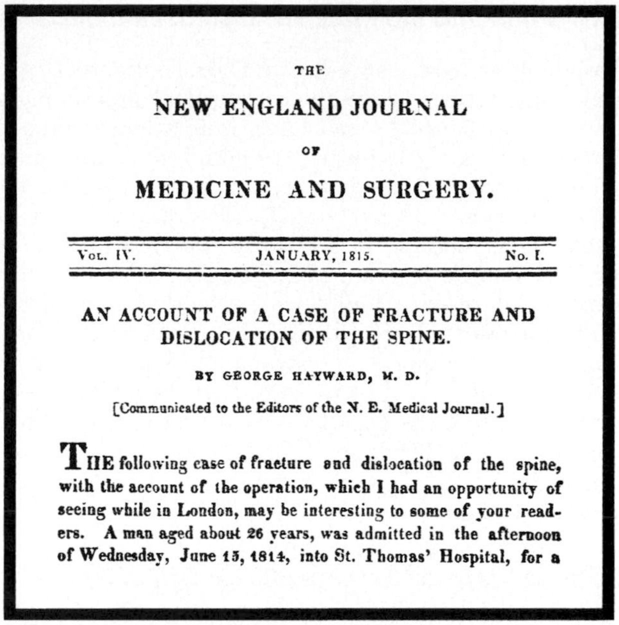
THE

NEW ENGLAND JOURNAL

OF

MEDICINE AND SURGERY.

VOL. IV. JANUARY, 1815. No. I.

AN ACCOUNT OF A CASE OF FRACTURE AND DISLOCATION OF THE SPINE.

BY GEORGE HAYWARD, M. D.

[Communicated to the Editors of the N. E. Medical Journal.]

THE following case of fracture and dislocation of the spine, with the account of the operation, which I had an opportunity of seeing while in London, may be interesting to some of your readers. A man aged about 26 years, was admitted in the afternoon of Wednesday, June 15, 1814, into St. Thomas' Hospital, for a

Figure 1.2 First page of H.J. Cline Jr.'s historic laminectomy, as reported by G. Hayward. *(From Cline HJ Jr [cited by Hayward G]: An account of a case of fracture and dislocation of the spine.* New Engl J Med Surg *4:13, 1815.)*

The Birth and Development of the Laminectomy

H.J. Cline, Jr. and the Argument Against Spinal Surgery

At the beginning of the nineteenth century, the prospects for spinal surgery appeared grim. The dismal results of a well-publicized operation for a traumatic spinal injury stimulated a heated debate over the "possibility" of spinal surgery that persisted for nearly a century. At the center of this debate was H.J. Cline, Jr., a little-known British surgeon.

In 1814, Cline performed a multilevel laminectomy for a thoracic fracture-dislocation associated with signs of a complete paraplegia (Figure 1.2).[23] The patient was a 26-year-old man who fell from the top of a house. "He was bled previous to his admission" to the St. Thomas's Hospital in London, "and some imprudent attempts were made to relieve him by pressing the knees against the injured part, which only increased the pain and inflammation."[23] Upon admission to the hospital the patient was examined by Cline, who "ascertained that some of the spinous processes . . . were broken off and were pressing upon the spinal marrow . . . [and] who resolved to cut down and remove the pressure from the spinal marrow."[23]

The patient was observed overnight in the hospital, and on the day following admission, Cline performed his proposed operation. Although the operation was performed within 24 hours of injury, Cline was unable to reduce the dislocation or to achieve a complete decompression of the neural elements. The patient survived for 3 days after surgery, with increasing pain and a steadily increasing pulse. On postoperative day 4, however, the patient died, "and on an examination of the body by Mr. Cline, it was found that the spinal marrow was entirely divided."[23] Despite the severity of the neural injury, and the complexity of the fracture-dislocation, the untoward outcome of this unfortunate case would remain a topic of conversation for almost a century, providing ample ammunition for the opponents of spinal surgery.

Of course, the case of Cline was not an isolated mortality. In 1827, for example, Tyrell[102] reported a 100% mortality for a small series of patients with spinal dislocation and neurologic injury treated surgically. Other reports (e.g., Rogers[92] in 1835) were often equally discouraging. Looking back on these early years of the debate about spinal surgery, the early twentieth century British surgeon Donald Armour[7] described the controversy this way:

> This [Cline's operation] precipitated and gave rise to widespread and vehement discussion as to its justification. This discussion, often degenerating into bitter and virulent personalities, went on many years. Astley Cooper, Benjamin Bell, Tyrell, South, and others favored it, while Charles Bell, John Bell, Benjamin Brodie, and others opposed it. The effect of so eminent a neurologist as Sir Charles Bell against the procedure retarded spinal surgery many years—the operation was described with such extravagant terms as "formidable," "well-nigh impossible," "appalling," "desparate [sic] and blind," "unjustifiable," and "bloody and dangerous."

Of course, surgical fatalities in this period were due as much to septic complications and anesthetic inadequacies as they were to surgical technique. The lack of an effective means of pain control during surgery intensified the problem of intraoperative shock and made speed essential. Furthermore, the problems of wound infection and septicemia were both predictable and frequently fatal. These hindrances to surgery were not ameliorated until the introduction of general anesthetic agents (i.e., nitrous oxide, ether, and chloroform) in the mid-1840s and the adoption of Listerian techniques (using carbolic acid) in the 1870s.

A.G. Smith and the First Successful Laminectomy

Despite these risks, a little-known Danville, Kentucky surgeon named Alban G. Smith performed a laminectomy in 1828 on a patient who had fallen from a horse and sustained a traumatic paraplegia. To Smith's credit, his patient not only survived the operation but achieved a partial neurologic recovery. The operative technique and surgical results were reported in the *North American Journal of Medicine and Surgery* in 1829 (Figure 1.3).[97] Smith's procedure comprised a multilevel laminectomy through a midline incision, involving removal of the depressed laminae and spinous processes, exploration of the dura mater, and closure of the soft tissue incision. Although the report of this landmark case appears to have attracted little attention at the time, it is a significant technical achievement and places Smith among the pioneers of the early modern period in spinal surgery.

Laminectomy for Extramedullary Spinal Tumor

During the half century after Smith's historic operation, the primary indication for laminectomy was spinal trauma. In the latter part of the nineteenth century, the indications for laminectomy were extended to tumor and infection. The first and most celebrated surgical case for spinal tumor in the nineteenth century, which was also the first successful one, played an important role in the rehabilitation of the laminectomy as a safe and effective procedure. This was the case of Captain Gilbey.

Captain Gilbey was an English army officer who suffered the misfortune of losing his wife in a carriage accident in which he also was involved. Although Gilbey himself escaped serious injury, he soon began to experience progressive dull back pain, which he attributed to the accident. As the pain became relentless, Gilbey sought the advice of a series of physicians, all of whom were unable to identify the source of his pain. Eventually, Gilbey was referred to the eminent London neurologist, William Gowers, who elicited from the patient a history of back pain, urinary retention, paraplegia, and a thoracic sensory level (Figure 1.4).[41]

The neurologist's diagnosis was immediate and unequivocal: the cause of Gilbey's symptoms was located in his spine, where a tumor was causing compression of the thoracic spinal cord. Although no intraspinal tumor had ever been resected successfully, Gowers referred the patient to his London surgical colleague, Victor Horsley (Figure 1.5). After all, Gowers had himself asserted, in his authoritative textbook, *Manual of Diseases of the Nervous System*, that removal of an intradural spinal cord tumor was "not only practicable, but actually a less formidable operation than the removal of intracranial tumors."

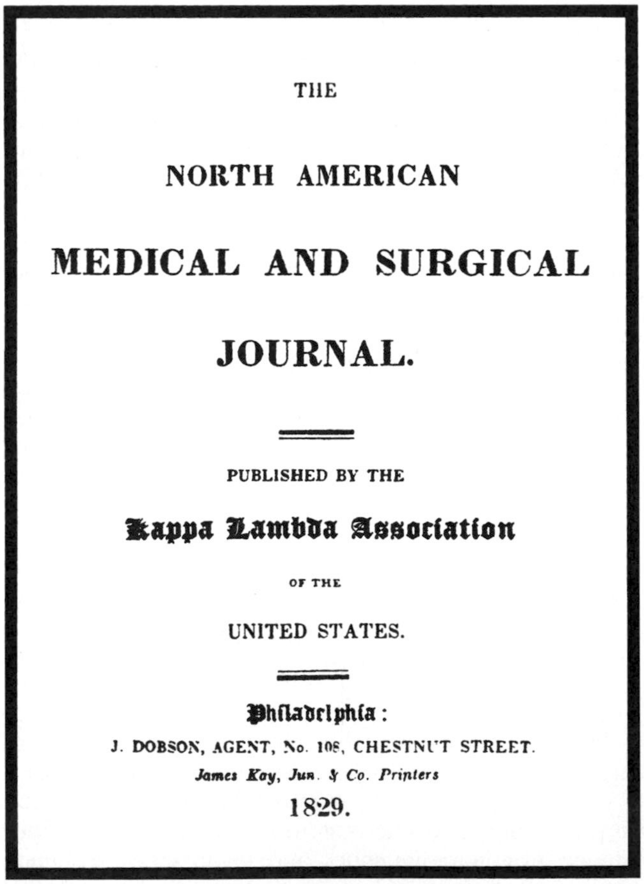

THE

NORTH AMERICAN

MEDICAL AND SURGICAL

JOURNAL.

PUBLISHED BY THE

𝕶𝖆𝖕𝖕𝖆 𝕷𝖆𝖒𝖇𝖉𝖆 𝕬𝖘𝖘𝖔𝖈𝖎𝖆𝖙𝖎𝖔𝖓

OF THE

UNITED STATES.

Philadelphia:

J. DOBSON, AGENT, No. 108, CHESTNUT STREET.

James Kay, Jun. & Co. Printers

1829.

Figure 1.3 Title page of journal that contains the first successful report of a laminectomy. The surgeon, and the author of the report, was Alban G. Smith of Danville, Kentucky. (*From Smith AG: Account of a case in which portions of three dorsal vertebrae were removed for the relief of paralysis from fracture, with partial success.* North Am Med Surg J 8:94-97, 1829.)

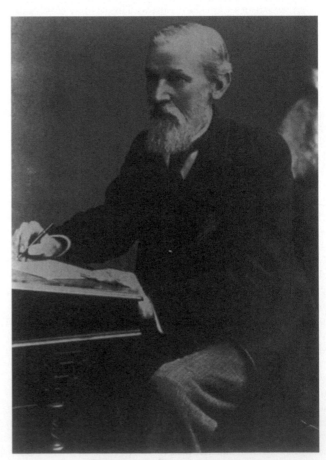

Figure 1.4 William R. Gowers.

Horsley acted quickly. Within 2 hours of the initial consultation, a skin incision was made at 1 PM, June 9, 1887 at the National Hospital, Queens Square, London. Despite his precipitous decision to undertake this dangerous operation, Horsley did not approach the operation unprepared. Although the Act of 1876 made it a criminal offense to experiment on a vertebrate animal for the purpose of attaining manual skill, Horsley had repeatedly practiced the proposed procedure in the course of his surgical experimentation. Despite some initial difficulty in locating the tumor, an intradural neoplasm in the upper thoracic spine causing compression of the spinal cord was identified and safely resected. The pathologic diagnosis was "fibromyxoma of the theca."

Follow-up 1 year later revealed almost complete neurologic recovery. The patient was ambulating without assistance and had returned to his premorbid work schedule. He remained well, with no evidence of tumor recurrence, up to the time of his death from an unrelated cause 20 years later.

Laminectomy for Intramedullary Spinal Tumor

In 1890, Fenger attempted to remove an intramedullary spinal tumor in an operation that resulted in the patient's death.[22] In 1905, Cushing[28,29] also attempted to remove an intramedullary spinal cord tumor but decided to abort the procedure after performing a myelotomy in the dorsal column. To Cushing's surprise, the patient improved after surgery. In 1907, von Eiselsberg[109] successfully resected an intramedullary tumor.

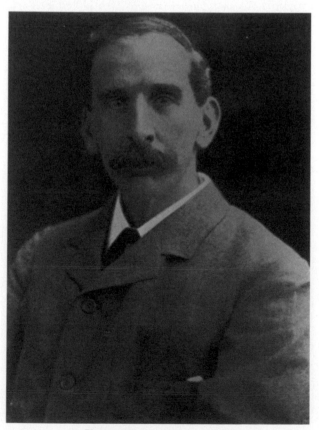

Figure 1.5 Sir Victor Horsley.

The unexpected improvement that was observed in the patient reported by Cushing attracted the attention of the New York surgeon Charles Elsberg. Elsberg[34] described the technique of Cushing, which he aptly named the "method of extrusion." The technique was intended to remove an intramedullary tumor by spontaneous extrusion of the tumor through a myelotomy made in the dorsal column. The rationale for this method was predicated on the theory that an intramedullary tumor was associated with an increase in intramedullary pressure. Release of this pressure by a myelotomy that extended from the surface of the spinal cord to the substance of the tumor was expected to provide a sufficient force to achieve spontaneous extrusion of the tumor. According to Elsberg, the advantage of this procedure over a standard tumor resection was that it required minimal manipulation of the spinal cord and therefore minimal spinal cord tissue injury.

Because the spontaneous extrusion of an intramedullary tumor occurred slowly, Elsberg performed these procedures in two stages. In the first stage, a myelotomy was fashioned in the dorsal column, extending from the surface of the spinal cord to the tumor (Figure 1.6A).

When the tumor was identified and observed to begin to bulge through the myelotomy incision, the operation was concluded, the dura mater left opened, and the wound closed. In the second stage of the procedure, which was performed approximately 1 week after the first stage, Elsberg reopened the wound and inspected the tumor (Figure 1.6B). Typically, the tumor was found outside the spinal cord, and the few adhesions that remained between the spinal cord and the tumor were sharply divided. After the tumor was removed, the wound, including the dura mater, was closed.

Variations in Laminectomy Technique

By the last decade of the nineteenth century, after the case of Captain Gilbey, the possibility of safely performing a spinal operation was embedded in the collective surgical consciousness. Furthermore, new anesthetic techniques and aseptic methods had become available to most practicing surgeons.[5] All of these factors served to increase the appeal of the laminectomy to surgeons and to widen its range of application. For example, after Horsley's widely publicized surgical success for spinal tumor, many similar operations were soon described in the literature,* and in 1896, Makins and Abbott[74] reported 24 cases of laminectomy for vertebral osteomyelitis.

Although the safety and efficacy of the laminectomy had convinced many proponents of the utility of the procedure, surgeons toward the end of the century began to worry about postoperative instability. Advances in operative technique and perioperative management meant that more and more patients survived the operation and ultimately became ambulatory, which further heightened concern about stability.

In 1889, Dawbarn[31] described an osteoplastic method of laminectomy that addressed this concern about postoperative spinal stability. Instead of a midline incision, Dawbarn described two lateral incisions that were carried down to the

*References 1,19,27,39,66,93.

transverse processes. The lateral incisions were connected in an H-like fashion, and a superior and inferior flap— including skin, muscle, fascia, and bone—was then turned. In closing the wound, the intact flaps were reflected back and reapproximated in their normal anatomic positions.

Although not all surgeons subscribed to the osteoplastic method, many turn-of-the-century surgeons were largely preoccupied with modifications of this procedure.[77] At the same time, however, a more important innovation in laminectomy technique, the hemilaminectomy, was developed independently in both Italy[4,108] and the United States.[100]

In 1910, A.S. Taylor of New York described the hemilaminectomy: a midline incision, a subperiosteal paraver-

tebral muscle takedown, and the removal of a hemilamina with a Doyen saw. The advantages of the hemilaminectomy over the cumbersome osteoplastic method were obvious, and Taylor argued that compared with the laminectomy, the hemilaminectomy interfered less with the mechanics of the spine. Despite such detractors as Charles Elsberg, who responded that the field of view was narrow and the effect of laminectomy on spinal mechanics negligible, Taylor successfully championed its use.

Charles A. Elsberg: The Laminectomy in Stride

Charles A. Elsberg was one of the most influential writers on spinal decompression (Figure 1.7). Working at the Neurological Institute of New York, which he had helped to found, Elsberg[36] published his first series of laminectomies in 1913. In 1916, he published his classic text, *Diagnosis and Treatment of Surgical Diseases of the Spinal Cord and Its Membranes.*[35] Although these publications represent landmarks in the history of spinal surgery, they comprise more of a culmination than an innovation in spinal surgery. Elsberg's work on spinal surgery, coming as it did at the end of a century of evolution of the decompressive laminectomy, effectively codified nineteenth and early twentieth century developments.

In his textbook, Elsberg outlined the surgical indications and contraindications for laminectomy. He noted the beneficial effects in his own large series of laminectomies and puzzled over the benefits that may occur in the absence of

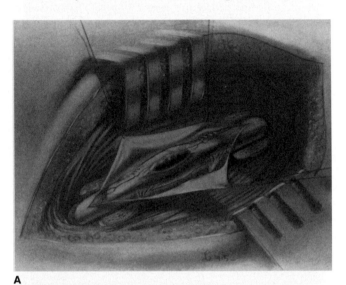

A

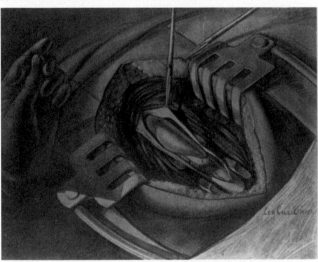

B

Figure 1.6 **(A)** The first stage in an intramedullary spinal cord tumor resection by the extrusion method. Note that the tumor is bulging through the myelotomy incision. The wound was subsequently closed. **(B)** The second stage in an intramedullary spinal cord tumor resection by the extrusion method, 1 week after the first stage. Note that the tumor has spontaneously extruded since the first operation, and now may be removed easily. *(From Elsberg CA, Beer E: The operability of intramedullary tumors of the spinal cord. A report of two operations with remarks upon the extrusion of intraspinal tumors. Am J Med Sci 142:636-647, 1911.)*

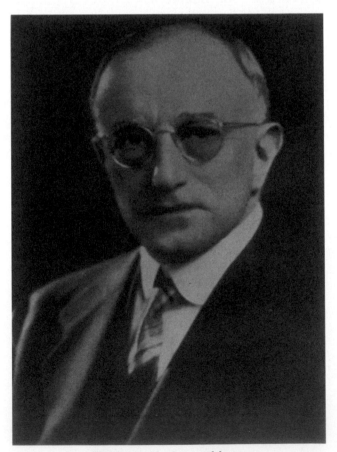

Figure 1.7 Charles A. Elsberg.

evident increased intradural pressure, such as in patients with multiple sclerosis. He argued that the primary indications for operation were cases of tumor, trauma, and infection that were associated with symptoms localized to a spinal level. Patients with progressive symptoms should be operated on quickly, in the absence of contraindications such as metastatic cancer or advanced Pott's disease.

Given the exhaustive scope of these early Elsberg publications—which, in addition to tumor, trauma, and infection, also review the management of congenital spine disease—conspicuously little is said about the most common late twentieth century indication for laminectomy: degenerative spine disease. The tardy development of a treatment for degenerative spine disease should be understood in the larger context of nineteenth and early twentieth century knowledge of spinal pathology.

Unlike degenerative disease, tumor, trauma, and infection were already well-known in antiquity. Although the concept of localization of function in the nervous system was undeveloped during the nineteenth century, the diagnosis and localization of tumor, trauma, and infection, particularly in their late stages, was not especially difficult. Degenerative disease, on the other hand, possessed a more subtle pathophysiology that was not as easily characterized, especially without the help of radiography. Thus recognition of degenerative spine disease eluded the nineteenth-century surgeon. This tardy appreciation for the clinical, surgical, and pathologic importance of degenerative spine disease deserves further mention.

Laminectomy for Intervertebral Disc Herniation. Intervertebral disc pathology was first described by Rudolph Virchow[108] in 1857 (Figure 1.8). Virchow's description of a fractured disc was made at autopsy on a patient who had suffered a traumatic injury.

In 1896, T. Kocher,[61] a Swiss surgeon identified and described a traumatic disc rupture in an autopsy of a patient who had fallen 100 feet and landed on her feet. Although Kocher recognized that the L1-L2 disc was displaced dorsally, no clinical correlation was suggested.

The first transdural intervertebral discectomy was reported by Oppenheim and Krause[89] in 1908. However, they reported the disc as "enchondroma."

In 1911, George Middleton,[81] a practicing physician, and John Teacher, a Glasgow University pathologist, described two cases of ruptured intervertebral disc observed at autopsy. Like Virchow and Kocher before them, however, Middleton and Teacher, although they described the pathology, failed to postulate its connection with radiculopathy or back pain.

In 1911, Joel Goldthwaite[39] made this connection. In an article on the lumbosacral articulation, Goldthwaite described and illustrated how weakening of the anulus fibrosus could result in dorsal displacement of the nucleus pulposus. The nucleus pulposus, he argued, could in turn result in low back pain and paraparesis. What eluded Goldthwaite and the surgeons before him, however, was the connection between a herniated disc and radiculopathy.

In a 1929 issue of the *Archives of Surgery*, Walter E. Dandy[30] published a description of two cases of herniated lumbar discs causing a cauda equina syndrome (Figure 1.9). Dandy correctly described how "loose cartilage from

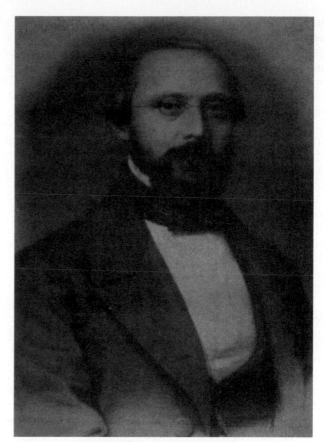

Figure 1.8 Rudolph Virchow.

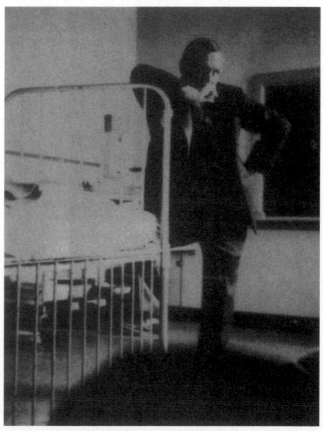

Figure 1.9 Walter E. Dandy.

the intervertebral disc" produced the symptoms of cauda equina compression that were relieved after surgical decompression. He considered that in the second decade of the twentieth century, more than 20 years after the first spinal fusion operations, intervertebral disc disease could be added to the list of indications for decompressive laminectomy.

Despite the several aforementioned publications on intervertebral disc herniation, the concept of disc herniation and its relationship to radiculopathy was defined by Mixter and Barr.

While several studies were performed in North America, an anatomic, radiologic and microscopic study was performed on 5000 human spines in Dresden Pathology Institute by *Schmorl* and *Junghanns*. The results of this study were published in a book entitled *"The Human Spine in Health and Disease."* In 1932, Barr, an orthopedic surgeon from Massachussets General Hospital, was assigned to write a critique of this study.

In June of 1932, Barr attempted to treat a patient with an extruded disc herniation. Following a 2-week unsuccessful course of nonoperational treatment, Barr consulted with Mixter. Mixter recommended a myelogram. The myelogram revealed a filling defect. Mixter operated on the patient and removed the "tumor." Barr studied the "tumor" specimens. Because Barr contributed to Schmorl's study published in German, he remembered the microscopic appearances of Schmorl's study and realized that the specimen from this index patient was the nucleus pulposus. After this finding, Mixter, Barr, and Mallory (pathologist) reevaluated all the cases that were diagnosed (or misdiagnosed) as chondroma in recent years at Massachusetts General Hospital. They retrospectively diagnosed most of these cases as ruptured intervertebral discs. Mixter and Wilson operated on the first ruptured disc herniation diagnosed preoperatively on December 31, 1932. Mixter and Barr reported the case in *New England Surgical Society* in September 30, 1933.[83,113]

In the late 1930s Love[69] from Mayo Clinic reported on an extradural laminectomy technique. In 1967, Yasargil[114] used the microscope for discectomy. The first results of the lumbar microdiscectomy were reported by Yasargil[114] and Caspar.[20]

Laminectomy for Cervical Disc Herniation. In 1905 Watson and Paul[110] performed a negative exploration for cervical spinal cord tumor. They found an anterior extradural mass in the intervertebral disc at autopsy. This may be the first reported case of cervical disc herniation. The first dorsal approach was performed by Elsberg[37] in 1925. He found a "chondroma" in a quadriparetic patient.

Laminectomy for Spinal Stenosis. Unlike the herniated intervertebral disc, the stenotic spinal canal was described comparatively early in the nineteenth century. Portal,[90] in 1803, observed that a small spinal canal may be causally related to spinal cord compression, leading to paraplegia. No clinical reports of this entity were published, however, until 1893 when William A. Lane[64] described the case of a woman aged 35 years with a progressive paraplegia and a degenerative spondylolisthesis. The patient improved after a decompressive laminectomy.

Further demonstration of the efficacy of decompressive laminectomy for spinal stenosis came from Sachs and Frankel[94] in 1900. They published an account of a man aged 48 years with neurogenic claudication and spinal stenosis whose symptoms improved after a two-level laminectomy. Recognition of the degenerative nature of the clinical entity of spinal stenosis was established by Bailey and Casamajor[8] in 1911 in a report on a patient who was successfully decompressed by Charles Elsberg. In his 1916 textbook, Elsberg[35] later wrote, "a spinal operation may finally be required in some cases of arthritis or spondylitis on account of compression of the nerve roots or the cord by new-formed bone. . . ."

In 1945, Dr. Sarpyener, a Turkish orthopedic surgeon, described congenital lumbar spinal stenosis.[95] This report was followed by a report on adult spinal stenosis from Dr. Verbiest.[105] In 1973 Hattori[48] described the technique of laminoplasty.

Approaches to the Spine
Dorsolateral Approaches to the Spine

In 1779, Percival Pott described a condition involving spinal kyphosis and progressive paraplegia in a now-classic monograph titled *"Remarks on that kind of palsy of the lower limbs which is frequently found to accompany a curvature of the spine and is supposed to be caused by it; together with its method of cure; etc."* (Figure 1.10). For the management of this condition, which now bears his name, Pott recommended the use of a paraspinal incision to drain pus from the invariably present paraspinal abscess. For almost a century, this simple surgical procedure became a standard part of the treatment of Pott's paraplegia.

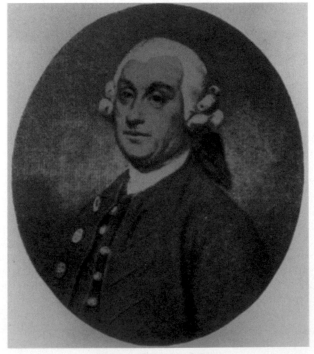

Figure 1.10 Percival Pott.

By the late nineteenth century, however, the laminectomy had received widespread acceptance as a safe and effective method of spinal decompression. This was in part related to the decrease in surgical mortality associated with the adoption of the Listerian methods beginning in the 1870s, and it was only natural then that the laminectomy would play a role in the management of Pott's disease. As in many of its applications, however, disenchantment arose with the results of laminectomy, and alternative approaches were therefore sought.[115] The most promising of these approaches was the so-called "costotransversectomy" of Ménard.

Ménard's Costotransversectomy

Like many surgeons at the turn of the century, Ménard[79] was disappointed by the surgical results of the laminectomy. In 1894, he described the costotransversectomy as an alternative method to achieve the goal of Pott, namely, drainage of the paraspinal abscess. The advantage of the costotransversectomy over the laminectomy lay in the improved exposure that it provided of the lateral aspect of the vertebral column. The procedure was also known as the "drainage latéral," emphasizing that the goal of the procedure was to drain the lateral, paravertebral tubercular abscess.

As described by Ménard, the costotransversectomy involved an incision overlying the rib that was located at the apex of the kyphos. The rib was then skeletonized and divided about 4cm distal to the articulation with its corresponding vertebra, from which it was disarticulated and removed. These maneuvers provided access to the tuberculous focus, which was exposed and then decompressed directly (Figure 1.11). Ménard did not intend to totally remove the lesion, but rather to simply decompress the abscess.

The surgical results of Ménard's costotransversectomy far surpassed the results obtained with the

laminectomy. There were several successes among his first few cases, including significant motor improvement among his first 23 cases.[98] Regrettably, these promising initial surgical results began to sour with time, as it became increasingly clear that two major complications were occurring with increasing frequency. These complications comprised the postoperative development of secondary infections and the postoperative formation of draining sinus tracts, both of which were created as a result of opening up the abscess. Because no antitubercular chemotherapeutic agents were available at the time, the consequences of the infections that ensued after surgery were frequently disastrous, resulting in significant surgical mortality. As Calot[16] grimly put it in 1930, "The surgeon who, so far as tuberculosis is concerned, swears to remove the evil from the very root, will only find one result waiting him: the death of his patient." The operation of Ménard thus fell into disrepute, and in time even Ménard abandoned it.

Capener's Lateral Rhachotomy

Like Ménard, Norman Capener of Exeter and Plymouth, England, attempted to find a surgical solution to the problem of Pott's paraplegia. Capener modified Ménard's costotransversectomy in a procedure that he developed and began using in 1933, which was first reported by H.J. Seddon[96] in 1935. Departing from the emphasis of Pott and Ménard, who simply decompressed the tubercular abscess, Capener attempted to directly remove the lesion, which typically consisted of a ventral mass of hardened material. To achieve his more radical goal of spinal decompression, Capener required a more lateral or ventral view of the vertebrae than was afforded by Ménard's costotransversectomy.

Capener's solution was to adopt Ménard's costotransversectomy with this difference: whereas Ménard approached the spine via a trajectory that was medial to the erector spinae muscles, Capener[18] transversely divided the muscles and retracted them rostrally and caudally (Figure 1.12). He named his new approach the *lateral rhachotomy* to distinguish it from Ménard's *costotransversectomy*. The simple change in dissection planes that distinguishes the

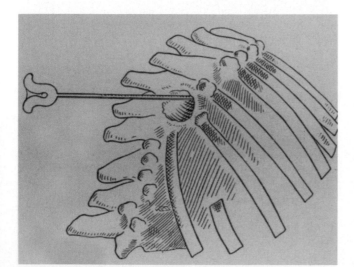

Figure 1.11 Drainage of a tubercular abscess via the costotransversectomy of Ménard. (*From Ménard V: Causes de la paraplegia dans le mal de Pott. Son traitement chirurgical par l'ouverture direct du foyer tuberculeux des vertebras.* Rev Orthop 5:47-64, 1894.)

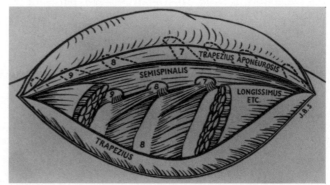

Figure 1.12 Dorsolateral exposure via Capener's lateral rhachotomy. Note that the exposure requires a transverse division of the paraspinal muscles. (*From Capener N: The evolution of lateral rhachotomy.* J Bone Joint Surg 36B:173-179, 1954.)

costotransversectomy from the lateral rhachotomy produces a significantly different trajectory and surgical exposure. Although the operation was designed for the surgical treatment of Pott's paraplegia, Capener later drew attention to the versatility of the approach, and its appropriateness for a variety of pathologic processes, including "the exploration of spinal tumors, the relief of certain types of traumatic paraplegia, and the drainage of suppurative osteitis of the vertebral bodies."[18]

It was perhaps unfortunate that for 19 years the only description of Capener's lateral rhachotomy was in a single case report published by another surgeon.[96] Not until 1954 did Capener himself describe the procedure, and even then he still chose not to publish the results of his 23 cases.[18]

In the interval between Seddon's 1935 description of the lateral rhachotomy and Capener's 1954 report of the same operation, the emergence of a new treatment, antitubercular chemotherapy, was to transform the history of the treatment of Pott's paraplegia. In 1947, streptomycin first became available for clinical use. This was followed by the introduction of para-aminosalicylic acid (PAS) in 1949 and isoniazid (INH) in 1952. The effect of the introduction of these new chemotherapeutic agents on the treatment of tuberculosis was spectacular. With the addition of streptomycin alone, the average relapse rate of tuberculosis was decreased by 30% to 35%. Although the effect of antitubercular chemotherapy was not as substantial for the treatment of spinal tuberculosis as for the pulmonary form, its mere availability raised new questions about the optimal management of Pott's paraplegia and, in particular, about the indications for surgical intervention.

Larson's Lateral Extracavitary Approach

In 1976, Sanford J. Larson and his colleagues[67] at the Medical College of Wisconsin published an influential article that helped to popularize Capener's lateral rhachotomy, which they modified and renamed the *lateral extracavitary approach* (Figure 1.13). This approach has been used more for trauma and tumor than for tuberculosis. The technical difference that distinguishes the lateral rhachotomy from the lateral extracavitary approach lies primarily in the treatment of the paraspinous muscles.

Whereas the procedure of Capener involves transversely dividing these muscles and reflecting them rostrally and caudally, the procedure of Larson involves a surgical exposure with a trajectory ventral to the paraspinous muscles, which are then reflected medially to expose the ventrolateral aspect of the spine. Later in the procedure these muscles are redirected laterally to provide access for instrumentation of the dorsal aspect of the spine using the same surgical exposure as that during the ventrolateral approach. Although neurosurgeons, as spine surgeons, had traditionally emphasized spinal decompression over spinal stabilization, an essential aspect of the significance of Larson's overall contribution to the discipline of spinal surgery lies in the fact that, as a neurosurgeon, he dedicated his career to the advancement of reconstructive spinal surgery.

Spinal Stabilization and Deformity Correction

The history of surgical stabilization and deformity correction must include a description of the birth and evolution of spinal fusion and spinal instrumentation. Special emphasis must be given to the role of spinal biomechanics and its influence on the development of internal fixation. Many factors hindered the development of surgical approaches to the decompression, stabilization, and deformity correction of the ventral spine. The development and mastery of the special techniques that were required to safely manage ventral spinal pathologies did not appear until after the turn of the century, in part because they depended on advances in anesthetic techniques and a more sophisticated approach to perioperative management.

Except for degenerative disease, the technique and indications for the decompressive laminectomy were well established by the turn of the century. The idea of spinal decompression, previously the exclusive province of surgical pioneers, had demonstrated its clinical utility with results that fully justified its acceptance into standard surgical practice. However, the idea of decompression, which had dominated spinal surgery during the nineteenth century, did not exist alone. Indeed, before the dawn of the twentieth century, attention had already turned to another surgical idea: spinal stabilization. Of course, many attempts at surgical stabilization of the unstable spine had been made during the nineteenth century and before. However, the ancient admonition that vertebral fractures comprised an "ailment not to be treated" was reinforced by the surgeon's singular lack of success. And, thus, despite early attempts at spinal stabilization in the latter part of the nineteenth century, spinal decompression

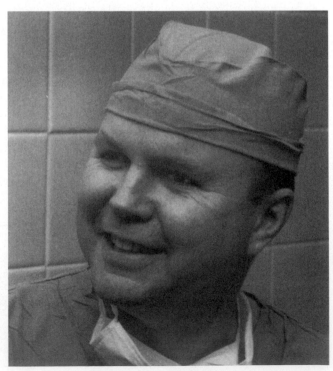

Figure 1.13 Sanford J. Larson.

remained the primary indication for surgery of the spine, until World War II.

Recognition of the idea that compression of the neural elements, in cases of tumor, trauma, and infection, could be responsible for neurologic compromise was the crucial first step needed to develop the idea that spinal decompression could improve neurologic outcome. The invention of a technical means to achieve decompression, namely by laminectomy, represented the next necessary step in bringing this concept to clinical practice. Similarly, the idea of spinal stabilization arose from the observation that the unstable spine was at risk for the development of progressive deformity and that surgical intervention might prevent this. Of course, bringing this concept into practice depended on achieving an adequate technical means. And indeed, two technical advances were developed around the turn of the century that provided a means for spinal stabilization that would revolutionize the practice of modern spinal surgery.

The Birth and Development of Spinal Fusion and Spinal Instrumentation

Both spinal fusion and spinal instrumentation were born around the turn of the century as methods of stabilizing the unstable spine. For many years, these two technical advances were developed and applied essentially independently, with results that were often complicated by pseudarthrosis. Early attempts at spinal instrumentation in particular failed to gain popularity because of their inability to maintain more than immediate spinal alignment. Spinal

fusions were often used to achieve stabilization, but these also frequently suffered a similar fate: pseudarthrosis.[101]

By the 1960s, however, a half century of experience with spinal fusion and instrumentation suggested the concept of the "race between bony fusion and instrumentation failure." The improved surgical results that arose from the application of this important surgical concept provided support for the successful strategy of combining spinal instrumentation with meticulous fusion.

Spinal Fusion

The idea of using spinal fusion for stabilization is attributed to Albee[3] and Hibbs,[49] who, in 1911, independently reported its use (Figure 1.14). Although these early operations were performed to prevent progressive spinal deformation in patients with Pott's disease, the procedure was later adopted in the management of scoliosis and traumatic fracture. The method of Hibbs, which was most frequently used, comprised harvesting an autologous bone graft from the laminae and overlaying the bone dorsally. Despite later improvements in this technique, however, such as the use of autologous iliac crest graft, the rate of pseudarthrosis, particularly in scoliosis, remained unacceptably high.[11]

In the 1920s Campbell[17] described trisacral fusion and iliac crest grafting. In 1922 Kleinberg[59] used xenograft for spinal fusion. ALIF was described by Burns[14] in 1933, and PLIF was performed by Cloward[24] in 1940. In the late 1990s TLIF was described. In 1977 Callahan *et al.*[15] used bone for lateral cervical facet fusion.

Several ventral cervical fusion techniques were described in 1950s. Robinson and Smith[91] described their

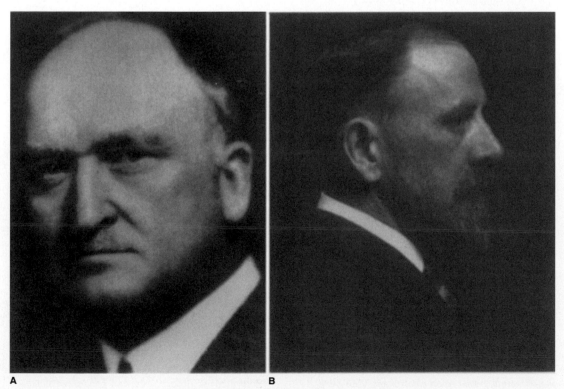

A **B**

Figure 1.14 (**A**) Fred Albee. (**B**) Russell Hibbs.

technique in 1955, and Cloward[25] described his cervical fusion technique in 1958.

Spinal Instrumentation and Clinical Biomechanics

Like spinal fusion, internal fixation was first applied around 1900. These early constructs comprised tension-band fixators that were applied dorsally, primarily in cases of trauma. The limitation of the constructs, however, soon became apparent because the metals they contained were subject to the corrosive effects of electrolysis.

With the introduction of vitallium by Venable and Stuck[104] in the 1930s, a metal was found that was previously used successfully as a dental filling material and that had proven resistant to electrolysis (Figure 1.15).[103] Further attempts at internal fixation during the 1930s and 1940s included fixed-moment arm cantilever constructs. These also failed to maintain alignment.[58,77,111]

F.W. Holdsworth

In the 1950s, the British orthopedic surgeon Sir Frank W. Holdsworth[51] performed perhaps the first large systematic study of the problem of internal fixation for the treatment of posttraumatic fracture. Although the constructs he used, which comprised cantilever beams attached to the spinous processes, were traditional, Holdsworth's emphasis on patient selection brought the process of surgical spinal stabilization to a new, more sophisticated, level. His rationale for patient selection was based on a biomechanical definition of instability that Holdsworth derived from a study of a large number of spinal-injured patients.

In 1963, Holdsworth[52] published his results and proposed a classification scheme of subaxial spinal fractures based on a two-column model of spinal stability. Four categories of fractures were identified on the basis of the mechanism of injury and on the presence or absence of spinal stability. The latter determination rested significantly on the integrity of the dorsal ligaments. Holdsworth categorized the fractures as follows:

1. Pure flexion: A pure flexion mechanism is usually associated with an intact dorsal ligamentous complex and no evidence of spinal instability. The vertebral body absorbs the greater part of the impact, and the result is a wedge compression fracture (Figure 1.16A).
2. Flexion-rotation: A rotation or flexion-rotation mechanism causes disruption of the dorsal ligamentous complex and results in an unstable fracture-dislocation. It is usually associated with paraplegia (Figure 1.16B).
3. Extension: An extension mechanism, which is usually stable, most frequently occurs in the cervical spine. It may be associated with a fracture of the dorsal elements, with an intact dorsal ligamentous complex (Figure 1.16C).
4. Compression: A compression or "burst" fracture is caused by forces transmitted directly along the line of the vertebral bodies. All of the ligaments are usually intact, and the fracture tends to be stable (Figure 1.16D).

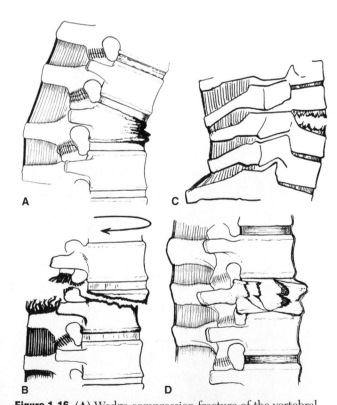

Figure 1.16 **(A)** Wedge compression fracture of the vertebral body. Pure flexion mechanism. Note that the posterior ligamentous complex is intact. **(B)** Rotational fracture-dislocation of the lumbar spine. The posterior ligamentous complex is disrupted. This is a very unstable injury. **(C)** Extension injury. The anterior longitudinal ligament is ruptured. The posterior ligamentous complex is intact. **(D)** Burst fracture. All ligaments are intact. (*From Holdsworth FW: Fractures, dislocations, and fracture-dislocation of the spine. J Bone Joint Surg 45B:6-20, 1963.*)

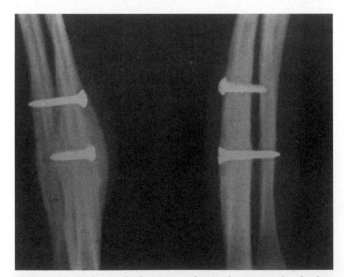

Figure 1.15 Radiograph showing no bone changes in dog limb about vitallium screws (*right*), but erosion of bone around steel screws (*left*). (*From Venable CS, Stuck WG, Beach A: The effects on bone of metals; based upon electrolysis.* Ann Surg 105:917-938, 1937.)

Holdsworth's classification was important, as he himself observed, not as a biomechanical theory (although it was this too), but because it had implications for treatment. At around the same time that Holdsworth's article appeared, several other classifications of spinal fractures were proposed. With the introduction of modern spinal biomechanics, a new era in spinal surgery had begun.[9,57]

Paul Harrington and the Birth of Modern Surgical Stabilization

In his 1891 report of a case of interspinous wiring for cervical fracture, Berthold Hadra[43] considered in what circumstances his newly described procedure would be indicated (Figure 1.17). Hadra concluded that his procedure might be indicated for "any deviation of a vertebra."[43] Despite the prescience of his innovation, the substance of Hadra's comment is remarkable, not so much for what it contains, as for what is missing from it; namely, any hint of consideration of biomechanical principles. When one considers the importance of biomechanical principles in Holdsworth's 1963 classification of spinal fractures, Hadra's turn-of-the-century approach to spinal stabilization serves to underline how much progress was made in the interval. The significance of this new (biomechanic) approach to spinal stabilization, which was heralded by Holdsworth, was brought home in the 1960s with the work of the father of modern spinal stabilization, Paul Harrington (Figure 1.18).

In 1945, after military service in World War II, Paul Harrington[47] entered into orthopedic practice in Houston, Texas. Within 2 years of beginning his practice in Houston, Harrington was faced with the orthopedic problems of a large population of poliomyelitis patients, which at that time had reached epidemic proportions. The involvement of the trunk, which afflicted many of these patients, often resulted in scoliotic spinal deformity in association with cardiopulmonary compromise. The presence of cardiopulmonary compromise in a patient with scoliosis often meant that the standard cast corrective measures could not be applied safely. Furthermore, in 1941, the American Orthopaedic Association[6] published a report on the results of treatment in 425 cases of idiopathic scoliosis. The report was quite discouraging. Among those patients treated by exercises and braces, but without spinal fusion, 60% progressed in their deformity, and 40% remained unchanged. In another group of patients who underwent surgical correction and fusion, 25% (54 of 214) developed pseudarthrosis and 29% had lost all correction. Among the entire group, the end result for 69% was considered fair or poor, and only 31% were rated good to excellent. It was against this backdrop of dismal results from nonoperative treatment and dorsal spinal fusion that Harrington began his seminal work.

After an initial (unsuccessful) trial of internal fixation with facet screw instrumentation,[46] the method was abandoned in favor of a combination of compression and distraction hooks and rods made of stainless steel. The advantages of these instruments in the establishment of deformity correction became obvious: for the first time in

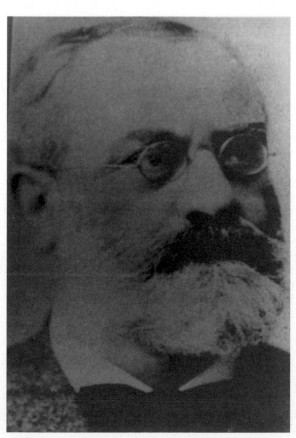

Figure 1.17 Berthold Hadra.

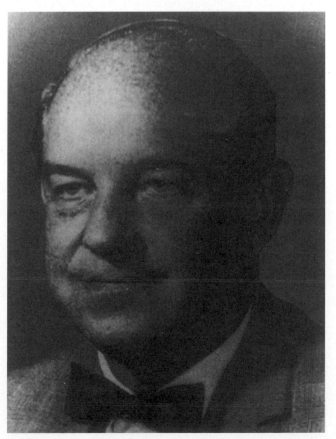

Figure 1.18 Paul Harrington.

the history of spinal stabilization, spinal instruments provided compression, distraction, and three-point bending forces, which proved equally useful in deformity correction as it did in the maintenance of post-traumatic stability. There were 19 patients observed during the early phase of Harrington's investigation of dorsal instrumentation. The results of this investigation were published in 1962.[47] The longevity of Harrington's spinal instrumentation system, which remains in use today, is a testimony to both its safety and its efficacy.

Nevertheless, despite a frequent and gratifying correction of the poliomyelitis curvature, the loss of that correction was commonly discovered within 6 to 12 months after surgery. In part, the failure to maintain the alignment achieved at surgery was the result of frequent instrument failure, most commonly instrument fracture and disengagement of the hooks. However, more fundamentally, Harrington recognized that the concept of a dynamic correction system was inherently flawed: the complication of instrument failure would be far less significant if a spinal fusion could maintain the deformity correction achieved by the placement of the implant.

The underlying principles that emerged from Harrington's early failures, then, became clear: (1) because spinal instruments fail over time, they should be applied as a strictly temporary measure; and (2) after instrumentation failure, a successful spinal fusion will maintain stabilization. As a corollary to these principles, Harrington acknowledged that there is a "race between instrumentation failure and the acquisition of spinal fusion." It stands to reason that if fusion is attained before instrumentation failure, the maintenance of deformity correction and stabilization will have been achieved. An understanding of the importance of a successful fusion in an instrumented spine is one of Harrington's most significant contributions to spinal surgery and marks the birth of the modern era of spinal stabilization and deformity correction.

Ventral Approaches to the Spine

Dorsal decompression via the laminectomy had become well-established by the turn of the century and was codified by Charles Elsberg in his 1916 textbook, *Diagnosis and Treatment of Surgical Diseases of the Spinal Cord and Its Membranes*. Interestingly, whereas the turn of the century marked the culmination of dorsal decompression in spinal surgery, it also signified the beginning of procedures for dorsal stabilization and deformity correction, as pioneered by Hadra (1891), Albee (1911), and Hibbs (1911). The groundwork for further development in this area was laid with the classification scheme of spinal fractures by mechanism and stability, as initially proposed by Holdsworth in 1963. This introduction into clinical practice of the principles of spinal biomechanics is also found in the work of Harrington in the 1950s and 1960s in his development of a novel system of dorsal thoracolumbar instrumentation. Although Harrington later recognized the need to supplement his instrumentation with meticuluous spinal fusion, and many modifications and innovations have since been made in dorsal instrumentation, successful outcomes in dorsal decompression, stabilization, and deformity correction had been achieved by the 1960s.

Nothing, however, has been said so far about the achievement of these goals in the ventral spine, where a significant portion of spinal pathology is located. As it happens, the first successful interventions for stabilization of the ventral spine were achieved in the same time frame as the dorsal ones (that is, in the first half of the twentieth century). What is peculiar about surgery of the ventral spine is that a decompressive procedure must be accompanied almost invariably by simultaneous stabilization, which often includes measures taken to obtain deformity correction. Therefore the history of the major goals of ventral spine surgery—that is, decompression, stabilization, and deformity correction—has been one of parallel developments, not serial ones, as was the case for the dorsal spine. In other words, the history of stabilization and deformity correction of the dorsal spine developed in the half century following the establishment of dorsal decompression. All three goals, in the ventral spine, were achieved during the same 50 years.

Ventral Decompression and Stabilization

The primary difficulty in applying ventral techniques to the spine was in the surgical approach. The relative technical ease and low morbidity associated with a dorsal approach to the dorsal spine provided ample opportunity for the early development of dorsal spinal techniques. By contrast, ventral approaches to the ventral spine required transgression of the abdomen or chest, which (similar to the head) up until the 1880s remained sanctuaries not to be opened, except by accident.[78]

In part, the late development of abdominal and thoracic surgery was a product of the problem of infection: cognizant of the morbidity and mortality related to hospital-acquired gangrene, few of those who entered a surgical ward in the nineteenth century did so with the hope of leaving alive. The reluctance to adopt the principles of antisepsis as first enunciated by Lister[68] in 1867 and a slowness to accept its theoretical foundation—the germ theory of disease—meant delays for the development of abdominal and thoracic surgery. However, even after the practice of antiseptic surgery became generally accepted, turn-of-the-century surgeons still approached abdominal surgery with trepidation.

Anyone who would contemplate surgically violating the thoracic cavity had to face the technical problem of the pressure relationships in the chest.[80] Beginning in 1903, Ferdinand Sauerbruch of Breslau conducted a series of experiments that led to the development of an apparatus in which negative pressure for the open thorax could be maintained, and around 1910, endotracheal or insufflation anesthesia became available (Figure 1.19). This alleviated one of the major technical difficulties confronted by would-be thoracic surgeons, but even then, good control of respiration by a reliable apparatus was not widely available until the late 1930s.

W. Müller

The first report of a successful attempt to approach the ventral thoracic or lumbar spine is attributed to Müller.[84] In 1906, Müller performed a transperitoneal approach to the lumbosacral spine in a patient with a suspected sarcoma. At operation, Müller found tuberculosis. After curetting the infected bone, Müller applied iodoform powder and closed. The surgical result was excellent. Notwithstanding the success of this initial operation, however, later attempts at the same procedure failed miserably. After several misadventures that ended in disaster, Müller was forced to abandon further attempts at a ventral exposure.

B.H. Burns

Perhaps the next published report of a successful ventral exposure did not appear until 1933, when B.H. Burns[14] of Great Britain performed a ventral interbody fusion of the lumbosacral spine for an L5-S1 spondylolisthesis (Figure 1.20). Before the Burns procedure, the only method available to stabilize an unstable spondylolisthesis was a dorsal fusion. However, the results of dorsal fusion for ventral instability, as Burns himself learned firsthand, proved unsound both in theory and in practice. Faced with a high incidence of failed dorsal fusions, Burns chose to take a transabdominal, transperitoneal approach to the lumbosacral spine, which he first investigated on three cadavers before operation. The first operation involved a 14-year-old boy who presented with low back pain and neurogenic claudication after jumping from a height. A radiograph of the lumbosacral spine showed an L5 spondylolysis and a Grade II, L5-S1 spondylolisthesis. A tibial autograft was taken and was tamped into a hole drilled obliquely from L5 to S1. Convalescence was uneventful and pain relief was achieved, even on ambulation at 2 months postoperatively.

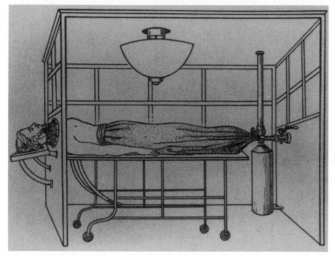

Figure 1.19 An early version of Sauerbruch's negative-pressure chamber.

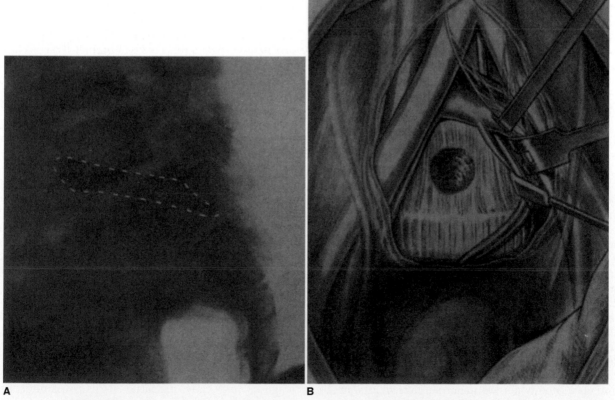

A   B

Figure 1.20 **(A)** Lateral radiograph of lumbar spine showing the graft placement in B.H. Burns' operation for spondylolisthesis. (*From Burns BH: An operation for spondylolisthesis.* Lancet 1:1233, 1933, *with permission.*) **(B)** Illustration of Burns' operation. Ventral view.

Ito and Others

Like the landmark operations of Albee and Hibbs, the first reported series of ventral spinal operations comprised a group of surgical treatments for spinal tuberculosis. In their 1934 article, "A New Radical Operation for Pott's Disease," Ito and others[54] observed that the surgical stabilization procedure described by Albee and Hibbs did not differ significantly from nonoperative immobilization; the goal in both instances was to rest and unload the diseased spine. Ito, on the other hand, a professor of orthopedic surgery from Kyoto, Japan, proposed a decompressive procedure, which he believed provided a definitive surgical treatment.

Of course, the obstacles that Ito confronted in devising a ventral approach to the spine were considerable. In addition to the obvious anatomic obstacles, all turn-of-the-century spine surgeons faced the seemingly intractable problem of infection. Although postoperative infections posed major difficulties for the development of (clean) abdominal and thoracic surgical procedures, these difficulties were compounded when the surgical indication *was* infection, as in the case of Pott's disease. Indeed, previous attempts to surgically decompress tuberculosis of the ventral spine via a lateral approach (i.e., a costotransversectomy) met with a high incidence of complications from postoperative secondary infection, permanent fistulas, or persistent spinal tuberculosis resulting from incomplete removal of infected bone.[60,79,106,107]

In part, these operations failed because they were performed prior to 1910, in the age of antiseptic, rather than aseptic, surgery. Perhaps they also failed in part because they predated the introduction of antimicrobial chemotherapy. However, the unsatisfactory results that these operations yielded was also importantly attributed to the poor surgical exposure of the vertebral bodies that the lateral approach provided. Recognizing this, Ito proposed a decompression operation that would adequately resect infected vertebrae in order to fully eradicate the presence of tuberculosis in the spine. Drawing on experience with the transabdominal approach, which he had previously used for another purpose, Ito reported his operative technique and surgical results on 10 patients with moderately advanced Pott's disease. The possibility of approaching the ventral spine occurred to Ito and his colleagues after repeated operations using their original technique for lumbosacral sympathetic ganglionectomy. In 1923, Ito and his colleagues[53] originated this technique for the purpose of improving lower extremity circulation and reported their results to the Japanese Surgical Society in 1925. The technique was subsequently modified to provide an extraperitoneal approach to the lumbar spine and was adopted for their radical operation for Pott's disease (Figure 1.21).

The significance of the work of Ito was beneficial for several reasons. First, Ito and his colleagues recognized the need to address the pathology directly, despite the technical difficulties that such an approach presented. Second, at a time when the major surgical treatment for Pott's disease was dorsal fusion, Ito proposed a radical new surgical therapy: decompression. An attempt to eradicate spinal infection by surgical decompression represented an

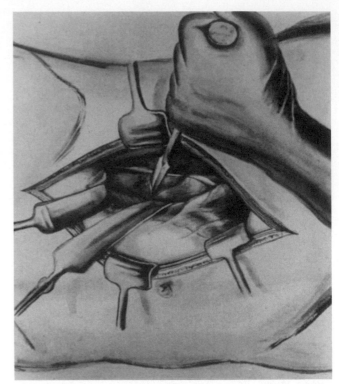

Figure 1.21 Extraperitoneal exposure of the body of the lumbar vertebra and resection of the body with a chisel. *(From Ito H, Tsuchiya J, Asaini G: A new radical operation for Pott's disease.* J Bone Joint Surg *16:499-515, 1934.)*

alternative approach to the standard stabilization procedure originated by Albee and Hibbs. In another sense, the idea of decompression harked back to the nineteenth century laminectomy for Pott's disease, which was largely abandoned because of disappointing results, after the introduction of dorsal spinal fusion.[88] Finally, Ito recognized the need, and established the technique, to stabilize the spine, which if not already unstable, was certainly rendered unstable by resection of the major load-bearing element. He accomplished this goal by fashioning a ventral interbody fusion, which both provided significant stability and facilitated spinal fusion (Figure 1.22). However, despite Ito's successes—all except two of Ito's ten cases showed a healing by primary intention and despite his acknowledgment of the inadequacies of the dorsolateral approach—Ito himself used the costotransversectomy approach in the two cases of thoracic Pott's disease included in his series.

Hodgson and Stock

Thus, it fell to another group of surgeons treating Pott's disease to develop a true ventral approach to the thoracic spine. In 1956, Hodgson and Stock[50] published their first report on ventral spinal fusion for Pott's disease. These authors acknowledged the contributions of Ito and his colleagues, and they repeated Ito's assessment of the restricted field of view afforded by the costotransversectomy. They noted that this field of view provided insufficient exposure to determine the extent of the lesion or to

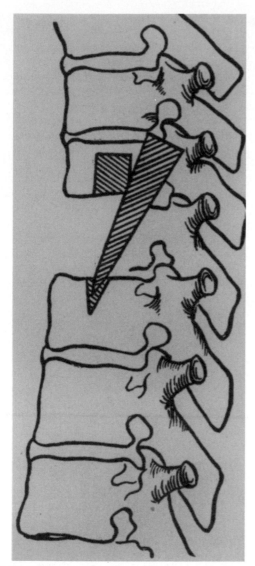

Figure 1.22 Schematic illustration of the insertion of ventral bone graft. *(From Ito H, Tsuchiya J, Asaini G: A new radical operation for Pott's disease.* J Bone Joint Surg *16:499–515, 1934.)*

confidently undertake its complete resection. What is more, the limited exposure of the costotransversectomy left no room to accurately insert a ventral bone graft, which they considered offered the best chance for fusion because the bone graft would be placed in a compression mode.

Hodgson and Stock also joined Ito and others in emphasizing decompression, rather than simple stabilization, as a method to arrest further vertebral destruction (which may be responsible for neural element compression and progressive kyphotic deformity), and as a means to eradicate the spinal focus of disease. Their approach to the thoracic spine via a thoracotomy, the first significant series of such an approach described, was facilitated by developments in the medical management of tuberculosis, including the introduction of chemotherapeutic agents (not available to Ito and others), and safer, more effective anesthetic techniques. The benefits of this approach, then, despite its technical difficulties, were

incontrovertible; it facilitated decompression, stabilization, and deformity correction through a single incision and surgical exposure, providing excellent neurologic and anatomic results. The authors took account of the unique anatomic features of the cervicothoracic and thoracolumbar junctions, where the approach was appropriately modified.

Ventral Deformity Reduction and the Development of Ventral Instrumentation

The contributions of Burns, Ito and associates, and Hodgson and Stock were seminal in the history of spinal surgery. They opened new vistas in the management of spinal pathologies, and their techniques were later applied to an increasingly wide range of pathologic conditions, including tumor, trauma, disc disease, and spinal deformity. The methods of Ito and associates were particularly prescient. They accomplished, with a single incision, the goals of both decompression and spinal stabilization, and they achieved both of these goals in the most effective possible manner. The establishment of deformity correction was addressed in the report by Hodgson, who confronted the problem of severe kyphotic deformity causing cardiopulmonary compromise.

On a larger scale, however, the problem of progressive spinal deformity did not receive the attention of these early authors, and no method of ventral internal fixation was yet available to spinal surgeons who wished to establish and maintain a deformity correction via a ventral approach. As mentioned, Paul Harrington addressed the problem of scoliotic deformity by the development of dorsal thoracolumbar distraction rods in the 1960s, and in doing so he initiated the modern instrumentation revolution.

Harrington's method of scoliosis reduction was based on the principle of lengthening the short (concave) side of the curve. After the introduction of a meticulous fusion technique to supplement the immediate rigid internal fixation achieved by the implant, the Harrington instrumentation system proved both a safe and effective corrective measure, an assessment that is corroborated by its long and successful history of clinical application. Nevertheless, the principle of simple dorsal distraction had its drawbacks. First, the Harrington method requires that the fusion be extended at least two levels above and below the extent of the spinal curvature, thus decreasing mobility in otherwise normal spinal motion segments. Second, in most instances, the distribution of force application with the Harrington instrumentation system is uneven, such that the total force applied is borne only by the two vertebrae attached to the upper and lower hooks. Finally, for patients who require a simultaneous ventral decompression and dorsal stabilization procedure, this could be accomplished only through a two-stage operation involving two separate incisions and surgical exposures. Thus, the arrival of a ventral instrumentation system, introduced by Dwyer[32] in 1969, proved an important addition to the spinal surgeon's surgical armamentarium.

A.F. Dwyer

A.F. Dwyer was an orthopedic surgeon from Australia who appears to have originated his method in an effort to provide an alternative to the Harrington technique of scoliotic deformity reduction. In his initial report of 1969, Dwyer described a method of ventral instrumentation in which compressive forces are applied to the convex side of the curve at each segmental level. The technique comprises excision of the discs at the motion segments involved, and the insertion of vertebral body screws into the convex aspect of the curve. A titanium cable is then threaded through the heads of the inserted screws and a tension force is applied, providing corrective bending moments at the intervertebral spaces. The tension is maintained by swaging the threaded cable on the screw heads (Figure 1.23).

In a follow-up article published in 1974, Dwyer and Schafer[33] reported their results of treatment in 51 cases, which demonstrated a generally favorable record of deformity correction and only a 4% rate of pseudarthrosis.[3] Furthermore, some of the disadvantages of the Harrington dorsal instrumentation system were overcome—fusion could be restricted to the motion segments of the curve only; the load borne by the instrumentation device was evenly distributed over the curve; and the exposure necessary for ventral decompression, stabilization, and deformity correction was achieved using a single incision. Although the initial enthusiasm for the Dwyer device was later diminished by the recognition that it encouraged the tendency of the spine toward progressive kyphosis and that it provided no resistance to axial loading, the generally successful application of this ventral instrumentation system stimulated the development of additional ventral implants, such as the instrumentation systems of Zielke and Pellin[116] and Kaneda and associates.[56]

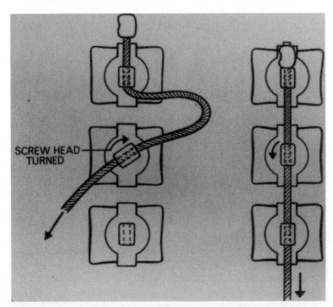

Figure 1.23 Dwyer's ventral short segment fixation device. *(From Dwyer AF, Schafer MF: Anterior approach to scoliosis. Results of treatment in fifty-one cases.* J Bone Joint Surg *56B:218-224, 1974.)*

Summary

The technical accomplishment of performing surgery on the ventral spine provides perhaps a useful marker for the endpoint of the history of "early modern" spinal surgery. By 1970, it may be argued, the basic groundwork had been laid for the subsequent advances, particularly in spinal instrumentation, that have been made over the last 25 years. These advances include an emphasis on location-appropriate decompression; the development of segmental spinal instrumentation by E.R. Luque in the early 1970s[70-73]; the refinement and proliferation of pedicular instrumentation techniques, first described by Harrington in 1969[45,112]; the introduction of universal spinal instrumentation by Cotrel and associates[26]; the further development of ventral thoracolumbar instrumentation by Zielke, Kostuik,[62] and Kaneda; the introduction of ventral cervical instrumentation by Caspar and associates in 1989[21]; and most recently, the application of endoscopic techniques.[55]

In conclusion, this essay has sought to organize and present the history of spinal surgery as a series of attempts to improve the surgeon's ability to more safely and effectively achieve spinal decompression, stabilization, and deformity correction—the three major goals of spinal surgery. The occasionally formidable obstacles encountered by those surgeons who have participated in this century-long odyssey were frequently managed, if not overcome, by concentrated and indefatigable effort. Alas, many of the same obstacles that faced the early spinal surgeons—including blood loss, pseudarthosis, instrumentation failure, and neurologic injury—continue to challenge and vex even the best-equipped contemporary spinal surgeons.

REFERENCES

1. Abbe R: Spinal surgery: Report of eight cases. *Med Rec* 38:85-92, 1890.
2. Adams F: *The Genuine Works of Hippocrates.* Baltimore, Williams & Wilkins, 1939.
3. Albee FH: Transplantation of a portion of the tibia into the spine for Pott's disease. *JAMA* 57:885-886, 1911.
4. Alessandri R: Laminectomia della terza e quarta vertebre lombre per lesione della cauda equina. *Riv Patol Nerv* 10:86-92, 1905.
5. Alessandri R: Processo osteoplastico modificato di laminectomia, con due casi operati. *Arch Ed Atti Soc Ital Chir* 18:135B154, 1905
6. American Orthopaedic Association Research Committee: End-result study of the treatment of idiopathic scoliosis. *J Bone Joint Surg* 23:963-977, 1941.
7. Armour D: Surgery of the spinal cord and its membranes. *Lancet* 1:423-430, 1927.
8. Bailey P, Casamajor C: Osteoarthritis of the spine as a cause of compression of the spinal cord and its roots. *J Nerv Mental Dis* 38:588-609, 1911.
9. Bailey RW: Fractures and dislocations of the cervical spine: orthopedic and neurosurgical aspects. *Postgrad Med* 35:588-599, 1964.
10. Benini A, Bonar SK: Andreas Vesalius 1514-1564. *Spine* 21:1388-1393, 1996.

11. Boucher HH: A method of spinal fusion. *J Bone Joint Surg* 41B:248-259, 1959.

12. Brasted JH: The Edwin Smith Papyrus. In: Wilkins RH (compiled): *Neurosurgical Classics.* Park Ridge, Ill, American Association of Neurologic Surgeons, 1992, pp 1-5.

13. Brok AJ: *Greek Medicine.* J.M. Dent & Sons. London, 1929.

14. Burns BH: An operation for spondylolisthesis. *Lancet* 1:1233, 1933.

15. Callahan RA, Johnson RM, Margolis RN, *et al.*: Cervical facet fusion for control of instability following laminectomy. *J Bone Joint Surg* 59(A):991-1002, 1977.

16. Calot T: Sur le meilleur traitement localdes tuberculoses doses articulations et ganglions lymphatiques. *Acta Chir Scand* 67:206-226, 1930.

17. Campbell WC: An operation for extra-articular fusion of sacroiliac joint. *Surg Gynecol Obstet* 45:218-219, 1927.

18. Capener N: The evolution of lateral rhachotomy. *J Bone Joint Surg* 36B:173-179, 1954.

19. Caponotto A, Pescarolo B: Estirpazione di un tumore intradurale del canale rachideo. *Riforma Med* 8:543-549, 1892.

20. Caspar W. A new surgical procedure for lumbar disc herniation causing less tissue damage through a microsurgical approach. *Adv Neurosurgery* 4: 77-80, 1977.

21. Caspar W, Barbier DD, Klara PM: Anterior cervical fusion and Caspar plate stabilization for cervical trauma. *Neurosurgery* 25:491 502, 1989.

22. Church A, Eisendrath DW: A contribution to spinal cord surgery. *Am J Med Sci* 103:395-412, 1892.

23. Cline HJ Jr (cited by Hayward G): An account of a case of fracture and dislocation of the spine. *New Engl J Med Surg* 4:13, 1815.

24. Cloward RB: The treatment of ruptured intervertebral disc by vertebral body fusion. *Ann Surg* 136: 987-992, 1952.

25. Cloward RB. The anterior approach for removal of ruptured cervical disks. *J Neurosurg* 15:602-617, 1958.

26. Cotrel Y, Dubousset J, Guillaumat M: New universal instrumentation in spinal surgery. *Clin Orthop* 227:10-23, 1988.

27. Cushing H: Intradural tumor of the cervical meninges with early restoration of function in the cord after removal of the tumor. *Ann Surg* 39:934-955, 1904.

28. Cushing H: The special field of neurological surgery. *Bull Johns Hopkins Hosp* 16:77-87, 1905.

29. Cushing H: The special field of neurological surgery: five years later. *Bull Johns Hopkins Hosp* 21:325-329, 1910.

30. Dandy WE: Loose cartilage from the intervertebral disc simulating tumour of the spinal cord. *Arch Surg* 19: 660-672, 1929.

31. Dawbarn RHM: A successful case of spinal resection. *New York Med J* 49:711-715, 1889.

32. Dwyer AF, Newton NC, Sherwood AA: An anterior approach to scoliosis. A preliminary report. *Clin Orthop* 62:192-202, 1969.

33. Dwyer AF, Schafer MF: Anterior approach to scoliosis. Results of treatment in fifty-one cases. *J Bone Joint Surg* 56B:218-224, 1974.

34. Elsberg CA, Beer E: The operability of intramedullary tumors of the spinal cord. A report of two operations with remarks upon the extrusion of intraspinal tumors. *Am J Med Sci* 142:636-647, 1911.

35. Elsberg CA: *Diagnosis and Treatment of Diseases of the Spinal Cord and Its Membranes.* Philadelphia, WB Saunders, 1916.

36. Elsberg CA: Experiences in spinal surgery. *Surg Gynecol Obstet* 16:117-132, 1913.

37. Elsberg CA: The extradural ventral chondromas (enchondroses), their favorite sites, the spinal cord and root symptoms they produce, and their surgical treatment. *Bull Neurol Inst NY* 1: 350-388, 1931.

38. Eskridge JT, Freeman L: Intradural spinal tumor opposite the body of the fourth dorsal vertebra; complete paralysis of the parts below the lesion; operation; recovery; with ability to walk without assistance within three months. *Phil Med J* 2:1236-1243, 1898.

39. Goldthwaite JE: The lumbosacral articulation. An explanation of many cases of "lumbago," "sciatica," and paraplegia. *Boston Med Sci J* 164:365-372, 1911.

40. Gower W: *A Manual of Diseases of the Nervous System,* 2 volumes. London, J & A Churchill, 1886-1888.

41. Gowers WR, Horsley VA: A case of tumour of the spinal cord. Removal; recovery. *Med Chir Trans* 53:379-428, 1888.

42. Gurunluoglu R, Gurunluoglu A: Paul of Aegina: landmark in surgical progress. *World J Surg* 27:18-25, 2003.

43. Hadra BE: Wiring the spinous processes in Pott's disease. *Trans Am Orthop Assoc* 4:206-210, 1891.

44. Harrington PR, Tullos HS: Reduction of severe spondylolisthesis in children. *South Med J* 62:1-7, 1969.

45. Harrington PR, Tullos HS: Spondylolisthesis in children. *Clin Orthop* 79:75-84, 1971.

46. Harrington PR: The history and development of Harrington instrumentation. *Clin Orthop Rel Res* 93:110-112, 1973.

47. Harrington PR: Treatment of scoliosis. *J Bone Joint Surg* 44A:591-610, 1962.

48. Hattori S. A new method for cervical laminectomy. *Central Jap J Orthop Traum Surg* 16:792-794, 1973.

49. Hibbs RA: An operation for progressive spinal deformities. *NY Med J* 93:1013-1016, 1911.

50. Hodgson AR, Stock FE: Anterior spinal fusion. A preliminary communication on the radical treatment of Pott's disease and Pott's paraplegia. *Br J Surg* 44:266-275, 1956.

51. Holdsworth FW, Hardy A: Early treatment of paraplegia from fractures of the thoraco-lumbar spine. *J Bone Joint Surg* 35B:540-550, 1953.

52. Holdsworth FW: Fractures, dislocations, and fracture-dislocation of the spine. *J Bone Joint Surg* 45B:6-20, 1963.

53. Ito H, Asami G: Lumbosacral sympathetic ganglionectomy. Its value as a therapeutic measure for thromboangiitis obliterans. *Am J Surg* 15:26, 1932.

54. Ito H, Tsuchiya J, Asaini G: A new radical operation for Pott's disease. *J Bone Joint Surg* 16:499-515, 1934.

55. Kambin P, Gellman H. Percutaneous lateral discectomy of the lumbar spine. *Clin Orthop* 174:128-132, 1983.

56. Kaneda K, Abumi K, Fujiya K: Burst fractures with neurologic deficits of the thoraco-lumbar spine. Results of anterior decompression and stabilization with anterior instrumentation. *Spine* 9:788-795, 1984.

57. Kelly RP, Whitesides TE: Treatment of lumbodorsal fracture-dislocations. *Ann Surg* 167:705-717, 1968.

58. King D: Internal fixation for lumbosacral fusion. *J Bone Joint Surg* 30A: 560-565, 1948.

59. Kleinberg S: The operative treatment of scoliosis. *Arch Surg* 5: 631-645, 1922.

60. Kocher T: *Chirurgische Operationslehre*. G Fischer, Jena, 1892.

61. Kocher T: Die Verletzungen der Wirbelsule zugeleich als Beitrag zur Physiologie des menschlichen Ruckenmarks. *Mitt Grenzgeb Med Chir* 1:415-480, 1896.

62. Kostuik JP: Anterior fixation for fractures of the thoracic and lumbar spine with or without neurologic involvement. *Clin Orthop* 189:103-115, 1984.

63. Kumar K: Historical perspective: spinal deformity and axial traction. *Spine* 21:653-655, 1996.

64. Lane WA: Case of spondylolisthesis associated with progressive paraplegia; laminectomy. *Lancet* 1:991, 1893.

65. Lang JK, Kolenda H: First appearance and sense of the term "spinal column" in ancient Egypt. Historical vignette. *J Neurosurg* 97(1 Suppl):152-155, 2002.

66. Laquer L: Ueber Compression der Cauda equina. Compressions-Erscheinungen im Gebeite der lumbal und Sacral wurzeln. Eroffnung des Canalis sacralis. Exstirpation eines Lymphangioma cavernosum. Beseitigung fast aller Beschwerden. *Neurol Centralbl* 10:193-204, 1891.

67. Larson SJ, Holst RA, Hemmy DC, Saiices A Jr: Lateral extracavitary approach to traumatic lesions of the thoracic and lumbar spine. *J Neurosurg* 45:628-637, 1976.

68. Lister J: *Six Papers. Selected by Sir Rickman J. Godley.* London, 1912.

69. Love JG: Removal of intervertebral discs without laminectomy. Proceedings of staff meeting. *Mayo Clinic* 14:800, 1939.

70. Luque ER, Cassis N, Ramirez-Wiella G: Segmental spinal instrumentation in the treatment of fractures of the thoracolumbar spine. *Spine* 7:256-259, 1982.

71. Luque ER: The anatomic basis and development of segmental spinal instrumentation. *Spine* 7:256-259, 1982.

72. Luque ER: Interpeduncular segmental fixation. *Clin Orthop* 203:54-57, 1986.

73. Luque ER: Segmental spinal instrumentation of the lumbar spine. *Clin Orthop* 203:126-134, 1986.

74. Makins GH, Abbott FC: On acute primary osteomyelitis of the vertebrae. *Ann Surg* 23:510-539, 1896.

75. Maquet P: Iatrophysics to biomechanics. From Borelli (1608-1679) to Pauwels (1885-1980). *J Bone Joint Surg Br* 74:335-339, 1992.

76. Marketos SG, Skiadas PK: Galen. A pioneer of spine research. *Spine* 24:2358-2362, 1999.

77. Markham JW: Surgery of the spinal cord and vertebral column. In Walker AE (ed): *A History of Neurological Surgery*. New York, Hafner Publishing Company, 1967, pp 370-371.

78. Matas R: Surgical operations fifty years ago. *Am J Surg* 82:111, 1951.

79. Ménard V: Causes de la paraplegia dans le mal de Pott. Son traitement chirurgical par l'ouverture direct du foyer tuberculeux des vertebras. *Rev Orthop* 5:47-64, 1894.

80. Meyer HW: The history of the development of the negative differential pressure chamber for thoracic surgery. *J Thor Surg* 30:114, 1955.

81. Middleton GS, Teacher JH: Injury of the spinal cord due to rupture of an intervertebral disc during muscular effort. *Glasgow Med J* 76:1-6, 1911.

82. Middleton WEK: A little-known portrait of Giovanni Alfonso Borelli. *Med Hist* 18:94-95, 1974.

83. Mixter WJ, Barr JS: Rupture of the intervertebral disc with involvement of the spinal canal. *N Engl J Med* 211: 210-215, 1934.

84. Müller W: Transperitoneale Freilegung der Wirbelsaule bei Tuberkuloser Spondylitis. *Deutsche Ztschr Chir* 85:128, 1906.

85. Naderi S, Acar F, Arda MN: History of spinal disorders and cerrahiyetülhaniye: a review of a Turkish treatise written by serefeddin Sabuncuoglu in 15th century. *J Neurosurg* 96:352-356, 2002.

86. Naderi S, Acar F, Mertol T, Arda MN: Functional anatomy of the spine by Avicenna in his eleventh century treatise Al-Qanun fi al-Tibb (The Canons of Medicine). *Neurosurgery* 52:1449-1453, 2003.

87. Novell JR: From Da Vinci to Harvey: The development of mechanical analogy in medicine from 1500 to1650. *J R Soc Med* 83:396-398, 1990.

88. Ollier L: *Traite des resections et des operations conservatrices qu'on peut pratiquer sur le systeme osseux.* Vol 3. G Masson, Paris, 1891, pp 833-857.

89. Oppenheim H, Krause F: Über Einklemung bzw. Strangulationbder Cauda Equina. *Dtsch Med Wochenschrift* 35: 697-700, 1909.

90. Portal A: *Cours d'Anatomie Medicale ou Elements de l'Anatomie de l'Homme.* Vol. 1. Baudouin, Paris, 1803.

91. Robinson RA, Smith GW. Anterolateral cervical disc removal and interbody fusion for cervical disc syndrome. *Bull John Hopkins Hosp* 96:223, 1955.

92. Rogers DL: A case of fractured spine with depression of the spinous processes, and the operation for its removal. *Am J Med Sci* 16:91-94, 1835.

93. Roy CD: Report of a case of spinal exsection and removal of a tumor from the cord. *South Med Rec* 20:564-566, 1890.

94. Sachs B, Frankel J: Progressive ankylotic rigidity of the spine. *J Nerv Ment Dis* 27:1, 1900.

95. Sarpyener MA. Congenital stricture of the spinal canal. *J Bone Joint Surg* 27: 70-79, 1945.

96. Seddon HJ: Pott's paraplegia: prognosis and treatment. *Br J Surg* 22:769, 1935.

97. Smith AG: Account of a case in which portions of three dorsal vertebrae were removed for the relief of paralysis from fracture, with partial success. *North Am Med Surg J* 8:94-97, 1829.

98. Sorrel-Dejerine Y: *Contribution a l'Etude des Paraplegies Pottiques.* Paris, 1925.

99. Spink MS, Lewis GL: *Albucasis, On Surgery and Instruments. A Definitive Edition of the Arabic text with English translation and Commentary.* London, The Wellcome Institute of the History of Medicine, 1973.

100. Taylor AS: Unilateral laminectomy. *Ann Surg* 51:529-533, 1910.

101. Thompson WAL, Ralston EL: Pseudoarthrosis following spine fusion. *J Bone Joint Surg* 31A:400-405, 1949.

102. Tyrell F: Compression of the spinal marrow from displacement of the vertebrae, consequent upon injury. Operation of removing the arch and spinous processes of the twelfth dorsal vertebra. *Lancet* 11:685-688, 1827.

103. Venable CS, Stuck WG, Beach A: The effects on bone of metals: based upon electrolysis. *Ann Surg* 105:917-938, 1937.

104. Venable CS, Stuck WG: Electrolysis: controlling factor in the use of metals in treating fractures. *JAMA* 3:349, 1939.

105. Verbiest H. A radicular syndrome from developmental narrowing of the lumbar vertebral canal. *J Bone Joint Surg (Br)* 36:230-237, 1954.

106. Vincent E: Contribution a la chirurgie rachidienne du drainage vertebral dans le mal de Pott. *Rev Chir* 1273-1294, 1892.

107. Vincent E: Chirurgie rachidienne et mal de Pott. *Rev Chir* 18:47-54, 1898.

108. Virchow R: *Untersuchungen uber die Entwickelung des Schadelgruendes im gesunden und krankhaften Ziistande, etc.* Berlin, G Reimer, 1857.

109. von Eiselsberg AF, Ranzi E: Ueber die chirurgische Behandlung der Him-und Rückenmarkstumoren. *Arch Klin Chir* 102:309-468, 1913.

110. Watson GL, Paul WE: Contribution to the study of spinal surgery: One successful and one unsuccessful operation for the removal of the tumor. *Boston Med Surg J* 153: 114-117, 1905.

111. Wilson PD, Straub LR: The use of a metal plate fastened to the spinous processes. American Academy of Orthopaedic Surgeons Instructional Course Lecture, Ann Arbor, MI, 1952.

112. Wiltse LL: History of pedicle screw fixation of the spine. *Spine: State of the Art Rev* 6:1-110, 1992.

113. Wiltse LL. The history of spinal disorders.Frymoyer JW (ed): *The Adult Spine. Principles and Practice.* Philadelphia, Lippincott-Raven, 1997, pp 3-40.

114. Yasargil MG. Microsurgical operation of herniated lumbar disc. *Adv Neurosurg* 4: 81, 1977.

115. Zavaleta MA: Resecion de vertebras. *Ann Circ Med Argent* 15:497-502, 1892.

116. Zielke K, Pellin B: Neue Instrumente und Implantate zur Erganzung des Harrington Systems. *Z Orthop Chir* 114:534, 1976.

CHAPTER 2

History of Spinal Instrumentation: The Modern Era

John K. Houten and Thomas J. Errico

The use of internal fixation as a tool for both stabilization and correction of deformity was a major advance in modern spinal surgery. A wide experience in the use of internal fixation in the treatment of the appendicular skeleton was extrapolated to the axial skeleton. This experience has culminated in the wide range of surgical implants currently available to the modern spinal surgeon. A thorough understanding of the evolution of spinal instrumentation should yield a better understanding of both present and future developments.

Dorsal Thoracolumbar Instrumentation

In 1975, the Harrington rod represented the "state of the art" in spinal instrumentation. The rod system, originally developed by Paul Harrington for the correction of spinal deformities, was soon used in the treatment of traumatic injuries[3,53] (Figure 2.1), degenerative disease,[42] and metastatic disease.[35,51] The system provided both distraction rods as well as compression rods and hooks. Over the years however, their widespread use led to recognition of their limitations. The use of a distraction system provided excellent correction of coronal plane deformities (scoliosis). Unfortunately, the use of distraction as the sole correction tool resulted in the loss of normal sagittal plane alignment. The loss of normal lumbar lordosis was associated with "flat back syndrome."[12,34] Hook dislodgement and rod breakage also proved to be troublesome complications.[22,50] In addition, casting or bracing was generally required in the postoperative period, and this proved to be difficult or impractical in some patients.[37]

In response to the difficulties encountered with Harrington rods, Eduardo Luque advanced a major concept in the mid-1970s that quietly pushed the future direction of spinal instrumentation: segmental spinal fixation. The issue of bracing was of particular importance to Luque. Practicing in the warm climate of Mexico City, it was difficult for Luque, from a practical standpoint, to use the postoperative casting required in Harrington rod instrumentation. In addition, a large number of his patients, who were from homes of low socioeconomic status, would travel a great distance to seek treatment and would not comply with bracing or would get lost to follow-up.

Luque popularized the use of a ³⁄₁₆-inch steel rod secured at each spinal level with sublaminar wires

(Figure 2.2). Luque reasoned that increasing the number of fixation points along a construct would reduce the force placed upon each individual point and obviate the need for a postoperative cast or brace. Additional beneficial effects of segmental fixation were that it increased the potential corrective power of instrumentation, reduced the potential for construct failure, and resulted in improved fusion rates.

The concept of segmental fixation to a contoured rod was widely embraced because it produced greater construct rigidity and allowed for improved control of the sagittal plane. The use of sublaminar wires was adopted by some users of Harrington rod instrumentation. A hybrid form of Paul Harrington's technique (from Texas) and Eduardo Luque's technique (from Mexico) was sometimes referred to as the "Tex-Mex" operation.

Although the corrective power of sublaminar wires was well-appreciated, many surgeons had reservations in using them because of reports of neurological injury resulting either from direct trauma or from epidural hematoma.[32,54] In addition, revision surgery after sublaminar wiring is problematic because scarring may preclude the passage of new wires at the same laminae. In response to these concerns, Drummond[18] developed a method for segmental fixation using a button-wire implant passed through the base of the spinous process. This technique does not provide as strong fixation as do sublaminar wires. It avoids, however, passing anything into the spinal canal and thus reduces the risk of direct neurological injury. This compromise of fixation for less risk of neurological injury was seen as a prudent choice by many surgeons operating on healthy, neurologically normal adolescents with idiopathic scoliosis. Nevertheless, some pundits referred to the procedure as the "chicken-Luque" procedure.

Increasingly sophisticated multiple hook-rod systems appeared in the 1980s that provided much of the strength of wire fixation but with greater flexibility to address deformities in both the sagittal and the coronal dimensions. The Cotrel Dubousset (CD) system was introduced into the United States in 1986 using a ¼-inch rough-surfaced rod.[14] Multiple hooks allowed spinal surgeons to apply compression and distraction over different areas within the same rod. The multiple hook design applied the principles of segmental fixation without the need for sublaminar wires. Significantly, the system provided for a unique mechanism for deformity correction: rod rotation. This proved a powerful force in the correction of scoliosis. Further stability was provided by cross-linking the two parallel rods together.

The advantages of the CD system were partially offset, however, by the difficulty of removing the system. The locking mechanism of the hooks was irreversible without destroying the hook or cutting the rod. The Texas Scottish Rite Hospital (TSRH) system was a design advance that addressed the issue of revision surgery. It was similar to the CD system in having multiple hooks and cross links but was designed to allow the removal of the system's individual components if necessary. Although the features of the TSRH system simplified revision surgery, the top-loading side-tightened system was not universally appreciated. After maturation of the fusion mass, the side-tightened bolts were not always

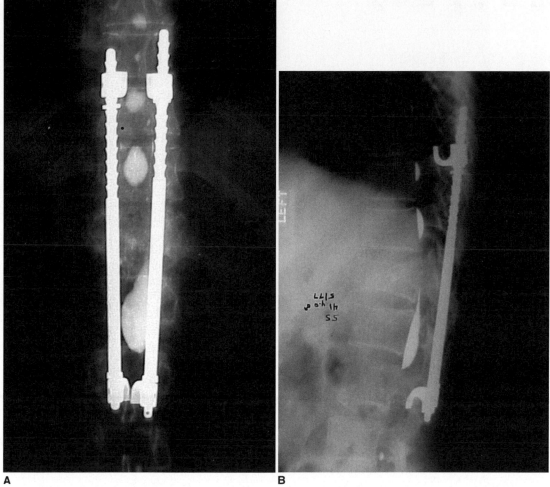

Figure 2.1 (**A**) AP and (**B**) lateral radiographs after surgical stabilization of a burst fracture of L3 with Harrington rod internal fixation.

accessible. The following decade saw the introduction of numerous, similar dual-rod systems like Moss-Miami and Isola.[12,49] The major variations revolved around the leading and locking mechanisms: side loading, top loading, side tightening, or top tightening. The last decade has seen the introduction of numerous systems that operate with the same design principles, with a shift toward the use of polyaxial screws that make coupling of the fixation points to the rods easier.

A major advance that became available with these spinal systems was the exploitation of the pedicle as a site for segmental fixation. This innovation is generally credited to Roy-Camille of Paris. Roy-Camille performed his first operation in 1963 but did not publish the results until 1970.[43] Pedicle screws presented many advantages when compared with other tools for spinal fixation. Pedicle screws are biomechanically superior as a point of fixation[1] compared with hook- or wire-rod constructs and can be placed into the sacrum, an area to which fixation is otherwise difficult. In addition, they can be placed even after a laminectomy has been performed and can be positioned without entering the spinal canal.[17] This advantage allowed for the massive proliferation of spinal instrumentation into the area of degenerative spinal disorders. Prior to the advent of pedicle-screw

instrumentation systems, there had been only sporadic reports of the use of instrumentation for degenerative spinal disorders. The Knodt rod (a small distraction rod system) had been used previously in degenerative disease but was associated with localized loss of lordosis and device dislodgement. In addition, the system needed some lamina for device fixation. Pedicle screw systems, however, can be used after a total laminectomy.

Arthur Steffee popularized the use of pedicle screws in the United States in 1984 using a contourable plate. At about the same time, a screw-rod system was in use in Europe, developed by Yves Cotrel of France, that became incorporated into the "Universal" CD system. Controversy soon followed, with both the screw-plate and screw-rod constructs developing a group of proponents.[23] Proponents of plates noted that plates were stronger. Most surgeons were ultimately attracted, however, to rods because their use provides greater flexibility, reduces encroachment upon the adjacent facet joints, and leaves more surface area for fusion. The marriage of the long dual-rod constructs to lumbar pedicle screws was an important development that enhanced the surgeon's ability to accomplish increasingly difficult and complex spinal reconstructions. The use of the polyaxial

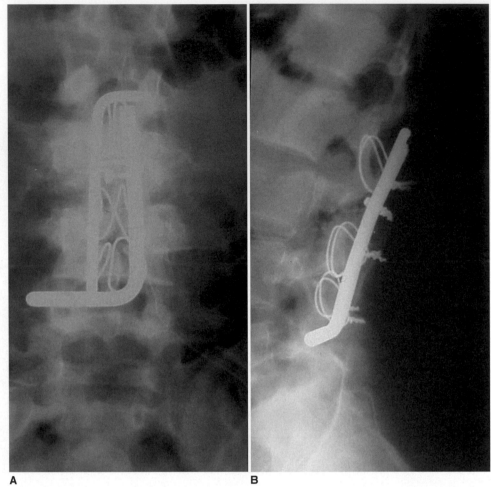

Figure 2.2 (**A**) AP and (**B**) lateral radiographs after surgical stabilization of a burst fracture of L3 with segmental sublaminar wire fixation to an angled rod using the technique described by Eduardo Luque.

pedicle screw has further advanced the ease of spinal reconstructions.

Ventral Thoracolumbar Instrumentation

Successful use of the Harrington instrumentation kindled interest in developing a ventral system to address neuromuscular scoliosis. Dwyer developed a ventral system for internal fixation using screws connected by a cable.[46] Winter attempted a combined ventral and dorsal approach with Harrington and Dwyer instrumentation to treat painful adult idiopathic scoliosis.[55] This concept was of particular interest in that these patients were at high risk for pseudoarthrosis and tended to tolerate bracing less well than adolescents.[55]

The Zielke system, developed in 1975, was the next step in the development of ventral instrumentation. The Zielke device connected transvertebral screws with a threaded rod and nuts and was more rigid than the Dwyer cables. This added both strength and the capacity for incremental correction and derotation, permitting a more powerful correction. The Zielke system produced a lower pseudoarthrosis rate and somewhat lower recurrence of the flat-back syndrome. In spite of these benefits, the system had many shortcomings. The pseudoarthrosis rate remained high when the system was used as a stand-alone device but was lowered with supplementation of dorsal fixation. This system also suffered from the tendency to shorten the anterior columns and to produce kyphosis.

The Dunn device was a ventral implant that consisted of two rods that spanned the distance between two vertebral body bridges: one placed ventrolaterally with a vertebral body staple and the other placed more dorsolaterally with an intervertebral body screw.[19] This system was not widely accepted because it was bulky and was associated with vascular complications.[25]

The ventral Kostuik Harrington instrumentation was an adaptation of short Harrington rods used in conjunction with a pedicle screw developed by Paul Harrington for the use in myelomeningocele. Introduced by John Kostuik in the early 1980s, it was an innovative short-segment ventral fixation device. The screw, when placed ventrolaterally in the vertebral bodies, allows for short-segment ventral correction of the kyphotic deformity associated with burst fractures. A second neutralization rod was placed parallel to the first rod to enhance stability (Figure 2.3). Over time, cross-fixators were added in an attempt to further enhance stability. Two parallel rods rigidly cross-linked are the biomechanical equivalent of a plate. Most ventral short-

segment constructs subsequently used plates with vertebral body screws.

Several other plate designs soon followed that were lower profile. Ryan introduced a plate secured by a rostral and caudal bolt inserted through the vertebral body. The

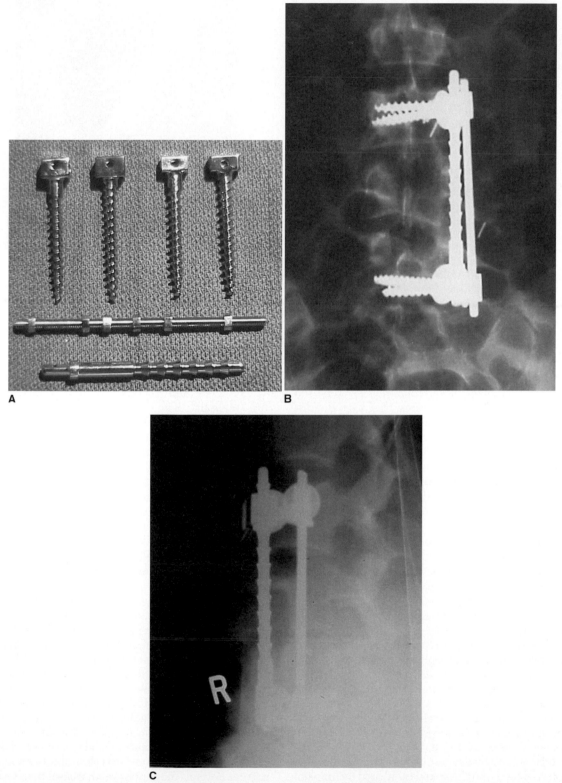

Figure 2.3 (**A**) Kostuik-Harrington screws sand rods. (**B**) AP and (**C**) lateral radiographs after surgical stabilization of a burst fracture of L4 with Kostuik-Harrington instrumentation.

single bolt design, however, offered less resistance to rotation than the designs that used two screws or bolts above and below.[45] The Yuan I-Plate was an alternative design that consisted of a 3.5-mm stainless steel plate secured with transvertebral screws.[56] Black *et al.*[8] published his experience with a low-profile, rectangular, stainless steel plate that had multiple holes that allowed for the placement of three screws at each vertebral level. The Kaneda device represented another stage in development of anterior thoracolumbar instrumentation because it allowed reduction of kyphotic deformities after ventral decompression while providing good strength without incidence of vascular injury.[25]

The next generation of ventral plates, including the Z-Plate™ (Medtronic/Sofamor Danek, Memphis, TN) and the Anterior Thoracolumbar Locking Plate System (Synthes, Paoli, PA), further improved implant design by providing a lower profile and changing the composition to titanium alloys. In addition, the newer systems allow for both the distraction of kyphotic deformities and the compression of the graft.

Dorsal Cervical Instrumentation

The earliest methods used to provide internal fixation for posterior cervical fusions involved the use of spinous process wiring. These techniques, however, are limited in that they often do not provide adequate stiffness or sufficient resistance to rotational movement and extension and cannot be used when the spinous processes have been removed.

For internal fixation of C1-2, the Brooks and Gallie techniques use sublaminar wires to compress an autologous bone graft. Although these techniques are reported to be associated with high fusion rates, they have the disadvantages of potentially producing neurological injury from the placement of sublaminar wires and the problem that wires may pull through osteoporotic bone. In addition, there is a small but persistent failure rate associated with the Gallie fusion that may be caused by inadequate immobilization allowing for "grinding down" of the graft.

Several instrumentation systems were devised as adjuncts or alternatives to wiring. The Daab plate was a stainless-steel implant shaped like an elongated "H" that could be compressed at either end to fixate it to a spinous process.[10,31] This instrumentation represented no significant advantage over the available wiring techniques, and it was probably inferior considering that it typically needing the resection of an intervening spinous process and the associated interspinous ligaments.

Halifax clamps are a pair of upgoing and downgoing sublaminar hooks tightened together with a screw that is then secured in position with a locking mechanism (Figure 2.4).[15,31] Halifax clamps have the advantage of relatively simple and rapid application. In addition, the area of bone contact is broader than that with wiring and is less likely to pull out of soft bone. They offer C1-2 fixation comparable with that achieved with the Brooks technique.[26] Relative disadvantages of the system are that hooks are introduced into the spinal canal, and the implant is relatively "high profile" and has limited application when stabilization is needed over multiple segments.

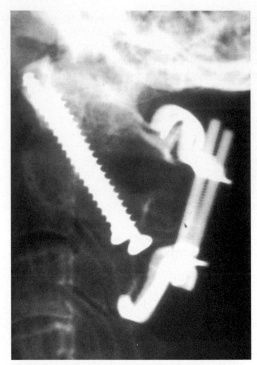

Figure 2.4 Postoperative lateral cervical radiograph demonstrating C1-2 internal fixation with Halifax Clamps. In this patient, the posterior clamps were placed to supplement fixation with C1-2 transarticular screws.

In the mid-1980s, Mager introduced transarticular screw placement for internal fixation of C1-2. This is a technically demanding procedure compared with wiring that achieves improved C1-2 stability to flexion-extension and rotation[27] than wiring procedures and is associated with the highest published C1-2 fusion rates.[28] This technique is not always feasible if there is anatomical variation in the course of the vertebral artery, although there is still benefit in unilateral placement.[28] Many practitioners supplement transarticular screws with posterior instrumentation as broken screws have been seen when used as a stand-alone procedure.

Lateral mass plate fixation with screws was introduced by Roy-Camille *et al.*[44] This technique of internal fixation is ideal in instances in which the laminae and spinous processes have been removed or fractured. The first technique for screw placement was modified by Magerl and Seeman,[38] Heller,[29] and An *et al.*[2] The original lateral mass plates were an application of preexisting bone plates with a distance between plate holes of 13mm. The Haid Plate and Synthes reconstruction plates were soon marketed, each offering a choice of two interhole distances. These systems all suffered from insufficient versatility in accommodating the wide variety of interhole differences often needed.[13] The AXIS™ system (Medtronic/Sofamor Danek, Memphis, TN) offers plate holes at intervals of 11, 13, and 15mm and a slotted hole design to allow for limitless interhole variations as well as improved ability to contour the plates.

The Cervifix™ system (Synthes Spine, Paoli, PA) consists of lateral mass screws that are inserted through clamps along a contourable titanium rod. This provides the flexibility to address variations in anatomy beyond that offered by the AXIS system. In addition, a hybrid plate-rod implant is available for occipital screw placement in occipital-cervical fusions. The Starlock™ instrumentation (Synthes Spine, Paoli, PA) is a newer system that allows independent insertion of lateral mass screws, which are then attached to clamps along a contourable titanium rod. Additionally, a tapered rod is available to cross the cervicothoracic junction. Cross-links and laminar hooks are also available. The Summit™ system (Depuy Acromed, Rayham, MA) is another newer design for lateral mass fixation that offers polyaxial screw heads and a top-loading 3-mm titanium rod for increased ease of rod insertion. It has the advantage of approximating the ease of use and flexibility of the lumbar pedicle screw systems presently available.

Ventral Cervical Instrumentation

Since the time that the first system was developed by Bohler in the mid 1960s, anterior cervical plating has become a popular means of supplementing a ventral cervical fusion.[52] Early in the development of this instrumentation, the potential for screw back-out was recognized as a serious concern for possible complications, including tracheal or esophageal erosion. The first systems widely available were the Caspar™ (Aesculap, San Francisco, CA) and the Orozco (Figure 2.5) (Synthes, Paoli, PA). Both of

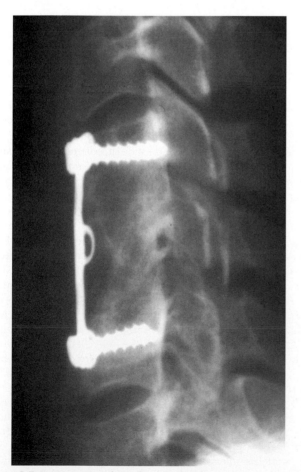

Figure 2.5 Postoperative lateral cervical radiograph demonstrating anterior internal fixation with the Orozco plate.

these systems consisted of simple plates with slots or holes but without any locking devices. Constraint of the screws depended upon obtaining bicortical purchase and "blocking" backout by screw angulation.

The rate of screw backout or breakage and graft subsidence was high with the first generation of anterior cervical plates. This led to the development of the Cervical Spine Locking Plate (CSLP) (Synthes, Paoli, PA)[41] first introduced in North America in 1991. The CSLP used a titanium expansion screw that secured the screwhead to the plate and, thus, allowed for unicortical purchase without the risk of screw backout. The substitution of titanium for stainless steel allowed for postoperative magnetic resonance imaging. The CSLP reduced the incidence of screw backout[48]; however, its limitations were a rigid screw trajectory and the fact that the plate was wide and difficult to contour.

The Orion™ ventral cervical plate (Medtronic/Sofamor Danek, Memphis, TN) represented the next major product introduction for anterior cervical plating. The plate was manufactured "prelordosed" with a wide variety of screw lengths to allow for unicortical or bicortical purchase. The drill guide was fixed to the plate, providing 15 degrees of rostral and caudal angulation and 6 degrees of medial angulation. Locking screws were added to fix the screws to the plate by overlapping the screw heads. Although the Orion plate saw widespread use and had good reported surgical results,[40,47] some surgeons felt that the system was too rigid and shielded the graft from stress, thereby promoting a significant rate of peudoarthrosis.[36]

Interest in avoiding stress-shielding of a graft while preventing screw backout led to the development of "semiconstrained" plate designs that would allow the graft to share stress with the plate. The A-line™ Cervical Plating System (Surgical Dynamics, Norwalk, CT) and the Codman Anterior Cervical Plate System (Codman & Shurtleff, Raynham, MA) both allow variability in screw direction and are then fixed to the plate with a locking system. Once locked, however, the screws can pivot within the plate hole in response to sufficient force, allowing for slight graft subsidence and maintenance of stress sharing with the graft. The Atlantis™ Plate (Medtronic/Sofamor Danek, Memphis, TN) provides the option of fixed or variable angle screws, making it possible to fashion a "hybrid" construct using both screw types.

An additional innovation directed at maintaining load sharing between the graft and plate to create a more optimal fusion environment is the development of slotted plates. Examples of available products applying this design include the ABC™ Plating System (Aesculap, Center Valley, PA), the Premier™ Anterior Cervical Plate System (Medtronic/Sofamor Danek, Memphis, TN), and the DOC™ Ventral Cervical Stabilization System (Depuy Acromed, Rayham, MA). Constructs made with these plates allow the screws to remain in essentially the same position within the vertebra while the screw head moves along a slot in response to graft subsidence. There is some evidence that the ability of the screw to "translate" within the plate is leading to a lower incidence of graft and plate failure in multilevel fusions.[21] The success of this technique is fueling sustained interest in these plate designs.

Ventral fixation of odontoid fractures can be achieved with the placement of one or multiple screws. Although the technique was published in 1971 by Barbour,[7] it did not achieve popularity until the late 1980s.[9] Controversy developed over whether one or two screw placements is optimal for fixation.[20] Several recent papers, however, have not shown improved results with multiple screw placement.[4,5] Some surgeons have advocated the application of cannulated screws placed over K-wires in this procedure, citing improved accuracy and the ability to redirect the screw trajectory as technical advantages. Other surgeons, however, prefer the original noncannulated screws, noting the potential risks of K-wire breakage as well as unintended K-wire advancement during screw placement.[24]

Cage Technology

The development of cages to promote interbody fusion traces back to the veterinary work of Bagby in which stainless-steel baskets filled with bone were used to treat Wobbler-neck syndrome in race horses.[16] Bagby subsequently pioneered the development of a cage for use in human lumbar interbody fusions.[6,33] The implantation of cages as an interbody device through either an anterior or posterior approach has become a widely performed procedure. Titanium-threaded cages include the BAK™ cage (Sulzer Spine-Tech, Minneapolis, MN) and the Ray Threaded Fusion Cage (Surgical Dynamics, Norwalk, CT). Brantigan et al[11] introduced cages composed of a radiolucent carbon fiber that allowed for improved postoperative imaging. It is also argued that the carbon fiber material has a modulus closer to that of native bone and, thus, should theoretically be a better fusion substrate than metal.[11]

Although the initial cage development was done for the cervical spine, the technology was first widely implemented in the lumbar spine. In April 2002, the Food and Drug Administration (FDA) approved the use of the BAK-C™ device (Sulzer Spine-Tech, Minneapolis, MN) for cervical fusion.[39] Recent experience with these implants has indicated that fusion rates are achieved comparable with those seen after procedures using uninstrumented allograft.[27a]

To facilitate ventral vertebral reconstruction after anterior and middle column resection, Harms developed a titanium mesh cage that can be packed with bone and is seated into the endplates.[29] This implant has found application in cases of vertebral body destruction resulting from metastatic disease, degenerative conditions, and trauma. The Harms cage was considered a valuable innovation even to those surgeons who prefer using struts made of allograft or autograft because a suitable bone graft is sometimes unavailable.

Summary

The development of instrumentation for internal fixation of the spine has dramatically improved the ability to successfully provide surgical intervention for a wide variety of spinal disorders. Internal fixation leads to higher fusion rates and provides more powerful means to correct spinal deformities.

In addition, spinal instrumentation allows for reduction or elimination of the need for postoperative external bracing.

Over the past 25 years, there has been an amazing increase in the variety of instrumentation available to provide internal spinal fixation. Surgeons are now able to select a specific type of implant that is best suited to address an individual patient's problem. Improved understanding of biomechanics and clinical experience with today's instrumentation should promote further advancement in internal fixation and even better patient outcomes in the future.

REFERENCES

1. Abumi K, Panjabi MM, Duranceau J: Biomechanical evaluation of spinal fixation devices. Part III. Stability provided by six spinal fixation devices and interbody bone graft. *Spine* 14:1249-1255,1989.
2. An HS, Gordin R, Renner K: Anatomic considerations for plate-screw fixation of the cervical spine. *Spine* 16:S548-551, 1991.
3. Anden U, Lake A, Nordwall A: The role of the anterior longitudinal ligament in Harrington rod fixation of unstable thoracolumbar spinal fractures. *Spine* 5:23-25, 1980.
4. Apfelbaum R, Lonser R, Veres R, Casey A: Direct anterior screw fixation for recent and remote odontoid fractures. *J Neurosurg* 93:227-236, 2000.
5. Arand M, Lemke M, Kinzl L, Hartwig E: Incidence of complications of the screw osteosynthesis of odontoid process fractures. *Zentralbl Chir* 126:610-615, 2001.
6. Bagby GW: Arthrodesis by the distraction-compression method using a stainless steel implant. *Orthopedics* 11:931-934,1988.
7. Barbour J: Screw fixation in fracture of the odontoid process. *South Anst Clin* 5:20, 1971.
8. Black RC, Gardner VO, Armstrong GW, et al: A contoured anterior spinal fixation plate. *Clin Orthop* 227:135-142, 1988.
9. Bome GM, Bedou GL, Pinaudeau M, et al: Odontoid process fracture osteosynthesis with a direct screw fixation technique in nine consecutive cases. *J Neurosurg* 68:223-226, 1988.
10. Bostman O, Myllynen P, Riska EB: Posterior spinal fusion using internal fixation with the Daab plate. *Acta Orthop Scand* 55:310-314, 1984.
11. Brantigan JW, Steffee AD, Geiger JM: A carbon fiber implant to aid interbody lumbar fusion. Mechanical testing. *Spine* 16:S277-282, 1991.
12. Bridwell KH: Spinal instrumentation in the management of adolescent scoliosis. *Clin Orthop* Feb:64-72, 1997.
13. Cooper PR: The Axis Fixation System for posterior instrumentation of the cervical spine. *Neurosurgery* 39:612-614,1996.
14. Cotrel Y, Dubousset J: [A new technic for segmental spinal osteosynthesis using the posterior approach]. *Rev Chir Orthop Reparatrice Appar Mot* 70:489-494, 1984.
15. Cybulski GR, Stone JL, Crowell RM, et al: Use of Halifax interlaminar clamps for posterior C1-C2 arthrodesis. *Neurosurgery* 22:429-431, 1988.
16. DeBowes RM, Grant BD, Bagby GW, et al: Cervical vertebral interbody fusion in the horse: a comparative study of bovine xenografts and autografts supported by stainless steel baskets. *Am J Vet Res* 45:191-199, 1984.

17. Dickman CA, Fessler RG, MacMillan M, Haid RW: Transpedicular screw-rod fixation of the lumbar spine: operative technique and outcome in 104 cases. *J Neurosurg* 77:860-870, 1992.

18. Drummond D, Guadagni J, Keene JS, *et al*: Interspinous process segmental spinal instrumentation. *J Pediatr Orthop* 4:397-404, 1984.

19. Dunn HK: Anterior stabilization of thoracolumbar injuries. *Clin Orthop* Oct:116-124, 1984.

20. El Saghir H, Bohm H: Anderson type H fracture of the odontoid process: results of anterior screw fixation. *J Spinal Disord* 13:527-530, 2000.

21. Epstein N: Anterior approaches to cervical spondylosis and ossification of the posterior longitudinal ligament: review of operative technique and assessment of 65 multilevel circumferential procedures. *Surg Neurol* 55:313-324, 2001.

22. Erwin VVD, Dickson JH, Harrington PR: Clinical review of patients with broken Harrington rods. *J Bone Joint Surg Am* 62:1302-1307, 1980.

23. Esses ST, Bednar DA: The spinal pedicle screw: techniques and systems. *Orthop Rev* 18:676-682, 1989.

24. Fuji T, Oda T, Kato Y, *et al*: Accuracy of atlantoaxial transarticular screw insertion. *Spine* 25:1760-1764, 2000.

25. Ghanayem AJ, Zdeblick TA: Anterior instrumentation in the management of thoracolumbar burst fractures. *Clin Orthop* Feb:89-100, 1997.

26. Grob D, Crisco JJ 3rd, Panjabi MM, *et al*: Biomechanical evaluation of four different posterior atlantoaxial fixation techniques. *Spine* 17:480-490, 1992.

27. Grob D, Jeanneret B, Aebi M, Markwalder TM: Atlanto-axial fusion with transarticular screw fixation. *J Bone Joint Surg Br* 73:972-976, 1991.

27a. Hacker RJ, Cauthen JC, Gilbert TJ, Griffith SL: A prospective randomized multicenter clinical evaluation of an anterior cervical fusion cage. *Spine* 15; 25:2646-2654, 2000.

28. Haid RW, Jr., Subach BR, McLaughlin MR, *et al*: C1-C2 transarticular screw fixation for atlantoaxial instability: a 6-year experience. *Neurosurgery* 49:65-68; discussion 69-70, 2001.

29. Heller JG, Carlson GD, Abitbol JJ, Garfin SR: Anatomic comparison of the Roy-Camille and Magerl techniques for screw placement in the lower cervical spine. *Spine* 16:S552-557, 1991.

30. Heller JG, Zdeblick TA, Kunz DA, *et al*: Spinal instrumentation for metastatic disease: in vitro biomechanical analysis. *J Spinal Disord* 6:17-22,1993.

31. Holness RO, Huestis WS, Howes WJ, Langille RA: Posterior stabilization with an interlaminar clamp in cervical injuries: technical note and review of the long term experience with the method. *Neurosurgery* 14:318-322, 1984.

32. Johnston CE 2nd, Happel LT, Jr., Norris R, *et al*: Delayed paraplegia complicating sublaminar segmental spinal instrumentation. *J Bone Joint Surg Am* 68:556-563,1986.

33. Kuslich SD, Ulstrom CL, Griffith SL, *et al*: The Bagby and Kuslich method of lumbar interbody fusion. History, techniques, and 2-year follow-up results of a United States prospective, multicenter trial. *Spine* 23:1267-1278; discussion 1279, 1998.

34. Lagrone MO, Bradford DS, Moe JH, *et al*: Treatment of symptomatic flatback after spinal fusion. *J Bone Joint Surg Am* 70:569-580, 1988.

35. Livingston KE, Perrin RG: The neurosurgical management of spinal metastases causing cord and cauda equina compression. *J Neurosurg* 49:839-843, 1978.

36. Lowery GL, McDonough RF: The significance of hardware failure in anterior cervical plate fixation. Patients with 2- to 7-year follow-up. *Spine* 23:181-186; discussion 186-187, 1998.

37. Luque ER: Segmental spinal instrumentation for correction of scoliosis. *Clin Orthop* March:192-198, 1982.

38. Magerl F, Seeman P: Stable posterior fusion of the atlas and axis by transarticular screw fixation. In Kehr P, Weidner A (eds): *The Cervical Spine*. Wien, Springer Verlag, 1987, 322.

39. Matge G: Anterior interbody fusion with the BAK-cage in cervical spondylosis. *Acta Neurochir* 140:1-8, 1998.

40. Mayr MT, Subach BR, Comey CH, *et al*: Cervical spinal stenosis: outcome after anterior corpectomy, allograft reconstruction, and instrumentation. *J Neurosurg* 96:10-16, 2002.

41. Morscher E, Sutter F, Jenny H, Olerud S: [Anterior plating of the cervical spine with the hollow screw-plate system of titanium]. *Chirurg* 57:702-707, 1986.

42. Morscher E: [Two-stage reposition and fixation of spondyloptosis with Harrington instrumentation and anterior intercorporal spondylodesis (author's transl)]. *Arch Orthop Unfallehir* 83:323-334, 1975.

43. Roy-Camille R, Roy-Camille M, Demeulenaere C: [Osteosynthesis of dorsal, lumbar, and lumbosacral spine with metallic plates screwed into vertebral pedicles and articular apophyses]. *Presse Med* 78:1447-1448, 1970.

44. Roy-Camille R, Saillant G, Mazel C: Internal fixation of the cervical spine by a posterior osteosynthesis with plates and screws. In Sherk H, Dunn E, Eisment F (eds): *The Cervical Spine*. Philadelphia, JB Lippincott, 1989, pp 390-403.

45. Ryan MD, Taylor TK, Sherwood AA: Bolt-plate fixation for anterior spinal fusion. *Clin Orthop* Feb:196-202,1986.

46. Schafer MF: Dwyer instrumentation of the spine. *Orthop Clin North Am* 9:115-122, 1978.

47. Schultz KD, Jr., McLaughlin MR, Haid RW, Jr., *et al*: Single-stage anterior-posterior decompression and stabilization for complex cervical spine disorders. *J Neurosurg* 93:214-221, 2000.

48. Spivak JM, Chen D, Kummer FJ: The effect of locking fixation screws on the stability of anterior cervical plating. *Spine* 24:334-338, 1999.

49. Stambough JL: Posterior instrumentation for thoracolumbar trauma. *Clin Orthop* Feb:73-88, 1997.

50. Sturz H, Hinterberger J, Matzen K, Plitz W: Damage analysis of the Harrington rod fracture after scoliosis operation. *Arch Orthop Trauma Surg* 95:113-122, 1979.

51. Sundaresan N, Galicich JH, Lane JM: Harrington rod stabilization for pathological fractures of the spine. *J Neurosurg* 60:282-286, 1984.

52. Vaccaro AR, Balderston RA: Anterior plate instrumentation for disorders of the subaxial cervical spine. *Clin Orthop* 112-121, 1997.

53. Wang GJ, Whitehill R, Stamp WG, Rosenberger R: The treatment of fracture dislocations of the thoracolumbar spine with halofemoral traction and Harrington rod instrumentation. *Clin Orthop* Jul-Aug:168-175, 1979.

54. Wilber RG, Thompson GH, Shaffer JW, *et al:* Postoperative neurological deficits in segmental spinal instrumentation: a study using spinal cord monitoring. *J Bone Joint Surg Am* 66:1178-1187, 1984,

55. Winter RB: Combined Dwyer and Harrington instrumentation and fusion in the treatment of selected patients with painful adult idiopathic scoliosis. *Spine* 3:135-141, 1978.

56. Yuan HA, Mann KA, Found EM, *et al:* Early clinical experience with the Syracuse I-Plate: an anterior spinal fixation device. *Spine* 13:278-285, 1988.

The
Fundamentals

CHAPTER 3

Differential Diagnosis of Surgical Disorders of the Spine

W. Putnam Wolcott, Jacek M. Malik,
Christopher I. Shaffrey, Mark E. Shaffrey,
and John A. Jane

Back pain is the most common reason cited for work absence in the United States, affecting approximately 31 million people annually.[118,127,135,136] Low back pain (LBP) alone is estimated to cost society between $20 billion and $50 billion a year in the United States. This is a huge financial burden on an already taxed medical system.[189] Rapid diagnosis and treatment that result in a rapid return to a premorbid level of activity should greatly reduce costs to the patient and to society.

Patients presenting with pain related to the spine do not have a surgical condition in the majority of cases.[118,124,189] Only approximately 8% to 10% of those with neurogenic pain have a surgical lesion. These individuals can present with a myriad of symptoms, and the differential diagnosis of spinal disorders is lengthy.[189]

This chapter presents a logical approach to evaluate the patient who presents with spinal pain or neurologic deficit with a suspected spinal disorder. An algorithm proposed by Borenstein et al. is used as a functional guide and is expanded to include patients who present with a neurologic deficit related to spinal pathology, as well as those who present with pain as their initial complaint.[23,24]

The following observations are used to classify spinal pathology: (1) the presence or absence of spinal region pain, (2) the characteristics of the pain, (3) the presence or absence of neurologic deficit, (4) the characteristics of the deficit, and (5) the presence of systemic signs and symptoms. Each patient is entered into the algorithm after a thorough history and physical examination.

The differential diagnosis process begins with the characterization of back pain, discovery of systemic signs and symptoms, and evaluation for neurologic deficit. With this information, further laboratory and radiologic evaluation can proceed, and ultimately, a diagnosis with appropriate surgical or medical management usually can be achieved. There is some expected overlap between groups in patient presentation; however, the basic framework of the algorithm should help the clinician restrict the differential diagnosis and call attention to uncommon conditions.

The causes of spinal pain and neurologic deficit are vast. Therefore an attempt is made to delineate the most common causes by age, location, character, site of pain,

rapidity of onset, and severity of neurologic deficit and associated systemic illness. For instance, pain in conjunction with fever and weight loss, recumbent position, morning stiffness, acute onset, or visceral component allows for initial categorization. The first half of this chapter deals with those disorders that usually present with spinal pain, and the second portion deals with those conditions that present with pain and neurologic deficit. The choice of imaging studies, laboratory tests, and surgical or medical management is summarized in Figures 3.1 and 3.2.

Spinal Pain
Pain Associated with Fever and Weight Loss

Patients who present with fever and weight loss associated with spinal pain are at increased risk for an infectious or neoplastic process. Vertebral osteomyelitis, discitis, epidural abscess, and granulomatous processes are the most common infectious conditions affecting the spine. Neoplastic processes, specifically metastatic disease and lymphoma, are often associated with a similar presentation. Neurologic deficits can occur, but are usually present after a period of diagnostic delay that may last weeks to months after the pain and systemic symptoms occur.

Vertebral Osteomyelitis
Patient Population. This disease represents the most common of the pyogenic infections of the axial skeleton.[8,91,163] Vertebral osteomyelitis occurs in 2% to 19% of all cases of osteomyelitis, with the largest percentage occurring in the elderly and debilitated.[11,39] More than half of patients with vertebral osteomyelitis are older than age 50.[163] Often, this diagnosis is initially missed because of its relatively benign and nonspecific presentation. Time from initial presentation to diagnosis ranges from 2 weeks to 5 months, with a mean of 6 to 8 weeks.[39,163] Adults tend to demonstrate a more chronic and indolent course with longer delays, whereas the pediatric and immunocompromised groups present with a more acute picture, which results in an earlier diagnosis.

Sources of Infection. A definitive source of infection is found in only 40% of cases, with the most common foci being genitourinary, soft tissue, respiratory, and intravenous drug abuse (IVDA).[19,51,91] Other less commonly encountered sources include enteric disease, dental extractions, endocarditis, and penetrating trauma.

The most common organisms isolated are the gram-positive cocci (GPC), which constitute 60% to 70% of all cases of vertebral osteomyelitis[1,91,115,163]; *Staphylococcus aureus* is the most prevalent organism, representing 55% to 60% of all positive cultures.[51,91,105,163,183] There has been a relative increase (14% to 18%) in other bacteria in more recent series, specifically gram-negative rods (e.g., *Escherichia coli, Pseudomonas aeruginosa*, and *Proteus*), which are found predominantly in the parenteral drug abuser or immunocompromised patient.[*]

Signs and Symptoms. The virulence of an organism is related to the timing of diagnosis, which can range from

---

[*]References 11,51,111,112,153,191,193.

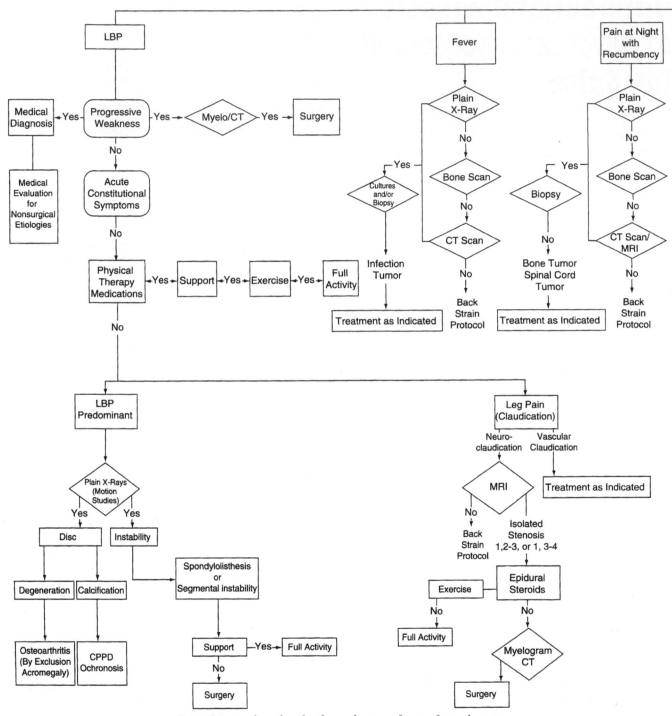

Figure 3.1 An algorithm for the evaluation of pain of spinal origin.

weeks to months after initial symptoms. The most common symptom is insidious diffuse back pain, which occurs in approximately 90% of patients.[91,115,163] Fever occurs in 40% to 52% of patients. Weight loss, radicular symptoms, myelopathy, spinal deformity, and meningeal irritation are less common presentations. Neurologic compromise and decreased mobility are late complications. Neurologic deficits are rare in the magnetic resonance imaging (MRI) era; however, neurologic sequelae were present in up to 50% of Hitchon and Yuh's original series.[91]

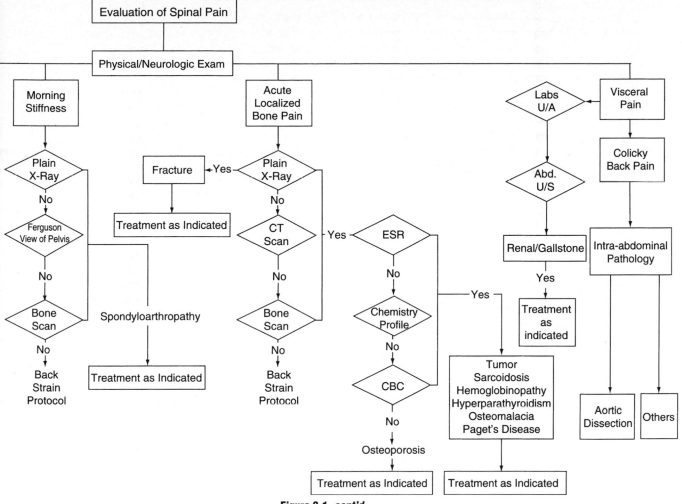

Figure 3.1 *cont'd*

Analysis of Findings. Diagnosis is based on pertinent laboratory findings, including an elevated erythrocyte sedimentation rate (ESR), blood and bone cultures, elevated white blood cell (WBC) count, and radiologic studies. The ESR is elevated in approximately 90% of patients. Positive blood cultures and an elevated WBC count are present in only 25% to 42% of adult cases. MRI with superior sensitivity and specificity of 89% to 100% is the gold standard for detection of osteomyelitis.[4,42,56,133] The characteristic changes observed on images can take from 2 to 3 weeks to become apparent.[4] Bone scans are useful for diagnosis secondary to high sensitivity (90%); however, they can be misleading because other inflammatory processes or neoplasia can mimic an infection on these scans.[45,60]

Patient Management. Management is based on biopsy results; the preferred method is a percutaneous aspiration and bone biopsy under computed tomography (CT) or fluoroscopic guidance.[35] An open biopsy is usually reserved for inadequate tissue acquired via percutaneous biopsy, neurologic compromise, and/or refractory disease.[73] Treatment entails bed rest and initiation of broad-spectrum antibiotics, followed by definitive antimicrobial therapy based on culture results.[11] Ventral decompression

and bone grafting may be required if neurologic sequelae ensue from excessive bone destruction or abscess formation.[11,51,91,98,111]

Epidural Abscess

Patient Population. The incidence of spinal epidural abscess (SEA), including all sources of infection, ranges from 1% to 10%.[7,8,11] Adults are primarily affected, with rare occurrences in children. Thoracic involvement is most common, followed closely by lumbar involvement. Cervical SEA occurs in less than 15% of cases[43,68,91]; dorsal location predominates in approximately two thirds of cases, with an occasional ventral abscess resulting from a direct extension of a located discitis or vertebral osteomyelitis.[68]

Sources of Infection. Epidural abscesses are usually caused by direct extension of a preexisting osteomyelitis in 20% to 60% of cases,[91] direct inoculation from surgical or procedural manipulation, or hematogenous spread from a distant focus. Trauma plays a role in the formation of late-onset abscesses secondary to formation of paraspinal hematomas that act as a physiologic culture medium. The bacteria in SEA are closely related to the organisms found

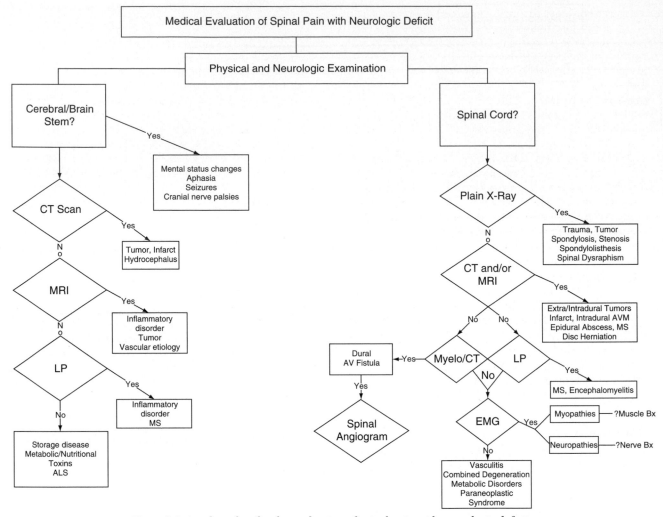

Figure 3.2 An algorithm for the evaluation of spinal pain with neurologic deficit.

in vertebral osteomyelitis, with gram-positive cocci also the most prevalent. *S. aureus* is isolated in 60% to 65% of the positive cultures, followed by other staphylococcal and streptococcal species.[91] Gram-negative rods, although uncommon, occurred with increasing frequency in recent series.

Signs and Symptoms. Spine pain is the initial clinical presentation in the majority of cases. There is a higher incidence of fever, leukocytosis, and neurologic compromise than in osteomyelitis[7,68,91,191]; meningeal signs may be present if the adjacent dura is violated. Misdiagnosis of SEA is common. This entity should be included in the differential diagnosis of any patient who presents with fever and spine pain.

Analysis of Findings. Laboratory studies, including ESR and WBC count, are elevated in the majority of patients. MRI is the diagnostic procedure of choice because of its ability to image multiple levels simultaneously.[68,109] The T_1-weighted images often reveal an isointense or hyperintense extradural lesion, with the T_2-weighted images showing a hyperintense collection with greater contrast enhancement.

Patient Management. Without surgical intervention, rapid neurologic deterioration occurs in approximately 10% to 15% of cases, even if the patient is given intravenous antibiotics.[91,163] Surgical debridement and decompression, with administration of applicable antibiotics, is appropriate; definitive antibiotic treatment should begin after cultures return.

Pediatric Discitis

Patient Population. Discitis represents two entirely different entities in the adult and pediatric populations.[39,41,50] Classically, discitis is a disease entity of the pediatric population, although it is an uncommon occurrence in the adult, except postoperatively.[47]

In children discitis has been described as either a chronic inflammatory disorder or a low-grade bacterial infection with a relatively benign course.[39,57] Early investigation and detection are important to prevent the progression to a devastating process, such as vertebral osteomyelitis. The incidence of pediatric discitis is unclear, but it has a peak age of occurrence at 6 years of age.[191]

Sources of Infection. The pediatric population is predisposed to discitis because of the vascular anastomotic network around and through the cartilaginous end-plates and discs; vascular obliteration of this surrounding vascular network occurs later in adolescence. The pediatric arterial network functions as a bacterial filter and endpoint.

Signs and Symptoms. The clinical presentation of back pain and painful ambulation is related to this entity's most common location in the lumbar spine.

Analysis of Findings. Diagnosis is made via an elevated ESR (in up to 75% of cases), a characteristic MRI or radionuclide bone scan, proper clinical setting, and appropriate age group. MRI, because of its ability to detect hydration changes in the disc, is the most sensitive and specific modality both to detect infection and to follow efficacy of treatment.[71,76,109] Gram-positive cocci, specifically staphylococcal and streptococcal species, predominate in positive cultures, occurring in more than 50% of reported cases.[50,51,151,191] Nondiagnostic biopsies and blood cultures are found in 20% to 30% of patients in most series.

Patient Management. Management consists of bed rest and a brief course of intravenous antibiotics until symptoms attenuate. Then oral antibiotic therapy is instituted. Prognosis is excellent in the uncomplicated case.

Adult Discitis

Spontaneous discitis is rare in the adult. It is encountered in 2% to 3% of surgical discectomy patients.[37,47,73] Clinical presentation reveals back pain at the operated level, usually from 1 to 3 weeks postoperatively. ESR is the most sensitive laboratory test for detection and monitoring of treatment progression. MRI is the investigative procedure of choice, because characteristic changes are visible with MRI well before plain radiographs.[4,133]

Granulomatous Infections

Granulomatous infections include all processes that produce the classic histologic granuloma. These processes include fungal; spirochete; uncommon bacterial organisms such as actinomycosis, nocardia, and brucellosis; and finally, the most common organism, *Mycobacterium tuberculosis* infections. It is emphasized that patients with other forms of granulomatous disease, such as Wegener's granulomatosis (a form of vasculitis), are at increased risk of an infectious disorder of the spine.[128]

Tuberculous Spondylitis

Although uncommon in developed countries, tuberculous spondylitis is the most common of the granulomatous infections that affect the axial skeleton.[*]

Patient Population. Although cases of tuberculosis declined in the United States until the mid-1980s, recent epidemiologic data suggest a current resurgence.[59,77] The

---

*References 17,19,43,62,77,196.

amount of extrathoracic involvement has increased from less than 8% to more than 18%.[17] In developed countries tuberculosis is a disease of the elderly, whereas in underdeveloped countries it predominates in children.[77] There are approximately 20,000 cases reported each year in the United States, with the immigrant, low socioeconomic, and immunocompromised populations representing the majority of cases.[17] Individuals infected with the human immunodeficiency virus (HIV) are responsible for 87% of matched registries of active tubercular infections in the United States. Skeletal involvement occurs in approximately 1% of all cases. Of those cases, 50% to 60% have an infection of the axial skeleton.[77]

Sources of Infection. Historically dubbed Pott's disease, tuberculous spondylitis is usually caused by *M. tuberculosis*; however, another species of mycobacteria may be the culprit. Tuberculosis spondylitis generally results from hematogenous spread of the pathogen via a pulmonary or genitourinary source. Other routes such as lymphatic dissemination or direct extension from adjacent areas of infection are less frequently encountered.

After the initial seeding from a primary focus elsewhere in the body, this granulomatous infection usually progresses via subligamentous spread across the disc space. This occurs along either the posterior or anterior longitudinal ligament, with relative disc-space sparing. Vertebral collapse, spinal deformity, epidural abscess, and subarachnoid seeding after dural erosion are late sequelae.

Signs and Symptoms. Clinical presentation involves bone pain over the affected site, most commonly the thoracolumbar spine, in conjunction with fever, malaise, and weight loss. Cervical and sacral involvement are rare, occurring in less than 0.03% of all reported cases.[177,196] In the progressive stages of disease kyphosis results from erosive bone destruction. Epidural abscesses are common sequelae, occurring in approximately 50% to 85% of cases.[59,62,97] Paraparesis caused by spinal tuberculosis has remained a constant, occurring in 20% of all cases of reported tubercular infections.[116]

Analysis of Findings. Diagnosis requires evaluation of a urine, sputum, or gastric specimen; a subcutaneous nodule; or bone biopsy to isolate the offending organism. A positive purified protein derivative (PPD) can be helpful, although false negatives can occur in the anergic patient because of age, malnutrition, or immunocompromise. A chest radiograph reveals no evidence of pulmonary disease in 40% to 50% of patients. Plain spine radiographs require 2 months of active tubercular osteomyelitis to become diagnostic.[59,77] Radiologic imaging, including MRI and CT/myelogram, is the basis for evaluating treatment progression and surgical planning. MRI is superior to evaluate soft tissue involvement and presence of abscess formation; CT provides better bone detail, especially in the dorsal elements.

Patient Management. Treatment modalities are based on positive biopsy and culture, degree of kyphosis, extent of neurologic compromise, and disease refractory to medical management. Neurologic sequelae occur in approximately 10% to 50% of cases of active disease, with 20% of cases of tuberculous spondylitis resulting in paraparesis.[116] Ventral decompression with spinal fusion, and debridement with initiation of proper antibiotic therapy, are the accepted modalities of treatment in the case of an evolving deficit. Prognosis, morbidity, and mortality are related to overall age, with children faring better than adults, and to the extent of systemic involvement and preoperative neurologic status.[67,85,97,187]

Actinomycosis

Patient management. Related morphologically to the fungi, *Actinomyces israelii* is an anaerobic gram-positive bacterium. An infection leads to purulent abscesses, external draining sinuses, and characteristic sulfa granules on microscopic examination. Actinomycosis is found most often in the cervical spine, because the majority of cases involve the mandible and supraclavicular areas with direct extension to the adjacent vertebra.[43,91] The actinomycosis infection clinically resembles tuberculous spondylitis, except with less vertebral destruction and disc space narrowing.

Signs and Symptoms. Clinical presentation includes neck pain with associated purulent sinus tracts. Diagnosis entails plain radiographs for bone erosion, MRI to evaluate associated abscess, and a biopsy to obtain a culture.

Patient Management. After diagnosis, medical treatment with penicillin is the mainstay, with a generally favorable outcome for uncomplicating abscesses.[163] Surgical intervention is required for abscess drainage, symptomatic epidural compression of neural structures, or instability that results from bone erosion.

Nocardia

Sources of Infection. *Nocardia asteroides*, a gram-positive bacterium, usually presents as a systemic illness, but can represent a rare cause of back pain secondary to involvement of the bony spinal column.[19,43] Nocardia usually spreads hematogenously from a pulmonary focus to the soft organ systems, but osteomyelitis has also been reported on rare occasions. There is a higher incidence of cervical and thoracic osseous involvement. This is related to the proximity of the pulmonary focus. Spread occurs through venous drainage of the retropharyngeal and mediastinal sites.[114]

Signs and Symptoms. Initial symptoms are constitutional with eventual radicular pain or myelopathy from extradural compression secondary to abscess formation.[114]

Patient Management. When there is no evidence of neurologic compromise or abscess formation, the patient is treated with sulfonamide antibiotics. Surgical intervention is warranted in the setting of epidural compression or bony instability.

Brucellosis

Brucella, a gram-negative rod, is extremely uncommon in developed countries, primarily because of milk pasteurization and uncontaminated food sources.

Source of Infection. A disease that affects farm animals, brucellosis is usually transmitted via ingestion of contaminated food or, reportedly, inhalation. Depending on the magnitude of the inoculum, incubation is a period of days to weeks.

Signs and Symptoms. The resultant illness usually presents as a systemic illness with indolent fever, lymphadenopathy, generalized malaise, and occasionally, back pain. Spinal involvement with a lumbar predilection is observed in 54% of cases.[132] Of those with spinal involvement, 12% present with some degree of spinal cord impingement.[19,43,91]

Analysis of Findings. Diagnosis can be made by blood culture, although half are negative; a positive *Brucella* agglutination test is diagnostic. Plain radiographs are usually nonproductive until late in the disease process. A technetium bone scan or MRI aids in the diagnosis of an active infection.

Patient Management. Early institution of treatment with appropriate antibiotics for 6 weeks is the rule for this curable disease.

Fungal Infections

Fungal infections of the axial skeleton are uncommon, even in endemic areas. Infection occurs by spore inhalation, with resultant pulmonic seeding and systemic spread. Fungal infections in patients with disseminated disease have varying degrees of spinal osseous involvement. This involvement with disseminated fungal infection occurs in 10% to 50% of patients with coccidioidomycosis and blastomycosis infections. There is a much lower incidence of axial involvement for candidiasis or aspergillosis.[19,43]

Coccidioidomycosis

Coccidioidomycosis, endemic to the southwestern United States, has a high rate of spinal involvement and occurs in 20% to 40% of cases of disseminated disease. Radiographs reveal that multiple simultaneous lytic lesions occur in up to 20% of patients with no specific predisposition to vertebral site involvement. Vertebral collapse and neurologic compromise are uncommon.[43] Diagnostic plain radiographs, immunodiffusion titers, and biopsy are used to determine treatment with appropriate antifungal pharmacotherapy.

Blastomycosis

The most virulent fungal agent for osseous involvement, and endemic to the Mississippi River valley, blastomycosis is spread via inhalation, with resultant pulmonary infection and focus. Blastomycosis is hematogenously spread, with a predilection for ventral vertebral involvement. This gives rise to vertebral collapse, joint erosion, and disc invasion. Clinical presentation and bone destruction resemble tuberculous spondylitis. However, blastomycosis more commonly has associated draining sinuses and a greater predisposition to include the dorsal elements.

Cryptococcus

Cryptococcus neoformans is a fungal infection more commonly known for central nervous system involvement in patients with acquired immunodeficiency syndrome (AIDS). It is usually inhaled in an aerosolized form and then spreads hematogenously from a pulmonary location. Osseous involvement occurs in only 10% of cases with the disseminated form.[50] Granuloma formation and cellular reaction are minimal. Radiographs reveal dorsal vertebral involvement and disc space sparing. The usual clinical presentation, which is a late sequela of disseminated cryptococcal meningitis, is swelling and pain of the affected vertebral site, as well as decreased spine mobility. Diagnosis is made via latex agglutination test, and positive cerebrospinal fluid (CSF) and blood cultures. Treatment is with amphotericin-B. Disease control, not eradication, is the goal in the immunocompromised host.

Candidiasis and Aspergillosis

Aspergillus, a mold, and *Candida*, a yeast, are extremely rare causes of vertebral osteomyelitis, with less than a total of 30 cases of both reported in the literature.[49] Both are pathogens of the immunocompromised host. Candidiasis is not as uncommon as other focal or systemic infections found in the intensive care unit (ICU) setting, secondary to the amount of invasive monitoring in critically ill patients.[112] Osseous involvement occurs during a prolonged hospitalization and inadequate treatment of a systemic infection.

Aspergillus is associated with sinus tract and abscess formation, as well as a radiographic picture similar to tuberculosis. Treatment of both of the aforementioned fungi is with amphotericin-B. Prognosis for aspergillosis spondylitis is poor, even after surgical debridement and drainage.[49]

Other Infections

Wegener's granulomatosis, syphilis, and parasitic infections, specifically echinococcosis of the spine, are also potential causes of back pain. Usually reported in patients with fulminant systemic infection, these infections must be included as potential sources of vertebral destruction and back pain associated with fever and weight loss.

Pain Associated with Recumbency and Night Pain
Tumor

Nocturnal pain and pain associated with recumbency are hallmarks of destructive lesions of the vertebral column, caused by either a skeletal metastasis or primary bone tumor.* Regrettably, the majority of spinal column tumors are malignant.

Patient Population. In the case of skeletal lesions, there are correlations between age, location, incidence, and presentation. Generally, age is directly correlated with the type of lesion. Younger patients tend to have a greater incidence of benign bone tumors, whereas those older than

age 30 are predisposed toward malignancy.[55,126] Malignant lesions of the axial skeleton, whether metastatic or primary, are found more often in ventral locations.[20,22,126] Benign processes tend to favor the dorsal elements. The incidence of skeletal metastases outweighs the incidence of primary bone tumors by a margin of 25 to 40:1.[12,20,126,140] The overall incidence of primary bone tumors is only 0.4%.[20,55,126]

Signs and Symptoms. The most frequent clinical presentation for spinal tumors is back pain occurring in up to 85% in the larger series.[20-55] The pain associated with neoplastic growth is usually secondary to one of several factors, which include pathologic fracture, tumor vascular engorgement, periosteal stretching, and impingement on nerve roots in the epidural space.[97]

Metastatic Disease

Cancer is the second leading cause of death in the United States, with approximately 1.3 million new cases per year.[126,140] Metastatic disease in the form of distant foci is evident at autopsy in 40% to 85% of cases of malignancy.[140]

The spine is the most common site of skeletal metastasis. At least 5% of patients with malignancies suffer from this condition.[140] In fact, epidural compression has been reported to be the presenting symptom in approximately 8% to 10% of patients with metastatic disease.[22,140] Of these patients nearly all initially complain of back pain, followed by weakness and ataxia. At the time of diagnosis more than 50% will have a paraparesis or bladder/bowel disturbance.[22,75,140]

The axial skeleton is the leading site of bone metastases that are caused by hematogenous spread through the rich venous network that drains the lungs, pelvis, and thorax. Breast, lung, prostate, and thyroid malignancies account for 50% to 60% of metastatic lesions.[22,126,140] Overall, epidural metastases are equally spread throughout the thoracic and lumbosacral spine. The number of symptomatic metastases, however, is highest in the thoracic region. In most series, symptomatic cervical lesions occur in only 6% to 8% of patients.[22]

Signs and Symptoms. On clinical presentation the patient's history reveals pain of an insidious, progressive nature, unrelated to mechanical activity unless caused by a pathologic fracture from trauma or an acute compressive axial load. Diffuse pain in the elderly, presumably caused by degenerative causes, can delay diagnosis. The axiom that acute neck or back pain in a patient with a known malignancy is metastatic disease until proven otherwise is a prudent guideline.[20]

Analysis of Findings. Ultimate diagnosis relies on radiographic studies, including plain radiographs. Bone scans are warranted for suspected occult lesions because approximately 30% to 50% of the trabeculated bone in a vertebral body must be destroyed before it is detected on plain radiography. However, Weinstein's cervical series detected 99% of metastatic lesions via plain radiographs alone.[140] Other radiographic modalities, including MRI and CT/myelography, are helpful in determining the

---

*References 20,26,58,79,118,124,149,178.

extent of bone destruction and epidural compression, as well as screening for other areas of involvement. In addition to superior sensitivity and specificity, the ability of MRI to scan large areas at once minimizes the chance of missing additional areas of neoplastic involvement.

Diagnostic regimens include laboratory studies demonstrating an elevated calcium level, prostate-specific antigen (PSA), or alkaline phosphatase (ALP), as well as pathologic confirmation via biopsy of a primary malignant focus (if present). Metastatic work-up, including both a plain chest radiograph and an enhanced abdominal/chest CT, determines the primary focus in the majority of cases.[12,22,140]

Patient Management. Treatment options for metastatic disease of the spine include both radiation and surgical intervention. Operative intervention is palliative, with pain control and maintenance of function and stability as the goals. It is usually reserved for neurologic compromise, radiation failure, spinal instability, or uncertain diagnosis.

The patient's preoperative functional status and level of activity directly correlate with the postoperative result.[12] Decompression and stabilization via a ventral approach is usually the route of choice; a review of dorsal decompression found an overall unfavorable result, with 12% to 40% below or at baseline preoperative function after surgery.[12,140] Rapid progression of neurologic deficit is also a poor prognostic indicator. Patients who suffer progressive neurologic deficits that occur over 24 hours have a 28% to 35% chance of permanent paraplegia, whereas those with slowly evolving deficits regain ambulatory function in approximately 60% to 76% of cases.[12,140] Overall, prognosis is directly related to neoplastic type, spinal location, and extent of systemic involvement.

Multiple Myeloma

Some controversy exists about whether multiple myeloma (MM) is a metastatic lesion or a primary bone malignancy. MM and solitary plasmacytoma account for 45% of all malignant bone tumors.[20,22,140,149] The overall incidence ranges from 2 to 5.4 per 100,000, with MM significantly more prevalent than solitary plasmacytoma.[20,22] These disorders are the result of abnormal proliferation of plasma cells, which are responsible for immunoglobulin and antibody production and affect the spine in 30% to 50% of reported cases. MM is primarily a disease of the sixth and seventh decades of life and has a predilection for the thoracic spine (50% to 60%), followed by the lumbar spine, and rarely (<10%), the cervical spine.

Signs and Symptoms. Initial clinical presentation reveals back pain in 75% of patients.[22,140] Unlike the classic metastatic disease presentation of pain with recumbency, the MM lesion is sometimes relieved by rest and aggravated by mechanical agitation that mimics other sciatic or neurogenic sources. The diagnosis of MM is usually made within 6 months of spinal or systemic symptomatology.

Systemic complications include hyperalbuminemia, renal insufficiency, nephrolithiasis, and characteristic serum protein abnormalities. Plain radiographs and CT can be solely diagnostic because of the characteristic osteolytic picture without sclerotic edges that involve the ventral portion of the vertebral body and usually spare the dorsal elements.

Patient Management. Treatment and prognosis vary greatly depending on whether the lesion is a solitary plasmacytoma or a manifestation of MM. Both conditions are exquisitely radiosensitive, but with different survival rates. The 5-year survival rate for the spinal disseminated variant of MM is 18% compared with more than 60% for the solitary lesion.[126] The solitary plasmacytoma lesion maintains a malignant potential and can develop into the disseminated variety up to 20 years later. In cases of rapid progressive neurologic compromise, radiation failure, or instability, surgical decompression and instrumentation are indicated.[22,140]

Chondrosarcoma

This malignant cartilage-forming primary bone tumor is an uncommon spinal neoplasm, and is primarily an adult appendicular lesion.[198] The spine is affected in only 6% of these cases,[1] although the incidence of spinal involvement in children is slightly higher.[1,176,198] There is an even distribution of tumor involvement among cervical, thoracic, and lumbar locations.[5] Chondrosarcomas arise either primarily or from a previously irradiated benign lesion. The secondary form occurs in approximately 26% of patients and is believed to be the result of irradiated Paget's disease or osteochondroma.[197]

At the time of clinical presentation, patients suffering from chondrosarcomas that affect the axial skeleton most commonly demonstrate pain (50%) and localized swelling (30%). Diagnosis is usually based on radiographic studies that reveal bone destruction, associated soft-tissue mass, and "fluffy" calcifications, especially in areas of a prior benign lesion and biopsy.[110] Treatment is en bloc resection, if feasible, because these tumors are usually radioresistant and have a high probability of local recurrence, if inadequate resection is performed. Prognosis correlates with tumor extension and grade. There is a linear relationship between degree of pain on presentation, a larger, more aggressive tumor, and decreased time of survival.[176] An individual with unresectable chondrosarcoma has a 5-year survival rate of only 20%.[1,198]

Chordoma

Originally described by Virchow as a tumor originating from the primitive notochord, chordoma is a tumor of the axial skeleton and the skull base that composes 1.4% of all skeletal sarcomas. It is a histologically low-grade, locally invasive tumor and the most common lesion of the sacrococcygeal region.[17,194] Metastases may occur in 5% to 43% of cases.[17,143,161,194] More than 50% of these lesions are located in the lumbosacral region, 35% are located in the clival and cervical area, and the remainder are spread throughout the rest of the vertebral column.[17]

A total of 90% of patients usually present with pain. A palpable mass is discovered in 10% to 20%.[162]

Neurologic deficit is usually found in the form of bowel/bladder dysfunction or less frequently, cauda equina symptoms (20%).[143] MRI is the imaging modality of choice to evaluate total tumor because of its ability to evaluate soft-tissue involvement.

Treatment is en bloc resection, when feasible. Radiation is usually reserved for local recurrence and inaccessible sites after surgery. There is considerable debate on pathologic subtypes with respect to grade, recurrence, and outcome. Age at presentation is probably the best prognostic indicator for disease-free survival after surgery, with younger patients having a better course.[194]

Lymphoma

Hodgkin's disease is a malignant disease of the reticuloendothelial system. Spinal involvement occurs in approximately 10% of all extranodal lymphomas.[126] The patient's age at presentation is bimodal, with those ages 15 to 35 and older than age 50 most frequently affected. Clinical presentation involves concurrent constitutional signs and symptoms of fever and night sweats with acute cord compression.

Lymphoma represents 75% of cases of the 10% to 15% of spinal neoplasms that present with epidural compression caused by extradural encroachment.[127] Spinal osseous involvement occurs at a decreasing frequency as one ascends the spine: lumbar, thoracic, and, uncommonly, cervical. The vertebral destruction is lytic. Treatment and prognosis are related to grade and stage of disease, even with appropriate institution of radiation and chemotherapy. Surgical intervention is warranted only when symptomatic neurologic compression occurs secondary to epidural compromise.

Osteogenic Sarcoma and Ewing's Sarcoma

Both osteogenic sarcoma, whether primary or secondary, and Ewing's sarcoma represent uncommon malignant lesions of the spinal column with a combined incidence of less than 3% to 4% of spinal column tumors.[20,55,120]

Osteogenic sarcoma is the most common primary malignant bone tumor, but is exceedingly rare in the spinal axis; the highest vertebral incidence reported is approximately 3%. Most cases of primary osteogenic sarcoma (50%) are present in the first 20 years of life. Secondary sarcomas arise in the fifth to sixth decades as a result of irradiated bone or a pre-existing pagetoid lesion. Almost 70% of clinical presentations are accompanied by a neurologic deficit secondary to epidural compression.[120] MRI is the initial modality of choice for diagnosis. Definitive diagnosis is dependent on CT-guided biopsy. Preoperative embolization, chemotherapy, and surgical extirpation, with adjuvant radiotherapy, are the current treatment modalities of choice. Overall prognosis is poor, with a life expectancy of 10 to 18 months. There are a few long-term survivors.[1,5,190]

Ewing's sarcoma affects the spinal axis in less than 3% of all cases. Primarily a disease of the pediatric population, the usual clinical presentation is pain. Diagnosis encompasses MRI and biopsy. Treatment involves a multidisciplinary approach that combines surgical extirpation, radiation, and chemotherapeutic protocols. Prognosis is poor when the spinal axis is involved, with death ensuing in most patients within 5 years.[121]

Benign Tumors

Benign tumors of bone are generally found in patients between ages 20 and 30, in a dorsal location, and a lumbar position. The more common types of benign lesions—osteochondroma, osteoid osteoma, and osteoblastoma—have a lower incidence of recurrence overall than malignant bone tumors in the axial skeleton. A guide to their characteristics and imaging function is provided in Table 3.1.

Osteochondroma

These lesions are the most common benign bone tumor, constituting 36% of all nonmalignant osseous tumors. Pathogenesis stems from a defect in the cartilaginous endplates during early spine development. Related to epiphyseal growth, these slow-growing tumors usually cease growing with epiphyseal closure.[30,190] The majority are asymptomatic lumbar spine lesions found on incidental radiographs.

Clinical presentation varies from patients who report a dull backache (smaller tumors) to decreased motion or deformity (larger tumors). Neurologic compromise is rare. However, when present, the cervical spine is the most common lesion location with resultant myelopathic symptoms. Plain radiographs demonstrate a protruding lesion with well-demarcated borders in the dorsal elements. Treatment for this condition is usually observation. On rare occasions pain, neurologic deficit, or an accelerated growth pattern may be related to malignant transformation. This necessitates surgical removal. Prognosis is usually excellent when complete curettage of affected periosteum and surrounding cartilage is performed.

Giant Cell Tumor

Unlike the majority of primary bone tumors, giant cell tumors (GCTs) are generally found in patients in their third decade of life, decreasing in occurrence in later years. These aggressive tumors carry some malignant potential and a high incidence of local recurrence. They are responsible for 21% of all primary benign bone tumors and affect the spinal axis in 8% to 11% of all cases. There is a 3% to 6% rate of concurrent aneurysmal bone cysts with a pre-existing GCT.[2] They most commonly occur in the sacral region when the spinal column is involved.

Pain, which can be radicular or diffuse, is usually followed by bowel or bladder dysfunction. Plain radiographs demonstrate cortical expansion with little reactive sclerosis or periosteal reaction.[2] Both T_1- and T_2-weighted MRI scans reveal homogeneous signals, whereas presurgical CT studies can better delineate the degree of vertebral bone involvement and define surgical margins. Because of the nondistinct histologic characteristics of GCTs, a thorough evaluation, including radiographic investigation coupled with intraoperative histology, is important to differentiate this condition from other primary bone tumors.

Treatment is usually en bloc resection. There is a relatively poor prognosis because of the high recurrence

TABLE 3.1

Benign Lesions of the Spine

Lesion	Incidence	Age/Sex	Location	Imaging
Hemangioma	Most common	All ages, both sexes	Vertebral body (T, L>C)	CT: "polka dot" body; MRI: "hot spot" on T_1W_1
Osteoid osteoma	Common (10% in spine)	10-20 years, M/F ratio 2–4:1	Neural arch (L, C>T)	Dense sclerosis, lucent nidua, lesion <2 cm
Osteoblastoma	Uncommon (40% in spine)	<30 years, M/F ratio 2.5:1	Neural arch (C>T, L)	Expansile lytic mass; +/– matrix mineralization
Giant cell tumor	Uncommon	10-50 years, most in 30s, slight female predominance, except in sacrum	Vertebral body (sacrum > vertebrae)	Lytic, expansile, highly destructive
Osteochondroma	Common, but rare in spine	5-30 years, M/F ratio 1.5:2.5:1	Spinous, transverse processes (10% to 20% multiple)	Pedunculated/sessile lesion; periosteum, cortex, marrow in continuity with host bone; cartilaginous cap +/– Ca^{++}
Aneurysmal bone cyst	Rare (20% in spine)	80% <20 years, slight female predominance	Posterior elements (C, T most common)	Multiloculated, expansile; eggshell-like rims; blood products with fluid-fluid levels; highly vascular
Eosinophilic granuloma	Very rare	Most 5-10 years, rarely >30 years	Any level; single level collapse; "vertebrae plana"	MRI: hyperintense on T_2, variable signal on T_1W_1

rates.[99] These tumors have the potential for malignant transformation, especially after local radiation, if surgical margins were inadequate.[99,190]

Osteoid Osteoma and Osteoblastoma

These two tumor types share a common pathologic origin, but differ in size and incidence of spinal involvement. Osteoid osteoma usually affects patients 20 to 30 years of age, accounting for 2.6% of all excised primary bone tumors and up to 18% of axial lesions. Approximately 40% of these axial lesions occur in the lumbar region. These tumors are thought to be a chronic inflammatory reaction rather than a true neoplasm; the majority are less than 2cm. On presentation, patients report a dull ache that is exacerbated at night. This condition is believed to be the result of prostaglandin production by the tumor; thus the classic pain relief with aspirin. Neurologic deficits are rare; nonstructural scoliosis is present in 40% to 63% of cases.[83] Plain films are pathognomonic, revealing a small radiolucent nidus of less than 2cm with an appropriate degree of surrounding sclerosis usually located in the posterior elements. Treatment is excision, instrumentation, and fusion if there is severe scoliosis, although minor deformities will resolve with resection alone. Overall, there is an excellent prognosis with marginal recurrence rates related to inadequate excision of nidus.

Osteoblastomas differ from osteoid osteomas in obtaining greater size (more than 2cm) and a greater propensity to produce spinal deformity. Less common than osteoid osteomas, osteoblastomas represent less than 3% of benign bone tumors, but have a greater propensity for axial involvement, which occurs in the vertebrae in 40% of cited cases. Approximately 90% of cases are in patients 30 years of age or younger.

Clinical presentation characteristically produces a higher degree of neurologic sequelae in the form of radicular pain (50%) secondary to lesion size, torticollis in 13% of cervical lesions, and pelvic pain from large sacral lesions. Treatment is en bloc resection with usual resolution of scoliotic deformity. Prognosis is favorable with adequate removal, with low recurrence rates of approximately 5%.

Aneurysmal Bone Cyst

Although only responsible for approximately 1% to 2% of all primary bone tumors, aneurysmal bone cysts (ABCs) affect the axial skeleton in 12% to 25% of all reported cases of ABC.[32,83,166,188] The incidence of ABC is greater in the thoracolumbar region (Figure 3.3). They occur more commonly in females and are a tumor of the young, with 75% to 80% of all cases occurring before age 20.[83] As in the majority of benign osseous lesions, dorsal element involvement predominates with 60% of spinal ABCs occurring there. The pathogenesis is unclear, but accepted theories include an underlying tumor or traumatic arterivenous malformation (AVM), with subsequent development of a cyst.[32]

Clinical presentation of patients harboring an ABC is related to location. This reveals that the more dorsally located lesion is largely asymptomatic, whereas one involving the pedicle or dorsal portion of the anterior column

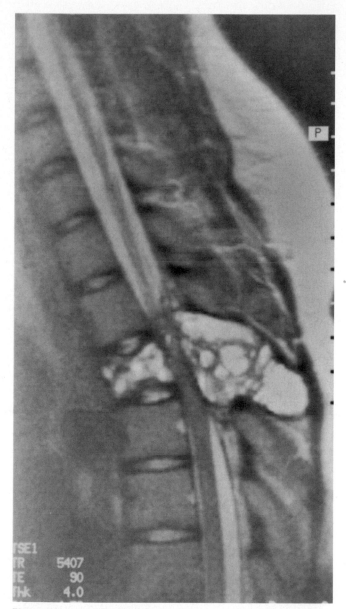

Figure 3.3 T_1-weighted MRI scan of an aneurysmal bone cyst with spinal cord compression.

produces myelopathic, or radicular, symptoms. Radiographs demonstrate a single osteolytic lesion with a thin, well-demarcated cortical rim; multiple vertebral involvement occurs in 40% of cases.[83,166]

Treatment is controversial but involves complete curettage of the involved site and possible postoperative radiation, if inadequate margins were obtained during resection. Recurrence rates vary from 6% to 70%, with a mean of 20%, depending on surgical resection and radiation.[166]

Hemangioma and Eosinophilic Granuloma

Hemangiomas and eosinophilic granulomas are uncommon lesions of the axial skeleton. Both account for less than 1% of primary benign bone tumors involving the spine and are generally located vertically. Characterized by slow growth and a female predominance, vertebral hemangiomas occur most commonly in the thoracolumbar spine and are found in 11% of general autopsies.[63] Symptomatic spinal hemangiomas are exceedingly rare, but when they do appear, the most common initial symptom in the case of a solitary lesion is back pain, with or without radiation into the lower extremities.[180] There is a loose relationship between pre-existing spinal hemangioma expansion and pregnancy that results in a neurologic deficit. This is believed to be caused by the physiologic volume increase of the circulatory system during pregnancy. This results in expansion of a previously asymptomatic vertebral hemangioma and resultant spinal cord compression.[63]

Diagnosis of symptomatic lesions is best made with MRI, whereas asymptomatic lesions are discovered incidentally during other radiographic investigations. Treatment for symptomatic lesions that involve the spine incorporates combinations of surgical curettage, embolization, and radiotherapy.[63,180]

Eosinophilic granuloma is the solitary osseous lesion version of a group of disorders characterized by an abnormal proliferation of Langerhans cells; it is termed histiocytosis X and includes both Letterer-Siwe and Hand-Schüller-Christian diseases.[*] The overall incidence for any variety of the histiocytosis X spectrum is one per million people. Eosinophilic granulomas most commonly occur in the pediatric population. The solitary variety is the most common version in the group under age 20.[169]

Clinical presentation most commonly involves pain in the thoracolumbar region, although cervical and clival lesions have been reported in the literature. MRI is the investigative procedure of choice, with ultimate diagnosis relying on biopsy.[49]

Treatment is somewhat controversial, but commonly includes surgical curettage and fusion for lesions that result in spinal instability; adjuvant radiotherapy or chemotherapy is reserved for disseminated versions.[3,169]

Spinal Cord Tumors

Intramedullary spine neoplasms represent 2% to 4% of all central nervous system tumors.[126,178] The majority of lesions that involve the cord and meninges occur in the epidural space in the form of metastatic disease.[22,140] The majority of nonmetastatic intraspinal neoplasms occur in adults between ages 30 and 50.[38,93,149,178] The largest group of neoplastic spinal lesions that involve the spinal cord and meninges occurs in the intradural-extramedullary space (40% to 50%), followed by the extradural space (30%) and the intramedullary space (20% to 25%).[178] In the pediatric patient the intradural space is involved in approximately 40% to 50% of cases.[38,178]

Back pain is the most common initial complaint in the adult population that harbors spinal neoplasms; the pediatric population with spinal tumors tends to present with neurologic deficit in the form of motor or gait disturbances.[*] The nature of back pain in the adult population is usually diffuse and unrelated to mechanical activity, thus prolonging diagnosis until the pain becomes radicular or

---

[*]References 3,46,49,99,162,169.
[*]References 22,26,93,140,149,178.

symptoms that are caused by cord or root compression ensue. Generally when the tumor is located in the spinal canal, there is an association between pain and neurologic deficit. For example, lesions located in the extradural space commonly produce pain without deficit, whereas neoplasms located within the intramedullary space will more often produce deficit at the time of diagnosis.

Extradural Lesions

Extradural lesions include all neoplasms, whether primary or metastatic, that abut the dura mater and affect the vertebrae, soft tissue, and vasculature. Symptoms may be caused by compression, invasion, or irritation of the involved anatomy. The majority of epidural lesions discussed earlier in the text are metastatic in origin. Other epidural pathologies, such as lipomatous masses that result from Cushing's disease or a hematoma (Figure 3.4), are also potential sources of pain but more often cause epidural cord compression with deficit.

The majority of vascular malformations present with an acute neurologic deficit secondary to an ischemic insult or compressive hemorrhage; these are addressed in later sections. The compressive epidural fatty mass present in Cushing's disease pursues a more indolent course. A clinical diagnosis of epidural lipomatosis is made in the proper clinical setting of a coexistent endocrine disorder with associated physical stigmata.[24] The radiologic procedure of

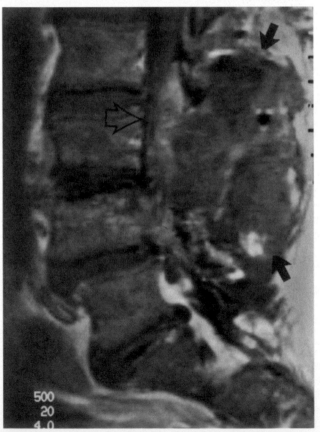

Figure 3.4 T$_1$-weighted MRI scan of an epidural hematoma (*black arrows*) compressing the thecal sac (*open arrow*), with resultant paraparesis after lumbar fusion.

choice is MRI for both the lipoma and acute epidural compression secondary to hematoma.

Intradural-Extramedullary Lesions

Meningiomas, schwannomas, and neurofibromas constitute more than 50% of all neoplastic processes in the intradural-extramedullary space. Nittner's review of 4885 adults with spinal cord tumors found schwannomas (23%) and meningiomas (22%) to be the most common lesion of the intradural-extramedullary space.[126,173] Symptoms may be nocturnal and most commonly involve pain caused by root irritation. Early neurologic compromise is uncommon because of the adaptive compressibility of surrounding fat, CSF, and adjacent vascular structures. Neurologic compromise occurs when the compliance of surrounding structures is at its nadir and extradural compression is directly transmitted to the spinal cord.

Although both meningiomas and nerve sheath tumors are benign lesions usually found in thoracic dorsal sites, neurofibromas are a common finding in phakomatoses. Almost always lesions of dorsal roots, neurofibromas present with radicular symptoms and are usually readily accessible to surgical excision via a dorsal route.[126,149] Although their malignant potential is low, nerve sheath tumors (NSTs) may be locally destructive if allowed to progress. Caudally located neurofibromas may displace adjacent nerve roots with possible bone erosion of nearby foramina as the neoplasm grows. Excision is recommended for symptomatic lesions and, with complete removal, recurrence is rare.

Schwannomas, commonly found with von Recklinghausen's neurofibromatosis, are usually solitary lesions found in thoracic sites in adults between 40 and 50 years of age. These tumors are most commonly found in the intradural-extramedullary space; however, approximately 20% will be found crossing the dura or to be solely extradural.

On clinical presentation patients with these tumors exhibit radicular symptoms, and the tumor is easily diagnosed with MRI. Surgical extirpation is the rule when symptomatic.

Meningiomas have a thoracic and female (4:1) predominance. More than 80% of meningiomas are located in the thoracic region[149] and occur in women at a 4:1 ratio to men.[93,94,126,149] Another benign tumor usually located dorsally, a meningioma commonly presents with pain from a compressed nerve root as it exits the neural foramina. Although less common in the cervical and lumbar spine, large, slow-growing meningiomas may produce myelopathic symptoms from spinal cord compression, especially at the craniocervical junction.[93] Meningiomas are the most common benign tumor at the foramen magnum.[93]

Age of presentation parallels that of intracranial meningiomas. Plain radiographs with subsequent CT/myelogram and/or MRI are the investigative modalities. Treatment is surgical excision with or without preoperative embolization.[149]

The remaining 30% of intradural-extramedullary tumors are composed of sarcomas (roughly 10%), followed by dermoids, epidermoids, arachnoid cysts, teratomas, ganglion cysts, and, rarely, spinal metastases.[126,149] These lesions possess characteristic features on MRI that help delineate them. The ultimate diagnosis relies on biopsy.

Arachnoiditis that presents with diffuse constant pain and associated paresthesias is the result of multiple operations on the back, or clumping of nerve roots after the administration of the outdated Pantopaque myelographic dye. The diagnosis is made via MRI or myelogram with visualization of characteristic nerve root clumping. Regrettably, there is no effective treatment.

Intradural-Intramedullary Tumors

Intramedullary spinal cord tumors (IMSCTs) account for 2% to 4% of central nervous system neoplasms[93,178] and are of neuroglial origin in 80% of cases, regardless of age. More than 90% of these tumors are rostral to the conus in patients under age 15. Children are predisposed to astrocytic tumors, whereas adult pathology is more evenly spread over the neuroglial spectrum.[38,173,178]

As age increases there is a shift in pathology, with ependymomas becoming more common than astrocytomas. The incidence of IMSCTs increases from rostral to caudal and may present with insidious pain, the most common finding in the adult population, or associated spinal cord dysfunction, in the form of band paresthesias or motor deficit. Typically, the pain associated with these lesions is unrelated to mechanical activity. Pediatric patients tend to present with gait or motor disturbances.[38,183] A delay of years in diagnosis is common.

Other intramedullary disorders such as AVM, syringomyelia, and metastases are potential, but extremely rare, causes of spinal pain. AVMs and hemangioblastomas of the spinal cord are potential causes of acute pain with subsequent neurologic sequelae secondary to rupture, resulting in hematoma formation or ischemic effects.

Diagnostic studies include plain radiographs that can reveal widened pedicles, or a myelogram that shows a diffuse enlargement of a cord segment. MRI is the gold standard to evaluate spinal cord dysfunction as a result of the aforementioned causes, with the exception of angiography, to evaluate AVMs. MRI is the procedure of choice for preoperative planning because of its multiple plane imaging and tumor localization. With the advent of microneurosurgery, resection margins are better with lower morbidity and mortality. Adjuvant radiation therapy for glial tumors is controversial, with some investigators finding no significant benefit.[173,178]

Pain Associated with Morning Stiffness

Persistent axial pain, with a prolonged tapering course after the initiation of increasing mechanical activity, heralds the possibility of an inflammatory disorder affecting the spine.[23,54,103,113] The two most common chronic inflammatory processes that involve the axial skeleton are rheumatoid arthritis (RA) and ankylosing spondylitis (AS). Although related, these diseases represent two vastly different pathologies with regard to gender, age, axial location, associated clinical findings, immunologic characterization, and indications for surgical intervention.

Ankylosing Spondylitis
Patient Population. The most prevalent of the seronegative spondyloarthropathies, with an incidence of up to 2% in the Caucasian population, AS is a common cause of axial pain in young adults.[28,78] Unlike RA, it has a male predominance and is most commonly found in the axial skeleton with a mild degree of peripheral involvement.

Pathogenesis is unclear, but there is a strong immunologic association with HLA-B27 positivity in approximately 95% of patients. The prototypical lesion is enthesopathic, affecting insertion sites of tendons and ligaments to bone, with characteristic radiologic changes of the sacroiliac joints and lumbosacral spine. The disease progresses in an ascending fashion from caudal to rostral, which results in severe flexion deformity if allowed to continue.[13]

Signs and Symptoms. Typical presentation is that of a young white male between ages 15 and 30, with insidious LBP in 80% to 90%, peripheral joint pain in the hip or shoulder in 20% to 40%, and sciatic pain in 5%.[28] Clinical diagnosis is based on a history of back pain and grades 3 to 4 bilateral sacroiliitis observed on plain radiographs. There have been several revisions of the original criteria for AS, but all accept the radiologic changes with a history of insidious onset of back pain, age younger than 40, persistence for greater than 3 months, morning stiffness, improvement with exercise, and limitation of chest expansion.[54,78] Because it takes from 3 to 7 years for the radiographic evidence of bilateral symmetric sacroiliitis to become evident, a loss of axial mobility, back pain, and morning stiffness are important signs and symptoms.[30,54,78] Associated fractures, spinal stenosis, and rotary instability are the end result of a fused vertebral column.[113,171] In the Fox and Kilgore series,[65] 28 of 33 cases presented with fractures and approximately 50% had a neurologic deficit associated with these traumatic lesions. The HLA-B27 positivity is suggestive, but inconclusive of disease diagnosis.

Patient Management. Prognosis and success of treatment relate directly to the time of diagnosis, initiation of physical therapy, and possible phenotypic expression. Treatment options for severely kyphotic deformities include cervical and lumbar osteotomies with subsequent traction and instrumentation for stabilization.[83,96,117,174,181]

The disease course predicts its progression in the first 10 years, with the more aggressive subtypes suffering the greatest amount of deformity. Approximately 92% of these patients will remain functionally active, whereas 40% will have some degree of immobility.[65]

Rheumatoid Arthritis
Patient Population. This chronic inflammatory process, which affects the synovium of peripheral joints, has a quoted prevalence of 1% for both genders by age 65, but is an uncommon cause of back pain.[107] Unlike AS, this disease affects an older patient population, has a female predominance, is found most often in the cervical spine, and necessitates a higher degree of surgical intervention secondary to instability.

Signs and Symptoms. RA affects the cervical spine most commonly in one of three ways: atlantoaxial subluxation, basilar invagination, and subaxial subluxation.

Craniocervical instability in the form of atlantoaxial subluxation (AAS) is present in 40% of cases.[34,103,107] Neurologic sequelae with AAS is extremely uncommon, even with up to 10mm of subluxation. Approximately 20% of patients with AAS will have some degree of basilar invagination. Basilar invagination is less common than AAS, but is more frequently associated with neurologic deficit. Kramer and colleagues[107,108] reported brain stem compression or myelopathy in 50% of patients with basilar invagination.

Diagnosis of RA is based on history, distribution of joint involvement, and positive rheumatoid factor. Neck pain should warrant a thorough radiographic evaluation, including flexion/extension radiographs and MRI for ligamentous viewing. Radiographic sequelae include soft-tissue swelling, narrowing of joint spaces, and ultimately, bone erosion.

Patient Management. Surgical intervention with fusion and/or traction is warranted for myelopathy, progressive subluxations, and severe pain.[34,103,107,137]

Other rheumatologic disorders of the spine include the remainder of the seronegative spondyloarthropathies such as Reiter's disease, Behçet's syndrome, Whipple's disease, and enteropathic arthritis, as well as osteoarthritis. These conditions represent other possible causes of back pain, with or without deformity, that may require either surgical intervention or, more commonly, conservative therapy for systemic symptoms.[100] There is an obvious overlap among most of the spinal arthropathies caused by the immunologic denominator, with some syndromes resulting in either instability or axial deformity.

Mechanical Pain

Pain without constitutional signs and symptoms that is initiated and exacerbated by activity is a large category that includes lumbar strain, disc protrusion and extrusion, spinal stenosis, spondylolisthesis, spondylolysis, and soft-tissue irritation disorders, such as in the piriform syndrome.* Other entities such as sacroiliac joint dysfunction, facet syndrome, dural ectasia, perineural or ganglion cysts, and collagen disorders (Ehlers-Danlos syndrome) are less well-differentiated causes of low back pain and are usually clinically diagnosed and conservatively managed.[52,87,95] The possibilities of differential diagnosis, with respect to the etiology of axial pain related to movement, can be numerous because most anatomic structures of the spine have been reported to be pain generators.[10,36,87]

Anywhere from 40% to 80% of the adult population has LBP sometime before age 50. Ninety percent of cases are a result of mechanical causes. The majority of cases improve with conservative therapy only. Although surgical intervention is relatively straightforward for a patient suffering from an acute deterioration with a progressive cauda equina syndrome, decisions regarding treatment of other areas of degenerative disease such as spinal stenosis and spondylolisthesis are not as clear. To evaluate degenerative spinal disorders it is necessary to determine the character of pain, whether it be LBP alone or associated with radicular symptoms, symptomatic neurogenic claudication, or rarely, myelopathy. Clinical history of onset and duration of symptoms, age, presence of a congenital disorder, and spinal deformity help differentiate among the more common degenerative lesions. MRI and CT/myelogram are most commonly used to evaluate degenerative spinal disorders.

Spinal Stenosis

Whether acquired as in the elderly or congenital (e.g., in the achondroplastic dwarf) patient, this condition has a common clinical presentation.* The classic bilateral low back, buttock, and thigh pain, consistent with neurogenic claudication associated with activity, can be present whether the patient is standing (94%) or has walked a short distance.[24]

Neurogenic claudication (NC) must be differentiated from vascular claudication (VC). The clinical picture of VC reveals progressive calf pain after ambulation, with associated decreased peripheral pulses and chronic tissue changes seen in cool distal extremities.

Spinal stenosis is a clinical entity with radiologic confirmation of a decreased spinal canal observed on axial MRI or CT/myelogram views. Surgical intervention for both cervical or lumbar stenosis encompasses decompression with or without fusion.†

Spondylolisthesis and Spondylolysis

Spondylolisthesis and spondylolysis are common causes of back pain in both the pediatric and adult population, with L5 the most common site of involvement.‡ Spondylolisthesis is the most common cause of back pain in patients younger than age 30.[24] Seitsalso and Hyvarinen's[167,168] series found that in the population younger than age 20 year with spondylolisthesis, 50% to 86% had LBP, 82% had radicular pain, and 74% had both conditions. Pain tended to correlate with the degree of lumbosacral kyphosis, not the extent of slippage.[168] Approximately 20% have spinal deformity that can be detected on physical examination.

The adult population had a more vague and insidious presentation with back pain as the most common complaint, followed by claudication and hamstring tightness, probably caused by concurrent spinal stenosis. Treatment varies depending on type of pain, degree of slip, and segmental instability. Surgical decompression and fusion are the mainstays for advanced disease.[29,90,164,165,167]

Herniated Nucleus Pulposus

Herniated nucleus pulposus (HNP) is a common cause of radicular pain in adults ages 30 to 40.[37,56,61,69,72] Only 35% of those who present with an HNP experience sciatica.[156,175,192] The pain is usually sharp and follows a dermatomal pattern. Diagnosis includes clinical findings

---

*References 24,36,56,61,90,95.

†References 21,64,90,111,118,125.
†References 15,29,64,90,102,106,122,138,154.
‡References 27,90,118,164,165,168.

consistent with the affected nerve root in the form of sensory, reflex, or motor deficits.[104]

The majority of herniated discs respond to conservative therapy, with surgical intervention reserved for neurologic deficit, severe pain, or severe spinal stenosis.[15,84,106,118,119] Other causes of back pain that may present in either a radicular pattern or with diffuse symptoms are a conjoined nerve root or perineural cyst; both may be detected by MRI.[136]

Scoliosis

Scoliosis represents another potential cause of back pain in adults who suffer from LBP. Lumbar degenerative rotating scoliosis, which is a result of either idiopathic or degenerative causes, with a Cobb angle of greater than 10 degrees is present in approximately 7.5% of the adult back pain population with an increasing prevalence with age.[82,148] As age increases, both the proportion of women and radicular symptoms increase.[82,148] The incidence of pain may be no greater in the adult scoliotic population, but clinical data suggest that when pain is present, it is greater in intensity and duration. Although the exact pain etiology is unclear, back pain is present in 86% of lumbar scoliotics.[148] The majority of cases of minor (less than 20 degree Cobb angle) lumbar scoliosis should be medically managed. Surgical intervention is reserved for progressive deformity, radicular pain, instability, neurologic deficit, and improvement of appearance.[148]

Acute Spinal Pain and Visceral Pain

The acute onset of localized spine pain can be related to the following causes: (1) fracture caused by trauma or an underlying systemic condition, (2) bone expansion with resultant periosteal stretching within a vertebral body, (3) adjacent encroaching soft-tissue process, (4) acute disc herniation, or (5) an acute vascular event that involves either spinal cord infarction or hemorrhage. In the case of an acute axial load traumatic fractures are usually suspected and detected with associated plain radiographs. The acute hemorrhage of either a vertebral body tumor, such as an aneurysmal bone cyst,[32] or the sudden rupture of a spinal AVM,[195] has rarely been associated with acute neck or back pain. The list of causes for pathologic fractures or vertebral body expansion that results from an underlying process is quite formidable and was reviewed in earlier sections.

The majority of metabolic and endocrinologic disorders are chronic processes that either affect bone mineralization and density or distort adjacent ligamentous structures by calcification or hypertrophy.[21,159,160] Although the majority of endocrinologic disorders such as osteomalacia, osteoporosis, and acromegaly predispose a patient to benign pathologic fractures, others such as Paget's disease can have malignant potential.[16,159] Individuals with metabolic disorders first present with systemic signs and symptoms before reporting progressive axial pain. Laboratory evaluation for abnormal hormone levels, electrolyte imbalances, elevated ESR or uric acid, and familial histories of phakomatosis or achondroplasia provide pertinent clues.

The etiology of back pain from both intrathoracic and abdominal pathologies encompasses every organ system, including common vascular entities. These include abdominal aortic aneurysm that can capture or erode adjacent vertebral bodies, esophageal perforation, cholelithiasis, nephrolithiasis, renal cancer, and uncommon entities such as hematocolpos.[40,70,86] In the proper clinical setting the nature of pain in these conditions, associated physical findings, and proper diagnostic tests help distinguish spinal from other nonaxial causes.

Neurologic Deficits

Spinal cord and column dysfunction can be manifested by a variety of pain, motor, sensory, muscle tone, and bladder disturbances; these neurologic changes fit specific spinal cord syndromes.[195] Pain can be of local, radicular, or a diffuse (dull ache) origin. Motor weakness can range from complete and acute to chronically progressive, taking the form of clumsiness. Sensory disturbances include dysesthesias, paresthesias, or complete anesthesia. Muscle tone abnormalities range from atonia to spasticity. A spinal lesion results in either a spastic or atonic bladder, depending on the level of the lesion. Pathologic processes of the spinal cord and column caused by congenital, traumatic, vascular, neoplastic, infectious or inflammatory, degenerative, or environmental causes generally reflect a spinal cord syndrome in the form of neurologic deficit with one or a combination of the aforementioned symptoms.

The time course of a neurologic deficit, in conjunction with a spinal cord syndrome, helps to formulate a differential diagnosis. This diagnosis of spinal cord dysfunction can then be grouped broadly into a compressive or noncompressive neurologic lesion that is further classified by the time course of deficit progression.[9]

A comprehensive history of symptom onset and physical examination, including a detailed neurologic evaluation, enables the clinician to ascertain anatomic lesion location, as well as associated syndromes. At this point further work-up, including radiographic and laboratory studies, helps limit the differential diagnosis.

A gross classification of disorders of neurologic function directly related to spinal pathology by etiology, associated dysfunction, and progression of symptoms is presented in the following pages. Other processes that mimic spinal pathology caused by intracranial, peripheral, or spinal nerves, neuromuscular junction, or metabolic causes are briefly reviewed.

Congenital Lesions

In the majority of significant neural tube developmental disorders a physical examination at birth reveals a spinal defect, with or without neurologic dysfunction. Other disorders such as tethered cord or congenital scoliosis may remain occult until symptoms present, secondary to spinal column growth.

Spinal Dysraphism

The variants of spina bifida and associated neural element herniation are the most common disorders of spinal dysraphism. Findings on incidental radiographs of spina bifida, or "split spine," can be either occult or overt (spina bifida aperta), with a resultant meningocele or meningomyelocele (MMC). Dorsal spina bifida occulta (SBO) usually remains asymptomatic. An overlying cutaneous abnormality often is the only indication of a developmental disturbance. When this condition becomes symptomatic, it is caused by an associated tethered cord, filum lipoma, or diastematomyelia. Symptomatology includes structural causes such as cavus deformities or scoliosis, and gait and bladder dysfunction caused by cord tethering. Surgical intervention is required only for symptomatic lesions.

In comparison, spina bifida aperta (SPA) (present in 0.6 per 1000 live births) has devastating neurologic effects that can include a complete spinal cord syndrome at the affected level.[31,44,94] MMC is associated almost universally with Arnold-Chiari type II malformation, as well as syringomyelia, hydrocephalus, diastematomyelia, and callosal dysgenesis. Spinal dysraphism should be considered with any child who initially presents with anal agenesis. A 9% incidence of spinal cord/column dysfunction is associated with the VATER (vertebral, anal, tracheoesophageal, renal) complex.[44] Neurosurgical intervention is required both for defect closure and possible decompression for both ventricular and cervical etiologies.

Diastematomyelia and diplomyelia are related congenital anomalies that refer to the sagittal division of the spinal cord into either two hemicords or two duplicated cords, respectively. Both are found in the thoracolumbar spine.

Diastematomyelia has an associated fibrous or bone spur that separates the two hemicords. A patient's condition when presenting with either entity ranges from asymptomatic to progressive spinal cord dysfunction, probably resulting from spinal cord tethering. A series by Miller and Bowen[129] on diastematomyelia cited these associated findings: musculoskeletal conditions (cavus foot, spinal dysraphism), 98%; congenital scoliosis, 79%; and cutaneous lesions, 56%. Neurologic deficit was present in 83% of patients in the form of weakness, and sensory or bladder disturbances. Radiographic evaluation includes both MRI, to evaluate for hydromyelia, and CT, to evaluate a bone ridge. Plain radiographs often demonstrate a widened interpeduncular distance. Surgical intervention is often required to prevent both further progression of neurologic deficit and deformity.

Tethered cord, often associated with an MMC, causes progressive neurologic deficits caused by traction on the conus medullaris. Occurring in approximately 15% of the MMC population, symptomatic tethered cords are diagnosed in patients with slowly progressive spasticity, bladder dysfunction, and sensory disturbances. Peterson[150] proposed a correlation between time of symptom onset and level of the lesion, age, and height. He concluded that lesions above L3 would become symptomatic before lesions located below L4, with age 6 as the cutoff point. MRI is the imaging investigation of choice. Release of the filum is indicated for symptomatic lesions.

Congenital syringomyelia and hydromyelia are disorders of the central canal. Hydromyelia (which is rarely symptomatic) is an incidental clinical finding at autopsy.

The most common form of syringomyelia is associated with Arnold-Chiari type II malformations.[57] The patient presents with bilateral sensory loss, usually of the upper extremities, pain, and later, spasticity. MRI is the procedure of choice to investigate the possibility of a syrinx. Other causes of secondary syringomyelia include traumatic, neoplastic, other congenital, and vascular disorders, and are reviewed in a later section. To prevent bulbar symptomatology, spasticity, or simply for pain relief, a posterior fossa decompression or shunting procedure is often required.

Scoliosis as a result of congenital causes has associated spinal cord abnormalities in 18% to 58% of cases.[82] These abnormalities include syringomyelia (25% to 62%), diastematomyelia (21%), neoplasm, tethered cords, and Arnold-Chiari type II malformations. Neurologic symptomatology in the form of spasticity, and sensory or bladder disturbances, is caused by the underlying disease and location.

Other congenital disorders such as Klippel-Feil syndrome (severely malformed cord), iniencephaly (downward displacement of cranial contents into a malformed cervical canal), and the prevalent Chiari malformations, with associated cervical or thoracic syringomyelia, present other causes of spasticity that require surgical intervention.

Trauma

Patients who present with a history of trauma provide an obvious clue to the differential diagnosis of acute spinal cord dysfunction. Traumatic injury of the spinal cord and column can be either direct or indirect. In direct trauma, often caused by a knife or gunshot injury, there is violation of the dura mater. In indirect trauma caused by fracture-dislocation, pure fracture, or pure dislocation, the dura mater is usually intact. Mechanisms of indirect trauma include flexion, extension, rotation, and compression. Other causes of spinal cord malfunction after trauma include spinal cord contusion, compression of adjacent vessels with resultant ischemia, and epidural compression caused by hemorrhage.

An adequate history, including mechanism of injury coupled with a detailed neurologic examination, pinpoints both the type and site of radiographic investigation. Traumatic fracture-dislocation has the highest incidence of neurologic deficit; the next highest is burst fracture. Traumatic fracture-dislocation of the cervical spine remains the most common cause of quadriplegia and paraplegia.[182] The greatest incidence of neurologically intact patients is found in compression and flexion injuries. The greatest incidence of complete spinal cord injury other than cervical pathology is found in thoracic spine injury, whereas injuries at the cauda equina level have a lower incidence of neurologic deficit. Of note is the acute onset of a central cord syndrome, most often caused by traumatic extension injuries of the cervical spine. Differential diagnosis includes bilateral brachial plexus injury or cruciate paralysis of Bell.[123]

Initial radiographic studies should contain appropriate plain radiographs, including anteroposterior/lateral radiographs of the spinal column. Other views such as a coneddown view are occasionally necessary for junctional areas of the spine. The entire spine needs to be radiographed because concurrent fractures are observed in 10% to 30% of trauma patients.[33] The majority of spinal fractures resulting from indirect causes are evident on plain radiographs alone. MRI is the study of choice for suspected traumatic discs and spinal cord and ligamentous injury, although CT is considered superior for anatomic bone detail.

Treatment of spinal fractures, including early versus late decompression, ventral versus dorsal approach, and stabilization, is discussed in another section.[75]

Post-traumatic syringomyelia (PTS) should be included in the differential diagnosis of any patient who develops deterioration of motor function, with an ascending sensory level after traumatic quadriparesis or paraparesis. Approximately 11% of all cases of syringomyelia are reported to be caused by trauma, whereas 3% of cases with severe cervical trauma with paraplegia/quadriplegia are said to result in post-traumatic syringomyelia.[9] Its course of symptom development ranges from 2 months to 36 years. It is found most often in the thoracolumbar region.[186]

Clinical presentation involves pain, ascending sensory level, motor deficits, and loss of reflexes above the previous lesion. MRI is the imaging procedure of choice to evaluate for a post-traumatic syrinx. Surgical intervention is required for pain, ascending deficits, or progressive spasticity.

Vascular Lesions

Acute or rapid subacute onset of paraplegia or quadriplegia, without evidence of trauma, suggests a vascular event involving the spinal cord. A slowly progressive myelopathy or radiculopathy can also be caused by vascular etiologies. These causes include occlusion, inflammatory disorders, hemorrhage, or vascular malformations. These etiologies in turn lead to acute or chronic symptomatology, caused by ischemic or compressive lesions. In the following sections vascular causes of cord malfunction are divided into ischemic, vascular malformation, and intracranial groups. Other rare causes of spinal cord malfunction from vascular etiologies are reviewed briefly.

Ischemia

Ischemia, whether a result of atherosclerotic, compressive, or traumatic causes, is probably the most common etiology for spinal cord compromise. Persons with circulatory insufficiency in the legs may harbor disease of the abdominal aorta with resultant spinal cord ischemia. Thromboembolic occlusion of spinal segmental arteries (e.g., the artery of Adamkiewicz), or dissection, clamping, or severe atheroma of the aorta are the most common causes of spinal cord infarction.[182] For example, clamping the aorta for intra-abdominal vascular surgery results in paraplegia in 0.5% to 38% of cases.[172] The anterior cord syndrome is a typical clinical presentation of ischemic spinal cord insult. The midthoracic level is the most common site of ischemia because it lies in a vascular watershed zone.

In less common cases of painless infarction of the spinal cord caused by systemic hypotension, low thoracic and lumbosacral spinal cord central gray matter involvement is observed.[18] Vasculitis and systemic embolism are rare causes of spinal cord ischemia. Polyarteritis nodosa and primary granulomatous angiitis, a neural vasculature disorder without systemic involvement often found with lymphoma, are rare causes of a sometimes painful acute or chronic myelopathy.[197]

The most important vascular input to the cervical spinal cord arises from the vertebral arteries that provide the cephalic origin of the anterior median and posterior lateral spinal arteries. The thoracic and lumbar spinal cord is supplied by segmental branches of the aorta and the branches of the internal iliac arteries. The segmental branches of the lateral sacral arteries nourish the sacral spinal cord. The segmental branches divide into anterior and posterior rami. The spinal artery, a branch of the posterior ramus, enters the vertebral foramen and divides into anterior and posterior medullary arteries that feed the anterior median spinal arteries and the posterior spinal arteries, respectively.

The chief blood supply to the spinal cord comes from the six to eight ventral and 10 or more dorsal medullary arteries that arise from the spinal arteries. The most important ventral medullary artery is the artery of Adamkiewicz, which usually approaches the spinal cord on the left side between the T10 and L3 cord segments. The major sources of the rostral spinal circulation are branches of the vertebral and ascending cervical arteries. The border zone between these main vascular systems is relatively vulnerable to ischemia, particularly in the midthoracic (T4-6) region of the spinal cord.

Among the vascular causes of paraplegia and quadriplegia, anterior spinal artery thrombosis is the most common. Although occlusion of the anterior spinal artery is uncommon, ischemia, in its region of supply, occurs relatively often. This is usually caused by disease of the aorta or segmental branches that supply the anterior spinal artery.

The anterior spinal artery syndrome, also known as anterior cord syndrome, consists of motor paralysis (upper and lower motor neuron), dissociated sensory loss (pain and temperature), and sphincter paralysis. It results from an infarction in the region of the anterior spinal artery that supplies the vertical two thirds of the spinal cord, and is usually the consequence of thrombotic atherosclerotic disease, aortic dissection, embolization, or vasculitis (particularly polyarteritis nodosa). The posterior columns are usually spared, which aids in the diagnosis. This syndrome may result as a complication of aortic angiography, cross-clamping of the aorta for more than 30 minutes, or spinal trauma with resulting direct compression of the ventral spinal cord and adjacent vessels.[6,173]

Spinal hemorrhages are usually apoplectic in nature, with rapidly developing paralysis and sensory loss. They may occur within the epidural or subdural spaces or within the spinal cord. Trauma, anticoagulant therapy, and vascular malformation are the primary causes.

Vascular Malformations

Spinal vascular malformations are an uncommon cause of neurologic deficit, representing only 10% of spinal epidural hemorrhage.[170] Spinal dural and extradural malformations usually present with chronic progressive myelopathy or radiculopathy and occasionally present acutely because of hemorrhage. Spinal vascular malformations are usually divided into three groups: dural arteriovenous fistulas, intradural vascular malformations, and cavernous angiomas (Box 3.1). A vascular malformation infrequently (in less than 3% of cases) may produce an audible bruit over the spinal cord. Dural arteriovenous fistulas occur most often in patients over age 40 who have a gradual onset and a progressive worsening of symptoms, and are exacerbated by changes in posture or activity. These lesions almost always affect the lower half of the spinal cord and produce symptoms only in the legs, bladder, and bowel.

In contrast, patients with intradural (AVMs) become symptomatic before the age of 40 and often present with an acute onset of symptoms caused by hemorrhage.[142] MRI has replaced myelography as the initial diagnostic study to evaluate these patients; intradural spinal AVMs present as serpentine areas of low-signal intensity in the subarachnoid space as a result of signal voids produced by blood flowing in the dilated tortuous vessels. T_1-weighted MRI images of intramedullary AVMs usually reveal a low-intensity signal that may be associated with focal widening of the cord.

Less specific findings of increased or decreased signal, associated with spinal cord expansion or evidence of venous congestion of the spinal cord, may be observed with a dural arteriovenous fistula.[53] Intradural AVMs enhance with gadolinium-DTPA, especially if imaging is delayed 40 to 50 minutes after contrast administration. In dural arteriovenous fistulas MRI findings may be normal or may reveal a nonspecific abnormal signal from the lower segments of the spinal cord.

In contrast to MRI, myelography findings are universally abnormal in these fistulas and demonstrate the presence of the lesion, with the exception of cavernous angiomas. In the search for a spinal AVM with a negative MRI and myelogram, arteriography would rarely be indicated. Spinal arteriography, however, should be performed in all patients with spinal AVMs that have been diagnosed by means of other studies.[142]

Similar histologically to their intracranial counterpart, cavernous angiomas are intramedullary lesions characterized clinically by sensorimotor disturbances over an acute or subacute period. These rare lesions of the spinal cord are characterized by acute neurologic dysfunction with intervening episodes of varying recovery.[141] They are found most often in thoracic and cervical locations. Cavernous angiomas may not be apparent on findings from myelography, CT imaging, or spinal arteriography. MRI remains the investigative procedure of choice,[142] usually revealing residual blood of subacute and chronic hemorrhage, characterized by mixed high- and low-signal components. It typically appears as a small high-signal focus on both T_1- and T_2-weighted or gradient-refocused images.[144]

Foix-Alajouanine syndrome is a rare form of necrotic myelopathy that results in slowly evolving myotrophic paraplegia in adult males. It has been attributed to spinal venous thrombosis, although its exact nature remains controversial.[173]

Trauma to the cervical column can also be a cause of vascular lesions of the spinal cord. These lesions include compression of adjacent vessels (ASA), dislocations with dissection or occlusion of the vertebral arteries, or spontaneous epidural hematomas caused by tearing of bridging veins.[146] The time course until the lesion appears ranges from acute to subacute, depending on the type of traumatic vascular injury.

Intracranial Lesions

Supratentorial vascular events are rarely confused with spinal disorders. An ischemic event such as the syndrome of infarction in the territory of the hemispheric branches of the anterior cerebral artery often results in contralateral weakness that involves primarily the lower extremity and, to a lesser extent, the arm (especially the shoulder). This is an example of intracranial pathology mimicking a spinal lesion. Paratonia is often present with bilateral damage to the mesial frontal region. From 24 to 48 hours after an ischemic event, CT is usually diagnostic for intracranial pathology. With intravascular arterial contrast enhancement, the more sensitive MRI scan shows immediate absence of normal "flow void."[134] Basilar artery occlusion can also mimic spinal pathology in the form of hemiplegia/quadriplegia; however, this occlusion will be accompanied by brain stem findings.

Neoplasm

Primary spinal tumors usually produce subacute or chronic evolution of symptoms over several months or even years. As mentioned earlier in this chapter, intramedullary spinal cord tumors usually present pain-

---

BOX 3.1

Classification of spinal vascular malformations

Type I
  Dural arteriovenous fistula
  Dorsal aspect of the lower thoracic cord and conus
  >50 years of age at presentation
  Draining vein can extend over multiple segments
  ~60% spontaneous

Type II
  Glomus malformation
  Dorsal aspect cervical cord
  <30-40 years of age at presentation
  Intramedullary location with multiple arterial feeders

Type III
  Juvenile type
  Extramedullary/extraspinal extension
  Multiple arterial feeders from several vertebral levels

Type IV
  Intradural/extramedullary
  Usually supplied by anterior spinal artery
  Conus medullaris location

lessly with deficit in the form of long tract signs, whereas patients with extramedullary lesions often present with pain and radicular symptoms. For all spinal cord tumors, however, pain is the most common presenting symptom.[53]

The most common extramedullary lesions are schwannomas, meningiomas, and neurofibromas; only 1% of spinal cord tumors involve multiple levels and, when present, suggest neurofibromatosis.[81] Neuroenteric cysts, especially in spina bifida, are a rare cause of acute progressive paraplegia or quadriplegia and should be considered with any intradural-extramedullary mass of the spinal cord.[25] Intramedullary spinal cord tumors (most commonly ependymomas and astrocytomas) usually present with myelopathy alone. It may assume the form of central cord syndrome. An MRI study will differentiate this condition from syringomyelia.

The location of the neoplasm in the spinal cord also affects the presenting symptomatology. Cervical lesions can cause weakness, fasciculations, and atrophy of the hand intrinsic muscles. Thoracic lesions tend to present with pain alone, whereas lumbar and conus lesions, in addition to the aforementioned cervical symptoms, present with bowel/bladder dysfunction. Metastatic lesions usually present with signs and symptoms of spinal cord compression in the form of long tract signs.[58]

Cerebral lesions (e.g., parasagittal meningiomas and brain stem gliomas) may mimic spinal pathology. However, metastatic lesions and gliomas occur most often in the differential diagnosis. The diagnosis of meningioma is made with CT and/or MRI of the head. On CT findings, meningiomas are hyperdense in 70% to 75% of cases, whereas 90% of meningiomas enhance strongly and uniformly. An MRI with enhancement demonstrates a typically isointense lesion, with respect to gray matter, in more than 95% of cases.[145]

Brain stem gliomas are the third most common childhood tumor of the posterior fossa, occurring most frequently between ages 5 and 10. The clinical evolution is relatively rapid. A neurologic examination may demonstrate cranial nerve abnormalities, evidence of increased intracranial pressure, and varying degrees of spastic hemiparesis or quadriparesis. A head CT scan reveals hypodensity throughout the pons, often extending rostrally into the midbrain with variable tumor enhancement. MRI is the diagnostic study of choice. What may appear "focal" on a CT scan is often revealed to be a diffuse neoplasm on an MRI scan.

Demyelinating Lesions

Although demyelination may not be the exact pathologic process encountered in the following diseases, this discussion includes disorders, whether inflammatory or destructive, that involve myelin. These disorders are central pontine myelinolysis (CPM), multiple sclerosis (MS), and transverse myelitis (TM).

Central Pontine Myelinolysis. This toxic, demyelinating disease without inflammation occurs in alcoholic, malnourished, or chronically debilitated adults. Over 75% of cases are associated with chronic alcoholism or rapid correction of hyponatremia.

The central pons is the most common site of pathologic changes that are characterized by myelin loss with relative neuronal sparing. In the pons, transverse pontine fibers are most severely affected, whereas the descending corticospinal tracts are often spared. Common clinical manifestations are spastic quadriparesis and pseudobulbar palsy.[101]

The diagnosis is based on the history of acutely corrected hyponatremia, confirmed with MRI findings that show hypointense areas on T_1-weighted images and hyperintense areas on T_2-weighted images, reflecting increased water content in the affected regions. These findings are not specific and have to be differentiated from infarct, metastasis, glioma, multiple sclerosis, encephalitis, and postradiation or chemotherapy changes.

Multiple Sclerosis. Multiple sclerosis (MS) is probably the best known of the demyelinating diseases. There are several clinicopathologic forms. The clinically definite diagnosis of MS requires the presence of six items: (1) objective central nervous system dysfunction, (2) two or more sites of central nervous system involvement, (3) predominant white-matter involvement, (4) relapsing-remitting or chronic (more than 6 months) progressive course, (5) age of onset between 10 and 50 years, and (6) no better explanation of symptoms. Poser and Scheinberg[155] modified these criteria by enhancing the clinical diagnosis with laboratory studies that include analysis of the spinal fluid, evoked potentials (EPs), and imaging studies.

The clinical picture of transverse myelitis related to MS accounts for only 0.6% of initial symptoms in these patients. In the majority of these cases symptoms other than impairment of spinal cord function precede the myelopathy. The most common initial symptoms are limb weakness, paresthesia, optic neuritis, diplopia, vertigo, and urinary difficulty.[66] These are followed by upper and lower motor neuron weakness, spasticity, increased or depressed muscle stretch reflexes, pain, L'hermitte's sign, intranuclear ophthalmoplegia and nystagmus, ataxia, impotence, hearing loss, affective disorder, and dementia. Bladder spasticity as an initial presenting symptom is also common. The symptoms and signs may be worsened by exercise or increased temperature (Uhthoff's phenomenon). Among neuroimaging studies, MRI is the modality of choice to confirm the diagnosis. In general, the MRI scan is positive in 85% to 95% of clinically definite MS patients.[147] In cases of progressive myelopathy, MS should be differentiated from compressive lesions, leukodystrophies (specifically adrenomyeloneuropathy), and familial spinal cerebellar degeneration.

While investigating the possibility of an MS plaque in the spinal cord, the practitioner should also obtain an MRI scan of the brain to rule out much more common and usually recognizable changes in the brain. The clinical diagnosis is supported by laboratory studies, including CSF examination, which may reveal a lymphocytic pleocytosis (usually less than 25 cells/mm^3), and normal or increased protein. Oligoclonal bands, lymphocytic reactivity to myelin basic protein, and an elevated IgG/A1b ratio are other laboratory findings that can support a diagnosis of MS.

EPs allow detection of central nervous system abnormality of function that may not be clinically detectable.

The multifocal nature of the disease may be supported by the discovery of a subclinical lesion in a site remote from the area of clinical dysfunction. The three most frequently used EPs are somatosensory evoked potentials (SSEPs), visual evoked responses (VERs), and brain stem auditory evoked responses (BAERs). In addition to their value to establish a diagnosis, EPs are useful in follow-up as they may be more sensitive indicators of change than the clinical examination or disability scales.[139] A variant of MS, neuromyelitis optica or Devic's disease, is a rare form of a rapidly progressive demyelination that is restricted to the optic nerves and the spinal cord.

Transverse Myelitis. Transverse myelitis (TM) is a nonhomogeneous group of idiopathic inflammatory processes defined as isolated spinal cord dysfunction over hours or days in patients who demonstrate no evidence of a compressive lesion[14,131] (Figure 3.5). TM can occur in acute, subacute, or chronic forms. Only the acute forms are discussed here. TM caused by other etiologies usually follows a longer time course, and is discussed in later text.

Acute transverse myelitis (ATM) can be subdivided into the autoimmune (ATMA) and necrotizing (ATMN) types. They are differentiated by acute versus subacute time course and associated illness.

ATMA usually occurs after a viral illness or in association with other autoimmune disorders, such as MS or lupus erythematosus. In several reviews of this process, 37% of patients reported a preceding febrile illness. The initial symptoms were paresthesias, back pain, or leg weakness. The maximal neurologic deficit developed within 1 day in 37% of the patients, 1 to 10 days in 45%, and more than 10 days in 18%. Outcome was rated as good in 42%, fair in 38%, and poor in 20%. In general, the results were worse in the group with a rapid onset of symptoms. About 7% of patients were eventually diagnosed with MS by clinical criteria.[66] According to Miller, cases of partial myelitis have a much higher frequency (50%) of subsequently developing MS.[130] Acute transverse myelitis has been associated with systemic vasculitis such as systemic lupus erythematosus, as well as with heroin abuse. Symptoms occur over days to weeks, most commonly in the thoracic spinal cord. Symptoms include ascending paresthesias, weakness, and urinary retention. The incidence is rare, occurring in only 0.13 per 100,000.[58]

ATMN (Foix-Alajouanine syndrome) is an acutely progressive necrotizing myelitis that occurs over hours to days. Clinical manifestations in the typical patient of adult years consist of severe paralysis, preceded by tingling or loss of sphincter control.[45] During the acute phase, MRI is normal in approximately half of the cases and is nonspecific in the remainder. Focal spinal cord enlargement on T_1-weighted and poorly delineated hyperintensities on T_2-weighted scans are the most commonly identified abnormalities. Occasionally, contrast enhancement is observed.[92] Diagnosis is based on clinical picture and absence of other potential causes of acute myelopathy on MRI, such as acute disc herniation hematoma, epidural abscess, or compression myelopathy. Electromyography (EMG) demonstrates motor unit denervation and, in about ohalf of the cases there is an increase in CSF pressure and leukocyte count.[184]

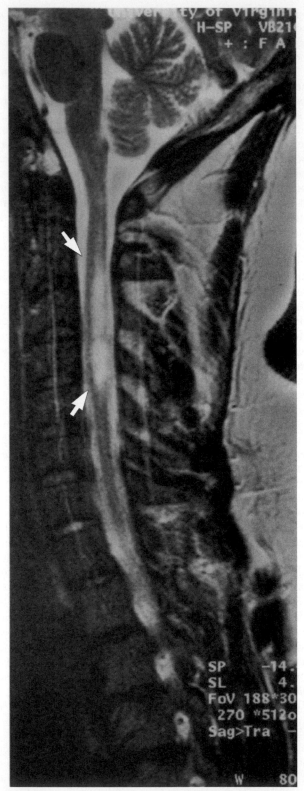

Figure 3.5 T_2-weighted MRI scan of transverse myelitis of the cervical spinal cord *(arrows)*. Patient presented with paresthesias in the right arm.

Inflammatory and Infectious Lesions

There is obvious overlap with several inflammatory and infectious disorders that affect the spinal cord. Infections that involve the spinal cord are predominantly viruses and are covered in this section. A clinical presentation for an individual with viral myelitis typically involves myelopathic symptoms. Inflammatory lesions include limbic encephalitis, brain stem encephalitis, poliomyelitis-like syndrome, and posterior root ganglionitis.

Inflammatory changes in the spinal cord involve either the anterior horn cell or the dorsal root ganglion. Prominent degeneration of the posterior columns may be observed.

Inflammatory myelopathies usually evolve over a few days. They may be caused by direct invasion of such neurotropic viruses as herpes zoster, poliomyelitis, cytomegalovirus, or herpes simplex. Approximately 20% of patients infected with HIV develop a vacuolar myelopathy. The evolution of symptoms in viral transverse myelitis takes from 1 to 10 days, during which the paraplegia or quadriplegia may be accompanied by an ascending sensory level. Inflammatory processes that occur in the epidural space may have a similar time course, but are usually accompanied by local back pain or radicular pain, local tenderness, and fever. Metastatic deposits, although progressing without fever, will also often produce pain. Subacute onset of generalized weakness may occur with inflammatory neuropathies.

Encephalomyelitis. A rare form of encephalomyelitis may present as a subacute poliomyelitis-like syndrome. It is often confused with amyotrophic lateral sclerosis (ALS) and progressive spinal muscular atrophy. This form of myelitis is associated with fasciculations, diminished or absent deep tendon reflexes, and profound weakness. The milder form of motor neuron involvement is observed in patients with lymphomas who have undergone spinal cord irradiation before the onset of weakness.

Different forms of encephalomyelitis may be accompanied by dorsal root ganglionitis (ganglioradiculitis) that rarely occurs in isolation.[89] This condition is manifested by disturbances of gait, paresthesias, numbness, and tingling in the limbs. Patients have loss of sensation and diminished reflexes, concomitant with an increase in gamma globulin levels.

Therapy is generally ineffective and prognosis is poor, with a mean survival from the time of diagnosis of less than a year. Pathology reveals neuronal loss, perivascular cuffing, microglial infiltrations, and gliosis. Extensive demyelination may also be observed. Other general symptoms and signs (e.g., fever, severe local back pain, and/or radicular pain associated with progressive paraplegia) suggest an infectious process in the epidural space. The vesicles or scars of a recent herpes zoster infection may provide a clue to the postzoster myelitis.

Degenerative Disorders

Degenerative disorders encompass a broad spectrum of diseases that affect the spinal cord and column. Diseases of the spinal column often present with a combination of pain and neurologic deficits; these were discussed in the section dealing with pain as a primary presenting symptom. Degenerative diseases of the neural tissue are generally referred to as motor neuron diseases and include upper motor neuron syndromes, lower motor neuron syndromes, and disorders that combine upper and lower motor neuron syndromes.

Upper Motor Neuron Syndromes. These rare diseases, which are both inherited and acquired, exhibit degeneration of the descending corticospinal or corticobulbar tracts, with variable involvement of the large pyramidal neurons in the motor cortex. The archetypical disorders in this group are hereditary spastic paraplegia (Strümpell's syndrome) and lathyrism, respectively. Hereditary spastic paraplegia (HSP) is a clinically and genetically heterogeneous disorder that presents with progressive spasticity and mild weakness in the lower extremities. It is inherited more commonly through the autosomal dominant trait. However, in some families autosomal recessive and rare forms of X-linked inheritance have been reported. Almost 75% of those affected demonstrate difficulty in walking at presentation. Lower extremity spasticity, hyperreflexia, and extensor plantar responses are usually encountered in established cases.

Diagnosis is based on the family history and physical findings and is supported by selected laboratory studies. Peripheral sensory and motor conduction studies, as well as myelography, are usually normal. The peroneal H-reflex, which is normally absent without reinforcement, is obtained in clinically definite cases and in most of those who may be affected. CSF is usually normal. However, elevated levels of protein (up to 100mg/dl) have been reported. Low amplitude or absent SSEPs from the upper and lower extremity nerves, and slowed spinal cord conduction are usually found. Differential diagnosis includes consideration of combined degeneration (caused by vitamin B_{12} deficiency), MS, and cervical spondylotic myelopathy, as well as intraspinal and slow-growing intracranial tumors, such as meningiomas, schwannomas, or neurofibromas.

Adrenoleukodystrophy should also be considered in cases of progressive paraplegia. This X-linked recessive disorder of males, manifested most commonly in children, may also be present in adults as adrenomyeloneuropathy (AMN), which is a related form. This condition is usually detected in patients older than age 20 who usually present with a progressive paraparesis. Unlike HSP, the onset of symptoms is usually abrupt. The motor findings are commonly accompanied by permanent sensory loss in the legs and sphincter dysfunction.

Lower Motor Neuron Syndromes. This group of diseases is dominated by inherited disorders. Spinal muscular atrophy (SMA) is the second most common childhood neuromuscular disease after Duchenne's muscular dystrophy, with an estimated 1 in 40 Caucasians harboring a gene for this condition. Degeneration of the anterior horn cells in this group of disorders leads to progressive weakness, characteristic muscle atrophy, and hyporeflexia. Fasciculations are occasionally observed, but sensory, corticospinal tract, and sphincter involvement are absent. In severe childhood cases contractures and skeletal abnormalities develop. Nerve conduction studies and EMG are diagnostic and allow differentiation from clinically similar disorders. Nerve conduction studies are usually normal in sensory and motor nerves. EMG reveals evidence of denervation in the form of fibrillations, fasciculation, and positive sharp waves. These findings are more prevalent in chronic cases. Neurogenic voluntary motor unit potentials, and in advanced atrophy, myopathic potentials, may be observed. Muscle histology shows group atrophy of type I and type II fibers, pyknotic nuclear clumps, and variable fiber hypotrophy.

Proximal spinal muscular atrophies account for nearly 80% of all SMA cases. Type I, acute infantile SMA (Werdnig-Hoffmann disease) is a progressive disease of infancy that accounts for about 25% of all SMA cases. Usually transmitted by an autosomal recessive gene, this condition presents in a third of the cases that demonstrate decreased fetal movements in the last trimester of pregnancy. The majority of affected infants are floppy at birth. The disease is almost uniformly fatal, usually in the sixth or seventh month of life. About 95% of affected children die by the age of 18 months.[179]

Type II (late infantile and juvenile-onset SMA) constitutes the largest group of these muscular atrophies, which accounts for 45% of all SMA cases. This group of childhood diseases includes cases of arrested Werdnig-Hoffmann disease, SMA type II and III of Emery, and Kugelberg-Welander disease. The disorder is probably inherited through a single autosomal recessive gene in about 90% of cases. The rest are caused by new dominant mutations.

In the majority of cases clinical onset occurs by 5 years of age and is often preceded by infection or immunization. Pelvic and pectoral girdle muscles are weak and atrophied almost universally; tongue and limb muscle fasciculations are common. There may be associated cranial nerve involvement, muscle pseudohypertrophy, mental retardation, hand tremor, and occasionally an eversion deformity of the feet. EMG is the study of choice to differentiate this disease from muscular dystrophies. The median survival is more than 12 years.

Type III (adult-onset SMA) accounts for 8% of all SMA cases. This genetically heterogeneous disorder of adult life is often confused with progressive muscular atrophy (PMA), a variant of adult ALS. The clinical symptoms usually develop usually between the ages of 20 and 50 with proximal symmetric muscle weakness, especially in the lower extremities. As in children with the disease, limb girdle weakness and muscle atrophy are typical. The involvement of the face and tongue is more common than in children and occurs in up to half of the cases, especially in those with a dominant genetic pattern for this disease. Unlike children with the disease, type III SMAs are usually benign, although the dominant form is more severe clinically. Progression is very slow, especially in recessive cases, with periods of stabilization and not much reduction of life span.

Distal spinal muscular atrophy (progressive) (Charcot-Marie-Tooth disease) is a genetically heterogeneous disorder, accounting for about 10% of all cases of SMA, and is mentioned here because it also accounts for 3% to 6% of all cases of the peroneal muscular atrophy syndrome. The scapular-peroneal form is an even less common disorder that belongs to this group, accounting for about 7% of all SMA cases.

Included among the acquired disorders in this group is a postpolio syndrome (postpolio muscular atrophy, late effects of poliomyelitis, and late progression of old polio). The postpolio syndrome (PPS) is defined as a new onset of muscle weakness, pain, and fatigue many years after recovery from acute paralytic poliomyelitis. The new symptoms usually occur 30 to 40 years after acute polio. The age at presentation is between 40 and 50 years. The female to male ratio is 1.5:1. Patients present with fatigue, joint pain, muscle pain, progressive weakness, and atrophy, particularly in previously affected muscles.

The following criteria for the diagnosis of postpolio muscular atrophy have been proposed: (1) documented past history of acute paralytic polio myelitis, (2) incomplete to fairly complete neurologic and functional recovery, (3) a period of neurologic and functional stability of at least 15 years, (4) documented new-onset muscle weakness and/or atrophy in an asymmetric distribution in previously involved and/or uninvolved muscles, usually with unaccustomed fatigue, (5) electrophysiologic evidence of acute denervation superimposed on chronic denervation-reinnervation, and (6) no other cause demonstrated. The disease is probably caused by premature aging that affects chronically overworked, surviving motor neurons. No evidence for reactivation of the old poliomyelitis has been found.[179]

Combined Upper and Lower Motor Neuron Syndromes. ALS (Charcot's disease, motor neuron disease) is found in adults and results from degeneration of the upper motor neuron and lower motor neuron.[185] The prevalence of ALS is four to six individuals per 100,000 and it is familial in 8% to 10% of cases. Familial cases usually follow autosomal dominant inheritance, but occasionally demonstrate a recessive pattern.[79] Mutations in the Cu-Zn superoxide dismutase gene are associated with familial ALS.[159]

The clinical picture of Charcot's disease usually consists of weakness and atrophy of the hands (lower motor neuron), with spasticity and hyperreflexia of the lower extremities (upper motor neuron). Voluntary eye muscles and urinary sphincter muscles are usually spared. If the involvement of lower motor neuron to lower extremities predominates, the hyperreflexia may be replaced by hyporeflexia. As the disease progresses, dysarthria and dysphagia ensue as a combination of upper and lower neuron pathology; tongue atrophy and fasciculations may be seen. Emotional lability is encountered, but only 1% to 2% of cases are associated with dementia. Approximately 20% of patients with corticospinal tract involvement show a Babinski sign. In the familial form, lower motor neuron involvement at presentation is more common (58%), particularly in the legs. Dementia is more often present (15%).

Clinical diagnosis is confirmed by electrophysiologic studies. EMG evidence of denervation is observed with reinnervation in the muscles from two or more extremities outside the distribution of a single peripheral nerve or nerve root in each extremity. The fasciculations fire at a lower frequency (0.3Hz) than those in the benign fasciculation syndrome (1.25Hz). Fibrillations and positive sharp waves are observed in advanced cases.[179]

ALS should be differentiated from cervical myelopathy related to cervical spondylosis. The following clinical features may be helpful. Atrophic weakness of the hands in ALS occurs early in the disease and does not follow a radicular pattern. Spasticity in the lower extremities is usually mild. Sensory changes are conspicuously absent. Typically, there is no involvement of the sphincters.

Progression of the disease may produce dysarthria or a hyperactive jaw jerk. With involvement of the lower motor neuron, this may produce tongue atrophy and fasciculation. Absence of sensory findings implies that the pain is usually present with cervical spondylomyelopathy. Neck pain is often accompanied by neck stiffness, limitation of movement, shoulder pain, sensory changes, more pronounced spasticity in the lower extremities, and better defined radicular symptoms in upper extremities.[80]

Miscellaneous

An acute or subacute course of paralysis may be observed in syndromes of tropical spastic paraparesis and tropical ataxic neuropathies; these conditions occur endemically in tropical regions. Attributed causes include nutritional deficiencies, toxins occurring in staple diets, malabsorption caused by tropical sprue, treponemal infections, and human T-lymphotropic virus type I (HTLV-1). These syndromes differ from lathyrism (a spastic paraparesis observed in southern India and other tropical countries that is caused by a toxin derived from *Lathyrus sativus*, a legume), as well as from myelopathies associated with *Schistosoma* infection that most commonly affect the conus medullaris.[182]

Subacute combined degeneration of the spinal cord (SCDSC), caused by a deficiency of B_{12}, is uncommon today because of the relative ease of diagnosis and treatment. However, when B_{12} levels are reduced for a prolonged period, neurologic sequelae ensue shortly after the anemia. Clinically, this condition presents with both sensory and motor symptoms consistent with thoracic dorsal column involvement, including paresthesias in the feet and loss of vibratory and positional sense. Diagnosis is made with laboratory studies that demonstrate a decreased B_{12} level and a neurologic examination consistent with a posterolateral syndrome. Treatment is with intramuscular B_{12} injections.[121] Incomplete paraplegia or quadriplegia may accompany myasthenia gravis, an autoimmune disease caused by a defect in neuromuscular transmission with an incidence of 3 per 100,000. Ocular, motor, and bulbar involvement, as well as preserved sensation, often point to the correct diagnosis. A rather stable, nonprogressive myelopathy is observed in degenerative spinal cord diseases, such as hereditary spastic paraplegia or spastic diplegia of cerebral palsy.

Guillain-Barré syndrome, diphtheria, acute intermittent porphyria, toxic peripheral neuropathies (thallium poisoning), or poorly understood immune response to malignant neoplasms (so-called paraneoplastic syndromes), may present in the form of a subacute myelopathy and evolve over weeks. The symptoms include an ascending or descending pattern and may produce a combination of upper and lower motor neuron signs. The prognosis for paraneoplastic syndromes is invariably poor.

Guillain-Barré syndrome, the most common acquired demyelinating neuropathy, is characterized by an acute onset of peripheral nerve dysfunction, usually after a viral illness. It presents clinically with symmetric limb weakness and/or paresthesias.[152] This disease is distinguished from the aforementioned causes of peripheral neuropathies by a history of toxin exposure or ingestion and its tendency to affect proximal muscles initially.

Another uncommon cause of slow progressive subacute or chronic myelopathy is postirradiation in nature. The myelopathy characteristically is a complication of radiotherapy when the spinal cord is included in the field of treatment. Radiation-induced myelopathy develops 6 months to several years after treatment with more than 3500rads. The symptoms evolve over several months to years, usually beginning with posterior column dysfunction, followed by corticospinal and spinothalamic tract signs.

Subacute progression of painless myelopathy, with sensory rather than motor symptoms, occurs commonly in so-called decompression sickness or Kesson's disease. The symptoms usually occur less than 6 hours after the patient's last dive.

Diseases that affect primary muscles are rarely acute in their onset. However, in so-called periodic paralysis attacks of generalized muscle weakness may evolve over minutes to hours. The patient with familial periodic paralysis usually has a medical history of similar attacks or a positive family history. This condition, which is associated with disturbances of serum potassium, is a disease of the young with initial attacks occurring around puberty.[158] It is extremely rare, with only a few cases reported each year. Clinically, patients present with weakness or paralysis of either the legs or all muscle groups usually after a period of rest.

Paraneoplastic syndromes are also common causes of neurologic deficit. Between 7% and 15% of patients with systemic cancer display remote effects of the malignancy known as paraneoplastic syndrome. In more than 50% of these patients the paraneoplastic symptoms precede diagnosis of the primary cancer. Underlying pathology includes inflammatory, vascular, and autoimmunologic changes. Vascular states are characterized by hypercoagulability, venous thrombosis, nonbacterial or marantic endocarditis, and intravascular coagulopathies. Autoimmune syndromes include myasthenia gravis, the myasthenic syndrome of Eaton-Lambert, and the polymyositis-dermatomyositis complex. The cerebellar syndromes with cortical cerebellar degeneration and myoclonic encephalopathies are thought to have underlying immunologic causes.

Frontal lobe tumors, hydrocephalus, parasagittal meningiomas, or bilateral anterior cerebral artery territory ischemia may cause paraparesis. Other symptoms and signs such as disturbances of mental status and language, seizures, and aberrant sphincter control may help localize the lesion in the intracranial portion of the central nervous system. There may be an element of ataxia and loss of postural reflexes in the cerebral paraparesis. Brain stem pathology usually affects additional cranial nerves, which localizes the lesion in the region above the foramen magnum. No sensory level is observed.

REFERENCES

1. Abdelwahab IF, Casden AM, Klein MJ, Spollman A: Chondrosarcoma of a thoracic vertebra. *Bull Hosp Jt Dis Orthop Inst* 51:34-39, 1991.
2. Abdelwahab IF, Kenan S, Hermann G, *et al:* Case report 845. Fluid-filling giant cell tumor with an aneurysmal bone

cyst component. *Skeletal Radiol* 23:317-319, 1994.

3. Acciarri N, Paganini M, Fonda C, *et al:* Langerhans cell histiocytosis of the spine causing cord compression: a case report. *Neurosurgery* 31:965-968, 1992.

4. Aliabadi P, Nikpoor N: Imaging osteomyelitis. *Arthritis Rheum* 37:617-622, 1994.

5. Alpaslan AM, Acaroglu RE, Kis M: Three-stage excision of recurrent cervical chondrosarcoma: a case report. *Arch Orthop Trauma Surg* 112:245-246, 1993.

6. Anderson NE, Willoughby EW: Infarction of the conus medullaris. *Ann Neurol* 21:470-474, 1987.

7. Ansari A, Yock DH, Seymour JL, Gilbert T: Acute pyogenic spondylodiscitis with epidural phlegmon. Diagnosis and management by MRI and multidisciplinary approach. *Minn Med* 76:21-24, 1993.

8. Anthony JP, Mathes SJ: Update on chronic osteomyelitis, review. *Clin Plast Surg* 18:515-523, 1991.

9. Anzil AP: Spinal cord pathology. *Neurosurg Clin North Am* 5:147-173, 1994.

10. Avrahami E, Frishman E, Fridman Z, Azor M: Spina bifida occulta of S1 is not an innocent finding. *Spine* 19:12-15, 1994.

11. Bamberger DM: Osteomyelitis: a commonsense approach to antibiotic and surgical treatment, review. *Postgrad Med* 94:177-182, 1993.

12. Bednar DA, Brox WT, Viviani GR: Surgical palliation of oncologic disease: a review and analysis of current approaches. *Can J Surg* 34:129-131, 1991.

13. Bennett GJ: Ankylosing spondylitis, review. *Clin Neurosurg* 37:622-635, 1991.

14. Berger JR LRM, Snodgrass S: Medical myelopathies. *Spine* 2:1553-1574, 1992.

15. Bernhardt M, Hynes RA, Blume HW, White AA 3rd: Cervical spondylitic myelopathy. *J Bone Joint Surg Am* 75A:119-128, 1993.

16. Bernstein J LJ: Metabolic bone disorders of the spine. In Rothman RH, Simeone FA (ed): *The Spine.* Philadelphia, WB Saunders, 1992, pp 1381-1428.

17. Bloch AB, Rieder HL, Kelly GD, *et al:* The epidemiology of tuberculosis in the United States. *Clin Chest Med* 10:297-313, 1989.

18. Blumbergs PC, Byrne E: Hypotensive central infarction of the spinal cord. *J Neurol Neurosurg Psychiatr* 43:751-753, 1980.

19. Boden SD, Laws ER: Infections of the spine. In Boden SD, Laws ER (eds): *The Aging Spine: Essentials of Pathophysiology, Diagnosis, and Treatment.* Philadelphia, WB Saunders, 1991, pp 205-219.

20. Boden SD, Laws ER: Tumors of the spine. In Boden SD, Laws ER (eds): *The Aging Spine: Essentials of Pathophysiology, Diagnosis, and Treatment.* Philadelphia, WB Saunders, 1991, pp 221-252.

21. Boden SD, Laws ER: Metabolic bone disease and the spine. In Boden SD, Laws ER (eds): *The Aging Spine: Essentials of Pathophysiology, Diagnosis, and Treatment.* Philadelphia, WB Saunders, 1991, pp 253-259.

22. Boogerd W, van der Sande JJ: Diagnosis and treatment of spinal cord compression in malignant disease. *Cancer Treat Rev* 19:129-150, 1993.

23. Borenstein DG, *et al:* Mechanical disorders of the lumbosacral spine. In Borenstein DG, Wiesel SW (eds): *Low Back Pain: Medical Diagnosis and Comprehensive Management.* Philadelphia, WB Saunders, 1989, pp 147-169.

24. Borenstein DG, *et al* : Rheumatologic disorders of the lumbosacral spine. In Borenstein DG, Wiesel SW (eds): *Low Back Pain: Medical Diagnosis and Comprehensive Management.* Philadelphia, WB Saunders, 1989, pp 175-235.

25. Brooks BS, Duvall ER, el Gammal T, *et al:* Neuroimaging features of neuroenteric cysts: analysis of nine cases and review of the literature. *AJNR Am J Neuroradiol* 14:735-746, 1993.

26. Burger EL, Lindeque BG: Sacral and non-spinal tumors presenting as backache. *Acta Orthop Scand* 65:344-346, 1994.

27. Burkus KJ, Lonstein JE, Winter RB, Denis F: Long-term evaluation of adolescents treated operatively for spondylolisthesis. *J Bone Joint Surg Am* 74A:693-704, 1992.

28. Cardenosa G, DeLuca SA: Ankylosing spondylitis. *Am Fam Physician* 42:147-150, 1990.

29. Caputy AJ, Luessenhop AJ: Long-term evaluation of decompressive surgery for degenerative lumbar stenosis, review. *J Neurosurg* 77:669-676, 1992.

30. Carbone LD, Cooper C, Michet CJ, *et al:* Ankylosing spondylitis in Rochester, Minnesota, 1935-1989. Is the epidemiology changing? *Arthritis Rheum* 35:1476-1482, 1992.

31. Castillo M, Hankins L, Kramer L, Wilson BA: MR imaging of diplomyelia. *Magn Reson Imag* 10:699-703, 1992.

32. Chakravarty LD, Brett F, Merry P: Aneurysmal bone cyst: an unusual presentation of neck pain in a young adult. *Br J Rheumatol* 33:597-598, 1994.

33. Chapman JR, Anderson PA: Thoracolumbar spine fractures with neurologic deficit. *Orthop Clin North Am* 25:595-609, 1994.

34. Clark CR: Rheumatoid arthritis: surgical considerations. In Rothman RH, Simeone FA (eds): *The Spine.* Philadelphia, WB Saunders, 1992, pp 1429-1445.

35. Cole WG: The management of chronic osteomyelitis, review. *Clin Orthop Relat Res* 264:84-89, 1991.

36. Collee GD, Vandenbroucke JP: Greater trochanteric pain syndrome (trochanteric bursitis) in low back pain. *Scand J Rheumatol* 20:262-266, 1991.

37. Connolly ES: Management of persistent or recurrent symptoms and signs in the post operative lumbar disc patient, review. *Neurosurg Clin North Am* 4:161-166, 1993.

38. Conrad EU 3rd, Olszewski AD, Berger M, *et al:* Pediatric spine tumors with spinal cord compromise. *J Pediatr Orthop* 12:454-460, 1992.

39. Correa AG, Edwards MS, Baker CJ: Vertebral osteomyelitis in children, review. *Pediatr Infect Dis J* 12:228-233, 1993.

40. Coscia MF, Hormuth DA, Huang WL: Back pain secondary to esophageal perforation in an adolescent. *Spine* 17:1256-1259, 1992.

41. Crawford AH, Kucharzyk DW, Ruda R, Smitherman HC Jr: Diskitis in children. *Clin Orthop Relat Res* 266:70-79, 1991.

42. Crim JR, Seeger LL: Imaging evaluation of osteomyelitis, review. *Crit Rev Diagn Imag* 35:201-256, 1994.

43. Currier BL EF : Infections of the spine. In Rothman RH, Simeone FA (eds): *The Spine.* Philadelphia, WB Saunders, 1992, pp 1319-1380.

44. Davidoff AM, Thompson CV, Grimm JM, *et al:* Occult spinal dysraphism in patients with anal agenesis. *J Pediatr Surg* 26:1001-1005, 1991.

45. Dawson DM, Potts F: Acute nontraumatic myelopathies. *Neurol Clin* 9:585-598, 1991.

46. DeCandido P, Resnik CS, Aisner SC: Case report 792. Eosinophilic granuloma of bone. *Skeletal Radiol* 22:371-373, 1993.

47. Dendrinos GK, Polyzoides JK: Spondylodiscitis after percutaneous discectomy. A case diagnosed by MRI. *Acta Orthop Scand* 63:219-220, 1992.

48. De Schepper AM, Ramon F, Van Marck E: MR imaging of eosinophilic granuloma: report of 11 cases. *Skeletal Radiol* 22:163-166, 1993.

49. D'Hoore K, Hoogmartens M: Vertebral aspergillosis. A case report and review of the literature, review. *Acta Orthop Belg* 59:306-314, 1993.

50. Dirschl DR: Acute pyogenic osteomyelitis in children, review. *Orthop Rev* 23:305-312, 1995.

51. Dirschl DR AL: Osteomyelitis. Common causes and treatment recommendations, review. *Drugs* 45:29-43, 1993.

52. DonTigny RL: Anterior dysfunction of the sacroiliac joint as a major factor in the etiology of idiopathic low back pain syndrome. *Phys Ther* 70:250-265, 1990.

53. Doppman JL DG, Dwyer AJ: Magnetic resonance imaging of spinal arteriovenous malformations. *J Neurosurg* 66:830-834, 1987.

54. Dougados M: Diagnosis and monitoring of spondylarthropathy. *Compr Ther* 16:52-56, 1990.

55. Dreghorn CR NR, Hardy GJ: Primary tumors of the axial skeleton: experience of the Leeds regional bone tumor registry. *Spine* 15:137-140, 1990.

56. Dubuisson A LJ, Stevenaert A: Soft cervical disc herniation: a retrospective study of 100 cases, review. *Acta Neurochir* 125:115-119, 1993.

57. du Lac P PM, Devred P: MRI of disc space infection in infants and children: report of 12 cases. *Pediatr Radiol* 20:175-178, 1995.

58. Elghazawi AK: Clinical syndromes and differential diagnosis of spinal disorders. *Radiol Clin North Am* 29:651-663, 1991.

59. Ellinas PA RF: Pott's disease in urban populations: a report of five cases and a review of the literature. *NY State J Med* 90:588-591, 1990.

60. Eschelman DJ BG, Naimark A: Pseudoarthrosis in ankylosing spondylitis mimicking infectious diskitis: MR appearance. *Am J Radiol* 12:1113-1114, 1991.

61. Fager CA: Identification and management of radiculopathy, review. *Neurosurg Clin North Am* 4:1-12, 1993.

62. Fam AG RJ: Another look at spinal tuberculosis. *J Rheumatol* 20:1731-1740, 1993.

63. Faria SL SW, Chiminazzo H: Radiotherapy in the treatment of vertebral hemangiomas. *J Radiat Oncol Biol Physi* 11:387-390, 1985.

64. Fisher WS III: Selection of patients for surgery, review. *Neurosurg Clin North Am* 4:35-44, 1993.

65. Fox MW OB, Kilgore JE: Neurological complications of ankylosing spondylitis. *J Neurosurg* 78:871-878, 1993.

66. Francis GS AJP, Duguette P: Inflammatory demyelinating diseases of the central nervous system. *Neurol Clin Pract* 2:1133-1166, 1991.

67. Freilich D, Swash M: Diagnosis and management of tuberculous paraplegia with special reference to tuberculous radiculomyelitis. *J Neurol Neurosurg Psychiatr* 42:12-18, 1979.

68. Friedman DP HJ: Cervical epidural spinal infection: MR imaging characteristics. *Am J Roentgenol* 163:699-704, 1994.

69. Frymoyer JW: Lumbar disc disease: epidemiology, review. *Instruct Course Lectures* 41:217-223, 1992.

70. Galassiere PF DA, Greenberg HM: Chronic, contained rupture of aortic aneurysms associated with vertebral erosion. *CJS* 37:23-28, 1993.

71. Garcia FF SC, Sartoris CC: Diagnostic imaging of childhood spinal infection, review. *Orthop Rev* 22:321-327, 1993.

72. Garrido E: Lumbar disc herniation in the pediatric patient, review. *Neurosurg Clin North Am* 4:149-152, 1993.

73. Gephard JS BJ: Percutaneous discectomy for the treatment of bacterial discitis. *Spine* 19:855-857, 1994.

74. Gertzbein SD: Multicenter spine fracture study. *Spine* 17:528-540, 1992.

75. Gilbert RW, Kim JH, Posner JB: Epidural spinal cord compression from metastatic tumour: diagnosis and treatment. *Ann Neurol* 3:40-51, 1978.

76. Gold R: Diagnosis of osteomyelitis, review. *Pediatr Rev* 12:292-297, 1991.

77. Gorse GF PF: Tuberculous spondylitis: a report of six cases and a review of the literature. *Medicine* 62:178-193, 1983.

78. Gran JT HG: The epidemiology of ankylosing spondylitis. *Semin Arthritis Rheum* 22:319-334, 1993.

79. Greenberg MS: Spine and spinal cord. In Greenberg MS (ed): *Handbook of Neurosurgery.* Lakeland, Fla., Greenberg Graphics, 1994, pp 463-518.

80. Greenberg MS: Differential diagnosis. In Greenberg MS (ed): *Handbook of Neurosurgery.* Lakeland, Fla., Greenberg Graphics, 1994, pp 177-209.

81. Greenburg JO: Neuroimaging of the spinal cord. *Neurol Clin* 9:679-703, 1991.

82. Gundry CR HK: Imaging evaluation of patients with spinal deformity. *Orthop Clin North Am* 25:247-263, 1994.

83. Gupta VK GS, Khosla VK: Aneurysmal bone cyst of the spine. *Surg Neurol* 42:428-432, 1994.

84. Haid RW DC: Instrumentation and fusion for discogenic disease of the lumbosacral spine. *Neurosurg Clin North Am* 4:135-148, 1993.

85. Hamada J SK, Seto H: Epidural tuberculoma of the spine: case report. *Neurosurgery* 28:161-163, 1991.

86. Harrison CS: Hematocolpos as a cause of low back pain. *Spine* 16:985-986, 1991.

87. Heary RF SS, Fobben ES: Preoperative diagnosis of an extradural cyst arising from a spinal facet joint: case report. *Neurosurgery* 38:415-418, 1992.

88. Hehne HJ ZK, Bohm H: Polysegmental lumbar osteotomies and transpedicled fixation for correction of long-curved kyphotic deformities in ankylosing spondylitis. *Clin Orthop Relat Res* 258:49-55, 1990.

89. Henson RA, Urich H: *Cancer and the Nervous System.* Oxford, England, Blackwell, 1982.

90. Herkowitz HN KL: Degenerative lumbar spondylolisthesis with spinal stenosis. *J Bone Joint Surg* 73A:802-808, 1991.

91. Hitchon PW OR, Yuh WT: Spinal infections, review. *Clin Neurosurg* 38:373-387, 1992.

92. Holtas S. BN, Frederiksson K: MRI in acute transverse myelopathy. *Neuroradiology* 35:221-226, 1993.

93. Honch GW: Spinal cord and foramen magnum tumors. *Semin Neurol* 13:337-342, 1993.

94. Hughes JT: Neuropathology of the spinal cord. *Neurol Clin* 9:551-571, 1991.

95. Jackson RP: The facet syndrome: myth or reality? *Clin Orthop Relat Res* 279:110-121, 1992.

96. Jaffrey D BV, Eisenstein S: Closing wedge osteotomy with transpedicular fixation in ankylosing spondylitis. *Clin Orthop Relat Res* 279:122-126, 1992.

97. Janssens JP DR: Spinal tuberculosis in a developed country: a review of 26 cases with special emphasis on abscesses and neurologic complications. *Clin Orthop Relat Res* 257:67-75, 1990.

98. Jeanneret B MF: Treatment of osteomyelitis of the spine using percutaneous suction/irrigation and percutaneous external spinal fixation. *J Spinal Disord* 7:185-205, 1994.

99. Johnson S KT, Weinstein A: Case report 768. *Skeletal Radiol* 22:63-65, 1993.

100. Kaplan JG, Rosenburg R, DeSouza T. *et al*: Atlantoaxial subluxation in psoriatic arthropathy. *Ann Neurol* 23:522-524, 1988.

101. Karp BI, Laureno R: Pontine and extrapontine myelinolysis: a neurologic disorder following rapid correction of hyponatremia. *Medicine* 72:359-373, 1993.

102. Katz JN DM, Stucki G: Diagnosis of lumbar spinal stenosis, review. *Rheum Dis Clin North Am* 20:471-483, 1994.

103. Katz JN LM: Differential diagnosis and conservative treatment of rheumatic disorders. In Frymoyer JW, *et al* (eds): *The Adult Spine: Principles and Practice*. Philadelphia, Lippincott-Raven, 1991, pp 699-718.

104. Kelsey JL GA, Mundt DJ: Low back pain/prolapsed lumbar intervertebral disc, review. *Rheum Dis Clin North Am* 16:699-716, 1990.

105. Koller WC, Wilson RS, Gla SL, *et al*: Senile gait: correlation with computed tomographic scans. *Ann Neurol* 13:343-344, 1983.

106. Kotilainen E: Microinvasive lumbar disc surgery. A study on patients treated with microdiscectomy or percutaneous nucleotomy for disc herniation, review. *Annal Chir Gynaecol* 209(suppl):1-50, 1994.

107. Kramer J JF, Kleefield J: Rheumatoid arthritis of the cervical spine. *Rheum Dis Clin North Am* 17:757-771, 1991.

108. Kramer J RC, Kleefield J: Degenerative disorders of the cervical spine. *Rheum Dis Clin North Am* 17:741-751, 1991.

109. Kramer J SR, Wimberger D: MRI of spondylitis. *Bildgebung* 59:147-151, 1992.

110. Kretzschmar HA EH: Mesenchymal chondrosarcoma of the craniocervical junction. *Clin Neurol Neurosurg* 92-4:343-347, 1990.

111. Krodel A SH, Siebert CH: Indications for and results of operative treatment of spondylitis and spondylodiscitis. *Arch Orthop Trauma Surg* 110:78-82, 1991.

112. Lafont A OA, Gelman M: *Candida albicans* spondylodiscitis and vertebral osteomyelitis in patients with intravenous heroin drug addiction. Report of 3 cases. *J Rheumatol* 21:953-956, 1994.

113. Laurent-Haupt L WK: Long-standing ankylosing spondylitis with back pain. *Rheum Dis Clin North Am* 17:813-816, 1991.

114. Laurin JM RC, Wheeler D: Vertebral osteomyelitis caused by *Nocardia asteroides:* report and review of the literature. *J Rheumatol* 18:456-458, 1991.

115. Lifeso RM: Pyogenic spinal sepsis in adults. *Spine* 15:1265-1271, 1990.

116. Lifeso RM WP: Tuberculous spondylitis in adults. *J Bone Joint Surg* 67A:1405-1413, 1985.

117. Lin SY WH, Chien SH: Correction osteotomy of flexion deformity of cervical spine in ankylosing spondylitis: a case report. *Kaohslung J Med Sci* 6:454-460, 1990.

118. Lindsley HB: Low back pain evaluation and management. *Compr The* 18:23-26, 1992.

119. Long DM: Decision making in lumbar disc disease, review. *Clin Neurosurg* 39:36-51, 1992.

120. Mameghan H FR, O'Gorman-Hughes D: Ewing's sarcoma: long term follow-up in 49 patients treated from 1967-1989. *Int J Radiat Oncol Biol Phys* 25:431-438, 1993.

121. Mancall E: Subacute combined degeneration of the spinal cord. In Rowland L (ed): *Merritt's Textbook of Neurology*. Philadelphia, Lea & Febiger, 1989, pp 691-694.

122. Markwalder T: Surgical management of neurogenic claudication in 100 patients with lumbar stenosis due to degenerative spondylolisthesis. *Acta Neurochir* 120:136-142, 1993.

123. Maroon JC AA, Wilberger JI: Central cord syndrome. *Clin Neurosurg* 37:612-621, 1991.

124. Martinelli TA WS: Low back pain: the algorithmic approach. *Compr Ther* 17:22-27, 1991.

125. Martinelli TA WS: Epidemiology of spinal stenosis: a review. *Instr Course Lect* 41:179-181, 1992.

126. Masaryk TJ: Neoplastic disease of the spine. *Radiol Clin North Am* 29:829-843, 1991.

127. McCowin PR BD, Wiesel SW: The current approach to the medical diagnosis of low back pain. *Orthop Clin North Am* 22:315-325, 1991.

128. Middleton G KD, Lee E: Wegener's granulomatosis presenting as lower back pain with prostatitis and ureteral obstruction. *J Rheumatol* 21:566-569, 1994.

129. Miller A GJ, Bowen R: Evaluation and treatment of diastematomyelia. *J Bone Joint Surg* 75A:1308-1317, 1993.

130. Miller DH MWI, Blumhardt LD: Magnetic resonance imaging in isolated noncompressive spinal cord syndromes. *Ann Neurol* 22:714-723, 1987.

131. Miller DH, McDonald WI, Blumhardt LD et al: Magnetic resonance imaging in isolated noncompressive compressive spinal cord syndromes. *Ann Neurol* 22:714-723, 1987.

132. Mir SA MS, Ahmed HA: Brucellosis as a cause of backache. *Trop Geogr Med* 148-151, 1990.

133. Morgenlander JC RM: Disc space infection: a case report with MRI diagnosis. *Am Fam Phys* 42:983-986, 1990.

134. Mueller DP YWTC, Fisher DJ: Arterial enhancement in acute cerebral ischemia: clinical and angiographic correlation. *AJNR* 14:661-668, 1993.

135. Nachemson AL: Newest knowledge of low back pain. *Clin Orthop Relat Res*, 1991.

136. Nachmeson AL: Spinal disorders: overall impact on society and the need for orthopedic resources. *Acta Orthop Scand* 62:17-22, 1991.

137. Nakano KK, Schoene WC, Baker RA, *et al*: The cervical myelopathy associated with rheumatoid arthritis: analysis of 32 patients with 2 postmortem cases. *Ann Neurol* 3:144-151, 1978.

138. Newcombe DS: Intermittent spinal ischemia: a reversible cause of neurologic dysfunction and back pain. *Arthritis Rheum* 37:142-144, 1994.

139. Nuwer MR PJW, Myers LW: Evoked potentials predict the clinical changes in a multiple sclerosis drug study. *Neurology* 37:1754-1761, 1987.

140. O'Connor MI CB: Metastatic disease of the spine. *Orthopedics* 15:611-620, 1992.

141. Ogilvy CS: Intramedullary cavernous angiomas of the spinal cord: clinical presentation, pathological features, and surgical management. *Neurosurgery* 31:219-230, 1992.

142. Oldfield EH: Spinal arteriovenous malformations. *Neurosurgery Update* 2:186-196, 1991.

143. O'Neill P GW: Fifty years of experience with chordomas in southeast Scotland. *Neurosurgery* 16:166-170, 1985.

144. Osborn AG: Nonneoplastic disorders of the spine and spinal cord. *Diagn Neuroradiol* 20:820-875, 1994.

145. Osborn AG: Meningiomas and other nonglial neoplasms. *Diagn Neuroradiol* 14:579-625, 1994.

146. Parent AD, Harkey HL, Touchstone DA et al: Lateral cervical spine dislocation and vertebral artery injury. *Neurosurgery* 31:501-507, 1992.

147. Paty DW OJJF, Kastrukott LF: MRI in the diagnosis of MS: a prospective study with compression of clinical evaluation, evoked potentials, oligoclonal banding, and CT. *Neurology* 38(2):180-184, 1988.

148. Perennou D SL: Adult lumbar scoliosis epidemiologic aspects in a low-back pain population. *Spine* 19:123-128, 1994.

149. Perrin RC MR: Thoracic spine tumors. *Clin Neurosurg* 38:353-372, 1991.

150. Peterson MC: Tethered cord syndrome in myelodysplasia: correlation between level of lesion and height at time of presentation. *Dev Med Child Neurol* 34:604-610, 1992.

151. Petty RE: Septic arthritis and osteomyelitis in children. *Curr Opin Rheumatol* 2:616-621, 1990.

152. Pleasure DE SD: Acquired neuropathies. In Rowland LP (ed): *Merritt's Textbook of Neurology*. Philadelphia, Lea & Febiger, 1989, pp 609-624.

153. Ponte CD MM: Septic discitis resulting from *Escherichia coli* urosepsis. *J Fam Pract* 34:767-771, 1992.

154. Porter RW: Central spinal stenosis: classification and pathogenesis. *Acta Orthop Scand Suppl* 251:64-66, 1993.

155. Poser CM PD, Scheinberg L: New diagnostic criteria for multiple sclerosis. *Ann Neurol* 13:227-231, 1983.

156. Rogers MA CH: Surgical treatment of the symptomatic herniated thoracic disc, review. *Clin Orthop Relat Res* 300:70-78, 1994.

157. Rosen DR, Siddique T, Patterson D, *et al*: Mutations in Cu/Zn superoxide dismutase gene are associated with familial amyotrophic lateral sclerosis. *Nature* 362:59-62, 1993.

158. Rowland LP: Familial periodic paralysis. In Rowland LP (ed): *Merritt's Textbook of Neurology*. Philadelphia, Lea & Febiger, 1989, pp 720-724.

159. Ryan MD TT: Spinal manifestations of Paget's disease. *Aust N Z J Surg* 62:33-38, 1992.

160. Salcman M KA, Symonds DA: Calcium pyrophosphate arthropathy of the spine: case report and review of the literature, review. *Neurosurgery* 34:915-918, 1994.

161. Sampson IR MH: Operative treatment of sacrococcygeal chordoma. *J Bone Joint Surg* 75A:1476-1484, 1993.

162. Sampson JH RE, Young JN: Solitary eosinophilic granuloma invading the clivus of an adult: case report. *Neurosurgery* 31:755-757, 1995.

163. Sapico FL MJ: Vertebral osteomyelitis, review. *Infect Dis Clin North Am* 4:539-550, 1990.

164. Saraste H: Spondylolysis and spondylolisthesis. *Acta Orthop Scand* 64:84-86, 1993.

165. Satomi K HK, Toyama Y: A clinical study of degenerative spondylolisthesis: radiographic analysis and choice of treatment. *Spine* 17:1329-1335, 1992.

166. Scully SP TH, O'Keefe RJ: Case report 830. *Skeletal Radiol* 23:157-160, 1994.

167. Seitsalso S OK, Hyvarinen H: Severe spondylolisthesis in children and adolescents. *J Bone Joint Surg* 72-:259-265, 1990.

168. Seitsalso S OK, Hyvarinen H: Progression of spondylolisthesis in children and adolescents: a long-term follow-up of 272 patients. *Spine* 16:417-421, 1991.

169. Sessa S SD, Lascombes P: Treatment of Langerhans-cell histiocytosis in children. *J Bone Joint Surg* 76A:1513-1524, 1994.

170. Sharma RR SF, Cast IP: Spinal extradural arteriovenous malformation presenting with recurrent hemorrhage and intermittent paraplegia: case report and review of the literature. *Surg Neurol* 41:26-31, 1994.

171. Shaw PJ AD, Bates D: Cauda equina syndrome associated with multiple lumbar arachnoid cysts in ankylosing spondylitis: improvement following surgical therapy. *J Neurol Neurosurg Psychiatr* 53:1076-1079, 1990.

172. Shenaq SA SL: Paraplegia following aortic surgery. *J Cardiothorac Vasc Anest* 7:81-94, 1993.

173. Simeone FA: Intradural tumors. In Rothman RH SF (ed): *The Spine*. Philadelphia, WB Saunders, 1992, pp 1515-1528.

174. Simmons EH: Ankylosing spondylitis: surgical considerations. In Rothman RH SF (ed): *The Spine*. Philadelphia, WB Saunders, 1992, pp 1447-1511.

175. Singounas EG KE, Kellerman AJ: Thoracic disc herniation: analysis of 14 cases and review of the literature, review. *Acta Neurochir* 116:49-52, 1992.

176. Slater G HR: Management of chondrosarcoma. *Aust N Z Surg* 63:587-589, 1993.

177. Slater RR BE: Pott's disease of the cervical spine. *South Med J* 84:521-523, 1991.

178. Stein BM MP: Intramedullary neoplasms and vascular malformations. *Clin Neurosurg* 39:361-387, 1992.

179. Tandan R: Disorders of the upper and lower motor neurons. In Bradley WG, Daroff RB, Fenichel GM, *et al* (eds): *Neurology in Clinical Practice*. London, Butterworth-Heinemann, 1991, pp 1687-1717.

180. Tekkok IH AB, Saglam S: Vertebral hemangioma symptomatic during pregnancy: report of a case and review of the literature. *Neurosurgery* 32:302-305, 1993.

181. Thiranont N NP: Transpedicular decancellation closed wedge vertebral osteotomy for treatment of fixed flexion

deformity of spine in ankylosing spondylitis. *Spine* 18:2517-2522, 1993.

182. Thompson PD: Paraplegia and quadriplegia. In Bradley WG, Daroff RB, Fenichel GM, *et al* (eds): *Neurology in Clinical Practice*. London, Butterworth-Heinemann, 1991, pp 261-273.

183. Torbiak R PR: Answer to case of the month: pyogenic discitis. Staphylococcal discitis complicated by bilateral psoas abscesses. *Can Assoc Radiol J* 41:49-50, 1990.

184. Tourtellotte WW, Shorr RJ: Cerebrospinal fluid. In Youmans JR (ed): *Neurological Surgery*. Philadelphia, WB Saunders, 1982, pp 423-486.

185. Tsubaki T, Toyokura Y: Amyotrophic lateral sclerosis (abstracted), 1978.

186. Umbach I HA: Post-spinal cord injury syringomyelia. *Paraplegia* 29:219-221, 1991.

187. Upadhyay SS HL: Surgical management of spinal tuberculosis in adults: Hong Kong operation compared with debridement surgery for short and long term outcome of deformity. *Clin Orthop Relat Res* 173-183, 1994.

188. Vandertop WP PJ, Snoeck IN: Aneurysmal bone cyst of the thoracic spine: radical excision with the use of the cavitron. *J Bone Joint Surg* 76A:608-611, 1994.

189. Vukmir RB: Low back pain: review of diagnosis and therapy. *Am J Emerg Med* 9:328-335, 1991.

190. Weinstein JN MR: Tumors of the spine. In Rothman RH SF (ed): *The Spine*. Philadelphia, WB Saunders, 1992, 1279-1319.

191. Wenger DR DJ, Ring D: Discitis and osteomyelitis. In Weinstein SL (ed): *The Pediatric Spine: Principles and Practice*. Philadelphia, Lippincott-Raven, 1994, pp 709-724.

192. Williams RW: Lumbar disc disease. Microdiscectomy, review. *Neurosurg Clin North Am* 4:101-108, 1993.

193. Wilson CM RE, Sturgess AD: *Haemophilus paraphrophilus* vertebral osteomyelitis, review. *Med J Austr* 160:512-514, 1994.

194. Wold LE Laws ER Jr: Cranial chordomas in children and young adults. *J Neurosurg* 59:1043-1047, 1983.

195. Woolsey RM YR: The clinical diagnosis of disorders of the spinal cord. *Neurol Clin* 9:573-581, 1991.

196. Wurtz R QZ: Cervical tuberculosis vertebral osteomyelitis: case report and discussion of the literature. *Clin Infect Dis* 16:806-808, 1993.

197. Yoong MF BP, North JB: Primary (granulomatous) angiitis of the central system with multiple aneurysms of the spinal arteries. *J Neurosurg* 79:603-607, 1993.

198. Young CL SF, Unni KK: Chondrosarcoma of bone in children. *Cancer* 66:1641-1648, 1990.

CHAPTER 4

Anatomy and Physiology of Congenital Spinal Lesions

Christopher I. Shaffrey, Andrew G. Chenelle, Mark F. Abel, Arnold H. Menezes, and Gregory C. Wiggins[°]

To understand the anatomy and pathophysiology of congenital and developmental spinal lesions, it is necessary to understand the normal embryologic process of spine development. Human spine embryology is complex, and much of the knowledge is derived from nonhuman vertebrates. Although it is difficult to transfer this knowledge to human conditions, modern cellular biologic techniques enhance our comprehension.

This chapter presents a brief review of the embryology of the spine and provides a background for understanding the anatomy and pathophysiology of congenital spinal lesions. Discussion covers overall spine embryology and the development of specialized regions (atlas, axis, sacrum), followed by developmental abnormalities of the spine. For additional reference, excellent reviews of spine embryology are available.[†]

General Principles of Spine Embryology

Embryogenesis

Human spine development begins when the primitive streak forms at day 15 of embryonic life. Before the primitive streak develops, the embryo is a bilaminar disc consisting of the epiblast (cellular layer of primitive ectoderm) and hypoblast (cellular layer that later forms part of the endoderm). The primitive streak consists of a thickened linear band of epiblast that appears caudally in the dorsal aspect of the embryonic disc. It elongates by adding cells at the caudal end as the rostral end thickens to form the primitive knot. Concurrently, a depression (primitive groove) forms in the primitive streak that is continuous with a depression (primitive pit) in the primitive knot. The rostrocaudal axis of the embryo is defined when the primitive streak develops.

At day 16, epiblastic cells invade the primitive groove, lose their attachments to the epiblastic tissue, and migrate between the epiblast and hypoblast to form the embryonic mesoderm. This migration of cells transforms the bilaminar embryo into a trilaminar embryo, made up of (1) the remnants of the epiblast forming ectoderm, (2) the newly formed mesoderm, and (3) the endoderm that is made up of invading mesodermal cells and the laterally displaced remnants of the hypoblast. The term for this process of transforming the bilaminar embryo to a trilaminar embryo is *gastrulation*. A group of genes that encode a zinc finger protein are believed to be necessary for appropriate mesenchymal cell migration from the primitive streak. Abnormalities in these genes may interfere with the process of formation of the mesoderm during gastrulation and with emigration of the neural crest from the neural tube.[3] Many congenital disorders of the spine involve malformations of tissues derived from all three embryologic layers. One might assume that many congenital spinal disorders arise from defects in gastrulation, when all three embryologic layers are available to the same insult.[51] Disorders in gastrulation can result in conditions such as sacral agenesis and imperforate anus.[1]

After the fourth week of gestation, the primitive streak ceases to produce mesodermal cells, greatly diminishes in size, and becomes an insignificant structure in the sacrococcygeal region of the embryo. Normally, the primitive streak undergoes degenerative changes and disappears.

Neurulation and Neurogenesis

The notochord is formed, at day 16, in the midline at the rostral end of the embryo by mesoblastic cells that migrate cranially from the primitive knot between the ectoderm and endoderm. The rostral ascent of these cells ends at the prochordal plate (a small collection of endodermal cells) that firmly adheres to the overlying ectoderm and is destined to become the oropharyngeal membrane. The notochord runs rostrally to the prochordal plate and caudally to the cloacal membrane. As the notochord develops, the primitive pit extends into it to form the notochordal canal (a lumen). Eventually, when the floor of the notochordal canal disappears, a notochordal plate is formed.

The primitive streak and the notochord are strong inductive tissues and play a critical role in induction and development of future organ systems. During formation, the notochord induces the overlying ectoderm to form the neural plate. Primary neurulation involves the formation and infolding of the neural plate to form the neural tube that eventually becomes the spinal cord down to the level of the lumbosacral junction and occurs days 18 to 27 after ovulation. The neural plate first appears rostral to the primitive knot. On day 18, the neural plate invaginates to form the neural groove with neural folds on both sides (Figure 4.1). By day 21, the neural folds have fused to form the neural tube. The neural tube then separates itself from the overlying ectoderm and the ectoderm fuses to become continuous over the dorsal aspect of the embryo.

The spinal cord distal to the second sacral vertebra develops by secondary neurulation.[115,157] This secondary neurulation begins by having neural crest cells migrate

[°]The views expressed in this material are those of the authors and do not reflect the official policy or position of the U.S. Government, the Department of Defense, or the Department of the Air Force.
[†]References 97,100,142,156,158,164,170,181,225

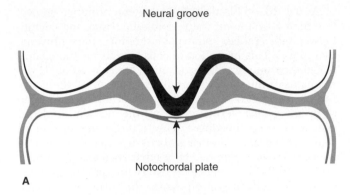

Neural groove

Notochordal plate

A

Neural crest cells

Neural tube

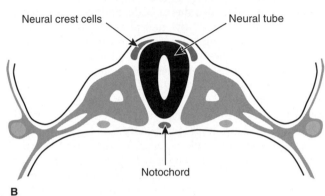

Notochord

B

Figure 4.1 Formation of the neural tube. (**A**) Axial section through notochordal tube. The notochordal tube has fused with the endoderm and is evaginating in the process of intercalation, forming the notochordal plate. (**B**) The neural tube. The ectoderm has separated from the neural crest and fused, reconstituting an intact layer. (*Modified from Moore KL, Persaud TVN: The* Developing Human: Clinically Oriented Embryology, *5th ed. Philadelphia, WB Saunders, 1993.*)

into the dorsal midline of the mesoderm and become identifiable as ependyma and later evolving into neural cells.[150] These cells then group together to form canals. They eventually fuse into one tubular structure that joins with the distal end of the spinal cord developing from the primary neurulation process.

Somite Formation and Skeletogenesis

As the notochord and the neural tube develop, the intraembryonic mesoderm on both sides begins to thicken and form paraxial mesoderm. At about 20 days of gestation, the paraxial mesoderm divides into paired cuboidal structures called *somites*. These somites are located laterally on both sides of the developing neural tube. The first pair of somites is near the rostral end of the neural tube. They then propagate in a rostral to caudal sequence. By 30 days, 38 pairs of somites, and eventually 42 to 44 pairs, have formed: 4 occipital, 8 cervical, 12 thoracic, 5 lumbar, 5 sacral, and 8 to 10 coccygeal. Eventually, the first occipital and the last 5 to 7 coccygeal pairs disappear. The process of secondary neurulation results in the development of the spinal cord segments below the lumbosacral junction and occurs during days 28 to 48 after ovula-

tion.[1,54] The caudal eminence is responsible for the development of the terminal spinal cord, vertebral segments S2 through the last coccygeal segment, and portions of the hindgut and lower urogenital systems. An embryologic insult to the caudal eminence has been implicated in a variety of disorders, including caudal agenesis, imperforate anus, cloacal exstrophy, and cloacal malformation.[70]

The true development of the vertebral column begins with these somites. As the cells in the somites proliferate, distinct cell masses appear. The dermatome is the most lateral cell mass, destined to become the skin and subcutaneous tissue. The medial cell mass differentiates into two components. The *myotome* is the dorsal aspect of the medial cell mass and differentiates into a cell aggregate destined to become striated muscle. The *sclerotome* is the ventral aspect of the medial somite cell mass and becomes an aggregate of cells destined to become the skeletal system.

These somites clearly have regional specificity early in development. Somites destined to become vertebrae in the thoracic region can be transposed to the cervical region and vertebrae resembling thoracic vertebrae and extrathoracic ribs result.[107] Some believe that the regional specificity of these somites is conferred by expression of "homeobox" (Hox) genes.[105] Additional developmental control of spinal development comes from "paired box" (Pax) genes.[37,203] In mice and chick embryos Pax gene expression has been shown to play a role in sclerotome patterning and in the development of the perinotochordal tube, and a late function in influencing the development of intervertebral discs during vertebral chondrification.[203,229] Signals from the developing notochord are necessary for normal Pax-1 expression.[224] Using antisense methodologies, Smith and Tuan[204] have shown that abnormal expression of Pax-1 during development results in complete loss and/or fusion of somites. Developmental abnormalities in the spine may arise from mistakes in expression of Pax and Hox genes or the influence of teratogens upon them.

By 35 days, the cells of the sclerotome condense to surround the notochord and neural tube, forming a mesenchymal vertebra. The ventral collection of mesenchymal cells condenses to form the mesenchymal centrum, the primitive vertebral body. The ventral aspect of the mesenchymal condensation occurs slightly before the development of the dorsal aspect, thus longitudinally separating in time the origins of the primitive vertebral body and neural arch. Differentiation of the part of the sclerotome destined to become the vertebral body appears to be under the influence of the neural tube. Differentiation of the parts of the sclerotome destined to become the neural arch appears to be influenced by the neural crest; thus the vertebral body and neural arch are under different inductive control. Developmental abnormalities that occur during early gestation may independently affect the vertebral body or the developing neural arch. In addition, developmental abnormalities may be limited to the ventral and dorsal elements because of the difference in the time course of their development.

The cells in each sclerotome form two distinct cell masses. There is a region of loosely packed cells in the rostral half of the sclerotome and a region of densely packed cells in the caudal half of each sclerotome. The densely packed cells evolve into intervertebral discs; the loosely packed cells eventually have chondrification centers develop within them and evolve into the bony elements of the spine.

Since 1855, Remark's[176] theory of resegmentation of the vertebrae had been universally accepted. Remark's theory suggests that the vertebral body forms when the rostral half of one somite migrates and joins with the caudal half of the somite above. This theory is appealing because it explains how intersegmental arteries cross the vertebral body and nerve roots exit between the bodies. Moreover, this theory has been used to explain developmental disorders of the spine such as hemivertebra and congenitally fused vertebra.[106] There is, however, some debate over the validity of this theory.[46,102]

This theory of resegmentation of the vertebrae was held as scientific dogma until it was called into question in 1985 by two separate investigators, Verbout and Dalgleish. Based on the histologic study of serial sections, Verbout[224] argued that the split between the dense (caudal) and the loose (rostral) halves of the somite are artifacts and that the vertebral bodies derive principally from an unsegmented *perichordal tube* and a loose column of axial mesenchyme, whereas the dorsal elements derive from caudal condensed mesenchyme. Dalgleish,[46] who studied the development of thoracic vertebrae in the mouse by autoradiographic means, confirmed Verbout's theory.

Recent experimental evidence, however, confirms the theory of resegmentation. Bagnall *et al*,[6] using the chick-quail chimera model, convincingly produced experimental evidence in support of the resegmentation theory. In an elegant study, Ewan and Everett[67] found further support for the resegmentation theory by using retroviral-mediated transfer of the lac Z gene to trace migration of the somites. In synthesizing the experimental evidence, a consensus seems to be emerging that the vertebral bodies are composed of the cranial and rostral halves of two adjacent somites, whereas the dorsal elements derive from the caudal somite.[43] One of the strongest arguments in favor of the resegmentation theory is the explanation of congenital malformations of the spine.

Nerve root relationships and vertebral muscle connections may be explained by considering the development of the dorsal elements. Dorsal element development is influenced by the neural crest and spinal ganglia. The neural arches develop between the spinal ganglia and thus are intersegmental with respect to the myotomes and are thus connected to two adjacent myotomal segments. This intersegmental orientation also explains the relationship of the nerve roots to the dorsal elements.

In addition to the usual spinal elements, the thoracic spine must develop ribs and rib articulations. There is experimental evidence indicating that the majority of the rib (dorsal or vertebral rib) originates from the somites.[213] All vertebrae have the potential to develop ribs as evidenced by the rib process equivalents on all vertebrae and yet only the thoracic vertebrae have a full complement of ribs. This is thought to be due to expression of Hox genes. The costal element derives from the aspect part of the anatomic transverse process.[36]

As the vertebral centra expand, the notochord gradually regresses within these expansions. Notochord cells tend to

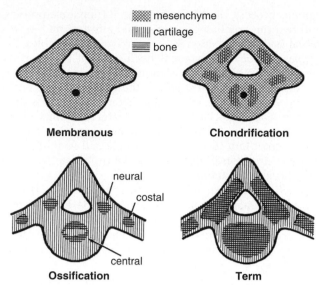

Figure 4.2 Schematic illustration of the sequential development of vertebral components: (**A**) membranous, (**B**) chondrification, (**C**) ossification, (**D**) term. *(From Parke WW: Development of the spine. In Herkowitz HN, Garfin SR, Balderston RA, et al [eds]: Rothman–Simeone: The Spine, 4th ed. Philadelphia, WB Saunders, 1999.)*

cluster in the eventual intervertebral spaces.[120,132,171] Notochord cells contribute significantly to the formation of the intervertebral disc, most notably the nucleus pulposus. Abnormal remnants of notochord can remain in the spinal axis most commonly in the coccygeal or basisphenoid regions, and give rise to chordomas. The vertebral matrix is conventionally understood to undergo three stages: membranous, chondrified, and ossified (Figure 4.2).

Chondrification begins at day 42 of embryonic life.[154] Chondrification centers appear in each mesenchymal vertebra and appear on both sides of the small remnant of notochord and coalesce toward the center. A chondrification center forms laterally in each vertebral arch and propagates dorsally to form a cartilaginous arch. This chondrification expands dorsally to form the spinous process. Late chondrification centers form at the junction of the centrum and neural arch and extend laterally to form the transverse processes. Concurrently, the dense mesenchymal part of the somite (that is to form the intervertebral disc) condenses to form the annulus fibrosus.

Ossification begins about day 72, enhanced by embryonic movement.[154] Ossification of the vertebrae, however, is not complete until age 25. Two primary ossification centers develop in the vertebral centrum. These are located dorsal and ventral to the notochord center, in contrast to the lateral chondrification centers. The dorsal and ventral ossification centers quickly fuse to form a single central ossification center. Ossification centers, which also form in each vertebral arch, grow into three regions: one each for the lamina, pedicle, and transverse process. At birth, each vertebra consists of three ossified bones connected by cartilage. The halves of the vertebral arch fuse between the ages of 3 to 5 years. First, the laminae fuse in the lumbar region and then progress rostrally. Five secondary ossification centers appear at puberty: one at the tip of the spinous process, one at the tip of each transverse process, and two rim epiphyses (superior and inferior) on the vertebral body. Ossification in the neural arch resembles diaphyseal ossification, whereas ossification of the centrum resembles epiphyseal ossification in long bones.

An adequate blood supply to the vertebrae is essential to the development and proliferation of the ossification centers. Cartilage canals are special structures that carry a vascular supply to the vertebral centrum.[228] Cartilage canals grow into the centrum dorsally and ventrally.[39] In contrast, the dorsal element vasculature enters from the peripheral periosteum.[39]

Each cartilage canal contains an artery, a vein, and associated surrounding capillary network. These end-artery systems have little or no anastomosis across the epiphyses. If a vascular network is compromised, rapid death of osteocytes occurs that can result in differential growth of the spine.

Development of the Occipital Complex

The occipital bone and the preotic regions of the skull are of somitic origin. There are at least four precervical myotomes in the human embryo.[197] DeBeer[50] argues that there are nine segments involved in skull formation; the first five are rudimentary and develop into the preotic cranium, and the last four develop into the occipital bone. The fate of these four sclerotomes is inferred from their relationships to the hypoglossal nerve. The hypoglossal nerve is multisegmented in origin, and at least four main roots can be identified.

The two most rostral occipital sclerotomes differentiate into the basiocciput (clivus). The third occipital sclerotome differentiates into the jugular tubercles. The fourth occipital sclerotome (proatlas) forms the occipital condyles; the ventral border of the foramen magnum; the rostral articulating facets of the atlas; and the apical, alar, and transverse ligaments of the dens.[142] The squamous portion of the occipital bone is membranous in origin.

Ossification of the occipital bone proceeds as follows: the two occipital squamous portions ossify from a single center, the clivus ossifies from a single center, the paired jugular tubercles ossify from individual centers, and the occipital condyles ossify from individual centers.[142]

Development of the Atlantoaxial Complex

The first and second cervical vertebrae develop from the fourth occipital somite through the second cervical somite (Figure 4.3). Parts of the axis develop from the fourth occipital somite; the remaining parts of the axis develop from the first cervical somite. The first cervical somite develops into the ventral arch of the atlas. The dorsal arch of the atlas most likely arises from the proatlantal sclerotome.[156] There is a contribution from the first cervical sclerotome to the midportion of the dens.[35,36]

The development of the axis is quite complex. The second cervical sclerotome forms the lower portion of the dens, the centrum, and the dorsal arch of the axis.[142] The dens has a contribution from three sclerotomes: the tip

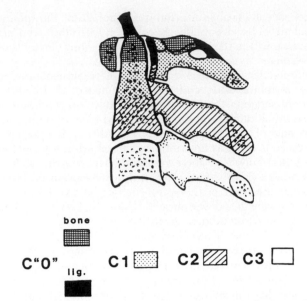

Figure 4.3 Schematic drawing of the contributions from the first three sclerotomes to the atlantoaxial complex. The proatlas (C"0") provides the tip of the odontoid process, the hypochordal anterior arch, and the dorsal part of the superior atlas facet as well as the upper half of the transverse ligament and the apical odontoid and retroarticular ligaments. *(From Parke WW: Development of the spine. In Herkowitz HN, Garfin SR, Balderston RA, et al [eds]: Rothman–Simeone: The Spine, 4th ed. Philadelphia, WB Saunders, 1999.)*

arises from the proatlantal sclerotome, the midportion from the first cervical sclerotome, and the base from the second cervical sclerotome.[156]

Ossification of the ventral arch of the atlas proceeds from a single ventral center of ossification, and the dorsal arch ossifies from two lateral ossification centers in the lateral masses.[7] Calcification of the arches of the atlas is usually complete by the third postnatal year and fusion of the ventral and dorsal arches usually is complete by age 7. The axis has five primary ossification centers at birth. There are two lateral ossification centers for the posterior neural arch and one ossification center for the axis body.[7] The neural arch is calcified by age 3 and the dorsal arch and body fuse by age 6. The body of the dens has two separate ossification centers that fuse by the seventh embryonic month.[142] The dens fuses to the body of the axis by age 6, and the synchondrosis between the tip and body of the dens fuses by age 12.

Development of the Sacrum

By the eighth postovulatory week, five cartilaginous sacral vertebrae are evident.[156] Each of these vertebrae goes on to form a centrum and bilateral neural processes. The base of each neural process consists of a ventrolateral alar process and a dorsolateral element consisting of a costal and transverse element.[156] At this point, the neural foramen face laterally. Much differential growth is required to turn these foramina to their eventual dorsal and ventral positions.[156]

Ossification of the sacrum is unique in that two epiphyseal plates provide additional ossification to the rostral and caudal surfaces of each segment. The ossification centers in the first three sacral vertebrae are evident by the ninth embryologic week. The centers in the fourth and fifth segments appear after week 24. The vertebral arches of the sacral vertebrae have the conventional bilateral centers, and six additional centers produce the sacral ala. The sacral vertebrae begin to fuse in the first postnatal year, and the last two sacral vertebrae fuse by adolescence. By age 18 epiphyseal plates have formed on the auricular surfaces of the sacral ala. By the third decade the entire sacrum is fused.

Disturbances of the normal embryologic development of the human vertebral column are relatively uncommon. Several of the most frequent "errors" of embryologic spinal maturation that manifest themselves as specific clinical disorders are discussed in the following sections.

General Epidemiology and Clinical Features of Congenital Spine Lesions

Congenital spinal anomalies are usually found as sporadic, isolated cases, with a 1% chance of transmission.[237,241] However, when the spinal anomaly is one of many organ system anomalies, the risk of transmission rises to 5% to 10%.[244] Teratogen exposure during the pregnancy should be sought in the history. Maternal diabetes is a well-recognized risk factor for the development of spinal dysraphism and sacral agenesis. A wide variety of associated anomalies can accompany the spinal deformity.[93,111,127,237,241] In fact, the incidence of associated renal abnormalities is 25% (18% to 40%) and cardiac abnormalities 5%.[54,93] Intraspinal anomalies such as stenosis, diastematomyelia, and tethering of the spinal cord may also occur (5% to 35%) in association with congenital spinal deformities.[127] Therefore, before treatment, the entire bony vertebral column and spinal cord must be thoroughly analyzed by radiographs and magnetic resonance imaging (MRI). These facts underscore the importance of obtaining a thorough genetic and family history and performing a meticulous physical examination. The uncovered organ system defect may be more significant to the patient's well-being than the spinal deformity.

The converse is also true. Any patient with a congenital organ system anomaly is at increased risk of having hidden vertebral anomalies. Certain syndromes are particularly apt to have associated congenital spinal deformities.[93,237] Facial and neck deformity often suggests anomalies of the cervical and cervicothoracic spine. Goldenhar syndrome (oculoauricular vertebral dysplasia) is associated with a constellation of anomalies including epibulbar dermoids of the eye, preauricular skin tags, and vertebral anomalies. The VATER complex is another group of syndromes that have congenital scoliosis as one component.[81] This acronym describes the common association of V (vertebral anomalies), A (anal atresia), and T (tracheoesophageal fistula) with E (esophageal atresia) and R (radial ray and renal defects). However, all of these defects may not be present, and others, such as the Sprengel anomaly (high scapula) or cardiac abnormalities, may accompany these anomalies. Therefore, although these syndromes have a high incidence of vertebral deformity, rarely will two patients with these syndromes have the exact same type of vertebral or associated organ anomalies. A spectrum of vertebral malformations can be found that involve a single segment, or many anomalies that encompass the entire spine; including deficient posterior elements, hemivertebrae, and vertebral fusions.

Congenital vertebral deformities are associated with renal abnormalities in 20% to 30% of cases.[59,93,127] Cardiac abnormalities, often associated with chest deformities (pectus carinatum or excavatum), occur in 10% of cases. Dorsal midline skin lesions (such as hairy patches or deep dimples), asymmetric foot deformities (cavus or flat feet), muscle weakness, or spasticity suggest underlying nervous system abnormalities. All of these systems must be thoroughly examined when a congenital spinal deformity is discovered. Renal ultrasound, cardiac consultation, and MRI of the entire brain stem and spinal cord are essential for the complete evaluation of patients with congenital spinal anomalies. Pulmonary function test and/or arterial blood gases should be obtained when a thoracotomy is planned or when severe thoracic lordosis is present. Conversely, when musculoskeletal abnormalities such as preaxial (radial) limb deficiencies or Sprengel's anomaly are present, radiographs of the spine are mandatory to rule out concomitant spinal anomalies.

Spinal Dysraphism

Generally, dysraphism refers to abnormal spinal cord and column development. Dysraphism is associated with malformations that most likely arise from the failure of normal embryologic structures to fuse in the midline. Conventionally, these malformations are somewhat artificially divided into two groups: spina bifida aperta and spina bifida occulta. The first group involves midline lesions that are *open*, or that might open, at birth. These lesions include spina bifida cystica (myelomeningocele, meningocele) and myelodysplasia. The second group has malformations that are hidden by complete layers of dermis and epidermis. These lesions include lipomyelomeningocele, neurenteric cyst, and diastematomyelia.[32,75]

In the United States, the incidence of neural tube defects declined from 1.3 per 1000 births in 1970 to 0.6 per 1000 births in 1989.[72,73,247] Worldwide, the incidence varies greatly; in Belfast, Northern Ireland, it approaches 8.7 per 1000 births.[102] Environmental factors that have been implicated include maternal hyperthermia; maternal deficiencies in folate, calcium, vitamin C, and zinc; and either lack of or overdose of vitamin A.[23,39,41,190,194,205,215] The level of the spinal dysplasia depends on the embryologic age at which the malformation is initiated. It is generally believed that neural tube defects follow a multifactorial inheritance pattern that interacts with environmental factors. The risk of having a child with spina bifida is approximately 0.1%, but if there is a sibling with spina bifida, the risk increases to 2.5% for subsequent children. There is also an increased risk of neural tube defects in the children of sisters and daughters of the mother who has a child with a myelomeningocele.

Malformations that begin before 28 days of gestation induce major defects in neurulation and cause a higher level of defects than malformations occurring after 28 days of gestation, when neurulation is complete. The higher the level of dysplasia, the less survivable the malformation.[11] In one study of 510 infants surviving the first day of life, approximately 5% of lesions were cranial/cervical, 5% were thoracic, 25% were thoracolumbar, 33% were lumbar, and 32% were sacral.[5] Detailed anatomical studies suggest a timetable for the formation of spinal dysraphism from 14 to 49 postovulatory days.[146]

The embryologic defects that cause spinal dysraphism are not entirely understood, and therefore many theories prevail. These theories may be broken into five groups: (1) simple nonclosure theory, (2) overgrowth and nonclosure theory, (3) so-called reopening theory, (4) overgrowth and reopening theory, and (5) primary mesodermal insufficiency theory. Experimental models have supported the possibility of all these hypotheses.[160,161,184]

Spina bifida aperta ranges from the exposure of the unfolded neural plate (myeloschisis) to various meningoceles that either involve the cord (myelomeningocele) or the subarachnoid space (meningocele). Theories abound regarding the defect in embryogenesis involved in dysplasia. The developmental arrest theory, first proposed by von Recklinghausen, states that myelodysplasia is due to the arrest of neural plate closure and a secondary failure of development of the dorsal spine elements.[137] The overgrowth hypothesis put forth by Ledeff in 1881 suggests that the failure of the neural tube to close results from the overgrowth of neural tissue in the lateral folds.[137] According to Gardner's[78] hydrodynamic theory, the neural tube closes normally, but increased hydrostatic pressure within the central canal causes the neural tube to reopen and the maldevelopment of elements.

There is experimental evidence to support these theories. In support of von Recklinghausen's simple nonclosure theory, Lendon[116] found, in studying the litters from 140 Wistar rats injected with Trypan blue during gestation, that a myelocele could result from faulty closure of the neural plate, and that this was often accompanied by blebs in the para-axial mesoderm. In support of the overgrowth and nonclosure theory, Smith et al.[205] studied dysraphic lesions in rat embryos from pregnant rats that were given vitamin A. They found that these embryonic lesions revealed hyperplasia of neural tube tissue that extended laterally to the edge of an epidermal defect. This defect consisted of the absence of fetal epidermis over the hyperplastic neural tissue. In support of the so-called reopening theory, Rokos et al.[183,184] studied congenital malformations in rats by applying trypan blue at variable times in development. They found that the presence of degenerative changes at the junction between ectoderm and neural tissue of early spina bifida indicated that a reopening of an already closed neural tube caused the malformation. Existence of heterotopic tubules in the same location at later stages of development led them to believe that previous damage had occurred. In support of the overgrowth and reopening theory, Oi et al.[160,161] studied the immunohistochemistry and histology of the exposed neural placode. In chick embryos they found that neuron-specific, enolase-positive elements were extremely active only in the overgrown placode. This was taken to support the overgrowth and reopening theory. In support of the primary mesodermal insufficiency theory, Marin-Padilla and Ferm[122] studied golden hamsters treated with a single dose of vitamin A. They found somite necrosis 12 to 24 hours after administration of vitamin A. The then-unprotected neural tissue secondarily degenerated. Given the range of spinal dysmorphisms, it is unlikely that one hypothesis can explain the full range of spinal dysmorphisms.

Characteristically in spinal dysraphism, the spinal column widens at the level of the defect. If the neural tube does not develop normally, it causes a deficiency of dorsal element formation and the lateral and ventral displacement of the pedicles and lateral elements of the spine. In addition, other abnormalities of the vertebrae can be associated with spinal dysraphism, such as wedge vertebrae and hemivertebrae. Occasionally, patients who have symptoms of what is thought to be idiopathic scoliosis in fact have some form of occult spinal dysraphism.[26] Additionally, the inductive effects of spinal dysraphism can cause multiple rib anomalies.[126]

Abnormal neural tube development prevents dermis and epidermis closure over the dorsal defect. Dura mater arises ventral to the deformed spinal cord, but then stretches laterally over the expanded pedicles and facets to join the lateral margins of the epidermis. A thin layer of pia/arachnoid and the zona epithelioma, an extremely thin layer of epithelium, covers the dorsal defect.

Usually, spina bifida aperta occurs in the craniocervical and lumbar areas of the spinal column. The morphogenesis of the dysraphism depends on the embryologic period in which the malformation occurs. If the insult occurs before the 28th day, myeloschisis (exposure of the malformed spinal cord) results from failure of neural tube closure. Myeloschisis is common at the thoracolumbar junction. If the insult occurs after 28 days of gestation, however, various forms of meningocele and myelomeningocele may develop.

Occult spinal dysraphism includes a variety of spinal malformations not immediately visible on the skin surface. Spina bifida occulta occurs from a maldevelopment of the dorsal neural arch structures. Some believe that this occurs when an already closed neural tube ruptures. Increased pressure inside of the central canal of the neural tube can cause a rupture that spills highly proteinaceous fluid from the canal into the surrounding tissue. With the decrease in pressure, the defect in the neural tube reanneals but the proteinaceous fluid inhibits normal development of the dorsal elements. Because the neural tube has closed, closure of the dermis and epidermis over the dorsal aspect of the spinal cord is not impeded.

Diastematomyelia

Diastematomyelia causes the spinal cord to develop into two hemicords, separated by a cartilaginous or bony septum[114,140] (Figure 4.4). In a study of 60 patients, Hood et al.[99] found that diastematomyelia occurs from the third thoracic to the fourth lumbar vertebrae. Approximately 50% of the lesions were associated with thoracic vertebrae, and 50% were associated with lumbar vertebrae.

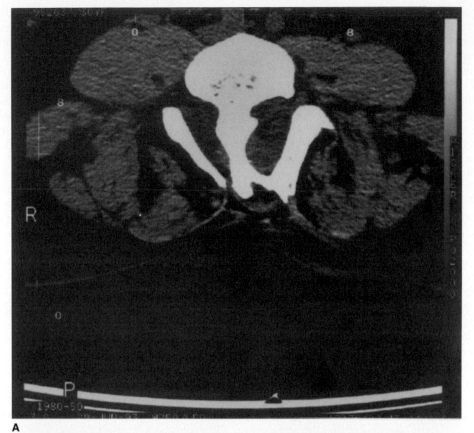

A

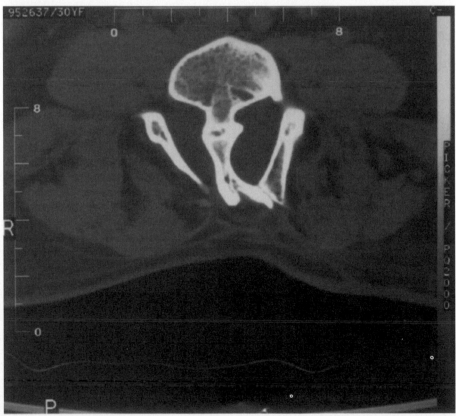

B

Figure 4.4 Diastematomyelia presenting in a female age 30 years with spasticity and long tract signs. (**A**) Soft tissue window. (**B**) Bone window.

In 1992, Pang et al.[167] presented a unified theory of diastematomyelia and diplomyelia embryogenesis that characterized these lesions as split cord malformations (SCMs). Type I SCMs consist of two hemicords, each contained in its own dural tube and separated by a dural sheathed rigid osseocartilaginous median septum. Type II SCMs consist of two hemicords housed in a single dural sheath and separated by a nonrigid, fibrous midline septum.[167] In their study of 39 patients, Pang and associates[165,167] found 19 patients with type I SCMs, 18 patients with type II SCMs, and 2 patients with composite SCMs in tandem.

Although the presence or absence of medial nerve roots has long been believed to aid in distinguishing diastematomyelia from simple diplomyelia, Pang et al.[167] found that medial nerve roots occur in 75% of both type I and type II SCMs. Notably, although most medial nerve roots were dorsal, ventral medial nerve roots were extremely rare.[167]

The SCM theory proposes that both types of SCMs originate from one embryologic error around the time of neural tube closure. The basic error occurs when the accessory neurenteric canal forms through the midline of the embryonic disc that maintains communication between endoderm and ectoderm.[167] While the abnormal fistula develops, mesenchyme condenses around it and the tract then splits the developing notochord and neural tube. The malformation phenotype depends on further spinal column/cord development. An SCM results if the embryo is able to heal around the tract. If the tract picks up primitive cells from the mesenchyme (destined to become the meninges), the two hemicords will each be invested in dura mater. The dura mater can stimulate bone growth that results in a midline spur (type I SCM).

There are many theories with various explanations of the embryology of diastematomyelia/diplomyelia/SCMs. For example, in 1940, Herren and Edwards[95] proposed the model of *twinning*, in which the lateral neural folds may roll to the midline and fuse with the neural plate (rather than with each other) and two hemicords result. Each hemicord may induce mesodermal formation of a protective matrix that results in the midline spicule.[95] Contrasting this hypothesis, Lichtenstein,[117] in 1940, proposed that diastematomyelia is primarily a defect in the mesoderm formation. He stated that when the maldeveloped midline septum splits the neural plate, two hemicords develop. Beardmore and Wigglesworth[14] proposed that diastematomyelia develops from an adhesion between the epiblast and hypoblast that forms before or during the outgrowth of the notochordal process. This adhesion provides a barrier to the developing and elongating notochord, which would then have to split around the lesion. Dias and Walker[51] have proposed that diastematomyelia arises early in development when all three germ layers are in close association (i.e., during gastrulation). They hypothesize that rather than integrating to form the notochord, individual germ layers remain separate and develop independently.

Neurenteric Cysts

If there is retained endoderm in the tract between hemicords, a neurenteric cyst can result.[61] These rare lesions are retained cystic structures, ventrally located in the spinal canal, derived from embryonic foregut.[28] These cysts occur most commonly in the thoracic and cervical spine.[98] In a meta-analysis of 23 reported cases, French[75] found that 40% occurred in the cervical spine and 50% occurred in the thoracic spine. The epithelium of these cysts varies from ciliated columnar lining that suggests a respiratory origin to linings that can resemble gut mucosa. Because of embryonic gut rotation, neurenteric cysts tend to lie to the right of the vertebral column.[201]

Most likely these lesions originate from communications between the yolk sac (eventual foregut) and the dorsal surface of the embryo. Normally, such a neurenteric canal is located in the region of the coccyx. Accessory neurenteric canals, however, can occur rostral to the coccyx, and if they persist, neurenteric cysts result.[25] This persistent neurenteric tract can result in vertebral abnormalities, such as a widened vertebral body (resulting from increased bone forming around the tract) and hemivertebrae. Neurenteric cysts can cause spinal cord compression usually appearing in childhood.

Lipomas

Lipomas of the spine are commonly observed in clinical practice, and may be considered a developmental abnormality. The most common form is a lipoma associated with occult spinal dysraphism.[40] They occur in the lumbosacral area 90% of the time.[76] In contrast, intraspinal lipomas not associated with spina bifida account for 4.7% of intraspinal tumors in children and show a predilection for the thoracic spine.[182] These lesions most likely result from inclusion of adipose cells from the overlying mesodermal tissue into the developing spinal canal or the folding neural tube.[34,58] A tethered spinal cord occurs when these lesions transverse both the bony and neural elements of the spine.[182]

Lipomas associated with spinal dysraphism take three principal forms: dorsal, terminal, or transitional. In the dorsal form, the lipoma extends from the subcutaneous space through incomplete neural arches and attaches to the dorsal spinal cord. It is rare for nerve roots to be contained within the substance of a dorsal lipoma. Terminal lipomas insert into the distal conus and may be entirely intraspinal, many times containing nerve roots. Features of both dorsal and terminal lipomas appear in transitional lipomas. The embryology of caudal lipomas most likely arises during secondary neurulation. During secondary neurulation the caudal end of the neural tube blends with a large collection of undifferentiated cells, the caudal cell mass. The last phase of secondary neurulation involves regression of the previously formed tail structures, leaving the filum terminale, coccygeal ligament, and the terminal ventricle of the conus as its only remnants. Cell rests with the potential for differentiation may be left in these elements and account for the development of lipomas, hamartomas, teratomas, and the rare malignancy.[114,115,139]

Dermoids and Dermal Sinus Tracts

Dermal sinus tracts are lined by squamous epithelium and may penetrate the spinal cord at any level in the midline from the lumbosacral spine to the occiput. They occur once in every 1500 births.[8] Dermoid and epidermoid nodules can frequently accompany dermal sinus tracts.[42] Dermoid and epidermoid tumors may arise within the tract in approximately half of all dermal sinuses.[8,9] These tumors are also encountered within the subarachnoid space arising from isolated congenital rests of cells derived from the multipotential caudal cell mass.[8,9] The embryology of dermal sinus tracts and dermoids of the spine is probably a result of incomplete dysjunction of ectoderm from endoderm during the fourth week of embryologic development. The dermal tract becomes elongated during ascent of the spinal cord within the spinal canal and may transverse several layers of dermis and epidermal space before entering the subarachnoid space. Dermal sinus tracts may frequently be missed on initial examination of the infant and only become apparent when the child has symptoms of recurrent meningitis.

Tethered Cord

Traditionally, the tethered cord syndrome has been defined as a low-lying conus medullaris because of a short and thickened filum terminale. Recently, the term has been expanded to include a spinal cord that is tethered by fibrous bands/adhesions or an intradural lipoma. The embryologic origin of the short and thickened filum terminale is not known. The pathophysiology of tethered cord syndrome has been postulated to involve hypoxic stress on the stretched spinal cord.[245,246] Clearly, by producing traction on the spinal cord, these lesions can cause profound neurologic deficits.

According to Pang and Wilberger[168] the degree of spinal cord traction, rather than the type or distribution of the tethering lesions, most likely determines the age of symptom onset. They contend that severe traction on the spinal cord results in presentation in childhood, whereas less severe traction is asymptomatic in childhood but appears later in life (because of repeated tugging of the conus during head and neck flexion), or when abnormal tension is aggravated by trauma or spondylotic spinal canal stenosis.[168]

Craniovertebral Junction Abnormalities

Craniovertebral junction abnormalities encompass a group of rare conditions that result from abnormal fetal development. In general, these disorders often remain dormant during childhood and manifest themselves during adulthood or after minor trauma. The close association between neural and vascular structures can result in compromise during the course of aging or after a traumatic insult. The craniovertebral junction includes the skull base, atlas, and axis, as well as the neural and vascular structures contained within them.

Basilar Invagination

Basilar invagination is the most common congenital anomaly of the atlanto-occipital articulation.[230] Basilar invagination results from a defect in the chondrocranium and is often associated with both skeletal and neural axis abnormalities. It results from deformation in all three parts of the occipital bone (basiocciput, exocciput, and squamous occipital bone).[133] Two types of basilar invagination have been identified: ventral and paramedian.[138,226] In ventral basilar invagination, the basiocciput is shortened and there is associated platybasia that raises the plane of the foramen magnum. In paramedian basilar invagination, hypoplasia of the exoccipital bone is present and there is a medial elevation of this portion of the occipital bone. Clinically, the distinction is not important and there is admixture between types.[152] There is an associated elevation of the floor of the posterior fossa that is most pronounced in the region of the foramen magnum. This anomaly may compromise the space available within the foramen magnum.[226,227]

Although the term *basilar impression* is often used synonymously with *basilar invagination,* this condition refers to an acquired form of basilar invagination that is caused by softening of the occipital bone that occurs in conditions such as rheumatoid arthritis, Paget's disease, hyperparathyroidism, achondroplasia, and osteogenesis imperfecta.[133] Associated skeletal developmental anomalies found with basilar invagination include occipitalization of the atlas and Klippel-Feil syndrome in addition to neural axis abnormalities such as Chiari malformation, syringobulbia, syringomyelia, and hydrocephalus.[10,49,56,125,145]

It has been reported that patients who are symptomatic from pure basilar invagination most commonly have complaints of weakness and paresthesias in the limbs, whereas those patients with symptomatic Chiari malformations have cerebellar and vestibular complaints. Both groups occasionally have evidence of lower cranial nerve dysfunction. Many patients do not develop symptoms until the second or third decade of life.[49] This may be related to increasing instability from ligamentous laxity caused by aging similar to delayed myelopathies reported after atlantoaxial dislocations.[77] If chronic instability is present, granulation tissue may develop and act as a space-occupying mass in the ventral portion of the foramen magnum. Fibrous bands and dural adhesions are common in the dorsal cervicomedullary junction and around the cerebellar tonsils in both primary and secondary basilar invagination.[136] There is a reported high incidence of vertebral artery anomalies in basilar invagination, and symptoms of vertebral artery insufficiency can occur.[16,125]

Diagnosis of basilar impression (or invagination) is based on radiographic evaluation that demonstrates the altered relationship between the occipital bone and the upper cervical spine. Classically, this diagnosis was made by radiographic evaluation of the craniovertebral junction. A series of reference lines have been described to assist with this evaluation. Recently, the trend has been toward the use of MRI and computed tomography (CT) as the diagnostic procedures of choice.[110,123] Although MRI delineates the relationship between the neural structures and the bony abnormalities superbly, it does not always define the osseous relationships adequately. Bony pathology should be evaluated with pluridirectional tomography or thin-section CT.

Basilar invagination can be inferred if the lateral atlantoaxial articulations cannot be visualized clearly on an open mouth (anteroposterior) odontoid radiograph.[214,226] Also, the tip of the dens should not exceed 10 mm rostral to the bimastoid line or cross the digastric line.[71]

Lateral radiographic evaluation uses multiple reference lines to determine normal and pathologic craniometric relationships of the craniovertebral junction. Chamberlain's palato-occipital line connects the dorsal hard palate to the dorsal border of the foramen magnum.[38,52] The tip of the odontoid process should lie below this line. McGregor's line is a modification of Chamberlain's line (which is more easily defined), which is drawn from the upper surface of the dorsal edge of the hard palate to the most caudal point of the occipital curve of the skull. A distance of 4.5 mm above McGregor's line is considered abnormal.[125] McRae's foramen magnum line connects the ventral and dorsal edges of the foramen magnum. The tip of the odontoid process should lie below it.[130,131] Wackenheim's clivus-canal line runs along the clivus into the cervical spinal canal, and the odontoid should lie ventral to this line.[227] Basilar invagination causes the odontoid process to lie within the foramen magnum, thus crossing Chamberlain's, McRae's, and Wackenheim's lines.

Assimilation of the Atlas

Assimilation of the atlas represents a failure of segmentation between the atlas and the base of the skull. Embryologically, this entity represents a failure of segmentation between the fourth occipital and first spinal sclerotomes. This condition occurs in 0.25% of the population.[226] The assimilation may be partial or complete and can involve the ventral arch of the atlas, the lateral masses, or the entire atlas. In many instances, assimilation of the atlas occurs with other spinal abnormalities, such as basilar invagination or the Klippel-Feil syndrome, systemic congenital abnormalities such as cleft palate, or urinary tract abnormalities.[19,131,207] Patients with atlanto-occipital fusion often present much like patients with classic Klippel-Feil syndrome with restricted motion, short neck, low hairline, and torticollis.[19,89,131,207] Menezes and colleagues[137] reported 96 patients with assimilation of the atlas who were detected among 890 patients with craniovertebral junction abnormalities. A Chiari malformation was seen in 42 of the 96 patients.[137]

An increased incidence of atlantoaxial instability occurs with assimilation of the atlas, especially if there is failure of segmentation between the second and third vertebrae.[131,133] McRae[130] noted the frequent association of assimilation of the atlas and congenital C2-3 fusion. Pang[167a] reported on patients with both assimilation of the atlas and fusion between the second and third vertebrae. All patients demonstrated instability between the atlas and axis that was generally reducible with traction in children under the age of 15 years. Fusion between the second and third vertebrae was present in 32 of the 96 patients with assimilation of the atlas reported by Menezes *et al.*[137]

Reducible atlantoaxial instability or reducible basilar invagination occurred in 15 of 18 children under the age of 14 years in this series.[137] With age progression, the reducibility decreased. This was most likely related to the formation of tough fibrotic granulation tissue around the dislocation.[133,136]

The onset of symptoms in assimilation of the atlas generally occurs between the ages of 20 and 40 years.[89] Dull headache and scalp tenderness in the distribution of the greater occipital nerve occurs frequently. Ventral compression of the brain stem from the odontoid processes is also a common finding. It can produce weakness, spasticity, gait disturbances, or cranial nerve dysfunction.[91] Neurologic symptoms have been related to the position of the odontoid process as an indication of the degree of actual or relative basilar impression.[90,130,131] Vertical and horizontal nystagmus is related to cerebellum and tonsillar abnormalities. Decreased posterior column function from dorsal compression by the foramen magnum or a dural band are less common findings.[206] Acute trauma and infection of the upper respiratory tract have been associated with the onset of symptoms of atlantoaxial instability.[136] Symptoms may develop precipitously, but in the majority of cases a gradual onset is observed.[85]

Atlantoaxial Instability

Atlantoaxial instability may result from aplasia or hypoplasia of the odontoid process, from laxity of the transverse ligament, or with assimilation of the atlas. Atlantoaxial instability is associated with Down syndrome, Klippel-Feil syndrome, numerous skeletal dysplasias, osteogenesis imperfecta, neurofibromatosis, and congenital scoliosis.[15,31,48,62,230] The clinical significance of this condition is the potential for neurologic compromise, which can range from pain and dysesthesias in the distribution of the greater occipital nerve to tetraplegia or death.[88] The articulation between the first and second cervical vertebrae is the most mobile segment in the vertebral column and has the least inherent stability.[94] The odontoid process acts as a bony buttress that prevents hyperextension. However, the remainder of the normal range of motion is maintained and is dependent on the integrity of the ligamentous and capsular structures.[94] Neurologic compromise can occur despite a normal odontoid process. With an attenuated or ruptured transverse atlantal ligament, a relative ventral shift of the atlas over the axis can result in spinal cord injury by impingement against the intact odontoid process such as occurs with atlantal assimilation.[88,179] The risk is less if the odontoid process is absent, fractured, or moves with the axis during flexion, as occurs with most cases of os odontoideum.[69]

The stability of the atlantoaxial joint can often be determined using lateral radiographs. The atlantodens interval (ADI) is the distance between the dorsal edge of the ventral ring of the atlas and the ventral edge of the odontoid process. The normal ADI is less than 3mm in adults and less than 4 mm in children.[68,98,119] Fielding *et al.*[68] suggested that an ADI greater than 3mm in adults indicates a disruption of the transverse ligament. An ADI of 5 to 10mm represents additional ligamentous damage with total ligamentous disruption occurring in patients with an ADI greater than 10mm.[68] In congenital anomalies, such as hypoplasia of the odontoid process or os odontoideum, the space available for the cord (SAC) is often a better predictor of potential for neurologic compromise. The SAC is the distance from the ventral edge of the dorsal ring of the atlas or foramen magnum to the dorsal aspect of the odontoid process or the dorsal aspect of axis (whichever is less). Greenberg[84] suggested that in the adult, spinal cord compression always occurred when the SAC was 14mm or less and never occurred if the SAC was 18mm or more. In cases of os odontoideum, a SAC of 13mm or less is associated with neurologic sequelae.[206] In cases with persistent concerns about atlantoaxial stability, flexion/extension lateral radiographs can be performed. An awake patient should voluntarily perform the flexion/extension movements. MRI should be considered for any patient with a neurologic deficit before obtaining flexion/extension radiographs. MRI with flexion and extension views provides an excellent method of determining the potential for neural impingement with movement.

Anomalies of the Odontoid Process

Aplasia-Hypoplasia of the Dens

Aplasia-hypoplasia of the dens is a rare condition that has a spectrum of presentations ranging from a hypoplastic rudimentary dens to complete absence of the dens. Usually, the rudimentary dens does not reach the upper edge of the ventral arch of the atlas, and there is an associated incompetence of the cruciate ligaments and alar ligaments resulting in atlantoaxial instability. This may be associated with the unusual occurrence of the developmental form of os odontoideum.[138,199] Distinguishing aplasia or hypoplasia is of limited clinical importance because both conditions can lead to atlantoaxial instability and treatment is identical.[92] Odontoid dysplasia may occur with various types of inborn errors of metabolism, especially dwarfing syndromes.[80,82,172]

Odontoid hypoplasia and os odontoideum are present in 30% to 35% of cases of atlantoaxial instability in patients with Down syndrome.[133] Vascular compromise from stretching and torsion of the vertebral arteries has been reported. Chronic atlantoaxial dislocation may provoke the formation of granulation tissue that can cause neurologic deficit because of constriction of the cervicomedullary junction.[134] Nagashima[147] evaluated patients with atlantoaxial dislocation with congenital anomalies of the odontoid process and divided the clinical presentation into three categories: acute, delayed, and chronic. Acute dislocation is related to a traumatic event; it may result in death if bony displacement is significant (via damage to the cervical spinal cord or vertebral arteries). In the delayed type, the onset of symptoms occurs months to years after the inciting trauma and often progresses to become disabling. In the chronic type, there is no history of trauma, but symptoms can also progress to chronic myelopathy.[147] The presentation in children with atlantoaxial dislocation and congenital anomalies is varied. Generalized weakness is common, but syncope, torticollis, dysesthesia, and tetraplegia have also been reported.[147]

Os Odontoideum

Os odontoideum is defined as an independent ossicle located rostral to the axis bone in the position of the odontoid process that is separated from a hypoplastic dens by a variable distance.* The space between the os odontoideum and the remnant of the odontoid process is above the level of the superior facet of the axis. This leads to potential incompetence of the transverse ligament, which can lead to atlantoaxial instability.[136] In children younger than 5 years of age, the normal epiphyseal line may be confused with the presence of an os odontoideum or a fracture. In os odontoideum, the free ossicle is rounded or oval, with a smooth cortical border. In the case of an odontoid fracture, the gap is usually narrow and irregular and often extends into the body of the axis at the level of the superior facet of the axis vertebra.[136] There is an increased incidence of os odontoideum in Down syndrome, spondyloepiphyseal dysplasia, Morquio's syndrome, and after upper respiratory tract infections.†

There are two types of os odontoideum: orthotopic and dystopic.[69] With the orthotopic variety, the ossicle lies in the location of the normal dens and moves with the axis body and the ventral arch of the atlas.[69,135,226] This type is often associated with an intact cruciate ligament.[133,136] In the dystopic variety, the os is located near the basion and is often fused to the clivus. The ventral arch of the atlas is hypertrophied and the dorsal arch is hypoplastic. Dystopic os odontoideum has a greater likelihood of causing neurologic compromise than the orthotopic variety.[133] This may occur because of dorsal compromise of the spinal cord by the ventrally located dorsal arch of the atlas during flexion and ventral compromise by the odontoid ossicle.[135] Evaluation of atlantoaxial instability should be performed with flexion extension MRI and polytomography. In cases of chronic subluxation, dense granulation tissue may form, leading to an irreducible state. Direct examination at the time of surgery for irreducible dislocations has demonstrated that the transverse portion of the cruciate ligament has slipped in front or behind the ossicle.[136]

The etiology of os odontoideum has been ascribed to congenital, vascular, and traumatic causes. Trauma or infection during childhood is the most likely etiology for the vast majority of cases of os odontoideum. Several cases have been reported in children with a normal odontoid process before trauma who subsequently developed os odontoideum.‡ Most patients have a significant episode of trauma before the diagnosis of os odontoideum.[69] After fracture or vascular compromise a separation of the bone fragments occurs, probably because of contracture of the apical ligaments. The ossicle continues to receive a blood supply via the apical arcade, but the blood supply in the region of the fracture is disrupted, resulting in poor healing. It is probable that there are congenital forms of os odontoideum. The congenital form results from failure of fusion of the portions of the dens derived from the proatlas and first cervical sclerotome. Dystopic os odontoideum is probably congenital in origin.

---

*References 5,52,55,69,84,86,211.
†References 15,45,48,79,118,121,208,209.
‡References 68,69,86,96,99,178.

Disorders of the Subaxial Cervical Spine
Klippel-Feil Syndrome

Klippel-Feil syndrome was first described as a case report with the clinical triad of a short neck, low dorsal hairline, and marked limitation of cervical range of motion resulting from single unsegmented vertebral mass extending from the craniocervical junction through the fourth thoracic vertebra.[108] Fewer than half of patients have all three signs.[93] The most consistent finding is limitation of cervical motion.[83] Currently, the term *Klippel-Feil syndrome* is used to describe any congenital fusion of the cervical spine with or without the clinical features of the original description (Figure 4.5).

The incidence of Klippel-Feil syndrome in the general population is not known. Brown *et al.*[30] reviewed 1400 skeletal specimens and found a 0.71% incidence of congenital fusions. They also reviewed all cervical radiographs performed at their institution during 1 year and found 0.6% congenital fusions.[30]

Often patients with Klippel-Feil syndrome have associated congenital abnormalities. These are often the conditions that prompt evaluation. Scoliosis is the most common associated condition, with 60% of patients having a signifi-

cant degree of scoliosis.[242] Careful monitoring is required because most of these patients required treatment with bracing or surgery.[93] The Klippel-Feil syndrome occurs in 25% of patients with congenital scoliosis.[242] Therefore, all patients with congenital scoliosis should have radiographs of the entire spine and skull to exclude the coexistence of the Klippel-Feil syndrome and, conversely, all patients with the Klippel-Feil syndrome should have radiographs of the lower spine. Approximately 50% of patients with congenital cervical or cervicothoracic scoliosis have associated Klippel-Feil anomalies. When cervical scoliosis is associated with Klippel-Feil anomalies, severe progressive lateral deviation of the neck and/or torticollis can develop.[202] Renal anomalies occur in over one third of patients. It has been suggested that routine screening ultrasonography be performed in all patients with Klippel-Feil syndrome.[53,93,143]

Sprengel's deformity (an abnormal elevation of the scapula) occurs in 25% to 35% of cases of Klippel-Feil syndrome. It may be unilateral or bilateral.[81,93,124,217] Other less-common associated anomalies include deafness, synkinesis (involuntary paired movements of the hands and occasionally the arms), congenital heart disease, cervical ribs, ptosis, Duane's contracture (an abducens nerve palsy in which the adducted eye becomes retracted), lateral rec-

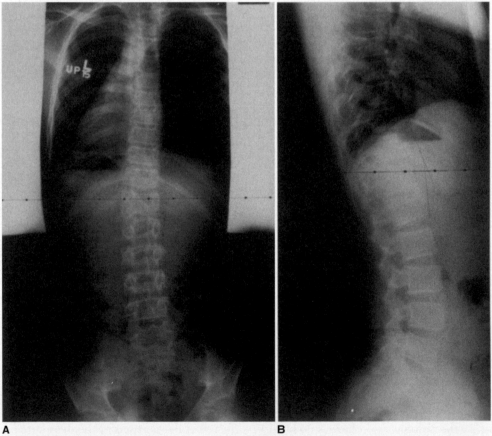

A   **B**

Figure 4.5 (**A**) Frontal and (**B**) lateral radiographs of a boy aged 12 years with a shortened neck and congenital hemivertebra at the thoracolumbar junction. Cervical films revealed a Klippel-Feil anomaly with fusion from C3-6. (**C**) Flexion and (**D**) extension radiographs demonstrated 10 mm of C1-2 instability; (**E** and **F**) treatment consisted of a dorsal C1-2 fusion. Lateral mass screws were used instead of sublaminar wires because the C1 lamina (**F**) was dysplastic.

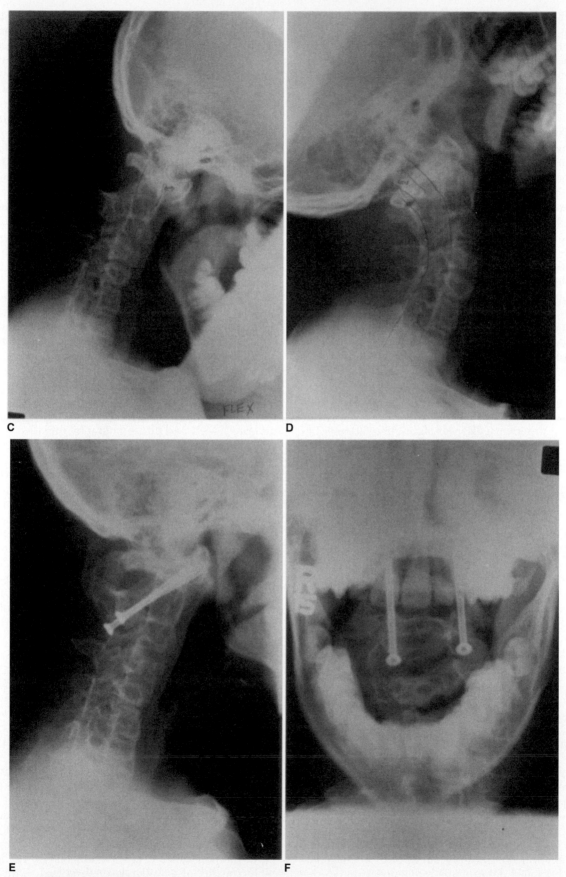

Figure 4.5 *cont'd*

tus palsy, facial nerve palsy, syndactyly, hypoplastic thumb, and upper extremity hypoplasia.[44,83,93,124,217]

Symptoms related to the Klippel-Feil syndrome can be classified as mechanical or secondary to neural compression. Cervical instability and stenosis are potential problems in Klippel-Feil patients. The spinal cord area adjacent to the vertebral fusion may be compressed because of cervical instability particularly at the occipital-C1 and C1-2 levels.[93,242] All of these patients should have flexion-extension cervical spine radiographs. Winter et al.[242] found, in their review of Klippel-Feil patients, that only 2% of the cervical anomalies required treatment, but that the associated scoliosis in the thoracic and lumbar spine was treated in the majority of cases. Neurologic deficits can range from radiculopathy to sudden death from minor trauma.* Overall, 20% of patients who develop neurologic symptoms do so during the first 5 years of life and 65% by the age of 30 years.[83] Neurologic symptoms detected during infancy are usually related to cranioverbtebral junction abnormalities. Children often have pain with atlantoaxial fusions; lower cervical fusions that are not massive often do not become problematic until the third decade or later, when degenerative changes begin to develop.[83,113] Patients with short segment fusions are less likely to develop symptoms, because of compensatory movement at uninvolved segments.[83]

Iniencephaly

Iniencephaly describes a disorder of the cervical spine consisting of congenital cervical synostoses, fixed retroflexion of the head, severe cervical lordosis, and varying degrees of deficits of the dorsal occiput and cervical vertebrae. This condition probably belongs to the spectrum of neural tube defects.[104,198,200] The majority of fetuses with this condition are not viable.[101,104,180] Parents of a child with iniencephaly have a 5% risk of having another child with a neural tube defect. Ultrasound and serum or amniotic α-fetoprotein can be used to detect this condition in utero.[144,189,198]

Surviving patients are often handicapped by the cervical lordosis and hyperextension of the head. This posture makes it impossible to see straight without flexing the low back and hips. Correction of this deformity with a dorsal suboccipital release, followed by bracing with a halo cast (with further correction through the use of turn-buckles) has been reported.[134,200]

Disorders of the Thoracolumbar Spine

Congenital Scoliosis

Congenital scoliosis is an abnormal curvature of the spine in the coronal plane that develops when anomalous vertebrae are present at birth. Congenital scoliosis is distinct from infantile idiopathic scoliosis, although both appear with deformity during childhood. Infantile idiopathic scoliosis has no structural vertebral abnormality. Although vertebral abnormalities are present at birth in congenital scoliosis, the spinal deformity is rarely noticeable during infancy, and usually presents during childhood or adoles-

---

*References 62,65,112,148,151,212.

cence. Patients with mild or compensated deformities are often diagnosed as adults when vertebral anomalies are discovered incidentally during routine radiographs. Congenital scoliosis can be associated with a variety of cardiac, genitourinary, and skeletal abnormalities.[59,93,127]

There is a wide spectrum of clinical presentations because of the range in number, location, and type of vertebral abnormalities that can exist in any individual. Certain vertebral anomalies result in rapidly progressive scoliosis during early childhood, resulting in severe morbidity, whereas other anomalies cause little or no deformity at any time.[129] In general, 25% of congenital scolioses do not progress, 50% progress slowly, and 25% progress rapidly.[241] Major advancements in the treatment of congenital scoliosis are improved imaging of the spine by CT and MRI, classification by type of vertebral anomaly, improved understanding of the natural history, and clarification of the indications and timing of surgery.

Advances in imaging have aided the diagnosis of associated neural axis abnormalities, such as occult spinal dysraphism and tethering of the spinal cord. Between 10% to 20% of all congenital scoliosis patients have some anomaly of the neural axis.[127] Dorsal midline skin lesions (such as hairy patches or deep dimples), asymmetric foot deformities (cavus or flat feet), muscle weakness, or spasticity all suggest underlying nervous system abnormalities. A thorough imaging evaluation is therefore indicated. MRI and ultrasonography provide the diagnosis of genitourinary abnormalities without an intravenous pyelogram.

Normal spine growth is a result of the total growth that occurs at the end-plates of the upper and lower surfaces of the vertebral bodies.[20] Congenital vertebral anomalies can cause absence, or functional deficiency, of the growth plates on one or both sides of the spine. Asymmetric spine growth results from a difference in growth between the greater and lesser affected sides of the spine. In some cases, normal growth occurs on one side and no growth on the other, producing a large deformity. The rate of deterioration and the final severity of the congenital scoliosis are proportional to the degree of growth imbalance produced by the vertebral anomalies. The location of the deficient growth plates determines whether a pure scoliosis exists or if some component of sagittal plane deformity is present, resulting in kyphoscoliosis or lordoscoliosis. Winter et al.[241] evaluated the prognosis for scoliosis progression for congenital vertebral abnormalities and devised a radiographic classification scheme.

Usually, the vertebral abnormalities can be classified by the anomaly in the mesenchymal precursor that results in either a failure of formation or a failure of segmentation. Failure of formation results from a defect in the developmental process that produces an absence of part or all of the vertebrae. The defects range from mild wedging to total absence of the vertebra. A hemivertebra occurs with the complete absence of half of a vertebra and is one of the most common causes of congenital scoliosis. The hemivertebra consists of a wedged vertebral body with a single pedicle and hemilamina (Figure 4.6).

Segmentation failure causes unilateral or bilateral bony fusion between vertebrae. The defect can involve ventral

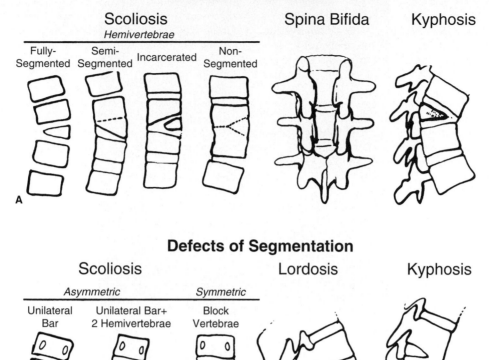

Figure 4.6 Structural abnormalities in congenital spine deformity. **(A)** Defects in formation resulting in congenital scoliosis, spina bifida, and congenital (type I) kyphosis. **(B)** Defects of segmentation that result in congenital scoliosis, congenital lordosis, and congenital (type II) kyphosis.

elements, dorsal elements, or both. The most common segmentation failure is the unilateral unsegmented bar, which results in a bony block that involves the disc spaces and facet joints (Figure 4.7). A combination of defects of formation and defects of segmentation can coexist in the same patient. An unsegmented bar with contralateral hemivertebrae can cause severe progressive scoliosis.[129,149]

Three major types of hemivertebrae are classified by the positioning of the hemivertebra and whether the disc spaces above and below the hemivertebra are morphologically normal (Figure 4.8). A *fully segmented hemivertebra* has a normal disc space above and below the vertebral body that allows near-normal longitudinal growth. There is an absence of a portion of the vertebral body and growth plates on the side of the unformed vertebra that results in limited growth potential. Because of full growth potential on one side of the spine and none on the other side at the level of the hemivertebra, there is a potential for significant deformity development. The hemivertebra is located at the apex of the scoliosis in these cases. The rate of progression and the need for treatment of the scoliosis caused by a fully segmented hemivertebra depends on its location

in the spine, with the thoracolumbar and the lumbosacral junction being the most problematic.[128] In general, these scoliotic curves progress at one to two degrees per year.[128,129]

The *incarcerated hemivertebra* is a variant of the fully segmented hemivertebrae. This type of hemivertebra is set into defects in the vertebrae above and below it. The incarcerated hemivertebra is small, oval, and with poorly formed disc spaces. The defects in the adjacent vertebrae tend to compensate for the hemivertebra, and the poor potential growth of the malformed growth plates results in less scoliotic deformity compared with the standard fully segmented vertebrae.[128]

A *semisegmented hemivertebra* is connected to either the vertebra above or below it and causes the absence of one disc space on the side of the hemivertebra with obliteration of two growth plates. Theoretically, this would result in similar growth on both sides of the spine because two active growth plates coexist on each side. However, the wedge shape of the hemivertebra and differences in growth (between sides) can result in some scoliosis.

A nonsegmented hemivertebra is connected to the vertebrae above and below, with no disc spaces and no growth

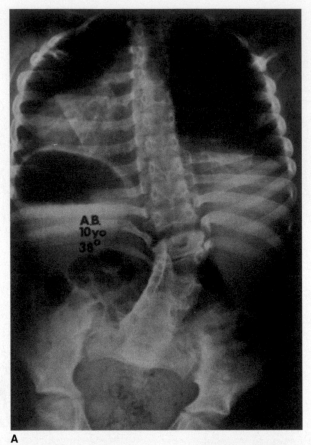

A

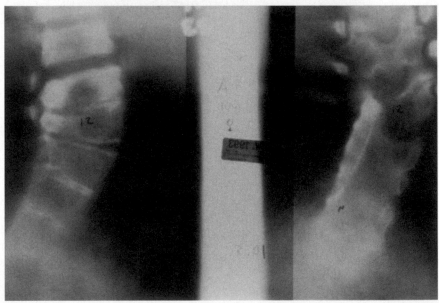

B

Figure 4.7 **(A)** A girl aged 4 years with congenital lumbar scoliosis (measuring 17 degrees) secondary to unilateral bar from T11 to the sacrum. **(B)** AP tomography showing the laminar synostosis.

potential. Although the wedge shape of the hemivertebra may cause some deformity, it is not progressive.

Another common cause of congenital scoliosis is a unilateral unsegmented bar.[129,240] This condition results from a failure of segmentation of two or more vertebrae. The unsegmented bar contains no growth plates but the unaf-

fected side of the spine continues to grow. The imbalance in growth results in the scoliosis with the unsegmented bar in the concavity. The rate of deterioration and final severity of scoliosis are determined by the number of vertebrae involved with the bar and the growth potential of the convexity. On average these curves deteriorate at a rate of

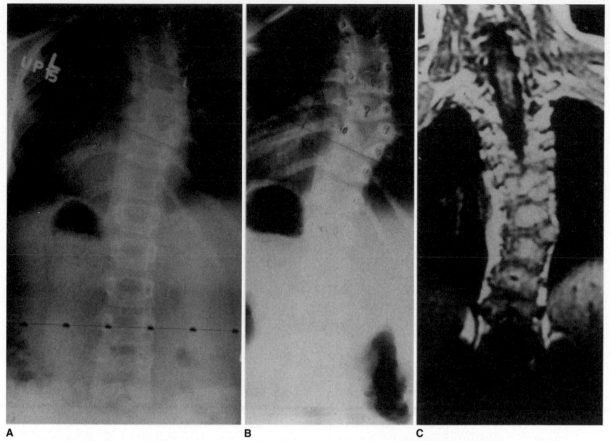

Figure 4.8 A girl aged 6 years presented with (**A** and **B**) 40 degree thoracic congenital scoliosis secondary to a right hemivertebra at T6 and T9, opposite the left rib and pedicle fusion from T4 to T6 (**C**). MRI revealed the fully segmented hemivertebra at T9 and semisegmented hemivertebra at T6.

5 degrees or greater per year and often result in a significant deformity.[129]

Congenital Kyphosis

Congenital kyphosis is an uncommon sagittal plane deformity that, if left untreated, is often associated with neurologic deficit.[141,243] As with congenital scoliosis, congenital kyphosis is caused by formation segmentation failure. Winter *et al.*[243] classified congenital kyphosis into three types: type I is the failure of formation of the vertebral body; type II is the failure of segmentation of the vertebral body, resulting in a ventral unsegmented bar; and type III is the mixed failure of formation and segmentation. The type I kyphosis is the most common and the most likely to develop both severe deformity and neurologic compromise.[141,243] The severity of type I kyphosis is directly proportional to the amount of vertebral body or bodies that fail to form.[243] The type II kyphosis is less common, produces less severe deformity, and is much less frequently associated with neurologic compromise than type I. The amount of kyphosis produced is proportional to the discrepancy between the ventral vertebral growth and the growth of the dorsal elements. Type III kyphosis is very rare and probably behaves like type I kyphosis.

Congenital Lordosis

Congenital lordosis is more rare than either congenital scoliosis or congenital kyphosis. This condition results from dorsal defects in segmentation, with normal ventral growth.[240] Often, it has some component of coronal plane deformity, leading to lordoscoliosis because of a dorsolateral location of the unsegmented bar. The most severe consequence of congenital lordosis is the development of an impairment of pulmonary function.[238,240]

Lumbar Spine Abnormalities

Congenital Spinal Stenosis

Congenital spinal stenosis occurs in a very small number of patients who present with spinal stenosis.[220] It results from a malformation present at birth that predisposes the patient to the development of stenosis, which often manifests itself later in life.[47] Verbiest described four patients whose first symptoms appeared between the ages of 45 and 50 years. Two of these patients had block vertebrae with hypoplastic articulations, and the other two had occult dysraphism with upward directed lamina, paramedial clefts, and narrowed interpedicular diameters.[220,222]

Verbiest described three types of congenital spinal stenosis. The first is a stenosis as a part of spinal dysraphism.[218-223] The signs and symptoms are usually not only the consequence of stenosis alone, but also of myelodysplasia. They eventually are associated with a lipoma. Serious radicular neurologic deficit occurs frequently in this condition.

The second type is a stenosis in an area of failure of vertebral segmentation (block vertebrae). Stenosis in the area of the block vertebrae was determined by a reduction of the midsagittal diameters of the vertebral canal. The signs and symptoms did not differ from those observed with idiopathic developmental stenosis.

The third type is an intermittent stenosis (De Anquin's syndrome) in which the spinous process of S1 is absent and the lamina of S1 has a large medial cleft. There may be a residual island of bone in the area of the cleft. This malformation is associated with a downward hooklike elongation of the spinous process of L5. The assumption of an increased lordotic posture during standing or walking, the tip of the hooklike spinous process of L5 presses directly on the ligamentum bridging the spina bifida occulta of S1 or on the rudimentary bony island in its central portion, thus reducing the midsagittal diameter of the upper sacral canal. This condition results in radicular pain during standing or walking and is relieved by sitting.[222]

Developmental Spinal Stenosis

Congenital spinal stenosis is differentiated from developmental spinal stenosis, which usually occurs as the result of an inborn chromosomal error or mutation that alters the fetal and postnatal spinal canal formation.[4] Developmental spinal stenosis commonly occurs in conditions such as achondroplasia, hypochondroplasia, diastrophic dwarfism, Morquio's syndrome, and hereditary multiple exostoses.[13,17,18,29,63] Idiopathic developmental spinal stenosis has been reported.[163,218,219,223] This condition may involve only the lumbar spine or can be associated with developmental stenosis of the cervical spine.[24,57,64]

Segmented Spinal Dysgenesis

Segmental spinal dysgenesis is a localized congenital defect in which severe stenosis occurs with malalignment and focal agenesis or dysgenesis in the thoracolumbar or lumbar spine.[192,193,195,239,242] This condition was initially described by Sarpyener.[192,193] Winter et al.[239] initially described this condition as congenital spinal stenosis and described nine patients with focal narrowing of the spinal canal in the area of the thoracolumbar junction. Neurologic deficits are often present at birth and may range from mild paresis to complete paraplegia. Patients may have congenital absence of nerve root or spinal cord segments. The spinal canal above and below the involved segment is usually normal and the sacrum is well formed, differentiating this condition from sacral agenesis. Winter et al.[239] described 20 patients with this condition. Localized spinal stenosis was a universal finding. The stenotic area ranged from three to six vertebral segments. Patients presented for medical evaluation from birth to 19 years of age, but the majority presented at 1 to 4 years. The majority of patients had involvement of the thoraco-

lumbar junction, but two had spinal dysgenesis of the upper thoracic spine, and one patient had extension to L4.[239] The etiology of this process is unknown.

Dysplastic (Congenital) Spondylolisthesis

Spondylolisthesis is the slippage of all or part of one vertebra onto another. A number of different etiologies have been identified. The role of upright posture contributing to this condition is well recognized. It has been stated that no known cases of spondylolysis or spondylolisthesis have been identified in nonambulatory patients.[185] Spondylolisthesis is extremely rare during infancy.[12,22,186] Newman[152] noted the association of spondylolysis with the onset of ambulation in early childhood. It has been suggested that spondylolisthesis results from a congenital defect or dysplasia that results in the development of a pars defect resulting from the stresses of upright posture and lumbar lordosis.[27]

The most widely accepted classification of spondylolisthesis is by Wiltse and colleagues.[235] They divided spondylolisthesis into five types: type I is dysplastic spondylolisthesis, type II is isthmic spondylolisthesis, type III is degenerative spondylolisthesis, type IV is traumatic spondylolisthesis, and type V is pathologic spondylolisthesis. Wiltse and Rothman[236] later suggested a common congenital component in the etiology of dysplastic and isthmic spondylolisthesis and further refined classification of spondylolisthesis.

Dysplastic spondylolisthesis accounts for 14% to 21% of the cases of spondylolisthesis with a 2:1 female to male ratio.[25,152,235] This type is characterized by structural anomalies of the lumbosacral junction, including dysplasia of the lamina and facet joints. The lack of the normal facet buttress provided by normal facet joints predisposes toward a slippage of the rostral vertebra on its caudal counterpart.[235] The dysplastic articular processes may be oriented in the axial or sagittal planes. In axial dysplasia, the articular processes have a horizontal orientation. This condition is often associated with spina bifida. In sagittal dysplasia the facet joints are often asymmetric, but the neural arch is usually intact. Therefore, high-grade slippage seldom occurs. Both types can present with hamstring spasm, back or leg pain, or neurologic deficit, including paresthesia, weakness, or, rarely, incontinence of the bowel or bladder. Neurologic deficits are usually associated with high-grade slips.

Axially oriented facet joints associated with spinal bifida have an increased risk for high-grade spondylolisthesis.[32] The pars interarticularis is often poorly developed and may elongate, develop a defect, or remain intact. If the pars interarticularis remains intact, neurologic symptoms usually occur only when the spondylolisthesis exceeds 35%.[32] Progression of spondylolisthesis is more likely in younger or skeletally immature patients and in patients with wide spina bifida. Initial treatment should be nonoperative unless progression is documented in younger patients or slippage greater than 50% is observed at the time of the initial evaluation. Fusion in situ is the most frequently performed surgical procedure, although some surgeons use reduction and fixation, especially with high-grade slips.

Spondylolisthesis in patients with sagittally oriented facet joints and an intact L5 lamina is frequently treated with decompression, along with fusion. Often, this results in a more rapid resolution of hamstring tightness and spasm.

Disorders of the Sacral Spine

Sacral Agenesis

Sacral agenesis has been defined as a group of disorders characterized by an absence of variable portions of the caudal spine. Williams and Nixon[234] coined the term *sacral agenesis* in 1957. Sacral agenesis belongs within the spectrum of aplastic vertebral malformations that are loosely grouped under the entity of caudal regression syndrome. It can range from agenesis of the coccyx to absence of sacral, lumbar, and lower thoracic vertebrae.[166]

The clinical severity parallels the number of spinal segments involved with the aplasia or dysplasia. With increasing severity, there are often associated anomalies of the genitourinary, gastrointestinal, and urinary systems.[210] Patients with sacral agenesis usually lack motor function below the level of the last normal vertebra. Of interest in sacral agenesis, compared with other dysplastic syndromes of the lower spine (e.g., myelomeningocele), is that sensation is relatively spared below the level of the lesion. In the development of the human embryo, the notochord induces the formation of the ventral spinal elements and cells derived from neural crest independently from the dorsal root ganglia. Thus an insult specific to the notochord/ventral spine could lead to the observed clinical picture in sacral agenesis.[103]

The exact incidence of sacral agenesis is difficult to determine because mild caudal agenesis is often not clini-cally apparent and severe cases can result in stillbirth or neonatal death.[166] Sacral agenesis is a relatively rare lesion. An incidence of 1 in 25,000 live births has been reported.[187] Sacral agenesis is considered to have a sporadic, nonfamilial inheritance pattern, although cases of siblings with the disorder have been reported.[66] Maternal diabetes appears to increase the risk of sacral agenesis.[21] Embryonal trauma producing longitudinal kinking of the long embryonic axis, dietary deficiencies, and teratogenic chemicals have caused caudal agenesis in experimental models.[1,66,166] Caudal agenesis, as well as other associated congenital anomalies such as imperforate anus and cloacal exstrophy, result from alterations in the normal formation and development of the caudal eminence.[66] The caudal eminence is a mass of undifferentiated cells at the caudal end of the embryo that gives rise to the distal spinal cord, the vertebral column, urogenital, and anorectal structures.[66]

Sacral agenesis has been classified into four types by Renshaw,[177] who based his classification on the amount of remaining sacrum and the orientation of the sacral articulation. Type I occurs in either partial or total unilateral agenesis of the sacrum. Type II is bilaterally symmetric partial agenesis of the sacrum, with a normal or hypoplastic first sacral vertebra and a stable articulation of the ilia with the first sacral vertebra. Type III is variable lumbar with total sacral agenesis. The ilia articulate with the lowest vertebra present in type III. Type IV is like type III lesions, except that the caudal end-plate of the lowest vertebra inserts on fused ilia or an iliac amphiarthrosis. Pang[166] recently devised a new classification scheme that combined salient features from other classification schemes (Figure 4.9). By this method, lumbosacral agenesis is divided into five types, with some of these

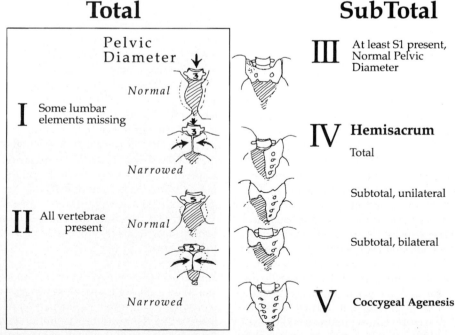

Figure 4.9 Classification of sacral agenesis. Types I and II have subtypes with normal and narrowed pelvic diameter. Type III is subtotal and S1 is at least present. Type IV consists of the varieties of hemisacrum possible, and type V splits into total and subtotal subtypes. (*Modified from Pang D: Sacral agenesis and caudal spinal cord malformations. Neurosurgery 32[5]: 755-779, 1993.*)

divided into subtypes. Type I is total sacral agenesis with some lumbar vertebrae also missing. Type II is total sacral agenesis with the lumbar vertebrae not involved. Type III is subtotal sacral agenesis with at least S1 present and the ilia articulate with the side of the rudimentary sacrum. Type IV is a hemisacrum, and type V is coccygeal agenesis.[166]

The clinical features of sacral agenesis can be quite severe. Because of the lack of motor innervation of the lower limbs, intrauterine contractures develop.[191] In severe forms of sacral agenesis, Renshaw III and IV, the malformation in the spine/pelvis articulation causes a severe kyphosis to develop. Affected children sit in the "Buddha" position with legs flexed and crossed and lean forward because of the kyphosis.[188] Other spinal deformities develop in children with sacral agenesis. Congenital and developmental scoliosis is common.[87,173] Klippel-Feil syndrome has also been reported.[175]

Multiple musculoskeletal deformities can present in patients with sacral agenesis. Hip dysplasia, club foot, and knee flexion contractures are common.[21,74,173] It appears that the etiologic factor responsible for sacral agenesis, such as an insult to the caudal eminence, occurs during the time of organogenesis. Therefore, children with sacral agenesis can present with multiple abnormalities of the gastrointestinal, cardiac, and renal systems.[70,166] There can be associated abnormalities of the terminal spinal cord associated with sacral agenesis. These include elongated conus medullaris with hydromyelia, tethering of the spinal cord by a thickened filum terminale, lipomas, split cord malformations, and terminal myelocystoceles.[166] Neurogenic bladder almost always results in cases of sacral agenesis above S2.[109]

Sacral Abnormalities

Teratomas

Teratomas in the spine almost exclusively occur in the sacrococcygeal region. This is due to their origin from pluripotent tissue derived from the area around Hensen's node.[2] This tissue migrates rostrally to lie in the coccyx. These usually benign tumors can undergo malignant transformation with delayed diagnosis or treatment.[216] In a recent series, 78% of sacrococcygeal teratomas (SCT) were benign and 22% malignant.[196]

Sacrococcygeal teratoma is the most common neoplasm in the newborn, with a reported incidence of 1 in 35,000 live births.[61,169] Of affected infants, 75% are female.[60] The majority of tumors are large, external, and cystic. The tumor mass usually protrudes from between the anus and the coccyx, although some tumors are located predominantly in the presacral space of the pelvis. Although the diagnosis is often possible prenatally by ultrasound, small presacral tumors can be missed in the newborn. The tumors range in size but average approximately 8.5 cm.[155,216] The cystic component is usually cerebrospinal fluid (CSF) but is not connected with circulating spinal fluid within the thecal sac. The spinal fluid arises from choroid plexus contained within the tumor mass.[60]

Sacrococcygeal teratomas have been classified into four types: type I tumors are totally external; type II tumors are almost totally external; type III tumors are almost completely internal; and type IV tumors are completely internal.[60] Symptoms are largely related to the degree of displacement or obstruction of the bladder, urethra, or rectum.

Surgical therapy by midline or chevron incision is the mainstay for benign SCT. After removal of the tumor with coccygectomy, survival is 95%.[196] Presacral tumors may require an abdominal approach combined with the usual sacral approach. Multiagent adjuvant chemotherapy is added to surgical therapy for malignant tumors with survival in up to 80% of cases reported.[196]

Syringomyelia

No discussion of congenital spinal lesions would be complete without including syringomyelia, a fluid-filled cavity of the spinal cord (Figure 4.10). Syringomyelia occurs frequently in the cervical and thoracic spine. Although not directly a congenital malformation, it may be considered a

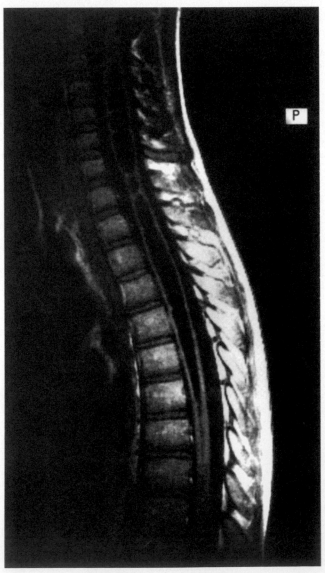

Figure 4.10 Congenital syrinx.

developmental abnormality because of its frequent association with malformations of the hindbrain (Chiari malformation).[137]

The Chiari I malformation is not associated with myelomeningoceles, as is the Chiari II malformation. It is not clear which embryologic miscues cause these conditions. It has been suggested that overgrowth of the cerebellum and medulla cause these malformations.[6] It has also been proposed that the Chiari I malformation is caused by difference in pressure between the cranial and spinal subarachnoid space. Patients who have undergone lumbar-peritoneal shunting occasionally develop Chiari I–like malformations. A higher incidence of traumatic delivery and presumed subarachnoid hemorrhage has been found in patients with Chiari I malformations.[153,231,233] This allows the formation of subarachnoid adhesions that impair CSF flow and thus allows a differential pressure between the cranial and spinal compartments to develop.

Concerning the pathophysiology of the hindbrain herniation in Chiari II malformations, some believe that spinal cord tethering, by the myelomeningocele, causes the herniation of the hindbrain. Research indicates that the presence of the meningocele predates the formation of the hindbrain hernia.[162]

Chiari malformations cause herniation of the cerebellar tonsils into the foramen magnum and scarring of the dura mater to the tonsils. There is a 50% to 75% incidence of cavitation (syrinx) of the spinal cord. The posterior fossa is small because of flattening of the squamous occipital bone. The foramen magnum is enlarged to accommodate the descended cerebellar tonsils.

Debate exists over the complex pathophysiology involved in syrinx formation in Chiari malformations.[233] The hydrodynamic theory, proposed by Gardner,[78] states that the arterial pulse is transmitted to the central canal of the spinal cord and creates distention by a "water hammer" effect. Williams' cranial-spinal pressure dissociation theory relies on the herniated tonsils to act as a one-way valve to allow fluid to pass easily from the spinal subarachnoid space to the cranial subarachnoid space, but prevent flow in the opposite direction.[233] This CSF then tracts into the fourth ventricle and outflows into the central canal because of a large craniospinal pressure difference. A combination of these two theories may explain syringomyelia associated with Chiari malformations.

Syringomyelia may present with pain in the spine, limb, and trunk. Radiographic features may be widening of the spinal canal and erosion of the vertebrae.[232] In support of the theories of misguided CSF flow around the herniated cerebellar tonsils, posterior fossa decompression without cyst drainage is usually curative.[33]

Summary

Many important embryologic events result in the development of the spine. The development of the human spinal column and its contents begins on day 15 postconception and continues through vertebral skeletal maturation at the age of 25 years. Spinal development usually proceeds in an ordered and systematic fashion. When breakdown occurs, spinal anomalies result.

REFERENCES

1. Alles AJ, Sulik K: Retinoic acid-induced spina bifida: evidence for a pathogenetic mechanism. *Development* 108:73-81, 1990.
2. Altman RP, Randolph JG, Lilly JR: Sacrococcygeal teratoma: American Academy of Pediatrics, Surgical Section, Surgery 1973. *J Pediatr Surg* 9:389-398, 1974.
3. Angela Nieto MA, Sargent MG, Wilkinson DG, Cooke J: Control of cell behavior during vertebrae development by Slug, a zinc finger gene. *Science* 264(5160):835-839, 1994.
4. Arnoldi CC, Brodsky AE, Cauchoix J, *et al:* Lumbar spinal stenosis and nerve root entrapment syndromes. Definition and classification. *Clin Orthop Rel Res* 115:4-5, 1976.
5. Bachs A, Barraquer-Bordas L, *et al:* Delayed myelopathy following atlantoaxial dislocation by separate odontoid process. *Brain* 78:537-553, 1955.
6. Bagnall KM, Higgins SJ, Sanders EJ: The contribution made by a single somite to the vertebral column: experimental evidence in support of resegmentation using the chick-quail chimaera model. *Development* 103:69-85, 1988.
7. Bailey DK: The normal cervical spine in infants and children. *Radiology* 59:712-719, 1962.
8. Bardell BS, Laurance B: Congenital dermal sinus associated with meningitis: report of a fatal case. *BMJ* 2:1558-1561, 1951.
9. Barkovich AJ, Edwards MSB, Cogen PH: MR evaluation of spinal dermal sinus tracts in children. *AJNR* 12: 123-129, 1991.
10. Barry A, Patten BM, Stewart BH: Possible factors in the development of the Arnold-Chiari malformation. *J Neurol* 14:285, 1957.
11. Barson AJ: Spina bifida: the significance of the level and extent of the defect to the morphogenesis. *Dev Med Child Neurol* 12:129-144, 1970.
12. Batts M: The etiology of spondylolisthesis. *J Bone Joint Surg* 21:879-884, 1939.
13. Beals RK: Hypochondroplasia: report of 5 kindreds. *J Bone Joint Surg* 51A:728-736, 1969.
14. Beardmore HE, Wigglesworth FW: Vertebral anomalies and alimentary duplications. *Pediatr Clin North Am* 5: 457-474, 1958.
15. Beighton P, Craig J: Atlanto-axial subluxation in Morquio syndrome. *J Bone Joint Surg* 55B:478-581, 1973.
16. Bernini F, Elefante R, Smaltino F, *et al:* Angiographic study on the vertebral artery in cases of deformities of the occipitocervical joint, abstracted. *Am J Roentgenol Radium Ther Nucl Med* 107:526, 1969.
17. Bethem D, Winter R, Lutter L, *et al:* Spinal disorders of the spine in diastrophic dwarfism. *J Bone Joint Surg* 62A:529-536, 1980.
18. Bethem D, Winter R, Lutter L, *et al:* Spinal disorders of dwarfism. *J Bone Joint Surg* 63:1412-1425, 1981.
19. Bharucha EP, Dastur HM: Craniovertebral abnormalities (a report of 40 cases). *Brain* 87:469-480, 1964.
20. Bick EM, Cogsel JW: Longitudinal growth of the human vertebrae: a contribution of human osteology. *J Bone Joint Surg* 32A:803-804, 1950.
21. Blummel J, Evans EB, Eggers GWN: Partial and complete agenesis or malformation of the sacrum with associated anomalies. *J Bone Joint Surg* 41A:497-518, 1959.

22. Borkow SE, Kleiger B: Spondylolisthesis in the newborn. *Clin Orthop* 81:73-76, 1971.

23. Bound JP, Francis BJ, Harvey PW: Neural tube defects, maternal cohorts, and age: a pointer to aetiology. *Arch Dis Child* 66:1223-1226, 1991.

24. Bowen V, Shannon R, Kirkaldy-Willis WH: Lumbar spinal stenosis. A review article. *Childs Brain* 4:257-277, 1978.

25. Boxall D, Bradford DS, Winter RB, *et al:* Management of severe spondylolisthesis in children and adolescents. *J Bone Joint Surg* 61A:479-495, 1979.

26. Bradford DS, Heithoff KB, Cohen M: Intraspinal abnormalities and congenital spine deformities: a radiographic and MRI study. *J Pediatr Orthop* 11:36-41, 1991.

27. Bradford DS, Hu SS: Spondylolysis and spondylolisthesis. In Weinstein SL (ed): *The Pediatric Spine*. Philadelphia, Lippincott-Raven, 1994, 585-601.

28. Bremer JL: Dorsal intestinal fistula; accessory neurenteric canal; diastematomyelia. *Arch Pathol* 54:132-138, 1952.

29. Brilsford JF: Chondro-osteo-dystrophy. *J Bone Joint Surg* 34B:53-63, 1959.

30. Brown MW, Templeton AW, Hodges FJ: The incidence of acquired and congenital fusions in the cervical spine. *Am J Roentgenol* 92:1255-1259, 1964.

31. Burke SW, French HG, Roberts JM, *et al:* Chronic atlanto-axial instability in Down syndrome. *J Bone Joint Surg* 67A:1356-1360, 1985.

32. Byrd SE, Darling CF, McLone DG: Developmental disorders of the pediatric spine. *Radiol Clin North Am* 29:711-752, 1991.

33. Cahan LD, Bentson JR: Considerations in the diagnosis and treatment of syringomyelia and the Chiari malformation. *J Neurosurg* 57:24-31, 1982.

34. Caram PR, Scarcella G, Carton CA: Intradural lipomas of the spinal cord. *J Neurosurg* 14:349-354, 1957.

35. Cave AJE: The morphological constitution of the odontoid process. *J Anat* 72:621, 1938.

36. Cave AJE: The morphology of the mammalian cervical pleurapophysis. *J Zool* 177:377-393, 1975.

37. Chalepakis G, Tremblay P, Gross P: Pax genes, mutants and molecular function. *J Cell Sci* 16(suppl):61-67, 1992.

38. Chamberlain WE: Basilar impression (platybasia). *Yale J Biol Med* 11:487, 1938.

39. Chandraraj S, Briggs CA: Role of cartilage canals in osteogenesis and growth of the vertebral centra. *J Anat* 158:121-136, 1988.

40. Chapman PH: Congenital intraspinal lipomas. Anatomic considerations and surgical treatment. *Childs Nerv Syst* 9:37, 1982.

41. Chatkupt S, Skurnick JH, Jaggi M, *et al:* Study of genetics, epidemiology, and vitamin usage in familial spina bifida in the United States in the 1990s. *Neurology* 44:65-70, 1994.

42. Cheek WR, Laurent JP: Dermal sinus tracts. In Marlin AD (ed): *Concepts in Pediatric Neurosurgery*. Basel, S. Karger, 1985, pp 63-75.

43. Christ B, Wilting J: From somites to vertebral column. *Ann Anat* 174:23-32, 1992.

44. Cross HE, Pfaffenbach DD: Duane's retraction syndrome and associated congenital malformations. *Am J Ophthalmol* 73:442-450, 1972.

45. Curtis BH, Blank S, Fisher RL: Atlantoaxial dislocation in Down's syndrome. *JAMA* 205:464-465, 1968.

46. Dalgleish AE: A study of the development of thoracic vertebrae in the mouse assisted by autoradiography. *Acta Anat* 122:91-98, 1985.

47. Dauser RC, Chandler WF: Symptomatic congenital spinal stenosis in a child. *Neurosurgery* 11:61-63, 1982.

48. Dawson EG, Smith L: Atlantoaxial subluxation in children due to vertebral anomalies. *J Bone Joint Surg* 61A:582-587, 1979.

49. De Barros MC, Farias W, Ataide L, *et al:* Basilar impression and Arnold-Chiari malformation: a study of 66 cases. *J Neurol Neurosurg Psychiatr* 1:596, 1968.

50. DeBeer GR: Skull. Oxford, 1-552, 1937.

51. Dias MS, Walker ML: The embryogenesis of complex dysraphic malformations: a disorder of gastrulation? *Pediatr Neurosurg* 18:229-253, 1992.

52. Dolan KD: Cervicobasilar relationships. *Radiol Clin North Am* 25:155-166, 1977.

53. Drvaric DM, Ruderman RJ, Conrad RW, *et al:* Congenital scoliosis and urinary tract abnormalities: are intravenous pyelograms necessary? *J Pediatr Orthop* 7:441, 1987.

54. Duhamel B: From the mermaid to anal imperforation: the syndrome of caudal regression. *Arch Dis Child* 30:152-155, 1961.

55. Dyck P: Os odontoideum in children: neurological manifestations and surgical management. *Neurosurgery* 2:93-99, 1978.

56. Dyste GN, Menezes AH: Presentation and management of pediatric Chiari malformations without myelodysplasia. *Neurosurgery* 23:589-597, 1988.

57. Edwards WC, LaRocca SH: The developmental segmental sagittal diameter in combined cervical and lumbar spondylosis. *Spine* 10:42-49, 1985.

58. Ehni G, Love JG: Intraspinal lipomas. *Arch Neurol Psychiatr* 53:1-28, 1945.

59. Eilers VE: Congenital scoliosis: a study of 234 patients treated and untreated. Part 1. Natural history. *J Bone Joint Surg* 50A:1-15, 1968.

60. Ein SH, Adeyemi SD, Mancer K: Benign sacrococcygeal teratomas in infants and children. A 25 years review. *Ann Surg* 191:382-384, 1980.

61. Ein SH, Mancer K, Adeyemi SD: Malignant sacrococcygeal teratoma-endodermal sinus, yolk sac tumor in infants and children: a 32-year review. *J Pediatr Surg* 20:473-477, 1985.

62. Elster AD: Quadriplegia after minor trauma in the Klippel-Feil syndrome. *J Bone Joint Surg* 66A:1473-1474, 1984.

63. Epstein JA, Malis LI: Compression of spinal cord and cauda equina in achondroplastic dwarfs. *Neurology* 5:875-881, 1955.

64. Epstein NE, Epstein JA, Carras R, *et al:* Coexisting cervical and lumbar spinal stenosis: diagnosis and management. *Neurosurgery* 15:489-496, 1984.

65. Epstein NE, Epstein JA, Zikha A: Traumatic myelopathy in a seventeen-year-old child with cervical spine stenosis (without fracture or dislocation) and a C2-C3 Klippel-Feil fusion. *Spine* 9:344-346, 1984.

66. Estin D, Cohen AR. Caudal agenesis and associated caudal spinal cord malformations. *Neurosurg Clin North Am* 6(2):377-391, 1995.

67. Ewan KBR, Everett AW: Evidence for resegmentation in the formation of the vertebral column using the novel approach of retroviral-mediated gene transfer. *Exp Cell Res* 198:315-320, 1992.

68. Fielding JW, Hawkins RJ, Ratzan SA: Spine fusion for atlanto-axial instability. *J Bone Joint Surg* 58A:400-407, 1976.

69. Fielding JW, Hensinger RN, Hawkins RJ: Os odontoideum. *J Bone Joint Surg* 62A:376, 1980.

70. Finer NN, Bowen P, Dunbar LG: Caudal regression anomalad (sacral agenesis) in siblings. *Clin Genet* 13:353-358, 1978.

71. Fischgold H, Metzger J: Etude radiotomographique de l'impression basilarie. *Rev Rheum* 19:261-264, 1952.

72. Spina bifida incidence at birth—United States, 1983-1990. *MMWR Morb Mortal Wkly Rep* 41:497-500, 1992.

73. Flood T et al: Spina bifida incidence at birth—United States. *JAMA* 268:708-709, 1992.

74. Freedman B: Congenital absence of the sacrum and coccyx. Report of a case and review of the literature. *Br J Surg* 37:299-303, 1950.

75. French BN: Midline fusion defects and defects of formation. In Youmans JR (ed): *Neurological Surgery*. Philadelphia, WB Saunders, 1990, pp 1081-1235

76. French BN: The embryology of spinal dysraphism. *Clin Neurosurg* 30:295-340, 1983.

77. Fromm GH, Pitner SE: Late progressive quadriparesis due to odontoid agenesis. *Arch Neurol* 9:291, 1963.

78. Gardner WJ: Hydrodynamic mechanism of syringomyelia: its relationship to myelocele. *J Neurol Neurosurg Psychiatr* 28:247-259, 1965.

79. Giblin PE, Mitchell LJ: The management of atlantoaxial subluxation with neurologic involvement in Down's syndrome: a report of two cases and review of the literature. *Clin Orthop* 140:66-71, 1979.

80. Goldberg MJ: Orthopedic aspects of bone dysplasias. *Orthop Clin North Am* 7:445-456, 1976.

81. Goldberg MJ: *The Dysmorphic Child: An Orthopedic Perspective*. Philadelphia, Lippincott-Raven, 1987.

82. Gorlin RJ, Cohen M, Wolfson J: Tricho-rhino-phalangeal syndrome. *Am J Dis Child* 118:595-602, 1969.

83. Gray SW, Romaine CB, Skandalakis JF: Congenital fusion of the cervical vertebrae. *Surg Gynecol Obstet* 118:373, 1964.

84. Greenberg AD: Atlanto-axial dislocations. *Brain* 91:655-684, 1968.

85. Hadley LA: *The Spine*. Springfield, IL, Charles C Thomas, 1956.

86. Hawkins RJ, Fielding W, Thompson WJ: Os odontoideum: congenital or acquired. A case report. *J Bone Joint Surg* 58A:413-414, 1976.

87. Helin I, Pettersson H, Alton D: Extensive spinal dysraphism and sacral agenesis without urologic disturbances. *Acta Radiol Diagn* 23:209-212, 1983.

88. Hensinger RN: Osseous anomalies of the cranio-vertebral junction. *Spine* 11:323, 1986.

89. Hensinger RN: Anomalies of the atlas. In *The Cervical Spine*. Philadelphia, Lippincott-Raven, 1989, pp 244-247.

90. Hensinger RN: Congenital anomalies of the cervical spine. In Rothman RH, Simeone FA (eds): *The Spine*. Philadelphia, WB Saunders, 1992, pp 288-289.

91. Hensinger RN: Congenital anomalies of the cervical spine—atlanto-occipital fusion. In Rothman RH, Simeone FA (eds): *The Spine*. Philadelphia, WB Saunders, 1992, pp 288-289.

92. Hensinger RN: Congenital anomalies of the cervical spine—anomalies of odontoid. In Rothman RH, Simeone FA (eds): *The Spine*. Philadelphia, WB Saunders, 1992, pp 279-289.

93. Hensinger R, Lang JE, MacEwen GD: Klippel-Feil syndrome: a constellation of associated anomalies. *J Bone Joint Surg* 66A:1246-1253, 1974.

94. Hensinger RN, MacEwen GD: Congenital abnormalities of the spine. In Rothman RH, Simeone FA (eds): *The Spine*. Philadelphia, WB Saunders, 1982.

95. Herren RY, Edwards JE: Diplomyelia (duplication of the spinal cord). *Arch Pathol* 30:1203-1214, 1940.

96. Hikuda S, Ota H, Okake N et al: Traumatic atlantoaxial dislocation causing os odontoideum in infants. Spine 5:207-210, 1980

97. Hinck VC, Hopkins CE, Savara BS: Sagittal diameter of the cervical spinal canal in children. *Radiology* 79:97-108, 1962.

98. Holcomb GW, Matson DD: Thoracic neurenteric cyst. *Surgery* 35:115-121, 1954.

99. Hood RW, Riseborough EJ, Nehme A, *et al:* Diastematomyelia and structural spinal deformities. *J Bone Joint Surg* 62A:520-528, 1980.

100. Hori A: A review of the morphology of spinal cord malformations and their relation to neuroembryology. *Neurosurg Rev* 16:259-266, 1993.

101. Hrgovic Z, Panitz HG, Kurjak A, *et al:* Contribution to the recognition of iniencephaly on the basis of a new case. *J Perinat Med* 17:375-379, 1989.

102. Humphreys RP: Current trends in spinal dysraphism. *Paraplegia* 29:79-83, 1991.

103. Ignelzi RJ, Lehman RAW: Lumbosacral agenesis: management and embryological implications. *J Neurol* 37:1273-1276, 1974.

104. Katz VL, Aylsworth AS, Albright SG: Iniencephaly is not uniformly fatal. *Prenat Diagn* 9:595-599, 1989.

105. Kessel M, Gruss P: Homeotic transformations of murine vertebrae and concomitant alteration of Hox codes induced by retinoic acid. *Cell* 67:89-104, 1991.

106. Keynes RJ, Stern CD: Mechanisms of vertebrate segmentation. *Development* 103:413-429, 1988.

107. Kieny M, Mauger A, Sengel P: Early regionalization of the somitic mesoderm as studied by the development of the axial skeleton of the chick embryo. *Dev Biol* 28:142-161, 1972.

108. Klippel M, Feil A: The classic. A case of absence of cervical vertebrae with the thoracic cage rising to the base of the cranium (cervical thoracic cage). *Clin Orthop Rel Res* 109:3-8, 1975.

109. Koontz WW, Prout GR: Agenesis of the sacrum and the neurogenic bladder. *JAMA* 203:139-144, 1968.

110. Kulkarni MV, Williams JC, Yeakley JW, *et al:* Magnetic resonance imaging in the diagnosis of the cranio-cervical manifestations of the mucopolysaccharidoses. *Magn Res Imaging* 5:317, 1987.

111. Kuhns JG, Hormell RS. Management of congenital scoliosis. *Arch Surg* 65:250-263, 1952.

112. Lebwohl NH, Eismont FJ: Cervical spine injuries in children. In Weinstein SL (ed): *The Pediatric Spine*. Philadelphia, Lippincott-Raven, 1994, pp 725-741.

113. Lee CK, Weiss AB: Isolated congenital cervical block vertebrae below the axis with neurological symptoms. *Spine* 6:118-124, 1981.

114. Lemire RJ, Beckwith JB: Pathogenesis of congenital tumors and malformations of the sacrococcygeal region. *Teratology* 25:201-213, 1982.

115. Lemire RJ, Loeser JD, Leech RW, *et al: Normal and Abnormal Development of the Human Nervous System.* Hagerstown, MD, Harper and Row, 1975.

116. Lendon RG: The embryopathogenesis of trypan-blue induced spina bifida aperta and short tail in the rat. *Dev Med Child Neurol* 35:3, 1975.

117. Lichtenstein BW: Spinal dysraphism, spina bifida and myelodysplasia. *Arch Neurol Psychiatr* 44:792-810, 1940.

118. Lipson SJ: Dysplasia of the odontoid in Morquio's syndrome causing quadriparesis. *J Bone Joint Surg* 59:340-344, 1977.

119. Locke GR, Gardner JL, Van Epps EF: Atlas-dens interval (ADI) in children: a survey based on 200 normal cervical spines. *Am J Roentgenol* 97:135-140, 1966.

120. Lohse CL, Hyde DM, Benson DR: Comparative development of thoracic intervertebral discs and intra-articular ligaments in the human, monkey, mouse and cat. *Acta Anat* 122:220-228, 1985.

121. MacRae DL: The significance of abnormalities of the cervical spine. *Am J Roentgenol* 84:3-25, 1960.

122. Marin-Padilla M, Ferm VH: Somite necrosis and developmental malformations induced by vitamin A in the golden hamster. *J Embryol Exp Morph* 13:1, 1965.

123. McAfee PC, Bohlman HH, Han JS, *et al:* Comparison of nuclear magnetic resonance imaging and computed tomography in the diagnosis of upper cervical spinal cord compression. *Spine* 11:295, 1986.

124. McElfresh E, Winter R: Klippel-Feil syndrome. *Minn Med* 56:353-357, 1973.

125. McGregor M: The significance of certain measurements of the skull in the diagnosis of basilar impression. *Br J Radiol* 21:1712, 1948.

126. McLennan JE: Rib anomalies in myelodysplasia. *Biol Neonate* 29:129-141, 1976.

127. McMaster MJ: Occult intraspinal anomalies and congenital scoliosis. *J Bone J Surg* 66A:588-601, 1984.

128. McMaster MJ, David CV: Hemivertebrae as a cause of scoliosis: a study of 104 patients. *J Bone Joint Surg* 68:588-595, 1986.

129. McMaster MJ, Oktsuka K: The natural history of congenital scoliosis: a study of 251 patients. *J Bone Joint Surg* 64A:1128-1147, 1982.

130. McRae DL: Bony abnormalities in the region of the foramen magnum: correction of the anatomic and neurologic findings. *Acta Radiol* 40:335, 1953.

131. McRae DL, Barnum AS: Occipitalization of the atlas. *Am J Roentgenol* 70:23-46, 1953.

132. Med M: Prenatal development of thoracic intervertebral articulation. *Folia Morphol* 25:175-177, 1975.

133. Menezes AH: Developmental and acquired abnormalities of the craniovertebral junction. In VanGilder JC, Menezes AH, Dolan KD (eds): *The Craniovertebral Junction and Its Abnormalities.* Karger, NY, 1987, pp 109-158.

134. Menezes AH: Bony abnormalities of the craniovertebral junction. In Pang D (ed): *Disorders of the Pediatric Spine.* Philadelphia, Lippincott-Raven, 1995, pp 97-110.

135. Menezes AH: Os odontoideum—pathogenesis, dynamics and management. In Marlin AE (ed): *Concepts in Pediatric Neurosurgery.* Basel, Karger, 1995, pp 133-145.

136. Menezes AH, Ryken TC: Craniovertebral junction abnormalities. In Weinstein SL (ed): *The Pediatric Spine: Principles and Practice.* Philadelphia, Lippincott-Raven, 1994, pp 307-321.

137. Menezes AH, Smoker WRK, Dyste GN: Syringomyelia, Chiari malformations, and hydromyelia. In Youmans JR (ed): *Neurological Surgery.* Philadelphia, WB Saunders, 1990, pp 1421-1459.

138. Menezes AH, VanGilder JC: Anomalies of the craniovertebral junction. In Youmans JR (ed): *Neurological Surgery.* Philadelphia, WB Saunders, 1990, pp 1359-1420.

139. Mickle J, McLennan J: Malignant teratoma arising within a lipomyelomeningocele. *J Neurosurg* 43:761-763, 1975.

140. Miller A, Guille JT, Bowen JR: Evaluation and treatment of diastematomyelia. *J Bone Joint Surg* 75A:1308-1317, 1993.

141. Montgomery SP, Hall JE: Congenital kyphosis. *Spine* 7:223-274, 1982.

142. Moore KL, Persaud TVN: The *Developing Human: Clinically Oriented Embryology,* ed 5. Philadelphia, WB Saunders, 1993.

143. Moore WB, Matthews TJ, Rabinowitz R: Genitourinary anomalies associated with Klippel-Feil syndrome. *J Bone Joint Surg* 57A:355-357, 1975.

144. Morocz I, Szeifert GT, Molnar P, *et al:* Prenatal diagnosis and pathoanatomy of iniencephaly. *Clin Genet* 30:81-86, 1986.

145. Muhonen MG, Menezes AH, Sawin PD, *et al:* Scoliosis in pediatric Chiari malformations without myelodysplasia. *J Neurosurg* 77:69-77, 1992.

146. Muller F, O'Rahilly RO, Benson DR: The early origin of vertebral anomalies, as illustrated by a "Butterfly Vertebra." *J Anat* 149:157-169, 1986.

147. Nagashima C: Atlanto-axial dislocation due to agenesis of the os odontoideum or odontoid. *J Neurosurg* 33:270-280, 1970.

148. Nagib MG, Maxwell RE, Chou SN: Identification and management of high-risk patients with Klippel-Feil syndrome. *J Neurosurg* 61:523-530, 1984.

149. Nasca RJ, Stilling FH, Stul HH: Progression of congenital scoliosis due to hemivertebrae and hemivertebrae with bars. *J Bone Joint Surg* 57A:456-466, 1975.

150. *Neural Tube Defects.* Ciba Foundation Symposium 181: West Sussex, England, John Wiley & Sons, 1994

151. Newman PH: The etiology of spondylolisthesis. *J Bone Joint Surg* 45B:39-59, 1963.

152. Newman PH: Stenosis of the lumbar spine in spondylolisthesis. *Clin Orthop* 115:116-121, 1976.

153. Newman PH, Terenty TR, Foster JB: Some observations on the pathogenesis of syringomyelia. *J Neurol Neurosurg Psychiatr* 44:964-969, 1981.

154. Noback CR, Robertson GG: Sequences of appearance of ossification centers in the human skeleton during the first five prenatal months. *Am J Anat* 89:128, 1969.

155. Noseworthy J, Lack EE, Kozakewich HPW, *et al:* Sacrococcygeal germ cell tumors in children: an updated experience with 118 patients. *J Pediatr Surg* 16(3):358-364, 1981.

156. O'Rahilly R, Meyer DB: The timing and sequence of events in the development of the vertebral column during the embryonic period proper. *Anat Embryol* 157:167-176, 1979.

157. O'Rahilly R, Muller F: The embryonic human brain. In *Atlas of Developmental Stages.* New York, Wiley-Liss, 1994.

158. O'Rahilly R, Muller F, Meyer DB: The human vertebral column at the end of the embryonic period proper 3. The thoracicolumbar region. *J Anat* 168:81-93, 1990.

159. Ogden JA, Ganey TM, Sasse J, *et al:* Development and maturation of the axial skeleton. In Weinstein SL (ed): *The Pediatric Spine: Principles and Practice.* Philadelphia, Lippincott-Raven, 1994, pp 3-69.

160. Oi S, Kokunai T, Okuda Y, *et al:* Identical embryopathogenesis for exencephaly and myeloschisis; an experimental study. *J Neurosurg* 72:450, 1990.

161. Oi S, Saya H, Matsumoto S: A hypothesis for myeloschisis: overgrowth and reopening. *J Neurosurg* 68:947, 1988.

162. Osaka K, Tanimura T, Hiragoma A, *et al:* Myelomeningocele before birth. *J Neurosurg* 49:711-724, 1978.

163. Paine KWE: Clinical feature of lumbar spinal stenosis. *Clin Orthop Rel Res* 115:77-82, 1976.

164. Pang D: Surgical complications of open spinal dysraphism. *Neurosurg Clin North Am* 6(2):243-257, 1995.

165. Pang D: Split cord malformation: Part II: clinical syndrome. *Neurosurgery* 31:481-500, 1992.

166. Pang D: Sacral agenesis and caudal spinal cord malformations. *Neurosurgery* 32(5):755-779, 1993.

167. Pang D, Dias MS, Ahab-Barmada M: Split cord malformation: Part I: a unified theory of embryogenesis for double spinal cord malformations. *Neurosurgery* 31:451-480, 1992.

167a.Pang D, Pollacv IF: Spinal cord injury within radiographic abnormality in children: The SCIOWORA syndrome. *J Trauma* 29:654-664, 1989.

168. Pang D, Wilberger JE: Tethered cord syndrome in adults. *J Neurosurg* 57:32-47, 1982.

169. Pantoja E, Llobert R, Gonzals-Flores B: Retroperitoneal teratoma: historical review. *J Urol* 115:520-523, 1976.

170. Parke WW: Development of the spine. In Herkowitz HN, Garfin SR, Balderston RA, *et al* (eds): *Rothman–Simeone: The Spine,* ed 4. Philadelphia, WB Saunders, 1999.

171. Peacock A: Observations on the pre-natal development of the intervertebral disc in man. *J Anat* 85:260-274, 1960.

172. Perovic NM, Kopits SE, Thompson RC: Radiologic evaluation of the spinal cord in congenital atlantoaxial dislocation. *Radiology* 109:713-716, 1973.

173. Phillips WA, Cooperman DR, Lindquist TC, *et al:* Orthopedic management of lumbosacral agenesis. *J Bone Joint Surg* 64A:1282-1294, 1982.

174. Powell KR, Cherry JD, Hougen TJ et al: A prospective search for congenital dermal abnormalities of the craniospinal axis. J Pediatr 87:744-750, 1975

175. Raas-Rothschild A, Goodman RM, Grunbaum M, *et al:* Klippel-Feil anomaly with sacral agenesis; an additional subtype, type IV. *J Craniofac Genet Dev Biol* 8:297-301, 1988.

176. Remark R: Untersuchungen uber die Entwicklung der Wirbeltiere. Berlin, Reimer, 1855.

177. Renshaw TS: Sacral agenesis: a classification and review of twenty-three cases. *J Bone Joint Surg* 60A:373-383, 1978.

178. Ricciardi JE, Kaufer H, Louis DS: Acquired os odontoideum following acute ligament injury. Report of a case. *J Bone Joint Surg* 58A:410-412, 1976.

179. Roach JW, Duncan D, Wenger DR, *et al:* Atlanto-axial instability and spinal cord compression in children. Diagnosis by computerized tomography. *J Bone Joint Surg* 66A:708, 1984.

180. Rodriguez MM, Reik RA, Carreno TD, *et al:* Cluster of iniencephaly in Miami. *Pediatr Pathol* 11:211-221, 1991.

181. Roessmann U: The embryology and neuropathology of congenital malformations. *Clin Neurosurg* 30:157-164, 1983.

182. Rogers HM, Long DM, Chou SN, *et al:* Lipomas of the spinal cord and cauda equina. *J Neurosurg* 34:349-354, 1971.

183. Rokos J, Cekanova E, Kithierova E: Pathogenesis of trypan-blue-induced spina bifida. *J Pathol* 118:25-34, 1976.

184. Rokos J, Knowles J: An experimental contribution to the pathogenesis of spina bifida. *J Pathol* 118:21-24, 1976.

185. Rosenberg NJ, Bargar WL, Friedman B: The incidence of spondylolysis and spondylolisthesis in nonambulatory patients. *Spine* 6:35-37, 1981.

186. Rowe GG, Roche MB: The etiology of separate neural arch. *J Bone Joint Surg* 35A:102-109, 1953.

187. Rusnak SL, Driscoll SG: Congenital spinal anomalies in infants of diabetic mothers. *Pediatrics* 35:989-995, 1965.

188. Russell HE, Aitken GT: Congenital absence of the sacrum and lumbar vertebrae with prosthetic management. *J Bone Joint Surg* 45A:501-508, 1963.

189. Sanders RC: Prenatal ultrasonic detection of anomalies with a lethal or disastrous outcome. *Radiol Clin North Am* 28:163-177, 1990.

190. Sandford MK, Kissling GE, Joubert PE: Neural tube defect etiology: new evidence concerning maternal hyperthermia, health and diet. *Dev Med Child Neurol* 34:661-675, 1992.

191. Sarnat HB, Case ME, Graviss R: Sacral agenesis: neurologic and neuropathologic features. *Neurology* 26:1124-1129, 1976.

192. Sarpyener MA: Congenital stricture of the spinal canal. *J Bone Joint Surg* 27A:70-79, 1945.

193. Sarpyener MA: Spina bifida aperta and congenital stricture of the spinal canal. *J Bone Joint Surg* 29:817-821, 1947.

194. Saunders RL: Combined anterior and posterior spina bifida in a living neonatal human female. *Anat Rec* 87:255-278, 1943.

195. Scott RM, Wolpert SM, Bartoshesky LE, *et al:* Segmental spinal dysgenesis. *Neurosurgery* 22:739-744, 1988.

196. Schropp KP, Lobe TE, Roa B, *et al:* Sacrococcygeal teratoma: the experience of four decades. *J Pediatr Surg* 27(8):1075-1079, 1992.

197. Sensenig EC: The development of the occiput and cervical segments and their associated structures in human embryos. *Contr Embryol Carneg Inst* 36:143-151, 1957.

198. Shands AR, Bundens WD: Congenital deformities of the spine: an analysis of the roentgenograms of 700 children. *Bull Hosp J Dis* 17:110-133, 1956.

199. Shapiro R, Robinson F: Anomalies of the craniovertebral border. *Am J Roentgenol* 127:281-287, 1976.

200. Sherk HH, Uppal GS: Congenital bony anomalies of the cervical spine. In Frymoyer JW (ed): *The Adult Spine,*

Principles and Practice. Philadelphia, Lippincott-Raven, 1991, pp 1015-1037.

201. Silvernail WI, Brown RB: Intramedullary enterogenous cyst. *J Neurosurg* 36:235-238, 1972.

202. Smith MD: Congenital scoliosis of the cervical or cervicothoracic spine. *Orthop Clin North Am* 25(2): 301-310, 1994.

203. Smith CA, Tuan RS: Human PAX gene expression and development of the vertebral column. *Clin Orthop* 302:241-250, 1994.

204. Smith CA, Tuan RS: Functional involvement of Pax-1 gene in somite development. Somite dysmorphogenesis in chick embryos treated with Pax-1 paired-box antisense oligonucleotide. *Teratology* 52:333-345, 1995.

205. Smith MT, Wissinger JP, Smith CG, *et al:* Experimental dysraphism in the rat. *J Neurosurg* 49:725-729, 1978.

206. Spierlings ELH, Braakman R: Os odontoideum: analysis of 37 cases. *J Bone Joint Surg* 64B:422-428, 1982.

207. Spillane JD, Pallis C, Jones AM: Developmental abnormalities in the region of the foramen magnum. *Brain* 80:11-48, 1957.

208. Spranger J, Langer LO, Wiedemann HR: Spondyloepiphyseal dysplasia congenita. In Fischer G (ed): *Bone Dysplasia.* Stuttgart, Verlag, 1974, pp 95-103.

209. Spranger JW, Langer LO: Spondyloepiphyseal dysplasia congenita. *Radiology* 94:313-322, 1970.

210. Stanley JK, Owen R, Koff S: Congenital sacral anomalies. *J Bone Joint Surg* 61B:401-409, 1979.

211. Stratford J: Myelopathy caused by atlantoaxial dislocation. *J Neurosurg* 14:97-104, 1957.

212. Strax TE, Baran E: Traumatic quadriplegia associated with Klippel-Feil syndrome: discussion and case reports. *Arch Phys Med Rehabil* 56:363-365, 1975.

213. Sweeney RM, Watterson RI: Rib development in chick embryos analyzed by means of tantalum foil blocks. *Am J Anat* 126:127-150, 1970.

214. Tanzer A: Die basilare impression. *Radiol Clin* 25: 135-142, 1956.

215. Urui S, Oi S: Experimental study of the embryogenesis of open spinal dysraphism. *Neurosurg Clin North Am* 6(2):195-202, 1995

216. Valdiserri RO, Eduardo JY: Sacrococcygeal teratomas: a review of 68 cases. *Cancer* 48:217-221, 1981.

217. VanKerckhoven MF, Fabry G: The Klippel-Feil syndrome: a constellation of deformities. *Acta Orthop Belg* 1981: 107-118, 1955.

218. Verbiest H: Further experiences on the pathological influence of a developmental narrowness of the bony lumbar vertebral canal. *J Bone Joint Surg* 37B:576-583, 1955.

219. Verbiest H: Pathomorphologic aspects of developmental lumbar stenosis. *Orthop Clin North Am* 6:177-196, 1975.

220. Verbiest H: Fallacies of the present definition, nomenclature and classification of the stenoses of the lumbar vertebral canal. *Spine* 1:217-225, 1976.

221. Verbiest H: Results of surgical treatment of idiopathic developmental stenosis of the lumbar vertebral canal. A review of twenty-seven years experience. *J Bone Joint Surg* 59B:181-188, 1977.

222. Verbiest H: Lumbar spinal stenosis. Morphology, classification and long-term results. In Weinstein JN, Wiesel SW (eds): *The Lumbar Spine.* Philadelphia, WB Saunders, 1990, pp 546-589.

223. Verbiest H: The significance and principles of computerized axial tomography in idiopathic developmental stenosis of the bony lumbar vertebral canal. *Spine* 4:546-589, 1990.

224. Verbout AJ: The development of the vertebral column. *Adv Anat Embryol Cell Biol* 90:1-122, 1985.

225. Vogter DM, Kaufman HH: Spinal dysraphism—a review. *W V Med J* 81:142-143, 1985.

226. VonTorkus D, Gehle W: The upper cervical spine. Regional anatomy, pathology and traumatology. In Georg, Thieme, Verlag (eds): *A Systemic Radiological Atlas and Textbook.* New York, Grune & Stratton, 1972, pp 2-77.

227. Wackenheim A: A radiologic diagnosis of congenital forms, intermittent forms and progressive forms of stenosis of the spinal canal of the level of the atlas. *Acta Radiol Diagn (Stockh)* 9:481-486, 1969.

228. Whalen JL, Parke WW, Mazur JM, *et al:* The intrinsic vasculature of developing vertebral end plates and its nutritive significance to the intervertebral discs. *J Pediatr Orthop* 5:403-410, 1985.

229. Whalin J, Whilting J, Koseki H, *et al:* The role of Pax-1 in axial development. *Development* 120:1109-1121, 1994.

230. Whitecloud TS, Brinker MR: Congenital anomalies of the base of the skull and the atlanto-axial joint. In Camins MB, O'Leary PF (eds): *Disorders of the Cervical Spine.* Baltimore, Williams & Wilkins, 1992, pp 199-211.

231. Williams B: Difficult labor as a cause of communicating syringomyelia. *Lancet* 2:51-53, 1977.

232. Williams B: Orthopaedic feature in the presentation of syringomyelia. *J Bone Joint Surg* 61B:314-323, 1979.

233. Williams B: On the pathogenesis of syringomyelia: a review. *J R Soc Med* 73:798-806, 1980.

234. Williams DI, Nixon HH: Agenesis of the sacrum. *Surg Gynecol Obstet* 105:84-88, 1957.

235. Wiltse LL, Newman PH, Macnab I: Classification of spondylolysis and spondylolisthesis. *Clin Orthop* 117: 23-29, 1976

236. Wiltse LL, Rothman LG: Spondylolisthesis: classification, diagnosis, and natural history. *Semin Spine Surg* 1:78-94, 1989.

237. Winter RB: *Congenital Deformities of the Spine.* New York, Thieme-Stratton, 1983.

238. Winter RB, Leonard AS: Case report: surgical correction of congenital thoracic lordosis. *J Pediatr Orthop* 10: 805-808, 1990.

239. Winter RB, Lonstein JE, Erickson D, *et al:* Congenital spinal stenosis. *Orthop Trans* 9:131, 1985.

240. Winter RB, Moe JH, Bradford DS: Congenital chronic lordosis. *J Bone Joint Surg* 60A:806-810, 1978.

241. Winter RB, Moe JH, Eilers VE: Congenital scoliosis: a study of 234 patients treated and untreated. *J Bone Joint Surg* 50A:1-47, 1968.

242. Winter RB, Moe JH, Lonstein JE: The incidence of Klippel-Feil syndrome in patients with congenital scoliosis and kyphosis. *Spine* 9:363-366, 1984.

243. Winter RB, Moe JH, Wang JF: Congenital kyphosis: its natural history and treatment as observed in a study of 130 patients. *J Bone Joint Surg* 55A:223-274, 1973.

244. Wynne-Davies R: Congenital vertebral anomalies: etiology and relationship to spina bifida cystica. *J Med Genet* 12:280-292, 1975.

245. Yamada S, Iacono RP, Andrade T, *et al:* Pathophysiology of tethered cord syndrome. *Neurosurg Clin North Am* 6(2):311-323, 1995.

246. Yamada S, Zinke DE, Sanders D: Pathophysiology of "tethered cord syndrome." *J Neurosurg* 54:494-503, 1981.

247. Yen IH, Khoury MJ, Erickson JD, *et al:* The changing epidemiology of neural tube defects, United States, 1968-1989. *Am J Dis Child* 146:857-861, 1992.

CHAPTER 5

Anatomy and Pathophysiology of Acquired Spinal Lesions

Nicholas N.M. Thomas, Gary L. Rea, and Philip R. Weinstein

One must understand the anatomy of the affected spinal region and the effects of a particular syndrome on that anatomy to understand the clinical presentation of a given spinal disorder, predict its natural history, and design treatment algorithms. Degenerative disc disease, rheumatoid arthritis, Scheuermann's disease, Paget's disease, ankylosing spondylitis, ossification of the posterior longitudinal ligament (OPLL), and spondylolisthesis lead to characteristic changes in spinal anatomy, and each results in characteristic radiographic findings that direct surgical therapy. Nonspecific symptoms common to these conditions are joint inflammation and nerve root entrapment.

Degenerative Disc Disease and Spondylosis

Degenerative disc disease (with its characteristic clinical syndromes of disc herniation, spondylosis, and radiculopathy) is associated with vascular, biochemical, and anatomic changes in the disc. There is a consistent anatomic pattern of disc degeneration in the spine, with most changes occurring in the midcervical, thoracolumbar, and lower lumbar regions. This pattern is thought to reflect the distribution of the mechanical stresses caused by spine movement and loading and an erect posture.[37]

The intervertebral disc consists of three components: (1) the nucleus pulposus; (2) the annulus fibrosus, which surrounds the nucleus pulposus; and (3) the cartilaginous end-plates, which attach these structures to the rostral and caudal vertebrae. The annulus is formed by a series of lamellae that have a high-collagen content and thereby provide significant resistance to tensile forces. The ventral annulus is usually wider and more organized than the dorsal annulus, which may even have discontinuous lamellae.[110] The nucleus pulposus, derived from the notochord,[104] has a much higher proteoglycan and water content than the annulus fibrosus. The hyaline cartilage end-plates are similar in collagen type to the inner annulus fibrosus and the nucleus pulposus.[52]

Proteoglycans contribute to osmotic pressure elevation, which results in the nucleus pulposus becoming turgid. This turgidity generates a swelling pressure that exerts radial stress, pushing the surrounding annular fibers outward and the end-plates apart, which in turn results in the development of circumferential tensile stress in the annular lamellae, particularly the inner lamellae. Stress also develops in the end-plates and is greatest over the nucleus pulposus, diminishing toward the outer annulus.

The disc acts as a deformable, fluidlike material, whose tendency to bulge is resisted by the tensile stress in the annular lamellae and the end-plates. Therefore a high intradiscal pressure is required to generate a high circumferential annular stress and thus prevent disc bulging. When disruption of the nucleus pulposus reduces the intradiscal pressure, bulging occurs.[20]

The disc receives its nutrients through small vessels in the cartilage end-plates and from the periphery of the annulus.[66] With aging, however, the end-plates calcify, and vessel loss occurs until nearly the entire disc is avascular.[105] With the loss of vasculature, there is increased anaerobic metabolism. This causes increased lactic acid production and cellular necrosis. The water content of the annulus fibrosus decreases from 78% at birth to 70% by the fourth decade, and the nucleus pulposus water content decreases from 90% to less than 70% with maturation.[40,72] With this change in vascularity, and with water loss in the region of the inner annulus and nucleus pulposus, there is a relative increase in fibrocytes and chondrocytes, which are more tolerant of a low pH environment.[104]

Until a subject is 2 years old, the nucleus pulposus is translucent and anatomically different from the annulus fibrosus.[125] By the second decade the inner annulus and nucleus grow increasingly fibrous and lose both height and proteoglycans.[72] In the third decade there is nuclear fragmentation and fibrosis. Progressive myxomatous degeneration, swelling, and fissure formation occur in the annulus by the fourth decade.[81,124] Eventually the nucleus pulposus may become disorganized, dehydrated, and fragmented with circumferential and radial tears.[81,125,126] Grading systems for these patterns of disc degeneration, using plain radiographs or magnetic resonance imaging (MRI) studies, have been published.[39,125]

On plain radiographs, the degenerative disc changes range from grade I to grade IV. Grade I is a normal disc. Grade II has minimal sclerosis with disc space narrowing or osteophyte formation. Grade III shows moderate sclerosis, and grade IV shows severe sclerosis with disc space narrowing or osteophyte formation.[39] Yu et al.[125] classified changes in the disc, with reference to the age of the subject and to the stage of degeneration, by comparing the anatomic characteristics with the appropriate MRI findings in cadaveric dissections (Figure 5.1 and Table 5.1).

The primitive notochord is present up to age 10. In the second decade of life a distinct fibrous band forms in the nucleus and disc height diminishes. In the third decade there is fragmentation and fibrosis of the nucleus. By the fourth decade there is swelling, separation, and myxomatous degeneration of the annular lamellae with fissure formation.[124]

One of the most common discogenic clinical syndromes is a herniated disc with sciatica. With degeneration there is fissure formation in a radial distribution. It is likely that the biomechanical cause of disc herniation is a combination of complex movements involving compression, lateral flexion, and/or rotation.[2-4,32]

With flexion the nucleus pulposus moves dorsally. The dorsal annulus has fewer and more disorganized lamellae and may be inherently weaker than the thicker ventral annulus. Degeneration of the annulus results in the development of peripheral, circumferential, and subsequently, radial tears. With complex stresses applied to the dorsally migrating nucleus, herniation may occur along a radial tear.

With herniation there can be nerve root impingement. The typical dorsolateral herniated disc affects the nerve root passing to the next lower foramen, but a more laterally herniated disc can affect the nerve root above. Masaryk et al.[69] used MRI findings to classify the stages of disc herniation. A bulging disc has an MRI signal similar to the rest of the disc, but the bulge is beyond the adjacent vertebral margin. A prolapsed or protruding disc has nearly breached the outer annular fibers and is barely contained. The disc remains contiguous with the rest of the nucleus pulposus by a pedicle that has a high signal on T_2-weighted MRI. The disc is extruded when it completely breaches the outer annular fibers and the posterior longitudinal ligament, but remains in continuity with the main part of the disc. If the fragment loses this continuity with the main part of the disc, it is a sequestered or "free" disc fragment situated in the epidural space. The International Society for the Study of the Lumbar Spine[113] classifies the disc as either contained or noncontained, with the latter group including extruded and sequestered discs.

Free fragments may migrate in a rostral or caudal direction. It appears that far-lateral herniated discs are more likely to migrate in a rostral direction to affect the nerve root above the disc space.[51]

Disc degeneration without herniation may also lead to changes affecting the biomechanical function and stability of the spinal joints. Although there are different opinions regarding whether facet or disc degeneration is the initial event that causes spondylosis, the three-joint, intervertebral-motion–segment concept emphasizes that disease in each component affects the others, which is to say that unilateral- or bilateral-facet disease or disc degeneration may lead to progressive changes in the other segmental units. Adjacent bone changes are associated with cartilaginous degeneration in these three joints; spurs or osteophytes

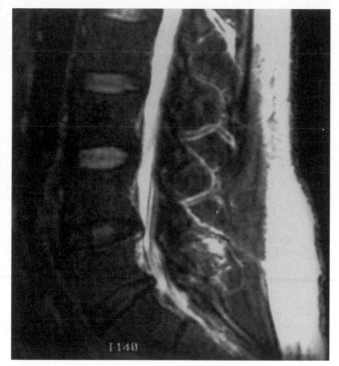

Figure 5.1 T_2-weighted MRI of lumbar spine demonstrating disc desiccation and herniation at the lower levels.

TABLE 5.1

Classification of Lumbar Discs

Type of Disc	Anatomic Characteristics	MRI Features
Immature	Nucleus pulposus and annulus fibrosus differentiated, primitive notochord may be present	High-signal intensity from nucleus and annulus
Transitional	Fibrous tissue in equator of annulus	High-signal intensity from nucleus and annulus, low-signal intensity in ventral and/or dorsal region of nucleus pulposus, corresponding to dense fibrous tissue
Adult	Annulus and nucleus not differentiated, annulus intact or marked by small concentric or transverse tears	Moderately high-signal intensity from nucleus and annulus, low-signal intensity from Sharpey fibers and fibrous tissue in midportion of disc
Early degenerated	Radial tear of annulus, diminishing amount and discoloration of fibrocartilage in nucleus	Diminishing signal intensity from nucleus pulposus, low signal from Sharpey fibers disrupted by region of higher signal intensity at location of annular tear, slightly diminished disc height
Severely degenerated	Replacement of nuclear and annular fibrocartilage with amorphous fiber and cysts	Severely reduced disc height, low (fibrous tissue) or high (fluid) signal intensity from intervertebral disc

From Yu S, Haughton VM, Sether LA, *et al*: Criteria for classifying normal and degenerated lumbar intervertebral disks. *Radiology* 170:523-526, 1989, with permission.

form where there is ossification at the peripheral annular attachment to the end-plates. These osteophytes are thought to be formed in regions of excessive motion. Kirkaldy-Willis[62] incorporated this concept into a theory regarding the natural history of spinal degeneration. He believed that there was facet and disc disease with progressive reciprocal dysfunction, which resulted in ligamentous laxity around the facet joint and increased stresses that lead to internal disc disruption. This condition causes subluxation, disc resorption, and finally, paradiscal osteophyte formation. Enlargement of the facets also occurs as a result of osteophyte formation. These changes may contribute to lumbar stenosis (Figure 5.2) or lateral recess syndrome.[77,83,122]

Patients with significant lumbar spinal canal narrowing, or stenosis patients, complain primarily of pain, weakness, and leg numbness while walking. This pain can be relieved when the patient flexes the spine by sitting, by leaning on shopping carts, or by leaning against counters. The symptomatic improvement is caused by increased spinal canal size, because flexion results in stretching of the protruding ligamentum flavum and posterior longitudinal ligament, as well as reduction of overriding laminae and facets.[84] This small amount of change in the spinal canal allows relief of the pressure on the nerve roots and provides the subsequent relief of symptoms. Returning to the erect posture leads to repeated compression and a further exacerbation of symptoms. During ambulation some patients experience the onset of symptoms because of increased metabolic demand in nerve roots that have become ischemic as a result of stenotic compression. Such neurogenic claudication is relieved when the subject sits down. Often, bicycling (with the lumbar spine flexed) is well tolerated.

Aging discs in the cervical spine cause characteristic spine alterations that may lead to cervical myelopathy or radicular pain and deficit. In young subjects there is a lordosis of the cervical spine, primarily a result of the greater ventral height of the annulus. With aging, however, there is loss of intradiscal water and narrowing of the disc. Thus progressive spine straightening occurs. In young patients the range of intervertebral motion is greatest at C5-6 and C6-7. Narrowing and degeneration with osteophyte formation is most marked at these levels (Figure 5.3). With these changes there is progressively less movement. In patients over age 60 more movement occurs at C3-4 and C4-5. Increased degenerative instability in older patients is associated with increased translational subluxation, especially retrolisthesis at C3-4 and C4-5.[50] In this scenario the spinal cord of the patient with cervical spondylotic myelopathy may not only be compressed by osteophytes, but may also suffer repeated injuries secondary to bony instability. A treatment protocol that does not take both these factors into account may have less than optimal success.

Rheumatoid Arthritis of the Spine

Rheumatoid arthritis affects both the spine and the peripheral joints. It has a prevalence of approximately 1%, with the greatest incidence in the fourth through sixth decades.[127] Rheumatoid arthritis is a disease of the synovial joints. The earliest change in the joints is synovitis, followed by an acute inflammatory response as a result of antibody-antigen complex formation. These formations activate the complement cascade and generate biologically

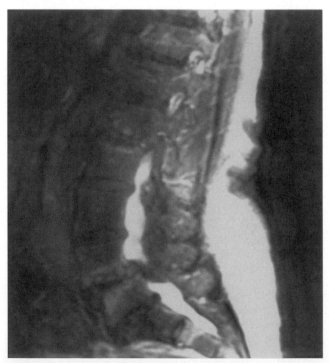

Figure 5.2 T$_2$-weighted MRI of lumbar spine demonstrating lumbar spinal canal stenosis, particularly at L4-5. There are osteophytic spurs ventrally and hypertrophied ligamentum flavum dorsally.

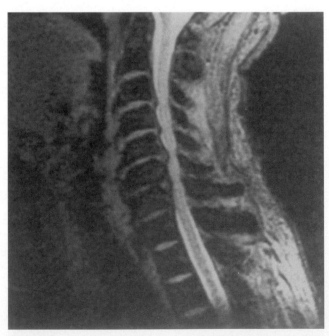

Figure 5.3 T$_2$-weighted MRI of cervical spine in a 72-year-old patient. Disc spaces are reduced in height, particularly at the C5-6 and C6-7 levels.

active substances, ultimately resulting in complete destruction of the joint. This acute process is followed by a chronic granulomatous process or pannus formation, which produces collagenase and other enzymes that destroy surrounding cartilage or bone.[28] This may lead to instability because of ligamentous incompetence.[86,127,128]

Considerable controversy regarding the pathogenesis of cervical spine rheumatoid joint disease revolves around whether the initial site of involvement is (1) the apophyseal joint, with resultant facet destruction and progressive secondary instability of the intervertebral disc, or (2) inflammation in the uncovertebral joint, which leads to primary disc destruction with secondary degenerative involvement of the apophyseal joints. Martel[68] examined 20 rheumatoid patients and found instability associated with apophyseal joint involvement. This leads to vertebral end-plate destruction, disc space narrowing, and erosion. At autopsy the discs showed evidence of necrosis and degeneration, with minimal inflammation. Martel proposed that apophyseal changes caused the instability with secondary disc destruction and end-plate microfractures. The relative infrequency of cervical spine disease in juvenile-onset arthritis was explained by the early bony ankylosis of the apophyseal joints observed in these subjects.

Ball[11] reviewed the pathology of 14 rheumatoid patients with no radiologic evidence of cervical rheumatoid disease and found that the earliest histologic lesions were in the uncovertebral joints. He suggested that the disc and adjacent bone are then secondarily involved with resultant inflammatory destruction and progressive instability. Because the uncovertebral joints are not completely developed in the first two decades of life,[30] this might also explain the infrequency with which cervical rheumatoid disease is seen in juvenile-onset rheumatoid arthritis.[6]

Cervical spine disease is observed in as many as 88% of patients with rheumatoid arthritis.[45] The manifestations include C1-2 instability, occipitocervical instability (with or without vertical displacement of the dens), and subaxial cervical rheumatoid arthritis.

C1-2 instability is the most common form of cervical rheumatoid involvement and may occur in up to 74% of the patients.[129] The dens is surrounded by two synovial joints, one ventrally, between the atlas and dens, and another between the transverse ligament and the dens. With involvement of the synovial joints there is progressive inflammation, destruction, and subsequent transverse ligament laxity, with destruction of the osseous attachments of the ligamentous complex. This loss of ligamentous integrity allows C1 to move ventrally on C2. If there is further significant disruption and osteomalacia of the dens itself, then dorsal C1-2 subluxation can also occur.[57] If the synovial apophyseal joints between C1-2 are involved as well, there may be lateral rotation in addition to subluxation at C1-2. Occipitocervical instability results from involvement of the atlanto-occipital articulations. With significant articular facet destruction, there is progressive collapse of the occiput at C1 and vertical displacement of the residual dens. This has also been termed *atlantoaxial impaction, vertical subluxation, cranial settling*, and *basilar invagination*.[57] Vertical displacement of the dens occurs in 5% to 32% of rheumatoid patients.[28,75,82]

In the subaxial region the levels most commonly involved with rheumatoid synovitis are C2-3 and C3-4. Subluxation (Figure 5.4) may occur in approximately 7% to 29% of the patients with rheumatoid arthritis.[57] These "staircase" subluxations are thought to be caused by significant ligamentous laxity and facet degeneration.[45,63] At

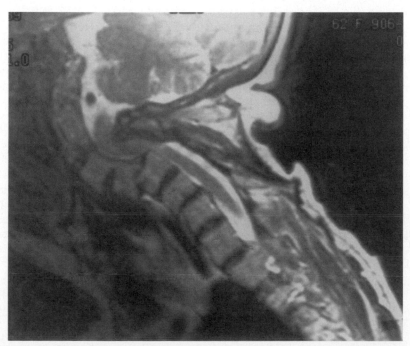

Figure 5.4 T$_2$-weighted MRI of cervical spine demonstrating C5-6 subluxation and spinal cord compression in a patient with rheumatoid arthritis. There is also marked vertical displacement of the dens.

any of the various sites of rheumatoid involvement, osseous erosion of adjacent bone, caused by osteoclastic resorption, occurs frequently.[21]

With the significant bony destruction, ligamentous laxity, and potential for neural compression observed in the rheumatoid cervical spine, the primary emphasis of treatment is reduction of subluxation and fusion/fixation to prevent spinal cord injury. After successful fusion, pain is often alleviated significantly. The chronic granulomatous pannus has also been shown to decrease in size with elimination of abnormal movement after successful arthrodesis.[119]

Scheuermann's Disease (Juvenile Kyphosis)

Scheuermann[93] first described the progressive dorsal kyphosis of adolescent children in 1920. The deformity is usually evident as a fixed thoracic kyphosis that does not correct with hyperextension, thereby differentiating it from a postural kyphosis. There may be compensatory hyperlordosis of the lumbar and cervical spine. A mild scoliosis is noted in 20% to 30% of patients.[19] Sorenson[99] described the characteristic features of ventral wedging of 5 degrees or more of at least three adjacent vertebrae. Other characteristics include kyphosis of greater than 40 degrees, vertebral end-plate irregularity, and disc space narrowing.[16] The prevalence of the disease ranges from 0.4% to 8%.[99] It occurs predominantly in males (91% in one series).[95]

Basic biomechanical factors and forces may play a role in this disorder. The thoracic spine has a natural kyphosis determined primarily by the shape of the vertebrae. The dorsal elements, including the ligamentum flavum and the laminae, resist forward flexion of the spine in tension, whereas the ventral bony elements and disc resist compression.[115] However, the facet joint capsules in the thoracic region are weaker than those in the lumbar region, so that any factor that increases the torque of the spine can result in greater deformity. The more marked the initial angulation of the spine, the larger the load (subject's weight), and the longer the duration of load application, the greater the likelihood of the progression of the deformity.

The pathogenesis of the disease remains unclear. Scheuermann believed that aseptic necrosis of the ring apophyses caused interruption of growth, which resulted in ventral vertebral body wedging.[13] Subsequent work has refuted this theory by demonstrating that the apophyses do not contribute to longitudinal growth. Such growth is now known to result from endochondral ossification of the end-plates.[13] Schmorl[94] felt that damage to the end-plate by herniated disc material was of importance. Schmorl's nodes are, however, not limited to the kyphotic region of the spine and are common in otherwise-normal patients. It has been postulated that osteoporosis is involved,[17,64] but recent investigations have found no differences in the trabecular bone density between patients with Scheuermann's disease and controls matched for age, gender, and race.[38,95] Other factors such as inflammation,[58] hormonal influences,[7] genetic factors,[44] altered calcium metabolism,[98] hypovitaminosis,[96] neuromuscular disorders,[59] extradural cyst formation,[24,118] defective collagen formation of the end-plate,[9] and a decrease in the colla-

gen/proteoglycan ratio of the end-plate[7] have been implicated, but their roles in the development of the disease have not been substantiated.

Recent research has concentrated on the ventral vertebra. There is a high association (greater than 90%) between ventral vertebral extensions and the diseased vertebrae, a feature that is absent in normal specimens.[95] Histologic examination of this area reveals disorganized endochondral ossification, which may be a result of abnormal stress. Traumatic features of vascular and fibrocartilage proliferation are evident in the ventral end-plates in Scheuermann's disease.[9,18,95] The dorsal vertebral height in cases of Scheuermann's disease is not significantly different from that of controls, implying that either the ventral and dorsal stresses are different or that the kyphotic changes occur after dorsal growth is completed (the normal pattern of ring apophysis closure starts dorsolaterally, then works ventrally).[95] Possibly, the natural thoracic kyphosis, being exacerbated by a rounded back, results in the development of the abnormal kyphosis.

Back pain is uncommon in the growing child with Scheuermann's disease. Low back pain has been reported to be common (up to 50%)[16] in adults with progressive, untreated dorsal kyphotic deformities. In other studies pain was not a significant problem.[99] Progression of deformity is documented in 80% of cases over 25 years, but the extent is generally not severe.[106] The kyphosis most commonly progresses before skeletal maturity, but can occur in adulthood.[101] Disc degeneration is also associated with the deformity. Development of neurological complications is rare.[121]

Treatment is indicated to correct the deformity, prevent its progression, and alleviate pain. The extent of the kyphosis and the age of the patient are important. The nonoperative forms of treatment such as the brace or cast are the first line of treatment for most cases in which the deformity is less than 65 degrees. These cases have a high success rate in correcting the deformity, especially if treatment begins before closure of the iliac apophyses (i.e., skeletal maturation).[74] Operative treatment with fusion is reserved for cases of a deformity that increases despite treatment for pain, for degenerative changes in adults associated with the kyphosis, and for a deformity greater than 65 degrees.[101]

Paget's Disease

Paget's disease is a metabolic bone disorder thought possibly to be viral in origin. Prevalence of the disease has marked geographical variation. In the United States, Paget's disease is found radiographically in 3% to 4% of patients older than age 40.[97] Histologically, the disease is characterized by areas of bone resorption and new bone deposition resulting from focal increases in the population of osteoclasts. The individual cells are larger than normal and contain inclusion bodies similar to paramyxovirus capsids. This suggests viral induction of the osteoclastic activity and results in a greater surface bone resorption. There is no disturbance of reactive bone formation; therefore increased osteoblastic activity compensates for the bone resorption and, in fact, produces a net-positive balance of bone. The bone is usually lamellar, and it is normally mineralized.[97] However, woven bone and occasionally, osteoid bone are also present, and result in reduced bone quality with disruption of the lamellar structure of both cortical and trabecular bone.

The pelvic bones are the most commonly affected, followed by the spine. Approximately 70% of patients have lumbar spine involvement, 45% have thoracic spine lesions, and the cervical spine is involved in 15% of cases.[73] The frequent involvement of the lumbar spine is thought to be caused by increased loading.[29] The lesions are primarily in cancellous bone. Approximately two thirds of the radiographically evident lesions are asymptomatic.[73] Back pain in Paget's disease is related to the combination of the bone deformity and subchondral bone enlargement that alters the contours of the joint surfaces and leads to joint degeneration. The subchondral changes include increased bone deposition and subchondral infarcts from abnormal pressure on expanded bone, each of which causes the bone to lose its normal flexibility and usual biomechanical properties.[97] Radiographically, there are localized osteolytic lesions, which may coalesce with time, in addition to sclerotic areas. As a result of the disorganized pattern of bone deposition, there is reduced biomechanical efficiency and an increased risk of fracturing. Healing of fractures is usually efficient. The histologic features of Paget's disease are observed in the fracture line.[97] Some authors have noted an increased incidence of neurologic sequelae with thoracic and cervical spine involvement, perhaps caused by the narrower diameter of the spinal canal in these regions.[29,43,70]

Neurologic sequelae have been reported in 25% to 30% of cases of Paget's disease.[43,49] The neurologic deficits are most often caused by bony compression of the spinal canal or the foramina, with the neural arch and the facet joints most commonly affected by the proliferative bone deposition.[43] Fractures and subluxations can also compromise the spinal canal, and platybasia can result in compression of the medulla. Vascular "steal," resulting from the increased vascularity of the pathologic bone, has also been implicated in the development of neurologic deficits.[23]

Ankylosing Spondylitis

Ankylosing spondylitis is an inflammatory disorder affecting synovial and cartilaginous joints, primarily in the axial skeleton. The most noticeable pathologic findings are inflammation of the ligamentous attachments (enthesopathy), diskovertebral erosions, and new bone formation that results in the bony ankylosis.

The etiology of the disease remains unknown, but appears to be multifactorial with both genetic and acquired factors playing a role. There is a male predominance, varying from 3:1 to 8:1.[41] Peak age of onset is between 15 and 29 years, with less than 5% beginning after age 50.[14] The prevalence in the United States population is about 0.1%.[22]

The earliest signs of ankylosing spondylitis occur in the region of ligamentous attachment to bone (the enthesis).[25,27] In ankylosing spondylitis the enthesis shows multiple, focal, microscopic inflammatory lesions that eventually destroy the ligament and erode the adjacent cortical bone. This process leads to an osteitis, primarily at the ventral and ventrolateral aspects of the attachment of the annulus fibrosus to the bone. This is the "anterior spondylitis," or Romanus lesion, that is observed radiographically.[87,88] As the reparative process occurs, woven bone replaces the cortical erosion (ossification in fibrous tissue without preceding cartilage formation). Ultimately this is replaced by lamellar bone.[11] Syndesmophytes are formed, most conspicuously on the ventrolateral aspects of the vertebrae. This results in new enthesis formation above the original level of cortical bone. Further thickening and growth of the syndesmophyte may be caused by inflammatory lesions in this new bone[11] or chondroid metaplasia with ossification.[26]

In the apophyseal joint, osteitis and enthesopathy occur at the junction of capsule and bone and result in reactive bone formation and ossification of the capsule,[8,12] usually in the presence of well-preserved articular cartilage, implying that the capsule-ligamentous attachment is of primary importance in the apophyseal joint pathology.[8,11] Ultimately the joint may become ankylosed by endochondral ossification. This may be the result of capsular ossification or the general immobility of the spine as a result of diskovertebral syndesmophytes, as described previously.[10,11] However, the observation that apophyseal joint ankylosis may occur in the absence of vertebral ankylosis at the same level makes the former more likely.[12]

There is also concomitant ossification of the supraspinous and interspinous ligaments where there is a nonspecific inflammatory process at the attachment of the ligaments.[88] The anterior longitudinal ligament, however, does not usually become ossified, except at its deep fibers adjacent to the annulus fibrosus.[26]

Bone resorption (resulting in squaring of the vertebrae), syndesmophyte formation, bony ankylosis of the intervertebral discs, and apophyseal joint and ligament ossification, complete the classic radiographic "bamboo-spine" appearance. Although there is increased bone formation at the attachments of the ligaments and at the apophyseal joints, the vertebrae in ankylosing spondylitis are generally osteoporotic. This may be a result of the systemic effects of the disease, immobilization of the vertebrae, the inflammatory process, or drug treatment.[46]

As the bony ankylosis in the discovertebral region and the apophyseal joints occurs, the normal flexibility of the spine is lost. The spine is much stiffer than normal and is unable to absorb and dissipate loading energy in an efficient manner. Because of these factors and osteoporosis, the bone is much more prone to fracture and subluxation after trivial trauma.[76] The spinal cord is significantly vulnerable in these fractures. The cervical spine appears to be particularly susceptible; approximately 75% of the spinal fractures occur in this region, primarily in the lower cervical spine.[54] These fractures tend to pass through the ventrodorsal width of the vertebra and may, additionally, involve the calcified ligaments in the spinous processes. This process may occur either at the level of the disc space or through the vertebral body.[76] There is often a cervical kyphosis, and the neck is especially vulnerable to hyperextension injuries.[47,54,60] Some authors have attempted to match the mechanism of injury to the fracture location, considering extension to cause transdiscal fractures and flexion to cause transvertebral fractures.[60] Others have not found this relationship.[47]

In spondylitic patients with cervical spine fractures the mortality rate is 35%, as compared with 20% for patients with a normal spine. Also, the risk of severe neurological sequelae in ankylosing spondylitis is 57% compared with 18% in the normal spine.[76] Without ligamentous support, and with multiple ankylosed vertebrae, any spinal movement is concentrated at the fracture site. Therefore fractures are usually very unstable. The increased risk of bleeding with fracture in ankylosing spondylitis is thought to be related to the enlarged diploic spaces of the pathologic cancellous bone, the extensive nature of the fracture, and damage to adjacent epidural veins.[47,53] Epidural hematomas have been reported to occur in 20% of cases.[86] This is especially problematic because fractures often occur after minor trauma, and often in the lower cervical region. This may be difficult to visualize radiographically, especially in osteoporotic bone. For these reasons there is greater potential for neurologic deficit.

When fractures occur, there is normal callus formation at the site, and although inadequate immobilization may lead to pseudarthrosis, healing is typically rapid.[54] Pseudarthrosis of transdiscal fractures in undiagnosed ankylosing spondylitis is often confused with disc space infection.

Although atlantoaxial instability is far less common in ankylosing spondylitis than in rheumatoid arthritis, it may occur.[67,114] Inflammation of the entheses, the apophyseal joints, and the synovial joint between the dens and the transverse ligament results in both bony and ligamentous damage, with subsequent instability similar to that observed in rheumatoid arthritis.

Ossification of the Posterior Longitudinal Ligament

Although OPLL was first reported in 1838 in England,[61] it has received increased attention because of the high incidence in Japanese and other Asian populations.[7,107] OPLL appears in approximately 2% of the cervical spine radiographs in the Japanese population, and autopsy studies show an incidence of 20% in subjects over age 60.[111] More recently it has been recognized in the non-Asian population, but the prevalence is lower in other countries: 0.1% in West Germany,[56] 0.12% to 0.7% in the United States,[34,56,71] and 1.7% in Italy.[5] The incidence appears to be higher in males, and it increases with age.[111] The pathogenesis of OPLL remains unclear. Routine tests, such as C-reactive protein, erythrocyte sedimentation rate, rheumatoid factor, and HLA-B27 are all normal.[107,111] HLA-Bw40 and SA5 are more common in OPLL patients, but there is no clear evidence of an inheritance pattern.[103,111] Metabolic abnormalities such as hypoparathyroidism and familial hypophosphatemic rickets may occur concurrently with OPLL,[111] implying a disturbance of calcium metabolism. However, the significance of these abnormalities in the pathogenesis of OPLL is unclear. In one series 28.4% of the OPLL patients were diabetic, and 17.7% had an impaired glucose tolerance test. Patients with diabetes mellitus also have an increased incidence of OPLL.[111]

Other hyperostotic conditions associated with OPLL are diffuse idiopathic skeletal hyperostosis (with a concomitance rate of 50%),[85] ankylosing spondylitis (with a 2% concomitance rate), and ossification of the yellow ligament (with a concomitance rate of 6.8%).[107,111]

Radiographically, this acquired spine abnormality is characterized by abnormal ossification along the dorsal border of the vertebral body. Over 90% of the disease occurs in the cervical spine. Thoracic or lumbar involvement is unusual. OPLL is classified according to its localization along the vertebrae. It has been classified into segmental, mixed, continuous, and localized forms.[111] The segmental type is characterized by calcification behind each vertebral body, with each segment separated by the uninvolved disc space. The continuous type extends over several vertebrae. The mixed type is a combination of these two types. The localized type demonstrates ossification limited to the ligament over the disc space. The vertebrae at C4, C5, and C6 are most affected, and the average number of vertebrae involved is 3.1.[111] Ligamentous ossification substantially reduces the size of the spinal canal, particularly in the mixed and continuous types.

Histologically, the normal posterior longitudinal ligament (PLL) contains both type I and type II collagen. In OPLL only type I collagen is identified, suggesting that the process of ossification involves replacement of the original collagen matrix.[123] The heterotopic bone formation observed with OPLL occurs in the superficial layer of the PLL, leaving an unossified gap between the dorsal aspect of the vertebral body and the ligament. The ossified ligament has a typical lamellar bone structure with Haversian canals and a few bone-marrow canals.[123] Calcification or ossification may also involve the dura mater.

The average radiographic narrowing of the anteroposterior diameter of the cervical spinal cord has been noted to be more than 40% for the mixed and continuous types.[111] The disease's progression in a single, small series has been documented as a mean annual increase of 4.07mm rostrocaudally and 0.67mm in the ventrodorsal direction.[92] Myelopathy is the most common neurologic abnormality. It is likely that a large proportion of cases are asymptomatic.[48] The relative paucity of symptoms has been attributed to the relatively slow rate of progression in most cases, as well as the lack of underlying developmental stenosis. However, a critical spinal canal diameter can be reached, where even minimal trauma can result in severe neurologic deficit.

The surgical treatment of OPLL has been aimed at enlarging the spinal canal by removing the vertebral bodies and the ossified ligament by ventral corpectomy and fusion. Internal fixation may obviate the need for postoperative halo or Minerva immobilization. The dorsal approach does not remove the primary pathologic lesion, and with rapid disease progression, ventral surgery may still be required as a secondary procedure.

Spondylolisthesis and Spondylolysis

Spondylolisthesis is the translational movement of one vertebra on another. Spondylolysis refers to a defect in the pars interarticularis and may or may not be observed in spondylolisthesis. Instability of the affected motion segment may cause back pain. Sciatica and radiculopathy are more likely caused by foramen stenosis than by spinal canal constriction. To understand the classification, implications, and radiographic findings of these conditions, the anatomy and biomechanics of the area of the lamina, known as the pars interarticularis, must be considered.

The pars interarticularis, or isthmus, is the bone between the lamina, pedicle, articular facet, and the transverse process. This region is able to resist significant forces in excess of 1251 newtons.[109] It has a cross-sectional area of about 0.75cm^2, with two layers of cortical bone and intervening trabecular bone.[55]

Flexion, extension, and rotation all have effects on the disc and, subsequently, the facet joints and pars interarticularis. With normal lumbar lordosis, with the discs inclined in a ventrocaudal direction, the load is transmitted by the discs.[1] Axial loading therefore places both the disc and the caudal facets under ventral shear stress.[33,108] This stress is parallel to the intervertebral disc and is resisted by the caudal facets of the apophyseal joints, the disc, and the muscles attached to the neural arch.[33,55,108] In the intact specimen under shear stress, approximately 60% of the stiffness is provided by the disc and 15% by the facet joints.[1] The lower lumbar level apophyseal joints lie directly across the plane of the disc and therefore may contribute more to resisting shear than the apophyseal joints in the upper lumbar region, which are at the level of the pedicles.[33] In addition, the upper lumbar disc spaces are more dorsocaudally inclined in the upright position, thus making the apophyseal joints less susceptible.

Exactly what movements cause the mechanical deformation and, ultimately, the failure of the pars interarticularis remains unclear. The contribution of flexion, extension, and rotatory movements has been reviewed.[33,108,109]

It can be demonstrated that as flexion occurs, compression and ventral shear stresses in the lower lumbar region increase.[33] Muscular, and then ligamentous, tension resists the shear stress. The simultaneous application of the shear stress and the resisting forces causes stress concentration at the caudal margin of the pedicle, which progresses across the pars.[33] The pars, not as strong as the pedicle, fails as the stress increases with greater flexion. Debate remains about whether a single episode of overload[33] or fatigue[117] causes microfractures that lead to a gross fracture with continuing overload. It is likely that a combination of both processes occurs.[108] The same mechanism that causes the fracture prevents complete healing, and fibrous nonunion results. This may allow progressive listhesis with elongation of the pars.[116]

Research and clinical information also implicate extension movement in generating stresses across the pars interarticularis that may lead to fracture.[108] It has been suggested that the frequency of spondylolisthesis in gymnasts is a result of hyperextension injuries occurring on landing in the upright position with accentuated lumbar lordosis. If the extended spine is in acceleration and is subjected to sudden deceleration, increased shear stress is generated along the disc space, which in the lower lumbar spine is at an angle to the line of deceleration. This results in further extension, increasing shear, and greater stress across the pars.[108] Also, the disc is less stiff in extension, making ventral translation even more probable.[109] Microfractures develop, and once the bone is defective, the forces acting on it result in further microfractures and progression of the lesion. Further support for the importance of lordosis in causing the pars defects is observed in patients with Scheuermann's disease in which a compensatory lumbar lordosis occurs. Asymptomatic lumbar spondylolysis has been reported in as many as 50% of these patients.[80]

Torque may also play a role in the development of spondylolisthesis, especially in the degenerative type. With disc degeneration the disc loses its ability to resist shear and torsional stresses.[32,33] Torsional stress, conveyed to the caudal facet, distorts the lamina-pedicle angle and results in the facet being less able to resist shear. The contralateral facet then has to resist more shear stress, and may also become damaged.[33] Stress concentration with injury to the pars may occur when torsional forces are applied to the neural arch, and ultimately, ventral subluxation may occur.[33]

The most widely used classification of spondylolisthesis is that of Wiltse *et al*.[116] Wiltse and colleagues divide the listhesis types into dysplastic, isthmic, degenerative, traumatic, and pathologic. Degenerative listhesis has a prevalence of 4% to 10%[31,112]; isthmic, 4%; and dysplastic, 1%.[120] Traumatic and pathological listhesis implies a history of localized trauma or generalized bony disease, which allows forward subluxation to occur.

Dysplastic Spondylolisthesis

Dysplastic spondylolisthesis, which is caused by a congenital defect of the upper sacrum, or the vertebral arch of L5, presents in young children and adolescents.[100] It has two subtypes: type "a," with the dysplastic articular facets oriented axially; and type "b," with dysplastic articular facets oriented sagittally. When the facets are dysplastic, the ability to resist the ventral shear stress is reduced and can result in listhesis. The pars may be initially intact or even remain intact, but in other cases the ventral shear stress results in microfractures of the pars, with subsequent pars elongation. Thus the pars is not the initiator of the listhesis.[65] In dysplastic cases with a subluxation of greater than 35%, there are likely to be neurological and muscular symptoms,[100] usually manifested as symptoms of cauda equina or nerve root compression. Paralysis and bowel dysfunction are uncommon. Hamstring tightness and abnormal gait, however, are common.[100]

Isthmic Spondylolisthesis

In isthmic spondylolisthesis there is a defect in the pars interarticularis (spondylolysis). Facet orientation is normal. There are three subtypes that depend on the integrity of the pars and the nature of the injury. In subtype "a" there is distinct separation of the pars interarticularis, as a result of fatigue fracture, a single traumatic episode, or a combination of both (Figure 5.5). In subtype "b" there is elongation of the pars, which actually appears intact and is thought to be a result of the healing of stress fractures of the pars. Fibrous nonunion is observed in these defects. This can appear similar to a dysplastic lesion with pars elongation. In subtype "c" there is an acute fracture of the pars, in addition to fractures elsewhere in the vertebra, usually a result of severe trauma.

Isthmic spondylolisthesis occurs at L5-S1 in approximately 82%, L4-5 in 11%, L3-4 in 0.5%, L2-3 in 0.3%, and in other levels, in approximately 6% of the cases.[42] The lesion does not appear in other primates, indicating that upright posture is important. Also, true lumbar lordosis, seen only in the human primate, may be a factor.[116]

Infant cadaveric dissections have demonstrated that lytic pars defects are not present at birth.[91] However, bilateral pars interarticularis defects have been documented in a 4-month-old.[15] The most common age for development and diagnosis of isthmic spondylolysis is between the ages of 5 and 7.[116] In a study of 500 children,[35] 4.4% of the 6-year-olds and 5.2% of the 12-year-olds had unilateral or bilateral pars defects, whereas the incidence is 6% in adults. It is postulated that with assumption of the upright sitting posture and lordosis of the lumbar spine, subluxation is most likely to develop.[102,116] In adolescent cases participation in contact sports may be significant.[116]

There is also evidence that genetic factors may play a role in isthmic spondylolisthesis.[36,117] White males have an incidence of 6.4%, compared with black women, who have

an incidence of 1.1%.[42] There is an association between the dysplastic and isthmic lesions and spina bifida occulta and hypoplasia of the sacrum.[90] The prevalence of spina bifida occulta of L5 or S1 and lumbosacral defects in one series was found to be 94% for the dysplastic type and 32% for the isthmic type.[120] The incidence of the two types of spondylolisthesis has been reported to be increased in first-degree relatives. Thirty-three percent and 15%, respectively, of first-degree relatives of patients with dysplastic and isthmic spondylolisthesis have radiographical evidence of subluxation.[120]

Although the initial degree of slip in isthmic spondylolisthesis can be marked, progression in adulthood is unusual. Slip is more prone to progress at L4-5 than L5-S1, and may be up to 28% in the teenage years..[35] Whether subluxation will progress, however, is difficult to predict. Treatment of each type of spondylolysis depends on the extent of neural compression and motion segment instability. Decompressive laminectomy, foraminotomies, and internal fixation may be required.

Degenerative Spondylolisthesis

Degenerative spondylolisthesis is more common in women than men,[78] with a ratio of 5:1. It is associated with spondylotic changes of the apophyseal joints and disc narrowing. Degeneration of the disc reduces its stiffness and places greater stress on the facets. When subjected to shear forces, this may lead to subluxation, without fracture of the pars. Subluxation does not usually exceed 30%.[79] Because of the greater inherent stability of L5 and the prevalence of L5 sacralization,[42] the L4-5 or L3-4 levels are more frequently affected.[89] Stabilization as a result of osteophyte formation usually occurs, and significant progression is rare without destabilizing surgical procedures. Degenerative spondylolisthesis is commonly associated with spinal stenosis and neurogenic claudication caused by lumbosacral radiculopathy. Decompression often relieves symptoms. Fusion with internal fixation may be required in cases with radiographic evidence of instability or severe back pain.

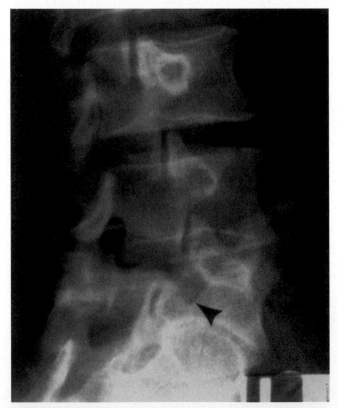

Figure 5.5 Oblique plain radiographs of the lower lumbar spine. Arrow indicates subtype "a" spondylolysis (absence of the neck of the Scotty dog).

REFERENCES

1. Adams MA, Hutton WC: The effect of posture on the role of the apophyseal joints in resisting intervertebral compressive forces. *J Bone Joint Surg* 62B:358-362, 1980.
2. Adams MA, Hutton WC: The relevance of torsion to the mechanical derangement of the lumbar spine. *Spine* 6:241-248, 1981.
3. Adams MA, Hutton WC: Prolapsed intervertebral disc. A hyperflexion injury. 1981 Volvo Award in Basic Science. *Spine* 7:184-191, 1982.
4. Adams MA, Hutton WC: Gradual disc prolapse. *Spine* 10:524-531, 1985.
5. Albisinni U, Merlini L, Terayama K, *et al*: X-ray epidemiology of ligaments, ossifications, and disc degeneration of the cervical spine [Italian]. *Chir Degli Organi Movimento* 70:15-22, 1985.
6. Ansell BM: The cervical spine in juvenile rheumatoid arthritis (International Congress Series, 61). In Carter ME

(ed): *Radiological Aspects of Rheumatoid Arthritis*. Amsterdam, Excerpta Medica, 1964.

7. Ascani E, Borelli P, LaRosa G, *et al*: Malattia di Scheuermann. I: studio ormonale, progressi in patologia vertebrale. In *Le Cifosi* vol 5. Bologna, Italy, Gaggi, 1982.

8. Aufdermaur M: The morbid anatomy of ankylosing spondylitis. *Doc Rheumatol Geigy* No. 2, 1957.

9. Aufdermaur M: Juvenile kyphosis (Scheuermann's disease): radiography, histology, and pathogenesis. *Clin Orthop Rel Res* 154:166-174, 1981.

10. Baker W, Thomas TG, Kirkaldy-Willis WH: Changes in the cartilage of the posterior intervertebral joints after anterior fusion. *J Bone Joint Surg* 51-:736-746, 1969.

11. Ball J: Enthesopathy of rheumatoid and ankylosing spondylitis. *Ann Rheum Dis* 30:213-223, 1971.

12. Ball J: Articular pathology of ankylosing spondylitis. *Clin Orthop Relat Res* 143:30-37, 1979.

13. Bick EM, Copel JW: The ring apophysis of the human vertebra. Contribution to human osteogeny II. *J Bone Joint Surg* 33A:783-787, 1951.

14. Blumberg B, Ragan C: The natural history of rheumatoid spondylitis. *Medicine* 35:1, 1956.

15. Borkow SE, Kleiger B: Spondylolisthesis in the newborn. A case report. *Clin Orthop Rel Res* 81:73-76, 1971.

16. Bradford DS: Juvenile kyphosis. *Clin Orthop Relat Res* 128:45-55, 1977.

17. Bradford DS, Brown DM, Moe JH, *et al*: Scheuermann's kyphosis: a form of osteoporosis? *Clin Orthop Relat Res* 118:10-15, 1976.

18. Bradford DS, Moe JH: Scheuermann's juvenile kyphosis. A histologic study. *Clin Orthop Relat Res* 110:45-53, 1975.

19. Bradford DS, Moe JH, Montalvo FJ, Winter RB: Scheuermann's kyphosis and roundback deformity: results of Milwaukee brace treatment. *J Bone Joint Surg* 56Λ:749, 1974.

20. Brinckmann P, Grootenboer H: Change of disc height, radial disc bulge, and intradiscal pressure from discectomy: an in vitro investigation on human lumbar discs. *Spine* 16:641-646, 1991.

21. Bywaters EG: Rheumatoid and other diseases of the cervical interspinous bursae, and changes in the spinous processes. *Ann Rheum Dis* 41:360-370, 1982.

22. Cardenosa G, Deluca SA: Ankylosing spondylosis. *Am Fam Phys* 42:147-150, 1990.

23. Chen JR, Rhee RS, Wallach S, *et al*: Neurologic disturbances in Paget disease of bone: response to calcitonin. *Neurology* 29:448-457, 1979.

24. Cloward RB, Bucy PC: Spinal extradural cyst and kyphosis dorsalis juvenilis. *Am J Roentgenol* 38:681, 1937.

25. Cooper RR, Misol S: Tendon and ligament insertion. A light and electron microscopic study, review. *J Bone Joint Surg* 52A:1-20, 1970.

26. Cruickshank B: Pathology of ankylosing spondylitis. *Clin Orthop Relat Res* 74:43-58, 1971.

27. Davies DV, Young L: The distribution of radioactive sulphur (35S) in the fibrous tissues, cartilages, and bones of the rat following its administration in the form of inorganic sulphate. *J Anat* 88:174, 1995.

28. Dirheimer Y: *The Craniovertebral Region in Chronic Inflammatory Rheumatic Diseases*. Berlin, Springer-Verlag, 1977.

29. Douglas DL, Duckworth T, Kanis JA, *et al*: Spinal cord dysfunction in Paget's disease of bone. Has medical treatment a vascular basis? *J Bone Joint Surg* 63B:495-503, 1981.

30. Ecklin U: *Die Altersveranderungen der Halswirbelsaule*. Berlin, Springer, 1960, pp 17, 28.

31. Farfan HF: The pathological anatomy of degenerative spondylolisthesis. A cadaver study. *Spine* 5:412-418, 1980.

32. Farfan HF, Cossette JW, Robertson GH, *et al*: The effects of torsion on the lumbar intervertebral joints: the role of torsion in the production of disc degeneration. *J Bone Joint Surg* 52A:468-497, 1970.

33. Farfan HF, Osteria V, Lamy C: The mechanical etiology of spondylolysis and spondylolisthesis. *Clin Orthop Relat Res* 8:40-55, 1976.

34. Firooznia H, Benjamin VM, Pinto RS, *et al*: Calcification and ossification of posterior longitudinal ligament of spine: its role in secondary narrowing of spinal canal and cord compression. *NY State J Med* 82:1193-1198, 1982.

35. Fredrickson BE, Baker D, McHolick WJ, *et al*: The natural history of spondylolysis and spondylolisthesis. *J Bone Joint Surg* 66A:699-707, 1984.

36. Friberg S: Studies on spondylolisthesis. *Acta Chir Orthop* (suppl 60): 1939.

37. Frymoyer JW, Moskowitz RW: Spinal degeneration. Pathogenesis and medical management. In Frymoyer JW (ed): *The Adult Spine: Principles and Practice*. Philadelphia, Lippincott-Raven, 1991, pp. 611-634.

38. Gilsanz V, Gibbens DT, Carlson M, King J: Vertebral bone density in Scheuermann disease. *J Bone Joint Surg* 71A:894-897, 1989.

39. Gordon SJ, Yang KH, Mayer PJ, *et al*: Mechanism of disc rupture: a preliminary report. *Spine* 16:450-456, 1991.

40. Gower WE, Pedrini V: Age-related variations in protein polysaccharides from human nucleus pulposus, annulus fibrosus, and costal cartilage. *J Bone Joint Surg* 51A: 1154-1162, 1969.

41. Gran JT: The epidemiology of rheumatoid arthritis. *Monogr Allergy* 21:162-196, 1987.

42. Grobler LJ, Wiltse LL: Classification, non-operative, and operative treatment of spondylolisthesis. In Frymoyer JW (ed): *The Adult Spine: Principles and Practice*. Philadelphia, Lippincott-Raven, 1991, pp 1655-1704.

43. Hadjipavlou A, Lander P: Paget disease of the spine. *J Bone Joint Surg* 73A:1376-1381, 1991.

44. Halal F, Gledhill RB, Fraser C: Dominant inheritance of Scheuermann's juvenile kyphosis. *Am J Dis Child* 132: 1105-1107, 1978.

45. Halla JT, Hardin JG, Vitek J, Alarcon GS: Involvement of the cervical spine in rheumatoid arthritis, review. *Arthritis Rheum* 32:652-659, 1989.

46. Hanson CA, Shagrin JW, Duncan H: Vertebral osteoporosis in ankylosing spondylitis. *Clin Orthop Relat Res* 74:59-64, 1971.

47. Harding JR, McCall IW, Park WM, Jones BF: Fracture of the cervical spine in ankylosing spondylitis. *Br J Radiol* 58:3-7, 1985.

48. Harsh GR, Sypert GW, Weinstein PR, *et al*: Cervical spine stenosis secondary to ossification of the posterior longitudinal ligament. *J Neurosurg* 67:349-357, 1987.

49. Hartman JT, Dohn DF: Paget's disease of the spine with cord or nerve-root compression. *J Bone Joint Surg* 48A:1079-1084, 1966.

50. Hayashi H, Okada K, Hamada M, *et al*: Etiologic factors of myelopathy. A radiographic evaluation of the aging changes in the cervical spine. *Clin Orthop Relat Res* 214:200-209, 1987.

51. Hood RS: Far lateral lumbar disc herniations. *Neurosurg Clin North Am* 4:117-124, 1993.

52. Hukins DWL: Disc structure and function.. In Ghosh P (ed): *The Biology of the Intervertebral Disc*, vol 1. Boca Raton, FL, CRC Press, 1988, pp 1-37.

53. Hunter T: The spinal complications of ankylosing spondylitis, review. *Semin Arthritis Rheum* 19:172-182, 1989.

54. Hunter T, Dubo H: Spinal fractures complicating ankylosing spondylitis. *Ann Intern Med* 88:546-549, 1978.

55. Hutton WC, Cyron BM: Spondylolysis. The role of the posterior elements in resisting the intervertebral compressive force. *Acta Orthop Scand* 49:604-609, 1978.

56. Isawa K: Comparative roentgenographical study on the incidence of ossification of the posterior longitudinal ligament and other degenerative changes of the cervical spine among Japanese, Koreans, Americans, and Germans. *Nippon Seikeigeka Gakkai Zasshi* (Japan) 54:461-474, 1980.

57. Katz JN, Liang MH: Differential diagnosis and conservative treatment of rheumatoid disorders. In Frymoyer JW (ed): *The Adult Spine: Principles and Practice*. Philadelphia, Lippincott-Raven, 1991, pp 699-718.

58. Kemp FH, Wilson DC: Some factors in the aetiology of osteochondritis of the spine. A report on two families. *Br J Radiol* 20:410-417, 1947.

59. Kewalramani LS, Riggins RS, Fowler WM, Jr: Scheuermann's kyphoscoliosis associated with Charcot-Marie-Tooth syndrome. *Arch Phys Med Rehab* 57:391-397, 1976.

60. Kewalramani LS, Taylor RG, Albrand OW: Cervical spine injury in patients with ankylosing spondylitis. *J Trauma* 15:931-934, 1975.

61. Key CA: On paraplegia depending on disease of the ligaments of the spine. *Guys Hosp Rep* (Series 1) 3:17-34, 1838.

62. Kirkaldy-Willis WH: *Managing Low Back Pain*. New York, Churchill Livingstone, 1983.

63. Komusi T, Munro T, Harth M: Radiologic review: the rheumatoid cervical spine, review. *Semin Arthritis Rheum* 14:187-195, 1985.

64. Lopez RA, Burke SW, Levine DB, Schneider R: Osteoporosis in Scheuermann's disease. *Spine* 13:1099-1103, 1988.

65. Macnab I: *Backache*. Baltimore, Williams & Wilkins, 1990, pp 84-103.

66. Maroudas A: Nutrition and metabolism of the intervertebral disc. In Ghosh P (ed): *The Biology of the Intervertebral Disc*, vol 2. Boca Raton, FL, CRC Press, 1988, pp 1-37.

67. Martel W: The occipito-atlanto-axial joints in rheumatoid arthritis and ankylosing spondylitis. *AJR* 86:223-240, 1961.

68. Martel W: Pathogenesis of cervical discovertebral destruction in rheumatoid arthritis. *Arthritis Rheum* 20:1217-1225, 1977.

69. Masaryk TJ, Ross JS, Modic MT, *et al*: High-resolution MR imaging of sequestered lumbar intervertebral disks. *Am J Roentgenol* 150:1155-1162, 1988.

70. Mawhinney R, Jones R, Worthington BS: Spinal cord compression secondary to Paget's disease of the axis. *Br J Radiol* 58:1203-1206, 1985.

71. McAfee PC, Regan JJ, Bohlman HH: Cervical cord compression from ossification of the posterior longitudinal ligament in non-Orientals. *J Bone Joint Surg* 69B:569-575, 1987.

72. McDevitt CA: Proteoglycans of the intervertebral disc. In Ghosh P (ed): *The Biology of the Intervertebral Disc*, vol 1. Boca Raton, FL, CRC Press, 1988, pp 151-170.

73. Meunier PJ: Bone histomorphometry and skeletal distribution of Paget's disease of bone. *Semin Arthritis Rheum* 23:219-221, 1994.

74. Montgomery SP, Erwin WE: Scheuermann's kyphosis: long-term results of Milwaukee brace treatment. *Spine* 6:5-8, 1981.

75. Morizono Y, Sakou T, Kawaida H: Upper cervical involvement in rheumatoid arthritis. *Spine* 12:721-725, 1987.

76. Murray GC, Persellin RH: Cervical fracture complicating ankylosing spondylitis: a report of eight cases and review of the literature, review. *Am J Med* 70:1033-1041, 1981.

77. Naylor A: Factors in the development of the spinal stenosis syndrome. *J Bone Joint Surg* 61B:306-309, 1979.

78. Newman PH: Surgical treatment for spondylolisthesis in the adult. *Clin Orthop Relat Res* 117:106-111, 1976.

79. Newman PH, Stone KH: The etiology of spondylolisthesis with a special investigation. *J Bone Joint Surg* 45B:39-59, 1963.

80. Ogilvie JW, Sherman J: Spondylolysis in Scheuermann's disease. *Spine* 12:251-253, 1987.

81. Osti OL, Vernon-Roberts B, Fraser RD: Annulus tears and intervertebral disc degeneration: an experimental study using an animal model. *Spine* 15:762-767, 1990.

82. Pellicci PM, Ranawat CS, Tsairis P, Bryan WJ: A prospective study of the progression of rheumatoid arthritis of the cervical spine. *J Bone Joint Surg* 63A:342-350, 1981.

83. Pennal GF, Schatzker J: Stenosis of the lumbar spinal canal. *Clin Neurosurg* 18:86-105, 1971.

84. Penning L, Wilmink JT: Posture-dependent bilateral compression of L4 or L5 nerve roots in facet hypertrophy. A dynamic CT-myelographic study. *Spine* 12:488-500, 1987.

85. Resnick D, Guerra J, Robinson CA, Vint VC: Association of diffuse idiopathic skeletal hyperostosis (DISH) and calcification and ossification of the posterior longitudinal ligament. *Am J Roentgenol* 1319:1049-1053, 1978.

86. Resnick D, Niwayama G: *Diagnosis of Bone and Joint Disorders*. Philadelphia, WB Saunders, 1988, pp 1103-1170.

87. Romanus R: *Pelvo-spondylitis Ossificans in the Male*. Stockholm, Aktiebolaget Godvil, 1953.

88. Romanus R, Yden S: Destructive and ossifying spondylitic changes in rheumatoid ankylosing spondylitis. *Acta Orthop Scand* 22:88-99, 1952.

89. Rosenberg NJ: Degenerative spondylolisthesis. Predisposing factors. *J Bone Joint Surg* 57A:467-474, 1975.

90. Rothman SLG, Glenn WV: Spondylolysis and spondylolysthesis. In Post JD (ed): *CT of the Lumbar Spine*. Baltimore, Williams & Wilkins, 1984, pp 591-615.

91. Rowe GG, Roche MB: The etiology of separate neural arch. *J Bone Joint Surg* 35A:102-110, 1953.

92. Sato M, Turu M, Yada K: The antero-posterior diameter of the cervical spinal canal in the ossification of the posterior longitudinal ligament. *No Shinkei Geka* 5:511-517, 1977.

93. Scheuermann H: Kyphosis dorsalis juvenilis. *Ugeskr Laeger* 82:385-393, 1920.

94. Schmorl G: Die Pathogenese der juvenilen Kyphose. *Fortschr Geb Rontgen* 41:359-383, 1930.

95. Scoles PV, Latimer BM, DiGiovanni BF, *et al*: Vertebral alterations in Scheuermann's kyphosis. *Spine* 16:509-515, 1991.

96. Simon RS: The diagnosis and treatment of kyphosis dorsalis juvenilis (Scheuermann's kyphosis) in the early stage. *J Bone Joint Surg* 24:681-683, 1942.

97. Singer FR, Mills BG: Primary bone cell dysfunction: I. Paget's disease of the bone. In Tam CS, Heersche JNM (eds): *Metabolic Bone Disease: Cellular and Tissue Mechanisms*. Boca Raton, FL, CRC Press, 1989, pp. 33-47.

98. Singh M, Riggs BL, Beabout JW, Jowsey J: Femoral trabecular pattern index for evaluation of spinal osteoporosis. A detailed methodologic description. *Mayo Clin Proc* 48:184-189, 1973.

99. Sorenson KH: *Scheuermann's Juvenile Kyphosis. Clinical Appearances, Radiography, Aetiology, and Prognosis*. Copenhagen, Munksgaard, 1964.

100. Stillerman CB, Schneider JH, Gruen JP: Evaluation and management of spondylolysis and spondylolisthesis. In Wilkins, Rengachery (eds): *Clinical Neurosurgery*. Baltimore, Williams & Wilkins, 1992, pp 384-415.

101. Sturm PF, Crawford-Dobson J, Armstrong GWD: The surgical treatment of Scheuermann's disease. *Spine* 18:685-691, 1993.

102. Taillard WF: Etiology of spondylolisthesis. *Clin Orthop Relat Res* 117:30-39, 1976.

103. Tanikawa E, Furuya K, Nakajima H: Genetic study on ossification of posterior longitudinal ligament. *Bull Tokyo Med Dent Univ* 33:117-128, 1986.

104. Taylor JR, Twomey LT: The development of the human intervertebral disc. In Ghosh P (ed): *The Biology of the Intervertebral Disc*, vol 1. Boca Raton, FL, CRC Press, 1988, pp 39-82.

105. Taylor JR, Twomey LT: Human intervertebral disc acid glycosaminoglycans. *J Anat* 180:137-141, 1992.

106. Travaglini F, Conte M: Progressi in patologia vertebrale. In *Le Cifosi*, vol 5. Bologna, Italy, Gaggi, 1982.

107. Trojan DA, Pouchot J, Pokrupa R, *et al*: Diagnosis and treatment of ossification of the posterior longitudinal ligament of the spine: report of eight cases and literature review. *Am J Med* 92:296-306, 1992.

108. Troup JD: Mechanical factors in spondylolisthesis and spondylolysis. *Clin Orthop Relat Res* 117:59-67, 1976.

109. Troup JDG: The etiology of spondylolysis. *Orthop Clin North Am* 117:59-67, 1977.

110. Tsuji H, Hirano N, Ohshima H, *et al*: Structural variation of the anterior and the posterior anulus fibrosus in the development of the human lumbar disc. *Spine* 18:204-210, 1993.

111. Tsuyama N: Ossification of the posterior longitudinal ligament of the spine. *Clin Orthop Relat Res* 184:71-84, 1984.

112. Valkenburg HA, Haanen HCM: The epidemiology of low back pain. In White AA, Gordon SL (eds): *The Proceedings of the American Association of Orthopedic Surgery Symposium on Low Back Pain*. 1982, pp 9-22.

113. Weinstein JN, Wiesel SW: *The Lumbar Spine: The International Society for the Study of the Lumbar Spine*. Philadelphia, WB Saunders, 1990, pp 394-395.

114. Weinstein PR, Karpman RR, Gall EP, Pitt M: Spinal cord injury, spinal fracture, and spinal stenosis in ankylosing spondylitis. *J Neurosurg* 57:609-616, 1982.

115. White AA, Punjabi MM, Thomas CL: The clinical biomechanics of kyphotic deformities. *Clin Orthop Relat Res* 128:8-17, 1977.

116. Wiltse LL, Newman PH, Macnab I: Classification of spondylolysis and spondylolisthesis. *Clin Orthop Relat Res* 117:23-29, 1976.

117. Wiltse LL, Widell EH, Jr, Jackson DW: Fatigue fracture: the basic lesion is isthmic spondylolisthesis. *J Bone Joint Surg* 57A:17-22, 1975.

118. Wise BL, Fostey JJ: Congenital spinal extradural cyst. *J Neurosurg* 12:421, 1955.

119. Wollin DG, Botterell EH: Symmetrical forward luxation of the atlas. *Am J Roentgenol Rad Nucl Med* 79:575-583, 1958.

120. Wynne-Davies R, Scott JHS: Inheritance and spondylolisthesis: a radiographic family survey. *J Bone Joint Surg* 61B:301-305, 1979.

121. Yablon JS, Kasdon DL, Levine H: Thoracic cord compression in Scheuermann's disease. *Spine* 13:896-898, 1988.

122. Yamada H, Oya M, Okada T, Shiozawa Z: Intermittent cauda equina compression due to narrow spinal canal. *J Neurosurg* 37:83-88, 1972.

123. Yasui N, Ono K, Yamaura I, *et al*: Immunohistochemical localization of types I, II, and III collagens in the ossified posterior longitudinal ligament of the human cervical spine. *Calcif Tissue Int* 35:159-163, 1983.

124. Yasuma T, Koh S, Okamura T, Yamauchi Y: Histological changes in aging lumbar intervertebral discs: their role in protrusions and prolapses. *J Bone Joint Surg* 72A:220-229, 1990.

125. Yu S, Haughton VM, Sether LA, *et al*: Criteria for classifying normal and degenerated lumbar intervertebral disks. *Radiology* 170:523-526, 1989.

126. Yu S, Haughton VM, Sether LA, Wagner M: Anulus fibrosus in bulging intervertebral discs. *Radiology* 169:761-763, 1988.

127. Zvaifler NJ: Rheumatoid arthritis: epidemiology, etiology, rheumatoid factor, pathology, pathogenesis. In Schumacher HR (ed): *Primer on Rheumatic Disease*. Atlanta, Arthritis Foundation, 1988.

128. Zvaifler NJ: Etiology and pathogenesis of rheumatoid arthritis. In McCarty, Hoopman (eds): *Arthritis and Allied Conditions*. Vol. 1. Philadelphia, Lea & Febiger, 1993, pp 723-726.

129. Zygmunt S, Saveland H, Brattstrom H, *et al*: Reduction of rheumatoid periodontoid pannus following posterior occipito-cervical fusion visualised by magnetic resonance imaging. *Br J Neurosurg* 2:315-320, 1988.

CHAPTER 6

Neural Injury at the Molecular Level

David H. Kim, Alexander R. Vaccaro,
Fraser C. Henderson, and Edward C. Benzel

The histopathological appearance of chronic cervical spondylotic myelopathy has been well described and includes the characteristic features of regional demyelination extending axially from the site of compression, preferential lateral column axonal loss, and anterior horn neuron dropout.[1-5] Recent studies are leading to a better understanding of myelopathy on a molecular level, and indicate that a significant portion of cell loss appears to be caused by the process of apoptosis. Although the intercellular and intracellular pathways regulating apoptosis are extremely complex, cell death ultimately affects a very restricted population of spinal cord cells, namely oligodendrocytes, suggesting the possibility that targeted anti-apoptotic therapy may be a reasonable goal for the treatment or prevention of myelopathy.

Microbiology of the Oligodendrocyte

Recent studies have revealed a pivotal role for the oligodendrocyte in several complex biological processes, including development, injury repair, and disease modulation, as well as the formation and maintenance of myelin.[6,7] A large oligodendroglial population is generated during the early course of human development, with an estimated 50% of these cells eventually disappearing in a process of programmed cell death, known as *apoptosis*.[8] With the maturation of the central nervous system, the oligodendroglia become responsible for the creation and maintenance of myelin sheaths which, although formed directly from oligodendroglial membrane, demonstrate key biochemical differences from the parent cell membrane in terms of chemical and protein composition.[9] Characteristics of the relatively small protein constituent are particularly important, and absence or alteration of the major protein components (i.e., proteolipid protein or myelin basic protein) can lead to the appearance of severe demyelinating disease.[10] The other salient feature of the oligodendrocyte is the extremely high concentration of microtubules, which contribute to formation of an elaborate cytoskeletal framework, allowing myelin sheath formation at remote distances from the cell karyon.[6]

Considerable progress has been made in understanding the response of oligodendroglial cells to injury, and a more complete understanding of this complex process may shed considerable light on the mechanism of injury in such processes as cervical spondylotic myelopathy. The oligodendrocyte appears to be exquisitely sensitive to a wide range of oxidative, chemical, radiation-induced, and mechanical injuries. High iron content and relatively inefficient antioxidant defense mechanisms appear to render the oligodendrocyte particularly vulnerable to oxidative stress.[11-14] Injury-related release of intracellular iron may contribute to the generation of damaging hydroxyl radicals via the Fenton reaction.[15] *In vitro* exposure of mature oligodendrocytes to hydrogen peroxide induces apoptotic cell death, whereas pre-incubation of these cells with the iron chelator deferoxamine appears to confer protection from oxidative cytotoxicity and apoptosis.[16,17]

Toxins such as cuprizone and ethidium bromide impair mitochondrial respiration and trigger apoptosis in oligodendroglial cells. These chemicals have been used to develop experimental models of demyelinating disease and injury. Radiation exposure directly damages DNA and is associated with apoptotic cell death. Several studies of delayed neurological injury after radiation therapy have revealed that oligodendrocytes are the most radiation-sensitive cell population in spinal cord tissue.[18,19]

Mechanical injury appears capable of triggering a specific immune response with generation of antibodies and cytotoxicity directed against oligodendrocyte markers.[20] This immune-mediated injury may be caused by macrophage activity and appears to involve several different cytokines, such as tumor necrosis factor, lymphotoxin, and gamma-interferon.[21-24] Activated macrophages also generate free radicals and nitric oxide, other potential mediators of apoptosis.[25,26] Immune complement activation may also lead to formation of the membrane attack complex, another product of macrophage activation that is also implicated in oligodendrocyte injury.

Besides the macrophage, at least two specific subpopulations of T cells may also be involved in oligodendroglial apoptosis. CD4-positive T cells adhere to target cells through the Fas transmembrane receptor identified on oligodendrocytic cells, thereby triggering apoptosis. Gamma-delta T cells have been found to co-localize with oligodendrocytes (expressing heat-shock protein 65), and may trigger cell death through production of gamma-interferon.[27]

Apoptosis

Apoptosis, also known as "programmed cell death," may be the primary cellular process underlying the disappearance of oligodendrocytes in the earliest histological stages of such processes as cervical spondylotic myelopathy. The process of apoptosis is distinct from necrosis and describes a stereotyped sequence of intracellular events that includes chromatin aggregation and internucleosomal DNA fragmentation, nuclear pyknosis, and cell shrinkage.[28,29] Apoptosis ultimately results in phagocytic engulfment of cells without extracellular discharge of cytosolic contents, and without generation of a local inflammatory response.[30]

In contrast to necrotic cell death, apoptosis is a much more abbreviated process that has made its study relatively difficult. Cells undergoing apoptosis initially shrink and lose contact with adjacent cells, forming membrane blebs and expressing prophagocytic cell surface signals.

The process then continues with chromatin condensation and fragmentation, and ends in compartmentalization of the entire cell into small, membrane-bound vesicles that are quickly phagocytized. By comparison, cell necrosis is a relatively prolonged affair that is characterized by cell membrane disruption, mitochondrial swelling, random DNA cleavage, and the generation of a local inflammatory reaction.[31]

Several molecular biology assays have been developed for identification of apoptosis in various settings. A marker of DNA cleavage, such as the terminal deoxynucleotidyl-transferase (TdT)–mediated nick-end labeling (TUNEL) technique, is a popular assay. Interpretation of studies relying on TUNEL staining may be limited by the observation that this method has been found to label cells undergoing necrosis as well and may not be as specific for apoptosis as once thought.[31] Internucleosomal DNA cleavage, the hallmark of apoptosis, can be revealed as a characteristic "laddering" pattern on gel electrophoresis, and this finding reinforces results of TUNEL staining. The most specific method for identifying apoptotic cells, however, remains direct histological examination and the identification of chromatin condensation along the nuclear periphery, condensation of the cytoplasm with intact organelles, and membrane blebbing.[32] A newly developed commercial assay is also available that uses monoclonal antibody to single-stranded DNA (Apostain). This method is purported to detect the earliest stages of apoptosis occurring before DNA fragmentation and supposedly has no cross-reactivity for necrotic cells.[33]

Molecular Mechanisms of Apoptosis

The molecular pathways involved in apoptosis have been extensively studied in the round worm, *Caenorhabditis elegans*, and one of the first genes associated with apoptosis was named for this worm, *CED 3*.[34] Subsequently, a homologous family of apoptosis-related protein products has been identified in mammals and termed the *CED 3/ICE* (interleukin-1ß-converting enzyme) family.[35-37] Also known as *caspases*, these proteins serve as functional cysteine proteases.[38] At least 10 distinct members of this gene family have been identified thus far with at least two proteins, caspase-3 and caspase-9, strongly associated with apoptosis in human cells.[39,40] The intracellular cascade involving caspase-3 ends in activation of specific endonucleases that cleave chromosomal DNA into internucleosomal fragments.[41] Production of these characteristic 185 base-pair fragments results in the DNA laddering that is one of the hallmarks of apoptosis. Activated caspase-9 appears to specifically induce mitochondrial release of cytochrome c, one of the earliest intracellular events in apoptosis.[42] Targeted inhibition of caspase-1 (ICE) and caspase-3 (CPP-32) in oligodendrocytes has been shown to prevent apoptotic death of these cells.[40]

As previously described, numerous chemical and biological triggers for apoptosis have been identified. Mature oligodendrocytes are particularly sensitive to oxidative stress.[11] Experimental exposure of oligodendroglial cells to hydrogen peroxide leads to increased expression and nuclear translocation of transcription factors NF-κB and AP-1, both implicated as critical elements in the apoptotic pathway.[17]

One of the most important biological triggers of oligodendrocyte apoptosis in spinal cord injury (SCI) may be tumor necrosis factor-α (TNF-α). TNF-α has been shown to induce apoptosis in oligodendrocytes, both *in vitro* and *in vivo*.[43-45] Designated death domains located on the intracellular side of the type I receptor for TNF-α (TNFR1) and related receptors have been associated with activation of caspase-3 and caspase-8 and apoptosis.[40] Gamma-interferon may further enhance susceptibility of oligodendrocytes to TNF-α triggered apoptosis through up-regulation of the so-called death receptor, fas.[46]

The oligodendrocyte apoptotic signal transduction pathway appears to begin with ligand binding to either fas (CD95 or Apo1) or p75 (low affinity neurotrophin receptors) cell-surface receptors. Both of these proteins are members of the tumor necrosis factor receptor (TNFR) family and co-localize with apoptotic cells in a rat model of cervical SCI.[32] Binding of fas ligand (fasL) to the extracellular cysteine-rich domain of fas results in formation of fas oligomers and allows interaction of the intracellular death domain with Fas-associated death domain protein (FADD).[47] The death domain of FADD, in turn, interacts with procaspases 8 and 10 and triggers a caspase activation cascade that ultimately ends in activation of at least three different effector enzymes, caspases 3, 6, and 7.[32] These effector molecules presumably interact with additional downstream targets, leading to cell apoptosis.[48] FLICE (FADD-like IL-1β-converting enzyme)–inhibitory proteins are proteins demonstrating sequence homology with the caspases, but acting as inhibitors of the apoptosis-triggering pathway.[49]

Another important apoptosis pathway involves the p53 tumor suppressor protein, as well as the proteins p21, Bcl-2, and Bax.[50] In a rat model of SPI, p53 protein appeared within 30 minutes of injury, co-localizing with glial cells and spreading in distribution over the course of 2 days.[50] Cellular studies have further demonstrated that exposure of oligodendroglial cells to hydrogen peroxide leads to rapid translocation of p53 from the cytosol to the nucleus and cell death by apoptosis.[51]

Apoptosis in Traumatic Spinal Cord Injury

It has been well established that cell loss in traumatic SCI occurs both at the time of injury and secondarily over a period of days to weeks after the traumatic event. At the epicenter of injury, most of the cell death occurs through necrosis, with macrophages and microglia becoming actively engaged in phagocytosis of necrotic cell debris.[52] However, cell loss in spinal cord white matter continues throughout a much more extensive axial section of the cord for up to several weeks in a process referred to as "secondary injury." Although it has become apparent that this continued cell loss significantly worsens neurological outcome in SCI, the underlying biological mechanisms remain poorly understood. Several recent studies suggest, however, that the primary process involves oligodendrocyte apoptosis.[53-58]

Initial evidence that apoptosis contributes to ongoing cell death after acute SCI came from animal studies in the rat.[59] Subsequently, it was demonstrated that compressive cord injury leads to preferential apoptosis of oligodendrocytes along degenerating longitudinal white-matter tracts.[54] These preliminary findings have been supported by similar results in other animal models, including primates.[55] In most animal studies visible signs of oligodendrocyte apoptosis appear within 24 hours and continue for at least 3 weeks after injury.[53-56,59-62]

A histopathological study of human SCI indicates that apoptotic oligodendrocyte cell death can continue from 3 hours to at least 8 weeks after injury.[63] In this study oligodendrocyte apoptosis appeared to correlate with specific patterns of wallerian degeneration and was associated with intracellular activation of caspase-3. Apoptosis was more pronounced in ascending white-matter tracts, and the authors speculated that this finding may reflect the pathological observation that wallerian degeneration affects ascending tracts before descending ones.[64] The extent of oligodendrocyte apoptosis correlated with the severity of neurological injury, being significantly less extensive in patients suffering incomplete neurological deficits. This correlation of apoptosis and neurological impairment is in agreement with previous findings from animal studies.[56] Of note, neuronal apoptosis was not seen, suggesting that neuronal loss occurs through the process of necrosis.

The biochemical trigger for oligodendrocyte apoptosis related to traumatic SCI is currently unknown but may be multifactorial. It has been observed that SCI is characterized by significant intracellular Ca^{2+} shifts, and several apoptotic processes are Ca^{2+} dependent, including DNA fragmentation and proteolysis.[65,66] Similarly, acute SCI has been associated with hypoxia and free-radical formation, which are also established triggers of apoptosis.[67,68] Glutamate excitotoxicity has also been implicated in secondary SCI and appears to lead to apoptotic cell death.[69]

Animal models have provided most of the information regarding biochemical responses to SCI. A rat model of SCI has demonstrated increased local TNF-α expression within 1 hour of injury, followed by increased nitric oxide levels at 4 hours.[70] In this model neutralizing antibody against TNF-α significantly reduced nitric oxide levels, as well as the extent of apoptosis. Similarly, addition of a nitric oxide synthase inhibitor, N^G-monomethyl-L-arginine acetate (L-NMMA) also reduced the number of apoptotic cells. The findings from this study suggest that TNF-α signaling triggers apoptotic cell death after SCI, and that this effect is mediated by nitric oxide. Of note, the amount of decrease in apoptosis after administration of L-NMMA (42%) was less than half that observed following TNF-α antibody administration (89%), implying the existence of multiple parallel apoptotic pathways.

Several studies of development suggest that specific trophic factors are produced by axons and that absence of these factors triggers oligodendrocyte apoptosis.[71-73] Members of the neuregulin ligand family, in particular the glial growth factor (GGF), bind to the HER4 receptor on the surface of oligodendrocytes and appear to play an important role in cell differentiation and survival.[74]

Alternatively, the traumatic event may result in direct release of pro-apoptotic factors into spinal cord tissue. It is well established that activated microglia release several factors that may cause apoptosis, including tumor necrosis factor-α, reactive oxygen intermediates, and nitric oxide.[75] A recent series of experiments in a rat model of SCI has identified consistent contact between microglia and apoptotic oligodendrocytes, suggesting that activated microglia

may be responsible for triggering apoptosis.[76] This interaction may be mediated by nerve growth factor (NGF).

Administration of exogenous thyroid hormone (triiodothyronine [T_3]) during the early period after acute SCI has also been found to increase the population of apoptotic cells.[77]

Apoptosis in Chronic Spinal Cord Compression

Several studies have suggested an important role for ischemic tissue injury in the pathogenesis of myelopathy occurring in the setting of cervical spondylosis. On the cellular level, the sensitivity of oligodendrocytes to hypoxic injury is well established and appears to support the possibility of an ischemic cause.[78] However, neurons are relatively more vulnerable to ischemic injury, and their sparing in early myelopathy makes a purely ischemic cause for cervical spondylotic myelopathy relatively unlikely.

Although necrosis and apoptosis often occur concurrently, distinguishing the two processes provides important information regarding the causes of specific disease processes. Although ischemia has been associated with apoptotic cell death, severe ischemia is more characteristically thought to result in cell necrosis. The fact that oligodendrocyte disappearance in both trauma and chronic spondylotic myelopathy is apoptotic in nature also suggests that mechanisms other than pure ischemia are involved.[54]

Animal models strongly support a role for apoptotic cell death in the tissue degeneration seen in chronic, compression-related cervical myelopathy. The tiptoe-walking Yoshimura (twy) mouse is a specific strain of inbred mouse that has been useful as a model for chronic spinal cord compression.[79] Twy mice become quadriparetic 4-8 months after birth because of the development of local hyperostosis along the dorsolateral margins of the C1-2 vertebrae and severe cord compression at this level.[80] Histological examination of spinal cord tissue from these mice has revealed a characteristic pattern of descending degeneration affecting the anterior and lateral columns and ascending degeneration along the posterior columns, in addition to severe tissue damage at the level of compression.[81] Cavity formation and myelin ovoids (representing myelin debris) were observed extending from the zone of compression into adjacent levels without gross deformation of the spinal cord. Detection of apoptotic cells using the TUNEL method assay revealed a distribution of glial apoptosis that appeared to mirror the pattern of degeneration while cell-specific staining confirmed that apoptotic cells were oligodendrocytes. The investigators included an autopsy study of a human patient dying with cervical myelopathy resulting from ossification of the posterior longitudinal ligament, in which a pattern of neuronal loss, demyelination, and apoptosis was observed that was similar to the findings in the twy mouse.

Oligodendrocyte survival depends on the presence of specific so-called survival factors elaborated by neighboring axons, leading to the possibility that oligodendroglial loss merely reflects antecedent neuronal injury. However, oligodendrocyte apoptosis likely precedes axonal degeneration in chronic myelopathy, as evidenced by both human and animal studies of spinal cord compression demonstrating apoptotic oligodendrocytes in the setting of intact demyelinated axons.[64,82,83]

Prevention of Apoptosis

Oxidative stress is a potent trigger for apoptotic death of oligodendrocytes.[16] Conversely, antioxidant therapy with pyrrolidine dithiocarbamate (PDTC) and vitamin E appears to moderate this effect considerably.[17] The asymmetrical distribution of phospholipid polar-head groups across the plasma membrane bilayer may play a role in determining vulnerability to oxidative stress.[84] Normally, there is an over-representation of choline phosphoglyceride and sphingomyelin in the outer leaflet, whereas the aminophospholipids, ethanolamine phosphoglyceride (EPG) and serine phosphoglyceride (SPG) are over-represented in the inner leaflet. Apoptosis has been associated with redistribution of SPG and EPG and loss of aminophospholipid asymmetry.[85] The large, polyunsaturated, fatty-acid content of both SPG and EPG makes them targets for propagating free-radical reactions, leading to generation of lipid peroxides and apoptosis.[15,86] Increasing polyunsaturated fatty-acid content through addition of docosahexaenoic acid enhances the sensitivity of oligodendrocytes to oxidative stress and results in increased rates of apoptosis.[84] Conversely, reducing EPG synthesis using N-monomethyl- and N,N-dimethylethanolamine supplements appears to rescue cells from apoptotic death.

Methylprednisolone treatment has been shown to protect the spinal cord from injury and has become a standard component of SCI protocols. The protective effect of steroid therapy may be mediated in part by an inhibitory effect on oligodendrocyte apoptosis. Intraperitoneal injection of rats with dexamethasone after SCI significantly decreases the extent of apoptosis in both neurons and glial cells.[87] At least part of this effect may be mediated through inhibition of TNF-α and NF-κB.[88]

The role of TNF-α in oligodendrocyte apoptosis appears complex and at times contradictory. Most studies have demonstrated primarily toxic effects, leading to apoptosis in several different models. This form of TNF-α–induced oligodendrocyte apoptosis can be inhibited *in vitro* by insulin-like growth factor I.[45] However, recent studies have revealed that TNF-α may, in certain instances, protect oligodendrocytes from apoptosis as well.[43,89,90]

The effects of TNF-α can be better understood through a description of its molecular mechanisms. TNF-α exerts biological effects through binding of two different cell surface receptors, the type I receptor (TNFR1) and the type 2 receptor (TNFR2).[91] TNFR binding has been shown to prevent neuronal apoptosis in several studies.[92-94] TNFR binding and activation leads to increased nuclear factor-κB (NF-κB) expression, and this TNFR-NF-κB signal transduction pathway has been identified as possibly a key endogenous, anti-apoptotic cellular mechanism.[95-98] NF-κB is a transcription factor that increases protein production of several genes, including cellular inhibitor of apoptosis protein 2 (c-IAP2).[99,100] C-IAP2, in turn, inhibits apoptosis through binding TNFR-associated factor 2.

Protein inhibitors of apoptosis have been studied in baculovirus, and homologs to these proteins, referred to as inhibitors of apoptosis proteins (IAPs), have been identi-fied in mammalian cells. IAPs appear to exert anti-apoptotic effects through caspase inhibition.[101-104]

Recent evidence suggests that activation of the TNFR-NF-κB pathway is important in protecting spinal cord cells from apoptosis after SCI. In an animal model of SCI, rats lacking TNFR1 demonstrated decreased spinal cord tissue levels of NF-κB activity, lower levels of c-IAP2, and increased caspase-3 activity. Apoptosis was significantly increased, the overall lesion size was larger with more extensive demyelination and axonal disruption, and functional recovery was significantly worsened.[105]

Pharmacologic modulation of TNF-α levels may yield benefits in patients with myelopathy or SCI. Interleukin-10 reduces TNF-α levels in the spinal cord and improves functional recovery from SCI in rats.[106]

Although inflammatory demyelinating disease represents a pathological process distinct from traumatic injury, the generation of high levels of TNF-α leading to oligodendrocyte apoptosis in both demyelinating disease and spinal cord injury implies potentially useful biochemical similarities.[107,108] Bcl-2 is a protein with anti-apoptotic properties that is produced by certain types of cells, including oligodendrocytes. The activity of bcl-2 has been studied in a rat model of human T lymphocyte virus type I (HTLV-I)-associated myeloneuropathy. In this model rats develop chronic progressive hind-limb weakness because of apoptotic oligodendrocyte death in the spinal cord.[109] A recent study using this rat model has associated oligodendrocyte apoptosis with enhanced sensitivity to exogenous TNF-α and strong down-regulation of bcl-2 in affected cells.[110] It is conceivable that endogenous production of anti-apoptotic proteins such as bcl-2 can be up-regulated therapeutically as a treatment strategy for SCI and cervical myelopathy.[*]

In the developing central nervous system, oligodendrocytes appear to be protected from apoptosis by molecular, and possibly electrical, signals provided through axonal contact.[115-117] Several studies have demonstrated that exposure to specific cytokines protects oligodendrocytes from apoptosis. Insulin-like growth factor I prevents TNF-α–triggered apoptosis in cell culture.[45] A study of transgenic mice expressing high levels of IGF-1 demonstrated decreased oligodendrocyte death after exposure to the demyelinating toxin cuprizone.[118] Basic fibroblast growth factor (FGF) triggers oligodendrocyte dedifferentiation and confers protection from apoptosis.[119-121]

Serum growth factor deprivation leads to apoptosis in cultured oligodendrocytes. This model of apoptosis has been recently used to study the role of the complement system in apoptosis. Although assembly of the membrane attack complex, C5b-9, on cell membranes typically leads to formation of transmembrane channels and cell death, sublytic levels of C5b-9 complement components activate the cell cycle and enhance cell survival by preventing apoptosis.[122,123] This anti-apoptotic effect appears to involve down-regulation of the proapoptotic cytosolic protein BCL-2 antagonist of cell death (BAD).[124] Studies suggest that a delicate balance exists between the protective anti-apoptotic effects of the membrane-bound BCL-2 and BCL-X$_L$ proteins and the proapoptotic cytosolic proteins BCL-2 associated X protein (BAX) and BAD.[125] This balance appears to determine

---

[*]References 54-56,63,76,111-114.

functional mitochondrial integrity and, consequently, whether a cell will undergo apoptosis.

Glutamate excitotoxicity represents yet another potential trigger for oligodendrocyte apoptosis.[126] Oligodendrocytes express α-amino-3-hydroxy-5-methyl-4-isoxazolpropionic acid (AMPA)/kainite-type glutamate receptors and have been shown to be exquisitely sensitive to glutamate toxicity.[127] The specific receptor antagonist 2,3-dihydroxy-6-nitro-7-sulfamyl-benzo(f)quinoxaline (NBQX) has been shown to protect oligodendrocytes from glutamate both *in vitro* and *in vivo*.[127,128]

Finally, the process of apoptosis requires active protein synthesis. Inhibition of protein synthesis in animal models using the chemotherapeutic agent cyclohexamide leads to a reduction in apoptotic cell death, less severe histopathology, and improved clinical recovery[56]

Discussion

Identification of apoptosis per se does not provide much insight into the causes of specific disorders, such as cervical myelopathy. Numerous potential factors can result in histologically identical apoptotic cell death, including both mechanical trauma and ischemia.[54,129,130] Various studies have identified oligodendrocyte apoptosis in response to axotomy, after exposure to specific cytokines, and caused by apparent genetic susceptibility.[72,89,131] Adding to the complexity, apoptotic pathways appear to interact with one another in reinforcing relationships. Products of lipid peroxidation-induced cell damage such as 4-hydroxynonenal (4-HNE) enhance extracellular concentrations of glutamate by reducing their uptake, and also appear capable of inducing apoptosis.[57,132]

Moreover, devising specific treatment strategies based on an incomplete understanding of the complex molecular mechanisms underlying apoptosis can be potentially hazardous. As previously discussed, several studies have pointed out the opposing effects of TNF-α on oligodendrocyte apoptosis.[133,134]

Nitric oxide is another example of a molecule with potentially activating and inhibiting effects on apoptosis. The observation that nitric oxide exposure can trigger apoptotic and necrotic cell death in oligodendrocytes has led to efforts to protect the spinal cord from secondary injury through modulation of nitric oxide levels.[26,135,136] However, a neurotoxicant-induced model of demyelination in genetically engineered mice lacking inducible nitric oxide synthase (iNOS) revealed significantly more extensive oligodendrocyte apoptosis after cuprizone exposure, compared to control animals.[137] This result warns of a potentially protective effect of nitric oxide in some cases of acute demyelination.

Finally, some investigators warn that attempts to block the wrong molecular events in a cell already committed to apoptosis may merely convert the process to one of necrosis. In conclusion, apoptosis is an important determinant of morbidity in cervical spondylotic myelopathy, as well as secondary SCI. Understanding the mechanism of cell death in these conditions will provide insight into potential targets for therapeutic intervention. Recognition that apoptosis plays a principal role in this process has introduced the possibility that the rational design of protease inhibitors active against specific proteins, such as caspase-3, may favorably modulate the response of spinal cord tissue to injury. Nevertheless, the molecular pathways governing apoptosis are extensive and interdependent, and a thorough understanding is required if any attempt at improving myelopathic outcome through modulation of this process is likely to succeed.

REFERENCES

1. Kameyama T, Hashizume Y, Ando T, et al: Spinal cord morphology and pathology in ossification of the posterior longitudinal ligament. *Brain* 118:263-278, 1995.
2. Mair WGP, Druckman R: The pathology of spinal cord lesions and their relation to the clinical features in protrusion of cervical intervertebral discs. *Brain* 76:70-91, 1953.
3. Ono K, Ota H, Tada K, *et al*: Cervical myelopathy secondary to multiple spondylotic protrusions: a clinicopathologic study. *Spine* 2:109-125, 1977.
4. Bohlmann HH, Emery S: The pathophysiology of cervical spondylosis and myelopathy. *Spine* 13:843-846, 1988.
5. Wilkinson M: The morbid anatomy of cervical spondylosis and myelopathy. *Brain* 83:589-617, 1960.
6. Pfeiffer SE, Warrington AE, Bansal R: The oligodendrocyte and its many cellular processes. *Trends Cell Biol* 3:191-197, 1994.
7. Ludwin SK: The pathobiology of the oligodendrocyte. *J Neuropath Exp Neurol* 56:111-124, 1997.
8. Barres BA, Raff MC: Control of oligodendrocyte number in the developing rat optic nerve. *Neuron* 12:935-942, 1994.
9. McLaurin JA, Yong VW: Oligodendrocytes and myelin. *Neurol Clin* 13:23-49, 1995.
10. Duncan ID. Inherited disorders of demyelination. In Kettenmann H, Ransom B (eds): *Neuroglia.* New York, Oxford University Press, 1995.
11. Smith KJ, Kapoor R, Felts PA: Demyelination: the role of oxygen and nitrogen species. *Brain Pathol* 9:69-92, 1999.
12. Gelman BB: Iron in CNS disease. *J Neuropath Exp Neurol* 54:477-486, 1995.
13. Connor JR, Menzies SL: Relationship of iron to oligodendrocytes and myelination. *Glia* 17:83-93, 1996.
14. Thorburne SK, Juurlink BHK: Low glutathione and high iron govern the susceptibility of oligodendroglial precursors to oxidative stress. *J Neurochem* 67:1014-1022, 1996.
15. Halliwell B: Reactive oxygen species and the central nervous system. *J Neurochem* 59:1609-1623, 1992.
16. Richter-Landsberg C, Vollgraf U: Mode of cell injury and death after hydrogen peroxide exposure in cultured oligodendroglia cells. *Exp Cell Res* 244:219-229, 1998.
17. Vollgraf U, Wegner M, Richter-Landsberg C: Activation of AP-1 and NF-κB transcription factors is involved in hydrogen peroxide-induced apoptotic cell death of oligodendrocytes. *J Neurochem* 73:2501-2509, 1999.
18. Li YQ, Wong CS: Apoptosis and its relationship with cell proliferation in the irradiated rat spinal cord. *Int J Radiat Biol* 74:405-417, 1998.
19. Li YQ, Jay V, Wong CS: Oligodendrocytes in the adult rat spinal cord undergo radiation-induced apoptosis. *Cancer Research* 56:5417-5422, 1996.

20. Brosnan CF, Raine CS: Mechanisms of immune injury in multiple sclerosis. *Brain Pathol* 6:243-257, 1996.

21. Hartung HP, Jung SF, Stoll G, et al: Inflammatory mediators in demyelinating disorders of the CNS and PNS. *J Neuroimmunol* 40:197-210, 1992.

22. Friede RL, Bruck W. Macrophage functional properties during myelin degradation. In Seil FJ (ed): *Advances in Neurology*. New York, Raven Press, 1993, pp. 327-336.

23. Selmaj K, Raine CS, Farooq M, et al: Cytokine cytotoxicity against oligodendrocytes: apoptosis induced by lymphotoxin. *J Immunol* 147:1522-1529, 1991.

24. McLaurin JA, D'Souza S, Stewart J, et al: Effect of tumor necrosis factor a and b on human oligodendrocytes and neurons in culture. *Int J Devl Neuroscience* 13:369-381, 1995.

25. Brett R, Rumsby M: Evidence of free radical damage in the central nervous system of guinea pigs at the prolonged acute and early relapse stages of chronic relapsing experimental allergic encephalomyelitis. *Neurochem Int* 23:35-44, 1993.

26. Merrill JE, Ignarro LJ, Sherman MP, et al: Microglial cell cytotoxicity of oligodendrocytes is mediated through nitric oxide. *J Immunol* 151:2132-2141, 1993.

27. Selmaj K, Brosnan CF, Raine CS: Colocalization of lymphocytes bearing gamma-delta T cell receptor and heat shock protein hsp65 oligodendrocytes in multiple sclerosis. *Proc Natl Acad Sci USA* 88:6452-6456, 1991.

28. Hockenberry D: Defining apoptosis. *Am J Pathol* 146: 16-19, 1995.

29. Kane AB: Redefining cell death. *Am J Pathol* 146:1-2, 1995.

30. Cohen JJ: Apoptosis. *Immunol Today* 14:126-130, 1993.

31. Majno G, Joris I: Apoptosis, oncosis, and necrosis: an overview of cell death. *Am J Pathol* 146:3-15, 1995.

32. Casha S, Yu WR, Fehlings MG: Oligodendroglial apoptosis occurs along degenerating axons and is associated with fas and p75 expression following spinal cord injury in the rat. *Neuroscience* 103:203-218, 2001.

33. Frankfurt OS, Robb JA, Sugarbaker EV, et al: Monoclonal antibody to single-stranded DNA is a specific and sensitive cellular marker of apoptosis. *Exp Cell Res* 226:387-397, 1996.

34. Horwitz HR, Ellis HM, Sternberg DW: Programmed cell death in nematode development. *Neurosci Comment* 1:56-65, 1982.

35. Fraser A, Evan G: A license to kill. *Cell* 85:781-784, 1996.

36. Martin SJ, Green DR: Protease activation during apoptosis: death by a thousand cuts? *Cell* 82:349-352, 1995.

37. Nagata S: Apoptosis by death factor. *Cell* 88:355-365, 1997.

38. Eldadah BA, Faden AI: Caspase pathways, neuronal apoptosis and CNS injury. *J Neurotrauma* 17:811-829, 2000.

39. Ellis RE, Yvan J, Horvitz HR: Sequential activation of ICE-like and CPP32-like proteases during Fas-mediated apoptosis. *Nature* 380:723-726, 1991.

40. Hisahara S, Shoji S, Okano H, et al: ICE/CED-3 family executes oligodendrocyte apoptosis by tumor necrosis factor. *J Neurochem* 69:10-20, 1997.

41. Janicke RU, Sprengart ML, Wati MR, et al: Caspase-3 is required for DNA fragmentation and morphological changes associated with apoptosis. *J Biol Chem* 273: 9357-9360, 1997.

42. Nicholson DW, Thornberry NA: Caspases: killer proteases. *Trends Biochem Sci* 22:299-306, 1997.

43. D'Souza S, Alinauskas K, McCrea E, et al: Differential susceptibility of human CNS-derived cell populations to TNF-dependent and independent immune-mediated injury. *J Neurosci* 15:7293-300, 1994.

44. Sipe KJ, Srisawasdi D, Dantzer R, et al: An endogenous 55 kDa TNF receptor mediates cell death in a neural cell line. *Mol Brain Res* 38:222-232, 1996.

45. Ye P, D'Ercole J: Insulin-like growth factor I protects oligodendrocytes from tumor necrosis factor-alpha-induced injury. *Endocrinology* 140:3063-3072, 1999.

46. Pouly S, Becher B, Blain M, Antel JP: Interferon-gamma modulates human oligodendrocyte susceptibility to Fas-mediated apoptosis. *J Neuropath Exp Neurol* 59: 280-286, 2000.

47. Ashkenazi A, Dixit VD: Death receptors: signaling and modulation. *Science* 281:1305-1308, 1998.

48. Muzio M, Salvesen GS, Dixit VM: FLICE induced apoptosis in a cell-free system. *J Biol Chem* 272:2952-2956, 1997.

49. Tschopp J, Irmler M, Thome M: Inhibition of fas death signals by FLIPs. *Curr Opin Immunol* 10:552-558, 1998.

50. Saito N, Yamamoto T, Watanabe T, et al: Implications of p53 protein expression in experimental spinal cord injury. *J Neurotrauma* 17:173-182, 2000

51. Uberti D, Yavin E, Gil S, et al: Hydrogen peroxide induces nuclear translocation of p53 and apoptosis in cells of oligodendroglia origin. *Brain Res Mol Brain Res* 65: 167-175, 1999.

52. Grossman SD, Rosenberg LJ, Wrathall JR: Temporal-spatial pattern of acute neuronal and glial loss after spinal cord contusion. *Exp Neurol* 168:273-282, 2001.

53. Katoh K, Ikata T, Katoh S, et al: Induction and its spread of apoptosis in rat spinal cord after mechanical trauma. *Neurosci Lett* 216:9-12, 1996.

54. Li GL, Brodin G, Farooque M, et al: Apoptosis and expression of Bcl-2 after compression trauma to rat spinal cord. *J Neuropath Exp Neurol* 55:280-289, 1996.

55. Crowe MJ, Bresnahan JC, Shuman SL, et al: Apoptosis and delayed degeneration after spinal cord injury in rats and monkeys. *Nat Med* 3:73-76, 1997.

56. Liu XZ, Xu XM, Hu R, et al: Neuronal and glial apoptosis after traumatic spinal cord injury. *J Neurosci* 17: 5395-5406, 1997.

57. Springer JE, Azbill RD, Knapp PE: Activation of the caspase-3 apoptotic cascade in traumatic spinal cord injury. *Nat Med* 5:943-946, 1999.

58. Barina M: Neuroscience's meeting of the minds in Washington. *Science* 274:1466, 1996.

59. Crowe MJ, Shuman SL, Masters JN, et al: Morphological evidence suggesting apoptotic nuclei in spinal cord injury. *Soc Neurosci Abstr* 21:232, 1995.

60. Beattie MS, Farooqui AA, Bresnahan JC: Review of current evidence for apoptosis after spinal cord injury. *J Neurotrauma* 17:915-925, 2000.

61. Nakahara S, Yone K, Sakou T, et al: Induction of apoptosis signal regulating kinase 1 (ASK1) after spinal cord injury in rats: possible involvement of ASK1-JNK and p38 pathways in neuronal apoptosis. *J Neuropath Exp Neurol* 15:1001-1011, 1999.

62. Wada S, Yone K, Ishidou Y, *et al:* Apoptosis following spinal cord injury in rats and preventative effect of *N*-methyl-D-aspartate receptor antagonist. *J Neurosurg* 91:98-104, 1999.

63. Emery E, Aldana P, Bunge MB, *et al:* Apoptosis after traumatic human spinal cord injury. *J Neurosurg* 89: 911-920, 1998.

64. Bunge RP, Puckett WR, Becerra JL, *et al:* Observations on the pathology of human spinal cord injury. *Adv Neurol* 59:75-89, 1993.

65. Kroemer G, Petit P, Zamzami N, *et al:* The biochemistry of programmed cell death. *Fedn Am Soc Exp Biol* J 9: 1277-1287, 1995.

66. Tymianski M, Tator CH: Normal and abnormal calcium homeostasis in neurons: a basis for the pathophysiology of traumatic and ischemic central nervous system injury. *Neurosurgery* 38:1176-1195, 1996.

67. Banasiak KJ, Haddad GG: Hypoxia-induced apoptosis: effect of hypoxic severity and role of p53 in neuronal cell death. *Brain Res* 797:295-304, 1998.

68. Griffiths IR: Spinal cord blood flow after acute experimental cord injury in dogs. *J Neurol Sci* 27:247-259, 1976.

69. Gwag BJ, Lobner D, Koh JY, *et al:* Blockade of glutamate receptors unmasks neuronal apoptosis after oxygen-glucose deprivation in vitro. *Neuroscience* 68: 615-619, 1995.

70. Lee YB, Yune TY, Baik SY, *et al:* Role of tumor necrosis factor-alpha in neuronal and glial apoptosis after spinal cord injury. *Exp Neurol* 166:190-195, 2000.

71. Raff MC, Barres BA, Burne JF, *et al:* Programmed cell death and the control of cell survival: lessons from the nervous system. *Science* 262:695-700, 1993.

72. Barres BA, Jacobsen MD, Schmid R: Does oligodendrocyte survival depend on axons? *Curr Biol* 3:489-497, 1993.

73. Warden P, Bamber NI, Li H, *et al:* Delayed glial cell death following Wallerian degeneration in white matter tracts after spinal cord dorsal column cordotomy in adult rats. *Exp Neurol* 168:213-224, 2001.

74. Vartanian T, Goodearl A, Viehover A, Fischbach G: Axonal neuregulin signals cells of the oligodendrocyte lineage through activation of HER4 and Schwann cells through HER2 and HER3. *J Cell Biol* 137:211-220, 1997.

75. Gehrmann J, Banati RB: Microglial turnover in the injured CNS: activated microglia undergo delayed DNA fragmentation following peripheral nerve injury. *J Neuropath Exp Neurol* 54:680-688, 1995.

76. Shuman SL, Bresnahan JC, Beattie MS: Apoptosis of microglia and oligodendrocytes after spinal cord contusion in rats. *J Neurosci Res* 50:798-808, 1997.

77. Beattie MS, Bresnahan JC, Masters JN, Crowe MJ: Incidence of apoptotic nuclear profiles in Xenopus laevis central nervous system is increased by exogenous thyroid hormone exposure. *Soc Neurosci Abstr* 21:1305, 1995.

78. Chuaqui R, Tapia J: Histologic assessment of the age of recent brain infarcts in man. *J Neuropathol Exp Neurol* 52:481-489, 1993.

79. Baba H, Maezawa Y, Imura S, *et al:* Quantitative analysis of the spinal cord motoneuron under chronic compression: an experimental observation. *J Neurol* 243:109-116, 1996.

80. Yamazaki M, Moriya H, Goto S, *et al:* Increased type XI collagen expression in the spinal hyperostotic mouse (twy/twy). *Calcif Tissue Intl* 48:182-189, 1991.

81. Yamaura I, Yone K, Nakahara S, *et al:* Mechanism of destructive pathologic changes in the spinal cord under chronic mechanical compression. *Spine* 27:21-26, 2002.

82. Bresnahan JC: An electron-microscopic analysis of axonal alteration following blunt contusion of the spinal cord of the Rhesus monkey. *J Neurol Sci* 37:59-82, 1978.

83. Blight AR: Delayed demyelination and macrophage invasion: a candidate for secondary cell damage in spinal cord injury. *CNS Trauma* 2:299-314, 1985.

84. Brand A, Yavin E: Early ethanolamine phospholipid translocation marks stress-induced apoptotic cell death in oligodendroglial cells. *J Neurochem* 78:1208-1218, 2001.

85. Emoto K, Toyama-Sorimachi N, Karasuyama H, *et al:* Exposure of phosphatidylethanolamine on the surface of apoptotic cells. *Exp Cell Res* 232:430-434, 1997.

86. Alexander-North LS, North JA, Kiminyo KP, *et al:* Polyunsaturated fatty acids increase lipid radical formation induced by oxidant stress in endothelial cells. *J Lipid Res* 35:1773-1785, 1994.

87. Zurita M, Vaquero J, Oya S, Morales C: Effects of dexamethasone on apoptosis-related cell death after spinal cord injury. *J Neurosurg* (Spine 1) 96:83-89, 2002.

88. Xu F, Fan G, Chen S, *et al:* Methylprednisolone inhibition of TNF-alpha expression and NF-κB activation after spinal cord injury in rats. *Mol Brain Res* 59:135-142, 1998.

89. Louis J-C, Magal E, Takayama S, Varon S: CNTF protection of oligodendrocytes against natural and tumor necrosis factor-induced death. *Science* 259:689-692, 1993.

90. Mayer M, Noble M: *N*-acetyl-L-cysteine is a pluripotent protector against cell death and enhancer of trophic factor-mediated cell survival in vitro. *Proc Natl Acad Sci USA* 91:7496-7500, 1994.

91. Smith CA, Farrah T, Goodwin RG: The TNF receptor superfamily of cellular and viral proteins: activation, costimulation, and death. *Cell* 76:959-962, 1994.

92. Glazner GW, Mattson MP: Differential effects of BDNF, ADNF9, and TNF-α on levels of NMDA receptor subunits, calcium homeostasis, and neuronal vulnerability to excitotoxicity. *Exp Neurol* 161:442-452, 2000.

93. Bruce AJ, Bolong W, Kindy MS, *et al:* Altered neuronal and microglial responses to excitotoxic and ischemic brain injury in mice lacking TNF receptors. *Nat Med* 2:788-794, 1996.

94. Scherbel U, Raghupathi R, Nakamura M, *et al:* Differential acute and chronic responses of tumor necrosis factor-deficient mice to experimental brain injury. *Proc Natl Acad Sci USA* 96:8721-8726, 1999.

95. Lenardo MJ, Baltimore D: NF-κB, a pleiotropic mediator of inducible and tissue-specific gene control. *Cell* 58: 227-229, 1989.

96. Wang CX, Nuttin B, Heremans H, *et al:* Production of tumor necrosis factor in spinal cord following traumatic injury in rats. *J Neuroimmunol* 69:151-156, 1996.

97. Tamatani M, Che YH, Matsuzaki H, *et al:* Tumor necrosis factor induces Bcl-2 and Bcl-x expression through NF-κB activation in primary hippocampal neurons. *J Biol Chem* 274:8531-8538, 1999.

98. Chen C, Edelstein LC, Gelinas C: The Rel/ NF-κB family directly activates expression of the apoptosis inhibitor Bcl-xL. *Mol Cell Biol* 20:2687-2695, 2000.

99. Chu ZL, McKinsey TA, Liu L, *et al*: Suppression of tumor necrosis factor-induced cell death by inhibitor of apoptosis c-IAP2 is under NF-κB control. *Proc Natl Acad Sci USA* 94:10057-10062, 1997.

100. Rothe M, Pan MG, Henzel WJ, *et al*: The TNFR2-TRAF signaling complex contains two novel proteins related to baculoviral inhibitor of apoptosis proteins. *Cell* 83: 1243-1252, 1995.

101. Xue D, Horvitz HR: Inhibition of the *Caenorhabditis elegans* cell-death protease CED-3 by a CED-3 cleavage site in baculovirus p35 protein. *Nature* 377:248-251, 1995.

102. Uren AG, Pakusch M, Hawkins CJ, *et al*: Cloning and expression of apoptosis inhibitory protein homologs that function to inhibit apoptosis and/or bind tumor necrosis factor receptor-associated factors. *Proc Natl Acad Sci USA* 93:4974-4978, 1996.

103. Roy N, Devereaux QL, Takahashi R, *et al*: The c-IAP-1 and c-IAP-2 proteins are direct inhibitors of specific caspases. *EMBO J* 16:6914-6925, 1997.

104. Wang CY, Mayo MW, Korneluk RG, *et al*: NF-κB anti-apoptosis: induction of TRAF1 and TRAF2 and c-IAP1 and c-IAP2 to suppress caspase-8 activation. *Science* 281:1680-1683, 1998.

105. Kim G-M, Xu J, Song S-K, *et al*: Tumor necrosis factor receptor deletion reduces nuclear factor-kappa B activation, cellular inhibitor of apoptosis protein 2 expression, and functional recovery after traumatic spinal cord injury. *J Neurosci* 21:6617-6625, 2001.

106. Bethea JR, Nagashima H, Acosta MC, *et al*: Systemically administered interleukin-10 reduces tumor necrosis factor-alpha production and significantly improves functional recovery following spinal cord injury in rats. *J Neurotrauma* 16:851-863, 1999.

107. Ruddle NH, Bergman CM, McGrath KM, *et al*: An antibody to lymphotoxin and tumor necrosis factor prevents transfer of experimental allergic encephalomyelitis. *J Exp Med* 172:1193-1200, 1990.

108. Selmaj K, Raine CS, Cannella B, Brosnan CF: Identification of lympotoxin and tumor necrosis factor in multiple sclerosis lesions. *J Clin Invest* 87:949-954, 1991.

109. Seto K, Abe M, Ohya O, *et al*: A rat model of HTLV-1 infection: development of chronic progressive myeloneuropathy in seropositive WKAH rats and related apoptosis. *Acta Neuropathol* 89:483-490, 1995.

110. Jiang X, Ikeda H, Tomaru U, *et al*: A rat model for human T lymphocyte virus type I-associated myeloneuropathy: down-regulation of bcl-2 expression and increase in sensitivity to TNF-alpha of the spinal oligodendrocytes. *J Neuroimmunol* 106:105-113, 2000.

111. Lou J, Lenke LG, Ludwig FJ, O'Brien MF: Apoptosis as a mechanism of neuronal cell death following acute experimental spinal cord injury. *Spinal Cord* 36:683-690, 1998.

112. Yong C, Arnold PM, Zoubine MN, *et al*: Apoptosis in cellular compartment of rat spinal cord after severe contusion injury. *J Neurotrauma* 15:459-472, 1998.

113. Abe Y, Yamamoto T, Sugiyama Y, *et al*: Apoptotic cells associated with Wallerian degeneration after experimental spinal cord injury: a possible mechanism of oligodendroglial death. *J Neurotrauma* 16:946-952, 1999.

114. Li GL, Faroque M, Holtz A, Olsson Y: Apoptosis of oligodendrocytes occurs for long distances away from the primary injury after compression trauma to rat spinal cord. *Acta Neuropathol* 98:473-480, 1999.

115. Trapp BD, Nishiyama A, Cheng D, Macklin W: Differentiation and death of premyelinating oligodendrocytes in developing rodent brain. *J Cell Biol* 137:459, 1997.

116. Tang DG, Tokumoto YM, Apperly JA, *et al*: Lack of replicating senescence in cultured rat oligodendrocyte precursor cells. *Science* 291:868, 2001.

117. Barres BA, Raff MC: Proliferation of oligodendrocyte precursor cells depends on electrical activity in axons. *Nature* 361:258, 1993.

118. Mason JL, Ye P, Suzuki K, *et al*: Insulin-like growth factor-1 inhibits mature oligodendrocyte apoptosis during primary demyelination. *J Neurosci* 20:5703-5708, 2000.

119. Grinspan JB, Stern JL, Franceshini B, Pleasure D: Trophic effects of basic fibroblast growth factor (bFGF) on differentiated oligodendroglia: a mechanism for regeneration of the oligodendroglial lineage. *J Neurosci Res* 36:672-680, 1993.

120. Yasuda T, Grinspan JB, Stern JL, *et al*: Apoptosis occurs in the oligodendroglial lineage and is prevented by basic fibroblast growth factor. *J Neurosci Res* 40:306-317, 1995.

121. Bansal E, Pfeiffer SE: FGF-2 converts mature oligodendrocytes to a novel phenotype. *J Neurosci Res* 50:215-228, 1997.

122. Rus HG, Niculescu F, Shin ML: Sublytic complement attack induces cell cycle in oligodendrocytes. *J Immunol* 156:4892-4900, 1996.

123. Halperin JA, Taratusca A, Nicholson-Weller A: Terminal complement complex C5b-9 stimulates mitogenesis in 3T3 cells. *J Clin Invest* 91:1974-1978, 1993.

124. Rus HG, Niculescu FI, Shin ML: Role of the C5b-9 complement complex in cell cycle and apoptosis. *Immunol Rev* 180:49-55, 2001.

125. Hengartner MO: The biochemistry of apoptosis. *Nature* 407:770-776, 2000.

126. Ellis RE, Yuan J, Horvitz HR: Mechanisms and functions of cell death. *Ann Rev Cell Biol* 7:663-698, 1991.

127. McDonald JW, Althomsons SP, Hyrc KL, *et al*: Oligodendrocytes from forebrain are highly vulnerable to AMPA/kainate receptor-mediated excitotoxicity. *Nat Med* 4:291-297, 1998.

128. Rosenberg LJ, Teng YD, Wrathall JR: 2,3-Dihydroxy-6-nitro-7-sulfamoyl-benzo(f)quinoxaline reduces glial loss and acute white matter pathology after experimental spinal cord contusion. *J Neurosci* 19:464-475, 1999.

129. Beilharz EJ, Williams CE, Dragunow M, *et al*: Mechanisms of delayed cell death following hypoxic-ischemic injury in the immature rat: evidence for apoptosis during selective neuronal loss. *Mol Brain Res* 29:1-14, 1995.

130. Hill IE, McManus JP, Rasquinha I, Tuor UI: DNA fragmentation indicative of apoptosis following unilateral cerebral hypoxia-ischemia in the neonatal rat. *Brain Res* 676:398-403, 1995.

131. Vela JM, Dalmau I, Gonzalez B, Castellano B: The microglial reaction in spinal cords of jimpy mice is related to apoptotic oligodendrocytes. *Brain Res* 712: 134-142, 1996.

132. Kruman I, Bruce-Kellar AJ, Bredsen D, *et al*: Evidence that 4-hydroxynonenal mediates oxidative stress-induced neuronal apoptosis. *J Neurosci* 17:5089-5100, 1997.

133. Gary DS, Bruce-Kellar AJ, Kindy MS, Mattson MP: Ischemic and excitotoxic brain injury is enhanced in mice lacking the p55 tumor necrosis factor receptor. *J Cereb Blood Flow Metab* 18:1283-1287, 1998.

134. Sullivan PG, Bruce-Kellar AJ, Rabchevsky AG, *et al*: Exacerbation of damage and altered NF-κB activation in mice lacking tumor necrosis factor receptors after traumatic brain injury. *J Neurosci* 19:6248-6256, 1999.

135. Boje KM, Arora PK: Microglial-produced nitric oxide and reactive nitrogen oxides mediate neuronal cell death. *Brain* Res 587:250, 1992.

136. Chao CC, Hu S, Molitor TW, *et al*: Activated microglia mediate neuronal cell injury via a nitric oxide mechanism. *J Immunol* 149:2736, 1992.

137. Arnett HA, Hellendall RP, Matsushima GK, *et al*: The protective role of nitric oxide in a neurotoxicant induced demyelinating model. *J Immunol* 168:427-433, 2002.

CHAPTER 7

Practical Anatomy and Fundamental Biomechanics

Narayan Yoganandan,
Andrea L. Halliday, Curtis A. Dickman,
and Edward C. Benzel

Vertebral Column

The human spinal column consists of 33 vertebrae interconnected by fibrocartilaginous intervertebral discs, by articular facet capsules, and by ligaments. Normally, there are 7 cervical (C1 to C7), 12 thoracic (T1 to T12), 5 lumbar (L1 to L5), 5 fused sacral (S1 to S5), and 4 separate coccygeal bones. The cervical, thoracic, and lumbar regions are flexible. The most common variations include sacralization of the fifth lumbar vertebra or lumbarization of the first sacral vertebra. Other variations are also common. Ventral and dorsal views of the vertebral column with the skull are shown in Figure 7.1.

The normal adult vertebral column has four curvatures; the cervical and lumbar regions have a lordosis; and the thoracic and lumbosacral regions have a kyphosis. The lordotic curvatures are convex ventrally. The kyphotic curvatures are concave ventrally. A thoracic and lumbosacral kyphosis exists in utero. Therefore they are called the primary curvatures. The cervical and lumbar lordotic curvatures develop with the raising of the head postnatally and the assumption of the erect posture. The cervical curvature is shallow; it begins at the dens of the axis and terminates at T2. The lumbar lordosis develops secondary to the upright position of the trunk. The sacral curvature is relatively smooth and concave. Variations in the intervertebral disc and vertebral body dimensions form and maintain these curvatures, which are often modified by age-related changes of the vertebra, osteophyte development, trauma, congenital malformations, neurological disorders, and imbalances of the paraspinal muscles. The center of gravity of the spinal column generally passes from the dens of the axis through the vertebra to the promontory of the sacrum.[52] The center of gravity of the body is located just ventral to the sacral promontory (Figure 7.2). The vertebral column has several different types of articulations: cartilaginous joints between the vertebral bodies, the apophyseal joints between the vertebral arches, unique articulations between the axis (C2) and atlas (C1), and the articulation of C1 with the skull.

Vertebra

The vertebra consists of a cylindrically shaped vertebral body ventrally, and a dorsal vertebral arch dorsally; all encase the spinal cord and nerve roots. The outer shell of the vertebral body consists of a thin layer of relatively rigid, compact cortical bone. This outer shell houses an inner core of soft and porous cancellous bone, which contains the bone marrow. The structure of cortical bone is aligned in vertical lamellae to resist compressive forces. The trabeculae of cancellous bone are ordered similar to columns, and they resist a variety of loads. The rostral and caudal surfaces of the vertebral body are generally concave, and are separated and bound together by the fibrocartilaginous intervertebral discs. The dorsal arch is composed of the laminae, the pedicles, the spinous processes, and the facet joints. Pedicles are stout bars of bone extending dorsolaterally from the rostral aspect of the vertebral body. The laminae extend dorsally, immediately from the pars interarticularis. They then fuse in the midline to form the dorsal wall of the spinal canal. The laminae are oblong plates with a sloping surface. The spinous process arises from the junction of the laminae. The orientation of the spinous process depends on the region of the spine (cervical, thoracic, and lumbar). The cervical transverse processes arise from each side of the vertebral body near the junction of the pedicle and the vertebral body. The thoracic and lumbar transverse processes arise from the junction of the pars interarticularis and the pedicle. The transverse and the spinous processes serve as attachments for muscles and ligaments. The articular processes arise from pars interarticularis, interposed between the pedicles, the laminae, and the facet joints. Generally the superior articular processes project cranially with the articulating surface of facet on the dorsal surface. Typically the inferior articular processes project caudally, with the articular surface facing ventrally. A thin layer of hyaline cartilage lines the surface of each facet, which is a synovial joint, lined with synovium, and surrounded by a joint capsule. Characteristic features of cervical, thoracic, and lumbar vertebrae are described in the next section.

Cervical Vertebrae

Cervical vertebrae are smaller than vertebrae in other regions. They are cylindrically shaped and are wider in the transverse than in the anteroposterior (AP) diameters. The size gradually increases from C3-7. The pedicles are short and project dorsolaterally. They arise from the vertebral body midway between the rostral and caudal surfaces. The arch is composed of paired pedicles and articular facets, the lamina, and the spinous processes. The laminae are narrow and overlap. The spinous processes are short and are usually bifid from C3-6. The transverse processes are unique and contain the transverse foramen from C1-6, which transmits the vertebral artery. The anatomy of a typical cervical vertebra (C3-7) is shown in Figure 7.3.

The pars interarticularis in the cervical spine has been termed the *lateral masses*. The superior and inferior facets extend from the lateral masses. The cervical facets from C2-3 to C6-7 are oriented approximately 45 degrees, with

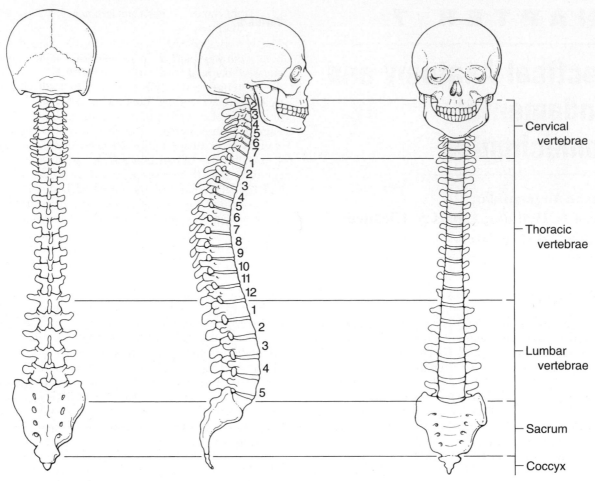

Figure 7.1 Human spinal column and skull. *Left*, dorsal view; *center*, right lateral view; *right*, anterior view, all illustrating the cervical, thoracic, and lumbar vertebrae, sacrum, and coccyx. *(From Sances AJ, Myklebust JB, Larson SJ*, et al*: Bioengineering analysis of head and spine injuries.* CRC Crit Rev Bioeng *2:1-79, 1981.)*

respect to the horizontal facets, and are aligned with a coronal orientation to their surfaces.

The first cervical vertebra (C1), or atlas, is ring shaped and supports the cranium. The atlas consists of a bony ring with stout lateral masses and anterior and posterior arches. It has large lateral masses containing the horizontally oriented facet surfaces. Rostral facets articulate with the occipital condyles of the skull, and the inferior facets articulate with the rostral facets of C2. The axis (C2) has a unique shape with a transitional morphology; it has a well-developed vertebral body with the odontoid process projecting rostrally. Its broad sloping superior facets extend laterally from the body.

Thoracic Vertebrae

Thoracic vertebrae are somewhat heart shaped and are intermediate in size between the lumbar and cervical vertebrae. The anatomy of a typical thoracic vertebra is shown in Figure 7.4A. They exhibit costal facets on each side at the junction of the vertebral body and the pedicle and on the transverse processes. These facets are unique to the thoracic vertebrae (Figure 7.4B). These costal facets are also observed on the thoracic transverse processes (except for the T10-12 vertebrae). The vertebrae at the

rostral and caudal regions have some transitional morphological features; that is, the T1-4 vertebrae have some cervical features, and T9-12 vertebrae have some lumbar features. The surface area gradually increases from T1-12. The middle four thoracic vertebrae have almost equal lateral and AP dimensions. Lateral dimensions increase toward the cervical and lumbar extremes of the thoracic region. The spinous processes of the first, second, eleventh, and twelfth thoracic vertebrae are horizontal; third, fourth, ninth, and tenth are oblique; and the fifth to eighth spinous processes overlap, and are long and vertical. The size of the transverse processes increases progressively from T1-12. The cervical features of T1 include the superior vertebral notch and the lumbar features of T12 include the lateral direction of the inferior articular processes. The laminae are broad and sloping and overlap one another similar to shingles on a roof. The thoracic facets are oriented along the coronal plane. At the thoracolumbar junction, they assume a more oblique, sagittal orientation.

Lumbar Vertebrae

Lumbar vertebral bodies are the largest and typically increase in diameter as one descends the lumbar spine.

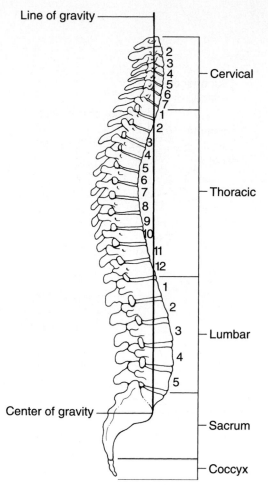

Figure 7.2 Human vertebral column showing the line of gravity. *(From Woodburne RT: Essentials of Human Anatomy, ed 7. Oxford, England, Oxford University Press, 1982.)*

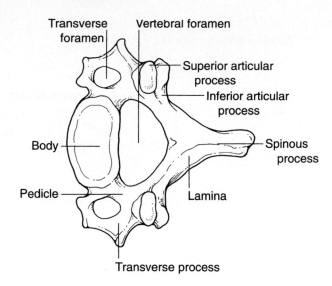

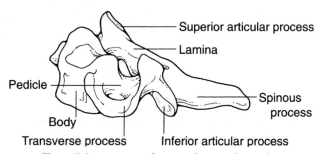

Figure 7.3 Anatomy of a typical cervical vertebra.

They are larger in transverse width than their AP diameter; a concavity of the vertebral body gives rise to an hourglass profile and a kidney-shaped cross section. The bodies of L1-2 vertebrae are deeper dorsally. The L4-5 vertebrae are deeper ventrally, whereas L3 vertebra is transitional. The lumbar laminae are relatively broad, wide, and overlap minimally. The interlaminar spaces are covered by the ligaments and by large, oblong, and horizontal spinous processes. Long, slender horizontal transverse processes incline slightly rostrally in the lower two lumbar segments. The transverse process of L3 projects the farthest and that of L5 spreads ventrally. The fifth lumbar vertebra represents the transition from the lumbar to the sacral spine. It is substantially taller ventrally. This contributes to the lumbosacral angle. The thick and conical transverse process arises from the junction of the pars and the pedicle of L5. The anatomy of a typical lumbar vertebra is shown in Figure 7.5.

Sacrum and Coccyx

The sacrum is triangular, concave, and relatively smooth on its pelvic surface. It is convex and highly irregular dorsally. It is formed by the fusion of the costal ligaments and the transverse processes. Five sacral bodies are demarcated by four transverse lines that end laterally in four pairs of ventral sacral foramina. The bilateral foramina are rounded laterally to indicate the courses of the emerging nerves. Coccyx may be a single bone fused from coccygeal elements, or the first segment may be separate from the other. These vertebrae are reduced in size; they have no laminae, pedicles, or spinous processes.

Vertebral End Plates

The vertebral end plates are formed by the rostral and caudal surfaces of the vertebral body. They are composed of concave surfaces of 1.3mm-thick cortical bone. The cartilaginous end plates are the superior and inferior thin planar surfaces of the intervertebral disc. They are the transition components between the fibrocartilaginous disc and the vertebral end plates. Each cartilaginous end plate is fused to the vertebral end plate by a calcium layer termed the *lamina cribrosa*, a sievelike surface that permits osmotic diffusion. Nutrients for the disc penetrate through the small pores at the lamina cribs.

Intervertebral Discs

The most rostral intervertebral disc space is located between the second and third cervical vertebrae, and the most caudal disc is between the L5 and S1 vertebrae. Twenty-three intervertebral discs span the vertebral column between C2 and S1. The intervertebral discs demonstrate regional geometric variations that parallel

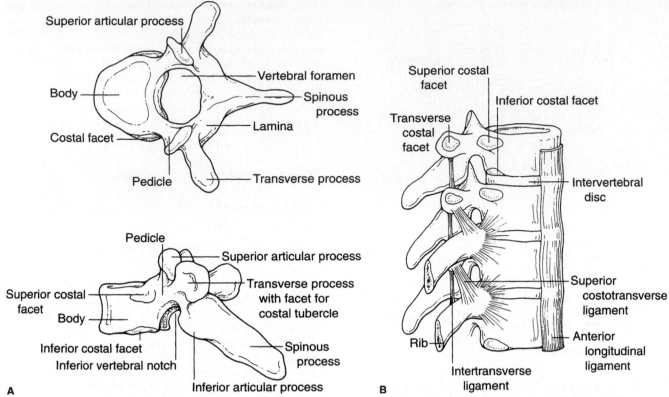

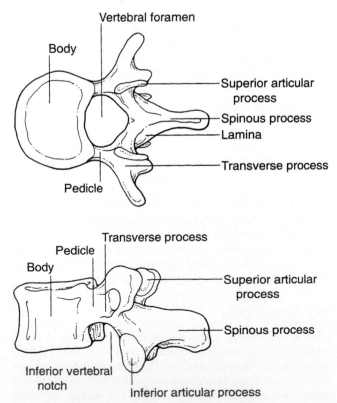

Figure 7.4 Typical thoracic vertebra. **(A)** In addition to the rib articulations, note the orientation of the articulating facets. **(B)** Drawing of thoracic spine showing nature of rib articulation to two vertebrae each.

Figure 7.5 Anatomy of lumbar vertebra.

morphological differences in the vertebral bodies. The discs account for approximately one third to one fifth of the total height of the vertebral column. The following four concentrically arranged components are often identified in the intervertebral discs:

1. An outer alternating layer of collagen fibers that forms the peripheral rim of the annulus fibrosus;
2. A fibrocartilage component that forms a major portion of the annulus fibrosus;
3. A transitional region between the central nucleus pulposus where the annulus and nucleus merge; and
4. The central nucleus pulposus.

The core of the intervertebral disc is termed the *nucleus pulposus*. This is made of a soft, pulpy, highly elastic mucoprotein gel. The nucleus contains various mucopolysaccharides, with relatively few collagen fibers and a large water content. The annulus fibers pass obliquely from the vertebral body above and below and are arranged in a helicoid manner. The annulus is composed of concentric layers of fibrous tissue. The orientation of the fibers within each layer is the same; the orientation of the fibers in adjacent layers differs by 30 degrees (Figure 7.6).

The intervertebral disc undergoes age-related changes. At birth the disc has four distinct anatomical regions. However, the distinguishing features disappear as age transforms the disc into fibrocartilage and the number and size of the collagen fibers increases. With age the macromolecular framework consists of collagen, proteoglycans, a noncollagenous matrix of proteins, glycol proteins, and

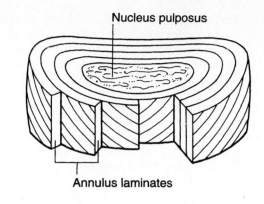

Nucleus pulposus

A

Annulus laminates

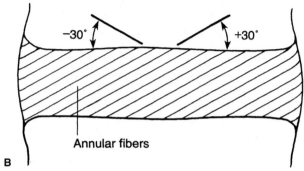

−30° +30°

Annular fibers

B

Figure 7.6 Intervertebral disk. (**A**) The nucleus and annulus fibrosus. The annulus is made of laminated bands of fibers arranged concentrically. (**B**) The annulus fibers and their orientation. (*From White AA, Panjabi MM:* Clinical Biomechanics of the Spine, ed 2. Philadelphia, *Lippincott, 1990.*)

small amounts of elastin. The elastic fibers are made of a central amorphous zone and a peripheral rim of dense microfibers. The arrangement of the fibers in the nucleus is irregular.

The intervertebral disc is approximately cylindrical with different ventral and dorsal heights. Typical cross-sections of the disc resemble an ellipse in the cervical region, a rounded triangle in the thoracic, and an ellipse in the lumbar region of the spine. Generally, midthoracic spine discs are mostly circular in cross section. In contrast midcervical intervertebral discs are less circular. Like the vertebral body, the cross section of the disc increases from C2 to T1.

Ligaments

Ligaments are multilayered and are composed primarily of two substances, elastin and collagen. Ligaments connect adjacent vertebrae and may extend over several segments along the spinal column. Ligaments and joint capsules provide the critical roles of allowing normal spinal motion to occur, and restricting excessive spinal motion.

Anterior Longitudinal Ligament

The anterior longitudinal ligament is continuous and spans the entire length of the spinal column. It begins at the occiput (as the anterior occipito-atlantal membrane) and continues down to the sacrum covering a fourth to a third

of the ventral circumference of the vertebral bodies and the intervertebral discs. It consists primarily of long-range collagen fibers aligned in interdigitizing layers. The deepest layer extends between the adjacent vertebrae binding to the edges of the intervertebral discs. The middle layer, on the other hand, binds the vertebral bodies and the discs over three levels and the superficial fibers extend approximately four to five levels. The ligament is thickest over the concavity of the vertebral body blending into the periosteum.

Posterior Longitudinal Ligament

The posterior longitudinal ligament also traverses the entire length of the spinal column like the anterior longitudinal ligament. It begins at C2 as the tectorial membrane and continues to the sacrum with fibers spreading out at the disc level and narrowing at the middle of the vertebral body. This ligament also consists of several layers with the deep fibers extending only to adjacent vertebrae and the stronger superficial fibers spanning several levels. Whereas the ligament closely adheres to the disc annulus, it attaches only marginally to the vertebral body. This ligament is also much thinner over the vertebral body and over the disc (by a factor of approximately half) and is thickest in the thoracic region. Both the posterior and anterior longitudinal ligaments have a longitudinal (rostral to caudal) fiber orientation.

Ligamenta Flava

The ligamenta flava are broad, paired ligaments that connect the spinal laminae. These ligaments arise from the ventral surface of the caudal lamina and attach to the dorsal border of the adjacent rostral lamina. Consequently, they are discontinuous at midvertebral levels and in the midline. They extend laterally to the joint capsules and become confluent. These ligaments extend from the C1-2 level to the L5-S1 level. They have a high elastin content and are yellow. In fact, the ligamenta flava are the most elastic tissues in the human body. The capsular ligaments attach the adjacent vertebra to the articular joints. The fibers are longer and more slack in the cervical than in the thoracic and lumbar levels of the spine. The fibers are perpendicular to the plane of the articular surfaces.

Interspinous and Supraspinous Ligaments

Interspinous and supraspinous ligaments connect the adjacent spinous processes. These ligaments are composed predominantly of elastin. The interspinous ligaments attach from the base to the tip of each spinous process. The interspinous ligaments start at C2-3 and terminate at L5-S1. Both ligaments are most prominent in the lumbar region. In contrast, the supraspinous ligament begins at the most dorsal aspect of the spinous process of C7 and continues into the lumbosacral region. The supraspinous ligament is primarily associated with the ligamentum nuchae of the neck contacting the spinous processes at their tips. It is the continuation of the elastic ligamentum nuchae in the cervical spine. The ligament fibers end between the L3-5 spinal levels. Figure 7.7A illustrates the ligamentous structures in the sagittal and axial planes.

Upper Cervical Spine Ligaments

Upper cervical spine ligaments span from the occiput to the C2 (Figure 7.7B). Beginning ventrally, the anterior longitudinal ligament is renamed as the anterior atlanto-occipital membrane from C1 to occiput. The apical ligament attaches from the tip of the odontoid process of C2 to the basion of the occiput. The alar ligaments connect the rostrolateral aspect of the odontoid process and run obliquely to the occipital condyles. The cruciate ligament has ascending and descending bands and a strong transverse portion that courses dorsally to the odontoid process and attaches to tubercles on the medial aspects of the lateral masses of the atlas. The vertical cruciate ligament attaches from the occiput, just dorsal to the apical ligament, and intertwines with its transverse portion. The descending band attaches to the dorsocaudal aspect of the body of C2. The tectorial membrane attaches to the ventral third of the basiocciput, just dorsal to the vertical cruciate ligament.

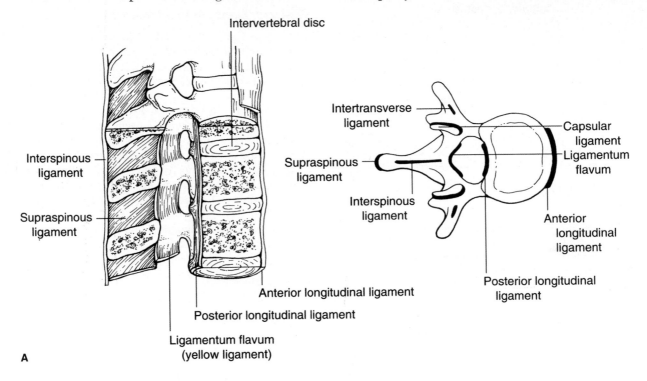

A

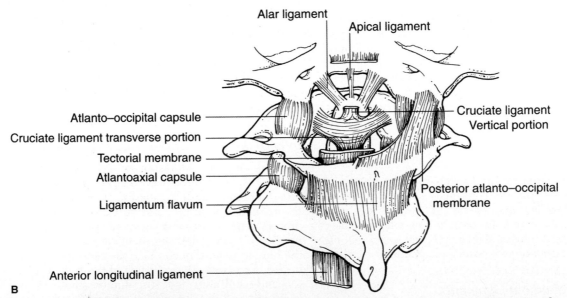

B

Figure 7.7 (A) Sagittal and axial section through the lumbar spine, demonstrating the associated ligaments. *(From Sances A, Myklebust JB, Maiman DJ, et al: The biomechanics of spinal injuries.* CRC Crit Rev Bioeng *11:1-76, 1984.)* **(B)** Schematic diagram of the upper cervical (OC-C1-C2) spinal region, emphasizing the ligaments. Cut-away posterolateral view showing the relative location of the major ligaments.

This ligament tapers caudally to become continuous with the posterior longitudinal ligament. Finally, there is the posterior atlanto-occipital membrane that connects the rostral aspect of the dorsal arch of C1 to the occiput.

Muscles

The superficial musculature of the rostral thoracic region and dorsal neck originate from thoracic spinous processes and insert laterally on the scapula. They are attached medially to the ligamentum nuchae, which is a fibrous intermuscular septum. The sternocleidomastoid muscles arise from the sternum and the clavicle, and insert into the mastoid process of the occipital bone. In the lower thoracic and lumbar regions, several muscles comprise the superficial layer; the most prominent muscle is the latissimus dorsi. This muscle arises from the spinous process of the lower thoracic vertebrae and extends as a sheet across to the ventral axilla. Both the intercostal muscles and serratus posterior muscles arise from the ribs in different directions. Muscles encircling the abdominal region include the external and internal obliques and the transversus abdominis. The rectus abdominis muscle is located in the ventral abdominal wall. Deeper muscles ventral to the vertebral column are less prominent than the dorsal muscles. In the cervical region the longus coli muscle passes from the atlas to the transverse processes of C3-6. Deep lateral muscles include the anterior scalenus, the longus capitis, and the intertransverse muscles. They also attach to the transverse processes.

In the thoracic region the longus coli muscle extends only a few segments. In the lower thoracic and upper lumbar region, however, the lateral muscle groups are prominent, especially the psoas, intertransverse, and quadratus lumborum muscles. The iliopsoas muscles originate from the lateral aspects of the vertebral bodies and extend to the femur. As in the rest of the spine, the intertransverse muscles extend between the transverse processes. The quadratus lumborum also originates from the transverse processes and runs obliquely to the lateral ileum.

Beneath the trapezius muscle, the splenius capitis muscle arises from the lower ligamentum nuchae, and the cervical and upper six thoracic transverse processes, to attach to the occiput. The narrowest muscle, the splenius cervicis originates only from the upper six thoracic spinous processes to insert on the dorsal tubercles of C1-3. The adjacent deeper layer includes the semispinalis capitis and semispinalis cervicis muscles. The more medial semispinalis cervicis arises from the transverse and articular processes of the upper thoracic vertebrae, inserting into the spinous process of the cervical spine. The lateral muscle originates from the transverse processes of C3-6 and inserts on the occipital bone. The deepest muscles of this group include the iliocostalis and longissimus cervicis, which arise from the upper thoracic ribs and transverse processes, respectively, to end on the transverse processes and facets of C4-7. Other deep muscles include the rectus capitis and capitis obliques, which serve as head extensors.

In the thoracic and lumbar regions the erector spinae muscle group lies in the vertebrocostal groove directly under the thoracolumbar fascia. This muscle group begins as a tendon attached broadly to the dorsocaudal sacrum and iliac crest and extends the entire length of the spine. Its columns are composed of shorter fascicles. The lateral column represents the iliocostalis muscles, the intermediate column represents the longissimus muscles, and the middle column represents the semispinalis muscles.

The iliocostalis muscles arise from the iliac crest and insert on the angles of each of the ribs (iliocostalis lumborum and thoracis), as well as the cervical transverse processes. The longissimus represents the largest column. It arises from the transverse process at the lowest spinal levels and inserts into the transverse processes rostrally with the most rostral fibers inserting onto the mastoid process of the skull. The narrow spinalis muscle arises from the spinous processes of the sacrum and inserts into the higher spinous processes.

Deep to the erector spinae muscle lies the paravertebral or transverse spinal muscles. These muscles, including the aforementioned semispinalis, have their origins primarily from the vertebral transverse process, and insert into the spinous process. The semispinalis group is continuous in the cervical and thoracic regions. The multifidus muscle is different in the cervical and lumbar areas, where the attachments are to the articular joint; in the thoracic region the attachments are to the transverse processes. This muscle is thickest in the lumbar region.

Spinal Cord

The spinal cord and the nerve roots traverse the spinal canal. The spinal cord is approximately 40- to 45-cm long in the adult and usually terminates at the L1-2 level. The rostral spinal cord at the level of the foramen magnum is continuous with the medulla oblongata. The dura mater, the pia mater, and the arachnoid are the three membranes that cover the spinal cord.

The spinal cord is suspended in the spinal canal by the dentate ligaments. These arise from the pia and are attached to the dura. Usually the spinal cord terminates approximately at the caudal aspect of the L1 vertebral body. The cauda equina consists of the nerve roots, which have not exited through their neural foramina. Spinal nerves are composed of a dorsal sensory root and a ventral motor root. With the exception of the C1 and C2 contributions to the spinal accessory nerve, nerve roots leave the spinal canal via the neural foramina. Anatomically, the spinal cord is divided into five sections: 8 cervical, 12 thoracic, 5 lumbar and 5 sacral, and 1 coccygeal. Figure 7.8A shows a schematic of the spinal cord, indicating the relationship among spinal segments, nerves, and vertebral bodies.

The tracts within the spinal cord in the cervical and thoracic regions, and the nerve roots in the lumbar region, are somatotopically oriented. The cortical spinal tracts are somatotopically arranged so that hand function is located more medially, whereas the foot function is located laterally. The spinothalamic tract is arranged so that hand sensation is located most medially and ventrally, and the sacral sensation is located most dorsally and laterally. The posterior columns are similarly arranged in a somatotopic manner. In the lumbar region the nerve roots are arranged so that the lower sacral segments are located most medially and the exiting upper lumbar regions most laterally (see Figure 7.8B).

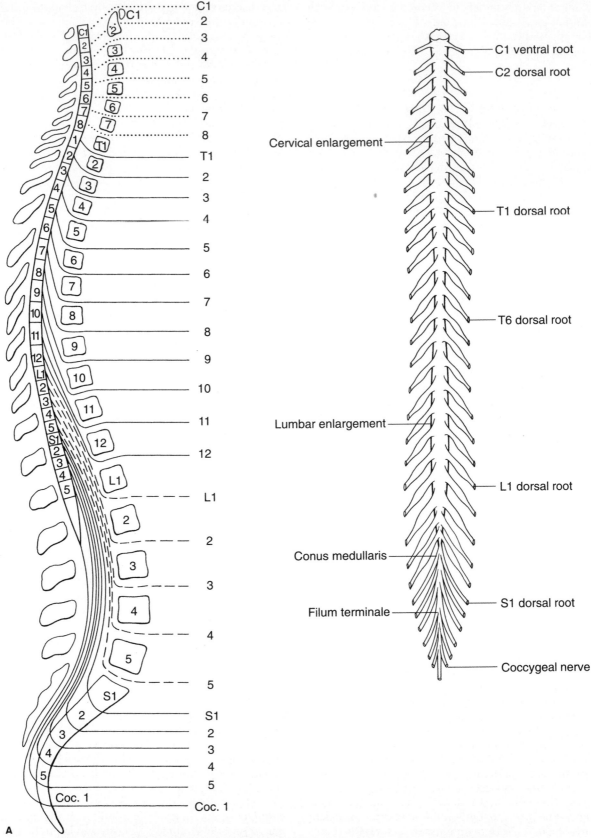

Figure 7.8 Diagrams of the human spinal cord. (**A**) *Left,* sagittal view showing relationships among spinal segments, spinal nerves, and vertebral bodies. *Right,* dorsal view illustrating various spinal land masses. (*From Haymaker W, Woodhall B:* Peripheral Nerve Injuries: Principles and Diagnosis. *WB Saunders, 1945.*)

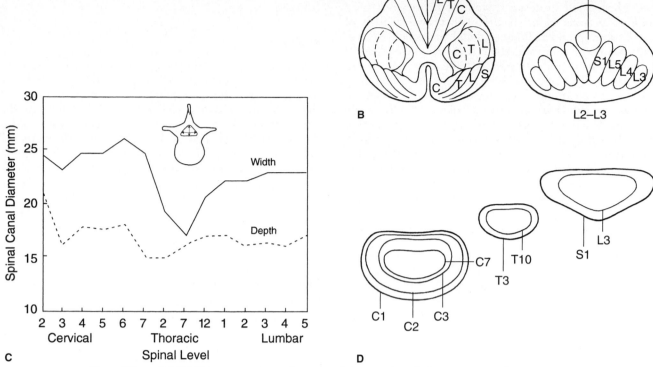

Figure 7.8 _cont'd_ (**B**) Diagrammatic axial section of the spinal cord, demonstrating the somatotopic orientation of spinal tracts (_left_). Diagrammatic axial section of the spinal canal at the level of the midlumbar spine (_right_). Note the orientation of the neural elements (depicted in clusters); the lower elements are situated most medially and those preparing to exit the spinal canal most laterally. (_From Benzel._[4]) (**C**) Spinal canal diameter versus spinal level. The width (_solid line_) and depth (_dashed line_) of the canal are depicted separately. (_Data from Berry_ et al.,[8] _Panjabi_ et al.,[34,37] _Reynolds_ et al.[43]) (**D**) A diagrammatic representation of the respective shapes and sizes of a typical spinal canal in the cervical (_left_), thoracic (_middle_), and lumbar (_right_) regions. (_From Sances_ et al.[46])

In a normal spine the spinal canal dimensions, and hence the subarachnoid space, are generous except in the midthoracic region (see Figure 7.8*C*). In the case of pre-existing spinal stenosis, however, the factor of safety is reduced. This is important during a spinal instrumentation procedure that might impinge on the neural elements (e.g., sublaminar wire or hook placement). The lumbar spinal canal depth does not change significantly as one descends from the upper to the lower lumbar regions; however, its width increases (see Figure 7.8*C*). The lumbar and sacral spinal canal cross-section area is also more generous than in other areas of the spine. It contains the cauda equina, which consists of peripheral nerves and is relatively resistant to traumatic insults. For both reasons, post-traumatic neural element injury in the lumbar region is less severe than that associated with comparable spinal column deformation in the other regions of the spinal column, particularly the midthoracic area. The respective shapes of the typical spinal canal in the cervical, thoracic, and lumbar regions are depicted in Figure 7.8*D*.

Fundamental Biomechanics

Biomechanics is often defined as the application of the principles of engineering and computers to solve biological problems. In particular, clinical biomechanics of the spine refers to the understanding of the normal and the pathological functions of the human vertebral column caused by the application of mechanical insult. The insult could be in the form of traumatic dynamic forces, deformations, or slowly applied loads to the spine.[59] Several terms must be explained to facilitate a better understanding of clinical spinal biomechanics.

Scalars and Vectors

A scalar is a quantity defined by its magnitude. It is directionally independent. Energy absorbed by the cervical spine secondary to the application of a load is an example of a scalar. In contrast, a vector possesses both magnitude and direction. Forces applied to the spine can be broken down into the components of vectors. To accomplish this a reference system must be chosen.

Force can be defined as an action that tends to change the state of the rest of the body to which it is applied. Force is a scalar. Force applied in a particular direction is often termed as the _force vector_ or _load vector_. In biomechanics, force and load are used synonymously. Because the spine is not a rigid entity, the application of force results in deformations.

Cartesian Coordinate System

The right-handed Cartesian system of reference is used routinely in spine biomechanics. The system consists of three axes: x, y, and z. Rotational and translational movements can occur along and about these axes. Translational movements are considered positive if the movements occur along the positive direction of the axis; it is considered negative if the moments are in the negative direction. Similarly, a clockwise rotation around an axis looking from the origin of the coordinate system toward the positive direction of the axis is termed *positive rotation*, whereas the counterclockwise rotation is termed *negative*. Figure 7.9 illustrates the right-handed Cartesian coordinate system of reference with the z axis oriented along the caudal to rostral direction, the x axis along the dorsal to ventral direction, and the y axis along the right-to-left direction. For the right-handed system, this results in a positive flexion moment (extension being negative), positive moment left-to-right lateral bending (right-to-left lateral bending is a negative moment), and positive twisting right axial rotation moment (left axial rotation is a negative moment). Recently, this reference system was adopted by the American Standard for Testing Materials. Once the coordinate system of reference is chosen, the force vector can be divided into its components.

Deformations

Deformation can be translational or rotational. Translational deformation results in a change in the length of the body; rotational deformation results in a change in the angle of the body to which the force is applied. Deformations result in strains.

Strain

Strain is defined as the change in unit length (linear) or change in unit angle (shear) in the body subjected to a force (vector). There are two types of strain: normal and shear. Normal strain is defined as "the change in the length divided by the original length." The shear strain is defined as "the change in the right angle (90 degrees)." When a deformable body is subjected to a load vector, deformations occur, resulting in strains. The deformation along the direction of the force application is termed *axial strain*, whereas the deformation transverse to the direction of application of the force is often termed the *transverse strain*. The ratio of the lateral (transverse) to the longitudinal (axial) strain is termed *Poisson's ratio*.

Kinetics and Kinematics

The study of the mechanics of the body in relation to the forces and the deformations is *kinetics*. In contrast, *kinematics* deals with the motion of the body (deformations) independent of the forces responsible for the deformations. Consequently, both the terms *kinetics* and *kinematics* are applicable to the biomechanics of the spine.

Force-Deformation Characteristics

Because of the deformability characteristics of the spine, the application of an external force or a load vector results in deformations. *Energy* is a term that is frequently used to relate the force and the deformation; it represents the amount of work done by a force load on a body. It is defined as the area under the force-deformation curve. In contrast, stiffness is defined as the ratio of force to the deformation. Because the force-deformation characteristics of a spinal structure are not always linear (Figure 7.10), the most linear portion of the curve is often selected for obtaining the maximum stiffness of the structure. Analysis

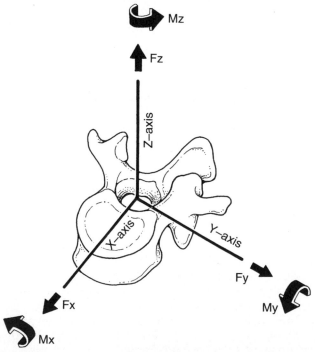

Figure 7.9 Schematic representation of the spine and three-dimensional coordinate axes. Linear forces are designated Fx, Fy, and Fz, and moments are designated Mx, My, and Mz. A positive x-force is dorsal to ventral, a positive y-force is from right to left, and a positive z-force is from caudal to rostral. A positive x-moment is right-lateral bending, a positive y-moment is flexion, and a positive z-moment is left-axial rotation.

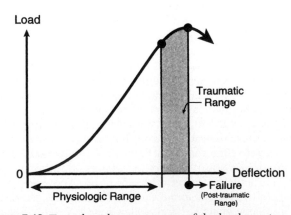

Figure 7.10 Typical nonlinear response of the lumbar spine, indicating the different stages in the biomechanical characteristics of the structure. (*From Yoganandan N, Larson SJ, Gallagher M, et al: Correlation of microtrauma in the lumbar spine with intraosseous pressures.* Spine *19:435-440, 1994.*)

of the typical force-deflection characteristics of the spinal structure (example of a functional unit) is given in the next section. Response is nonlinear; that is, force does not increase linearly with the deformation, or vice versa. Within the principles of structural mechanics, this biomechanical load-deflection response has been classified into the physiological loading phase, the traumatic loading phase, and the failure, or post-traumatic, loading phase. The stiffness response of the structure has been used to derive these biomechanical classifications. This system has been used to design a schema to evaluate the onset of spinal injury caused by external load. This may help define the mechanism of spinal disorders.

In the physiologic loading phase the spinal structure acts as an integral unit, and the stiffness increases gradually to a maximum value. During this phase, the structure obtains its highest stiffness; consequently, its resistance increases with the externally applied loads. This region represents the highest mechanical efficiency domain in the structural response. Trauma does not occur during this region of loading. With the increase in the application of load, yielding of the structures occurs. This is identified biomechanically by the onset of decreased stiffness for the first time during the loading process. Previous studies have demonstrated microfailures during this phase of loading.[58] The end of this traumatic range is characterized by changes in the stiffness that correspond to the ultimate load-carrying capacity of the structure. After reaching its peak during the physiologic loading phase, the stiffness gradually decreases to zero at the end of the traumatic loading phase, indicating that the structure has reached its ultimate load-carrying capacity. In the subsequent phase (i.e., the post-traumatic loading phase) the structure responds with negative resistance; that is, an increase in the deformation results in a decrease of the load. Trauma has been identified on radiographs when the structure has been loaded to this level. Based on the simple fundamental force-deformation response, and using the stiffness as a mechanics-based criterion, studies have indicated that microtrauma may initiate the loss of a local component before the structure has reached its ultimate load-carrying capacity.[65,66] In other words, even under subfailure loading the structure may exhibit signs of weakness or microfailure.

Flexibility, Stiffness, and Range of Motion

Flexibility is defined as the inverse of stiffness (i.e., the ratio of the deformation to an applied load input). Flexibility and stiffness are inversely interchangeable in spinal biomechanics. Another quantity, the range of motion, is frequently used in spinal biomechanics. This refers to the deformation from one extreme to the other extreme under the physiologic range of translation or rotation of an intervertebral joint.

Coupling

Because of the three-dimensionality of the spinal structure, motions are coupled. Coupling is defined as the capacity of the spine to move in translations and/or rotations independent of the principal motion. In other words, it represents obligatory movements of the spine (translations or rotations) that always accompany a primary motion. Both principal and coupled motions exist in the spine. Principal motion can be defined as the motion associated with the direction or the plane of application of the external force. Any out-of-phase motion is the coupled motion. For example, axial rotation of the upper cervical spine is usually coupled with lateral bending. Similarly, in the lower cervical spine, axial rotation and lateral bending of the vertebra in the opposite direction are usually coupled (Figure 7.11).

Bending Moment

The force vector may act on a lever arm to cause a bending moment. A diagram indicating the amount of bending moment at various sections of the structure is termed the *bending moment diagram*. Frequently in spinal biomechanics, three-point bending (Figure 7.12A) and four-point bending (Figure 7.12B) are used. In three-point bending the force is applied at the middle of the length of a structure (span) with the structure being supported at its two ends. This results in a triangular-shaped bending moment with the maximum moment occurring under the points-of-load application. In contrast, in four-point bending the spinal structure is subjected to two equal loads placed at equal distances from the center, and the structure rests on two simple supports. This results in a trapezoidal-shaped bending moment diagram wherein the bending moment is constant between the points-of-load application. In this region the shear force is zero. A pure moment is sustained by the structure between the points of loading, and consequently, the

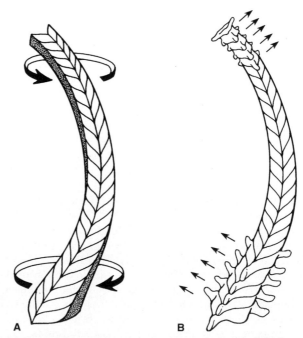

Figure 7.11 The coupling phenomenon is the relationship between lateral bending and rotation in the cervical and lumbar regions. This is depicted diagrammatically (**A**) and anatomically (**B**). The coupling phenomenon results in rotation in opposite directions of these two regions. The thoracic spine does not exhibit significant coupling. (*From Benzel E. Stability and instability of the spine. In Benzel E (ed):* Biomechanics of Spine Stabilization, Principles and Clinical Practice. *New York, McGraw Hill, Inc, 1995, pp 25-40.*)

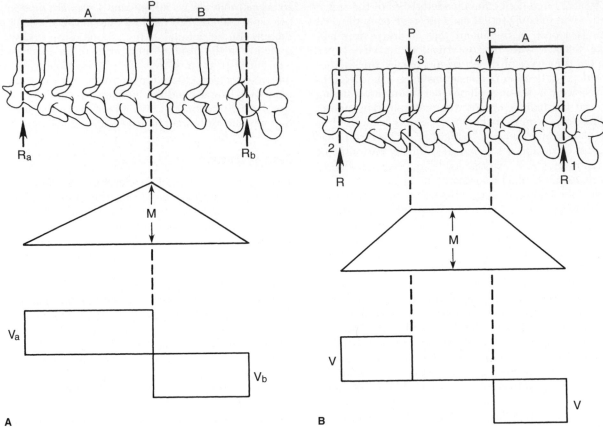

A   **B**

Figure 7.12 **(A)** Three-point loading diagram, in response to lateral bending *(upper)*. A bending moment diagram verifying that maximum moment is under the loading point *(middle)*. A shear diagram, depicting opposite but equal values *(lower)*. **(B)** Four-point bending diagram *(upper)*; bending moment *(middle)* is maximal between loading points. There is no shear force medial to loading points *(lower)*.

results obtained using a four-point bending technique can be applied for a pure bending moment situation.

Instantaneous Axis of Rotation

If the load is applied along the long axis of the spine, it is termed an *axial load* or a *longitudinal load*. This load may result in structural buckling. The buckling load represents the highest load that the column can sustain before failure, when the load is applied in the longitudinal manner. The instantaneous axis of rotation (IAR) is an important parameter that defines the characteristic movements during rotation of a vertebra. It is the central point about which the vertebra rotates. The IAR is defined as follows: The axis perpendicular to the plane of the motion of the body and passing through a point within the confines of the body or outside the body that does not move is the IAR for that motion at that point in time. Box 7-1 indicates these biomechanical terms and the associated units.

Clinical Biomechanics
Internal Deformations

The human spinal column resists external mechanical forces by undergoing internal deformations. The mechanical and structural changes depend on the type of force vector applied to the spine. The following terms are used routinely:

BOX **7.1**

Units of some commonly used parameters

Description	*Units*
Displacement	mm
Elastic modules	N/cm^2
Energy	N-m, joules
Force	N
Moment	N-m
Rotation	Degrees, radians
Strain	Nondimensional
Stress	N/cm^2, MPa
Torque	N-m
Stiffness	N/mm
Flexibility	mm/N

flexion, extension, subluxation, rotation, and distraction (Box 7.2). Flexion refers to a forward-bending moment. Extension refers to a backward-bending moment. Subluxation refers to anteroposterior or posteroanterior shear. Rotation refers to an axial twist or torsion. Distraction refers to stretch or tension. Because of the anatomical characteristics of the vertebral column, the human spine is under the action of compressive force applied in an eccentric manner. Depending on the location of the center of gravity

Terminologies used synonymously

Clinical	Bioengineering
Extension	Rearward bending
Flexion	Forward bending
Lateral flexion	Lateral bending
Angulation	Rotation
Rotation	Torque/twist
Stretch/distraction	Tension
Subluxation	Shear

(see Figure 7.2), this force generally induces a flexion moment. One of the principal actions of the vertebral body is to resist compressive forces. The compressive force resisted by the body gradually increases from the cervical to the lumbar levels. As described in the earlier section on anatomy, both the width and the depth, and the height of the vertebral bodies, increase as one descends from a rostral to a caudal direction. This geometric phenomenon permits an efficient load-carrying capacity of the structure of the lumbar region compared with the cervical region. The exception is the height of the C6 vertebral body, which is less than C5 and C7; the height of the lower lumbar vertebral body is usually less than that of L2. Although the general shape of the vertebral body is cylindrical, the concave geometry of the dorsal aspect of the vertebral body (the surface facing the spinal canal) is significant in ventral spinal operations in which screw purchase of the dorsal vertebral body cortex is critical. Misinterpretation of the lateral radiograph may lead to neural impingement by the screw. Figure 7.13A-C provides properties of the vertebrae, from the cervical to the lumbar region. The compression strength of the vertebral body shown in Figure 7.13C indicates the general trend. There are, however, wide variations. This is due principally to the sample size, sample population, and the age-dependent characteristics of the specimens tested in the literature. An understanding of the tolerance levels under compression for the vertebral bodies is also important from the fracture fixation technique viewpoint.

Facet Joints

The facet joints do not substantially support axial compressive loads unless the spine is in extension. Change in the orientation of the facet joints alters the mobility, and hence the load-carrying capacity, of the spinal column under different force vectors. For example, the primarily coronal orientation of the facet joints in the cervical spine, compared with an intermediate orientation in the thoracic region and a sagittal orientation in the lumbar region, account for the alterations in the magnitudes of the rotations of these regions. In particular, the facet joint orientation changes substantially from L1 (approximately 25 degrees) to L5-S1 (approximately 50 degrees). Figure 7.14 depicts the orientation of the facet joints in the cervical, thoracic, and lumbar regions. The general sagittal-plane orientation of the facet joints in the lumbar region renders the lumbar spine unable to resist flexion or translational movements, whereas the ability to resist rota-

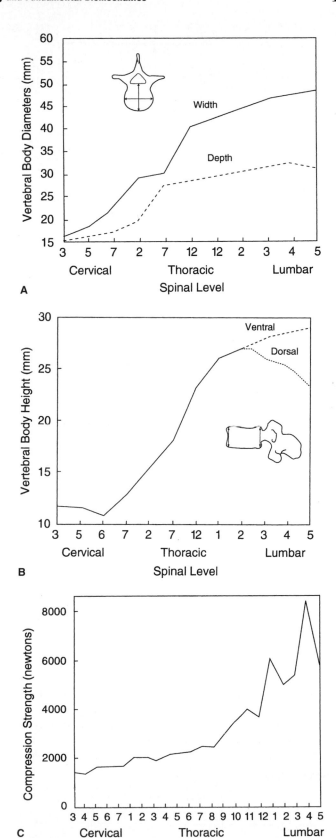

Figure 7.13 **(A)** Vertebral body diameters versus spinal level. The width (*solid line*) and depth (*dashed line*) of the vertebral bodies are depicted separately. **(B)** Vertebral body height versus spinal level. The dorsal height (*dotted line*) and ventral height (*dashed line*), where significantly different, are depicted separately. **(C)** Vertebral compression strength versus spinal level. (*Data from Berry et al.,[8] Panjabi et al.,[34,37] White and Panjabi.[51]*)

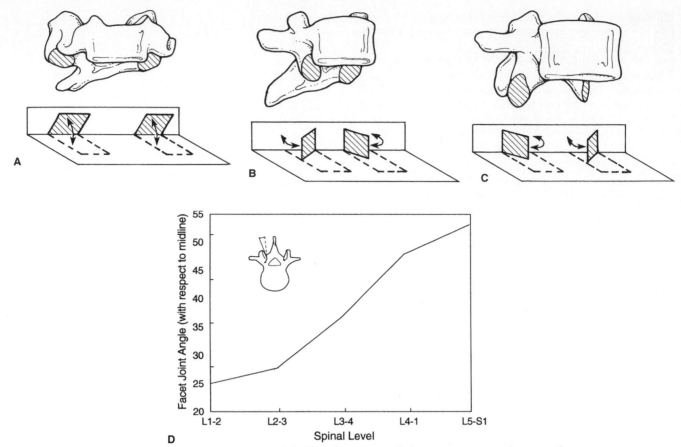

A   **B**   **C**

D

Figure 7.14 Facet joint orientation. **(A)** The relative coronal plane orientation in the cervical region. **(B)** The intermediate orientation in the thoracic region. **(C)** The relative sagittal orientation in the lumbar region. **(D)** The facet joint orientation changes substantially in the lumbar region; here the facet joint angle (with respect to midline) is depicted versus spinal level. (*Data from Ahmed et al.,[3] Taylor and Twomey,[47] Van Schaik et al.,[49] White and Panjabi.[51]*)

tion is substantial (Figure 7.15). Relatively decreased incidents of subluxation found clinically can be attributed to a nearly coronal facet orientation at the L5-S1 level. It is well known that the subluxation is more common at L4-5 than at L5-S1, despite the relative oblique orientation of the L5-S1 disc interspace. The ability of the cervical spine facet joints to resist flexion and extension, lateral bending, and rotation is relatively reduced because of the coronal plane orientation. Consequently, such movements are substantial in the cervical spinal region.

Spinal Cord

The spinal cord participates with the vertebral column in configurational changes secondary to changes in body positioning. The susceptibility to injury will vary with the specific abnormalities of the vertebral column. The physical properties of the spinal cord and the related nerve roots, dentate ligaments, and pia and dura mater have been reported.[10,11] The spinal cord is part of a continuous tract originating in the mesencephalon and extending to the point where the nerve roots exit. This structure participates in the physical alterations with the predominant

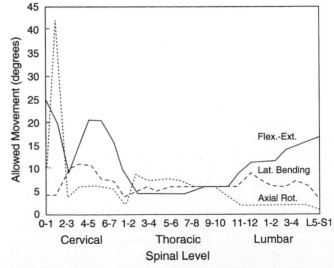

Figure 7.15 Segmental motions allowed at the various spinal levels. Combined flexion and extension (*solid line*), unilateral lateral bending (*dashed line*), unilateral axial rotation (*dotted line*). (*Data from Lin et al.,[26] Panjabi et al.,[35] White and Panjabi.[51]*)

effects occurring at the local level of distraction. Similar to the biomechanical response of a functional spinal unit, distraction in the cadaver spinal cord demonstrates a load-displacement curve with two distinct phases. Large initial displacements occur with small force levels demonstrating the elastic flexibility of the cord. However, this initial flexibility is followed by stiffening in which additional stretch or distraction requires higher load levels.[15]

In flexion the spinal cord elongates within the spinal canal and decreases in the AP diameter. This induces increased axial tension in the axon cylinders of the white matter tracts and lesions of the vertebral canal that compromise the cross-sectional area; especially those processes ventral to the spinal cord call for the local and generalized increases in axial tension within the spinal cord. In extension the spinal cord shortens and increases in the AP diameter with relative relaxation of the axon cylinders. The corresponding decreased cross-sectional area of the spinal canal, occurring from the dorsal bulging of the annulus, as well as the infolding of the ligamentum flavum and scaffolding of the lamina, may result in a "pincerlike" action on the cord. Studies indicate that irreversible spinal cord damage occurs when the compression exceeds approximately 30% of the initial cord diameter. Tensile forces applied to the spinal cord in the neutral position will produce a relatively even load distribution across the structure, but if the cord undergoes bending, compressive forces will increase on the concave side, causing increasing distractive forces on the convex side (Figure 7.16). Shear forces, in contrast to tensile forces, are maximal toward the center of the spinal cord. By definition, shear forces act in a perpendicular plane to the tensile forces. Interaction of these force vectors applied to the various regions of the spinal cord during flexion indicates the potential for a complex pattern of injury. During a sudden forceful hyperextension, marked increases in the shear stresses in the central region of the cord occur as a result of the pincerlike action.

Pedicle

The sagittal pedicle height increases gradually from the cervical to thoracolumbar region and decreases caudally in the lumbar spine. The transverse pedicle width decreases from the cervical to the midthoracic area and then increases caudally in the lumbar spine, favoring the placement of pedicle screws in the lumbar spine (Figure 7.17). Because of the already generous dimension, a small variation in the pedicle height in the lumbar region is not clinically significant (Figure 7.18). The decrease of the transverse pedicle angle from the cervical to the thoracolumbar region, and then a caudal increase in the lumbar spine, necessitates a wider angle of approach for the placement of pedicle screws in the lower lumbar spine (Figure 7.19). An appreciation of vertebral anatomy is important for pedicle screw placement in the sacral region. There is, however, usually a great margin of safety for screw placement in this region of the vertebral column.

Intervertebral Disc

Any load resisted by the vertebral body is transferred to the adjacent one (generally caudal) through the inter-

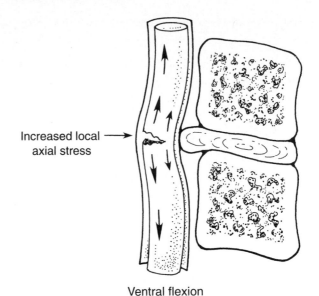

Ventral flexion

Figure 7.16 Illustration of the increased tensile stresses in the dorsal half of the spinal cord during flexion with an increasing compressive stress imposed by a ventrally placed osteophyte. (*From Cusick JF. Pathophysiology and treatment of cervical spondylotic myelopathy. In Black P (ed):* Clinical Neurosurgery. *Baltimore, Williams and Wilkins, 1991, pp 661-681.*)

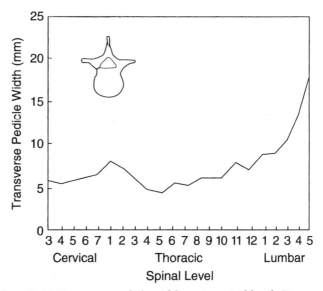

Figure 7.17 Transverse pedicle width versus spinal level. (*Data from Krag* et al.,[25] *Panjabi* et al.,[34] *Zindrick* et al.[67])

vertebral disc. Because of the nonhomogeneity and anisotropy of the material properties of the vertebral body and the intervertebral disc, the mechanism of load transfer is complex. Differences in the age-related changes between the intervertebral disc and the vertebral body also add to the complexity. Because of the relative flexibility of the intervertebral disc, compared with a very rigid cortical shell enclosing a relatively soft, cancellous core, the intervertebral disc resists compression, tension, shear, bending, and torsion forces. Depending on the age and magnitude of the external load vector, any combination of these forces resulting in complex three-dimensional deformations is possible. Consequently, this component of the spine has

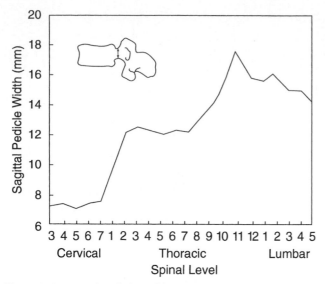

Figure 7.18 Sagittal pedicle width versus spinal level. (*Data from Krug* et al.,[25] *Panjabi* et al.,[34] *Zindrick* et al.[67])

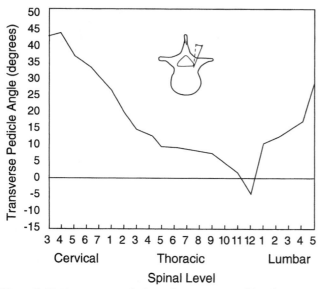

Figure 7.19 Transverse pedicle angle versus spinal level. (*Data from Krug* et al.,[25] *Panjabi* et al.,[34] *Zindrick* et al.[67])

received a great deal of attention by researchers. Similar to the vertebral body geometry, changes in the disc geometric properties account for the increases in the load to be resisted by the lumbar disc in contrast to the cervical intervertebral discs.

Unlike the vertebral body, intervertebral discs cannot be tested in isolation (i.e., the adjacent supports of the vertebra are necessary to determine the properties of the intervertebral discs as an entity). Routinely, functional segments (vertebra-disc-vertebra structure with or without the posterior complex) are used to determine the strength of the intervertebral discs.[51] Biomechanical testing has indicated that the first component to fail in a functional spinal unit is the end-plate.[38,58] In the lumbar spine normal intervertebral discs respond with higher load-carrying capacity and higher stiffness compared with degenerated intervertebral discs.[65] Studies have also demonstrated the

movement of the nucleus material into the cancellous core of the vertebral body under discographic techniques.[56] Initiation of trauma identified biomechanically by the first decrease of stiffness within the specimen still able to resist further increases of load, occurs with the movement of the nucleus pulposus into the vertebral end-plate, causing its rupture.[55] Under symmetric axial-compressive loading, the disc bulges in the transverse plane.[12] The compressive structural property of the disc does not contribute to the commonly observed disc herniation in the dorsal lateral direction; it depends primarily on the specific loading situations, which include compression, combined with other loading modes.[2] Although the disc is never subjected to a direct uniform tension along its entire cross section, certain modes of loading induce tensile forces in different regions of the disc. For example, under physiologic conditions, the annulus of the disc is subjected to tensile forces. Under flexion the dorsal aspect of the disc is subjected to tension; in extension the ventral part of the disc experiences tension. In right lateral bending, tensile forces are resisted by the disc on the left side; in left lateral bending, tensile forces are resisted on the right side of the disc. From this point of view the disc resists tensile forces locally, although the applied load vector may be in a different loading mode.

Depending on the level of the spine, the disc resists a considerable amount of rotation, or torsional forces. The average failure torque for a nondegenerated disc is 25% higher than a degenerated disc. Similar to the case of an axial compressive load-deflection curve on a spinal unit, the torque versus angle curves are nonlinear. With increasing rotation the torsional stiffness increases. Whereas the end-plate integrity alters in compression, under torsion the end-plates generally remain intact. In experimental *in vitro* human cadaver studies, cracking sounds emanate secondary to injury to the annulus. This may have a clinical correlation in the fact that patients with low back pain often report that they have experienced a "pop" in the back.

Ligaments

Although ligaments possess three-dimensional geometry, in terms of attachment and insertion, from a biomechanical perspective they are uniaxial structures; that is, they respond to tensile forces only. Figure 7.20 illustrates the tensile load-carrying capacity of spinal ligaments. The effectiveness of a ligament depends on the morphology and the moment arm through which it acts. To appreciate the contribution of a ligament to the load-carrying capacity of the spine, one must consider the anatomic location, as well as the strength of the ligament under tensile forces. A very strong ligament that functions through a relatively short lever arm may contribute less to the stability than a weaker ligament working through a longer lever arm (Figure 7.21). For example, although the posterior longitudinal ligament is relatively strong, it offers little resistance to flexion because of its ventral attachment. In other words, because the ligament is closer to the IAR than the interspinous ligament, it is less effective (Figure 7.22). This is similarly true for the ligamentum flavum. This ligament is deficient in the midline (i.e., a longitudinal midline cleavage plane exists). This property facilitates

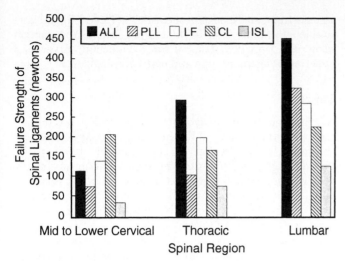

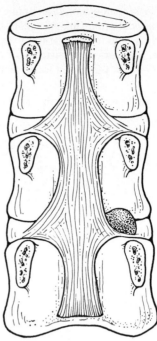

Figure 7.20 Failure strength of spinal ligaments versus spinal region. *ALL,* Anterior longitudinal ligament; *CL,* capsular ligament, *ISL,* interspinous ligament; *LF,* ligamentum flavum; *PLL,* posterior longitudinal ligament. *(Data from Chazal et al.,[14] Goel and Njus,[21] Myklebust et al.,[30] Nachemson and Evans,[32] Panjabi et al.,[36,37] Pintar et al.,[40] Traczuk,[48] White and Panjabi.[50,51])*

Figure 7.22 The posterior longitudinal ligament is narrow in the region of the vertebral body and attached laterally (at the level of its widest point) in the region of the disc interspace. The most common site of disc herniation is the dorsal paramedian region of the intervertebral disc. This injury has been reproduced by flexion, lateral bending (away from the side of the prolapse), and the application of an axial load. *(From Adams MA, Hutton WC: Prolapsed intervertebral disc. A hyperflexion injury.* Spine *7:184-191, 1982)*

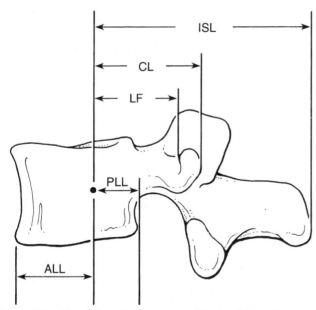

Figure 7.21 The relative lever arm (moment arm) length of ligaments causing flexion (or resisting extension). This length depends on the location of the IAR. An "average" location is used in this illustration. *Dot,* IAR; *ALL,* anterior longitudinal ligament; *CL,* capsular ligament; *ISL,* interspinous ligament; *LF,* ligamentum flavum; *PLL,* posterior longitudinal ligament.

surgical entrance to the epidural space. The ligamentum flavum is not lax except under hyperextension. This factor, along with its high elastin content, minimizes the likelihood of buckling during extension, which might result in dural sac compression. The dorsal location of the posterior longitudinal ligament relative to the IAR, combined with a shorter moment arm, renders it a weak resistor of flexion and for the retropulsion of bone and disc under distraction. Although the capsular ligaments have a shorter lever arm, particularly in the cervical spine, they play a large

role in the maintenance of spinal stability. This stems from their increase of strength compared with their counterparts in the thoracic and lumbar regions.

Biomechanical studies have shown that the ligaments farthest from the IAR, in general, demonstrate the highest amount of strength.[30,39] The variations of strength and stability can be related to spinal geometry and loading characteristics.[61] The failure deflection generally increases with the distance from the vertebral center of rotation, with a general increase in strength moving from cervical to lumbar levels. Ligaments in the convex side of the spinal curvature are generally stronger. Additional increases in the strength are observed at the thoracolumbar and cervicothoracic junctions. Based on an exhaustive study of 132 samples, Pintar *et al.*[40] determined the biomechanical parameters for the six major ligaments of the lumbar spine. Responses based on mechanical characteristics and anatomical considerations were grouped into T12 to L2, L2 to L4, and L4 to S1 levels, maintaining individuality and nonlinearities. Using the principles of nondimensionalization, which account for interspecimen variabilities,[40] the biomechanical parameters in terms of the stiffness, energy, stress, and strain to failure, along with the cross-sectional area and the original length, have been computed for the anterior and posterior longitudinal ligaments, joint capsules, ligamentum flavum, and interspinous and supraspinous ligaments (Figure 7.23 and Tables 7.1 to 7.3). Upper cervical ligament data are also available (Table 7.4).

Yoganandan *et al.*[54] conducted a similar analysis on the middle-lower cervical spine ligaments. Using *in situ* biomechanical testing and cryomicrotomy techniques, they determined the properties of the C2-5 and C5-T1 ligaments. Data were reported in the form of stiffness, energy, stress, strain, and modulus of elasticity (Table 7.5) and area and length (Table 7.6). In the original article, Yoganandan *et al.* also provided detailed force-deflection curves as a function of ligament type and cervical spinal lever.

Muscles

The internal force resisted by the muscle depends on factors such as its length at the initiation of contraction. The maximum force develops at approximately 125% of the resting length of the muscle; in contrast, at approximately half of its resting length the muscle develops very low force. The muscle stress (the maximum force per unit area) ranges from 30 to 90 Newtons/cm^2.[23] Electromyographic (EMG) studies are routinely used to determine muscle action. Generally the relationship between an EMG and a muscle's distractive force is monotonic. Whereas muscles contribute significantly to maintain the stability of the spinal column under physiologic conditions, the action of the muscles is not clearly understood under dynamic forces. During flexion, most of the back muscles are active; at full flexion, however, they often become inactive except for the iliocostalis dorsi. EMG activity in the back muscles occurs at the beginning and at the completion of the full extension from the neutral position, with only slight activity between these two extremes. The abdominal muscles, in contrast, respond with increasing activity during bending. During lateral bending, the activity of the muscle increases primarily on the ipsilateral side. During axial rotation, the erector spinae muscles on the ipsilateral side and musculi rotatores on the contralateral side are active. Abdominal muscles show only slight activity during rotation.

Regional Characteristics
Cervical Spine

The Upper Cervical Spine and Craniocervical Junction. The atlanto-occipital joints allow flexion-extension. Minimal degree of lateral bending, coupled with minimal rotation, is allowed. Most cervical rotation occurs about the OC-C1-2 complex. The movements allowed in the craniocervical region are shown in Table 7.7. Although movement in the upper cervical spinal region does not occur in all planes and in rotation at each spinal level, its sum from occiput to C2 exceeds that observed in any other

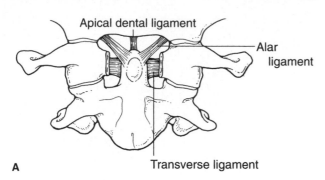

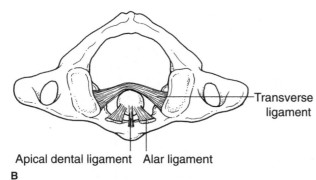

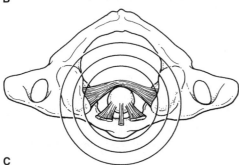

Figure 7.23 **(A)** The OC-C1-C2 ligaments, as viewed from a ventral orientation with the anterior arch of C1 removed. **(B)** The same ligaments viewed from a rostral orientation. **(C)** The predominance of rotation of the cervical spine is allowed between C1 and C2 about the odontoid process peg (IAR).

TABLE 7.1

Values of Cross-Sectional Area and Original Length for Ligaments of the Lumbar Spine (T12-S1)

Ligament	N	Cross-sectional area (mm²)		Original length (mm)	
		Range	Mean ± SD	Range	Mean ± SD
ALL	25	10.6-52.5	32.4 ± 10.9	30.0-48.5	37.1 ± 5.0
PLL	21	1.6-8.0	5.2 ± 2.4	27.8-36.7	33.3 ± 2.3
JC	24	19.0-93.6	43.8 ± 28.3	12.8-21.5	16.4 ± 2.9
LF	22	57.2-114.0	84.2 ± 17.9	13.0-18.0	15.2 ± 1.3
ISL	18	13.8-60.0	35.1 ± 15.0	6.7-20.0	16.0 ± 3.2
SSL	22	6.0-59.8	25.2 ± 14.0	17.0-33.5	25.2 ± 5.6

From Pintar FA, Yoganandan N, Myers T, et al: Biomechanical properties of human lumbar spine ligaments. *J Biomech* 25:1351-1356, 1992.
ALL, Anterior longitudinal ligament; *ISL,* interspinous ligament; *JC,* joint capsules; *LF,* ligamentum flavum; *PLL,* posterior longitudinal ligament; *SSL,* supraspinous ligament.

TABLE 7.2

Biomechanical Parameters of Human Lumbar Spine Ligaments

		Spinal level					
Parameter	Type	T12-L1	L1-L2	L2-L3	L3-L4	L4-L5	L5-S1
Stiffness (N/mm)	ALL	32.9 ± 20.9	32.4 ± 13.0	20.8 ± 14.0	39.5 ± 20.3	40.5 ± 14.3	13.2 ± 10.2
	PLL	10.0 ± 5.5	17.1 ± 9.6	36.6 ± 15.2	10.6 ± 8.5	25.8 ± 15.8	21.8 ± 16.0
	JC	31.7 ± 7.9	42.5 ± 0.8	33.9 ± 19.2	32.3 ± 3.3	30.6 ± 1.5	29.9 ± 22.0
	LF	24.2 ± 3.6	23.0 ± 7.8	25.1 ± 10.9	34.5 ± 6.2	27.2 ± 12.2	20.2 ± 8.4
	ISL	12.1 ± 2.6	10.0 ± 5.0	9.6 ± 4.8	18.1 ± 15.9	8.7 ± 6.5	16.3 ± 15.0
	SSL	15.1 ± 6.9	23.0 ± 17.3	24.8 ± 14.5	34.8 ± 11.7	18.0 ± 6.9	17.8 ± 3.8
Energy (J)	ALL	3.30 ± 2.01	3.88 ± 2.34	5.31 ± 1.98	5.35 ± 4.54	8.68 ± 7.99	0.82 ± 0.54
	PLL	0.22 ± 0.15	0.22 ± 0.21	0.33 ± 0.11	0.11 ± 0.04	0.07 ± 0.05	0.29 ± 0.27
	JC	1.55 ± 0.55	4.18 ± 2.15	3.50 ± 1.61	2.35 ± 1.88	2.05 ± 0.99	2.54 ± 1.31
	LF	2.18 ± 1.89	1.58 ± 0.93	0.56 ± 0.46	2.63 ± 2.09	3.31 ± 1.20	2.47 ± 0.60
	ISL	0.72 ± 0.47	2.65 ± 0.25	1.06 ± 0.73	0.59 ± 0.29	1.13 ± 0.91	0.78 ± 0.56
	SSL	3.75 ± 2.78	4.09 ± 2.00	4.72 ± 5.77	11.64 ± 5.39	3.40 ± 2.59	3.18 ± 1.94
Stress (MPa)	ALL	9.1 ± 0.6	13.4 ± 3.9	16.1 ± 6.2	12.8 ± 7.0	15.8 ± 1.9	8.2 ± 2.5
	PLL	7.2 ± 4.1	11.5 ± 10.0	28.4 ± 11.3	12.2 ± 1.9	20.6 ± 7.3	19.7 ± 7.1
	JC	13.2 ± 1.1	10.3 ± 2.9	14.4 ± 1.4	7.7 ± 1.6	3.5 ± 1.2	5.6 ± 2.5
	LF	4.0 ± 1.2	2.5 ± 0.8	1.3 ± 0.4	2.9 ± 1.7	2.9 ± 1.4	4.1 ± 0.5
	ISL	4.2 ± 0.2	5.9 ± 1.8	1.8 ± 0.1	1.8 ± 0.3	2.9 ± 1.9	5.5 ± 0.1
	SSL	8.9 ± 3.2	15.5 ± 5.1	9.9 ± 5.8	12.6 ± 2.7	12.7 ± 7.1	14.0 ± 1.7
Strain (%)	ALL	31.9 ± 24.5	44.0 ± 23.7	49.0 ± 31.7	32.8 ± 23.5	44.7 ± 27.4	28.1 ± 18.3
	PLL	16.2 ± 9.3	15.7 ± 7.4	11.3 ± 0.2	15.8 ± 3.7	12.7 ± 6.3	15.0 ± 8.4
	JC	78.2 ± 24.3	90.4 ± 17.7	70.0 ± 27.5	52.7 ± 7.2	47.9 ± 5.4	53.8 ± 28.8
	LF	61.5 ± 11.9	78.6 ± 6.7	28.8 ± 8.2	70.6 ± 13.6	102.0 ± 12.9	83.1 ± 19.3
	ISL	59.4 ± 36.1	119.7 ± 14.7	51.5 ± 2.9	96.5 ± 35.8	87.4 ± 6.7	52.9 ± 23.2
	SSL	75.0 ± 7.1	83.4 ± 21.4	70.6 ± 45.0	109.4 ± 2.5	106.3 ± 9.7	115.1 ± 49.1

From Pintar FA, Yoganandan N, Myers T, *et al:* Biomechanical properties of human lumbar spine ligaments. *J Biomech* 25:1351-1356, 1992.
ALL, Anterior longitudinal ligament; *ISL,* interspinous ligament; *JC,* joint capsules; *LF,* ligamentum flavum; *PLL,* posterior longitudinal ligament; *SSL,* supraspinous ligament.

TABLE 7.3

Overall Mean Values of Stiffness (N/mm⁻¹) for Ligaments of the Lumbar Spine (T12-S1)

Ligament	Mean ± SD
ALL	33.0 ± 15.7
PLL	20.4 ± 11.9
JC	33.9 ± 10.7
LF	27.2 ± 9.2
ISL	11.5 ± 6.6
SSL	23.7 ± 10.9

ALL, Anterior longitudinal ligament; *ISL,* posterior longitudinal ligament; *JC,* joint capsules; *LF,* ligamentum flavum; *PLL,* interspinous ligament; *SSL,* supraspinous ligament.
From Pintar FA, Yoganandan N, Myers T, *et al:* Biomechanical properties of human lumbar spine ligaments. *J Biomech* 25:1351-1356, 1992.

region of the spine (see Figure 7.23). The anatomical features of the upper cervical spine offer several points of fixation for instrumentation constructs and sites for bony fusion attachment. Upper cervical spine surgery is complicated by the difficulties associated with calvarial fixation, the unique anatomy of the upper cervical vertebrae, and the substantial spinal movement allowed in this region.

The atlantoaxial region represents a unique integration of anatomy and function, allowing three-dimensional movement of the head through both individual and coupled motions. At the atlanto-occipital joint, 13 to 16 degrees of flexion-extension occurs. In addition, over 8 degrees of lateral bending occurs without rotation. At the atlantoaxial junction, flexion-extension is significant (10 to 13 degrees). The most significant motion at C1-2 is 40 degrees of unilateral axial rotation, which represents 40% of the total rotation seen in the cervical spine. In any forced rotation of the entire cervical spine, maximum rotation occurs at C1-2 before use of potential rotation in the lower cervical spine.[29]

Translation also occurs in the upper cervical spine, although it is normally limited to approximately 2mm primarily because of the anatomical relation between the odontoid process, the arch of C1, and the transverse atlantal ligament. Other motion limiters include those that inhibit hyperflexion: the relationship between the anterior lip of the foramen magnum and the odontoid process at the occiput-C1 and the low elasticity of the tectorial membrane at C1-2. Extension limiters include the tectorial membrane, as well as the anterior longitudinal ligament. Rotation is contained by the contralateral C1-2 alar ligament.[29]

Middle and Lower Cervical Spine. Orientation of the facet joints in the coronal plane do not excessively limit spinal movement in any direction or in rotation; an exception is extension. This orientation facilitates spinal instrumentation in certain situations. With the integrity of the facet joints and pedicles maintained, the vertebral bodies are able to equally resist axial loading, and translation instability may be effectively managed by the application

TABLE 7.4

Mean and Standard Deviation Values of Force and Deflection at Failure for Human Upper Cervical Spinal Ligaments

Ligament Type	Spinal Levels	Failure Load (N)	Failure Deflection (mm)
Anterior atlanto-occipital membrane	OC-C1	233 (± 23)	18.9 (± 2.7)
Posterior atlanto-occipital membrane	OC-C1	83 (± 17)	18.1 (± 2.7)
Anterior longitudinal	C1-C2	281 (± 136)	12.3 (± 6.7)
Apical	OC-C2	214 (± 115)	11.5 (± 10.5)
Alar	OC-C2	357 (± 220)	14.1 (± 7.2)
Joint capsules	OC-C2	315 (± 134)	11.4 (± 7.2)
Ligamentum flavum	C1-C2	113 (± 85)	8.7 (± 5.2)
Vertical cruciate	OC-C2	436 (± 69)	25.2 (± 14.6)
Tectorial membrane	OC-C2	76 (± 44)	11.9 (± 2.5)

From Myklebust JB, Pintar FA, Yoganandan N, *et al.:* Tensile strength of spinal ligaments. *Spine* 13:526-531, 1988.

TABLE 7.5

(a) Biomechanical Data of C2-C5 Ligaments (*n* = 25), (b) Biomechanical Data of C5-T1 Ligaments (*n* = 25), (c) Bilinear Young's Modulus (MPa) of Cervical Ligaments (*n* = 25)

(a)

Type	Sample Size	Stiffness N/mm	Energy Nm	Stress MPa	Strain %
			Parameter		
ALL	10	16.0 ± 2.7	0.61 ± 0.25	8.36 ±1.76	30.8 ± 5.0
PLL	7	25.4 ± 7.2	0.21 ± 0.1	6.29 ± 2.28	18.2 ± 3.21
JC	8	33.6 ± 5.53	1.49 ± 0.54	5.67 ± 1.47	148 ± 28.5
LF	12	25.0 ± 7.04	0.49 ± 0.17	2.64 ± 0.79	77.0 ± 12.9
ISL	8	7.74 ± 1.61	0.13 ± 0.03	2.97 ± 0.76	60.9 ± 11.2

(b)

Type	Sample Size	Stiffness N/mm	Energy Nm	Stress MPa	Strain %
ALL	7	17.9 ± 3.44	0.54 ± 0.13	12.0 ± 1.41	35.4 ± 5.86
PLL	10	23.0 ± 2.39	0.4 ± 0.11	12.8 ± 3.38	34.1 ± 8.77
JC	11	36.9 ± 6.06	1.5 ± 0.37	7.36 ± 1.27	116 ± 19.6
LF	11	21.6 ± 3.65	0.91 ± 0.22	2.64 ± 0.34	88.4 ± 13.1
ISL	8	6.36 ± 0.69	0.18 ± 0.06	2.88 ± 0.74	68.1 ± 13.8

(c)

Type	C2-C5 E_1	E_2	ε_{12}	C5-T1 E_1	E_2	ε_{12}
ALL	43.8	26.3	12.9	28.2	28.4	14.8
PLL	40.9	22.2	11.1	23.0	24.6	11.2
JC	5.0	3.3	56.8	4.8	3.4	57.0
LF	3.1	2.1	40.7	3.5	3.4	35.3
ISL	4.9	3.1	26.1	5.0	3.3	27.0

From Yoganandan N, Kumaresan S, Pintar F: Geometric and mechanical properties of human cervical spine ligaments.
J Biomech Engr 122:623-629, 2000.
Note: ε_{12} denotes the strain transition between the two bilinear moduli (E_1 and E_2).

TABLE 7.6

Area (*n* = 4) and Length (*n* = 4) of Cervical Spine Ligaments

Type	C2-C5 Area (mm²)	Length (mm)	C5-T1 Area (mm²)	Length (mm)
ALL	11.1 ± 1.93	18.8 ± 1.04	12.1 ± 2.68	18.3 ± 0.5
PLL	11.3 ± 1.99	19.0 ± 1.04	14.7 ± 6.77	17.9 ± 0.54
JC	42.2 ± 6.39	6.92 ± 0.68	49.5 ± 12.28	6.72 ± 0.45
LF	46.0 ± 5.78	8.45 ± 0.85	48.9 ± 7.9	10.6 ± 0.64
ISL	13.0 ± 3.27	10.4 ± 0.77	13.4 ± 1.03	9.87 ± 0.69

From Yoganandan N, Kumaresan S, Pintar F: Geometric and mechanical properties of human cervical spine
ligaments. *J Biomech Engr* 122:623-629, 2000.

TABLE 7.7

Movements Allowed in the Craniocervical Region

Joint	Motion	Range of Motion (degrees)
Occiput-C1	Combined flexion/extension	25
	Lateral bending (unilateral)	5
	Axial rotation (unilateral)	5
C1-C2	Combined flexion/extension	20
	Lateral bending (unilateral)	5
	Axial rotation (unilateral)	40

From Maiman DJ, Yoganandan N: Biomechanics of cervical spine trauma. In Black P (ed): *Clinical Neurosurgery,* Baltimore, Williams & Wilkins, vol 37, 1991, pp 543-570.

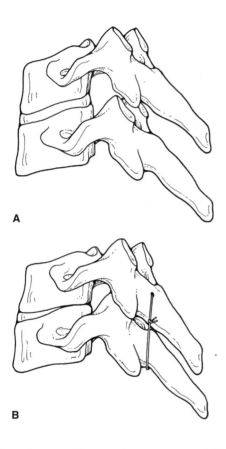

A

B

Figure 7.24 In the cervical spine, the orientation of the facet joints can be used to advantage via cerclage wiring techniques. **(A)** The compression of two spinous processes together in a tension-band manner prevents subluxation by bringing the rostral and caudal facets together. **(B)** Because the facet joints are oriented coronally, the close approximation of the superior and inferior facets causes them to abut each other and thus prevent translational deformation. *(From Benzel E. Stability and instability of the spine. In Benzel E (ed):* Biomechanics of Spine Stabilization, Principles and Clinical Practice. *New York, McGraw Hill, Inc, 1995, pp 25-40.)*

of a tension band fixation construct (Figure 7.24). Facets and the joint capsules are injured under internal tension secondary to spinal hyperflexion. Normally, they absorb approximately one fifth of the total compressive loads applied to the lumbar spine segment.[31] They also have an important role in resisting pathologic forces. In facetec-

TABLE 7.8

Normal Motion of the Cervical Spine

	Maiman *et al.*[28]	Johnson *et al.*[24]
Lateral bending	64.2 (± 6.8)	
Rotation	134.2 (± 17.1)	
Flexion-extension		
OC-C1	16.7 (± 10.0)	18.8 (± 2.2)
C1-C2	13.6 (± 6.0)	13.7 (± 1.7)
C2-C3	11.6 (± 4.7)	12.0 (± 1.2)
C3-C4	15.2 (± 3.8)	17.6 (± 1.5)
C4-C5	17.1 (± 4.5)	20.1 (± 1.6)
C5-C6	17.1 (± 3.9)	21.8 (± 1.6)
C6-C7	18.1 (± 6.1)	20.7 (± 1.6)

From Maiman DJ, Yoganandan N: Biomechanics of cervical spine trauma. In Black P (ed): *Clinical Neurosurgery,* Baltimore, Williams & Wilkins, vol 37, 1991, pp 543-570.

tomy studies the shear and combined compression flexion strength and kinematics of the spine are significantly compromised.[17,18,31,41,42]

In the lower cervical spine the primary spinal motions are related to the integrity of the intervertebral discs. Flexion-extension is distributed throughout the cervical spine a total of 60 to 75 degrees. Sagittal translation is limited to 2 to 3mm at all cervical spine levels. This is a function of the facets, ligaments, and the intervertebral discs. Consequently, even small increases in translations may be harmful. Lateral bending, on the other hand, is a prominent motion, particularly above C6; between C2 and C5 there is 10 to 12 degrees of lateral bending per spinal level, and at C7-T1 there is 4 to 8 degrees. Typically, lateral bending is coupled with other motions, particularly axial rotation. This coupling, in which the spinous processes are rotated in the opposite direction of the lateral bending, may be a consequence of muscle contraction or the three-dimensional spatial orientation of the spinous processes (Table 7.8).[29]

Thoracic Spine

The thoracic spinal cord is shielded from injury by the massive regional paraspinal muscle masses and by the thoracic cage. The narrow spinal canal diameter in the upper thoracic region, however, complicates the issue. The former protects the neural elements; the latter contributes to neural injury. This may explain the increased incidence of catastrophic neurologic injuries associated with thoracic spinal fractures. The significant paraspinal muscle mass protects the spine from injury. However, the narrow spinal canal leaves little room to spare for the spinal cord, which is easily compromised by malalignment of the spine or retropulsion of bone caused by a fracture[7] (Figure 7.25). The normal kyphotic posture of the thoracic spine, with its associated predisposition to spinal fracture, amplifies all of these factors. Biomechanical studies dealing with the effects of laminectomy on thoracic spine stability are reported.[57]

Lumbar Spine

Its relatively large proportions, and the resumption of the lordotic curvature, make this region relatively resistant to failure. Furthermore, the transition of the spinal cord into the cauda equina makes catastrophic spinal injury from trauma less likely. The caudal end of the spinal column is associated with significant logistical therapeutic dilemmas. Frequently, an inability to obtain a solid point of sacral fixation creates a multitude of surgical problems. Similarly, an appropriate bending moment is not often resisted by the instrumentation construct because of an inadequate length of the lever arm below the injury.[54-57] Furthermore, the relatively steep orientation of the lumbosacral joint exposes the lumbosacral spine to increases in translational deformations.[5]

Spinal Stability

The original concept describing stability in terms of the two columns was presented by Holdsworth.[22] This was based on the clinical experience of Holdsworth and

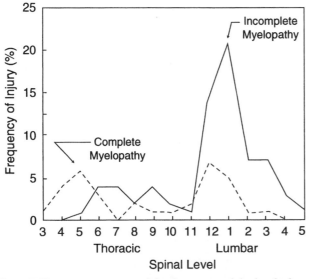

Figure 7.25 A representation of the frequency of the level of vertebral injury in patients with traumatic spinal cord injury, contrasting complete myelopathies (no function preserved below the level of injury) *(dashed line)*, and incomplete myelopathies (some function preserved below the level of injury) *(solid line)*. Note that in patients with complete myelopathies the curve is shifted to the left. *(From Benzel EC, Larson SJ: Functional recovery after decompressive operation for thoracic and lumbar spine fractures.* Neurosurgery 19:772-777, 1986.)

Nicoll,[22,33] and the experimental work of Roaf.[44] In this two-column definition, the dorsal column consists of the posterior ligamentous complex, that is, the interspinous and the supraspinous ligaments, the ligamentum flavum, and the apophyseal joints. The anterior column consists of the vertebral body, the intervertebral disc, and the anterior and posterior longitudinal ligaments. Holdsworth[22] contended that the stability of the spine depends principally on the integrity of the dorsal ligament complex. Consequently, a simple burst fracture with no dorsal involvement was considered stable. In addition, a compression burst fracture with an intact dorsal complex also is stable. Unstable fractures consist of the loss of integrity of the posterior ligament complex and at least one of the components of the anterior column.

The consideration of "columns" in defining the extent of stability helps the physician to conceptualize and categorize case-specific phenomena. The theory of Louis[27] is that the spine bears weight principally by sustaining axial loads along the vertebral body and intervertebral discs and the two facet joint complexes, at each segmental level (Figure 7.26). This concept assists in the instability assessment process only when predominantly axial loads are involved. Because of its obvious association with the bony columns of the spine (vertebral body and facet joints), this three-column concept by Louis[27] assesses the bony component failure more effectively than the soft-tissue damage. Conventional radiographs and computed tomography scans are excellent tools to assess this type of instability. However, except for the case of a significant vertebral body failure, a correlation between the external bony injury and the presence of chronic instability may be tenuous.[4] In addition, this theory does not facilitate the assessment of distraction, flexion, and extension components of injury. The three-column concept of Denis[19,20] is more applicable to this situation. The three-column theory assists in assessing the bony collapse associated with axial load bearing; it also provides insight into the assessment of the distraction, flexion, and extension components of injury (injury to the dorsal elements) of the spinal column. This three-column theory proposed by Denis[19,20] adds the concept of a middle column to the two-column theories of Holdsworth,[22] and allows specific assessment of that component to the spinal column in the region of the neutral axis.

The neutral axis is that longitudinal region of the spinal column that bears a significant portion of the axial load, and about which spinal distraction or compression does not necessarily occur with flexion or extension (Figure 7.27). Usually the neutral axis is located in the region of the midposterior aspect of the vertebral body (i.e., the middle column of Denis).[19] This also encompasses the IAR in the sagittal plane.

The middle column definition of Denis was based on experimental studies demonstrating that transection of the entire dorsal ligament complex alone was insufficient to produce instability. However, when the posterior longitudinal ligament and the dorsal portion of the disc were also transected, instability ensued. Therefore in the three-column spine of Denis, the middle column consists of the posterior longitudinal ligament, the dorsal annulus fibrosus, and the dorsal wall of the vertebral body; the anterior column consists of the anterior longitudinal ligament, the ventral annulus fibrosus, and the ventral wall of the vertebral body. The posterior column is the same as in the two-column approach of Holdsworth. Of the major spinal injuries defined by Denis, only minimal and moderate compression fractures with an intact posterior column should be considered stable. The two- and three-column theories differ in classifying burst fractures in terms of stability. Denis classifies the burst fracture as unstable because both the anterior and middle columns are affected. All of the fractures and fracture/dislocations categorized as unstable by Denis demonstrated trauma in at least two of three columns. Many other definitions of clinical instabil-

ity also exist. Clinical instability is also defined as the loss of the ability of the spine under physiologic loads to maintain its pattern of displacement, so that there is no initial or additional neurologic deficit, no major deformity, and no incapacitating pain.[51]

In the biomechanical literature, stability and instability are used interchangeably. Instability is the inverse of stability. Benzel[4] defined instability as the inability to limit excess or abnormal spinal displacement. The use of the word *excessive* reflects the difficulty of quantifying instability in clinical situations. Stability has also been classified as acute and chronic. Acute instability may be broken down into two subcategories: overt and limited. Chronic

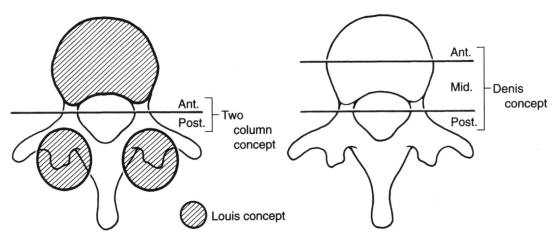

Figure 7.26 The "column" concepts of spinal instability. The concept described by Louis *(left)* assigns significance to the vertebral body and the facet joint complexes (lateral masses) on either side of the dorsal spine. Denis's three-column concept *(right)* assigns significance to the region of the neutral axis and the integrity of the posterior vertebral body wall (the middle column). The two-column construct *(right)* relies on anatomically defined structures, the vertebral body (anterior column), and the posterior elements (posterior column). Louis's three-column concept *(left)* similarly relies on anatomically defined structures. *(From White AA, Panjabi MM: Clinical Biomechanics of the Spine, ed 2. Philadelphia, Lippincott, 1990.)*

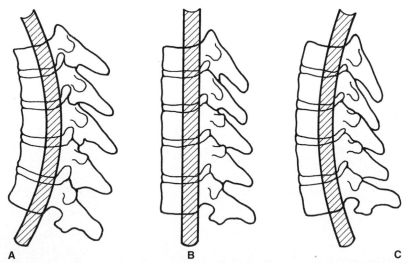

Figure 7.27 The depiction of the neutral axis *(shaded areas)*. The neutral axis is the longitudinal region of the spinal column that bears much of the axial load and about which spinal element distraction or compression does not significantly occur with the assumption of **(A)** flexed, **(B)** neutral, or **(C)** extension postures. *(From Benzel E. Stability and instability of the spine. In Benzel E (ed): Biomechanics of Spine Stabilization, Principles and Clinical Practice. New York, McGraw Hill, Inc, 1995, pp 25-40.)*

instability can similarly be broken into two subgroups: glacial instability and the instability associated with dysfunctional segmental motions.

Quantification of Acute Instability

Numerous authors have attempted to quantitate the degree or extent of acute instability by a point system approach. White and Panjabi[51] described a region-specific point system in which an accumulation of five or more points indicates an unstable spine. The system emphasizes the differences between the cervical, thoracic, and thoracolumbar and lumbar regions. These are the essential assessments of overt and limited instability as defined in the next paragraph. The primary purpose of a stability determination is to delineate the most appropriate management scheme for patient care. Recently, Benzel[4] presented the quantification of acute instability in subaxial cervical, thoracic, and lumbar regions based on the point system suggested earlier by White and Panjabi. In principle, the earlier classification was combined in such a way that regional differences were eliminated so that the point system was independent of spinal region.

The stretch test for the assessment of acute cervical spine instability by White and Panjabi involves a progressive addition of cervical traction up to 33% of the patient's weight with serial radiographic and clinical assessments. A positive test indicating the presence of instability is the one that shows a disc interspace separation of more than 1.7mm or a change in the angle between the vertebrae of more than 7.5 degrees between the prestretch and poststretch conditions. The merits of this test are debatable. First, it is clearly not without risk, whether those risks be immediately obvious or occult. Risk of tethering the spinal cord over a ventral mass may also exist. The most significant and least immediately recognized risk of this procedure is that of a false-negative test (i.e., the presence of stability in a really unstable circumstance). This test has been used as a determinant of eligibility for participation in contact sports.[4] It should be noted that the resistance of stretching by muscle action (voluntary or involuntary) may conceal ligamentous deficiencies, particularly in an athlete.

Flexion-extension radiographs may also not be helpful, and in certain cases, could be misleading, particularly after trauma. If pathology is observed and iatrogenic injury via the act of flexion and extension is not incurred, the radiographs are useful.[4] They are, however, not without risk, if spinal instability is present. A "normal" flexion-extension radiograph may not always indicate stability (i.e., the test may be a false negative). Incomplete patient cooperation and "guarding" against excessive spinal movement caused by underlying acute pathology can also disguise an injury process that, if not treated properly, may lead to catastrophe.

The definition of stability in clinical practice must address the integrity of each component. Whether the two-column or the three-column approach is used initially, each component must be subsequently analyzed to reach a clinical decision. The problem of simple definitions of stability is that clinical cases are not always simple.

Examination of a burst fracture should lend itself to additional questions, such as the nature and extent of vertebral body compression, and the number of ligament(s) in the posterior column stretched beyond their elastic limits, or even torn. These questions deal with component-related problems. Understanding of the biomechanical characteristics and an inter-relationship among spinal components is limited. Additional research that relates component attributes to acute and chronic instability must be undertaken. The clinician should have a detailed understanding of the biomechanical properties of the individual components (discs, ligaments, facet joints, vertebral bodies) and the relationship of their integrity to the overall stability and load-carrying capacity of the spine.

Anomalous Anatomy

Anomalous spinal anatomy is occasionally associated with structural, biomechanical, and neurological sequelae. For example, the Klippel-Feil anomaly in the cervical spine can place excessive stress on adjacent motion segments via the application of an abnormally lengthy moment arm. This, in turn, could result in the acceleration of degenerative changes at adjacent motion segments.

Similarly, the lumbarization of the L5 vertebral body (i.e., the presence of 4, instead of 5, lumbar segments) could place excessive stress at the L4-5 disci interspace. Conversely, the presence of six lumbar vertebrae could result in excessive lordosis and abnormal loading patterns that expose the lower lumber motion segments to significant stress that may lead to increased rates of disc herniation and degenerative changes.

Anomalous nerve root anatomy, such as conjoined nerve roots (Fig. 7.28), can expose the patient to injury from disc herniation or trauma, because of the restriction of normal nerve root motion and mobility. In addition, the unaware surgeon may cause intraoperative iatrogenic injury if the presence of this anomaly is not evident to the surgeon before surgery.

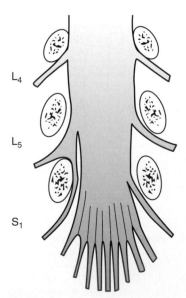

Figure 7.28 Anomalous nerve root.

Soft-Tissue Biomechanics

As discussed earlier in this chapter, the integrity of the soft tissues is vital to maintain spinal stability and physiologic function. Physiologic dysfunction in the form of pain to the neck or headache occurs secondary to low-speed motor vehicle rear impacts, and these injuries do not often result in osseous damage. These injuries, often termed *whiplash trauma*, are soft-tissue related.[9] Studies conducted by Yoganandan *et al.*[60,63] have explained the mechanisms of headache and neck pain, the two most common complaints of whiplash patients. Using biomechanical tests, Yoganandan *et al.*[53] documented soft-tissue injuries in the form of ligamentous and facet joint compromise, secondary to single rear impact acceleration using intact whole-body postmortem human subjects. Cusick *et al.*[16] and Yoganandan *et al.*[60,62-64] have discussed the formation of a reverse curve during the earlier stages of the rear impact acceleration wherein the spine attains a nonphysiologic curvature (i.e., upper cervical spine flexion associated with lower cervical spine extension). Using kinematic analysis as a biomechanical basis, these studies indicated that flexion at the upper segment may stretch the posterior suboccipital structures, creating tensile forces, which may affect the related neural structures and be responsible for suboccipital headaches. The local lower cervical spinal extension indicated that the facet joint slides from the anterior to the posterior direction and the joint stretches ventrally while compressing dorsally, indicating a pinching mechanism. The sliding and the pinching mechanism results in a stretch of the joint itself. This local stretch of the lower cervical spine facet joint may be responsible for neck pain in whiplash patients. A diagrammatic representation of the facet joint pinching mechanism resulting in a stretch of the facet joint is shown in Figure 7.29. Ongoing studies at the Medical College of Wisconsin have begun to indicate the differences between males and females with regard to cervical spine motions during rear impact, in particular, during the time of formation of the nonphysiologic S-curve. Specifically, female intervertebral joints have shown a higher degree of motion than male intervertebral joints at the lower cervical spine levels. These studies appear to support the clinical and epidemiological finding that females are more susceptible to soft-tissue–related injuries than males.

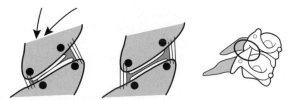

Figure 7.29 Diagrammatic representation of the facet joint-pinching mechanism occurring in the lower cervical spine under whiplash loading because the compression is more pronounced in the posterior facet joint and the sliding is approximately the same. This causes the posterior aspect of the facet to be pinched. *(From Cusick JF, Yoganandan N, Pintar FA: Whiplash syndrome: Kinematic factors influencing pain patterns.* Spine *2001;26:1252-1258, 2001.)*

ACKNOWLEDGMENTS

This research was supported in part by Grant PHS CDC R49CCR 515433, DOT NHTSA Grant DTNH22-93-Y-17028, and the Department of Veterans Affairs Medical Center Research Service.

REFERENCES

1. Adams MA, Hutton WC: Prolapsed intervertebral disc. A hyperflexion injury. *Spine* 7:184-191, 1982
2. Adams MA, Hutton WC: Gradual disc prolapse. *Spine* 10:524, 1985.
3. Ahmed AM, Duncan NA, Burke DL. The effect of facet geometry on the axial torque-rotation response of lumbar motion segments. *Trans Orthop Res Soc.* Atlanta, 1–10, 1988.
4. Benzel E. Stability and instability of the spine. In Benzel E (ed): *Biomechanics of Spine Stabilization, Principles and Clinical Practice.* New York, McGraw Hill, Inc, 1995, pp 25-40.
5. Benzel EC. Biomechanics of lumbar and lumbrosacral spine fracture. In Miller CA (ed): *Spinal Trauma: Current Evaluation and Management.* Rolling Hills, IL, American Association of Neurological Surgeons, 1993, pp 165-195.
6. Benzel EC, Kesterson L: Posterior cervical interspinous compression wiring and fusion for mid to low cervical spine injuries. *J Neurosurg* 70:893-899, 1989.
7. Benzel EC, Larson SJ: Functional recovery after decompressive operation for thoracic and lumbar spine fractures. *Neurosurgery* 19:772-777, 1986.
8. Berry JL, Moran JM, Berg WS, et al.: A morphometric study of human lumbar and selected thoracic vertebrae. *Spine* 12:362-366, 1987.
9. Bogduk N, Yoganandan N: Biomechanics of the cerviccal spine Part 3: Minor injuries. *Clin Biomech* 16:267-275, 2001.
10. Breig A. Biomechanics of the central nervous system. *Some Basic Normal and Pathological Phenomena.* Stockholm, Almqvist & Wiksell International, 1960.
11. Breig A, Turnbull IM, Hassler O: Effects of mechanical stress on the spinal cord in cervical spondylosis. A study of fresh cadaver material. *J Neurosurg* 25:45-56, 1966.
12. Brinckmann P, Horst M: The influence of vertebral body fracture, intradiscal injection, and partial discectomy on the radial bulge and height of human lumbar discs. *Spine* 10:138, 1985.
13. Carpenter MB. *Human Neuroanatomy.* Baltimore, Williams & Wilkins, 1976.
14. Chazal J, Tanguy A, Bourges M, *et al.*: Biomechanical properties of spinal ligaments and a histological study of the supraspinal ligament in traction. *J Biomech* 18:167-176, 1985.
15. Cusick JF. Pathophysiology and treatment of cervical spondylotic myelopathy. In Black P (ed): *Clinical Neurosurgery.* Baltimore, Williams and Wilkins, 1991, pp 661-681.
16. Cusick JF, Yoganandan N, Pintar FA: Whiplash syndrome: Kinematic factors influencing pain patterns. *Spine* 2001;26:1252-1258, 2001.
17. Cusick JF, Yoganandan N, Pintar FA, *et al.*: Biomechanics of cervical spine facetectomy and fixation techniques. *Spine* 13:808-812, 1988.
18. Cusick JF, Yoganandan N, Pintar FA, *et al.*: Biomechanics of sequential lumbar posterior surgical alteration. *J Neurosurg* 76:805-811, 1992.

19. Denis F: The three-column spine and its significance in the classification of acute thoracolumbar spinal injuries. *Spine* 8:817-831, 1983.

20. Denis F: Spinal instability as defined by the three-column spine concept in acute spinal trauma. *Clin Orthop* 189:65-76, 1984.

21. Goel VK, Njus GO: Stress-strain characteristic of spinal ligaments. 32nd Trans Orthop Res Soc, New Orleans, 1-2, 1986.

22. Holdsworth FW: Fractures, dislocations and fracture dislocations of the spine. *J Bone Joint Surg* 45B:6-20, 1963.

23. Ikegawa S, Tsunoda N, Yata H, *et al*. The effect of joint angle on cross-sectional area and muscle strength of human elbow flexors. In Winter DA, .Wells RP, Hayes KC, Patla AE (eds): *Human Kinetics, R.W.N.,* vol 5A, Biomechanics, Champaign, IL, 1979, pp 39-43.

24. Johnson RM, Hart DL, Simmons EF, *et al*: Cervical orthoses. A study comparing their effectiveness in restricting cervical motion in normal subjects. *J Bone Joint Surg* 56A:332-339, 1977.

25. Krag MH, Weaver DL, Beynnon BD: Morphometry of the thoracic and lumbar spine related to transpedicular screw placement for surgical spinal fixation. *Spine* 13:27-32, 1988.

26. Lin HS, Liu YK, Adams KH: Mechanical response of the lumbar intervertebral joint under physiological (complex) loading. *J Bone Joint Surg* 60A:41-55, 1978.

27. Louis R: Spinal stability as defined by the three-column spine concept. *Anat Clin* 7:33-42, 1985.

28. Maiman DJ, Millington DP, Novak S: The effect of thermoplastic Minerva jacket on cervical spine motion. *Neurosurgery* 25:363-368, 1989.

29. Maiman DJ, Yoganandan N: Biomechanics of cervical spine trauma. In Black P (ed): *Clinical Neurosurgery*, Baltimore, Williams & Wilkins, vol 37, 1991, pp 543-570.

30. Myklebust JB, Pintar FA, Yoganandan N, *et al*.: Tensile strength of spinal ligaments. *Spine* 13:526-531, 1988.

31. Nachemson A: Lumbar interdiscal pressure. *Acta Orthop Scand* 43 (Suppl), 1960.

32. Nachemson A, Evans J: Some mechanical properties of the third lumbar inter-laminar ligament (ligamentum flavum). *J Biomech* 1:211-217, 1968.

33. Nicoll EA: Fractures of the dorso-lumbar spine. *J Bone Joint Surg [Br]* 31:376-394, 1949.

34. Panjabi MM, Duranceau J, Goel V, *et al*: Cervical human vertebrae. Quantitative three-dimensional anatomy of the middle and lower regions. *Spine* 16:861-869, 1991.

35. Panjabi MM, Dvorak J, Duranceau J, *et al*: Three-dimensional movements of the upper cervical spine. *Spine* 13:726-730, 1988.

36. Panjabi MM, Hausfeld JN, White AA: A biomechanical study of the ligamentous stability of the thoracic spine in man. *Acta Orthop Scand* 52:315-326, 1981.

37. Panjabi MM, Takata K, Goel V, *et al*: Thoracic human vertebrae. Quantitative three-dimensional anatomy. *Spine* 16:888-901, 1991.

38. Perry O: Fracture of the vertebral end-plate in the lumbar spine. *Acta Orthop Scand* 125:157-165, 1957.

39. Pintar FA: *Biomechanics of Spinal Elements*. Milwaukee, Marquette University, 1986.

40. Pintar FA, Yoganandan N, Myers T, *et al*: Biomechanical properties of human lumbar spine ligaments. *J Biomech* 25:1351-1356, 1992.

41. Raynor RB, Moskovich R, Zidel P, *et al*: Alterations in primary and coupled neck motions after facetectomy. *Neurosurgery* 21:681-687, 1987.

42. Raynor RB, Pugh J, Shapiro I: Cervical facetectomy and its effect on spine strength. *J Neurosurg* 63:278-282, 1985.

43. Reynolds AF, Roberts A, Pollay M, *et al*: Quantitative anatomy of the thoracolumbar epidural space. *Neurosurgery* 17:905-907, 1985.

44. Roaf R: A study of the mechanics of spinal injuries. *J Bone Joint Surg* 42B:810, 1960.

45. Sances A, Myklebust JB, Maiman DJ, *et al*: The biomechanics of spinal injuries. *CRC Crit Rev Bioeng* 11:1-76, 1984.

46. Sances AJ, Myklebust JB, Larson SJ, *et al*: Bioengineering analysis of head and spine injuries. *CRC Crit Rev Bioeng* 2:1-79, 1981.

47. Taylor JR, Twomey LT: Age changes in lumbar zygapophyseal joints. Observations in structure and function. *Spine* 11:739-745, 1986.

48. Traczuk H: Tensile properties of human lumbar longitudinal ligaments. *Acta Orthop Scand* 115, 1968.

49. Van Schaik JPJ, Verbiest H, Van Schaik FDJ: The orientation of laminae and facet joints in the lower lumbar spine. *Spine* 10:59-63, 1985.

50. White AA, Panjabi MM: The basic kinematics of the human spine. A review of past and current knowledge. *Spine* 3:12-20, 1978.

51. White AA, Panjabi MM: *Clinical Biomechanics of the Spine*, ed 2. Philadelphia, Lippincott, 1990.

52. Woodburne RT: *Essentials of Human Anatomy*, ed 7. Oxford, England, Oxford University Press, 1982.

53. Yoganandan N, Cusick JF, Pintar FA, *et al*: Whiplash injury determination with conventional spine imaging and cryomicrotomy. *Spine* 26:2443-2448, 2001.

54. Yoganandan N, Kumaresan S, Pintar F: Geometric and mechanical properties of human cervical spine ligaments. *J Biomech Engr* 122:623-629, 2000.

55. Yoganandan N, Larson SJ, Gallagher M, *et al*: Correlation of microtrauma in the lumbar spine with intraosseous pressures. *Spine* 19:435-440, 1994.

56. Yoganandan N, Larson SJ, Pintar FA, *et al*: Intravertebral pressure changes caused by spinal microtrauma. *Neurosurgery* 35:415-421, 1994.

57. Yoganandan N, Maiman DJ, Pintar FA, *et al*: Biomechanical effects of laminectomy on thoracic spine stability. *Neurosurgery* 32:604-610, 1993.

58. Yoganandan N, Maiman DJ, Pintar FA, *et al*: Microtrauma in the lumbar spine: a cause of low back pain. *Neurosurgery* 23:162-168, 1988.

59. Yoganandan N, Myklebust JB, Ray G, *et al*: Mathematical and finite element analysis of spinal injuries. *CRC Review Biomed Eng* 15:29-93, 1987.

60. Yoganandan N, Pintar FA (eds): *Frontiers in Whiplash Trauma: Clinical and Biomechanical*. The Netherlands, IOS Press, 2001.

61. Yoganandan N, Pintar FA, Butler J, *et al*: Dynamic response of human cervical spine ligaments. *Spine* 14:1102-1110, 1989.

62. Yoganandan N, Pintar FA, Cusick JF: Cervical spine kinematics under inertial flexion extension. *North Am Spine Soc.* Vancouver, Canada, 1996:265-266.

63. Yoganandan N, Pintar FA, Cusick JF: Head-neck biomechanics in simulated rear impact. AAAM Conf. Charlottesville, VA, 1998:115-136.

64. Yoganandan N, Pintar FA, Larson S, *et al* (eds): *Frontiers in Head and Neck Trauma: Clinical and Biomechanical.* The Netherlands, IOS Press, 1998.

65. Yoganandan N, Ray G, Pintar FA, *et al*: Stiffness and strain energy criteria to evaluate the threshold of injury to an intervertebral joint. *J Biomech* 22:135-142, 1989.

66. Yoganandan N, Ray G, Sances AJ, *et al*: Assessment of traumatic failure load and microfailure load in an intervertebral disc segment. *Advances in Bioengineering* 130-131, 1985.

67. Zindrick MR, Wiltse LL, Doornik A, *et al*: Analysis of the morphometric characteristics of the thoracic and lumbar pedicles. *Spine* 12:160-166, 1987.

CHAPTER 8

Physical and Neurologic Examination

Paul J. Holman and Edward C. Benzel

In recent years, advances in medical technologies and changes in healthcare systems have dramatically altered the practice of medicine and the physician–patient relationship. One consequence of these changes, unfortunately, is that the physical examination is no longer the focus of many physician–patient encounters and is often overlooked when important clinical decisions are made. In the field of spinal surgery, the widespread availability of neuroimaging of the spinal column and modern health care policies regulating coverage of elective surgery are two factors that have contributed to this change. Patients who are often referred for their initial consultation with their MRI "in hand" worry more about the radiologist's interpretation of the scan than their symptoms. In many instances, patients are required to consult with multiple surgeons and receive conflicting recommendations regarding the appropriateness of surgical treatment. In this type of environment, it is essential for the surgeon to place a priority on the fundamentals of history taking and the neurologic examination to establish good relationships with patients and guide them in choosing the best therapy.

History Taking

A surgeon's ability to efficiently obtain a thorough history is the cornerstone of treating patients with spinal disorders. Communicating a genuine interest in the patient and a willingness to offer both surgical and nonsurgical treatment are of paramount importance, particularly in complicated patients, such as those suffering from chronic pain syndromes and those referred as part of workers' compensation. Using simple, open-ended questions early in the interview allows patients to articulate their perception of the problem and helps the physician identify treatment goals. The physician can then ask a patient more directed questions to obtain the necessary information to formulate a preliminary differential diagnosis. Careful review of the patient's past medical history is important to uncover conditions with symptoms commonly seen in patients with spinal pathology. Diabetes, peripheral vascular disease, inflammatory arthropathies, and neoplastic disorders are common examples. Any history of trauma involving the spine and related surgical procedures should be noted, in addition to injuries involving the shoulder, hip, and long bones. Unrecognized compression neuropathies secondary to casting, for example, can subsequently be confused with radiculopathy. It is also important to inquire about

a history of any psychiatric disorders, particularly those that may impact the patient's perception of pain.

Taking a good history regarding pain associated with spinal disorders deserves special attention. Radicular pain tends to be constant but may be exacerbated by movement or *Valsalva maneuvers*. The pain occurs in the distribution of the affected nerve root and may have dysesthetic qualities. Mechanical back pain resulting from degenerative disc disease, spondylotic changes of the facets, or gross instability from trauma or cancer tends to be worse with movement and is relieved with rest. The pain associated with neurogenic pseudoclaudication is typically an aching or cramping pain in the buttocks, thighs, or legs that becomes worse with standing and walking short distances and is relieved with sitting or reclining. Pain or paresthesia in the hands that awakens the patient at night and is relieved by shaking the hand is a red flag for nerve entrapment. Pain or paresthesia radiating to the upper extremities and that is associated with medial scapular pain is more likely to be radicular in origin.

General Physical Examination

Although a comprehensive general physical exam may not be feasible in every patient, details gathered from the patient's medical history serve as a guide to performing an examination of other organ systems. Basic vital signs should be recorded in most patients. Hypertension and atrial fibrillation are two examples of disorders easily identified by physical examination that could significantly impact diagnosis and operative risk in a patient with transient cerebral ischemia. Auscultation of the lungs and palpation of the abdomen are essential in the setting of metastatic spine disease. Pleural effusion, extensive atelectasis, and ascites impact anesthetic risk and may influence patient positioning and surgical approach. Examination of peripheral pulses and distal skin integrity is important in patients with diabetes and possible vascular claudication.

Components of the Neurologic Examination

After completing the relevant portions of the general examination, the neurologic examination is performed. The surgeon may choose to focus the exam on a particular spinal region, but patients often complain of symptoms referable to both the cervical and thoracolumbar spine, particularly those with extensive spondylosis. A comprehensive exam may also be beneficial, for example, by uncovering signs of cervical myelopathy in a patient who needs lumbar decompression and may be at risk for neurologic deterioration during positioning or intubation. Evaluation of cranial nerve function should be included in patients with bulbar symptoms or with coexisting head and spinal trauma. A comprehensive examination should include: (1) inspection and palpation of the entire spinal column, (2) range of motion (ROM) testing of both the spine and joints of affected extremities, (3) sensory and motor evaluation, (4) gait analysis, and (5) an assessment of normal and pathologic reflexes. The order in which these modalities is tested is dictated by surgeon preference, but minimizing patient movement and reserving maneuvers that may cause pain for the end of the exam are important considerations.

Inspection

A generalized inspection of the patient with emphasis on cutaneous features, posture, and gait begins as the patient first appears for evaluation and the history is reviewed.

Cutaneous Abnormalities

The skin should be inspected for café-au-lait spots and other sequela of neurofibromatosis, in addition to scars from old trauma or prior surgery. The dorsal midline skin should be carefully inspected for dimpling, abnormal pigmentation, fatty masses, and tufts of hair, all of which could signal an underlying congenital spinal anomaly. In patients with symptoms of claudication, the peripheral pulses are palpated and the skin of the distal extremities is inspected for edema, skin ulceration, loss of hair, and other signs of peripheral vascular disease.

Posture

Inspection of the spinal column as a single unit should be performed from both a lateral and posterior viewpoint. Abnormalities in "spinal balance," both in the sagittal and coronal planes can be pathologic and have important implications when considering surgical deformity correction. Coronal imbalance can be assessed clinically by examining the standing patient from behind and measuring the distance between a plumb line dropped from C7 and the gluteal cleft.

Gait Analysis

Examination of a patient's gait is an invaluable component of the neurologic exam. Watching patients walk as they appear for consultation, even before formal testing begins, can be of diagnostic value.

Alterations of Gait Associated with Cord Compression

A wide-based, unsteady gait is frequently seen in myelopathic patients and can be accentuated by evaluating tandem walk. Unfortunately, a wide-based gait is not specific for myelopathy and is common in patients with cerebellar pathology, decreased proprioception resulting from peripheral neuropathy, and conditions affecting posterior column function, such as tabes dorsalis and spinocerebellar ataxias. A spastic gait can be seen in stroke patients or in those with an old cord injury and is manifested by circumduction of a hemiplegic leg or "scissoring" of the legs in a paraparetic patient. The diagnosis of *Parkinson's disease* should always be kept in mind when patients referred for possible myelopathy display a shuffling gait (festination) with either forward (propulsion) or backward (retropulsion) walking.

Other Characteristic Gaits

Patients suffering from compression of neural elements of the lumbosacral spine often show characteristics of "antalgic gait." This term is somewhat nonspecific but involves alter-ation of the movement of the affected extremity in an attempt to silence the pain generator. Lumbar radiculopathy associated with weakness of several different muscles can alter gait. Weakness of ankle dorsiflexors and foot drop may cause a patient to walk with a "steppage gait." To clear the ground while the patient pushes off, the hip is flexed excessively and the foot may slap the ground. Weakness of gluteus medius (L5) hip abduction or gluteus maximus (S1) hip extension may cause the patient to rock the thorax, or "waddle," to compensate for poor hip fixation. Patients with advanced lumbar stenosis and neurogenic claudication tend to walk in a flexed–forward position, commonly referred to as the "anthropoid posture."

Palpation and Range of Motion (ROM) Testing of the Spine and Related Areas

Formal palpation and range of motion (ROM) testing of the spinal column, shoulders, hips, and pelvis are also included in a comprehensive exam. The spinous processes of the entire vertebral column are palpated and assessed for tenderness and associated paravertebral muscle spasm. Splaying of adjacent spinous processes or a palpable step off may indicate spondylolisthesis. Patients with fibromyalgia and related disorders frequently complain of pain exacerbated by stimulation of multiple "trigger points." Axial rotation, flexion, extension, and lateral bending are assessed for each region of the spine.

Cervical Spine

In the cervical spine the resting head position is noted before evaluation of ROM. A patient with a fixed rotation or tilt to one side may have an underlying unilateral facet dislocation. While precise quantitative evaluation of ROM is not typically performed, the clinician should note obvious limitations and which maneuvers generate pain. Pain or restricted rotation of the head, 50% of which occurs at C1-2,[11] may indicate pathology at this level. Head rotation associated with vertigo, tinnitus, visual alterations, or facial pain may be nonspecific, but occlusion of the vertebral artery should be included in the differential. Selecki[7] showed that rotation of the head more than 45 degrees could significantly kink the contralateral vertebral artery. Extension and rotation of the head can exacerbate preexisting nerve root compression, and flexion in the setting of cord compression often causes paresthesia in both the arms and legs (*L'hermitte's sign*).

Thoracic Spine

Examination of the thoracic spine should focus on the detection of scoliosis or a kyphotic deformity. The patient is observed from behind for symmetry in the level of the shoulders, scapulae, and hips. If a scoliotic deformity is noticed on inspection, flexion and lateral bending are assessed to further characterize the curve and determine its flexibility. Asymmetry in the paravertebral musculature with forward flexion can generate an angle in the horizontal plane that can be followed for progression.

In the upper thoracic spine, there are 4 degrees of sagittal plane rotation, 6 degrees of lateral bending, and 8 to 9 degrees of axial rotation at each segment. In the lower two to three segments, these median figures are 12 degrees, 8 to 9 degrees, and 2 degrees, respectively.[11]

Lumbar Spine and Related Areas

Palpation should include not only the spinous processes and paravertebral muscles, but also the greater trochanter, the ischial tuberosity, and the sciatic nerve itself. The greater trochanter is palpated for focal tenderness when the patient's chief complaint includes thigh discomfort. The bursa is usually not palpable unless it is boggy and inflamed. Acute trochanteric bursitis is included in the primary differential diagnosis of lumbar radiculopathy and can also be a chronic secondary pain generator. The sciatic nerve can be palpated at the midpoint between the greater trochanter and ischial tuberosity, when the patient's hip is maximally flexed. Tenderness can occur with peripheral nerve compression by a tumor or an enlarged pyriformis muscle or when the contributing roots are compressed in the spine.

The most important aspect of ROM testing in the lumbar spine is flexion–extension. A simple clinical test is to ask the patient to bend forward with the knees fully extended, and measure the distance from the patient's fingertips to the floor. Patients with facet arthropathy or spondylolisthesis often have back pain that is exacerbated by extension. Lateral bending and axial rotation are strongly coupled in the lumbar spine and more restricted because of sagittal facet orientation. It is critical to exclude the hip as a potential pain generator in the evaluation of possible lumbar spine disease. The *Patrick or Fabere test* is used to detect pathology in the hip or SI joint. The patient is tested in the supine position, and the extremity in question is flexed, abducted, and externally rotated at the hip. This can be accomplished by asking the patient to place the lateral aspect of the foot on the involved side on the opposite shin. Pain with this maneuver is likely from the hip joint. Pain from the SI joint itself is suspected when simultaneous downward pressure on the flexed knee and the opposite anterior superior iliac spine increases symptoms. The SI joint can also be tested as a pain generator by performing the *pelvic rock test.* The examiner places both hands around the iliac crest with the thumbs on the anterior superior iliac spine and compresses medially.

Motor Examination

Muscle weakness is frequently seen in patients suffering from compression of specific nerve roots or the spinal cord itself. Weakness may be the patient's primary symptom and discovered only after physical examination. Motor deficits may be acute and rapidly progressive (i.e., after traumatic disc herniation or more insidious in onset, similar to the setting of cervical myelopathy). A detailed motor examination and muscle grading (Table 8.1) of the key muscles innervated by the cervical and lumbar nerve roots should be performed in every patient. Evaluating strength systematically will allow the clinician to identify common patterns of muscle weakness seen in cord compression and

TABLE 8.1

Grading Motor Function

Grade	Description
0	No palpable/visible contraction
1	Muscle flicker
2	Movement with gravity eliminated
3	Movement against gravity with full range of motion
4	Movement against gravity and some resistance
5	Movement against full resistance

brachial plexus syndromes and reduce the likelihood of missing nonsurgical pathology.

Cervical Spine

Figure 8.1 and Table 8.2 summarize the motor tests used to grade muscle strength for the cervical nerve roots that contribute to motor function of the upper extremity. It is important to remember that the configuration of the brachial plexus (pre- or post-fixed) can alter the typical pattern of innervation by one level. The anatomical relationship of the cervical vertebrae and motor roots must be kept in mind when attempting to correlate motor deficits to nerve root compression seen on an MRI or myelogram. A C5-6 disc herniation, for example, typically compresses the origin of the C6 root before it exits the neural foramen above the C6 pedicle.

Lumbar Spine

Figure 8.2 and Table 8.3 summarize the motor tests used to grade muscle strength for the lumbar nerve roots commonly affected in clinical practice. Again, correlating clinical findings with radiographic abnormalities is imperative. With a typical paracentral L4-5 disc herniation, for example, the root of origin (L5) is compressed as it courses toward the undersurface of the L5 pedicle. A far lateral disc herniation at the same level may compress the root of exit (L4). Detecting motor deficits in lower extremity, particularly in a large, muscular patient, can sometimes be difficult. Testing the patient's ability to heel (tibialis anterior) and toe (gastrocnemius) walk, maneuvers that require a patient to overcome body weight, can uncover a subtle weakness.

Sensory Examination

The key sensory dermatomes of the upper and lower extremities are depicted in Figures 8.1 and 8.2. The nipple line (T4) and umbilicus (T10) are useful thoracic landmarks. It is emphasized, however, that these landmarks are variable. Of particular note is that the T2 dermatome may be as low as the nipple line, and that it demarcates the C4-T2 dermatome junction. The clinician should always compare dermatomes from one side to the other and ask the patient to quantify differences. Both light touch and pain perception should be tested, and proprioception and vibratory sense should be included in patients

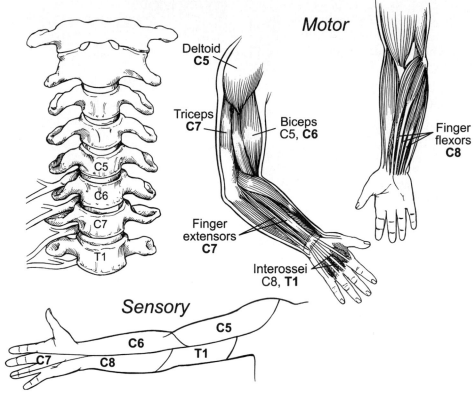

Figure 8.1 Examination of the cervical spine.

TABLE 8.2				
Clinical Examination for Cervical Radiculopathy				
Disc Herniation	**Affected Root**	**Motor Test/Muscle**	**Sensory Test**	**Reflex**
C4-5	C5	Shoulder abduction/ deltoid	Lateral deltoid	Biceps
C5-6	C6	a. Elbow flexion/biceps b. Radial wrist extension/ extensor.	Thumb and lateral forearm	Brachioradialis and biceps (< C5)
C6-7	C7	c. Carpi radialis longus a. Elbow extension/triceps b. Finger extension/ ext digitorum communis	Middle finger	Triceps
C7-T1	C8	a. Finger flexion/flexor digitorum superficialis and profundus b. Hand intrinsics/interossei (<T1)	Little finger	—
T1-2	T1	Hand intrinsics/ interossei	Medial arm	—

suspected of having cord compression, peripheral nerve entrapment, or sensory neuropathy. The sensory examination is particularly critical in the evaluation of the spinal cord-injured patient to determine the level of injury and to monitor for a progressing deficit. A rectal examination should usually be performed to assess for sphincter tone and perianal dermatomes. Preservation of perianal sensation in the presence of a discrete sensory level defines an incomplete lesion and may dramatically impact management and prognosis for recovery. Special mention should be made here of provocative sensory tests for nerve

entrapment syndromes that can occasionally be confused with cervical radiculopathy. Median nerve compression (C6) in the carpal tunnel, ulnar nerve entrapment (C8) in the cubital tunnel or *Guyon's canal*, and radial nerve compression (C7) in the forearm are important differential diagnoses and occasionally coexist with root compression in the neck, the "double crush phenomenon."[10] Tapping on the nerve proximal to the site of compression can reproduce symptoms (*Tinel's sign*) in middle course of nerve root compression while the nerve is attempting to regenerate. Sustained wrist flexion over 60 seconds can

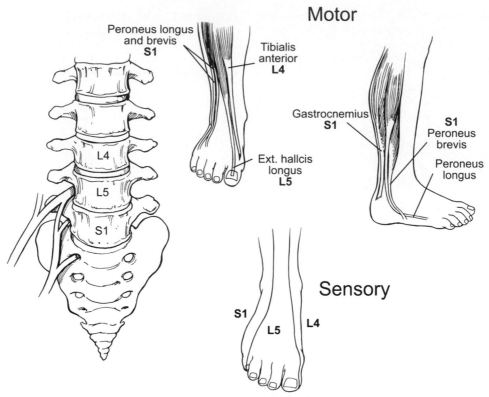

Figure 8.2 Examination of the lumbar spine.

TABLE 8.3

Clinical Examination for Lumbar Radiculopathy

Herniated Disc	Affected Root (Root of Origin)	Motor Test/Muscle	Sensory Test	Reflex
L3–4	L4	a. Knee extension/quadriceps b. Ankle dorsiflexion (>L5)	Posteromedial leg	Patellar
L4–5	L5	a. Great toe extension/extensor hallucis longus b. Ankle dorsiflexion (<L4)	Anterolateral leg and dorsum of foot	—
L5–S1	S1	Ankle plantar flexion/gastrocnemius, soleus	Lateral malleolus and lateral and plantar foot	Achilles

---

produce signs of median nerve compression (*Phalen sign*), and similar testing can be done by flexing the elbow (ulnar nerve compression) or pronating the forearm (radial nerve compression).

Reflex Examination

The neurologic examination also includes an evaluation of the deep tendon (stretch) and superficial reflexes.

Deep Tendon Reflexes

The deep tendon reflexes are used to assess the integrity of a monosynaptic reflex arc at various levels of the cord. Table 8.4 depicts the common system for grading deep tendon reflexes. Hyperactive reflexes generally indicate an

TABLE 8.4

Grading of Deep Tendon Reflexes

Grade	Description
0	No response
1	Diminished
2	Normal
3	Increased
4	Hyperactive (with clonus)

upper motor neuron lesion, and diminished or absent reflexes can be seen in lower motor neuron lesions. Metabolic abnormalities such as hypothyroidism or hyperthyroidism should always be excluded as an etiology for abnormal reflexes. Reflexes are compared from one side to another, and reinforcement maneuvers that require isometric contraction of other muscle groups can be used to eliminate cortical modulation of the reflex arc. The Jendrassik maneuver can accentuate lower extremity reflexes and requires the patient to pull interlocked fingers apart while the reflex is tested. Asking the patient to clench the teeth or push down on the examination table with the thighs can accentuate upper extremity reflexes. Although the commonly tested reflexes are truly mediated by multiple nerve roots, Tables 8.2 and 8.3 outline the dominant nerve roots involved.

Superficial Reflexes

The superficial reflexes are mediated by the cerebral cortex with the afferent limb being supplied by cutaneous stimulation. The absence of a normal cutaneous reflex may signal an underlying upper motor neuron lesion. In the thoracic spine, the *upper abdominal* (T5-8), *mid abdominal* (T9-10), and *lower abdominal* (T11-12) superficial reflexes can be used to assess the integrity of motor efferents from these levels. As the appropriate dermatome is stroked from lateral to medial, the ipsilateral abdominal muscles will contract. In a thin, muscular patient the examiner will occasionally observe movement of the umbilicus toward the stimulated side. In the lumbar spine, the *superficial cremasteric reflex* is mediated by L1 and L2. Stimulating the upper medial thigh in a male patient will cause elevation of the testicle on the ipsilateral side. The *superficial anal reflex,* or "anal wink," is used to assess S2-4 and involves contraction of the external anal sphincter in response to stimulation of the perianal skin. The importance of testing this reflex in the setting of spinal cord injury has been previously mentioned.

Pathologic Reflexes

Upper motor neuron lesions should be suspected in patients harboring the classic pathologic reflexes. These include the plantar response in the lower extremity and a positive *Hoffmann's sign* in the hand. The plantar reflex is typically assessed by the *Babinski test*. The surgeon uses a sharp instrument to stroke the plantar surface of the foot from lateral to medial, a maneuver that usually results in flexion of all the toes. A positive test involves dorsiflexion of the great toe alone or in combination with ankle dorsiflexion and hip flexion ("triple response"). The same reflex can be elicited by stroking the lateral side of the foot (*Chaddock test*) or the crest of the tibia (*Oppenheim test*).

The upper extremity analogue of the plantar response is *Hoffmann's sign*. The palmar surface of the hand is lightly supported as the patient's middle finger is flicked into extension or flexion at the distal interphalangeal joint. A positive response involves reflex flexion of the thumb and fingers and is commonly seen in myelopathic patients with cervical spinal cord compression. A recent study[8] of 536 patients with spine-related problems found 16 patients with a positive Hoffmann's sign and no pain or neurologic symptoms referable to the cervical spine. Interestingly, ¹⁵⁄₁₆ (94%) of these patients had some degree of cord compression on cervical MRI. The clinical significance of this study is unclear, however, because prior studies[1] have documented cervical cord impingement in up to 20% of asymptomatic adults over age 40.

Provocative Nerve Root Testing

If the history and basic physical examination raise the clinical suspicion of a radiculopathy, performing a series of provocative nerve root tests can further improve diagnostic accuracy. These tests were designed to reproduce clinical symptoms by accentuating nerve root irritation by compressive pathology.

Cervical Spine

Patients with cervical radiculopathy often complain of worsening pain with Valsalva activities or when rotating the head toward the symptomatic extremity. A foraminal closing test (Figure 8.3) is performed by hyperextending the patient's head and rotating it toward the affected side, decreasing the size of the intervertebral foramen. A positive test reproduces the patient's radicular symptoms and is often referred to as *Spurling's sign*. A recent review of the Spurling test,[9] which was administered prior to EMG testing of 255 patients referred for possible cervical radiculopathy, found poor sensitivity (30%) but excellent specificity (93%). Similar maneuvers can be used to reproduce radicular symptoms, including pure axial compression followed by traction, but these tend to be poorly

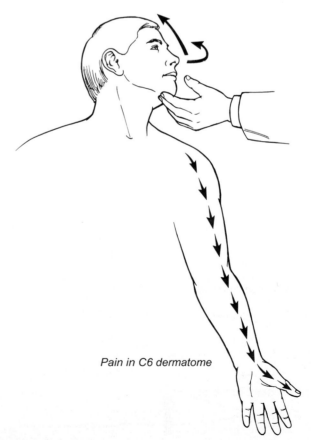

Pain in C6 dermatome

Figure 8.3 Foraminal closing maneuver positive for a C6 radiculopathy.

tolerated by patients. Patients with cervical radiculopathy may also get relief by placing the affected extremity behind the head: shoulder abduction relief sign.[3]

Lumbar Spine

There are several well described nerve root tension signs that are useful when testing for lumbar radiculopathy.[6]

Straight Leg Raising Test (SLR, or Lasègue's sign)

The most widely used test to differentiate leg pain resulting from hip pathology versus nerve root irritation is the Straight Leg Raising Test (SLR). The test was discovered by the French pathologist Ernest Charles Lasègue[2] and described in 1881 by one of his pupils, J. J. Forst. In the supine position, the patient's fully extended leg is slowly raised and the patient reports any pain that is elicited. The SLR is considered positive if pain or paresthesia occurs in a radicular distribution at less than 60 degrees of elevation

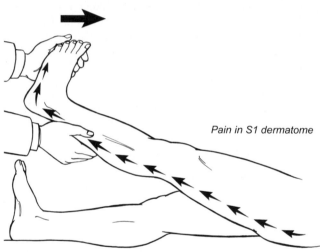

Pain in S1 dermatome

Figure 8.4 Positive straight leg raising for an S1 radiculopathy.

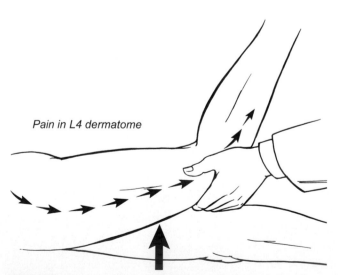

Pain in L4 dermatome

Figure 8.5 Positive reverse straight leg raising for an L4 radiculopathy.

(Figure 8.4). Lowering the affected leg and dorsiflexing the ankle will exacerbate the pain. Allowing the foot to rest on the examining table by flexing the knee will typically ease the pain (*bowstring sign*). Pain limited to the low back, hip, or posterior thigh is not indicative of a radiculopathy. SLR is most specific for L5 or S1 radiculopathy.

Reverse Straight Leg Raising (Femoral Stretch Test)

This test is more sensitive for pain caused by radiculopathy involving L2, L3, and L4. In the prone position, the patient's knee is maximally flexed as the hip is extended (Figure 8.5). A positive test involves pain in the distribution of the affected nerve root.

Crossed Straight Leg-Raising Test (Well Leg/Straight Leg Raising Test)

This test is performed by raising the unaffected leg with the patient in the supine position and is positive when radicular pain occurs in the clinically affected extremity. This phenomenon is also referred to as *Fajersztajn's sign,* in honor of the Polish neurologist who first described it[5] and, interestingly, also suggested that foot dorsiflexion would aggravate sciatica. The test is typically positive when the patient has a large central disc herniation. It is more specific but less sensitive than SLR.[4]

Hoover Test

This test is included to exclude weakness of nonorganic origin and should be performed in series with SLR. After placing both hands under the patient's heels, the patient is asked to raise one leg. If the examiner cannot feel downward pressure in the resting leg, the patient is not likely giving a true effort.

Summary

Meticulous history taking and physical examination skills are critical to the surgeon caring for patients with spinal disorders.

REFERENCES

1. Boden DS, McGowin PR, Davis DO, *et al*: Abnormal magnetic-resonance scans of the cervical spine in asymptomatic subjects. *J Bone Joint Surg Am* 72:1178-1183, 1990.
2. Chabrol H, Corraze J: Charles Lasegue, 1809–1863. *Am J Psychiatry* 158(1):28, 2001.
3. Davidson RI, Dunn EJ, Metzmaker JN: The shoulder abduction test in the diagnosis of radicular pain in cervical extradural compressive monoradiculopathies. *Spine* 6:441-446, 1981.
4. Hudgins, WR. The crossed straight leg raising test: A diagnostic sign of herniated disc. *J Occup Med* (6): 407-408, 1979.
5. Karbowski, K. History of the discovery of the Lasègue phenomenon and its variants. *Schweiz Med Wochenschr* 114(27-28):992-995, 1984.

6. Scham, SM, Taylor, TKF. Tension signs in lumbar disc prolapse. *Clin Orthop* 75:195-204, 1971.
7. Selecki BR: The effects of rotation of the atlas and axis: Experimental work. *Med J Aust* 1:1012-1015, 1969.
8. Sung RD, Wang JC: Correlation between a positive Hoffmann's reflex and cervical pathology in asymptomatic individuals. *Spine* 26(1):67-70, 2001.
9. Tong HC, Haig AJ, Yamakawa K: The Spurling test and cervical radiculopathy. *Spine* 27(2):156-159, 2002.
10. Upton ARM, McComas AJ: The double crush in nerve entrapment syndromes. *Lancet* 2:359-362, 1973.
11. White AA III, Panjabi, MM: Basic biomechanics of the spine. *Neurosurgery* 7(1):76-93, 1980.

CHAPTER 9

Spinal Masqueraders

Nonspinal Conditions Mimicking Spine Pathology

Rick J. Placide and Daniel J. Mazenac

It is not rare for spinal pathology to refer pain to other parts of the body. In fact, conditions of the spine can present with a multitude of signs and symptoms masquerading as any number of pathological conditions. A classic example is a C5 radiculopathy from a disc herniation that presents as shoulder pain. Conversely, nonspinal disorders may present with pain thought to be of spinal origin. For example, trochanteric bursitis commonly presents with pain or dysfunction that appears to be originating from the lumbar spine. This chapter reviews a number of nonspinal conditions that produce symptoms seemingly of spinal origin, but that actually originate from some structure not directly related to the spine. These conditions mimicking spine pathology range from the relatively benign to those that are life threatening and may present as axial spine pain, radiculopathy, or myelopathy.

Musculoskeletal System

A variety of conditions involving the musculoskeletal system are known to mimic spine pathology.[25,28,39,40,46,47] Typically, degenerative conditions in the upper and lower extremities such as arthritis, tendonitis, and bursitis are the primary culprits bringing the patient to the spine specialist with a suspicion that their complaints are of spinal origin (Box 9.1). There are many musculoskeletal structures in the extremities that can present with signs and symptoms that seem to be originating from the spine; however, the most common extraspinal musculoskeletal masqueraders of spine disease are the shoulder, hip, and sacroiliac joints.

Shoulder

The term shoulder describes a region of the body and not a specific joint. In fact, the shoulder complex includes four separate articulations: the glenohumeral, scapulothoracic, sternoclavicular, and acromioclavicular joints. Any of these joints are subject to trauma and degenerative changes and can therefore cause pain and dysfunction that can be confused with cervical spine pathology. Two of the more common conditions involving the shoulder are impingement syndrome and osteoarthritis. The presenting signs and symptoms will often overlap with those of cervical radiculopathy. A thorough history and physical examination is often required to differentiate between cervical spine and shoulder pathology. Recall that pain coming from shoulder pathology typically does not radiate distal to the elbow and that shoulder and cervical spine disease may coexist.

Impingement Syndrome

Impingement syndrome is a condition caused by repeated mechanical insult to the rotator cuff, with the tendons forced against the overlying coracoacromial arch as the arm is elevated overhead. There are a variety of anatomical, biomechanical, and neurological causes that either narrow the space available for the rotator cuff or cause abnormal arthrokinematics leading to impingement of the tendons. Classically, there are three stages of impingement (described by Neer). Stage 1 is characterized by subacromial edema and hemorrhage, stage 2 progresses to tendonitis and fibrosis, and, ultimately, stage 3 results in tearing of the rotator cuff, either partially or completely.[43]

The patient with impingement generally complains of activity-related shoulder pain that extends from the top of the shoulder into the arm laterally—to the level of the deltoid tuberosity. This is especially true with overhead activities. Night pain and the inability to lie on the affected side may be additional complaints, particularly if a rotator cuff tear is present. Ultimately, the patient develops movement compensation patterns that place abnormal stresses on associated structures, leading to symptoms such as scapular and cervical muscle strain. While cervical spine provocative maneuvers such as Spurling's test, are negative[44] (Figure 9.1), a variety of physical examination maneuvers have been developed to diagnose shoulder impingement and are designed to reproduce the patient's symptoms by compressing the rotator cuff under the subacromial arch.[43] The Neer impingement sign and the Hawkins sign are two such tests (Figures 9.2 and 9.3). The Neer impingement sign can be particularly useful as this overhead position is not well tolerated in the patient with impingement syndrome, but may bring relief to the patient with cervical radiculopathy, since this position decreases neural tension. Palpation may elicit tenderness over the rotator cuff tendons or the acromioclavicular joint. This joint can be a source of impingement due to degenerative changes, such as spurring and synovitis. In the presence of a rotator cuff tear, weakness of abduction (supraspinatus) and external rotation (infraspinatus) may be noted. However, other structures innervated by C5 and C6, such as the deltoid and bicep muscles, remain intact. In addition, impingement syndrome is not typically associated with sensory loss or reflex changes that are found in cervical radiculopathy.

A subacromial injection of local anesthetic can implicate or rule out impingement as the cause of the patient's symptoms. Plain radiographs including anteriorposterior, lateral, axillary, and scapular outlet views can be helpful, as are advanced imaging techniques such as magnetic resonance imaging (MRI). Care must be taken in interpreting the MRI scans in the absence of a quality physical examination because the prevalence of abnormal studies in asymptomatic subjects is in the range of 15% to 25% for the cervical spine and from 4% to 54% for rotator cuff tears, depending on the age of the patient.[2,37]

BOX 9.1

Selected conditions of the musculoskeletal system with potential to mimic cervical or lumbar radiculopathy

Upper extremity

Shoulder
- Impingement syndrome
- Rotator cuff tear/tendonitis
- Osteoarthritis (glenohumeral, acromioclavicular)
- Glenoid labral tear, glenoid cyst

Elbow
- Lateral/medial epicondylitis

Wrist/Hand
- DeQuervain's tenosynovitis
- Flexor/extensor tendonitis

Lower extremity

Hip
- Osteoarthritis, avascular necrosis (AVN)
- Greater trochanteric bursitis
- Abductor/adductor/iliopsoas tendonitis
- Acetabular labral tear
- Femoral neck fracture

Knee
- Pes anserine bursitis
- Iliotibial band friction syndrome

Leg/ankle/foot
- Exertional compartment syndrome
- Plantar fasciitis

General
- Polymyalgia rheumatica
- Fibromyalgia
- Myofascial pain syndrome

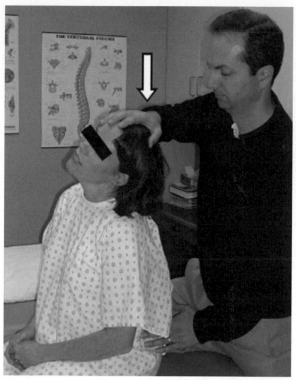

Figure 9.1 Spurling examination. Rotation and lateral flexion to the involved side with mild extension and axial load reproduces upper extremity radicular symptoms.

Glenohumeral Osteoarthritis

Osteoarthritis (OA), also known as degenerative joint disease (DJD) of the glenohumeral (GH) joint is not as common as knee or hip OA but is by no means rare. There are primary (idiopathic) and secondary causes of GH OA. Examples of secondary causes are posttraumatic, infectious, metabolic, and inflammatory. The patient with early GH OA presents with activity-related pain that is relieved by rest. The pain is generally located about the shoulder and there may be mild range of motion (ROM) restrictions. The distribution of pain is similar to that which a patient with a C5 radiculopathy might present. As the disease progresses, pain may persist at rest and night pain may become a complaint. ROM becomes more restricted, particularly external rotation, due to anterior capsular and subscapularis contracture. Motion restrictions will be similar for active and passive ROM. Rotator cuff strength is usually maintained, but may seem limited secondary to pain. Palpation may demonstrate tenderness, especially about the posterior GH joint line and crepitus may be noted with ROM activities. Plain radiographs (anteroposterior[AP], lateral, and axillary views) of the shoulder are usually conclusive in the case of GH OA. Diagnostic intraarticular injections can help differentiate shoulder OA from cervical spine disease.

Hip

The hip joint is the articulation between the head of the femur and the acetabulum. However, when patients refer to the "hip," they may be referring to any number of associated and neighboring structures. Due to the proximity of the hip to the lumbar spine, conditions about the hip are often confused with lumbar spine pathology, particularly radiculopathy. When discussing pathology around the hip, it is sometimes useful to separate the conditions into intraarticular and extraarticular processes. Examples of intraarticular pathology include OA and a torn acetabular labrum whereas extraarticular examples are greater trochanteric bursitis and piriformis syndrome.

Hip Osteoarthritis

OA of the hip, as in the shoulder, can be primary or secondary. It can be unilateral or bilateral. When systemic or inflammatory disease processes are responsible for the condition, involvement is more likely to be bilateral. Primary OA is by far the most common form of hip OA. It increases in frequency with increasing age, although the precise interrelationship between aging and arthritis is not clear. The patient with primary hip arthritis will complain of activity-related pain that is relieved by rest. Those with severe degenerative changes may even have pain at rest. Their ambulation distance will be decreased due to pain and the patient may develop an antalgic gait pattern. As the disease progresses, the patient may complain of difficulty with tasks such as donning shoes and socks due to limitation in hip ROM. As with any intraarticular hip pathology,

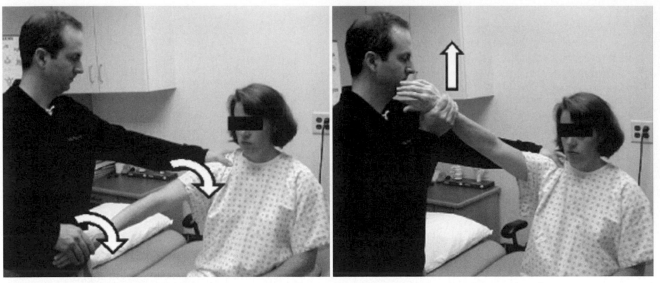

Figure 9.2 Neer's impingement test: causes rotator cuff impingement against the anterior edge of the acromion with shoulder flexion.

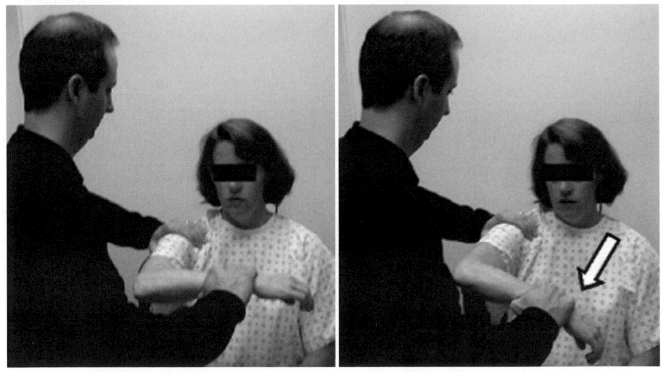

Figure 9.3 Hawkins impingement test: causes rotator cuff impingement against the coracoacromial ligament in this position.

OA causes groin pain that can radiate down the ventromedial thigh to the knee. Secondary involvement of the gluteus musculature and trochanteric bursa due to an altered gait pattern may cause lateral hip and thigh pain as well.

Physical examination may demonstrate gait abnormalities such as a trunk lean over the affected hip during weight bearing (to decrease the abductor moment about the hip). The patient may display apparent and/or true leg length discrepancy due to hip flexor/adductor contractures

and/or hip joint cartilage loss, respectively. There may be weakness of the hip abductors and they may be tender to palpation. ROM tends to be limited, primarily in hip internal rotation. The most provocative maneuver with hip OA is to flex the hip of the supine patient to at least 90 degrees and then apply adduction and internal rotation. In the case of unilateral disease, this motion is restricted and painful on the involved side. Patients with OA of the hip do not typically have sensory or reflex changes as part of their

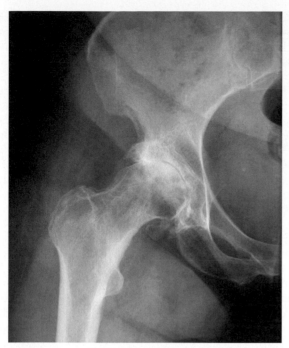

Figure 9.4 Radiograph demonstrating hip osteoarthritis. Note the joint space narrowing, osteophytes, subchondral sclerosis, and subchondral cysts, which are the hallmark signs of osteoarthritis.

clinical picture unless there is coexisting neuropathy or spinal pathology. Uncommonly, a diagnostic, intraarticular hip injection with local anesthetic is required to differentiate hip and spine symptomatology. The standard radiographic work-up for primary hip OA is an AP pelvis radiograph and AP and lateral radiographs of the involved hip. This is usually confirmatory (Figure 9.4).

Greater Trochanteric Pain Syndrome

Greater trochanteric pain syndrome (GTPS) is a term that has been used to describe lateral hip pain of soft tissue origin in the region of the greater trochanter. Trochanteric bursitis is the most common etiology of this syndrome. However, other conditions have been described such as tendonitis or tears of the gluteus medius and iliotibial band (ITB) irritation.[28,46] These conditions are likely related to overuse, abnormal biomechanics, or local trauma. Patients with GTPS complain of pain about the hip laterally that may radiate proximally to the buttock and distally along the lateral aspect of the thigh to the lateral knee. Several lumbar dermatomes share this distribution, allowing GTPS to mimic lumbar radiculopathy. It has been reported that up to 20% to 25% of patients being evaluated for lumbar spine pathology were found to have GTPS as the source of their complaints. In addition, greater trochanteric bursitis has been found in 25% to 35% of patients with low back pain.[28,46]

Physical examination of the patient with GTPS reveals local tenderness to palpation of the involved structure (tendon or bursa). Tenderness may be ventral, dorsal, rostral, or directly over the greater trochanter, depending on the structure involved. Similarly, the patient complains of increased symptoms when sleeping on the involved side

due to direct pressure on the inflamed structures. Resisted hip abduction or external rotation also compresses or stresses the tissues in GTPS, reproducing the patient's symptoms. Once the physical examination has implicated a particular structure but lumbar radiculopathy has not been ruled out, an injection of a local anesthetic can help in the differentiation between local pathology and referred pain. Plain radiographs are useful to help to rule out hip arthritis and other local pathology such as a fracture of the greater trochanter. Often, the patient complains of tenderness upon palpation in this region, even when this is not the presenting complaint. Recognizing the existence of the various conditions under the umbrella of GTPS, coupled with a careful history and physical exam is usually sufficient to differentiate between hip and lumbar spine disease. One must realize, however, that these conditions can coexist.

Sacroiliac Joint

The sacroiliac joint (SIJ) is certainly capable of producing pain locally. SIJ pain is also in the differential diagnosis as an extraspinal cause of low back and lower extremity pain. A variety of pathological processes can affect the SIJ, including sacroiliac joint pain syndrome, osteoarthritis, sacroiliitis (as in ankylosing spondylitis and Reiter's syndrome), septic arthritis, and traumatic SIJ instability or dislocation. Many of these conditions have an obvious history as well as objective radiographic findings, implicating the SIJ as a pain generator. However, in the absence of "hard" findings on examination or radiographs, attributing a patient's pain to the SIJ has in recent decades been met with skepticism due to the controversy over the joint's ability to be a source of pain and the thought that the SIJ did not move in most individuals. Recent injection studies have demonstrated the SIJ to be a potential source of pain in the low back, buttock, and lower extremity and studies involving radiostereometric analyses have shown small but definite motion at the SIJ.[18,40]

Sacroiliac Pain Syndrome

The clinical presentation of the patient with sacroiliac pain syndrome (SIPS) can be highly variable. In patients with a diagnosis of low back pain, the prevalence of this syndrome has been reported to range from 13% to 30%. Injection studies of the SIJs of asymptomatic volunteers produced pain in the low back, posterior superior iliac spine (PSIS) area, buttock, and thigh. Further studies on symptomatic subjects demonstrated that SIJ injection with a local anesthetic relieved a variety of pain patterns including pain in the low back, PSIS region, abdomen, buttock, groin, thigh, leg, and foot.[40] Clearly, SIPS can mimic lumbar spine pathology including discogenic pain and radiculopathy.

The patient with SIPS typically presents with pain in the lateral low back, in the parasacral region with radiation to the buttock and posterolateral proximal thigh. They may complain of tenderness in the area of the sacral sulcus. Some authors have suggested that a painful SIJ can refer pain into the calf and foot, although much less commonly. There are many tests described in the literature to test for

SIJ dysfunction and to review all of these is not within the scope of this chapter. Two categories of SIJ testing include tests designed to stress the SIJ and reproduce the patient's symptoms and those designed to detect abnormal or asymmetrical motion by palpation of certain anatomical landmarks about the pelvis.[8] Some tests used to stress the SIJ include Gaenslen's test, FABER test, and SIJ compression/distraction maneuvers. Motion palpation tests include the standing flexion test and Gillet test. However, the use of the physical examination tests to provoke SIJ pain through manually stressing the joint, to detect motion abnormalities by palpation or to rely on features of the patient history have all correlated poorly with the response of fluoroscopically guided intraarticular SIJ injections.[40] Currently, the diagnostic test of choice for SIPS seems to be a fluoroscopically guided intraarticular SIJ injection of a local anesthetic.

Peripheral Neuropathy

Peripheral neuropathy is one of the more common masqueraders of spinal pathology, particularly radiculopathy and myelopathy. There are many etiologies of peripheral neuropathy including compression or entrapment, metabolic, nutritional, toxic, hereditary, autoimmune, neoplastic, and those associated with neuromuscular disease[4,9,19,22,23,35] (Box 9.2). Even in the face of an extensive work-up, the etiology of peripheral neuropathy is frequently not identified. When this is the case, the initial serological studies should include vitamin B_{12}, folate, hemoglobin A_{1C}, erythrocyte sedimentation rate, and thyroid stimulating hormone. There are certainly many more causes of peripheral neuropathy than are discussed in this section. The list is too exhaustive to review in this chapter. The authors suggest a neurology text for further detail.

Compression Neuropathy

Compression or entrapment neuropathy is a type of mononeuropathy resulting from local compression on a peripheral nerve. One well-known example is carpal tunnel syndrome. Compression neuropathies can present with varying degrees of motor, sensory, and autonomic disturbances and can be confused with myelopathy and radiculopathy. However, a careful history, physical examination, and special studies such as electromyography and nerve conduction velocity (EMG/NCV) help localize the site of compression. Injections of local anesthetics at the suspected site of compression can be performed easily in the office and can often help to differentiate between several diagnoses. There are numerous peripheral nerve compression syndromes of the upper and lower extremities. Therefore, only a select few are discussed in detail with others represented in table format (Tables 9.1 and 9.2).

Upper Extremity Compression Neuropathies

Thoracic Outlet Syndrome. Thoracic outlet syndrome (TOS) is a controversial diagnosis. Some authors even question the existence of this condition. The terminology

describing this entity is confusing, as well. In fact, there are over 10 different terms used to describe this syndrome in the literature.[38] In any event, TOS has persisted as the most widely recognized term for this condition and will therefore be used in the following discussion.

TOS has been divided into two major categories based on clinical presentation: vascular and neurogenic. The vascular syndrome can be further divided into arterial and venous. The neurovascular structures primarily involved in TOS include the subclavian artery and vein and the brachial plexus. The neurogenic form is caused by brachial plexus entrapment. It is the most common type encountered clinically.

Coursing from proximal to distal, the neurovascular bundle first passes between the anterior and middle scalene muscles. This is referred to as the scalene triangle, with the first rib forming the base of the triangle. The subclavian vein is the exception, since it usually passes ventral to the anterior scalene muscle. Next, the neurovascular structures pass through the costoclavicular space, bordered by the clavicle rostrally and the first rib caudally. Finally, the neurovascular bundle passes beneath the coracoid process of the scapula through the subcoracoid space. This space is bordered by the coracoid process rostrally,

---

BOX 9.2

Selected conditions associated with peripheral neuropathy

Metabolic
- Diabetes
- Hypothyroidism
- Uremia
- Combined subacute system degeneration

Nutritional
- Pyridoxine (vitamin B_6), cobalamin (vitamin B_{12}), and vitamin E deficiency
- Alcoholism
- Generalized malnutrition

Toxicity
- Lead
- Mercury
- Isoniazid
- Cisplatin

Infection
- Diphtheria
- Lyme disease
- Herpes zoster

Autoimmune disease
- Rheumatoid arthritis
- Systemic lupus erythematosus
- Polyarteritis nodosa
- Sjögren disease

Neoplastic
- Paraneoplastic syndromes
- Pancoast tumor

Hereditary
- Hereditary sensory-motor neuropathy (Charcot-Marie-Tooth)
- Amyloidosis

Idiopathic
- Brachial neuritis (Parsonage-Turner syndrome)

TABLE 9.1

Compression Syndromes of the Upper Extremity

Compressive Syndrome	Anatomy	Masquerading As...
Thoracic outlet syndrome	Brachial plexus compression at the level of the scalenes, clavicle, first rib, or coracoid process	Cervical radiculopathy, primarily C8, T1
Suprascapular nerve compression	Suprascapular nerve compression at the transverse scapular ligament or at the spinoglenoid notch	C5, (C6) radiculopathy
Carpal tunnel syndrome	Median nerve compression at the wrist	C6 radiculopathy
Pronator syndrome	Median nerve compression about the anteromedial elbow	C6 radiculopathy
Anterior interosseous nerve (AIN) syndrome	AIN compression in the proximal volar forearm	This syndrome not commonly confused with cervical radiculopathy because there are no sensory disturbances, only motor abnormalities (weakness of the flexor digitorum profundus to the index finger, flexor pollicus longus and pronator quadratus)
Cubital tunnel syndrome	Ulnar nerve compression about the medial elbow	C8, T1 radiculopathy
Ulnar tunnel syndrome	Ulnar nerve compression in the canal of Guyon at the wrist	C8, T1 radiculopathy
Wartenberg's syndrome	Superficial radial nerve compression between the brachioradialis and extensor carpi radialis longus in forearm	C6 radiculopathy
Posterior interosseous nerve (PIN) syndrome	PIN compression in the proximal forearm	C6, C7 radiculopathy
Radial tunnel syndrome	Radial nerve compression at or distal to the elbow	C6 radiculopathy

TABLE 9.2

Compression Syndromes of Lower Extremity

Compressive Syndrome	Anatomy	Masquerading As...
Piriformis syndrome	Sciatic nerve compression at the level of the piriformis muscle	S1 radiculopathy
Meralgia paresthetica (lateral femoral cutaneous nerve)	LFCN compression at the level of the inguinal ligament	L2, L3 radiculopathy
Obturator neuropathy	Compression due to many intrapelvic and hip pathologies	L1, L2, L3 radiculopathy
Saphenous neuropathy	Saphenous nerve compression at Hunter's canal or from direct trauma	L4 (L3, L5) radiculopathy
Peroneal neuropathy	Common peroneal nerve compression at the level of the fibular head	L4, L5 radiculopathy
Tarsal tunnel syndrome (tibial nerve)	Tibial nerve compression at the posteromedial ankle	L5, S1 radiculopathy

the scapula dorsally, and the tendon of the pectoralis minor and costocoracoid ligament ventrally.

Etiologies of TOS can be divided into congenital, traumatic, and acquired categories.[38] An example of a congenital anomaly causing TOS is the presence of a cervical rib or fibrous cervical band. The presence of this anomaly causes the neurovascular structures to be stretched and kinked as they are draped over the extra rib or cervical band on their way to the upper extremity. Cervical ribs can be noted on careful inspection of plain radiographs of the cervical spine (Figure 9.5). An unusually large C7 transverse process seen on AP cervical spine radiographs suggests the presence of a cervical band[26] (Figure 9.6). Traumatic factors can also play a role in developing TOS. One example is a clavicle fracture that heals in a mal-reduced position or one that develops a significantly large callus. This can decrease the size of the costoclavicular space, leading to compression of the neurovascular structures. The most common cause of TOS, which falls into the acquired category, is posture related. Upper thoracic and cervical spine posture influences the flexibility and tone of the scalene muscles. Forward shoulder posture with scapular depression narrows the costoclavicular space and causes adaptive shortening of the pectoralis minor muscle and the costocoracoid ligament.

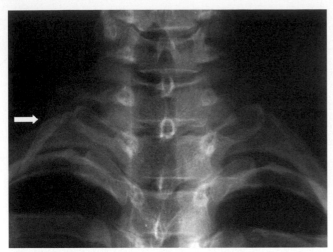

Figure 9.5 Anteroposterior cervical spine radiograph demonstrating a unilateral cervical rib *(arrow)*.

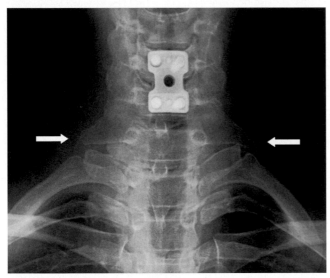

Figure 9.6 Anteroposterior cervical spine radiograph demonstrating large C7 transverse processes *(arrows)*. In the right clinical setting, this may suggest the presence of cervical fibrous bands. This patient underwent C5-6 anterior cervical discectomy and fusion and bilateral carpal tunnel releases without resolution of her bilateral upper extremity paresthesias. Her symptoms finally resolved after surgical release of left and right fibrous cervical bands.

Signs and symptoms in the patient with TOS include pain, paraesthesias, motor weakness, and autonomic disturbances in the involved upper extremity. Pain can be reported from the supraclavicular and periscapular regions down the arm to the fingers, and not necessarily in a dermatomal pattern. Paresthesias including tingling or numbness may be more often described in the C8-T1 distribution. Motor deficits may be noted in the hand, particularly the intrinsic muscles. Even without objective weakness or visible atrophy, the patient may complain of hand weakness and poor dexterity. Chronic cases of TOS have been known to cause trophic changes in the hand. Vasomotor signs and symptoms, including periodic pallor

or cyanosis, may indicate involvement of the sympathetic fibers or vascular compression.[38]

Many cases of TOS are diagnoses of exclusion. However, once other diagnoses have been ruled out and TOS is being considered, there are several physical examination maneuvers to assist in establishing the diagnosis. Unfortunately, none of these tests are specific or sensitive. They, however, are used together along with clinical judgment and other tests (radiographs, EMG/NCV) to rule out related pathology. The physical examination maneuvers are designed to reproduce the patient's symptoms by compressing the brachial plexus at various points. Adson's maneuver is probably the most recognized physical examination method of testing for TOS. With the patient standing or seated, the examiner locates the radial pulse and then extends, externally rotates, and slightly abducts the shoulder while keeping the elbow straight. The patient is then instructed to rotate the cervical spine toward (or away from) the test extremity, then take a deep breath in and hold it. Disappearance of the pulse indicates a positive test, as does the reproduction of paresthesias. Unfortunately, some individuals with no symptoms will lose their pulse with this maneuver, so interpretation of this test must be made in the context of the entire clinical picture. Additional tests for TOS include the Roos test, the Wright test, and the costoclavicular syndrome test. Finally, tapping or gently applying pressure to the supraclavicular fossa may reproduce the patient's upper extremity paresthesias. Eliciting a positive Tinel's in this manner is consistent with TOS.

Median Neuropathy. The most common peripheral neuropathy of the upper extremity is compression of the median nerve at the level of the wrist, known as carpal tunnel syndrome. The median nerve is formed by the lateral and medial cords of the brachial plexus and therefore carries fibers from C5, C6, C7, C8, and T1. The carpal tunnel is a fibro-osseous channel containing nine flexor tendons and the median nerve. The causes of carpal tunnel syndrome are too numerous to mention, but can be divided into two major categories: those conditions that decrease the size of the carpal tunnel such as distal radius fracture, and those that take up space in the tunnel such as flexor tenosynovitis and ganglion cysts. Additional median nerve compression neuropathies that occur about the elbow and proximal forearm include the pronator syndrome and the anterior interosseous syndrome (see Table 9.1).

Carpal Tunnel Syndrome. The clinical picture of CTS includes pain and paresthesias in the palmar-radial aspect of the hand, often worse at night and aggravated by repetitive use of the hand. Occupational and recreational risk factors should be elicited in the history, including vibration exposure and repetitive use of the hands and wrists. The most common pattern of median nerve sensory distribution in the hand is shown in Figure 9.7A compared with the typical C6 and C7 dermatomes (Figure 9.7B). EMG/NCV testing can help delineate anomalies such as Martin-Gruber anastomosis. The physical examination may demonstrate decreased sensation in the median nerve distribution, particularly

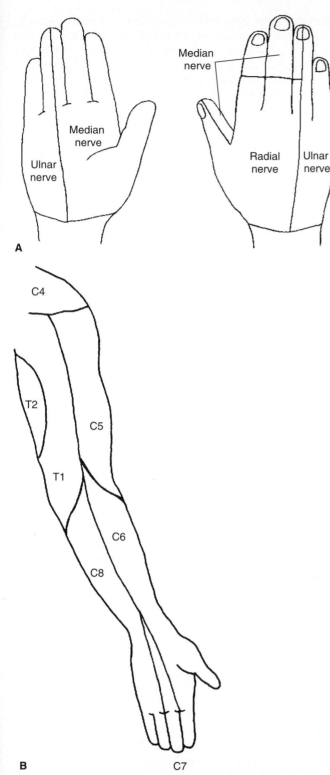

Figure 9.7 A representation of peripheral nerve sensory distribution (**A**) versus dermatomal distribution (**B**) for the upper extremity.

formed test. The examiner uses a finger to lightly tap over the carpal tunnel in an effort to reproduce paresthesias in the median nerve distribution, indicating a positive test (sensitivity 0.60, specificity 0.67). The tapping should be performed from the wrist to the proximal forearm to rule out more proximal sites of median nerve compression. Phalen's test requires maintaining the wrist flexed to 90 degrees. Numbness and tingling in the median nerve distribution within 60 seconds is considered a positive test (sensitivity 0.75, specificity 0.47). The carpal compression test is performed when the examiner applies direct pressure over the median nerve at the wrist. Paresthesias within 30 seconds is considered a positive response (sensitivity 0.87, specificity 0.90).[42]

When the diagnosis of carpal tunnel syndrome is suspected, cervical radiculopathy (C6) and proximal median nerve compression should be ruled out. Cervical (C6) radiculopathy can be placed higher or lower on the differential diagnosis list by a careful examination of hand and forearm sensation, wrist extensor strength, deep tendon reflexes (brachioradialis), Spurling test, and cervical spine ROM. Certainly cervical radiculopathy and carpal tunnel syndrome can coexist, making EMG/NCV testing an invaluable part of the work-up. When a patient presents with signs and symptoms of bilateral carpal tunnel syndrome, systemic and metabolic etiologies such as hypothyroidism, diabetes, and amyloidosis (to mention a few) should be considered.

Ulnar Neuropathy. The ulnar nerve is prone to compression at several sites in the upper extremity and can mimic lower cervical spine radiculopathy. The ulnar nerve is a terminal branch of the medial cord of the brachial plexus and usually carries spinal levels C8 and T1. The most common site of ulnar nerve compression in the upper extremity is at the dorsomedial elbow, referred to as cubital tunnel syndrome. Cubital tunnel syndrome can be caused by fascial and anomalous muscle tissue, various soft tissues such as tumors and ganglion cysts, subluxating ulnar nerve, bone spurs, and cubitus valgus deformity. The ulnar nerve can also be compressed in the canal of Guyon at the wrist, a condition called ulnar tunnel syndrome. The canal of Guyon is a fibro-osseous tunnel where the ulnar nerve and artery pass from the forearm into the hand. Several of the more common pathologies implicated are ganglion cysts, ulnar artery aneurysm (or thrombosis), and fractures of the hook of the hamate.[42]

Cubital Tunnel Syndrome. The patient with cubital tunnel syndrome complains of numbness and/or paresthesias in the ulnar side of the hand. There will also be numbness in the distribution of the dorsal sensory branch of the ulnar nerve but a lack of sensory disturbance in the medial forearm, which is supplied by the C8 dermatome (see Figure 9.7B). This helps differentiate cubital tunnel syndrome from cervical radiculopathy. The patient may also complain of worsening symptoms when the elbow is in a flexed position for a prolonged period, such as when driving or sleeping. This is due to increased intraneural pressure and decreased cubital tunnel space with elbow flexion or from subluxation of the ulnar nerve over the medial epicondyle as the elbow is flexed. Tapping over

with threshold testing using Semmes-Weinstein monofilament. A late finding may be thenar muscle atrophy and weakness, particularly of the abductor pollicis brevis. Additional physical examination maneuvers are directed at reproducing the patient's hand paresthesias. Tinel's percussion test is probably the most commonly per-the cubital tunnel (Tinel's sign) can often reproduce the patient's paresthesias. In addition to sensory changes, there may also be interosseous wasting and related weakness, which is usually a late finding. The more common sites of ulnar nerve compression about the elbow, from proximal to distal are: Arcade of Struthers, medial intermuscular septum, medial epicondyle, cubital tunnel, and proximal edge of the pronator aponeurosis. A careful physical examination can usually differentiate cervical radiculopathy from cubital tunnel syndrome. EMG/NCV can confirm the level of compression and plain radiographs of the elbow can rule out bony pathology as a source of compression.[42]

Radial Neuropathy. The radial nerve has several regions of potential compression in the upper extremity, rarely proximal to the elbow and more commonly in the forearm. The radial nerve carries fibers from C5, C6, C7, C8 and inconsistently T1 and is one of the terminal branches of the posterior cord. Syndromes involving compression of the radial nerve include radial tunnel syndrome, Wartenberg's syndrome, and posterior interosseous nerve (PIN) compression syndrome. These are compression neuropathies of the forearm and can usually but not always be differentiated based on patient complaints and careful physical examination. Radial neuropathy is most likely to be confused with a C6 or C7 radiculopathy (see Figure 9.7).

Lower Extremity Compression Neuropathies

Piriformis Syndrome. Piriformis syndrome refers to entrapment of the sciatic nerve as it passes beneath or through the piriformis muscle, causing pain along the distribution of the sciatic nerve (buttock, dorsal thigh, and dorsal leg). This distribution is also a common source of pain in a patient with lower lumbar intervertebral disc herniation, thereby causing a diagnostic dilemma. The piriformis syndrome is a controversial diagnosis such that some authors deny its existence; others feel it should be a diagnosis of exclusion, while others consider it a primary diagnostic entity.[12] The sciatic nerve is the largest nerve in the body and is actually composed of two nerves: the common peroneal and the tibial nerves. The peroneal portion arises from the ventral rami of spinal levels L4-S2 where the tibial portion arises from the ventral rami of L4-S3. The sciatic nerve exits the pelvis, coursing through the greater sciatic foramen, usually caudal to the piriformis muscle; however, great variability exists in the relationship between the piriformis muscle and the sciatic nerve. The sciatic nerve exits the pelvis caudal to the piriformis approximately 85% of the time. The peroneal portion passes through while the tibial portion passes caudal to the piriformis muscle about 12% of the time and the peroneal portion travels rostral to the piriformis muscle with the tibial portion caudal to the piriformis muscle in about 3% of cases. Additional variations in this relationship have been described as well.

There are many reported etiologic factors associated with sciatic nerve compression at the level of the piriformis muscle. As mentioned, anatomic anomalies altering the relationship between the piriformis muscle and the sciatic nerve may increase the potential for nerve entrapment.[36] Abnormal mechanics about the lumbar spine,

pelvis, and hips has also been implicated in piriformis syndrome due to chronic stretching of the piriformis muscle or chronic overuse of the muscle, both of which can increase compression of the nerve. Patients' symptoms can be intermittent and dynamic, precipitated by particular activities and positions.[34]

The patient with piriformis syndrome will usually complain of unilateral buttock, posterior thigh, and trochanteric pain. The pain will occasionally refer distal to the knee. Physical examination may demonstrate an antalgic gait and the affected side may be held in an elevated and externally rotated position, a so-called positive piriformis sign. Palpation of the piriformis region may elicit tenderness and may precipitate pain in the distribution of the sciatic nerve. The patient with piriformis syndrome may also have a positive straight-leg raising test or worsening of their symptoms as the piriformis muscle is stretched with hip adduction and internal rotation. In fact, Freiburg's sign is manifested by reproduction of the patient's pain upon forced internal rotation of the hip. Resisting hip abduction and external rotation while the patient is in the seated position, known as Pace's sign, may also reproduce symptoms in the patient with piriformis syndrome. Most patients with piriformis syndrome will be diagnosed on physical examination, with or without the use of a diagnostic injection. The role of imaging studies in the work-up of piriformis syndrome seems to be most important for ruling out other causes of "sciatica-type" pain. Special testing such as EMG/NCV may demonstrate abnormalities in the patient with piriformis syndrome, but negative electrical studies do not rule out the condition.

Meralgia Paresthetica. Meralgia paresthetica is a term used to describe pain, paresthesias, and/or numbness in the ventrolateral thigh due to neuropathy of the lateral femoral cutaneous nerve (LFCN) and is also referred to as Bernhardt disease. The term *meralgia* comes from the two Greek words, *meros* (thigh) and *algos* (pain). The LFCN typically originates from the dorsal branches of the ventral rami of L2, L3, and occasionally L1 and therefore has the ability to mimic lumbar radiculopathy. The most common site of entrapment is thought to be the site at which the nerve passes above, below, or through the inguinal ligament just medial to the anterior superior iliac spine (ASIS). There is considerable anatomic variation as the nerve courses past the inguinal ligament from the pelvis to the thigh.[16]

Some authors have divided the etiology of meralgia paresthetica into spontaneous and iatrogenic forms, but this section will discuss only the spontaneous etiologies. Most noniatrogenic causes of LFCN neuropathies are either mechanical compression or metabolic neuropathy. Mechanical compression can be from external causes such as obesity and pregnancy due to increased intraabdominal pressure and direct compression at the level of the inguinal ligament, as well as from wearing tight, low-lying pants or belts. Compression can also come from within by way of intraabdominal and intrapelvic tumors, for example. The LFCN bypasses many potentially entrapping structures prior to reaching the level of the inguinal ligament. Several metabolic conditions, including diabetes mellitus and alcoholism, can be causative or at least associated with neuropathy of the LFCN.

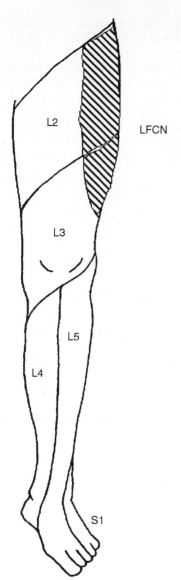

Figure 9.8 A representation of lower extremity dermatomal sensory patterns of innervation versus that of the lateral femoral cutaneous nerve (LFCN, *shaded region*).

ropathies, injection of a local anesthetic at the site of compression can be used as a diagnostic test.

Metabolic Neuropathy

Diabetic Neuropathy

The patient with diabetes mellitus may present with a wide variety of signs and symptoms with respect to peripheral neuropathy as their disease process can affect sensory, motor, and autonomic fibers. Although the causative factors for neuropathy in diabetics are multiple and complex, several studies support hyperglycemia as having an important role in the development of neuropathy.[3] Classifying neuropathy in diabetes is difficult. However, one simple classification distinguishes between mononeuropathy (isolated or multiple) and polyneuropathy. This section discusses the three most common presentations: sensory mononeuropathy, proximal motor neuropathy, and distal sensory neuropathy.

In the mononeuropathy category, there are several common peripheral compression neuropathies that the patient with diabetes is at greater risk of developing more frequently than the nondiabetic patient. Some examples are carpal tunnel syndrome, cubital tunnel syndrome, meralgia paresthetica, and peroneal neuropathy near the head of the fibula. Additionally, the patient with diabetes (and other endocrinopathies) may present more commonly with bilateral symptoms due to the systemic nature of the neuropathy. These sensory mononeuropathies are not limited to the periphery, as the patient with diabetes can suffer from truncal neuropathy. The patient describes pain and paresthesias in a band-like distribution about the chest and abdomen. As far as the spine specialist is concerned, these neuropathies can certainly mimic extremity and truncal radiculopathy.

Proximal motor neuropathy (also known as diabetic amyotrophy or diabetic polyradiculopathy) is another clinical presentation in the diabetic patient, typically in the older patient with type II diabetes. Presenting signs and symptoms include pain, weakness and atrophy of the proximal lower extremity musculature.[28] It can present unilaterally or bilaterally, with bilateral findings being asymmetrical. These clinical findings can be similar to those found in the patient with lumbar spinal stenosis and coexisting pathology makes diagnosis and treatment more difficult.

The most common neuropathy found in the diabetic population is the distal sensory neuropathy. These patients can present with a wide variety of symptoms ranging from significant burning pain, paresthesias, and numbness to an insensate foot with Charcot arthropathy. Distal sensory neuropathy usually develops gradually. However, there is an acute form that may develop during a period of poor glycemic control. The legs and feet are commonly involved in a stocking-like distribution and less commonly the hands are affected in a glove-like distribution. Proprioception may also be impaired, as the patient may complain of progressively worsening balance with increasing falls as well as demonstrating increased sway with Romberg testing.[3] Many of these signs and symptoms overlap with those of spinal stenosis.

The patient with meralgia paresthetica complains of pain, burning, paresthesias, numbness, or hypersensitivity in the distribution of the LFCN, which overlaps the dermatomal distribution supplied by L2 and L3 (Figure 9.8). The LFCN carries only sensory fibers. Therefore weakness on examination should raise suspicion of conditions other than meralgia paresthetica to explain the patient's symptoms.[11] Physical examination may demonstrate decreased sensation in the LFCN distribution, which is different than the true L2 or L3 dermatome distribution. Extending the hip, which places the nerve under tension, increases intraneural pressure and exacerbates the compressive pathology; this maneuver may reproduce the patients' paresthesias and pain. Additionally, palpation or Tinel's percussion about the site of compression may also reproduce their symptoms. If the history and physical examination are equivocal, electrodiagnostic testing can be helpful and as with most peripheral compression neu-

9.3

Visceral organ conditions known to mimic spine pathology

Cardiovascular
- Myocardial ischemia
- Aortic aneurysm
- Vascular claudication
- Infectious endocarditis

Pulmonary
- Pancoast tumor
- Lung carcinoma with paraneoplastic syndromes (peripheral neuropathy)

Gastrointestinal
- Peptic ulcer disease
- Cholecystitis
- Pancreatic disease (pancreatitis, carcinoma)
- Colon disease, carcinoma (lumbosacral radiculopathy)

Genitourinary
- Urolithiasis
- Pyelonephritis, polycystic kidney disease, renal infarct
- Prostate disease
- Malignancy

Gynecological
- Ovarian cyst
- Endometriosis
- Uterine malpositioning
- Carcinoma

Visceral Organs and Related Systems

The visceral organs of the thoracic, abdominal, and pelvic cavities are associated with pathological conditions that may present with signs and symptoms that can be confused with spine pathology (Box 9.3). The mechanism responsible for this is generally thought to be through a referred pain mechanism. Although the majority of patients with these conditions have signs and symptoms related to the organ system involved, back pain or radiculopathy could be the sole presenting complaint. This section discusses the cardiovascular, pulmonary, gastrointestinal, genitourinary, and gynecological systems.

Cardiovascular System

Myocardial Ischemia

Cardiac ischemia can present with multiple signs and symptoms, occurring either together or in isolation. Ischemic heart disease can present with any combination of the following signs and symptoms: retrosternal pain; pressure, tightness or burning; nausea; diaphoresis; epigastric discomfort; pain and numbness in the shoulder, arm, or hand; and interscapular, neck, jaw, or face pain. Many of these signs and symptoms are referred to as angina "equivalents."[45] In fact, there are several case reports of patients presenting to their dentist with complaints of jaw or tooth pain, ultimately discovered to be of cardiac origin.

Of particular interest to the spine surgeon is the upper extremity and interscapular back pain that can be of cardiac origin. The prevalence of arm pain or numbness

has been reported as high as 46% to 67% and back pain approximately 6% in patients with myocardial ischemia.[13,14] When arm pain does occur due to cardiac ischemia, it is more common on the left and typically refers to the shoulder, medial arm, and forearm. An additional useful aspect of the patient's history is that the symptoms are exertional. Fortunately, the majority of patients with ischemic heart disease have more than just arm pain and an appropriate history and review of systems (ROS) will help lead to the correct diagnosis.

Abdominal Aortic Aneurysm

The patient with abdominal aortic aneurysm (AAA) can present with back pain. AAA may be asymptomatic and studies have indicated the prevalence of asymptomatic AAAs (>3 cm) is 3% to 10% in patients over 50 years of age in the western world, with an increasing incidence partly related to an aging population and improved detection methods.[5] When symptoms are present, this is likely related to aneurysm leaking, rupture or acute expansion. Most AAAs rupture dorsally, where the retroperitoneal space provides a tamponade effect to slow or contain the hemorrhage, which can produce chronic low back pain. When they rupture ventrally, the peritoneal cavity provides little tamponade, resulting in significant hemorrhage and acute patient deterioration. The classic triad of abdominal or back pain, pulsatile abdominal mass and hypotension is present in only about 25% of cases with confirmed AAA rupture.[27] AAAs will increase in diameter approximately 0.2 to 0.5 cm per year on average.[32]

The most common complaint is an acute onset of abdominal or back pain, which may radiate to the groin or flank. Other symptoms include those related to aneurysm compression of neighboring structures. Duodenal compression can lead to nausea and vomiting and compression of the ureter(s) may cause hydronephrosis and urinary tract symptoms. Dorsal aneurysm expansion can erode adjacent vertebral bodies, causing back pain. Additionally, aortic aneurysms may compromise blood flow to the spinal cord by aneurysm location and/or thrombus formation. These patients can present with back pain, radicular complaints, and varying degrees of myelopathy or paralysis from spinal cord ischemia.[24] Even in the absence of bony erosion and spinal cord ischemia, AAA can cause chronic back pain that is quite vague.

Diagnosing an asymptomatic AAA on physical examination is difficult. Variables making this difficult include the skill and experience of the examiner, size of the patient, size of the aneurysm, and whether the examination is focused or not. Diagnosing symptomatic AAA can also be difficult. In a study looking specifically at misdiagnoses of ruptured AAAs, 30% were initially misdiagnosed. Misdiagnoses included renal colic, diverticulitis, gastrointestinal hemorrhage, myocardial infarction, and idiopathic back pain. Fifty-four percent of the patients complained of back pain and it was the second most common complaint after abdominal pain.[27]

Since physical examination for diagnosing AAA is not reliable, imaging becomes crucial. Ultrasound, CT, and MRI are all useful in certain situations, but CT is the most utilized because of its rapidity, availability, cost, and ability to provide detail for surgical planning. Plain radi-

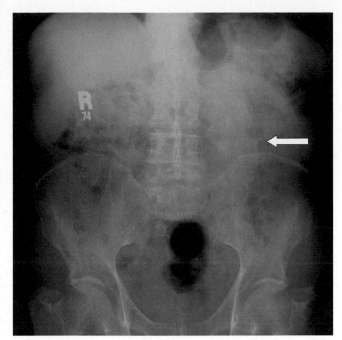

Figure 9.9 Anteroposterior lumbar spine radiograph demonstrating lumbar spondylosis as well as an abdominal aortic aneurysm. Note the enlarged calcified aortic wall. This patient had a 3-month history of low back pain prior to presentation. Vascular surgery consultation resulted in an aortic grafting procedure.

ographs occasionally demonstrate an AAA (Figure 9.9). The calcified aneurysmal vessel wall may be seen as well as softer signs such as loss of the psoas or kidney shadow. If an AAA is discovered or suspected, a prompt vascular surgery consult is in order. Aneurysms less than 5 cm in diameter can be followed with ultrasound every 4 to 6 months with a risk of rupture ranging from 0% in 5 years to 6% per year. In aneurysms greater than 5 cm, the risk of rupture is approximately 25% at 5 years.[32]

Vascular Claudication

Intermittent vascular claudication is a disease of the cardiovascular system that must be distinguished from neurogenic claudication due to central spinal stenosis and is a symptom of chronic arterial insufficiency. Chronic arterial insufficiency can be categorized into two major groups: (1) aortoiliac disease affecting the distal aorta and iliac arteries or (2) femoral-popliteal-tibial disease affecting the arteries of the leg. Chronic arterial insufficiency of the lower extremities may have two distinct presentations: intermittent claudication and ischemic rest pain. Ischemic rest pain is typically nocturnal, diffusely involving the forefoot. In this case, the patient soon learns that the pain is relieved through dependency (effect of gravity on perfusion pressure) of the involved limb and sleeps with the involved foot in a dependent position.

The more common condition mimicking spine pathology is intermittent vascular claudication. These patients can present with buttock, thigh, calf, and/or foot claudication, depending on the site of the occlusion. Calf claudication is the most common presentation. Like any of the lower extremity vascular claudication symptoms, they are reliably reproduced after a certain amount of exercise or ambulation distance and are relieved after a few minutes of rest. This is also seen in spinal stenosis with neurogenic claudication symptoms. However, there are signs and symptoms that are useful in differentiating these two conditions.

Generally, either disease can present with a variety of lower extremity complaints, including numbness, weakness, cramping sensation, pain and, a feeling of tiredness in the legs. In the case of foraminal stenosis, the findings may include a dermatomal distribution of sensory changes and a myotomal pattern of weakness. Numbness is a common complaint in either condition. A complaint of weakness in arterial insufficiency is typically a sense of hip and thigh weakness, especially with proximal occlusion. Cramping in the calves is a classic complaint of vascular insufficiency but will present in either disease as will the vague complaint of lower extremity fatigability and tiredness with ambulation. The lower extremity symptoms caused by arterial insufficiency are relieved with rest (stopping ambulation) whether standing or sitting. That is to say, a change in patients' spine posture does not affect their symptoms. In patients with spinal stenosis, standing itself may produce symptoms and sitting (lumbar spine flexion) relieves the symptoms.[21] Some patients with neurogenic claudication volunteer that they can walk further when shopping and leaning on a cart. This position allows the lumbar spine to flex, which will increase the dimensions of the spinal canal and intervertebral foramen, thereby relieving neural element compression. When impotence is a complaint, it is commonly associated with buttock and thigh claudication as a result of aortoiliac insufficiency.

In addition to presenting symptoms, there are some physical examination findings unique to each condition. In neurogenic claudication, the involved spinal levels may correspond to diminished deep tendon reflexes and positive nerve root tension tests. Physical examination maneuvers associated with lumbar spinal stenosis include a wide-based gait, abnormal Romberg test, thigh pain after 30 seconds of lumbar extension, and neuromuscular deficits.[21] Intermittent vascular claudication may present with diminished pulses (femoral, popliteal, dorsalis pedis, and posterior tibial) and bruits. Ankle-brachial indices (ABI) will also be diminished. Normal ABI is 1 while vascular "claudicators" have an ABI between 0.6 and 0.9. An ABI less than 0.5 may be associated with rest pain and ulceration. Realize that the calcified vessels in the patient with diabetes yield a falsely elevated ABI. In those patients with vascular claudication, there may also be trophic changes in the feet and distal legs (thin, shiny, atrophic skin, thickened and ridged nails and loss of hair) and they may feel cool. One may also find that elevating the limb produces pallor (cadaveric) of the foot and a dusky rubor when placing the foot in the dependent position (Buerger's sign). Finally, the van Gelderen bicycle test can help differentiate vascular and neurogenic claudication.[15] Exercising on a stationary bike should reproduce the symptoms of vascular disease more rapidly and reliably because the disease is one of ischemia, so the type of exercise (walking or cycling) should not matter. However, in spinal stenosis, sitting or positions of lumbar spine flexion (as on a stationary bike) often relieves the lower extremity symptoms and therefore patients with spinal stenosis will be able to ride a stationary bike without necessarily reproducing their symptoms. Certainly, a patient can have both spinal stenosis and arterial occlusive disease; therefore, consultation with a vascular surgeon may be warranted in this situation.

Infective (Bacterial) Endocarditis

The term infective endocarditis (IE) is used to describe an infection of the endocardial surface of a heart valve. The clinical picture of IE can be extremely varied and of all the potential presenting symptoms, musculoskeletal complaints are frequent and often the initial complaint.[6,17,30] Several series have reported that greater than 40% of patients with IE will manifest musculoskeletal signs and symptoms, and as many as 25% of patients will have musculoskeletal complaints as the initial symptom.[6] Of particular interest to the spine specialist are the complaints of neck and back pain and lower extremity myalgias in the thighs and calves. As many as 5% to 20% of patients with IE will have back pain as their presenting symptom and this may be the only complaint for several months, delaying the correct diagnosis. Lower extremity myalgias, while not radicular in distribution, may be severe enough to make the clinician consider radiculopathy in the differential diagnosis, particularly when accompanied by back pain.[17]

The low back pain associated with IE can be quite severe and can present with paraspinal tenderness, muscle spasm, and decreased ROM. The pain may be accentuated by straight leg raising and Valsalva maneuvers, and may be accompanied by lower extremity myalgias, all suggesting a herniated lumbar intervertebral disc.[6] Generally, in the patient with complaints of back pain, they are unable to obtain positional relief. Some patients with low back pain and IE will have a disc space infection or vertebral osteomyelitis; however, the majority of the musculoskeletal manifestations are thought to be related to arterial emboli containing bacteria and immune complexes causing a vasculitic reaction. It has also been suggested that the low back pain in some patients may be a nonspecific manifestation of the infection. Other common symptoms of IE include fever, chills, weakness, anorexia, and headache. Additional signs include heart murmur (changing or new) and dermatological manifestations such as splinter hemorrhages and petechiae.

Pulmonary System

Pancoast Tumor

The most significant pulmonary condition to present with signs and symptoms seemingly of spinal origin is a tumor at the superior pulmonary sulcus (Pancoast tumor). This region lies in close proximity to the C8 and T1 nerve roots and the lower trunk of the brachial plexus, making cervical radiculopathy as well as peripheral neuropathy high on the differential diagnosis in the patient with a Pancoast tumor. There are several signs and symptoms that can help raise suspicion of a superior sulcus tumor. First, the majority of patients with a Pancoast tumor are smokers. Unfortunately, respiratory

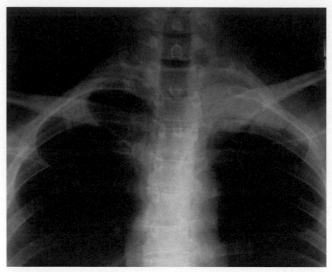

Figure 9.10 Anteroposterior chest radiograph demonstrating left upper lobe opacity: an expected appearance with a Pancoast tumor.

symptoms rarely dominate the initial clinical picture. One of the first and most significant symptoms is shoulder pain and this will be the presenting symptom in greater than 90% of patients.[48] The lower trunk of the brachial plexus, the subclavian artery and vein, and the sympathetic chain and stellate ganglia are a few of the important structures in close proximity to the superior pulmonary sulcus that help explain some of the signs and symptoms in these patients. In addition to shoulder pain and lower plexus neuropathy, other findings include Horner's syndrome, supraclavicular fullness, upper extremity swelling or discoloration, and hand intrinsic wasting. Many authors state Pancoast tumor should be in the differential diagnosis whenever lower brachial plexopathy exists, and some include this in their differential even with C8 and T1 radiculopathy. If the diagnosis of Pancoast tumor is entertained, chest-imaging beginning with routine chest radiographs, including an apical lordotic view, remains a crucial step in the work-up (Figures 9.10 through 9.13). Unfortunately, the average lag time between the onset of symptoms and definitive diagnosis is 7 to 7.5 months.[48]

Gastrointestinal System

Although not common, patients with gastrointestinal (GI) pathology present with pain referred to the spine. Pathology of the stomach/small intestine (ulcer disease), gall bladder, pancreas, and large intestine can all mimic spine pathology.[1] Peptic ulcer disease, cholecystitis, and pancreatic conditions can all refer pain to the mid-back region while diseases of the colon can refer pain to the back or can cause compression on the lumbosacral plexus, mimicking lumbar radiculopathy.* Although there are usually signs or symptoms related to the primary structure involved, there are occasions when back pain or radiculopathy will be the presenting symptom.

---

*References 1,7,20,29,31,41,49.

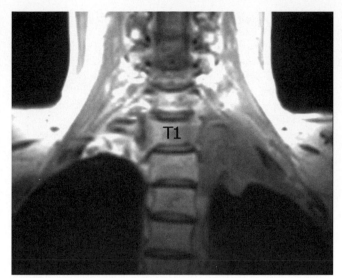

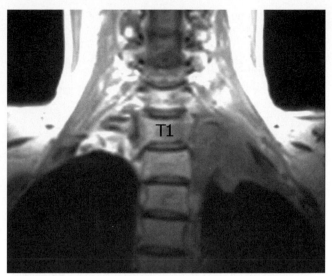

Figure 9.11 Magnetic resonance image: coronal image of the patient in Figure 9.10. Note the left upper lobe tumor encroaching upon the lower portion of the brachial plexus. When upper extremity paresthesias continued after cervical spine surgery, additional work-up revealed the Pancoast tumor.

Figure 9.13. MRI scan: coronal image of the patient in Figures 9.10, 9.11, and 9.12. Note the left upper lobe tumor, encroaching upon the lower trunks of the brachial plexus. When upper extremity paresthesias continued after spine procedures, additional work-up revealed the Pancoast tumor.

Genitourinary System

The kidneys, ureters, and bladder can be a source of referred pain to the abdomen, flank, back, and groin and can therefore mimic spine disease.[1,33] Several conditions known to cause either flank, back, or groin pain include urolithiasis, pyelonephritis, and neoplasm. Disease of the prostate has also been associated with low back pain. As with most organ systems, these conditions will usually have presenting complaints other than referred pain such as abdominal pain, abdominal mass, dysuria, hematuria, nausea, and/or fever, depending on the underlying process.

Urolithiasis (Kidney Stones)

Urolithiasis is a condition describing the presence of calculi within the urinary system. This condition will affect 2% to 5% of the population in their lifetime with males being affected more often than females. Depending on the location of the calculi in the urinary system, the patient may complain of dermatomal pain about the thoracolumbar region, flank and back pain, or groin pain. Kidney pain of visceral origin follows a dermatomal pattern from T10 to L1 and tends to be dull and poorly localized because it is mediated by slow C-type fibers. Parietal pain is usually located adjacent to the affected organ, so in the case of kidney pathology the pain will be located about the flank and back with the presence of costovertebral angle tenderness. This pain is usually sharp and well localized. Pain originating from the ureters may refer to the low back and groin.[33] The onset of pain in the patient with urolithiasis is usually sudden and is not mechanical, that is, they cannot find a comfortable position. There may be urinary symptoms such as urgency, frequency, and dysuria and signs such as hematuria (most if not all will have at least microhematuria).[1] Plain radiographs such as kidney, ureter, and bladder (KUB) may demonstrate calculi but intravenous

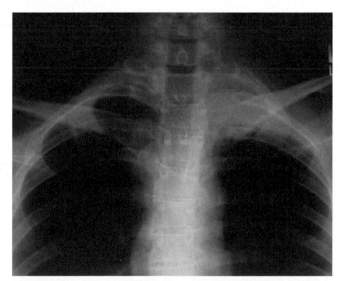

Figure 9.12. Anteroposterior chest radiograph demonstrating left upper lobe opacity: an expected appearance with a Pancoast tumor.

The patient with peptic ulcer disease (PUD) and biliary colic due to cholelithiasis may present with back pain, from the interscapular to the thoracolumbar region. In fact, a German gastroenterologist named Ismar Boas (1858-1938) described a tender spot (Boas' point) to the left of the T12 vertebrae dorsally in patients with gastric ulcer disease. The literature reflects this with cases of patients being treated for musculoskeletal thoracic spine problems only to have resolution of their pain after diagnosis and treatment for PUD. In patients with cholelithiasis and biliary colic, one half complain of periscapular back pain. Often, these patients will complain of intermittent abdominal pain and nausea and may have a positive Murphy's sign.[20]

pyelogram and ultrasound are two of the more reliable studies in detecting calculi.

Gynecological System

Although the pelvic organs are an infrequent cause of low back pain, various pathological conditions of the ovaries, fallopian tubes, and uterus have been associated with low back and sacral pain.[1,29] Conditions that involve the uterosacral ligament are thought to be an important source of low back pain. This can occur due to ligament strain from a malpositioned uterus or from carcinoma invading the ligament. Menstrual pain may be felt in the sacral region as a dull, cramping, poorly localized pain and may radiate into the lower extremities.[10] In this case, the pain has a temporal relationship with the menstrual cycle.

Summary

The evaluation of a patient with neck or back pain, radiculopathy, or myelopathy usually reveals a spinal source to explain their complaints. It is not rare, however, to have their symptoms stemming from a condition unrelated to the spine. This chapter is not intended to be all-inclusive, but hopefully it will serve as an initial source of information and as a reminder that not all patients present the same and that there are many masqueraders of spine disease.

REFERENCES

1. Borenstein DG, Wiesel SW, Boden SD (eds): *Low Back Pain: Medical Diagnosis and Comprehensive Management*. Philadelphia, WB Saunders, 1995.
2. Boden SD, McCowin PR, Davis DO, *et al:* Abnormal magnetic resonance scans of the cervical spine in asymptomatic subjects: a prospective investigation. *J Bone Joint Surg Am* 72A:1178-1184, 1990.
3. Boulton AJM, Malik RA: Diabetes mellitus: neuropathy. In DeGroot LJ and Jameson JL (eds): *Endocrinology*, ed 4. Philadelphia, WB Saunders, 2001, pp 868-876.
4. Busis NA: Femoral and obturator neuropathies. *Neurol Clin* 17(3):633-653, 1999.
5. Cronenwett JL, Krupski WC, Rutherford RB: Abdominal aortic and iliac aneurysms. In Rutherford RB (ed): *Vascular Surgery*, ed 5. Philadelphia, WB Saunders, 2000, pp 1246-1280.
6. Churchill MA, Geraci JE, Hunder GG: Musculoskeletal manifestations of bacterial endocarditis. *Ann Intern Med* 87:754-759, 1977.
7. Doran FSA: The sites to which pain is referred from the common bile-duct in man and its implication for the theory of referred pain. *Br J Surg* 54 (7):599-606, 1967.
8. Dreyfuss P, Michaelsen M, Pauza K, *et al:* The value of medical history and physical examination in diagnosing sacroiliac joint pain. *Spine* 21(22):2594-2602, 1996.
9. Dropcho EJ: Remote neurological manifestations of cancer. *Neurol Clin* 20(1):85-122, 2002.
10. Engstrom JW: Back and neck pain. In Fauci AS, Braunwald E, Jameson JL, Kasper DL, Hauser SL, Longo DL (eds): *Harrison's Principles of Internal Medicine*, ed 15. New York, McGraw-Hill, 2001, pp 79-90.
11. Erbay H: Meralgia paresthetica in differential diagnosis of low back pain. *Clin J Pain* 18:132-135, 2002.
12. Fishman LM, Dombi GW, Michaelsen C, *et al:* Piriformis syndrome: diagnosis, treatment, and outcome—a 10-year study. *Arch Phys Med Rehabil* 83: 295-301, 2002.
13. Goff DC, Sellers DE, McGovern PG, *et al:* Knowledge of heart attack symptoms in a population survey in the United States: the REACT trial. Rapid Early Action for Coronary Treatment. *Arch Intern Med* 158 (21):2329-2338, 1998.
14. Goldberg R, Goff D, Cooper L, *et al:* Age and sex differences in presentation of symptoms among patients with acute coronary disease: the REACT trial. Rapid Early Action for Coronary Treatment. *Coron Artery Dis* 11 (5):399-407, 2000.
15. Gray JC: Diagnosis of intermittent vascular claudication in a patient with a diagnosis of sciatica. *Phys Ther* 79:582-590, 1999.
16. Grossman MG, Ducey SA, Nadler SS, Levy AS: Meralgia paresthetica: diagnosis and treatment. *J Am Acad Orthop Surg* 9(5):336-344, 2001.
17. Härkönen M, Olin P, Wennström J: Severe backache as a presenting sign of bacterial endocarditis. *Acta Med Scand* 210:329-331, 1981.
18. Harrison DE, Harrison DD, Troyanovich SJ: The sacroiliac joint: a review of anatomy and biomechanics with clinical implications. *J Manipulative Physiol Ther* 20(9):607-617, 1997.
19. Harvey G, Bell S: Obturator neuropathy: An anatomic perspective. *Clin Orthop* 363:203-211, 1999.
20. Horton JD, Bilhartz LE: Gallstone disease and its complications. In Feldman M, Friedman LS and Sleisenger MH (eds): *Sleisenger and Fordtran's Gastrointestinal and Liver Disease: Pathophysiology/Diagnosis/Management*, ed 7. Philadelphia, WB Saunders, 2002, pp 1065-1090.
21. Katz JN, Dalgas M, Stucki G, *et al:* Degenerative lumbar spinal stenosis: diagnostic value of the history and physical examination. *Arthritis Rheum* 38(9):1236-1241, 1995.
22. Kleiner JB, Donaldson WF, Curd JG, Thorne RP: Extraspinal causes of lumbosacral radiculopathy. *J Bone Joint Surg Am* 73-A(6):817-821, 1991.
23. Krarup C, Crone C: Neurophysiological studies in malignant disease with particular reference to involvement of peripheral nerves. *J Neurol* 249:651-661, 2002.
24. Larsson EM, Heiling M, Holtås S: Aortic pathology revealed by MRI in patients with clinical suspicion of spinal disease. *Neuroradiology* 35:499-502, 1993.
25. Lauder TD: Musculoskeletal disorders that frequently mimic radiculopathy. *Phys Med Rehabil Clin N Am* 13: 469-485, 2002.
26. Liu JE, Tahmoush AJ, Roos DB, Schwartzman RJ: Shoulder-arm pain from cervical bands and scalene muscle anomalies. *J Neurol Sci* 128:175-180, 1995.
27. Marston WA, Ahlquist R, Johnson G, et al: Misdiagnosis of ruptured abdominal aortic aneurysms. *J Vasc Surg* 16: 17-22, 1992.
28. Mazanec DJ: Differential diagnosis of low back pain and sciatica. *Seminars Spine Surg* 6(3):180-185, 1994.

29. Mazanec DJ: Pseudospine: conditions that mimic spine pain. In Cole AJ, Herring SA (eds): *The Low Back Pain Handbook: A Guide for the Practicing Clinician,* ed 2. Philadelphia, Hanley & Belfus, 2003, pp 117-131.

30. Meyers OL, Commerford PJ: Musculoskeletal manifestations of bacterial endocarditis. *Ann Rheum Disease* 36:517-519, 1977.

31. Murtagh J: Three unusual presentations of interscapular back pain. *Aust Fam Physician* 22(6):1000-1004, 1993.

32. Nevitt MP, Ballard DJ, Hallett JW: Prognosis of abdominal aortic aneurysms: a population study. *N Engl J Med* 321:1009-1014, 1989.

33. Quast MS, Goldflies ML: A new differential diagnosis for musculoskeletal posterior thoracic wall pain: a case report. *Orthop Rev* 18(4):461-465, 1989.

34. Rodrique T, Hardy RW: Diagnosis and treatment of piriformis syndrome. *Neurosurg Clin North Am* 12(2): 311-319, 2001.

35. Saal JA, Dillingham MF, Gamburd RS, Fanton GS: The pseudoradicular syndrome: lower extremity peripheral nerve entrapment masquerading as lumbar radiculopathy. *Spine* 13(8):926-930, 1988.

36. Sayson SC, Ducey JP, Maybrey JB, *et al:* Sciatic entrapment neuropathy associated with an anomalous priformis muscle. *Pain* 59:149-152, 1994.

37. Sher JS, Uribe JW, Posada A, *et al:* Abnormal findings on magnetic resonance images of asymptomatic shoulders. *J Bone Joint Surg* 77A:10-15, 1995.

38. Sheth RN, Belzberg AJ: Diagnosis and treatment of thoracic outlet syndrome. *Neurosurg Clin North Am* 12(2):295-309, 2001.

39. Slipman CW, Rogers DP, Lipetz JS: An unusual extraspinal cause of bilateral leg pain. *Arch Phys Med Rehabil* 80: 721-724, 1999.

40. Slipman CW, Jackson HB, Lipetz JS, *et al:* Sacroiliac joint pain referral zones. *Arch Phys Med Rehabil* 81:334-338, 2000.

41. Spoelhof GD, Bristow M: Back pain pitfalls. *Am Fam Physician* 40(4):133-138, 1989.

42. Szabo RM: Nerve compression syndromes. In Manske PR (ed): *Hand Surgery Update.* Rosemont, IL, American Academy of Orthopaedic Surgeons, 1996, pp 221-231.

43. Tifford CD, Plancher KD: Nonsurgical treatment of rotator cuff tears. In Norris TR (ed): *Orthopaedic Knowledge Update Shoulder and Elbow.* Rosemont, IL, American Academy of Orthopaedic Surgeons, 1997, pp 135-149.

44. Tong HC, Haig AJ, Yamakawa K: The Spurling test and cervical radiculopathy. *Spine* 27(2): 156-159, 2002.

45. Topol EJ: The history. In Topol EJ (ed): *Textbook of Cardiovascular Medicine,* ed 2. Philadelphia, Lippincott Williams and Wilkins, 2002, pp 265-272.

46. Tortolani PJ, Carbone JJ, Quartararo LG: Greater trochanteric pain syndrome in patients referred to orthopedic spine specialists. *The Spine Journal* 2:251-254, 2002.

47. Uppal GS, Uppal JA, Dwyer AP: Glenoid cysts mimicking cervical radiculopathy. *Spine* 20(20):2257-2260, 1995.

48. Vargo MM, Flood KM: Pancoast tumor presenting as cervical radiculopathy. *Arch Phys Med Rehabil* 71:606-609, 1990.

49. Weiss DJ, Conliffe T, Tata N: Low back pain caused by a duodenal ulcer. *Arch Phys Med Rehabil* 79(9):1137-1139, 1998.

CHAPTER 10

Pathophysiology of Cervical Myelopathy: Biomechanical Concepts

Fraser C. Henderson, Edward C. Benzel, David H. Kim, and Alexander R. Vaccaro

Cervical spondylotic myelopathy (CSM) is a well-described clinical syndrome that evolves from a combination of etiologic mechanisms. The strong association between a narrowed, spondylotic cervical spinal canal and the development of CSM has previously led to the formulation of a relatively simple pathoanatomic concept: a narrowed spinal canal causes compression of the enclosed cord, leading to local tissue ischemia, injury, and neurologic impairment. However, this simple mechanism fails to explain the entire spectrum of clinical findings observed in CSM, particularly the development of significant neurologic signs in patients without evidence of static cord compression.

Current support for a biomechanical etiology of CSM comes from three areas: clinical studies of cervical mobility in patients with CSM, histopathologic studies of spinal cord tissue from CSM patients, and biomechanical studies that have led to an improved understanding of the material properties and biomechanical behavior of spinal cord tissue under various physiologic and pathologic conditions. A growing body of evidence indicates that spondylotic narrowing of the spinal canal results in increased strain and shear forces, and that these pathologic forces cause both diffuse and focal axonal injuries within the spinal cord. This biomechanical theory appears to more fully address the clinical and pathologic findings in various studies of spinal cord injury, and better explains the occurrence of clinical myelopathy in patients without static cord compression.

Clinical Patterns of Cervical Spondylotic Myelopathy

Clinical myelopathy typically appears in late adulthood in the setting of progressive degenerative changes, including cervical disc degeneration, osteophytic spur and transverse bar formation, posterior longitudinal ligament (PLL) calcification, ligamentum flavum thickening, and osteoarthritic facet hypertrophy.[1-3] Progressive encroachment on the spinal canal by anterior and posterior anatomic structures may first lead to spinal cord compression that occurs only transiently during physiologic cervical range of motion.

The appearance of clinical signs and symptoms arising from this condition has been described as "dynamic stenosis." With progressive narrowing of the spinal canal, dynamic compression may eventually evolve into static compression of the enclosed spinal cord and the appearance of classic CSM.

Retrospective observational studies indicate that development of CSM is more common in patients with underlying congenital stenosis of the spinal canal. A sagittal spinal canal diameter of less than 12mm is strongly associated with signs and symptoms of myelopathy, whereas a diameter greater than 16mm appears to confer a relatively low risk.[4-8]

Histopathology of Cervical Spondylotic Myelopathy

The theory that ischemic injury is the pathophysiologic basis of CSM originates in early histologic studies of cervical myelopathy, which revealed several changes consistent with ischemic tissue damage. These include cystic cavitation, gliosis, anterior horn cell dropout, and prominent involvement of the central gray matter, as well as Wallerian degeneration of the posterior columns and corticospinal tracts.[2,9-11] In these studies the most severe histologic changes were observed at the level of ventral spondylotic bars, with the most visible histologic changes occurring in the lateral funiculi of the spinal cord, particularly the corticospinal tracts. The anterior columns and dorsal region of the dorsal columns appeared to demonstrate the least extent of injury-related change.

Attempts have been made to correlate the severity of histopathologic findings with the range of clinical findings in patients with CSM. In general, less severe myelopathy has been associated with changes confined largely to the lateral funiculi, whereas more severe cases appear to be associated with involvement of the medial gray area and ventral aspect of the dorsal columns, as well as gliosis and anterior horn cell dropout. In cases of severe CSM there is extensive Wallerian degeneration, proceeding proximally and distally from the site of spinal cord compression.

Spinal Cord Ischemia and Cervical Spondylotic Myelopathy

The anatomic basis for the ischemic insult proposed in CSM has been attributed to various mechanisms, including compression of radicular feeders within the neuroforamina, compromise of venous drainage by ventral spondylotic bars, and compression of the anterior spinal artery, as well as its ventral branches.[12,13] Several animal studies support the concept of a potential role for compressive ischemia in the pathogenesis of CSM.[14-16]

Cadaver studies have demonstrated that flattening of the cervical spinal cord is associated with elongation of the laterally directed terminal branches of the central arteries arising from the anterior spinal artery, as well as elongation of the penetrating branches of the lateral pial plexus (corona radiata). It is hypothesized that attenuation of these transversely directed arteries results in decreased arterial blood flow to the corticospinal tracts. Shortening of the ventral-dorsal dimension of the spinal cord, however, results in widening of the arteries directed in the ventral-dorsal direction and relative preservation of blood flow to the anterior columns. These findings might explain the relative vulnerability to injury of the laterally positioned corticospinal tracts, compared with the anterior columns.[17]

Recent clinical studies strongly suggest that compression and ischemia alone do not fully explain the pathogenesis of CSM. Despite observational studies associating CSM with various anatomic factors, such as the presence of decreased ventral-dorsal spinal canal diameter, subluxation, and dorsal osteophytes, at least one study has demonstrated that these factors hold no significant predictive value in terms of identifying which patients are at risk for clinical progression of their myelopathy.[18] Several other studies have also failed to identify an association between the degree of spinal stenosis and spinal cord compression and clinical prognosis.[7,12,19]

Moreover, surgical decompression that results in expansion of the spinal canal and relief of compressive pressures does not consistently alter the natural history of CSM.[20] Ebersold *et al.*[21] performed a retrospective review of 100 CSM patients undergoing surgical decompression, with an average 7-year follow-up, and concluded that decompression alone resulted in no clear, long-term improvement. Two thirds of patients experienced initial clinical improvement, but half of these demonstrated subsequent clinical deterioration. At final follow-up, only a third of the original group were improved, leading the authors to conclude that long-term outcome was not predicated on the presence or severity of spinal cord compression and ischemia, but on other "nonvascular" factors.

Biomechanical Factors and CSM

There is a growing body of evidence indicating that abnormal or excessive motion of the cervical spine is strongly associated with clinical progression of CSM. Adams and Logue performed a retrospective clinical review that demonstrated a cervical flexion/extension arc in excess of 40 degrees was the most significant variable in predicting poor clinical outcome in patients with CSM.[12] Similar retrospective studies have been performed by Barnes and Saunders,[18] as well as by Yonenobu *et al.*,[19] in which patients with a flexion/extension arc of greater than 60 degrees after laminectomy were at increased risk for developing progressive myelopathy.

In contrast to the relatively poor results following simple decompression for CSM, several studies demonstrate excellent clinical results associated with the elimination of abnormal cervical motion. Using a simple neck brace to restrict cervical motion often leads to improvement in patients suffering cervical myelopathy from disc protrusions.[22] The largest series of patients undergoing ventral decompression and fusion for CSM demonstrated an 86% improvement rate, with no significant deterioration.[23] Overall, surgical fusion through a variety of approaches has also been associated with favorable clinical results, including ventral decompression and fusion without instrumentation,[21] with ventral plating,[24-28] and dorsal decompression with instrumented fusion.[29-32]

The significant clinical recovery experienced by most myelopathic patients after decompression and fusion indicates that neurologic deficits resulting from cervical myelopathy are recoverable.[23-25,28-30] Moreover, the rapid improvement experienced by many patients after surgery suggests that these patients do not have the apparently irreversible, histologic changes demonstrated in many pathologic studies. In contrast, failure of some patients to improve clinically after decompression and fusion may be a result of irreversible spinal cord injury. Histologic examination of spinal cord tissue from these patients may reveal severe ischemic injury, as previously described by histologic studies.

Pathology of Spinal Cord Stretch Injury

The significance of spinal stenosis and spinal cord compression in early CSM may not be caused by the generation of local ischemia, but rather the creation of a tethering effect, which results in production of local, potentially injurious, tissue strain and shear forces. The concept that increased cervical mobility, coupled with kyphotic deformity, results in spinal cord elongation and increased axial strain forces is not new.[17,33] Several studies have demonstrated the adverse effects of even low-grade mechanical stretching on neural tissues. During normal motion, large axial strains occur in the cervical spinal cord.[34] The white matter of the spinal cord can be viewed as an axial array of parallel fibers with individual fibers demonstrating variable levels of crimping. As a whole the cord is initially compliant to stretch, but it becomes progressively stiffer as the fibers straighten out and begin to bear tensile load.[35] Rapid occurrence of these strains can exceed the material properties of the tissue, leading to tissue disruption and transient or permanent neurologic injury. The degree of injury appears to be related to the peak strain of the tissue and the loading rate.[36]

Cadaver studies suggest that even physiologic flexion of the cervical spine leads to stretching and the production of strain forces within the neuraxis.[17] Flexion of the spinal column has been found to result in significant elongation of the spinal canal, with concomitant stretching of the spinal cord. During physiologic flexion of the head and trunk in rhesus monkeys, net movement of the spinal cord occurs from the upper spine downward to the level of C4-5, whereas net movement of the spinal cord occurs upward below this level.[33] Net movement occurs to a greater extent below C4-5, with 1.6mm of movement at C1 and 6mm of movement at T3. The amount of spinal cord stretch occurring at each level is proportional to the degree of flexion at the adjacent intervertebral disc space. For example, at the lower cervical and upper thoracic spine, where the amount of flexion tends to be greatest, local spinal cord strain can reach 24%. A separate study has measured a 17.6mm length increase at the level of the cervicothoracic junction, which was translated into a strain of 10% of resting spinal cord length (Reid *et al.*). This phenomenon might explain the clinical observation that signs that are often localized to levels apparently remote from the level of stenosis (e.g., hand intrinsic muscle wasting with high cervical stenosis).

In the absence of compressive pathology the natural elongation of the spinal cord that occurs with neck flexion and hyperextension is distributed over the entire length of the spinal cord. However, with tethering of the spinal cord, as a result of local compression, the axial strain cannot be distributed throughout the cord and is instead limited to the segment of cord between the distracting force and the tethering point. Local spinal cord degenerative changes are frequently identified adjacent to thickened dentate ligaments, which suggests that localization of injurious mechanical forces at these levels may be associated with the tethering effect of the ligaments.[33,37] A biomechanical study of the material properties of the dura mater indicates that elastic behavior is uniform throughout the length of the spinal canal; however, strain forces are significantly greater in the cervical region than in either the thoracic or lumbar regions.[38]

The tethering action of the dentate ligaments may be responsible for accentuating the effect of tensile spinal cord stress and exacerbating local tissue injury. Moreover, it has been suggested that dorsal displacement of the spinal cord, as a result of the presence of ventral spondylotic bars, may lead to stretching of the dentate ligaments and tethering of the cervical cord via the ventrolaterally positioned nerve root sleeves. Repetitive and persistent microtrauma to these nerve root sleeves may lead to the progressive thickening that has been observed with age.[37] Therefore axial tension generated within the spinal cord during physiologic motion may be amplified at certain levels, as a result of two separate factors—overall spinal canal lengthening and the local tethering effects of the dentate ligaments.

Several investigators have attributed delayed, progressive cervical myelopathy to a combination of underlying structural kyphosis and abnormal or excessive cervical motion. Dynamic lengthening of the cervical spinal cord that occurs during neck flexion is magnified in patients with cervical kyphosis. Conversely, kinematic magnetic resonance imaging studies have demonstrated that lengthening of the spinal cord also occurs during neck extension in some patients with fixed kyphotic deformity of the cervical spine. In the setting of static spinal cord compression and superimposed instability, cervical extension can also lead to aggravation of the cord impingement and significant upper cervical cord elongation.[39]

Models of Spinal Cord Stretch Injury

A mathematic model for spinal cord stretch injury has been developed. Levine.[40] represented the spinal cord as a simplified solid material with uniform elastic properties in order to predict the three-dimensional stresses experienced during physiologic motion and in spondylosis. According to this model, flattening of the cord is not a result of ventral-dorsal compression, but rather the consequence of laterally directed tension arising from the dentate ligaments, which tighten in flexion. This model, with a ventral spondylotic bar and tethering dentate ligaments predicts maximal stresses in the lateral funiculi. The model provides a possible explanation for the characteristic histologic findings in CSM, in which there is relative sparing of the anterior and posterior funiculi. It also explains why histopathologic changes are found over a relatively extended segment of spinal cord tissue, as opposed to being limited to the point of compression. However, the importance of the dentate ligaments in the etiology of CSM is brought into question by the inconsistent results of sectioning these ligaments at the time of surgery.[41]

Breig[58] also developed a mechanical model that seeks to explain some of the apparent inconsistencies found in histologic studies of CSM. For instance, in addressing the question of why some chronic, ventral compression injuries result in predominantly dorsal cord injury, cadaver models demonstrate that a compression force applied ventrally to the spinal cord in the presence of stenosis creates a pincer mechanism, resulting in increased axial tension in the cord and fissuring opposite the side of compression. In this model the spinal cord is represented as a viscoelastic cylinder which, when compressed from the sides, exhibits net tissue creep to the free ends of the cylinder. As a result, tension forces are created perpendicular to the plane of compression. With mild compressive deformation of the spinal cord, elastic stretch of the axis cylinders occurs. However, when the ventral-dorsal diameter of the spinal cord is reduced by 20% to 30%, axial tension forces exceed the material properties of the tissue and result in tearing of axial fibers. The stress field produced by this pincer mechanism is multidirectional, and secondary shearing forces are also created. This model explains how ventral compression of the spinal cord in the presence of stenosis might result in stretch and shear injury to myelin and neural elements.

Spinal Cord Tethering and Shear Injury

Studies involving the tethered spinal cord syndrome may also contribute to a better understanding of the pathogenesis of CSM. Stretch injury is now widely accepted as the principal cause in developing myelopathy in the tethered cord syndrome. The symptoms and clinical findings of pain, numbness, weakness, pes cavus, scoliosis, and bowel and bladder dysfunction have all been attributed to stretching injury of the spinal cord.[42-48] The degree or amount of traction on the conus medullaris determines the age or onset of symptoms. Extensive tethering and severe stretching of the conus medullaris results in neurologic disturbances in infancy, whereas a lesser degree of tethering often remains subclinical until adulthood, when symptoms may become manifest in the setting of an acute event (i.e., hyperflexion injury) or chronic process (e.g., development of ventral disc or bone protrusions).[49] Although the clinical manifestations of the tethered cord syndrome are most commonly referable to the lumbosacral spinal cord, patients often exhibit neurologic signs and symptoms that originate from the cervical cord. For example, long tract involvement may lead to interscapular pain, hand numbness and poor coordination, as well as upper extremity hyperreflexia. Quadriparesis has also been reported.[50] This phenomenon supports the hypothesis that tension within the spinal cord might be transmitted to remote segments of the cord, where the lateral columns are fixed in position by the dentate ligaments. It has been suggested that injury to the large-diameter fibers of the corticospinal tracts occurs some distance from the actual tethering and results in the clinical picture of mixed upper and lower motor neuron deficits.[49] Significant spinal cord stretching has been observed up to five segments from the site of tethering in one study.

Experimental studies involving the lumbar and sacral spinal cord of cats have demonstrated that acute tethering is very traumatic to spinal cord tissue, particularly when stretching occurs repeatedly.[51] Although these studies were designed to investigate the mechanics of the tethered cord syndrome, some interesting findings may be applicable to CSM. Spinal cord elongation is most pronounced immediately adjacent to the point of application of the tethering force. Under low levels of tension the spinal cord demonstrates purely elastic behavior and returns to normal resting length. At greater tension plastic deformation occurs. Portions of the spinal cord near the point of application of stretch remain elongated 7% over the original length, even after release of tension.

Tissue dysfunction in the tethered cord syndrome has been associated with impairment of oxidative metabolism. The relationship of tissue ischemia to spinal cord stretching in this syndrome is unclear. Although a tethered cord may result in permanent neurologic deficit, the fact that surgical untethering usually results in significant improvement of sensorimotor and bladder function indicates a degree of reversibility that militates against a purely ischemic cause.

A guinea pig model of spinal cord stretch injury has been developed in which the filum terminale was tethered and attached to a 5g weight. Tethering resulted in significant delay and decreased amplitude of somatosensory evoked potentials. Lipid peroxidation and hypoxanthine levels were significantly increased. Electron microscopic examination of tissue revealed potentially reversible histologic changes, such as edema, destruction of the gray-white junction, axonal injury with loss of neurofilaments, and evidence of myelin sheath damage.[52]

The localization of demyelinating injury to the corticospinal tracts in cases of trauma is suggestive of the demyelination and edema seen in the posterolateral funiculi of CSM patients.[11,13,53-56] Autopsy studies of rheumatoid arthritis patients with myelopathy have revealed edema localized to the posterolateral funiculi, as well as axonal retraction balls, suggestive of stretch-related injury without evidence of significant ischemia.[57]

The finding that tethering of the spinal cord in one region leads to generation of stretch and shear forces remote from the site of tethering or compression is directly applicable to numerous pathologic processes throughout the spine. The spinal cord can be tethered at any level by scarring, external compression, or spinal deformity. Spinal cord deformation over a large disc herniation at the apex of a kyphosis can contribute to stretch and shear injury, remote from the locus of deformation.[58] Similarly, deformation of the brainstem or medullospinal junction over the odontoid process in basilar invagination results in both local and remote neurologic dysfunction (e.g., diplopia, dysphagia, dysarthria, vertigo), as well as sensorimotor deficits.[59] Although these effects may also be explained by ischemic injury, local ischemia has not been found.[57] Again, correction of brainstem deformity through surgical removal of the odontoid process or occipitocervical stabilization typically results in significant clinical recovery.[60] Simple decompression appears to be inadequate if significant ventral medullary deformity persists.[61,62] Disturbances of sleep and alterations in central respiratory function have been attributed to medullary deformity secondary to basilar invagination, and these disturbances have been reversed by correction of ventral medullary deformity.[63] The neurologic dysfunction observed in association with basilar invagination may therefore be a result of deformation and stretch injury of the neuraxis.

Histopathology of Spinal Cord Shear Injury

If neuraxial deformation, abnormal motion, and stretch injury are the primary causes of CSM and similar neurologic syndromes, then the histopathologic manifestations appear to be myelin edema and reactive axonal changes. A form of spinal axonal injury has been observed that is similar to the diffuse axonal injury (DAI) seen in the brain after deceleration injuries.

DAI is the most common brain injury resulting from blunt head trauma, and patient morbidity has been directly associated with the extent of DAI.[64,65] Experimental primate models have demonstrated that the location and quantity of axonal changes directly correlate with observed morbidity.[66,67] Clinical and pathologic studies have revealed that axonal injury is a component of traumatic brain injury throughout the spectrum of severity, from concussion to severe forms of prolonged coma.[68] Despite these histopathologic observations, the pathogenesis of DAI remains unclear. An early hypothesis speculated that tearing of the axon at the time of injury resulted in expulsion of a ball of axoplasm into the brain parenchyma.[69,70] However, recent DAI studies have demonstrated that axons undergoing shear strain do not undergo immediate disruption, but rather a nondestructive injury manifests as axonal swelling in internodal regions.[71] Axonal stretch at the time of injury results in axolemmal damage, disruption of axon transport and metabolism, and the delayed formation of a retraction ball or reactive axonal swelling.[71,72] This focal swelling is thought to be a pre-stage secondary axotomy.[73-76]

Studies have demonstrated that traumatic axonal injury results in impairment of anterograde axonal transport. In a guinea pig optic nerve model, 17% of axons demonstrated injury within 15 minutes of an applied stretch injury. The cell body of injured axons retained the ability to incorporate and transport horseradish peroxidase, but local interruption of axonal transport was demonstrated.[77] In a separate study axonal injury was localized to the nodes of Ranvier, where histologic changes were noted, consisting of axolemmal blebs, loss of subaxolemma density, loss of nodal gap substance, and neurofilament disarray.[75] Although distended, the axolemma remained intact. These findings suggest the possibility that stretch injury disrupts unidentified structural elements located at the node (i.e., membrane-associated proteins), which associate with the cytoskeleton and maintain nodal architecture. Furthermore, the study investigators speculated that nodal disruption leads to local cytoskeletal collapse and impairment of anterograde transport in a grossly intact axon.[75] The study also identified evidence of localized myelin injury with thinning and myelin profiles within the sheath adjacent to the axolemma.

The cell ultrastructural events proceeding from axonal injury have been well characterized.[73] Continued anterograde transport to the site of focal impairment appears to result in localized ballooning of the axon and formation of a reactive axon bulb, or "Strich ball." Over the ensuing 1 to 3 days, the proximal axon segment containing the axon bulb continues to expand, because of persistent anterograde transport and deposition of smooth endoplasmic reticulum and other intracellular organelles. These deposits become dispersed peripherally around an enlarged neurofilamentous core within the axon bulb. With further enlargement of the bulb, thinning of the overlying axolemma and myelin sheath occurs. Eventually, anatomic disconnection occurs between axonal segments proximal and distal to the original site of injury. The overlying myelin sheath is disrupted, and then reforms to enclose the axon bulb, while the distal axonal segment undergoes wallerian degeneration. Meanwhile the proximal axon bulb continues to expand, as a result of continued anterograde transport of intracellular contents from the neuronal soma. In rodent studies, by 14 days, most reactive axons degenerate, become electron dense, and are eventually phagocytized by microglia. By contrast, in studies of mild to moderate head trauma in cats, some reactive axons have been observed to undergo a regenerative process, with outgrowth of regenerative sprouts and growth cones. The growth cones can be identified for several months as they grow into surrounding parenchyma, and there is a concomitant decrease in the extent of axonal swelling, presumably as a result of axoplasm flow into the new growth.[78,79]

Axon cytoskeletal collapse and rapid loss of the microtubular network appear to underlie the observed impairment of axoplasmic transport after injury.[80] A quantitative analysis of injury-associated changes within the axoskeleton identified evidence of injury throughout the length of the axon, but maximal changes were in the midportion of the stretched nerve. Small axons demonstrated compaction of neurofilaments. Larger axons demonstrated one of two observed responses. Those axons with enlargement of the para-axonal space demonstrated compaction of neurofilaments, loss of microtubules, and reduction in axonal caliber. Those axons with formation of intramyelinic spaces demonstrated decreased numbers and increased spacing between neurofilaments and microtubules. Neurofilaments have been implicated in maintenance of axon caliber, whereas microtubules are thought to provide the mechanism for fast axonal transport. Neurofilament compaction is thought to precede the cytoskeletal disappearance accompanying wallerian degeneration. Collapse of neurofilaments into tightly packed bundles in the center of the axon may precede secondary axotomy in nondisruptive stretch injury of central nerves.[81]

Injury-associated changes in the axonal cytoskeleton are preceded by alterations in axolemmal permeability. Intra-axonal accumulation of calcium has been demonstrated in focal spinal cord injury.[82-85] Recently, increased calcium influx has been demonstrated in axons suffering stretch injury.[86] Using a guinea pig optic nerve model, a characteristic sequence of cellular events has been observed to occur over 24 hours. Initially, tensile strain leads to mechanical disruption of the myelin lamellae surrounding the nerve. Presumed loss of activity of the ecto-Ca-ATPase pump at sites of myelin disruption are then thought to allow increased calcium influx into the myelin, possibly mediating myelin dissociation, and increased periaxonal space over several hours. Increased calcium influx into the injured axon results in proteolysis of neurofilaments and dephosphorylation of neurofilament sidearms.[87] In severe spinal cord injury, calcium-induced neurofilamentous degradation can be detected within 30 minutes.

Although increased calcium influx has been strongly implicated in neurofilamentous degradation via calcium-activated neutral proteases, some investigators question the relationship between calcium influx and the reactive axonal changes seen in stretch-related injury.[73] Povlishok contends that neurofilamentous disarray is either a direct mechanical effect of trauma on the cytoskeleton or the result of increased neurofilament subunit exchange between stable neurofilaments and a pool of soluble kinetically active subunits.

Although changes in axolemmal permeability and cytoskeletal disruption appear to trigger a cascade of intra-axonal changes in moderate to severe injury, in mild injury reactive axonal changes and retraction balls have been demonstrated in the absence of any change in axolemmal permeability and without evidence of neurofilament or microtubule loss. In these instances it has been speculated that a "focal misalignment" occurs at the time of injury, resulting in impaired axoplasmic flow and delayed axotomy.[88] It is conceivable that two different injury patterns exist and that the specific mechanism depends on the severity of tensile strain. In vitro studies have shown that axons under low tensile load undergo disruption of axoplasmic flow without evidence of axolemmal permeability change. High-tensile loading leads to immediate changes in axolemmal permeability and rapid disruption of axoplasmic flow.[89]

Anatomically, axons appear to be disrupted at sites of maximal tension. Large-caliber axons with a long intra-axial course appear to be more susceptible to tensile injury.[49] Reactive changes have been observed in which axons change course, cross blood vessels, and decussate.[90]

Relationship Between Ischemia and Shear Injury

Stretch injury renders axons more susceptible to secondary injury from other processes, including ischemia.[90] However, the role of ischemia in stretch-related injury is unclear. Reactive axonal swelling occurs in a histologic background that lacks strong evidence of ischemic change. Microscopic studies have failed to identify correlative changes in microvasculature or ischemia-related changes in the neuronal soma, axonal processes, or dendritic processes.[71] Iodoantipyrine studies have revealed no significant changes in regional blood flow.[91,92] Moreover, axons undergoing reactive change are frequently found surrounded by intact neurons, without any evidence of ischemia or injury. When axonal injury is observed in proximity to the soma, central chromatolysis has been observed but may be secondary to pathologic processes within the axon. The rapidity of onset of axonal changes weighs heavily against a process originating in the neuronal soma.

The fact that some axons undergo reactive change while immediately adjacent axons appear uninjured is difficult to explain. It is conceivable, as Povlishok speculates, that specific differences in axonal anatomy, such as location of intra-axial turns, crossing points, and decussations, may make certain axons uniquely susceptible to injury at specific levels.

In the peripheral nervous system, axonal swelling can be seen in response to various insults (e.g., ischemia, severance, and crushing).[73] Caution must be used before assigning a given etiology to the morphologic finding of axonal swelling.

Apoptosis

The pathogenesis of myelopathy is beginning to be dissected on a molecular level. Recent studies suggest that a significant portion of cell loss in chronic compression-related myelopathy is caused by apoptosis.[93] The process of apoptosis is biologically distinct from necrosis and refers to a well-defined sequence of intracellular events that are characterized by internucleosomal chromosome fragmentation, membrane blebbing, and phagocytosis, without generation of an inflammatory response.[94] In contrast, cell necrosis typically involves random DNA cleavage, membrane disruption, mitochondrial swelling, and local inflammation.[95]

Although necrosis and apoptosis often occur concurrently, identifying the dominant biologic process can provide important insight into the causes of specific disorders. In the case of CSM the identification of primarily apoptotic cell death is significant. Although ischemia is one of numerous triggers associated with apoptotic cell death, severe ischemia such as that implied in the pathogenesis of CSM is more characteristically thought to cause cell death through necrosis. Therefore the fact that oligodendrocyte disappearance in CSM appears to be apoptotic in nature suggests that a mechanism other than pure ischemia is involved.[96]

A prominent role for apoptosis has already been implicated in the secondary cell loss that occurs after traumatic spinal cord injury.[96-100] Cell loss occurs in spinal cord injury, both at the time of injury and secondarily over a period lasting days to weeks. At the injury epicenter, most cell death occurs through necrosis, and leads to active clearance of necrotic cell debris through macrophage and microglial phagocytosis.[101] However, white-matter cell loss continues through a longer segment of the spinal cord for several weeks in a process called "secondary injury." Animal studies have demonstrated that compressive cord injury leads to apoptosis of oligodendrocytes along degenerating white-matter tracts.[96,98] These studies indicate that apoptosis begins within 24 hours of injury and continues for at least 3 weeks.

Strong evidence for the occurrence of apoptotic cell death in chronic compression-related cervical myelopathy comes from studies of an animal model of chronic compression-related cervical myelopathy, the tiptoe-walking Yoshimura mouse.[102] The Yoshimura mouse is an inbred strain that characteristically develops quadriparesis 4-8 months after birth because of severe spinal cord compression, a result of hyperostosis along the posterolateral margins of the C1 and C2 vertebrae.[103] Histopathologic examination of cord tissue from Yoshimura mice has demonstrated descending degeneration, affecting the anterior and lateral columns as well as ascending degeneration along the posterior columns, in addition to severe

injury at the level of compression.[93] Moreover, cavity formation and myelin ovoids representing myelin debris were identified extending from the zone of compression into adjacent levels lacking evidence of gross cord deformation. The terminal deoxynucleotidyl transferase (TdT)-mediated dUTP nick-end labeling (TUNEL method) assay was used to reveal a pattern of glial cell apoptosis mirroring the pattern of white column degeneration. Histologic staining using cell type-specific markers confirmed that the apoptotic cells were oligodendrocytes. The study investigators also performed an autopsy of a patient with cervical myelopathy from ossification of the PLL, and reported discovering a similar pattern of neuronal loss, demyelination, and apoptosis.

Summary

The presence of cervical spine mobility, instability, and kyphosis is strongly predictive of clinical progression in patients with cervical spondylotic myelopathy. Deformation of the spinal cord by the presence of spondylotic transverse bars, and tethering of the cord by local stenosis appear to be major underlying factors that lead to abnormal stretch of the cord with movement. Stretching of the deformed or tethered cord leads to the generation of injurious tensile and shear forces in constituent axons.

Strong support for the shear and strain injury theory of CSM pathogenesis comes from several recent developments, including the concept of "dynamic stenosis," an increased understanding of the pathogenesis of neurologic injury in other syndromes associated with spinal cord tethering, histologic studies revealing reactive axonal injury in the spinal cord of patients with CSM, and a more sophisticated understanding of the pathophysiology of stretch-related myelin and axonal injury.

Axonal injury reproducibly occurs at sites of maximal tensile loading and mechanical injury to the neuronal axon triggers a well-defined sequence of intracellular and paracellular events. Myelin stretch injury leads to changes in axolemmal permeability. Histologically, cytoskeletal collapse is observed in neural cells in association with alterations in anterograde and retrograde axonal transport. Eventually, delayed axotomy occurs. The stretch and shear model may account for the clinical presentation and recovery potential of milder forms of CSM. More importantly, a greater understanding of the deleterious effects of stretch and shear on the cervical spinal cord may improve treatment strategies for CSM and other spinal cord injuries.

REFERENCES

1. Taylor AR: The mechanism of injury to the spinal cord in the neck without injury to the vertebral column. *J Bone Joint Surg* [Br] 33B:543-547, 1951.
2. Payne EE, Spillane JD: The cervical spine: an anatomico-pathological study of 70 specimens (using a special technique) with a particular reference to the problem of cervical spondylosis. *Brain* 80:571-617, 1957.
3. Stoltman HF, Blackwood W: The role of the ligamenta flava in the pathogenesis of myelopathy in cervical spondylosis. *Brain* 87:47-50, 1964.

4. Arnold JG: The clinical manifestations of spondylochondrosis (spondylosis) of the cervical spine. *Ann Surg* 141:872-889, 1955.

5. Crandall PH, Batzdorf U: Cervical spondylotic myelopathy. *J Neurosurg* 25:57-66, 1966.

6. Dunsker SB: Cervical spondylotic myelopathy: pathogenesis and pathophysiology. In Dunsker SB (ed): *Cervical Spondylosis*. New York, Raven Press, 1981, pp 119-134.

7. Hayashi H, Okada K, Hashimoto J, *et al*: A radiographic evaluation of the aging changes in the cervical spine and etiologic factors of myelopathy. *Spine* 13:618-625, 1988.

8. Wolf BS, Khilnani M, Malis L: The sagittal diameter of the bony cervical canal and its significance in cervical spondylosis. *J Mt Sinai Hosp* 23:283-292, 1956.

9. Hoff J, Nishimura M, Pitts L, *et al*: The role of ischemia in the pathogenesis of cervical spondylotic myelopathy: a review and new microangiopathic evidence. *Spine* 2: 100-108, 1972.

10. Hughes JT: *Pathology of the Spinal Cord*. Philadelphia, Saunders, 1978, pp 176-179.

11. Ogino H, Tada K, Okada K, *et al*: Canal diameter, antero-posterior compression ratio, and spondylitic myelopathy of the cervical spine. *Spine* 8:1-15, 1983.

12. Adams CBT, Logue V: The movement and contour of the spine in relation to the neural complications of cervical spondylosis. *Brain* 94:569-586, 1971.

13. Mair WGP, Druckman R: The pathology of spinal cord lesions and their relation to the clinical features in protrusion of cervical intervertebral discs. *Brain* 76:70-91, 1953.

14. Al-Mefty O, Harkey HL, Marawi I, *et al*: Experimental chronic compressive cervical myelopathy. *J Neurosurg* 79:550-561, 1993.

15. Doppman JL: The mechanism of ischemia in anteroposterior compression of the spinal cord. *Invest Radiol* 10:543-551, 1975.

16. Gooding MR, Wilson CB, Hoff JT: Experimental cervical myelopathy: effects of ischemia and compression on the canine cervical spinal cord. *J Neurosurg* 43:9-17, 1975.

17. Breig A, Turnbull I, Hassler O: Effects of mechanical stresses upon the cervical cord in cervical spondylosis: a study on fresh cadaver material. *J Neurosurg* 25:45-56, 1966.

18. Barnes MP, Saunders M: The effect of cervical mobility on the natural history of cervical spondylotic myelopathy. *J Neurol Neurosurg* Psych 47:17-20, 1985.

19. Yonenobu K, Okada K, Fuji T, *et al*: Causes of neurological deterioration following surgical treatment of cervical myelopathy. *Spine* 11:818-823, 1986.

20. Nurick S: The pathogenesis of the spinal cord disorder associated with cervical spondylosis. *Brain* 95:87-100, 1972.

21. Ebersold MJ, Pare MC, Quast LM: Surgical treatment for cervical spondylitic myelopathy. *J Neurosurg* 82:745-751, 1995.

22. Campbell AMG, Phillips DG: Cervical disc lesions with neurologic disorder. *Br Med J* 2:481-485, 1960.

23. Eleraky MA, Llanos C, Sonntag VKH: Cervical corpectomy: report of 185 cases and review of the literature. *J Neurosurg* 90:35-41, 1999.

24. Saunders RL, Bernini PM, Shireffs TGJ, *et al*: Central corpectomy for cervical spondylotic myelopathy:

a consecutive series with long-term follow-up evaluation. *J Neurosurg* 74:163-170, 1991.

25. Zdeblick TA, Bohlmann HH: Cervical kyphosis and myelopathy: treatment by anterior corpectomy and strut grafting. *J Bone Joint Surg* (Am) 71:170-182, 1989.

26. Bernard TNJ, Whitecloud TSI: Cervical spondylotic myelopathy and myeloradiculopathy: anterior decompression and stabilization with autogenous fibular strut graft. *Clin Orthop Rel Res* 128:149-160, 1987.

27. Seifert V, Stolke D: Multisegmental cervical spondylosis: treatment by spondylectomy, microsurgical decompression and osteosynthesis. *Neurosurg* 29:498-503, 1991.

28. Kojima T, Waga S, Kubo Y, *et al*: Anterior cervical vertebrectomy and interbody fusion for multilevel spondylosis and ossification of the posterior longitudinal ligament. *Neurosurgery* 24:864-872, 1989.

29. Maurer PK, Ellenbogen RG, Ecklund J, *et al*: Cervical spondylotic myelopathy: treatment with posterior decompression and Luck rectangle bone fusion. *Neurosurgery* 29:680-684, 1991.

30. Kumar VGR, Rea GL, Mervis LJ, McGregor JM: Cervical spondylotic myelopathy: functional and radiographic long-term outcome after laminectomy and posterior fusion. *Neurosurgery* 44:771-777, 1999.

31. Cusik JF, Steiner RE, Berns T: Total stabilization of the cervical spine in patients with cervical spondylitic myelopaty. *Neurosurgery* 18:491-495, 1986.

32. Gonzalez-Feria L: The effect of surgical immobilization after laminectomy in the treatment of advanced cases of cervical myelopathy. *Acta Neurotic* (Wien) 31:185-193, 1975.

33. Smith CG: Changes in the length and position of the spinal cord with changes in posture in the monkey. *Radiology* 66:259-266, 1956.

34. Margulies S, Meaney DF, Bilston LB, *et al*: In vivo motion of the human cervical spinal cord during extension and flexion. Proceedings of the IRCOB Conference. Verona, Italy, 1992, pp 213-224.

35. Bilston LE, Thibault LE: The mechanical properties of the human cervical spinal cord in vitro, *Ann Biomed Eng* 24:67-74, 1996.

36. Galbraith JA, Thibault LE, Matteson DR: Mechanical and electrical responses in the giant squid axon to simple elongation. *J Biomech Eng* 115:13-22, 1993.

37. Bedford PD, Bosanquet FD, Russell WR: Degeneration of the spinal cord associated with cervical spondylosis. *Lancet* 55-59, 1952.

38. Tencer AF, Allen BL, Ferguson RL: A biomechanical study of thoracolumbar spine fractures with bone in the canal. III. Mechanical properties of the dura and its tethering ligaments. *Spine* 10:741-747, 1985.

39. Muhle C, Metzner J, Weinert D, *et al*: Kinematic imaging in surgical management of cervical disc disease, spondylosis and spondylotic myelopathy. *Acta Radiologica* 40:146-153, 1999.

40. Levine DN: The pathogenesis of cervical spondylotic myelopathy. *J Neurol Neurosurg Psych* 62:334-340, 1997.

41. Bishara SN: The posterior operation in treatment of cervical spondylosis with myelopathy: a long-term follow-up study. *J Neurol Neurosurg Psychiatry* 34:393-398, 1971.

42. Sostrin RD, Thompson JR, Roue SA, *et al*: Occult spinal dysraphism in the geriatric patient. *Radiology* 125: 165-169, 1977.

43. Kaplan JO, Quencer RM: The occult tethered cord syndrome in the adult. *Radiology* 137:387-391, 1980.
44. Hoffman HJ, Hendrick EB, Humphreys RP: The tethered spinal cord: its protean manifestations, diagnosis and surgical correction. *Childs Brain* 2:145-155, 1976.
45. Garceau JG: The filum terminale syndrome. *J Bone Joint Surg [Am]* 35:711-716, 1953.
46. Fitz CR, Nash DC: The tethered conus. *Am J Neuroradiol* 125:515-523, 1975.
47. Breig A: Overstretching of an circumscribed stretching in the spinal cord—a basic cause of symptoms in cord disorders. *J Biomech* 3:7-9, 1970.
48. Pierre-Kahn E, Lacombe J, Pichon J, *et al*: Intraspinal lipomas with spina bifida. *J Neurosurg* 65:756-761, 1986.
49. Pang D, Wilberger JE: Tethered cord syndrome in adults. *J Neurosurg* 57:32-47, 1982.
50. Rogers HR, Long DM, Chou SN, French LA: Lipomas of the spinal cord and the cauda equina. *J Neurosurg* 34: 349-354, 1971.
51. Tani S, Yamada S, Knighton RS: Extensibility of the lumbar and sacral cord: pathophysiology of the tethered spinal cord in cats. *J Neurosurg* 66:116-123, 1987.
52. Kocak A, Kilik A, Nurlu G, *et al*: A new model for tethered cord syndrome: a biochemical, electrophysiological and electron microscopic study. *Pediatr Neurosurg* 34:120-126, 1997.
53. Wilkinson M: The morbid anatomy of cervical spondylosis and myelopathy. *Brain* 83:589-617, 1960.
54. Dastur DK, Wadia NH, Desai AD, Sinh G: Medullospinal compression due to atlantoaxial dislocation and sudden hematomyelia during decompression. *Brain* 88:897-927, 1965.
55. Wadia NH: Myelopathy complicating congenital atlantoaxial dislocation. *Brain* 90:449-470, 1967.
56. Nakano KK, Schoene CW, Baker RA, Dawson DM: The cervical myelopathy associated with rheumatoid arthritis: analysis of 32 patients with two postmortem cases. *Ann Neurol* 3:144-151, 1978.
57. Henderson FC, Geddes JF, Crockard HA: Neuropathology of the brainstem and spinal cord in end stage rheumatoid arthritis: implications for treatment. *Ann Rheum Dis* 52:629-637, 1993.
58. Breig A: *Adverse Mechanical Tension in the Central Nervous System*. New York, Wiley, 1978.
59. Menezes AH, van Gilder JC, Clark CR, El-Khoury G: Odontoid upward migration in rheumatoid arthritis. *J Neurosurg* 63:500-509, 1985.
60. Kohno K, Sakaki S, Shiraishi T, Okumura H: Successful treatment of Arnold-Chiari malformation associated with basilar impression and syringomyelia by the transoral approach. *Surg Neurol* 33:284-287, 1990.
61. Levy WJ, Mason L, Hahn JF: Chiari malformation presenting in adults: a surgical experience in 127 cases. *Neurosurgery* 12:377-390, 1983.
62. Paul KS, Lye RH, Strange FA, Dutton J: Arnold-Chiari malformation: review of 71 cases. *J Neurosurg* 58:183-187, 1983.
63. Howard RS, Henderson FC, Hirsch NP, *et al*: Respiratory abnormalities due to craniovertebral junction compression in rheumatoid disease. *Ann Rheum Dis* 53:134-136, 1994.
64. Adams JH, Mitchell DE, Graham DI, Doyle D: Diffuse brain damage of intermediate impact type: its relationship to "primary brainstem damage" in head injury. *Brain* 100:487-502, 1977.
65. Adams JH, Graham DI, Murray LS, Scott G: Diffuse axonal injury due to non-missile injury in humans: an analysis of 45 cases. *Ann Neurol* 12:557-563, 1982.
66. Gennarelli TA, Thibault LE, Adams JH, *et al*: Diffuse axonal injury and traumatic coma in the primate. *Ann Neurol* 12:564-574, 1982.
67. Adams JH, Doyle D, Ford I, *et al*: Diffuse axonal injury in head injury: definition, diagnosis, and grading. *Histopathology* 15:49-59, 1989.
68. Gennarelli TA: Cerebral concussion and diffuse brain injuries. In Cooper PR (ed): *Head Injury*. Baltimore, Williams and Wilkins, 1993, pp 137-158.
69. Cajal SRY: *Degeneration and Regeneration of the Central Nervous System*. Oxford, Oxford University Press, 1928.
70. Strich SJ: Shearing of nerve fibers as a cause of brain damage due to head injury. *Lancet* 2:443-448, 1961.
71. Povlishok JT, Becker DP, Cheng CLY, Vaughn GW: Axonal change in minor head injury. *J Neuropath Exp Neurol* 42:225-242, 1983.
72. Erb DE, Povlishok JT: Axonal damage in severe traumatic brain injury: an experimental study in cat. *Acta Neuropathologica* 76:347-358, 1988.
73. Povlishok JT: Traumatically induced axonal injury: pathogenesis and pathobiological implications. *Brain Path* 2:1-12, 1992.
74. Christman CW, Grady MS, Walker SA, *et al*: Ultrastructural studies of diffus axonal injury in humans. *J Neurotrauma* 11:173-186, 1994.
75. Maxwell WL, Irvine A, Graham DI, *et al*: Focal axonal injury: the early response to stretch. *J Neurocytol* 20: 157-164, 1991.
76. Pettus EH, Povlishok JT: Characterization of a distinct set of intraaxonal ultrastructural changes associated with traumatically induced alteration in axolemmal permeability. *Brain Res* 722:1-11, 1996.
77. Gennarelli TA, Thibault LE, Tipperman R, *et al*: Axonal injury in the optic nerve: a model of diffuse axonal injury in the brain. *J Neurosurg* 17:244-253, 1989.
78. Lampert PW: A comparative electron microscopic study of reactive, degenerating, and dystrophic axons. *J Neuropath Exp Neurol* 26:345-368, 1967.
79. Friede RL, Bischausen R: The fine structure of stumps of transected nerve fibers in subserial sections. *J Neurol Sci* 44:181-187, 1980.
80. Maxwell WL: Microtubular changes in axons after stretch injuries. *J Neurotrauma* 12:363, 1995.
81. Jafari S, Maxwell WL, Neilson M, Graham DI: Axonal cytoskeletal changes after non-disruptive axonal injury. *J Neurocytol* 26:207-221, 1997.
82. Schlaepfer: Calcium induced degeneration of axoplasm in isolated segments of rat peripheral nerve. *Brain Res* 69:203-215, 1974.
83. Ballentine JD, Spector MS: Calcification of axons in experimental spinal cord trauma. *Ann Neurol*:520-523, 1977.
84. Ballentine JD: Pathology of experimental spinal cord trauma. II. Ultrastructure of axons and myelin. *Lab Invest* 39:254-266, 1978.

85. Ballentine JD: Spinal cord trauma in search of the meaning of granular axoplasm and vesicular myelin. *J Neuropath Exp Neurol* 47:77-92, 1988.

86. Maxwell WL, McGreath BJ, Graham DI, Gennarelli TA: Cytochemical evidence for redistribution of membrane pump calcium-ATPase and ecto-Ca-ATPase activity, and calcium influx into myelinated nerve fibers of the optic nerve after stretch injury. *J Neurocytol* 24:925-942, 1995.

87. Hall GF, Lee VM: Neurofilament sidearm proteolysis is a prominent effect of axotomy in lamprey giant central neurons. *J Comp Neurol* 353:38-49, 1995.

88. Pettus EH, Christman CW, Giebel ML, Povlishok JT: Traumatically induced altered membrane permeability: its relationship to traumatically induced reactive axonal change. *J Neurotrauma* 11:507-522, 1994.

89. Galant PE: The direct effects of graded axonal compression on axoplasm and fast axoplasmic transport. *J Neuropath Exp Neurol* 51:220-230, 1992.

90. Povlishok JT, Jenkins LW: Are the pathobiological changes evoked by traumatic brain injury immediate and reversible? *Brain Pathol* 5:415-426, 1995.

91. Povlishok JT: Diffuse deafferentation as the major determinant of morbidiy and recovery following traumatic brain injury. *Advances Neurotrauma Res* 2:1-11, 1990.

92. Povlishok JT: Current concepts on axonal damage due to head injury. Proceedings of the 11th International Congress of Neuropathology, 1991, pp 749-753.

93. Yamaura I, Yone K, Nakahara S, *et al*: Mechanism of destructive pathologic changes in the spinal cord under chronic mechanical compression. *Spine* 27:21-26, 2002.

94. Cohen JJ: Apoptosis. *Immunol Today* 14:126-130, 1993.

95. Majno G, Joris I: Apoptosis, oncosis, and necrosis: an overview of cell death. *Am J Pathol* 146:3-15, 1995.

96. Li GL, Brodin G, Farooque M, *et al*: Apoptosis and expression of Bcl-2 after compression trauma to rat spinal cord. *J Neuropathol Exp Neurol* 55:280-289, 1996.

97. Katoh K, Ikata T, Katoh S, *et al*: Induction and its spread of apoptosis in rat spinal cord after mechanical trauma. *Neurosci Lett* 216:9-12, 1996.

98. Crowe MJ, Bresnahan JC, Shuman SL, *et al*: Apoptosis and delayed degeneration after spinal cord injury in rats and monkeys. *Nat Med* 3:73-76, 1997.

99. Liu XZ, Xu XM, Hu R, *et al*: Neuronal and glial apoptosis after traumatic spinal cord injury. *J Neurosci* 17: 5395-5406, 1997.

100. Springer JE, Azbill RD, Knapp PE: Activation of the caspase-3 apoptotic cascade in traumatic spinal cord injury. *Nat Med* 5:943-946, 1999.

101. Grossman SD, Rosenberg LJ, Wrathall JR: Temporal-spatial pattern of acute neuronal and glial loss after spinal cord contusion. *Exp Neurol* 168:273-282, 2001.

102. Baba H, Maezawa Y, Imura S, *et al*: Quantitative analysis of the spinal cord motoneuron under chronic compression: an experimental observation. *J Neurol* 243:109-116, 1996.

103. Yamazaki M, Moriya H, Goto S, *et al*: Increased type XI collagen expression in the spinal hyperostotic mouse (twy/twy). *Calcif Tissue Intl* 48:182-189, 1991.

CHAPTER 11

Biology of Spine Fusion

L. Brett Babat and Scott D. Boden

Biology of Spine Fusion

More than 185,000 spinal arthrodeses are performed in the United States each year, the majority of which are posterolateral lumbar intertransverse process fusions. Nonunion rates for single-level fusions have been reported to be as great as 35% and higher in multiple-level procedures.[138] Pseudarthroses frequently result in less than optimal outcomes, and often necessitate further surgery. Clearly the physiologic, molecular, and mechanical requirements for successful fusion have yet to be fully elucidated.

To obtain a successful fusion, multiple factors must work in concert. These include the local environment of the fusion, systemic factors, and the possible use of fusion enhancers (Box 11.1). Mechanical and biologic factors are closely linked; any cogent discussion of the biology of spinal fusion must be limited to a particular mechanical situation. Because lumbar intertransverse process arthrodesis is the most commonly performed, this chapter focuses on fusion in this environment.

Local Factors
Graft Properties

The choice of graft material has profound implications for the success or failure of an arthrodesis. The ideal graft is osteogenic, osteoinductive, and osteoconductive.

Osteoinduction

Osteoinduction is the stimulation of multipotential stem cells to differentiate into functioning osteogenic cells. This is mediated by growth factors in the bone matrix itself. Urist introduced this concept[145,147] in his studies of the osteoinductive properties of demineralized bone matrix (DBM). Both autogenous and allograft bone are osteoinductive.

Osteogenicity

Osteogenicity refers to the presence of viable osteogenic cells, either predetermined or inducible, within the graft. These cells are important in the early stages of the fusion process, uniting graft and host bone. Only fresh autologous bone and bone marrow are osteogenic.

Osteoconduction

Osteoconductivity refers to a material's capacity to foster neovascularization and infiltration by osteogenic precursor cells via creeping substitution. A material may lack induc-

tive stimuli and viable bone precursor cells, but still be osteoconductive. Such grafts act only as scaffolding for bone healing. Calcium phosphate ceramics, coral, and collagen are such materials, whereas allograft bone is osteoconductive and osteoinductive, and autograft bone is osteoconductive, osteoinductive, and osteogenic.

Connectivity

Connectivity is the ability of an osteoconductive graft material to be "connected" to local bone. This is determined by the surface area available for incorporation into the fusion mass.

Graft Material
Autograft

Autogenous iliac crest bone is the gold standard of graft material. Historically, it has been the most successful graft source in spinal fusion.* Cancellous autograft has the requisite matrix proteins, mineral, and collagen for the ideals of osteoinductivity, osteogenicity, and osteoconductivity. Its large trabecular surface makes it highly connective as well. However, donor site complication rates as high as 25%-30% have been reported,[82] although an 8% incidence is a more commonly cited number.[150] Causes of morbidity include increased blood loss, chronic donor site pain, increased operative time, infection, and nerve injury. Furthermore, the quantity of bone is limited, and may be insufficient for long fusions, or in patients who have had previous graft harvests.

Autogenous cortical bone may be useful when structural support is needed at the graft site. Otherwise it is less desirable than cancellous bone. Because of the lack of bone marrow, there are fewer osteogenic cells. Because these cells are embedded in a compact matrix, they are less likely to survive, as diffusion of nutrients is somewhat impeded. Cortical bone has less surface area per unit weight, so there are fewer matrix proteins exposed, and connectivity is marginal. Also, vascular ingrowth is slower; the graft is therefore incorporated more slowly, and mechanical strength lags. Cancellous bone is fairly rapidly incorporated and remodeled, whereas portions of cortical graft may remain necrotic for extended periods.

When the likelihood of avascular graft healing is low, such as in previously irradiated tissue beds, vascularized grafts may be desirable. Because perfusion is interrupted for only a brief period, more osteogenic cells remain viable, and fusion occurs more readily.

Allograft

The desire to avoid donor site morbidity led to increased use of allograft bone in spine surgery. This was made practical by advances in procurement, sterilization, preparation, and storage.[46] Though widely used in spine surgery, concerns regarding fusion rates and disease transmission remain. Allograft is not osteogenic, as there are no surviving cells in the graft. Because of the processing and storage requirements of allograft, some of the osteoinductive poten-

---

*References 40,62,69,106,118,142,149.

tial of allograft is lost. Allograft carries a small but real risk of disease transmission,[20,26,32,97] and it may elicit an immune response from the recipient.[21,45]

Sterilization is not a substitute for donor screening and sterile harvesting of donor bone. The most common sterilization methods are high-dose gamma irradiation and ethylene oxide gas sterilization.[32] Both methods alter the structure of matrix proteins, decreasing the osteoinductive capacity and mechanical strength of the bone.[112] Other sterilization methods such as autoclaving are even more destructive, and are generally not used.

Before bone is harvested from a donor, a complete social and medical history must be obtained. The cause of death must be determined, and serologic and other laboratory tests need be performed. Bone must then be sterilely harvested within 24 hours of death, cultured, and processed for storage.

Immunogenicity and maintenance of osteoinductive and osteoconductive properties are affected by processing and preservation techniques. Bone is generally frozen or freeze-dried as soon as possible after harvest. Both methods decrease immunogenicity and allow for extended storage. Freezing does not diminish the mechanical properties of the bone, and it may be stored at −70°C for 5 years. Freeze-drying further reduces immunogenicity and inactivates viral agents, but reduces the mechanical strength of the graft.[111-113] However, freeze-dried bone may be stored under vacuum, at room temperature, for an indefinite period.

Although allograft has generally performed well in both cervical and lumbar interbody fusions,° in which the graft is subject to compression, the results in the posterolateral lumbar environment, in which primarily tensile forces exist, have not been as favorable.[74,88] This has led many surgeons to use allograft as an autograft expander rather than substitute, at least in posterolateral arthrodeses.

Xenograft

Bone graft taken from other species has been reported in the orthopedic literature. Despite processing, xenografts remain immunogenic and provoke a host response. The graft may be encapsulated, with resultant blockade to revascularization. Ivory and cow horn resist incorporation into host bone, and are no longer used. Bovine bone, both freeze-dried[3,61,63,116] and deproteinized,[99,126] remains weakly antigenic. Both types of this xenograft have been used in spine surgery, with mixed success. Xenograft is not generally recommended as graft material.

Ceramics

Calcium phosphate ($CaPO_4$) ceramics, including hydroxyapatite (HA) and tricalcium phosphate (TCP), have been widely used in orthopedic and spine surgery.[19] These osteoconductive, biodegradable materials are compatible with the remodeling of bone necessary to achieve optimal strength. Other, nonresorbable materials remain in the fusion mass, leaving permanent stress risers and prolonging strength deficiencies.

To be useful as a graft material, synthetics must have several properties. They must be compatible with local tissues, remain chemically stable in body fluids, and be able to withstand sterilization. Furthermore, they must be available in useful shapes and sizes, be cost-effective, and have reliable quality control. $CaPO_4$ ceramics qualify,[45,71,107] and have been widely used in dentistry and maxillofacial surgery,[30,35,71,77] as well as in animal models.[65-69,101] They have also been used in humans.°

Both HA and TCP ceramics are brittle. They may be prepared as either compact or porous materials. The greater crystallinity and density of the compact forms results in greater strength and resistance to dissolution *in vivo*. However, the more porous versions more nearly approximate the interconnectivity of cancellous bone, enhancing bone ingrowth at the expense of more rapid degradation. Under physiologic conditions, HA is resorbed very slowly, whereas TCP is generally resorbed within 6 weeks of implantation.[74]

Natural coral has been used to augment or even replace autograft, with some success.[27,54,117,124] The calcium carbonate ($CaCO_3$) in coral is hydrothermally converted to $CaPO_4$. The structural geometry of coral is similar to cancellous bone, making it highly osteoconductive and connective. There is no risk of disease transmission.

$CaPO_4$ ceramic use as a spine fusion bone graft substitute has been studied in animal models. Flatley *et al.*[45] used porous blocks of a 1:1 ratio of calcium HA and TCP ceramic in a rabbit posterolateral fusion model. At 12 weeks, histologic sections demonstrated bone ingrowth reaching the central portion of the block. There was no fibrous barrier between the new bone and the ceramic. Holmes *et al.*[67] used coralline HA in a canine posterior/facet model. Although the distribution of bone ingrowth was similar to that seen in autograft controls, Holmes *et al.* reported no solid fusions, even at 6 months. Using coral porites (calcium carbonate) and a 65:35 HA:TCP biphasic ceramic, Guigui and colleagues[53] found a 100% rate of fusion in a sheep model. These results must be carefully interpreted in light of a 100% rate of fusion with autograft in that same model.[52]

°References 8,17,29,59,89,92,121.

°References 18,19,67,108,123,132.

The use of composites of ceramic and an osteoinductive agent such as DBM, autograft, or recombinant bone morphogenetic protein (BMP) has also been investigated.[101,141,146] Ragni and Lindholm,[119] in a rabbit interbody fusion model, found that the addition of DBM enhanced the incorporation of an HA block. Animals treated with an HA/DBM composite showed significantly earlier fusion consolidation than those treated with autograft or either HA or DBM alone. By 6 months, however, results of autograft were comparable to those with the composite. Zerwekh et al.[154] compared a collagen/HA-TCP ceramic/autograft composite with autograft alone in a canine posterior fusion model. Histologic comparisons of bone ingrowth were similar in both groups at 12 months, as were the results of biomechanical testing. Working in a canine segmental posterior spine fusion model, Muschler and colleagues[102] compared fusions with autograft, collagen/HA-TCP ceramic composite, collagen/HA-TCP ceramic/autograft composite, collagen/HA-TCP ceramic/ bone matrix protein composite, and with no graft. Autograft had a significantly superior union score. Ceramic composite alone performed no better than the no-graft control. The addition of bone matrix protein, however, improved the union score, making it comparable to the composite/autograft treatment.

The clinical efficacy of ceramics, either alone or as part of a composite, has not been established. Passuti et al.,[108] in a study of 12 severely scoliotic patients, used internal fixation and blocks of 3:2 HA-TCP ceramic alone or mixed with autogenous cancellous bone. After 15 months' average follow-up, radiographs demonstrated fusion in all patients. Histologic examination of biopsy material from two of the subjects revealed new bone formed directly on the ceramic surface, and ingrowth into the macropores. Similarly, Pouliquen et al.[117] successfully used natural coral as a graft substitute in 49 patients with idiopathic scoliosis. Although the results were favorable, their small patient populations, single diagnosis, and average patient age of 14 limited these studies. The use of ceramics and composites as a graft replacement or extender holds promise in spinal fusion. More work is needed to determine the efficacy in both anterior and posterior fusion environments, especially in primates, and, ultimately, in human beings.

Mechanical Stability

Fusion rate is affected by the mechanical stability of the involved segments.[57,93-95,104,153] Therefore internal fixation has been the most commonly used approach to increase fusion rates. Several studies have demonstrated more frequent union with the use of instrumentation.* However, nonunion still occurs in 10% to 15% of patients so treated,[16,98,149,151] especially when hardware loosening or failure occurs.[4] Fusion level, number of segments involved, patient weight and activity level, and postoperative bracing[131] all influence the rate of fusion.

The effects of spinal instrumentation and stability have most commonly been investigated with in vitro models.[55,56,73,96,148] Although this approach can tell us much about short-term effects, caution must be exercised in

extrapolating to the clinical situation. Bench-top testing cannot account for the interaction of instrumentation with the biology of fusion. Animal models provide a method to study this complex relationship in vivo.

McAfee et al. created a canine instability model to study both the effect of spinal instrumentation on fusion success[57,93,153] and the radiographic incidence of fusion with respect to spinal stability.[57,93-95] At 6 months, radiographs revealed a greater probability of fusion in the instrumented animals than in the noninstrumented animals. The instrumented fusions were also more rigid. Likewise, Zdeblick et al.[153] demonstrated both an increased rate of fusion and a more rigid fusion when anterior instrumentation was used in a coonhound model of an unstable L5 burst fracture. These results were replicated by Shirado.[133] Kotani et al.[78] showed that, even after solid posterolateral arthrodesis was achieved in a sheep model, transpedicular fixation continued to provide mechanical support.

The biologic activity of the graft material may partly determine the need for internal fixation. Fuller et al.[39,48] showed that rigid fixation improved bone ingrowth into a calcium carbonate block in a canine anterior thoracic interbody fusion model. Because ceramics are not osteoinductive, a mechanically stable environment is crucial for ingrowth. Osteoinductive graft substitutes may not be as reliant on construct rigidity.

Nagel et al.[104] developed a sheep model of delayed union and nonunion. Posterior lumbar laminar and facet fusions with iliac crest graft were performed on seven sheep. Six of the seven sheep developed nonunions at the L6-S1 interspace; all cephalad interspaces fused (21 of 21). Eight normal sheep underwent in vivo flexion/extension radiographs. Five normal sheep spines were studied ex vivo, using displacement transducers to test stiffness, displacement, and strain in flexion/extension. The lumbosacral level demonstrated significantly more motion than the other levels, suggesting that motion was a major factor in determining the success of fusion in this sheep model. Similar observations have been made in dogs.[70] The increased stability and decreased motion that instrumentation provides would seem valuable in such instances.

Fusion success is also affected by the physical stresses placed on the graft.[41] In human beings, 80% of the load at a motion segment is transmitted through the intervertebral disc. Graft placed ventrally, in the interbody region, is thus primarily subjected to compression. This compressive force promotes fusion, presumably by stimulating vascular ingrowth and the proliferation of mesenchymal cells. Dorsally placed graft experiences tensile forces, as does graft placed in the intertransverse process region, though less so. Under these less favorable mechanical conditions, fusion is more dependent on biologic factors.

Facet preparation for fusion has been shown to increase motion of the involved segment. Although many surgeons routinely include facet fusion in posterolateral intertransverse process arthrodeses, biomechanical studies have demonstrated a resultant decrease in stability[1,12] The developing fusion mass is thus subjected to increased strain, perhaps predisposing to nonunion. However, exclusion of the facets from fusion preparation decreases the surface area incorporated into the fusion mass, and may result in a less rigid fusion. Rigid instrumentation allows

*References 16,57,93,94,151,153.

the facets to be prepared and incorporated, without sacrificing stability. However, in the osteoporotic patient, the screw/bone interface is often weak. Even with instrumentation, facet preparation may not be appropriate in these individuals.

Contradictory human studies of the effects of spinal instrumentation have been widely reported. Zdeblick[151] discussed 124 patients fused for different conditions. Patients were randomized into three groups, all having dorsolateral autograft fusions. Patients in group 1 were not instrumented, those in group 2 were instrumented with a semirigid pedicle screw system, and individuals in group 3 had rigid pedicle screw instrumentation implanted. The rigid group had a significantly higher fusion rate (95%) than the noninstrumented group (65%). The instrumented groups together had 95% excellent or good results, whereas the noninstrumented patients had only 71% good or excellent outcomes, a significant difference.

Bridwell et al.[16] described 44 patients with degenerative spondylolisthesis. Patients were individualized into three groups: no fusion; noninstrumented posterolateral fusion; and pedicle screw instrumented posterolateral fusion. Patients with more than 10 degrees or 3mm of motion were automatically assigned to the instrumentation group. There was an 87% fusion rate in the instrumented group, versus a 30% rate in the noninstrumented patients. There was no significant clinical difference in successful outcomes between the noninstrumented and unfused group (30% versus 33%). Successful outcomes in the instrumented group, 83%, were significantly greater. This is in stark contrast to the report of Fischgrund et al.[43] Although they demonstrated a markedly increased rate of fusion in their instrumented patients (83% versus 45% in the noninstrumented fusions), they found no difference in clinical outcome.

The meta-analysis of Mardjetko et al.[90] reviewed 25 papers describing 889 patients with degenerative spondylolisthesis. Five of the included studies described patients undergoing decompression and posterolateral arthrodesis with pedicle screw instrumentation. Although there was a trend toward an increased rate of fusion in the instrumented versus noninstrumented patients (93% versus 86%), it did not reach significance ($p = .08$). The clinical outcome was better in the uninstrumented group: 90% versus 86%. However, the authors acknowledged several limitations of their review: data from different treatments over 20 years, variable study designs and quality, and possible dilution of data from the stronger, better-designed studies that suggested an advantage to instrumentation.

Overall, it is generally agreed that spinal instrumentation decreases the rate of pseudarthrosis. However, there are situations, especially with single-level fusions, in which there may be no significant clinical benefit obtained.

Graft Site Preparation

Preparation of the bony anatomy into which the graft is placed is of paramount importance to achieving a successful fusion. The exposed area of viable, vascular bone should be maximized. This is done by decortication, which may be accomplished with curettes, rongeurs, osteotomes, or a power burr. Use of a high-speed burr may result in thermal

necrosis. This may be minimized with continuous irrigation, use of a burr with deep flutes, and minimizing contact time between burr and bone. As the surface area of decorticated bone increases, so, too, do connectivity and the availability of osteogenic cells and exposed matrix proteins. Furthermore, a large surface is helpful in forming a bony bridge strong enough to carry the mechanical load.

Soft-Tissue Bed

Spine fusion depends on the influx of osteoprogenitor and inflammatory cells. The local soft tissues must support bone graft healing. An adequate blood supply is a critical requirement for success. Fusion bed vasculature supplies nutrients to the maturing fusion, provides endocrine stimuli, and is a source of inflammatory and osteoprogenitor cells. Nonviable and traumatized tissues should be removed from the graft site.

Hurley et al.[70] evaluated the role of local soft tissues in a canine dorsal spine fusion model. Thirty-seven animals underwent a modified Hibbs fusion (control), a Hibbs fusion with a fluid-permeable, cell impermeable membrane interposed between fusion site and muscle mass, or with a membrane impermeable to both cells and fluids. All 12 animals with the semipermeable membrane fused; none of the 10 animals with the impermeable membrane did so.

Radiation has a detrimental effect on a healing spine fusion, especially in the first few postoperative weeks. This effect may be caused by cytotoxicity, but is probably also the product of the resultant intense vasculitis and inhibition of angiogenesis. Even after the acute injury, radiation-induced osteonecrosis and dense, hypovascular scars make for a poor fusion environment. Studies suggest that a 3- to 6-week delay in radiation would be beneficial to the fusion process.[15,38] Use of vascularized grafts anastomosed to nonirradiated vessels may also increase the chance of successful fusion.

Systemic Factors
Nicotine

Smokers have a higher rate of pseudarthrosis than do nonsmokers.[8,17,60,81,98] Cigarette smoke retards osteogenesis and inhibits graft revascularization. Tobacco smoke extracts cause calcitonin resistance,[64] increase fracture end resorption,[82] and interfere with osteoblastic function.[34]

A direct relationship between systemic nicotine and spinal pseudarthrosis has been demonstrated in a rabbit model. Silcox et al.[134] performed L5-6 posterolateral intertransverse process arthrodeses with autologous iliac crest graft in 28 rabbits. The animals were implanted with osmotic mini-pumps, delivering either saline (control), or nicotine equivalent to a human who smokes one to one-and-a-half packs per day. At 5 weeks, 56% of control animals had a solid fusion by manual palpation; no solid fusions were seen in the nicotine-exposed animals ($p = .02$).

Drugs

Drugs taken during the perioperative period can have a detrimental effect on the process of fusion. Chemotherapeutic agents administered in the early postoperative period inhibit bone formation and arthrodesis.[22,47,105] Nonsteroidal anti-inflammatory drugs (NSAIDs) suppress the inflammatory response, and may inhibit spinal fusion.[83]

Dimar and colleagues[36] performed three-level dorsal fusions in 39 rats. Half the animals received indomethacin, 3mg/kg/day, 6 of 7 days, and the other animals received saline. Treatment was started one week preoperatively, and continued for 12 weeks after surgery. In the control rats 27 of 60 levels achieved solid or moderate fusions, whereas only four of 42 levels were similarly fused in the indomethacin group ($p < .001$). However, the model that was used had not been well characterized, assessment of fusion was not rigidly defined, and the indomethacin dose was significantly greater on a mg/kg basis than that used in human beings.

Glassman et al.[49] performed a retrospective review of 288 patients who had undergone L4-S1 instrumented, autologous iliac crest graft spinal fusions. Ketorolac had been administered to 167 of them; the remaining 121 did not receive NSAIDs. Using surgical exploration, hardware failure, and tomograms to determine fusion, they found 4% pseudarthroses in the control group, versus 17% in the ketorolac group ($p < .001$). The odds ratio indicated that nonunion was approximately five times more likely in those individuals who received ketorolac. There are several problems with this study, however. Among them, it is unclear whether one or multiple surgeons were involved. Also, patients received varying numbers of ketorolac doses, beginning at different postoperative times. However, their results are supported by Martin and colleagues,[91] who, working in a rabbit model, compared fusion in animals receiving ketorolac or saline. They found 35% fusions in the ketorolac-treated animals versus 75% in the controls ($p = .037$).

Recently, a new class of NSAIDs has been introduced. These new drugs are specific for the cyclo-oxygenase 2 (COX-2) isoform of the enzyme targeted by NSAIDs. Long and colleagues[86] investigated the effect of orally administered celecoxib (a COX-2 inhibitor) on spinal fusion in the rabbit model. They compared rabbits receiving celecoxib 10mg/kg daily with groups receiving either indomethacin 10mg/kg or saline. They found a significant difference between the rate of fusion in controls and that in the indomethacin group. Celecoxib animals fused at an intermediate rate. Although the celecoxib rate was not significantly different from saline controls (45% versus 64%), it was not significantly different from indomethacin (18%) either. Regardless, the study is limited by its small size, as well as the relatively high dose of indomethacin. Furthermore, as celecoxib is more rapidly metabolized in rabbits than in human beings, the dose used was low relative to the clinical situation.

Osteoporosis

The most common metabolic bone disease in the United States, osteoporosis is commonly assumed to be a negative factor in bone healing. The decreased bone density that is the hallmark of osteoporosis makes stabilization with instrumentation difficult in this population. Additionally, there may be changes in marrow quality and bone turnover rate. Older animals have a decreased capacity for osteoin-duction.[72] In terms of fusion potential, a decrease in the number of osteogenic stem cells in the elderly may be more important than absolute bone mass.

Hormones

Hormones affect bone formation both directly and indirectly, and are likely to influence spinal fusion as well. These chemical messengers have complex interactions with bone-forming and absorbing cells, both positive and negative.

Growth hormone, via somatomedins, exerts a stimulatory effect on cartilage and bone formation.[114,115] In vivo growth hormone stimulates bone healing by increasing gastrointestinal absorption of calcium, as well as by increasing bone formation and mineralization.[100,143] Thyroid hormone, which acts synergistically with growth hormone, is required for somatomedin synthesis by the liver. Furthermore, thyroid hormone has a direct stimulatory effect on cartilage growth and maturation, thereby positively influencing bone healing.

Corticosteroids have been shown both experimentally and clinically to be detrimental to bone healing, increasing bone resorption and decreasing formation. Corticosteroids have been shown to both inhibit and to promote osteoblastic differentiation,[58,75] as well as to decrease the synthesis of bone matrix.[31]

Estrogens and androgens play important roles in skeletal maturation, as well as in the prevention of age-associated bone loss. Their effects on bone healing, however, remain controversial. Some studies indicate they may stimulate bone formation,[5] whereas most others do not support this.[80,120] Neither affects bone collagen synthesis,[25] but estrogens may increase bone mineralization by increasing serum levels of parathyroid hormone and vitamin D_3.

Fusion Enhancers
Electrical Stimulation

Since 1974, when Dwyer et al.[37] first demonstrated improved spinal fusion rates, electrical stimulation has been increasingly accepted as an aid to spinal fusion. Since that time, direct current electrical stimulation (DCES), pulsed electromagnetic fields (PEMFs), and combined magnetic fields (CMFs) have been shown to have varying effectiveness.

DCES uses an implanted generator that delivers a constant 20 to 40 microampere current to the fusion bed, for 6 to 9 months. The effective stimulation area is 5 to 8mm from the cathode. Although the exact mechanism of action is not fully understood, several physiologic effects have been demonstrated. The current attracts charged proteins by electrophoresis, bone, cartilage, and endothelial cells by galvanotaxis, and depolarizes cell membranes. Faradic reactions at the bone/electrode interface reduce oxygen tension and increase pH, similar to that seen at the growth plate and in healing fractures. Increased pH has been shown to increase osteoblastic bone formation and to inhibit resorption by osteoclasts.[6,144]

PEMF devices generate an electromagnetic field across the fusion area via external coils that are worn from

3 to 8 hours per day for 3 to 6 months. A varying magnetic field induces an electric current, which is hypothesized to stimulate bone healing, possibly by depolarizing cell membranes and increasing calcium influx into bone cells.[24,42,44] Regardless of the exact mechanism, PEMFs have been shown to increase the levels of BMP-2 and BMP-4 in rat calvarial cells.[9,125]

The CMF device is also worn externally, usually for 30 minutes per day. It combines a static magnetic field with a time-variable field. Although animal data showed increased bone stiffness at the 30-minute dose, the effect was far greater with 24-hour per day treatment.[137]

Kane[76] published the first large multicenter study of the use of DCES in dorsolateral spinal fusion. Eighty-two patients treated with DCES were compared to a historical control population of 150 patients fused without electrical stimulation. The DCES group had a 91% fusion rate, significantly higher than the 81% in the controls. Of note, the DCES group had a significantly higher rate of revision surgery for pseudarthroses. The report also described a prospective, randomized control study in a "difficult to fuse" population of patients who had failed one or more previous attempts at fusion, were undergoing multilevel arthrodeses, had grade II or higher spondylolisthesis, or had other risk factors. The 31 patients in the stimulation group had a significantly higher fusion rate of 81%, compared with 54% of the 28 patients in the control population.

Recent work has lent further support to the use of DCES in dorsolateral spinal fusion. Reports indicate that DCES increases the percentage rate of fusion in dorsolateral, pedicle screw instrumented fusions, from the mid-80s to the mid-90s.[79,122] Furthermore, DCES has been shown to increase the fusion rate in smokers from 66% to 83%.[79]

Simmons[135] was the first to report on the use of PEMF in spinal fusion. He described treatment of pseudarthroses after posterior lumbar interbody fusion in 13 patients, 77% of whom progressed to fusion without further surgery. In the more demanding environment of posterior pseudarthroses Lee[84] reported a 67% success rate with PEMF.

Linovitz et al.[85] recently reported a double-blind, randomized, placebo-controlled trial of the use of CMF in noninstrumented fusions. The study found 64% of patients with active devices had fused by 9 months, compared with 43% of patients with placebo devices. However, stratification by gender showed that the difference was only significant for the female patients in the study. The reasons for this remain unclear.

Although there seems to be support for the use of electrical stimulation in spine fusion, not all modalities are equally effective. Currently, DCES appears to have the greatest effect. Furthermore, all these devices carry a substantial monetary cost. The determination of the patients that would best be served by their use has yet to be fully elucidated.

Growth Factors

BMPs are a group of proteins belonging to the TGF-β family. During the more than 35 years since they were first described by Urist,[145] they have been found to play important roles in both endochondral and intramembranous bone formation, as well as in fracture healing. Recently, there has been much attention paid to a possible role for these proteins in spinal fusion.

BMPs bind to receptors on multiple cell types, including osteoblasts, osteoclasts, and mesenchymal stem cells. Their effects are exerted through a second messenger system, leading to, at low concentrations, cartilage formation; at higher levels, direct bone formation is fostered. This bone is histologically and mechanically normal.

Several BMP preparations are in or are nearly in clinical evaluation. Recombinant human BMP-2 (rhBMP-2) and BMP-7 (rhBMP-7), which is more commonly termed osteogenic protein-1 (OP-1), are manufactured by recombinant DNA techniques, and are pure preparations. A third preparation, bovine BMP extract (bBMPx), is derived from bovine bone, and thus contains several different BMPs, along with other proteins.

Animal Studies

There have been many studies evaluating the feasibility and efficacy of achieving spinal arthrodeses with BMPs.[129] Cook et al.,[28] using OP-1 in a canine facet and interlaminar fusion model, obtained solid fusions in 12 weeks, as compared with 26 weeks for autogenous graft. In a similar model Muschler et al.[103] found no difference between autograft and rhBMP-2 at 3 months, though the model was criticized for its intrinsic high-fusion rate.

A canine intertransverse-process fusion model demonstrated solid fusion with rhBMP-2 within 3 months, whereas autologous iliac crest graft animals had not fused at this point.[127] This same model was used to demonstrate that rhBMP-2 could produce solid fusions *without decortication*.[128] Using the rabbit intertransverse-process fusion model they developed, Schimandle and Boden[130] achieved 100% fusion with rhBMP-2, compared with 42% fusion in the autograft group. rhBMP-2 was further able to overcome the inhibitory effect of ketorolac in the same model.[91] Working in the same model, Grauer et al.[51] and Patel et al.[110] established that OP-1 has the same effects, but required a higher dose of BMP.

Several studies have examined the effectiveness of these agents in nonhuman primates. Boden et al.[13] tested bBMPx in the lumbar spine of adult rhesus monkeys. Four of the four animals implanted with 3mg or more of the bovine protein achieved a posterolateral intertransverse process fusion, whereas none of the six animals implanted with a lower dose fused. However, a second study[33] demonstrated only 40% fusion with this same dose, and 54% with a 5mg dose, though the autograft animals showed only 21% fusion.

Boden et al.[11] reported the use of rhBMP-2 with a hydroxyapatite/tricalcium phosphate carrier for posterolateral fusions in the rhesus monkey. All rhBMP-2 concentrations resulted in solid fusions, whereas none of the autograft animals fused. They have since developed carriers with better handling characteristics, with the same excellent results in the rabbit and monkey models.[139,140]

Human Studies

A safety and efficacy study of OP-1 for posterolateral spinal arthrodesis has been completed in human beings.[109]

Sixteen patients with degenerative spondylolisthesis, undergoing noninstrumented posterolateral fusion, were randomized to receive either autograft and OP-1, or autograft alone. At 6 months, nine of the 12 autograft/OP-1 patients had fused, versus only two of four autograft alone patients, though the difference was not statistically significant. Clinically, 83% of the OP-1 patients had 20% or better improvement in their Oswestry score, whereas only 50% of the autograft alone patients had this level of success. Again, the difference was not statistically significant. Of note, OP-1 had no adverse effects.

Speck[136] presented preliminary results of an ongoing Australian OP-1 study in which patients with degenerative spondylolisthesis undergo decompression, followed by noninstrumented posterolateral fusion with autograft on one side, and OP-1 putty contralaterally. Computed tomographic (CT) scans of the fusion masses of five patients at 6 months show equal or greater bone formation on the OP-1 side than seen on the autograft side.

Several clinical studies of rhBMP-2 in human beings have either been completed or are ongoing.* Only Luque[87] and Boden et al.,[10] however, have published clinical studies of rhBMP-2 in the posterolateral fusion environment. Luque examined two patient cohorts in a prospective, randomized, open-label trial of rhBMP-2, with a biphasic calcium phosphate (BCP) carrier in patients undergoing single-level lumbar fusions for degenerative instability. The first group (seven patients) received rhBMP-2/BCP unilaterally, with autograft on the contralateral side. Eighty-six percent of the rhBMP-2 sides fused by 12 months, whereas only 57% of the autograft-treated sides fused. The second group received a higher rhBMP-2/BCP dose bilaterally, without autograft; at 12 months, 100% had fused. Oswestry scores improved by 15 or more points in 85.7% of Cohort 1 patients and in 100% of Cohort 2 individuals. Boden et al.[10] performed a prospective randomized clinical pilot trial of rhBMP-2 with BCP carrier versus autograft. All 20 patients with BMP-2 and the BCP carrier had solid fusions judged by CT scans, as evaluated independently. Nine of these patients had no internal fixation. The BMP-2 patients did better than autograft patients, in terms of fusion success and clinical outcome.

The use of osteoinductive factors in spine surgery is in its infancy. It appears that they may provide an effective alternative to the current gold standard, autograft, and may perhaps improve on it. The role these factors will play in spine surgery will be increasingly elucidated in the near future.

---

*References 2,7,12,14,23,50,152.

REFERENCES

1. Abumi K, Panjabi MM, Kramer KM, et al: Biomechanical evaluation of lumbar spinal stability after graded facetectomy. *Spine* 15(11):1142-1147, 1990.
2. Alexander J, Branch C, Haid R, et al: An analysis of the use of rhBMP-2 in PLIF constructs: Clinical and radiographic outcomes. Presented at the 18th Annual Meeting of the American Association of Neurological Surgeons and Congress of Neurological Surgeons Section on Disorders of the Spine and Peripheral Nerves. Orlando, Fl, Feb 27-Mar 2, 2002, p26.
3. Anderson K, LeCocq J, Mooney J: Clinical evaluation of processed heterologous bone transplants. *Clin Orthop* 29:248-263, 1963.
4. Aurori B, Weierman R, Lowell H, et al: Pseudarthrosis after spinal fusion for scoliosis: a comparison of autogeneic and allogeneic bone grafts. *Clin Orthop* 199:153-158, 1985.
5. Baran D, Bergfeld M, Teitelbaum S, et al: Effect of testosterone therapy on bone formation in an osteoporotic hypogonadal male. *Calcif Tissue Res* 26:103-106, 1978.
6. Baranowski T, Black J: The mechanism of faradic stimulation of osteogenesis. In Blank M, Findle E (eds): *Mechanistic Approaches to Interactions of Electrical and Electromagnetic Fields with Living Systems*. New York, Plenum Press,1987, p. 399.
7. Baskin D, Ryan P, Westmark R, et al: ACDFP with Cornerstone-SR (allograft and plate: rhBMP-2 vs. autograft). Presented at the 18th Annual Meeting of the American Association of Neurological Surgeons and Congress of Neurological Surgeons Section on Disorders of the Spine and Peripheral Nerves. Orlando, Feb 27-Mar 2, 2002:26.
8. Blumenthal, Baker, Dossett, et al: The role of anterior lumbar fusion for internal disc disruption. *Spine* 13: 566-569, 1988.
9. Bodamyali T, Bhatt B, Hughes F, et al: Pulsing electromagnetic fields simultaneously induce osteogenesis and upregulate transcription of bone morphogenetic proteins 2 and 4 in rat osteoblasts in vitro. *Biochem Biophys Res Commun* 250:485-491, 1998.
10. Boden SD, Kang J, Sandhu H, Heller JG: Use of recombinant human bone morphogenetic protein-2 to achieve posterolateral lumbar spine fusion in humans: a prospective and randomized clinical pilot trial: 2002 Volvo Award in clinical studies. *Spine* 27:2662-2673, 2002.
11. Boden S, Martin G, Morone M, et al: Posterolateral lumbar intertransverse process spine arthrodesis with recombinant human bone morphogenetic protein-2/hydroxyapatite-tricalcium phosphate after laminectomy in the nonhuman primate. *Spine* 24: 1179-1185, 1999.
12. Boden S, Martin C, Rudolph R, et al: Increase of motion between lumbar vertebrae after excision of the capsule and cartilage of the facets. *J Bone Joint Surg (Am)* 76:1847-1853, 1994.
13. Boden S, Schimandle J, Hutton W: Evaluation of a bovine-derived osteoinductive bone protein in a non-human primate model of lumbar spinal fusion. *Trans Orthop Res Soc* 21:118, 1996.
14. Boden S, Zdeblick T, Sandhu H, et al: The use of rhBMP-2 in interbody fusion cages. *Spine* 25:376-381, 2000.
15. Bouchard J, Koka A, Bensusan J, et al: Effects of irradiation on posterior spinal fusions: a rabbit model. *Spine* 19:1836-1841, 1994.
16. Bridwell K, Sedgewick T, O'Brien M, et al: The role of fusion and instrumentation in the treatment of degenerative spondylolisthesis with spinal stenosis. *J Spinal Disord* 6:461-472, 1993.

17. Brown M, Makanin T, Davis P: A roentgenographic evaluation of frozen allografts versus autografts in anterior cervical spine fusions. *Clin Orthop* 119:231-236, 1976.

18. Bucholz R Clinical experience with bone graft substitutes. *Orthop Clin North Am* 18:323-334, 1987.

19. Bucholz R, Carlton A, Holmes R Hydroxyapatite and tricalcium phosphate bone graft substitutes. *Orthop Clin North Am* 18:323-334, 1987.

20. Buck B, Malinin T, Brown M: Bone transplantation and human immunodeficiency virus. *Clin Orthop* 240:129-136, 1989.

21. Burchardt H, Enneking W: Transplantation of bone. *Surg Clin North Am* 58:403-427, 1978.

22. Burchardt H, Golwczewskie F, Enneking W: The effect of adriamycin and methotrexate on the repair of segmental cortical autografts in dogs. *J Bone Joint Surg* 65:103-108, 1983.

23. Burkus J, Transfeldt E, Kitchel S, *et al*: *A Prospective Randomized Study Assessing the Clinical and Radiographic Outcomes of Patients Treated with Rhbmp-2 and Threaded Cortical Bone Dowels in the Lumbar Spine*. New Orleans, NASS, 2000, p 1114.

24. Cain C, Adey W, Luben R: Evidence that pulsed electromagnetic fields inhibit coupling of parathyroid hormone in bone cells. *J Bone Joint Surg* 30:302-312, 1948.

25. Canalis E, Raisz L: Effect of sex steroids on bone collagen synthesis in vitro. *Calcif Tissue Res* 25:105-110, 1978.

26. Centers for Disease Control. Transmission of HIV through bone transplantation: Case report and public health recommendations. *JAMA* 260:2487-2488, 1988.

27. Chiroff R, White E, Weber J, *et al*: Tissue ingrowth of replamineform implants. *J Biomed Res Symp* 6:29-45, 1975.

28. Cook S, Dalton J, Tan E, *et al*: In vivo evaluation of recombinant human osteogenic protein (rhOP-1) implants as a bone graft substitute for spinal fusions. *Spine* 19:1655, 1994.

29. Cloward R: Gas-sterilized cadaver bone grafts for spinal fusion operations: a simplified bone bank. *Spine* 5:4-10, 1980.

30. Coviello J, Brilliant J: A preliminary study on the use of tricalcium phosphate as an apical barrier. *J Endocrinol* 5:6-13, 1979.

31. Cruess R, Sakai T: Effect of cortisone upon synthesis rates of some components of rat matrix. *Clin Orthop* 86: 253-259, 1972.

32. Czitrom A: Principles and techniques of tissue banking. In Heckman J (ed): *AAOS Instructional Course Lectures*, ed 42. Rosemont, IL, AAOS, 1993, pp 359-362.

33. Damien C, Grob D, Boden S, *et al*: Purified bovine BMP extract and collagen for spine arthrodesis: Preclinical safety and efficacy. *Spine* 27(16S):S50-S58, 2002.

34. de Vernejoul M, Bielakoff J, Herve M, *et al*: Evidence for defective osteoblastic function: a role for alcohol and tobacco consumption in osteoporosis in middle-aged men. *Clin Orthop* 179:107-115, 1983.

35. Denissen H, deGroot K: Immediate dental root implants from synthetic dense calcium hydroxylapatite. *J Prosthet Dent* 42:551-556, 1979.

36. Dimar J, Ante W, Zhang, *et al*: The effects of nonsteroidal anti-inflammatory drugs on posterior spinal fusions in the rat. *Spine* 21:870-876, 1996.

37. Dwyer AF, Yau AC, Jefcoat KW: Use of direct current in spine fusion. *J Bone Joint Surg* (A) 56:442, 1974.

38. Emery S, Brazinski M, Koka A, *et al*: The biological and biomechanical effects of irradiation on anterior spinal bone grafts: a canine model. *J Bone Joint Surg (Am)* 76:540-548, 1994.

39. Emery S, Fuller D, Stevenson S: Ceramic anterior spinal fusion: biological and biomechanical comparison in a canine model. *Spine* 22:2713-2719, 1996.

40. Enneking W, Burchardt H, Puhl J, *et al*: Physical and biological aspects of repair in dog cortical bone transplants. *J Bone Joint Surg (Am)* 57:237-252, 1975.

41. Evans J: Biomechanics of lumbar fusion. *Clin Orthop* 193:38-46, 1985.

42. Fernier R, Ross S, Kanehisa J, *et al*: Osteoclasts and osteoblasts migration in opposite directions in response to a constant magnetic field. *J Cell Physiol* 129:283-288, 1986.

43. Fischgrund J, Mackay M, Herkowitz H, *et al*: Degenerative lumbar spondylolisthesis with spinal stenosis: a prospective, randomized study comparing decompressive laminectomy and arthrodesis with and without spinal instrumentation. *Spine* 22:2807-2812, 1997.

44. Fitzsimmons R, Strong D, Mohan S, *et al*: Four-amplitude, low frequency electrical field-stimulated bone cell proliferation may in part be mediated by increased IGF-II release. *J Cell Physiol* 150:84-89, 1992.

45. Flatley T, Lynch K, Benson M: Tissue response to implants of calcium phosphate ceramic in the rabbit spine. *Clin Orthop* 179:246-252, 1983.

46. Friedlander G: Current concepts review: bone banking. *J Bone Joint Surg (Am)* 48:915-923, 1966.

47. Friedlander G, Tross R, Doganis A, *et al*: Effects of chemotherapeutic agents on bone. I. Short-term methotrexate and doxorubicin (Adriamycin) treatment in a rat model. *J Bone Joint Surg (Am)* 66:602-607, 1984.

48. Fuller D, Stevenson S, Emery S: The effects of internal fixation on calcium carbonate: Ceramic anterior spinal fusion in dogs. *Spine* 21:2131-2136, 1996.

49. Glassman S, Rose S, Dimar J, *et al*: The effect of postoperative anti-inflammatory administration on spinal fusion. *Spine* 23:834-838, 1998.

50. Gornet M, Burkus K, Dickman C, *et al*: rhBMP-2 with tapered cages: a prospective randomized lumbar fusion study. NASS, 2001.

51. Grauer J, Patel T, Erulkar J, *et al*: Evaluation of OP-1 as a graft substitute for intertransverse process lumbar fusion. *Spine* 26:127-133, 2001.

52. Guigui P, Plais P, Flautre B, *et al*: Experimental model of posterolateral spinal arthrodesis in sheep. Part 1. Experimental procedures and results with autologous bone graft. *Spine* 19:2791-2797, 1994.

53. Guigui P, Plais P, Flautre B, *et al*: Experimental model of posterolateral spinal arthrodesis in sheep. Part 2. Application of the model: Evaluation of vertebral fusion obtained with coral (Porites) or with a biphasic ceramic (Triosite). *Spine* 19:2798-2803, 1994.

54. Guillemin G, Meunier A, Dallant P, *et al*: Comparison of coral resorption and bone apposition with two natural corals of different porosities. *J Biomed Mater Res* 23: 765-779, 1989.

55. Gurr K, McAfee P, Shih C: Biomechanical analysis of anterior and posterior instrumentation systems after

corpectomy: a calf spine model. *J Bone Joint Surg (Am)* 70:1182-1191, 1988.

56. Gurr K, McAfee P, Shih C: Biomechanical analysis of posterior instrumentation systems after decompressive laminectomy. *J Bone Joint Surg (Am)* 70:680-691, 1988.

57. Gurr K, McAfee P, Warden K, *et al*: Roentgenographic and biomechanical analysis of lumbar fusions: a canine model. *J Orthop Res* 7:838-848, 1989.

58. Hahn T: Corticosteroid-induced osteopenia. *Arch Intern Med* 138:882-885, 1978.

59. Hanley E Jr, Harvell J, Shapiro, *et al*: Use of allograft bone in cervical spine surgery. *Sem Spine Surg* 1:262-270, 1989.

60. Hanley E Jr, Levy J: Surgical treatment of isthmic lumbosacral spondylolisthesis: Analysis of variables affecting results. *Spine* 14:48-50, 1989.

61. Harmon P: Processed heterologous bone implants (Boplant, Squibb) as grafts in surgery. *Acta Orthop Scand* 35:98-116, 1964.

62. Heiple K, Chase S, Herndon C: A comparative study of the healing process following different types of bone transplantation. *J Bone Joint Surg (Am)* 45:1593-1616, 1963.

63. Heiple K, Kendrick R, Herndon C, *et al*: A critical evaluation of processed calf bone. *J Bone Joint Surg* 49:1119-1127, 1967.

64. Hollo I, Gergely I, Boross M: Smoking results in calcitonin resistance. *JAMA* 237:2470, 1977.

65. Holmes R: Bone regeneration within a coralline hydroxyapatite implant. *Plast Reconstr Surg* 63:626-633, 1979.

66. Holmes R, Bucholtz R, Mooney V: Porous hydroxyapatite as a bone graft substitute in diaphyseal defects. *J Bone Joint Surg (Am)* 68:904-911, 1986.

67. Holmes R, Mooney V, Bucholtz R, *et al*: A coralline hydroxyapatite bone graft substitute. *Clin Orthop* 188:252-262, 1984.

68. Holmes R, Slayer K: Bone regeneration in a coralline hydroxyapatite implant. *Surgical Forum* 29:611-612, 1978.

69. Hoogendoorn H, Renooij W, Akkermans L, *et al*: Long-term study of large ceramic implants (porous hydroxyapatite) in dog femora. *Clin Orthop* 187:281-288, 1984.

70. Hurley L, Stinchfield F, Bassett A, *et al*: The role of soft tissues in osteogenesis: an experimental study of canine spine fusions. *J Bone Joint Surg (Am)* 41:1243-1254, 1959.

71. Jarcho M: Calcium phosphate ceramics as hard tissue prosthetics. *Clin Orthop* 157:259-278, 1981.

72. Jergesen H, Chua J, Kao R, *et al*: Age effects on bone induction by demineralized bone powder. *Clin Orthop* 268:253-259, 1991.

73. Johnston C, Ashman R, Sherman M, *et al*: Mechanical consequences of rod contouring and residual scoliosis in sublaminar segmental instrumentation. *J Orthop Res* 5:206-216, 1987.

74. Jorgenson S, Lowe T, France J, *et al*: A prospective analysis of autograft versus allograft in posterolateral lumbar fusion in the same patient: a minimum of 1 year follow-up in 144 patients. *Spine* 19:2048-2053, 1994.

75. Jowsey J, Riggs B: Bone formation in hypercortisonism. *Acta Endocrinol* (Copenh) 63:21-28, 1970.

76. Kane W. Direct current electrical bone growth stimulation for spinal fusion. *Spine* 13:363-365, 1988.

77. Kent J, Quinn J, Zide M, *et al*: Alveolar ridge augmentation using nonresorbable hydroxylapatite with or without autogenous cancellous bone. *J Oral Maxillofac Surg* 41:629-642, 1983.

78. Kotani Y, Cunningham B, Cappuccino A, *et al*: The role of spinal instrumentation in augmenting lumbar posterolateral fusion. *Spine* 21:278-287, 1996.

79. Kucharzyk D: A controlled prospective outcome study of implantable electrical stimulation with spinal instrumentation in a high-risk spinal fusion population. *Spine* 24:465-469, 1999.

80. Lafferty F, Spencer G, Pearson O: Effects of androgens, estrogens, and high calcium intakes on bone formation and resorption in osteoporosis. *Am J Med* 36:514-528, 1964.

81. Lau G, Luck J, Marshall G, *et al*: The effect of cigarette smoking on fracture healing: an animal model. *Clin Res* 37:132A, 1989.

82. Laurie S, Kaban L, Mulliken J, *et al*: Donor site morbidity after harvesting rib and iliac bone. *Plast Reconstr Surg* 73:93393-8, 1984.

83. Lebwohl N, Starr J, Milne E, *et al*: Inhibitory effect of ibuprofen on spinal fusion in rabbits (abstract). American Academy of Orthopaedic Surgeons annual meeting, 1994, p 278.

84. Lee K: Clinical investigation of the spinal stem system, open trial phase: pseudarthrosis stratum. Presented at the Annual Meeting of the AAOS, Las Vegas, Feb 1989.

85. Linovitz R, Pathria M, Bernhardt M, *et al*: Combined magnetic fields accelerate and increase spine fusion: a double-blind, randomized, placebo-controlled study. *Spine* 27(13):1383-1388, 2002.

86. Long J, Lewis S, Kuklo T, *et al*: The effect of cyclooxygenase-2 inhibitors on spinal fusion. *J Bone Joint Surg (Am)* 84(a):1763-1768, 2002.

87. Luque E: Latest clinical results using demineralized bone materials and rhBMP-2: the Mexican experience. In *Total Spine*. Advanced Concepts and Constructs. Cancun, Mexico, Feb 2000.

88. Malanin T, Brown M: Bone allografts in spinal surgery. *Clin Orthop* 154:68-73, 1981.

89. Malanin T, Rosomoff H, Sutton C: Human cadaver femoral head homografts for anterior cervical spine fusions. *Surg Neurol* 7:249-251, 1977.

90. Mardjetko S, Connolly P, Shott S: Degenerative lumbar spondylolisthesis: a meta-analysis of the literature 1970-93. *Spine* 10:2256S-2265S, 1994.

91. Martin G, Boden S, Titus L: Recombinant human bone morphogenetic protein-2 overcomes the inhibitory effect of ketorolac, a nonsteroidal anti-inflammatory drug (NSAID), on posterolateral lumbar intertransverse process spine fusion. *Spine* 24(21):2188-2194, 1999.

92. May V, Mauck W. Exploration of the spine for pseudarthrosis following spinal fusion in the treatment of scoliosis. *Clin Orthop* 53:115-122, 1967.

93. McAfee P, Farey I, Sutterlin C, *et al*: Device-related osteoporosis with spinal instrumentation. *Spine* 14:919-926, 1989.

94. McAfee P, Farey I, Sutterlin C, *et al*: The effect of spinal implant rigidity on vertebral bone density: a canine model. *Spine* 16:S190-S197, 1991.

95. McAfee P, Regan J, Farey I, *et al*: The biomechanical and histomorphometric properties of anterior lumbar fusions: a canine model. *J Spinal Disord* 1:101-110, 1988.

96. McAfee P, Werner F, Glisson R: A biomechanical analysis of spinal instrumentation systems in thoracolumbar fractures: comparison of traditional Harrington distraction instrumentation with segmental spinal instrumentation. *Spine* 10:204-217, 1985.

97. McCarthy R, Peek R, Morrissy R, *et al*: Allograft bone in spinal fusion for paralytic scoliosis. *J Bone Joint Surg (Am)* 68:370-375, 1986.

98. McGuire R, Amundson G: The use of primary internal fixation in spondylolisthesis. *Spine* 18:162-172, 1993.

99. McMurray G: The evaluation of Kiel bone in spinal fusions. *J Bone Joint Surg* (Br) 64:101-104, 1982.

100. Misol S, Samaan N, Ponseti I: Growth hormone in delayed fracture union. *Clin Orthop* 74:206-208, 1971.

101. Moore D, Chapman M, Manske D: The evaluation of a biphasic calcium phosphate ceramic for use in grafting long-bone diaphyseal defects. *J Orthop Res* 5:356-365, 1987.

102. Muschler G, Huber B, Ullman T, *et al*: Evaluation of bone grafting materials in a new canine segmental spinal fusion model. *J Orthop Res* 11:514-524, 1993.

103. Muschler G, Hyodod A, Manning T, *et al*: Evaluation of human bone morphogenetic protein 2 in a canine spinal fusion model. *Clin Orthop* 308:229, 1994.

104. Nagel D, Kramers P, Rakn B, *et al*: A paradigm of delayed union and nonunion in the lumbosacral joint: a study of motion and bone grafting of the lumbosacral spine in sheep. *Spine* 16:553-559, 1991.

105. Nilsson O, Bauer H, and Brostrom L: Methotrexate effects on heterotopic bone in rats. *Acta Orthop Scand* 58:47-53, 1987.

106. Nisbet N: Antigenicity of bone. *J Bone Joint Surg (Br)* 59:263-266, 1977.

107. Osborn J, Newesely H: The material science of calcium phosphate ceramics. *Biomaterials* 1:108-111, 1980.

108. Passuti N, Daculsi G, Rogez J, *et al*: Macroporous calcium phosphate ceramic performance in human spine fusion. *Clin Orthop* 248:169-176, 1989.

109. Patel T, Vaccaro A, Truumees E, *et al*: A safety and efficacy study of OP-1 (rhBMP-7) as an adjunct to posterolateral lumbar fusion. Presented at the North American Spine Society Meeting, Seattle, 2001.

110. Patel T, Erulkar J, Grauer J, *et al*: Osteogenic protein-1 overcomes the inhibitory effect of nicotine on posterolateral lumbar fusion. *Spine* 26:1656-1661, 2001.

111. Pelker R, Friedlander G: Biomechanical aspects of bone autografts and allografts. *Orthop Clin N Am* 18:235-239, 1987.

112. Pelker R, Friedlander G, Markham T: Biomechanical properties of bone allografts. *Clin Orthop* 174:54-57, 1983.

113. Pelker R, Friedlander G, Markham T, *et al*: Effects of freezing and freeze-drying on the biomechanical properties of rat bone. *J Orthop Res* 1:405-411, 1984.

114. Phillips L, Vassilopoulou-Sellin R: Somatomedins I. *N Engl J Med* 302:371-380, 1980.

115. Phillips L, Vassilopoulou-Sellin R: Somatomedins II. *N Engl J Med* 302:371-380, 1980.

116. Pieron A, Bigelow D, Hamonic M: Bone grafting with Boplant: results in thirty-three cases. *J Bone Joint Surg (Am)* 50:364-368, 1968.

117. Pouliquen J, Noat M, Verneret C, *et al*: Coral as a substitute for bone graft in posterior spinal fusion in childhood. *French Journal of Orthopaedic Surgery* 3: 272-280, 1989.

118. Prolo D, Rodrigo J: Contemporary bone graft physiology and surgery. *Clin Orthop* 200:322-342, 1985.

119. Ragni P, Lindholm S: Interaction of allogeneic demineralized bone matrix and porous hydroxyapatite bioceramics in lumbar interbody fusion in rabbits. *Clin Orthop* 272:292-299, 1991.

120. Riggs B, Jowsey J, Goldsmith R, *et al*: Short- and long-term effects of estrogen and synthetic anabolic hormone in postmenopausal osteoporosis. *J Clin Invest* 51:1659-1663, 1972.

121. Rish B, McFadden J, Penix J: Anterior cervical fusion using autologous bone grafts: a comparative study. *Surg Neurol* 5:119-121, 1976.

122. Rognozinski A, Rognozinski C: Efficacy of implanted bone growth stimulation in instrumented lumbosacral spinal fusion. *Spine* 21:2393-2398, 1996.

123. Rokkanen P, Vainionpaa S, Tormala P, *et al*: Biodegradable implants in fracture fixation: Early results of treatment of fractures of the ankle. *Lancet* 1422-1424, 1985.

124. Roux F, Brasnu D, Loty B, *et al*: Madreporic coral: A new bone graft substitute for cranial surgery. *J Neurosurg* 69: 510-513, 1988.

125. Sahinoglu T, Bhatt B, Gullett L, *et al*: Pulsed electromagnetic fields induce osteogenesis and upregulate transcription of bone morphogenetic protein-2 and 4 mRNA in rat osteoblasts in vitro. Presented at the 42nd Annual Meeting of the Orthopaedic Research Society, Atlanta, Feb 19-22, 1996.

126. Salama R: Xenogeneic bone grafting in humans. *Orthop* 174:113-121, 1983.

127. Sandhu H, Kanim L, Kabo J, *et al*: Effective doses of recombinant human bone morphogenetic protein-2 in experimental spinal fusion. *Spine* 21:2115, 1996.

128. Sandhu H, Kanim L, Toth J, *et al*: Experimental spinal fusions with recombinant human bone morphogenetic protein-2 without decortication of osseous elements. *Spine* 22:1171, 1997.

129. Sandhu H, Khan S: Animal models for preclinical assessment of bone morphogenetic proteins in the spine. *Spine* 27 (16S):32-38, 2002.

130. Schimandle J, Boden S, Hutton W: Experimental spinal fusion with recombinant human bone morphogenetic protein-2. *Spine* 20:1326, 1995.

131. Schimandle J, Weigel M, Edwards C: Indications for thigh cuff bracing following instrumented lumbosacral fusions. North American Spine Society 1993, p 41.

132. Shima T, Keller J, Alvira M, *et al*: Anterior cervical discectomy and interbody fusion. *J Neurosurg* 51:533-538, 1979.

133. Shirado O, Zdeblic T, McAfee P, *et al*: Quantitative histological study of the influence of anterior spinal instrumentation and biodegradable polymer on lumbar interbody fusion after corpectomy. *Spine* 17:795-803, 1992.

134. Silcox D, Daftari T, Boden S, *et al*: The effect of nicotine on spinal fusion. *Spine* 20:1549-1553, 1995.

135. Simmons J: Treatment of failed posterior lumbar interbody fusion (PLIF) of the spine with pulsing electromagnetic fields. *Clin Orthop* 183:127-132, 1985.

136. Speck G: Posterolateral fusion using OP-1: a model using degenerative spondylolisthesis. Presented at the Australian Spine Meeting, Adelaide, Australia, 2000.

137. SpinaLogic. Summary of safety and effectiveness, PMA No. P910066/S11, 1999.

138. Steinmann JC, Herkowitz HN: Pseudarthrosis of the spine. *Clin Orthop* 284:80-90, 1992.

139. Suh DY, Boden S, Ugbo J, *et al*: Evaluation of rhBMP-2 with various ceramic/collagen sponge carriers in posterolateral spinal fusion in the rabbit and nonhuman primate. *AAOS*, 2002:88.

140. Suh DY, Boden S, Ugbo J, *et al*: Delivery of recombinant human morphogenetic protein-2 (rhBMP-2) using a compression-resistant matrix in posterolateral spinal fusion in the rabbit and in the nonhuman primate. *Spine* 27: 353-360, 2002.

141. Takaoka K, Nakahara H, Yoshikawa H, *et al*: Ectopic bone induction on and in porous hydroxyapatite combined with collagen and bone morphogenetic protein. *Clin Orthop* 234:250-254, 1988.

142. Tuli S: Bridging of bone defects by massive bone grafts in tumorous conditions and in osteomyelitis. *Clin Orthop* 87:60-73, 1972.

143. Udupa K, Gupta L: The effect of growth hormone and thyroxine in healing of fracture. *Ind J Med Res* 53: 623-628, 1965.

144. Urban M, Brighton C, Black J: Dose response relationship for Faradic stimulation of osteogenesis in the rabbit tibia by use of a single-strand platinum cathode. In Brighton C, Pollock S (eds): *Electromagnetics in Biology and Medicine*. San Francisco, San Francisco Press, 1999, p. 199.

145. Urist M: Bone: formation by autoinduction. *Science* 150:893-899, 1965.

146. Urist M, Lietze A, Dawson E: Beta-tricalcium phosphate delivery system for bone morphogenetic protein. *Clin Ortho* 187:277-280, 1984.

147. Urist M, Silverman B, Buring K, *et al*: The bone induction principle. *Clin Orthop* 53:243-283, 1967.

148. Wenger D, Carollo J, Wilkerson J, *et al*: Laboratory testing of segmental spinal instrumentation versus traditional Harrington instrumentation for scoliosis treatment. *Spine* 7:265-269, 1982.

149. West J III, Bradford D, Ogilvie J: Results of spinal arthrodesis with pedicle screw plate fixation. *J Bone Joint Surg (Am)* 73:1179-1184, 1996

150. Younger EM, Chapman MW: Morbidity at bone graft donor sites. *J Orthop Trauma* 3:192-195, 1989.

151. Zdeblick T: A prospective randomized study of lumbar fusion: preliminary results. *Spine* 18:983-991, 1993.

152. Zdeblick T, Heim S, Kleeman T, *et al*: Laparoscopic approach with tapered metal cages: rhBMP-2 vs. Autograft. *NASS*, 200, 2001.

153. Zdeblick T, Shirado O, McAfee P, *et al*: Anterior spinal fixation after lumbar corpectomy: a study in dogs. *J Bone Joint Surg (Am)* 73:527-534, 1991.

154. Zerwekh J, Kourosh S, Scheinberg R, *et al*: Fibrillar collagen-biphasic ceramic calcium phosphate composite as a bone graft substitute for spinal fusion. *J Orthop Res* 10:562-572, 1992.

CHAPTER 12

Spine Fusion: Anatomy and Biomechanics of Bone-Bone Interface

Ajith J. Thomas, Russ P. Nockels, and Christopher I. Shaffrey

In the late nineteenth century, Sir William Macewen firmly established bone grafting as a treatment option to replace missing bone and to enhance bone formation. His interest in bone grafting led him to perform allografts and autografts in his patients.[39] In the United States, spinal fusion was first reported in the early 1900s by Albee[1] for the treatment of Pott's disease, and by Hibbs[30] who used fusion surgery to halt the progression of scoliotic deformity. Since that time the number of cervical and lumbar fusions has increased. In fact, it doubled between 1980 and 1990.[16] Spinal arthrodesis is now one of the most common surgical procedures performed in the United States.

Unfortunately, a number of complications have been associated with spinal fusion. Pseudarthrosis can occur in up to 35% to 40% of multilevel lumbar fusions.[14] Donor site morbidity can also be considerable.[2] To achieve successful bony fusion, minimize complications, and achieve a good functional outcome, it is important to understand the various structural, biologic, and biomechanical aspects of bone fusion.

Anatomy of the Bone-Bone Interface
Histologic Components

On a gross level, all bones are composed of two basic components: cortical (compact) bone and cancellous (trabecular) bone. Cortical bone is a dense, solid mass, except for its microscopic channels, and contains parallel stacks of curved sheets called "lamella," which are separated by bands of interlamellar cement. Regularly spaced throughout lamella are small cavities, or lacunae. Lacunae are interconnected by thin, tubular channels called "canaliculi." Entrapped bone cells (osteocytes) are located in the lacunae, and their long, cytoplasmic processes occupy canaliculi. The cell processes within canaliculi communicate by gap junctions, with processes of osteocytes lying in adjacent lacunae. Canaliculi open to extracellular fluid at bone surfaces, thus forming an anastomosing network for the nutrition and metabolic activity of the osteocytes. Cortical bone possesses a volume fraction of pores less than 30% and has an apparent density up to about 2g/ml. Its compressive strength is approximately tenfold that for a similar volume of cancellous bone.

Cancellous bone is porous and appears as a lattice of rods, plates, and arches individually known as "trabeculae." It has a greater surface area and can be readily influenced by adjacent bone marrow cells. Because of this structural difference, cancellous bone has a higher metabolic activity and responds more readily to changes in mechanical loads.[59]

Cortical and cancellous bone may consist of woven (primary) or lamellar (secondary) bone. Woven bone forms the embryonic skeleton and is then resorbed and replaced by mature bone as the skeleton develops.[52] In the adult, woven bone is found only in pathologic conditions, such as fracture healing and in tumors. Woven and lamellar bone differ in formation, composition, organization, and mechanical properties. Woven bone has an irregular pattern of collagen fibers, contains approximately four times as many osteocytes per unit volume, and has a rapid rate of deposition and turnover. The osteocytes of woven bone vary in orientation, and the mineralization of woven bone follows an irregular pattern in which mineral deposits vary in size and in their relationship to collagen fibrils. In contrast, the osteocytes of lamellar bone are relatively uniform, with their principle axis oriented parallel to that of other cells and to the collagen fibrils of the matrix. The collagen fibrils of lamellar bone lie in tightly organized, parallel sheets, with uniform distribution of mineral within the matrix.[8,15]

The irregular structure of woven bone makes it more flexible, more easily deformed, and weaker than lamellar bone.[59] For these reasons the restoration of normal mechanical properties to bone tissue at the site of a healing fracture requires eventual replacement of the woven bone of the fracture callus with mature lamellar bone.[8]

Biomechanical Properties of Graft Material

There are important differences in the biomechanical properties of graft material. Comparison testing of various graft material shows allograft or fresh-frozen cancellous bone to be the weakest, failing at 863 Newton (N) of compression. Air-dried, ethylene-oxide sterilized, tricortical bone failed at an average load of 2308N, and fresh-frozen, tricortical allograft bone failed at an average load of 2257N. Freeze-drying, air-drying, or ethylene-oxide sterilization was found to have little effect on the strength of bone when subjected to compression.[6]

Iliac crest wedges are the most commonly used graft material. The percentage of cortical and cancellous bone remains constant at 41% and 59%, respectively, regardless of the total cross-sectional area of the wedge. Donor age also does not affect this physical parameter.[64] Gamma radiation does not have any effect on the mechanical or material properties of the iliac crest wedges.[68] Rehydrated iliac crest wedges are more deformable than freeze-dried wedges.[65] During loading, freeze-dried wedges fail dramatically, fracturing into many small pieces, which is secondary to its "brittle nature." Rehydrated wedges fail with a circumferential fracture along the side of the wedge where the cortical bone is thinnest. It has been recommended that freeze-dried wedges be rehydrated in a vacuum before clinical use.[65] Water or saline can be added to the vacuum-sealed container holding the wedge; the wedges gain 100% of their wet weight within 5 minutes of addition of water or saline. Graft collapse occurred more frequently with freeze-dried allografts (30%) than with autografts in anterior cervical fusions.

The loads at the lumbar spine have been well documented in various positions and levels of activity.[61] Either autograft or allograft iliac crest wedges are biomechanically sound in an interbody fusion of the lumbar spine, since it would provide load-bearing capacities approximately fourfold greater than would be applied in vivo. Specimens from the anterior-superior iliac spine could bear substantially greater axial loads (average 3230N) in comparison to specimens from the posterior superior iliac spine (average 1458N).[54] Fibular strut grafts are the strongest and have been shown to have a compressive strength of 5070N.[63] However, their cross-sectional area, which is important in preventing telescoping of the graft, is much smaller. In interbody fusion the cross-sectional area of the graft should be substantially greater than 30% of the end-plate to provide a margin of safety.[12]

Incorporation of Bone Graft

Incorporation is defined as the process of envelopment of a complex of necrotic old bone with viable new bone.[10] The complex develops through resorption of the necrotic old bone with viable new bone being laid down. The incorporation of the bone graft is a dynamic process and involves the equilibrium of the following processes: (1) proliferation of the osteoprogenitor cells, (2) differentiation of osteoblasts, (3) osteoinduction, (4) osteoconduction, and (5) the biomechanical properties of the graft.[36,45] The process of incorporation is tightly regulated by cytokines, termed "bone growth factors." Cytokines are small proteins that serve as signaling agents for cells.

The process whereby a tissue is influenced to form osteogenic elements is termed "osteoinduction." Induction requires an inducing stimulus, such as a piece of bone or an osteogenic cell, and an environment favorable for osteogenesis. Osteoconduction is the process by which capillaries, perivascular tissue, and osteoprogenitor cells from the recipient bed grow into the graft. It can occur within a framework of nonbiologic materials or nonviable biologic materials. In viable bone grafts osteoconduction is facilitated by osteoinductive processes and therefore occurs more rapidly than in nonviable or nonbiologic materials.[60]

Differences in Cancellous and Cortical Bone Graft Incorporation

Cancellous grafts are revascularized more rapidly and completely than cortical grafts. The open trabecular pattern of cancellous bone facilitates vessel ingrowth. Revascularization has been reported to begin within a few hours after grafting,[17] and may be complete by 2 weeks. In contrast, the dense structure of cortical bone prevents neovascular penetration during the first several weeks after grafting, and hence revascularization of cortical bone may take several months. Because of the dense architectural structure of cortical bone, new vessel incorporation follows pre-existing haversian and Volkmann's canals.[21]

Several differences exist between cancellous and cortical grafts regarding the cellular process of repair. With cancellous grafts, primitive mesenchymal cells that originate in the trabecula may differentiate directly into osteoblasts, thereby resulting in relatively early new bone formation. The new bone forms on the dead trabeculae of the graft. This is followed by a resorptive phase. Cancellous bone initially undergoes an appositional new bone formation phase called "creeping substitution," which is the process of new tissue invading along channels made by invasive blood vessels or along pre-existing channels in the transplanted bone.[46] The necrotic areas within the cancellous bone graft eventually are entirely resorbed by osteoblastic activity and totally replaced with new viable bone. As the revascularization of cancellous bone graft proceeds, primitive mesenchymal cells differentiate into osteogenic cells. These osteogenic cells form osteoblasts that line the edges of dead trabeculae and deposit a seam of osteoid that is annealed to, and eventually surrounds, a central core of dead bone. This process of alignment of osteoblasts on existing bone surfaces, with the synthesis of osteoid in successive layers to form lamellae, is termed "appositional bone formation." Thus initially, there is an increase in the size of the graft. Cancellous grafts tend to repair completely with time. The areas of entrapped necrotic bone are resorbed by osteoclasts. In time the cancellous bone graft is completely replaced by viable new bone.

Cortical grafts must undergo osteoclastic resorption before osteoblastic new bone formation occurs. In cortical grafts the repair process is initiated by osteoclasts with preferential early resorption of the external cortical surface. Osteoblasts appear only after bone resorption has begun, and the initial deposition of osteoid usually occurs in resorbed areas. Cortical grafts remain as admixtures of necrotic and viable bone. In cortical grafts, revascularization is primarily the results of vascular infiltration through the Volkmann's and haversian canals.[45] Osteoclasts initiate resorption of bone approximately 2 weeks after vascularization. Resorption is maximal at 6 weeks, and then gradually the graft recovers normal strength by 1 year. New bone formation takes place, and the newly formed bone seals off the remaining necrotic bone from further encroachment beginning at around 12 weeks. Thus if a biopsy specimen is obtained from a cortical graft years after placement, it demonstrates an admixture of necrotic and viable bone.

Biomechanics of Graft Incorporation

Cancellous grafts are incorporated by an early appositional phase. New bone formation onto the necrotic trabeculae of the graft tissue leads to an early increase in graft strength. It has been shown that necrotic bone maintains its mechanical strength.[21] Hence cancellous grafts initially strengthen with the addition of new bone. As the necrotic cores are resorbed, the mechanical strength of the graft area normalizes.

Cortical bone grafts first undergo osteoclastic bone resorption, which significantly increases graft porosity and thus decreases the graft strength. In the canine model of autogenous cortical transplant, the greatest compromise in mechanical strength occurs at 12 weeks[21] (Figure 12.1). The strength returns to normal between 1 and 2 years post-transplantation. Human being data suggest that cortical grafts lose approximately half their biomechanical strength during the first 6 months, and this will persist for another 6 months.[20] This process is related to osteoclastic graft resorption, and is slowly reversed during the second year after implantation. These observations correlate with the highest incidence of mechanical graft failure between 6 and 8 months after transplantation. If the graft is allogenic, this process is further prolonged. Hence it is important to protect segmental grafts during the critical phase when the resorptive phase outstrips the appositional phase. This is usually accomplished by load sharing with spinal instrumentation or a spinal orthosis.

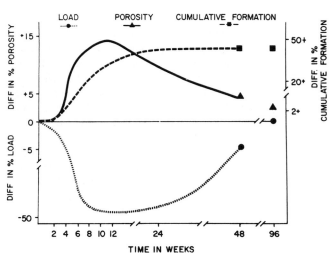

Figure 12.1 Graph illustrating the quantitative temporal interrelationships between the physical integrity and the biologic processes of repair within a segmental autogenous cortical bone transplant. The initial persistence of strength (0–4 weeks after transplantation) indicates the subsequent loss was caused by reparative processes, rather than to any intrinsic weakness in the material. The sudden loss in strength at 6 weeks is caused by the increased internal porosity. From 6 to 12 weeks, the decrease in mechanical strength is reduced by 50%. The level of porosity continues to increase until week 12, because of the temporal lag in the apposition of new bone formation. At 24 weeks, there is no significant improvement in strength, despite the beginning reduction in the porosity of the transplant and maturation of the callus. At 48 weeks, however, the physical integrity of the transplant has returned toward normal, primarily the result of decreased material porosity, since the amount of callus has not increased. By two years, the physical integrity of the transplant has returned toward normal, primarily the result of decreased material porosity, since the amount of callus has not increased. By 2 years the physical integrity of the transplant and the internal porosity of the remaining transplanted material is normal. The biologic completeness of repair (i.e., approximately 50% of the graft is viable) is not significant because mechanical strength has been retained. The admixture of necrotic and viable bone remains for the life of the individual's skeletal metabolic activity. *(From Burchardt H: Biology of cortical bone graft incorporation. In Friedlaender GE, Mankin HJ, Sell KW [eds]: Osteochondral Allografts: Biology, Banking, and Clinical Applications. Boston, Little, Brown and Company, 1983, p 55.)*

Temporal Profile of Graft Incorporation

During the first week after grafting, both cancellous and cortical grafts have similar histologic features. Both are surrounded by coagulated blood, and the graft is the focus of a tissue response characterized by vascular buds infiltrating the grafted bed. By the second week, fibrous granulation tissue becomes increasingly dominant in the graft bed, the number of inflammatory cells decrease, and osteoclastic activity increases. Within the confines of the graft, osteocytic autolysis proceeds, resulting from anoxia and injury by surgery, with necrosis delineated by vacant lacunae. Some cells, however, survive by diffusion of nutrients from surrounding host tissues. Creeping substitution of cortical bone grafts progresses transversely and parallel to the long axis of the transplanted segment. Thus the repair is found to be greater at the graft-host junctions.[56]

The histologic sequence of healing in spine fusion has not been studied in detail. A recent study elaborated on the process of dorsolateral intertransverse fusion in rabbits,[3] describing three phases. The early reparative phase (1 to 3 weeks) consists of hematoma formation and granulation tissue. There is minimal ossification. This is followed by the middle reparative phase (4 to 5 weeks), when the fusion solidifies, and the late remodeling phase (6 to 10 weeks).

Both membranous and enchondral ossification play a role in the fusion process. Membranous ossification is the predominant mechanism that begins at the termini of the fusion mass, and emanates from the decorticated transverse process. The central portion of the fusion mass, where the vascular supply is poorer and movement is greater, heals by cartilage formation and enchondral ossification.

Host Response and Incorporation of Autograft and Allograft

Autograft remains the "gold standard" in most fusion applications. In certain situations in which there is insufficient autologous bone or when large structural grafts are needed, allograft fusion rates can approach or equal those of autograft rates, without donor site morbidity. A successful spinal fusion requires a sufficient area of decorticated host bone, ample graft material, minimal motion at the fusion site, and a rich vascular supply.[55]

Histocompatibility matching has an important influence on the process of incorporation. Allografts of bone that is mismatched for major histocompatibility complex antigens functions poorly compared with autogenous grafts.[11,57] Bone cells display class I and class II histocompatibility antigens, and there are both cellular and humoral responses to bone allografts.[58] Syngeneic grafts are the most successful. Grafts with major histocompatibility mismatch have delayed and incomplete revascularization, compared to syngeneic grafts. In addition, there is often marked resorption of bone, resulting in almost complete loss of graft.[57] Freezing the graft, followed by thawing, disrupts and kills the cells. It mutes the antigenicity in major mismatches and thus enhances incorporation of such grafts. However, the killing of cells also diminishes the biologic activity of the graft. It is the osteoinductive component that is mainly affected. The function of an allograft as an osteoconductive system seems virtually unimpaired.

In fresh cancellous allografts, the initial phase consisting of hemorrhage and necrosis is identical to that of the autograft. The fibrin clot and the same inflammatory response develops. However, in the allograft the fibrin clot breaks down and the granulation tissue, which provides nutrition to the repair site, is invaded by chronic inflammatory cells rather than fibroblasts and blood vessel elements. The major portion of the delay appears to occur in osteoclastic resorption and new bone formation. Final graft incorporation remains incomplete.

In cortical allografts the length of time of creeping substitution is greatly prolonged. The invasion by host vessels, and recruitment and differentiation of cellular elements to become osteoblastic and osteoclastic cells, are greatly diminished. The proportion of necrotic graft bone to viable host bone is much greater in allogeneic grafts. In fact, the active process of graft substitution may last several years.

Modeling and Remodeling Associated with Spine Fusion

The bone modeling associated with spinal fusion is extremely complex. Variables that may affect bone remodeling after graft insertion include: (1) those related to the design of implant, materials used, and methods of fixation; (2) those related to the local bone, including its density and shape; and (3) those related to the patient, including age, gender, hormonal balance, and activity.[9] Osteoblasts and osteoclasts are influenced by the magnitude and state of strain imposed on them by load applied to the bone. Stresses or strains within a given range seem to be required to maintain a steady-state remodeling of bone in which the rate of bone formation equals the rate of resorption. Stresses below the optimum are often associated with stress shielding, leading to bone resorption. Stresses and strains exceeding upper limits can also produce resorption of bone as a result of pressure necrosis. Cyclic stresses are required to maintain osseous homeostasis. Constant loads, even when within the desired range, can result in insufficient stimulus to maintain bone mass. Observations of strain-related electric potentials in bone, biopotentials, and electrical stimulation of osteogenesis have resulted in the suggestion that bioelectric phenomena function as the regulators of adaptive remodeling of bone.

Growth Factors and Cytokines in Regulating Bone Remodeling

Bone cells carry out diverse functions and are mainly derived from two cell lines: mesenchymal and hematopoietic. The mesenchymal stem-cell line consists of undifferentiated cells, or preosteoblasts, that differentiate into osteoblasts, bone-lining cells, and osteocytes. The hematopoietic stem-cell line consists of circulating marrow monocytes that differentiate into preosteoclasts and osteoclasts. These cells are regulated by various cytokines.

Bone formation in spinal fusion is a complex and regulated process. The cellular events involved in bone formation include chemotaxis of osteoblast precursors, proliferation of committed osteoblast precursors, and differentiation and expression of regulatory factors and structural proteins of bone and mineralization.[42] These processes require tight regulatory control. They may be modulated by systemic hormones, such as parathyroid hormone, but predominant control is by local factors or cytokines. Cytokines are small proteins that serve as signaling agents for cells. Cytokines are classified based on their cellular origin and principal biologic activities.[26] The main families include interleukins, tumor necrosis factors, growth factors, colony-stimulating factors, interferons, and chemokines.

Bone morphogenetic protein (BMP) is a member of the transforming growth factor-B (TGF-B) superfamily. The BMP constitutes a growth family of more than 12 proteins, nine of which have been shown individually to induce ectopic bone formation.[47] They seem to have as their target the undifferentiated mesenchymal-type perivascular cell. BMP-2 is the most widely investigated osteoinductive growth factor in spinal fusion.[47,49] It is involved in the differentiation of osteoblasts from progenitor cells that reside in the bone marrow. Several animal studies have shown that recombinant human (rh) BMP-2 induces bone formation at an orthotopic site at which the integration with the pre-existing bone is structurally sound. It has also been shown that BMP plus marrow yields the highest union rates (100%) and is three times superior to autogenous cancellous graft.[66]

In animal studies rhBMP-2 has been used in dorsal spinal fusion models[13,38] and dorsolateral intertransverse fusion,[49-51] with the demonstration of increased new bone formation. In a canine model, in which lumbar fusion was performed at three levels, autologous grafting was compared with a synthetic graft material impregnated with rhBMP.[43] At 12 weeks, the union score and mechanical strength of the fusion were the same in both groups. Subsequent studies have examined enhancement of fusion with rhBMP in combination with autograft.[29,53] Although they demonstrated significantly increased amounts of new bone formation in comparison to the autograft alone group, no increase in biomechanical strength was shown. Thus the use of BMP with autograft has not been studied. No studies have yet reported the efficacy of allogeneic graft with BMP. However, if it were to provide efficacy equivalent to autogenous cancellous bone, the morbidity associated with the harvest of an autogenous graft could be avoided.

Dorsolateral transverse process fusion is frequently used for achieving primary lumbar intersegmental arthrodesis. Use of rhBMP-2 with synthetic grafts has been superior to autogenous iliac bone for producing radiographically and mechanically solid transverse process fusion in canines by 3 months.[50] Similar results have also been reported in rabbit and primate models.[5]

In lower vertebrates there appears to be a minimum threshold dose of rhBMP-2, above which a consistent fusion is achieved,[49] and additional increases in dosage does not produce further mechanical, radiographic, or histologic differences. This has been corroborated in nonhuman primates.[4] However, other factors may play a role in the biologic response to rhBMP in vivo, including the time course activity of rhBMP on the bone-formation process, its interaction with other growth factors, and the influence of delivery vehicles. The biocompatibility of polylactic acid polymers has been questioned and could produce an immune response. The role of instrumentation remains to be resolved.

Other bone-inducing proteins such as recombinant human osteogenic protein (rhOP) have been used in dorsal spinal fusions with type I collagen as a carrier.[13] These also seem superior to autogenous iliac bone.

Biomechanics of Fusion

There is a wealth of literature on the biomechanics of fusion, but the vast majority involve in vitro models. In an in vivo situation, a variety of biologic factors influence the mechanical properties of fusion mass. The type of surgical construct and choice of bone graft selected should be individualized, based on the biologic and mechanical considerations. The main indications for a spinal fusion are listed in Box 12.1.

Biomechanics of the Fusion Mass

In dorsal and dorsolateral fusion, healing occurs through callus formation. As ossification proceeds the callus is converted from a low stiffness, rubbery quality to a hard-tissue type of resiliency. The mineralization of the callus progressively increases its tensile strength. The fusion site during all stages of the reparative process is highly susceptible to mechanical factors, directly related to the amount of motion between the graft fragment and host surface. The amount of relative motion determines the morphologic patterns of fracture repair. As healing proceeds there is a decrease in the amount of motion. When mechanical stability is compromised, there is always more cartilage formation, and occasionally, an exuberant callus. Frequently, with excessive motion the fusion mass is incomplete and a pseudarthrosis develops. Rigid internal fixation has been demonstrated to reduce pseudarthrosis rates in most clinical applications.

Positioning of Bone Graft

As White and Panjabi[61] describe, "The placement of a fusion mass at the maximum distance from the instantaneous axes of rotation will be more effective in preventing the movement around those axes" (Figure 12.2). The instan-

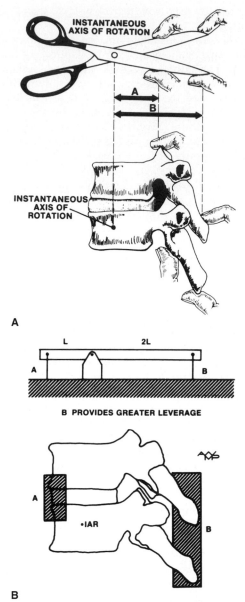

Figure 12.2 **(A)** To prevent the opening of the blades of the scissors by holding them together, it is distinctly easier to pinch the blades together at the tips (*distance B*) rather than at the midpoint of the blade (*distance A*). Because distance B is further from the instantaneous axis of the rotation (IAR), there is greater leverage. The same concepts apply to the vertebral functional spinal unit. Flexion, separation, or opening of the spinous processes, is more readily prevented by placing the fingers at the tips of the spinous processes (*distance B*) rather than at the facet joints (*distance A*). Thus with regard to a flexion movement, a healed bone graft at distance B, at the tips of the spinous processes, is more effective than one closer to the IAR, other factors being constant. These concepts partially explain the efficacy of the rather delicate interspinous and supraspinous ligaments. **(B)** The concept of leverage is shown again here. The anterior bone graft A is a short distance (analogous to *L*) form the IAR and therefore provides less leverage than bone graft B, which is a greater distance (analogous to *2L*) from the instantaneous axis of rotation. (*From White AA, Panjabi MM: Clinical Biomechanics of the Spine. Philadelphia, JB Lippincott, 1990, p 533.*)

taneous axis of rotation (IAR) is defined as the point in the body, or some hypothetical extension of it, that does not move when a rigid body moves in a plane. An axis perpendicular to the plane of motion and passing through the point is the IAR for that motion at that instant (Figure 12.3). It can be defined more simply as the axis around which the vertebral body rotates. It is like a fulcrum. Usually, but not always, the IAR passes through the confines of the vertebral body. With isolated destruction of columns of the spine, the IAR migrates to the remaining intact structures, as shown in Figure 12.4.

The greater the distance of the fusion mass from the IAR, the greater the leverage in preventing motion around those axes of rotation. Examples include dorsal, dorsolateral, and intertransverse lumbar fusion, in which the fusion mass is located at a distance from the IAR (which is located in the region of the vertebral body). A ventrally placed graft is closer to the IAR and applies less leverage, but can still be extremely effective, especially in cases of anterior column deficiency.

The concept of rigidity is also important. A fusion mass that involves all the dorsal elements and transverse processes provides more rigidity than a fusion that only involves the spinous process. In some situations it can be disadvantageous to place the graft at a distance from the IAR. For example, after a dorsal fusion for discogenic pain, motion may still occur at the disc interspace, even when all dorsal elements except the pedicle are fixed.[25,48] In such situations an interbody fusion may be considered[24] (Figure 12.5).

The biomechanics of different types of lumbar fusion, regarding the production of biomechanical changes, have been studied.[22,37] The three types of fusion evaluated included dorsal, bilateral lateral, and ventral. All types of fusion increased bending and axial stiffness. There is

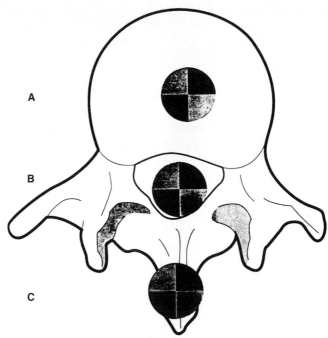

Figure 12.4 Location of the axis. The location of the IAR for the intact and compromised specimens. (**A**) Facet joints compromised. (**B**) Intact spine. (**C**) Facet joints and annulus compromised. *(From Haher TR, O'Brien M, Felmly WT, et al: Instantaneous axis of rotation as a function of the three columns of the spine. Spine 1992;17(6S):S153. Reprinted with permission.)*

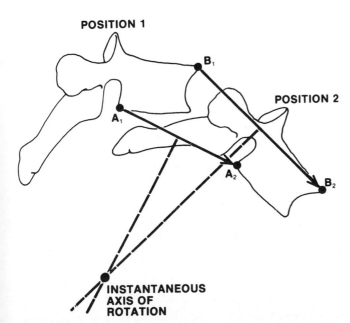

Figure 12.3 Instantaneous axis of rotation (IAR). A construction for determining the IAR is shown. A_1-A_2 and B_1-B_2 are translation vectors of points A and B. *(From White AA, Panjabi MM: Clinical Biomechanics of the Spine. Philadelphia, JB Lippincott, 1990, p 660. Reprinted with permission.)*

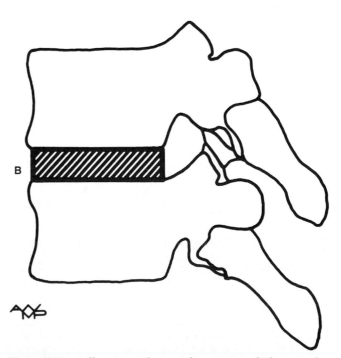

Figure 12.5 An illustration showing the position of a bone graft (B), which can provide maximum rigidity by eliminating interbody motion. *(From White AA, Panjabi MM: Clinical Biomechanics of the Spine. Philadelphia, JB Lippincott, 1990, p 535. Reprinted with permission.)*

increased stress on the adjoining segments that were not fused, especially the facet joints. Overall, bilateral intertransverse fusion is a superior method because it provides good stabilization to the fused segments and has less effect on adjacent, unfused segments, especially the facet joints. Dorsal (intraosseous) fusion is the least beneficial, producing the highest amount of stress in adjoining segments and allowing superficial motion in the disc space.

The spine experiences compressive forces on the concave side and tensile forces on the convex side of a curve. In the lumbar spine, if the graft material is placed in the intervertebral disc space, it is subjected to compressive loading. It is believed that compressive forces acting on the graft will promote fusion by stimulating the osteoconductive healing process. In contrast, a graft placed in a dorsal location experiences only tensile forces and will not be stimulated in a similar manner (Figure 12.6).

Kyphotic Deformity and Bone Graft Positioning

At the IAR, there is neither compression nor tension. The farther instrumentation or bone graft is placed from the IAR, the greater the stress. For instance, in a kyphotic deformity, dorsal instrumentation is subjected to severe tensile stress. To reduce stress on a dorsal implant some structural graft should be placed as ventrally as possible, away from the IAR. This counteracts the tensile stress dorsally. At times, with severe kyphotic deformity, multiple ventral grafts may be required (Figure 12.7). It has been demonstrated that ventral and dorsal fusions are associated with a better correction, and maintenance of correction, than the dorsal group, only with congenital kyphosis.[62]

Load Sharing

Denis[18] introduced the three-column theory of the spine to classify and assist with the management of thoracolumbar spine injuries. Of these three columns the anterior and posterior columns are the principle support structures.[32] The anterior column resists compression and axial loading, while the posterior column maintains the tension. To maintain an erect posture, all forces and movements must be balanced about the IAR. The IAR is located dorsal to the annulus fibrosus in the intact spine.[28]

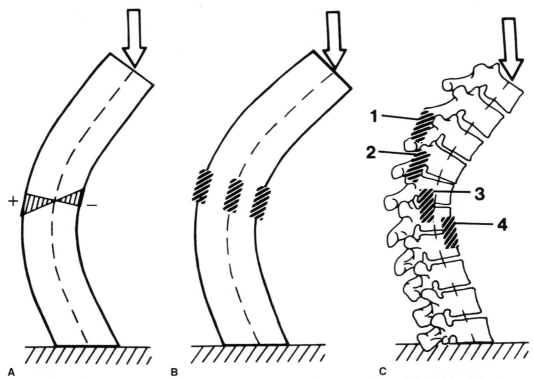

Figure 12.6 (**A**) The spinal column may be analyzed by regarding it to be similar to a beam. There is tension on the convex side of the curve and compression on the concave side. The dashed line is the neutral axis, and there is neither tension nor compression along this line. (**B**) Bone grafts inserted at the various points tend to behave as follows. The graft on the convex side of the curve is mainly under tension and cannot resist deforming forces until fully attached at both interfaces. The graft at the dashed line (neutral axis) provides little or no resistance to bending in the plane of the page. (**C**) In the spine the graft at position *1* is well away from the neutral axis, and when biologically fused at both interfaces can offer effective tensile resistance against progressive kyphosis. The graft at position *2* can do the same but is less effective because it is closer to the neutral axis. The graft at position *3* is not likely to be as effective as *1* or *2* in preventing progression of deformity, because it is even closer to the neutral axis. Graft *4* is effective because it immediately begins to resist compressive forces, which tends to prevent additional deformity and angulation at that point. The graft is also some distance away from the neutral axis, giving it mechanical advantage. (*From White AA, Panjabi MM, Thomas CL: The clinical biomechanics of kyphotic deformities.* Clin Orthop 8:128, 1977.)

Deficiencies in the anterior or posterior column in the thoracolumbar spine usually lead to kyphosis.[7] Kyphosis is corrected by lengthening the anterior column or shortening the posterior column. If the anterior or middle column is destroyed, alignment can be restored by a ventral structural graft and the resulting fusion. In this situation the axial load is shared by both anterior and posterior columns. When deciding on whether to perform a ventral or dorsal fusion, or a combination of both, the principles of load sharing should be considered. If both the ventral and dorsal elements are involved, both columns usually have to be instrumented and fused. For example, a burst fracture will compromise if the dorsal elements frequently require both ventral and dorsal spine reconstruction. With persistent post-traumatic kyphosis after a dorsal instrumentation procedure for a cervical or thoracolumbar fracture, there is an elimination of anterior column load sharing. Instrumentation, such as a pedicle screw implant, is exposed to high cantilever bending loads, and may fail.[41] With correction of a kyphotic deformity, ventral surgery may not be necessary if the weight-bearing line is shifted behind the axis of rotation.[19] By shifting the center of gravity dorsally, the anterior column does not have to support as much axial load. The prerequisites for such a strategy include: (1) correction or overcorrection, if surgically feasible; (2) intact dorsal elements; and (3) good osteogenic potential. If sagittal correction is not accomplished, the load on the anterior column is high and anterior column reconstruction is needed to prevent dorsal instrumentation failure.

Ventral instrumentation, without structural bone grafting, will usually fail. A strong structural graft is required to resist axial loading and flexion.[27] Tricortical ilium, fibula, humerus, or titanium cages packed with autogenous graft provide excellent anterior column support. Single rib grafts do not provide adequate structural support. Load sharing, in this case, implies that a balance between ventral structural bone grafts and ventral or dorsal instrumentation exists. As the fixation length of ventral and dorsal constructs is reduced, load sharing with the anterior column has become increasingly important regarding the reduction of the incidence of failure of the shorter devices. The conditions frequently requiring both ventral and dorsal reconstruction include tumors involving both anterior and posterior columns, fractures involving all three columns, and post-laminectomy kyphosis.[7]

In dorsolateral spinal fusion, instrumentation adds to the stability of the fusion by significant load sharing. In a human spine model where bilateral facetectomies were performed and transpedicular screws were used to restore stability, the spinal instrumentation provided 68% of the load sharing, along with the anterior and middle columns.[34] As the fusion mass develops in vivo the load-sharing component of the instrumentation decreases. If an adequate fusion mass does not develop, the cyclical stresses placed on the instrumentation will lead to hardware failure (Figure 12.8).

Stress Shielding

In a canine model dorsolateral fusion without instrumentation resulted in fusion in only 57%, compared to a 100% fusion rate with pedicle screw fixation and a 71% fusion rate with Luque rods. Histologic evaluation of the vertebral body at the level of the fusion demonstrated osteoporosis

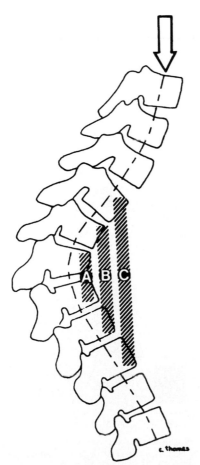

Figure 12.7 This illustration shows the various locations of ventral bone grafts for kyphotic deformity. The biomechanical considerations involved in choosing graft *A*, *B*, or *C* are discussed in the text. (*From White AA, Panjabi MM, Thomas CL: The clinical biomechanics of kyphotic deformities.* Clin Orthop 1977;8:128.)

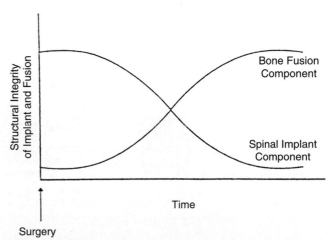

Figure 12.8 The relationship between bone fusion acquisition and spinal implant integrity changes with time after surgery. (*From Benzel EC:* Biomechanics of Spine Stabilization. *New York, McGraw-Hill, 1994, p 104.*)

in animals that had been instrumented. This has been corroborated in human beings.[44] Patients who had undergone instrumented dorsolateral lumbar fusion were found to have decreased vertebral body mineral density at the level of fusion, compared to matched controls. This phenomenon has been termed "stress shielding." However, in animal models the spine fusions that had been instrumented demonstrated increased areas of bone incorporation and biomechanical stability,[23,33,40] and any pre-existing osteoporosis was more than adequately compensated. In general, rigid fixation results in better union. Ventral interbody fusions are more prone than dorsal onlay fusions to the negative effects of stress shielding.

Biomechanical Consideration at Specific Sites

Ventral cervical spine fusions are commonly performed using the Smith-Robinson technique. It achieves a wide decompression and provides an optimal load-bearing capacity (Figure 12.9). The end plates are left intact. The cancellous portion of the graft is in contact with the verte-bral end plates and readily permits revascularization. It is important to remember that transplanted bone weakens as resorption proceeds and consequently, the graft is weaker at 6 months than at the time of implantation.

In the thoracic spine, segments of ribs may be used to provide structural support. However, they have a low compressive strength, which is related to their unfavorable length-to-width ratio, curvature, and small area of contact with the end plate. Fibular strut grafts or iliac crest grafts can be used, if structural support is important. Figure 12.10 demonstrates the relative strengths of various grafts used in ventral thoracic/lumbar fusion.

In the lumbar spine, despite the potential for surgical complications, interbody fusions are being increasingly performed. The lumbar spine experiences static loads in the 759-1600lb range and up to 2000lb for high loading. The compressive strength of iliac allografts ranges from 396 to 1475lb, whereas femoral cortical rings have a strength in excess of 15,000lb. Some surgeons thus prefer femoral cortical allografts.[35] Interbody cages are another option. They eliminate the associated iliac crest harvest complications.

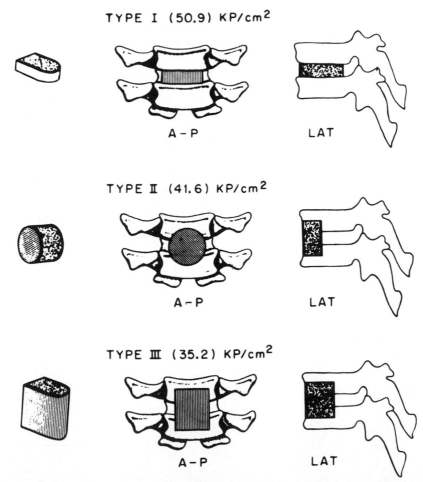

TYPE I (50.9) KP/cm^2

A-P   LAT

TYPE II (41.6) KP/cm^2

A-P   LAT

TYPE III (35.2) KP/cm^2

A-P   LAT

Figure 12.9 Graft configuration: how the graft fits into vertebrae, and how the vertebrae are altered to receive it. *Type I*: Smith-Robinson. *Type II*: Cloward. *Type III*: Bailey-Badgeley (modified). The numbers are mean values for load-bearing capacity of each of the three surgical constructions. (*From White AA, Jupiter J, Southwick WO, Panjabi MM: An experimental study of the immediate load-bearing capacity of three surgical constructions for anterior spine fusions.* Clin Orthop 91:21, 1973.)

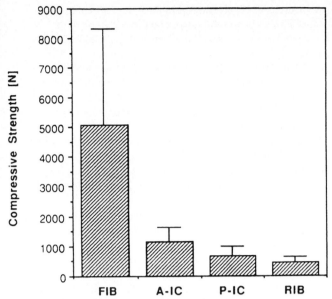

Figure 12.10 Compressive strength of anterior thoracic/lumbar grafts. The fibular graft *(FIB)* was significantly stronger in compression *(P = .05)* than the anterior *(A-IC)* and posterior *(P-IC)* grafts and the rib *(RIB)* graft. *(From Wittenberg RH, Moeller J, Shea M, et al: Compressive strength of autologous and allogenous bone grafts for thoracolumbar and cervical spine fusion. Spine 1990;15:1076.)*

The dorsolateral intertransverse fusion is the most commonly performed fusion procedure. It involves the facet joints, the pedicles, the transverse process, and the gutter between them. There is greater stability with axial rotation and lateral bending. Motion can persist, even after solid fusion, and can cause discogenic pain, particularly when the facet joints are not included in the arthrodesis. This motion occurs through the pedicles and can be minimized by augmenting the fusion with spinal instrumentation.[31,67]

Summary

Bone is a complex and constantly changing structure. The dynamic nature of bone and its remarkable healing potential determines the final outcome of spinal fusion. The surgeon's technical skill and implant design only facilitate this healing process. An augmented understanding of the basic structure and biomechanics of bone interfaces is advantageous to the surgeon in choosing appropriate grafts for specific situations, and in minimizing the risk of late complications, such as pseudarthrosis. There is currently an explosion of knowledge regarding the mechanisms of bone formation and the control of bone cell function. In the near future we will have the opportunity to exploit this to significantly enhance the outcomes of fusion procedures.

REFERENCES

1. Albee FH: Transplantation of a portion of the tibia into the spine for Pott's disease. *JAMA* 57:885-886, 1911.
2. Banwart JC, Asher MA, Hassanein RS: Iliac crest bone graft harvest donor site morbidity. A statistical evaluation. *Spine* 20(9):1055-1060, 1995.
3. Boden SD, Schimandle JH, Hutton WC, Chen MI: The use of an osteoinductive growth factor for lumbar spinal fusion. Part 1: The biology of spinal fusion. *Spine* 20:2626-2632, 1995.
4. Boden SD, Schimandle JH, Hutton WC: The use of an osteoinductive growth factor for lumbar spinal fusion. Part 11. Study of dose, carrier, and species. *Spine* 20: 2633-2644, 1995.
5. Boden SD, Moskovitz PA, Morone MA, Torbitake Y: Video-assisted lateral intertransverse process arthrodesis. Validation of a new minimally invasive lumbar spinal fusion technique in the rabbit and nonhuman primate (rhesus) models. *Spine* 21:2689-2697, 1996.
6. Brantigan JW, Cunningham BW, Warden K, *et al*: Compression strength of donor bone for posterior lumbar interbody fusion. *Spine* 18:1213-1221, 1993.
7. Bridwell KH: Load sharing principles. The role and use of anterior structural support in adult deformity. *Instructional Course Lectures* 45:109-115, 1996.
8. Buckwalter JA, Glimcher MJ, Cooper RR, Recker R: Bone Biology 1: structure, blood supply, cells matrix and mineralization. *Instructional Course Lectures* 41:371-386, 1996.
9. Buckwalter JA, Glimcher MJ, Cooper RR, Recker R: Bone Biology 11: formation, form, modeling, remodeling and regulation of cell function. *Instructional Course Lectures* 42:387-399, 1996.
10. Burchardt H: The biology of bone graft repair. *Clin Orthop Rel Res* 174:28-42, 1983.
11. Burchardt H, Enneking WF: Transplantation of bone. *Surg Clin North Am* 5 8:403-427, 1978.
12. Closkey RF, Parsons R, Lee CK, *et al*: Mechanics of interbody spinal fusion: analysis of cortical bone graft area. *Spine* 18:1011-1015, 1993.
13. Cook SD, Dalton JE, Tan EH, *et al*: In vivo evaluation of recombinant human osteogenic protein (rhOP-1) implants as bone graft substitute for spinal fusions. *Spine* 19: 1655-1663, 1994.
14. Cotler JM, Star AM: Complications of spinal fusion. In Cotler JM, Cotier HM (eds): *Spinal Fusion: Science and Technique*. New York, Springer Verlag, 1990, pp. 361-87.
15. Currey JD: Function and form of bone. In Mow VC, Ratcliffe A, Woo SL-Y (eds): *Biomechanics of Diarthrodial Joints*, vol 2. New York, Springer-Verlag, 1990, pp 3-30.
16. Davis H: Increasing rates of cervical and lumbar spine surgery in the United States, 1979-1990. *Spine* 19: 1117-1124, 1994.
17. Deleu J, Trueta J: Vascularization of bone grafts in the anterior chamber of the eye. *J Bone Joint Surg* 4OA:187, 1965.
18. Denis F: The three column spine and its significance in the classification of acute thoracolumbar spinal injuries. *Spine* 8: 817-831, 1983.
19. Edwards CC, Osbome VA: Correction of chronic post traumatic kyphosis with the kyphoreduction construct and stress relaxation (abstract). Proceedings of the American Academy of Orthopaedic Surgeons 61st Annual Meeting, New Orleans. Rosemont, IL, Amercian Academy of Orthopedic Surgeons, 1994, p 160.
20. Enneking WF, Morris JL: Human autologous cortical bone transplants. *Clin Orthop* 87:28, 1972.

21. Enneking WF, Burchardt H, Puhl JJ, Piotrowski G: Physical and biologic aspects of repair in dog cortical bone transplants. *J Bone Joint Surg* 57A:232, 1975.

22. Esses SI, Doherty BJ, Crawford MJ, Dreyzin V: Kinematic evaluation of lumbar fusion techniques. *Spine* 21(6): 676-684, 1996.

23. Feighan JE, Stevenson S, Emery SE: Biologic and biomechanic evaluation of posterior lumbar fusion in the rabbit. The effect of fixation rigidity. *Spine* 20:1561-1567, 1995.

24. Fraser RD: Interbody, posterior and combined lumbar fusions. *Spine* 20:167S-177S, 1995.

25. Goel VK, Kim YE, Lim TH, Weinstein JN: An analytical investigation of spinal information. *Spine* 13:1-11, 1988.

26. Goldring SR, Goldring MB. Cytokines and skeletal physiology. *Clin Orthop Related Res* 324:13-23, 1996.

27. Gurr KR, McAfee PC, Shih CM: Biomechanical analysis of anterior and posterior instrumentation systems after corpectomy: a calf-spine model. *J Bone Joint Surg* 7OA:1182-1191, 1988.

28. Haher TR, O'Brien M, Felmly WT, *et al*: Instantaneous axis of rotation as a function of the three columns of the spine. *Spine* 17(suppl 6):S149-S154, 1992.

29. Helm GA, Sheehan JM, Sheehan JP, *et al*: Utilization of type I collagen gel, demineralized bone matrix, and bone morphogenetic protein-2 to enhance autologous bone lumbar spinal fusion. *J Neurosurg* 86:93-100, 1997.

30. Hibbs RA: An operation for progressive spinal deformities. A preliminary of three cases from the service of the Orthopedic Hospital. *NY State J Med* 93:1013-1016, 1911.

31. Jacobs RR, Montesano PX, Jackson RP: Enhancement of lumbar spinal fusion by use of translaminar facet joint screws. *Spine* 14:12-15, 1989.

32. James KS, Wenger KH, Schlegel JD, *et al*: Biomechanical evaluation of the stability of thoracolumbar burst fractures. *Spine* 19:1731-1740, 1994.

33. Johnston CE, Welch RD, Baker KJ, Ashman RB: Effect of spinal construct stiffness on short segment fusion mass incorporation. *Spine* 20:2400-2407, 1995.

34. Kotani Y, Cunningham BW, Cappuceino A, *et al*: The role of spinal instrumentation in augmenting lumbar posterolateral fusion. *Spine* 21:278-287, 1996.

35. Kozak JA, Heilman AE, O'Brien JP: Anterior lumbar fusion options. *Clin Orthop Rel Res* 300:45-51, 1994.

36. Lane K, Sandhu HS: Current approaches to experimental bone grafting. *Orthop Clin North Am* 18:213-225,1987.

37. Lee KC, Langrana NA: Lumbosacral spinal fusion. A biomechanical study. *Spine* 9:574-581, 1984.

38. Lovell TP, Dawson EG, Nilsson OS, Urist MR: Augmentation of spinal fusion with bone morphogenetic protein in dogs. *Clin Orthop* 243:266-274, 1989.

39. Macewen W: *The Growth of Bone*. Glasgow, James Maclehose and Sons, 1912.

40. McAfee PC, Farey ID, Sutterlin CE, *et al*: Device related osteoporosis with spinal instrumentation. *Spine* 14:919-926, 1989.

41. McCormack T, Karikovic E, Gaines RW: The load sharing clssification of spine fractures. *Spine* 19:1741-1744, 1994.

42. Mundy GR: Regulation of bone formation by bone morphogenetic proteins and other growth factors. *Clin Orthop Rel Res* 323:24-28, 1996.

43. Muschler GF, Hyodo A, Manning T, *et al*: Evaluation of human bone morphogenetic protein in a canine spinal fusion model. *Clin Orthop Rel Res* 308:229-240, 1994.

44. Myers MA, Casciani T, Whitbeck MG Jr, Puzas JE: Vertebral body osteopenia associated with posterolateral spine fusion in humans. *Spine* 21:2368-2371, 1996.

45. Prolo DJ, Rodrigo JJ: Contemporary bone graft physiology and surgery. *Clin Orthop* 200:322-342, 1991.

46. Ray RD. Bone grafts and bone implant. *Otolaryngol Clin North Am* 5:389-398, 1972.

47. Riley EH, Lane JM, Urist MR, *et al*: Bone morphogenetic protein-2. Biology and applications. *Clin Orthop Rel Res* 324:39-46, 1996.

48. Rolander SD: Motion of the lumbar spine with special reference to the stabilizing effect of posterior fusion. *Acta Orthop Scand* (Suppl) 90:1, 1966.

49. Sandhu HS, Linda EA, Kabo JM, *et al*: Effective doses of recombinant human morphogenetic protein-2 in experimental spinal fusion. *Spine* 21: 2115-2122, 1996.

50. Sandhu HS, Kanim LEA, Kabo JM, *et al*: Evaluation of rhBMP-2 with an OPLA carrier in a canine posterolateral (transverse process) spinal fusion model. *Spine* 20: 2669-2682, 1995.

51. Schimandle JH, Boden SD, Hutton WC: Experimental spinal fusion with recombinant human bone morphogenetic protein-2. *Spine* 20:1326-1337, 1995.

52. Sevitt S (ed): *Bone Repair and Fracture Healing in Man*. Edinburgh, Scotland, Churchill Livingstone, 1981, pp 1-24.

53. Sheehan JP, Kallmes DF, Sheehan JM, *et al*: Molecular methods of enhancing lumbar spine fusion. *Neurosurgery* 39:548-554, 1996.

54. Smith MD, Cody DD: Load bearing capacity of corticocancellous bone grafts in the spine. *J Bone Joint Surg (Am)* 75:1206-1213, 1993.

55. Steiranan JC, Herkowitz HN: Pseudarthrosis of the spine. *Clin Orthop* 284:80-90, 1992.

56. Stevenson JS, Bright RW, Dunson GL, Nelson FR: Technetium-99m phosphate bone imaging: A method for assessing bone graft healing. *Radiology* 110:391-394, 1973.

57. Stevenson S, Li XQ, Davy DT, *et al*: Critical biological determinants of incorporation of nonvascularized cortical bone grafts. *J Bone Joint Surg* 79A:1-16, 1997.

58. Stevenson S: The immune response to osteochondral allografts in dogs. *J Bone Joint Surg* 69A:573-582, 1987.

59. Torzilli OA, Burstein AH, Takebe K, *et al*: The material and structural properties of maturing bone. In Cowin SC (ed): *Mechanical Properties of Bone*. New York, American Society of Mechanical Engineers, 1981, pp 145-161.

60. Urist MR: Osteoinduction in undemineralized bone implants modified by chemical inhibitors of endogenous matrix enzymes. *Clin Orthop* 87:132, 1972.

61. White AA, Panjabi MM: *Clinical Biomechanics of the Spine*. Philadelphia, JB Lippincott, 1990.

62. Winter RB, Moe JH, Lonstein JE: The surgical treatment of congenital kyphosis. A review of 94 patients age 5 years or older with 2 years or more follow-up in 77 patients. *Spine* 10:224-231, 1984.

63. Wittenberg RH, Moeller J, Shea M, White AA III, Hayes C: Compressive strength of autogenous bone grafts for thoracolumbar and cervical spine fusion. *Spine* 15: 1073-1078, 1990.

64. Wolfinbarger L Jr, Zhang Y, Adam BT, *et al*:
A comprehensive study of physical parameters,
biomechanical properties and statistical correlations of iliac
crest bone wedges used for spinal fusion surgery. I.. Physical
parameters and their correlations. *Spine* 19:277-283, 1994.

65. Wolfinbarger L Jr, Zhang Y, Adam BT, *et al*:
A comprehensive study of physical parameters,
biomechanical properties and statistical correlations of
iliac crest bone wedges used for spinal fusion surgery.
II. Mechanical properties and correlation with physical
parameters. *Spine* 19:284-295, 1994.

66. Yasko AW, Cole BJ, Lane JM, *et al*: Comparison of
recombinant human BMP-2 versus cancellous bone to heal
segmental bone defects. *Trans Orthop Res Soc* 17:100, 1993.

67. Zdeblick TA: A prospective, randomized study of lumbar
fusion: preliminary results. *Spine* 18:983-991, 1993.

68. Zhang Y, Wolfinbarger L Jr: A comprehensive study of
physical parameters, biomechanical properties and
statistical correlations of iliac crest bone wedges used for
spinal fusion surgery III. Multivariable regression analysis
and practical formulas for strength prediction. *Spine*
19:296-303, 1994.

CHAPTER 13

Bone Void Fillers: Bone and Bone Substitutes

Edward C. Benzel, Isador H. Lieberman, and Lisa A. Ferrara

One of the most common types of graft (second only to blood) is bone, with over 450,000 procedures using bone, performed annually in the United States, and 2.2 million worldwide.[47] Spine arthrodesis is the most common reason for autogenous bone harvest, with approximately 250,000 spinal fusions performed in the United States each year.[63] It is axiomatic that autogenous cancellous bone is the gold standard against which all other bone graft materials are compared. The osteogenic, osteoinductive, and osteoconductive properties of autograft are unequaled in stimulating bone repair. The procurement site of choice is the iliac crest because of the quantity and quality of available bone. Nevertheless, there are significant drawbacks to autograft, including procurement morbidity, limited availability, and increased operative time. In fact, iatrogenic complications originating from the graft procurement site represent a significant source of patient and physician concern. The primary operation may be successful, but the secondary procedure can result in increased patient recovery time and disability.[24,32,35,39]

Allograft is a commonly chosen alternative to autograft, especially when autografting is either impractical or impossible. However, this convenience comes at a price. Just like any organ allograft transplant, the allograft has the potential to transfer disease and trigger a host immune response. The allograft is heavily processed to mitigate these risks at the expense of impaired osteoinductivity and diminished mechanical properties. This renders allograft inferior to autograft as a bone graft material. In addition, processing adds to the already significant procurement costs.

Because of these drawbacks to both autograft and allograft, synthetic alternatives have been a very active area of research over the past 20 years. Nevertheless, only about 10% of the 2.2 million worldwide bone graft procedures involve synthetics because of perceived inferiority to native autograft and allograft.[47] Drawbacks of many synthetics include poor resorbability, inclusion of animal or marine-derived components, variable handling characteristics, limited availability, and added cost. Until recently, synthetic grafts provided only osteoconductive properties, lacking osteoinductive and osteogenic potential. However, composite grafts that combine a synthetic osteoconductive matrix with osteoinductive growth factors and osteogenic cells have the potential to provide the advantages of autogenous bone graft—without its disadvantages. Numerous preclinical and clinical trials are under way to determine whether this potential can be realized.

The Use of Cancellous Bone Grafts Versus Substitutes

The Role of Cancellous Bone

Cancellous bone can be considered a scaffold within which a variety of cell types interact to perform a wide array of essential functions, in addition to its importance as the nurturing microenvironment for hematopoiesis, myelogenesis, and platelet formation. Cancellous bone serves as an incubator that protects and grows the sources of its own maintenance and renewal of pluripotent osteoprogenitor stem cells. The growth, migration, and differentiation of these bone-forming cells are regulated by local growth factors elaborated by the cells and platelets within the cancellous bone.[48] In line with its role as a cell incubator, cancellous bone is highly porous and vascular. It demonstrates a limited weight-bearing function and is susceptible to collapse under compressive forces. Surrounding and protecting the cancellous bone is cortical bone. This dense structural material makes up the bulk of the skeleton and provides for the axial load-bearing capabilities of the skeleton.

General Characteristics of a Successful Bone Graft

A bone graft functions in a manner similar to cancellous bone, supporting new tissue growth by providing the bone and blood cells with a matrix substrate. For a bone graft to be successful, three processes—osteogenesis, osteoconductivity, and osteoinductivity—that mimic natural events in cancellous bone must take place.

Osteogenesis

Osteogenesis is the process of bone formation through cellular osteoblastic activity, which depends, in turn, upon the presence of osteoprogenitor stem cells. Osteogenic grafts provide cells with the direct ability to form new bone.

Osteoinduction

Osteoinduction is the biologically mediated recruitment and differentiation of cell types essential for bone formation. Osteoinductive grafts supply factors that induce undifferentiated tissue to differentiate into bone.

Osteoconduction

Osteoconduction involves the apposition of growing bone to the three-dimensional surface of a suitable scaffold provided by the graft.[3] Osteoconduction requires the structural and chemical environments that simulate those found in cancellous bone.[15] The ideal scaffold provides dimensional stability and degrades at a rate commensurate to the speed of new bone formation.[47]

In addition, material for a successful bone graft must have good handling characteristics, be nontoxic (e.g., not leach chemicals into the circulation), and exhibit biomechanical characteristics (e.g., tension, compression, modules of elasticity) similar to those of cancellous bone. Spine surgeons are currently using a variety of materials, both stand-alone and in combination. Table 13.1 summarizes the biologic properties that constitute a graft's osteointegrative capabilities (the formation of bony tissue around the implant without growth of fibrous tissue at the bone-implant interface).[37,65]

Potential Uses of Natural and Synthetic Bone Grafts

Surgeons introduce bone graft, natural or synthetic, for many types of repair procedures, namely, in fusion (e.g., cervical fusion after discectomy, as an onlay lumbar graft, an interbody lumbar graft, and in fractures) and as a bone void filler (e.g., collapsed vertebral body, autograft donor site repair, bony defects as a result of trauma or tumor resection, osteonecrosis). Synthetic graft material can also be used in conjunction with either autograft or allograft as a bone graft extender.

Graft Materials

Autograft

Pro

Autograft includes osteogenic bone and marrow cells as well as an osteoconductive matrix of cartilage, minerals, matrix proteins, and osteoinductive proteins associated with the matrix.[2] Neither host rejection nor disease transmission is an issue with an autograft. The combination of these properties can result in high graft success rates. Many spinal fusion procedures (i.e., dorsal cervical and thoracic and intervertebral) that use autogenous graft produce fusion rates over 90%.[63]

Con

The separation of body tissue from its blood supply results in cell death.[63] The viability of autogenous bone as a living graft and host is severely compromised when it is harvested. Furthermore, the quality of the donor stock is not constant; it is dependent upon many factors such as the patient's age, gender, health, and genetic disposition. Thus, the potential of autograft to effect repair is not always achieved. This opens the door for alternatives. Although some spinal fusion procedures result in high fusion rates, this is not uniformly so. Many common procedures, such as dorsolateral lumbar fusion, produce fusion rates as low as 56%.[63,66] Although regarded as the gold standard, autogenous bone demonstrates less than ideal biologic performance.[6]

However, probably the greatest drawback to autograft use is the need for a second fascial incision and surgical dissection with its attendant complication potential. In fact, minor complications such as superficial infection, seroma/hematoma, temporary sensory loss, and mild or transient pain are common. Major complications at the donor site range in incidence from 0.7% to 25%.[63] These include infection, prolonged wound drainage, herniation of muscle and abdominal contents through the donor defect, deep hematomas, need for reoperation, pain lasting longer than 6 months, profound sensory loss, vascular and neurologic injury, unsightly scars, subluxation, gait disturbances, sacroiliac joint destabilization, enterocutaneous fistula, pelvic or iliac fracture, and heterotopic bone formation.[11,17,23] Life-threatening complications include major vessel or visceral injury.

TABLE 13.1			
Osteointegrative Properties of Bone Graft Materials[25,45,59,63,70]			
Graft Material	**Osteogenesis**	**Osteoinduction**	**Osteoconduction**
Autograft	2	2	2
Allograft	0	1	2
Xenograft	0	0	2
α-TCP	0	0	1
β-TCP (porous)	0	0	2
Hydroxyapatite	0	0	1
Injectable calcium phosphate cement (e.g., Norian SRS®°)	0	0	1
BMA	3	2	0
β-TCP plus BMA	3	2	2
DBM	0	2	1
Collagen	0	0	2
BMP	0	3	0
Hyaluronic acid	0	0	0
Bioactive glasses	0	0	1
Degradable polymers	0	0	1
Porous metals	0	0	1

Score range 0 (none) to 3 (excellent).
α-*TCP*, α-tricalcium phosphate; β-*TCP*, β-tricalcium phosphate; *BMA*, bone marrow aspirate; *BMP*, bone morphogenetic protein; *DBM*, demineralized bone matrix.
°Synthes-Stratec, Oberdorf, Switzerland.

Neurologic injury may occur from dissection close to several nerves in the area (sciatic, lateral femoral cutaneous, and cluneal).[39] Vascular injury to the superior gluteal vessels may occur from dissection too close to the sciatic notch. Chronic pain at the donor site, present in up to 25% of cases,[68] may be attributable to excessive removal of bone from the sacroiliac region with violation of the sacroiliac joint.[39]

Hu[39] reported a series of 14 patients who suffered a fracture at the iliac bone graft procurement site after spine fusion. The majority of these patients were elderly women with chronic medical diseases. The authors, therefore, recommend iliac bone graft procurement with caution in this group to minimize the potential for these iatrogenic fractures. Based on subsequent cadaver studies, the authors recommend at least a 3cm distance between the anterosuperior iliac crest and the graft procurement site[38] and a 3cm maximum distance from the dorsal ilium.[71]

Although risk of surgical complications can theoretically be minimized, certain procurement issues remain. These include increased operative time and blood loss, temporary disruption of donor-site bone structure, pain, vascular injuries, and cosmetic defects.[2,68]

Bone can also be obtained from the local decompression site or from a remote site such as the rib or tibia. These have their own problems and are typically a choice of last resort.

Osteoconductive Matrices

Most other bone grafts serve primarily as an osteoconductive matrix, with minimal to no self-supplied osteogenic or osteoinductive properties. The trade-off is greater source availability and no second operative site. The structural properties of the three-dimensional scaffold matrix (especially the degree of porosity) are the primary determinants of the speed and completeness of incorporation and remodeling. The osteoconductive scaffold provides an appropriate environment into which bone cells and bone morphogenetic proteins (BMPs) can migrate, adhere, and proliferate.

Allograft

Allografts were initially used only for massive grafting where autograft use was impossible. However, by 1996 allografts constituted 34% of all bone grafts performed in the United States, increasing in use more than 14-fold compared with just a decade earlier.[6] Allograft has become the most common autograft substitute or extender for autograft.

Pro

Three factors have led to the surge in popularity of allograft.[6] First, the National Organ Transplant Act increased overall availability. Second, donor screening and tissue processing have improved safety and quality of donated tissue. Third, the manufacture of new allograft forms (e.g., dowels) has greatly improved overall allograft utility and versatility. Perhaps the greatest advantage of allograft is its wide availability in a variety of physical forms that can be customized to specific applications. Machine tooling to shape structural allograft into forms such as wedges or threaded bone dowels can allow allograft to function as both bone graft and a fixation device.[63] Other advantages include the reduction of procurement morbidity, the potential for immediate structural support, and a reasonable success rate (greater than 60%) reported for specific procedures (e.g., hip revision surgery, management of tumors in bone).[28] Success rates for ventral-spinal lumbar fusions with allograft are comparable to those with autograft.[19]

Con

Allografts do not generate equivalent results with those of autografts.[19] Allografts can vary greatly in initial bone quality, be of higher initial expense, transmit disease, and evoke immunogenic reactions.[25] Processing constraints, required for patient safety, do not guarantee the absence of disease transmission or immunogenic reaction, but they do minimize risks posed by these adverse responses. One study of 1146 femoral heads considered suitable for bone-bank donation found unexpected disease in 8%, including three undiagnosed malignant bone tumors.[56] Minimal processing of allograft (i.e., freezing freshly obtained bone) is not sufficient to inactivate the AIDS virus, as HIV transmission has been reported by this means.[19]

Processing renders the graft nonviable and mitigates osteoinduction potential by destroying proteins useful in recruiting bone cells and inducing new bone formation. Since the processed allografts are less representative of human tissue relative to autografts, allografts are not as readily received and incorporated by the host. Allografts are slower to be resorbed and not as completely replaced by new bone as are autografts.[19] The structural integrity of the processed bone complex is also compromised, and stability at the defect site, critical for rapid healing and return to function, is more difficult to achieve.[58,63] Results are especially poor for dorsal lumbar fusion,[19] and lower reported fusion rates for allograft implants compared with autograft-only implants were found in two studies.[63]

Quantity of allograft material is constrained by limited supply; tissue banks report difficulty with procurement because of fear of gross disfigurement at the donor site.[9] Donor-to-donor variation results in uncertain, nonuniform quality.[36] Bone quality varies with donor age and gender; even same-size bones from different anatomic sites in a single donor can vary in strength by up to 20%.[58]

A low-grade inflammatory reaction is typically associated with allograft.[25] This immune response may contribute to allograft failure (i.e., fracture and nonunion).[19,27,31] Because of an initial intense inflammatory reaction, new capillaries are easily thrombosed, resulting in a delay in vascularization and osteoinduction.[19] Even at maturation, necrotic bone can comprise as much as 50% or more of the graft.[19]

A literature review of animal studies suggests a correlation between histocompatibility difference and allograft failure, both biologically and biomechanically.[27] In a mouse model, the immunologic reaction appears to be specific to donor antigen and is comprised of killer/suppressor T cells, cells that are associated with soft-tissue rejection.[27] In humans, alloreactivity appears similar to the animal findings, resulting in an overall sensitization rate of 67%, higher than that seen after blood transfusion (12% to 50%).[28,67] The immune response system may share common bone marrow-derived precursors and cytokines with the bone remodeling system, explaining the potential interaction of the immune response with bone remodeling.[27] The most convincing evidence of a causal relationship between immunogenicity and poorer outcome is that among 29 patients studied who received allograft, those lacking sensitization to class II antigens achieved better clinical results than did sensitized patients.[28]

The two types of allograft in common use, fresh-frozen and freeze-dried, differ in their processing. Each has its advantages and disadvantages. Fresh-frozen allografts retain BMP, are stronger and more completely incorporated in host bone than freeze-dried grafts,[19] but are also the most immunogenic and have produced documented HIV transfer. Freeze-dried allograft is the least immunogenic and has caused no documented HIV or viral disease transmission. However, its BMP is destroyed and it has the most compromised mechanical integrity, with decreased graft strength of up to 50% relative to freshly frozen allograft.[58,63]

In summary, although allograft tissue processing is necessary, it adds expense, reduces graft function both biologically and mechanically, and does not eliminate allograft risks entirely. Despite processing, histologic evidence of a low-grade inflammatory reaction is typical. These factors indicate that allograft is an inferior graft compared with autograft.

Demineralized Bone Matrix

Demineralized bone matrix (DBM) is thought to possess more osteoinductive properties than regular allograft because of enhanced bioavailability of growth factors following the demineralization process.[25,63] DBM gels and putties have become widely used in spinal fusion surgery since 1990, with about 500,000 mL used for implants each year in the United States.[63] The first widely available DBM preparation was Grafton gel (Osteotech Inc., Eatontown, NJ), consisting of DBM combined with a glycerol carrier. One retrospective study assessed the augmentation of local bone autograft with a DBM/glycerol composite for dorsolateral lumbar spine fusion as a means to avoid second-site autologous bone harvest. The control group used iliac crest autograft alone. The percentage of patients fused was similar in both groups (60% and 56% for DBM and controls, respectively; P = .83).[64] Although prospective clinical studies are under way, available data suggest a role for DBM as a bone-graft extender, rather than as a bone-graft substitute, in spinal surgery.[63] Other physical forms of DBM are being evaluated.

Xenograft

Xenograft bone tissue is harvested from animals. Because of their immunogenicity, xenograft preparations have generally proven impractical for clinical use. Removal of proteinaceous and fatty materials during processing, as what is done in the preparation of Kiel bone, Bio-Oss, or Oswestry bone, reduces immunogenicity to a degree.[20] However, the processing required to produce this type of graft removes the osteoinductive matrix proteins. To guarantee viral inactivation, all such proteins must be removed. Processing strategies, such as freezing and freeze-drying, are less common today than in the past because of unacceptable disease-transmission risk. Chemical washes have become more prevalent, but these tend to reduce or eliminate osteoinductivity.

Noninjectable Ceramics

Synthetic ceramics are osteoconductive but do not intrinsically possess any osteoinductive potential. The most common ceramics in current use are hydroxyapatite $[Ca_{10}(PO_4)_6(OH)_2]$, tricalcium phosphate $[Ca_3(PO_4)_2]$, calcium sulfate dihydrate $[CaSO_4 2(H_2O)]$, and combinations thereof.

Although exhibiting different chemical properties from tissue grafts, ceramics provide off-the-shelf availability of consistently high-quality synthetic materials that have no biologic hazards. After incorporation, the strength of the repaired defect site is comparable to that of cancellous bone.[30] Therefore, ceramics can be used as an alternative or as an addition to either cancellous autograft or allograft[7] or as a cancellous bone void filler, bone graft extender, or in sites where compression is the dominant mode of mechanical loading.

A randomized, prospective study of 341 patients undergoing dorsal spinal fusion for idiopathic scoliosis was undertaken in which patients received autograft or synthetic porous ceramic blocks (macroporous biphasic calcium phosphate [MBCP], Triosite™, Zimmer, Inc., Warsaw, IN; a mixture of hydroxyapatite and tricalcium phosphate).[60] Curve correction, curve maintenance, pain, and function were comparable between the two groups 18 months postoperatively. However, wound complications were more frequent in the autograft group; 14 patients experienced delayed healing, infection, or hematoma compared with only 3 wound complications in the MBCP group. In addition, 15 autograft patients had pain at the donor site at 3 months. In addition, other donor-site complications at 3 months included seven infections, two hematomas, and four delayed healing. Histologic findings showed new bone incorporating into the MBCP—evidence of good osteoconduction. These results suggest that synthetic porous ceramic is a safe and effective substitute for iliac graft autograft in this patient population.

Another prospective study of 106 cases in lumbar spinal fusion used MBCP granules mixed with autogenous bone chips and bone marrow obtained from the local spine.[10] Dorsal deformity correction involving the semi-rigid New Orleans instrumentation was performed in all patients. Only six nonunions were observed (three resulting from primary spondylolisthesis), suggesting a high success rate for MBCP in spinal fusion involving a semi-rigid instrumentation. The authors conclude that because the degenerative spine is not favorable to fusion, this technique offers an alternative to autograft to reduce patient morbidity from iliac bone harvest.[10]

Cost may become prohibitive in selected cases. This and unproven clinical efficacy make assumptions regarding widespread clinical applications tenuous.

Rapidly Resorbing Ceramics

Scaffolds of tricalcium phosphate (the α and β forms have different crystalline structures but the same elemental and stoichiometric characteristics; the α form is formulated at 1200°C and the β form is formulated at 800°C) and calcium sulfate have been used as synthetic bone void fillers for more than 20 years.[18,52] Calcium phosphate contains stoichiometric amounts of calcium and phosphorus, 39% and 20% by weight, respectively, similar to those found in natural bone.[46] It produces calcium-phosphate rich microenvironments that stimulate osteoclastic resorption and then osteoblastic new bone formation, resulting in new bone formed within the resorbed implant.[14] Less porous formulations resorb prior to achieving complete bone ingrowth.[25] The rate of resorption and the porosity of several bone substitutes are presented in Tables 13.2 and 13.3.

Calcium sulfate (plaster of Paris) is available in the form of pellets (OsteoSet, Wright Bio-Orthopedics, Arlington, TN). Calcium sulfate is nonporous and is rapidly removed from the surface site by chemical dissolution. Its removal is much more rapid than the bone formation process.

Intermediate Resorbing Ceramics

b-Tricalcium phosphate

An ultraporous β-tricalcium phosphate (β-TCP) formulation (Vitoss, Orthovita, Malvern, PA), engineered using nanoparticle technology, has a porosity comparable to natural cancellous bone. This involves a range of porosities (1 μ–1000 μ): 75% is greater than 100-μ pore size (critical for osteoconduction and resorbability); 25% is less than 100-μ pore size (critical for nutrient flow and oxygen transport). Smaller particles improve osteoconductive perform-

ance.[43] β-TCP particles average 100nm in diameter,[22] small enough for normal osteoclastic digestion during bone remodeling. The sponge-like porosity (90% void space) wicks cells and nutrients into the implant via enhanced capillarity. Because of its high porosity, β-TCP can be manipulated at surgery, poured as morsels or sculpted as blocks. Even after compression, β-TCP retains significant porosity. Like all ceramics, β-TCP is neither osteogenic nor osteoinductive.

Slowly Resorbing Ceramics

Hydroxyapatite is another ceramic that, although readily available, is associated with extremely slow remodeling. Slowly resorbing or nonresorbing material can interfere with remodeling and be the nidus of a mechanical stress point. The slow resorption and brittleness of hydroxyapatite make it less than ideal for clinical use. Therefore, hydroxyapatite is often used in modified forms, for example, combining it with calcium carbonate to speed the rate of resorption.[25]

In a study of 12 adolescent patients with scoliosis, spinal fusions were obtained after a follow-up mean time of 15 months in all patients randomized to treatment with either hydroxyapatite/tricalcium phosphate composite alone or in combination with autograft.[57] New bone ingrowth into ceramic pores was observed in two patients biopsied.

Injectable Ceramics (Calcium Phosphate Cement)

In contrast to preformed, solid constructs of calcium phosphate (so formed outside the body by manufacturing methods and subsequently placed by surgical intervention), liquid components can be injected directly into a bone defect site. This can then set into a solid, defect-filling, cement-like mass of calcium phosphate. It then slowly transforms into bone in 3 to 4 years (Norian SRS®, Norian Corp, Cupertino, CA) (Ed Norian SRS is now owned and marketed by Synthes).[13,41,62] The transformation of liquid components into a solid mass of calcium phosphate is achieved by well-known chemical reactions with a low-temperature exotherm. The resulting bone filler has a biologic response and compressive strength similar to cancellous bone,[13] and has promise for some clinical applications such as adjunct treatment of vertebral body compression fractures and possibly for the augmentation of pedicle screw fixation.

The primary drawbacks to injectable calcium phosphate are slow resorption, low porosity, and high commercialization costs. A potential risk to patients relates to one of the advantages of calcium phosphate: As calcium phosphate is applied in a liquid state and hardens in situ, its components may flow into and set within an unrecognized intraarticular extension of a fracture, causing an undesirable fusion of joint surfaces.[59] Another potential issue related to the calcium phosphate cements relates to the toxicity of calcium phosphate ions. Because these are true cements, that is, ions in suspension, when the material is deposited into a blood-filled cavity it may become diluted and the calcium phosphate ions are free to circulate, potentially generating cardiac arrhythmias or pulmonary mast cell-type reactions.

TABLE 13.2

Resorption Characteristics of Ceramics

Ceramic	Speed of Resorption
Hydroxyapatite	Slow
β-Tricalcium phosphate	Intermediate
α-Tricalcium phosphate	Rapid
Calcium sulfate	Very rapid

TABLE 13.3

Porosity and Osteoconductivity of Ceramics

Ceramic	Porosity/osteoconductivity
Calcium phosphate	Very little
Hydroxyapatite	Little
α-Tricalcium phosphate	Intermediate
β-Tricalcium phosphate	Very high

Collagen

Animal-derived collagen has been used with synthetic calcium phosphate bone fillers to modulate physical properties of bone-filling agents and to deliver factors that stimulate bone formation.[40] The admixture of collagen imparts a putty-like consistency to the bone graft that facilitates handling and placement at the time of surgery. The rationale for this combination rests in the approximation of bone minerals with collagen in normal bone matrix and the plentiful supply and low immunogenicity of processed xenographic collagen.

A composite of processed bovine dermal collagen and a biphasic (i.e., nonstoichiometric) calcium phosphate mixture of hydroxyapatite and TCP have been investigated in two canine spinal fusion models. In a dorsal segmental spinal fusion, the collagen/calcium phosphate mixture was inferior to autogenous bone,[55] whereas in a ventral segmental spinal fusion, the collagen/calcium phosphate mixture served as an effective autogenous bone extender when three parts of the mixture were mixed with one part of autogenous bone.[73] In the latter study, 12-month histologic and mechanical data were comparable between animals treated with autogenous bone and with 3:1 mixtures of the collagen/calcium phosphate composite and autogenous bone.

Nonbiologic Osteoconductive Substrates

The advantages of nonbiologic osteoconductive substrates include absolute control of the final structure, no immunogenicity, and excellent biocompatibility.[14] Examples include degradable polymers, bioactive glasses, and porous metals such as tantalum.

Qualitative Assessment of Ceramics

A summary of the overall advantages and disadvantages of various bone graft materials is presented in Table 13.4. The table provides an overview of the clinical and economic aspects of the ceramics available today. These ceramics can perhaps be best judged by their resorption and porosity characteristics (see Tables 13.2 and 13.3). Of particular note in this regard is the importance of using a bone substitute that resorbs (and remodels) at a rate similar to that of cancellous bone (intermediate; see Table 13.2) and that is highly porous (see Table 13.3).

Comparative Studies

A canine study was undertaken to determine the rate of new bone ingrowth into defect sites repaired with either porous β-TCP synthetic cancellous bone void filler or hydroxyapatite-coated calcium carbonate.[21] Cylindrical canine metaphyseal defects measured 10 mm × 25 mm in canine humeri. Bone ingrowth and scaffold resorption were quantified using standard histomorphometric techniques for specimens examined up to 1 year postimplantation.

Approximately 80% of the implanted β-TCP resorbed at 12 weeks, compared with only 34% of hydroxyapatite-coated calcium carbonate ($P < .05$). By 24 and 52 weeks, the remaining β-TCP implant volume was 3% and 1% of original implant size, respectively.

As early as 3 weeks, β-TCP showed resorption (clearing) from the center outward and some immature bone formation (Figure 13.1). At 6 weeks, the volume of new bone formed throughout the implants exceeded, by approximately 20%, the volume of original bone in areas adjacent to the defects (Figure 13.2). Remodeling was

---

TABLE 13.4

Summary of the Defining Advantages and Disadvantages of Bone Graft Materials[14,25,45,59,63,70]

Graft Material	Advantages	Disadvantages	Clinical Results*
Autograft	Osteogenic, osteoinductive, osteoconductive	Procurement morbidity, limited availability	56%–100%[63]
Allograft	Osteoconductive, weakly osteoinductive	Immunogenic, disease transfer risk	60%–90%*[28]
DBM	Osteoconductive, osteoinductive	Lacks structural strength[69]	60%[64]
Ceramics	Osteoconductive, limitless supply, biocompatible	Not osteogenic or osteoinductive, expensive	Equivalent to autograft in scoliosis, but decreased complications[57,60]
β-TCP/BMA composite	Osteogenic, osteoinductive, osteoconductive, limitless supply, biocompatible	R&D, commercialization costs	Not available
Collagen	Good delivery vehicle for other synthetic graft materials	By itself, a poor graft material	Preclinical only
Nonbiologic substrates	Osteoconductive	Foreign body reaction with degradable polymers	Preclinical only
BMP/synthetic composite	Osteogenic, osteoinductive, osteoconductive, limitless supply, biocompatible	R&D, commercialization costs	Ongoing clinical studies using rhBMP-2 combined with either ceramic or collagen sponge show results comparable to autograft[2]

β-TCP, β-Tricalcium phosphate; BMA, bone marrow aspirate; BMP, bone morphogenetic protein; DBM, demineralized bone matrix.
*Numeric clinical results are the overall incidence of vertebral body fusion in spine surgery, except for the entry for allograft, which represents the clinical, radiographic, and biologic assessments of massive osseous and osteochondral allografts as quoted in the cited reference.

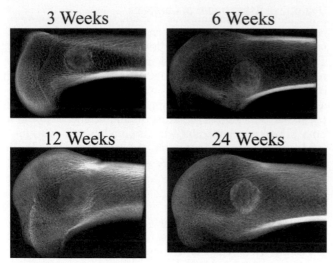

Figure 13.1 Radiograph of β-TCP implant from 3 to 24 weeks.

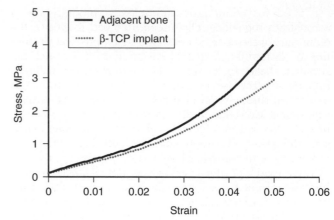

Figure 13.3 Results of compression testing of the β-TCP implant compared with adjacent bone at 52 weeks.

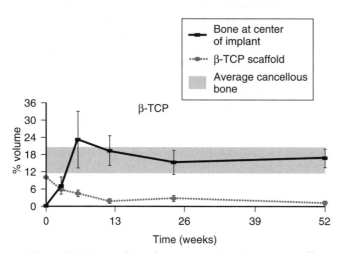

Figure 13.2 Rates of new bone ingrowth and resorption.[21]

essentially complete in 6 to 12 weeks, with bone density in the normal range and the scaffold almost completely resorbed by the end of the period. By 24 weeks, the implant trabecular orientation approximated the normal stress patterns of adjacent bone. Serial histologic and radiographic assessments made at 12, 24, and 52 weeks demonstrated comparable architecture and density between new bone within the defect sites and the adjacent original bone. The stress-strain curve of β-TCP was nearly identical to bone at 24 weeks and at 52 weeks (Figure 13.3). In contrast, the calcium carbonate stress-strain curve differed markedly from bone at 24 weeks. X-ray diffraction data of the β-TCP implants confirmed a 95% match to normal bone at 1 year.[51]

The study suggested that normal bone remodeling occurred with the β-TCP scaffold within 6 to 12 weeks after implantation. In contrast, about one third of the hydroxyapatite-coated calcium carbonate–implanted defect showed new bone formation (mainly at the periphery). No foreign-body response to either ultraporous β-TCP or hydroxyapatite-coated calcium carbonate was observed. The ultraporous β-TCP was manipulated easily at surgery, despite its very high porosity.

These results were superior to those of prior similar studies using other ceramics in several respects. Bruder[8] had found that a ceramic composed of hydroxyapatite and β-TCP produced no callus around the defect site or the host bone in the first 16 weeks after implantation, indicating inadequate bone healing. Both Bruder[8] and Kon[43] found that, using traditional synthetics, bone formation was most prevalent at the periphery of the defect. Bruder[8] noted that the only new bone that formed as a result of the osteoconductivity of the porous ceramic was an extension of the outgrowth from the cut ends of the host bone. In contrast, one of the striking observations about β-TCP is the initiation of resorption and osteogenesis at the center of the repaired defect site.

In summary, Bruder[8] found that hydroxyapatite bone substitute was not ideal for the treatment of segmental defects because of its brittle nature, susceptibility to fracture, and lack of completely interconnected pores.

Biologic/Synthetic Composite Grafts

A composite graft can be defined as any combination of materials that includes both an osteoconductive matrix and an osteogenic or osteoinductive material. The carrier matrix could be any of the osteoconductive materials listed in Table 13.1. When the osteoconductive scaffold is mixed with bone marrow aspirate (BMA), the newly formed composite graft may acquire osteogenic and osteoinductive potential, thus providing a competitive alternative to autograft. Other biologic agents that may impart this potential include osteoblastic progenitor stem cells, blood, platelet-rich fraction, and osteoinductive growth factors such as BMP, TGF (transforming growth factor), and FGF (fibroblast growth factor).[49]

Osteogenic and Osteoinductive Bone Marrow Aspirate

Background

In theory, osteoblast progenitor cells could be obtained from the periosteum of long bones, the peritrabecular connective tissue, or the bone marrow, and combined with a synthetic scaffold. This strategy is designed to minimize the need for chemotaxis and massive proliferation of osteoblast progenitor cells into the defect. Logically, the direct implantation of progenitor cells should lead to more rapid, uniform, and reliable healing of bone defects. A major challenge to this approach is the need to more fully identify the proper type and source of cells for autologous cell therapy.[8] However, for now, extensive clinical experience with bone marrow transplantation makes bone marrow a practical choice as a source of progenitor and osteoinductive cells.[53]

A number of studies exist that look at BMA and its positive effects on bone formation both *in vitro*[50] and *in vivo*.[16,50] The critical cellular components that contribute to bone growth are present in BMA. Identifiable cell types include both fibroblasts and undifferentiated stromal cells. Osteoprogenitor stem cells are estimated to constitute 1 in 50,000 bone marrow cells in young patients and 1 in 2,000,000 cells in elderly patients. They are the most useful of bone tissue cells because they can differentiate into four other cell types (osteoblasts, adipose cells, chondroblasts, and fibroblasts) and modify their morphologic/ functional attributes as needed.[1] The mesenchymal stem cells have the potential to differentiate into a variety of tissues, including bone, cartilage, tendon, ligament, and adipose aggregations. Consequently, BMA is an abundant source of osteogenic cells for immediate transplantation. Animal research suggests that precursor cells in bone marrow proliferate and differentiate after transplantation. Among the cells derived from such proliferation are active osteoblasts that drive the process of new bone formation.[26,53]

Many investigators are engaged in characterizing the progenitor populations present in bone marrow, and *in vitro* studies of bone marrow–derived osteoblastic progenitors have helped define the potential role of the many growth factors involved in regulating osteoblast differentiation.[49] Uncontrolled clinical trials suggest that mixtures of aspirated bone marrow and autograft may be effective in treating nonunions,[29,34] but prospective trials using bone marrow alone have not been performed.[3]

Another advantage of BMA is its availability and the relative safety of its harvest. It is the only source that requires neither an open surgical procedure nor the added time and cost of *in vitro* cell growth.[25] Cell progenitors derived from bone marrow can be harvested by aspiration from patients, with limited dilution by peripheral blood as long as the volume of aspirate from a single site is held to 2 mL or less.[53] Furthermore, the number of progenitors available in a graft site can be increased by concentration, if necessary, to further enhance the biologic result of bone grafting.[11,44] For subsequent use in transplantation, stem cells can also be cultured and expanded to many times their original number.

BMA/Bone composites

Bone marrow has been successfully used to stimulate healing in tibial fractures, suggesting a promptly renewable and reliable source of osteogenic cells without the disadvantages of standard open-grafting techniques.[11] In a study using human BMA taken from the femoral head and the iliac crest, the recovered cells demonstrated osteogenic potential *in vivo* in nude mice. The osteogenic potential was maintained as the cells were expanded in culture and enriched for grafting purposes.[33] Autologous bone marrow aspirated from the iliac crest had a beneficial effect upon osteogenesis in 25 of 28 patients when implanted with xenograft bone graft material (Kiel bone).[61] The addition of bone marrow to autograft iliac crest bone graft facilitated greater bone formation and fusion success rates than did autograft alone ($P < .05$) in a rabbit dorsolateral spine fusion model.[16] Furthermore, a study of 23 pediatric patients found that xenograft bone and other bone substitutes could be rendered osteogenic by combining these materials with fresh autologous bone marrow.[72]

BMA/Synthetic composites

A number of studies have assessed composites of bone marrow and synthetics for bone grafting.[8,40,43] Ceramics of tricalcium phosphate, hydroxyapatite, and collagen hydroxyapatite were evaluated alone and with added BMA to assess their ability to heal defects created surgically in the canine radius. These implants were also compared with a graft of autogenous cancellous bone. The addition of BMA was essential for tricalcium phosphate and hydroxyapatite to achieve results comparable to those obtained with cancellous bone at 24 weeks.[40]

Studies on healing of canine femoral defects with implanted calcium phosphate cylinders loaded with cultured autologous mesenchymal stem cells showed that the addition of the cells augmented the development of new periosteal bone around the implants.[8] Similarly, although porous hydroxyapatite bioceramic (HAC) alone was effective for repair of tibial defects (at 6 months), the introduction of bone marrow stromal cell populations into the composite resulted in far more extensive bone defect repair over a 2-month period.[43] However, in both studies, even in the cell-loaded scaffold, a higher concentration of new bone began in the periphery. The authors speculate that this is the result of better survival of loaded cells within the outermost portions of the HAC cylinder, which are probably vascularized faster and more efficiently than more internal regions. They note that this may be related to the design of the implant device. The β-TCP animal study, which showed bone formation initiating within the center of the β-TCP carrier, supports this explanation. As early as 3 weeks post-implantation, β-TCP showed resorption beginning from the center of the implant, perhaps because of the concentration of nutrients in the center.

The new generation of β-TCP implants brings unique biomechanical properties that make them particularly well suited for use with BMA in a composite graft. The broad range of interconnected porosity (1μm–1mm) allows nutrient fluids to percolate throughout the structure and to support the migration of parenchyma into the scaffold, enhancing the processes of new bone development and scaffold resorption. The unique structure of ultraporous β-TCP is thus conducive to rapid vascularization that is necessary for nourishing the seeded bone marrow, including bone-forming cells. In this respect, a β-TCP/BMA composite may be superior even to autograft, which suffers from anoxic cell death in the center of the graft, owing to the absence of vascularization (Figure 13.4). One of the

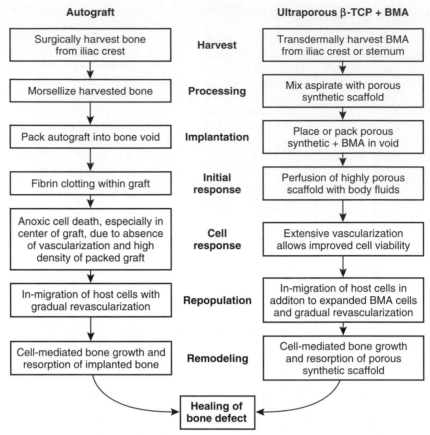

Figure 13.4 Processes in filling bone voids with either autograft or porous synthetic (i.e., β-TCP) seeded with BMA. Both are expected to support the osteogenesis, osteoconduction, and osteoinduction needed for healing. *β-TCP,* Beta-tricalcium phosphate; *BMA,* bone marrow aspirate.

striking features of grafting with β-TCP compared with other synthetic constructs is the central pattern of bone formation, suggesting penetration of cells and nutrients.

Thus, a composite made up of ultraporous β-TCP seeded with aspirated autologous bone marrow could deliver many of the positive qualities of an autograft and avoid most of the negative ones. The β-TCP scaffold supplies an osteoconductive surface for bone and tissue ingrowth. Ultraporosity facilitates infusion of bone matrix proteins and growth factors, making the β-TCP osteoinductive. Local and recruited osteogenic cells penetrate the composite and interact with the seeded bone-forming cells to impart osteogenic properties to β-TCP (Figure 13.5). β-TCP seeded with BMA can thus provide all three properties necessary for a successful bone graft that were previously satisfied by autografts, namely, osteogenesis, osteoinduction, and osteoconduction.

BMP/Synthetic composites

Based on favorable preclinical studies, three pilot human trials of purified recombinant human bone morphogenetic protein-2 (rhBMP-2) in spinal fusion have been launched over the past 4 years.[63] In the first trial, patients were randomized to receive threaded interbody fusion cages filled with either rhBMP-2/collagen sponge (11 patients) or autograft (3 patients). By 6 months, all patients in the

rhBMP-2/collagen sponge treatment group had achieved fusion compared with two of the three patients in the autograft treatment group. Reductions in the number of hospital days of patients treated with the composite sponge (2 days vs. 3.3 days) was attributed to the lack of secondary bone-harvesting procedures in patients in the composite-sponge treatment group.[4,63]

In the second trial, fusions of dorsal transverse processes were attempted with rhBMP-2/biphasic ceramic block composites on one side versus autograft on the contralateral side (seven patients). Initial results indicate that incidences of fusion are similar between treatment groups.[63] An additional trial is planned to determine the efficacy of the composite graft alone.

In the third trial (ongoing), cervical disks were removed and adjoining vertebrae were fused with autogenous bone harvested from the iliac crest. The resulting defects in the ilium were filled with rhBMP-2/collagen sponges (45 patients). This study is designed to investigate dose-response, with four different rhBMP-2–dose implants and a sham implant. The osteoinductive influence of BMP is to be determined by serial pelvic CT scans.

Collectively, the results of these trials will help confirm the applications of BMP in spine surgery.

Degradable polymers have almost no osteoconductive potential and are associated with an adverse foreign body reaction.[5,42] Nevertheless, because they are so versatile

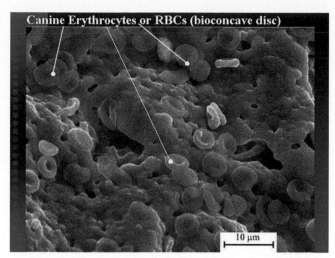

Figure 13.5 Scanning electron microscopy (SEM) image at magnification × 2000, showing a large number of canine erythrocytes (approximately 4 to 5μm diameter) in the center of the β-TCP scaffold. Cells can be transported via β-TCP; this includes mesenchymal stem cells, which are approximately 15 μm in diameter.

(a potential growth factor delivery vehicle with customized degradation rates and three-dimensional structure), research in this area remains active.

A porous biodegradable copolymer, poly (DL-lactide-coglycolide) (PLGA), was evaluated as a carrier for rhBMP-2, using a canine posterior segmental spinal fusion model.[54] The rhBMP-2/PLGA was compared with autogenous cancellous bone and with PLGA alone. Grafts were implanted in 33 fusion sites in 11 beagle dogs. At 12 weeks, sites were examined for union and assessed for strength with mechanical tests to failure. No significant difference in union score, stiffness, or strength was found for autogenous cancellous bone compared with rhBMP-2/PLGA; both scored higher for union than PLGA alone ($P = .001$ and $P = .0007$, respectively). The authors suggest that use of the composite material may provide efficacy equivalent to autogenous cancellous bone for dorsal spinal fusions and avoid the morbidity associated with autogenous graft procurement.

Summary

Bone is the most commonly transplanted tissue, except for blood. Autogenous bone grafting is one of the most common orthopedic procedures, performed in about 200,000 cases annually in the United States.[70] Although materials of biologic origin are now generally used, their preference may diminish as well-characterized inorganic materials with off-the-shelf availability offer potential to eliminate procurement morbidity associated with autograft and to eliminate risk of disease transmission associated with allograft.

However, the development of a usable osteoconductive carrier has lagged behind the isolation and synthesis of osteoinductive growth factors. Preclinical data indicate that the enhanced capillarity of such ceramics as

β-TCP may bring these bone-healing elements together in better balance. Advances in tissue engineering of synthetic composite grafts should demonstrate a synergy between components with results superior even to autogenous bone grafts.[45] The improved understanding of osteoprogenitor cell function, and advances in procurement and cell separation, will provide for increased osteogenic capabilities with negligible harvest morbidity. Finally, BMPs and synthetic composites show significant promise in the bone healing and bone fusion arenas. Pending clinical information regarding BMA/bone composites, BMPs, and synthetic composites is eagerly awaited.

REFERENCES

1. Anonymous Bone. In Ross MH, Romrell LJ, Kaye GI (eds): *Histology: a Text and Atlas,* ed 3. Baltimore: Williams & Wilkins, 1995, pp 150-187.
2. Arrington ED, Smith WJ, Chambers HG, *et al:* Complications of iliac crest bone graft harvesting. *Clin Orthop* 329:300-309, 1996.
3. Bauer TW, Muschier GF: Bone graft materials: an overview of the basic science. *Clin Orthop* 371:10-27, 2000.
4. Boden SD, Martin GJJ, Morone M, *et al:* The use of coralline hydroxyapatite with bone marrow, autogenous bone graft, or osteoinductive bone protein extract for posterolateral lumbar spine fusion. *Spine* 24:320-327, 1999.
5. Bostman O, Hirvensalo E, Makinen J, Rokkanen P: Foreign-body reactions to fracture fixation implants of biodegradable synthetic polymers. *J Bone Joint Surg Br* 72:592-596, 1990.
6. Boyce T, Edwards J, Scarborough N: Allograft bone: the influence of processing on safety and performance. *Orthop Clin North Am* 30:571-581, 1999.
7. Browner BD, Jupiter JB, Levine AM, *et al* (eds): *Skeletal Trauma: Fractures, Dislocations, Ligamentous Injuries,* ed 2, vol 2. Philadelphia, WB Saunders, 1998.
8. Bruder SP, Kraus KH, Goldberg VM, Kadiyala S: The effect of implants loaded with autologous mesenchymal stem cells on the healing of canine segmental bone defects. *J Bone Joint Surg Am* 80A:985-996, 1998.
9. Carter G: Harvesting and implanting allograft bone. *AORN J* 70:660-670, 1999.
10. Cavagna R, Daculsi G, Bouler JM: Macroporous calcium phosphate ceramic: a prospective study of 106 cases in lumbar spinal fusion. *J Long Term Eff Med Implants* 9:403-412, 1999.
11. Connolly J, Guse R, Lippiello L, Dehne R: Development of an osteogenic bone-marrow preparation. *J Bone Joint Surg Am* 71:684-691, 1989.
12. Connolly JF, Guse R, Tiedeman J, Dehne R: Autologous marrow injection as a substitute for operative grafting of tibial nonunions. *Clin Orthop* 266:259-270, 1991.
13. Constantz BR, lson IC, Fulmer MT, *et al:* Skeletal repair by *in situ* formation of the mineral phase of bone. *Science* 267:1796-1799, 1995.
14. Cornell CN: Osteoconductive materials and their role as substitutes for autogenous bone grafts. *Orthop Clin North Am* 30:591-598, 1999.

15. Cornell CN, Lane JM: Current understanding of osteoconduction in bone regeneration. *Clin Orthop* 7(355S):S267-S273, 1998.

16. Curylo LJ, Johnstone B, Petersilge CA, *et al:* Augmentation of spinal arthrodesis with autologous bone marrow in a rabbit posterolateral spine fusion model. *Spine* 24:434-438, 1999.

17. Dosoglu M, Orakdogen M, Tevruz M, *et al:* Enterocutaneous fistula: a complication of posterior iliac bone graft harvesting not previously described. *Acta Neurochir (Wien)* 140:1089-1092, 1998.

18. Doursounian L, Cazeau C, Touzard RC: Use of tricalcium phosphate ceramics in tibial plateau fracture repair: results of 15 cases reviewed at 38 months. Available at http://bhd.online.fr/framesus.htm. Accessed Sept 10, 2003.

19. Ehrler DM, Vaccaro AR: The use of allograft bone in lumbar spine surgery. *Clin Orthop* 371:38-45, 2000.

20. Elves MW, Salama R: A study of the development of cytotoxic antibodies produced in recipients of xenografts (heterografts) of iliac bone. *J Bone Joint Surg Br* 56: 331-339, 1974.

21. Erbe E, Clineff T, Lavagnino M, *et al:* Comparison of Vitoss™ and ProOsteone 50OR in a critical-sized defect at 1 year [abstract]. Presented at Annual Meeting of the Orthopaedic Research Society, February 25-28, 2001. San Francisco. Abstract 975.

22. Erbe E: Chemistry and resorption characteristics of a synthetic cancellous bone void filler, an ultraporous beta-tricalcium phosphate scaffold (abstract), 2000. Presented at World Spine 1. First Interdisciplinary World Congress on Spinal Surgery, August 28-September 1, 2000. Berlin, Germany.

23. Fernando TL, Kim SS, Mohler DG: Complete pelvic ring failure after posterior iliac bone graft harvesting. *Spine* 24:2101-2104, 1999.

24. Fernyhough JC, Schimandle JJ, Weigel MC, *et al:* Chronic donor site pain complicating bone graft harvesting from the posterior iliac crest for spinal fusion. *Spine* 17(12): 1474-1480, 1992.

25. Fleming JE Jr, Cornell CN, Muschier GF: Bone cells and matrices in orthopedic tissue engineering. *Orthop Clin North Am* 31:357-374, 2000.

26. Friedenstein AJ, Petrakova KV, Kurolesova Al, Frolova GP: Heterotopic transplants of bone marrow. *Transplantation* 6:230-247, 1968.

27. Friedlaender GE: Bone allografts: the biological consequences of immunologic events. *J Bone Joint Surg Am* 73A:1119-1122, 1991.

28. Friedlaender GE, Strong DM, Tomford WVV, Mankin HJ: Long-term follow-up of patients with osteochondral allografts: a correlation between immunologic responses and clinical outcome. *Orthop Clin North Am* 30:583-588, 1999.

29. Garg NK, Gaur S: Percutaneous autogenous bone-marrow grafting in congenital tibial pseudarthrosis. *J Bone Joint Surg Br* 77B:830-831, 1995.

30. Gazdag AR, Lane JM, Glaser D, Forster RA: Alternatives to autogenous bone graft: efficacy and indications. *J Am Acad Orthop Surg* 3:1-8, 1995.

31. Goldberg VM, Powell A, Shaffer JW, *et al:* Bone grafting: role of histocompatibility in transplantation. *J Orthop Res* 3:389-404, 1985.

32. Gupta AR, Shah NR, Patel TCh, Grauer JN: Perioperative and long-term complications of iliac crest bone graft harvesting for spinal surgery: a quantitative review of the literature. *Int Med J* 8(3):163-166, 2001.

33. Haynesworth SE, Goshima J, Goldberg VM, Caplan Al: Characterization of cells with osteogenic potential from human marrow. *Bone* 13:81-88, 1992.

34. Healey JH, Zimmerman PA, McDonnell JM, Lane JM: Percutaneous bone marrow grafting of delayed union and nonunion in cancer patients. *Clin Orthop* 256:280-285, 1990.

35. Heary RF, Schlenk RP, Sacchieri TA, *et al:* Persistent iliac crest donor site plan: Independent outcome assessment. *Neurosurgery* 50(3):510-516, March 2002.

36. Henman P, Finlayson D: Ordering allograft by weight: suggestions for the efficient use of frozen bone-graft for impaction grafting. *J Arthroplasty* 15:368-371, 2000.

37. Higuchi KW: Osseointegration or osteointegration? [letter]. *Oral Surg Oral Med Oral Path Oral Radiol Endod* 89:132, 2000.

38. Hu R, Hearn T, Yang J: Bone graft harvest site as a determinant of iliac crest strength. *Clin Orthop* 310:252-256, 1995.

39. Hu RW, Bohlman HH: Fracture at the iliac bone graft harvest site after fusion of the spine. *Clin Orthop* 309:208-213, 1994.

40. Johnson KD, Frierson KE, Keller TS, *et al:* Porous ceramics as bone graft substitutes in long bone defects: a biomechanical, histological, and radiographic analysis. *J Orthop Res* 14:351-369, 1996.

41. Jupiter JB, Winters S, Sigman S, *et al:* Repair of five distal radius fractures with an investigational cancellous bone cement: a preliminary report. *J Orthop Trauma* 11:110-116, 1997.

42. Kadilaya S, Lo H, Leong KVV, *et al:* Biodegradable polymers and synthetic bone graft in bone formation and repair. 1994. Presented at American Academy Orthopaedic Surgeons Symposium. Park Ridge, IL 11:317-324, 1994.

43. Kon E, Muraglia A, Corsi A, *et al:* Autologous bone marrow stromal cells loaded onto porous hydroxyapatite ceramic accelerate bone repair in critical-size defects of sheep long bones. *J Biomed Mater Res* 49:328-337, 2000.

44. Krzymanski G, Kalozak M, Wiktor-Jedrzejczak W: The use of bone-marrow-derived fibroblastoid cells and fresh bone marrow in the treatment of bone defects: an experimental study. *Int J Oral Maxillofac Surg* 26:55-60, 1997.

45. Lane JM, Tomin E, Bostrom MPG: Biosynthetic bone grafting. *Clin Orthop* 367S:S107-S117, 1999.

46. LeGeros RZ: Calcium phosphates in oral biology and medicine. *Monogr Oral Sci* 15:1-201, 1991.

47. Lewandrowski KU, Gresser JD, Wise DL, Trantolo DJ: Bioresorbable bone graft substitutes of different osteoconductivities: a histologic evaluation of osteointegration of poly(propylene glycol-cofumaric acid)-based cement implants in rats. *Biomaterials* 21: 757-764, 2000.

48. Lowery GL, Kulkarni S, Pennisi AE: Use of autologous growth factors in lumbar spinal fusion. *Bone* 25(suppl): 47S-50S, 1999.

49. Ludwig SC, Boden SD: Osteoinductive bone graft substitutes for spinal fusion: a basic science summary. *Orthop Clin North Am* 30:635-645, 1999.

50. Majors AK, Boehm CA, Nitto H, *et al:* Characterization of human bone marrow stromal cells with respect to osteoblastic differentiation. *J Orthop Res* 15:546-557, 1997.

51. Marx J, Erbe E, Mesropian C: Structural evolution of Vitoss™ scaffold to bone in canine humeral defect at 1 year (abstract). Presented at Annual Meeting of the Orthopaedic Research Society, February 25-28, 2001. San Francisco, CA.

52. McAndrew MP, Gorman PW, Lange TA: Tricalcium phosphate as a bone graft substitute in trauma: a preliminary report. *J Orthop Trauma* 2:333-339, 1989.

53. Muschler GF, Boehm C, Easley K: Aspiration to obtain osteoblast progenitor cells from human bone marrow: the influence of aspiration volume. *J Bone Joint Surg Am* 79A:1699-1709, 1997.

54. Muschler GF, Hyodo A, Manning T, *et al:* Evaluation of human bone morphogenetic protein 2 in a canine spinal fusion model. *Clin Orthop* 308:229-240, 1994.

55. Muschler GF, Negami S, Hyodo A, *et al:* Evaluation of collagen ceramic composite graft materials in a spinal fusion model. *Clin Orthop* 328:250-260, 1996.

56. Palmer SH, Gibbons CL, Athanasou NA: The pathology of bone allograft. *J Bone Joint Surg Br* 81B:333-335, 1999.

57. Passuti N, Daculsi G, Rogez JM, *et al:* Macroporous calcium phosphate ceramic performance in human spine fusion. *Clin Orthop* 248:169-176, 1989.

58. Pelker RR, Friediaender GE: Biomechanical aspects of bone autografts and allografts. *Orthop Clin North Am* 18:235-239, 1987.

59. Perry CR: Bone repair techniques, bone graft, and bone graft substitutes. *Clin Orthop* 360:71-86, 1999.

60. Ransford AO, Morley T, Edgar MA, *et al:* Synthetic porous ceramic compared with autograft in scoliosis surgery: a prospective, randomized study of 341 patients [published erratum appears in *J Bone Joint Surg Br* May;80(3):562, 1998]. *J Bone Joint Surg Br* 80:13-18, 1998.

61. Salama R, Weissman SL: The clinical use of combined xenografts of bone and autologous red marrow: a preliminary report. *J Bone Joint Surg Br* 60:111-115, 1978.

62. Sanchez-Sotelo J, Munuera L, Madero R: Treatment of fractures of the distal radius with a remodellable bone cement: a prospective, randomised study using Norian SRS. *J Bone Joint Surg Br* 82:856-863, 2000.

63. Sandhu HS, Grewal HS, Parvataneni H: Bone grafting for spinal fusion. *Orthop Clin North Am* 30:685-698, 1999.

64. Sassard WR, Eidman DK, Gray PMJ, *et al:* Augmenting local bone with Grafton demineralized bone matrix for posterolateral lumbar spine fusion: avoiding second site autologous bone harvest. *Orthopedics* 23:1059-1065, 2000.

65. Siegel MA: Osseointegration or osteointegration? [letter]. *Oral Surg Oral Med Oral Pathol Oral Radiol Endod* 89:132, 2000.

66. Steinmann JC, HerkoWtz HN: Pseudarthrosis of the spine. *Clin Orthop* 284: 80-90, 1992.

67. Strong DM, Friedlaender GE, Tomford WW, *et al:* Immunologic responses in human recipients of osseous and osteochondral allografts. *Clin Orthop* 326:107-114, 1996.

68. Summers BN, Eisenstein SM: Donor site pain from the ilium: a complication of lumbar spine fusion. *J Bone Joint Surg Br* 71B:677-680, 1989.

69. Truumees E, HerkoWtz HN: Alternatives to autologous bone harvest in spine surgery. *Univ Penn Orthop J* 12: 77-88, 1999.

70. Van Heest A, Swiontkowski M: Bone-graft substitutes. *Lancet* 353(*suppl I*):28-29, 1999.

71. Varga E, Hu R, Hearn TC, Woodside T, Yang J: Biomechanical analysis of hemipelvic deformation after corticospongious bone graft harvest from the posterior iliac crest. *Spine* 21:1494-1499, 1996.

72. Wientroub S, Goodwin D, Khermosh O, Salama R: The clinical use of autologous marrow to improve osteogenic potential of bone grafts in pediatric orthopedics. *J Pediatr Orthop* 186-190, 1989-1990.

73. Zerwekh JE, Kourosh S, Scheinberg R, *et al:* Fibrillar collagen-biphasic calcium phosphate composite as a bone graft substitute for spinal fusion. *J Orthop Res* 10:562-572, 1992.

CHAPTER 14

Osteointegration (Osseointegration)

Daisuke Togawa, Thomas W. Bauer, Lisa A. Ferrara, Jason Eckhardt, Isador H. Lieberman, and Edward C. Benzel

Osteointegration (Osseointegration)

Recent advances in spine surgery have led to expanded use of synthetic biomaterials. The interface between host bone and a synthetic device has an important influence on the clinical efficacy of that device. These interfaces have been described as abutting (e.g., interbody bone graft, interbody cement), penetrating (e.g., nail, staple, screw), gripping (e.g., hook, wire), conforming (e.g., polymethylmethacrylate [PMMA]), and osteointegrating (e.g., some forms of biologic bond to metal or ceramics).[5] With regard to the root of the word *osteointegration*, the word *integrate* is derived from Latin, and so is the prefix *osseo-*, whereas *osteo-* is derived from Greek.[77] Therefore the term *osseointegration* is often (or preferably) used, instead of *osteointegration*.

Since Branemark, a Swedish dentist, introduced the term *osseointegration* to describe the process by which some oral implants interface with bone,[9] this term has been widely used in the dental and orthopedic arenas. Branemark originally defined osseointegration as "direct structural and functional connection between ordered, living bone and the surface of a load carrying implant."[9] During the past 30 years, however, the term has been used in a number of scientific publications regarding both structural (morphologic) and functional (physiologic) senses. Various factors influence this process at the implant-bone interface, including preparation of the surrounding bone, the surface preparation and sterilization procedures to remove organic residues from the implant, surface topography, overall implant design, and load transmission. The term *osseointegration* therefore has been used in a broad sense in the aforementioned publications.

With maturation and consolidation of the bone-implant interface, the bone and implant function as a biomechanic unit. This implies that load transfer from implant to bone is distributed more evenly over a much larger surface area. Most surgeons expect direct bone apposition for interbody fusion devices, artificial discs, pedicle screws, and various spacers. However, it remains unclear how often and to what extent this is achieved.

Osteoconductivity

An osteoconductive material promotes bone apposition along its surface. The term *osteoconduction* is not absolute, and is best understood when used in the context of a comparative study in which variables of the substrate material, porosity, surface geometry, and surface chemistry are highly controlled and defined.[2] For example, when matched by size, shape, and surface texture, hydroxyapatite (HA) is more osteoconductive than titanium, but titanium is more osteoconductive than a similar segment of cobalt-chromium alloy, or stainless steel; and rough stainless steel is more osteoconductive than polished stainless steel. Thus there are several different factors that influence the extent to which osteoblasts bind to a surface and produce bone matrix.

Biomaterials
Metals

Metals have been used in various forms as implants, including stainless steels, cobalt-based alloys, and pure titanium and titanium-based alloys. Each metal has different characteristics and behaves differently *in vivo*. For example, titanium alloy differs from stainless steel by having less resistance to abrasive wear, but providing better corrosion resistance, biocompatibility, less magnetic resonance imaging (MRI) distortion, and increased modulus of elasticity. Because of these advantages, titanium alloy is often used for orthopedic and spine implants. As described by Wolff's law, bone grows in response to applied stress and often is resorbed if a mechanical stimulus is lacking.[72] Of importance, the stiffness of many metals may shield the underlying bone from stress. Alloys with elastic moduli less than that of stainless steel, such as Ti6Al4V, have been successfully used in fracture fixation, but stress shielding is still observed.[73,78] At the implant-bone interface, most of these metals demonstrate variable osteoconductivity. Titanium implants generally have a better biocompatibility and osteoconductivity than many other metals, and their surface chemistry and texture is more influential regarding bone ingrowth.

Surface Texture

Early investigations were undertaken by Smith in the 1960s, using a porous surface ceramic.[53] Currently a wide variety of surface textures have been used to help achieve bone ingrowth into prosthetic devices, in both dental and orthopedic implant applications. Three-dimensional, porous surfaces of sintered beads or wire, roughened surfaces created by etching the implant surface, and rough surfaces created by the application of metal by plasma spray or other methods have been tested in a number of animal and clinical studies (Figures 14.1 and 14.2).[17,21,41,66] For example, Friedman *et al.* tested various biomaterials with different surfaces in the rabbit femur and showed that the shear strength and bone apposition of implants with arc-deposited titanium coating, and with one and three layers of cobalt-chromium beads, were significantly greater than those of implants with plasma-sprayed cobalt-chromium texture and grid-blasted titanium alloy.[22] Moreover, previous studies have suggested that the metal surface texture of a biomaterial can influence cell attachment and bone apposition. Martin *et al.*[42] showed that surface texture affects cell attachment, as well as cell morphology, proliferation, and differentiation. Thomas and Cook[59] showed that roughened implants yielded more direct bone apposition *in vivo* when compared to smooth implants of the same materials. Similarly, Turner *et al.*[70] demonstrated greater bone apposition to titanium canine hip implants with an average texture of 45μm compared to implants with texture of 8, 4, and 1μm.

Excellent clinical results (joint surgery) have been reported with several surface treatments.[21,41] However, the optimal surface texture for each implant remains controversial. A number of medical device manufacturers continue to investigate new surfaces in an attempt to improve fixation and lower cost. Thus a surface topography that incorporates such surface modifications can alter the tissue and/or cell interactions with bone, and appears to affect biomechanical interactions as well.[28] Still to be determined, however, is the contribution of bone type and location to the extent of osseointegration (i.e., vertebral body end plates osseointegrate as well as tibial plateau).

Other Materials

Various other biomaterials have been used at the bone-implant interface for spine surgery, including PMMA, calcium phosphate cement, ceramics (HA, bioactive glasses), and polymers (polylactic acid [PLA]), polyglycolic acid (PGA), hydrogels, carbon fiber-reinforced polymer, and polyetheretherketone (PEEK). All foreign materials

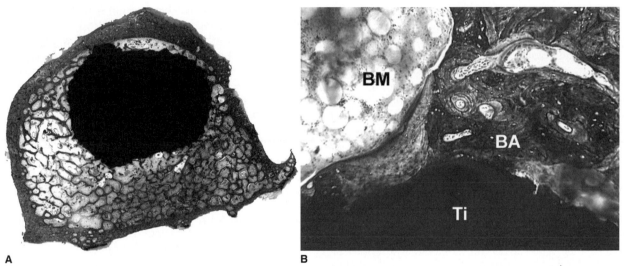

Figure 14.1 Direct bone apposition to metal hip implant. **(A)** Gross view. **(B)** Direct bone apposition *(BA)* and healthy bone marrow *(BM)* are observed without an intervening layer of fibrous tissue on this experimental canine femoral titanium implant *(Ti;* surface: arc apatitic titanium). *(From Togawa D,* et al: *Lumbar intervertebral body fusion cages—histological evaluation of clinically failed cages retrieved from humans,* J Bone Joint Surg 86A(1):70-79, 2004.)

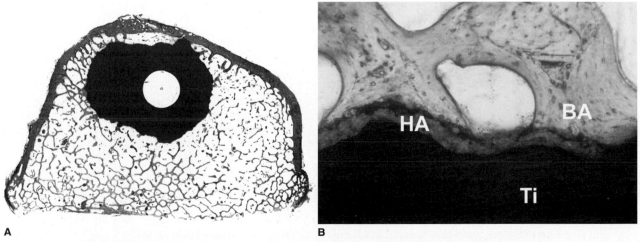

Figure 14.2 Direct bone apposition to hydroxyapatite coated titanium implant. **(A)** Gross view. **(B)** Hydroxyapatite *(HA)*-coated titanium femoral stems *(Ti)* show extensive bone apposition *(BA)* compared to non-HA–coated stems (canine total hip arthroplasty model). *(From Togawa D, Bauer TW, Mochida Y, et al.[66])*

induce some response when implanted in a host; so strictly speaking, all materials are bioactive. This response is often inflammatory, but some materials induce relatively little inflammation and instead promote bone formation by osteogenic, osteoconductive, or osteoinductive processes. Although PMMA and carbon have excellent biocompatibility, both are less osteoconductive than calcium phosphates or some metals. PMMA has been used for years to help stabilize pathologic fractures, but its exothermic curing and poor osteoconductivity are disadvantages for some clinical applications. Carbon fiber-reinforced polymer and PEEK can yield wear debris,[31,61,63,64] but in the spine, carbon fiber-reinforced polymer has been used as an interbody stabilization device, and has been associated with clinically successful outcomes without significant particle-induced osteolysis.[11,26] Nevertheless, there is no evidence that these cages have direct bone apposition around them.

Hydroxyapatite is an osteoconductive calcium phosphate that can be prepared as granules, blocks, or as coating on implants.[3] When placed in a suitable host site, HA is osteoconductive and has some compressive strength, but in general, blocks of sintered HA are difficult to machine. In addition, they are brittle and very slow to resorb. Injectable cements are composed of either calcium phosphates or bioglass derivatives. The calcium phosphate cements are highly osteoconductive, develop about 55Mpa compressive strength, cure isothermically, are very slow to resorb, and are very weak in tension and shear. The bioglass cements are not as osteoconductive, but offer greater shear strength.[4] Bioabsorbable materials such as PLA and PGA are less osteoconductive in general. But since Kulkarni *et al.* introduced resorbable polymers for use in surgical implants, these materials have been used successfully in various surgical applications.[8,12,14,16,36] The use of these materials in spine surgery has only been advocated recently. The main advantage of a resorbable material is that it confers initial and intermediate stability without having any of the long-term complications, such as stress shielding or migration of the implant. The gradual degradation of bioabsorbable spinal implants allows axial loads that were initially borne by the implant, to be progressively transferred to the bone.[15] Another advantage of such materials is that there is no interference with radiographic studies. These materials have been used as plates and interbody fusion devices,[74-76] but again there is little histologic evidence of direct bone apposition to the implant.

Surgical Applications

Osseointegration of spinal implants is desirable for many clinical applications. A variety of biomaterials have been used in spine surgery with the hope of achieving osseointegration.

Interbody Fusion

Interbody fusion devices are widely used for spinal arthrodesis and have demonstrated their clinical effectiveness for various degenerative disorders of the spine. Numerous types of spinal fusion cages have been developed from titanium, or carbon fiber-reinforced or bioabsorbable polymer composites.[10,37,49,55,67] They also have been created in many shapes—horizontal cylinders, vertical rings or mesh, rectangular, and open boxes. All shapes can be packed with bone graft or graft materials to promote interbody fusion. With respect to cage design, a difference in the extent of end-plate, material stiffness, and other characteristics may be factors associated with success. Successful spinal fusion with interbody cage devices has been radiographically confirmed in a number of clinical studies.[11,38,43,49] The results of some animal studies have shown histologic evidence of bone graft incorporation and good connectivity between the bone inside the cages and adjacent vertebral bodies.[7,19,67,68] However, the extent of direct bone apposition to clinically satisfactory cages is unknown, but clinically failed cages show no direct bone apposition, even when viable bone is present in the center of the cages (Figures 14.3 and 14.4).[60,64]

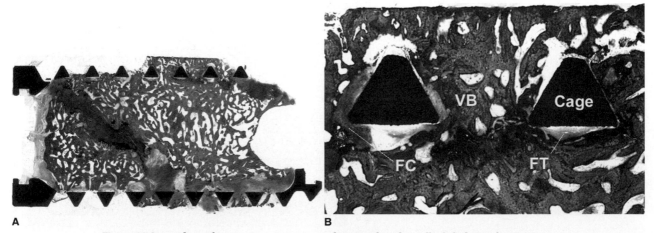

Figure 14.3 No direct bone apposition to metal cage. This clinically failed metal cage (**A**) contained viable bone (*VB*) extending through the openings along one side. (**B**) The bone must have connected to bone outside the cage, but there is no direct bone apposition to the metal of the cage. Instead, fibrous tissue (*FT*) and fibrocartilage (*FC*) surround each strut of metal. (*From Togawa D, Bauer TW, Lieberman IH, et al.*[66])

Pedicle Screws

Pedicle screw, rod, or plate systems used in conjunction with a dorsal intertransverse bone graft maintain spinal alignment and provide immediate structural stability, thereby allowing early mobilization of the patient while promoting arthrodesis. However, pedicle integrity is poor in osteoporotic vertebrae, in part because of low screw-bone interface strength. Different methods of improving the purchase of these screws have been investigated, including modifications of the design of the thread, the shape, and their surface.* Sanden *et al.*[50] investigated the effects of both partial and total HA coating of pedicle screws on purchase in a series of the patients with lumbar and lumbosacral degenerative disorders. Approximately 1 year after the surgery, the instruments were removed in some patients, and the authors measured both insertion and extraction torques during the procedure. The results demonstrated that both insertion and extraction torques for fully coated screws were significantly higher than for uncoated or partly coated screws. Of particular note, the extraction torques exceeded the upper limit of the torque wrench (600Nm) for many HA-coated screws, suggesting that HA-coated pedicle screws improved fixation with reduced risk of loosening of the screw.

Another strategy to improve the chances of successful fixation with pedicle screws in weakened cancellous bone is to augment the pedicle screw tract with cement to increase its stiffness and strength.[5,46,69] Turner *et al.*[69] tested HA composite resin cement (Kuraray Co., Krashiki, Japan) to determine whether it could stiffen the screw-bone interface in a human cadaveric study. Cement augmentation significantly improved the initial load-carrying capacity (116%), the load-carrying capacity after mechanical testing (165%), and the initial rate of decrease of the implant-bone interface (159%). These results suggested

that cement augmentation of pedicle screws increased the stiffness and stability of the screw-bone interface. Furthermore the partially pressurized injection of cement into the screw hole causes the cement to distribute itself into the trabecular bone. This effectively increases the diameter of the screw as well.[5] What remains to be determined is whether the significant improvement in fixation improves the fusion rate or causes late osteoporosis as a result of stress shielding.

Spacers, Carriers, and Scaffolds

In spine surgery HA is widely used as a spacer, especially for ventral cervical spine fusions and laminoplasty procedures.* HA spaces are reported to have excellent osteoconductivity regarding radiographic studies, with good clinical results and few complications. Histologic evaluation of three spinous processes of the cervical spine removed from a patient with a recurrent intramedullary tumor at the time of revision laminectomy, 1 year after laminoplasty, confirmed direct bone apposition of bone to an HA spacer at three of the six bone-hydroxyapatite interfaces.[32]

Clinically, HA and tricalcium phosphate (TCP) have been shown to be effective as bone graft expanders in dorsal spinal fusion surgery,[23,54] but it may be difficult to distinguish bone from residual synthetic calcium phosphates when radiographs are used as an outcome measure in fusion studies. Human biopsies obtained from fusion mass 1 year after dorsolateral fusion that used HA/TCP granules show extensive bone apposition (Figure 14.5).[62]

HA, TCP, and collagen can be used as carriers of bone morphogenetic proteins (BMPs).[6,27,45,51] The combination matrices, mixed with HA, could have some compression resistance and act as carriers for BMPs.[1] Akamaru *et al.*[1] used biphasic ceramic phosphate (BCP) granules (15% HA, 85%

---

*References 18,20,34,39,40,52.

*References 24,29,30,32,35,47,57.

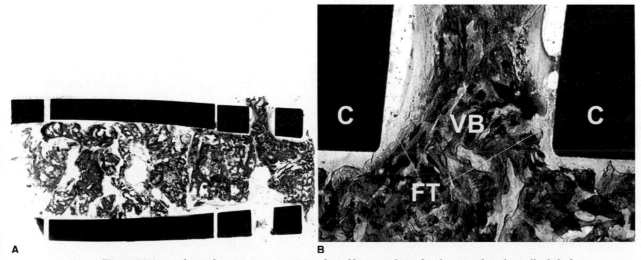

A   **B**

Figure 14.4 No direct bone apposition to carbon fiber reinforced polymer. This clinically failed carbon-fiber reinforced polymer cage (**A**), retrieved from the cervical spine, showed no direct bone apposition to the carbon fiber polymer (*C*) (**B**), even if most of the bone inside the cage was viable bone (*VB*). The viable bone extends through the lateral hole, but fibrous tissue (*FT*) separates bone from the cage. (*From Togawa D, Bauer TW.*[60])

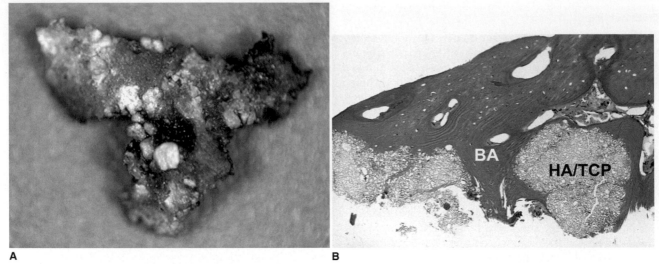

A   **B**

Figure 14.5 Direct bone apposition to hydroxyapatite/tricalcium phosphate (*HA/TCP*) granules. (**A**) Gross view. (**B**) Biopsy specimens obtained from human dorsolateral fusion with HA/TCP mixed with autograft showed partial direct bone apposition (*BA*) to the residual HA/TCP granules approximately 1 year after the surgery. (*From Togawa D, Bauer TW, Kanayama M, et al.*[62])

TCP), combined with human recombinant BMP-2, for an adult monkey dorsolateral spinal fusion model. Histologic results revealed that most of the ceramic had resorbed 24 weeks after surgery, but some was still present and encased in normal bone, suggesting that the ceramic served as a scaffold and became incorporated with new bone before it could be resorbed.

Artificial Disks

Functional disk interspace prostheses have been sought since the 1950s. Although there were a few early attempts, disk replacement did not become a viable therapy until the late 1980s. Several devices currently available in Europe are undergoing evaluation in the United States in clinical trials.[25] The SB Charite disk prosthesis (Waldemar Link, Hamburg, Germany) was created in Germany in the early 1980s.[13] The third generation of the SB Charite lumbar total disk replacement prosthesis has been used in more than 5000 patients worldwide since 1987. A porous ingrowth coating has been widely available outside the United States since 1998. Theoretically the unconstrained characteristic of the prosthesis should reduce the stress at the bone-metal interface and lead to more favorable porous ingrowth characteristics than a constrained prosthesis. In their baboon study, McAfee *et al.*[44] reported that 14 of 14 HA-coated SB Charite prosthetic vertebral end-plates were well fixed, with no evidence of loosening.[44] A coronal histologic section of the SB Charite prosthesis in their study shows excellent bone ingrowth into the HA-coated end-plates without evidence of fibrous tissue or synovium 6 months after surgery. Among several types of total disk prostheses, a triaxial three-dimensional fabric woven from a high-molecular–weight polyethylene fiber is under study.[33] The superior and inferior surfaces are coated with bioactive materials to promote bony ingrowth to anchor the device. Recently Takahata *et al.*[56] reported on the mechan-

ical properties and histologic appearance of this disk material, compared to a glass ceramic spacer in an *in vivo* sheep model. The results showed that bone tissue grew into the space between the ultrahigh-molecular–weight polyethylene fibers beginning at 4 months after surgery. The interfacial tensile strength at 6 months was significantly higher in the total disk material group than in the glass ceramic spacer group ($p < .05$).

Vertebral Augmentation

Vertebral augmentation has been extensively used to treat vertebral bodies involved with osteolytic metastases, myeloma, and osteoporotic compression fractures. PMMA is the most common material used for such procedures. Because PMMA is not as osteoconductive as HA, it cannot be expected to promote bone apposition. Technically, under fluoroscopic guidance, PMMA is injected into the weakened vertebrae until the cement is interdigitated into trabecular bone within the vertebrae, so that the cement is locked within the vertebrae. A recent report describing the histology of excised human specimens shows that there was no direct bone apposition to the cement. Instead, a thin membrane of fibrous tissue separated bone from the PMMA (Figure 14.6).[65] To bypass perceived limitations of PMMA, alternative cements that have variable osteoconductive properties have been tested. For example, several animal studies with injectable calcium phosphate cements confirm their feasibility, mechanical effectiveness, biocompatibility, and osteoconductivity (Figure 14.7).[58,71] Moreover, Nakano *et al.*[48] reported good clinical results of percutaneous vertebral augmentation using calcium phosphate cement in the treatment of osteoporotic vertebral compression fractures. Composite cements (acrylic cements in conjunction with ceramics) are bioactive, highly radiopaque, and feature excellent mechanical properties. One such cement, Cortoss (Orthovita, Malvern, PA), is

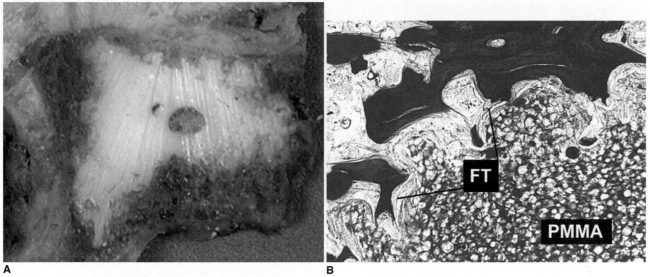

Figure 14.6 Interface between polymethylmethacrylate *(PMMA)* and bone. **(A)** Gross view. **(B)** Although PMMA interdigitated into trabecular bone of this vertebral body obtained after kyphoplasty, there is no direct bone apposition to the PMMA. Instead a thin fibrous tissue *(FT)* separates bone from the PMMA. *(From Togawa D, Bauer TW, Lieberman IH, Takikawa S.[65])*

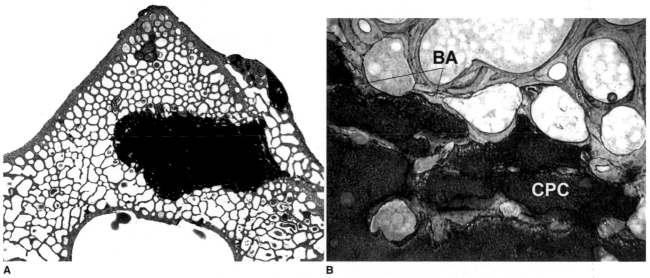

Figure 14.7 Interface between calcium phosphate cement and bone. **(A)** Gross view. **(B)** Calcium phosphate cement (CPC, BoneSource®, Howmedica Osteonics, Mahwah, NJ) injected into a defect in a vertebral body showed extensive bone apposition *(BA)* 24 months after the surgery. *(From Takikawa S, Bauer TW, Turner AS, et al: Comparison of injectable calcium phosphate cement and polymethylmethacrylate for use in vertebroplasty: In-vivo evaluation using an osteopenic sheep model. Trans Society for Biomaterials 231, 2002.)*

currently undergoing clinical trials for vertebroplasty, and so far, has been shown to be a potentially valuable alternative to PMMA. It is emphasized, however, that composite cement's osteoconductivity in human vertebrae is still unknown.

Summary

In this chapter the terminology of osseointegration and osteoconductive materials and their clinical applications were discussed. The term *osteointegration (osseointegration)* has

been used in both structural and functional applications. To satisfy both conditions the material must achieve complete direct bone apposition and be clinically effective. Most types of spine implants have been associated with clinical success, which suggests that such implants may have achieved osseointegration in the broadest sense. However, it is often unknown if complete and direct bone apposition to the implant has been morphologically achieved; or for that matter, if it is even necessary. Thus osseointegration is desirable but it may not always be necessary. It must be emphasized that it is necessary for surgeons to understand the importance of material properties, implant characteristics, implant design, and the characteristics of the local environment (e.g., blood flow, load transmission) to achieve clinically successful osseointegration in spine surgery.

REFERENCES

1. Akamaru T, Suh D, Boden SD, *et al*: Simple carrier matrix modifications can enhance delivery of recombinant human bone morphogenetic protein-2 for posterolateral spine fusion. *Spine* 28:429-434, 2003.
2. Bauer TW, Muschler GF: Bone graft materials. An overview of the basic science. *Clin Orthop* 371:10-27, 2000.
3. Bauer TW, Smith ST: Bioactive materials in orthopaedic surgery: overview and regulatory considerations. *Clin Orthop* 395:11-22, 2002.
4. Bauer TW, Togawa D: Bone graft substitutes: toward a more perfect union. *Orthopedics* 26:925-926, 2003.
5. Benzel EC: Implant-bone interface. In *Biomechanics of Spine Stabilization*. New York, Thieme New York, 2001, pp 155-170.
6. Boden SD, Kang J, Sandhu H, Heller JG: Use of recombinant human bone morphogenetic protein-2 to achieve posterolateral lumbar spine fusion in humans: a prospective, randomized clinical pilot trial: 2002 Volvo Award in clinical studies. *Spine* 27:2662-2673, 2002.
7. Boden SD, Martin GJ Jr, Horton WC, *et al*: Laparoscopic anterior spinal arthrodesis with rhBMP-2 in a titanium interbody threaded cage. *J Spinal Disord* 11:95-101, 1998.
8. Bostman OM: Absorbable implants for the fixation of fractures. *J Bone Joint Surg Am* 73:148-153, 1991.
9. Branemark PI, Zarb G, Albrektsson T: *Tissue Integrated Prosthesis; Osseointegration in Clinical Dentistry*. Chicago, Quintessence Publishing, 1985.
10. Brantigan JW, Steffee AD: A carbon fiber implant to aid interbody lumbar fusion. Two-year clinical results in the first 26 patients. *Spine* 18:2106-2107, 1993.
11. Brantigan JW, Steffee AD, Lewis ML, *et al*: Lumbar interbody fusion using the Brantigan I/F cage for posterior lumbar interbody fusion and the variable pedicle screw placement system: two-year results from a Food and Drug Administration investigational device exemption clinical trial. *Spine* 25:1437-1446, 2000.
12. Bucholz RW, Henry S, Henley MB: Fixation with bioabsorbable screws for the treatment of fractures of the ankle. *J Bone Joint Surg Am* 76:319-324, 1994.
13. Buttner-Janz K, Schellnack K, Zippel H: [An alternative treatment strategy in lumbar intervertebral disk damage using an SB Charite modular type intervertebral disk endoprosthesis]. *Z Orthop Ihre Grenzgeb* 125:1-6, 1987.
14. Caborn DN, Coen M, Neef R, *et al*: Quadrupled semitendinosus-gracilis autograft fixation in the femoral tunnel: a comparison between a metal and a bioabsorbable interference screw. *Arthroscopy* 14:241-245, 1998.
15. Ciccone WJ II Motz C, Bentley C, Tasto JP: Bioabsorbable implants in orthopaedics: new developments and clinical applications. *J Am Acad Orthop Surg* 9:280-288, 2001.
16. Cizek GR, Boyd LM: Imaging pitfalls of interbody spinal implants. *Spine* 25:2633-2636, 2000.
17. Collier JP, Mayor MB, Chae JC, *et al*: Macroscopic and microscopic evidence of prosthetic fixation with porous-coated materials. *Clin Orthop* 235:173-180, 1988.
18. Cook SD, Salkeld SL, Whitecloud TS III, Barbera J: Biomechanical evaluation and preliminary clinical experience with an expansive pedicle screw design. *J Spinal Disord* 13:230-236, 2000.
19. Cunningham BW, Kanayama M, Parker LM, *et al*: Osteogenic protein versus autologous interbody arthrodesis in the sheep thoracic spine. A comparative endoscopic study using the Bagby and Kuslich interbody fusion device. *Spine* 24:509-518, 1999.
20. DeCoster TA, Heetderks DB, Downey DJ, *et al*: Optimizing bone screw pullout force. *J Orthop Trauma* 4:169-174, 1990.
21. Engh CA, Hooten JP, Zettl-Schaffer KF, *et al*: Porous coated total hip replacement. *Clin Orthop* 298:89-96, 1994.
22. Friedman RJ, An YH, Ming J, *et al*: Influence of biomaterial surface texture on bone ingrowth in the rabbit femur. *J Orthop Res* 14:455-464, 1996.
23. Fujibayashi S, Shikata J, Tanaka C, *et al*: Lumbar posterolateral fusion with biphasic calcium phosphate ceramic. *J Spinal Disord* 14:214-221, 2001.
24. Goro T, Ohata K, Takami T, *et al*: Hydroxyapatite laminar spacers and titanium miniplates in cervical laminoplasty. *J Neurosurg* 97:323-329, 2002.
25. Guyer RD, Ohnmeiss DD: Intervertebral disc prostheses. *Spine* 28:S15-S23, 2003.
26. Hashimoto T, Shigenobu K, Kanayama M, *et al*: Clinical results of single-level posterior lumbar interbody fusion using the Brantigan I/F carbon cage filled with a mixture of local morselized bone and bioactive ceramic granules. *Spine* 27:258-262, 2002.
27. Hassan AH, Evans CA, Zaki AM, George A: Use of bone morphogenetic protein-2 and dentin matrix protein-1 to enhance the osteointegration of the Onplant system. *Connect Tissue Res* 44:30-41, 2003.
28. Hayashi K, Matsuguchi N, Uenoyama K, *et al*: Evaluation of metal implants coated with several types of ceramics as biomaterials. *J Biomed Mater Res* 23:1247-1259, 1989.
29. Hirabayashi S, Kumano K: Contact of hydroxyapatite spacers with split spinous processes in double-door laminoplasty for cervical myelopathy. *J Orthop Sci* 4:264-268, 1999.
30. Iguchi T, Kanemura A, Kurihara A, *et al*: Cervical laminoplasty: evaluation of bone bonding of a high porosity hydroxyapatite spacer. *J Neurosurg* 98:137-142, 2003.
31. Jockisch KA, Brown SA, Bauer TW, Merritt K: Biological response to chopped-carbon-fiber-reinforced PEEK. *J Biomed Mater Res* 26:133-146, 1992.
32. Kokubun S, Kashimoto O, Tanaka Y: Histological verification of bone bonding and ingrowth into porous hydroxyapatite spinous process spacer for cervical laminoplasty. *Tohoku J Exp Med* 173:337-344, 1994.
33. Kotani Y, Abumi K, Shikinami Y, *et al*: Artificial intervertebral disc replacement using bioactive three-dimensional fabric: design, development, and preliminary animal study. *Spine* 27:929-935; discussion 35-36, 2002.
34. Krag MH, Beynnon BD, Pope MH, *et al*: An internal fixator for posterior application to short segments of the thoracic, lumbar, or lumbosacral spine. Design and testing. *Clin Orthop* 75-98, 1986.

35. Kubo S, Goel VK, Yang SJ, Tajima N: Biomechanical evaluation of cervical double-door laminoplasty using hydroxyapatite spacer. *Spine* 28:227-234, 2003.

36. Kulkarni RK, Pani KC, Neuman C, Leonard F: Polylactic acid for surgical implants. *Arch Surg* 93:839-843, 1966.

37. Kuslich SD, Danielson G, Dowdle JD, *et al*: Four-year follow-up results of lumbar spine arthrodesis using the Bagby and Kuslich lumbar fusion cage. *Spine* 25:2656-2662, 2000.

38. Kuslich SD, Ulstrom CL, Griffith SL, *et al*: The Bagby and Kuslich method of lumbar interbody fusion. History, techniques, and 2-year follow-up results of a United States prospective, multicenter trial. *Spine* 23:1267-1278; discussion, 79, 1998.

39. Kwok AW, Finkelstein JA, Woodside T, *et al*: Insertional torque and pull-out strengths of conical and cylindrical pedicle screws in cadaveric bone. *Spine* 21:2429-2434, 1996.

40. Lapresle P, Missenard G: Hydroxylapatite-coated Diapason screws: first clinical report. *J Spinal Disord* 8(Suppl 1): S31-S9, 1995.

41. Mallory TH, Head WC, Lombardi AV, *et al*: Clinical and radiographic outcome of a cementless, titanium plasma spray-coated total hip arthroplasty femoral component. *J Arthroplasty* 11:653-660, 1996.

42. Martin JY, Schwartz Z, Hummert TW, *et al*: Effect of titanium surface roughness on proliferation, differentiation, and protein synthesis of human osteoblast-like cells (MG63). *J Biomed Mater Res* 29:389-401, 1995.

43. McAfee PC, Boden SD, Brantigan JW, *et al*: Symposium: a critical discrepancy—a criteria of successful arthrodesis following interbody spinal fusions. *Spine* 26:320-334, 2001.

44. McAfee PC, Cunningham BW, Orbegoso CM, *et al*: Analysis of porous ingrowth in intervertebral disc prostheses: a nonhuman primate model. *Spine* 28:332-340, 2003.

45. Minamide A, Kawakami M, Hashizume H, *et al*: Evaluation of carriers of bone morphogenetic protein for spinal fusion. *Spine* 26:933-939, 2001.

46. Moore DC, Maitra RS, Farjo LA, *et al*: Restoration of pedicle screw fixation with an in situ setting calcium phosphate cement. *Spine* 22:1696-1705, 1997.

47. Nakano K, Harata S, Suetsuna F, *et al*: Spinous process-splitting laminoplasty using hydroxyapatite spinous process spacer. *Spine* 17:S41-S43, 1992.

48. Nakano M, Hirano N, Matsuura K, *et al*: Percutaneous transpedicular vertebroplasty with calcium phosphate cement in the treatment of osteoporotic vertebral compression and burst fractures. *J Neurosurg* 97:287-293, 2002.

49. Ray CD: Threaded titanium cages for lumbar interbody fusions. *Spine* 22:667-679; discussion, 79-80, 1997.

50. Sanden B, Olerud C, Petren-Mallmin M, Larsson S: Hydroxyapatite coating improves fixation of pedicle screws. A clinical study. *J Bone Joint Surg Br* 84:387-391, 2002.

51. Schimandle JH, Boden SD, Hutton WC: Experimental spinal fusion with recombinant human bone morphogenetic protein-2. *Spine* 20:1326-1337, 1995.

52. Sell P, Collins M, Dove J: Pedicle screws: axial pull-out strength in the lumbar spine. *Spine* 13:1075-1076, 1988.

53. Smith L: Ceramic-plastic material as a bone substitute. *Arch Surg* 87:653-661, 1963.

54. Spivak JM, Hasharoni A: Use of hydroxyapatite in spine surgery. *Eur Spine J* 10(Suppl 2):S197-S204, 2001.

55. Steffen T, Tsantrizos A, Fruth I, Aebi M: Cages: designs and concepts. *Eur Spine J* 9(Suppl 1):S89-S94, 2000.

56. Takahata M, Kotani Y, Abumi K, *et al*: Bone ingrowth fixation of artificial intervertebral disc consisting of bioceramic-coated three-dimensional fabric. *Spine* 28: 637-644; discussion, 44, 2003.

57. Takayasu M, Takagi T, Nishizawa T, *et al*: Bilateral open-door cervical expansive laminoplasty with hydroxyapatite spacers and titanium screws. *J Neurosurg* 96:22-28, 2002.

58. Takikawa S, Bauer TW, Turner AS, *et al*: Comparison of injectable calcium phosphate cement and polymethyl-methacrylate for use in vertebroplasty: In-vivo evaluation using an osteopenic sheep model. *Trans Society for Biomaterials* 231, 2002.

59. Thomas KA, Cook SD: An evaluation of variables influencing implant fixation by direct bone apposition. *J Biomed Mater Res* 19:875-901, 1985.

60. Togawa D, Bauer TW: The histology of human retrieved body fusion cages: good bone graft incorporation and few particles. *Trans 47th Annual Meeting of Orthopaedic Research Society, in San Francisco* 950, 2001.

61. Togawa D, Bauer TW, Brantigan JW, Lowery GL: Bone graft incorporation in radiographically successful human intervertebral body fusion cages. *Spine* 26:2744-2750, 2001.

62. Togawa D, Bauer TW, Kanayama M, *et al*: Histological evaluation of human posterolateral lumbar fusion mass induced by Osteogenic Protein-1. *Trans 71st Annual Meeting of American Academy of Orthopaedic Surgeons, San Francisco, CA* Poster, 396, 2004.

63. Togawa D, Bauer TW, Lieberman III, *et al*: Histology of tissues within retrieved human titanium mesh cages. *Spine* 28:246-253; discussion, 54, 2003.

64. Togawa D, Bauer TW, Lieberman IH, Sakai H. Lumbar intervertebral body fusion cages: Histological evaluation of clinically failed cages retrieved from humans. *J Bone Joint Surg Am* 86:70-79, 2004.

65. Togawa D, Bauer TW, Lieberman IH, Takikawa S: Histologic evaluation of human vertebral bodies after vertebral augmentation with polymethyl methacrylate. *Spine* 28:1521-1527, 2003.

66. Togawa D, Bauer TW, Mochida Y, *et al*: Bone apposition to three femoral stem surfaces in canine total hip arthroplasty. *Trans Soc for Biomaterials* 251, 2001.

67. Toth JM, Estes BT, Wang M, *et al*: Evaluation of 70/30 poly (L-lactide-co-D,L-lactide) for use as a resorbable interbody fusion cage. *J Neurosurg* 97:423-432, 2002.

68. Toth JM, Seim HB III Schwardt JD, *et al*: Direct current electrical stimulation increases the fusion rate of spinal fusion cages. *Spine* 25:2580-2587, 2000.

69. Turner AW, Gillies RM, Svehla MJ, *et al*: Hydroxyapatite composite resin cement augmentation of pedicle screw fixation. *Clin Orthop* 253-261, 2003.

70. Turner TM, Urban RM, Hall DJ, *et al*: The effect of femoral stem surface roughness on the extent of fibrous membrane formation and bone in a canine total hip replacement model. *Trans of 27th annual meeting of Society for Biomaterials* 298, 2001.

71. Turner TM, Urban RM, Lim TH, *et al*: Vertebroplasty using injectable calcium phosphate cement compared to polymethylmethacrylate in a unique canine vertebral body large defect model. *Trans 49th Annual Meeting of Orthopaedic Research Society, in New Orleans,* Paper no. 0267, 2003.

72. Uhthoff HK, Dubuc FL: Bone structure changes in the dog under rigid internal fixation. *Clin Orthop* 81:165-170, 1971.

73. Uhthoff HK, Finnegan M: The effects of metal plates on post-traumatic remodelling and bone mass. *J Bone Joint Surg Br* 65:66-71, 1983.

74. Vaccaro AR, Carrino JA, Venger BH, *et al*: Use of a bioabsorbable anterior cervical plate in the treatment of cervical degenerative and traumatic disc disruption. *J Neurosurg* 97:473-480, 2002.

75. van Dijk M, Smit TH, Arnoe MF, *et al*: The use of poly-L-lactic acid in lumbar interbody cages: design and biomechanical evaluation in vitro. *Eur Spine J.* 2003;12: 34-40.

76. Warren SM, Hedrick MH, Sylvester K, *et al*: New directions in bioabsorbable technology. *J Neurosurg* 97:481-489, 2002.

77. Watts TL: Osseointegration is Latin. *Oral Surg Oral Med Oral Pathol Oral Radiol Endod* 89:532, 2000.

78. Woo SL, Lothringer KS, Akeson WH, *et al*: Less rigid internal fixation plates: historical perspectives and new concepts. *J Orthop Res* 1:431-449, 1984.

CHAPTER 15

Materials and Material Properties

Edward H. Scheid, Jr., James S. Harrop,
Ashwini Sharan, Gregory Bennett,
and Vijay K. Goel

The goals of the majority of spine surgeries consist of decompressing the neural elements and restoring the spinal alignment and stability. Previously, spinal reconstructive or stabilizing materials consisted only of autograft, allograft, or in limited circumstances, polymethylmethacrylate (PMMA). Through a better understanding of spinal alignment, bone healing, and fusion principles, and an improvement in implant technology, there has been significant advancement in the field of biomaterials for bone fusion. Traditionally, stabilizing implants had been made of surgical grade stainless steel. The favorable properties of this material included strength, corrosion resistance, and toughness, but, regrettably, this impaired imaging quality, since stainless steel causes extensive magnetic resonance imaging artifacts.

The next generation of spinal implants consisted of titanium alloys. These implants provided better corrosion resistance, less magnetic resonance imaging distortion, and a decrease in ductility and scratch sensitivity but with less strength.

Spine surgeons must be aware of these general differences in implants in order to maximize outcomes. A decreased risk of implant failure can be achieved by making an educated decision as to what material would best suit an individual patient. A practical knowledge of the principles of materials is helpful to evaluate the design of new implants, to anticipate design limitations, and to further lessen the risk of implant failure. For example, allograft bone is a composite material with widely varying properties, depending on its composition and configuration. In the future, ceramic and composite materials for use as bone substitutes may be increasingly available. These materials have properties that are very different from metals and require different considerations in design as well as surgical application.

The first recorded use of a metallic implant device was in 1804 when a steel implant was used in a fracture repair.[6,12] Later, in 1924, stainless steel, which contains 18% chromium and 8% nickel, was first applied for medical purposes. The next major advance in metallurgy was the aircraft industry's development of light-weight but resilient metals known as titanium alloys.[6,12] In the 1950s, the biomedical field began to make use of titanium. Presently, titanium is one of the most advantageous metals because of its high strength, low modulus, and high corrosion resistance.[6]

The majority of spinal implants used today include either a stainless steel (iron-based) or titanium-based alloy. This chapter reviews the forces and physical properties of implants, terminology for material properties, the nature of atomic bonds and various strengthening mechanisms of alloys, the nature of biologic materials, and biocompatibility. In addition, properties of specific spinal implant alloys will be explored.

Forces

The International System, or SI units, which is based on the metric system, is the nomenclature used by the biomedical engineering profession. The newton (N) is a direct measure of force and is recorded as intrinsic units: kg(m)/sec2. As defined by Newton's Second Law, force is equivalent to the product of mass and acceleration. Forces, when applied to the spine, not only consist of a magnitude but also have a directional component. The combination of a force with direction is a vector. Vectors can be displayed graphically or by trigonometric relationships. Vectors can be used to analyze biomechanical forces acting simultaneously on a biologic structure or implant material by making a free body diagram that assumes a state of equilibrium, thereby defining the forces inside the structure or implant material to be dependent and proportional to those outside the structure (Figure 15.1).

A very important principle for the spine surgeon to understand is the Force/Deformation relationship (Figure 15.2). When force and deformation are graphically displayed, the result is a characteristic curve. The force deformation curve has a straight or elastic region in which materials can deform and recover to its original shape (Figure 15.2, first portion of curve). As the load increases beyond the elastic region, the deformation increases into the curved or plastic region (Figure 15.2, second portion of curve); when the specimen is unloaded, it will be permanently deformed. If deformation is continued, the specimen will eventually fail (e.g., fracture) (Figure 15.2, third portion of curve).

Atomic Bonds, Structures, and Property Relationships

All materials are composed of molecules that interact via intermolecular forces. These bonds determine the properties of the material as a whole. If materials were composed of only one type of molecule and these molecules were perfectly consistent in their orientation, then chemistry alone would be sufficient for deriving all of the element's properties. However, materials are typically composed of numerous molecules of considerable diversity. Nevertheless, despite the variety of molecules in metals, certain observations can be made from their chemical composition.

Metals are created through the interaction of crystals. These crystals are formed when the electrons that surround the atoms in clouds are given up and conducted as electricity. Metal structures are polycrystalline (i.e., they are formed by a multitude of crystals). Atoms within a crystal can form one of several relationships. These relationships define the crystal structure. They include body-centered cubic (BCC), face-centered cubic (FCC), and hexagonal close packed (HCP) (Figures 15.3 to 15.5).

In addition to variations in the unit cell of crystals, metals have many imperfections in the crystals, consisting of line defects, point defects, missing atoms, additional atoms, and impurities with foreign atoms. Metals can be further contaminated with larger impurities from nonmetallic elements such as oxides and sulfides.

Point defects occur when a lattice site within a crystal is empty and not occupied by an atom.[6,14] Point defects are present in all metals and provide a mechanism for diffusion, which is the movement of solute through a solvent.

Line defects are microscopic dislocations and are the major defect affecting a given metal's mechanical proper-

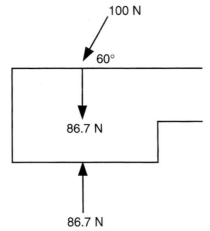

Figure 15.1 Free body diagram of a lumbar vertebrae with an externally applied load of 100N at an incident angle of 60 degrees. The vertebra will have to resist the shear component as well (horizontal component—not shown in the figure—of the incident force). The resultant downward force on the vertebral body is sin (60) × 100N = 86.7N. The vertebra is in equilibrium with its surroundings and not moving. Therefore, a force of the same magnitude is acting on the caudal end plate.

ties. Line defects occur when there is an incomplete chain of atoms inside a crystal. This results in a local distortion of the structure of the crystal because of the resultant dislocation. There is considerable internal strain in the immediate vicinity of the dislocation. When a force is applied, the line defect can propagate through the crystal structure, resulting in a permanent structural change (Figures 15.6 and 15.7). This is termed *plastic deformation*. When a metal is plastically deformed, a permanent structural change persists after the force is removed from the metal.[6]

An example of an area defect is a grain boundary.[6] When metal begins the solidification process, crystals form independently of one another. Each crystal grows into a crystalline structure, or grain. The size and number of grains developed by a certain amount of metal depend on the rate of nucleation, which is the initial stage of formation of a crystal. Rapid cooling usually produces smaller grains, while slower cooling produces larger grains. The orientation of crystal boundaries (grain boundaries) is very influential in the spread of dislocations that become cracks.

A high nucleation rate yields a high number of grains for a given amount of metal. Therefore, the grain size will be small. However, if the rate of growth of the crystals is high relative to their nucleation rate, fewer grains will develop, but they will be of larger size.

As a grain grows, it eventually comes in contact with another grain. The surfaces that separate grains are termed *grain boundaries*. Grain boundaries are the junction areas of the many metal crystals that compose an implant. The grain size has a significant effect on the mechanical properties of a metal. A higher number of grain boundaries increases strength. Grain boundaries prevent line defects from propagating from one grain to another. A higher number of grain boundaries necessitates a higher force required to induce a plastic deformation. Since a higher number of grain boundaries occurs in alloys with smaller grains, smaller grains yield an increase in strength and larger grains are generally associated with low strength and ductility.

The many ways in which a metal can acquire defects affecting its strength has led to the development of various

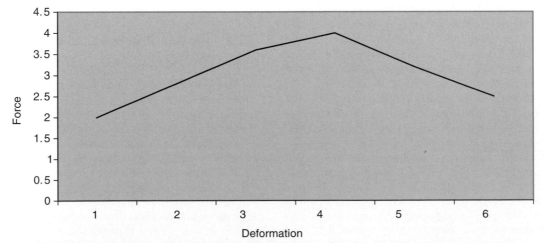

Figure 15.2 Force versus Deformation curve. The force has a straight or elastic region in which materials can deform and recover to their original shape. As load increases beyond the elastic region, the deformation increases in to the plastic region; when the specimen is unloaded, it will be permanently deformed. If the deformation is limited, the specimen will eventually fail (e.g., fracture).

strengthening mechanisms to improve the performance of a metal or alloy. All strengthening mechanisms act on the theory that impeding line defects results in increased strength.

Solid solution strengthening occurs when one or more elements are added to a metal. Atoms of the solute will

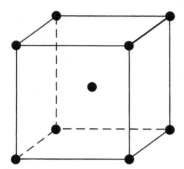

Figure 15.3 The unit cell is the smallest group of atoms showing a characteristic structure. The body-centered cube is the most ductile.

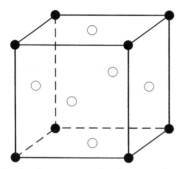

Figure 15.4 The face-centered cube is moderately ductile.

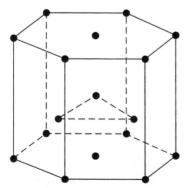

Figure 15.5 The hexagonal close-packed cube is the least ductile.

take places within the crystalline lattice by substituting for a solvent (metal) atom. Alternatively, the solute atom may occupy a site not previously occupied by a solvent atom by lying in an interstitial site. Interstitial atoms are usually much smaller than the solvent, whereas substituting elements are often similar in size to the solvent. Interstitial solid solution strengthening is often more effective. The effect of solid solution strengthening is to stop line defects from spreading a dislocation by developing solute-rich regions in the area surrounding the line defect. The result is a requirement for an increased force to induce a plastic deformation.

Cold working deforms the metal and results in an increase in strength. Deformation of a metal increases the amount of line defects within the metal. These dislocations then entangle with one another. The result is an increasing amount of energy that continues to move these line defects within the grain. The increase in strength from cold working comes at the expense of a decrease in ductility.

Hot working involves the use of high temperature to deform the metal. This is often used to allow a metal to form a shape while altering the microstructure of the alloy. It is possible to obtain a reduction in grain size by hot working. By increasing the temperature to a level that causes a deformation, the dislocations become disentangled. The metal then undergoes recrystallization, and new dislocation-free grains are formed.

Mechanical Properties

Knowing the dimensions of a material, when a force is applied, permits the stress or load per unit area to be determined. Stress is recorded as newton/meter^2 (N/m^2) (Pascal) and is a small quantity. Therefore, most materials are tested with thousands of N/m^2, or megaPascals. Strain is a dimensionless unit that is the percentage of elongation (or shortening) during application of force. When both the load and the deformation are divided by the original area or length of the specimen respectively, the result is stress and strain, which can be displayed graphically (Figure 15.7).

Spinal surgeons should have a basic understanding of the typical stress-strain curve (see Figure 15.2). The stress-strain curve defines the mechanical behavior of a metal under various degrees of stress and strain. The ratio of stress to strain is the modulus, or elastic modulus. The relationship is as follows:

$$E = stress/strain$$

The modulus (E) reflects the stiffness of the material. Stiffness, in turn, is dependent on the relative difficulty of

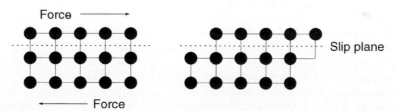

Figure 15.6 During stress, individual atomic bonds are disrupted and the atoms slip along a plane.

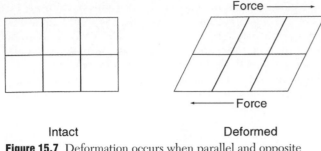

Figure 15.7 Deformation occurs when parallel and opposite forces are applied to a structure with one side immobilized.

stretching atoms from their resting position in a crystal lattice. It is important to note that the modulus is not affected to a significant degree by line defects.

At a certain amount of stress, a plastic deformation occurs. At this point, line deformations begin to cause deformations, which propagate through the grain. The linear relationship between stress and strain breaks down, and the slope of the modulus decreases. The point at which this occurs is the proportional limit. Yield stress is arbitrarily defined as the point at which permanent deformation reaches 0.2% of the metal. Ultimate stress is defined as the highest stress reached during testing of the metal. Percent elongation, a measure of ductility, is the degree of plastic deformation acquired prior to failure.

Fatigue strength is another property of metal that is important when considering bioimplantation. Fatigue is a process whereby repetitive stress or strain is applied to a metal, eventually leading to breakdown, crack formation, and eventual failure of the metal. By definition, the fatigue strength is the cyclic stress required to cause failure of the metal at a given number of cycles. When a metal fails from fatigue, it usually takes much longer and a greater number of cycles to form the initial crack than to achieve complete failure. As such, any material that acts to prevent crack formation will improve the metal's resistance to fatigue.

Fatigue failures have become less frequent in implants because of improved materials and strengthening processes. When they do occur, crack formation is usually the inciting factor. Most of these cracks form at the alloy surface. Therefore, surface conditions become very important in preventing fatigue failure.

Spinal Implants: Rigid Versus Dynamic

Spinal implants can be described as rigid, dynamic, or hybrid. Dynamic implants provide for some subsidence between segments. The advantage of a dynamic implant is that it is capable of offsetting stress at the implant-bone interface and therefore does not provide stress shielding of the bone graft.

The purpose of a rigid construct is to completely immobilize the spine. Because of the properties of bone, this is rarely achieved. The movement in a rigid system often increases with the passage of time, through weakening of the implant-bone interface. Repetitive movement under sufficient stress will eventually lead to failure at the interface, unless bony fusion first occurs.

It is important to realize that rigid fixation does not completely optimize bony fusion acquisition because of stress shielding. The goal of rigid fixation is only to hold long enough for bony fusion to take place.

The purpose of a dynamic construct is to provide for intersegmental subsidence. While excessive movement can inhibit fusion, the minimal intersegmental movement (which facilitates compression), increases the rate of bone fusion. Also, the minimal intersegmental movement absorbs some of the strain that is encountered at the implant-bone interface.

Biologic Materials

Bone is the "gold standard" of implant materials as a biologic material. It consists of a framework of type I collagen fibers, a matrix of calcium hydroxyapatite, and small amounts of protein polysaccharides and mucopolysaccharides (ground substance or cement). The organic content of bone is relatively constant at 0.6 g/ml, whereas the mineral content varies (up to 2 g/ml). Bone is slightly viscoelastic, in that rapid deformations result in 95% of the eventual displacement caused by slow deformations. Because of this difference, the energy required for fracture is higher under rapid loading conditions. Under very rapid (ballistic) conditions, bone shatters into comminuted fragments. The total energy required to create a fracture is thus reduced. Bone is anisotropic, with a fiber pattern that is parallel to the predominant axis of loading. It displays both elastic and plastic behavior.

The stiffness of bone is approximately 10% stainless steel and 20% titanium alloy (Ti-6Al4V, or simply Ti6-4). This means that the stiffness of bone is closer to titanium than steel implants. This fact has been used to suggest that there is a better "match" between titanium and bone than between stainless steel and bone. In certain circumstances this might be important, such as when a permanently implanted device will be subjected to repeated deformations while the bone-implant juncture could loosen. Alternatively, the use of steel implants creates a construct of higher stiffness. Surgical constructs of higher stiffness have been associated with higher fusion rates, both clinically and experimentally. Because the optimal stiffness of a surgical construct for bone healing is unknown, the selection of implant material should not be influenced by minor variations in the stiffness of materials.

Stainless Steel

Stainless steel implants are iron- and carbon-based alloys. Medical grade stainless steel alloys typically contain chromium (18%-22%), nickel (18%-22%), molybdenum (2.5%), manganese (2.5%), and carbon (0.03%-0.08%), by weight.

Initial trials of stainless steels, as an implant, showed that to resist corrosion by aiding resistance to chloride degradation was insufficient. The addition of molybdenum and chromium reduced the incidence of corrosion and pitting by aiding the defense against chloride degradation.[6,14]

The 316 stainless steels, which have a face-centered cubic structure, are the most common steels that are used for spinal implants. There are two grades, grade 1 (316) and grade 2 (316L)—grade 2 having the lower carbon content. The lower carbon content aids in reducing the formation of metal carbides, which leads to a decrease in the corrosion resistance of the alloy.[6,23] These 316 alloys are commonly used in fracture fixation devices. They are commonly hot- or cold-worked and solid solution-strengthened.

Titanium-Based Alloys

Titanium-based alloys are currently the most commonly used alloys for bioimplantation. Titanium, either pure (cP-Ti) or an alloy with aluminum and vanadium (Ti-6Al-4V), are the most common compositions for titanium in the United States.[6,14]

Titanium-based alloys are advantageous for several reasons. They have both high strength and fatigue resistance. Commercially pure titanium has a hexagonal close-packed structure; various grades differ in their oxygen concentration. In small quantities, oxygen serves to solid-solution strengthen the alloy by interstitial placement of the atom. However, in excessive amounts, oxygen can lead to the alpha-case, thereby weakening the material by decreasing the number of grain boundaries. This results in a much lower fatigue strength and surface ductility.[6,14,23] Titanium-based alloys also have decreased stiffness when compared to stainless steel. The reduction in stiffness facilitates transfer of the stress at the bone-implant interface to the alloy; this minimizes bone resorption at the interface. Titanium-based alloys have higher fatigue strength when compared to stainless steel. However, titanium alloys are vulnerable to any surface flaws. Any scratch or notch can rapidly accelerate the fatigue failure process. Titanium, in its pure form, is generally weaker than stainless steel, but it can be cold-worked to increase its strength.[6,12] Titanium alloys also lack any known immunogenicity. This is an important advantage for any foreign body implant.

Surface Structure and Modifications of Alloys

As discussed previously, any surface component that prevents crack formation will decrease an alloy's sensitivity to fatigue. Implant alloys typically use an oxide film for their surfaces. These oxide films are considered passive films because they are the result of oxidation of the outermost metal atoms on the surface of the alloy.[6]

Corrosion is an oxidative process that is a threat to alloys. Corrosion would ensue rapidly without passive films. Stainless steels have oxide films composed of Cr_2O_3, FeO, and Fe_2O_3. This thin film separates the metal from its surrounding, corrosive environment and is the major factor in the resistance to decay. Titanium alloys form TiO_2, which plays a similar role as chromium oxide does for stainless steel. Oxide films also serve as a protective barrier on articulating surfaces of the alloy.

Immersion of steel alloy surfaces in nitric acid baths also delays corrosion. Nitric baths dissolve impurities anywhere where they exist on the surface of the metal implants, thereby ensuring an intact oxide film.

Surface modification is a technique used to increase local strength and hardening of implants. Two types of surface modifications include ion implantation and vapor

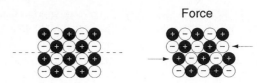

Figure 15.8 Ceramics have strong ionic bonds that deter slops when like charges repel one another.

deposition.[6,14] Ion implantation involves the acceleration of ions toward the surface of the alloy. It is the direct implantation of gas phase ions into the alloy. The ions penetrate and increase the number and type of subsurface defects and dislocations. This leads to an increase in the durability of the metal surface and a reduction in its susceptibility to corrosion.[6,24]

Another method of surface modification is either chemical or physical vapor deposition. This technique adds a new hardened coating to the alloy surface, usually composed of CrN or TiN. One shortcoming of hardened coatings is that they have variable adhesion with the alloy.

Last, nitriding is a process that modifies the surface of a material by a chemical reaction with nitrogen, which places nitrides on the surface. Stainless steel or titanium can have a portion of their surface undergo nitriding by reacting the surface with either gaseous ammonia or molten potassium cyanate.[6,14] The result is a great increase in surface hardness of the alloy.

Ceramics

By comparison to metals, ceramics have chemical bonds that are predominantly ionic, with a densely packed array of oppositely charged atoms (Figure 15.8). These atoms have limited mobility because of the interaction of charges of nearby atoms. This charge interaction results in a stiff material with low ductility and no plasticity. Ceramics are a group of substances that are composed of crystals oriented randomly in a dense framework that consists of metallic oxides. They may have inorganic chain molecules, such as silicon dioxide in a glass phase. Traditional ceramic materials frequently have impurities and internal microporous inclusions that limit the strength to less than the theoretical maximum. Newer ceramics are synthesized with chemically pure materials with high densities or as composites with greatly increased strength.[11,21,27]

An advantage of oxide ceramics is their wear reduction compared to that of alloys.[6,11] Metals and alloys have a protective oxide film that can be peeled off by adherence to opposing surface polymers.[6,11] This causes local ion release from the alloy. This loss and reformation of the oxide film is a repetitive process that can accelerate degradation of the surface of the alloy implant. Oxide ceramics do not have a passive oxide film and may, as a result, have less long-term breakdown.

Synthetic Polymers

Synthetic polymer production is a field of implant technology that is rapidly expanding. Polymers, commonly known as plastics, are typically very large molecules made from a large number of individual subunits called monomers. Polymers are chemical compounds that are formed by combining these smaller, repeating structural units. The subunits repeat in various patterns, following principles similar to those of molecular biology. The covalent bonds in polymers have a fixed length. The complex folding of polymers is created by weak hydrogen bond cross-links that permit unfolding and elongation. The two most commonly used polymers are polymethylmethacrylate (PMMA) and ultra-high molecular weight polyethylene (UHMWPE).[6]

Stiffening the "backbone" molecular chain and increasing the cross-links, the polymer can be made less flexible. Numerous other properties can be influenced by chemical changes, including density, crystallization, solubility, thermal stability, and strength. Ultra-high molecular weight polyethylene has been extensively used for artificial joints because of its favorable surface wear and creep properties. In spine surgery, PMMA has been used extensively because of the additional polymerization that occurs when the powder and liquid are mixed.

The intermediate phase of polymerization yields a doughy material that can be worked and shaped into complex defects before it hardens. PMMA has many molecular and macroscopic defects that contribute to its characteristically weak tensile strength. These defects originate in the powder phase that consists of microspheres. The microspheres are bound together as the methylmethacrylate monomer (liquid phase) polymerizes into a matrix that incorporates the microspheres. Even after hardening, the juncture between the powder phase microspheres and the liquid phase remains relatively weak. Additionally, the polymer chains have very few cross-links. For all these reasons, the polymerized PMMA has a low tensile strength.

Composite materials are a combination of a filler and matrix. Traditionally, the filler is glass or carbon fibers, whereas the matrix is epoxy, carbon, UHMWPE, PMMA, or a variety of other materials. The fibers can be particulate or relatively large and stiff, in which case they are termed *whiskers*. Composites with whiskers have high tensile strength but can be brittle. Fiber orientation in relation to the direction of loading is important. A complex variety of stress responses can be obtained in polymer matrix composites, making these materials anisotropic. Biologic materials such as bone, ligament, and tendon are also composites with anisotropy. An example of a composite used in spine surgery is the carbon fiber cage for interbody fusion. It is composed of long-fiber carbon and Ultrapek (poly ether ether ketone).[3]

Biocompatibility

All surgical procedures are associated with a disruption of normal anatomic tissue planes. This results in an accumulation of exudative fluid, fibrin, platelets, and polymorphonuclear leukocytes. From days 3 to 5 postsurgery, macrophages accumulate and remove the surgical debris. By 10 days the macrophages are no longer present, and lymphocytes predominate. This is followed by fibroblasts, which complete the cellular phase of healing. Ceramic implants are very biocompatible, since the cellular response to wound healing is not significantly altered.

However, in the presence of a metal implant, the immune system is activated, with the production of protein-metal hapten complexes, complement activation, and the resultant cellular and humoral immune responses. A chronic inflammatory state with sustained populations of macrophages, lymphocytes, and occasional plasma cells persists for several weeks or months. Eventually, these foreign bodies are sequestered by dense fibrous tissue, as the inflammatory response subsides. Direct apposition of bone to an implant, without an interposed fibrous layer, is very rare, with the exception of titanium and bioactive ceramics, such as calcium hydroxyapatite.

In total joint replacement, wear debris accumulates as a function of the force across the joint, the relative displacements of the articular surfaces, and a variety of wear mechanisms, including abrasion, corrosion, fretting (micromotion), and third-body wear resulting from wear debris between the articular surfaces. Wear debris can also cause adverse local responses to the implant, such as osteolysis and regional lymphadenopathy. These phenomena will be of increasing interest to neurosurgeons if articulating artificial discs become more widely used as an alternative to spinal fusion.[16]

For most surgical constructs, stainless steel implants are sufficiently nonreactive to permit bone fusion before the deleterious consequences of the normal inflammatory response, such as severe pain or loosening. The presence of a metal implant may lead to an increased risk of infection. *In vitro* testing of stainless steel and cobalt alloy materials has shown inhibition of macrophage chemotaxis and phagocytosis, which may contribute to the increased risk of infection. The avascular fibrous layer that accumulates around metal implants in bone may also contribute to this risk. Sites associated with PMMA are especially vulnerable, most likely due to the 0.1- to 0.5-mm layer of necrotic bone that is created by the direct toxicity of the methacrylate monomer and the heat released during hardening.

The fibrous layer around implants may be associated with painful late loosening of the device. For example, after an intertransverse lumbar fusion has occurred, micromotions may persist between the vertebral bodies and result in painful movements of vertebral bone in relation to pedicle screws. In theory, bone ingrowth and direct adhesion to an implant (such as what occurs with titanium) may lessen the risk of infection and painful late loosening.

Metal allergy is widely prevalent and well recognized but a poorly understood occurrence. Metal ions alone will not stimulate the immune system. When linked with proteins, metals such as cobalt, chromium, and especially nickel are immunogenic. The immune response to metals is characteristically delayed hypersensitivity. This has been proposed as the cause of premature loosening in total hip arthroplasties. Delayed development of sensitivity after prolonged exposure to a metal implant has been well documented, using the leukocyte migration inhibition test.[20] The clinical significance of metal allergy in spinal surgery is unknown, but these data suggest that patients reporting skin sensitivity to metal should be considered for titanium implants (rather than stainless steel) before elective spinal surgery.

Osteolysis, or periprosthetic bone loss may occur at the site of an implant. Structural remodeling of surrounding bone occurs in response to stress shielding. This bone destruction can lead to loosening and possible failure of the implant. Factors that are thought to play a role in osteolysis include the formation of particulate debris and loosening, or motion, of the implant.[6] Once the particles are generated, macrophages proliferate and attack the periprosthetic space. This leads to activation of an inflammatory cascade and the induction of osteoclastic pathways.

Summary

Contemporary spinal surgeons are faced with the task of making informed decisions regarding a choice of implant for stabilization. It is important for the spinal surgeon to have an understanding of the physical and chemical properties of any material that the surgeon is contemplating implanting into the patient. Various advantageous properties of alloys, and biomaterials in general, include strength, ductility, modulus, hardness, and biocompatibility. Each material possesses different advantages and disadvantages. It is up to the surgeon to understand this increasingly complex aspect of the field and to make decisions accordingly.

REFERENCES

1. Adams MS, Benzel EC, Baldwin NG: Metal corrosion of implanted spinal instrumentation. Abstract. Joint Section on Disorders of the Spine and Peripheral Nerves, Annual Meeting, Orlando, FL, 1996.
2. Agins JH, Alcock NW, Bansal M, et al: Metallic wear in failed titanium alloy total hip replacements: a histological and quantitative analysis. *J Bone Joint Surg* 63B:435, 1981.
3. Albrektsson T, Branemark PI, Hansson HA, Lindstrom J: Osteointegrated titanium implants. *Acta Orthop Scand* 52:155, 1981.
4. Black J: Orthopaedic biomaterials in research and practice (151-154). New York: Churchill Livingstone, 1988.
5. Black J: Systemic effects of biomaterials. *Biomaterials* 5:11, 1984.
6. Bradley RJ, Chaoi EYS, Friedman J: Biomechanics and biomaterials (151-174). In Dee R, Hurst L, Gruber M, Kottmaier S (eds): *Principles and practice of orthopaedics.* 2nd ed. New York: McGraw-Hill, 1997.
7. Brantigan J, Steffee A: A carbon fiber implant to aid interbody lumbar fusion. *Spine* 14:2106-2117, 1993.
8. Brantley AGU, Mayfield JK, Koeneman JB, Clark KR: The effects of pedicle screw fit: an in vitro study. *Spine* 19:1753-1758, 1994.
9. Bunshah RF: PVD and CVD coatings. ASM handbook: friction, lubrication and wear technology. 18:840, 1992.
10. Coe JD, Warden KE, Herzig MA, McAfee PC: Influence of bone mineral density on the fixation of thoracolumbar implants. *Spine* 15:902-907, 1990.
11. Cooke FW: Ceramics in orthopedic surgery. *Clin Orthop* 276: 135, 1992.
12. Friedman DW, Orland PJ, Greco RS: Biomaterials: an historical perspective. In Greco RS, (ed): *Implantation biology: the host response and biomedical devices.* Boca Raton, FL: CRC Press, 1994:1-12.
13. Friedman RJ, Black J, Galante JO, *et al*: Current concepts in orthopaedic biomaterials and implant fixation. In Heckman JD (ed): *Instr Course Lect*, vol 43. Rosemont, IL: The American Academy of Orthopaedic Surgeons, 1994.
14. Gilbert JL: Metals (123-134). In Callaghan JJ, Rosenberg AG, Rubash HE (eds): *The adult hip.* Philadelphia: Lippincott-Raven Publishers, 1998.
15. Gilbert JL, Stulberg SD: Fatigue fracture of titanium alloy (Ti-6Al-4V) knee prosthesis in vivo. ASM handbook of case histories in failure analysis, Vol 2. Metals Park, OH: ASM International, 1994:2.
16. Hedman T, Kostuik J, Fernie G, Hellier W: Design of an intervertebral disc prosthesis. *Spine* 16:S256-S260, 1991.
17. Kalpakjian S: Manufacturing engineering and technology (50-51). Reading, MA: Addison-Wesley, 1995.
18. Lim T-H, An HS, Evanich C et al: Strength of anterior vertebral screw fixation in relationship to bone mineral density. *J Spinal Disord Tech* 8:121-125, 1995.
19. McElhaney JH: Dynamic response of bone and muscle tissue. *J Appl Physiol* 21:1231-1236, 1996.
20. Merritt K, Brown SA: Biological effects of corrosion products from metals (195-206). In Fraker AC, Griffin CD (eds): *Corrosion and Degradation of Implant Materials.* ASTM STP 859. American Society for Testing and Materials, Philadelphia, 1985.
21. Park JB, Lakes RS: *Biomaterials. An Introduction.* ed 2. Plenum Press, New York, 1992, pp 117-140.
22. Posner AS: The structure of bone mineral. *Clin Orthop* 9:5-14, 1957.
23. Rae T: The toxicity of metals used in orthopaedic prosthesis. An experimental study using cultured human synovial fibroblasts. *J Bone Joint Surg* 63B:435, 1981.
24. Reinsch WA. Terminology for titanium microstructure. In: *Titanium and Titanium Alloys: Source Book.* ASM. Metals Park, OH: American Society for Metals, 1982, p 47.
25. Soshi S, Shiba R, Kondo H, Murota K: An experimental study on transpedicular screw fixation in relation to osteoporosis of the lumbar spine. *Spine* 16:1335B1341, 1991.
26. Spector M. Biomaterial failure. *Orthop Clin North Am* 23: 211-217, 1992.
27. White A, Panjabi M: *Clinical Biomechanics of the Spine.* pp. 86B87. Lippincott-Raven, Philadelphia, 1990.
28. Williams DF: Consensus and definitions in biomaterials, in de Putter C, de Lange GL, de Groot K, Lee AJC (eds): *Advances in Biomaterials.* Amsterdam, Elsevier, 1988, pp 11-16.
29. Williams DF: Titanium as a metal for implantation. *J Med Engl Technol* 1: 266, 1977.
30. Zdeblick TA, Kunz DN, Cooke ME, McCabe R: Pedicle screw pull-out strength. *Spine* 18:1673B1676, 1993.

CHAPTER 16

Biomechanical Testing

Jean-Valéry C.E. Coumans, Lisa A. Ferrara, Tunc Oktenoglu, Robert F. McLain, and Edward C. Benzel

Biomechanics is a science that combines classical physics and engineering for the study of the structural aspects of a biologic system. Since it bridges two distinct fields, it requires a knowledge of anatomy, physiology, and engineering methods. Biomechanical testing enables one to quantitatively determine the displacement of a structure in response to an applied force or stimulus. From biomechanical experiments, quantification of strength, stiffness, fatigue, and other variables is obtainable. In pathologic conditions of the spine, or following surgery such as a multilevel laminectomy, the mechanical properties of the spine are altered. Such alterations can be precisely characterized with biomechanical testing. Biomechanical testing also enables the testing of new spinal implants. Biomechanical testing allows a new device to be compared to existing devices prior to its use in patients.

Ideally, *in vivo* biomechanical testing is performed, but this is not feasible in human beings, except for intraoperative measurements,[3,13] intradiscal pressure measurements,[38,44] or with the implantation of telemeterized load sensors.[36,37] *In vitro* testing of cadaveric human or animal specimens is therefore used as a surrogate measure of *in vivo* load/displacement data. This involves assumptions that must be defined because they pertain to the particular experiment. More recently, mathematic models have been employed in an attempt to predict the behavior of the spine in response to a load. Table 16.1 summarizes the different types of biomechanical testing and their advantages and disadvantages.

Application of Biomechanical Testing

Many different biomechanical testing systems exist, some proprietary, and the common denominator shared by all devices is the ability to measure displacement in response to an applied load, or the ability to measure load in response to displacement. The devices themselves generally consist of a hydraulic arm or actuator, load cell, loading jig, and potting fixture (Figure 16.1). Systems involving pulleys and cables are also used to apply moments.

Types of Tests

Biomechanical tests can be divided into static and dynamic tests (Table 16.2).[31] A strength test is a type of static test that involves the application of a load or displacement until failure occurs, providing information on the mechan-

ical properties of a specimen or construct. It allows the determination of parameters such as the elastic modulus, the yield strength (the stress at which the onset of plastic deformation occurs), the ultimate strength (the stress just prior to failure), and the energy absorbed at failure (toughness). Each specimen can be used only once since it is a destructive test. One example of its use involves the evaluation of new spinal implants and facilitating their comparison to existing instrumentation.[9,32]

Stability tests entail the application of a load of sufficiently low magnitude to avoid permanent deformation. Viewed another way, the specimen is only tested on the elastic segment of the stress versus strain curve. The test is not destructive and may be repeated under varying conditions. It permits characterization of the stiffness, creep, and the viscoelastic properties of the material.

Fatigue testing involves cyclical loading with subfailure loads until failure occurs, providing information about the longevity of a construct under certain load conditions. This test, like strength testing, is destructive. When it is repeated with different specimens under different loading parameters, a fatigue curve can be plotted.

Load Control Versus Displacement Control

In vitro biomechanical testing can be divided into load control and displacement control testing. In load control testing, also known as *flexibility testing*, the specimen is mounted onto the actuator, a fixed load is applied, and the resultant displacement is measured. The advantage of this method is that it permits a greater freedom of movement of the specimen, since only the base of the tested specimen requires immobilization. No constraints are applied to the spinal segment. In other words, a spinal segment is free to move in any axis in response to a constant applied load.[17,31] This may reveal complex or coupled motions in response to a load. Alternatively, displacement control testing, also known as *stiffness testing*, relies on the displacement of the motion segment over a given distance, and on the resulting force. This type of testing is difficult with stiff specimens and artificially constrains the imparted motion but has the advantage of allowing the application of translational or rotational input.

Cyclic Loading

In life, the spine is exposed to a variety of cyclic frequencies that range from 0.5 cycles per second to 25 cycles per second when exposed to vibration during activity.[12] It is estimated that over the time needed for fusion to occur, the spine will experience 1 million cycles.[12] A load that does not cause failure with a single application may do so when applied repeatedly. Thus fatigue testing is an important part of the evaluation of spinal constructs. The number of cycles required for failure to occur depends on the magnitude of the load, its method of application, and the physical properties of the specimen, including its size, its material properties, and the integrity of its surface.[30]

When fatigue testing is undertaken, the frequency and load must be predetermined. A greater frequency speeds up the testing process. However, biologic and even inert materials behave differently with different rates of loading,

TABLE 16.1

Biomechanical Testing Methodologies

Method	Advantages	Disadvantages	References
Synthetic support	Ideal for the study of spinal implants	Limited use	2, 9, 25
Cadaveric, animal	Availability, price, specimen homogeneity	Additional assumptions necessary when generalizing to human beings	10, 29, 43
Cadaveric, human	More closely resembles clinical scenario than animal or mathematic model	Lack of availability, specimen heterogeneity, expense, potential for disease transmission	4, 7, 11, 21, 32, 34, 40
In vivo, animal	More physiologic than a cadaveric spine	Expense, variables difficult to control, nonhuman	20, 23, 24, 26
In vivo, human	Applicability	Limited tests possible, ethical concerns, more difficult control of variables	13, 28, 36, 37, 38, 44
Mathematic	Reproducibility, noninvasive, rapidly decreasing cost	Multiple assumptions needed that require experimental verification, not yet reliable for predictions	15, 16, 18, 42, 45

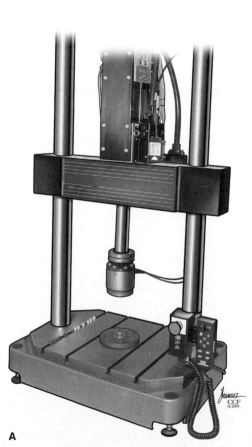

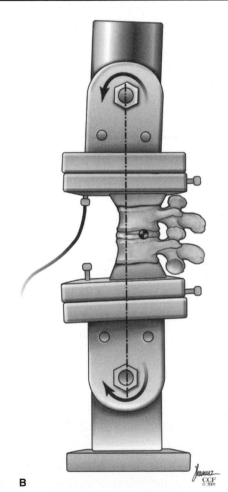

A   B

Figure 16.1 (**A**) A typical biomechanical materials testing apparatus used to apply physical loads to tissue with feedback that measures the response. (**B**) Depiction of a specimen mounted onto a materials test machine using customized gripping fixtures that will measure angles of deflection and overall displacements.

and erroneous conclusions might be reached with excessive, nonphysiologic frequencies. Additionally, one must decide, based on the hypothesis to be tested, whether to test the specimen in compression, in tension, in torsion, or with a combination of forces.

Mathematic Testing

The mathematic or computer testing of the biomechanical properties of the spine relies on a method termed *finite element analysis*.[15,16,18,27,39,45] This process has proven itself in engineering and design applications and is finding

TABLE 16.2			
Types of Tests			
Test	**Method**	**Static**	**Destructive**
Stability	Evaluation of load-deformation characteristics. Loads are "physiologic" and do not induce permanent deformation.	Yes	No
Strength	Load applied to failure.	Yes	Yes
Fatigue	Load applied repeatedly, often until failure occurs	No	Yes

increasing use in biomechanical applications.[18] The finite element method breaks down the structure to be studied into a finite number of geometric shapes or "elements," which are interconnected by "nodes." The geometric information can be derived from computed tomography (CT) of human spines. The material properties of the various components, such as the modulus of elasticity, the shear modulus, density, and Poisson's ratio are ascribed based on a library of predetermined values.[16] The greater the number of elements, the more detailed the representation and the more computer intensive the process. "Simple" approaches reduce each spinal motion segment to a few elements and allow the analysis of multiple segments and their associated musculature, rib cage, and so forth. Complex approaches, employing a large number of elements and nodes, are used to model the stress and strain of a single or a few motion segments.[15] The advantage of finite element analysis is its reproducibility and the ability to noninvasively study the effects of a multitude of manipulations, such as laminectomy or facetectomy.[45] The rapid evolution of computing capabilities along with their declining cost is allowing increasingly complex models to be considered. However, at the present time, numerous assumptions derived from experimental data still need to be made, producing solutions, which in turn require experimental verification. Nonetheless, validation has been demonstrated in the determination of fracture patterns in a finite element model of C3,[18] and in the response of the intervertebral disc to dynamic loading, for example.[27] With further refinements it should be possible to design models to predict results that are not readily determined experimentally,[39] such as the effect of bone remodeling.

Experimental Design and Considerations

The experimental method must be chosen in light of the hypothesis. Although there is no perfect substitute for studying the spine *in vivo*, *in vitro* studies provide an alternative, which can be tailored to the particular hypothesis and standardized. After formulating a hypothesis, one identifies a testing paradigm and defines its characteristics and assumptions. The mode of testing is also anticipated. If one phase of the analysis examines a highly unstable construct incapable of resisting physiologic loads, a displacement-controlled test may be selected. If, on the other hand, small displacements were anticipated after implant placement, load-controlled analysis would be preferred. The type of specimen, its preparation, length, fixation into the testing apparatus,

the method of load application, and the end points are defined prior to the start of the study.

Specimen Selection

For *in vitro* testing, one has the option of using human, animal, or synthetic specimens. One can further select fresh or thawed specimens. Fresh human specimens pose an availability problem and the added risk of disease transmission. Most biomechanical experiments conducted on human tissue are done in thawed spines, which raises concerns about the effect of freezing, storage, and subsequent thawing on the specimens. Fortunately, this question has been addressed in experiments specifically designed to assess the effect of prolonged freezing.[4,14,34,40] In one experiment involving prolonged freezing of human thoracic spines,[34] no significant differences were found between fresh specimens and specimens stored for up to 7 months at −18°C in the amount of displacement in response to a physiologic load. Furthermore, no change occurred with daily testing for 14 days. The specimens consisted of two adjacent thoracic vertebrae and the associated disc, ligaments, and facet joints. These results are in agreement with those from another laboratory, looking at the effect of freezing on the compressive stiffness and hysteresis of the human lumbar spine.[40] Another experiment, published 10 years later by other investigators,[14] compared the effect of physiologic loads applied to sheep spines before and after 3 months of freezing. No statistically significant differences were found. Using porcine cervical spines, however, others observed an increase in ultimate compressive load and energy to failure following 1 month of freezing at −20°C.[6] There was no difference, however, in the stiffness and displacement at failure.

Cadaveric animal spines are frequently used in biomechanical tests. They are easier to obtain and more affordable than human spines. They are also more uniform in size and bone density. Wilke[43] has shown that sheep spines are similar to human spines in their biomechanical properties. Others have advocated the use of baboon spines for the study of the atlantoaxial complex, citing similarities to human spines.[10] Another advantage of using animal spines is the uniformity of the specimens. Unlike cadaveric human spines, the specimens are free of degenerative disease. Synthetic spines are also used for the testing of instrumentation (Figure 16.2).[9] This method is appropriate when the implant itself is under evaluation and inherent assumptions are recognized. It is highly reproducible and lends itself to the evaluation of novel implants and components, allowing a comparison to be made between systems. This

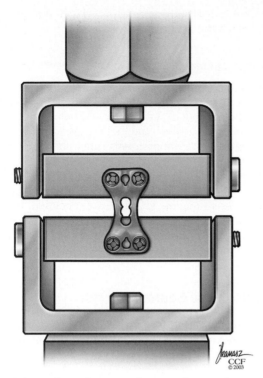

Figure 16.2 Mechanical testing of a ventral-cervical construct using fixation of the implant to ultra-high molecular weight polyethylene cylinders that function as artificial vertebral bodies. This paradigm, devoid of biology, can readily be standardized for the testing of spinal implants.

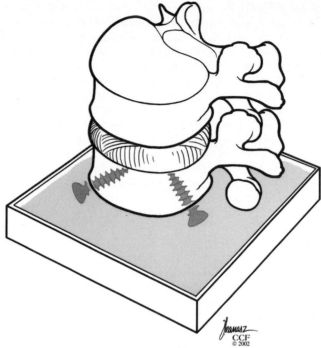

Figure 16.3 The process of affixing the specimen to the mold is often achieved with a polyester resin or polymethylmethacrylate. In this illustration, the specimen is embedded into the viscous material and held in place with a custom jig until the material has cured.

type of test necessarily negates the bone-implant interface but allows a greater degree of reproducibility than with the inclusion of biologic material. The implant is affixed to ultra-high molecular weight polyethylene cylinders that are machined to match the size of vertebral bodies. The construct is placed in the actuator, and load-displacement curves are obtained. Models have thus been developed for lumbar pedicle screw constructs,[9] anterior thoracolumbar instrumentation,[25] and standardization in the testing methodology has been obtained in the case of anterior cervical instrumentation.[2] From a purely semantic point of view, such experimentation is more suitably referred to as mechanical testing than biomechanical testing.

Specimen Preparation

Essential to the preparation of a specimen is the selection of an appropriate spinal level and specimen length. A functional unit or motion segment is the smallest repeating unit of the spine, consisting of two vertebrae, their associated disc, facet joints, and ligaments: the capsular ligament, the anterior and posterior longitudinal ligaments, and the interspinous and supraspinous ligaments. If one elects to use a single motion segment in biomechanical testing, the tensile strength provided by ligaments, such as the anterior and posterior longitudinal ligaments, which span multiple levels, will be underestimated.[1] The deepest fibers of the anterior and posterior longitudinal ligaments extend only to the adjacent vertebra. However, more superficial fibers extend two to three vertebrae, and the most superficial fibers extend across four vertebrae. Using a single motion segment also ignores the

loading above and below by the adjacent discs. Conversely, the use of an excessively long spinal segment predisposes to "snaking," another source of error. A long spinal segment devoid of musculature can buckle. As a result, nonphysiologic movement will occur in the middle vertebrae.[1] Thus, selecting the smallest specimen that will allow the hypothesis to be tested will minimize this variable.

Preparation of the specimen also entails removal of the extraneous soft tissues and musculature and careful preservation of the ligamentous and osseous structures.

Specimen Fixation

The process of affixing the specimen to the testing apparatus is known as *potting*. The specimen is attached to a potting fixture, which is fastened to a loading jig. Central to this procedure is minimizing damage to the specimen, especially when high moments are used.[1] Some investigators have reported good success with the use of dental plaster,[1] a combination of wood screws and polyester resin,[32] polymethylmethacrylate,[8,43] or a low melting point bismuth alloy.[0] Figure 16.3 illustrates this process. Recently, investigators reported on the use of freezing the spine in a particular alignment to achieve a desired posture during testing.[29]

Environmental Conditions

Temperature and humidity affect the mechanical properties of the spine.[1] With warmer temperatures, ligaments expand and the creep rate of discs increases. However, the strength of bone and the energy absorbed at failure are unaffected.[1] There are no appreciable differences between room temperature and body temperature; therefore, testing at room temperature is acceptable.[1] Hydration of tissues, however, has a profound effect on their mechanical properties. The intervertebral discs, in particular, are dependent on hydration to maintain their volume. They contain abundant quantities of proteoglycans, which increase their osmolarity, causing them to imbibe water. The intradiscal water is lost in response to loading, and the disc height decreases. This process is reversible with unloading. Therefore, discs should be kept at 100% humidity prior to and during testing. However, they should not be stored at 100% humidity while unloaded to prevent excessive swelling.

Preloading

When the intervertebral disc is unloaded, its water content increases. It has been demonstrated that axial loading of the lumbar spine increases its stiffness.[21] In cadaveric experiments, the discs are unloaded from the time of death to the time of testing, which alters their biomechanical properties. This effect may be circumvented in part by preloading the spine prior to conducting a test. Some authors have advocated the application of 300N for a minimum of 15 minutes,[1] or the application of 1-2 kN for 2 to 6 hours to simulate the hydration level of a disc late in the day.

The loads that are applied to the human spine include postural loads and loads due to movement and activity.[35] The preloads can be significant and have been measured at 1.4 kN for a 70kg man in the sitting position at the L3-4 disc.[28] Even when supine, the L3-4 load in a 70kg person is approximately 0.2 kN.[28] The intradiscal pressure is greater in healthy discs than in degenerated ones. A study recently demonstrated a highly significant correlation between the grade of disc degeneration, as assessed by MRI scanning, and *in vivo* intradiscal pressure measurements.[38] In *in vitro* biomechanical testing, the effect of preloading on the load/displacement curve of a spinal segment following the subsequent application of physiologic loads is significant.[35] Thus, preloading the specimen during biomechanical testing may provide a closer approximation of the *in vivo* behavior of the spine.

Application of Simple or Complex Loads

In the simplest case, one can subject the specimen to a pure axial load. The amount of deformation that results is dependent on the elastic modulus of the structure, its size, and its shape.[5] The stiffness of a material can be calculated by dividing the applied load by the displacement. In the case of a pure material, it is also equal to the elastic modulus multiplied by the cross-sectional area and divided by the length. This axial load application has been used, for example, in comparing the effect of posture (straight vs. lordotic) on the load-bearing ability and failure modes of the cervical spine.[29] Devices have been constructed to enable the application of complex loads, for example, to reproduce the effect of spinal muscles. When such an experiment is conducted, one does not need to replicate the force imparted by each muscle on the vertebrae. Rather, the coordinated action of muscles can be approximated with the application of force along the appropriate vector.

Application of Force Versus Moment

A force applied to an object will cause its acceleration. Moment is a force applied about an axis. Its magnitude is equal to the product of the force and the distance from the point of rotation, at which the force is applied: the moment arm (Figure 16.4). Pure moments cannot be easily applied, except for torsion. Flexion/extension and lateral bending are, for example, frequently approximated by the eccentric application of an axial load.[31] When this is done, the moment varies along the length of the specimen. In theory, the application of a pure moment occurs uniformly along the specimen.[8] Attempts to approximate this ideal situation have been made, using systems of cables and pulleys.[8]

Limitations and Sources of Error

A biomechanical study is of little value to the clinician if its results cannot be extrapolated in some way to the treatment

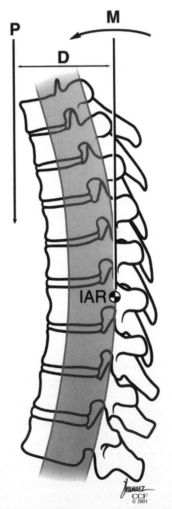

Figure 16.4 Inducing a bending moment through the application of a force at a particular offset from the center of rotation of the spine. Moment = Force × Distance. The IAR designates the instantaneous axis of rotation.

of patients. A potential pitfall is the over-generalization of cadaveric or animal data to clinical practice. This can be avoided only with a characterization of the assumption associated with a study.

Specimen Variability

When human cadaveric tissue is used, there is variability among the specimens. Cadavers vary according to size, age, bone density, and hydration status.[22] Additionally, disease conditions and the use of steroids can affect the characteristics of the specimen. The mechanical properties of bone vary as a function of bone density. Experiments have shown that the compressive strength of bone is proportional to the square of the apparent density, defined as the mineralized tissue mass per volume.[7] The elastic modulus is itself proportional to the cube of bone density.[7] Given the increase in bone porosity with advancing age, it is not surprising that studies have demonstrated a significant decrease in elastic modulus, yield strength, and energy absorbed at failure with age.[4] To complicate matters, this effect is different for different bones.[4] In some cases, it has been argued that the inhomogeneity of human specimens might be desirable because it reflects more accurately the anatomic variability encountered clinically.[33]

The normal aging process is also associated with degeneration of the intervertebral disc. One observes decreased motion, increases in creep rate, and reduced fatigue strength.[19] This alteration occurs in both human beings and animals.[24] It is probably the result of desiccation of the nucleus pulposus and the accumulation of tears in the annulus fibrosus. An *in vivo* porcine study demonstrated the effect of degeneration on the creep rate and elastic modulus of the disc. Compared to an uninjured disc, chemonucleolysis decreased the elastic modulus 23% and resulted in a 15% increase in the average creep rate.[23] In *in vivo* measurements of intradiscal pressure in 28 patients with back problems, the intradiscal pressure was shown to be related to the degree of disc degeneration as assessed by an MRI scan. Severe disc degeneration was associated with less intradiscal pressure than in normal discs.[38] Thus, when biomechanical data is acquired in "healthy spines," the results may not be directly applicable to patients with degenerated discs.

Extrapolating from Cadaveric and Animal Data

When animal tissue is used, assumptions regarding differences in anatomy must be defined prior to extrapolating the results to human beings. Additionally, the use of cadaveric material may not adequately reflect the *in vivo* scenario. Indeed, differences have been observed in the properties of porcine intervertebral discs between live and recently sacrificed animals.[24] Measurements were taken in anesthetized animals and the experiment repeated *in situ* 5 minutes after sacrificing the animal. Significant differences in stiffness, viscosity, and creep rates were observed. Although some of the effects are ascribable to incomplete disc recovery after the first test,[1] even the depth of respiration had an effect on disc pressure. Similarly, another group of investigators found significant load differences on implants fitted with a telemeterized fixation device, between awake and anesthetized

patients.[36] It is likely that even more profound differences exist between *in vivo* and *ex vivo* biomechanical testing.

The Effect of Musculature

Although most biomechanical tests of the spine do not take muscles into account, the effect of musculature is significant. Muscles stabilize the spine by limiting vertebral motion. In fact, muscles continually load the spine. This can be demonstrated by measuring the intradiscal pressure at rest. In the prone position, the intradiscal pressure is 144 N.[38] An exact quantification of the effect of muscles is at present not possible because a direct measurement of muscle load is not feasible. The effect of the musculature must be derived through indirect means, such as electromyography, through measurement of intradiscal or intraabdominal pressure,[28,38] or through mathematic models.[36,42]

The spine is subject to complex loads that involve shear, bending, and torsion moments. A single direction of testing, such as the application of a pure axial load, does not replicate a clinical situation. Furthermore, one cannot simply sum individual moments in order to predict the effects of multiple loads, since the load/displacement curves are nonlinear and time-dependent.

Creep and the Viscoelastic Response

The material properties of the spine and of biologic materials, in general, depend on the rate and history of loading or loading frequency. A constant applied load causes a deformation over time or creep response (Figure 16.5).[19] The faster a disc is loaded, the stiffer it becomes and the greater its capacity to absorb energy. Since the mechanical properties of biologic materials (and therefore the results of biomechanical studies) depend on the rate of load application, the data must be interpreted in light of the physiologic rate of loading. In other words, is the experiment designed to replicate physiologic or traumatic load application? Similarly, during fatigue testing, one must achieve a balance between the frequency of loading and the duration of the test. With prolonged testing, significant soft tissue degradation can occur.[25] This is avoidable with testing at higher frequencies, but excessively high frequencies may not allow the tissues to return to their native states.

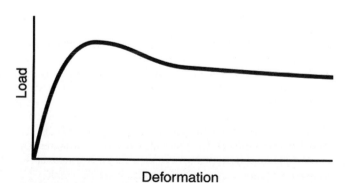

Figure 16.5 Illustration of a typical viscoelastic response or creep curve, with respect to the biomechanical nature of soft tissues.

Data Interpretation

The quality of the data is affected by the preparation of the specimen (testing conditions), and its usefulness is determined by the relevance of the experimental design to the hypothesis. Was the ideal specimen selected? Were the appropriate loads applied and in the correct direction? Even in properly conducted studies, it is difficult to compare similar experiments performed in different laboratories because of the different testing methodologies and the absence of standardization.[41] The exception to this has been the development of a standard for the testing of instrumentation in corpectomy models.[2]

Another significant hurdle in bridging data from the laboratory to the care of patients is in extrapolating animal or cadaveric data to patients. False conclusions can be minimized with a careful characterization of the assumptions. *In vitro* testing, for example, necessarily excludes the effects of inflammation, healing, and remodeling. Additionally, the data obtained *in vitro* with the application of separate loads cannot necessarily be summed to derive the response of a segment to the application of a complex load. This nonlinear summation makes predictions of *in vivo* responses difficult.[12]

Finally, the relevance of the data to clinical applications must be scrutinized.[41] The common goal of spinal instrumentation is to limit movement across the instrumented segment. When biomechanical testing reveals a particular construct to be stiffer than another, one should ask whether a more rigid construct is necessarily better. In the end, biomechanical data requires validation through clinical experimentation and serves as an adjunct to the decision-making process.

REFERENCES

1. Adams MA: Mechanical testing of the spine: an appraisal of methodology, results and conclusions. *Spine* 20:2151-2156, 1995.
2. American Society of Testing and Materials. Standard test for PS5-94 static and dynamic spinal implants assembly in a corpectomy model. West Conshohocken, PA: American Society of Testing and Materials, 1997:1-11.
3. Buhler DW, Berlemann U, Oxland TR, Nolte LP: Moments and forces during pedicle screw insertion. *Spine* 23:1220-1228, 1998.
4. Burstein AH, Reilly DT, Martens M: Aging of bone tissue: mechanical properties. *JBJS* 58A:82-86, 1976.
5. Burstein AH, Wright TM: Mechanical behavior of materials (133-137). In *Fundamentals of Orthopaedic Biomechanics*. Baltimore: Williams & Wilkins, 1994.
6. Callaghan JP, McGill SM: Frozen storage increases the ultimate compressive load of porcine vertebrae. *J Orthop Res* 13:809-812, 1995.
7. Carter DR, Hayes WC: The compressive behavior of bone as a two-phase porous structure. *JBJS* 59A:954-962, 1977.
8. Crawford NR, Brantley AGU, Dickman CA, Koeneman EJ: An apparatus for applying pure nonconstraining moments to spine segments in vitro. *Spine* 20:2097-2100, 1995.
9. Cunningham BW, Sefter JC, McAfee PC: Static and cyclical biomechanical analysis of pedicle screw spinal constructs. *Spine* 18:1677-1688, 1993.
10. Dickman CA, Crawford NR, Tominaga T, *et al*: Morphology and kinematics of the baboon upper cervical spine: a model of the atlantoaxial complex. *Spine* 19:2518-2523, 1994.
11. Dimar JR, Voor MJ, Zhang YM, Glassman SD: A human cadaver model for determination of pathologic fracture threshold resulting from tumorous destruction of the vertebral body. *Spine* 23:1209-1214, 1998.
12. Edwards WT: Biomechanics of posterior lumbar fixation: analysis of testing methodologies. *Spine* 16:1224-1232, 1991.
13. Frank E, Chamberland D, Ragel B: A proposed technique for intraoperative measurement of cervical spine stiffness. *Neurosurgery* 39:147-150, 1996.
14. Gleizes V, Viguier E, Feron JM, *et al*: Effects of freezing on the biomechanics of the intervertebral disc. *Surg Radiol Anat* 20:403-407, 1998.
15. Goel VK, Gilbertson LG: Application of the finite element method to thoracolumbar spinal research: past, present and future. *Spine* 20:1719-1727, 1995.
16. Goel VK, Lim TH, Gilbertson LG, Weinstein JN: Clinically relevant finite element models of a ligamentous lumbar motion segment. *Semin Spine Surg* 5:29-41, 1993.
17. Goel VK, Wilder DG, Pope MH, Edwards WT: Biomechanical testing of the spine: load-controlled versus displacement-controlled analysis. *Spine* 20:2354-2357, 1995.
18. Graham RS, Oberlander EK, Stewart JE, Griffiths DJ: Validation and use of a finite element model of C-2 for determination of stress and fracture patterns of anterior odontoid loads. *J Neurosurg (Spine1)* 93:117-125, 2000.
19. Hansson T: The intervertebral disc: dynamic changes during loading. *Semin Spine Surg* 5:17-22, 1993.
20. Hult E, Ekstrom L, Kaigle A, *et al*: In vivo measurement of spinal column viscoelasticity—an animal model. *Proc Inst Mech Eng [H]* 209:105-110, 1995.
21. Janevic J, Ashton-Miller JA, Schultz AB: Large compressive preloads decrease lumbar motion segment flexibility. *J Orthop Res* 9:228-236, 1991.
22. Kaab MJ, Putz R, Gebauer D, Plitz W: Changes in cadaveric cancellous vertebral bone strength in relation to time: a biomechanical investigation. *Spine* 23:1215-1219, 1998.
23. Keller TS, Hansson TH, Holm SH, *et al*: In vivo creep behavior of the normal and degenerated porcine intervertebral disk: a preliminary report. *J Spinal Disord Tech* 1:267-278, 1989.
24. Keller TS, Holm SH, Hansson TH, Spengler DM: The dependence of intervertebral disc mechanical properties on physiologic conditions. *Spine* 15:751-761, 1990.
25. Kotani Y, Cunningham BW, Parker LM, *et al*: Static and fatigue biomechanical properties of anterior thoracolumbar instrumentation systems. *Spine* 24:1406-1413, 1999.
26. Ledet EH, Sachs BL, Brunski JB, *et al*: Real-time in vivo loading in the lumbar spine. *Spine* 25:2595-2600, 2000.
27. Lee CK, Kim YE, Lee CS, *et al*: Impact response of the intervertebral disc in a finite-element model. *Spine* 25:2431-2439, 2000.
28. Nachemson A: The load on lumbar disks in different positions of the body. *Clin Orthop* 45:107-122, 1966.
29. Oktenoglu T, Ozer F, Ferrara LA, *et al*: Effects of cervical spine posture on axial load bearing ability: a biomechanical study. *J Neurosurg (Spine1)* 94:108-114, 2001.

30. Ozkaya N, Nordin M: Introduction. In *Fundamentals of Biomechanics, Equilibrium, Motion, and Deformation,* ed 2. New York: Springer-Verlag, 1999, p 13.

31. Panjabi MM: Biomechanical evaluation of spinal fixation devices: I. a conceptual framework. *Spine* 13:1129-1134, 1988.

32. Panjabi MM: Biomechanical evaluation of spinal fixation devices: II. stability provided by eight internal fixation devices. *Spine* 13:1135-1140, 1988.

33. Panjabi MM: Cervical spine models for biomechanical research. *Spine* 23:2684-2700, 1998.

34. Panjabi MM, Krag MH, Summers D, Videman T: Biomechanical time-tolerance of fresh cadaveric human spine specimens. *J Orthop Res* 3:292-300, 1985.

35. Panjabi MM, Krag MH, White III AW, Southwick WO: Effects of preload on load displacement curves of the lumbar spine. *Orthop Clin North Am* 8:181-192, 1977.

36. Rohlmann A, Bergmann G, Graichen F, Mayer HM: Influence of muscle forces on loads in internal spinal fixation devices. *Spine* 23:537-542, 1998.

37. Rohlmann A, Graichen F, Weber U, Bergmann G: Monitoring in vivo implant loads with a telemeterized internal spinal fixation device. *Spine* 25:2981-2986, 2000.

38. Sato K, Kikuchi S, Yonezawa T: In vivo intradiscal pressure measurement in healthy individuals and in patients with ongoing back problems. *Spine* 24:2468-2474, 1999.

39. Shirazi-Adl A: Models of the functional spinal unit. *Semin Spine Surg* 5:23-28, 1993.

40. Smeathers JE, Joanes DN: Dynamic compressive properties of human lumbar intervertebral joints: a comparison between fresh and frozen specimens. *J Biomech* 21:425-433, 1988.

41. Stokes IA: Mechanical testing of instrumentation: a test of mechanics. *Spine* 23:2263-2264, 1998.

42. Vasavada AN, Li S, Delp SL: Influence of muscle morphometry and moment arms on the moment-generating capacity of human neck muscles. *Spine* 23:412-422, 1998.

43. Wilke HJ, Kettler A, Claes LE: Are sheep spines a valid biomechanical model for human spines? *Spine* 22: 2365-2374, 1997.

44. Wilke HJ, Neef P, Caimi M, Hoogland T, Claes LE: New in vivo measurements of pressures in the intervertebral disc in daily life. *Spine* 24:755-762, 1999.

45. Yoganandan N, Kumaresan S, Voo L, Pintar FA: Finite element application in human cervical spine modeling. *Spine* 21:1824-1834, 1996.

CHAPTER 17

Fundamentals of Spine Surgery

James S. Harrop, Cary D. Alberstone, and Edward C. Benzel

Decision-Making Process

Clinical decision making is one of the most challenging tasks for any physician, particularly for spine surgeons. Multiple factors influence the surgical and medical decision-making process. Although the patient is the surgeon's first priority, other factors such as financial and social pressures affect this process. This chapter addresses some of the fundamentals of this process, including patient selection, informed consent, surgical planning, biomechanics, technology, and medical economics.

Patient Selection

Patient selection is the most important and difficult task in the surgical treatment of spinal disorders. A technically perfect operation in the wrong patient might fulfill the surgical goals of the procedure but is unlikely to resolve the patient's initial complaints and deficits. Unfortunately a proper study of spine surgery indications is not only difficult to design, but is also equally difficult to execute. Therefore there is little evidence to guide the spine surgeon concerning operative indications, techniques, and timing of surgery. This has impeded physicians' abilities to collect and analyze clinically relevant data. Without this data to guide clinical decision making, the problem of patient selection and management strategy determination will remain difficult.

Spine surgeons have realized the limited use of previous attempts at analyzing the natural history and postsurgical outcome of spinal disorders. Therefore there is presently a drive in the spine community to provide more prospective analyses, comparing treatment strategies along with outcome analyses using recognized scales, such as the Oswestry and SF-36. These analyses report patient satisfaction and quality of life after procedures, rather than fusion rate and neurologic recovery. The former are the ultimate goals and the true determinants of treatment efficacy.

Besides increasing patient satisfaction and quality of life, other factors such as personal, financial, and defensive practice strategies, and third-party payers have motivated surgeons to address the challenges and difficulties of patient selection. In particular, third-party payers are reluctant to reimburse physicians, hospitals, and patients for procedures that lack clear indications or documented evidence of efficacy. In the current environment of cost-containment, surgeons are increasingly pressured by outside influences to demonstrate that they practice safe and appropriate surgery, by documenting their surgical outcomes. Although the motivations that underlie these powerful forces are frequently not altruistic, it should be evident that the results of so-called outcome research will benefit both the patient and the surgeon.

The excellent design and timely execution of carotid endarterectomy studies provides a paradigm for the potential benefits of outcomes research.[3,6] These studies clearly defined objective criteria for surgical treatment, based on risk and benefit ratios. Although outcome assessment is obviously more straightforward for carotid endarterectomy than spinal surgery, the carotid endarterectomy trials nevertheless serve as a reminder of the powerful influence such trials can exert on surgical practice. These trials have not only proven the safety and efficacy of the procedure itself, but have provided unambiguous guidelines for patient selection. However, the suboptimal prospective study of extracranial to intracranial (EC-IC) bypass for ischemic stroke, which concluded surgical treatment was less effective than medical therapy, illustrates some weaknesses of these studies.[2]

Consent for Surgery

When the clinical judgment of the surgeon supports surgical treatment for a disorder, the traditional relationship between the patient and the surgeon has been such that the surgeon recommends surgery and the patient, if willing, agrees. The modern "legal" contract that attempts to formalize this interaction is the consent for surgery form. This form is used to document that the patient has agreed to allow the surgeon to perform an operation, with an understanding of the risks, benefits, and alternative treatment options. This form is what most patients and surgeons conceptualize as *consent for surgery*.

However, this consent for surgery form is not just a piece of paper. It manifests the patient's right to determine how he or she will be treated. Physicians' recognition of this distinction has led to a more thoughtful and meaningful agreement or consent that satisfies stringent ethical and legal requirements. This is what is presently referred to as *informed consent*.

Informed Consent

Patient autonomy, the most fundamental of all patients' rights, is portrayed through the informed consent. It is the permission a patient grants to a physician to administer a treatment. The patient should understand the rationale for the treatment, the alternatives to the treatment, the nature of the treatment, the intended result of the treatment and its chances for success, and the nature and risks of adverse consequences of the treatment. During the interval of informed consent the physician is able to define the problem facing the patient, based on limited prospective studies, suspected natural history course, alternative treatments, and risks and benefits, along with goals of surgical treatment. This conference also allows the physician to address any fears and expectations the patient might have about his or her disease process and possible treatment schemes.

In the context of clinical decision making several objections have been raised regarding the logic, and even the possibility, of informed consent. The defense of the doctrine of informed consent is beyond the scope of this chapter. However, a few points in response to objections about informed consent are worthy of consideration. Some argue that since the physician possesses a superior knowledge of the medical situation and proposed procedures, the patient cannot properly decide about informed consent. This argument is based on a misconception that gives undue primacy to patient understanding. In fact, one's right not to be assaulted is not conditional on one's understanding of the motivation for the assault. In the context of clinical decision making, then, it seems reasonable to argue that a patient's limited understanding of the consequences of the choice does not abrogate the right to decide what is to be done.

Several studies have shown that patients are frequently unable to recall the content of the information that the physician conveyed during the session at which informed consent was supposedly obtained.[1,4,5] Sometimes these scenarios are the basis for legal claims against unsuspecting physicians, who are accused of not adequately informing the patient of potential complications. Physicians can avoid these confrontations by carefully documenting their conversations with patients and their families in the medical record, indicating both the time and the date of the conversation as evidence that it occurred before any intervention. However, legal repercussions aside, the demonstration that patients frequently do not remember information provided by physicians is certainly not a logical argument against the virtue of informed consent. There are many instances in life when one is unable to recall the reasons or motivations for making even the most important decisions.

Finally, there is no reason why a patient should be disallowed the right to make a decision that is not consistent with the best medical prognosis. Many factors must be considered in every medical decision. This is especially true of such an important decision as the one to undergo surgery, which is influenced by a wide array of circumstances and beliefs, such as occupation, lifestyle, state of health, family, and the patient's idea of what constitutes a life that is worth living.

Beyond Informed Consent

What informed consent implies, but does not explicitly state, is that medical decisions should be a cooperative effort between the patient, his or her family, and the physician. This combined effort has the goal of effectively managing the patient's pathologic process in a timely and efficient manner. The fragile interaction between patient and physician in this decision process can be interrupted if the physician dominates the relationship. Physicians are naturally more knowledgeable than patients about medical matters. Therefore physicians can influence the decision of a patient by creating a sense of urgency or necessity to accept their preferred course of action. This manipulation of the decision is typically an unconscious act. The result is a course of treatment for which the patient indirectly may have hesitancy or may be reluctant to pursue.

The responsibility of the physician is to help the patient make a decision that is truly in the patient's best interest, and not simply the one that matches the physician's preference. There is a natural tendency among patients to experience fear and intimidation if they choose to defy the physician's implied or stated wishes. This is not to say that the physician is obligated to refrain from stating or implying his or her preference, but rather that the patient should be made to feel comfortable to inquire and engage in the decision-making process.

This process by which a decision is reached, and the decision itself, should be documented in the medical record, and the time and date should be recorded. This serves to protect the physician in case of future litigation, and to solidify in the physician's mind the rationale for the course of action that is taken. The importance of engaging the patient in the process of clinical decision making cannot be overemphasized.

Surgical Considerations

Spinal Anatomy and Biomechanics

Once the physician and the patient have decided to pursue surgical treatment of the spinal disorder, the surgeon must define the goal of the procedures and a course to obtain that goal. A surgical approach and objectives are defined during this interval. Because of the lack of prospective data on surgical treatments, the spine surgeon must frequently rely on personal experiences, along with common sense, in the treatment of spinal disorders.

Spine surgeons have a fund of knowledge that is based on common teachings and practice. Included in this knowledge base is a basic understanding of what may be termed the fundamentals of spinal surgery, which includes spinal anatomy and biomechanics. It is efficient for the surgeon to think in terms of principles. To illustrate how spinal anatomy and biomechanics can be applied to the process of clinical decision making, 10 principles of spinal biomechanics, and their implications for clinical practice, are provided in the following examples:

1. PRINCIPLE 1. *The ventral surgical approach is generally the preferred approach in patients with a loss of cervical lordosis.* The ventral approach decompresses ventral mass and tends to preserve the dorsal tension band. This minimizes the risk of further kyphotic deformation. Conversely, the dorsal approach is relatively contraindicated in patients with a loss of cervical lordosis, because it weakens the dorsal tension band, which tends to exacerbate progressive spinal deformity.
2. PRINCIPLE 2. *Dorsal distraction of the lumbar spine is an undesirable force application because it tends to produce a flattened back.* The loss of lordosis is not an uncommon complication of lumbar spine surgery. The flattened back is a common cause of chronic low back pain, because it alters the normal spinal sagittal balance. Fortunately, this problem is nearly always avoidable if the surgeon obeys this principle.
3. PRINCIPLE 3. *With a dorsal fusion operation, a more dorsally placed fusion mass more*

effectively resists kyphotic deformation. The dorsal fusion mass resists kyphotic deformity in direct proportion to the length of the moment arm through which it acts. The moment arm is defined as the distance between the fusion mass and the more ventrally located instantaneous axis of rotation (IAR). Therefore the greater the distance the fusion mass is from the IAR, the longer the moment arm available for the resistance of kyphotic deformation.

4. PRINCIPLE 4. *The effectiveness of a spinal brace is inversely proportional to the axial distance between the spine and the inner shell of the brace, and is directly proportional to the length of the brace.* These relationships are explained by the theoretical principle that the efficacy of bracing is related to the cosine of the angle defined by the edge of the brace, the IAR at the unstable segment, and the long axis of the spine. The implication is that a long and tight-fitting spinal brace will result in more effective spinal stabilization than a short and loose-fitting brace.

5. PRINCIPLE 5. *With a three-point bending construct, the ability of the implant to maintain spinal alignment is directly related to the length of the implant.* The implication of this principle for clinical practice is that increasing the length of the longitudinal member of a dorsal hook-rod system will increase its ability to maintain spinal alignment. This relationship does not apply to short-segment fixators, such as pedicle screw devices that function as cantilevers. This is because the moment arm of the force application of a three-point bending construct is measured along the long axis of the spine, whereas the moment arm of a short-segment fixator is equal to the perpendicular distance between the longitudinal member and the IAR.

6. PRINCIPLE 6. *In general a ventrally placed short-segment fixation device should be applied in a compression mode.* This mode of force application allows the fixation device to share the axial load with its associated interbody strut. Conversely, when such an implant is placed in the distraction mode, there is an undesirable allocation of forces. In this case the spinal implant bears all of the load, which greatly increases the chance of implant failure. The principle of load sharing versus load bearing is a key principle in the practice of spinal stabilization.

7. PRINCIPLE 7. *Three-column spinal injury (circumferential injury) indicates overt spinal instability, which generally requires spinal stabilization.* This principle is based on the three-column theory of spinal stability. The three columns are divided into: (1) an anterior column, which consists of the ventral half of the vertebral body, (2) a middle column, which consists of the dorsal half of the vertebral body, and (3) a posterior column, which consists of all of those elements that are dorsal to the vertebral body. Interruption of any one, or even two, of these columns does not necessarily lead to spinal instability. However, significant interruption of all three columns almost invariably destabilizes the spine. In these cases surgical spinal stabilization helps protect the neural elements from initial or progressive injury, and facilitates early mobilization of the patient.

8. PRINCIPLE 8. *With time, spinal instrumentation will almost certainly fail without the acquisition of a concomitant bony fusion.* This principle emphasizes the limited role of spinal instrumentation in maintaining spinal alignment. As a corollary to this principle, it is often said that there is a "race between spinal implant failure and the acquisition of a bony fusion." The implication is that the surgeon must be cognizant that the goal of spinal instrumentation is to maintain spinal alignment only as long as it takes to acquire an adequate fusion. It follows from this that the execution of a meticulous arthrodesis procedure is imperative.

9. PRINCIPLE 9. *Spinal decompression procedures that decompress the neural elements are performed at the expense of spinal stability.* This principle does not imply that neural element decompression (such as is accomplished by lumbar discectomy) invariably results in spinal instability. It should, however, serve as a reminder to the surgeon that the question of spinal stability must always be included in the process of surgical decision making and surgical planning. Appropriate measures must always be taken to avoid or to compensate for this problem.

10. PRINCIPLE 10. *The surgeon should violate any of the aforementioned principles if they conflict with more reasonable or more general principles, or if they conflict with what is obvious (common sense).*

Technology and the Spine

There is concern for the unmitigated application of spinal instrumentation, in which little data is available to support their clinical application. The increasingly rapid development of expensive implants, with little documented efficacy, should cause surgeons to pause and reflect on basic surgical goals and principles. Typically goals include neural decompression, the acquisition of surgical spinal stability, and the correction of spinal deformity. These goals should be formulated without an emphasis on using newer technology or techniques. Therefore the surgeon should not formulate the surgical goals based on how he or she can use technology to benefit the patient. Rather the directive of the treatment should be what is best for the patient, and only secondarily on the technology that best achieves this goal.

Economics

Managed care and third-party payers have directed physicians to analyze cost and benefits for not only the individual patient, but also for society as a whole, while still achieving the highest quality of care for the individual. Society aims to achieve a health care system with the highest value to the individuals, in which value is equated to quality, divided by cost.

$$\text{Value} = \text{quality/cost}$$

In spine surgery over the last several decades, the quality of patient care has improved drastically, because of a better understanding of biomechanical principles and the use of sophisticated spinal implants for stability augmentation during fusion. However, surgeons must be cognizant of the cost of spinal implants and the true quality (of life) these devices afford the patient. Does the use of a device that raises the cost of the implant 200% improve the quality twice as much? In most instances the answer is: most likely not. Therefore the overall value, based on the aforementioned equation, is decreased. This is not to say new technology should not be used, but rather the surgeon should evaluate its indications and goals individually for each surgical procedure. Once again this emphasizes the importance of prospective outcome assessments to evaluate these devices in an unbiased manner.

Economic assessments in the spine surgery arena are difficult, because of multiple available treatment options and strategies. The managed-care environment is based on the objective of cost-containment. This emphasizes economic efficiency at the expense of clinical outcome. Therefore surgery may be underused because of its high cost. Unfortunately this fails to recognize the overall goal of achieving high quality and of the value of health care for the patient. A dangerous situation may be created in this manner (i.e., clinical decisions may be predominantly motivated by cost, rather than by value). Ultimately, physicians and payers must assess both cost and quality to establish an appropriate approach to patient management.

The importance of clinical outcome studies can never be overemphasized; however, similar to any research material, their results should not be taken for granted. This could happen in a health care system that is driven solely by cost and not value or quality of health care. Conversely, the quality of a health care service cannot be assumed just because the service is expensive. Physicians should strive to be cost-effective, and to simultaneously produce high-quality outcomes, which results in higher quality of care for the patient and society. If cost and quality of information were available for large populations of patients with well-defined medical problems, who received care via similar medical management algorithms, both quality and cost-efficiency could be assessed and hence optimized.

The use of actuarial-derived data as the sole data influencing clinical decision making is ill-advised and perhaps dangerous, since it is based only on cost and resource use. This point can be emphasized through the following example:

A surgical procedure is determined, on the basis of actuarial-derived data, to be "optimally performed" at an annual rate of 50 procedures per 100,000 cared lives. In the managed care environment "optimally performed" is defined as the lowest achievable utilization rates. However, the annual community surgical rate for this procedure is 100 procedures per 100,000 cared lives. The implication of this discrepancy is that the community surgery rate is twice that which it should be (100 procedures versus 50).

This analysis fails to take into account two very important factors: (1) the quality of clinical outcome, and (2) financial savings associated with surgery via indirect costs. Indirect costs are herein defined as costs that cannot be specifically traced to an individual service or product.

The maximization of net revenue and the minimization of the cost of operative management are important to the spine surgeon. An analysis of the overall cost of a procedure must consider not only the cost of performing the procedure (direct costs), but also the cost of *not* performing the procedure (hidden cost or indirect costs). The determination of the savings associated with not performing a procedure is not as simple as computing the cost of the procedure. The surgical procedure may obviate the need for additional nonsurgical care, which may be more costly than the operation alone. The actuarial-derived data (on which many attempts at cost-containment are based) merely provide information about the number of procedures performed (and secondarily, their direct costs). What is not readily obvious is that if surgery were not performed, nonsurgical management would be provided instead, at an additional cost (indirect). The economic relationship between surgical and nonsurgical care may be depicted as follows:

Cost of Surgical Management = Surgical management costs + *Routine* nonsurgical management costs

Cost of Nonsurgical Management = *Routine* nonsurgical management costs + *Additional* nonsurgical management costs°

Savings Associated with Surgical Management = Additional nonsurgical management costs† − Surgical management costs

The withholding of surgical treatment eliminates the cost of surgical management. However, the indirect and hidden cost must be calculated, along with social costs (e.g., loss of work and function), before the actuarial-data–derived treatment can be declared a strategy success, both from a financial and a social perspective. The hidden costs and indirect costs associated with additional nonsurgical management must also be considered in the overall financial benefit. The aforementioned example can be extended further to emphasize this point.

Assume that 50 of the 100 patients who normally would have undergone surgery did not undergo the procedure. Of the 50 patients denied surgery, assume 25 received nonsurgical care that was more expensive than the surgical care (e.g., physical therapy, pain management schemes, and chiropractic treatments for the management of a cervical disc herniation). In this scenario we may conclude that the so-called optimal rate of surgery was not cost-effective. If we assume that the cost of additional nonsurgical management for the remaining patients was less expensive than surgical care would have been, the surgical rate that results in the minimum overall cost is about 75 cases per 100,000 cared lives per year, not 50.

°Hidden cost is associated with not performing an operative procedure.
†Nonsurgical management provided in lieu of surgery, if surgery was not performed.

The analysis previously described considers neither quality of patient care, nor outcome or value. It is merely a cost analysis that considers the effects of savings. However, if surgeons can demonstrate cost-effective and favorable outcomes, then patients, third-party payers, and surgeons all stand to benefit.

Summary

Clinical decision making in spine surgery is affected by a myriad of influences. This chapter has attempted to describe only a few of these influences. It is emphasized that the surgeon should be cognizant of the complexities that affect such important decisions as informed consent, the use of technology, patient selection, surgical planning, and cost. In the presence of an ever-increasing number of threatening influences, surgeons must remain focused on their principal goal (i.e., optimizing patient care).

REFERENCES

1. Byrne DJ, Napier A, Cuschieri A: How informed is signed consent? *Br Med J* 296:839-840, 1988.
2. EC-IC Bypass Study Group: Failure of extracranial-intracranial arterial bypass to reduce the risk of ischemic stroke: results of an international randomized trial. *N Engl J Med* 313:1191-1200, 1985.
3. Executive Committee for the Asymptomatic Carotid Atherosclerosis Study: Endarterectomy for asymptomatic carotid artery stenosis. *JAMA* 273:1421-1428, 1995.
4. Herz DA, Looman JE, Lewis LK: Informed consent: Is it a myth? *Neurosurg* 30:453-458, 1992.
5. Kekuchi K, Hara T, Hara T: Patient understanding of the informed consent for cataract surgery. *J Ophthalmic Nurs Technol* 15:216-219, 1996.
6. North American Symptomatic Carotid Endarterectomy Trial Collaborators: Beneficial effect of carotid endarterectomy in symptomatic patients with high-grade carotid stenosis. *N Engl J Med* 325:445-453, 1991.

CHAPTER 18

Preoperative and Surgical Planning for Avoiding Complications

**Mehmet Zileli, Sait Naderi,
and Edward C. Benzel**

Technical complications in spine surgery usually arise from the overaggressive handling of soft tissue, or from hardware failure. Other reasons include poor patient selection, an incorrect diagnosis, an ill-chosen approach, an inadequate operation (e.g., incomplete decompression of a compressive lesion), and injury to normal anatomic structures.

The surgeon should have a clear idea of the diagnosis, and a clear, three-dimensional understanding of the pathologic anatomy, as demonstrated by imaging studies. Finally, an astute surgeon should use common sense by "measuring twice, cutting once, and paying meticulous attention to detail."

General Precautions
Antibiotics

The role of preoperative and perioperative antibiotics in spine surgery remains controversial. The average infection rate for spine operations is less than 2%. Evidence suggests that the incidence of infections may be decreased further if antibiotics are administered before the operation.[11,18,32,33] Indeed a review of the literature provides support for the use of perioperative antibiotics.[18] Because the most frequently detected organism is a *Staphylococcus* species, a first-generation cephalosporin is usually satisfactory, unless an allergic propensity is recognized.[14]

Steroids

The role of perioperative steroids in spine surgery is also controversial. The administration of steroids before spinal cord injury confers greater benefit than administration after injury.[7,14] Although the literature is inconclusive, some surgeons choose to administer 4 to 8mg of dexamethasone (or an equivalent dosage of methylprednisolone) preoperatively, and to continue steroid administration for 24 hours postoperatively. Because short-term use of steroids is effective in experimental studies,[7,19] and long-term administration is associated with increased risks, its use for more than 24 hours seems unnecessary, and possibly harmful.

Intubation

Neck positioning during intubation is important in patients with cervical spinal cord compression. C1-2 extension is most commonly associated with intubation, and is usually well tolerated by the patient. In patients with severe stenosis at or above the level of C3-4, intubation with fiber optic system guidance, while the patient is awake and under local anesthesia, is usually preferred. Preoperative skull or halter traction may facilitate intubation and surgery by providing gentle traction and extension. Some surgeons suggest that patients with severe cervical myelopathy should be positioned before the induction of general anesthesia.[11]

Positioning

Numerous complications are associated with improper positioning, including air embolism, quadriplegia, peripheral nerve palsies, pyriformis syndrome, posterior compartment syndrome, and excessive bleeding.

Elastic bandages or sequential compression devices should be placed on the lower extremities before the induction of anesthesia. The legs must not be lower than the hips in the sitting position. Great care should be taken in moving the patient to the prone position. Three-point skull fixation in the prone position may be used, although it is associated with potential complications.

Extreme rotation, extension, or flexion of the head may cause cervical spinal cord damage and resulting quadriplegia. Older patients with cervical spondylotic bars are more inclined to this complication. Awake positioning, awake intubation, or evoked-potential monitoring may be helpful. Loss of somatosensory evoked potentials, with neck flexion and recovery with repositioning, has been reported.[42] In patients with severe spinal canal narrowing the neutral or near-neutral position is preferred.

A stretch injury of the brachial plexus may occur in both the prone and supine positions, by abducting the arm greater than 90 degrees. An axillary roll should be used to prevent injury, with the lateral decubitus position when the dependent arm is compressed. The ulnar nerve could be injured because of its superficial position at the elbow. A pad under an extended elbow helps prevent this injury. Elbow extension minimizes exposure of the ulnar nerve to compression. The radial nerve may be injured if the arm hangs over the operating table edge. Padding under the arm may prevent compressive injury. Common peroneal nerve injury with resulting foot drop may occur in the supine, the sitting, and the lateral decubitus positions. The superficial location of the nerve at the head of the fibula may increase the risk of compression. The superficial femoral nerve may be compressed in the prone position and cause a postoperative transient meralgia paresthetica.

Compression and stretch injury of any nerve is possible during positioning. A general rule of thumb is to use a position without excessive compression of the extremities, and to place appropriate pads beneath potentially exposed nerves. If the patient appears comfortable, nerve injury is less likely. Injury to the lateral femoral cutaneous nerve was reported as high as 20%.[25] External pressure at the anterior superior iliac spine during prone position is the main reason for the injury of the nerve. The nerve can also be injured at the retroperitoneum by hematoma or traction, and during bone graft harvesting at the anterior iliac crest.

Compression of the eyes, with resulting blindness, has been reported with the use of the horseshoe headrest.[20,26,35] The head should be positioned to prevent it from slipping on the horseshoe headrest. Three-point skull fixation is a viable alternative to the horseshoe, and should significantly reduce the incidence of this complication.

Air Embolism

Air embolism is one of the most serious complications encountered. It is predominantly related to operations performed above the level of the heart.[28] Two precautions to avoid air embolism are suggested: (1) if possible, avoid the sitting position, and (2) monitor the patient at risk meticulously with Doppler ultrasound and end-tidal P_{CO_2}. In such patients a central venous catheter should be used so that air can be emergently evacuated from the right atrium, if an air embolism is detected. The central venous pressure should be maintained at greater than 10cm, so that the pressure in epidural veins does not decline. Do not use nitrous oxide when using the sitting position.

The incidence and clinical importance of air embolism is greater in the sitting position than in other positions.[1] Its incidence has been reported to be as high as 50%.[28] If air embolism occurs, a central venous catheter may be used to withdraw air from the left atrium. At the same time the surgeon should flood the wound with Ringer's solution and inspect and control any open veins with bipolar coagulation. Bleeding bone surfaces should be treated with wax, and the wound should be precisely packed with wet gauze. If signs of air embolism persist, the position of the patient should quickly be changed to the right-side-up position to aid the removal of air via the central venous catheter from the right atrium.

Paradoxic Air Embolism

A patent foramen ovale, or another right-to-left shunting, causes paradoxic air embolism. It is optimally prevented by an accurate preoperative diagnosis with an echocardiogram. Saline injection during echocardiography (if performed) is suggested for the patients in whom a sitting-position operation is considered. If shunting from right to the left atrium is encountered, the sitting position should not be used.[22] If the patient is placed in the sitting position, positive end-expiratory pressure should not be used, because it increases the right atrial pressure, which increases the risk of paradoxic air embolism. In this case air may enter the cerebral arteries, resulting in coma, quadriplegia, or death.

Intravascular Volume Control

Central and arterial lines should be placed preoperatively, if there is a risk of excessive bleeding. If the sitting position is used, adequate hydration of the patient is imperative. If sympathetic tone is diminished or lost as a result of severe spinal cord compression, a central catheter should be placed. The sitting position in such patients is particularly troublesome.

Doppler and End-Tidal CO$_2$ Monitoring

Both Doppler and end-tidal CO_2 monitoring are useful in all sitting-position operations. Although the Doppler is not necessarily a vital monitoring technique (i.e., it may show very small volumes of air that do not change P_{CO_2} and vital signs), the surgeon should immediately search for a source of air entrance into the venous system. If a vessel is identified, it should be coagulated. If not, the wound should temporarily be packed with wet sponges. If the end-tidal CO_2 drops, the wound must be packed; if hemodynamic stability is diminished, the wound must be closed.

Intraoperative Radiographs

Intraoperative imaging can ensure the correct level of the operation, and may provide information about the degree of decompression, realignment, or stabilization.

Incidental Durotomy

Unintended tear of the dura mater is a common complication of the spine surgery. Its incidence has been reported between 3.1% and 14% in different series.[8,21,38] Immediately after surgery, a tear causes headaches, wound infection, and cerebrospinal fluid (CSF) fistulae. In long-term, persistent CSF leak, pseudomeningocele, neurologic deficit, and arachnoiditis are common problems associated with durotomy.[8] It should be better recognized and treated appropriately.

Operative Technique

General techniques for complication avoidance include: (1) adequate visualization, (2) use of a high-speed drill, (3) use of microcurettes with varying angles and sizes, and (4) adequate positioning. The decision to operate, the approach, operation technique, and the use of internal fixation and fusion are each important considerations.

Complication Avoidance in the Upper Cervical Spine

The reducibility of the lesion is an important consideration for upper cervical spine pathologic processes. If the lesion is reducible, only a dorsal fixation and fusion procedure may be indicated. If the lesion is not reducible, the optimal operation depends on the localization of the compression.

For an extradural lesion located between the midclivus and the C3 vertebral body, a transoral approach may provide the trajectory and exposure of choice. If the lesion is intradural, a dorsal or lateral transcondylar approach may be more appropriate. Complex pathologic lesions with lateral extension that are located between the C1 and midcervical levels may be approached via a transmandibular, transglossal approach. For more limited pathologic lesions located between the lower clivus and the C2 vertebral body, a ventrolateral or ventromedial retropharyngeal approach may be used. In general, if stabilization is required, a dorsal or lateral transcondylar approach with instrumentation should be considered.

Transoral Approach
Cerebrospinal Fluid Fistula

For intradural pathology a lateral, transcondylar or dorsal approach is associated with a significantly lower risk of a CSFCSF fistula, compared with the transoral approach. If the latter approach is used and a CSF leak occurs, the dural leaves may be covered with fascia and fibrin glue. A lumbar drain is usually placed postoperatively to treat a CSF fistula.

Severe Tongue Swelling

Intermittent release of the tongue retractor may prevent severe tongue swelling. Other methods to avoid tongue swelling include the intravenous administration of dexamethasone and postoperative massaging of the tongue to reconstitute venous and lymphatic flow.[24] Patients who are candidates for tongue swelling should not be extubated before complete resolution of the tongue swelling.

Hemorrhage

Because bleeding may accumulate in the deep and narrow wound, meticulous hemostasis is imperative. The careful control of bleeding should be maintained throughout the operation. Injury to the vertebral artery may require clipping or compression occlusion of the artery.

Meningitis

Meningitis is commonly associated with intradural operations. Mouth irrigation with an antibiotic solution may be used preoperatively for 2 to 3 days, after preoperative cultures of the oropharynx are obtained. Intraoperatively the mouth is swabbed with Betadine solution. The presence of a retropharyngeal abscess is a contraindication to surgery. In patients with meningitis, postoperative antimicrobial therapy is administered.

Retropharyngeal Abscess and Palatal and Pharyngeal Wound Dehiscence

In the presence of late wound dehiscence a retropharyngeal abscess should be sought. Palatal and pharyngeal wound dehiscence is often related to inadequate wound closure. If complications develop, they commonly occur 1 week after the operation.

Neurologic Worsening and Instability

Neurologic worsening is often related to inadequate decompression. It may also be caused by loss of alignment, or an iatrogenic injury. Injury during surgical positioning or intubation may be avoided by the use of fluoroscopy during positioning, and an awake fiberoptic intubation. Instability can be investigated with postoperative dynamic

(flexion/extension) radiographs. If instability is present, an occipitocervical fusion may be necessary.[24]

Median Labiomandibular Glossotomy

Median labiomandibular glossotomy is a very morbid operation that requires a preoperative tracheotomy or the maintenance of tracheal intubation, until the edema of the tongue, palate, and pharynx resolve. If the dura mater is opened, meticulous closure with the application of fibrin glue is useful to avoid CSF fistulae and resulting meningitis. To obtain optimal cosmetic results, the assistance of a plastic surgeon may be appropriate.

Transcervical Retropharyngeal Approach

Hypoglossal nerve injury and carotid artery injury are commonly observed with a transcervical retropharyngeal approach. To avoid intraoperative stroke via embolization, some surgeons use preoperative angiography or Doppler examination of the carotid artery.[24]

Lateral Transcondylar Approach

The most feared complications of the lateral transcondylar approach are vertebral artery injury, air embolism, CSF leakage, and hypoglossal nerve injury. Appropriate decompression and protection of the vertebral artery minimizes the risk of injury. Air embolism may be prevented by the aforementioned neuroanesthetic techniques. To prevent CSF leakage, an inverted J-shaped incision may provide a more precise closure of the muscle flaps than that achieved with a paramedian vertical incision. A CSF fistula is a less common, and less treacherous complication of this procedure, compared with the transoral approach. The hypoglossal nerve injury is another complication of transcondylar approach. The hypoglossal nerve may be injured during a condylectomy procedure. Preoperative bone window, computed tomographic (CT) images of the occipital condyle may help to localize the hypoglossal canal and its inner and outer orifices.

Complication Avoidance in the Subaxial Cervical Spine

Surgical intervention in a patient with a complete traumatic spinal cord lesion and overt instability may be necessary to re-establish spinal stability. Systemic complications of trauma such as hypotension, respiratory difficulties, and metabolic derangements should be well controlled before embarking on a stabilization procedure.

For cervical spondylotic disease the shape of the cervical curvature should be considered in deciding on the operative approach. In general, cervical kyphosis is a specific indication for a ventral approach, to avoid postoperative instability and to provide adequate ventral decompression.[4]

Often, intradural tumors are optimally approached dorsally, whereas vertebral body tumors are best approached ventrally. A burst or wedge fracture with spinal canal compromise is best approached ventrally. However, severe three-column instability may require both a ventral and a dorsal approach. The indications for the ventrolateral approach are laterally situated tumors, nerve root decompression,[23,37] and the rarely observed symptomatic vertebral artery compression.

Potential Injuries Associated with Ventral Approaches
Spinal Cord Damage

To avoid spinal cord damage, attention should be paid to: (1) patient positioning, (2) illumination and visualization, (3) anesthetic and surgical techniques, (4) position of the surgeon, and (5) evoked-potential monitoring.

It is perhaps best to place the patient in a neutral position, although mild extension may aid exposure. Care must be taken to avoid hyperextension, which may cause or exacerbate already existing spinal cord compression. Neurologic examination in a test-extension posture in the awake patient before surgery may help avoid neurologic injury related to positioning.

For optimum illumination and visualization an operating microscope may help avoid injury to neural and vascular structures, especially in narrow surgical fields, such as those associated with the transoral approach.[3,5,10,30]

An anesthetic technique without paralytic agents may be useful to monitor motor responses from unwanted irritation of the spinal cord or nerve roots. Only bipolar coagulation should be used. It may be helpful to avoid using Kerrison rongeurs for bone removal, and instead to use a Leksell rongeur or a high-speed drill. Curettes may be used for the last pieces of bone. To avoid injury to the spinal cord and nerve roots, the graft should not be impacted into the recess with great force, and its depth should not be greater than 13mm.

Frequently the surgeon inadvertently obtains a more extensive decompression on the side opposite the side of the approach.[12] This may be prevented by either working alternately from both sides of the patient, or by using the correct angle of view of the operating microscope.

Although its use is controversial, evoked-potential monitoring is considered helpful by some surgeons.[42,44]

Cervical Nerve Root Injury

A cervical nerve root may be injured during far-lateral dissection as a part of the ventrolateral approaches. Therefore lateral dissection should not be carried dorsal to the anterior tubercle of transverse process.

C5 Radiculopathy

The C5 motor nerve root is most frequently affected by surgery. This may occur in association with both ventral and dorsal operations. Because its mechanism of injury is not well understood, its prevention is also controversial. It has been suggested that excessively wide exposures result in tethering of the nerve roots. Saunders[31] recommends that the ventral cervical decompression should not exceed 15 to 16mm in diameter, because an excessive degree of spinal cord displacement may cause traction on a relatively fixed cervical nerve root. The natural history

of this complication is spontaneous resolution in most cases.[31]

Dural Tears

Dural tears, CSF fistulae, and pseudomeningoceles may occur, especially in cases of ossification of the posterior longitudinal ligament (OPLL) or severe trauma. Using good illumination, the operating microscope, and diamond-tip burrs in the vicinity of the dura mater may decrease the frequency of these complications. Remember that the posterior longitudinal ligament thins out laterally, and therefore the spinal cord is relatively less protected.

If a violation of the dura mater occurs, repair from a ventral approach is not always possible. A tear is best managed with a piece of fascia with Gelfoam and fibrin glue application, and with a lumbar drain placed postoperatively (for 48 to 72 hours). If the dura mater has been excised, a Gelfoam and fascia application under the bone graft, without suturing, together with lumbar drainage, may be used. Prophylactic insertion of a lumbar drain before surgery should be considered in high-risk patients.

Major Vessel Injury

Brachiocephalic Vein and Vertebral Artery Injuries. The brachiocephalic vein may bleed during dissection for low cervical and upper thoracic inlet exposures. Vertebral artery injury occurs in approximately 1% of cases and is usually caused by lateral use of the cutting burrs. The surgeon should respect the midline. Longus colli muscles and uncovertebral joints are the key structures for the identification of the midline. Because the uncinate processes are the lateral borders of the spinal canal, bony removal or dissection lateral to the uncinate processes may cause damage to the vertebral artery and nerve roots. Therefore the uncinate processes should be clearly defined, and careful high-speed drilling of the uncinate processes should be just medial to the vertebral artery.

Ventral cervical bone resection should not be carried out wider than 18 to 20mm. The medial border of the foramen transversarium from one side to the opposite side is 30mm. An anomalous position of the vertebral artery should be carefully sought on the preoperative CT and magnetic resonance imaging (MRI) scans. During the ventrolateral approach the vertebral artery may be displaced laterally with a narrow-tipped retractor, but not more than 1 to 2mm.[30]

Carotid Artery Injury. The risk of carotid artery injury is greater with a ventrolateral approach than with the more common ventromedial approach. To avoid an injury to the carotid artery and internal jugular vein, it is necessary to identify the artery before retraction, to retract the artery laterally without opening its sheath, and to place the blades of the self-retaining retractors under the longus colli muscles. Inspection of the carotid sheath and the jugular vein should be conducted before closure to detect inadvertent injury of these structures.

Esophagus and Trachea Injury

Injury to the esophagus is a rare, but devastating complication. Some suggest the use of finger dissection below the superficial cervical fascia, rather than a sharp dissection. The surgeon should be aware of any preoperative problems with esophageal dysmotility (observed in 10% of patients; mostly in the elderly), and avoid injury to the pharyngeal muscles during dissection in the upper cervical region. During lengthy operations the medial blades perhaps should be released regularly to avoid esophageal necrosis. Inspection of the esophagus and the trachea should be conducted before closure, to detect inadvertent injury to these structures.

Recurrent Laryngeal Nerve Injury

Hoarseness after surgery is usually related to traction of the recurrent laryngeal nerve. It occurs in 3% to 11% of patients. It is usually transient. The recurrent laryngeal nerve passes under the subclavian artery on the right side and under the aorta on the left side. Although the right recurrent laryngeal nerve was thought to be more susceptible to stretch as midline structures are retracted, a recent study comparing the incidences of recurrent laryngeal nerve injury in right- and left-sided surgeries showed that there is no difference in incidence of recurrent laryngeal nerve injury with the side of surgical approach.[6] The same study also showed that re-operative surgery causes significantly more injuries than primary surgery.

Although recurrent laryngeal nerve palsy after anterior cervical spine surgery was thought to be the result of direct injury to the nerve, there is no data to support this hypothesis. Apfelbaum *et al.*[2] have proven that the most common cause of vocal cord paralysis after anterior cervical spine surgery is compression of the recurrent laryngeal nerve within the endolarynx. We recommend monitoring the endotracheal cuff pressure and release after retractor placement. In the series of Apfelbaum *et al.*[2] on instituting this maneuver, the rate of temporary paralysis has decreased from 6.4% to 1.69%.[8]

Excessive retraction of the medial structures may result in postoperative stridor, hoarseness, and dysphagia. A rare complication is an esophageal fistula. To prevent excessive medial retraction, the following suggestions are made: (1) rostral and caudal dissection should be greater than is needed, (2) retraction should be relaxed on an hourly basis, and (3) the medial retractor should be inserted under the longus colli muscles, if possible.

Hypoglossal Nerve Injury

Twelfth cranial nerve injury is rare, but possible, during high cervical dissections. Knowledge of its anatomy and course should minimize its injury. The hypoglossal nerve runs downward, lateral to the internal and external carotid arteries. Lateral to the occipital artery, the nerve usually turns forward a little above the level of the hyoid bone to disappear deep to the suprahyoid muscles. As it turns around the occipital artery, it gives off the superior root of the ansa cervicalis.

Thoracic Duct Injury

The thoracic duct is on the left side. Because this structure is located laterally, it is uncommon to injure the thoracic duct, at least in exposures medial to the sternocleidomastoid muscle.

Sympathetic Chain Injury

Injury to the sympathetic chain is associated with an ipsilateral Horner's syndrome. It is usually attributed to dissection of the longus colli muscles too far from the midline. They are easily injured during the ventrolateral approach. The sympathetic chain is located between the carotid sheath and the longus colli muscles in the midcervical region. Lateral retraction of the longus colli muscle during transverse foramen, or uncovertebral joint exposition at the lower cervical levels, may injure the sympathetic chain.[15] Horner's syndrome, visual symptoms, and an odd sense over the face may result. To avoid this complication the sympathetic chain and longus colli muscle should be mobilized over the length of the exposure, and the medial retraction blade should be inserted after the lateral blades.

Other Potential Complications with Ventral Approaches
Bone, Epidural Space, and Posterior Longitudinal Ligament Bleeding

Because extensive bone waxing may prevent fusion, it is often better to use Gelfoam, even for bone bleeding. Bipolar coagulation and Gelfoam may be useful to control bothersome epidural bleeding. Venous bleeding from the plexus around the vertebral artery is a common nuisance. Care must be taken to avoid injury to the vertebral artery during control of venous bleeding.

Postoperative Hematoma

To prevent postoperative hematomas, suction drains may be kept in place for 24 hours postoperatively. The use of drains for this purpose, however, is controversial.

Graft Bed Preparation

If a fibular graft is to be used, the ventral width of the decompression should be no more than the greatest diameter of the graft to ensure a good lateral bony approximation.[30] This is not usually necessary for the iliac crest graft, which may be fashioned to fit the decompression site.

Graft Complication and Dislocation

Allografts have a higher incidence of pseudarthrosis and an associated small risk of transmitting viral infections. Although autografts may also be complicated by pseudarthrosis, they are preferred in most instances. The graft should not be placed deeper than 13mm. It should distract the intervertebral space approximately 2mm, and be recessed approximately 3mm.[30] Excessive end-plate removal may increase the incidence of graft subsidence.

Graft dislocation may occur ventrally or dorsally. Dorsal dislocation is rare but more serious, because it may cause significant compression of the spinal cord. Partial graft extrusion is of little consequence and usually does not require treatment. Three technical considerations may help prevent graft dislocation: (1) Contour the graft into a shape that fits snugly into the mortise of the graft bed. The graft should be recessed so that the ventral cortical bone is a few millimeters dorsal to the ventral vertebral body. This border, however, should not be confused with the ventral vertebral osteophytes. An obsessive tailoring of grafts is appropriate. (2) Placement of a ventral cervical plate may help avoid graft dislocation. (3) Postoperative bracing may decrease the risk of graft dislocation.

Graft Pseudarthrosis

The pseudarthrosis rate, using different graft techniques, varies between 0% to 26%.[3,10,29,34] The risk of pseudarthrosis increases, if more than one level is fused. If one long piece of cortical-cancellous graft or cortical bone is used, however, the risk is lowered.[10,40] It should be emphasized that the presence of pseudarthrosis does not necessarily compromise the clinical results of surgery.[9]

Vertebral Avascular Necrosis

Avascular necrosis of the vertebrae is encountered with the use of grafts at individual interspaces.[26] The Cloward technique for a ventral cervical fusion at two adjacent levels may cause avascular necrosis. If a multilevel fusion is needed, Cloward[9] suggests that a Smith-Robinson graft may be inserted at one disc level, and a bone dowel may be inserted at an adjacent level.[9]

Ventral Plating Complication

Screw breakage, plate breakage, esophageal erosion, pain, and difficulty swallowing may complicate the results of ventral plating. Many surgeons do not advocate placing a screw into a graft, for fear that such a screw may dislodge or weaken the graft.

Failure to Improve Postoperatively

Most patients should improve neurologically after surgery. If no improvement occurs, but is expected, the use of CT or MRI is prudent. The most likely reason for lack of improvement is an inadequate decompression. It is common for a right-handed surgeon operating from the right side to leave residual compression on the right side. Another cause of failure to achieve neurologic improvement may be OPLL, which may easily be overlooked on the preoperative MRI scan. Obtaining a preoperative CT scan is helpful in ruling out the possibility of OPLL.

Dorsal Approaches
Neurologic Deterioration

Patients with cervical kyphosis are poor candidates for cervical laminectomy. A lordotic or neutral position is preferred. Instrumentation under the lamina in the cervical region can cause neurologic damage. The predominant risk during the keyhole foraminotomy is direct nerve root trauma. To avoid this, dissection should only be performed from the axilla of the root.

Lateral mass plating may also cause nerve root injury, and occasionally, vertebral artery injury. With transarticular screw fixation, if a vertebral artery injury is detected after a screw is placed, a second one should be placed. The screw causing the vertebral artery injury may be left in place. It may effectively serve to tamponade vertebral artery bleeding. Residual bleeding may be effectively managed with oxidized cellulose (Surgicel).

Postoperative Instability and Kyphosis

Respect for the facet joints and joint capsules is necessary to prevent postlaminectomy instability.[41] Two additional precautions may be taken to prevent this complication: (1) the use of laminoplasty instead of laminectomy may decrease the risk of instability (although this is not proven); and (2) lateral mass plating and fusion may be carried out to prevent deformity, minimize instability, and decrease the movement associated with the degenerative process.

Complication Avoidance in the Cervicothoracic Junction (C7-T3)

Because degenerative diseases in this region are rare, and surgical indications most commonly comprise tumor, trauma, and infection, decision making is usually not difficult. Dorsal pathology located at the cervicothoracic junction is usually exposed with the standard dorsal midline approach.

Ventral approaches to the cervicothoracic junction are technically demanding. Because the kyphotic angle of the upper thoracic spine may compromise the surgical view, the need to access lesions at and below T1 and T2 necessitates a more caudal exposure than is afforded by the ventromedial cervical approach in most patients. Although surgery to the T3 vertebral body is feasible with the ventromedial approach, the surgical view is so limited that only a biopsy of a tumor or partial decompression may be possible. With adequate extension of the neck, it is possible to perform a T1-2 discectomy in nonobese patients with long necks.

If only a partial decompression or biopsy without instrumentation is anticipated in a nonobese patient, the standard ventromedial cervical approach with mild neck extension is appropriate for ventral pathologies in the cervicothoracic region.

If, however, extensive resection, with or without instrumentation is required, an upper sternal osteotomy, with or without a medial claviculotomy, may be performed. Another option is transpleural thoracotomy through the fourth rib. Because the latter approach is associated with high morbidity, sternotomy is a last-resort option.

Potential Injuries and Other Complications Associated with Ventral Surgery
Recurrent Laryngeal Nerve Injury

When using a right-sided approach, the surgeon can identify the recurrent laryngeal nerve between the trachea and the esophagus. The right recurrent laryngeal nerve exits the carotid sheath at a variable level, coursing medially and entering the tracheoesophageal groove behind the upper pole of the thyroid gland. Because its highly variable course on this side increases its risk of injury, a left-sided approach for cervicothoracic lesion is warranted.[35]

Thoracic Duct Injury

With left-sided incisions, the thoracic duct may be identified as it enters the dorsal aspect of the subclavian vein. Injury to thoracic duct results in chylothorax. If this occurs, the duct should be ligated.[35,39]

Major Vessel, Lung Apex, and Gland Injuries

Major vessel injury may occur via coarse-tissue manipulation or excessive traction.[13,36] Lung apex injury may be detected by filling the wound with saline solution and applying positive pressure ventilation.

If a ventromedial exposure is used, the esophagus, trachea, and thyroid gland are susceptible to injury and should be carefully inspected before wound closure.

Brachial Plexus Injury

The brachial plexus may be injured during the transaxillary and supraclavicular approaches. Stretch injuries of the plexus may be sustained by improper surgical positioning. Meticulous attention paid to surgical positioning helps prevent the occurrence of these injuries. Any change in patient positioning during the course of surgery, whether inadvertent or intentional, should prompt a re-evaluation of the patient's position.

Intercostal Neuralgia

Intercostal neuralgia may occur as a complication of the transaxillary injury. Incision of the nerve proximal to the dorsal root ganglion (disrupting the nerve by destroying the cell body) should eliminate this complication.

Chest Wall Deformity and Scar

Chest wall deformities and scars are particularly associated with trans-sternal and transmanubrial approaches. This must be considered during preoperative planning and when obtaining patient's consent.

Complication Avoidance in the Thoracic, Lumbar, and Sacral Spine

If thoracic, lumbar, and sacral lesions are completely dorsal, a dorsal approach with laminectomy is appropriate. A vertebral body lesion between L1 and L4 may be exposed via a retroperitoneal ventrolateral approach. If the lesion is located between the L5 and S1 levels, and a limited operation such as a biopsy or simple discectomy and interbody fusion is required, a pelvic brim extraperitoneal approach may be suitable. If the lesion is located between the L5 and S1 levels and requires extensive exposure (e.g., a high-grade spondylolisthesis or an L5 tumor), a direct ventral approach such as the transperitoneal approach may be suitable.

Potential Injuries Associated with Dorsal Surgery

Some of the complications frequently encountered during dorsal spine surgery were discussed previously in the section on posterior cervical spine surgery. Neurologic deterioration, incidental durotomy, and postoperative instability can also be seen during dorsal, thoracic, and lumbar spine surgery.

The lateral extracavitary approach has been reported to have a high incidence rate (55%) of complications, and pulmonary complications are predominant.[27]

Instability and Deformity

Instability and deformity after surgery depend on the level and amount of decompression and preoperative instability. Disruption of the dorsal ligaments and facet capsules and extensive laminectomy are the main reasons of instability. Avoiding excessive facetectomy and laminectomy in children, and using alternative methods such as microdiscectomy and costotransversectomy may prevent postoperative instability.

Potential Injuries Associated with Ventral Surgery

To avoid complications during the thoracotomy or retroperitoneal approach, one should have a firm grasp of the retroperitoneal anatomy. The incidence of intraoperative soft-tissue injuries is increased by the use of high-speed drills.

Pulmonary Injury

Atelectasis, pneumothorax, pneumonia, and pleural effusions may occur after thoracotomy. A tube thoracostomy may be necessary to treat these complications. It should be removed only after drainage diminishes significantly. A pneumothorax usually clears in 2 to 3 days.

Lumbar Sympathetic Plexus Injury

The lumbar sympathetic plexus, located on the lateral aspects of the lumbar vertebrae, are fine structures, and may be stretched and injured during ventral spine dissection. This will often cause a warm leg on the ipsilateral site. This is reported in 10% of ventral lumbar surgeries.[43] It usually resolves spontaneously.

Superior Hypogastric Plexus Injury

Superior hypogastric plexus injury may result in bladder dysfunction in females and either retrograde ejaculation or sterility, or both, in males. The superior hypogastric plexus is situated in the bifurcation of the aorta on the fifth lumbar vertebral body and the sacrum. This sympathetic plexus innervates the smooth muscles of the seminal vesicle, which contracts as the bladder neck closes during ejaculation. It also activates the transport of spermatozoa from the testes to the seminal vesicles. Thus injury can cause a retrograde ejaculation and sterility. Although it is rare (0.42%),[16,17] careful dissection of the fascia ventral to the promontory, and avoidance of electrocautery in this region, may help prevent this complication.

Great Vessel Injury

Iliac vessel mobilization is usually difficult with retroperitoneal dissections at lower lumbar levels. Care should be taken to protect the iliolumbar veins that emerge from the iliac veins laterally. An experienced surgeon with a good knowledge of vascular anatomy is a prerequisite for ventral lumbar surgery. At the L5-S1 level, working between two iliac arteries and veins may be easier for disc surgery and cage insertion. However, L4-5 and upper levels sometimes need excessive retraction of great vessels. Fine retractors and meticulous use of high-speed drills are necessary for protection of the vessels.

Major vascular injury may also occur during a dorsal approach (lumbar disc surgery). The mortality of such complications may be as high as 50%.[13] Most frequently, vascular injury is caused by pituitary forceps during over-aggressive disc resection. Up-angled pituitary forceps and marked instruments may help avoid penetration beyond the anterior longitudinal ligament. Decompression of the abdomen by proper positioning facilitates displacement of the great vessels away from the spine.[36]

Visceral Injury

Injury to the liver, spleen, or kidney is a severe complication. This occurs most commonly with transdiaphragmatic approaches to the thoracolumbar spine. Because handheld retractors are responsible for some of these injuries, meticulous care must be taken during their use.

Ureteral Injury

The ureter may be difficult to identify, particularly in obese patients. The anatomy may also be obscured in patients with metastatic cancer. In these circumstances the preoperative placement of a ureteral catheter or stent may help the surgeon identify the ureter intraoperatively.

Artery of Adamkiewicz

The artery of Adamkiewicz plays an important role in the vascular supply of the thoracic spinal cord. It is usually found on the left side at the level of T9. Some surgeons routinely obtain a preoperative angiogram to identify its anatomy and location. Based on this information, the surgeon may prefer to approach the spine from the side opposite the artery.[4]

Other Potential Complications with Ventral Surgery
Deep Vein Thrombosis

Deep vein thrombosis is a common problem related to retraction of the venous structures. Careful vessel retraction, avoidance of vessel injury, and use of a compressive

stocking intraoperatively may prevent this complication. Perioperative prophylactic anticoagulants or intermittent compression boots may help avoid this complication, if used routinely.

Abdominal Incisional Hernia, Prolonged Ileus, and Hemorrhage

Abdominal wall hernias can be avoided by meticulous reapproximation of the muscle layers at closing. After the retroperitoneal approach, a postoperative ileus may last 24 to 48 hours. After the transperitoneal approach, an ileus may last even longer.

Blood loss may be reduced during dorsal exposures by anticipating the presence of the dorsal branch of the interarticular artery, which emerges just lateral to the facet joints in the thoracic and lumbar regions.

Shoulder-Girdle Dysfunction

Dorsal surgery in the cervicothoracic region involves the division of strong scapular and latissimus dorsi muscles. They should be closed in a thorough manner to prevent postoperative shoulder-girdle dysfunction.

REFERENCES

1. Albin MS, Carroll RG, Maroon JC: Clinical considerations concerning detection of venous air embolism. *Neurosurgery* 3:380-384, 1978.
2. Apfelbaum RI, Kriskovich MD, Haller JR: On the incidence, cause, and prevention of recurrent laryngeal nerve palsies during anterior cervical spine surgery. *Spine* 25:2906-2912, 2000.
3. Aronson N, Filtzer DL, Bagan M: Anterior cervical fusion by the Smith-Robinson approach. *J Neurosurg* 29:397-404, 1973.
4. Batzdorf U, Batzdorff A: Analysis of cervical spine curvature in patients with cervical spondylosis. *Neurosurgery* 22:827-836, 1988.
5. Benzel EC: *Surgical Exposure of the Spine: An Extensile Approach.* Park Ridge, IL, AANS Publishing, 1995.
6. Beutler WJ, Sweeney CA, Connolly PJ: Recurrent laryngeal nerve injury with anterior cervical spine surgery risk with laterality of surgical approach. *Spine* 26:1337-1342, 2001.
7. Braughler JM, Hall ED: Current application of "high dose" steroid therapy for CNS injury. *J Neurosurg* 62:806-810, 1985.
8. Cammisa FP, Girardi FP, Sangani PK, *et al*: Incidental durotomy in spine surgery. *Spine* 25:2663-2667, 2000.
9. Cloward RB: The anterior surgical approach to the cervical spine: the Cloward approach: past, present and future. *Spine* 13:823-827, 1988.
10. Connolly ES, Seymore RJ, Adams JE: Clinical evaluation of anterior cervical fusion for degenerative cervical disc. *J Neurosurg* 23:431-437,1965.
11. Dempsey R, Rapp RP, Young B, *et al.* Prophylactic parenteral antibiotics in clean neurosurgical procedures. *J Neurosurg* 69:52-57, 1988.

12. DePalma AF, Rothman RH, Lewinneck RE, Canale S: Anterior interbody fusion for severe cervical disc degeneration. *Surg Gynecol Obstet* 134:755-758, 1972.

13. DeSaussure RL: Vascular injury coincident to disc surgery. *J Neurosurg* 16:222-229, 1959.

14. Ducker TB: Cervical radiculopathies and myelopathies— posterior approaches. In Frymoyer JW (ed): *The Adult Spine: Principles and Practice.* New York, Raven Press, 1991, pp 1187-1205.

15. Ebraheim NA, Lu J, Yang H, *et al*: Vulnerability of the sympathetic trunk during the anterior approach to the lower cervical spine. *Spine* 25:1603-1606, 2000.

16. Esses SI, Botsford DJ: Surgical anatomy and operative approaches to the sacrum. In Frymoer (ed): *The Adult Spine: Principles and Practice.* New York, Raven Press, 1991, pp 2095-2106.

17. Flynn JC, Price CT: Sexual complications of anterior fusion of the lumbar spine. *Spine* 9:489-492, 1984.

18. Haines SF: Systemic antibiotic prophylaxis in neurological surgery. *Neurosurgery* 6:355-361, 1980.

19. Hall ED, Wolf MS, Braughler MJ: Effects of a single large dose of methylprednisolone sodium succinate on experimental post-traumatic spinal cord ischemia. *J Neurosurg* 61:124-130, 1984.

20. Jampol LM, Goldbaum M, Rosenberg M, *et al*: Ischemia of ciliary arterial circulation from ocular compression. *Arch Ophthalmol* 93:1311-1317, 1975.

21. Jones AAM, Stambough JL, Balderston RA, *et al*: Long-term results of lumbar spine surgery complicated by unintended incidental durotomy. *Spine* 14:443-446, 1989.

22. Lynch JJ, Scuchard GH, Gross CM, *et al*: Prevalence of right-to-left atrial shunting in a healthy population: detection by Valsalva maneuver contrast echocardiography. *Am J Cardiol* 53:1478-1480, 1984.

23. Manabe S, Tateishi A, Ohno T: Anterolateral uncoforaminotomy for cervical spondylotic myeloradiculopathy. *Acta Orthop Scand* 59:669-674, 1988.

24. Menezes AH: Surgical approaches to the craniocervical junction. In Frymoyer JW (ed): *The Adult Spine: Principles and Practice.* New York, Raven Press, 1991, pp 967-985.

25. Mirovsky Y, Neuwirth M: Injuries to the lateral femoral cutaneous nerve during spine surgery. *Spine* 25:1266-1269, 2000.

26. Mosdal C: Cervical osteochondrosis and disc herniation. eighteen years' use of interbody fusion by Cloward's technique in 755 cases. *Acta Neurochir* (Wien) 70: 207-255,1 984.

27. Resnick DK, Benzel EC: Lateral extracavitary approach for thoracic and thoracolumbar spine trauma: operative complications. *Neurosurgery* 43:796-803, 1998.

28. Roberts MP: Complications of positioning for neurosurgical operations on the spine. In Tarlov EC (ed): *Complications of Spinal Surgery.* Park Ridge, IL, AANS Publishing, 1991, pp 1-13.

29. Robinson RA, Walker AE, Ferlic DC, *et al*: The results of an anterior interbody fusion of the cervical spine. *J Bone Joint Surg* (Am) 44:1579-1586, 1962.

30. Saunders RL: Anterior reconstructive procedures in cervical spondylotic myelopathy. *Clin Neurosurg* 37: 682-721, 1991.

31. Saunders RL: On the pathogenesis of the radiculopathy complicating multilevel corpectomy. *Neurosurgery* 37: 408-413, 1995.

32. Savitz MH, Katz SS: Rationale for prophylactic antibiotics and neurosurgery. *Neurosurgery* 9:142-144, 1981.

33. Shapiro M, Wald U, Simchen E, *et al*: Randomized clinical trial of intra-operative antimicrobial prophylaxis of infection after neurosurgical procedures. *J Hosp Infect* 8:283-295, 1986.

34. Simmons EH, Bhalla SK: Anterior cervical discectomy and fusion: a clinical and biomechanical study with eight-year follow-up. *J Bone Joint Surg* (Br) 51:225-237, 1969.

35. Sundaresan N, DiGiancinto GV: Surgical considerations and approaches. In Sundaresan N, Schmidek HH, Schiller AL, *et al* (eds): *Tumors of the Spine: Diagnosis and Clinical Management.* Philadelphia, WB Saunders, 1990, pp 358-379.

36. Tarlov EC: Major vascular injury secondary to spine surgery. In Tarlov EC (ed): *Complications of Spinal Surgery.* Park Ridge, IL, AANS Publishing, 1991, pp 23-27.

37. Verbiest H: Anterolateral operations for fractures and dislocations in the middle and lower parts of the cervical spine. Report of a series of forty-seven cases. *J Bone Joint Surg* (Am) 51:1489-1530, 1969.

38. Wang JC, Bohlman HH, Riew DK: Dural tears secondary to operations on the lumbar spine: Management and results after a two-year-minimum follow-up of eighty-eight patients. *J Bone Joint Surg* (Am) 80:1728-1732, 1998.

39. Watkins RG: Cervical, thoracic and lumbar complications -anterior approach. In Garfin SR (ed): *Complications of Spine Surgery.* Baltimore, Williams & Wilkins, 1989, pp 29-52.

40. White AA III, Hirsch C: An experimental study of the immediate load bearing capacity of some commonly used iliac grafts. *Acta Orthop Scand* 42:482-490, 1971.

41. Whitecloud TS, Kelley LA: Anterior and posterior surgical approaches to the cervical spine. In Frymoyer JW (ed): *The Adult Spine: Principles and Practice.* New York, Raven Press, 1991, pp 987-1013.

42. Wilder BL: Hypothesis: the etiology of midcervical quadriplegia after operation with the patient in the sitting position. *Neurosurgery* 11:530-351, 1977.

43. Zdeblick TA: The treatment of degenerative lumbar disorders. A critical review of the literature. *Spine* 20: 1265-1269, 1995.

44. Zileli M, Coskun E, Özdamar N, *et al*: Surgery of intramedullary spinal cord tumors. *Eur Spin J* 5:243-250, 1996.

CHAPTER 19

Data Management

Michael J. Speck, Mary B. Bondy, and Robert J. Morlock

The development of a systematic approach to the capture and analysis of key spine patient outcomes data has become critical as the treatment of spinal disorders, especially surgical treatment, has grown increasingly complex and expensive. Coupling the complexity and expense of treatments with the fact that very little (if any) objective information exists regarding the appropriateness of various treatment modalities for various spine conditions, leads to the obvious conclusion that well-documented, observable evidence is needed (for purposes of this discussion, patient outcome is defined as patient-reported levels of pain, disability, and occupational/functional status). Data must be collected that provide clinicians, as well as other major stakeholders in the healthcare system, with needed information to make better clinical and business decisions. This imperative has led to the initial development of many outcomes assessment information systems in the last 10 years. The ultimate goal of these efforts, through their assistance to clinicians, is to improve the health status of the population with respect to spinal conditions.

Hence those in the spinal disorders field have become increasingly aggressive regarding the pursuit of an objective assessment of outcomes in recent years. Such an endeavor hinges on the effective capture, storage, retrieval, and analysis of data as it relates to spine patients and their treatment. The relational database has been established as a reliable mechanism for achieving these goals. The nature and characteristics of the data storage paradigm (i.e., a relational database versus a set of text files) will have an enormous impact on the credibility and quality of the research. Therefore a keen understanding of this component of the outcomes assessment system development effort is paramount.

Background

Insurance companies, employers, state and federal governments, healthcare providers, and consumers are all looking to outcomes research efforts to provide information that will assist them in making better decisions, particularly regarding the appropriateness of medical surgical care and patient selection.[1] The economic and psychosocial costs of spine procedures are substantial. The medical cost alone of treating low-back problems is increasing at an accelerated rate. Estimates of the total societal cost of back pain in the United States have exceeded $50 billion annually.[7] Although medical costs are high, loss of time from work, as well as workers' compensation payments for work-related low-back problems, can cost up to three times as much as medical treatment.[3] This places the employers' focus on the ability

of a patient to return to work, regardless of the type of injury and the type of treatment received. A worker's level of pain and disability post-treatment has often been seemingly independent of the type of treatment (including surgery) received. Additionally, outcomes data are critical in assessing the costs and benefits of new technologies. Finally, and perhaps most importantly, nonmonetary costs to the patient and society can be substantial. The inability to function normally at work and in other daily activities has an impact on the quality of life of both patients and their families. This is a major focus of patient outcomes assessment.

Marked regional variations occur in the rates of hospitalization, surgery, and the use of diagnostic tests for low-back problems.[8] Some patients appear to be more disabled after treatment than at presentation, which is another potential indicator of ineffective care.[2] Despite evidence that demonstrates the risk associated with repeat surgical procedures for low-back problems, there are patients who have had as many as 20 spine operations.[6] Other treatment methods such as extended bed rest or long-term use of high-dose opiates can prolong symptoms and further debilitate patients.

To provide truly meaningful outcomes information, data must be gathered from many sources, including the patient (demographic information, pain and disability indicators, work limitations, indirect costs, quality of life, and general health status), the physician (signs and symptoms, diagnosis, treatment(s) provided, physician referrals, tests ordered), and internal information (from information systems within the provider organization [e.g., procedures provided, direct costs for outpatient and inpatient care]).

Introduction to Information Systems: Human Resources, Technology and Processes

Information systems consist of three major interrelated and interdependent components: technology, people, and processes. Although the technology component is by far the most obvious, visible, and recognized aspect of an information system, it is a mistake to view technology as having greater importance than either of the other two.

Cleveland Clinic Experience

At the Cleveland Clinic a team of clinical, technical, and administrative staff has embraced the challenge of creating a spine patient outcomes information system, and has been actively developing such a system since early 2000. The patient population treated by the Cleveland Clinic Back and Neck Center, the patient care arm of the Cleveland Clinic Spine Institute, is extremely complex from a clinical analysis perspective because of the diverse nature of the spinal disorders encountered. The analysis of patient data is further complicated by the numerous treatment options, both surgical and nonoperative, considered by the multidisciplinary team of clinicians during each episode of care. A structured approach to this dilemma requires a refined and sophisticated patient classification scheme. The Spine Clinical Outcomes Information System (SCOIS) at the Cleveland Clinic is designed to create patient profiles that are to be used in building a classification scheme that clearly stratifies and categorizes patients; in other words, a "diagnostic fingerprint" or patient profile is created for each patient.

The patient profile is built from data that are collected from both clinicians and patients, combined with details of any medical or surgical intervention from other hospital or clinic information systems. Data collection forms are to be completed by the physician at the time of each clinical encounter. Data collected includes each patient's diagnoses, symptoms, physical and neurologic findings, diagnostic tests, referrals, and treatment plan. At the initial encounter patients are asked to complete a questionnaire detailing some of their personal characteristics and demographic information. They are asked to complete standardized questionnaires that address their general health and spine care history.

By studying aggregates of these profiles the efficacy of various treatment strategies can be analyzed from both clinical and research perspectives. Objective contrasts and comparisons between and among the medical and surgical treatment strategies proposed for a multitude of spinal disorders will become possible; thus leading to the ultimate goal of clinical behavior modification based on concrete, objective intelligent outcomes information. Ultimately, SCOIS will provide a generalized research platform that can be used for more specialized or specific research projects.

Building a Successful Outcomes Information System

The database itself is but one component of an efficient scheme for data collection, storage, and retrieval. At this point it is necessary to highlight a crucial aspect of understanding outcomes information systems (outcomes systems). The word "system" is used herein to accent the simple distinction between the data "store," or database (i.e., the electronic data storage *mechanism*), and its functional environment. Although each system typically has a database at its core that is responsible for data storage, the overall system is much broader, including database management software, data processing software, presentation applications (i.e., browsers), user interfaces (i.e., input and output screens), and the hardware on which it operates (Figure 19.1). The term "database" simply refers to the data storage mechanism. Within the context of an overall information system the database can perform properly, but the database is entirely useless outside of the system. Ideally a well-designed database will drive the development of its interrelated technical components (i.e., hardware and software), resulting in an efficient and elegant solution for outcomes research.

Too often the term "database" is used to describe not only the database, but also the database management software used to create and administer it. Although the difference is subtle, it is an important one. Database management software has drastically simplified the database administration process (maintenance and data management) in recent years, and this has fostered the idea that the underlying databases are simple as well. This is a common and costly misconception. A poorly designed database that is at the heart of an outcomes system will invariably lead to faulty data processing and an unsuccess-

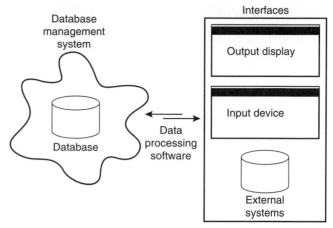

Figure 19.1 Schematic of database management.

ful project. Unfortunately, poor database design is not always immediately evident, and a substantial amount of time, effort, and resources can be wasted before the inherent problems manifest themselves.

This discussion is intended to help bridge the divide between those who desire a medical outcomes information system and those who possess the knowledge and skills to build and maintain it. There is often a significant gap between the perceived resource requirements, in terms of time, technology, and human resources, to create such a system, and what is actually required. This is especially true with respect to the time necessary for design and development. However, effective communication between the users and the technical staff (i.e., those commissioned to build and maintain a system) can drastically shorten the development cycle. Therefore this relationship is herein analyzed throughout all of the system development stages, beginning with the initial conceptual development and finishing with implementation. The system development process is deconstructed into three key stages: definition, design, and deployment.

System (Project) Definition

Defining the Research Focus

Defining the research focus of the outcomes information system must be a thoughtful, deliberate exercise by the principal investigator, co-investigators, and clinical project leadership. Concentration, thorough investigation, and consensus building, with respect to defining the research question(s) that is to be answered by the data collected, stored, and ultimately retrieved from the outcomes system, is both necessary and critical. A clear vision of the research questions at hand, the statistical analysis, and hence the system purpose will establish a solid platform on which the entire system can be built. The result of the definitional phase is the determination of the system/project size and scope from a clinical, technologic, and operational standpoint. Once defined, the research purpose serves as the benchmark against which the final system will be evaluated.

A common approach to system development that yields little success is to, consciously or unconsciously, postpone the process of defining the research goals. Those electing this approach treat the definitional phase for the outcomes research information system as an evolutionary process in which the defining elements will theoretically become evident as the project takes shape, rather than taking specific steps to determine them explicitly. This consistently and inevitably leads to a poorly designed database at the heart of the outcomes system, which functions neither efficiently nor appropriately. Conversely, thorough investigation and due diligence during the definitional phase of the outcomes research project fosters the establishment of a blueprint from which the entire system can be built, thus maximizing the systems efficiency and its ability to achieve the stated objectives.

Understanding the Clinical and Operational Environment

It is impossible to design an appropriate model for data management without a clear understanding of the physician's working environment. This includes cataloging the types of disorders that are treated, the available treatment options, the factors that influence treatment decisions (i.e., patient age, comorbidities, medical history), the myriad of possible outcome patterns, the nature and impetus of patient/physician interactions, and measures by which treatments are validated. Clearly it is the clinician who can best describe this environment, and the transfer of this information to the information technology personnel on the project team is critical. Any disconnect between the clinician and the analyst is most damaging during this phase. However, if this divide can be overcome in the early stages of the process, subsequent tasks become increasingly more manageable.

The establishment of clear project objectives primarily provides a blueprint for the information system, and also delivers a number of secondary benefits. It is during this phase that the original concept is validated; participants (e.g., clinicians, nurses, administrators, analysts) have the opportunity to consider every aspect of the project; and most importantly, the outcomes information system will have a distinct model for comparison. Without this objective model there is no clear way to determine whether the overall project goals have been satisfied.

Patient Population

The first definitional requirement relates to the description of the patient population. A method by which the individual patients and their associated treatments can be compared as a subset of a heterogeneous patient population needs to be established. Some of the critical metrics such as age and gender are universal and relatively straightforward, whereas others such as education level and workers compensation status are more directed and often relate to specific research questions. Core elements that indicate the patient's pathologic profile include diagnoses, symptoms, and physical signs.

Data Elements

Pursuant to the definition of the outcomes model, difficult decisions surrounding the inclusion of data elements need to be made. The natural tendency is to attempt to collect enough data to potentially answer any research question that may surface. This, however, becomes very onerous for both clinician and patient. In this arena, considering patient and clinic burden, brevity is preferred. Therefore careful consideration must be given to each item that is presented for inclusion.

Input from multiple participants is important during this phase of the process so that critical data elements are not overlooked. However, the exclusion of data elements that will not contribute significantly to the overall goals of the project is equally important. Great attention to detail is a requirement in the definitional phase to achieve a proper balance in the data model. The inclusion of too many data elements will add unnecessary strain on the system's resources (both human and technologic), and the exclusion of critical data elements will render the system ineffective.

Beyond the selection process all of the data elements must be presented in a standardized, concise manner that can be readily adopted by all of the system participants (health care providers). Standardizing the terms used to describe spinal disorders and their manifestations makes the categorization of patients according to each specific disorder a possibility. Standardization also allows patients and the available treatment options to be matched in a consistent and reliable manner. This standardization process is essentially the process of establishing the common language that will subsequently be used by all participants to describe their patients, treatment options, pathologies, and patient symptoms throughout the course of treatment.

System Design

Once the nature of the data to be gathered has been defined, the source of the data must be determined. Direct data collection (i.e., patients and clinicians) and electronic sources (i.e., cost and procedure-related data from the operating room and financial systems) must be considered. The availability and accessibility of these resources varies among institutions. Hence data acquisition must be tailored to fit. Efficient data acquisitions can be realized through the automation of the data collection process. Such automated processes should be introduced to the model wherever and whenever possible. This, of course, is dependent on the availability of data "feeds" from alternate information systems (i.e., patient demographic data can be retrieved from a patient scheduling system). However, not all of the data requirements can be satisfied from outside the system. Some information will need to be collected directly from clinicians, patients, or both. Outcomes systems must merge all of the data sources gracefully to succeed.

Data sources are not nearly as important, however, as the data destinations. The most critical aspect of system design is found in the modeling of data. Because the components of the clinician's environment have been clearly outlined during the initial (definitional) phase of the project, their definitions are now readily available for use while designing the outcomes information system. Most effective information systems are merely reflections of real-world models. The outcomes information system is no exception. The entire process shifts from a definitional into a translational role, as the description of real-world entities become definitions used in the construction of a virtual model. This process is not academic, but accurate descriptions of the data, the environment, and the relationships among them, can markedly simplify the process.

In the initial phase, definitions of the patients and of their diagnoses, symptoms, and treatments, deal directly with the observable aspects of the clinician's environment. In the design phase these definitions are abstracted, assuming a role of data description within the database. Hence the definitional phase deals with *what* data should be stored, and the design phase determines *how* it should be stored. The design phase is also the point at which the primary responsibility shifts from the clinician to the system analyst. The system analyst, working from the model constructed by the medical and administrative staff, must develop a data model suitable for accurate, meaningful data processing. The data elements selected and defined earlier must now be organized logically into an overall data design that facilitates consistent data storage and retrieval. New questions will be considered for the same data elements determined in the definitional phase. These are directed at defining the *nature* of the data.

For instance, if a patient's medical record number is to be used as the main form of identification, a series of questions about the data element itself need to be addressed. First and foremost, is the medical record number an appropriate identifier? Is it truly unique, or are there circumstances in which multiple patients can share a medical record number? Will the medical record number be readily available at the time the information is collected? Are there any legal or business constraints on the use of a medical record number as a tracking measure within the information system? In this example, although medical record numbers are suitable for identifying specific patients, there are a number of privacy issues surrounding their use. Current law requires the use of a separate, unique identifier for each patient that is independent of the medical record number. As a result, sensitive information cannot be directly linked back to a given patient outside of the outcomes system itself. Consequently, even though the medical record number is an *effective* identification technique for patients (and patient records), it is not an *appropriate* identifier in the overall data model.

Additional questions regarding the information pertain to the *type* of the data to be acquired. Drawing from the previous example, is the medical record number numeric, or can alphabetic characters be included? If character data can be used, the medical record number must be stored in a character format; otherwise, it could make sense to store the data numerically (character formats can include numeric data, but numeric formats cannot accommodate alphabetic characters; for example, 123456 can be stored numerically, whereas 4B3R589 cannot). Once this distinction has been made it is still necessary to decide *which* character or numeric format should be implemented. For instance, if a data element will be used in any mathematical calculations, a numeric data type is necessary. However, numeric data types can be further subdivided into integer, long, float, and double, each with its own range of values, storage space requirements, and functionality (i.e., the float data type typically requires more storage space than an integer

data type, but it permits the use of decimal places, whereas integers will not).

Columns are assigned specific data types during the database design process. Data type assignment is based on the data storage requirements of each column, and valid data entries must conform to their data type designations. The data type selection effectively restricts the allowable values in a given column (i.e., a column storing "date of service" will only allow date values). In relational databases (defined later in this chapter), data types provide an excellent example of how the data is controlled implicitly through the actual structure of the data. As a result, it is important to consider current and future data needs while selecting the data type for any column. If used effectively, data typing protects the quality of the data and reduces data entry vulnerabilities.

On a grander scale, the system analyst must also consider established protocols for patient care to design a system that can be incorporated into the treatment course with the least amount of resistance. This includes assessing the physical layout of clinical areas, clinical and support staff availability for outcomes system functions, patient flow throughout the clinical areas, etc. If workstations are available in a waiting area, perhaps the patient can complete an electronic survey while he or she is waiting to see the physician. Otherwise, paper surveys can be used, but it must be determined whether the surveys will then be scanned into the data store or if a staff person is to be responsible for data entry once collected.

The most fundamental questions in the design phase address the type of database appropriate for the outcomes research project. If the study includes one clinician and a small patient population, a simple desktop database will be more than adequate. In this case the data store might even take the form of a series of files saved on the investigator's computer in lieu of a traditional database. However, if the data store must be accessed from numerous physical locations, or if there are many users sending and consuming data, the desktop approach quickly becomes unmanageable. Clearly, quantitative information, including the number of unique patients and patient visits anticipated in a given time will have significant implications concerning the type of database that is to be used. As the demands (i.e., number of data elements, number of users, number of simultaneous research queries) on the data collection and storage system increase, the viable options are narrowed to the realm of database servers, in which the data are centrally stored and managed, and access can be offered over a network (whether it be local or global). Regardless of the type of database implemented in the outcomes information system, the core principles of database design are applicable. Because the relational database model is the *de facto* standard in this arena, it is the focus of this discussion.

Relational Database

The relational model takes its name from the mathematical term "relation," which can roughly be translated to mean *table*, the building block for relational databases. Regardless of the method by which the relational system stores the data, presentation to the user for viewing and modification takes a tabular form, constructed of tuples (pronounced like *couples*) and attributes, commonly referred to as rows and columns, respectively. Although the mathematical terms (i.e., relation, tuple, and attribute) provide the greatest precision in database description, this discussion uses the more familiar terms (i.e., table, row, and column) for greater clarity and comprehension. The relational model presents information stored in each table in such a way that every column contains "like data." More formally, the data contained in each column are of the same *domain*, or data type. The data type selection actually restricts the possible values of a column. For instance, the selection of an integer data type prohibits the entry of alphabetic characters in that column. The use of a character format permits both numeric and alphabetic values to be entered, but the values are stored in such a manner that calculations are not possible without first converting them to a numeric data type. For this reason, character formats should not be selected for any columns that store data that may be used in any type of calculations (i.e., scores, ages). However, they are appropriate for identification numbers or text fields.

Each row groups attributes of a specific *entity*. In a table that stores patient information, every row stores attributes of a specific patient. This contrasts the columnar view, which provides a longitudinal perspective of one specific attribute across the entire population (i.e., all of the ages of patients are stored in the same column). Consequently, the intersection of a row and column is a special occurrence within each table. The intersection represents a specific characteristic of the entity being defined by the row. For example, the patient table in Figure 19.2 contains the columns "LastName," "FirstName," "Birthdate," "Physician," "AppointmentDate," and "Diagnosis." The intersection of the first row and the column called "FirstName" indicates that the entity being described (in this case, a patient) has the first name "Jane."

The reliability of these intersections is inextricably bound to the ability to distinguish each row from every other row. This requires the assignment of a unique identifier, or *primary key*, to every row within the table. A common instinct for the row identification in a table that houses patient information is to use the patient's name as the primary key. This solution, however, breaks down as soon as two different patients with the same name are entered. The medical record number is usually a better alternative, providing a completely unique value for identifying each patient. However, for reasons discussed previously (patient privacy law), the medical record number is not a viable option. A more appropriate method is to assign an independent, arbitrary value as a primary key for the row. One column within the table is dedicated to the primary keys, and will be structured to require that each value is unique. The resulting table will look like Figure 19-2, with a column called "PatientKey" used to store the primary keys.

By assigning a distinct value as primary key for each row, two different patients with the same name can now be identified unambiguously. The uniqueness of the primary key is important because it serves as a device to connect different tables within the database. Establishment of these connections, or *relationships*, across tables becomes essential as the database is normalized (a process of "tuning" the data storage system, discussed later in this chapter). If each row cannot be identified and referenced individually, relationships between separate tables become confused and unreliable. In the relational model a table's primary key provides a means for other tables to reference its information. When the primary key of one table is stored in another as a link between them, it is called a *foreign key*, and it establishes the relationship between the two tables. As a result, data elements that are stored in separate tables in a database can be combined to form new tables (called *derived tables*), as Figure 19.3 demonstrates. By linking records from the patient and physician tables through the "PhysicianForeignKey" column, a derived table is created that contains the relevant data from both tables.

Although this example is somewhat trivial, the ability of the primary/foreign key model to connect otherwise disjointed tables is clear. As the discussion develops, the importance of this concept will become more evident. The application of the primary/foreign key model is one of the building blocks for normalizing the relational system.

Normalization

The rules of normalization, originally defined by Dr. E.F. Codd, deal primarily with the elimination of data redundancies that lead directly to flawed data and impractical, inefficient data management in relational systems.[4] The rules of normalization provide solid guidelines for building effective relational database systems. Normalization leverages the actual structure of the database to improve the integrity of the data. In practice, normalization is manifested as a "spreading" of the data, as information is stored throughout the database in many separate tables that are interrelated. Entities should be grouped and related in the

Patient Table

PatientKey	LastName	FirstName	Birthdate	Physician	AppointmentDate	Diagnosis
1	Smith	Jane	01/01/1950	Jones	02/01/2003	Spondylolisthesis
2	Smith	Jane	02/01/1960	White	03/01/2003	Scoliosis
3	West	Robert	03/01/1970	Jones	04/01/2003	Rheumatoid Arthritis
4	Smith	Jane	02/01/1960	White	03/01/2003	Kyphosis

Two different patients with the same name can be distinguished by using a unique key value.

Figure 19.2 The relational model—patient table.

same manner that they would be observed in their real-world roles. In the same way, the differences should be maintained by using separate tables (i.e., a patient table should not contain information concerning the physician). Although this idea is fairly simple, it is the foundation of normalizing the database.

The rules of normalization are ordered by their degree of specificity, and each higher-order rule is contingent on compliance with each of the previous rules. A database that is in second normal form (term used to describe a database that complies with the second rule of normalization) must also be in first normal form. There were originally only three rules of normalization, but subsequent rules have been added. Each rule is more rigid than its predecessor and more difficult to employ. The highest-order rules, in fact, are so strict that they can actually cause a decline in the performance of a relational system. It is uncommon for a production database to achieve anything higher than third normal form.

First Rule of Normalization

The first rule of normalization is somewhat academic: each column in a given row will contain one—and only one—value. Violation of this principle is relatively easy to recognize and correct. It would seem unnatural, for instance, to include a column called "Physician/Diagnosis" that contains both the name of the patient's physician and the patient's diagnosis. This problem is easily resolved by separating the two independent values into two distinct columns, "Physician" and "Diagnosis." A subtler example is demonstrated in the storage of a patient's name in a single column, rather than creating one column for the first name and another for the last name. Arguments can be made that this is not truly a violation of first normal form, but the two-attribute approach is more suitable because of the common use of last name as an identifier and sort item for groups of patients.

The higher-order rules of normalization deal more specifically with the reduction of data in the relational system. The storage of duplicate information in multiple locations causes the process of modification to become unruly. For example, in the database depicted in Figure 19.2, if Dr. Jones gets married, triggering a name change, two rows are affected (those with values of 1 and 3 in the "PatientKey" column). As a result, the physician value stored in the "Physician" column of each record must be updated, signaling a data storage redundancy. In Figure 19.3 this redundancy is corrected by isolating the physician information into its own table ("Physician"). The data have been effectively *reduced*, so that the same change requires the update of only one row. This type of data reduction demonstrates the importance of the primary key in the relational model. Separate, related tables are "bridged" by storing the primary key from one table (i.e., "PatientKey") as a foreign key in another (i.e., "PatientForeignKey").

Second Rule of Normalization

Although this design strengthens the overall structure of the database, Figure 19.3 has yet to satisfy the standard set by the second rule of normalization: every non-key attribute must be irreducibly dependent on the primary key.[5] The second rule deals with the logical grouping of data elements. Tables should be designed to mirror their real-world counterparts. A table commissioned to store patient data

Patient Table

PatientKey	LastName	FirstName	Birthdate	PhysicianForeignKey	AppointmentDate	Diagnosis
1	Smith	Jane	01/01/1950	1	02/01/2003	Spondylolisthesis
2	Smith	Jane	02/01/1960	2	03/01/2003	Scoliosis
3	West	Robert	03/01/1970	1	04/01/2003	Rheumatoid Arthritis
4	Smith	Jane	02/01/1960	2	03/01/2003	Kyphosis

The Key/Foreign Key relationship allows data from separate tables to be "joined" in the creation of derived tables.

Physician Table

PhysicianKey	Physician
1	Jones
2	White

Derived Table (Join of Patient and Physician Tables)

LastName	FirstName	Birthdate	AppointmentDate	Diagnosis	Physician
Smith	Jane	01/01/1950	02/01/2003	Spondylolisthesis	Jones
Smith	Jane	02/01/1960	03/01/2003	Scoliosis	White
West	Robert	03/01/1970	04/01/2003	Rheumatoid Arthritis	Jones
Smith	Jane	02/01/1960	03/01/2003	Kyphosis	White

Data from patient table   Data from physician table

Figure 19.3 Derived tables.

should contain attributes of the patient only, completely separate from other entities, such as diagnosis or physician.

To achieve second normal form the tables must be restructured. Duplication can be easily identified while reviewing the content of the database shown in Figure 19.3. The patient named Jane Smith, who was born Feb. 20, 1960, has two rows in the "Patient" table. As a result, her name and date of birth are repeated unnecessarily. This repetition is caused by the inclusion of the attribute "Diagnosis" as part of the "Patient" table, even though it is functionally independent. To rectify this situation the "Patient" table must be separated again into a set of smaller tables. This process, known as decomposition, must be "lossless" to maintain the integrity of the data. Just as the term implies, lossless decomposition is a process that retains all essential data and removes redundant values while preserving the ability to reproduce the content of the original table, as needed. This process is demonstrated in Figure 19.3, in which the "Patient" and "Physician" tables are stored separately, but can be joined to form a derived table that contains the data from both. It should be noted that derived tables are temporary, and should not be included in the long-term data storage design. Derived tables simply provide a convenient, short-term view of related data from separate tables.

In the current example (Figure 19.3), the "Diagnosis" column is the source of the redundancy and must be sequestered to its own table. However, this separation must be done without any data loss. To accomplish this, an "Appointment" table should be added to serve as a bridge between each patient and their associated diagnoses. The "Appointment" table will also connect patients and physicians.

The relationship between patients and appointments is established by storing the "PatientKey" for each patient in the "PatientForeignKey" column. The relationship between the "Patient" and "Appointment" tables in the database mirrors the relationship between patients and appointments in reality. The relationship can be best described as "one-to-many" in which one patient can have many appointments. If this relationship is built into the database design, a patient can have multiple appointments (requiring multiple entries in the "Appointment" table), but only one entry is required in the "Patient" table. As a result, the data redundancy visible in Figure 19.3 (in columns "LastName," "FirstName," and "Birthdate") is eliminated.

The process of decomposition continues as the diagnosis and physician information are also separated. The relationships between the patient and the associated physician and diagnoses must be maintained. The "Appointment" table is used to connect the "Patient," "Physician," and "Diagnosis" tables. Once again, the database design draws from a real-world example. An appointment is the point in the treatment process at which the patient meets with the physician and the physician determines the diagnosis. The database model is a natural extension of this relationship. The restructured database is shown in Figure 19.4.

Two tables worth mentioning have been introduced into the model "Physician Appointment" and "Diagnosis Appointment."[11] Up to this point all of the tables included in the database have been based in the real world, but the new tables are more abstract. Their sole function is to

establish a link between tables in such a way that the principles of normalization will not be compromised. As a result, they do not have real-world counterparts.

The new tables are necessary because of the nature of the relationships between both appointments and diagnoses and appointments and physicians. These relationships are best described as "many-to-many." For example, every appointment can be associated with multiple diagnoses, and every diagnosis can be associated with multiple appointments. "Junction" tables must be included in the database model to account for this interaction and eliminate data redundancy. In the absence of these tables multiple diagnoses in any given appointment would cause the unnecessary repetition of appointment data.

Third Rule of Normalization

Third normal form addresses redundancies that stem from transitive data elements (information from one table is implied by information stored in another table). The specific details of third normal form reach beyond the scope of this discussion, but the possibility of higher forms of normalization is noteworthy. The underlying and driving force in normalization is the minimization of redundancies in the relational model. A glaring exception to this rule is the primary/foreign key relationship, in which the redundancy itself is the mechanism by which relationships among tables are established. This anomaly is a necessary byproduct of normalization, and is the only desirable form of redundancy in the relational model. However, if the effectiveness of the database would be compromised through compliance with any of the rules of normalization, that rule must be breeched. The effectiveness of the database should outweigh all other considerations.

Technologic Vulnerabilities

The most important factor when considering system vulnerabilities is the protection of data. Access to the database should be restricted to legitimate users, and the nature of access should be structured to fit the use patterns of each specific user. Full permission to every component of the database should be limited to the database administrator. Read-only access for all other users is preferred, reserving write access (update) for situations that require it. For example, a physician will need to update the tables used for any direct data entry (i.e., symptoms, diagnosis), implying write access. However, the same physician will not need permission to update a patient survey table, in which read-only access will suffice. Provision of full access to the database for all users can easily result in the corruption of data.

Control over permissions to the database can be managed with the database management systems built into most commercial database packages. Access can be restricted on a table-by-table basis (by the administrator), allowing for access customizations to fit the use patterns, as previously discussed. Additional layers of software can also be built on top of the database to further control access. Customized software applications can be written to limit user interaction with the database and provide data verification functions. These added tiers act as a buffer for

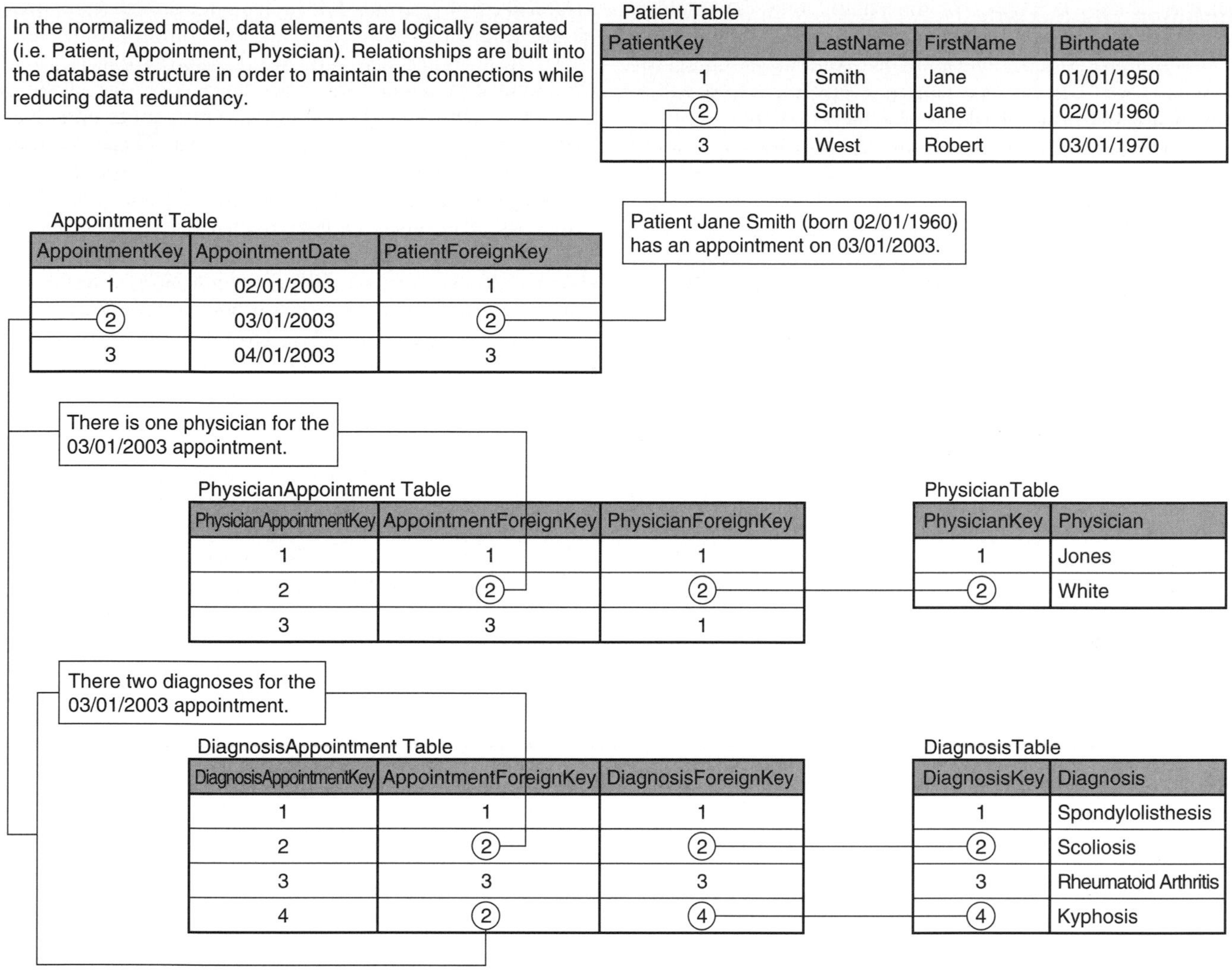

In the normalized model, data elements are logically separated (i.e. Patient, Appointment, Physician). Relationships are built into the database structure in order to maintain the connections while reducing data redundancy.

Patient Table

PatientKey	LastName	FirstName	Birthdate
1	Smith	Jane	01/01/1950
2	Smith	Jane	02/01/1960
3	West	Robert	03/01/1970

Patient Jane Smith (born 02/01/1960) has an appointment on 03/01/2003.

Appointment Table

AppointmentKey	AppointmentDate	PatientForeignKey
1	02/01/2003	1
2	03/01/2003	2
3	04/01/2003	3

There is one physician for the 03/01/2003 appointment.

PhysicianAppointment Table

PhysicianAppointmentKey	AppointmentForeignKey	PhysicianForeignKey
1	1	1
2	2	2
3	3	1

PhysicianTable

PhysicianKey	Physician
1	Jones
2	White

There two diagnoses for the 03/01/2003 appointment.

DiagnosisAppointment Table

DiagnosisAppointmentKey	AppointmentForeignKey	DiagnosisForeignKey
1	1	1
2	2	2
3	3	3
4	2	4

DiagnosisTable

DiagnosisKey	Diagnosis
1	Spondylolisthesis
2	Scoliosis
3	Rheumatoid Arthritis
4	Kyphosis

Figure 19.4 Appointment tables.

the outcomes system and can effectively monitor the quality of the information before it reaches the database.

A subtler vulnerability relates to the timeliness of the data. The timing and availability of information stored in the database varies significantly, depending on the method of data collection. This becomes critical when some data elements are reliant on the presence of others. For example, an outcomes system that tracks patients by appointment creates such a scenario. At each appointment the patient completes a survey and the physician completes an assessment of the patient's health. In the database model for such a system the appointment provides the bond between the patient survey and the physician assessment. Relationships will have been established in the database design that link the table of appointments with the tables for surveys and assessments. If a particular appointment is not present in the appointment table, it cannot be referenced by either of the other tables, and any attempt to do so will result in an error, preventing the database from being updated.

Participation provides another interesting challenge in the pursuit of an outcomes system. Data collection systems that are too costly in terms of time, effort, or resources will not succeed. A successful model is one that leaves the smallest possible footprint, a prospect that is best realized through collaboration. In the healthcare industry, the availability of information has increased exponentially in recent years. Pursuant to this, outcomes systems are afforded the opportunity to draw from many sources within the organization. Data are collected and retained for every patient throughout the scheduling, registration, treatment, and billing processes as the trend of paperless patient care continues. Consequently, information is typically stored in many different systems throughout the organization, and effective outcomes systems will draw from these disparate data sources whenever possible. Not only does the sharing of data reduce the possibility of errors stemming from data entry, but it also minimizes the level of effort necessary from the participants (both patients and physicians). For example, if a patient's demographic information is gathered for the registration process, it should not be necessary to collect it again when the patient completes a survey. As multiple systems are leveraged within the outcomes system, the resulting automation can significantly reduce the risk of unverified data. Moreover, participation levels improve as the required effort decreases.

Building The System

As mentioned previously, the three major components of any electronic information system are technology, people, and processes in which the human and technologic components interact. It is useful in analyzing the requirements for building a system, and in diagnosing any shortfalls or failures of a system once it is built, to categorize the required inputs and/or desired outputs (i.e., expectations) among these three component parts. The preceding sections of this chapter have been devoted primarily to technology and processes; therefore this section focuses on understanding the people involved and their roles in creating the system.

Resource Requirements

As a prerequisite for success, human resources from the clinical, information technology, and administrative areas of the organization must be dedicated to the project. These individuals must be highly skilled in their respective disciplines, and ideally (to help champion the project) they should command a high degree of respect among their peers before joining the project team. Further, they should be able to sustain a high degree of personal commitment to the success of the project over the long range (typically a period of 3-5 years), and possess excellent interpersonal and team-building skills (i.e., listening, speaking, demonstrating a collaborative work-style, showing sensitivity to individual differences). Each member of the project team must fully understand and agree to accept a defined role in the process of system development and implementation. First and foremost, a project leader, director, or manager must be identified. The project leader is responsible for the overall success of the system via effective management of all aspects of the project.

It is recommended that a clinician fill this role in any healthcare information system project, because clinicians are the key stakeholders in these projects. Clinical support, guidance, and direction are vital to the development of a system that will actually meet the needs of physicians and nurses. This is true from both an input (i.e., the data elements to be collected and collection process requirements in the clinical setting) and output (i.e., the data and information produced and provided to clinicians by the system) perspective. If the end result of all of the time, money, and effort invested in the system does not satisfy the clinical participants and stakeholders, the project surely has failed. If the perceived benefits do not outweigh the actual and perceived costs of participating in the system, it has failed as well.

All project team members are expected to take responsibility for ensuring the success of the system as it relates to their respective disciplines. For example, the physicians and nurses are responsible for the clinical success of the system. As such, they must ascertain that the data elements to be collected and information outputs are meaningful and relevant to clinicians, that the collection process is user-friendly to their colleagues and patients, and that the data collected will produce appropriate, clinically valid, and meaningful output for clinical outcomes measurement and research. The entire team relies exclusively on the clinical contingent to assess and decide all clinical parameters.

A system analyst is required to assume responsibility for the technical success of the system. Regardless of his or her actual title or position within the organization, this person must be highly skilled and knowledgeable, with respect to efficient and effective data management strategies, project management strategies, and the fundamental principles of information systems. Most importantly, relationships must be fostered between the technical and clinical personnel, so that each has a keen understanding of the other's working environment. The system analyst will not be able to build a system tracking clinical activity and patient outcomes without a clear description of the physician's working environment. Inefficiencies in the project will develop if the clinician cannot describe this setting in a manner that the system analyst can comprehend.

Finally, an administrative representative is relied on to manage the operational and financial aspects of the project. For the project to be successful, the system must ultimately "fit" into the constraints of a busy and demanding clinical setting, especially since it requires collecting data from both physicians and patients at the time of an outpatient visit. This is typically the greatest challenge in developing such systems, and has been noted as a major obstacle to outcomes measurement systems development. Data collection methods must be evaluated from a cost-benefit perspective and for user-friendliness. Securing "buy in" from affected operational and clinical personnel is essential, and is a task that is typically shared by the entire team, although the administrative representative carries the main responsibility for this function throughout the project. The administrator also handles tasks such as securing copyright permission for patient surveys or Institutional Review Board (IRB) approval of clinical studies when applicable, preparing a budget and securing approvals, informing clinical and operational personnel as to project milestones, implementation schedules, etc. It is recommended that at least one management representative join the team for the entire duration of the project, whereas other operational or financial personnel may be called on to participate in or consult with the project team for defined project tasks.

Deployment

Successful deployment of the system is predicated on clear communication about the implementation schedule, tasks, and implications for all involved. This includes communication among the team members, and perhaps most importantly, between the team and all affected parties. Advanced notification and discussion of timeframes, expectations, and the roles of all operational and clinical personnel in assisting patients and physicians in data collection are needed. The establishment of feedback loops for communicating implementation problems and issues is essential to the deployment process. People need to know, on a real-time basis, how to report technical malfunctions or process issues. In turn, responsive troubleshooting by members of the project team is equally essential. It is suggested that the project leader or his or her designee feed back timely project updates and process statistics to key stakeholders, including clinical departments, medical staff, and management, to keep people informed of the implementation schedule and milestones.

Measuring Success

Both objective and subjective indicators can gauge the success of an outcomes information system. Establishing the metrics by which the system's success will be measured is ideally done early in the project development phase. This ensures that the system created is, in fact, that which is desired by the stakeholders. A simple report that presents the results of objective and subjective evaluations is useful and recommended. Ideally, monthly reports are generated during the first year or two of implementation.

Objective Metrics

- The number/percentage of all patients seen, in the target population, from whom *patient*-reported data is collected. Example: 89 (89%) of 100 patients seen in March 2002 completed the required data collection survey.
- The number/percentage of all patients seen, in the target population, for whom *physician*-reported data was collected. Example: Physicians submitted data on 90 (90%) of 100 patients seen in March 2002.
- The number/percentage of survey "matches" between physician and patient collected data. Example: For the 200 surveys collected from patients during March 2002, there were 190 (95%) surveys collected on the same patients by physicians.
- The number/percentage of surveys (either physician or patient) completed entirely (no questions or sections left blank or illegibly marked). Example: 95 (95%) of 100 surveys completed by physicians (or patients) were complete.
- The average and range of time required for patients to complete a survey. Example: It was observed that patients spent between 10 and 35 minutes to complete a survey, with the average being 15 minutes.
- The average and range of time required for physicians to complete a survey. Example: Physicians spent between 5 and 15 minutes to complete a survey, with the average being 7 minutes.
- Based on a random cross-check of selected fields from 20 completed physician-reported surveys with the corresponding patient medical record, the number and percentage of surveys in which the survey data were in agreement with the medical record. Example: In 16 of 20 physician surveys the selected data fields were in complete agreement with the medical record.
- Quantification of individual physician participation relative to other physicians within the department (e.g., Physician A provided data on 62% of her

patients compared with a department-wide percentage of 84%).

Subjective Metrics

- Patient-reported perceptions of the time required and user-friendliness of the surveys.
- Perceptions of the operational and clinical personnel with respect to the ease of administration of the patient surveys, user-friendliness, etc.
- Patient expectations about treatment.
- Patient satisfaction with staff.
- Measures of pain and functional limitation.
- Usefulness and appropriateness of output reports that are produced and provided to the clinicians, as well as the clinicians' impressions about the data.
- Clinicians' impressions and those of the entire project team, as to the cost-benefit ratio of system inputs versus outputs.

In the final evaluation of any outcomes system, both objective and subjective measures must be considered. Both measures combine to form a critical component of an ongoing monitoring and evaluation of the system. Feedback will not only help to determine the effectiveness and relevance of the outcomes project, but will also be used as the primary tool to develop enhancements and refinements as the system evolves.

REFERENCES

1. Andersson GBJ, Weinstein JN: Introduction to health outcomes related to low back pain. *Spine* 19(18Suppl):2026S-2027S, 1994.
2. Bigos S, Bowyer O, Braen G, *et al*: Overview. Purpose and rationale. In Agency for Health Care Policy and Research, Public Health Service USD, editors. Acute low-back problems in adults. Clinical practice guideline No. 14. Pub. No. 95-0642 ed. Rockville, MD: AHCPR, 5-6, 1994.
3. Cunningham LS, Kelsey JL: Epidemiology of musculoskeletal impairments and associated disability. *Am J Public Health* 74:574-579, 1984.
4. Codd, EF: A relational model of data for large shared data banks. *Communications of the ACM*, Association for Computing Machinery, 13(6):377-387, 1970.
5. Date, CJ: *Introduction to Database Systems*. Reading, Mass., Addison Wesley Longman, 2000.
6. Deyo RA, Cherkin D, Conrad D, Volinn E: Cost, controversy, crisis: low-back pain and the health of the public. *Ann Rev Public Health* 12:141-156, 1991.
7. Frymoyer JW, Cats-Baril WL: An overview of the incidences and costs of low-back pain. *Orthop Clin North Am* 22: 263-271, 1991.
8. Taylor VM, Deyo RA, Cherkin DC, Kreuter W: Low-back pain hospitalization: Recent United States trends and regional variations. *Spine* 19:1207-1213, 1994.

CHAPTER 20

Education and Knowledge-Base Acquisition and Retention

Chima Ohaegbulam, Gregory R. Trost,
Isador H. Lieberman, and Marc E. Eichler

Introduction

Relatively little attention is paid by most teachers and students in clinical medicine, in general, and in spine surgery, in particular, to a formal analysis of the learning process. This chapter aims to examine this in some detail to improve the efficiency of the "educational machine."

In all learning situations, there should be established objectives. In the specific context of spine surgery, these might include the following (modified from Douglas et al.[5]):

For the learner:

1. Acquisition of cognitive, attitudinal, and psychomotor skills needed to care for patients
2. Management of patients in a setting that maximizes learning and minimizes risk to the patients
3. Familiarity with personnel management and the structure of the health care system
4. Understanding of the realities of being a physician in the present climate of litigation and third-party payment

For the teacher:

1. Supervision of learners to maximize their learning and minimize risk to patients
2. Facilitation of clinical reasoning by learners
3. Demonstration and supervision of procedures
4. Act of role modeling for learners
5. Provision of feedback on diagnostic and management skills
6. Introduction of concept of a changing organizational construct in medical care delivery
7. Evaluation of the learners' performance with regard to cognitive, attitudinal, and psychomotor skills.

The North American Spine Society[9] (NASS) has published guidelines for training in spinal surgery. For residency training, five categories of education are defined:

1. Core knowledge
2. Clinical evaluation
3. Operative management
4. Postoperative care
5. Rehabilitation

In each of these categories, more specific details are listed in the published guidelines. A set of criteria of what the educational program should consist of is also specified for fellowship training. This covers:

1. Hospital resources
2. Teaching faculty
3. Educational program
4. Resources for research
5. Evaluation of the process

Elements of learning

Learning cannot be directly measured, but its occurrence can be inferred when outcomes of the learning process are measured. Observable or measurable changes in performance should result from learning.

Adults (as opposed to children) are interested in concepts, principles, and the application of knowledge, as opposed to simply learning the facts. The most productive learning occurs when concepts and principles are linked to existing knowledge and experiences.[5]

The following describes the increasing efficiency with which learning occurs, with increasing participation in the learning process: People generally remember (1) 20% of what they hear, (2) 30% of what they see, (3) 50% of what they hear and see, (4) 70% of what they say, and (5) 90% of what they do.[2,5] This hierarchy should be borne in mind with the planning of the learning environment for trainees.

It is now widely accepted that there are three major domains involved in learning: the cognitive, affective, and psychomotor domains. These domains are often more commonly referred to as *knowledge, attitude,* and *skills.*

The Cognitive Domain

The cognitive domain emphasizes remembering, understanding, reordering information, and combining ideas and concepts. It is the largest proportion of learning and has several progressive levels:

1. Knowledge to recall information
2. Comprehension to understand or know the meaning
3. Application to use the information or to apply it in its proper context
4. Analysis to be able to break the information into components
5. Synthesis to combine ideas and concepts resulting in new ideas
6. Evaluation to judge the value of information

Each of these levels is a prerequisite of the next. Unfortunately, traditional teaching in the clinical settings tends to remain in the lower levels of this hierarchy, with an emphasis on the memorization of minute details. This may be, in part, because of the emphasis on the use of formal examinations as the major source of evaluation.

The Affective Domain

This domain emphasizes feelings, emotions, or a degree of acceptance or rejection. It is probably the most difficult to assess.[6] Attitudes are usually described as being in the affective domain and are based on complex sets of values and beliefs. They are acquired throughout life and are based on a wide range of influences.

The affective domain concerns the application of knowledge and skills. It can be divided into a number of discrete areas, including:

1. Clinical judgment
2. Interaction with patients and relatives
3. Ethics
4. Reliability
5. Professional development
6. Teamwork
7. Image or appearance

The Psychomotor Domain

This domain emphasizes motor skills. Unfortunately, standards for learning skills may not always be evident, and a stepwise learning sequence may not be possible to follow. Ideally, the learner is able to go in a stepwise fashion, from the basic information about a procedure or skill to seeing an expert perform the task, being able to practice the skill on a model, if available, and then performing the skill under supervision before being asked to attempt it independently.

In the context of spine surgery, as in most of clinical medicine, the skills that are learned during residency training form a foundation for more complex skills. This can have significant effects on the effectiveness with which one learns during subspecialty fellowship training. An inadequate foundation that is established earlier in one's career can become very difficult to rectify.

Teaching-Learning Plan

There are three components to a teaching-learning plan: (1) objectives or goals for teaching, (2) teaching methods, and (3) an evaluation to determine whether the goals for teaching have been met. These components are interdependent.

Establishing Objectives

The definition of objectives or learning outcomes describes in specific terms how the learner is to perform after instruction. In addition to the depiction of specific outcomes, it should also describe the conditions, how well the objectives should be performed, and in what time frame they should be achieved.

Objectives should be categorized in the three areas of focus for learners: cognitive, affective, and psychomotor.

Cognitive objectives call for mastery of information and are often the easiest to specify.

Affective objectives are the most difficult to specify. This is particularly so because attitudes are difficult to observe accurately. The goals associated with affective objectives include stipulations about professional attitude (i.e., attendance, punctuality, and appearance), and attitude toward patients (i.e., appreciation of family, work, or psychologic dynamics in illness behavior) is behavior that is established earlier in life.

Psychomotor (or skill) objectives are easier to specify because observable behavior is the outcome. Objective means of evaluating these types of behaviors, however, is an area of general medical education that is only slowly becoming more widespread in surgical education.

Teaching Strategies for Cognitive Learning

Different strategies have specific advantages and disadvantages. The choice of strategy should pertain to the goals and objectives of the learning experience, as well as the number of teachers and students. Available methods include self-directed learning, one-on-one tutorials, lectures, and discussion groups. Strategies may be split into two groups: learner-based and teacher-based methods.

Learner-Based Strategies

Self-directed learning is the most important strategy for cognitive learning. It requires a commitment to the task and has reading as its cornerstone. Although it is an effective and efficient way of learning factual information, it has the disadvantage of being largely passive. Retention of content may be lower than with other types of learning. A plan for such learning is valuable, where the learner asks the following questions:

1. What is the desired body of knowledge?
2. Where is the knowledge available?
3. What is the most efficient way of acquiring such knowledge?
4. How should the data be analyzed?
5. How should the efficiency of acquisition and retention be tested?

The self-directed learner should also use a teacher to guide the collection of information or test conclusions.

The one-on-one tutorial is the classic method for clinical teaching. It has the advantage of being individualized and learner-centered within a mentor-student relationship. Feedback is immediately available. Its effectiveness can be dependent on the personal rapport between teacher and learner.

Such learner-based strategies are especially important as more advanced levels in surgical training are achieved, for several reasons. Class size becomes smaller such that the individual student plays a larger role in directing the training. Personal interests on the student's role also begin to play larger roles in defining the knowledge and skill and achieving goals for the later stages in training, where the basic knowledge foundation is presumably already well established.

Teacher-Based Strategies

Lectures are an effective method of presenting factual information. They can be developed around the steps of planning, preparation, presentation, and a post-lecture analysis. Planning should assess the learners' baselines and specify goals for the lecture. Preparation should define a structural plan and integrate appropriate lecture aids such as audiovisual material. Presentation should be in a format that actively involves learners and take into account the average attention span of about 20 minutes (regarding lecture assimilation) and actively use questions or brainstorming to maintain interest. The importance of repetition of core concepts cannot be overemphasized. A post-lecture analysis evaluation is essential. It should monitor the learner's questions, individual interests, and material retention. Criticism and feedback should be invited regarding style and content.

Integrated lecture/discussions can be based on clinical cases to provide points of focus for discussion. Developing these points of focus should use the same format as the lecture, but planning and preparation can be more difficult and require a thorough grasp of the subject by the teacher. It requires careful thought to ensure that a plan is in place to cover all of the important points of the subject.

Discussion groups function best when they are small and teacher-intensive. Subject reviews or case discussions are two of many ways of planning such groups.

The latter two strategies are more commonly available on a day-to-day basis during residency or fellowship training. It should be possible to integrate these, to some extent, into other activities such as clinics and operations.

A definite relationship exists between the quality of teaching and student performance.[3] It has been shown that higher board scores have been achieved by students who rated their attending surgeons higher than the teachers of lower-scoring residents. This encourages an arrangement in which residents are exposed proportionally to the most effective educators[2] and infers that the most effective educators should teach the most.

Teaching Strategies for Affective Learning

Methods that are available for enhancing affective learning include videotape review and peer discussion groups.

Role modeling by teaching physicians is also important in the teaching of appropriate behavior, appearance, attitudes, and approach to patients and staff. Attitudes are not taught; they must be experienced.

Teaching Strategies for Psychomotor Skills

Planning strategies for the development of skills requires an analysis by the teacher of the skills to be taught. These skills must be broken down into their component parts and each part analyzed. The most difficult parts will demand the most time and effort to teach. Teaching plans must take this into account.

Available strategies include models and simulations, clinical demonstration, videotape or computer review, and practice of skills during supervised patient care. The teacher must select the optimal tools from the armamentarium for each educational situation.

Models have the obvious advantages. They facilitate practice of a skill set that does not affect patient care and that provides immediate feedback regarding performance. They may be part of an incremental step-by-step process that approaches the clinical performance of a task. For example, the benefit of using simplified models, with tasks broken down into constituent steps that are dealt with one at a time, has been shown in a urologic surgery paradigm.[10]

Clinical demonstrations are important, prior to having a trainee perform a procedure without supervision. Videotapes are very helpful, especially with less commonly performed procedures, for illustrating specific techniques.

Evaluation

There must be a means for evaluating the acquisition of skills to assess the effectiveness of the teaching-learning process and make adjustments where necessary. The NASS guidelines[8] suggest that evaluations of a fellow's performance should be communicated with the fellow, including an assessment of cognitive, motor, and interpersonal skills, attitude, and surgical judgment. The guidelines also suggest that the fellow should have an opportunity to periodically assess the training program in terms of meeting the educational goals.

It is ideal for specific goals to be set for each stage or point in the trainee's course through a program. Several training programs use evaluation forms that use rating scales to score the attainment of goals. The reliability of these scores increases as the number of people scoring the trainee and the number of discrete goals increase.

Evaluation of Cognitive Skills

Tests of knowledge must (1) measure whether objectives for learning have been met and be (2) valid measures of the learning that has occurred.

The tests can use short-answer, true-false, multiple-choice, or essay-type questions. True-false items are popular but difficult to effectively use for evaluation because guessing is always a factor, and there is a 50% chance of choosing the right answer. With multiple-choice questions, asking "how" or "why" is generally better for measuring understanding than asking "who," "what," or "where" questions. Reliability is generally increased with larger numbers of questions per test topic.[1]

The essay format is the oldest form of written evaluation, but it is the most subjective. The primary objection to the essay format is the poor reliability with associated scoring, both interscorer and intrascorer. It also discriminates against learners with poor verbal abilities, but it is useful for testing higher cognitive skills and, if designed well, tests synthesis and judgment.

Oral examinations are advantageous in situations where flexibility must be maintained because areas to be covered cannot be predicted in advance. Learners can be probed in particular areas as the need arises; however, establishing criteria for performance is difficult, and some of the difficulties that apply to scoring an essay format also apply here. With careful case selection and pre-definition of scoring rules, examination score reliabilities of up to 0.88 can be achieved.[1]

Validity and reliability must be assured to the extent possible in evaluating cognitive skills.

Evaluation of Attitudes and Skills

Attitudes are clearly more difficult to measure than skills. However, it is important to have an objective means of measuring the achievement of attitude goals to establish a basis for providing constructive feedback and, potentially, the basis for future recommendations. Goals for minimum attendance and punctuality are the easiest to establish. The monitoring of specific behaviors, such as inquiry into patients' relevant family and social structures, interpersonal skills, and listening ability, are no less important. Skills are more easily measured because they can be directly observed. Methods for doing so in clinical education include structured types, such as checklists and rating scales, to less structured types such as chart reviews.

Assessing operative skills objectively and effectively remain a challenge. It has been suggested that such assessments may be easier in a surgical skills laboratory than in the operating room.[4] However, abstract tests of manual dexterity are unreliable. Dental and laparoscopic surgery have developed the most extensive literature on the formal evaluation of surgical skills. It is not positive in this regard.

Objective Structured Clinical Examinations (OSCEs) were first used in medical schools in the late 1970s and early 1980s, and their use is spreading to residency.[7] With these tests, various clinical skills are broken down into their constituent parts, and candidates rotate around various bench stations completing set tasks at each station. The reliability of well-constructed OSCEs appears to be at least 0.8. These have been further modified into Objective Structured Assessment of Technical Skills (OSATs), which have been described by Winckel, Reznick, and others.[11] These tests use bench models of surgical tissues to assess performance. Where OSCEs evaluate successful completion of an entire task, OSATs evaluate elements of a simulated operation that are selected for the test. These tests are scored with check lists or rating scales.

Although OSCEs are useful for measuring specific clinical skills and abilities, they are difficult to create and administer. Also, they are cost-effective only when there are many candidates to be examined simultaneously.[1]

Portfolios are another means by which cognitive or psychomotor skills can be measured.[1] These are collections, by the trainee, of evidence of learning and achievement related to the training plan. The portfolio might include, for example, logs of procedures and operations. It is possible to have reproducible assessment of portfolios when an agreement of criteria and standards for contents exists.

Surgical models are also useful, and virtual reality (VR) simulations are likely to become increasingly popular in the training and evaluation of surgeons.

Summary

The three major domains in learning include cognitive (knowledge), affective (attitude), and psychomotor (skills) domains. Effective teaching and learning involve setting objectives by using appropriate methods and evaluating both the teacher and learner across each of the respective domains.

REFERENCES

1. ABMS: Toolbox of assessment methods. 2003: 2000.
2. Benzel E: *Teaching and learning the fundamentals.* Lecture at Joint Section on Disorders of the Spine and Peripheral Nerves, 2003.
3. Blue AV, Griffith CH, III, Wilson J, *et al*: Surgical teaching quality makes a difference. *Am J Surg* 177:86-89, 1999.
4. Darzi A, Smith S, Taffinder N: Assessing operative skill: needs to become more objective. *BMJ* 318:887-888, 1999.
5. Douglas KC, Hosokawa MC, Lawler FH: *A Practical Guide to Clinical Teaching in Medicine.* Springer series on medical education. New York, Springer, 1988, p 11:xiii, 191.
6. Evans AW: Assessing competence in surgical dentistry. *Br Dent J* 190:343-346, 2001.
7. Harden RM, Gleeson FA: Assessment of clinical competence using an objective structured clinical examination (OSCE). *Med Educ* 13:41-54, 1979.
8. Herkowitz HN, Connolly PJ, Gundry CR, *et al*: Educational guidelines for orthopaedic and neurosurgical spinal fellowship training. *Spine* 25:2704-2705, 2000.
9. Herkowitz HN, Connolly PJ, Gundry CR, *et al*: Resident and fellowship guidelines: educational guidelines for resident training in spinal surgery. *Spine* 25:2703-2707, 2000.
10. Katz R, Nadu A, Olsson LE, *et al*: A simplified 5-step model for training laparoscopic urethrovesical anastomosis. *J Urol* 169:2041-2044, 2003.
11. Winckel CP, Reznick RK, Cohen R, Taylor B: Reliability and construct validity of a structured technical skills assessment form. *Am J Surg* 167:423-427, 1994.

Anatomy and Surgical Approaches and Exposures of the Vertebral Column

CHAPTER 21

Occipital Cervical Region

Robert A. McGuire, Jr., and Ashraf A. Ragab

Although fewer procedures are performed at the occipital cervical junction when compared with subaxial cervical procedures, there are specific indications where the exposure of the occipital cervical region is needed for surgical intervention. Indications include trauma, which may lead to instability or compressive lesions arising from tumors or infection. Vague symptoms such as pain, headaches, or limitations of motion may develop as a result of these lesions. Once the origin of these symptoms is correctly identified and the indications for surgery arise, the remaining challenge is the surgical approach. In order to approach these lesions safely, a thorough understanding of the anatomy, the surgical approaches available, and the complications that may occur is mandatory. This chapter discusses the surgical anatomy and the ventral and dorsal approaches to the occipital cervical region.

Surgical Anatomy

Dorsal Surgical Anatomy of the Occipital Cervical Region

Dorsal approaches to the occipitocervical area are most commonly used for occipitocervical fusions. During the approach, dissection through several muscular layers is necessary. The trapezius muscle constitutes the first superficial layer. The trapezius arises from the external occipital protuberans, the ligamentum nuchae and the spines of the seventh cervical and all thoracic vertebrae.[13] The upper fibers insert into the lateral third of the clavicle and form the curve of the shoulder. The middle fibers insert into the medial edge of the acromion and the superior margin of the spine of the scapula, and the lower fibers ascend also onto the scapular spine (Figure 21.1). The nerve supply of the trapezius muscle is the accessory nerve.

The second muscle layer consists of the levator scapulae. This muscle originates as slips from each of the transverse processes of the upper four cervical vertebrae. The muscle inserts onto the medial border of the scapula and is supplied by the ventral rami to the third and fourth cervical nerves and the fifth through the dorsal scapular nerve. The splenius muscle originates from the lower aspect of the ligamentum nuchae and the spines of the seventh cervical and upper six thoracic vertebrae. Its fibers pass rostrally, and it is divided into cervical and cranial components. The splenius cervicis is the lateral component, which inserts into the transverse processes of the

upper three cervical vertebrae, deep to the levator scapulae muscle. Meanwhile, the splenius capitis muscle inserts on the lower aspect of the mastoid process of the temporal bone. Its nerve supply is the dorsal rami of the cervical nerves. Beneath the splenius lies the cervical component of the erector spinae muscle. The erector spinae muscle is composed of three main columns: the iliocostalis, longissimus, and spinalis muscles (from lateral to medial). The longissimus capitis muscle is a long muscle that lies under the splenius muscle immediately dorsal to the transverse processes. It arises from the transverse processes of the upper four thoracic vertebra and passes upward to be inserted into the back of the mastoid process. The ligamentum nuchae is a strong fibrous substance, which is median between the muscles of the two sides. It is considered a continuation of the superior spinous and interspinous ligaments from the spine of the seventh cervical vertebra through the external occipital protuberans.

The main vessels in the dorsal occipital cervical area are the occipital artery and the vertebral artery. The occipital artery arises from the external carotid artery in the front of the neck and runs dorsally and rostrally deep to the mastoid process and then courses dorsally immediately deep to the muscles attached to the superior nuchal line. It then pierces the trapezius muscle 2.5cm from the midline to ramify on the back of the head (Figure 21.1). As for the vertebral artery, only the third part of this artery is significant during the approach. It emerges from the foramen and the transverse process of the atlas and hooks dorsomedially around the dorsal surface of the lateral mass of the atlas (Figure 21.1). It is partly separated from the arch of the atlas by the first cervical nerve (Figure 21.2; see also Figure 21.1). It then passes ventromedially in front of the thickened lateral edge of the dorsal atlanto-occipital membrane, which forms an arch over the artery. In some occasions this arch may be ossified. The artery then pierces the dura mater and enters the vertebral canal. The suboccipital plexus of veins is a network of veins that drains into the deep cervical vein and into the vertebral venous plexus around the vertebral artery. The greater occipital nerve is the medial branch of the dorsal ramus of the second cervical nerve, which is the thickest cutaneous nerve in the body. It appears at the middle of the lower border of the inferior oblique muscle and curves superior medially across the suboccipital triangle. It runs rostrally on that muscle and then pierces the trapezius muscle about 2cm lateral to the occipital protuberans. (see Figure 21.1).

Ventral Anatomy of the Occipital Cervical Junction

From the ventral aspect of the atlas originate three muscles. These are the longus colli, rectus capitis anterior, and rectus capitis lateralis (Figure 21.3).

1. The longus colli muscle is the longest and most medial of the muscles. It extends from the anterior tubercle of the atlas to the lower part of the body of the upper thoracic vertebrae. Between these points it is attached to all the vertebral bodies and into the third to sixth cervical transverse processes.

2. Rectus capitis anterior, which is a short, wide muscle that originates from the ventral surface of

the lateral mass of the atlas and is inserted into the base of the skull ventral to the occipital condyle.

3. Rectus capitis lateralis is a short muscle that runs vertically between the rostral surface of the transverse process of the atlas and jugular process of the occipital bone. It lies dorsal to the jugular foramen and is separated from the rectus capitis anterior by the ventral ramus of the first cervical nerve, which supplies both muscles. The function of these muscles is to stabilize the skull on the vertebral column (Figure 21.3).

Ventral to the prevertebral muscles is the retropharyngeal space. The anterior tubercle of the atlas may be palpated through the dorsal pharynx during a transoral approach.

The Vertebral Artery

The anatomy of the vertebral artery must be understood, because injury to this artery may have dire consequences. The artery starts as a branch of the subclavian artery and passes to the transverse process of the sixth cervical vertebra.[13] The artery then ascends vertically through the foramina transversaria accompanied by the vertebral veins and plexus of sympathetic nerve fibers derived from the cervicothoracic ganglion of the sympathetic trunk. Between the transverse processes, it lies medial to the intertransverse muscles and ventral to the ventral rami of the cervical nerves. Upon entering the axis it turns laterally under the superior articular facet in the foramen transversarium and enters the foramen transversarium of the atlas, which is placed farther laterally than the others. Therefore, at this level, the artery takes a lateral course (Figure 21.2). The artery then emerges on the rostral surface of the atlas between the rectus capitis lateralis muscle and the superior articular process of the atlas. Here it lies with the ventral ramus of the first cervical nerve and curves with it horizontally around the lateral and dorsal aspect of the superior articularis process. It then traverses the articular process and the dorsal arch of the atlas where it lies rostrally to the dorsal ramus of the first cervical nerve. The artery then turns rostrally and pierces the dura and arachnoid mater. It enters the cranial cavity through the foramen magnum. It then runs ventrally and rostrally over the ventral surface of the medulla oblongata to meet and join the opposite vertebral artery at the inferior border of the pons to form the basilar artery. Through the branches of these vessels, blood is supplied to the hindbrain, midbrain and the dorsal aspect of the cerebrum and the rostral aspect of the spinal medulla. The vertebral vein originates from a plexus of veins that is formed by the union of veins from the internal

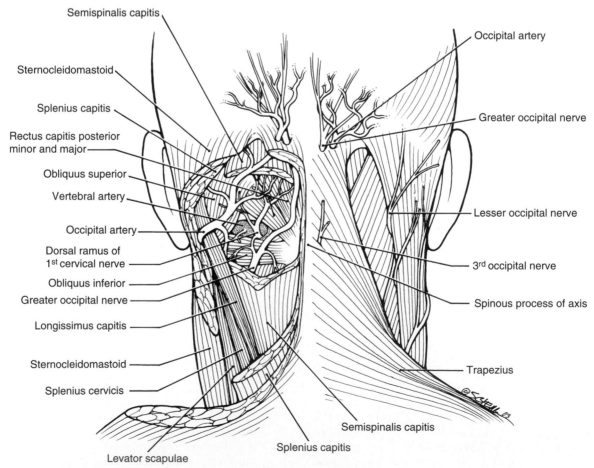

Figure 21.1 Dorsal surgical anatomy of the occipital cervical region. Superficial (*right*) and deep (*left*).

venous plexus and suboccipital triangle. It accompanies the vertebral artery through the foramina transversaria and exits the sixth cervical transverse process. It passes ventral to the subclavian artery and ends by entering the dorsal surface of the brachiocephalic vein near its origin.

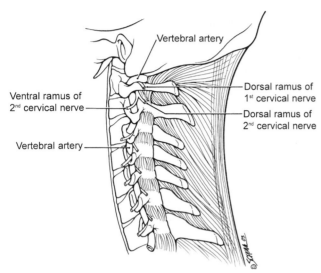

Figure 21.2 Course of the vertebral artery. The dorsal ramus of the first cervical nerve runs between the arch and the vertebral artery.

The Atlanto-Occipital Joint

The atlas is a ring of bone with a lateral mass on each side (Figure 21.4, *top*).[13] The lateral masses are articulated rostrally with the occipital condyles and caudally with the superior articular facets of the axis. Each has a transverse process projecting laterally from it. The atlas is attached to the occiput by strong ligaments, which hold these bones together. However, the articular surfaces, which the atlas has with the skull and with the axis, are of two different configurations. The kidney-shaped occipital condyles lie on the ventrolateral aspect of the foramen. They fit into the superior articular facets of the atlas which are also kidney shaped (see Figure 21.4). The joint allows flexion and extension and slight side-to-side rocking of head motion, but no rotation. The stability of these joints depends on the aid of ligaments, the tectorial membrane, and the longitudinal bands of the cruciate ligament, which all bind the skull to the axis. The ligaments of the joints of the atlas include the anterior longitudinal ligament, which tapers rostrally to be attached to the tubercle of the axis and continues as a narrow band to the base of the skull. The dorsal atlanto-occipital membrane is a rostral continuation of the ligamentum flavum. This membrane passes from the dorsal arch of the atlas to the margin of the foramen magnum dorsal to the atlanto-occipital joint. The lateral margins of the membrane arch over the corresponding vertebral artery and the first cervical nerve. In some cases, these margins may be ossified. The tectorial membrane is a broad ligamentous sheet, which is the rostral continuation

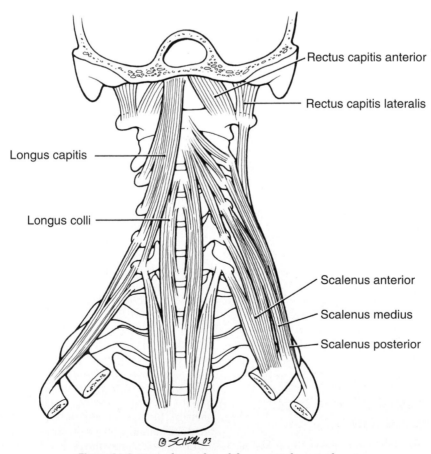

Figure 21.3 Ventral muscles of the occipital cervical region.

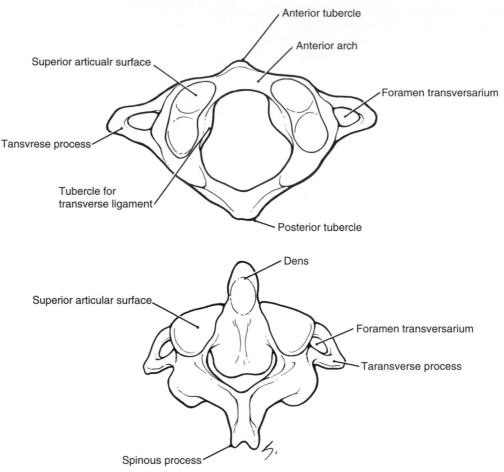

Figure 21.4 Bony anatomy of the atlas *(top)* and the axis *(bottom)*.

of the posterior longitudinal ligament. It passes from the dorsal surface of the body of the axis to the cranial surface of the occipital bone, and it holds the axis to the skull and covers the dorsal surfaces of the dens with its ligaments and the ventral margin of the foramen magnum. The cruciate ligament is formed by rostral and ventral longitudinal bands, which pass from the transverse ligament to the cranial surface of the occipital bone and the body of the axis, respectively. The apical ligament of the dens is a cord-like ligament, which stretches from the apex of the dens to the cranial surface of the occipital bone, immediately above the foramen magnum. The alar ligaments are strong ligaments that arise from the sloping sides of the dens (Figure 21.5). They pass laterally and upward to the medial sides of the occipital condyle and tighten when the atlas, carrying the skull, rotates around the dens. They are the main factor in limiting rotation of the atlantoaxial joint. The first and second cervical spinal nerves pass dorsally to the occipitocervical and C1-2 joint capsules, respectively, and not ventral to the articular facets, as is the case with the remaining subaxial cervical vertebrae.

Approaches to the Occipital Cervical Region
Dorsal Approach to the Occipital Cervical Region

The dorsal approach is most commonly used when fusion of the occipitocervical region is indicated. This approach

has been described by different authors in the past, including Grantham *et al.*[8] and Wertheim and Bohlman.[18] Key in the approach is positioning of the patient to allow safe intubation and protect the neural elements. Longitudinal traction should be applied preoperatively to provide stability during the intubation process. The patient is then logrolled into the prone position. Support for the head may also be provided using a Mayfield three-point headrest. Radiography or intraoperative fluoroscopy is used to confirm the alignment of the occiput to the atlas and the remainder of the cervical spine. The skin is then prepared and the subcutaneous tissues injected with a solution of epinephrine 1:500,000. A midline incision is made, extending from the external occipital protuberance to the spinous process of the fourth or fifth cervical vertebra. The spinous process of the C2 is the most prominent of the spinous processes encountered during the approach. The spinous process of C2 is bifid, allowing the short external rotators of the head to be attached to the cervical spine. Once the skin is incised, the incision is extended into the deep fascia and into the ligamentum nuchae. It is of great importance to remain in the midline to avoid excessive bleeding. This can be confirmed by palpating the alignment of the spinous processes and by visualizing the avascular midline plane of the ligamentum nuchae. By staying in the midline, the paramedian venous plexuses are avoided. The paravertebral muscles are stripped off the spinous processes and the lamina subperiosteally to avoid excessive bleeding.

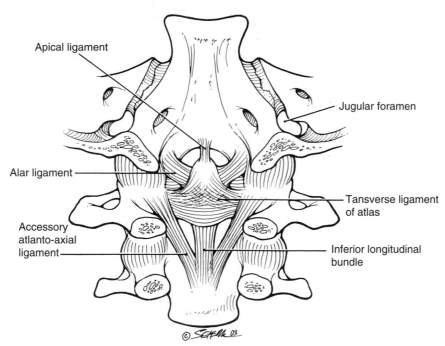

Figure 21.5 Ligamentous anatomy of the occipital cervical region.

Although some may feel that it is safe to use Cobb elevators in dissecting the muscles subperiosteally off the lamina, the authors do not recommend this. The fact that the laminae are weaker in this region than in the lumbar spine may lead to fracture of the lamina because of excessive force, as well as increased blood loss caused by uncontrolled stripping of the musculature. However, a Cobb elevator may be used to retract the muscles while the muscles are stripped off of the lamina using a freer elevator or cautery in a controlled manner. At the base of the skull, full-thickness scalp flaps are reflected along the occipital ridge about 2 to 3cm laterally. The extensive lateral dissection along the lamina of the cervical spine should be to the groove, which indicates the junction of the lamina along with the articular facet. Once the occipital exposure is completed, special care must be taken during the dissection of the arches of C1. The vertebral artery runs on the rostral surface of the arch and the lateral third of the arch (Figures 21.1 and 21.2). To expose this area safely, only 1cm on each side of the dorsal arch of C1 is dissected. In this area, it is important to elevate the muscles subperiosteally. Cauterizing in this area is not recommended because of the thin membrane that attaches the base of the skull to the arch of atlas. Once exposure of the bony occipital protuberance, the dorsal arch of the atlas, and the remainder of the laminae of the cervical spine is accomplished, arthrodesis may be completed. This may be performed using the technique described previously by Grantham or modifications that were introduced by other authors.[8] With this technique, 24-gauge stainless-steel wires are used along with iliac crest bone graft that is contoured to span the distance from the occiput and the upper cervical lamina after the laminae and occiput are decorticated with a burr. Occipital plates or rods that are inserted into the lateral mass of C1 and C2 using screws may also be used to provide more rigid fixation.

Ventral Approaches

Indications for ventral approaches include ventral bony tumors with neural compression, extradural tumors, intradural midline lesions, and irreducible subluxations.[3,4,6,7,12] The ventral approach may also be used for repair of nonunion of C2 odontoid fractures and for odontoid resection.[16] The ventral aspect of the occipital-cervical junction may be approached via an extension of the ventral retropharyngeal/extrapharyngeal approach to the upper cervical spine or via a transoral approach.

Ventral Retropharyngeal Approach

The ventral retropharyngeal approach to the upper cervical spine has been described by Whitesides[19] and McAfee *et al.*[11] This approach allows exposure of the ventral aspect of the axis and atlas and also may allow exposure of the clivus and ventral aspect of the foramen magnum. Decompression and occipitocervical fusion may be performed through this approach.

Cortical somatosensory-evoked potentials may be measured. The patient is positioned on the operative wedge frame and the neck extended as far as allowed while the patient is awake without signs of neurological compromise. A modified transverse submandibular incision is used (Figure 21.6). The incision is made on the patient's right side, if the surgeon is right handed. This exposure is the rostral extension of the ventral lateral exposure to the mid-part of the cervical spine. The fascial planes that are dissected through are the same as that described in the ventral approach to the cervical spine, consisting of the superficial fascia and the deep fascia layers. The submandibular incision is made through the platysmal muscle, and the superficial fascia and skin is immobilized in the platysmal plane of the superficial fascia. The marginal mandibular branch of the fascial nerve is

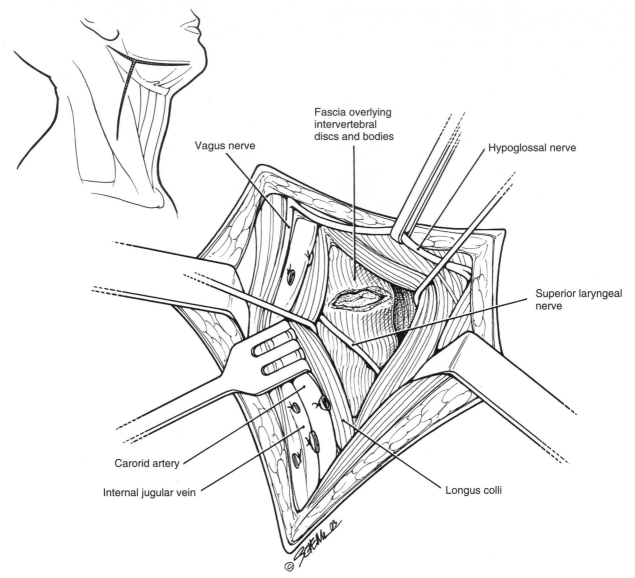

Figure 21.6 Surgical exposure of the occipital cervical region through an anterior retropharyngeal approach.

found with the aid of the nerve stimulator by ligating and dissecting the retromandibular veins superiorly. The common fascial vein is continuous with the retromandibular vein, and the branches of the mandibular nerve usually cross the latter vein superficially and superiorly. The superficial branches of the fascial nerve are protected. The ventral border of the sternocleidomastoid muscle is mobilized by longitudinally transecting the superficial layer of deep cervical fascia. The submandibular salivary gland is resected and the duct is sutured adequately to prevent the formation of a salivary fistula. The jugular-digastric lymph node from the submandibular and carotid angles can be resected and sent for frozen section if a neoplasm is in question. The dorsal belly of the digastric muscle and the stylohyoid muscle are identified and the digastric tendon is divided and tagged for later repair. As described by Whitesides[19] rostral traction at the base of the origin of the stylohyoid muscle can cause injury to the facial nerve as it exits from the skull. After the digastric and stylohyoid

muscles are divided, the hyoid bone and the hypopharynx are mobilized medially. The hypoglossal nerve, which is identified with a nerve stimulator, is then completely mobilized from the base of the skull to the anterior border of the hypoglossal muscle (Figure 21.6). It is retracted rostrally through the remainder of the procedure. The dissection then proceeds to the retropharyngeal space between the carotid sheath laterally and the pharynx medially. Rostral exposure to the atlas and the base of the skull is facilitated by ligating the branches of the carotid artery and internal jugular vein (Figure 21.6). The vessels to be ligated include, from caudally and progressing rostrally, the superior thyroid artery and vein, lingual artery and vein, ascending pharyngeal artery and vein, and facial artery and vein. After ligation, the carotid sheath is easily mobilized laterally. The superior pharyngeal nerve, which is also identified with the help of the nerve stimulator, is mobilized from its origin near the nodose ganglion to the entrance into the larynx. The alar and prevertebral fascia are transected longitudinally to expose the longus coli muscle that runs longitudinally. It is important at this point to maintain the orientation of the anterior tubercle of the atlas since rotation and lateral dissection may endanger the vertebral artery. The dissection along the prevertebral fascia may be extended cranially to reach the base of the skull and the clivus through this approach. Once this exposure is achieved, ventral decompression and, if needed, fusion of the occipital cervical junction may be initiated.

Transoral Approach

The transoral procedure allows exposure of the clivus, the arches of the atlas, and the ventral aspect of C2 (Figure 21.7). Adequate interdental distance (at least 25mm) is necessary for this exposure. If this is not achievable or there is a disease involving the temporal-mandibular joint, a transmandibular splitting approach or other more extensive approaches may be necessary.[17]

Preoperative management includes assessment of the interdental space. After this is found to be adequate, the dorsal pharynx should be cultured to allow adequate pre-operative antibiotic coverage. Palpation of the dorsal pharynx is then performed to identify the landmarks. This is performed after the dorsal pharynx is anesthetized with topical anesthetic to prevent the gag reflex. The anterior tubercle of C1 and the ventral body of C2 are palpable because they are directly dorsal to the mucous membrane. A tracheotomy is performed. Some authors avoid tracheotomy by using a nasal tracheal fiberoptic intubation while the patient is awake. The nasal tracheal tube does not impinge on the surgical field for lesions below the foramen magnum. They reserve tracheotomy for patients for whom long-term ventilatory problems are expected.[5,6] A nasogastric tube may be used to retract the uvula and soft palate to allow adequate exposure (Figure 21.8). The nasogastric tube is passed through the nose and out of the mouth to elevate the soft palate. Intraoral retractors are used to depress the tongue to allow better exposure. The uvula of the palate may also be sutured to the roof of the mouth, and the tongue is retracted inferiorly (Figure 21.8). Before the midline incision of the mucosa is made, the area is infiltrated with a 1:600,000 solution of epinephrine. The midline incision is then made, extending about 2cm above the anterior arches of the atlas and 2cm below the prominence of the arch. The desired structures can be accessed by retracting the mucosa laterally. This facilitates exposure of the clivus of the occiput, C1 and C2. The rotation of the atlas may be deceiving and the ventral aspect of the lateral mass may be mistakenly perceived as the anterior tubercle of the C1.[5] This will place the vertebral artery at risk of being injured; it also will come closer to the midline because the atlas is rotated. If access to the clivus more superiorly is needed, the hard palate may be split with a reciprocating saw to allow more access to the clivus. When access to the retropharyngeal space using the transoral approach is limited due to a transdental distance of less than 25mm or due to severe macroglossia, other approaches may be used. These include extended maxillotomy or mandibular osteotomy approaches.[9,10,17]

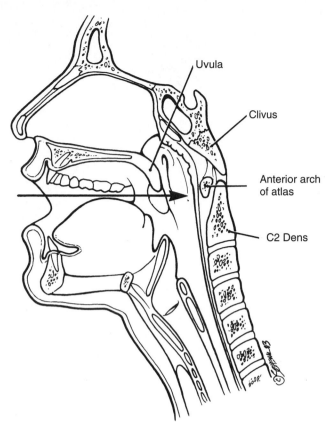

Figure 21.7 The clivus, ventral arch of C1, and dens are accessible through the transoral approach.

Extended Approaches to the Cranio-Cervical Junction

Extended Maxillotomy

James and Crockard[10] described surgical access to the base of the skull and upper cervical spine by extended maxillotomy. This provides a much wider surgical access to the base of the skull. With this technique, a tracheotomy and placement of the gastric tube is performed first. Next, the patient is positioned in the supine or the three-quarter supine position with some degree of neck extension to facilitate access to the palate. Surgical exposure of the cranial base is performed through an incision made above the mucogingival reflection from the first molar tooth on either side, and the soft tissues are reflected subperiosteally to expose the anterior and lateral walls in the maxilla (Figure 21.9). The osteotomy sites include (1) a transverse standard LeFort osteotomy cut that is made using an air-powered reciprocating saw, and (2) a sagittal cut that separates the two parts of the maxilla by sawing to the side of the midline suture (Figure 21.9). The bone between the central and incisor teeth is divided using a fine osteotome to avoid damage to the adjacent dental roots. This median section is completed with division of the soft palate in the midline. This exposure allows larger access to the clivus through which a clivectomy can be performed. Excision of tumors and approaches to aneurysms can also be performed through this exposure. Complete details of the procedure may be found in the technique described by James and Crockard.[10]

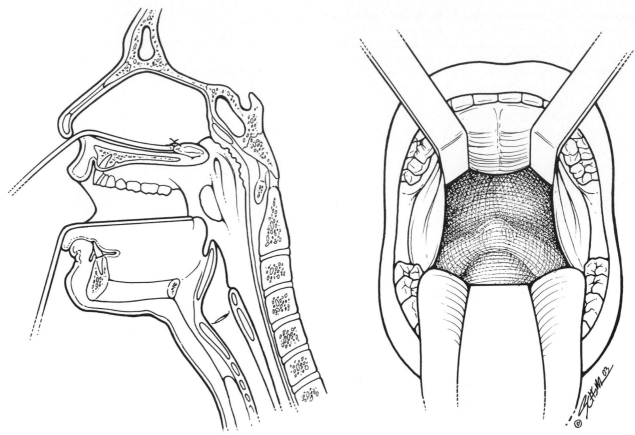

Figure 21.8 Placement of retractors for exposure during the transoral approach. The ventral arch of C1 and the dens may be palpated through the pharynx *(right)*.

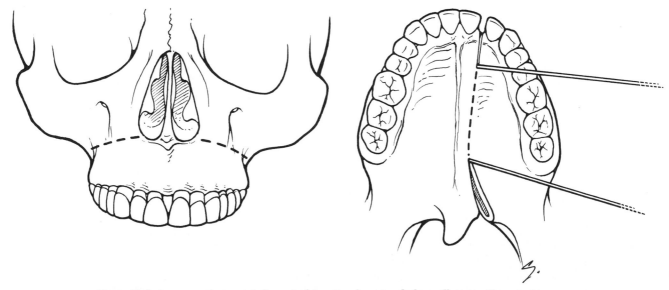

Figure 21.9 Access to the occipital cervical junction by extended maxillotomy. Transverse standard LeFort osteotomy *(left)* and sagittal cut to maxilla *(right)*.

Bilateral Sagittal Split Mandibular Osteotomy

Another approach that may be of use in gaining access to the retropharyngeal space when there is limited exposure may be the bilateral sagittal split mandibular osteotomy (as described by Vishteh *et al.*[17]). In their technique, the sagit-tal split mandibular osteotomy is performed on both sides of the mandible, as an adjunct to the transoral approach to the anterior cranio-vertebral junction. They described the osteotomy as a stair-step split mandibulotomy (Figure 21.10). Before the osteotomy is performed, a plate is

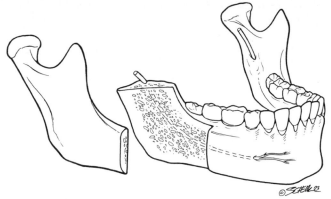

Figure 21.10 Bilateral sagittal split mandibular osteotomy.

placed in the appropriate position across the lateral osteotomy site on which the procedure is to be performed. A drill hole is made on each side and screws are placed. The remaining drill holes are drilled and the plate is removed and set aside. The osteotomy site courses through the lateral cortex medially above the lingula along the anterior border of the ramus lateral to the second and third molars and through the lateral cortex.

Transcondylar Approach to Cranial Vertebral Junction (Extreme Radial Cranial Cervical Approach)

Access to the cranial vertebral junction through a ventral approach sometimes has it limitations, including inadequate exposure, or inability to perform cranial cervical fusion; difficulty in reaching lateral located lesions; narrowing of the interdental distance less than 25mm and thereby limiting the exposure; and the risk of infection from a contaminated field. The extreme lateral/transcondylar approach has been described by al-Mefty et al[1] and Bejjani et al[2] to access extradural nonneoplastic lesions of the anterior cranial vertebral junction where decompression and stabilization are needed. The advantages of this approach include a more direct access to the lesion and direct visualization of the dural sac, eliminating manipulation of the brain stem or upper spinal cord. Identification and control of the ipsilateral vertebral artery is also facilitated, along with direct visualization and protection of the lower cranial nerves. This approach also provides a more sterile field than the transoral approach. Occipital cervical fusion and instrumentation can be performed during the same procedure as opposed to the transcondylar approach.

The patient is placed in a halo brace with his neck and head in the neutral position. The positioning of the patient is in the supine position with the entire body being rotated 45 degrees to the opposite side. Intubation is performed while the patient is awake. Intraoperative monitoring is also recommended, including bilateral somatosensory-evoked potentials, bilateral brain stem auditory-evoked response, and the cranial nerves 10, 11, and 12.[1] The skin incision begins behind the ear at the level of external auditory canal and extends medial to the midline and inferiorly to level of C4, where it curves anteriorly to reach the anterior border of the sternomastoid muscle. The skin flap is elevated ventrally. This exposes the greater auricular nerve

and the sternomastoid muscle. Blunt dissection is performed along the anterior border of the sternomastoid muscle and falls superiorly to the mastoid process where it is attached. The sternomastoid, splenius capitis, longissimus, and semi-spinalis muscles are detached from the mastoid in one layer and retracted. The eleventh cranial nerve must be identified and preserved where it enters the middle third of sternomastoid muscle. The dorsal belly of the digastric muscle is kept in place to protect the facial nerve as it exits the stylomastoid foramen. The deep muscular layer forms the suboccipital triangle, which is delineated by the major and minor rectus capitis muscles medially, the superior oblique muscle superiorly, and the inferior oblique muscle inferiorly. The apex of the triangle is the transverse process of C1. The horizontal segment of the vertebral artery and C1 root can be seen in this triangle. The C2 nerve root can be followed laterally where it crosses over the vertebral artery and its vertical segment between C1 and C2. The nerve root is protected. The vertebral artery is then identified from the transverse foramen of C2 to its entry to the dura mater. The vertebral artery is moved out of the foramen of C1 after this foramen is opened with a diamond drill, and the artery is then held inferomedially. The C1 nerve root may be sacrificed. After exposure is complete, the mastoid tip is drilled to expose the occipital condyle and the jugular bulb. The occipital condyle and the condylar surface of C1 are exposed widely and drilled out. The hypoglossal canal is then identified and the twelfth nerve is preserved. After the lateral bone structures are resected, the odontoid process and the surrounding ligaments are clearly seen. The odontoid process is drilled until the contralateral condyle is identified. In patients with severe odontoid invagination, the jugular bulb must be skeletonized to permit a more superior extension. Complete details of the procedure may be found in the technique described by al-Mefty et al.[1]

Salas et al.[14] described variations of the extreme lateral cranial cervical approach in an anatomical study and clinical analysis of 69 patients. The variations include the transfacet oral approach, the retrocondylar approach, the partial transcondylar approach, the complete transcondylar approach, the extreme lateral transjugular approach, and the transtubercular approach.[14,15] These are all variations to allow improved assess and exposure to the pathology, depending on the location of the pathology.

In summary, approaches to the cranio-cervical junction are not as frequent as surgery to the subaxial cervical spine. However, when the indication for surgery at the cranio-cervical junction arises, a thorough understanding of the anatomy and techniques of exposure is necessary to avoid injury of vital neurovascular structures that may be encountered during the approach. The approach will vary according to the location and type of the pathology and the need for stabilization.

REFERENCES

1. Al-Mefty O, Borba LA, Aoki N, *et al:* The transcondylar approach to extradural nonneoplastic lesions of the craniovertebral junction. *J Neurosurg* 84(1):1-6, 1996.

2. Bejjani GK, Sekhar LN, Riedel CJ: Occipitocervical fusion following the extreme lateral transcondylar approach. *Surg Neurol* 54(2):109-115, 2000.

3. Clark CR: Occipitocervical fusion for the unstable rheumatoid neck. *Orthopedics* 12:469-473, 1989.

4. Crockard HA: Midline ventral approaches to the craniocervical junction and upper cervical spine. *The Cervical Spine: An Atlas of Surgical Procedures,* Philadelphia, Lippincott, 1994, pp 93-112.

5. Crockard, HA: Anterior approaches to lesion of the upper cervical spine. *Clin Neurosurg* 34:389-416, 1988.

6. Crockard HA, Calder I, Ransford A: One-stage transoral decompression and posterior fixation in rheumatoid atlanto-axial subluxation. *J Bone Joint Surg* 72-B:682-685, 1990.

7. Crockard HA, Pozo JL, Ransford AP, *et al:* Transoral decompression and posterior fusion for rheumatoid atlanto-axial subluxation. *J Bone Joint Surg Br* 68(3):350-356, 1986.

8. Grantham SA, Dick HM, Thompson RC Jr, Stinchfield FE: Occipitocervical arthrodesis. Indications, technic and results. *Clin Orthop* 65:118-129, 1969.

9. Hall JE, Denis F, Murray J: Exposure of the upper cervical spine for spinal decompression by a mandible and tongue-splitting approach. *J Bone Joint Surg* 59:121-123, 1977.

10. James D, Crockard A: Surgical access to the base of skull and upper cervical spine by extended maxillotomy. *Neurosurgery* 29:411-416, 1991.

11. McAfee PC, Bohlman HH, Riley LH Jr, *et al:* The anterior retropharyngeal approach to the upper part of the cervical spine. *J Bone Joint Surg Am* 69:1371-1383, 1987.

12. Menezes AH, Traynelis VC, Gantz BJ: Surgical approaches to the craniovertebral junction. *Clin Neurosurg* 41:187-203, 1994.

13. Romanes GJ: *Cunningham's Manual of Practical Anatomy. Head and Neck and Brain.* London, Oxford University Press, 1967.

14. Salas E, Sekhar LN, Ziyal IM, *et al:* Variations of the extreme-lateral craniocervical approach: anatomical study and clinical analysis of 69 patients. *J Neurosurg* 90(4 Suppl):206-219, 1999.

15. Ture U, Pami MN: Extreme lateral-transatlas approach for resection of dens of the axis. *J Neurosurg* 96(1 Suppl): 73-82, 2002.

16. Vender JR, Harrison SJ, McDonnell DE: Fusion and instrumentation at C1-3 via the high anterior cervical approach. *J Neurosurg* 92(1 Suppl):24-29, 2000.

17. Vishteh AG, Beals SP, Joganic EF, *et al:* Bilateral sagittal split mandibular osteotomies as an adjunct to the transoral approach to the anterior craniovertebral junction. Technical note. *J Neurosurg* 90(4Suppl):267-270, 1999.

18. Wertheim SB, Bohlman HH: Occipitocervical fusion. Indications, technique, and long-term results in thirteen patients. *J Bone Joint Surg Am* 69(6):833-6, 1987.

19. Whitesides TE, Jr: Lateral retropharyngeal approach to the upper cervical spine. *Cervical Spine,* Philadelphia, Lippincott, 1983:517-527.

CHAPTER 22

The Cervical Spine and Cervicothoracic Junction

John W. German, Alexander J. Ghanayem, Edward C. Benzel, and Joseph T. Alexander

Cervical and Nuchal Anatomy

An understanding of anatomy is the most basic tenet of surgery. Because both ventral and dorsal approaches are commonly used when operating on the cervical spine, it is essential that the spine surgeon be familiar with the anatomy of both the cervical and nuchal regions.

Anatomic Overview of the Neck

Frick et al.[2] have presented an overview of the anatomy of the neck with the cervical spine as the centerpiece. Dorsal to the cervical spine lies the nuchal musculature, which is covered superficially by two large muscles: trapezius and the levator scapulae. Just ventral to the vertebral bodies lies the visceral space that contains elements of the alimentary, respiratory, and endocrine systems. The visceral space is surrounded by the cervical musculature and portions of the cervical fascia. Dorsolateral to the visceral space but separated from the visceral space, as well as the cervical musculature, lie the paired neurovascular conduction pathways. Thus, in this scheme, the neck may be divided into five distinct regions: cervical spine, nuchal musculature, visceral space, cervical musculature, and neurovascular conduction pathways.

Surface Anatomy of the Neck

Knowledge of the surface anatomy of the neck is essential when planning cervical spine surgery. These relationships help establish the site of the skin incision and dictate which vertebral level(s) may be approached.

The most prominent structure of the upper dorsal surface of the nuchal region is the inion. This may be palpated in the midline and is a part of the occipital bone. The spinous processes of the cervical vertebrae may then be followed caudally to the vertebrae prominence, variably corresponding to the spinous process of C7 (most common), C6, or T1.

The prominent surface structure of the ventral neck is the laryngeal prominence, which is produced by the underlying thyroid cartilage. The thyroid cartilage is composed of two broad plates that are readily palpable. This cartilage protects the vocal cords, which lie at the midpoint of the

ventral surface. Rostral to the thyroid cartilage lies the horseshoe-shaped hyoid bone, which is easy to palpate with the neck extended. The hyoid bone lies in the mouth-cervical angle[3] and mediates the muscular attachments of the muscles of the floor of the mouth (middle pharyngeal, hyoglossus, and genioglossus muscles) as well as those of the six hyoid muscles (stylohyoid, thyrohyoid, geniohyoid, omohyoid, mylohyoid, and sternohyoid). The hyoid bone provides some movement during swallowing. This, however, is limited caudally to the fourth cervical vertebral body by the stylohyoid ligament.[2] The transverse process of the atlas may be palpated at a point marked by a line between the angle of the mandible and a point 1cm ventrocaudal to the tip of the mastoid process.[3]

Caudal to the thyroid cartilage lies the signet-ring-shaped cricoid cartilage. The cricoid cartilage marks the laryngotracheal transition of the respiratory system and the pharyngoesophageal transition of the gastrointestinal system. Caudal to the cricoid cartilage lies the trachea. The isthmus of the thyroid gland overlies the first few rings of the trachea. This may make palpation of these rings difficult. The trachea may be followed caudally to the jugular notch, which is the rostral depression of the manubrium. Dorsally, the trachea may be palpated, while laterally the sternal heads of the sternocleidomastoid muscle may be palpated. The sternocleidomastoid muscle is the key landmark of the ventral neck, with respect to the traditional division of the neck into triangles.

Triangles of the Neck

The sternocleidomastoid muscle divides the neck into two large triangles: anterior and posterior, which are respectively subdivided into four and two triangles each. Knowledge of these triangles includes a definition of the borders and the contents of each triangle (Figure 22.1).

The borders of the posterior or dorsal triangle are the dorsal edge of the sternocleidomastoid muscle, the ventral edge of the trapezius muscle, and the middle third of the clavicle. The deep cervical fascia covers the dorsal cervical triangle, thus forming its roof. The floor of the dorsal cervical triangle is formed by the scalenus posterior, scalenus medius, levator scapulae, and splenius capitis muscles, as well as the lateral extension of the prevertebral fascia that overlies these muscles. The dorsal belly of the omohyoid muscle partitions the dorsal cervical triangle into a large rostral occipital triangle named for the occipital artery exiting at its apex and a small caudal subclavian triangle named for the subclavian artery, which lies deep to it.

The spinal accessory nerve leaves the deep surface of the sternocleidomastoid muscle to enter the dorsal triangle of the neck, which it crosses to innervate the trapezius muscle. The two important structures found in the dorsal cervical triangle, which arise above the spinal accessory nerve, are the occipital artery and the lesser occipital nerve. The occipital artery leaves the dorsal cervical triangle at its apex where the sternocleidomastoid and trapezius muscles approach one another on the superior nuchal line. This artery then ascends to supply the dorsal scalp. The lesser occipital nerve ascends along the dorsal surface of the sternocleidomastoid muscle before ramifying into several superficial branches that supply the scalp dorsal to the ear.

Caudal to the spinal accessory nerve are many important anatomic structures. The external jugular vein, which is formed by the confluence of the posterior auricular and the posterior division of the retromandibular vein at the angle of the mandible, courses over the sternocleidomastoid muscle obliquely to enter the dorsal cervical triangle caudally, en route to joining the subclavian vein approximately 2cm above the clavicle.[3] Two branches of the thy-

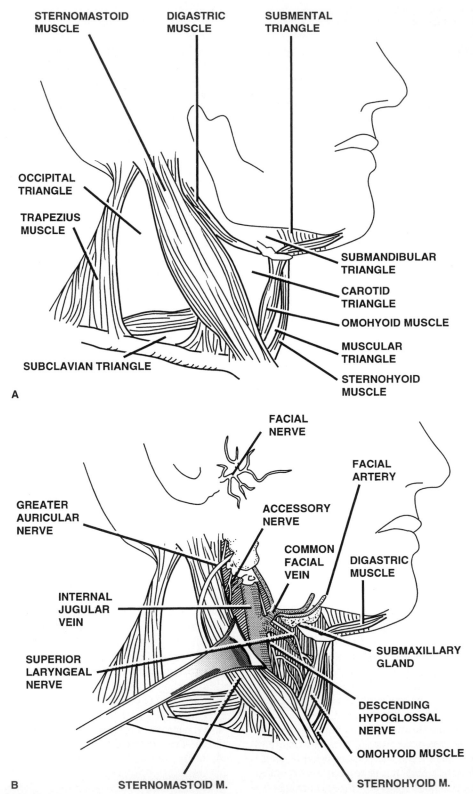

Figure 22.1 (**A**) Cervical triangles. (**B**) Carotid triangle and its contents. (*Copyright University of New Mexico, Division of Neurosurgery, Albuquerque, NM, with permission.*)

rocervical trunk cross the dorsal cervical triangle. The suprascapular artery runs rostral to the clavicle before passing deep to the clavicle to supply the periscapular muscles. The transverse cervical artery lies 2 to 3cm rostral to the clavicle and also runs laterally across the dorsal cervical triangle to supply the periscapular muscles.

Three superficial nerves also exit the dorsal triangle below the spinal accessory nerve. In all cases, these nerves arise from the cervical plexus, which is formed by the ventral rami of the rostral four cervical spinal nerves. The plexus lies within the lateral neurovascular conduction pathways located between the internal jugular vein and the sternocleidomastoid muscle. The superficial nerves then arise along the middle portion of the dorsal border of the sternocleidomastoid muscle to supply the skin of the neck and scalp between the mastoid process and the inion. The great auricular nerve crosses the sternocleidomastoid muscle and ascends toward the parotid gland, branching into dorsal and ventral rami that supply the skin in an area stretching from the angle of the mandible to the mastoid process and the skin of the neck. The transverse cervical nerve also crosses the sternocleidomastoid muscle to supply the skin overlying the ventral cervical triangle. The supraclavicular nerves arise from a single trunk that trifurcates into lateral, intermediate, and medial branches that innervate the skin of the neck, ventral chest, ventral shoulder, sternoclavicular joint, and acromioclavicular joint. The phrenic nerve arises, in part, from the cervical plexus and, in part, from the brachial plexus. The brachial nerve arises near the scalenus anterior muscle, where it crosses ventromedially and deep to the transverse cervical and suprascapular arteries and the prevertebral fascia, to descend through the superior thoracic aperture near the origin of the internal mammary artery. The upper, middle, and lower trunks of the brachial plexus lie deep to the floor of the posterior cervical triangle. They emerge between the scalenus medius and scalenus anterior muscles and cross deep to the transverse cervical and suprascapular arteries to descend under the clavicle to enter the axilla.

The borders of the anterior or ventral cervical triangle are the ventral edge of the sternocleidomastoid muscle, the inferior border of the mandible, and the midline of the neck. The ventral cervical triangle may be subdivided into four smaller triangles: submental, submandibular, carotid, and muscular.

The submental triangle is bounded by the hyoid body and laterally by the ventral bellies of the right and left digastric muscles. This triangle has, as its floor, the two mylohyoid muscles that connect to each other in the midline by forming a median raphe. Within this triangle lie the submental lymph nodes that drain the ventral tongue, the floor of the oral cavity, the middle portion of the lower lip and the skin of the chin, and several small veins that ultimately converge to form the anterior jugular vein.

The boundaries of the submandibular triangle are the anterior and posterior bellies of the digastric muscle and the inferior border of the mandible. The floor of the submandibular triangle is formed by the mylohyoid, hyoglossus, and middle constrictor muscles. The submandibular gland fills a significant portion of this triangle, and its duct passes parallel to the tongue to open into the mouth. The

hypoglossal nerve also passes into this triangle along with the nerve to the mylohyoid muscle, a branch of the inferior alveolar nerve, and portions of the facial artery and vein.

The carotid triangle is bounded by the ventral border of the sternocleidomastoid muscle, the rostral edge of the rostral belly of the omohyoid muscle, and the caudal edge of the dorsal belly of the digastric muscle. Within the carotid triangle lie the bifurcation of the common carotid artery, the internal jugular vein laterally, the vagus nerve dorsally, and the ansa cervicalis (Figure 22.1B).

The muscular triangle is bounded by the median plane of the neck, the caudal edge of the rostral belly of the omohyoid muscle, and the medial border of the sternocleidomastoid muscle. Within this triangle lie the infrahyoid muscles and neck viscera.

Cervical Fascia

An understanding of the cervical fascia aids the surgeon approaching a targeted cervical spine level by providing an avascular plane of dissection. There are three layers of the cervical fascia: investing, visceral, and prevertebral (Figure 22.2). The investing fascia surrounds the entire neck, splitting to enclose the sternocleidomastoid and trapezius muscles and the submandibular and parotid glands. Rostrally, the investing fascia is connected to the hyoid bone, the caudal border of the mandible, the zygomatic arch, the mastoid process, and the superior nuchal line. Caudally, the investing fascia splits to attach to the ventral and dorsal surfaces of the sternum, thus forming the suprasternal space.[3] The investing fascia forms the roof of both the ventral and dorsal cervical triangles.

The visceral, or pretracheal, fascia courses deep to the infrahyoid muscles and surrounds the visceral space, including the thyroid gland, trachea, and esophagus. The visceral fascia is attached to the hyoid bone and the thyroid cartilage rostrally and extends caudally to the dorsal surface of the clavicles and sternum and into the mediastinum. Laterally, this layer blends into the carotid sheath. The thyroid vessels are located deep to this layer.

The prevertebral layer of cervical fascia surrounds the vertebral column and its musculature, including the scalene and longus groups of muscles. Ventral to the vertebral bodies, the prevertebral fascia splits into a ventral alar layer and a dorsal prevertebral layer, forming a potential space. This space is referred to as the "danger zone" because it extends from the skull base rostrally to the level of T12 caudally and communicates with the mediastinum. Within the prevertebral fascia, and in front of the longus colli muscle, lies the cervical portion of the sympathetic chain. This usually consists of three cervical ganglia that lie at the levels of the first rib, the transverse process of C6, and the atlantoaxial complex. Fibers from the superior cervical ganglia pass to the internal carotid artery to innervate the pupil. Interruption of the sympathetic trunk in the neck results in an ipsilateral Horner's syndrome.

Cervical Musculature

The cervical musculature is divided into two layers: superficial and deep. The muscles of the superficial layer

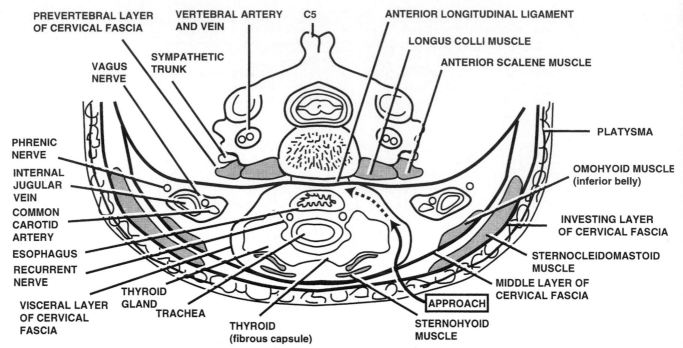

Figure 22.2 Cervical fascia. (*Copyright University of New Mexico, Division of Neurosurgery, Albuquerque, NM, with permission.*)

include the platysma, the sternocleidomastoid, and the infrahyoid group. The platysma lies just under the surface of the skin and is one of the muscles of facial expression, innervated by the cervical ramus of the seventh cranial nerve. It is draped like an apron from the mandible to the level of the second rib and laterally as far as the acromion processes. The sternocleidomastoid muscle arises from the region of the jugular notch and courses rostrolaterally to the mastoid process. It is dually innervated by the 11th cranial nerve, and ventral branches of the C2-4 spinal nerves. The spinal accessory nerve enters the deep surface of the muscle at the border of the middle and rostral thirds. The two main actions of the sternocleidomastoid muscle are to turn the head to the contralateral side and to flex the head ipsilaterally. The infrahyoid group represents the rostral continuation of the rectus muscular system of the trunk.[2] This group contains four muscles: sternohyoid, sternothyroid, omohyoid, and thyrohyoid. The first three members of this group are innervated by the ansa cervicalis, and the thyrohyoid receives its innervation from the C1 spinal nerve via the hypoglossal nerve. The main actions of the infrahyoid group are to assist in swallowing and mastication. This group, together with the suprahyoid group, determines the rostrocaudal location of the larynx between the hyoid bone and the rostral thoracic aperture and can help flex the cervical spine and lower the head.

The deep layer of cervical musculature includes two groups: scalene and longus groups. The scalene group includes three muscles: anterior, medius, and posterior. These muscles form a roof over the cupula of the lung. As a group, these muscles arise from the transverse processes of the subaxial cervical spine and project to the first and second ribs. The scalene muscles are innervated by the ventral rami of C4-8. They help to elevate the rib cage during respiration. The longus group also includes three

muscles: rectus capitis anterior, longus capitis, and longus colli (Figure 22.3). As a group, these muscles arise from the ventral vertebral body, transverse processes, and basilar portion of the occiput, and project caudally along the ventrolateral aspects of the cervical and upper thoracic vertebral bodies. These muscles are innervated by the ventral rami of C1-6, and their main action is to flex the head and the cervical spine.

Cervical Viscera

The cervical viscera are arranged in three layers: a deep gastrointestinal layer, containing the pharynx and esophagus; a middle respiratory layer, containing the larynx and trachea; and a superficial endocrine layer, containing the thyroid and parathyroid glands. These structures are not covered in detail and much of the anatomy of the larynx and trachea has already been described in other sections of this chapter. As previously noted, these structures are contained within the visceral or pretracheal fascia.

The pharynx is a fibromuscular tube that projects from the pharyngeal tubercle of the clivus to its transition into the esophagus near the level of C6. The dorsal surface of the pharynx lies on the prevertebral fascia and must be mobilized during ventral approaches to the cervical spine. The muscles of the pharynx may be divided into two groups: constrictors and internal muscles of the pharynx. The constrictor group includes three muscles whose main action is to sequentially constrict the pharynx during swallowing, thus propelling food caudally. All of the constrictors are innervated by the pharyngeal plexus, which receives its branches from both the glossopharyngeal and vagus nerves. The constrictors do not form a continuous tube but are open at four points, allowing certain structures to pass into the pharynx. Rostral to the superior con-

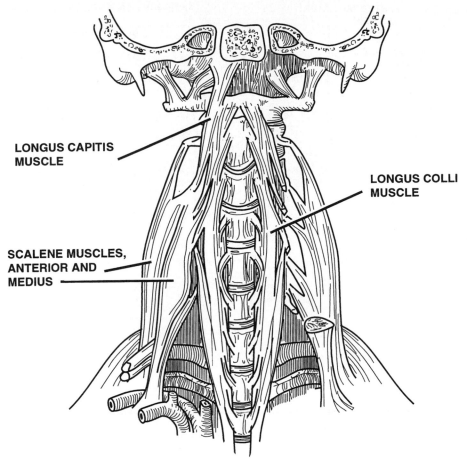

Figure 22.3 The scalene and longus muscles. (*Copyright University of New Mexico, Division of Neurosurgery, Albuquerque, NM, with permission.*)

strictor, the ascending palatine artery, the eustachian tube, and the levator veli palatini muscles pass to enter the pharynx. Between the superior and inferior constrictors pass the glossopharyngeal nerve, the stylohyoid ligament, and the stylopharyngeus muscle. In the gap between the middle and inferior constrictors pass the internal laryngeal nerve and the superior laryngeal artery and vein. Caudal to the inferior constrictor pass the recurrent laryngeal nerve and the inferior laryngeal artery. The internal muscle groups of the pharynx have a common function of elevating the larynx and pharynx during swallowing and a common innervation by the glossopharyngeal nerve. At the level of C6, the pharynx blends into the esophagus, which passes through the superior thoracic aperture to the stomach. In the root of the neck, the esophagus is in close approximation to the thoracic duct as it empties into the left subclavian vein.

The isthmus of the thyroid gland usually overlies the first two or three tracheal rings. The isthmus is the center bridge of glandular tissue that connects the right and left lobes. The entire gland is surrounded by a fibrous capsule, which should be differentiated from the pretracheal fascia. The thyroid gland is heavily vascularized and receives its blood supply from the superior and inferior thyroid arteries, which are branches of the external carotid and thyrocervical arteries, respectively. The recurrent laryngeal nerve is in close approximation to the inferior thyroid

artery, and if this artery must be ligated, it is best ligated at a distance from the thyroid gland to avoid the nerve. A similar relationship exists between the superior thyroid artery and the external laryngeal nerve, again dictating arterial ligation distal from the substance of the gland. The thyroid gland is drained by the superior, middle, and inferior thyroid veins. The inferior thyroid veins may cover the ventral surface of the trachea and represent a potential source of bleeding during tracheotomy.

Conduction Pathways

There are two major neurovascular conduction pathways within the neck: cervicocranial and cervicobrachial (Figure 22.4). The cervicocranial neurovascular bundle is outlined by the carotid sheath, which contains the common carotid artery medially, the internal jugular vein laterally, the vagus nerve dorsally, and the lymphatic plexus. As a whole, the cervicocranial neurovascular bundle lies lateral to the visceral space and ventral to the prevertebral fascia. The bundle passes rostrally from the thorax and enters the carotid triangle, where the common carotid artery bifurcates into the internal carotid artery dorsolaterally and the external carotid artery ventromedially. Within the carotid triangle, the external carotid artery provides a total of eight branches: three ventral, one medial, two dorsal, and two terminal. The ventral

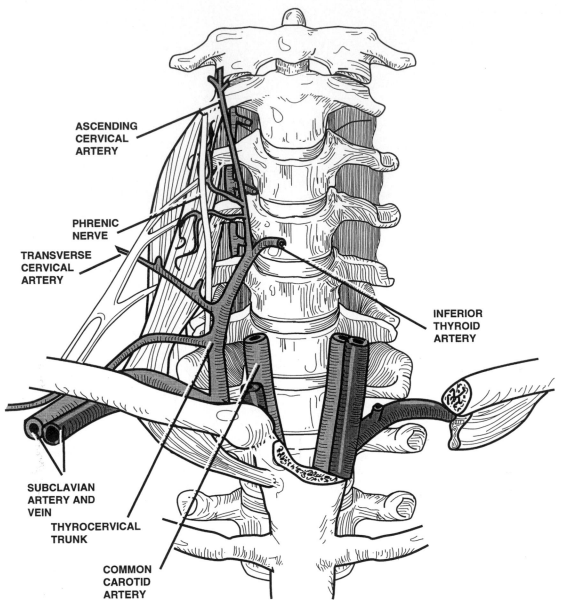

Figure 22.4 The conduction pathways. (*Copyright University of New Mexico, Division of Neurosurgery, Albuquerque, NM, with permission.*)

branches include the superior thyroid, lingual, and facial arteries. The superior thyroid artery descends from its origin caudal to the greater cornu of the hyoid to supply the thyroid gland. The lingual artery also arises at the level of the greater cornu of the hyoid bone and crosses under the hyoglossus muscle to supply the tongue. The facial artery is the final ventral branch of the external carotid artery. It runs under the submandibular gland before crossing the mandible and arriving to supply the face at the ventral surface of the masseter muscle. The sole medial branch is the ascending pharyngeal artery, which arises from the medial external carotid artery to supply the pharyngeal wall. The two dorsal branches are the posterior auricular and occipital arteries. The posterior auricular artery runs from underneath the parotid gland to the mastoid process. The occipital artery also reaches the mastoid but on its medial aspect in the groove named for the artery. The two termi-

nal branches are the superficial temporal and maxillary arteries. The internal jugular vein originates in the jugular foramen as the superior bulb turns dorsolaterally to enter the carotid sheath lateral to the common carotid artery. It eventually drains into the subclavian vein.

Five of the cranial nerves—the facial, glossopharyngeal, vagus, spinal accessory, and hypoglossal—traverse the neck. The facial nerve exits the skull at the stylomastoid foramen and ramifies into five branches within the parotid gland. The most caudal branch, the marginal mandibular, courses under the mandible and may be encountered in retropharyngeal approaches. Damage to this ramus results in the drooping of the ipsilateral lip. Arising from the jugular foramen are the vagus, glossopharyngeal, and spinal accessory nerves. The vagus travels dorsally in the carotid sheath and gives off two important branches that run in the neck to supply the larynx.

The superior laryngeal nerve exits just below the inferior vagal ganglion and bifurcates into a small external laryngeal nerve that supplies the motor innervation to the inferior pharyngeal constrictor and cricothyroid muscles. This nerve also bifurcates into a large internal laryngeal branch that receives the sensory input of the laryngeal mucosa above the glottis. Damage to the superior laryngeal nerve results in early fatigue of voice, difficulty in producing high notes, and decreased gag reflex resulting in a risk of aspiration. Both inferior laryngeal nerves ascend from the thorax in the tracheoesophageal groove, enter the inferior pharyngeal constrictor to supply motor innervation to the intrinsic laryngeal muscles, and receive all sensory innervation below the glottis. Damage to the inferior laryngeal nerve results in hoarseness. The glossopharyngeal nerve exits the skull from the jugular foramen in close approximation to the vagus nerve and courses between the internal carotid artery and the internal jugular vein before passing between the stylopharyngeus and styloglossus muscles to enter the base of the tongue. The caudal ganglion of the glossopharyngeal nerve has two branches. The tympanic nerve, which supplies sensory innervation to the tympanic mucosa, divides into the tympanic plexus, from which the lesser petrosal parasympathetic fibers form to supply the otic ganglion. The communicating rami join the auricular ramus of the vagus. Below the inferior ganglion, the glossopharyngeal divides into the following branches: the stylopharyngeus ramus, the carotid sinus ramus, the tonsillar ramus, the lingual ramus, and the pharyngeal ramus. Both the vagus nerve and the glossopharyngeal nerve contribute to the pharyngeal plexus, which mediates motor and sensory innervation of the pharynx. The spinal accessory nerve traverses the rostrodorsal corner of the carotid triangle to reach the deep surface of the sternocleidomastoid muscle one third of the distance from the mastoid to the clavicle and then continues through the occipital triangle to supply the trapezius muscle. The hypoglossal nerve exits the skull from the hypoglossal canal, enters the carotid triangle deep to the dorsal belly of the digastric, and courses between the carotid artery and the internal jugular vein before turning medially to enter the substance of the tongue. The hypoglossal nerve gives off the superior branch to the ansa cervicalis, which innervates the strap muscles and may be divided at the time of surgery.

The other major neurovascular conduction pathway is the cervicobrachial pathway, which supplies the upper extremities. The subclavian artery and the components of the brachial plexus exit the neck over the first rib and between the anterior and middle scalene muscles and then proceed through the posterior triangle of the neck to enter the axilla. The subclavian artery gives off the following arteries: vertebral, thyrocervical, internal thoracic, costocervical, and dorsal scapular. The vertebral artery is the vessel of most interest to the spine surgeon (Figure 22.5). It arises from the dorsal aspect of the subclavian artery and courses medial to the anterior scalenus to enter the foramen transversarium of the sixth cervical vertebra. It then ascends in the foramen transversarium until the level of the axis, where it courses medially in a groove bearing its name and through the atlantooccipital membrane to enter the cranial cavity. The subclavian vein runs ventral to the artery and to the scalenus anterior muscle just under the clavicle.

Nuchal Musculature

The intrinsic musculature of the dorsal neck may be divided into three layers: superficial, intermediate, and deep (Figure 22.6). All of these muscles are innervated by the dorsal rami of several consecutive spinal nerves. The superficial layer contains the splenius capitis and the splenius cervicalis, which take their origin from the ligamentum nuchae and the spinous processes of C6-T1. The splenius capitis inserts along the lateral third of the superior nuchal line and on the mastoid process. The splenius cervicalis muscle inserts into the posterior tubercles of the transverse processes of C1-4. These muscles may produce extension, lateral bending, and rotation of the head or neck.

The intermediate layer is composed of the massive erector spinae group, of which there are three columns: spinalis medially, iliocostalis laterally, and longissimus muscle between. All three columns share a common origin from the iliac crest, sacrum, and caudal lumbar spinous processes. The spinalis group inserts along the spinous processes of the cervical spine. The longissimus group inserts onto the mastoid process, and the iliocostalis group inserts into the posterior tubercles of the transverse processes of C4-6. As a group, the erector spinae muscles may extend or laterally bend the head or neck.

The deep layer of spinal musculature is also termed the transversospinalis group because it lies in the angle of the spinous and transverse processes. This layer is divided into three groups of muscles. The semispinalis group lies most superficially and has both capitis and cervicalis divisions. The semispinalis capitis muscle arises from the transverse processes of T1-6 and inserts medially between the superior and inferior nuchal lines. The semispinalis cervicalis muscle originates from the transverse processes of the lower cervical and upper thoracic spine and inserts on the cervical spinous processes. Beneath the semispinalis division lies the multifidus division, which are short muscles that span only one to three spinal segments. These muscles pass from the lamina caudally to the spinous process of adjacent levels. The deepest division of the transversospinalis group are the rotators that arise from the transverse process of one vertebral level and insert on the base of the spinous process at the adjacent rostral level. As a group, the transversospinalis muscles may rotate and extend the head or neck.

Spinal Anatomy

The upper cervical spine is characterized by the axis and its "anatomical neighbors"(Figure 22.7). The subaxial cervical spine varies minimally from level to level, and is discussed as a single unit (Figure 22.8). The components of the subaxial vertebrae include: body, upper and lower articular processes, pedicles, lamina, and spinous process. The vertebral bodies are the axial load-bearing elements of the spine. In the subaxial cervical spine the vertebral body height increases as the spine is descended with a slight reversal of this relationship at C6, which is usually shorter than either C5 or C7. Each body has a dorsally directed concavity, which forms the ventral spinal canal.

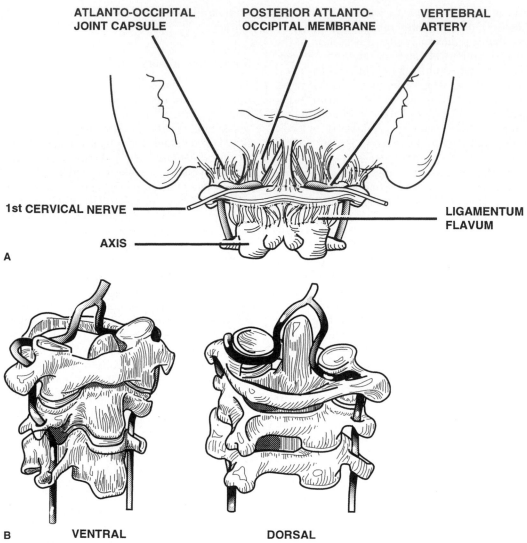

ATLANTO-OCCIPITAL
JOINT CAPSULE

POSTERIOR ATLANTO-
OCCIPITAL MEMBRANE

VERTEBRAL
ARTERY

1st CERVICAL NERVE

AXIS

LIGAMENTUM
FLAVUM

A

B   VENTRAL   DORSAL

Figure 22.5 The cervicocranium and the vertebral artery relationships. **(A)** Dorsal soft tissue and bony relationships of the vertebral artery and **(B)** ventral *(left)*, dorsal *(right)*, and bony relationships of the vertebral artery. *(Copyright University of New Mexico, Division of Neurosurgery, Albuquerque, NM, with permission.)*

From each body arise three body projections: rostrally the uncus, laterally the ventral ramus of the transverse process, and dorsolaterally the pedicle.

The rostral aspect of each of the lower cervical vertebral bodies contains the uncus, a dorsolateral bony projection. The uncus gives the body a rostrally concave shape in the coronal plane and enables the vertebral body to receive the rounded caudal aspect of the immediately adjacent vertebrae body, sometimes overlapping the next level by a third of the vertebral body height. The uncovertebral joints limit lateral translation and contribute to the coupling of lateral bending and rotation of the cervical spine.

The anterior tubercle arises from the rostral vertebral body and projects laterally while the posterior tubercle arises from midportion of the lateral mass and projects ventromedially to join the anterior tubercle. The lateral surface of the pedicle, the dorsal surface of the anterior tubercle, and the ventral surface of the posterior tubercle form the foramen transversarium that transmits the vertebral artery from C6 to the atlas. The anterior scalene,

longus colli capitis, longus colli cervicalis, and ventral intertransversus muscles take their origin from the anterior tubercles. The splenius cervicalis, longissimus, levator scapulae, middle scalene, posterior scalene, and iliocostalis take their origin from the posterior tubercle. On the rostral surface of each transverse process there is a prominent groove carrying the exiting nerve root.

The pedicles of the subaxial cervical spine connect the vertebral bodies with the lateral masses and are small and medially oriented. The lateral masses of the subaxial cervical spine consist of a superior and inferior articulating surface that form the facet joint. The facet joint is a coronally oriented synovial joint that is protected by a thin capsule. The vascular supply to the joint capsule arises from the vertebral, ascending pharyngeal, deep transverse cervical, supreme intercostal, and occipital arteries. The facet joints are innervated by the dorsal branches of the spinal nerves, which enter the joint at the center of the dorsal capsule. The laminae are thin and the spinous processes of the midcervical spine are small and often bifid.

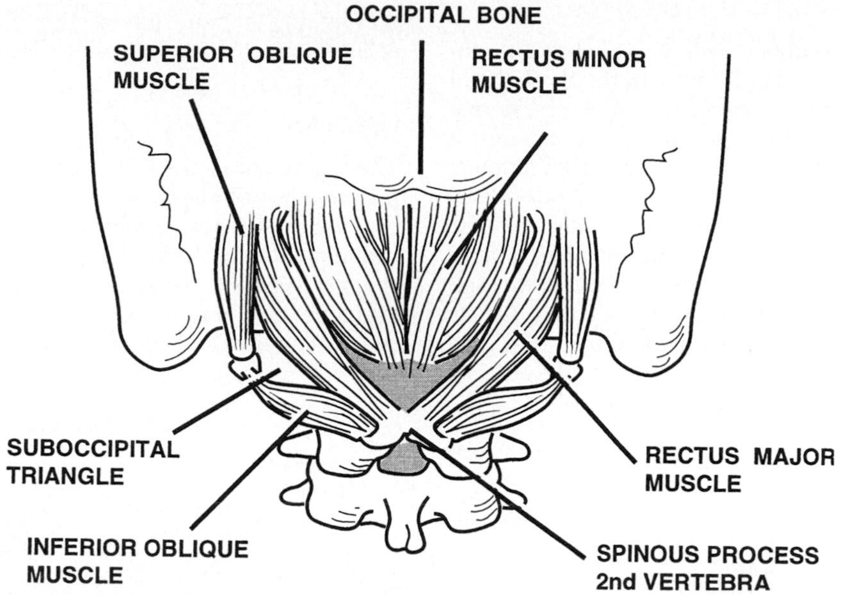

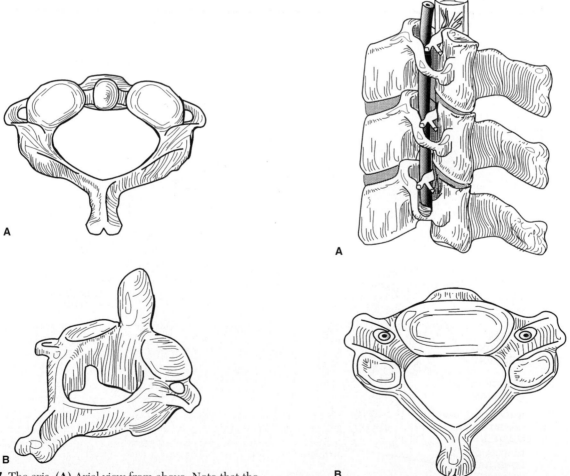

OCCIPITAL BONE

SUPERIOR OBLIQUE MUSCLE

RECTUS MINOR MUSCLE

SUBOCCIPITAL TRIANGLE

RECTUS MAJOR MUSCLE

INFERIOR OBLIQUE MUSCLE

SPINOUS PROCESS 2nd VERTEBRA

Figure 22.6 The suboccipital region. (*Copyright University of New Mexico, Division of Neurosurgery, Albuquerque, NM, with permission.*)

A

B

Figure 22.7 The axis. (**A**) Axial view from above. Note that the articular facets and odontoid are anterior to the spinal canal. (**B**) Posterior view. (*Copyright University of New Mexico, Division of Neurosurgery, Albuquerque, NM, with permission.*)

A

B

Figure 22.8 The subaxial spine. (**A**) Lateral and (**B**) axial views. (*Copyright University of New Mexico, Division of Neurosurgery, Albuquerque, NM, with permission.*)

Discs

The intervertebral discs adjoin each of the subaxial verte-bral bodies and contribute significantly to the flexibility of the spine. The cartilaginous end plates of the bordering vertebral bodies are the rostral and caudal boundaries of the disc space, and the anterior and posterior longitudinal ligaments overlie, respectively, the ventral and dorsal sur-faces of the intervertebral disc space. Laterally, the disc space is limited by the uncal process. The end plate is more substantial on its periphery than centrally and is composed of hyaline cartilage. The disc itself is composed of the gelat-inous nucleus pulposus surrounded by a fibrous ring. The fibrous ring contains intersecting layers of predominantly collagen and, to a lesser extent, elastin fibers.

Ligaments

The ligaments of the cervical spine are essential for the maintenance of alignment and stability. The ligaments of the subaxial spine include the anterior longitudinal ligament, the posterior longitudinal ligament, the inter-spinous ligament, the supraspinous ligament, the capsular ligaments, ligamentum flavum, and the intertransverse lig-aments (Figures 22.9 and 22.10). The anterior longitudinal

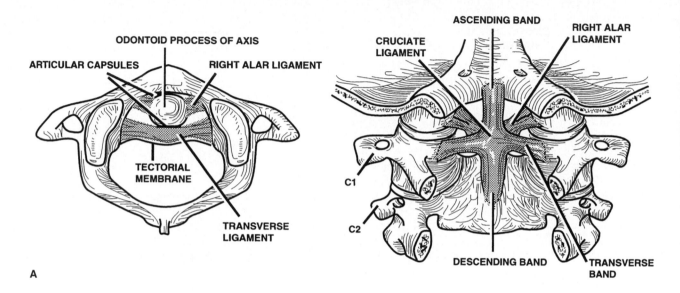

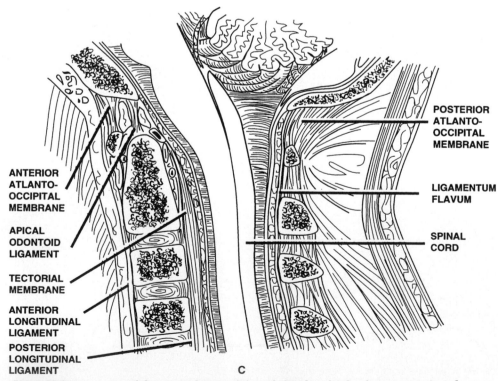

Figure 22.9 Ligaments of the cervical spine: (**A**) axial, (**B**) dorsal (after laminectomy), and (**C**) midsagittal views. (*Copyright University of New Mexico, Division of Neurosurgery, Albuquerque, NM, with permission.*)

ligament is attached to the ventral surfaces of the vertebral bodies and the intervening discs. It spans the entire length of the spine from the skull base to the sacrum. The main biomechanical feature of the anterior longitudinal ligament is resistance of hyperextension. The superficial fibers extend four or five vertebral bodies and the deep fibers span two vertebral bodies.

The posterior longitudinal ligament is attached to the discs on the dorsal surface of the vertebral bodies and rostrally fans out to become continuous with the tectorial membrane. The main biomechanical effect of the posterior longitudinal ligament is resistance of hyperflexion. The interspinous and supraspinous ligaments attach adjacent spinous processes and are represented in the cervical region as the ligamentum nuchae, which runs from the inion to the spinous process of C7. This fibromuscular septum divides the paraspinal muscles and serves as an attachment site for the nuchal musculature. This represents the midline avascular plane, which may be transversed when exposing the dorsal cervical spine. These ligaments can limit flexion to a significant degree because of their long lever arm, with respect to the instantaneous axis of rotation. The capsular ligaments are loose under normal cervical spine movement and become taut with movement, thus limiting excessive flexion and rotation. The ligamentum flavum is an elastic ligament that traverses adjacent lamina in a shingle-like fashion, arising from a ridge on the inner surface of the lamina and projecting to the inner surface of the next rostral lamina. The intertransverse ligaments connect adjacent transverse processes, which have little biomechanical effect in the cervical spine.

Intervertebral Foramen

The cervical spinal nerves exit from the spinal canal through the intervertebral foramen. True foramina, with four distinct walls, are found in the subaxial cervical spine, and partial foramina are present at the atlantooccipital and atlantoaxial levels.

The pedicles form the rostral and caudal boundaries of each foramen. The cervical spinal nerves exit above the like-numbered pedicle in close proximity to both the cervical disc and the uncovertebral joint at that level. The ventral wall of the intervertebral foramen is formed rostrally by the vertebral body and caudally by the uncovertebral joint that overlies the disc space. The dorsal wall is formed by the capsule of the facet joint, which covers the underlying superior articular process. The superior articular process often projects above the uncal process of the same intervertebral foramen. Degeneration of either the uncovertebral joint or the facet joint can cause stenosis of the intervertebral foramen, resulting in radiculopathy. The spinal nerve crosses dorsally to the vertebral artery as it ascends in the foramen transversarium.

Blood Supply

The blood supply of the subaxial cervical spine is derived mainly from the vertebral artery with additional and variable contributions from the ascending pharyngeal, occipital, and deep cervical arteries.

The vertebral artery branches segmentally to supply the cervical spine through two main branches: ventral branch and dorsal branch. The ventral branch is transmitted

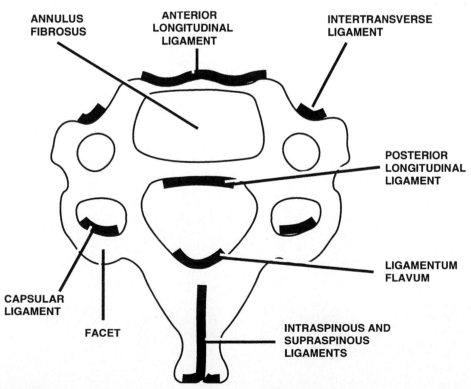

ANNULUS FIBROSUS

ANTERIOR LONGITUDINAL LIGAMENT

INTERTRANSVERSE LIGAMENT

POSTERIOR LONGITUDINAL LIGAMENT

LIGAMENTUM FLAVUM

CAPSULAR LIGAMENT

FACET

INTRASPINOUS AND SUPRASPINOUS LIGAMENTS

Figure 22.10 Ligaments of the subaxial cervical spine (axial view). (*Copyright University of New Mexico, Division of Neurosurgery, Albuquerque, NM, with permission.*)

across the midportion of the lateral surface of the vertebral bodies below the transverse process and below the longus colli muscles. It contributes to the blood supply of the ventral vertebral body through the accompanying ventral vertebral body arterial plexus.

The dorsal branch enters the intervertebral foramen and, in turn, gives off three branches. The first is transmitted along the nerve roots and supplies the spinal cord itself, anastomosing with the anterior and posterior spinal arteries. The second branch supplies the inner surface of the lamina and the ligamentum flavum. The third branch contributes to the blood supply of the dorsal vertebral body through the accompanying dorsal vertebral body arterial plexus, which passes underneath the posterior longitudinal ligament.

The venous drainage of the cervical spine includes an internal and external system. The internal vertebral venous plexus (Batson's plexus) extends from the coccyx to the occiput. It consists of numerous small valveless veins that run ventral and dorsal to the thecal sac and merge at the intervertebral foramen. The internal system then exits the spinal canal along the nerve roots and flows into the external vertebral plexus, which is represented in the cervical region by the vertebral veins. The vertebral veins form a peripheral veil around the vertebral artery and, subsequently, anastomose with the condylar, mastoid, occipital, and posterior jugular veins.

REFERENCES

1. Alexander JT: Cervical spine and skull base anatomy. In Benzel EC (ed): *Surgical Exposures of the Spine: An Extensile Approach*. AANS, Park Ridge, IL, 1995, pp 1-19.
2. Frick H, Leonhardt H, Starck D: *Human Anatomy 1*. Stuttgart, Thieme, 1991.
3. Lang J: *Clinical Anatomy of the Cervical Spine*. Stuttgart, Thieme, 1993.
4. Moore KL: *Clinically Oriented Anatomy*. Baltimore, Williams & Wilkins, 1992.

CHAPTER 23

Thoracic Spine

Stephen M. Papadopoulos and Richard
G. Fessler

Traumatic vertebral fractures, spinal metastases, bacterial and tuberculous infections, primary bone tumors, meningeal tumors, vascular malformations, primary bone disease, and congenital connective-tissue or skeletal disorders commonly affect the thoracic spine.[1-6] Such disorders commonly cause compressive myelopathy or radiculopathy. Therefore surgical approaches to this region have become a vital component of the spine surgeon's armamentarium.

Anatomy of the Thoracic Spine

The anatomy of the thoracic spine contrasts with that of the cervical and the lumbar spine because of the complex osteoligamentous articulation with the thoracic rib cage. Each rib of the thoracic spine articulates with its adjacent intervertebral disc and vertebral bodies by a radiate ligament ventrally and by costovertebral ligaments dorsolaterally. The ventral costovertebral ligament joins the rostral portion of the rib neck to the caudal portion of the rostral transverse process. The middle costovertebral ligament attaches the dorsal neck of each rib to the ventral surface of its adjacent transverse process. Finally, the dorsal costovertebral ligament joins the rostral portion of the rib neck to the caudal base of the transverse process.[7] The costotransverse ligaments run from the transverse process of each vertebra to the rib and are divided into superior, posterior, and inferior costotransverse ligaments. In addition, the capsular ligaments secure the neck of the rib ventral to the transverse process (Figure 23.1).

An understanding of the complex three-dimensional anatomy of the head of the rib, the transverse process, the pedicle, the neuroforamen, the rib articulation with the vertebral body and disc, and the intercostal neurovascular bundle is essential to proper, safe exposure of this region. The dorsal, ventral, and lateral diameters of the vertebral bodies increase from T2 through T12. Physiologic kyphosis of the thoracic spine results from a relatively greater height of the dorsal vertebral wall compared with the ventral vertebral wall, observed between the thoracolumbar junction and the cervicothoracic junction. Pedicle dimensions vary significantly over the levels of the thoracic spine. Transverse pedicle diameters decrease from approximately 9mm at T1 to 5mm at T5, and then increase again at T12. Sagittal width increases from T1 to T11. Pedicle angles decrease from T1 to T12, with an angle of 25 degrees at T1 and 0 degrees at T12.

Facet orientation in the thoracic spine is primarily in the coronal plane, which allows significant rotational motion. Laminae overlying the facets increase in width and thickness from the cervicothoracic junction to the thoracolumbar junction. The relatively short, broad laminae in the upper and middle thoracic spine prevent hyperextension. Additional stability is provided to the thoracic spine by the anterior longitudinal ligament. This ligament increases in tensile strength from the cervicothoracic junction to the thoracolumbar junction and is firmly attached to the annulus fibrosus.

Surgical Approaches and Methods of Neural Decompression

Until recently, traditional operative decompressions in the thoracic spine have consisted of dorsal laminectomy.[8,9] However, discogenic, traumatic, or metastatic neural compression is most frequently ventral, and traditional laminectomy is less frequently used in these clinical settings, except for the rare instances in which there is dorsal compression. In fact, laminectomy alone is associated with a significant incidence of neurologic injury when it is used in the treatment of anterior pathology.[5,10]

Several techniques have been used to expose and decompress the ventral thoracic spine from T1 to T10. These fall into three general categories: ventral, dorsolateral, and dorsal approaches.[11] The advantages and disadvantages of the various approaches for neural decompression are reviewed in Table 23.1. In general the approach should be selected that best addresses the pathology.

Ventral approaches from T4 to T11 are through a standard thoracotomy incision with the patient in the lateral decubitus position. The lung is retracted to expose the vertebral column. The parietal pleura, segmental vessels, and periosteum are mobilized to expose the thoracic pathology completely. Spinal cord decompression and vertebrectomy, with bone strut grafting and instrumentation, may be performed.[12-14]

The dorsolateral approaches include the parascapular, extracavitary, and costotransversectomy techniques.[8,15] Both are performed with a back incision and require removal of the rib and transverse process to gain a lateral view of the vertebral body. Neural decompression and vertebrectomy may be followed by strut grafting. The exposure with costotransversectomy is more limited, so decompression of large fragments that compress the spinal cord and strut grafting may be difficult. Dorsal instrumentation may be performed simultaneously through the same incision with either technique.

The transpedicular, or dorsal, approach typically consists of a laminectomy and removal of one or both facets and pedicles with a drill. The surgeon then works lateral to the thecal sac to dissect fragments off the cord or reimpact bone fragments into the vertebral body. This approach is indicated when spinal cord compression is accessible and ventral strut grafting is not essential. Intraoperative ultrasonography is helpful to confirm neural decompression if visualization is poor.

Ventral Surgical Approaches

Ventral surgical approaches of the thoracic spine provide excellent visualization and access to the ventral spinal elements, with minimal manipulation of the neural structures, and with an opportunity for direct reconstruction of

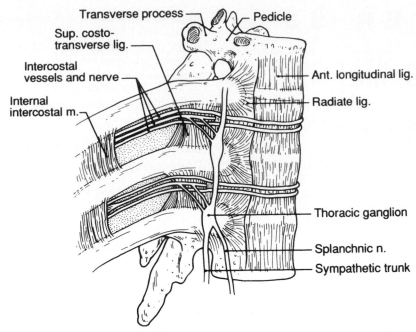

Figure 23.1 Ventral lateral view of the thoracic vertebral column depicting the relationship of the bony, ligamentous, vascular, and neural structures.

the anterior column in instances of trauma, tumor, or infection, or in the treatment of scoliosis.[16] Hodgson and Stock provided the first extensive description of the ventral exposure of the thoracic spine via thoracotomy to debride tuberculous abscesses in the treatment of Pott's disease.[1] They reported a mortality and morbidity rate of 2.9%, providing the impetus for other surgeons to use this approach in a variety of pathologic conditions (Table 23.2).

Approaches to the ventral thoracic spine may be classified into three general strategies (Table 23.3). The lower cervical and upper three cervical thoracic vertebrae may be exposed by a direct ventral cervical approach, extended caudally with a median sternotomy or upper sternal resection. This is particularly useful in the setting of direct ventrally situated disease without significant paraspinal or lateral involvement. In the treatment of thoracic disc disease the lowest disc space that may be routinely approached is T2-3, because of the sweeping kyphosis of the upper thoracic spine and the inclination of the disc space. In the treatment of vertebral disease (i.e., tumor or infection) adequate exposure for a T3 corpectomy with subsequent reconstruction may be accomplished by this approach. The second through sixth thoracic segments should be approached through a right dorsolateral thoracotomy. The left side of the upper thoracic spine is relatively less accessible because of the location of the aortic arch and great vessels. Although the right side may provide some additional hemostatic difficulties because of the fragility of venous structures, exposure of the sixth through the eleventh thoracic segments may be achieved through either a left or right thoracotomy. Many authors prefer the left side because mobilization of the aorta is technically easier and safer than mobilization of the vena cava or azygos venous system. However, one should be guided by the optimal approach for neural decompression, if that is the primary goal of the operative procedure. With scoliosis or other deformities, the choice would be the side of the apex or convexity of the curve. In cases of severe aortic atherosclerosis or aortic aneurysm the left side should be avoided.[10] Exposure of the thoracolumbar junction can be achieved through a left thoracotomy, combined with a dorsal detachment of the diaphragm and entrance into the retroperitoneal abdominal space. Again, the left side is preferred because the vascular anatomy is favorable and retraction of the liver is avoided.

Median sternotomy

Ventral lesions from C7 to T3 may be approached by combining standard ventral cervical exposure paralleling the medial border of the sternocleidomastoid muscle with a rostral sternal osteotomy to approximately T2, or a median sternotomy to T4.[17] This allows the optimal exposure of this level without significant risk to surrounding structures. The left side is preferred because of the lower "recurrence" on the left side of the recurrent laryngeal nerve (aorta on the left versus innominate on the right; Figure 23.2).[18] Median sternotomy allows for a direct ventral approach to the spine, but it may be limited if there is significant lateral or paravertebral involvement.[19]

Surgical anatomy

The thoracic inlet is oval shaped with a dorsoventral diameter of approximately 5cm and a transverse diameter of approximately 10cm in adults. The sternocleidomastoid muscle attaches to the sternum and clavicle by two heads. The oblique sternohyoid muscle arises from the dorsal surface of the medial portion of the clavicle and sternoclavicular junction. Key vascular structures in the rostral mediastinum include the innominate vein and artery, common carotid and left subclavian arteries, internal jugular vein, and the arch of the aorta. The innominate artery and vein and the aortic arch limit the caudal extent of

TABLE 23.1

Surgical Approaches to the Thoracic Spine

Approach	Type	Incision/Position	Indications	Contraindications	Advantages	Disadvantages
Anterior	Anterior cervicothoracic	(1) supine (2) anterolateral cervical/median sternotomy	(1) anterior compression of the spinal cord or roots, T1-3	(1) posterior or posterolateral neural compression (2) medical complications are relative contraindications	(1) excellent anterior exposure of the dura (2) may use anterior instrumentation	(1) limited to T1-3 (2) risk of recurrent laryngeal nerve and esophageal injury
	Transthoracic	(1) lateral decubitus position (2) thoracotomy incision	(1) anterior compression of the spinal cord or roots (2) anterior release in the treatment of thoracic scoliosis	(1) posterior neural compression (2) medical complications are relative contraindications	(1) good anterior exposure of the dura (2) procedure of choice for correction of thoracic scoliosis (3) excellent control of radicular vasculature (4) may use anterior instrumentation	(1) morbidity of thoracotomy (2) staged posterior instrumentation may be needed (3) requires diaphragm mobilization for access to T10-L1
Posterolateral	Lateral parascapular extrapleural approach (T1–4) Costotransversectomy	(1) prone position (2) paramedian incision	(1) accessible anterolateral neural compression without significant anteromedial component	(1) marked deformity and extensive vertebral body fractures (2) anterior neural compression are relative contraindications	(1) less surgery (2) posterior instrumentation may be performed simultaneously	(1) risk of incomplete decompression as a result of limited exposure (2) anterior strut grafting is difficult
	Lateral extracavitary	(1) prone position (2) "hockeystick"-shaped incision	(1) accessible lateral neural compression without significant anterior component	(1) polytrauma and medical complications are relative contraindications	(1) lateral and posterior neural exposure (2) posterior instrumentation may be performed simultaneously (3) minimal risk of injury to lung, great vessels, and diaphragm	(1) extensive muscle dissection (2) difficult to visualize the ventral dura and contralateral pedicle

Continued

TABLE 23.1

Surgical Approaches to the Thoracic Spine _cont'd_

Approach	Type	Incision/Position	Indications	Contraindications	Advantages	Disadvantages
Posterior	Laminectomy	(1) prone position (2) midline thoracolumbar incision	(1) posterior laminar fractures with neural entrapment or posterior epidural hemorrhage, with incomplete cord or cauda equina injury	(1) anterior neural compression	(1) less surgery (2) dural tears easier to repair posteriorly (3) posterior instrumentation may be performed simultaneously	(1) cord compression is typically anterior (2) may be destabilizing with anterior pathology
	Transpedicular decompression	(1) prone position (2) midline thoracolumbar incision	(1) accessible far-lateral anterior neural compression	(1) medial pathology requiring manipulation of the spinal cord for exposure (2) marked deformity and extensive vertebral body fractures are relative contraindications	(1) less surgery (2) posterior instrumentation may be performed simultaneously (3) some access to lateral vertebral body	(1) risk of incomplete decompression as a result of limited exposure (2) risk of deformity without anterior strut grafting

exposure. The recurrent laryngeal nerve arises from the vagus nerve, courses under the innominate artery on the right, and under the aortic arch on the left, and typically courses obliquely and ascends in the tracheoesophageal groove. The known incidence of nonrecurrence of the laryngeal nerve on the right side is 1%. For these reasons some surgeons prefer a left-sided approach for this exposure. The only significant disadvantage of the left-side exposure is the position of the thoracic duct.

TABLE 23.2

Historical Aspects of Ventral Thoracic Spinal Surgery		
Reference	**Year**	**Approach**
Cauchoix[13]	1957	Median sternotomy for C7-T4
Nanson[25]	1957	Neck approach for T1-3
Sundaresen[6]	1984	Clavicular resection for T1-3
Lesoin[19]	1986	Trans-sternal approach for T1-Tr
Hodgson[1,2]	1956,1960	Transthoracic approach
Perot[3]	1969	Transthoracic approach (disc)
Dwyer[26]	1969	Transthoracic approach (scoliosis)
Harrington[27]	1981	Transthoracic approach (cancer)
Heitmiller[23]	1988	Thoracolumbar approach
Leventhal[7]	1992	Thoracolumbar approach

TABLE 23.3

Ventral Approaches to the Thoracic Spine	
Level	**Approach**
C7-T3	Ventral cervical/median sternotomy
T2-6	Right thoracotomy
T6-11	Left (or right) thoracotomy
T10-L2	Left (or right) thoracoabdominal/retroperitoneal

The blood supply of the spinal cord in the cervicothoracic region is derived from radicular arteries that originate from the vertebral, thyrocervical, and costocervical branches of the subclavian artery. These vessels should not be encountered with a ventral midline approach.

Operative approach

The patient is positioned supine with the neck slightly extended and the chin up. The skin incision is made parallel to the ventral border of the sternocleidomastoid muscle. It is then carried caudally along the midline over the sternum to approximately the level of the angle of Lewis. The platysma muscle is divided along the fibers in the direction of the incision. A plane is developed along the anterior border of the sternocleidomastoid muscle by retracting the carotid sheath laterally and the trachea and esophagus medially (Figure 23.3). The sternohyoid muscle is identified and then detached from the medial clavicle and sternum. A plane is then developed by finger dissection underneath the sternum and into the upper mediastinum. Thymus tissue may be encountered, and can be swept away. The superior thyroid artery should be identified and ligated. A median sternotomy is then performed with an oscillating saw, down to the angle of Lewis, and the mediastinum is opened with a crank retractor. The pleura is then carefully dissected on both sides and retracted. It is essential to stay within the confines of the mediastinal space. The left innominate vein may need to be divided with ligatures for adequate caudal exposure. A plane is developed beneath the esophagus and above the prevertebral fascia. Self-restraining mediolateral retractors are placed under the elevated longus colli muscles. These muscles atrophy in the upper thoracic spine, and good footing of the retractor blades may be difficult. A table-mounted retractor may be very helpful in achieving and maintaining proper exposure. Great care must be taken not to place undue stretch on the recurrent laryngeal nerve at

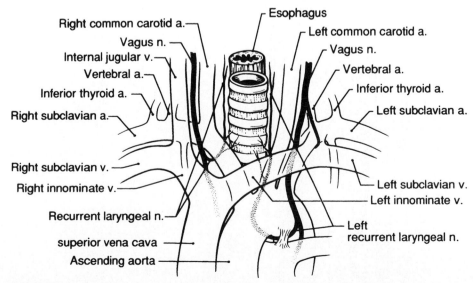

Figure 23.2 Ventral anatomy of the cervicothoracic junction. Note the differential relationship of the recurrent laryngeal nerve on the left versus the right side.

this level. The prevertebral fascia is then cleared of all surrounding connective tissue. The proper level can generally be identified by counting rib heads, which are palpable lateral to the ventral spine; however, this should be confirmed with intraoperative radiographs. The appropriate resection or reconstruction is then performed.

Right upper thoracic dorsolateral thoracotomy

Lesions from T2 to T6 are best approached through a right dorsolateral thoracotomy, through the interspace above the rib localized to the appropriate level of spinal pathol-

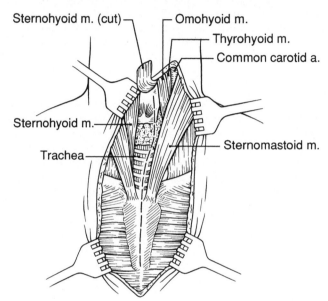

Figure 23.3 Operative exposure for the ventral cervicothoracic junction.

ogy.[20] For example, exposure of the T3-4 disc space would be approached through a right T3-4 intercostal space exposure. In general the intercostal space entered should represent the rostral margin of the spinal pathology. The left-sided exposure of the rostral portion of the thoracic spine is limited by the position of the aortic arch and great vessels.

Surgical anatomy

The right upper dorsolateral thoracotomy requires the identification and division of several important structures. The trapezius muscle extends from the spinous processes and attaches to the spine of the scapula throughout the length of the cervical and thoracic spine. Its fibers run obliquely and laterally to the scapular spine. Deep to the trapezius muscle is the rhomboid muscle group. The latter arises from the spinous processes of C6 to T5. Midline attachment of the latissimus dorsi muscle is also deep to the trapezius muscle from approximately T6 through T12. The serratus posterior inferior muscle arises as muscular bundles from the lower four ribs, whereas the serratus posterior superior muscle arises from the upper three ribs medially (Figure 23.4).[10]

In addition to the muscles, a series of ligaments join the ribs, transverse processes, and vertebral bodies. The head of the rib articulates with the corresponding vertebral body, as well as with the disc space adjacent to the body above. In the lower thoracic spine the rib heads articulate with the corresponding vertebral body, but the level of rib articulation changes to a position that overlaps the upper adjacent disc space in the middle and upper thoracic spine. The pedicle lies directly ventral to the base of the transverse process and directly medial to the head of the rib. The neuroforamen is bounded by the rostral margin of the pedicle

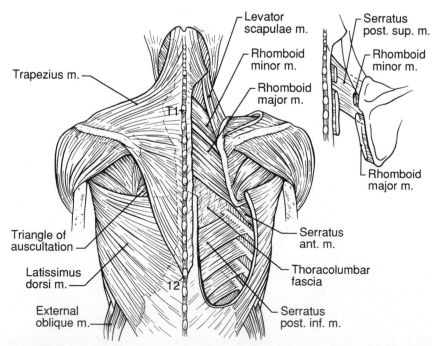

Figure 23.4 Superficial muscular anatomy of the dorsal thorax and the thoracic spine.

below, the caudal margin of the pedicle above, the dorsal margins of the vertebral body and disc, and the ventral portion of the corresponding facet joint (Figure 23.5). The corresponding intercostal vein and artery arise from the aorta and the azygos vein on the right. This arterial/venous bundle lies in the midportion of the body. The disc space may be identified as the intervening space between the intercostal vessels and directly beneath the rib head. The intercostal vessels join with the neurovascular bundle exiting the neuroforamen and with the subcostal neurovascular bundle below the corresponding rib. The sympathetic trunk runs parallel to the thoracic spine, splaying over the area of the rib heads.

Operative technique

The patient is placed in a lateral decubitus position and tilted forward approximately 15 degrees. An axillary roll is placed beneath the axilla and a pillow is placed between the legs. The lower leg is kept extended and the upper leg is flexed slightly. A "vacuum bean bag" is molded around the body. Tape is placed over the hip and secured to the table on both sides.

A double-lumen endotracheal tube may be used to achieve selective lung deflation, if necessary. The skin is prepared over the shoulder so that the shoulder and scapula can easily be mobilized within the sterile field. The skin incision is carried medial to and below the angle of the scapula (Figure 23.6).[21] Careful sequential identification of the muscle layers is necessary for proper closure. The trapezius muscle is divided lateral to its midline attachment. The rostral portions of the latissimus dorsi, rhomboid major, and serratus posterior muscles are also divided. As the muscle layers are divided the scapula is further retracted rostrally to identify medial muscular tissue "on stretch." This requires division for proper scapula retraction and exposure of the upper ribs. A plane is then developed deep to the scapula, and the first rib is located

with a gloved hand. It is essential to identify and palpate the first rib, which can be recognized by its downward and inward slope. The ribs are then sequentially counted until the appropriate space is identified. The interspace should be confirmed with a radiopaque marker and intraoperative radiographs. The periosteum of the appropriate rib is then stripped circumferentially. This is accomplished with the Doyan periosteum elevator and is carried as medial as possible. The rib is then cut approximately 3 to 4cm from the rib head, and the interspace is opened above the cut rib. For example, to expose the T3-4 interspace, the T4 rib is cut, and the chest is entered at the T3-4 intercostal space.

The parietal pleura may be opened at this juncture, or if limited exposure is needed, the operation may be performed extrapleurally. If the pleura is opened, the right lung is deflated and the ventrolateral portion of the thoracic spine is identified. The azygos vein is easily identified along the ventrolateral border of the spine (Figure 23.7).

To expose the pertinent paravertebral structures, a pleural flap is made adjacent to the spine. The pleura is raised with a medial base (Figure 23.8), and the intended ribs and vertebral bodies to be exposed are identified subpleurally when the pleural flap is raised. It is important to have a clean subpleural exposure so that the intercostal vessels, sympathetic trunk, rib head, and neuroforamen may be identified. The appropriate intercostal vessels are then ligated close to the origin of the azygos vein and aorta. This provides appropriate collateral flow to the radicular and subcostal vascular bundles. The corresponding rib heads are removed to identify disc space, pedicle, and transverse processes. When the appropriate disc space

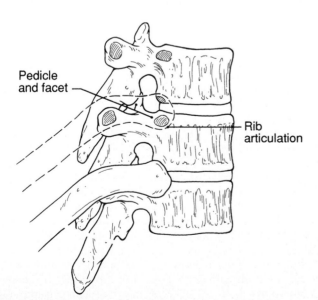

Figure 23.5 Bony anatomic relationship of the ventrolateral aspect of the midthoracic spine.

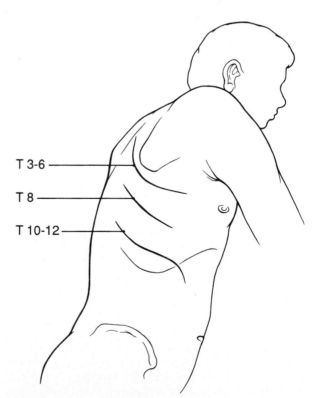

Figure 23.6 Typical skin incisions used for exposure of the ventrolateral thoracic spine.

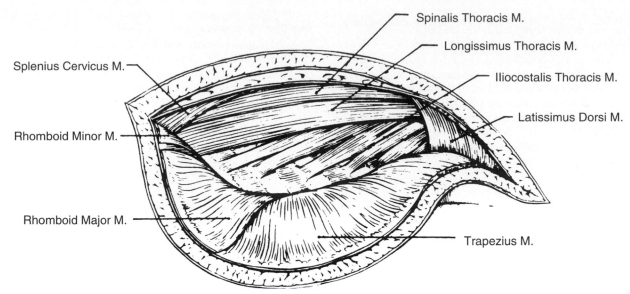

Figure 23.7 Right-sided intrathoracic exposure of the midthoracic spinal column.

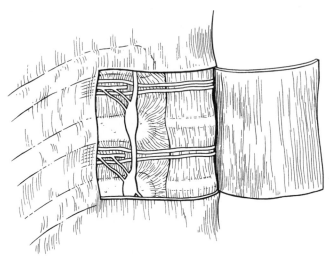

Figure 23.8 Right ventral lateral exposure of the costovertebral junction after elevation of the parietal pleura.

is identified, a discectomy is the initial step, after which appropriate decompression and reconstruction may be performed. Sequential ligation of intercostal vessels should be limited to the minimum needed for appropriate exposure.

When the operation is completed, the pleural flap is replaced and tacked with sutures. A tube thoracostomy is placed, the chest is closed, and the wound is closed in the usual fashion.

Left Dorsolateral Thoracotomy
Surgical anatomy

The pertinent surgical anatomy on the left side, compared with that on the right, is related to the aorta and great vessels. On the left the aortic arch reaches the level of the fourth thoracic vertebra and is closely applied to the ventral lateral aspect of the vertebral bodies on the left of the midline. In addition, rostral to the arch, the esophagus,

thoracic duct, and subclavian artery are in proximity to the vertebral body. In the lower thorax the aorta lies to the left of the midline, with short radicular vessels coursing across the midbody and anastomosing with the intercostal vessels at the level of the neuroforamen (Figure 23.9). Exposure of the thoracic spine uses a similar technique of ligation of the radicular vessels close to the aorta and vena cava. The aorta is then raised and elevated from the anterolateral aspect of the vertebral body.

Operative technique

The patient's position is similar to that in the right-sided approach, with the patient being placed in a lateral decubitus position and being tilted forward approximately 15 degrees. The bed may be flexed but must be returned back to neutral position before reconstruction of the spine. Axillary rolls are placed beneath the lower axilla, and a pillow is placed beneath the legs. Generally the lower leg is kept extended at the knee, and the upper leg is flexed. The patient is again secured to the operating table with wide adhesive tape across the hip. If lung retraction is anticipated, a double-lumen endotracheal tube may be used for anesthesia. The skin incision should be overlying the level of intended rib resection. Both the latissimus dorsi muscle and the serratus anterior muscles are mobilized by blunt dissection with the finger underneath the muscles. They are then transected with electrocautery along the line of the incision. Dorsally it may be necessary to divide the trapezius and rhomboid muscles for higher exposures. The scapula is retracted and a plane is developed beneath the scapula and above the chest wall. The first rib is generally inside the second rib and may be difficult to identify when palpated from the dorsal chest. The level must be confirmed with intraoperative radiographs. The rib below the interspace to be entered is then cut approximately 3 to 4cm from the rib head. A choice may be made whether to perform an extrapleural operation or an intrapleural operation. If an extrapleural operation is preferred, the pleura is dissected off the

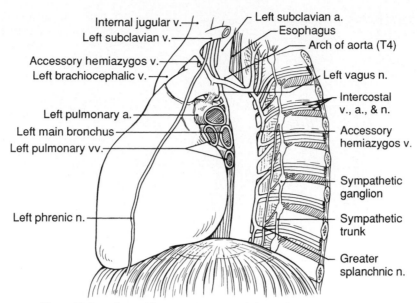

Internal jugular v.
Left subclavian v.
Accessory hemiazygos v.
Left brachiocephalic v.
Left pulmonary a.
Left main bronchus
Left pulmonary vv.
Left phrenic n.

Left subclavian a.
Esophagus
Arch of aorta (T4)
Left vagus n.
Intercostal v., a., & n.
Accessory hemiazygos v.
Sympathetic ganglion
Sympathetic trunk
Greater splanchnic n.

Figure 23.9 Left intrathoracic exposure of the midthoracic spine.

medial portion of the rib and vertebral body to be exposed. This gives direct exposure of the radicular vessels, sympathetic chain, rib head, and vertebral bodies. If the chest is entered and the spine is observed from the pleural side, a pleural flap is gently elevated to expose the underlying structures. The parietal pleura is typically quite delicate and should be carefully reflected. When the pleura is reflected, the intercostal vessels (as they course over the vertebral body) should be identified and ligated, as previously described. Disc spaces are then identified, and a resection is carried out that is appropriate for the operation. After the procedure the pleural flap is laid back and tacked in place and the wound is closed in the usual fashion.

Thoracoabdominal Approach
Surgical anatomy

For surgical approaches to the thoracolumbar junction, any of a variety of transthoracic, extrapleural, and retroperitoneal approaches may be employed.[22] For thoracolumbar exposure, the dorsolateral costal attachment of the diaphragm may be divided to allow entrance into the retroperitoneal space and exposure of the anterior spine. The typical approach involves thoracotomy with resection of the tenth or eleventh rib; the dorsolateral portion of the diaphragm is detached from the lower costal attachment, and a plane is developed in continuity with the retroperitoneal space.

The diaphragm is a dome-shaped muscle that is muscular at its periphery and tendinous centrally. Ventrally and laterally it attaches to the lower six ribs and xiphoid cartilage. Dorsally it originates from the upper lumbar vertebrae through the crura and the arcuate ligaments of the twelfth rib. The medial arcuate ligament arises from the crura and crosses over the psoas muscle to insert into the transverse process of the first lumbar vertebra. The lateral arcuate ligament arises from the transverse process of the first lumbar vertebra and extends over the quadratus lumborum muscle to the tips of the twelfth rib. The

right crus extends down the right side of the bodies of L1, L2, and L3; the left crus attaches to the bodies of L1 and L2 on the left side. The esophagus, vena cava, azygos vein, and thoracic aorta ascend through the diaphragm near the ventrolateral portion of the spine. The esophageal hiatus is at the level of the tenth thoracic vertebra (Figure 23.10).

Operative procedure

After positioning and preparing the patient, as described for a left thoracotomy, the skin incision is made in the region of the tenth or eleventh rib. The incision is carried more ventrally, depending on the extent of caudal exposure required (Figure 23.6).[23] Subperiosteal dissection is then carried out exposing the tenth or eleventh rib, which is then cut approximately 4cm from the rib head. The endothoracic fascia and pleura are carefully stripped from the inner surface of the rib to minimize the actual pleural opening, which is gradually spread with a crank retractor. With blunt dissection the diaphragm is kept under tension, and a circumferential incision is made in the medial portion of the diaphragm adjacent to the costal margin. This allows exposure of the rostral retroperitoneal space, which is gradually developed by blunt dissection. The spleen, kidneys, and stomach are retracted medially and caudally using a broad, malleable retractor. The ventral surface of the thoracolumbar junction, the vertebral bodies, and the aorta can be visualized (Figure 23.11). Again, the aorta may be mobilized after selective division of the segmental vessels near the aorta. The crus of the diaphragm is stripped from the anterior longitudinal ligament with a periosteum elevator. The arcuate ligament is divided at its insertion into the lumbar transverse process at the twelfth rib. The anterior longitudinal ligament and the ventrolateral surface of the vertebral bodies are carefully stripped of all soft tissue and are exposed for appropriate resection. After the operation is completed the diaphragm is reattached to its costal margin and the wound is closed in the usual fashion.

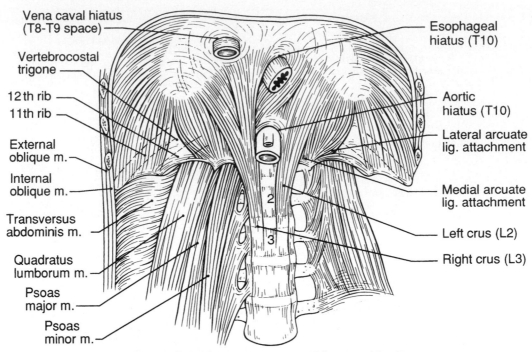

Figure 23.10 Infradiaphragmatic anatomy of the ventral lumbar spine.

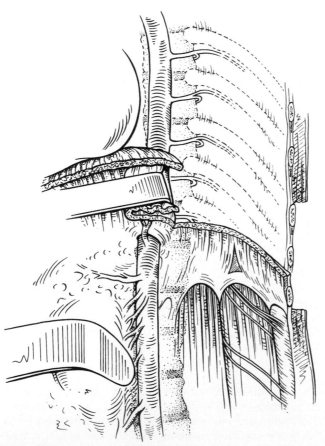

Figure 23.11 Left intraoperative exposure of the thoracolumbar junction with diaphragmatic incision.

Dorsolateral Surgical Approaches
Lateral Parascapular Extrapleural (Lateral Extracavitary) Approach to the Upper Thoracic Spine
Surgical anatomy

The upper thoracic vertebrae (T1-4) present unique anatomic challenges for surgical access. The thoracic cage narrows to reach the thoracic inlet, regaining intimate associations between the rostral mediastinal structures and the vertebral column. Techniques that have been described to expose these vertebrae include the supraclavicular, transmanubrial, and transthoracic (through the third rib) approaches.[24] All of these techniques provide excellent access to a limited section of the rostral thoracic spine, but none provide access to all of the vertebrae. The lateral parascapular extrapleural (lateral extracavitary) approach to the upper thoracic spine allows excellent exposure of each vertebra for neural decompression, corpectomy, and vertebral reconstruction and allows simultaneous dorsal spinal fixation.[8,15]

Operative procedure

A midline incision is made extending from three spinous processes above, to three spinous processes below the level of the lesion, which is then curved gently to the scapular line on the side of the desired surgical approach (Figure 23.12). The deep fascia is incised over the spinous processes and sharply dissected off them so that the trapezius muscle can be identified. The trapezius and rhomboid muscles are then dissected off the spinous processes in the subperiosteal plane, and the muscle layers

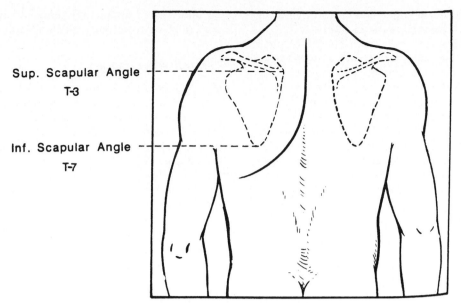

Figure 23.12 Skin incision used for the lateral parascapular extrapleural approach. *(From Fessler RG, Dietze DD Jr, Millan MM, Peace D: Lateral parascapular extrapleural approach to the upper thoracic spine. J Neurosurg 75:349-355, 1991.)*

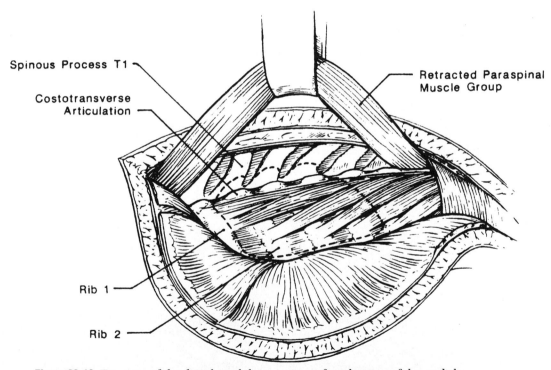

Figure 23.13 Exposure of the dorsolateral thoracic spine after elevation of the medial paraspinous muscle group and the lateral trapezius. *(From Fessler RG, Dietze DD Jr, Millan MM, Peace D: Lateral parascapular extrapleural approach to the upper thoracic spine. J Neurosurg 75:349-355, 1991.)*

are identified on edge as they are stripped. The skin and the trapezius and rhomboid muscles are reflected together toward the medial border of the scapula as a musculocutaneous flap (Figure 23.13). This provides the surgeon with excellent exposure of the dorsal rib cage and dorsal vertebral elements. The thoracic cage is opened dorsally by

removing two or three ribs from the costotransverse and costovertebral articulations to the dorsal bend of each rib. To expose a vertebral body, the corresponding rib and the rib below must be removed (thus to expose T3, the third and fourth ribs must be removed). The intercostal muscles and neurovascular bundles are stripped subperiosteally off the ribs, and the costotransverse and costovertebral ligaments are excised to free the rib head and neck. The ipsilateral lung is collapsed to minimize the risk of pleural injury. The dorsal rib is cut as far laterally as possible, generally just lateral to the dorsal bend. With the cut end protected, the rib head and neck are worked free. The intercostal veins are sacrificed, and the intercostal nerves and arteries are ligated and transected, leaving the sutures long for later retraction. The intercostal nerves and arteries are traced to the vertebral foramen, the sympathetic chain and dorsal intercostal vasculature are identified on the lateral vertebral surface, the rami communicantes are transected, and the segmental vasculature is sacrificed. The sympathetic chain is displaced ventrolaterally in a subperiosteal dissection, revealing the vertebral body, pedicle, and foramina. The pathologic process becomes clearly visible and a biopsy specimen may be sent for pathologic identification, if indicated. Excellent access to the ventrolateral aspect of the spinal canal and dural sac is achieved (Figure 23.14). Before wound closure, the operative field is filled with saline to check for an air leak. A layered wound closure is performed.

Costotransversectomy

The costotransversectomy approach to the thoracic spine provides a dorsolateral exposure to the thoracic spinal column. The limitations of this technique are limited access and limited visualization of the ventral dural sac. It is ideal for anterolateral and lateral exposure of the spinal column, canal, and dura.

The anatomic principles and relationships are essentially the same as those considered for the anterior thoracotomy approach. In fact, there is little difference (except for position of the patient and orientation of the incision) between an intercostal, extrapleural thoracotomy approach and a posterolateral costotransversectomy approach.

Operative procedure

The patient is placed prone on unequal rolls. A large roll is placed on the "up" side of the exposure; and a smaller roll is placed on the "down" side of the exposure. The table is tilted so that at the initiation of the operation the back is parallel to the floor. After appropriate exposure is achieved the table can be tilted in the other direction, resulting in a nearly 45-degree tilt of the patient. This allows excellent access and visualization of the lateral and ventrolateral portions of the spine. The patient should be secured to the table with heavy tape.

Two incisions may be used: (1) a midline incision with a "T" over the rib to be resected or (2) a curvilinear incision that should have a midportion approximately 6 to 7mm from the midline, with the distal and proximal tips of the incision approximately 3cm from midline. Surgical dissection is achieved to expose the rib transverse process, facet joint, and lamina, if needed. The rib is then dissected subperiosteally with a Doyan subperiosteum elevator, and is cut approximately 6cm from the rib head. The level should be identified and confirmed with intraoperative radiographs. The pleura is gently swept away from the underside of the rib head and the anterolateral portion of the spine. A broad, malleable retractor may be placed on the pleura to retract the pleura and lungs. The anatomic principles are similar to those described for the dorsolateral thoracotomy. The rib head is then removed to identify the disc space. Segmental vessels may be identified and ligated, if necessary, and the transverse process can be removed, allowing exposure of the pedicle, disc space, and the neuroforamen above and below the pedicle. The

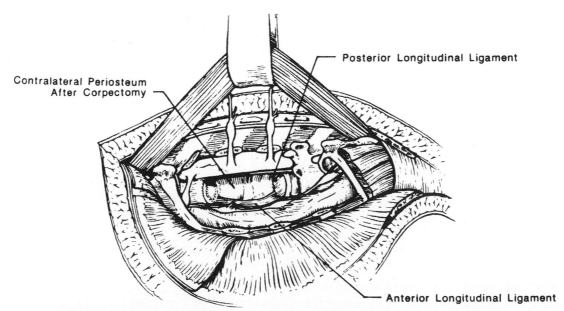

Contralateral Periosteum
After Corpectomy

Posterior Longitudinal Ligament

Anterior Longitudinal Ligament

Figure 23.14 Complete exposure and decompression of the ventrolateral thoracic spine after decompression via the lateral parascapular extrapleural approach. *(From Fessler RG, Dietze DD Jr, Millan MM, Peace D: Lateral parascapular extrapleural approach to the upper thoracic spine.* J Neurosurg *75:349-355, 1991.)*

appropriate resection is done, and closure is performed in the routine fashion.

REFERENCES

1. Hodgson AR, Stock FE: Anterior spinal fusion: a preliminary communication on radical treatment of Pott's disease and Pott's paraplegia. *Br J Surg* 44:266-275, 1956.
2. Hodgson AR, Stock FE, Fang HSY, Ong GB: Anterior spinal fusion: the operative approach and pathologic findings in 412 patients with Pott's disease of the spine. *Br J Surg* 48:172-178, 1960.
3. Perot PL Jr, Munro DD: Transthoracic removal of midline thoracic disc protrusions causing spinal cord compression. *J Neurosurg* 31:452-458, 1969.
4. Richardson JD, Campbell DL, Grover FL, *et al*: Transthoracic approach for Pott's disease. *Ann Thorac Surg* 21:552-556, 1976.
5. Standefer M, Hardy RW Jr, Marks K, Cosgrove DM: Chondromyxoid fibroma of the cervical spine—a case report with a review of the literature and a description of an operative approach to the lower anterior cervical spine. *Neurosurgery* 11:288-292, 1982.
6. Sundaresan N, Shah J, Foley KM, Rosen G: An anterior surgical approach to the upper thoracic vertebrae. *J Neurosurg* 61:686-690, 1984.
7. Leventhal MR: Spinal anatomy and surgical approaches. In Crenshaw R (ed): *Campbells Operative Orthopaedics*. St Louis, Mosby, 1992, pp 3493-3516.
8. Fessler RG, Dietze DD Jr, Millan MM, Peace D: Lateral parascapular extrapleural approach to the upper thoracic spine. *J Neurosurg* 75:349-355, 1991.
9. Tator CH, Duncan EG, Edmonds VE, *et al*: Comparison of surgical and conservative management in 208 patients with acute spinal cord injury. *Can J Neurol Sci* 14:60-69, 1987.
10. Smith TK, Stallone RJ, Yee JM: The thoracic surgeon and anterior spinal surgery. *J Thorac Cardiovasc Surg* 77: 925-928, 1979.
11. Johnson RM, Southwick WD: Surgical approaches to the spine. In Rothman RH, Simeone FA (eds): *The Spine*, ed 2. Philadelphia, WB Saunders, 1982, pp 147-171.
12. Anderson TM, Mansour KA, Miller JI Jr: Thoracic approaches to anterior spinal operations: anterior thoracic approaches. *Ann Thorac Surg* 55:1447-1452, 1993.
13. Cauchoix J, Binet J: Anterior surgical approaches to the spine. *Ann R Coll Surg Engl* 27:237-243, 1957.
14. Erickson DL, Leider LL, Brown WE: One-stage decompression-stabilization for thoracolumbar fractures. *Spine* 2:53,1977.
15. Larson SJ, Holst RA, Hemmy DC, Sances A Jr: Lateral extracavitary approach to traumatic lesions of the thoracic and lumbar spine. *J Neurosurg* 45:628-637, 1976.
16. Cook WA: Transthoracic vertebral surgery. *Ann Thorac Surg* 12:54-68, 2001.
17. Fielding JW, Stillwell WT: Anterior cervical approach to the upper thoracic spine. A case report. *Spine* 1:158-161, 1976.
18. Micheli LJ, Hood RW: Anterior exposure of the cervicothoracic spine using a combined cervical thoracic approach. *J Bone Joint Surg Am* 65:992-997, 1983.
19. Lesoin F, Thomas CE 3rd, Autricque A, *et al*: A transsternal biclavicular approach to the upper anterior thoracic spine. *Surg Neurol* 26:253-256, 1986.
20. McElvein RB, Nasca RJ, Dunham WK, Zorn GL Jr: Transthoracic exposure for anterior spinal surgery. *Ann Thorac Surg* 45:278-283, 1988.
21. Crawford FA, Kratz JM: Thoracic incisions. In Sabiston DC Jr, Spencer FC (eds): *Surgery of the Chest*, ed 4. Philadelphia, WB Saunders, 1983, pp 143-145.
22. Burrington JD, Brown C, Wayne ER, Odom J: Anterior approach to the thoracolumbar spine: technical consideration. *Arch Surg* 111:456-463, 1976.
23. Heitmiller RF: The left thoracoabdominal incision. *Ann Thorac Surg* 46:250-253, 1988.
24. Charles R, Govender S: Anterior approach to the upper thoracic vertebrae. *J Bone Joint Surg Br* 71:81-84, 1989.
25. Nanson EM: The anterior approach to upper dorsal sympathectomy. *Surg Gynecol Obstet* 104:118-120, 1957.
26. Dwyer AF, Newton NC, Sherwood AA: An anterior approach to scoliosis. A preliminary report. *Clin Orthop* 62:192-202, 1969.
27. Harrington KD: The use of methylmethacrylate for vertebral-body replacement and anterior stabilization of pathologic fracture-dislocations of the spine due to metastatic malignant disease. *J Bone Joint Surg Am* 63:36-46, 1981.

CHAPTER 24

The Lumbar and Sacral Spine

Robert E. Isaacs and Richard G. Fessler

Surgical approaches to the lumbar and sacral spine should be dictated by the location and extent of the pathology to be addressed. Knowledge of the pertinent adjacent structures, whether neural, visceral, muscular, or vascular, aids in limiting potential complications while facilitating the procedure. Complex spine reconstruction and minimally invasive techniques require the surgeon to use this knowledge, given limited information. For these reasons, surgical decision making begins with an appropriate overview of anatomy.

Anatomy
Osseous Anatomy

In the lumbar spine, the large osseous ring that surrounds the spinal canal is bordered ventrally by a cancellous cylindric mass (the vertebral body), dorsally by the vertebral arch, and dorsolaterally by the pedicles. Three other key vertebral elements are located near the pedicle and laminae: transverse process and superior and inferior articular processes. With its neural and bony relationships, the pedicle is key to conceptualizing the lumbar spine. The pedicles are wide and thick and are widely spaced on the rostral dorsolateral aspect of the body. In the rostral/caudal dimension, their height is one-half that of the vertebral body. The angles in the transverse and sagittal planes increase and decrease respectively as the lumbar spine is descended (Figure 24.1).[2]

The transverse processes are flat and long in the first four lumbar vertebrae; they are small stubs at the fifth lumbar vertebra. The mamillary processes are large in the lumbar area, providing attachment sites for the origins of the thick lumbar muscles.

The articular processes bear complementary relationships rostrally and caudally. The rostral facet is concave and faces dorsomedially to meet the caudal facet from above. The caudal facet, an extension of the laminae, faces ventrolaterally and complements the superior articulating facet of the vertebral body below. The junction of the two facets forms the roof of the neural foramina (Figure 24.2).

The sacrum consists of five fused vertebrae. It has a triangular shape and forms the dorsal aspect of the pelvis. It joins with the fifth lumbar vertebra via the L5-S1 disc and facets. The five fused vertebrae have homologous structures referable to the lumbar spine. The transverse processes are the laterally projecting alae that articulate with the pelvis. A prominent midline dorsal ridge represents the fused spinous processes. More laterally, another ridge forms the sacral articular crest with a functional superior articular process at S1. This facet faces caudally and dorsally. Because of the sacrovertebral angle created by the tilt of the sacrum as it joins the fifth lumbar vertebra, this joint functions to prevent ventral displacement of the lumbar spine on the sacrum. Ventrally, transverse ridges represent fused vertebrae and enclose remnants of intervertebral discs. Foramina dorsally and ventrally provide sites of exit for the ventral and dorsal divisions of the sacral nerves. The sacrum is the most variable portion of the spine. Lengthening or shortening of the lumbar spine by deletion or addition of segments to and from the sacrum is not uncommon (Figure 24.3).[22]

Thoracic vertebrae T2-9 have points of articulations for each rib: one on the vertebral body and the other on the corresponding transverse process. T11 and T12 have a single costal facet on their pedicles (Figure 24.4). The typical rib has a head, a neck, a tubercle, and a shaft or body. The crest of the head is joined to the intervertebral disc by an intraarticular ligament with two surface articulations: one on the numerically corresponding vertebra and one on the vertebra above it. The neck is the nonarticulating portion of rib between the head and tubercle. The tubercle is on the dorsal portion of the rib at the junction of the neck and shaft. The tubercle of most ribs has a smooth convex facet that articulates with the transverse process of the corresponding vertebra and a rough nonarticular surface to which the lateral costotransverse ligament attaches. The body of the rib is thin and flat, with its greatest in the diameter in the rostral to caudal orientation. The point of greatest curvature is called the angle of the rib. The costal groove and the flange formed by the caudal border of the rib accommodate and protect the intercostal vessels and nerve that accompany the rib. The eleventh and twelfth ribs are short and capped with cartilage. They have a single facet on their heads and no neck or tubercle. The eleventh rib has a slight angle and a shallow costal groove. The twelfth rib has neither of these features. Minet[16] classifies the twelfth rib as long, medium, or short. The long type is parallel to the eleventh rib, and the short is horizontal and less oblique than the long type. For thoracolumbar surgery, it is important to understand the relationship of the pleural sac to the twelfth rib. The pleural sac passes caudally over the inferior border to the twelfth rib and continues in this direction for 1 to 2cm. From there it passes horizontally, crossing caudally, and 3 to 4cm lateral to the twelfth rib head, it continues to pass along the twelfth rib for another 7 to 8cm (Figure 24.5).[16]

Soft-Tissue Anatomy

Around the bony cylindric canal of the lumbar spine and triangular sacrum, soft-tissue structures have intimate and crucial anatomic relationships. These include: (1) synovial and nonsynovial tissue, (2) muscles and ligaments that attach directly or indirectly to the spine, (3) exiting nerve roots that form a plexus of nerves in and around muscle structures or important autonomic plexuses, and (4)

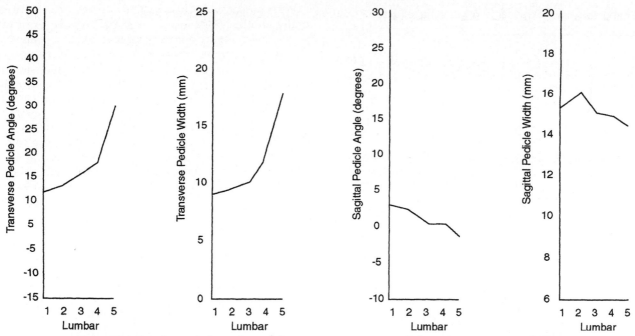

Figure 24.1 Lumbar pedicle angles and dimensions: transverse pedicle angle, transverse pedicle width, sagittal pedicle angle, and sagittal pedicle width. (*Data from Panjabi* et al.,[21] *Krag* et al.,[13] *and Zindrick* et al.[27])

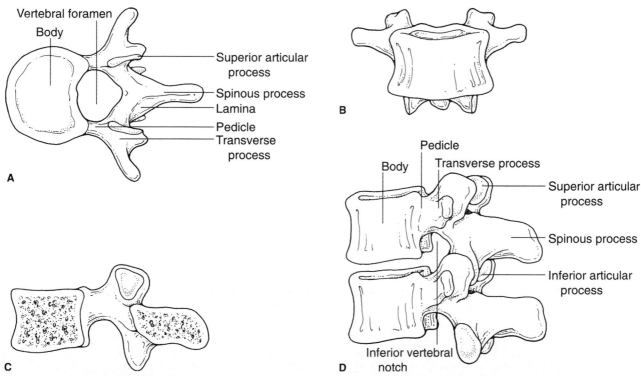

Figure 24.2 (**A**) Lumbar vertebra viewed from above. (**B**) Ventral. (**C**) Median sagittal. (**D**) In articulation.

soft-tissue structures, such as vasculature and viscera that are adjacent to bony structures.

Lumbar Spine

Muscles and Ligaments. The ligaments important to the lumbar spine include the ligamentum flavum (which bridges the space between adjacent laminae, attaching to the ventral surface of the upper lamina and rostral lip of the lower one), the intertransverse ligaments, the interspinous ligaments, and the unpaired supraspinous ligament.

The intrinsic and extrinsic musculature adjacent to the spine is commonly dissected in approaches to the spine

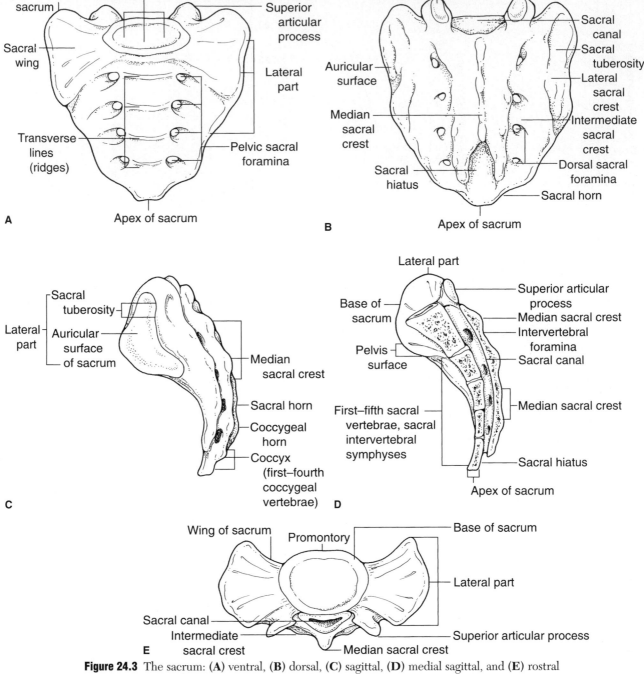

Figure 24.3 The sacrum: (**A**) ventral, (**B**) dorsal, (**C**) sagittal, (**D**) medial sagittal, and (**E**) rostral views.

and provides important landmarks in specific approaches. Intrinsic muscles consist of the erector spinae, multifidus, quadratus lumborum, and deep muscles. The large erector spinae muscle is divided into three columns: iliocostalis, longissimus, and spinalis muscles. The iliocostalis muscle, as its name indicates, is the most lateral of the group and arises from the iliac crest and inserts into the ribs. The longissimus muscle, intermediate in the column, runs between the transverse processes of the vertebrae. The spinalis muscle, the most medial, inserts and attaches to spinous processes in the lumbar and thoracic region. All three columns of the erector spinae muscle extend the vertebral column and bend the vertebral column laterally.

Central to the erector spinae muscles are several short muscles that interconnect adjacent and nearby vertebral bodies. This group of small muscles, called the multifidus muscles, originates on the mamillary processes of the rostral facets and runs rostrally and medially to insert on the spinous processes of vertebrae two to four segments above. The quadratus lumborum muscle is located ventral and lateral to the erector spinae muscles. This muscle originates on the iliac crest and iliolumbar ligament and runs obliquely to insert ventrally on the lowest rib and transverse processes of the upper four lumbar vertebrae. Ventral and medial to this muscle are the small intertransversarius muscles that span the transverse processes.

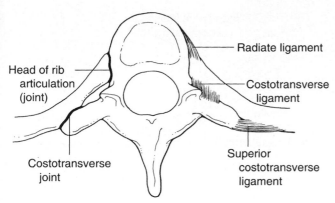

Figure 24.4 Cross-section through thoracic vertebra and costovertebral joints.

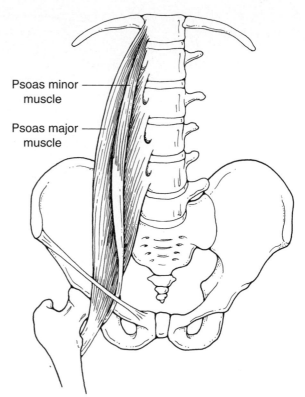

Figure 24.6 Psoas muscle relationships to lumbar and sacral vertebrae and pelvis.

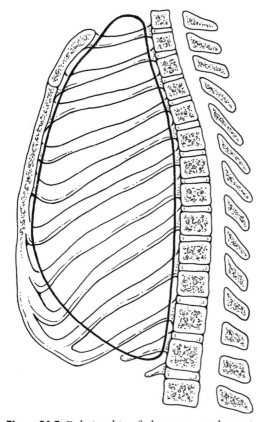

Figure 24.5 Relationship of pleura to costal margin.

Ventrolateral and adjacent to the lumbar vertebral bodies are the psoas muscles, which originate from the lateral aspects of the vertebral bodies and transverse processes of L1-5 and pass through the pelvis and into the thigh dorsal to the posterior inguinal ligament (Figures 24.6 and 24.7).

The extrinsic musculature consists of the rectus abdominis, external oblique, internal oblique, transversalis, latissimus dorsi, and serratus dorsalis caudalis muscles (Figure 24.7). The rectus muscles run bilaterally on the ventral abdominal wall from the pubis to the middle ribs. The internal and external oblique muscles and the transversalis muscles are layered superficial to deep as

described. They arise from the ribs and thoracodorsal fascia dorsally and insert on the iliac crest caudally and the linea alba medially. The latissimus muscle is a large and diffuse muscle that originates on the sacrum, dorsal iliac crest, and tenth, eleventh, and twelfth ribs. The fibers in the costoiliac interval run rostrally and laterally. The serratus dorsalis caudalis muscle originates from the lower four ribs, runs caudally and medially, and inserts on the thoracolumbar fascia ventral to the latissimus dorsi muscle.

Exiting Nerve Roots. The lumbar plexus is formed within the psoas major muscle. The largest and most important branches of the lumbar plexus are the obturator and femoral nerves (L2, L3, and L4). The ilioinguinal and iliohypogastric nerves are derived from L1, enter the abdomen dorsal to the medial arcuate ligament and pass inferolaterally, ventral to the quadratus lumborum muscle, piercing it near the anterior superior iliac spine. The genitofemoral nerve (L1 and L2) pierces the fascia iliaca and the ventral surface of the psoas major muscle and divides lateral to the common and external iliac arteries into two femoral and genital branches. The lumbosacral trunk (L4 and L5) is a large flat nerve, from which the L4 component descends through the psoas major muscle on the medial part of the transverse process of the L5 vertebra and passes closely over the ala of the sacrum to join the first sacral nerve (Figure 24.8).

The sympathetic and parasympathetic nerves are distributed to the abdominal viscera via a tangle of plexuses

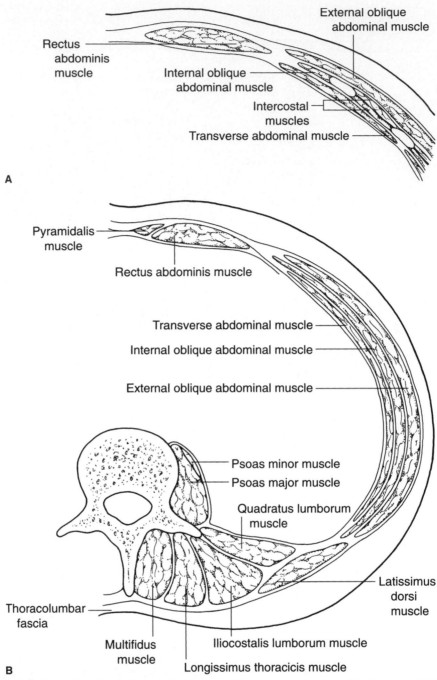

Figure 24.7 Coronal sections through the thoracoabdominal musculature: **(A)** above and **(B)** below the umbilicus.

and ganglia located on the ventral surface of the aorta. The principal components of this system are the celiac plexus ganglia, which are located on each side of the celiac trunk at the level of the rostral aspect of the first lumbar vertebra. The greater, lesser, and lowest splanchnic nerves are branches of thoracic sympathetic ganglia 5 to 12. The hypogastric plexus runs on the ventral surface of the aorta. It receives contributions from the lateral rami of the right and left lumbar sympathetic trunks and from median rami of the celiac plexus and the superior and inferior mesenteric plexuses. It spans the distance from the fourth lumbar to the first sacral vertebra. Its shape and bifurcations can be variable.[13] In males the

plexus innervates the bladder, vas deferens, and seminal vesicles and is important in the neurophysiology of ejaculation (Figure 24.9).

Soft-Tissue Structures. The thoracolumbar junction is one of the more complicated areas of the vertebral column and has important soft-tissue anatomic structures that require special attention. The thoracolumbar fascia is made up of dorsal, intermediate, and ventral layers. The dorsal layer surrounds the erector spinae muscles dorsally. It arises with the tendon of the latissimus dorsi on the sacrum and iliac crest and attaches on the spinous processes of the lumbar vertebrae. The intermediate layer

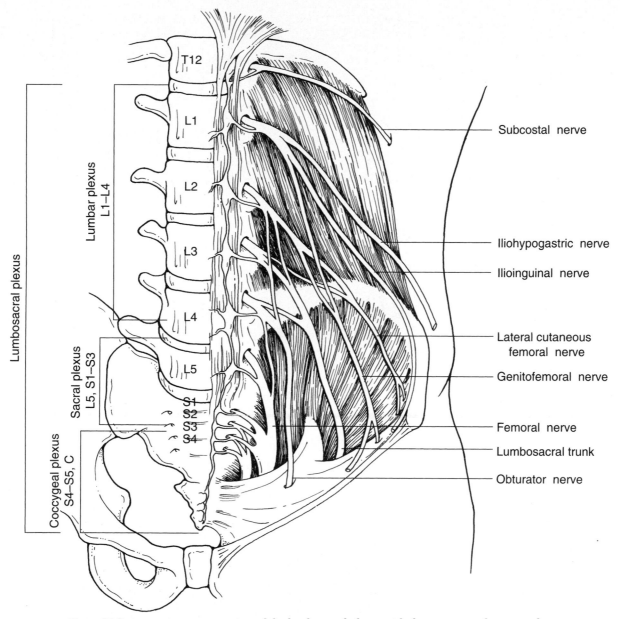

T12

L1

L2

L3

L4

L5

S1
S2
S3
S4

Lumbar plexus L1–L4

Lumbosacral plexus

Sacral plexus L5, S1–S3

Coccygeal plexus S4–S5, C

Subcostal nerve

Iliohypogastric nerve

Ilioinguinal nerve

Lateral cutaneous femoral nerve

Genitofemoral nerve

Femoral nerve

Lumbosacral trunk

Obturator nerve

Figure 24.8 Anatomic representation of the lumbosacral plexus with the psoas muscle removed on one side.

of the thoracolumbar fascia attaches to all of the transverse processes of the lumber vertebrae and to the caudal border of the twelfth rib. The lumbocostal ligament of Henle arises from the transverse process of L1 and runs rostrolaterally, inserting to the caudal border of the twelfth rib close to its medial end. The ventral layer of the thoracolumbar fascia is attached to the lateral arcuate ligament rostrally, to the iliac crest caudally, to the transversalis fascias laterally, and to the psoas fascia medially. This layer covers the quadratus lumborum muscle and is in contact with the retroperitoneal contents (Figure 24.10; see also Figures 24.6 to 24.9).[17]

The lateral arcuate ligament arises from the L1 transverse process and crosses the proximal portion of the quadratus lumborum muscle to attach to the lower border of the twelfth rib lateral to the insertion of the quadratus lumborum muscle.

The diaphragm consists of a muscular portion and a central aponeurosis termed the *central tendon*, upon which the muscular portion converges (Figure 24.11). The muscular portion is divided into three parts based on the origins of its fibers: sternal, costal, and lumbar. The sternal part of the diaphragm arises from the xiphoid process. The costal part of the diaphragm arises from the internal surface of the caudal six ribs at the costal margin. The lumbar part of the diaphragm arises from the lumbar vertebrae by two crura and three arcuate ligaments. The musculotendinous crura envelop the aorta and attach ventrolaterally to the rostral two lumbar vertebral bodies on the left and the upper three on the right. The crura blend with the anterior longitudinal ligament of the lumbar spine. Three arcuate ligaments give rise to fibers of the diaphragm. The median arcuate ligament unites the medial sides of the two crura. The medial arcuate ligament on each side is a

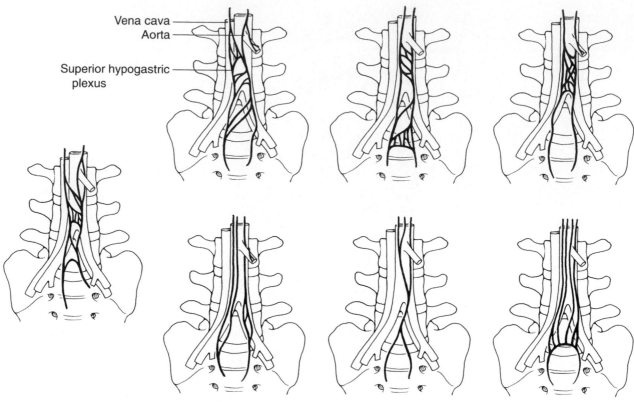

Figure 24.9 Variations of the superior hypogastric plexus.

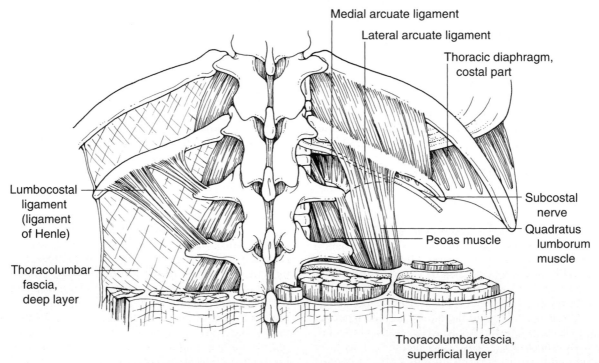

Figure 24.10 Fascial planes of thoracolumbar junction: dorsal view.

thickening of the ventral thoracolumbar fascia over the rostral part of the psoas muscle. From the crus it runs over the psoas and has an attachment to the transverse process of the first lumbar vertebra. The lateral arcuate ligament is a thickening of the anterior thoracolumbar fascia running

over the rostral aspect of the quadratus lumborum muscle forming attachments to the twelfth rib and transverse process of the first lumbar vertebra.[18]

The abdominal aorta begins at the aortic hiatus in the diaphragm at the level of the T12-L1 intervertebral disc

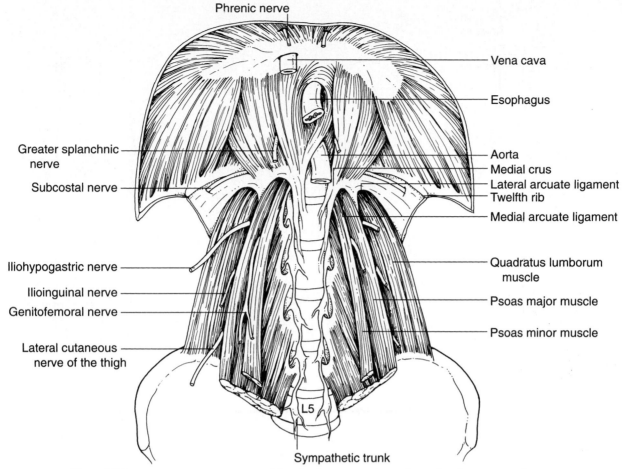

Figure 24.11 Anatomic representation of the diaphragm in relationship to lumbar spine and intimate structures.

and ends at about the level of L4 by dividing into the two common iliac arteries. The inferior vena cava begins ventral to the fifth lumbar vertebra by the union of the common iliac veins and ascends to the right of the median plane and pierces the central tendon of the diaphragm at the level of the eighth thoracic vertebra. Five anatomic variants of the aortocaval axis are outlined according to the level of bifurcation and origin of the aorta and vena cava, respectively (Figure 24.12).[14] The aorta is ventral to the vena cava and lumbar vertebral bodies and sits slightly to the left, and the vena cava is located slightly to the right.

The branches of the abdominal aorta may be grouped into four types: (1) those arising rostrally to the celiac (T12), superior mesenteric (L1), and inferior mesenteric (L3) arteries; (2) those arising laterally—the renal (L1), the middle suprarenal (L1), and the testicular or ovarian (L2) arteries; (3) those arising dorsolaterally—the parietal branches of the inferior phrenic arteries, which give rise to the superior suprarenal arteries and the four pairs of lumbar arteries; and (4) an unpaired parietal artery, the sacral artery, which arises from the dorsal surface of the aorta just proximal to its bifurcation (Figure 24.13). The lumbar arteries pass dorsomedially. On the right they run dorsal to the inferior vena cava, dividing between the transverse processes into the ventral and dorsal branches. The ventral branch passes deep to the quadratus lumborum muscle to anastomose with the inferior epigastric arteries. Each dor-

sal branch passes dorsally lateral to the articular processes and supplies the spinal cord, cauda equina, meninges, erector spinae muscles, and overlying skin.[5] The radicular arteries, which supply blood to the posterior and anterior spinal arteries, arise from these dorsal branches. The largest of these, the arteria radicularis magna (spinal artery of Adamkiewicz), supplies most of the blood to the caudal spinal cord, including the lumbosacral enlargement (Figures 24.14 and 24.15).

Tributaries of the inferior vena cava are the common iliac veins (L5), the lumbar veins, the right testicular or ovarian vein (the left drains into the left renal vein), the renal veins, the azygos vein, the right suprarenal vein (the left also drains into the renal vein), the inferior phrenic veins, and the hepatic veins. The lumbar veins consist of four or five segmental pairs. They may drain separately into the inferior vena cava or the common iliac vein, but they are usually united on each side by a vertical connecting vein, the ascending lumbar vein that lies dorsal to the psoas major muscle. Each ascending lumbar vein passes dorsal to the medial arcuated ligament of the diaphragm to enter the thorax. The right ascending lumbar vein joins the right subcostal vein to form the azygos vein, and the left subcostal vein forms the hemiazygos vein.[18]

The cisterna chyli is saclike and is located between the origin of the abdominal aorta and the azygos vein. It lies on the right sides of the bodies of the first two lumbar

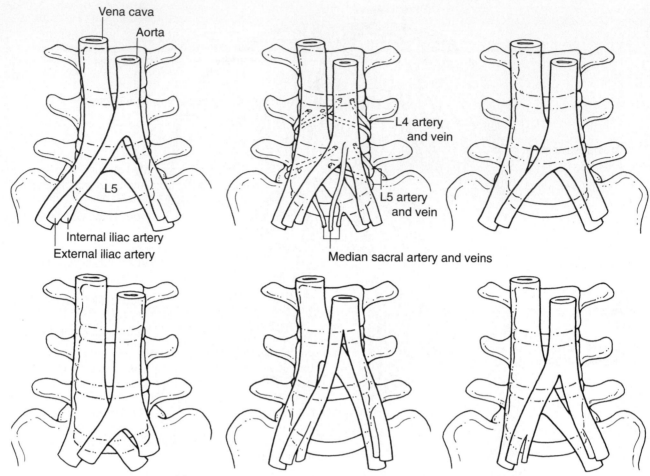

Figure 24.12 Variations of the aortocaval junction and tributary vessels.

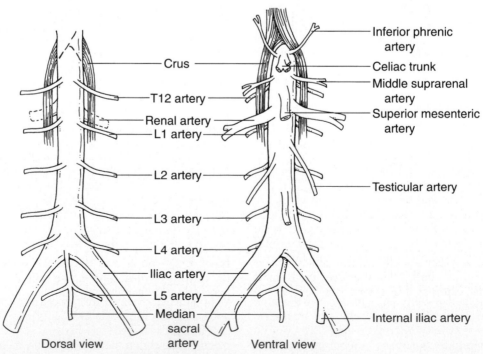

Figure 24.13 Abdominal aorta and its branches.

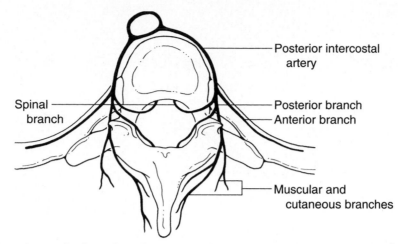

Figure 24.14 Blood supply to the spinal cord and vertebral canal in transverse section.

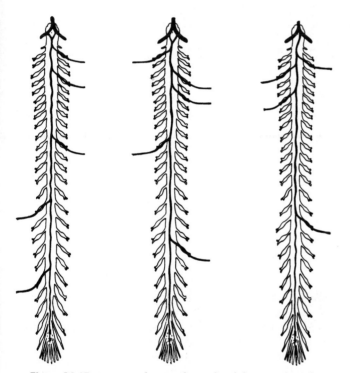

Figure 24.15 Segmental arterial supply of the spinal cord.

vertebrae and is located dorsal to the right crus of the diaphragm. The thoracic duct begins in the cisterna chyli.

Each kidney lies dorsal to the peritoneum on the dorsal abdominal wall. The kidneys lie along the vertebral column against the psoas muscle. The ureter is retroperitoneal throughout its length. It adheres to the peritoneum and is usually retracted with it during retroperitoneal approaches to the spine. The ureter descends nearly vertically along the psoas major muscle. On the right, it is next to the vena cava, and on both sides, it crosses the brim of the pelvis and the external iliac artery, just beyond the bifurcation of the common iliac artery.

Sacral Spine
Synovial and Nonsynovial Tissue. The joints of the sacrum consist of the superior bilateral facet joints with the fifth lumbar vertebrae, the sacrococcygeal joint, caudally with the coccyx via the cornua, and the sacroiliac joints laterally with the innominate bone. The anterior longitudinal ligament passes over the sacral promontory. The posterior longitudinal ligament runs across the dorsal surface of the lumbosacral disc, forming the ventral margin of the sacral canal. The sacrococcygeal joint contains a disc and is secured by four ligaments (ventral, dorsal, and two lateral ligaments). The sacroiliac joint is strengthened ventrally by ventral and lumbosacral ligaments. Other accessory ligaments are the sacrospinous, sacrotuberous, and iliolumbar ligaments.

Nerve Roots. The sacral canal contains sacral and coccygeal nerve roots. The filum terminale consists of two parts: interna and externa. The interna extends from the tip of the conus to the level of the second sacral neuroforamen. The externa begins at the level of the second sacral neuroforamen and attaches to the first coccygeal vertebra. The dorsal root ganglia lie in the sacral canal, central and rostral to the foramina from which their respective rami emerge. The sacral plexus is complex (Figure 24.16).[20] The predominant nerves of the plexus are the superior and inferior gluteal, sciatic, posterior, femoral, and pudendal nerves. The sympathetic trunk passes deep to the common iliac artery to run on the ventral surface of the sacrum. Each trunk continues caudally to the coccyx to form a single ganglion, the ganglion impar. The pelvic plexus lies embedded in the subperitoneal serosa lateral to the sacrum on the rostral surface of the obturator internus (Figure 24.17).

Soft-Tissue Structures. Important muscles in the sacral region include the gluteal, piriformis, and levator ani muscles. The floor of the pelvic cavity is made up mainly of the levator ani muscle. This muscle originates on the body of the pubis and the ischial spine and inserts on the central perineal tendon, the wall of the anal canal, the anococcygeal ligament, and the coccyx. It forms a sheet extending from the pubis ventrally, ischium laterally, and coccyx dorsally and encircles the urethra and anus in the middle. It is divided into three parts: pubococcygeus, puborectalis, and iliococcygeus muscles. The anococcygeal raphe of the ligament is the median fibrous intersection

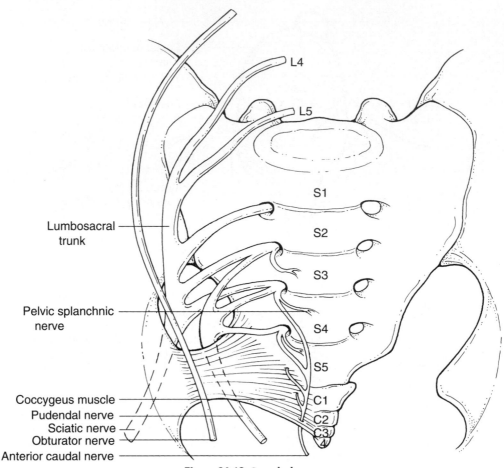

Figure 24.16 Sacral plexus.

of the pubococcygeus muscle from each side and extends between the anal canal and the coccyx. Muscles in the gluteal region that become important are the gluteus maximus and the piriformis. The gluteus maximus originates on the external surface of the ileum (including the iliac crest), dorsal surface of the sacrum and coccyx, and sacrotuberous ligament. The piriformis muscle originates on the ventral surface of the sacrum and the sacrotuberous ligament.

The common iliac arteries pass caudally and laterally to bifurcate into the external and internal iliac arteries at the level of the lumbosacral disc. The right common iliac artery crosses over the right common iliac vein to lie lateral and ventral to it at the point of bifurcation of the artery. The left iliac artery runs parallel and lateral to the left iliac vein. Branches of the common and internal iliac arteries are the iliolumbar, lateral sacral, and superior and inferior gluteal arteries (Figure 24.18). The venous anatomy is also variable but on the whole, it mirrors the arterial anatomy.

In adults, the bladder lies in the pelvis minor, dorsal to the pubic bone. The pelvic part of the ureter courses dorsocaudally, external to the parietal peritoneum on the lateral wall of the pelvis and ventral to the internal iliac artery. In males, the ureter enters the bladder dorsorostrally, just above the seminal vesicle. In females, its entrance to the bladder is the same, but it is in close proximity to the uterine artery and fornix.

Surgical Approaches
Dorsal Approach

After endotracheal intubation, the patient is carefully log rolled onto a spinal table. Pressure points (i.e., eyes, elbows, genitalia, and abdomen) should be routinely checked and padded as necessary. The abdomen should hang freely in order to decrease intraabdominal pressure. This will decrease venous bleeding intraoperatively. Fluoroscopy or plain radiography may be used to mark the level and to plan the appropriate incision length.

After a thorough preparation, the usual incision is in the midline over the previously palpated spinous processes. Fatty tissue is dissected with a sharp scalpel or Bovie. Achieving hemostasis early prevents "rundown" later in the case. Once the thoracoabdominal fascia is reached, it is precisely incised over the spinous processes to allow optimal closure at the end of surgery. The muscle attachments to the spinous processes, laminae, and facet joints are then dissected subperiosteally. This can be achieved with a Cobb elevator or a Bovie. In this manner, the lamina can be exposed for laminectomy or laminotomy to gain access to the conus medullaris, cauda equina, and disc interspace. With further lateral muscle dissection over the facet joint, the erector spinae muscles can be fully removed from their attachments, and the facets, pedicle, and transverse processes can be fully exposed. Care must be taken to avoid disrupting the facet joint capsule.

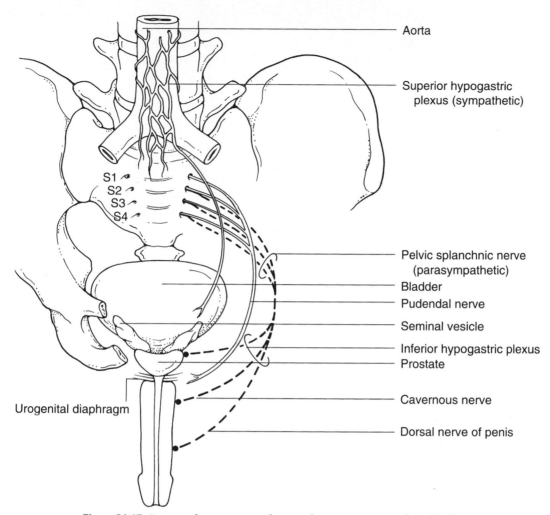

Aorta

Superior hypogastric plexus (sympathetic)

S1
S2
S3
S4

Pelvic splanchnic nerve (parasympathetic)

Bladder

Pudendal nerve

Seminal vesicle

Inferior hypogastric plexus

Prostate

Cavernous nerve

Dorsal nerve of penis

Urogenital diaphragm

Figure 24.17 Superior hypogastric and sympathetic innervation of the bladder.

The ligamentum flavum is found between the laminae originating in the middle of the undersurface of the rostral laminae and inserting under the rostral edge of the caudal laminae. It is thinnest in the midline and is made up of two layers that extend laterally to the facet joint to form the ventral portion of the facet capsule.

Depending on the goals of surgery, partial or complete removal of laminae, facet joints, and pedicles can be performed. An ability to mentally visualize the location of the pedicle from dorsal bony structures is crucial to successful bony dissection and preservation of neural structures.

The disc space at L5-S1 is located at the level of the interlaminar space. As one proceeds rostrally, each disc space becomes more rostral in relation to the interlaminar space. As a rule, one-half of the laminae must be removed to approach the L3-4 or L4-5 discs (Figure 24.19).

The lumbar epidural plexus can be a source of profuse bleeding. Proper visualization using appropriate lighting, bone removal, and retraction will generally enable adequate hemostasis with bipolar electrocautery or direct compression.

The dorsal exposure of the sacrum is the same as that described above, except that as one dissects laterally over the sacrum, the dorsal foramina can be inadvertently entered, causing damage to the dorsal nerve roots. En bloc and combined procedures for approaching tumors of the sacrum are discussed below.

The closure is performed in multiple layers, with special attention being paid to tight closure of the fascia.

Ventral Approach

Although most approaches are dorsal, in selected cases a ventral approach is indicated. This approach has been used for lumbar sympathectomy, osteomyelitis, and ventral interbody fusion for many years.[3,5,8,12,19,21]

The location of the lesion dictates the exposure. For T12-L1, a thoracoabdominal or lateral extracavitary approach is preferred. For L2 to L5, a retroperitoneal approach through the flank is optimal, if the pathology can be addressed from one side. If bilateral L2-5 exposure is required, a transperitoneal approach can be used. The best exposure of the L5-sacrum complex can be achieved through a transperitoneal ventral midline approach. Occasionally, this can be combined with a perineal approach for greater sacral exposure. Combined approaches are dictated by the surgical goals and the need for stabilization. A complete sacrectomy may require ventral, dorsal, and perineal exposures, and a ventral T12-L1 decompression

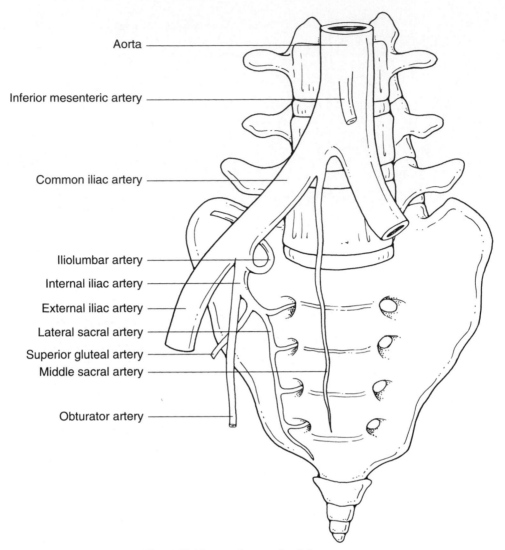

Aorta

Inferior mesenteric artery

Common iliac artery

Iliolumbar artery

Internal iliac artery

External iliac artery

Lateral sacral artery

Superior gluteal artery

Middle sacral artery

Obturator artery

Figure 24.18 Vascular supply of the sacrum.

may require a simultaneous dorsal exposure for placement of instruments.

Approach to T12-L1

The patient is placed in the right lateral decubitus position. Pressure points are checked, including elbows and knees. A right-sided approach can also be used if dictated by the pathology, but the left side is preferred to avoid retraction of the liver and the fragile vena cava.

The length of the incision is dictated by the number of vertebrae to be exposed, and the thoracic ribs guide the rostral aspect of the incision. If the T11 body is to be adequately visualized, the T10 rib should be removed. If the body of T12 is to be exposed, the T11 rib should be removed, and for L1, the T12 rib should be removed. The incision is begun dorsally, near the midline, and it follows the appropriate rib ventrally and obliquely downward on the upper middle abdomen. Its endpoint is determined by the number of lumbar vertebrae to be exposed (Figure 24.20).

The abdominal muscle layers are transected in line with the skin incision. Beginning superficially they are tran-

sected in the following order: (1) latissimus dorsi and external oblique, (2) serratus posterior inferior and internal oblique, (3) transversus abdominis, and (4) sacrospinalis and multifidus. The latter muscles are transected at the spinous process level of T12, perpendicular to the muscle fiber direction, and are elevated subperiosteally 2.5cm rostrally and caudally for facilitating medial exposure. At times, the sacrospinalis muscle can be retracted medially without transecting it. The transversalis fascia is opened and the peritoneum identified. Usually, there is a certain amount of fat in the preperitoneal space. A history of abdominal surgeries dictates that great care be taken to not open adherent peritoneum or bowel. Once a plane is established, and the peritoneum is bluntly dissected from the transversalis fascia, the rest of the transversalis muscle is opened. Retractors are placed, and the peritoneum is sharply separated from the abdominal wall with finger or sponge dissection. For difficult adherent areas, sharp dissection may be carefully performed.

With retraction of the sacrospinalis muscle, the intermediate layer of the thoracolumbar fascia is identified and followed to the ligament of Henle. This ligament is detached from the L1 transverse process at its lower

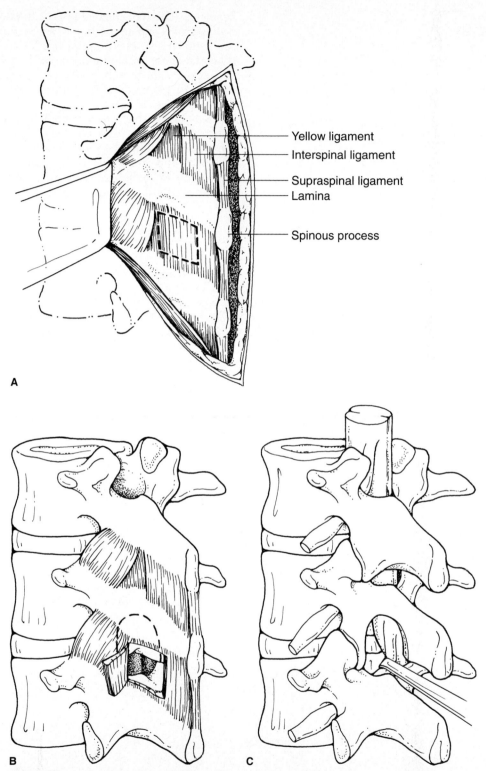

Figure 24.19 **(A)** Dorsal subperiosteal exposure of the lumbar spine. **(B)** Removal of the ligamentum flavum. **(C)** Exposure of the lumbar disc.

border that is contiguous with the rostral insertion of the quadratus lumborum muscle, the parietal pleura is gently separated from the ventral surface of the quadratus lumborum muscle and retracted above the twelfth rib. The medial half of the rib is resected after detaching the quadratus lumborum muscle from the twelfth rib. The pleura is retracted upward with the periosteum of the twelfth rib,

and the quadratus lumborum muscle is retracted downward with the lower half of the periosteum of the twelfth rib. The insertion of the lateral arcuate ligament is also detached from the transverse process of L1, leaving enough for reattachment. After verification that the pleura and peritoneum have been freed, the diaphragm is transected above the arcus lumbocostalis (medial arcuate

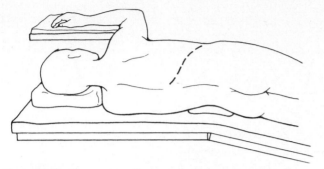

Figure 24.20 Skin incision for extrapleural retroperitoneal approach.

ligament). The right medial crus of the diaphragm is also divided, following application of stay sutures. Phrenic and subcostal vessels may require ligation and incision. The subcostal nerve should be preserved (Figure 24.21).

To expose the vertebrae, the retroperitoneal tissue and the parietal pleura are split at the thoracolumbar junction. The psoas muscle is retracted medially. A plane is established between the vertebral body and the psoas attachment to the bodies. If a body is collapsed or filled with tumor, it is important to locate normal landmarks above and below this body, since tissue planes may be disrupted at the site of pathology. The psoas muscle is dissected medially until the base of the pedicle is palpated, and the

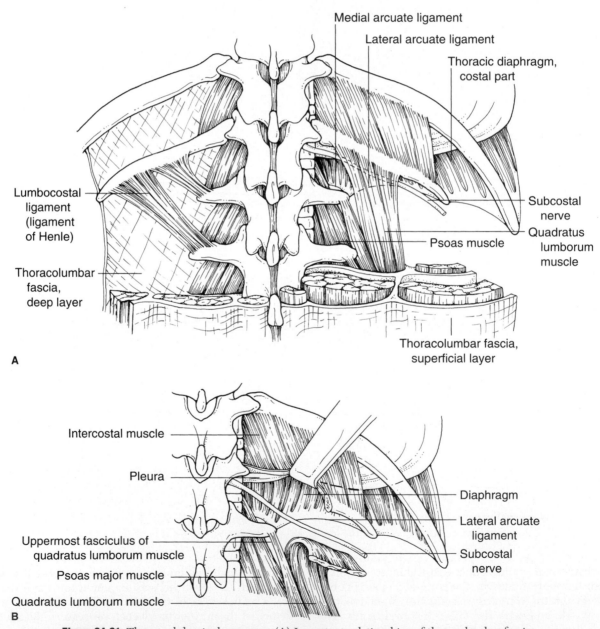

Figure 24.21 Thoracoabdominal exposure. **(A)** Important relationships of thoracolumbar fascia and lumbocostal ligament of Henle, quadratus lumborum, and diaphragm. **(B)** Sectioning of quadratus lumborum, medial 12th rib, and diaphragm.

ventral neural foramen is exposed. Transecting the parietal pleura in line with the vertebral bodies exposes the segmental vessels that run transversely over the vertebral bodies. They are mobilized, ligated, and transected as needed. The anterior longitudinal ligament can then be loosened with a periosteal elevator to establish the ventral plane in front of the pathologic site. When exposing the vertebral bodies, dissection should begin over the intervertebral discs, using the hinged anterior longitudinal ligament and the medially placed psoas muscle to protect the sympathetic chain and great vessels. If a more rostral exposure is required, the parietal pleura can be further retracted and the medial half of the eleventh rib can be resected. During this dissection, it is important to recall the location of the ascending lumbar vein, azygos vein, thoracic duct, splanchnic nerves, and sympathetic plexus.

Closure is performed in multiple layers with careful reapproximation of the diaphragmatic crus. The diaphragm above the medial arcuate ligament is closed using the stay sutures. The quadratus lumborum muscle is resutured to the rostral half of the periosteum of the twelfth rib. The abdominal musculature is closed in multiple layers and the iliocostal, serratus posterior, serratus inferior, and latissimus dorsi muscles are sutured.

Retroperitoneal Approach to L2-5

The patient is placed in the lateral decubitus position, with the side of surgery dictated by the pathology. If one has a choice of sides, the left side is preferred to avoid liver retraction and manipulation of the vena cava. The spleen is smaller and can be easily retracted, although injury has been reported.[9] The table is angled so that the middle of the patient's body is concave and arched downward. This opens the space between the ribs and the iliac crest, and allows the viscera to fall away. The upper hip should be flexed to relax the psoas muscle. The incision is dictated by the level to be exposed (Figure 24.22). The umbilicus can be used as a guide. To expose L5-S1, an incision is made between the symphysis pubis and umbilicus. A slightly higher incision is made for L4-5, the incision for L3-4 is made at the umbilicus, and for L2-3, above the umbilicus. If L2 exposure is desired, the skin incision begins near the midline at the level of the spinous process of T11 and continues along the twelfth rib before running obliquely and vertically toward the rectus sheath. The caudal distance of the incision is dictated by the number of vertebral bodies to be exposed.

The latissimus dorsi, external oblique, internal oblique, and transversus muscles should be cut in line with the skin incision. The transversalis fascia is opened, and the retroperitoneal space is entered. The peritoneum is thin and blue and needs to be dissected thoroughly from the abdominal wall in all directions. The peritoneum is thickest laterally and is easier to separate from the transversalis in this location; toward the midline, it is thinner and more attached. A sponge or sharp dissection for adhesions can be used as needed. The correct plane of dissection may not be clearly obvious. The dissection follows dorsal to the kidney in the potential space between the renal fascia and quadratus lumborum and psoas muscles. The retroperitoneal fat and contents, along with the ureter (identified

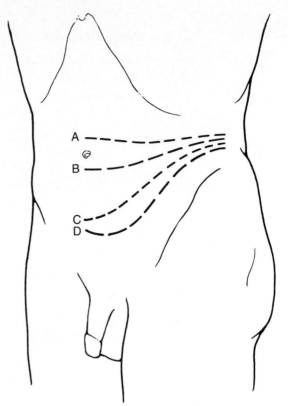

Figure 24.22 Retroperitoneal incisions: **(A)** L2-3, **(B)** L3-4, **(C)** L4-5, and **(D)** L5-S1.

by its cylindric shape and peristaltic movements), are gently retracted medially. The quadratus lumborum muscle is identified. When palpating through this muscle, the transverse processes can be mistaken for the vertebral bodies. If in the correct plane, the psoas muscle will come into view. A common mistake is to enter the retropsoas space, which is a blind pouch between the psoas and the quadratus lumborum muscles (Figure 24.23). On the surface of the psoas muscle, the genitofemoral nerve is noted as a small white structure lying on the belly of the psoas muscle. This nerve should be protected. The lumbar spine is immediately medial to the psoas muscle and can be obscured by this muscle. If access to L2 is required, it is helpful to resect the twelfth rib. The periosteum is incised over the twelfth rib, and the peripheral portion of the rib is resected, with care taken to not open the pleural cavity.

A Finochietto rib retractor or Bookwalter retractor is used to open the wound longitudinally, and a padded Deaver retractor is used to retract the kidney and peritoneal contents medially. To expose the ventrolateral borders of L2-5, the psoas muscle can be mobilized dorsally with a Cobb elevator or Bovie. The sympathetic trunk, which lies just medial to the psoas muscle, should be preserved as much as possible. It should be remembered that the ascending iliolumbar vein crosses the L4-5 disc space and needs to be ligated and separated to expose the disc space and the L5 vertebral body. The segmental vessels located at the midportion of each vertebral body should be isolated, ligated, and cut outside the neuroforamina without retraction of the vessels. Once the segmental vessels have been incised, the aorta can be mobilized medially to

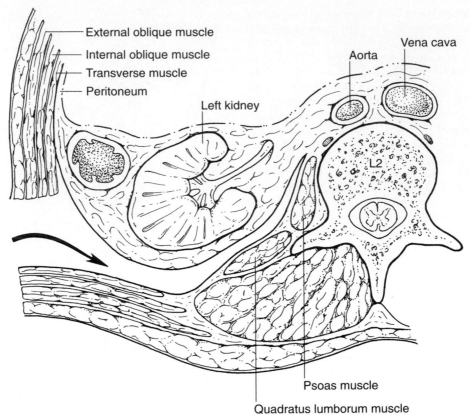

Figure 24.23 Retroperitoneal approach in the coronal plane and anatomic relationships to muscle and retroperitoneal contents.

expose the ventral aspect of the vertebral bodies. Next, the Cobb elevator can be used to separate the anterior longitudinal ligament from the ventral vertebral bodies. This provides a barrier of protection as the surgeon works on the selected vertebral body. If the pathology is not obvious or the sacral promontory is not evident, a radiograph should be obtained to determine the appropriate level.

The closure begins with the rib bed, which is reapproximated. The muscle closure is undertaken in multiple layers.

Transperitoneal or Retroperitoneal Paramedian Rectus Approach

Although L4-5 can be approached retroperitoneally, exposure of L5 and the sacrum can be achieved more readily through a direct ventral approach. Before surgery, the patient should be prepared with a bowel cathartic. The supine position is augmented with a sacral bolster to elevate the sacrum and provide better exposure. The Trendelenburg position allows the peritoneal contents to rest upward. The level of incision should be subumbilical, several centimeters above the pubis. If exposure of more rostral vertebral bodies is desired, the length of the incision can be extended to the umbilicus. The abdominal wall is opened para midline at the border of the left rectus muscle. If the midline is used and the linea alba opened, the preperitoneal fat will be identified immediately.

One can decide at this point whether to use a transperitoneal or a retroperitoneal approach. A retroperitoneal approach on the left side is safe, with the viscera and hypogastric plexus being protected, but it has the disadvantage of a less direct route and less than maximal exposure of the spine.[7] The parietal peritoneum can be retracted from the lateral abdominal wall with a swab stick or blunt hand dissection. Once the retroperitoneal contents are packed and retracted upward and lateral, the psoas muscle and genitofemoral nerves are visualized. The common iliac artery ventral to the vein can be seen through a layer of retroperitoneal fatty tissue. At the caudal margin of L4, the ureter and testicular vessels cross the common iliac artery laterally to medially. Midway above the aortic bifurcation runs the superior hypogastric plexus that fans out ventrally to the promontory. For exposures above L5, the plexus is retracted medially; for exposures below L5, it is retracted laterally (Figure 24.24). The psoas muscle is detached laterally, and the iliolumbar and segmental vessels are ligated and separated as necessary. For lower lumbar access, the iliac vessels are freed from the anterior longitudinal ligament and mobilized contralaterally.

Transperitoneally, the peritoneum is a thin, blue membrane that is freed from the abdominal wall and opened in a linear fashion. The greater omentum, small bowel, and the mesenteric root are retracted rostrally. The mesocolon is retracted laterally, and the sigmoid colon retracted caudally. After the bowel is mobilized, the aortic bifurcation and sacral promontory are identified through the dorsal peritoneum. The dorsal peritoneum is opened in a linear fashion along the right common iliac artery from the aortic bifurcation to the bifurcation of the internal and external iliac arteries. Care should be taken to identify the

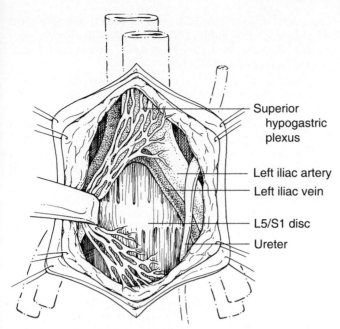

Figure 24.24 Superior hypogastric plexus laterally retracted.

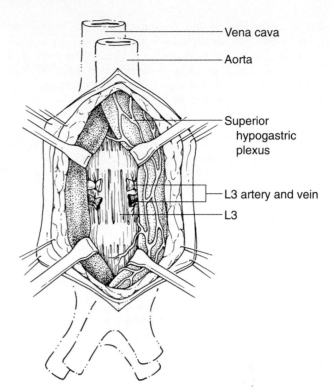

Figure 24.25 Transperitoneal L3-4 exposure with the segmental vessels ligated and aorta and common iliac arteries retracted laterally.

ureter, which should cross the right external iliac artery and the hypogastric plexus, which is directly ventral to the fifth lumbar vertebra and the L5-S1 disc space. To aid in dissection, saline solution is infiltrated into the dorsal peritoneal tissue before incision. This elevates the peritoneal tissue while leaving the superior hypogastric plexus adherent to the aorta.[17] The plexus is best preserved by finding the plane between the anterior longitudinal ligament and the prevertebral tissue and mobilizing the structures en bloc. The sacral vein and artery may be adherent to the sacrum. Ligation and incision may be necessary to mobilize the large vessels laterally. L3 and L4 may also be exposed in this dissection by ligating and transecting appropriate segmental vessels to allow lateral retraction of the aorta and common iliacs arteries (Figure 24.25). If the aortic bifurcation is located more rostral than usual, an interiliac approach may be used.

The parietal peritoneum is closed with running absorbable suture. Before the omentum is pulled down, one must ensure that no torsion is present on the mesenteric root. The ventral peritoneum is also closed, as was the dorsal peritoneum. The rectus and skin are closed in multiple layers.

Laparoscopic Transperitoneal Approach

Especially for the case of disc pathology at L5-S1, a laparoscopic approach allows for a direct ventral exposure without the need for open laparotomy. As with the standard open procedure, a routine bowel prep, a Foley catheter, and an orogastric tube are utilized. The patient is positioned supine in steep Trendelenburg to aid in retracting the peritoneal contents toward the upper abdomen. Portals are placed in a diamond shape, with the superior/periumbilical portal being used for the camera, the middle or lateral portals for dissection and retraction, and the suprapubic for the spinal instrumentation (Figure 24.26). The spinal working portal is not placed until the

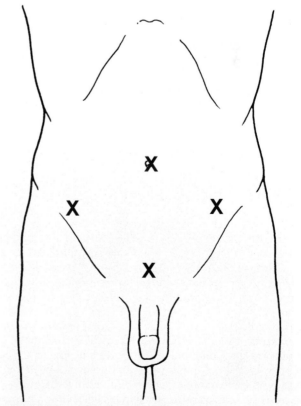

Figure 24.26 Ventral abdominal wall showing the configuration of the laparoscopic portals.

disc space is defined and the dorsal peritoneum and vasculature has been dissected free from it.

Dissection of the peritoneum is performed through a right-sided vertical incision as described above, with care taken to avoid coagulating on or near the hypogastric plexus. For exposure to the L5-S1 disc space, the middle sacral artery and several small veins may need to be clipped and then ligated. Once the disc space has been exposed, a long needle may be used to determine the angle of the L5-S1 disc space. This technique allows for optimal positioning for the spinal working portal, and it greatly facilitates the procedure (Figure 24.27).

Once completed, each portal is removed and each incision is closed in layers.

Approaches to the Sacrum

Surgical approaches to the sacrum vary according to the location of the pathologic lesion and according to whether debulking or en bloc resection is the surgical goal. This area is surgically challenging because of (1) its relationship to the pelvis, (2) dorsal tilt, (3) concavity, (4) long intraosseous course of the vertically positioned sacral nerve roots, and (5) approximation to the iliac wings and overhang of the superior iliac crests.[15] Often, combined approaches are necessary because of these anatomic constraints. Ventral and dorsal approaches that have been described for the low lumbar spine are often applicable to the sacrum. Other approaches that are useful are the lateral sacroiliac approach and the perineal approach (if the pathology is caudal or extending laterally outside of the sacrum into the iliac wings). A combined ventral/dorsal abdominosacral approach or a radical sacrectomy are useful if en bloc resection is desired.[15,23]

The dorsal transsacral approach is indicated for lesions contained within the sacral canal (no presacral extension). Incisional biopsy or intralesional debulking is easily performed via the dorsal approach. Routine subperiosteal dissection and sacral laminectomy, followed by intraspinal or

intrasacral tumor removal using standard microsurgical technique, is the method of choice. For marginal resection of tumors with presacral extension, a combined dorsal/ventral approach is indicated.

The ventral approach is preferred for complete visualization of the presacral space and can be achieved with either a transabdominal or retroperitoneal exposure.[10] The former is preferred if bilateral visualization of the sacrum is desired, as in the case of large tumors. Ventral access allows exposure of the iliac and sacral vessels and other viscera for early control of the vascular supply of the tumor and for dissection of the tumor-viscera junction. These approaches provide good exposure of the mid sacrum and upper sacrum. Intradural or intraspinal tumors cannot be adequately exposed from a ventral approach.[11] The main advantage of the retroperitoneal approach is the option for a combined retroperitoneal/dorsal exposure for intraspinal en bloc tumor resection.

For lesions below the mid sacrum or upper sacrum (Figure 24.28), the perineal approach is indicated.[14] The patient is positioned in the flexed prone (i.e., Kraske) position. A single, longitudinal incision is made that extends below the coccyx. Separating the anococcygeal raphe and releasing the gluteal and levator ani muscles exposes the presacral space. The anal canal and rectum are bluntly dissected from the tumor surface. After the tumor margins are identified, the lateral sacral attachments of the piriformis muscle and the sacrospinous and sacrotuberous ligaments are incised bilaterally. A laminectomy is performed dorsally at the foramina, one space above the lesion. The filum externa and nerve roots caudal to the determined level are divided and sectioned. An osteotome is used to section the sacrum ventrally through the perineal opening

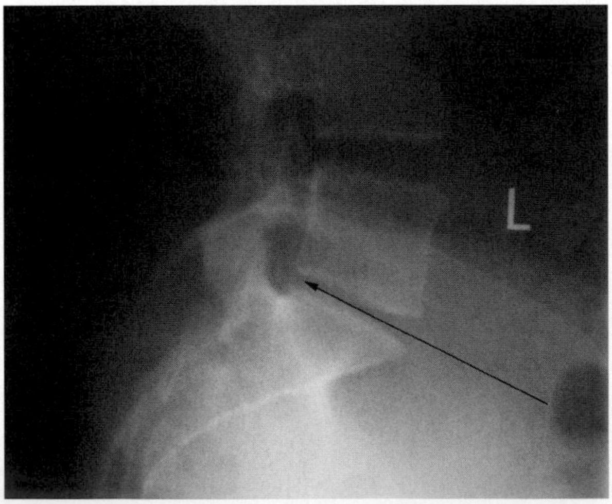

Figure 24.27 Lateral radiograph showing the correct working angle *(arrow)* for the suprapubic portal to allow entry into the L5-S1 disc space.

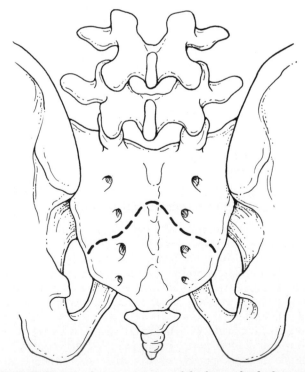

Figure 24.28 Dorsal representation of the lower third of sacrum that can be removed through a perineal approach.

at the appropriate level, usually below S3. The tumor can then be removed en bloc or with wide margins. The wound is closed in layers over a suction drain.

The lateral approach to the sacroiliac joint allows simultaneous exposure of the dorsal and ventral surface of the sacroiliac joint for resection of tumors that involve the sacroiliac joint, lateral ala, and the medial iliac wing. The incision is shaped like a hockey stick, starting over the sacrum and curving laterally over the iliac crest (Figure 24.29). The muscular attachments of the abdominal, erector spinae, and gluteus muscles and the lumbodorsal fascia are detached and reflected. The gluteus muscles are elevated using a subperiosteal technique down to the sciatic notch. The gluteal vessels and nerves should be preserved. Ventrally, subperiosteal elevation of the iliac and psoas muscles exposes the sacroiliac joint. Care must be taken to not injure the lumbosacral nerve trunk as it passes ventral to the surface of the sacroiliac joint. The osteotomy is performed in a dorsoventral direction. The sacral osteotomy is begun lateral to the upper three dorsal neuroforamina and directed ventrally. Laterally, the iliac osteotomy is carried down to the sciatic notch. The entire specimen is removed en bloc. The bony margins are covered with bone wax and Gelfoam, as desired, and closed in layers over drains.[15]

The abdominosacral approach is a combination of a low ventral sacral approach and the dorsal sacral approach.[8] It is also used for the sacrectomy, if en bloc resection is indicated.[23] The incision for the ventral approach varies, depending on whether rectum resection is required. If it can be preserved, the peritoneum need not be opened. A generous, semicircular incision provides adequate exposure of the sacrum after retracting the peritoneal contents rostrally. The patient is positioned supine with legs bent and flexed. The semicircular incision is made just above the pubis bone, cutting through the tendon of the rectus muscle, 1cm above its attachments bilaterally (Figure 24.28). The peritoneum is swept upward to expose the common and external and internal iliac vessels. Vessel loops are applied for vascular control. This dissection is performed medially under the dorsal parietal peritoneum, preserving the superior hypogastric plexus and ureter, and meets in the midline behind the rectum.

If the rectum is resected, the peritoneal cavity is opened through a caudal midline incision. It will be necessary to ligate the superior rectal vessels, cut the bowel through the ureterosigmoid junction, and invaginate the tissue of incised bowel. The peritoneum is incised through the bottom of the rectovesical pouch, and the rectum is released ventrally. With the patient in the lithotomy position, an inverted U incision is made around the anus, and the anal canal and rectum are dissected free.

The internal iliac arteries and veins are separated and controlled with vessel loops. The lateral and medial sacral veins and arteries are incised and ligated. If a sacrectomy above S1 is to be performed, iliolumbar vessels must also be taken. The periosteum is stripped and the sympathetic nerve trunk is incised ventral to S1. Lateral to the sympathetic trunk, the lumbosacral nerves L4 and L5 pass ventral to the sacral wing and the sacroiliac joint. These must be released and protected. Finally, the sacrum is removed via osteotomy. It is advised that the osteotomy line be carried past the sacroiliac joint so that it can be palpated during the dorsal approach (Figure 24.30). Also, if an en bloc resection is desired, the osteotomy should be performed one level

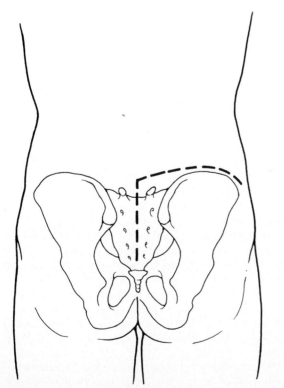

Figure 24.29 Hockey-stick incision for the lateral approach to the sacroiliac joint.

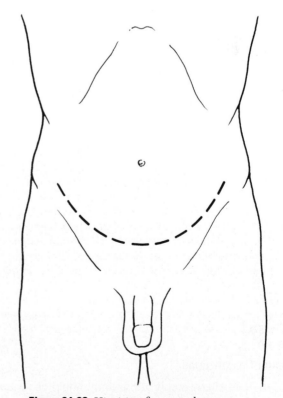

Figure 24.30 Uincision for ventral sacrectomy.

above the tumor. The wound is closed in multiple layers or is closed temporarily, if the rectum is to be resected.

For a combined procedure, the patient is turned and a dorsal midline incision is made from L5 to the coccyx. The iliac attachments of the gluteus muscles are transected, leaving a cuff for reattachment. The sacral attachments of the gluteus maximus and underlying piriformis muscles and the anococcygeal, sacrospinous, and sacrotuberous ligaments are transected, also leaving a cuff. The gluteal nerves and vessels are preserved, if possible. The sciatic nerves are dissected through the sciatic notch and preserved. A partial lower L5 and upper sacral laminectomy is performed to expose the dural sac, which is ligated just below the last nerve root to be preserved. The ventral osteotomy line is then palpated, and the dorsal osteotomy is performed. This should extend from the midline through the sacroiliac joint. Stabilization of the lumbar spine to the ileum may be required, if the L5-S1 joints are taken. However, if the S1 vertebral body is left intact, stabilization is usually not necessary. Once the osteotomy is complete, the distal end of the sacrificed sacral nerve roots are divided just proximal to their entry into the sciatic nerve. Bleeding is usually profuse. Hemostasis should be quickly achieved with bone wax and electrocautery. If the rectum can be preserved, the anal region is released from the dissecting bands that attach it to the coccyx. However, if it is to be included, the levator ani is transected on each side. In an en bloc procedure, the sacrospinal muscles are taken with the specimen to avoid violating the tumor wall. The wound is closed in multiple layers over a drain. If the rectum has been included in the specimen, the patient is placed in the supine position and the abdomen is opened again. The sigmoid colon is removed from its mesentery, a colostomy is performed, and the pelvic peritoneum is closed. The wound is again closed in a standard fashion.

Complications
Visceral Complications

Perforation of the peritoneum is common, especially if there has been previous surgery, scarring, or infection. If this should happen, immediate repair is indicated. With the retroperitoneal approach, the abdominal wall is well developed laterally and, therefore, the transverse abdominus muscle and peritoneum can be readily identified and separated. For a pararectus retroperitoneal approach, the peritoneum can be identified just lateral to the rectus sheath.

With the retroperitoneal approach, the ureter is usually identified on the undersurface of the peritoneal sac. It should be swept medially and ventrally. With the transperitoneal approach, the ureter is lateral and is usually not a problem. If the ureter was incised, primary repair is indicated.

Injury to bowel, bladder, kidneys, spleen, or any other visceral organ during direct or retroperitoneal approaches should be dealt with by the appropriate surgical specialist.

Vascular Complications

To prevent vascular complications, one should be aware of the variations in vascular anatomy, for example, a large left iliac vein, an unusual bifurcation of the aorta or vena cava, or atypical positions of the lumbar veins. In addition, osteophytic spurs associated with reactive changes in the disc can cause the vena cava to become adherent to the disk. Because most vascular structures are injured during disc removal, a layer of tissue is left between the disc (or disc/vertebral body) and the great vessels.

Lumbar veins can be variable in location, especially the fifth, or iliolumbar, vein. This vein drains into either the vena cava or left iliac vein and can become a tether, if it becomes necessary to move the vena cava from left to right. The risk of avulsion of the vein directly off the vena cava exists and can cause rapid blood loss. As the left iliac vein courses over the disc space at L5-S1, it can be stretched and flat. It must be identified and controlled to avoid injury when opening the L5-S1 disc space.[24] This vein can also be large, bulbous, and difficult to retract. If it is lacerated, proximal and distal control must be obtained prior to repair.

Arterial injury can occur in the form of clot formation or laceration. The most common injury reported is to the left iliac artery during an approach to the L4-5 disc space. This vessel must be partially mobilized to approach the disc space. Once it is mobilized, retractors must be carefully positioned and checked periodically to avoid kinking or compressing the large vessels.

Pulmonary Complications

Pleural tears should be treated with a tube thoracostomy. Chylothorax has been reported because of damage to the thoracic duct during ventral surgery while mobilizing the right crus of the diaphragm.[6]

Neural Complications

Neural injury can occur to the superior hypogastric plexus, sympathetic chain, cauda equina, or lumbosacral plexus. The superior hypogastric plexus is responsible for closure of the bladder neck during ejaculation. If the plexus is damaged, the result may be retrograde ejaculation.[11] This may be avoided by careful dissection of structures within the bifurcation of the aorta. By entering this area to the right of the left iliac artery and vein and sweeping the tissue from left to right, one can retract this tissue en bloc to preserve the plexus (see Figure 20.24). Blunt dissection with gentle retraction of the prevertebral tissue must be used and excessive electrocautery avoided.

The paraspinous sympathetic lumbar chain must usually be stretched or cut in the normal course of the ventral approach. Usually, the patient complains of a cold foot on the opposite side of the dissection. In fact, the ipsilateral foot is abnormally warm because of the lack of vasoconstrictive ability on the side of the surgery.

Cauda equina damage results from direct penetration into the spinal canal. Correct graft measurement, controlled impaction technique, and good visualization of pathologic anatomy, should minimize risk of cauda equina injury.

The lumbosacral plexus is located in the psoas muscle. Penetration or aggressive retraction must be avoided to prevent significant plexus damage. Often the psoas muscle is markedly enlarged and bulging over the spine. Psoas muscle dissection should begin at the midline (at the disc space). A pin retractor can be used to hold the muscle away from the surgical site after dissection is completed.

Summary

Adequate exposure of ventral lumbosacral anatomy is limited by the physical impediments imposed upon this region by the thoracic cage and pelvis, thoracic and abdominal viscera, and the great vessels. Because of these constraints, a number of specific surgical approaches have been designed to maximize exposure of specific regions. To perform these operations safely and effectively, the surgeon must have a thorough understanding of the three-dimensional anatomy of the lumbosacral region, the potential anatomic variants, and a detailed plan for achieving the surgical goal within existing constraints. In addition, by understanding where the majority of complications arise and how to avoid them, the safety of these procedures can be improved significantly.

REFERENCES

1. Bauer R, Kerschbaumer F, Poisel S, Harle A: Approaches. In Bauer R (ed): *Atlas of Spinal Operations*, ed 1. New York, Thieme, 1993, p 52.
2. Benzel EC: Biomechanically relevant anatomy and material properties of the spine and associated elements. In Benzel EC (ed): *Biomechanics of Spine Stabilization: Principles and Clinical Practice*, ed 1. New York, McGraw-Hill, 1995.
3. Blumenthal SL, Baker J, Dossett A, Selby KD: The role of anterior lumbar fusion for internal disc disruption. *Spine* 13:566, 1988.
4. Burrington JD, Brown C, Wayne ER, Odom J: Anterior approach to the thoracolumbar spine. *Arch Surg* 111:456, 1976.
5. Crock HV: Anterior lumbar interbody fusion. *Clin Orthop* 82:157, 1980.
6. Eisenstein S, O'Brien JP: Chylothorax: a complication of Dwyer's anterior instrumentation. *Br J Surg* 64:339, 1977.
7. Found EM, Weinstein JN: Surgical approaches to the lumbar spine. In Frymoyer JW (ed): *The Adult Spine: Principles and Practice*, ed 1. Philadelphia, Lippincott-Raven, 1991, p 1522.
8. Freebody D, Bendall R, Taylor RD: Anterior transperitoneal lumbar fusion. *J Bone Joint Surg* 53B:617, 1971.
9. Hodge DW, DeWald RL: Splenic injury complicating the anterior thoracoabdominal surgical approach for scoliosis. *J Bone Joint Surg* 65A:396, 1983.
10. Huth JF, Dawson EG, Eilber FR: Abdominosacral resection for malignant tumors of the sacrum. *Am J Surg* 148:157, 1984.
11. Johnson RN, McGuire EJ: Urogenital complications of anterior approaches to the lumbar spine. *Clin Orthop* 154:114, 1981.
12. Kirkaldy-Willis WH, Thomas GT: Anterior approaches in the diagnosis and treatment of infections of the vertebral bodies. *J Bone Joint Surg* 47A:87, 1965.
13. Labate JS: The surgical anatomy of the superior hypogastric plexus—"presacral nerve." *Surg Gynecol Obstet* 67:199, 1938.
14. Louis R: Chirurgie de rachis. *Anatomie Chirurgicale et Voles D'Abord.* Berlin, Springer-Verlag, 1982.
15. McCormick PC, Post KD: Surgical approaches to the sacrum. In Doty JR, Rengachry SS (eds): *Surgical Disorders of the Sacrum*, ed 1. New York, Thieme, 1994, p 257.
16. Minet J: Etude de la 12 cote et de 3 ses variations: application a la incision lombaire. *Arch D Mald* 9:47, 1935.
17. Mirbaha MM: Anterior approach to the thoraco-lumbar junction by a retroperitoneal-extrapleural technic. *Clin Orthop* 91:41, 1973.
18. Moore K: The abdomen. In *Clinically Oriented Anatomy*, ed 2. Baltimore, Williams & Wilkins, 1985, p 268.
19. Newman MH, Grinstead GL: Anterior lumbar interbody fusion for internal disc disruption. *Spine* 17:831, 1992.
20. Rengachry SS: Surgical anatomy of the sacrum. In Doty JR, Rengachry SS (eds): *Surgical Disorders of the Sacrum*, ed 1. New York, Thieme, 1994, p 31.
21. Sterner B, Gunterberg B: High amputation of the sacrum for extirpation of tumors. *Spine* 3:351, 1978.
22. Stephen EI, Botsford DJ: Surgical anatomy and operative approaches to the sacrum. In Frymoyer JW (ed): *The Adult Spine: Principles and Practice*, ed 1. Philadelphia, Lippincott-Raven, 1991, p 2099.
23. Sacks S: Anterior interbody fusion of the lumbar spine. *J Bone Joint Surg* 47B:211, 1965.
24. Watkins R: Anterior lumbar interbody fusion surgical complications. *Clin Orthop* 284:47, 1992.

Surgical Procedures

3.1 DECOMPRESSION AND ARTHRODESIS OF THE CERVICAL SPINE

CHAPTER 25

Upper Cervical and Craniocervical Decompression

Christopher G. Paramore, Volker K.H. Sonntag, and Robert F. Spetzler

The decision to operate on the craniovertebral junction must be individualized and is based on the patient's history, physical examination, and radiographic studies. Major factors to be considered are the presence of spinal canal compromise and instability. In the presence of a clear neurologic deficit with radiographic confirmation of compression, the decision to operate is easy (Figure 25.1). More thought is required for patients who may be only mildly symptomatic or have only minor radiographic evidence of compression or instability. In these instances other factors, such as the natural history of the underlying pathology, the reliability of the patient, and the risk of surgical morbidity, must be scrutinized seriously. In the patient deemed to be a surgical candidate, the approach to the lesion should be dictated by the location of the compression. The following is a synopsis of various approaches to compressive pathology of the craniovertebral junction.

Ventral Approaches

The transoral transpharyngeal approach has become an accepted technique for removal of ventral extradural pathology located from the lower clivus to the upper cervical spine. Pharyngeal abscesses have been drained by this route since antiquity,[37] but the first description of a transoral operation directed at a lesion, a bullet, was reported by Kanavel[22] in 1917. Southwick and Robinson[37] removed an osteoid osteoma from C2 via this route in 1944. Fang and Ong,[16] in the first major treatise on this subject, reported six patients who underwent transoral decompression for irreducible atlantoaxial instability or congenital anomalies. The high complication rate reported contributed to the slow acceptance of this procedure by the neurosurgical community. However, the safety and efficacy of this technique are now well established.*Although the transoral approach provides a relatively straight pathway to the anterior craniover-

*References 11,13,19, 23,26,38.

tebral junction, it has the downside of exposing the operative field to bacterial contamination. This may become an issue if one attempts to place a bone graft and/or instrumentation[24] or if an intradural exposure is required. Thus, others have developed approaches that allow access to this area by an extrapharyngeal exposure.[40] Although technically challenging, this is a viable alternative approach to the transoral approach, if careful technique is used. At the authors' institutions, most patients requiring ventral craniovertebral decompression have been treated by the transoral method.

Technique

The patient is placed under general anesthesia and intubated with a reinforced endotracheal tube. Fiber optic endoscopy and awake intubation are used when neck extension is not possible or if the patient is already in a halo or other traction device. The patient is placed supine and the head is immobilized via the Mayfield headrest (Codman, Inc., Randolph, MA) or halo adapter. The Spetzler-Sonntag transoral retractor (Aesculap, San Francisco, CA), or an equivalent device, is positioned. The endotracheal tube and tongue are retracted caudally while the palate is elevated, using a self-retaining flexible spatula. Palatal retraction with suture and transnasal catheters may be required if the Spetzler-Sonntag retractor is not used (Figure 25.2). Ventilation via tracheostomy may be required, although rarely, if splitting of the mandible is required to facilitate exposure.[41] This may be necessary if the patient is unable to open the mouth wide enough to accomplish the procedure.

The oral cavity is prepared with Betadine solution, and the operating microscope is brought into the field. A lateral radiograph is obtained to confirm the position of the retractor and to verify the angle of approach toward the pathology. A midline incision is made and carried down to the bone with electrocautery. A subperiosteal dissection of the pharyngeal tissues is performed, and self-retaining retractors are placed to expose the lower clivus, C1, and C2. Although commonly reported in the literature, division of the soft palate has rarely been necessary in our experience.

Using a high-speed air drill the ventral arch of C1 is removed, as needed, to gain exposure to the lesion. If possible, a portion of the ventral arch of C1 is preserved to prevent spreading of the lateral masses of C1 and to denote the anatomic midline. Furthermore, the anterior tubercle of C1 serves as a target for the placement of posterior C1-C2 transfacet screws if atlantoaxial fusion is performed, as is often necessary.[14] Frequently, a large amount of pannus is present between the arch of C1 and the dens in rheumatoid arthritis patients. This is removed with cautery, curettes, and rongeurs. No more than 1.5cm should be exposed on either side of the midline. Further dissection endangers the vertebral arteries, hypoglossal nerves, and cervical neurovascular bundle (Figure 25.3).[17]

319

Several factors must be considered when removing the dens. Rostrally, the alar and apical ligaments must be sectioned in order to remove the tip of the dens. This region is often adherent to the dura mater, making it prone to a cerebrospinal fluid (CSF) fistula.[28] Section of these ligaments is best achieved while the base of the dens is still intact and

the tip is not "floating." As the decompression proceeds, the dura tends to billow into the operative field, often in duplicated folds, making dissection difficult. Leaving a thin shell of bone along the length of the dens delays this phenomenon until the end of the decompression. The completeness of decompression can be ascertained using a lateral image

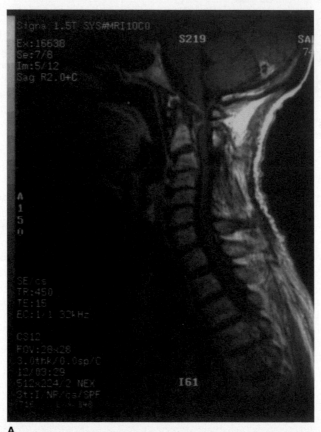

A

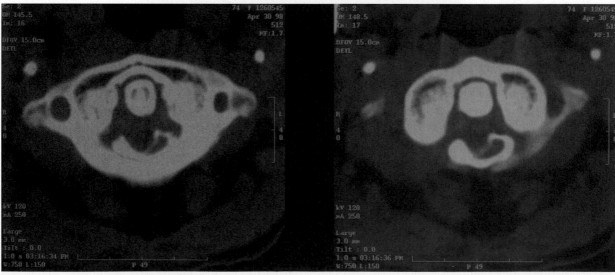

B

Figure 25.1 This 71-year-old female had symptoms of progressive myelopathy secondary to a retroodontoid mass, without evidence of C1-2 instability, basilar invagination, or rheumatoid arthritis. (**A**) MRI revealed an isointense mass with peripheral gadolinium enhancement. (**B**) Postmyelogram computed tomography scans revealed a large retrodental soft tissue mass compressing the spinal cord. The patient underwent transoral decompression followed by C1-2 posterior fusion with autograft, interspinous cable fixation, and transarticular screw fixation.

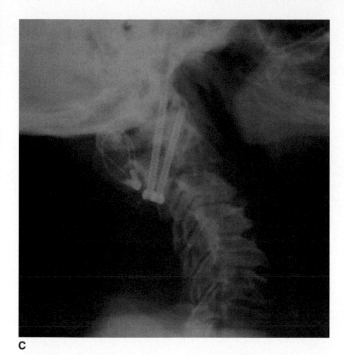

C

Figure 25.1 *cont'd* (**C**) Reveals a solid fusion. Pathologic examination of the specimen revealed fibrocartilage consistent with exuberant transverse ligament degeneration. *(From Cai CY, Palmer CA, Paramore CG: Exuberant transverse ligament degeneration causing high cervical myelopathy.* J Spinal Disord *14(1):84-88, 2001.)*

intensifier and locally applied iodinated contrast material. More recently, frameless stereotactic assistance has made determination of the extent of resection easier.[31]

After the decompression is completed, hemostasis is achieved. A Valsalva maneuver is performed to evaluate for an occult CSF leak. A single-layer closure of the pharynx is accomplished with absorbable sutures. A feeding tube is placed before the anesthetic agents are reversed. The endotracheal tube is retained for 24 to 48 hours and then removed if no complications ensue. Swelling of the tongue and airway obstruction are the primary concerns. Fluids are allowed per mouth after 1 week. Dorsal stabilization may be performed immediately during the same sitting or on a delayed basis of 2 to 3 days.

Complication Avoidance

Most patients suffering from irreducible compression of the craniovertebral junction are debilitated. In severe cases, a short course of parenteral nutrition prior to surgery may improve postoperative wound healing. Inadequate decompression of the cervicomedullary junction may occur if the depth of dissection is not clearly appreciated. The use of radiography augmented with iodinated contrast material, or frameless stereotaxy, will help ascertain the extent of decompression. For patients with large amounts of pannus, a clear plane between the dura and dens may not emerge. Careful dissection on a

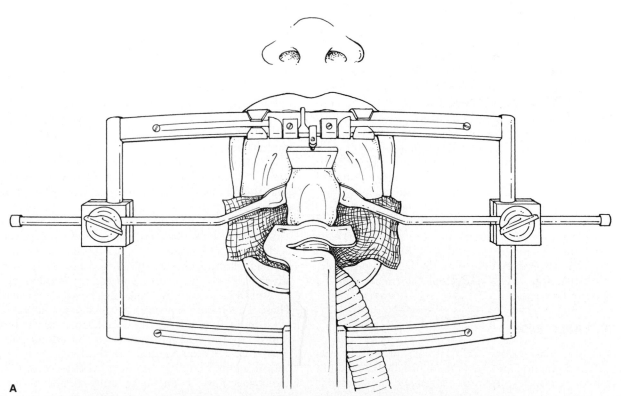

A

Figure 25.2 Transoral approach to ventral C1-2 compressive pathology. (**A**) Position of the Spetzler-Sonntag retractor system (Aesculap, San Francisco, CA). A contoured blade retracts both the tongue and the endotracheal tube. A thin blade elevates the palate, eliminating the need for rubber catheter transnasal retraction. Lateral pharyngeal retractors are adjusted by peripherally located knobs.   *Continued*

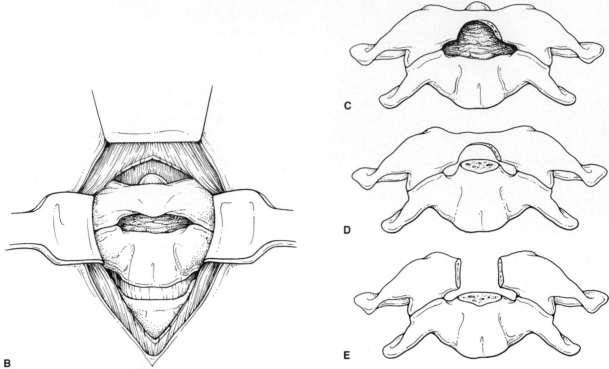

B

C

D

E

Figure 25.2 *cont'd* (**B**) The mucosa and musculature of the posterior pharynx are split and retracted, exposing the atlas and axis. Pannus is visible at the interface of the atlas and dens. (**C**) The caudal half of the anterior arch of the atlas has been removed, exposing pannus overlying the dens. Typically this is enough exposure to adequately decompress the spinal cord. (**D, E**) The pannus and odontoid have been resected, thereby decompressing the dura. (*Modified from Barrow Neurological Institute, Phoenix, AZ, with permission.*)

layer-by-layer basis, using microdissectors and microscapels, is often necessary to fully decompress the dura. However, such maneuvers may put the dura at risk for laceration. If the dura is breached during a transoral procedure, the subarachnoid space may become contaminated with bacteria, leading to meningitis. Thus, prophylactic use of antibiotics, particularly those covering mouth flora, is indicated. Prompt placement of a lumbar drain at the end of the surgical procedure is indicated if a tear in the dura occurs. A primary closure of the dural defect should be attempted, and augmentation of the dural closure with fibrin glue and autologous or donor fascia should be considered. Postoperatively, it is essential to ensure that tongue and airway swelling have abated before the patient is extubated. Reintubation of a patient with respiratory failure on the basis of postoperative obstruction may be difficult or impossible—a situation to best avoid.

Lateral Approaches

Compressive bony lesions at the lateral aspect of the craniovertebral junction are rare and are usually the result of congenital anomalies. In our experience, and others', these lesions have been associated with assimilation of the atlas to the occiput.[27] This condition is believed to result from failed segmentation of the first cervical and last cranial sclerotomes.[9,27,34] Assimilation of the atlas is associated with congenital fusion of C2 and C3.[33] Neurologic

compromise results from stenosis of the foramen magnum, manifested by unilateral overgrowth of the lateral masses and facet joints. For these lesions, a true lateral approach is required because a transoral procedure does not allow enough access dorsally and laterally, and a dorsal decompression does not allow resection of the lesion without unacceptable retraction of the spinal cord and medulla.

The traditional ventrolateral approaches to the cervical spine[4,10,37] offered only a very limited view of the craniovertebral junction. Whitesides and Kelly[42] described an operation designed to circumvent this limitation, which was based on Henry's[21] approach to the vertebral artery. This technique emphasized a dorsal reflection of the sternocleidomastoid muscle after its division at the mastoid process, allowing direct lateral exposure of the vertebral artery via blunt dissection. Recently, a number of variations of these pioneering exposures have been described.* These techniques emphasize removal of the lateral masses of C1 and C2, as well as the dorsal aspect of the occipital condyle, permitting the removal of intradural pathology located laterally and ventrally to the brain stem. Tumors, both intradural and extradural, as well as vertebrobasilar aneurysms have been successfully removed via these approaches.[1,7,18,33] These approaches are equally suited to laterally located compressive lesions arising from the bony articulations. Access to this region may be gained through

---

*References 1,7,15,18,33,35,39.

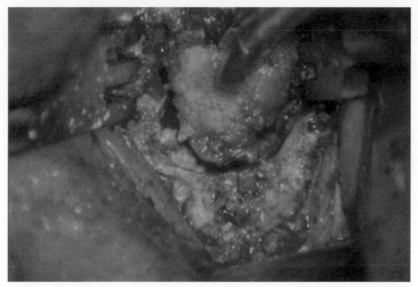

Figure 25.3 Transoral removal of the dens. Removal of the odontoid remnant after drilling and release of the ligamentous attachments is demonstrated. The self-retaining blades are visible, retracting the pharyngeal tissues. The atlas, at the lower aspect of the image, has been only partially removed.

either a laterally or medially based incision, with the muscle flap retracted medially or laterally, respectively. Either provides adequate access to the lateral craniovertebral junction. The approach described here is based on the dorsal midline approach, which is familiar to all spine surgeons.

Technique
The Far-Lateral Approach for Lateral Bony Compression of the Craniovertebral Junction

In this approach,[39] the patient is placed in a modified park-bench position, with the lower arm placed off the head of the table and cradled in padding. The head is suspended by the Mayfield head holder. The axilla is well padded. The head is flexed, then rotated contralaterally to bring the lesion up. Finally, lateral bending away from the side of the lesion maximally opens the angle between the occiput and upper cervical spine. The upper shoulder is then pulled caudally and the body is taped securely, thus permitting full lateral and vertical rotation of the table.

The incision is begun at the mastoid tip and curved rostromedially just below the superior nuchal line to the midline. It is then taken caudally to C4. A cuff of fascia and muscle is left superiorly to aid in closing. Subperiosteal dissection of the remaining muscle is performed from the occiput to C2, and the entire muscle mass is retracted laterally, using a Leyla bar, or an equivalent device, and fish hooks. The ganglion of the C2 root as it exits above its lamina is preserved. The remainder of the operation is performed under the operating microscope (Figure 25.4).

The lateral mass of C1 is exposed, and the vertebral artery is identified from the transverse foramen of C1 to its entry into the dura. Bleeding from the vertebral venous plexus can be troublesome but can usually be controlled with bipolar cautery and packing. A laminec-

tomy of C1 is performed from beyond the midline to the ipsilateral sulcus arteriosus. The vertebral artery is unroofed in its foramen to allow for mobilization. A lateral suboccipital craniectomy is performed with a foot–plated drill or rongeurs. Additional bone is then removed until the lateral mass of C1, the occipital condyle, and the bony abnormality are exposed. A decompression of the anomaly is then performed, with care taken to protect the vertebral artery. Usually, a high-speed, high-performance air drill is preferred. A diamond burr and upbiting curettes are used to complete the decompression. If the dura mater is breached, the rent is closed primarily with sutures or with a patch graft, if primary closure is not feasible. A stabilization procedure is performed if indicated. The wound is closed in anatomic layers, and a lumbar drain is placed if the integrity of the dura is violated.

Up to two thirds of the medial occipital condyle may be removed without compromising mechanical stability or risking neurologic injury. Brisk venous bleeding may be encountered if the posterior condylar emissary vein is breached. This can usually be controlled with bone wax and Nu-knit surgical gauze. The hypoglossal canal is situated in the ventral medial one third of the occipital condyle and is not threatened unless the site of compression dictates dissection in this region. Likewise, the stability of the occiput-C1 articulation is not compromised unless the ventral portion of the condyle must be resected to effect an adequate decompression. In such circumstances, bone grafting and instrumentation are indicated.

Several patients at the authors' institutions have undergone this procedure for removal of laterally situated bony abnormalities that distorted the cervicomedullary junction. Patients have presented with neck pain and varying degrees of neurologic deficit. All underwent successful decompression of their lesions via the far lateral approach, with no neurologic worsening and no complications (Figure 25.5). Potential complications of this operation are directly related to the angle of approach. Because it traverses the operative field, the vertebral artery is vulnerable to damage. During the decompression it is necessary to gently retract the vessel, and care must be taken not to harm it with traction or pressure. Rents in the vessel should be sutured primarily if possible; excision of the damaged segment with end-to-end anastomosis is also an option. Permanent occlusion of the vessel, although tolerated by most patients, should be avoided if practical.

Other complications reported with this technique or its variants[7,18,33] include brain stem edema, air embolism, lower cranial nerve palsies, hydrocephalus, CSF leak, and death. Most of the reported complications involved patients with ventrally and laterally placed tumors, thus requiring concomitant brain retraction and cranial nerve dissection. For patients requiring the resection of extradural bony anomalies, the incidence of hydrocephalus and cranial nerve palsies should be reduced. Because of the uncertain relationship between craniocervical anomalies and hydrocephalus,[2] external ventricular or lumbar drainage should be considered in these patients, if the dura is breached, in order to lessen the likelihood of CSF fistula.

Dorsal Approaches

During the formative years of neurosurgery and the discipline of spine surgery, a dorsal decompression of the foramen magnum and upper cervical spine was the procedure of choice for all types of craniocervical compression. It soon became clear, however, that laminectomy and suboccipital craniectomy, in the face of ventrally placed pathology, were seldom effective. In some cases it worsened the neurologic status of the patient. Currently, surgical approaches are targeted directly at the offending pathology. However, there remain a number of conditions in which dorsal decompression is the procedure of choice.

Achondroplasia is the most common form of dwarfism, and it commonly appears with symptomatic spinal stenosis. Abnormalities of the craniovertebral junction can lead to stenosis of the foramen magnum with resultant cervicomedullary compression.[32] Thick epidural banding at the level of the foramen magnum frequently accompanies the bony changes and may contribute to alteration of CSF dynamics and hydrocephalus.[2,32] The constellation of findings that define Chiari I malformation represents another set of anatomic anomalies that are best treated by a dorsal decompression. Neurologic function may be jeopardized both by direct compression at the level of the foramen magnum and by the deleterious effects of altered CSF

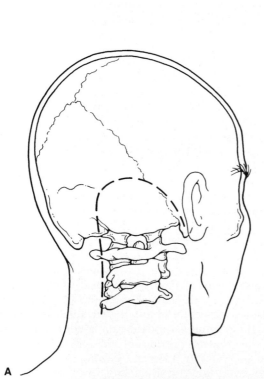
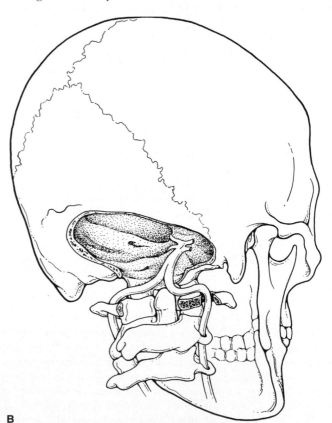

Figure 25.4 Far-lateral approach to craniovertebral pathology. **(A)** The skin incision extends from the midline to the inion, then across to the mastoid tip. Subperiosteal dissection allows the entire muscle mass to be retracted laterally. **(B)** Bony removal includes the arch of C1 from the midline to the sulcus arteriosus of the vertebral artery. A standard suboccipital craniectomy is enlarged to include up to two thirds of the occipital condyle. Laterally based compressive lesions can thus be resected with a minimum of brain retraction. (*Modified from Barrow Neurological Institute, Phoenix, AZ, with permission.*)

flow patterns. Syringomyelia, hydrocephalus, or both are commonly associated with Chiari I malformation and, in many instances, these conditions may improve after dorsal decompression and duraplasty.[6] Finally, chronic C1-2 subluxation or basilar settling, secondary to several degenerative diseases, often leads to irreducible medullary compression. Laminectomy of C1 is often used as an adjunct to dorsal stabilization in these instances.

Technique

The patient is placed in the prone position. If the neck is stable, the head is flexed forward to no farther than a fin-ger-width from the sternum. Otherwise, the patient is operated on in the neutral position in either traction or halo immobilization. A midline incision is made from the inion to C3 or C4. A relatively bloodless plane exists in the midline, and dissection is carried through this plane to the occiput and spinous process of C2. The dorsal and lateral muscular attachments to C2 are left intact unless a full laminectomy of C2 is required for an adequate decompression. The deepest part of the exposure is the foramen magnum/C1 region. Dissection is carried down the occiput in a subperiosteal fashion until the bone begins to curve sharply ventrally, indicating the margin of the foramen magnum. The dorsal ring of C1 is identified

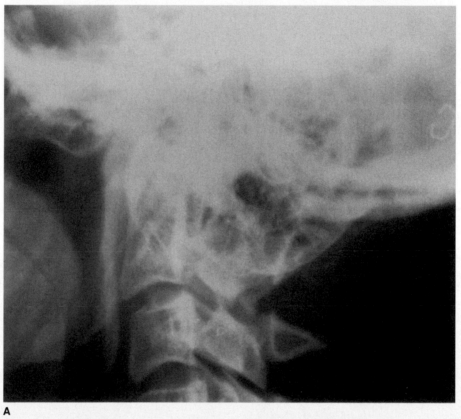

A

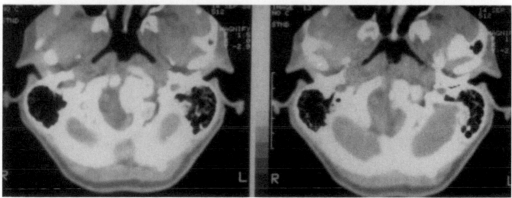

B

Figure 25.5 Decompression of the craniovertebral junction via the far lateral approach. A 41-year-old woman had complained of headaches since age 6. Examination revealed severely restricted neck motion and early myelopathy. (**A**) Lateral cervical spine film demonstrates assimilation of the atlas to the occiput. (**B**) Axial CT scans reveal lateral compression of the cervicomedullary junction from a bony mass arising from the occipitoatlantal articulation.

Continued

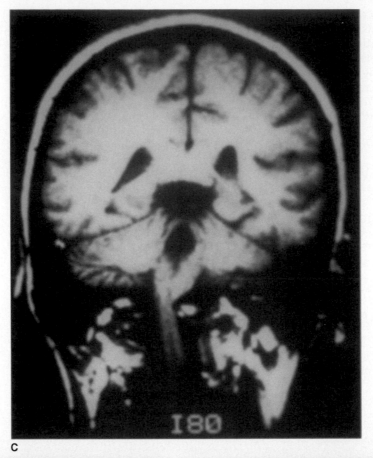

C

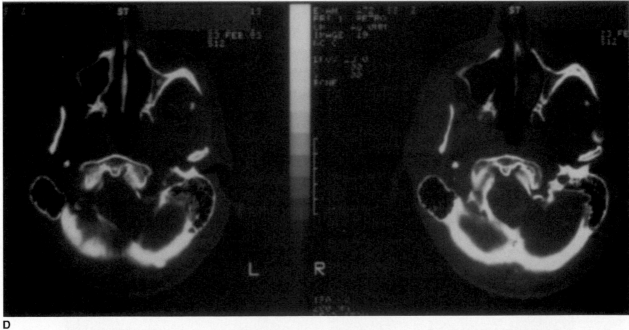

D

Figure 25.5 *cont'd* (**C**) Coronal MRI reveals the degree of cord compression. (**D**) Postoperative axial CTs reveal resolution of the compression.

and cleaned of muscular attachments, using periosteal elevators and curettes. As the dissection proceeds later-ally, it is not uncommon to encounter brisk bleeding from the paravertebral venous complex. This is usually easily controllable with bipolar diathermy and Surgicel. The

foramen magnum is similarly exposed and self-retaining retractors placed. If necessary, craniocervical alignment is verified or corrected, using fluoroscopy.

The amount of bone removed depends on the anatomy of the deformity. In cases of irreducible atlantoaxial subluxation, it may be necessary to perform only a laminectomy of C1 before a definitive dorsal fusion and instrumentation. For more complex craniocervical anomalies, such as those associated with Chiari I malformation or achondroplasia, suboccipital craniectomies with one- or two-level cervical laminectomies are required. Because the foramen magnum is often misshapen in these conditions, it is important to perform a generous dorsolateral decompression. Duraplasty has been advocated for many of these conditions, and opening the dura provides the added advantage of lysing arachnoidal adhesions and exploring the foramen of Magendie for a "veil" obstructing the flow of CSF. A graft for duraplasty may be obtained from the paravertebral fascia, fascia lata, cadaveric dura, or pericardium. The wound is closed in layers, with careful attention to close the junction of the galea and fascia overlying the inion. Most CSF leaks result from inadequate closure of this region.

Complications

Reported complications for this procedure stem mainly from the dural closure. Aryanpur et al.[2] reported four cases of CSF leaks in a series of 15 achondroplastic patients; one of these developed meningitis. Another patient without a documented CSF leak also went on to develop meningitis. Three of these patients required postoperative shunting for unsuspected hydrocephalus. Authors recommend the routine placement of ventriculostomies in these patients at the time of surgery, with the decision to shunt based on the postoperative pressure measurements. Ryken and Menezes[32] reported no CSF leaks in a series of six patients with achondroplasia undergoing posterior fossa decompression; however, they performed duraplasty in only three patients. One of these patients required multiple lumbar punctures for a pseudomeningocele. Keiper et al.[23] reported four patients treated with suboccipital craniectomy, laminectomy, removal of epidural bands, and preservation of the dura. None of these patients required shunting. Batzdorf[6] reported two pseudomeningoceles in five patients undergoing decompression for Chiari I malformation.

Clearly, a patient's preoperative neurologic status weighs heavily on the surgical outcome. Patients with longstanding cervicomedullary compression often have respiratory compromise and swallowing difficulty, making them susceptible to postoperative pneumonia. Diligent respiratory care is mandatory to reduce the morbidity in these frail patients.

Summary

Advances in neuroradiologic technology and microneurosurgical techniques have combined to provide diagnostic and therapeutic modalities undreamed of 30 years ago. Compressive pathology can be safely and expertly removed from the front, side, or rear of the craniovertebral junction. Each of these procedures has well-recognized complications, and prudent preoperative planning includes strategies for avoiding and, if necessary, dealing with them safely. As with all operations, patient selection is crucial to determining outcome. A technically excellent operation leads to a satisfactory outcome only if the clinical presentation correlates well with the physical examination and radiographic studies.

REFERENCES

1. Al-Mefty O, Borba LAB, Aoki N: The transcondylar approach to extradural noneoplastic lesions of the craniovertebral junction. *J Neurosurg* 84:1-6, 1996.
2. Aryanpur J, Hurko O, Francomano C *et al:* Craniocervical decompression for cervicomedullary compression in pediatric patients with achondroplasia. *J Neurosurg* 73:375, 1990.
3. Ashraf J, Crockard HA: Transoral fusion for high cervical fractures. *J Bone Joint Surg* 72B:76, 1990.
4. Bailey RW, Badgley CE: Stabilization of the cervical spine by anterior fusion. *J Bone Joint Surg* 42A:565, 1994.
5. Baldwin HZ, Miller CG, Van Loveren HR *et al:* The far lateral/combined supratentorial and infratentorial approach: a human cadaveric prosection model for routes of access to the petroclival region and ventral brain stem. *J Neurosurg* 81:60, 1994.
6. Batzdorf U: Chiari I malformation with syringomyelia: evaluation of surgical therapy by magnetic resonance imaging. *J Neurosurg* 68:726, 1988.
7. Bertalanffy H, Seeger W: The dorsolateral, suboccipital, transcondylar approach to the lower clivus and anterior portion of the craniocervical junction. *Neurosurgery* 29:815, 1991.
8. Cai CY, Palmer CA, Paramore CG: Exuberant transverse ligament degeneration causing high cervical myelopathy. *J Spinal Disord* 14(1):84-88, 2001.
9. Chandraraj S, Briggs CA: Failure of somite differentiation at the cranio-vertebral region as a cause of occipitalization of the atlas. *Spine* 17:1249, 1992.
10. Cloward RB: The anterior approach for removal of ruptured cervical disks. *J Neurosurg* 15:602, 1958.
11. Crockard HA, Calder I, Ransford AO: One-stage transoral decompression and posterior fixation in rheumatoid atlanto-axial subluxation. *J Bone Joint Surg* 72B:682, 1990.
12. Delgado TE, Garrido E, Harwick RD: Labiomandibular, transoral approach to chordomas in the clivus and upper cervical spine. *Neurosurgery* 8:675, 1981.
13. Di Lorenzo N: Craniocervical junction malformation treated by transoral approach: a survey of 25 cases with emphasis on postoperative instability and outcome. *Acta Neurochir (Wien)* 118:112, 1992.
14. Dickman CA, Locantro J, Fessler RG: The influence of transoral odontoid resection on stability of the craniovertebral junction. *J Neurosurg* 77:525, 1992.
15. Dowd GC, Zeiller BA, and Awasthi D: Far lateral transcondylar approach: dimensional anatomy. *Neurosurgery* 45:95-100, 1999.
16. Fang HSY, Ong GB: Direct anterior approach to the upper cervical spine. *J Bone Joint Surg* 44A:1588, 1962.
17. Fasel J, Morscher E: A contribution to the anatomic basis of the transoral approach to the atlas and axis. *Surg Radiol Anat* 10:15, 1988.
18. George B, Dematons C, Cophignon J: Lateral approach to the anterior portion of the foramen magnum: application to surgical removal of 14 benign tumors. Technical note. *Surg Neurol* 29:484, 1988.

19. Hadley MN, Martin NA, Spetzler RF, *et al:* Comparative transoral dural closure techniques: a canine model. *Neurosurgery* 22:392, 1988.

20. Hadley MN, Spetzler RF, Sonntag VKH: The transoral approach to the superior cervical spine: a review of 53 cases of extradural cervicomedullary compression. *J Neurosurg* 71:16, 1989.

21. Henry AK: *Extensile Exposure.* Edinburgh, London, Churchill Livingstone, 1973.

22. Kanavel AB: Bullet located between the atlas and the base of the skull: technique of removal through the mouth. *Surg Clin North Am* 361, 1917.

23. Keiper GL Jr., Koch B, Crone KR: Achondroplasia and cervicomedullary compression: prospective evaluation and surgical treatment. *Pediatr Neurosurg* 31:78-83, 1999.

24. Kerschbaumer F, Kandziora F, Klein C, *et al:* Transoral decompression, anterior plate fixation, and posterior wire fusion for irreducible atlantoaxial kyphosis in rheumatoid arthritis. *Spine* 25(20):2708-2715, 2000.

25. Kratimenos GP, Crockard HA: The far lateral approach for ventrally placed foramen magnum and upper cervical spine tumours. *Br J Neurosurg* 7:129, 1993.

26. Marks RJ, Forrester PC, Calder I, *et al:* Anaesthesia for transoral craniocervical surgery. *Anaesthesia* 41:1049, 1986.

27. Menezes AH: Primary craniovertebral anomalies and the hindbrain herniation syndrome (Chiari I): data base analysis. *Pediatr Neurosurg* 23:260-269, 1995.

28. Menezes AH: Complications of surgery at the craniovertebral junction: avoidance and management. *Pediatr Neurosurg* 17:254, 1991.

29. Menezes AH, VanGilder JC: Transoral-transpharyngeal approach to the anterior craniocervical junction: ten-year experience with 72 patients. *J Neurosurg* 69:895, 1988.

30. Merwin GE, Post JC, Sypert GW: Transoral approach to the upper cervical spine. *Laryngoscope* 101:780, 1991.

31. Pollack IF, Welch W, Jacobs GB, *et al:* Frameless stereotactic guidance: an intraoperative adjunct in the transoral approach for ventral cervicomedullary junction decompression. *Spine* 20(2):216-220, 1995.

32. Ryken TC, Menezes AH: Cervicomedullary compression in achondroplasia. *J Neurosurg* 81:43, 1994.

33. Sen CN, Sekhar LN: An extreme lateral approach to intradural lesions of the cervical spine and foramen magnum. *Neurosurgery* 27:197, 1990.

34. Shapiro R, Robinson F: Anomalies of the craniovertebral border. *Am J Roentgenol* 127:281, 1976.

35. Shucart WA, Kleriga E: Lateral approach to the upper cervical spine. *Neurosurgery* 6:278, 1980.

36. Smith GW, Robinson RA: The treatment of certain cervical-spine disorders by anterior removal of the intervertebral disc and interbody fusion. *J Bone Joint Surg* 40A:607, 1958.

37. Southwick WO, Robinson RA: Surgical approaches to the vertebral bodies in the cervical and lumbar regions. *J Bone Joint Surg* 39A:631, 1957.

38. Spetzler RF, Dickman CA, Sonntag VKH: The transoral approach to the anterior cervical spine. *Contemp Neurosurg* 13:1, 1991.

39. Spetzler RF, Grahm TW: The far-lateral approach to the inferior clivus and the upper cervical region. Technical note. *BNI Quarterly* 6:35, 1990.

40. Vender JR, Harrison SJ, and McDonnell DE: Fusion and instrumentation at C1-3 via the high anterior cervical approach. *J Neurosurg (Spine 1)* 92:24-9, 2000.

41. Vishteh AG, Beals SP, Joganic EF, *et al:* Bilateral sagittal split mandibular osteotomies as an adjunct to the transoral approach to the anterior craniovertebral junction. *J Neurosurg (Spine 2)* 90:267-70, 1999.

42. Whitesides TE, Jr., Kelly RP: Lateral approach to the upper cervical spine for anterior fusion. *South Med J* 59:879, 1966.

CHAPTER 26

Upper Cervical and Occipitocervical Arthrodesis

H. Alan Crockard, Volker K.H. Sonntag, and Nicholas Theodore

Stabilization and arthrodesis at the cervicomedullary junction (CMJ) provide the surgeon with a variety of challenging problems that should be considered before embarking on any procedure in the area. Because 80% of all head movements occur at the most rostral of the spine's two joints, there will be considerable stresses on any construct and a tendency to nonfusion. Conversely, for the patient, immobilization of these joints may cause a significant disability. Apart from acute trauma, much of the pathology in this region progresses slowly. If there is a tumor and region that deforms slowly over many years, as with a bony abnormality, the molding and alternation of joint surfaces produce secondary subaxial deformities, such as kyphosis or increased lordosis. The effect of the fusion on this factor must also be considered. Knowledge of the anatomy in this region is paramount. Thus, detailed multiplanar imaging to show the vertebral artery, distortion of the neuraxis, and soft-tissue interpositions must be available.

There are a variety of means to treat instability at the CMJ, ranging from external orthosis to reduction and bone grafting with external immobilization, and to a wide selection of implantable instrumentation, with or without external immobilization. It is important to remember that only patients with spinal instrumentation are potentially stable, and though bone and wire may feel rigid at the time of surgery, this type of fixation is most successful in combination with a Minerva or halo vest immobilizer. Whether to depend on internal fixation alone or combine it with some external orthosis is a matter of individual circumstances and the surgeon's preferences and experience.

In this chapter, the technical aspects of the various types of arthrodesis of the upper cervical spine and CMJ are emphasized. There are, however, certain principles that should influence the situation. With acute deformity, arthrodesis of the normal anatomy is desirable. However, over-vigorous corrections may damage an already compromised neuraxis. In this latter situation, decompression and fixation of deformity may be the best option. The type of stabilization offered to the young, healthy athlete may be too aggressive to the debilitated rheumatoid or to the patient with metastatic bone disease.

All screw systems are basically "one shot" techniques, and although rescue screws can be used, the bone/metal interface is compromised by repositioning. Sublaminar wiring techniques have the potential for compression of the neuraxis at the time of passage. These have been largely replaced by sublaminar cable systems. Because of the importance of postoperative imaging, nonferrous implants must be considered and titanium screw-plate implants and cables are to be highly recommended.

Odontoid Screw Fixation and Ventral Atlantoaxial Facet Screw Fixation

Odontoid or atlantoaxial facet screw fixation may be performed via a ventral operative approach.* These techniques are suitable for unstable odontoid fractures or for atlantoaxial instability in which the dorsal arches of C1-2 cannot be directly incorporated into a fusion (Figures 26.1 and 26.2).

Both methods of screw fixation are performed through an identical operative exposure with the patient in a supine position. Lateral and anteroposterior fluoroscopic guidance are necessary to provide precise intraoperative visualization of the upper cervical spine. Preoperative computed tomography (CT) studies are required to determine the position of the vertebral arteries, to evaluate the bony architecture, and to assess for abnormalities that would preclude screw placement.

Odontoid screw fixation is ideal for acutely fixating unstable odontoid fractures, since it preserves normal C1 motion. This technique can be used only if the transverse atlantal ligament is intact. If the transverse atlantal ligament is disrupted, fixating the odontoid does not stabilize the atlas. The integrity of the transverse atlantal ligament can be directly assessed with magnetic resonance imaging (MRI).[8] Odontoid screw fixation can be problematic for odontoid fracture nonunions. It is difficult to remove scar tissue from a nonunion and to reduce the fracture to facilitate a bony union. Odontoid screw fixation is performed with the patient positioned supine on the operating table with the head extended.

Operative Technique

A transverse skin incision is made at the level of C5-6, using the cricothyroid junction as a superficial landmark (Figure 26.3). This incision is carried down through the platysma muscle, which is widely undermined to allow optimal retractor placement. The ventral border of the sternocleidomastoid muscle is identified and mobilized laterally, along with the carotid sheath. The esophagus, trachea, and infrahyoid (strap) muscles are reflected medially, using a handheld retractor. The ventral border of the cervical spine is identified, and using Kittner dissectors, the retropharyngeal space is opened to the level of C2. The medial borders of the longus colli muscles are coagulated, and their bellies are elevated laterally. Caspar-toothed self-retaining retractors are then introduced under the longus colli muscles to maintain exposure. The authors angle the Caspar retractor rostrally, using lateral C-arm fluoroscopy to confirm the position at the C2-3 interspace. A handheld retractor or malleable

*References 2,3,9,10,12,19.

retractor easily elevates any soft tissue obscuring the exposure. The next goal is to definitively demonstrate the midline ventral/caudal aspect of the body of C2. This usually requires that a midline trough be created through the annulus and disc at the C2-3 interspace. Frequently, a midline gutter must be cut into the ventral body of C3 to provide adequate visualization of the ventral/caudal end plate of C2. A Synthes® drill guide (authors' choice) is placed on the anterior/inferior lip of C2 in the midline. Using the 2mm bit on a Synthes® air drill, real-time biplanar fluoroscopy (Figure 26.4) is used to monitor progress until the drill bit approaches the cortex of the odontoid tip.[1] The drill bit is then backed out of the pilot hole, and a tap for use with a 4mm screw is advanced under fluoroscopic control until it approaches the distal cortex of the dens. At this point, a partially threaded nonself-tapping cancellous titanium lag screw is selected. The screw length forms scored markings on the tap. If the odontoid fracture is widely separated from the body of the axis, the screw length is adjusted accordingly. The authors

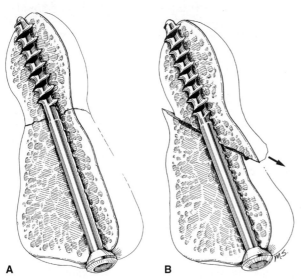

Figure 26.1 Ventral odontoid screw fixation of the odontoid. The ideal odontoid fracture is (**A**) a horizontal fracture through the bone of the odontoid. (**B**) An oblique fracture can become malaligned secondary to shearing forces generated during screw fixation. (*Reprinted with permission of Barrow Neurological Institute, Phoenix, AZ.*)

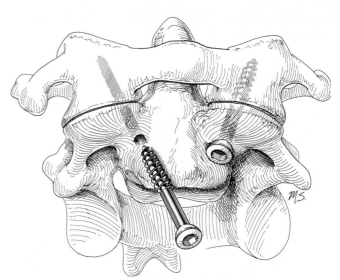

Figure 26.2 Ventral C1-2 transarticular screw. Lag screws are placed bilaterally through the anterior portion of the C1-2 joint. The use of a C1 lag screw allows the facet to be compressed under tension after the articular cartilage is scraped with a curette prior to screw placement. (*Reprinted with permission of Barrow Neurological Institute, Phoenix, AZ.*)

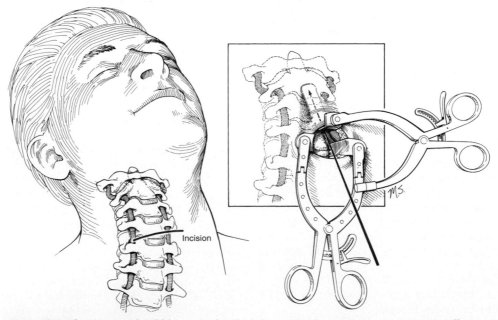

Figure 26.3 The incision should be at the level of about C5. The patient's anatomy must allow proper trajectory to the tip of the dens. (*Reprinted with permission of Barrow Neurological Institute, Phoenix, AZ.*)

frequently customize the lag screw by clipping the distal 2 to 3mm to provide the perfect length for the patient's individual anatomy and to achieve the appropriate lag effect. The screw is advanced under fluoroscopic control and tightened until the screw head is just countersunk with respect to the body of C2 (Figure 26.5). It is important that the screw head does not protrude into the C2-3 interspace, since this can provide a lever effect resulting in screw loosening or failure. The wound is copiously irrigated, and meticulous hemostasis is obtained prior to closure of the platysma and skin.

Ventral atlantoaxial facet screw fixation is similar to odontoid screw fixation. The operative exposure is identical; however, the screw insertion and trajectory differ. Before the screws are placed, the facet joints are decorticated with a bone curette to enhance fusion. Screws enter the C2 vertebral body in the recess between the vertebral body and the superior C2 facet. The screws are directed rostrally into the lateral masses of C1 (Figure 26.2). The screws are shorter than the screws used for odontoid fixation (i.e., 20 to 25mm).

A pilot hole is made with a 2.5-mm diameter drill. The drilling begins in the groove between the C2 vertebral body and the C2 superior facet. A single 3.5-mm diameter screw is placed into each facet under fluoroscopic guid-ance. Nonself-tapping or self-tapping screws can be used. A lag effect is preferred so that the C1-2 facets will be compressed. This technique stabilizes C1-2 rigidly but sacrifices all C1-2 motion.

The ventral operations for C1-2 facet or odontoid screw fixation are limited by the difficulties of high cervical exposure and soft-tissue retraction and by the inability to add grafts to enhance fusion. Ventral upper cervical screw fixation is technically more demanding than dorsal cervical fixation.

Ventral upper cervical screw fixation requires a thin body habitus and extension of the head to facilitate screw placement. The trajectory of the drill must be almost parallel to the ventral surface of the cervical spine. Short necks and barrel-shaped chests hinder operative access. These techniques should be performed only if C1-2 alignment can be restored before screw insertion; otherwise, the fixation will be malaligned.

Upper Cervical Spine (C1-2)

Screw-plate fixation systems have found wide applications in the lower cervical spine. Ventral cervical plating after trauma or after complex ventral decompressive procedures has become a standard in the armamentarium of the spine

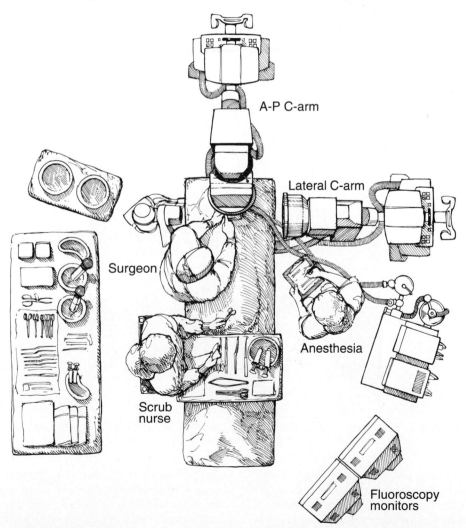

Figure 26.4 Biplanar fluoroscopy is very useful for safe and efficient placement of the screw or screws. (*Reprinted with permission of Barrow Neurological Institute, Phoenix, AZ.*)

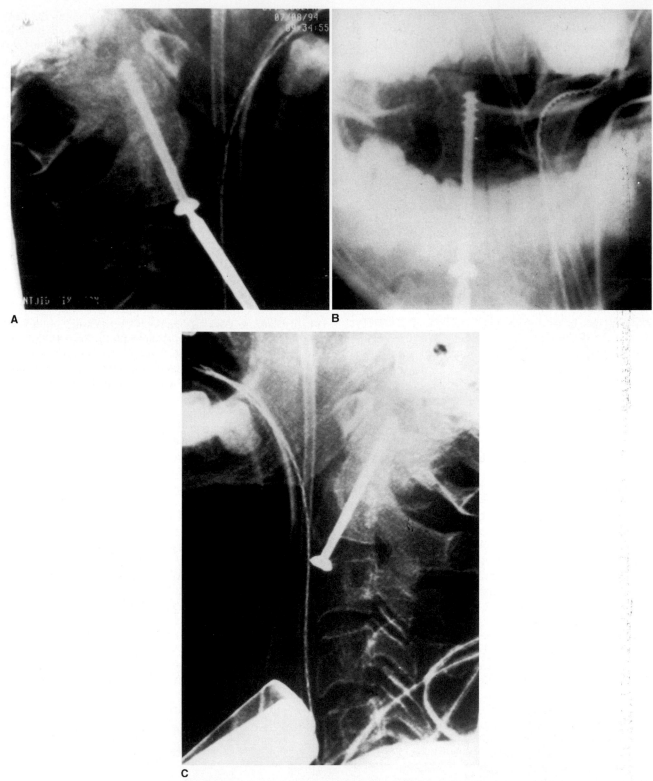

Figure 26.5 The screw is advanced with the aid of (**A**) lateral and (**B**) AP fluoroscopy until the (**C**) screw head is countersunk with respect to the body of C2.

surgeon. In the last several years, advances in screw-plate technology have made these operations safer and easier.[27]

The traditional ventral screw-plate system for the cervical spine developed by Caspar[5] depends on bicortical purchase to prevent the screw from "toggling" and backing out. Precise fluoroscopic guidance is required. Major dif-

ficulties can be encountered in imaging the lower cervical spine sufficiently because shoulders can impede fluoroscopic visualization of C6, C7, and T1. Also, dural penetration with resultant spinal cord injury, a cerebrospinal fluid (CSF) leak, or both are possible when bicortical purchase is required. Despite these limitations, the Caspar

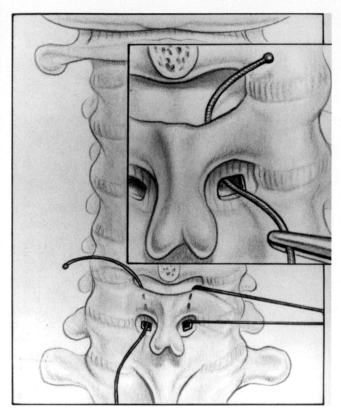

Figure 26.6 The safest place to pass a sublaminar cable is at the junction of laminar and spinous process. *(From Codman.)*

technique has proved reliable in experienced hands in large clinical series.[23,28]

A major innovation in screw-plate design was the locking screw plate.[18] Locking the screw head to the plate eliminated toggling and reduced backout, thereby making the need for bicortical purchase unnecessary. The commercial Synthes® system uses this method with screws that require only cancellous purchase. A disadvantage of the system is that the locking-head mechanism predetermines the trajectory of the screws, and few options are available in each plate. Additionally, only one length of screw is offered; in some stout patients with large vertebrae, it would be desirable to use longer screws for better purchase. However, this system has been embraced broadly by the spinal surgery community.[4,18] Other equivalent systems may be used.

Other advances include the development of C1 lateral mass and C2 pedicle screw fixation, using a connecting rod.[17,24,26] When anatomically feasible, this type of construct avoids some of the potential pitfalls inherent in transarticular screw fixation. Like standard atlantoaxial transarticular fixation, however, preoperative CT is necessary to confirm anatomic suitability. Although evidence suggests that this method is not as robust as standard techniques, it does represent a feasible alternative to transarticular fixation.[25]

Ventral C2-3 Plating

A C2-3 fusion using plates is usually done for trauma such as hangman's fracture.[29] The plating is not done routinely after cervical discectomy unless it is associated with trauma. The incision is centered over the C2-3 interspace and verified with lateral fluoroscopy, which is used throughout the procedure. After routine dissection to the upper vertebral column has been carried out, the C2-3 interspace is identified and a discectomy, often with the aid of the microscope, is done. Alignment is carried out at this time, if indicated, under gentle traction. A tricortical iliac crest autograft or an appropriate shaped allograft is placed in the interspace. An appropriate sized plate is selected and placed under fluoroscopy guidance. Two screws are placed in C2, two screws in C3, and usually one screw into the graft. The wound is closed and the patient is placed in a hard collar for approximately 6 weeks.

Sublaminar Cable Techniques

For the safe passage of sublaminar cables it is essential to perform an adequate flavumectomy. Any obstruction to a wire or cable places the neuraxis in danger.[6] Great care is taken to avoid CSF leak; the hydrodynamic buffer of an intact dural sac also prevents spinal cord damage. The safest place to pass the cable is in the midline directly under the spinous process (Figure 26.6). Prior to the passage of any cables and after the flavumectomy, the exposed bone surfaces are decorticated to allow for bone fusion; attempting this maneuver with the air drill after passage of the cables will risk their damage.

To include the occiput, it is usually easier and safer to make two 3mm diameter drill holes on each side of the proposed site of the implant and gently separate the dura. In the elderly patient, it may be difficult to maintain an intact dura in the occipital region. Cable passage around the foramen magnum may be difficult because the dura is most adherent in this area. In addition, the inner aspect of the bone may curve inward and obstruct cable passage.

In general terms, with the elderly patient's osteoporotic bone, the more bone/metal contacts the less the loading and the "pullout" risk is reduced. The occipital bone may be very thin in some places, and some ingenuity is required to secure the implant successfully.

The difference between monofilament wire and cable fixation is that the latter requires some form of cinch which can be crimped onto the tightened cables. With a multilevel construct the wound can become somewhat crowded if the tightening is adjusted to give a balanced construct. The alternative of tightening and crimping one level at a time has the disadvantage of removing the ability to adjust the construct's position or improve the reduction.

Bone Grafting

In general, the authors' preference is to use iliac crest either as tricortical, bicortical, or cancellous chips in this region. Fibula provides apparent strength, but the disparity between its rigidity and osteoporotic vertebral body may lead to "cutout" or pistoning. In addition, recent studies have shown that provided stability can be maintained; the amount of surface area contact is the predominant factor that provides for a more speedy osteosynthesis, thus, the advantage of morcellated cancellous bone.

In the young child, the iliac crest is largely cartilaginous. This is particularly true in the dwarfing syndromes where ossification is delayed. The authors'[15] preference in these circumstances is to harvest parietal skull bone through a bicoronal flap. If identical free flaps are taken and carefully split, half thickness skull bone replacements at both sites facilitate solid and cosmetically pleasing skull reconstruction within 3 months and provide a good harvest of bone that can be shaped or morcellated (Figure 26.7).

The strategic placement of the bone graft in an area where there will be the greatest mechanical stress is more important than the total amount of bone. Obviously, complete immobilization of the joint during osteosynthesis should reduce the nonfusion rate. In certain conditions, however, nonfusion occurs despite internal and external fixation. Patients with end-stage rheumatoid arthritis or immunosuppressive therapy are examples of high-risk patients for pseudarthrosis.

In dorsal occipitocervical fixation, the skull bone adjacent to the foramen magnum and the lateral masses of atlas and axis should be well prepared and bone graft impacted into this area to obtain the best fusion. With atlantoaxial fusion, a Gallie/Brooks/Sonntag type of bone graft interposed between the dorsal lamina of C1 and C2 is essential. However, decortication of the lateral mass joints under the C2 nerve root is also important to encourage joint arthrodesis. This can be difficult to achieve and can be dangerous because of the potential for damage to the vertebral artery. In conditions that have destroyed lateral mass substance, iliac crest between the skull and along the lateral mass area will restore the biomechanical strut.

Occipitocervical Fixation

A variety of methods use implant and sublaminar cables or wire. An inverted U-shaped loop can be manufactured at surgery from a Wisconsin rod using standard rod bending techniques (Figure 26.8).[22] This process requires experience to shape the construct satisfactorily. A preformed implant of various sizes (Hartshill Ransford loop), whose flare around the axis counters a tendency to translocation, is popular (Figure 26.9).[7,20] Spinal rectangles (Luque or Hartshill) have been used but conform poorly. The Ti-Frame™ is an improvement that allows

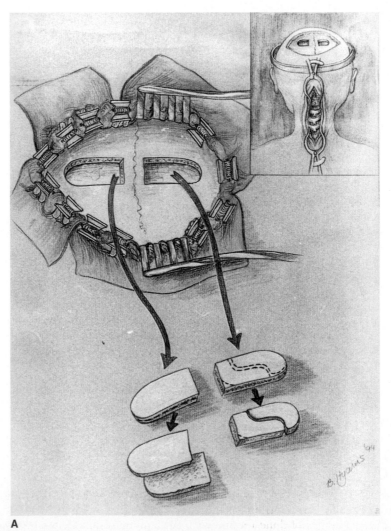

A

Figure 26.7 Bone graft harvest from the parietal bone. **(A)** Through a bicoronal skin flap, identical bone shapes are removed.

excellent fixation and good conformance (Figure 26.10). Newer screw-fixation systems, using improved occiput fixation techniques and polyaxial lateral mass screws, have become popular (see following). For all systems, it is essential that the implant be shaped for the ideal position with the head in the reduced or best achievable position prior to fixation.

During preparation of the area, the spinous processes are removed from the levels to be included in the fixation, with the exception of the lowest level, where care is taken to preserve the interspinous ligaments to prevent the subsequent development of a kyphos below the fused segment.

In general, subperiosteal resection of the muscle attachments using a large Cobb elevator will strip the muscles and the veins with minimal bleeding. The facet joints are the lateral extent of the exposure and at C1-2 the post primary ramus of the C2 nerve root points to the position of the vertebral artery.

Fixation of the craniovertebral junction with transarticular screws is an option to the aforementioned techniques.[13,14,16] This method requires the placement of bilateral transarticular screws from C1 into the occipital condyle. This method provides rigid stabilization and may be a suitable alternative to occipitocervical arthrodesis when there is no significant instability of C1-2.

Grob Plate

A variety of plate and screw constructs can be used for dorsal occipitocervical fusion. As in cabling technology, the ultimate point of failure is the thickness of the occipital bone. Grob[4] invented a Y-shaped construct that allows screws to be placed in the thickest part of the occiput, the midline crest (Figure 26.11). Occasionally, a large median occipital venous sinus may complicate the situation. The lower limbs are shaped to lie over the lateral masses of the upper cervical vertebral and fixed in the standard fashion (vide infra). Newer renditions and modifications are available.

Gallie/Brooks/Sonntag Fusion

Perhaps one of the earliest attempts at secure atlantoaxial instability involved preparation of the dorsal laminar of the atlas and axis with preservation of the C2-3 interspinous

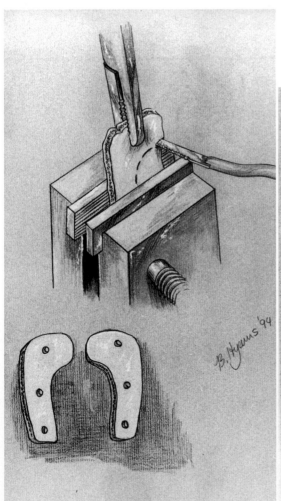

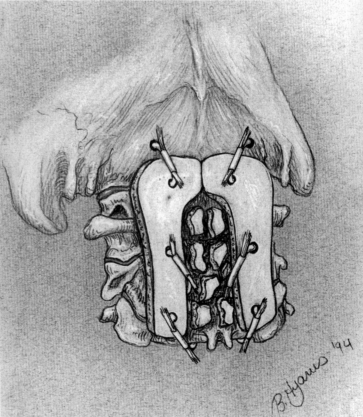

B **C**

Figure 26.7 *cont'd* (B) The bicortical bone is split and shaped to conform to the implant site.
(C) The half thickness remaining is reinserted onto the cranial defect and the wound is closed.

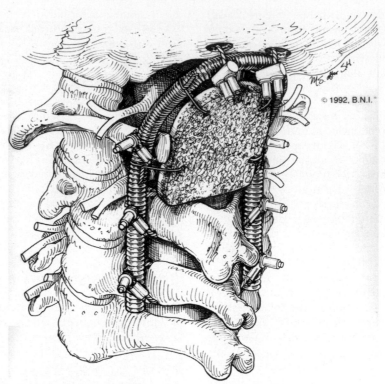

© 1992, B.N.I.

Figure 26.8 Occipitocervical fixation using a customized bent Wisconsin rod. (*Reprinted with permission of Barrow Neurological Institute, Phoenix, AZ.*)

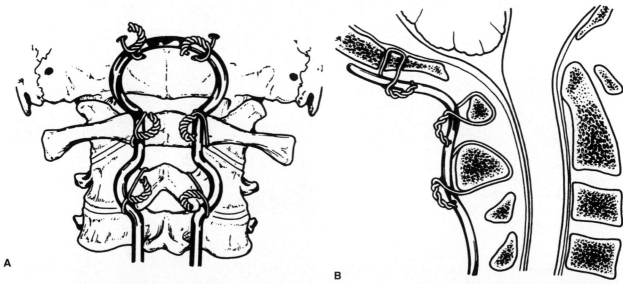

A

B

Figure 26.9 Various sizes of Hartshill Ransford loop with a "flare" designed to fit over C2 will counter the tendency to translocate. (**A**) Posterior view. (**B**) Later aspect. The legs are cut to 1cm below the most caudad cable loops.

ligament. A carefully crafted bone graft is inserted between the adjacent arches, which ideally should be in their normal anatomic position. The tightened cable "holds" the position. Although widely used, this fixation has a potential for nonunion for a variety of reasons. The construct is a one-point fixation and will not counter rotatory or translatory movements. Therefore, it should not routinely be used alone and is recommended that it be

used in combination with another form of fixation, such as C1-2 transarticular screws (Figure 26.12).

C1-2 Transarticular Screws

The technique originally described by Magerl and associates involves the passage of long screws (40 to 50mm)

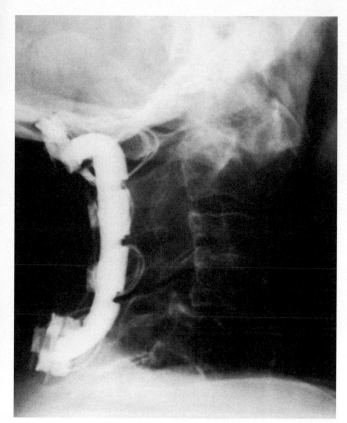

Figure 26.10 A lateral view of a Ti-Frame™ inserted so that the square end lies against the occiput. Cable is passed through the notches, which provides fixation almost as rigid as a plate and screw device.

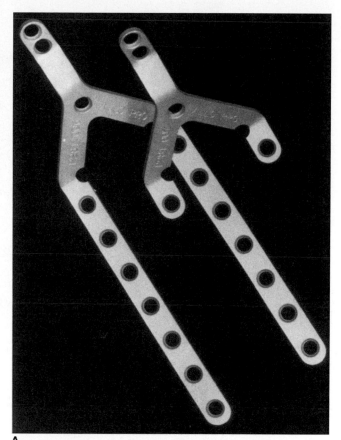

A

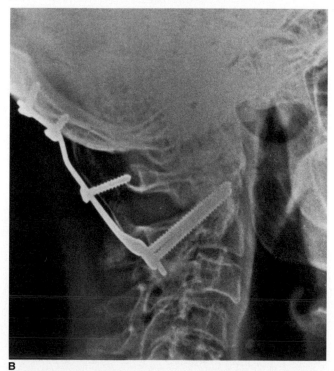

B

Figure 26.11 (A) The Y-plate, made out of titanium, is commercially available in two sizes: the short one for the C0-1 fixation, and the long one can be cut at any desired level or used for the fusion of the entire cervical spine. **(B)** The Y-plate has been combined with a transarticular C1-2 screw fixation. The graft is fixed with an additional screw. (*Reproduced with permission by D. Grob.*)

from the posterior aspect of the C2 facet laminar junction parallel to the dural sac but aimed ventrally to transverse the C1-2 joint and engage in the anterior combined bone surface of the C1 lateral mass (Figure 26.13). Either by "overdrilling" the track through C2 or by the use of a lag screw, a compression fixation of the joint can be effected. With good bone quality and perfect trajectory, it is perhaps one of the most rigid fixations of this joint. It is, however, technically demanding and there are significant hazards and potentials for complication.

Careful preoperative evaluation of the patient and detailed imaging are essential. If there is a congenital malformation or a long-standing irreducible deformity, this fixation may be unsuitable. Lateral mass destruction, torticollis, or a rotatory subluxation of the joint will preclude its use. The position and size of the vertebral arteries determine the technique's feasibility. High definition, thin-cut CT scan studies are essential. Recent software additions, make it possible to calculate the optimal track for the screw.

As in ventral odontoid screw fixation, patient positioning and the ability to easily perform bipolar imaging are mandatory. With the patient in the prone position, the planned trajectory of the drill is checked fluoroscopically to ensure that the drill will not be obstructed by the shoulders. Although the drill guard may be introduced through separate stab incisions in the neck parallel to the midline exposure, too much head extension results in a low drill line that may be obstructed by the shoulders. The

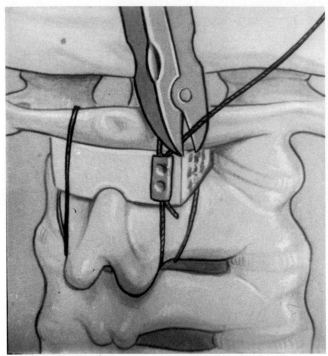

Figure 26.12 A Sonntag C1-2 interlaminar fixation using bone graft and cable. It should be combined with some other form of fixation such as posterior C1-2 transarticular screws or an external arthrosis.

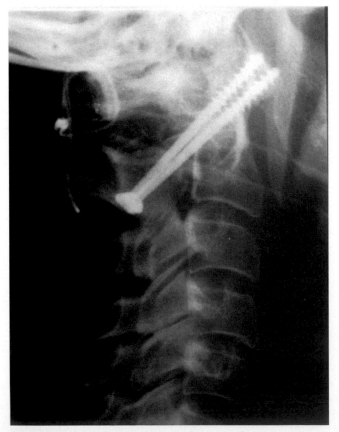

Figure 26.13 Dorsal C1-2 transarticular screw fixation. (A) Anteroposterior. (B) Lateral projection. Biplanar imaging is essential to avoid the dura or the vertebral artery.

importance of this planning prior to the incision cannot be overemphasized.

Preparation of the area involves exposure of the laminae and lateral masses of the first two vertebrae. Again, the surgical key is identification of the C2 nerve root as it emerges from the dural sac (Figure 26.14). Subperiosteal dissection will often strip the numerous epidural veins associated with the nerve and minimize bleeding. Alteration of body position with more "head up" position is also useful in reducing venous bleeding. Deep to the nerve lies the C1-2 joint, and its medial limit in the spinal canal is a useful landmark. The vertical component of the vertebral artery is about 8mm lateral; the foramen transversarium can be located with a blunt hook.

If there is significant instability or persisting deformity, the authors' practice is to pass the cables around C1 so that the atlas can be manipulated into reduction and held firmly in that position during the drilling. The authors prefer is to use K-wires and cannulated drills. Both K-wires are passed prior to any drilling. This way the joint is immobilized at an early stage. Also, the potential injury by a K-wire is significantly less than a cutting drill. Prior to fixation, curettes are used to remove some of the joint surfaces and encourage subsequent arthrodesis.

With the drills in position, the current preference is to use a titanium lag screw of suitable length with its lagged component only in the C1 portion to provide compression fixation. "Three-point" fixation using a dorsal type cable and bony "third point" provides very firm fixation and significantly increases the incidence of bony fusion.

Damage to the vertebral artery is the most dangerous complication, and a bilateral injury may result in death. If the vessel becomes injured, it is essential that good hemostasis be achieved. If the vessel is injured within the bone, insertion of the screw may completely occlude the damaged vessel. Damage to the "free" horizontal or vertical portions necessitates proximal and distal vessel control. Whether a vascular bypass is constructed depends on the skills available at the institute where the accident has occurred. An attempted vascular bypass by an inexperienced surgeon may cause some complication. Provided there is a good contralateral vertebral artery, there may be no brain stem damage with its loss. If the vertebral artery becomes damaged with the placement of the first screw, it is highly recommended not to proceed with the placement of the second screw.

Intralaminar Clamps (Halifax)

The idea of a compression clamp holding adjacent lamina together without having to dissect the dura sac is attractive and, like the plate and hook systems used subaxially, may provide firm fixation. However, at the craniovertebral junction, the construct cannot counter translation or rotational forces, and there is a very high incidence of construct failure.[21]

The atlantoaxial region is exposed the usual way, and adjacent surfaces of C1 and C2 are decorticated and prepared for the insertion of a triangulated graft placed under the clamp (Figure 26.15).

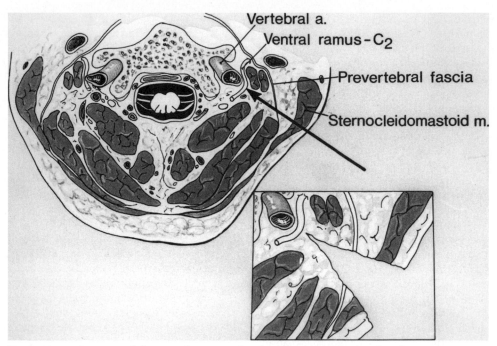

Vertebral a.
Ventral ramus – C₂
Prevertebral fascia
Sternocleidomastoid m.

Figure 26.14 The surgical "key" to the area is the identification of the C2 dorsal primary ramus. Ventral to it lies the vertical component of the vertebral artery.

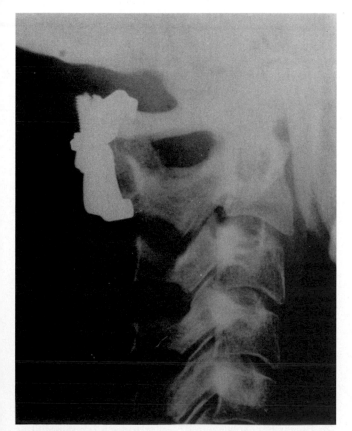

Figure 26.15 Lateral radiograph of a C1-2 Halifax clamp and bone graft.

The idea is to provide a "spacer" so that the joint will be in anatomic alignment, and, at the same time, compress the bone graft. There are a variety of clamp sizes and shapes. It is essential to use those that conform exactly to the bony contours. Cross-banding with cable will improve

the stability and counter rotatory forces. Screw "back out" has been reduced with improved construction of the instrumentation.

Lateral Mass Fixation (C2-3)

With this construct, a titanium plate is placed over the facet joints, and screws 14 to18mm long are placed through the lateral mass of C3 and into the pedicle of C2, respectively. The trajectory into C3 is 20 degrees dorsal and 20 degrees lateral to avoid the root and vertebral artery. (The entire facet is exposed, and a "hillock" is identified close to its center point.) The entry point into C2 is determined after dissecting the medial superior aspect of pedicle. The drill is aimed 20 degrees midline and 40 degrees caudally.

The technique is particularly useful in trauma with facet dislocation. After reduction, it provides firm dorsal tension-band fixation. It is most useful in the situation of instability at the level of a laminectomy.

Good bone quality is essential, and anything less than firm screw fixation may result in early "pullout" of the screws. Marked long-standing irreducible deformity may cause difficulties with correct screw placement. There is strong potential for damage to a nerve root or the vertebral artery.

Atlantoaxial Rotatory Subluxation and Dislocation

In children, a very minor injury may cause rotatory subluxation at the C1-2 joint causing pain with a characteristic "cock robin" deformity.[11] Many are undiagnosed and reduce spontaneously. Some become a recurrent problem and others become irreducible because of discontinuity of joint-surface contact (dislocation). It occurs in children because their joint surface is less curved than that of adults. With a relatively large head-to-body size ratio, the joint is particularly susceptible to rotational damage. Failure to reduce this joint results in permanent loss of head movement, torticollis, and, in the very young child, asymmetrical facial development. Early diagnosis and skilled closed reduction are the treatment of choice. If the situation is neglected, it may become irreducible within a few weeks. With CT, the detail of the deformity can be clearly understood. In the past, a Minerva jacket was reported to reduce the deformity. CT has shown that this is often true because of compensation of the subaxial spine with little change in the atlantoaxial deformity. In the authors' view, complete dislocation of the joint becomes irreducible within a very short time. Unless reduction is successful in the first few days postinjury, open reduction is the only course. The structure most at risk is the vertebral artery.

A lateral approach to the dislocated joints allows early identification and protection of the vertebral artery and, at the same time, ventral and dorsal access to the dislocated joint. Usually, there is soft tissue interposition (the explanation for the irreducibility of recurrent subluxation). Occasionally, a portion of the transverse ligaments is noted.

In bilateral facet dislocation, open reduction is often required. A small amount of bone graft can be inserted in the joint, and the patient is maintained in a halo, body jacket, or equivalent arthrosis. In some patients with a unilateral dislocation, no bone graft has been used, and external immobilization after open reduction has restored full neck movement.

REFERENCES

1. Apfelbaum RI: Anterior screw fixation of odontoid fractures. In Rengachary SS, Wilkins RH (eds): *Neurosurgical Operative Atlas*. Chicago, Williams & Wilkins, 1989, pp 189-199.
2. Barbour JR: Screw fixation in fracture of the odontoid process. *South Aust Clin* 5:20-24, 1971.
3. Borne GM, Bedou GL, Pinaudeau M, *et al:* Odontoid process fracture osteosynthesis with a direct screw fixation technique in nine consecutive cases. *J Neurosurg* 68: 223-226, 1988.
4. Casey AT, Hayward RD, Harkness WF, Crockard HA: The use of autologous skull bone grafts for posterior fusion of the upper cervical spine in children. *Spine* 20:2217-2220, 1995.
5. Caspar W, Barbier DD, Klara PM: Anterior cervical fusion and Caspar plate stabilization for cervical trauma. *Neurosurgery* 25:491-502, 1989.
6. Crockard HA: Evaluation of spinal laminar fixation by a new, flexible stainless steel cable (Sof'wire): early results. *Neurosurgery* 35:892-898, 1994.
7. Crockard HA, Calder I, Ransford AO: One-stage transoral decompression and posterior fixation in rheumatoid atlanto-axial subluxation. *J Bone Joint Surg Br* 72:682-685, 1990.
8. Dickman CA, Mamourian A, Sonntag VKH, Drayer BP: Magnetic resonance imaging of the transverse atlantal ligament for the evaluation of atlantoaxial instability. *J Neurosurg* 75:221-227, 1991.
9. Dickman CA, Sonntag VKH, Marcotte PJ: Techniques of screw fixation of the cervical spine. *BNI Quarterly* 8:9-26, 1992.
10. Etter C, Coscia M, Jaberg H, Aebi M: Direct anterior fixation of dens fractures with a cannulated screw system. *Spine* 16:S25-S32, 1991.
11. Fielding JW, Hawkins RJ, Ratzan SA: Spine fusion for atlanto-axial instability. *J Bone Joint Surg Am* 58:400-407, 1976.
12. Geisler FH, Cheng C, Poka A, Brumback RJ: Anterior screw fixation of posteriorly displaced type II odontoid fractures. *Neurosurgery* 25:30-38, 1989.
13. Gonzalez LF, Crawford NR, Chamberlain RH, *et al:* Craniovertebral junction fixation with transarticular screws: biomechanical analysis of a novel technique. *J Neurosurg* 98:202-209, 2003.
14. Grob D: Transarticular screw fixation for atlanto-occipital dislocation. *Spine* 26:703-707, 2001.
15. Grob D, Dvorak J, Panjabi M, Antinnes JA: The role of plate and screw fixation in occipitocervical fusion in rheumatoid arthritis. *Spine* 19:2545-2551, 1994.
16. Grob D, Dvorak J, Panjabi M, *et al:* Posterior occipitocervical fusion: a preliminary report of a new technique. *Spine* 16:S17-S24, 1991.
17. Harms J, Melcher RP: Posterior C1-C2 fusion with polyaxial screw and rod fixation. *Spine* 26:2467-2471, 2001.
18. Kostuik JP, Connolly PJ, Esses SI, Suh PB: Anterior cervical plate fixation with the titanium hollow screw plate system. *Spine* 18:1273-1278, 1993.
19. Lesoin F, Autricque A, Franz K, *et al:* Transcervical approach and screw fixation for upper cervical spine pathology. *Surg Neurol* 27:459-465, 1987.
20. Malcolm GP, Ransford AO, Crockard HA: Treatment of non-rheumatoid occipitocervical instability: internal fixation with the Hartshill-Ransford Loop. *J Bone Joint Surg Br* 76:357-366, 1994.
21. Moskovich R, Crockard HA: Atlantoaxial arthrodesis using interlaminar clamps: an improved technique. *Spine* 17: 261-267, 1992.
22. Papadopoulos SM, Dickman CA, Sonntag VKH: Atlantoaxial stabilization in rheumatoid arthritis. *J Neurosurg* 74:1-7, 1991.
23. Randle MJ, Wolf A, Levi L, *et al:* The use of anterior Caspar plate fixation in acute cervical spine injury. *Surg Neurol* 36:181-189, 1991.
24. Resnick DK, Lapsiwala S, Trost GR: Anatomic suitability of the C1-C2 complex for pedicle screw fixation. *Spine* 27:1494-1498, 2002.
25. Richter M, Schmidt R, Claes L, *et al:* Posterior atlantoaxial fixation: biomechanics in vitro comparison of six different techniques. *Spine* 27:1724-1732, 2002.
26. Stokes JK, Villavicencio AT, Liu PC, *et al:* Posterior atlantoaxial stabilization: new alternative to C1-2 transarticular screws. *Neurosurg Focus* 12:Article 6, 2002.
27. Suh PB, Kostuik JP, Esses SI: Anterior cervical plate fixation with the titanium hollow screw plate system: a preliminary report. *Spine* 15:1079-1081, 1990.
28. Tippets RH, Apfelbaum RI: Anterior cervical fusion with the Caspar instrumentation system. *Neurosurgery* 22: 1008-1013, 1988.
29. Tuite GF, Papadopoulos SM, Sonntag VKH: Caspar plate fixation for the treatment of complex hangman's fractures. *Neurosurgery* 30:761-765, 1992.

CHAPTER 27

Ventral and Ventrolateral Subaxial Decompression

Fadi Hanbali, Ziya L. Gokaslan, and Paul R. Cooper

Over the past few decades, several techniques have been developed in which a direct ventral or ventrolateral approach was used to gain access to the cervical spine to treat a variety of clinical conditions. All allowed access to the ventral aspect of the dura mater, the nerve roots, and the vertebral arteries, and all provided for considerable flexibility in the approach available to remove lesions, stabilize the cervical spine, or both.[47]

Ventral compression of the spinal cord or the nerve roots is the most common indication for ventral decompression. Clinical conditions like cervical trauma with ventral disc herniation or bone fragments, acute cervical disc herniation, cervical spondylosis, ossification of the posterior longitudinal ligament, neoplastic processes, and infection can all be successfully managed by a ventral decompressive technique. Ventrolateral decompression may be required for vertebral artery stenosis secondary to tumor, spondylosis, or compression of the cervical nerve roots.[48] Although these decompressive measures are quite effective and generally safe, they, nevertheless, may be associated with a number of complications that can be quite serious and even devastating. Ventral cervical discectomy, although considered relatively safe and simple, is one of the most common procedures involved in malpractice litigation.

General Considerations

The first step for avoiding complications associated with any surgical procedure is to perform the appropriate operation on the appropriate patient. Although a detailed discussion of various indications for surgery and criteria for patient selection is beyond the scope of this chapter, the importance of correlating the clinical picture with the imaging abnormalities cannot be overemphasized. The majority of middle-aged patients will have at least some degree of degenerative changes of the cervical spine, but only a few will have symptomatic spinal cord or nerve root compression. Therefore, a careful analysis of patient history and meticulous neurologic examination are essential to accurately correlate the imaging abnormalities with the patient's clinical picture.

The ventral approach to the cervical spine is performed through a plane between the sternocleidomastoid muscle and the carotid sheath laterally and the strap muscles and tracheoesophageal viscera medially. This approach is appropriate for ventral cervical discectomy, vertebrectomy, fusion, and instrumentation (Figure 27.1).

The ventrolateral approach, however, is more suitable for decompression of the vertebral artery in the transverse foramen or between the foramina or spinal nerve roots outside the spinal canal. Two different techniques are described in the literature. Verbiest's[55,56] technique is performed through the same plane as is the ventral approach. However, further exposure is performed lateral to the longus colli muscle on the ipsilateral side. This allows the visualization of the costotransverse lamella, which forms the roof of the foramen transversarium that covers the vertebral artery. Hodgson,[31] on the other hand, approached the cervical spine lateral to the sternocleidomastoid muscle and the carotid sheath. These structures, along with the musculovisceral column, are retracted medially (Figure 27.2). The remainder of the exposure is similar to that described by Verbiest, with the exception that the longus colli muscles are retracted medially to laterally in order to gain access to the vertebral artery.

Essentially, the structures at risk of injury are the same with either the ventral or the ventrolateral approach. In the Hodgson approach, tracheoesophageal viscera and the recurrent laryngeal nerve (RLN) are protected, whereas the nerve roots, sympathetic chain, and the vertebral artery are at greater risk.

Specific Complications, Avoidance, and Management
Preoperative Period

In patients with a significant neurologic deficit, the preoperative use of corticosteroids may be considered. However, there is no convincing data in the literature to support the efficacy of the routine use of corticosteroids in patients undergoing decompressive operation.

Although hyperextension of the neck usually facilitates exposure during the operation and restores normal lordotic curvature of the cervical spine, excessive hyperextension during intubation or during the operative procedure may further narrow the spinal canal and exacerbate a preexisting neurologic deficit, especially in patients with spinal canal compromise. Some authors[7] claim that the amount of hyperextension that can be tolerated by the patient can be assessed in the preoperative period by placing the neck in the amount of extension anticipated during the operation and/or intubation. If the patient can maintain this position for 30 minutes without motor or sensory symptoms, the operation can be performed safely in that position. If, however, any symptoms are induced during the testing, the neck must be kept neutral throughout surgery, and the patient should be intubated fiberoptically.

Some authors[24] advocate the use of intraoperative evoked-potential monitoring as a means to identify and avoid dangerous manipulation of the neural tissue during surgery. However, there is currently no convincing evidence that the use of intraoperative evoked-potential monitoring improves outcome after decompressive surgery. Somatosensory evoked potentials (SSEP) are most

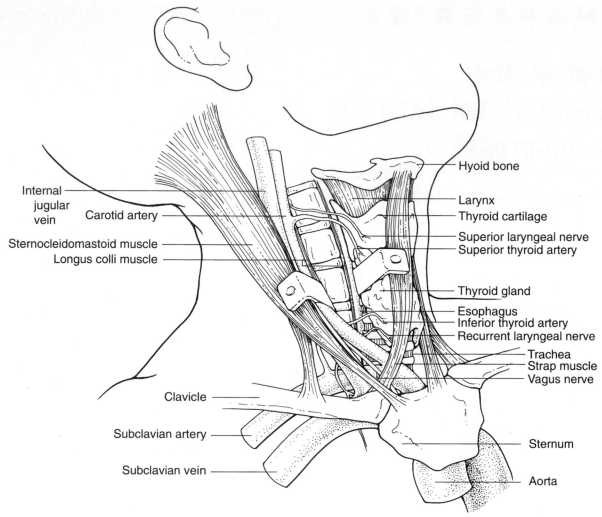

Figure 27.1 Ventral exposure of the cervical spine and anatomic structures of surgical importance.

commonly used for this purpose. However, this type of monitoring may be associated with false-positive intraoperative SSEP changes, thus creating significant anxiety for the surgeon and possibly unnecessary anesthetic and surgical maneuvers. Motor evoked-potential monitoring reflects the function of the ventral spinal cord tracts more reliably than does SSEP monitoring and may avoid some of the false-positive intraoperative changes observed with SSEPs.

To facilitate identification of the lower cervical segments on the localizing radiograph, wide adhesive tapes may be applied over the shoulders for caudal traction. In this case, excessive traction should be avoided because there is potential risk for traction injury of the upper brachial plexus.

Intraoperative Period

A right-sided approach is generally recommended because it is easier for the right-handed surgeon. Some authors, however, believe that a right-sided approach is associated with higher risk of injury to the RLN, especially in the lower cervical spine. The risk, however, is low.

The risk is probably balanced by the convenience of the position for right-handed surgeons. A left-sided approach, on the other hand, carries the risk of injury to the thoracic duct during exposure of the lower cervical spine.[21] A recent review of 328 patients who underwent ventral cervical spine fusion procedures showed no association between the side of the approach and the incidence of RLN symptoms.[8]

The skin incision is usually transverse and localized in a skin crease. A diagonal skin incision along the medial border of the sternocleidomastoid muscle may be alternatively used for multilevel disease. After the skin incision is made, the platysma muscle is dissected both rostrally and caudally. One should look for branches of the external jugular vein because these may be inadvertently transected with sharp scissors during the dissection. If identified, the blood vessels can be coagulated and sharply divided. The platysma is then incised vertically parallel to its fibers throughout the limits of the exposure to prevent undue traction.

For a ventrolateral approach, more complete exposure of the sternocleidomastoid muscle is required. During the opening of the ventral cervical fascia, the greater auricular

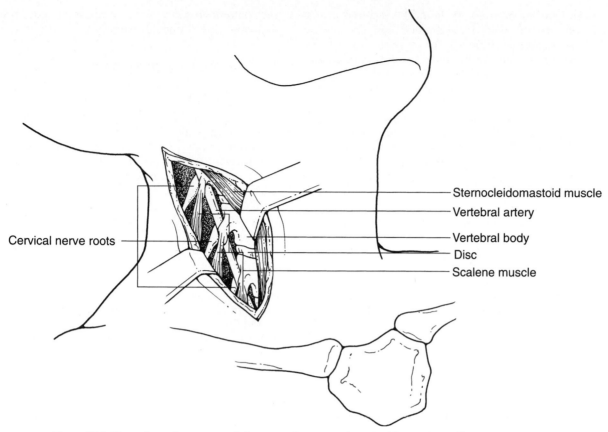

Figure 27.2 Ventrolateral exposure of the cervical spine as described by Hodgson.[31]

nerve and other ventral cutaneous nerves are at risk of injury.[57] Injury of the greater auricular nerve results in decreased sensation of the skin of the face in the area of the parotid gland. This nerve penetrates the deep fascia on the dorsal surface of the sternocleidomastoid muscle at approximately midbelly and travels rostrally on the surface of sternocleidomastoid muscle toward the ear. The anterior cutaneous nerve, on the other hand, takes a more horizontal course across the sternocleidomastoid muscle before dividing into the ascending and descending branches. The ascending branch provides cutaneous innervation of the skin overlying the mandible. Damage to this nerve can result in decreased sensation over the mandible. The key to avoiding these injuries is to identify these structures and to be aware of their anatomic location.

During the lateral retraction of the sternocleidomastoid muscle for a ventrolateral approach, the eleventh cranial nerve is also at risk of injury and must be identified. This nerve enters the sternocleidomastoid muscle two- to three-finger widths below mastoid tip and exits the muscle obliquely, caudally passing across the posterior triangle of the neck to the ventral border of the trapezius muscle.

After the superficial cervical fascia is incised and the plane is developed between the sternocleidomastoid muscle laterally and the strap muscles medially, certain structures are at risk of injury. These include the larynx and trachea, esophagus and pharynx, laryngeal nerves, carotid artery, internal jugular vein, vagus nerve, sympathetic chain, and pleura. The complications related to these structures are discussed separately.[57]

Injury to the Larynx and Trachea

Perforation of the trachea, though a rare and unusual complication of this procedure, can occur during the medial dissection. If it does occur, direct repair is usually possible. Severe laryngeal retraction can result in significant laryngeal edema that may appear as an immediate postoperative emergency. Many measures can be undertaken to reduce the severity of the postoperative glottic edema, including systemic corticosteroids, cold mist, and inhalation of racemic epinephrine. If these measures are not successful, reintubation may be attempted. If these maneuvers fail, a tracheotomy should be performed.[4]

Injury to the Esophagus and Pharynx

Dysphagia is a common problem after ventral cervical surgery and is usually secondary to edema from retraction. This symptom usually resolves within a few days without any treatment. In certain cases, however, it may persist as long as several weeks and, in rare cases, it may be permanent.[15,17,25] It is more common in elderly patients and in those who have had extensive mobilization of the upper esophagus or hypopharynx. In a questionnaire mailed to 497 patients who had undergone ventral cervical fusion procedures, 60% reported some dysphagia after the surgical procedure compared to 23% in the control group.[59]

Esophageal or pharyngeal lacerations can occur, especially in the upper cervical region where the hypopharynx is thinner, either from sharp dissection or from the teeth of self-retaining retractors. If esophageal perforation is recognized intraoperatively, it should be repaired prima-rily.[53] The wound should be drained and the patient placed on nasogastric drainage for at least 7 to 10 days. Fusion in these circumstances is contraindicated.[47] Subsequently, a swallow study with a water-soluble con-trast agent should be obtained to confirm that the perfo-ration has sealed. In the majority of the cases, the injury to the esophagus is not recognized during surgery and shows symptoms later as a local infection, fistula, sepsis, or mediastinitis.[15,26,41] The presence of crepitus or enlarg-ing mass in the neck or mediastinal air on a chest radio-graph usually suggests the strong possibility of an esophageal perforation.[41] Diagnosis can be confirmed with an esophagogram. However, this test may not always be positive when esophageal injury is present. Esophagoscopy or a postesophagogram computed tomog-raphy (CT) scan may also demonstrate a perforation.[41] The treatment of a delayed perforation consists of naso-gastric drainage, antibiotics, and reexploration of the inci-sion. If a defect is found, it should be repaired and a wound drain placed. To avoid this complication, the longus colli muscles should be freed enough, rostrally, caudally, and laterally, so that the sharp teeth of the self-retaining retractors can be placed safely under them with-out risk of dislodgment during the procedure (Figure 27.3). In addition, the esophagus and other soft-tissue structures should be hidden by the retractors to avoid injury by the high-speed drill during bone removal.

Occasionally, perforation of the esophagus can result from a displaced graft.[38,39] To avoid this problem, some surgeons recommend reapproximation of the longus colli muscles over the graft. When a displaced graft perforates the esophagus, reexploration is required. Either replace-ment or removal of the graft may be indicated, depending upon the need for the graft to maintain stability. The esophageal perforation should be repaired, if possible, and

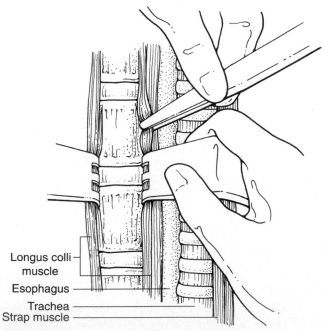

Figure 27.3 Placement of self-retaining retractors under the longus colli muscle to prevent dislodgment during surgery.

Longus colli muscle
Esophagus
Trachea
Strap muscle

the patient treated with antibiotics and nasogastric drainage, as described previously.

Injury to the Laryngeal Nerves

Both the superior and inferior (recurrent) laryngeal nerves are at risk during the exposure of the ventral cervical spine.[10,29] Flynn[26] noted that RLN injury is the "... single largest complication ... that has ... frequently resulted in litigation." Some proposed mechanisms of this complica-tion include direct surgical trauma, nerve division or liga-ture, pressure or stretched-induced neurapraxia, and postoperative edema.[29,40,50]

The superior laryngeal nerve is a branch of the inferior ganglion of the vagus nerve and innervates the cricothy-roid muscle. The superior thyroid artery is encountered above C4 and is an important anatomic landmark for the superior laryngeal nerve. Damage to this nerve may result in hoarseness, but it often produces symptoms such as easy voice fatigue.[10] In order to avoid injury to this nerve, one should be aware of its anatomic location.

On the left side, the inferior (recurrent) laryngeal nerve loops under the arch of the aorta and is protected in the left tracheoesophageal groove. On the right side, however, it travels around the subclavian artery, passing dorsomedi-ally to the side of the trachea and esophagus. It is vulner-able as it passes from the subclavian artery to the right tracheoesophageal groove.[2] Damage to the RLN may result in hoarseness, vocal breathiness or fatigue, weak cough, dysphagia, or aspiration.[40]

On the right side, the inferior thyroid artery is an anatomic marker for the RLN. The nerve usually enters the tracheoesophageal groove, the point at which the infe-rior thyroid artery enters the lower pole of the thyroid. Ligation of this artery without identifying the course and position of the RLN may jeopardize the integrity of this nerve.[37] Another possible mechanism of injury to the RLN is inadvertent dissection in the plane between the trachea and esophagus.[2] Preoperative insertion of a nasogastric tube not only allows easier identification of the esophagus for protection against an esophageal injury, but it also allows the localization of the tracheoesophageal groove and the avoidance of the plane. Endotracheal tube related RLN injury has also been cited.[5,13,36,52] Monitoring of the endotracheal cuff pressure and its release after retractor placement has decreased the rate of RLN temporary paralysis from 6.4% to 1.7% in one series.[3]

One should also be aware of the anatomic variations, especially on the right side where the RLN may be nonre-current. However, the frequency of this aberrancy is well below 1%.[11] In this situation, it travels directly from the vagus nerve and the carotid sheath to the larynx. If a sus-pected nonrecurrent nerve is encountered, it may be iden-tified with a nerve stimulator and a laryngoscopic examination of the vocal cords.[10] If it cannot be retracted safely, it is best to abandon the procedure and use a left-sided approach.

The RLN is better protected during Hodgson's[57] approach than it is during a standard ventral cervical approach. However, it should be kept in mind that this nerve is still vulnerable at the position at which it enters the right tracheoesophageal groove. It is important to remember that during the Hodgson procedure, the midline is first identified after the prevertebral fascia is incised and the longus colli muscle retracted from medial to lateral position. The key to avoiding injury to the important anatomic structures during the Hodgson approach is to recognize that the approach is lateral to the sternocleidomastoid muscle, as well as to the carotid sheath. However, during the opening of the prevertebral fascia, the midline is identified, and the longus colli muscles are retracted medially to laterally.

Minor hoarseness or sore throat after a ventral cervical operation is common and has been reported in approximately one-half of patients.[2] It resolves without further intervention in weeks or months in the majority of patients. The cause is usually edema from tracheal intubation. However, injury to the laryngeal nerves can also occur and may result in permanent laryngeal dysfunction. The true incidence of injury to the recurrent laryngeal nerve is difficult to determine but is probably about 1% to 2%.[8,10,16] In one series, an incidence of early impairment of vocal cord mobility has been reported to be as high as 11%.[29] Beutler et al.[8] reported that the incidence of RLN symptoms was 2.1% with anterior cervical discectomy, 3.5% with corpectomy, 3% with instrumentation, and 9.5% with reoperative anterior surgery.

Because many patients have some degree of voice change after ventral cervical operations, a thorough investigation is not required in most cases. However, a laryngoscopic examination should be performed in persistent cases. If there is an RLN palsy, the vocal cord will be faced in the paramedian position. Immediate treatment is not usually required for a paralyzed vocal cord because, in most instances, the nerve has not been severed, and the condition will resolve with time. In some patients, hoarseness or voice dysfunction may be minimal and not require treatment. However, patients with persistent hoarseness after several months can be treated with injections of Gelfoam or Teflon into the vocal cord. Gelfoam produces a temporary improvement and may be used as an interim measure pending spontaneous return of function. Teflon injection is a permanent treatment modality that is used in patients in whom no recovery is expected.[10]

Injury to the Structures in the Carotid Sheath

Care must be taken to not enter the carotid sheath laterally in order to avoid injury to the carotid artery, internal jugular vein, or the vagus nerve. Laceration of the carotid artery may result from the sharp teeth of retractor blades or during the dissection with sharp instruments.[58] It is important to recognize that manipulation of the carotid artery may result in an embolic stroke resulting from dislodgment of debris from a preexisting carotid plaque.[20,58] In some cases, it may be useful to monitor the temporal artery pulse after placement of the self-retaining retractors in order to avoid the risk of stroke as a result of carotid occlusion from retraction. In most cases, carotid artery lacerations can be repaired primarily. However, one may consider abandoning the procedure if such an injury occurs early in the course of the operation.

Injury to the internal jugular vein results from either sharp dissection or the sharp teeth of a dislodged self-retaining retractor. This usually causes a significant amount of bleeding, and it can compromise the exposure of the other important anatomic structures. Bleeding should be controlled, and either the laceration should be repaired or the jugular vein should be ligated.

Injury to the vagus nerve can result from entry into the carotid sheath. This is a very unusual complication, but if transection is observed intraoperatively, primary anastomosis should be attempted.

Injury to the Vertebral Artery

Injury to the vertebral artery may result from asymmetric and far lateral bone removal and is most likely to occur on the left side during a standard right-sided approach (Figure 27.4).[18] In a cadaveric study, the course of the vertebral artery was analyzed in 222 cervical spines. A 2.7% incidence of tortuous vertebral artery was identified.[19] Injury to the vertebral artery can also result from an aggressive dissection of the longus colli muscles, which injures the vascular structures between the transverse processes. Although primary repair of the vertebral arteries has been recommended, this is usually very difficult. No clear-cut evidence is available to enable decision making in this regard. Commonly, bleeding can be controlled with gentle compression using a muscle pledget, Gelfoam, or Surgicel, after which an angiogram should be obtained to check whether an arteriovenous fistula or pseudoaneurysm has developed after vertebral artery injury.[18] In some cases, ligation is required to control bleeding.[54] The risk of neurologic deficit after a unilateral vertebral artery occlusion is low.[49] However, a case of Wallenberg's syndrome has been described, resulting from thrombosis of the vertebral artery after the use of a vertebral spreader.[32] To avoid this injury, one should identify the midline carefully and proceed with drilling accordingly.

Occasionally, transection of the vertebral artery can occur inadvertently during decompression of the vertebral artery, via an anterolateral approach. This requires control of the bleeding by a ligature at the level above and below the lesion.[7] Thorough mobilization of the vertebral artery invariably causes bleeding from the surrounding venous plexus. Vigorous retraction and aggressive mobilization of the vertebral artery should be avoided to minimize hemorrhage.

Injury to the Sympathetic Chain

The sympathetic chain may be more vulnerable to damage during ventral lower cervical spine procedures because it is situated closer to the medial border of the longus colli muscles at C6 more than at C3. The longus colli muscles diverge laterally and the sympathetic chain converges medially at C6.[22] Injury to the cervical sympathetic chain, which results in Horner's syndrome, is unusual but can result from either transection or retraction of the sympathetic chain. The incidence of permanent injury is less than 1%.[26] To avoid this injury during a ventral approach, the soft-tissue dissection should be limited to the medial aspect of the longus colli muscles.

During a ventrolateral approach, the sympathetic chain is particularly at risk of injury. The sympathetic chain is located ventral to the transverse processes. It is either embedded in the dorsal carotid sheath or lies on the

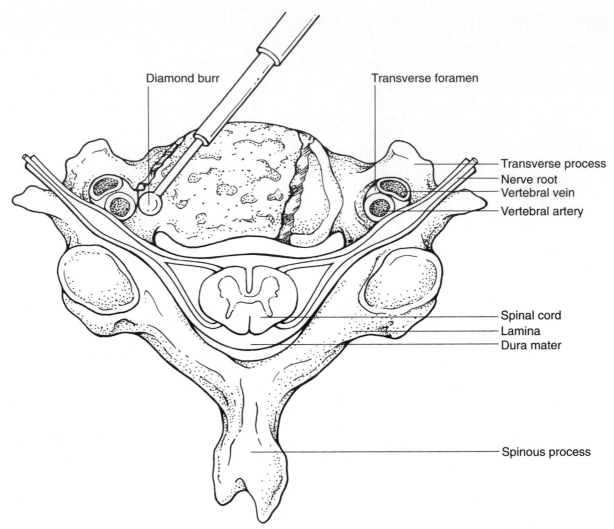

Figure 27.4 Mechanism of injury at the vertebral artery as a result of misassessment of the midline or asymmetric drilling.

connective tissue between the sheath and the longus colli muscle. To avoid injury, the superior cervical ganglion at C1 and the middle cervical ganglion at C6 should be included with the sympathetic chain as it is retracted laterally to medially together with the longus colli muscle.

Increased Neurologic Deficit

Increased neurologic deficit after a ventral cervical operation is unusual. Most spinal cord or nerve root injuries are associated with technical mishaps (excepting most C5 deficits). Although the exact figure is difficult to determine, Flynn[26] reported a 1.3% incidence of additional radicular dysfunction and a 3.3% incidence of worsening myelopathy. If neurologic deficit becomes apparent immediately after the surgery, the most likely causes are direct surgical trauma to the neural elements or problems related to positioning or manipulation of the neck during incubation.

To avoid neurologic injury, certain measures should be undertaken at every step of the procedure. Important precautionary measures regarding positioning, neck hyperextension, intubation, and electrophysiologic monitoring

have been described in the previous paragraphs. During intraoperative localization, the localizing needle in the disc space (18-gauge spinal needle) should be bent at the tip as shown in Figure 27.5, so that inadvertent advancement of the needle into the spinal canal is impossible.

During the removal of spondylotic ridges, it is important that osteophytes not be disconnected from the vertebral bodies until they have been thinned sufficiently to permit removal with fine curettes. Otherwise, further attempts to drill may result in compression of the spinal cord (Figure 27.6). Achieving a complete decompression before placement of the bone graft is also crucial. As shown in Figure 27.7, in instances of incomplete decompression, tapping of the bone graft may result in compression of the spinal cord. During the final advancement of the bone graft, a bone tamp should be positioned in such a way that one-half of the surface of the tamp is against the remaining rostral or caudal vertebral body (Figure 27.8). This prevents an inadvertent advancement of the graft into the spinal canal, resulting in spinal cord compression. Countersinking of the bone graft can be accomplished by angling the tamp but maintaining the position of the tamp relative to the vertebral body (Figure 27.8). Occasionally,

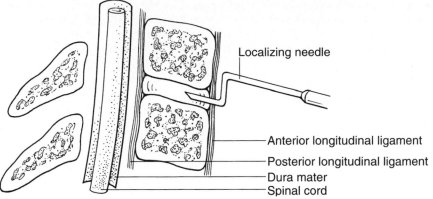

Figure 27.5 The localizing needle (18-gauge spinal needle) should be bent at the tip to prevent inadvertent penetration of the spinal cord.

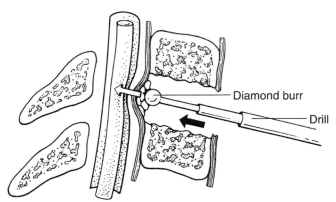

Figure 27.6 Possible mechanism of injury if the bone fragments become disconnected from the vertebral bodies before they have been completely thinned out during the removal of the spondylotic ridges. In this case, the remaining mobile fragment may cause neural impingement during further drilling.

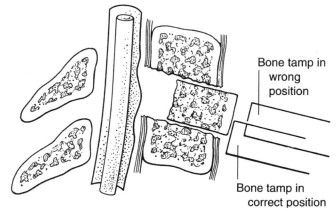

Figure 27.8 Recommended position of the bone tamp during the final positioning of the bone graft to prevent inadvertent advancement into the spinal cord. The tamp cannot pass beyond (dorsal) to the ventral margin of the vertebral body. The seating of the bone graft into a recessed position may require the angling of the tamp, while maintaining the obligatory positioning of the tamp partially over the vertebral body (*inset*).

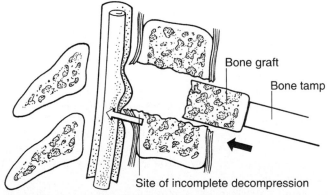

Figure 27.7 Possible mechanism of spinal cord injury in cases of incomplete decompression as a result of "water hammer" effect during the placement of bone graft. Impaction of the bone graft may result in transmission of force vectors to the spinal cord via the persistent osteophyte.

an anteroposterior plane is limited to 13mm, penetration of the spinal canal is very unlikely. Nerve root injuries are less common than spinal cord injuries, but for unclear reasons, the C5 nerve root is very sensitive to trauma.[51]

If a neurologic deficit is not present immediately after the patient awakens but appears within hours, the possibility of an epidural hematoma should be considered. In the case of suspected epidural hematoma with rapidly deteriorating neurologic function, the patient should be returned to the operating room for immediate exploration, without delay for diagnostic studies. In patients who have neurologic deficits immediately after surgery, one should consider administering glucocorticoids and should obtain lateral cervical spine radiographs to determine the position of the bone graft. If the patient's neurologic status is stable, magnetic resonance imaging (MRI) may be valuable to determine the cause of the deterioration. If a hematoma or bone graft misplacement is suspected, expeditious reexploration is required as described above.

misplacement or displacement of a bone graft may cause nerve or cord compression. To avoid this injury, the depth of the graft should be measured very carefully, and the depth of the vertebral body should be measured on preoperative imaging studies. If the depth of the bone graft in

If neurologic worsening occurs within days after the operation, an epidural abscess must be considered in the differential diagnosis. Obviously, the abscess should be drained as soon as possible, and the patient should be treated with appropriate antibiotics.[7]

Sleep-induced apnea has been reported as an unusual complication of ventral cervical spine surgery. It is usually a self-limited process. Supportive respiratory therapy is occasionally needed.[34]

Dural Laceration and Cerebrospinal Fluid Fistula

Dura mater laceration and cerebrospinal fluid leak may occur during removal of the posterior longitudinal ligament or during drilling. Direct repair is usually not feasible. A piece of gelatin foam should be placed over the dural defect, and lumbar subarachnoid drainage should be performed for 4 to 5 days. To minimize the chance of dural laceration from the drill bit, one should consider switching to a diamond drill when the dorsal cortex or the slope of the uncovertebral joints is encountered. The surgeon must also be aware that the nerve roots are more ventrally located than the spinal cord. Therefore, if one were to continue drilling laterally at the same ventrodorsal depth as the midline dura mater, violation of the dural sleeves of the nerve roots (and vertebral artery) could occur.

Postoperative Period
Soft-Tissue Hematomas and Respiratory Problems

Cervical soft-tissue hematomas after ventral cervical operation are unusual,[7,57] and many can be managed nonoperatively. However, a large hematoma may lead to airway obstruction and is a potentially life-threatening complication. To avoid this problem, careful hemostasis before closure is imperative. A Jackson-Pratt drain, inserted in the prevertebral space before closure, should be left in place for 24 hours in case hemostasis was not achieved adequately. The patient should be monitored very carefully in the recovery room after the operative procedure for signs of respiratory insufficiency or cervical swelling. Some surgeons advocate not using the cervical collar in the immediate postoperative period because of the risk of masking the signs of an expanding cervical hematoma.[54] If a palpable hematoma is noted immediately after the cervical procedure, but the patient does not have any respiratory compromise, the hematoma may be treated expectantly. However, a large or expanding hematoma should be drained, even if the patient is otherwise asymptomatic. If respiration is compromised, emergency treatment is required. The patient should be reintubated, if possible, and the wound opened. If intubation is not easily accomplished, the wound should be reopened in the recovery room and, if necessary, the airway reestablished via a tracheotomy or cricothyroidotomy.

Postoperative Infection

Infectious processes can occur after a ventral cervical operation and may affect only the superficial layers or involve the deeper structures. These are reported in 0.4% to 2% of patients with spinal complications.[38,45] Superficial infections external to the platysma muscle can be treated by simple opening of the incision, followed by dressing changes and administration of appropriate antibiotics and secondary closure.

Cellulitis or abscess in the deeper tissues, however, requires a more thorough evaluation. Perforation of the esophagus or pharynx should always be considered a possibility and a potential source of infection. This is especially true when an unusual mixture of organisms is identified. In such instances, the incision should be explored under general anesthesia to drain the abscess and investigate the possibility of an esophageal perforation with intraoperative inspection. Subsequently, a postoperative esophagogram and CT should be obtained to assess the status of the perforation.

The issue of bone graft removal in the presence of infection is complex.[23] The authors chose to leave the graft in place, treat with antibiotics, and follow the status of the graft with cervical spine films. If the graft is collapsing, removal and replacement with autograft would be indicated; in most cases, bone healing will take place.

Epidural abscesses and meningitis have also been reported in association with ventral cervical operations. However, these complications are quite rare.[7] If a patient has progressive postoperative spinal cord dysfunction, with or without evidence of osteomyelitis or systemic signs of sepsis, epidural abscess should always be considered in the differential diagnosis. Either MRI or CT myelography should be used to establish the diagnosis. Meningitis should be considered in a septic patient if a dural laceration was observed or suspected intraoperatively. Lumbar puncture is required to confirm the suspicion.

Graft Complications

The predominant complications related to the bone graft are graft collapse, extrusion and migration, and nonunion. These may occur from suboptimal sizing, vertebral end plate fracture, postoperative trauma, or inadequate immobilization. Graft collapse is most frequently observed in elderly patients with osteoporotic bone.[15] If there is any question regarding the structural integrity of autologous bone, an allograft should be used. However, in younger patients, autologous graft is stronger than allograft in resisting axial compression. The majority of patients with graft collapse are asymptomatic and do not require reoperation.

Graft extrusion and migration is reported in 2.1% to 4.6% of single-level fusions and in 10% to 29% of multilevel fusions with bony or ligamentous instability after ventral cervical discectomy and fusion. Graft displacement may require reoperation if the patient reports dysphagia, respiratory compromise, or neurologic deficits.[46,60,61] A well-fitting graft and placement with compression may help reduce this complication.

Graft pseudoarthrosis has been reported in 5% to 10% of patients who undergo single-level fusion, in 15% to 20% of two-level fusions, and in 30% to 63% of three-level fusions.[28,39,43,60] Despite radiographic nonunion, the majority of these patients are clinically asymptomatic, and reoperation is not indicated. However, persistent neck pain, progressive angulation, and subluxation mandate graft revision.

Instrumentation Complications

Between 1985 and 1996, the number of cervical spine fusion procedures performed increased by 310%.[1] Most patients undergoing a ventral cervical spinal cord decompression and fusion are stabilized using plates and screws. The advantages of instrumentation include more consistent fusion, particularly in patients undergoing multiple-level fusion, decreased time to fusion, reduced graft-related complications, and maintenance of intraoperative sagittal alignment correction.[12,27,30,33,60]

The overall incidence of instrumentation-related complications ranges from 0% to 33%.[44] Screw loosening and backout develops when the bone-screw interface deteriorates as a result of cyclic loading. To circumvent this problem, screws with bicortical purchase and superior holding strength can be used, but these have a greater potential for neurologic injury. Locking screws have also been developed for use with unicortical screws to overcome this complication.[14,60] Some biomechanical studies have shown that plate fixation results in increased rigidity at the fused levels, causing acceleration of degenerative changes at adjacent uninstrumented and unfused levels by increasing the shear stresses at these levels.[35,42] In addition, some authors[60] argue that the increased duration of surgery with possible augmented blood loss and the implantation of foreign material theoretically increases the risk of postoperative infection.

Failure to Improve

The patient with nerve root compression should have immediate or nearly immediate relief of arm pain after the surgical procedure. There is a group of patients, however, who do not follow this pattern but who ultimately have a good result. Some patients may have arm discomfort persisting for several weeks. Usually, immediate imaging studies are not required in such cases. However, if the pain is very severe or increases during the period of observation, one should obtain cervical spine radiographs to be certain that the surgical level is correct and the graft has been properly placed. If the symptoms persist for more than 3 months, the patient will require reevaluation using MRI or CT myelography.

The patient with persistent or worsened myelopathy presents a more difficult problem. Although most patients, after a satisfactory decompression, should have immediate improvement of some of the symptoms, overall improvement of myelopathic symptoms may take longer than recovery from radicular symptoms. If a patient does not have any significant neurologic recovery, imaging studies should be obtained at some point to rule out the possibility of an inadequate decompression. More recent experience with multilevel median corpectomy has suggested that the majority of patients whose myelopathy fails to improve after surgery have had an inadequate decompression of the spinal cord.[6,9,51] In such instances, reoperation may then be considered.

REFERENCES

1. Abraham DJ, Herkowitz HN: Indications and trends in use in cervical spinal fusions. *Orthop Clin North Am* 29: 731-744, 1998.
2. An HS: Surgical exposure and fusion techniques of the spine. In An HS, Cotler JM (eds): *Spinal Instrumentation*. Baltimore, Williams & Wilkins, 1992, pp 1-32.
3. Apfelbaum RI, Kriskovich MD, Haller JR: On the incidence, cause, and prevention of recurrent laryngeal nerve palsies during anterior cervical spine surgery. *Spine* 25:2906-2912, 2000.
4. Aronson NI: The management of the soft cervical disc protrusion using the Smith-Robinson approach. *Clin Neurosurgery* 20:253-258, 1973.
5. Benninger MS, Gillen JB, Altman JS: Changing etiology of vocal fold immobility. *Laryngoscope* 108:1346-1350, 1998.
6. Bernard TN, Jr., Whitecloud TS, III: Cervical spondylotic myelopathy and myeloradiculopathy: anterior decompression and stabilization with autogenous fibula strut graft. *Clin Orthop* Aug:149-160, 1987.
7. Bertalanffy H, Eggert HR: Complications of anterior cervical discectomy without fusion in 450 consecutive patients. *Acta Neurochir (Wien)* 99:41-50, 1989.
8. Beutler WJ, Sweeney CA, Connolly PJ: Recurrent laryngeal nerve injury with anterior cervical spine surgery risk with laterality of surgical approach. *Spine* 26: 1337-1342, 2001.
9. Boni M, Cherubino P, Denaro V, Benazzo F: Multiple subtotal somatectomy: technique and evaluation of a series of 39 cases. *Spine* 9:358-362, 1984.
10. Bulger RF, Rejowski JE, Beatty RA: Vocal cord paralysis associated with anterior cervical fusion: considerations for prevention and treatment. *J Neurosurg* 62:657-661, 1985.
11. Cannon RC: The anomaly of nonrecurrent laryngeal nerve: identification and management. *Otolaryngol Head Neck Surg* 120:769-771, 1999.
12. Caspar W, Barbier DD, Klara PM: Anterior cervical fusion and Caspar plate stabilization for cervical trauma. *Neurosurgery* 25:491-502, 1989.
13. Cavo JW, Jr.: True vocal cord paralysis following intubation. *Laryngoscope* 95:1352-1359, 1985.
14. Clausen JD, Ryken TC, Traynelis VC, et al: Biomechanical evaluation of Caspar and Cervical Spine Locking Plate systems in a cadaveric model. *J Neurosurg* 84:1039-1045, 1996.
15. Cloward RB: Complications of anterior cervical disc operation and their treatment. *Surgery* 69:175-182, 1971.
16. Cloward RB: New methods of diagnosis and treatment of the anterior cervical spine. *Clin Neurosurg* 8:93-132, 1962.
17. Connolly ES, Seymour RJ, Adams JE: Clinical evaluation of anterior cervical fusion for degenerative cervical disc disease. *J Neurosurg* 23:431-437, 1965.
18. Cosgrove GR, Theron J: Vertebral arteriovenous fistula following anterior cervical spine surgery: report of two cases. *J Neurosurg* 66:297-299, 1987.
19. Curylo LJ, Mason HC, Bohlman HH, Yoo JU: Tortuous course of the vertebral artery and anterior cervical decompression: a cadaveric and clinical case study. *Spine* 25:2860-2864, 2000.
20. Dohn DF: Anterior interbody fusion for treatment of cervical-disk conditions. *JAMA* 197:897-900, 1966.

21. Ebraheim NA, Lu J, Skie M, *et al:* Vulnerability of the recurrent laryngeal nerve in the anterior approach to the lower cervical spine. *Spine* 22:2664-2667, 1997.

22. Ebraheim NA, Lu J, Yang H, *et al:* Vulnerability of the sympathetic trunk during the anterior approach to the lower cervical spine. *Spine* 25:1603-1606, 2000.

23. Emery SE, Chan DP, Woodward HR: Treatment of hematogenous pyogenic vertebral osteomyelitis with anterior debridement and primary bone grafting. *Spine* 14:284-291, 1989.

24. Epstein NE: Somatosensory evoked potential monitoring in cervical spine surgery. In Cooper PR (ed): *Degenerative Diseases of the Cervical Spine.* Park Ridge, IL, American Association of Neurological Surgeons, 1992, pp 73-90.

25. Esperson JO, Buhl M, Erikson EF: Treatment of cervical disc disease using Cloward's technique. I. General results, effects of different operative methods and complications in 1106 patients. *Acta Neurochir (Wien)* 70:97-114, 1984.

26. Flynn TB: Neurologic complications of anterior cervical interbody fusion. *Spine* 7:536-539, 1982.

27. Geisler FH, Caspar W, Pitzen T, Johnson TA: Reoperation in patients after anterior cervical plate stabilization in degenerative disease. *Spine* 23:911-920, 1998.

28. Graham JJ: Complications of cervical spine surgery. In The Cervical Spine Research Society Editorial Committee (eds): *The Cervical Spine,* ed 2. Philadelphia, Lippincott-Raven, 1989, p 831.

29. Heeneman H: Vocal cord paralysis following approaches to the anterior cervical spine. *Laryngoscope* 83:17-21, 1973.

30. Heidecke V, Rainov NG, Burkert W: Anterior cervical fusion with the Orion locking plate system. *Spine* 23:1796-1802; discussion 1803, 1998.

31. Hodgson A: Approach to the cervical spine C3-C7. *Clin Orthop* 39:129-134, 1965.

32. Horwitz HN, Rizzoli HV: Herniated intervertebral discs and spinal stenosis. In Horwitz HN, Rizzoli HV (eds): *Postoperative Complications of Extracranial Neurological Surgery.* Baltimore, Williams & Wilkins, 1987, pp 30-98.

33. Katsuura A, Hukuda S, Imanaka T, *et al:* Anterior cervical plate used in degenerative disease can maintain cervical lordosis. *J Spinal Disord* 9:470-476, 1996.

34. Krieger AJ, Rosomoff HL: Sleep-induced apnea. II. Respiratory failure after anterior spinal surgery. *J Neurosurg* 40:181-185, 1974.

35. Lee CK: Accelerated degeneration of the segment adjacent to a lumbar fusion. *Spine* 13:375-377, 1988.

36. Lim EK, Chia KS, Ng BK: Recurrent laryngeal nerve palsy following endotracheal intubation. *Anaesth Intensive Care* 15:342-345, 1987.

37. Lu J, Ebraheim NA, Nadim Y, Huntoon M: Anterior approach to the cervical spine: surgical anatomy. *Orthopedics* 23:841-845, 2000.

38. Lunsford LD, Bissonette DJ, Jannetta PJ, *et al:* Anterior surgery for cervical disc disease. Part I: Treatment of lateral cervical disc herniation in 253 cases. *J Neurosurg* 53:1-11, 1980.

39. Lunsford LD, Bissonette DJ, Zorub DS: Anterior surgery for cervical disc disease. Part II: Treatment of cervical spondylotic myelopathy in 32 cases. *J Neurosurg* 53:12-19, 1980.

40. Netterville JL, Koriwchak MJ, Winkle M, *et al:* Vocal fold paralysis following the anterior approach to the cervical spine. *Ann Otol Rhinol Laryngol* 105:85-91, 1996.

41. Newhouse KE, Lindsey RW, Clark CR, *et al:* Esophageal perforation following anterior cervical spine surgery. *Spine* 14:1051-1053, 1989.

42. Panjabi MM: Biomechanical evaluation of spinal fixation devices. I. A conceptual framework. *Spine* 13:1129-1134, 1988.

43. Parsons IM, Kang JD: Mechanisms of failure after anterior cervical disc surgery. *Curr Opin Orthop* 9:2-11, 1998.

44. Rappaport LH, O'Leary PF: Cervical disc disease. In Bridwell KH, Dewald RL (eds): *Textbook of Spinal Surgery.* Philadelphia, Lippincott-Raven, 1997, pp 1371-1396.

45. Salcman M: Complications of cervical spine surgery. *Crit Care Med* 29:2027-2028, 2001.

46. Saunders RL, Bernini PM, Shirreffs TG, Jr., Reeves AG: Central corpectomy for cervical spondylotic myelopathy: a consecutive series with long-term follow-up evaluation. *J Neurosurg* 74:163-170, 1991.

47. Schmidek HH, Smith DA: Anterior cervical disc excision in cervical spondylosis. In Schmidek HH, Sweet WH (eds): *Operative Neurosurgical Techniques,* ed 3, vol 2. Philadelphia, WB Saunders, 1995, pp 1783-1804.

48. Schneider RC: Treatment of cervical spine disease: cervical herniated pulposus, spondylosis and stenosis. In Schneider RC, Kahn EA, Crosby EC (eds): *Correlative Neurosurgery,* ed 3. Springfield, IL, Charles C. Thomas, 1982, p 13.

49. Shintani A, Zervas NT: Consequence of ligation of the vertebral artery. *J Neurosurg* 36:447-450, 1972.

50. Sperry RJ, Johnson JO, Apfelbaum RI: Endotracheal tube cuff pressure increases significantly during anterior cervical fusion with the Caspar instrumentation system. *Anesth Analg* 76:1318-1321, 1993.

51. Sugar O: Spinal cord malfunction after anterior cervical discectomy. *Surg Neurol* 15:4-8, 1981.

52. Terris DJ, Arnstein DP, Nguyen HH: Contemporary evaluation of unilateral vocal cord paralysis. *Otolaryngol Head Neck Surg* 107:84-90, 1992.

53. Tew JM, Jr., Mayfield FH: Complications of surgery of the anterior cervical spine. *Clin Neurosurg* 23:424-434, 1976.

54. Tew JM, Jr., Mayfield FH: Surgery of the anterior cervical spine: preventions of complications. In Dunsker SB (ed): *Cervical Spondylosis.* New York, Raven Press, 1981, pp 191-208.

55. Verbiest H: Anterolateral operations for fractures and dislocations in the middle and lower parts of the cervical spine: report of a series of 47 cases. *J Bone Joint Surg Am* 51:1489-1530, 1969.

56. Verbiest H: A lateral approach to the cervical spine: technique and indications. *J Neurosurg* 28:191-203, 1968.

57. Watkins R: Lateral approach to the cervical spine (Hodgson). In Watkins R (ed): *Surgical Approach to the Spine.* New York, Springer Verlag, 1983, p 39.

58. Whitecloud TS, II: Cervical spondylosis: the anterior approach. In Frymoyer JW (ed): *The Adult Spine: Principles and Practice,* vol 2. New York, Raven Press, 1978, pp 1165-1185.

59. Winslow C, TJ W, Wax M: Dysphonia and dysphagia following the anterior approach to the cervical spine. *Arch Otolaryngol Head Neck Surg* 127:51-55, 2001.

60. Zaveri GR, Ford M: Cervical spondylosis: the role of anterior instrumentation after decompression and fusion. *J Spinal Disord* 14:10-16, 2001.

61. Zdeblick TA, Cooke ME, Wilson D, *et al:* Anterior cervical discectomy, fusion, and plating: a comparative animal study. *Spine* 18:1974-1983, 1993.

CHAPTER 28

Single and Multiple-Single Interbody Fusion Techniques

Robert F. Heary, Edward C. Benzel, and Ceslovas Vaicys

Cervical discectomy via ventral approach, better known as anterior cervical discectomy (ACD) or anterior cervical discectomy and fusion (ACDF), is one of the most common procedures performed by spine surgeons. Complication rates are low and the clinical results are gratifying. Some surgical complications are treatable at the time of their detection intraoperatively or in the immediate postoperative period, and other complications may have no reasonable treatment once detected. Avoiding irreversible complications is the only logical solution to their treatment. Overall, complication rates for ACDF operations vary from approximately 5%[9,59,64,80] to 15%.[4,26,54,67,75] The operation itself is divided into stages, including general surgical considerations, discectomy, donor site considerations, and bony fusion.

Surgical complications may be categorized as occurring in the preoperative, intraoperative, or postoperative period. A majority of the complications that occur during an ACD and ACDF are avoidable with appropriate patient selection, careful preoperative planning, meticulous surgical technique, and close follow-up and monitoring.

A brief history of ACD and ACDF surgery is useful. More than 400 years ago, Vesalius described the intervertebral disc.[20] It was not until 1928 that Stookey described a number of clinical syndromes that result from disc protrusions. These protrusions were thought to be neoplasms of notochordal origin and were incorrectly identified as chondromas.[77] During this same era other investigators provided a more precise understanding of the pathophysiology of the intervertebral disc.[50,58,70]

In the 1950s the first reports of ventral approaches to cervical disc pathology appeared. The two most common methods for ACDF were described by Robinson and Smith in 1955[66] and by Cloward in 1958.[17] Robinson and Smith described an operation for removal of cervical disc material with replacement of a rectangular bone graft, obtained from the iliac crest, to allow for the development of a cervical fusion.[66] With Cloward's method, the discectomy was performed by a dowel technique.[17] Although numerous modifications have been developed since the 1950s, the great majority of spine surgeons currently use either the Cloward or the Smith-Robinson technique.*

Preoperative Considerations

The best predictor of a good postoperative clinical result is proper preoperative patient selection. ACD and ACDF are indicated for myelopathy, radiculopathy, and for degenerative disc disease with mechanical pain. The presence of clinical symptoms, a consistent physical examination, and confirmatory imaging studies leads to the best postoperative result. In addition, a meticulous evaluation of the general overall medical condition of the patient is mandatory. Postoperative mortality may be caused by myocardial infarction,[8,20,26,30] respiratory failure,[62] pulmonary embolism,[53] or laryngeal edema,[30] among many other potential complications.

General considerations that may directly affect ACDF include the presence of diabetes mellitus or immunocompromised states. The immunocompromised states include acquired immune deficiency syndrome (AIDS), autoimmune disturbances, or systemic medical conditions that require corticosteroid administration. A history of smoking is associated with diminished postoperative fusion rates.*

The deleterious effects of smoking are manifested by inhibition of the neovascularization necessary for incorporation of a bone graft.[23] A current preoperative recommendation is cessation of smoking for a minimum of 8 weeks before surgery and for a minimum of 12 weeks postoperatively. A preoperative dependence on narcotic analgesics has been associated with suboptimal outcome. This is particularly true if the clinical surgical indication is axial neck (mechanical) pain in the absence of radiculopathy or myelopathy. Of note is preoperative difficulty with swallowing. This is more common in the elderly and should be investigated, as necessary, before surgical intervention. If possible, the use of estrogen replacements or oral contraceptive pills in female patients should be discontinued preoperatively. These medications are known to increase the development of deep vein thromboses in the postoperative period.

Preoperative radiographic imaging studies are necessary to confirm the history and physical examination findings. Plain radiographs remain a cornerstone of the preoperative radiographic evaluation. Lateral cervical spine radiographs allow for an assessment of the sagittal plane alignment. Flexion and extension views are useful to establish the presence of spinal instability that may alter the surgical decision-making process. Finally, the dorsal elements should be assessed for splaying of the spinous processes or for facet joint abnormalities.

The gold standard imaging study for ventral cervical surgery remains the myelogram, followed by a postmyelogram computed tomographic (CT) scan. This study provides excellent anatomic detail of both the spinal cord and the cervical nerve root sleeves. Recently, magnetic resonance imaging (MRI) has been popularized. MRI allows for greater soft-tissue detail and is very useful for identifying disc degeneration. However, MRI is extremely sensitive and may overestimate the extent of surgical pathology. A recent study has demonstrated a significant incidence of abnormal MRI findings in asymptomatic patients.[46] As a result it is important to remember that an abnormal MRI

---

*References 7,10,11,15,28,32,34,48,57,75.

*References 1,8,12,16,42,87.

is not necessarily an indication for surgery. However, note that MRI allows for the evaluation of pathology in a sagittal plane. Finally, reports of lower cervical spine ACD performed in patients with significant pathology of the foramen magnum and the upper cervical spine region should increase the surgeon's index of suspicion for such lesions.[4,59]

Intraoperative Considerations

The majority of intraoperative complications may be avoided by careful preoperative planning and meticulous intraoperative technique. If intraoperative complications occur, they are usually best managed at the time of detection. However, some may not be detected until the postoperative period. Thus there is considerable overlap between the management of intraoperative and postoperative complications. Intraoperative considerations include positioning, incision, dissection, retraction, distraction, discectomy, donor site considerations, and fusion.

Positioning

The patient is positioned supine on the operating table, and general endotracheal anesthesia is administered. If significant spinal cord compression or myelopathy is present, consideration should be given to a fiber optic, awake, nasotracheal intubation. After successful intubation, the patient's neurologic examination is confirmed before the induction of general anesthesia.

The patient's head should be supported with either a donut or a Mayfield horseshoe headrest. The neck should be supported dorsally with a firm support to prevent intraoperative motion. In addition, an attempt at achieving a normal lordotic cervical curvature should be made to optimize the postoperative sagittal plane alignment. Ordinarily, a degree of neck extension is preferable to improve the lordotic curvature, as well as to aid in the dissection process. This is particularly true for upper cervical dissections. It is important to evaluate the patient's ability to extend the neck preoperatively and to not exceed this degree of extension intraoperatively. Hyperextension of the neck in a narcotized patient may lead to spinal cord compression.[80]

The operating table is flexed slightly at its midpoint, and a sandbag or other bolster is placed beneath the iliac crest to facilitate bone graft harvesting. All bony prominences must be padded, with particular attention paid to the protection of the ulnar nerves at the elbow. The knees are flexed and the heels are padded. Antiembolic stockings may be placed, and sequential compression devices are used to prevent the development of an intraoperative deep vein thrombosis.

After patient positioning and before preparation, the endotracheal cuff is deflated for 5 seconds and then reinflated. This maneuver was described by Apfelbaum[2] and has been used to limit compression of the vocal cords at the level of the arytenoid cartilage in the larynx. The recurrent laryngeal nerve terminates at the arytenoid cartilage, and if it is compressed by the endotracheal tube, a recurrent laryngeal nerve palsy may result.

A Doppler probe may be used to auscultate a baseline signal for the superficial temporary artery. During intraoperative retraction (of the carotid artery), the Doppler pulse can be re-evaluated. If tongs are to be used, they are placed at this stage.

Incision

The side of approach is based on the preference of the operating surgeon. There are advocates for both right- and left-sided approaches. As a general rule a right-handed surgeon can approach the operation more easily from the patient's right side. With a right-sided approach the recurrent laryngeal nerve is more vulnerable. This is particularly true with lower cervical dissections (Figure 28.1) The reported incidence of postoperative recurrent laryngeal nerve palsies presenting as postoperative hoarseness varies between 0.8% and 3.7%.[*] Likewise, from a left-sided approach, the recurrent laryngeal nerve has a longer course and may be less likely to be injured. Conversely, the thoracic duct is vulnerable with the left-sided approaches to the lower cervical spine (Figure 28.2).[75] In addition, the thoracic duct may be bifid, and injury to one of the limbs of the thoracic duct may not be recognized intraoperatively. If chyle is observed, simple ligation of the thoracic duct is usually all that is necessary. With lower cervical discectomies there is a theoretic risk of pneumothorax or mediastinitis from either side.[17,19,20,85]

It is essential to make the skin incision at the proper level. The most common error in this case is to place the incision too caudal, thereby obligating the physician to operate at an awkward, oblique angle. This can limit visibility during the discectomy. It is much easier to gain access caudally from a rostrally placed incision than the converse.

With one- or two-level discectomies a transverse incision is most commonly used. This is placed in a skin fold that allows for a more cosmetic postoperative result. If three or more discectomies are to be performed, an oblique incision that parallels the medial border of the sternocleidomastoid muscle is necessary. This incision is commonly used for carotid endarterectomies, because it allows for a better exposure of multiple spinal levels.

Dissection

The dissection is carried sharply through the subcutaneous tissue and the platysma muscle. The platysma muscle may be sharply divided in a transverse fashion or split longitudinally for access to the subplatysmal space. As a general rule, transecting the platysmal muscle is preferable for exposures of two or more levels. If access to multiple levels of the upper cervical spine is necessary, a generous subplatysmal dissection is used to limit the extent of soft-tissue retraction required to gain adequate exposure. After the subplatysmal dissection is completed the fascia overlying the medial border of the sternocleidomastoid muscle is sharply divided, and the deep dissection is performed, either sharply or bluntly. The plane of the deep dissection is between the sternocleidomastoid muscle and carotid

---

[*]References 4,5,22,26,30,35,38,43,54,75,80,90.

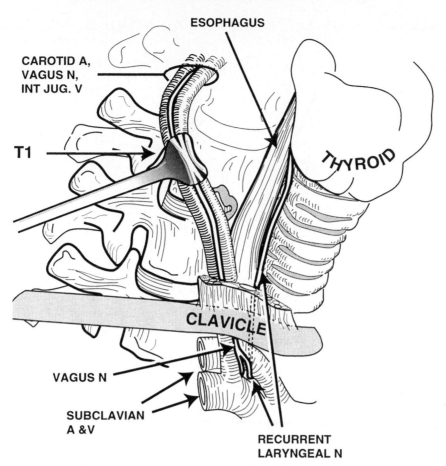

Figure 28.1 Right-sided low cervical exposure places the right recurrent laryngeal nerve at risk. The regional anatomy is depicted. (*Copyright University of New Mexico, Division of Neurosurgery.*)

sheath laterally, and between the trachea, esophagus, and strap muscles of the neck medially. Careful dissection, with identification of the carotid artery by palpation and gentle finger dissection, is required to avoid carotid artery injuries.[24,26,41,53] This trajectory allows for exposure of the prevertebral fascia. In patients who have not undergone previous ventral cervical surgery, blunt dissection is easily and safely accomplished. Excessive soft-tissue stretching should be avoided because occasionally, recurrent laryngeal nerve injury has been hypothesized to be secondary to stretching. In this case, avoiding high endotracheal cuff pressures may reduce the incidence of recurrent laryngeal nerve injuries.[2]

In patients who undergo reoperation sharp dissection may be necessary. It is important to confirm that the dissection remains dorsal to the hypopharynx and the esophagus. With reoperation, a nasogastric tube should be placed. This may be palpated to confirm the location of the esophagus and hypopharynx. The incidence of hypopharynx perforation during upper cervical discectomies varies between 1%[5,22,67,76] and 5%.[35,49,73] Esophageal perforation has also been reported in lower cervical discectomies.* If the hypopharynx or esophagus is penetrated, a drain should be placed, a layered closure performed, and a nasogastric

feeding tube inserted. The latter must be maintained for at least 1 week postoperatively.

If there is a question of perforation of the alimentary tract, the nasogastric tube should be withdrawn so that the tip of the tube is in the esophagus. After this maneuver instillation of a colored inert dye, such as methylene blue or indigo carmine, should assist with the demonstration of the violation. Unrecognized esophageal perforations can lead to the development of deep soft-tissue infections (including mediastinitis). These manifest as high fevers, severe retrosternal pain, and subcutaneous emphysema. Other severe complications of esophageal perforation include esophagocutaneous fistula[49] and even death.[36]

Retraction

On entering the prevertebral space a radiographic marker must be placed, and a lateral cervical spine radiograph obtained. This mandatory step ensures that the correct level is operated on. There have been reports of ACDs being performed at the wrong levels.[59,75]

When the appropriate level has been identified, it is useful to mark the true anatomic midline. This is best accomplished by marking a point midway between the most medial borders of the longus colli muscles. After the midline is identified, the longus colli muscles are elevated

---

*References 14,18,22,36,52,61,86.

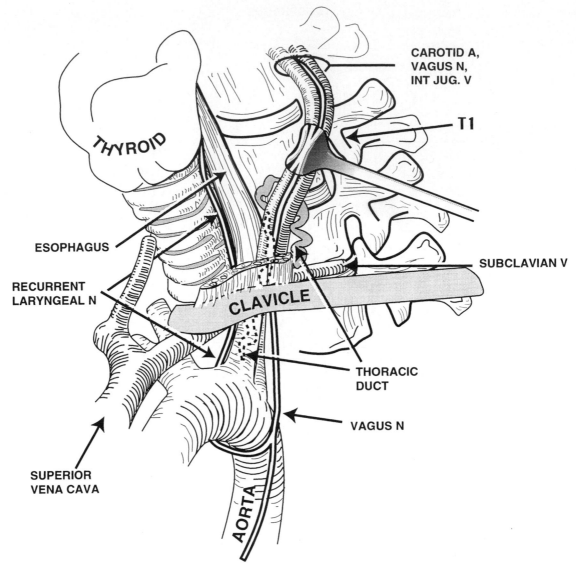

Figure 28.2 Left-sided low cervical exposure places the thoracic duct at risk. The regional anatomy is depicted. *(Copyright University of New Mexico, Division of Neurosurgery.)*

from the vertebral bodies and discs bilaterally. Longus colli dissection should be limited to 3mm of muscle. If the longus colli muscles are dissected excessively, Horner's syndrome may result. Horner's syndrome presents as the triad of ipsilateral ptosis, myosis, and anhydrosis. The incidence of postoperative Horner's syndrome varies from 0.2% to 2%.*

After the longus colli muscles are elevated a self-retaining retractor system is used. Toothed retractors are placed under the longus colli muscles bilaterally. With single-level discectomies there is rarely a need to place vertical self-retaining retractors. When operating on the lower cervical spine, it is essential to avoid retraction of the recurrent laryngeal nerve. This is particularly problematic when a right-sided cervical approach is used. If necessary, vertical retractors should be smooth at the tips, and care should be taken to avoid excessive retraction.

The self-retaining lateral retractors should be carefully placed to avoid excessive retraction on the esophagus, which may lead to postoperative dysphagia. A mild, transient, postoperative dysphagia is common after ventral cervical surgery. Dysphagia rates have been reported to vary from 1.8% to 7.7%,* to between 21.2% and 35%.[4,5,75] Intermittently releasing the retractor pressure during prolonged surgical procedures avoids this complication. Most dysphagia episodes are transient and do not require a gastrostomy tube. In cases of severe postoperative dysphagia, a gastrostomy tube may be needed for enteral feedings.

Excessive lateral retraction may also compress the carotid sheath. In patients with significant preoperative atherosclerosis, prolonged pressure against the carotid artery can lead to thrombosis with cerebral ischemia. To avoid this problem, after the lateral self-retaining retractors have been placed, the pulse of the superficial temporal

---

*References 4,5,22,25,26,59,69,80,88.

*References 3,8,9,20,30,35,54,72,85.

artery above the level of the zygoma may be auscultated with a Doppler probe or palpated by the anesthesiologist intraoperatively. This measure confirms blood flow in the external carotid artery. Because the common carotid artery bifurcates into its external and internal branches at the C3-4 level, this maneuver increases the degree of confidence (indirectly) that blood flow in the internal carotid artery has not been significantly compromised. In addition, the retractors may alter the position of the endotracheal tube. Release of the endotracheal tube cuff for 5 seconds, followed by reinflation to the lowest pressure that eliminates air leak, confirms that the vocal cords are not being excessively compressed.[2]

Distraction

After the retractors have been firmly positioned the annulus fibrosus is incised and the ventral two thirds of disc material is removed with a combination of rongeurs and curettes. Distraction techniques may improve the visualization of the disc interspace. Commonly, Gardner-Wells tongs are placed before draping, and additional weights may be added to augment distraction. Holter distraction may also be used. Improved visualization may be achieved by the use of intervertebral body disc spreaders. Alternatively, posts may be placed into the vertebral bodies above and below the desired disc exposure, with a distractor placed over the posts.

After the distractor is placed an operating microscope may be used to improve the magnification and lighting. Alternatively, a head light or high-quality overhead light, with or without loupe magnification, may be used. Adequate visualization is essential for performing the discectomy procedure safely.

Discectomy

The adequacy of neural decompression is directly related to the completeness with which the discectomy itself is performed. In addition, most neurologic complications occur at this stage of the procedure. The disc is removed, including the entirety of the dorsal annulus fibrosus in the midline. The depth of the dissection necessary to achieve this may be estimated from the preoperative MRI and CT scans. Small, upbiting microcurettes and rongeurs allow for removal of the annulus fibrosus. Hemostasis is achieved with bipolar electrocautery, Gelfoam soaked in thrombin, and cotton patties. After removal of the annulus fibrosus, the underlying posterior longitudinal ligament (PLL) can be seen.

The need to open the PLL is debated. Numerous authors recommend routine opening of the PLL after removal of the dorsal annulus fibrosus.[*] However, others do not agree with the routine sectioning of the PLL after good quality preoperative radiographic imaging studies.[60,84,89] Although preoperative imaging studies may suggest that the disc material has not protruded dorsally, the PLL may be safely sectioned to allow for entry into the epidural space. On entry a blunt nerve hook may be used to search for disc material. In addition, the PLL itself may

be thickened and responsible for ongoing neural compression. As a result, if there is any doubt about the adequacy of decompression, the PLL should be opened sharply to allow a direct look at the underlying dura mater. Likewise, ridges from dorsal osteophytes may compress the spinal cord or nerve roots. If osteophytes are detected, either by preoperative imaging studies or during the surgical procedure, they should be resected.[*]

Tearing of the underlying dura mater is possible during the opening of the PLL. This is particularly likely in cases of ossification of the PLL and in patients who have undergone previous ventral procedures.[55,74] In a series of 450 patients who underwent ventral cervical surgery Bertalanffy and Eggert reported eight patients (1.8%) who sustained damage to the dural sac. Of these eight patients, one developed meningitis.[5] If a dural tear occurs, it is usually impossible to repair the defect primarily. The methods used to prevent egress of cerebrospinal fluid (CSF) include placing free muscle and fascial grafts and using Gelfoam soaked in thrombin or fibrin glue. With a dural tear, placing a lumbar subarachnoid drain must be considered to divert CSF in the immediate postoperative period. Once the PLL is opened, instead of electrocautery, thrombostatic agents such as Gelfoam and cotton patties should be used for hemostasis.

The width of the decompression is determined on a case-by-case basis. Care must be taken to maintain the orientation of the midline, which is essential when determining the width of decompression. Useful techniques include referring to the marking of the true bony midline made before the longus colli muscle dissection, as well as being aware of the anatomic bony structures, such as the uncovertebral joints. As a general rule a 15-mm bony dissection centered over the midline is necessary for an adequate decompression.[68] If nerve root compression is present, the dissection may be extended laterally. The medial border of the uncovertebral joint serves as a bony anatomic marker of the lateral extent of a cervical discectomy. Limiting the dissection to this point will allow for a good decompression of the shoulder of the nerve root. Once again the majority of intraoperative neurologic injuries that occur are the result of loss of orientation of the bony anatomic midline. A useful intraoperative maneuver to prevent an excessively wide discectomy is frequent placement of a cotton patty in the discectomy defect. A standard cotton patty measures 13mm and allows for reorientation throughout the procedure.

As mentioned earlier in this chapter, it is during the deep portion of the discectomy procedure that the majority of neurologic injuries occur. The most common complications include dural tears, damage to the neural elements, and vertebral artery injuries. Intraoperative nerve root injuries and spinal cord contusions occur in less than 1% of ACDs.[†]

If the discectomy is too wide, the vertebral artery may be injured. The vertebral artery and its accompanying venous plexus are at risk during removal of the lateral disc material.[‡] Profuse arterial bleeding occurs after a vertebral

---

[*]References 5,27,35,63,82,90.

[*]References 9,29,34,40,43,54,56,60,65.
[†]References 5,17,30,51,54,59,78,80.
[‡]References 13,21,24,26,41,67.

artery injury. If the patient's head was rotated as part of the initial operative positioning, the head should be immediately returned to the midline before attempts are made to control bleeding.[37] Immediate tamponade should be used for the initial management of vertebral artery injuries.. If the tamponade maneuver is unable to curtail bleeding successfully, either direct ligation or primary repair of the vertebral artery may be necessary.[24] These maneuvers are technically demanding and require extension of the exposure in both a rostral and a caudal direction.

In patients with two functional vertebral arteries and an intact circle of Willis, the majority of vertebral artery injuries are asymptomatic. As a result, the actual incidence of vertebral artery injuries may be underappreciated. However, if one vertebral artery is thrombosed, or if a hypoplastic artery is present, occlusion of the dominant vertebral artery may be catastrophic.[74] Shintani and Zervas reviewed the results of 100 patients whose vertebral arteries were ligated for a variety of reasons and found a 12% mortality rate.[71] A useful note is that each vertebral artery is ordinarily accompanied by one to three paravertebral veins that are generally located medial to the vertebral arteries. If paravertebral vein bleeding is encountered, hemostasis should be attained, and further lateral dissection should not be attempted.[37] Injuries to these paravertebral veins are not associated with a postoperative neurologic deficit. The venous bleeding simply serves as a warning that the vertebral artery may be in proximity.

If the discectomy is performed for myelopathy or degenerative disc disease, the width of the discectomy should be more limited. Saunders has stated that a width of 15mm is adequate for decompression.[68] However, if nerve root compression is part of the preoperative diagnosis, a wider discectomy on one or both sides may be necessary. When performing the dissection in the lateral portion of the disc space, the use of dissectors such as blunt nerve hooks should limit the possibility of direct nerve root trauma. Nerve root injuries may result from direct trauma or from excessive manipulation of the nerve root during the discectomy. Manipulation of the nerve root is particularly problematic with the C5 nerve root, which appears to be more vulnerable to injury, and therefore extreme care should be taken to avoid manipulating it when performing C4-5 discectomies. If a nerve root injury occurs, there is no effective intraoperative management.[68]

Donor Site Considerations

The skin incision for harvesting an autologous bone graft from the iliac crest should be at least 2cm lateral to the anterior superior iliac spine. An incision placed medial to this point may result in an injury to the lateral femoral cutaneous nerve. If direct transection of the nerve occurs, permanent numbness in the ventrolateral thigh results. Lateral femoral cutaneous nerve dysfunction may be transient when it occurs secondary to excessive retraction of the nerve.

Numbness of the skin that immediately surrounds the iliac incision is a common complaint and is usually transient. The skin incision should also be placed approximately 0.5cm below the most prominent edge of the iliac ridge. In this manner the incision does not lie over the iliac crest, thus minimizing irritation from belts and other items. Also the fascial plane between the inner and outer musculature inserting on the iliac crest may be dissected with the least amount of muscle destruction.

Autologous iliac crest bone grafts for ACDF are usually tricortical. When the iliac crest is being exposed for the removal of the bone graft the medial musculature must be dissected free from the most medial border of the iliac crest. If the transversalis fascia is violated during this medial dissection, a hernia may occur. If this fascial violation is detected intraoperatively, it should be repaired immediately to prevent the hernia.

Tricortical iliac crest bone grafts may be obtained by using an oscillating sagittal saw. The use of an osteotome produces microfractures in the bone graft,[47] which as hypothesized by some, may lead to graft collapse. Many surgeons, however, successfully use osteotomes for this purpose.

After the removal of the bone graft, hemostasis is obtained with unipolar electrocautery for soft-tissue hemostasis. Frequently, bleeding of the exposed cancellous portion of the iliac crest may occur. This is controlled best by irrigating the wound generously, followed by firmly packing the wound with laparotomy pads soaked in thrombin. The wound is copiously irrigated again. After adequate hemostasis has been obtained a drain may be placed in the bed of the wound and brought through a separate stab wound in the skin. Foreign bodies such as bone wax should be used minimally and only when necessary.

The major complications associated with iliac crest bone graft sites include lateral femoral cutaneous nerve palsies, postoperative hematomas, and postoperative wound infections. Appropriately placed skin incisions should prevent nerve palsies, and good surgical technique should prevent the development of hematomas. The incidence of donor site hematomas ranges from 2%* to 7%.[25,72,85,88] Donor site infections may be limited by the use of perioperative antibiotics, generous irrigation, and preventing wound hematoma accumulation. The incidence of donor site infections has been reported to be between 0.2%[†] and 5%.[20,84] Finally, it is important to limit the subperiosteal dissection when removing an iliac bone graft, because hematomas may develop in the subperiosteal space and lead to persistent hip pain or meralgia paresthetica. The latter occurs in 0.6% to 5.8%.[‡]

Fusion

The majority of difficulties with postoperative axial neck pain result from inadequate bony fusion. Regardless of whether the discectomy was performed for myelopathy, radiculopathy, or degenerative disc disease, a solid bony fusion is optimal. Some authors use allograft bone,[12,19,91] methylmethacrylate,[31] or coral[81] as a spacer after discectomy. A recent prospective study has shown that long-term bony fusion results obtained with autologous iliac crest bone grafts are superior to results with allografts.[6] However, some authors cite donor site complications as a reason to avoid autologous iliac bone grafts.[39,84] In patients

---

*References 8,10,26,33,42,44,45,64,84,91.
†References 3,6,26,32,33,45,54,59,64,72,80,88.
‡References 3,10,26,54,80,84.

without immunocompromise, who are nonsmokers and who undergo single-level discectomy, long-term fusion rates are high, regardless of the fusion substrate used.[8,20,67,85,91] In smokers, immunocompromised patients, and patients who undergo multilevel discectomies, autologous bone graft yields the best long-term fusion results.[6]

Experience from the treatment of long bone fractures has shown two elements to be of greatest importance in achieving a bony fusion—compression and immobilization. After distraction of the disc space a bone graft that is slightly larger than the interspace should be placed. This allows for the bone graft to be seated under a compressive load.

Before placement of a bone graft, the recipient site must be meticulously prepared. This includes removal of all articular cartilage from the bony end plates above and below, with care taken to preserve the actual end plates. In addition, ventral osteophytes should be resected. The graft should be aligned between the vertebral bodies above and below so that the cancellous portion of the vertebral body is in direct alignment with the cancellous portion of the bone graft proper. Before placing the bone graft, small perforations of the vertebral body end plates above and below with a high-speed drill allow for exposure of bleeding cancellous bone. These end plate perforations should be aligned with the cancellous portion of the iliac bone graft.

A slightly oversized bone graft should be centered over the midline with a minimum width of 10mm and a maximum width of 15mm. The depth of the bone graft should be determined by a careful review of the preoperative imaging studies, and it should be confirmed by intraoperative visual inspection. In general, bone graft depth should measure between 12 and 15mm.

The bone graft is oriented with the open end of the tricortical graft directed dorsally. This allows maximum cortical bone at the most ventral aspect to provide a stable strut ventrally, thereby minimizing kyphotic angular deformation. The bone graft should be gently impacted into place and countersunk so that the most ventral aspect of the bone graft is 1mm below the most ventral surface of the vertebral bodies above and below. Attempts to reduce segmented kyphotic deformation or preserve normal lordotic posture should be aggressive. Kyphotic deformities predispose to further degenerative changes at adjacent levels.

After the graft is placed, a blunt nerve hook should be used to confirm that the graft is not seated too deeply. If the bone graft is seated too deeply or too far laterally, the spinal cord or nerve roots may be compressed. If this is identified intraoperatively, the graft should be removed, and either replaced or modified, to fit the interspace accordingly. After the bone graft is in place, all distraction devices are removed, all traction is discontinued, and a lateral cervical radiograph is obtained. The radiograph should be studied to confirm the depth of the bone graft, and to reconfirm that the facet joints are not overdistracted (Figure 28.3A).

The most common complication of the fusion portion of the operation is the development of a delayed nonunion, or pseudarthrosis. Complications related to improper positioning of the bone graft are less common.

Useful intraoperative maneuvers to avoid nonunion include placement of the graft under tension and the use of an adequately sized bone graft. Preservation of the vertebral body end-plates above and below minimize the chance of collapse or pistoning (Figure 28.3B). Graft collapse has been detected on follow-up imaging studies in 0.8% to 5.8% of cases.* Foreign bodies should be avoided at all times. Bone wax limits bony fusion rates and should be avoided.

After the bone graft is placed, hemostasis must be attained. Generous irrigation is performed. A drain may be placed in the prevertebral space, ventral to the bone graft, and it is brought out through a separate stab wound in the skin. However, as with the iliac donor site, drains are not mandatory.

Complications

Postoperative complications are categorized as problems related to the decompression (neurologic) and those related to the fusion (pain). In the immediate postoperative period, neurologic complications are the most common.

The most catastrophic immediate postoperative complication is the development of an epidural hematoma, with an accompanying neurologic dysfunction. Symptomatic epidural hematomas occur in 0.2% to 0.9% of cases.[5,13,41,59,82] This complication is managed by immediate surgical evacuation of the hematoma. Any unnecessary delay in the evacuation of an epidural hematoma may lead to an irreversible neurologic deficit. If a postoperative neurologic decline that suggests an epidural hematoma is observed, either a CT scan and a myelogram, or an MRI study should be performed immediately. If an epidural hematoma is identified, the patient is immediately returned to the operating room, the bone graft is removed, and the hematoma is evacuated. If there is no evidence of compression of neural tissue on the neuroimaging study, expectant observation is proper. In the absence of imaging evidence of neural compression, the majority of neurologic deficits recover.

An additional complication during the postoperative period is an unrecognized dural tear. If this occurs, a lumbar drain, placed for 1 week, may divert the flow of CSF and allow the durotomy to spontaneously close. If this is unsuccessful, surgical re-exploration and direct operative treatment of the durotomy may be necessary.

Wound infections may occur at variable periods during the postoperative course. These are best identified by persistent pain, as well as by an elevation of the erythrocyte sedimentation rate. Fever or an elevated white blood cell count are not reliable indicators of postoperative wound infections. Wound infections occur in 0.1% to 2% of cases.[†] If a cervical wound infection is identified, the treatment is prompt surgical re-exploration, culture, irrigation, and closure of the wound, with the placement of a drain. Appropriate antibiotics are used postoperatively. If an iliac crest wound infection occurs, the wound must be reopened and drained. Prevention of cervical and iliac crest wound infections is accomplished best by avoiding

---

*References 3,8,25,83,84,91.
†References 3,4,5,30,40,42,54,56,59,79,88,89.

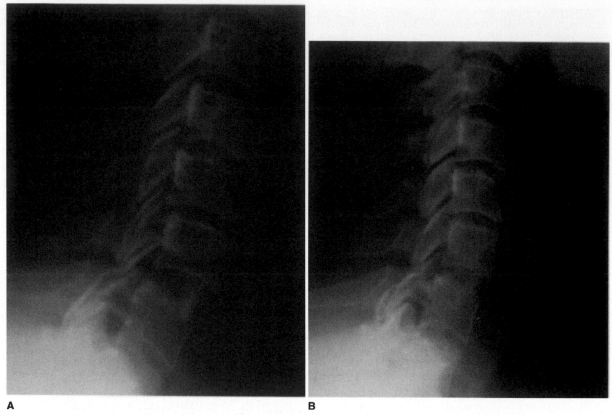

A   **B**

Figure 28.3 Generous oversized bone graft with the crest portions of the graft oriented ventrally. Note that the graft is seated 1 to 2mm below the most ventral surface of the vertebral bodies above and below (**A**). A subsequent radiograph (3 months' postoperatively) demonstrates an acceptable degree of subsidence (**B**).

the use of foreign bodies (e.g., bone wax) and by obtaining meticulous hemostasis. Some surgeons argue that the use of drains may decrease the development of hematomas and, subsequently, decrease the wound infection rates. Others argue that they provide an access route for microorganisms.

Iliac region pain is ordinarily secondary to the development of a subperiosteal hematoma. The majority of these resolve spontaneously. If the hematoma is excessively large or painful, surgical re-exploration and evacuation of the hematoma may be necessary. Persistent occult blood loss during the postoperative period may be secondary to enlargement of a retroperitoneal hematoma. This may dictate the need for re-exploration of the iliac crest graft harvest site. A wound infection must also be ruled out. In questionable situations, obtaining a bone scan and a C-reactive protein level may be helpful in establishing the diagnosis. A postoperative hernia secondary to violation of the transversalis fascia may present with chronic donor site pain postoperatively. This may be diagnosed by an intraluminal contrast study, such as a barium enema. If a painful hernia is present, or if a bowel obstruction occurs, surgical reexploration, with closure of the hernia defect, is often successful.

Postoperative neck pain in the first few weeks is usually transient and self-limited. Persistent postoperative pain in the neck, arm, and interscapular region pain has been observed in 4% to 20% of cases.[5,33,35,40,54] Wound infec-

tions, or the development of a deep hematoma, should be ruled out.

A bony nonunion, or pseudarthrosis, after an ACDF often presents with persistent axial neck pain. This may or may not be associated with radicular symptoms. Bony fusion is typically well under way by 12 weeks postoperatively. This may be delayed in smokers, immunocompromised patients, or patients undergoing multilevel discectomies. A pseudarthrosis is diagnosed by persistent axial neck pain with evidence of a radiographic lucency at the vertebral body-graft junction at 6 or more months after surgery. Bone graft collapse is diagnosed by a 2-mm or greater loss of graft height detected on radiographs taken 12 months postoperatively.[42]

If a pseudarthrosis develops, imaging studies should be performed to confirm whether neural compression is also present. If neural compression is present, a repeat ventral operation is necessary to remove the bone graft, perform a neural element decompression, and re-fuse the cervical spine. If axial neck pain is present, and neuroimaging studies do not demonstrate evidence of neural compression, a cervical pseudarthrosis is best treated with a dorsal fusion of the involved motion segment. A successful dorsal fusion for the treatment of a pseudarthrosis secondary to an ACDF most often results in a stable circumferential fusion. In exceptional cases it may be necessary to revise a pseudarthrosis ventrally and perform a dorsal fusion at the same time. This leads to a higher fusion rate, but is considered excessive by some.

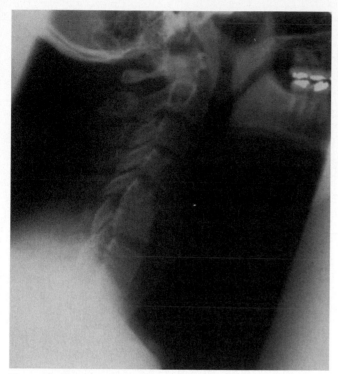

Figure 28.4 An undersized graft that pistoned before fusion. A kyphotic deformity resulted, as depicted above.

If the patient develops persistent axial neck pain, and plain radiographs are unable to demonstrate a lucency suggestive of a pseudarthrosis, further diagnostic studies may be necessary. Tomograms are more sensitive than plain radiographs for detecting pseudarthroses. In addition, flexion and extension views may help confirm the diagnosis.

The issue of postoperative immobilization is controversial. Some authors use no postoperative bracing after a single-level ACDF. Others use a cervical collar for a variable period of 6 to 12 weeks. In rare circumstances a postoperative Minerva jacket or halo vest may be used for prolonged immobilization. A spinal implant may be indicated in a patient who is likely to suffer fusion failure. Such patients include smokers, immunocompromised patients, and those undergoing multilevel discectomies.

In the postoperative period, serial radiographs are obtained until a bony fusion is confirmed. Patients should be followed for a minimum of 12 months postoperatively and should only be discharged after evidence of a successful clinical and radiographic fusion.

Other delayed complications that may occur after an ACDF include a loss of cervical lordosis. This is most commonly observed after the use of undersized grafts, graft material of insufficient integrity, or excessive end-plate removal, possibly leading to the development of a kyphotic deformity (Figure 28.4).[49,59,83,91] In general, no surgical intervention is necessary for this problem, unless it is severe. Graft subsidence, without angulation, may also occur.

Some neck motion is lost postoperatively. As a general approximation, there is a 10-degree loss of cervical motion for each fused motion segment. For a single-level discectomy this loss of motion is not ordinarily discernible. With multilevel discectomies the patient and physician may notice a loss of neck motion.

Graft protrusions or dislodgements occur in 0.4% to 4.6% of cases.* The treatment of a graft dislodgement involves a surgical re-exploration and fusion.

Discitis or osteomyelitis may also occur as a delayed complication.† This warrants antibiotic therapy and usually, surgical debridement.

Some patients (as many as 50%) develop persistent radiographic nonunion without clinical symptoms. Lateral radiographs from these patients have a persistent lucency, but there are no clinical neck pain or radicular symptoms. Such patients should be followed clinically with serial imaging studies. Delayed radiographic fusion may occur in some of these cases. If radiographic fusion is not demonstrable, but no clinical symptoms are present, there is no indication for surgical re-exploration.

After an ACDF, there is an increased risk of disc degeneration at the levels adjacent to the fused segments (accelerated degenerative changes). This is most common and is clinically significant at the interspace immediately rostral to the fusion. Adjacent level disc degenerations are most common after longer cervical fusions and may necessitate revision surgery. Longer-term follow-up is necessary after a multiple-level ACDF, both to monitor the fusion itself and to monitor for degenerative changes at adjacent levels.

Multiple-Level ACDF

The complications associated with multiple-level discectomies and fusion are similar to those for single-level operations, with respect to each fused segment. However, certain complications are more prevalent with multiple-level operations. The rate of pseudarthrosis increases with the addition of each fused segment.[8,20,67,85,91] Thus the indication for each fused level must remain as strict as the indications for a single-fused level. In addition, longer fusions are associated with an increased rate of disc degeneration in adjacent segments. With respect to operative considerations, dysphagia rates are higher. This is because of the longer duration of surgery with prolonged retraction of the esophagus. Similarly, the incidence of hoarseness secondary to recurrent laryngeal nerve dysfunction is higher with multiple-level discectomies. This is particularly true if the C6-7 space is fused. Multiple-level discectomies require a longer operative time. This increases the complications related to anesthesia, as well as general medical problems. In addition, larger iliac crest bone grafts are necessary for multiple-level discectomies. The incidence of bleeding, pain, and infections at the iliac crest donor site may thus be increased. The strategies for avoiding and managing each of the individual complications are identical for multiple-level and single-level discectomies.

Summary

Many of the complications associated with ACDF can be avoided by performing properly indicated surgery,

---

*References 10,25,26,33,54,57,59,64,72,80,84,85.
†References 5,9,25,35,49,69,84.

employing careful preoperative planning, and using meticulous surgical technique. When intraoperative complications occur, many of them can be managed immediately. However, some complications do not develop until the postoperative period. When postoperative complications are detected, immediate imaging studies and treatment, as necessary, are warranted. As a rule, the postoperative neurologic results depend on the adequacy of the decompression. Pain relief depends on the adequacy of the bony fusion, as well.

Long-term follow-up is essential to confirm both the clinical and radiographic successes of the ACDF. With proper preoperative patient selection, careful preoperative planning, meticulous intraoperative surgical technique, and diligent postoperative follow-up, the incidence of complications after ACDF can be minimized.

REFERENCES

1. An HS, Silveri CP, Simpson JM: Comparison of smoking habits between patients with surgically confirmed herniated lumbar and cervical disc disease and controls. *J Spinal Disord* 7:369-373, 1994.
2. Apfelbaum RI, Johnson JO, Sperry RJ: Prevention of recurrent laryngeal nerve palsies in anterior cervical surgery. *Neurosurgery* 37:518, 1995.
3. Aronson N, Filtzer DL, Bagar M: Anterior cervical fusion by the Smith-Robinson approach. *J Neurosurg* 29:397-404, 1968.
4. Bertalanffy H, Eggert H-R: Clinical long-term results of anterior discectomy without fusion for treatment of cervical radiculopathy and myelopathy: a follow-up of 164 cases. *Acta Neurochir (Wien)* 90:127-135, 1988.
5. Bertalanffy H, Eggert H-R: Complications of anterior cervical discectomy without fusion in 450 consecutive patients. *Acta Neurochir (Wien)* 99:41-50, 1989.
6. Bishop RC, Moore KA, Hadley MN: Anterior cervical interbody fusion using autogeneic and allogeneic bone graft substrate: a prospective comparative analysis. *J Neurosurg* 85:206-210, 1996.
7. Bohler J, Gaudernak T: Anterior plate stabilization for fracture: dislocations of the lower cervical spine. *J Trauma* 20:203-205, 1980.
8. Bohlman HH, Emery SE, Goodfellow DB, Jones PK: Robinson anterior cervical discectomy and arthrodesis for cervical radiculopathy: long-term follow-up of 122 patients. *J Bone Joint Surg* 75A:1298-1307, 1993.
9. Bollati A, Galli G, Gandolfini M: Microsurgical anterior cervical disc removal without interbody infusion. *Surg Neurol* 19:329-333, 1983.
10. Brigham CD, Tsahakis PJ: Anterior cervical foraminotomy and fusion. *Spine* 20:766-770, 1995.
11. Brodke DS, Zdeblick TA: Modified Smith-Robinson procedure for anterior cervical discectomy and fusion. *Spine* 17:427-430, 1992.
12. Brown CW, Orme TJ, Richardson HD: The rate of pseudarthrosis (surgical nonunion) in patients who are smokers and patients who are nonsmokers: a comparison study. *Spine* 11:942-943, 1986.
13. Busch G. Anterior fusion for cervical spondylosis. *J Neurol* 219:117-126, 1978.
14. Capen DA, Garland DE, Waters RL. Surgical stabilization of the cervical spine: a comparable analysis of anterior and posterior spine fusions. *Clin Orthop* 196:229-237, 1985.
15. Chang KW, Lin GZ, Liu YW, et al: Intraosseous screw fixation of anterior cervical graft construct after diskectomy. *J Spinal Disord* 7:126-129, 1994.
16. Clerny G: Smokers suffer impaired bone healing. *Science News* 141:133, 1992.
17. Cloward RB: The anterior approach for removal of ruptured discs. *J Neurosurg* 15:602-614, 1958.
18. Cloward RB: A new method of diagnosis and treatment of cervical disc disease. *Clin Neurosurg* 8:93-132, 1962.
19. Cloward RB: Gas-sterilized cadaver bone grafts for spinal fusion operations. *Spine* 5:4-10, 1980.
20. Connolly ES, Seymour RJ, Adams JE: Clinical evaluation of anterior cervical fusion for degenerative cervical disc disease. *J Neurosurg* 23:431-437, 1965.
21. Cosgrove GR, Theron J: Vertebral arteriovenous fistula following anterior cervical spine surgery: report of two cases. *J Neurosurg* 66:297-299, 1987.
22. Cuatico W: Anterior cervical discectomy without interbody fusion: an analysis of 81 cases. *Acta Neurochir (Wien)* 57:269-274, 1981.
23. Daftari TK, Whitesides TE, Heller JG, et al: The effect of nicotine on the revascularization of bone graft: an experimental study in rabbits. *Spine* 19:904-911, 1994.
24. de los Reyes RA, Moser FG, Sachs DP, Boehm FH: Direct repair of an extracranial vertebral artery pseudoaneurysm: case report and review of the literature. *Neurosurgery* 26:528-533, 1990.
25. DePalma AF, Rothman RH, Lewinnek GE, Canale ST: Anterior interbody fusion for severe cervical disc degeneration. *Surg Gynecol Obstet* 134:755-758, 1972.
26. Dohn DF: Anterior interbody fusion for treatment of cervical-disk conditions. *JAMA* 197:897-900, 1966.
27. Dunsker SB: Anterior cervical discectomy with and without fusion. *Clin Neurosurg* 24:516-521, 1977.
28. Emery SE, Bolesta MJ, Banks MA, Jones PK: Robinson anterior cervical fusion: comparison of the standards and modified techniques. *Spine* 19:660-663, 1994.
29. Epstein JA, Carras R, Lavine LS, Epstein BS. The importance of removing osteophytes as part of the surgical treatment of myeloradiculopathy in cervical spondylosis. *J Neurosurg* 30:219-226, 1969.
30. Espersen JO, Buhl M, Eriksen EF, et al: Treatment of cervical disc disease using Cloward's technique: general results, effect of different operative methods and complications in 1106 patients. *Acta Neurochir (Wien)* 70:97-114, 1984.
31. Fathie K: Anterior cervical diskectomy and fusion with methyl methacrylate. *Mt Sinai J Med* 61:246-247, 1994.
32. Galera R, Tovi D: Anterior disc excision with interbody fusion in cervical spondylotic myelopathy and rhizopathy. *J Neurosurg* 28:305-310, 1968.
33. Gore DR, Sepic SB: Anterior cervical fusion for degenerated or protruded discs: a review of one hundred forty-six patients. *Spine* 9:667-671, 1984.
34. Hakuba A: Trans-unco-discal approach: A combined anterior and lateral approach to cervical discs. *J Neurosurg* 45:284-291, 1976.
35. Hankinson HL, Wilson CB: Use of the operating microscope in the anterior cervical discectomy without fusion. *J Neurosurg* 43:452-456, 1975.

36. Harrington KD: Anterior decompression and stabilization of the spine as a treatment for vertebral collapse and spinal cord compression from metastatic malignancy. *Clin Orthop* 233:177-197, 1988.

37. Heary RF, Albert TJ, Ludwig SC, *et al*: Surgical anatomy of the vertebral arteries. *Spine* 21:2074-2080, 1996.

38. Heeneman H: Vocal cord paralysis following approaches to the anterior cervical spine. *Laryngoscope* 83:17-21, 1973.

39. Hirsch C: Cervical disk rupture: diagnosis and therapy. *Acta Orthop Scand* 30:172-186, 1960.

40. Hoff JT, Wilson CB: Microsurgical approach to the anterior cervical spine and spinal cord. *Clin Neurosurg* 26:513-528, 1978.

41. Hohf RP: Arterial injuries occurring during orthopaedic operations. *Clin Orthop* 28:21-37, 1963.

42. Howard SA, Simpson JM, Glover JM, Stephany J: Comparison between allograft plus demineralized bone matrix versus autograft in anterior cervical fusion. *Spine* 20:2211-2216, 1995.

43. Husang L, Probst C: Microsurgical anterior approach to cervical discs: review of 60 consecutive cases of discectomy without fusion. *Acta Neurochir (Wien)* 73:229-242, 1984.

44. Jacobs B, Krueger EG, Leivy DM: Cervical spondylosis with radiculopathy: results of anterior diskectomy and interbody fusion. *JAMA* 211:2135-2139, 1970.

45. Jeffreys RV: The surgical treatment of cervical spondylotic myelopathy. *Acta Neurochir (Wien)* 47:293-305, 1979.

46. Jensen MC, Brant-Zawadzki MN, Obuchowski N, *et al*: Magnetic resonance imaging of the lumbar spine in people without back pain. *New Engl J Med* 331:69-73, 1994.

47. Jones AA, Dougherty PJ, Sharkey NA, Benson DR: Iliac crest bone graft: osteotome versus saw. *Spine* 18:2048-2052, 1993.

48. Kambin P: Anterior approach to the cervical disk with bone grafting. *Mt Sinai J Med* 61:243-245, 1994.

49. Kewalramani LS, Riggins RS: Complications of anterior spondylodesis for traumatic lesions of the cervical spine. *Spine* 2:25-38, 1977.

50. Keyes DC, Compere EL: The normal and pathological physiology of the nucleus pulposus of the interretebral disc: an anatomical, clinical, and experimental study. *J Bone Joint Surg* 14:897-938, 1932.

51. Kraus DR, Stauffer ES: Spinal cord injury as a complication of elective anterior cervical fusion. *Clin Orthop* 112:130-141, 1975.

52. Kuriloff DB, Blaugrund S, Ryan J, O'Leary P: Delayed neck infection following anterior spine surgery. *Laryngoscope* 97:1094-1098, 1987.

53. Lesoin F, Bouasakao N, Clarisse J, *et al*: Results of surgical treatment of radiculomyelopathy caused by cervical arthrosis based on 1000 operations. *Surg Neurol* 23:350-355, 1985.

54. Lunsford LD, Bissonette DJ, Jannetta PJ, *et al*: Anterior surgery for cervical disc disease. I. Treatment of lateral cervical disc herniation in 253 cases. *J Neurosurg* 53:1-11, 1980.

55. Marshall LF: Cerebrospinal fluid leaks: etiology and repair. In Rothman RH, Simeone FA (eds): *The Spine*. Philadelphia, WB Saunders, 1992, pp 1892-1898.

56. Martins AN: Anterior cervical discectomy with and without interbody bone graft. *J Neurosurg* 44:290-295, 1976.

57. McGuire RA, St. John K: Comparison of anterior cervical fusions using autogenous bone graft obtained from the cervical vertebrae to the modified Smith-Robinson technique. *J Spinal Disord* 7:499-503, 1994.

58. Mixter WJ, Barr JS: Rupture of the intervertebral disc with involvement of the spinal canal. *N Engl J Med* 211:210-215, 1934.

59. Mosdal C: Cervical osteochrondrosis and disc herniation: eighteen years' use of interbody fusion by Cloward's technique in 755 cases. *Acta Neurochir (Wien)* 70:207-225, 1984.

60. Murphy MG, Gado M: Anterior cervical discectomy without interbody bone graft. *J Neurosurg* 37:71-74, 1972.

61. Newhouse KE, Lindsey RW, *et al*: Esophageal perforation following anterior cervical spine surgery. *Spine* 14:1051-1053, 1989.

62. Onji Y, Akiyama H, Shimomura Y, *et al*: Posterior paravertebral ossification causing cervical myelopathy: a report of eighteen cases. *J Bone Joint Surg* 49A:1314-1328, 1967.

63. Reynolds AF: Epidural bleeding in anterior discectomy (letter). *J Neurosurg* 50:126, 1979.

64. Riley LH, Robinson RA, Johnson KA, Walker AE: The results of anterior interbody fusion of the cervical spine. *J Neurosurg* 30:127-133, 1969.

65. Robertson JT, Johnson SD. Anterior cervical discectomy without fusion: long-term results. *Clin Neurosurg* 27:440-449, 1980.

66. Robinson RA, Smith GW: Anterolateral cervical disc removal and interbody fusion for cervical disc syndrome (abstract). *Bull John Hopkins Hosp* 96:223-224, 1955.

67. Robinson RA, Walker AE, Ferlic DC, Wieckling OK: The results of anterior interbody fusion of the cervical spine. *J Bone Joint Surg* 44A:1569-1587, 1962.

68. Saunders RL: On the pathogenesis of the radiculopathy complicating multilevel corpectomy. *Neurosurgery* 37:408-413, 1995.

69. Savitz MH: Minimalist approach to anterior cervical diskectomy. *Mt Sinai J Med* 61:239-242, 1994.

70. Schmorl G. Uber Verlagerung von Bandscheiloengewebe und ihre Folgen. *Arch Klin Chir* 172:240-276, 1932.

71. Shintani A, Zervas NT: Consequence of ligation of the vertebral artery. *J Neurosurg* 36:447-450, 1972.

72. Simmons EH, Bhalla SK, Butt WP: Anterior cervical discectomy and fusion: A clinical and biomechanical study with eight-year follow-up. (With a note on discography: technique and interpretation of results.) *J Bone Joint Surg* 51B:225-237, 1969.

73. Smith GW, Robinson RA: The treatment of certain cervical spine disorders by anterior removal of the intervertebral disc and interbody fusion. *J Bone Joint Surg* 40A:607-623, 1958.

74. Smith MD, Emery SE, Dudley A, *et al*: Vertebral artery injury during anterior decompression of the cervical spine. *J Bone Joint Surg* 75B:410-415, 1993.

75. Snyder GM, Bernhardt M: Anterior cervical fractional interspace decompression for treatment of cervical radiculopathy: a review of the first 66 cases. *Clin Orthop* 246:92-99, 1989.

76. Stombaugh JL, Simeone FA: Neurogenic complications of spinal surgery.. In Rothman RH, Simeone FA (eds): *The Spine*. Philadelphia, WB Saunders, 1992, pp 1885-1891.

77. Stookey B. Compression of the spinal cord due to ventral extradural cervical chondromas: diagnosis and surgical treatment. *Arch Neurol Psychiat* 20:275-291, 1928.

78. Sugar O: Spinal cord malfunction after anterior cervical discectomy. *Surg Neurol* 15:4-8, 1981.

79. Taheri ZE, Gueramy M: Experience with calf bone in cervical interbody spinal fusion. *J Neurosurg* 36:67-71, 1972.

80. Tew JM, Mayfield FH: Complications of surgery of the anterior cervical spine. *Clin Neurosurg* 23:424-434, 1976.

81. Thalgott JS, Fritts K, Giuffre JM: The use of coral bone replacement in anterior cervical interbody fusions. Presented at the twenty-third Annual Meeting of the Cervical Spine Research Society, Santa Fe, New Mexico, 1995.

82. U HS, Wilson CB: Postoperative epidural hematoma as a complication of anterior discectomy: report of three cases. *J Neurosurg* 49:288-291, 1978.

83. Villas C, Martinez-Peric R, Preite R, Barrios RH: Union after multiple anterior cervical fusion: 21 cases followed for 1-6 years. *Acta Orthop Scand* 65:620-622, 1994.

84. Watters WC, Levinthal R: Anterior cervical discectomy with and without fusion: results, complications, and long-term follow-up. *Spine* 19:2343-2347, 1994.

85. White AA III, Southwick WO, Deponte RJ, *et al*: Relief of pain by anterior cervical-spine fusion for spondylosis: a report of sixty-five patients. *J Bone Joint Surg* 55A:525-534, 1973.

86. Whitehill R, Sirna EC, Young DC, Cantrell RW: Late esophageal perforation from an autogenous bone graft: report of a case. *J Bone Joint Surg* 67A:644-645, 1985.

87. Whitesides TE, Hanley EN, Fellrath RF: Smoking abstinence: is it necessary before spinal fusion? *Spine* 19:2012-2014, 1994.

88. Williams JL, Allen MB Jr., Harkess JW: Late results of cervical discectomy and interbody fusion: some factors influencing the results. *J Bone Joint Surg* 50A:277-286, 1968.

89. Wilson DH, Campbell DD: Anterior cervical discectomy without bone graft: report of 7 cases. *J Neurosurg* 47:551-555, 1977.

90. Yamamoto J, Ikeda A, Stibuya N, *et al*: Clinical long-term results of anterior discectomy without interbody fusions for cervical disc disease. *Spine* 16:272-279, 1991.

91. Zdeblick TA, Ducker TB: The use of freeze-dried allograft bone for anterior cervical fusions. *Spine* 16:726-729, 1991.

CHAPTER 29

Threaded Interbody Cage Fixation for Cervical Spondylosis and Ossification of the Posterior Longitudinal Ligament

Hiroshi Nakagawa and Junichi Mizuno

With advances in neuroimaging using computed tomography (CT) and magnetic resonance imaging (MRI), the diagnosis of cervical disc herniation and spondylosis, as well as associated ligamental ossification, has become more precise and less invasive. In addition, routine microsurgery and refined drills and instruments have facilitated the performance of less invasive and more efficient ventral cervical spine procedures.

Special Consideration in Japan

In Japan there are two factors that differ from North America and Europe, which significantly affect the surgical strategies for cervical discogenic diseases.

One is that cervical spondylosis and disc degeneration are often associated with segmental or the local type of ossification of the posterior longitudinal ligament (OPLL) and hypertrophy of the posterior longitudinal ligament (HPLL).[8,23,25,35,37]

Therefore, simple discectomy or simple ventral fusion is usually not sufficient for decompression of the dura mater and spinal cord, which are ventrally compressed beyond the disc level by OPLL or HPLL. Therefore, a corpectomy is often necessary to achieve reasonable ventral decompression and, subsequently, a good outcome.[1,4,14,21,22]

Routine evaluation by dynamic radiographs, CT, and MRI for patients with cervical myelopathy and radiculopathy, therefore, seems appropriate in this clinical environment.

Prominent OPLL of continuous or mixed type is readily diagnosed by plain radiographs. However, a small segmental or local OPLL is difficult to detect and easily missed by plain radiographs alone but can be easily and definitively diagnosed by thin-slice CT. Recent further advancements of sagittal CT reformation and 3-D CT have almost totally replaced the usage of polytomography for the diagnosis of OPLL.

MRI is superior in delineating the extent of spinal cord compression and possible disc protrusions, as well as high signal intensity areas within the cord, but it is unable to detect small calcified or ossified lesions, such as OPLL. It is important to understand the advantages and disadvantages of each study to establish the correct diagnosis and to facilitate the decision-making process.

Allograft bone is not available in Japan. Vertebral grafts, ceramics, and, most recently, titanium cages have become popular adjuncts to ventral fusion, in addition to conventional iliac grafts.[13,28,29]

The Evolution of Surgical Technique

Over the last 20 years, the authors'[21,22,26,28] surgical techniques for cervical spondylosis and OPLL have significantly changed from a more invasive to a less invasive technique.

Corpectomy with Iliac Graft

In 1991 and previous years, multilevel corpectomy with iliac crest interbody graft was used for multilevel OPLL and spondylosis, but graft problems, donor-site discomfort, and the necessity of postoperative application of a halo brace were drawbacks of this method, although ventral plate fixation dramatically reduced the usage of halo brace application.[1,14,26]

Corpectomy with Vertebral Graft

From 1992 to 1997, limited or keyhole corpectomy with vertebral graft, using Williams'[9,28,38] microsurgical saw (Ace Medical Co., Los Angeles, CA), was carried out with reasonable results in 60 patients with cervical spondylosis associated with segmental OPLL.

One of the pitfalls of this method is that the bone grafts taken from the cervical spine are more fragile than iliac grafts, especially in heavy smokers, aged women with osteoporosis, and patients on long-term hemodialysis.

Interbody Cage Fixation

Threaded titanium cages were first used for posterior lumbar interbody fusion (PLIF) of lumbar spine instability.[32] In 1997, the interbody cage BAK/C (Spine Tech, Minneapolis, MN) became available in Japan for ventral cervical fusion. However, these instruments were made for macrosurgery and were too large and difficult to use under the operating microscope. Therefore, the authors[22,29,30] developed smaller and more slender instruments for microsurgical procedures, so that the entire procedure of decompression and cage fixation could be done under microsurgical control as a less invasive procedure.

Keyhole Approach Without Grafting

A microsurgical keyhole ventral approach without bone grafting, which consisted of medial microdiscectomy of 10mm width for central and paramedian discs and spurs and transuncal foraminotomy for lateral or foraminal spur and discs has been used with satisfactory results.[6,10,27] This keyhole microdiscectomy is a less invasive and more effective ventral approach and yielded favorable results.[17,24] The small exposure, however, is often not adequate to fully decompress the spinal cord and nerve roots that were compressed by bilateral spur and/or OPLL.

Modified Microsurgical Approach

By using the advantages of keyhole discectomy and limited corpectomy with vertebral graft and, at the same time, avoiding the pitfalls of the aforementioned procedures, a modified microsurgical technique for interbody cage fixation for cervical spondylosis and OPLL was developed. In this chapter the surgical indications and techniques for the single-cage method and twin-cage method (Figure 29.1) are presented.[29,30]

Surgical Technique

Under general endotracheal anesthesia, the patient is placed supine with the head slightly extended. The ventral cervical procedure is usually approached from the right side of the neck, except for left transuncal foraminotomy in which a left-sided approach is mandatory. The skin incision is made transversely along the crease for cosmetic reasons, even in a three-level approach. The subcutaneous tissue is dissected rostrally and caudally, and the platysma muscle is sectioned obliquely along the ventral border of the sternocleidomastoid muscle.

The ventral aspect of the cervical spine is then approached by dissecting the deeper fascia, usually rostral to the omohyoid muscle, while the right carotid tubercle of C6 is palpated as a landmark with the surgeon's left index finger. The level of the intervertebral disc space is identified by portable radiograph or by fluoroscopy, with a needle inserted into the disc space at one or two levels, and a small amount of dye, usually indigo carmine, is injected through the needle for even further confirmation of level location. The blue coloring of the disc is quite useful in contrasting the bony spur with the disc when drilling the spur. After the introduction of the operating microscope with a dual eye-piece system in which the surgeon and an assistant are able to see the operative field in the same depth, discectomy is carried out.

Single-Cage Method for OPLL

In cases of OPLL, usually segmental or local, some degree of corpectomy is often necessary to remove the ossified ligament which extends behind the vertebrae.

For this reason, a larger cage of porous CCM (A-Spine, Tokyo, Japan) with mean of 10, 12, or 14mm in inner diameter is usually used in the single-cage method. After complete discectomy, Williams' microsurgical saw with a straight blade of 0.35mm in thickness is used to perform a 10-mm square corpectomy for a 12-mm cage followed by reaming to make a round hole (Figure 29.2A,B). Bone chips are saved for packing into the cage.

If a Williams' saw is not available, another straight surgical saw can be used carefully, or a round hole can be made stepwise by using progressively larger reamers. Through this hole, the remaining vertebral body, spur, and ossified ligament are drilled out with great care, making the OPLL paper-thin by using a high-speed drill with regular and diamond burs. The thinned-out OPLL, hypertrophied ligament, and herniated disc are then excised mostly en-bloc by using a microknife, curette, and Kerrison rongeurs to make the dura bulge and well decompressed (Figure 29.2B,C). Most of the ossified ligament behind the vertebrae can be removed from these limited holes rostrally and caudally to the lesion by drilling a tunnel in the dorsal portion of the vertebral body.

After achieving good hemostasis with a bipolar coagulator and gentle compression with Surgicel or Oxycel,

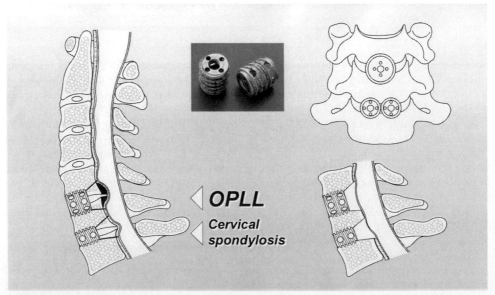

Figure 29.1 Interbody cage fixation for cervical spondylosis and ossification of the posterior longitudinal ligament (OPLL). Single-cage method with a larger cage at 10, 12, or 14mm in inner diameter is used for cervical OPLL. Twin-cage method with smaller cages at 6, 7, or 8mm is applied to cervical spondylosis and discs. Center photo shows porous CCM.

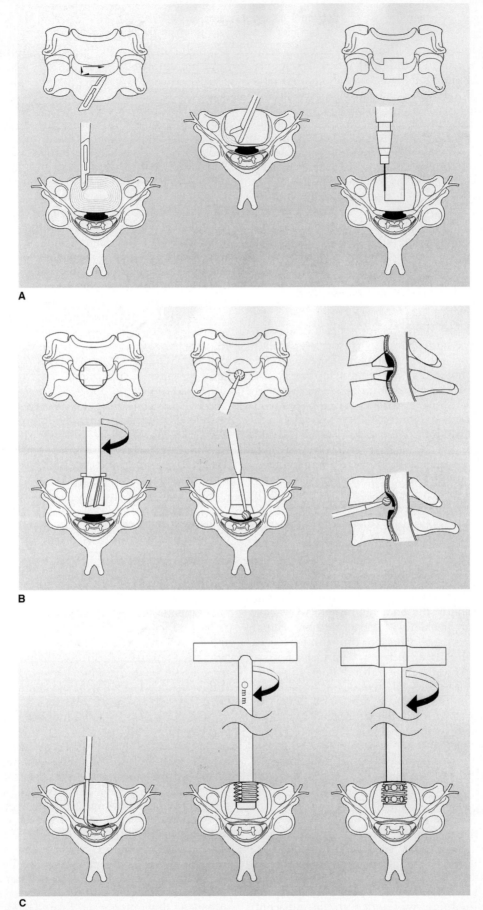

Figure 29.2 Single-cage method for cervical ossification of the posterior longitudinal ligament (OPLL). **(A)** Square corpectomy using Williams' saw following total discectomy. **(B)** Drilling of OPLL through a round space enlarged with a reamer. **(C)** Following ventral decompression by removal of thinned-out OPLL, one cage is inserted after tapping.

a single cage of, for example, 12mm packed with vertebral bone chips is carefully inserted following tapping (Figure 29.2C). Copious bleeding from the lateral portion of the posterior longitudinal ligament is relatively rare but sometimes occurs just laterally to prominent OPLL and from the interligamental sinus between the superficial and deep layers.[15] Leakage of cerebrospinal fluid (CSF) from the torn or defective dura may occur, especially in the case of prominent OPLL, and is usually managed locally with a fascia graft taken from the longus colli and fibrin glue and, if necessary, with lumbar drainage.

In the case of multilevel OPLL, single-cage and twin-cage methods are combined at adjacent levels tailored to each case.

Twin-Cage Method for Cervical Spondylosis and Herniated Discs

In cases of spondylosis with bilateral prominent spur and/or instability or large herniated discs two smaller cages 6, 7, and 8mm in inner diameter of porous CCM are used side by side. Following complete discectomy laterally extended to the uncinate process, a binocular-shaped hole is made by using reamers of 6, 7, or 8mm on the right and left sides (Figure 29.3A). Spreaders are effectively applied when the disc space is collapsed and narrowed, and spurs are drilled out far laterally enough to decompress the medial portion of the foramina containing the nerve root. This is important, particularly when the spur and disc in the far lateral portion and in the intervertebral foramen are responsible for radiculopathy of the patients (Figure 29.3B). The posterior longitudinal ligament is then incised with a microknife to expose the dura and to remove possible free fragments of the disc materials which are sometimes located in the epidural space but more often between the two layers of the ligament. After fine adjustment by drilling of the medial portion of the uncinate process, 6-, 7-, or 8-mm cages, usually packed with vertebral bone chips, are snugly inserted side by side into the reamed space, while the space is slightly retracted by a spreader for the first cage insertion (Figure 29.3C). If the bone chips are not sufficient, the cage is supplemented with hydroxyapatite granules (Bonfil, Mitsubishi PC, Osaka, Japan). It is important to pay attention to the direction of the cages during insertion, and symmetrical insertion is preferred. The ventral surface of the cage is usually leveled to the ventral cortex of the vertebral body or slightly dorsal to it to avoid subsidence of the cages.

Combined Method

In cases of multilevel spondylosis and OPLL, single-cage and twin-cage methods are carefully applied to each level and tailored to the pathology of each case. In 17% of the cases, a keyhole approach without bone graft, such as oblique discectomy, medial discectomy, or transuncal foraminotomy, was added to the adjacent level to try to reduce the level of cage fixation. Recently, oblique microdiscectomy through a 6- to 7-mm hole made at the medial insertion of the longus colli has often been used for a central or paramedian disc to preserve the majority of the disc material and to avoid kyphotic deformity.

Case

Between August 1997 and April 2000, a series of 144 consecutive cases was operated on with cervical interbody cage fixation with more than a 1½-year follow-up. There were 106 (74%) men and 38 (26%) women, with ages ranging from 24 to 84 years (mean, 56.4 years). The average duration of symptoms was 2 years and 1 month. The main symptom was myelopathy in 119 (83%) and radiculopathy in 25 (17%). Twenty-two (15%) had a history of recent minor trauma and 14 (10%) had previous surgery of the cervical spine. Seventy (49%) received a one-level procedure; 66 (46%), two-level; and 8 (5%), three-level. Based on the neuroimaging and operative findings, cervical spondylosis associated with segmental or local OPLL was disclosed in 55 (38%) and cervical spondylosis and/or discs without OPLL in 89 (62%). Initially, BAK/C was used in 61 cases, NOVUS CT-Ti (Sofamor Danek, Memphis, TN) in four cases, and, lately, porous CCM (A-Spine, Tokyo, Japan) was applied in 79 cases.

Surgical results were satisfactory (excellent and good) in 130 of 144 cases (90%), judging from the Neurosurgical Cervical Spine Scale (NCSS). Seventy-three (51%) went back to the previous work and 57 (39%) to lighter work.[11] There were no significant differences between patients with cervical spondylosis and those with OPLL. The aged group of 70 years and over had less favorable results compared with the younger group but showed significant neurologic improvement in as much as 78%. The most influential factor for poor prognosis was the severity of preoperative neurologic status. Of 35 patients with severe myelopathy, only 22 (63%) improved satisfactorily, and 83 (97%) of 84 with mild to moderate myelopathy demonstrated satisfactory recovery. All 25 patients with radiculopathy had good prognoses.

It is difficult to evaluate complete bony fusion within and around the cages on follow-up radiographs, although new bone formation can be visualized surrounding the cages. An unchanged distance between the spinous processes at the operated level in dynamic lateral radiographs seems to be a reliable sign of solid fusion. On follow-up radiographs more than 1 year after operation, 78 (97.5%) of 80 cases showed solid fusion.

Postoperative wound hematoma causing acute respiratory distress is a rare but serious complication of the cervical ventral approach. This unfortunate accident occurred in one patient 3 hours postoperatively but was properly managed by emergent tracheotomy, followed by reexploration of the wound. The patient was discharged within 3 weeks with good neurologic improvement. In two cases of prominent OPLL, CSF leakage resulting from dural tear and defect occurred but was well managed with local repair and lumbar drainage. There were three cases of temporary recurrent laryngeal nerve disturbance. Regarding cage-related complications, there were three cases of cage subsidence in early cases without any effect on outcome. There were no dislodgments or fractures of the cages, cord or nerve root injury, or wound infection.

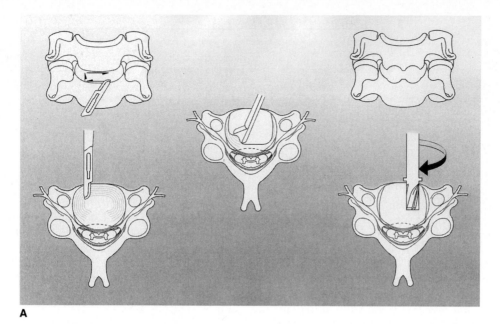

A

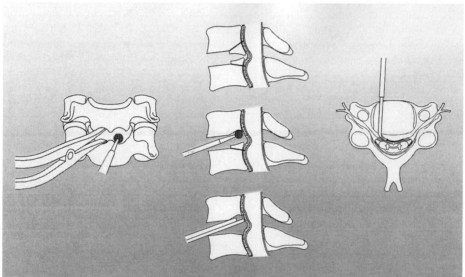

B

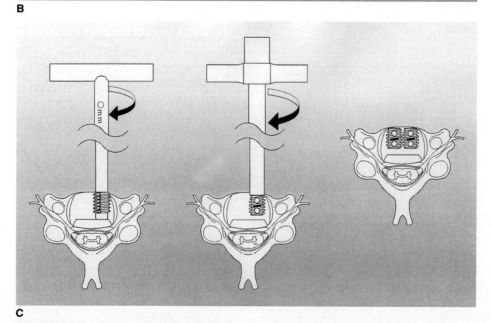

C

Figure 29.3 Twin-cage method for cervical spondylosis and discs. **(A)** Binocular-shaped space is made by a reamer on both sides of the disc space following total discectomy. **(B)** Bilateral osteophytectomy with drills and Kerrison punch followed by removal of herniated discs. **(C)** Two smaller cages inserted side by side while the disc space is slightly retracted with a spreader.

Summary

Since the ventral approach with interbody fusion for cervical discs was introduced by Cloward[2,33] and Smith and Robinson[2,33] in 1958, ventral discectomy with iliac bone graft, with or without the help of an operating microscope, has been the standard procedure with reasonably satisfactory results. However, kyphotic deformity, graft collapse, and donor-site discomfort cannot be totally disregarded.[22,28] To avoid these disadvantages, microdiscectomy without bone graft has been advocated by many authors,[17,24,27] with excellent results. This method, however, is often not appropriate for spondylosis with prominent bilateral spurs and OPLL. In addition, teaching this keyhole approach to younger surgeons is not really easy or practical because of limited exposure. Allografting is one solution to the problems of the autograft but is reported to have a lower fusion rate compared with the autograft.[16] Moreover, allografting is not available in many countries. Porous hydroxyapatite, synthetic or coralline, has also been introduced as a substitute for autogenous graft for cervical interbody fusion, with satisfactory results.[13,36] In the last decade, various threaded cages have been used for posterior and anterior lumbar interbody fusion, with or without pedicle-screw fixation for lumbar instability and spondylolisthesis.[19] In experiments using the equine cervical spine by DeBowes et al.,[2] osseous union was prevalent at 6 months after cage implantation by a reduction in the range of motion at the site of cage fixation.

OPLL of the cervical spine, which was first reported in an autopsy study by Tsukimoto[37] in 1960, has been extensively studied for its pathophysiology and surgical management over the last 30 years, especially in Japan. OPLL is one of the major causes of cervical compressive myelopathy in Japan and is often associated with cervical spondylosis.° Therefore, it is absolutely vital to establish the precise diagnosis in patients with cervical myelopathy or radiculopathy by using routine radiographs, CT and MRI, and to define whether or not cervical spondylosis is associated with OPLL and/or HPLL.[23]

If OPLL is segmental or local type and is localized at one, two, or even three intervertebral levels, the ventral approach is often selected by the surgeon.[1,4,14,22,26] In extensive OPLL of continuous or mixed type over four levels, expansive laminoplasty (open-door or double-door) is commonly used because multilevel decompression is readily obtained, and the procedure is less risky compared with the ventral approach.[8] As discussed, corpectomy with direct removal of OPLL and onlay iliac graft had been the standard procedure but was discontinued nearly 10 years ago because of drawbacks, such as graft problems, donor-site pain, and the necessity of a halo brace.

Since August 1997, ventral interbody cage fixation with autogenous vertebral graft became the authors' standard surgical technique for cervical spondylosis and OPLL because this method provides immediate stabilization, rare cage-related complications, and no donor-site problems, in addition to sufficient space for microsurgical decompression. However, the surgeon's microsurgical technique must be more refined and adjusted to the relatively smaller keyhole corpectomy, compared with wide corpectomy, to perform safe decompression. In cervical spondylosis, the twin-cage method is commonly used, and, if associated with OPLL or HPLL, the single-cage method with a larger cage is the procedure of choice to access OPLL behind the vertebral body. For multilevel lesions, a combined method is applied depending on the pathology at each level. The majority of the cases (95%) were one-level or two-level, but three-level cage fixation was performed in eight cases (5%) with multilevel OPLL, with reasonable results. Surgical results were generally satisfactory with rare complications and early ambulation, short hospital stay, and early return to work.° Biomechanical testing of cervical interbody cages has indicated better stability (predominantly with the twin-cage method, compared with the single-cage method) and no significant difference in design variation between the cages.[12] Animal studies have demonstrated good bony fusion.[3,39]

In conclusion, interbody cage fixation with autogenous vertebral graft following microsurgical decompression is a safe and effective method for the ventral approach of cervical spondylosis and OPLL, with few complications. The single-cage method is commonly used for OPLL and HPLL, and the twin-cage method is normally used for cervical spondylosis. The surgical method is tailored to the pathology of each level. This procedure facilitates early ambulation, short hospital stay, and early return to work.

ACKNOWLEDGMENT

The authors wish to thank Mr. Shunji Ono for preparing the figures and Ms. Emiko Nagase for her editorial assistance.

°References 5,18,22,29,30,31.

REFERENCES

1. Abe H, Tsuru M, Ito T, et al: Anterior decompression for ossification of the posterior longitudinal ligament of the cervical spine. *J Neurosurg* 55:108-116, 1981.
2. Cloward RB: The anterior approach for removal of ruptured cervical disks. *J Neurosurg* 15:602-617, 1958.
3. DeBowes RM, Grant BD, Bagby GW, et al: Cervical vertebral interbody fusion in the horse: a comparative study of bovine xerografts and autografts supported by stainless steel baskets. *Am J Vet Res* 45:191-199, 1984.
4. Epstein N: The surgical management of ossification of the posterior longitudinal ligament in 51 patients. *J Spinal Disord* 6:432-455, 1993.
5. Hacker RJ: A randomized prospective study of an anterior cervical interbody fusion device with a minimum of 2 years of follow-up results. *J Neurosurg* 93(suppl 2): 222-226, 2000.
6. Hakuba A: Trans-unco-discal approach: a combined anterior and lateral approach to cervical discs. *J Neurosurg* 45:284-291, 1976.
7. Hashizume Y, Iijima S, Kishimoto H, et al: Pathology of spinal cord lesions caused by ossification of the posterior longitudinal ligament. *Acta Neuropathol* 63:123-130, 1984.
8. Hirabayashi K, Watanabe K, Wakano K, et al: Expansive open-door laminoplasty for cervical spinal stenotic myelopathy. *Spine* 8: 693-699, 1983.

°References 1,4,7,8,14,20,21,26.

9. Isu T, Kamada K, Kobayashi N, *et al:* The surgical technique of anterior cervical fusion using bone grafts obtained from cervical vertebral bodies. *J Neurosurg* 80:16-19, 1994.

10. Jho HD: Microsurgical anterior cervical foraminotomy for radiculopathy: a new approach to cervical disc herniation. *J Neurosurg* 84:155-160, 1996.

11. Kadoya S: Grading and scoring system for neurological function in degenerative cervical disease: neurosurgical cervical spine scale. *Neurol Med Chir* (Tokyo) 32:40-41, 1992.

12. Kandziora F, Pflugmacher R, Schafer J, *et al:* Biomechanical comparison of cervical spine interbody fusion cage. *Spine* 26:1850-1857, 2001.

13. Kim P, Wakai S, Matsuo S, *et al:* Bisegmental cervical interbody fusion using hydroxyapatite implants: surgical results and long-term observation in 70 cases. *J Neurosurg* 88:21-27, 1998.

14. Kojima T, Waga S, Kubo Y, *et al:* Anterior cervical vertebrectomy and interbody fusion for multilevel spondylosis and ossification of the posterior longitudinal ligament. *Neurosurgery* 24:864-872, 1989.

15. Kubo Y, Waga S, Kojima T, *et al:* Microsurgical anatomy of the lower cervical spine and cord. *Neurosurgery* 34:895-902, 1994.

16. Martin GJ, Haid RW, MacMilan M, *et al:* Anterior cervical discectomy with freeze-dried fibula allograft: overview of 317 cases and literature review. *Spine* 24:852-859, 1999.

17. Martins AN: Anterior cervical discectomy with and without interbody bone graft. *J Neurosurg* 44:290-295, 1976.

18. Matge G: Anterior interbody fusion with the BAK-Cage in cervical spondylosis. *Acta Neurochir* (Wien) 140:1-8, 1998.

19. Matge G, Leclercq TA: Rationale for interbody fusion with threaded titanium cages at cervical and lumbar levels: results on 357 cases. *Acta Neurochir* (Wien) 142:425-434, 2000.

20. Mizuno J, Nakagawa H, Iwata K, *et al:* Pathology of the spinal cord lesions caused by ossification of the posterior longitudinal ligament, with special reference to reversibility of the spinal cord lesion. *Neurol Res* 14:312-314, 1992.

21. Mizuno J, Nakagawa H, Isobe M: Surgical results of anterior approach in ossification of the posterior longitudinal ligament in the cervical spine. *Spinal Surg* (Japan) 11:39-46, 1997.

22. Mizuno J, Nakagawa H: Outcome analysis of anterior decompressive surgery and fusion for cervical ossification of the posterior longitudinal ligament: report of 107 cases and review of the literature. *Neurosurg Focus* 10:Article 6, 2000.

23. Mizuno J, Nakagawa H, Hashizume Y: Clinicopathological analysis of hypertrophy of the posterior longitudinal ligament of the cervical spine based on clinical and pathological study. *Neurosurgery* 49:1091-1098, 2001.

24. Murphy MG, Gado M: Anterior cervical discectomy without interbody bone graft. *J Neurosurg* 37:71-74, 1972.

25. Nagashima C: Cervical myelopathy due to ossification of the posterior longitudinal ligament. *J Neurosurg* 37:653-660, 1972.

26. Nakagawa H, Mizuno J: The pathophysiology and management of ossification of the posterior longitudinal ligament. In Barrow DL (ed): *Perspectives in Neurological Surgery.* St Louis, Quality Medical, 1992, pp 38-48.

27. Nakagawa H, Yamamoto H, Mizuno J, *et al:* Microdiscectomy and osteophytectomy without bone graft in cervical spondylosis and herniated discs: long-term follow-ups. *Spinal Surg (Japan)* 6:33-39, 1992.

28. Nakagawa H, Mizuno J, Tamai K, *et al:* Anterior approach with autogenous vertebral bone graft in ossification of the posterior longitudinal ligament of the cervical spine. *Spinal Surg* (Japan) 9:37-42, 1995.

29. Nakagawa H, Mizuno H, Chang HS, *et al:* Minimally invasive methods in anterior approach for cervical discogenic disease. *Jpn J Neurosurg (Tokyo)* 8:189-193, 1999.

30. Nakagawa H, Sang-Don Kim, Jimichi Mizuno, *et al:* Microsurgical interbody cage fixation for cervical spondylosis and OPLL: clinical experience of 301 cases. Submitted for publication.

31. Profeta G, de Falco R, Ianniciello G, *et al:* Preliminary experience with anterior cervical microdiscectomy and interbody titanium cage fixation (Novus CT-Ti) in patients with cervical disc disease. *Surg Neurol* 53:417-426, 2000.

32. Ray CD: Threaded titanium cages for lumbar interbody fusions. *Spine* 22:667-680, 1997.

33. Smith GW, Robinson RA: The treatment of certain cervical spine disorders by anterior removal of intervertebral disc and interbody fusion. *J Bone Joint Surg Am* 40:607-624, 1958.

34. Takahashi T, Tominaga T, Yokobori T, *et al:* In vitro biomechanical evaluation of interbody fusion cage for anterior cervical fusion in a caprine model. *Spinal Surg (Japan)* 15:1-6, 2001.

35. Terayama K, Maruyama S, Miyashita R, *et al:* Ossification of the posterior longitudinal ligament in the cervical spine. *Orthop Surg (Japan)* 15:1083-1095, 1994.

36. Thalgott JS, Fritts K, Giuffre JM, *et al:* Anterior interbody fusion of the cervical spine with coralline hydroxyapatite. *Spine* 24:1295-1299, 1999.

37. Tsukimoto H: A case report: autopsy of syndrome of compression of spinal cord owing to ossification within spinal canal of cervical spines. *Nippon Geka Hokan (Japan)* 29:1003-1007, 1960.

38. Williams RC: Anterior cervical fusion utilizing autogenous bone graft from the cervical vertebrae. *Neurosurgery* 11:339-342, 1992.

39. Zdeblick TA, Ghanayem AJ, Rapoff AJ, *et al:* Cervical interbody fusion cages: an animal model with and without bone morphogenic protein. *Spine* 23:758-766, 1998.

CHAPTER 30

Interbody Strut Techniques

Richard L. Saunders, Vincent C. Traynelis, and Sanford E. Emery

Since 1985, techniques for extensive ventral decompression for spondylotic spinal cord syndromes have approached a standard level of care.[6] Few, if any, series fail to exceed the outcomes associated with multiple-level discectomy or laminectomy. Although such enthusiasm may reflect selection bias and the optimism associated with a new procedure, the complete spine surgeon must be comfortable with anterior decompression by corpectomy and with the requisite strut grafting. This chapter focuses on the latter.

There are two seemingly different approaches to strut grafting: (1) the bone interlocking method and (2) the more recent use of plates and screws (see Chapters 77 and 116). There are clear indications for each method, and the modern surgeon should not be polarized. This chapter focuses on the noninstrumented graft, including situations in which hardware is to be considered.

Fundamentals of Grafting

Three fundamental concepts with regard to strut grafting need to be recognized. First and foremost is an understanding of the factors affecting spinal stability. Problems can result if these factors are ignored. An uninstrumented, unstable spine requires extensive external bracing (e.g., the halo or Minerva techniques). This is relatively independent of the surgical fusion technique. Ordinarily the stable spine requires no hardware and little or no external bracing. As indicated in Box 30.1, the trough decompression used in cervical spondylotic myelopathy does not compromise stability.[7] On the other hand, a laminectomy probably does.

The second essential component of strut grafting is that the goal of the surgical procedure should be clear. This should be the amelioration of stresses placed on the spinal cord by disease, compression, distortion, stretching, and movement. Although this is not the topic of this chapter per se, if these primary goals are subverted with an eye to subsequent reconstruction, the essential purpose of the surgical undertaking may be compromised. One must design the surgery with the principal focus on the nervous system (Figure 30.1).

The third fundamental concept of strut grafting is a knowledge of the characteristics of the reconstruction material. The choices are limited, and in practice, surgeons have only the iliac crest and fibular allograft or autograft as options. Autograft calvarium has been used for struts. However, this source has not been embraced widely.

Bone Graft

Perhaps more important than the origin of the graft material is the selection and handling of the graft itself. Autogenous iliac crest incorporates rapidly, which is an important advantage. Its use, however, can be compromised by sloppy harvesting techniques (see Chapter 64), osteoporosis, and injudicious tailoring. We usually limit its use to two or three vertebral segments. In fashioning iliac crest to the bony defect, it is critical to preserve two contiguous cortical surfaces, which include the ends of the graft, to maintain as much strength as possible. The use of allograft iliac crest, with or without hardware, is illogical.

Using the fibula has several advantages: (1) it is a robust construct, to the extent that the surgeon must be cautious with its use in the osteoporotic spine; (2) it allows the struts to be any length; (3) it is strong; and (4) it provides a central channel for the packing of autograft cancellous bone to enhance early incorporation and fusion. An arguable disadvantage of the fibula is the mismatch of the densities with that of the vertebral body. The vertebra will always fail before the fibula graft does. In practical terms this problem is principally that of "pistoning," in which the fibula penetrates through the vertebral body, and may actually enter the next motion segment. Some pistoning is unavoidable, especially in osteoporosis, but it is usually of no significant consequence (Figure 30.2). Two critical ways to limit pistoning are to use minimal distraction during graft placement, and to use an orthotic fit to limit flexion. Too much graft loading and excessive neck flexion early in convalescence almost guarantees pistoning. Minimizing dissection of the vertebral body graft bed site is important in regard to the preservation of ultimate vertebral body height. This accommodates for the inevitable penetration of the graft into the vertebral body. Preservation of vertebral height may require total resection of the rostral subaxial vertebra, if it is involved in the compressive process. A partially resected vertebral body and a fibula graft are a dangerous combination.

Fibula, though robust, has the disadvantage of being extremely slow to be incorporated; the time required for incorporation is several times longer than that for iliac crest. This raises concerns about pseudarthrosis, although it has not been documented. We have attempted to decrease graft harvest morbidity by using allograft fibula packed with autograft cancellous bone, taken through the top of the iliac crest. Because allograft fibula alone is not unacceptable for strut grafting, the addition of an autograft core enhances the construct. Iliac crest graft morbidity associated with a limited cancellous graft harvest is less than that associated with a simple Smith-Robinson graft harvest. Autogenous cancellous bone is accessed via the superficial surface of the iliac crest through a 3-cm skin incision. The medial and outer surfaces of the iliac crest are not disturbed, as is necessary with the harvest of tricortical grafts. This minimizes postoperative pain. Through a cauterized area of the crest, a 1cm cortical defect is created with a high-speed cutting burr, and cancellous bone is taken with a large curette. This, in turn, is packed into the central canal of the allograft fibula with a 3mm-diameter rod. No bone is placed around the outside of the fibula strut.

Another obvious difference between iliac crest and fibula is the level of accommodation to the cervical lordosis, the former being fairly natural, and the latter, by comparison, being poker straight. Whether this has any practical importance after graft incorporation is questionable. Because fibula definitely heals slower than iliac crest, a significant difference in the pseudarthrosis rate might be expected; this, however, has not been observed.

30.1

Factors influencing stability

Ventral element integrity
Dorsal element integrity
Dynamic radiographic elements
    Sagittal plane translation greater than 3.5 mm
    Sagittal plane rotation greater than 20 degrees

(From White AA, Panjabi MM: *Clinical Biomechanics of the Spine*, ed 2. Philadelphia, Lippincott-Raven, 1990, p 314.)

Strut Graft
Soft-Tissue Management

The soft tissues of the ventral neck contain structures that may be injured by prolonged retraction. Because extensive anterior decompression and strut grafting are time consuming, one must assume an inherent, ischemic, soft-tissue morbidity proportional to the duration of retraction. Accordingly, regular relaxation of retractors is important to avoid hoarseness, stridor, and swallowing dysfunction. This measure virtually eliminates soft-tissue morbidity.

Preparation of Vertebral Defect for Strut Grafting

Perhaps as important as the pathophysiologic process that causes myelopathy is the prevention of graft displacement. Although plates and screws prevent graft displacement and improve graft incorporation, they should never be relied on to prevent graft impaction against the spinal cord. The bed for the graft must be prepared in such a manner that the avenue toward the spinal canal is shorter or narrower than the graft itself. If graft migration were to occur, the direction should be away from the spinal cord. When hardware is to be employed, the use of deep slots or mortises in the vertebral body is limited by the need for adequate remaining vertebral body volume for screw purchase. When

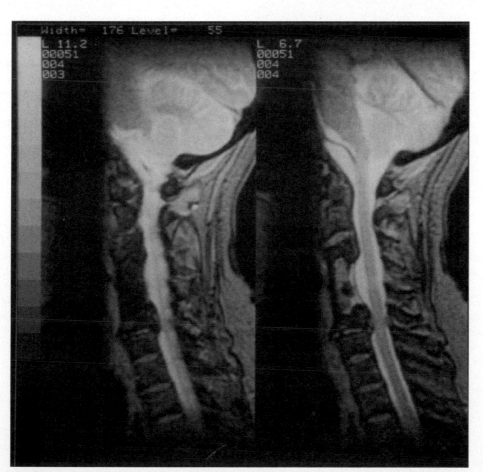

Figure 30.1 Postoperative magnetic resonance imaging scan of a two-level decompression. Note the persisting spinal canal stenosis.

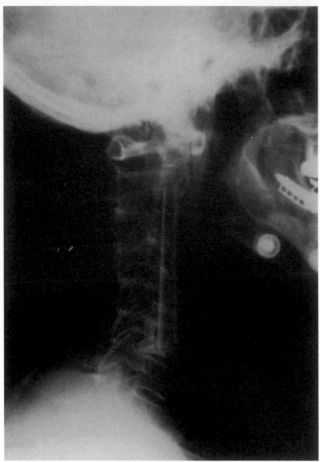

Figure 30.2 Fibula strut graft. Note the penetration of the caudal mortise (i.e., "pistoning"). Pistoning through next motion segment is observed 3 years postsurgery. No symptoms were present and no further treatment was rendered.

hardware employment is not anticipated, spinal canal protection is attained by one or more of three strategies (Figure 30.3A-C): (1) the keystone mortise and tenon, (2) the dovetail technique, and (3) the lateral step method.

Keystone technique

The keystone graft method places the graft close to the middle column of the vertebral body. It is secured by means of mortises or slots in the opposing vertebral end-plates (Figure 30.3A).

Proper preparation of the mortises in the keystone technique requires consideration of the angling of the cervical disc space (Figure 30.3D). This disc space angling is the consequence of the ventral vertebral surface being slightly more caudal than the dorsal vertebral surface. The caudal mortise can be fashioned into the face of the vertebral end-plate, without removal of the anterior cortical corner of the vertebra. Thus the sloping of this end-plate away from the spinal canal provides the opportunity for creating the ideal mortise. The dorsal mortise lip is longer than its ventral counterpart. This ensures that any potential displacement of the graft occurs across the shallower ventral mortise lip. Because the caudal vertebral mortise

can be readily fashioned with preservation of the cortical vertebral margins, this is the strongest mortise construct (Figure 30.3D).

The creation of the ideal caudal mortise is simple, whereas that of the rostral mortise is not. Again, the critical consideration is the disc space angle. At the caudal end plate of the rostral mortise, the angle is such that to ensure a shorter ventral mortise lip, a portion of the anterior vertebral body must be resected. To avoid undue anterior resection, while ensuring adequacy of the posterior mortise lip, appreciable resection of the dorsal vertebral margin in the decompression is precluded. Should any dorsal vertebral body decompression be pursued, the remaining vertebral body may be inadequate for proper mortising (Figure 30.3D).

Dovetail technique

The dovetail grafting method refers to fashioning a segment of the graft that is placed ventral to the anterior vertebral surfaces, and that is longer than the length of the decompression defect. "Dovetail" refers to the bipartite shape of both ends of the graft, one slightly longer than the other. This is not unlike the tail of a dove (Figure 30.3B). The shorter of the two "tail feathers" at both ends is placed into matching slots, which are drilled into the opposing end-plates of the cephalic and caudal vertebra. The rostral slot is of a depth such that the respective dovetail can be inserted to a depth that allows the clearance of the distal "tail" into its respective slot with moderate cervical traction. The graft, thus in place, is then shifted distally for a final locking-in position. The advantage of this construct is that it can be prepared in such a way that it is unequivocally too large to be displaced into the spinal canal. The disadvantages are that it can place excessive vertical loads on the ventral vertebral body cortex and may not allow significant impaction of the cancellous components of the graft and vertebra. In theory the graft is located within the anterior column. Therefore vertebral failure may not be via impaction but via displacement. Obviously this construct does not lend itself to plating.

Lateral bone step technique

As described by Awasthi and Voorhies,[1] lateral bone steps on either side of the decompression can be fashioned on either side of the anterior spinal canal, after completion of decompression by widening of the trough superficially (Figure 30.3C). The graft is then tailored to so that it is wider than the width of the decompression, and it is placed superficial to the lateral steps.

Preparation of the Strut Graft

The keystone graft (Figure 30.3A) is tailored for intimate lateral surface contact with the sides of the decompression trough. This fit should not require more than firm pressure for positioning. Forcefully hammering a slightly wide graft past a tight lateral contact point risks subsequent displacement by a lateral levering mechanism that may occur with minimal neck movement. Width tailoring is usually accomplished with a high-speed burr or oscillating saw.

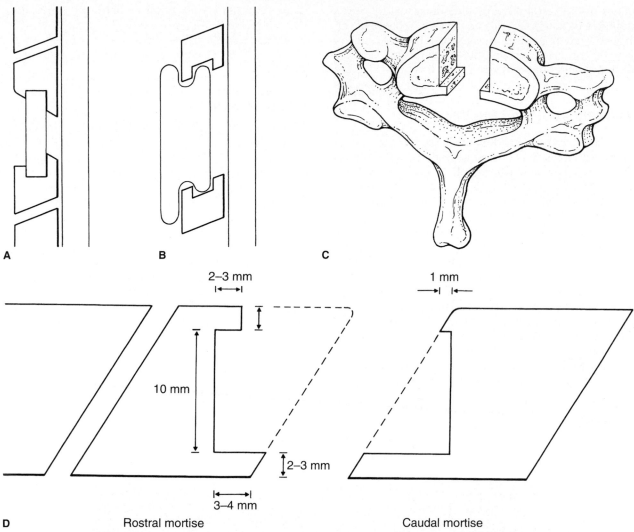

Figure 30.3 Schematics of keystone (**A**), dovetail, and Voorhies lateral step (**B** and **C**) techniques, and the measurement details of keystone mortises (**D**).

A rongeur may cause cortical microfractures, which may lead, especially in the osteoporotic patient, to subsequent postoperative midshaft graft fracture. The width is repeatedly checked by placing both ends of the graft into the vertebral trough until a fit that allows no lateral play is achieved. By a similar tailoring sequence, the rostral tip of the graft is fashioned to fit its mortise exactly. Because the ventral mortise lip is foreshortened deliberately, the strut can be angled into the mortise, and the fit can be assessed before the final determination of the strut length. After the exact graft width and rostral fit have been determined, the length is ascertained by marking the caudal aspect of the graft with the graft fully positioned rostrally, while manual cervical traction is applied. Traction will usually provide at least 1mm of trough distraction. This, in turn, results in the graft marked 1mm longer than the defect. The caudal mortise graft fit is then tailored, as was the rostral end. The graft can now be forced into place, rostral end first, using firm pressure or very light hammer tapping. It is important to force the caudal portion of the graft into the trough until it contacts the posterior mortise and lies deep to the anterior mortise lip. Caution should be

used to avoid overdistracting the spine, resulting in "too tight" a fit, because this may predispose it to increased axial loading and fracture of the caudal vertebrae.

Once in place, the graft is stressed with a flexion and then an extension movement of the neck by the circulating nurse in collaboration with the anesthesiologist. This forces the graft into the mortises and determines whether levering will cause displacement. It is done under direct vision after removal of the interfering retractors. In cases in which this stress test is uneventful, subsequent displacement has not been observed.

Similarly, the dovetail graft (Figure 30.3B) is fastidiously tailored. However, as already noted, the strategy of locking the graft by caudal engagement requires a greater vertebral slot or mortise depth. Because tailoring of the anterior mortise lips, as in the keystone method, is not necessary with the dovetail technique, the anterior vertebral cortical edges should assure the utmost vertebral resistance to fracture. A cortical surface of the iliac crest graft should be placed toward the depth of the decompression to ensure a strong graft construct. The positioning of the cortical margin of the bone graft within the confines of the vertebral body (i.e., dorsal to the ventral vertebral body margins) helps minimize the chance of ventral bone graft migration. Because the fibula has a tendency to cut or penetrate into its receiving vertebral bodies, it should be used sparingly for this purpose.

Complications of Strut Grafting

It has not been determined whether strut grafting across the cervicothoracic junction is associated with additional limitations. Whereas a short graft is probably inconsequential, the potential for fracture (either immediate or late fracture of the vertebra, strut, or both) with the use of a long construct may be significant.

Also unknown is the necessity, if any, for the correction of a kyphotic curve.[4] In practice, the draping of the spinal cord over the ventral fulcrum that is associated with a kyphosis should be corrected by the decompression. Spine straightening may not be as critical under these circumstances. Such correction would load the graft substantially, thereby risking graft or hardware complication.

Techniques for avoiding morbidity have been defined in the discussions in this chapter. Fortunately, hematoma and infection of the anterior neck are uncommon, but there are no specific management schemes unique to strut grafting for preventing these complications. The use of a suction drain for 24 hours may lessen their incidence.

Persistent neck pain should raise concern for infection. Infection, especially after the first convalescent week, should prompt suspicion of esophageal leakage. Infection

alone does not require graft or hardware removal; however, drainage is usually necessary.

Graft complications take the form of displacement, midgraft fracture, mortise fracture, pistoning, and angulation.

Graft Displacement

Displacements and graft fracture with displacement almost always occur within days of surgery and are usually best handled by repeat surgery. Usually displacement alone reflects a technical error. The principal concern is for an associated vertebral fracture consequent to graft displacement (Figure 30.4). Vertebral fractures are usually caudal and, unless minor, will require extending the fusion across the next motion segment. This does not require further decompression, but does require a new strut and the creation of a bed across the fractured vertebra. Unless the problem stemmed from unrecognized instability, the revised graft does not necessarily require plating or aggressive bracing. Many surgeons, however, having had one construct fail, would opt for circumferential stabilization in this situation.

Graft Pistoning

Pistoning usually occurs, to some degree, when fibula is used (Figure 30.2). It is important to avoid circumferential sharpening of the fibula strut ends. Similarly, more than 1mm of distraction should be avoided. The degree of penetration may appear alarming on a radiograph. One series

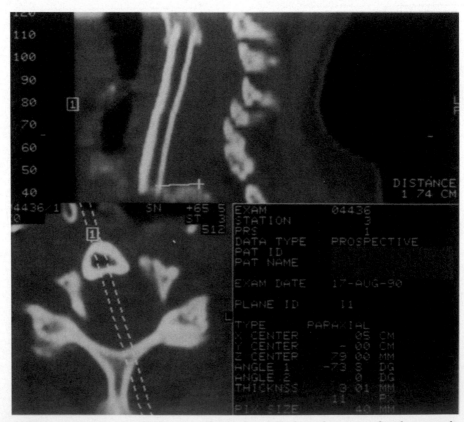

Figure 30.4 Computed tomographic scan of a displaced fibula graft associated with a ventral fracture of the caudal vertebral body.

documented an average of 6 to 7mm of fibula strut graft settling in two- or three-level corpectomy patients without adverse outcomes.[4] Even when there is entrance into the next disc space (usually the caudal disc space), the authors have not surgically intervened and have observed no consequences.

Graft Angulation

Graft angulation, usually at the rostral mortise, occurs in less than 10% of grafts. The incidence of this complication is not necessarily proportional to strut graft length (Figure 30.5). This may be a result of inadequate orthotic support or technical problems. Clearly, plating should minimize the incidence of this problem. The revision of an angulated graft is infrequently necessary. More extensive bracing such as with a halo vest or Minerva jacket may be the most appropriate first line of treatment.

Pseudarthrosis

Late sequelae of strut grafts, pseudarthrosis (Figure 30.6), and midshaft graft fracture (Figure 30.7), appear to be unavoidable. If these are associated with a potentially compressive osteophyte or persistent neck pain, a dorsal interspinous fusion, with or without lateral mass plates, is a treatment option. Late fractures may heal with the passage

of time alone (Figure 30.7A-B). Ventral revision of a pseudarthrosis is feasible if a compressive osteophyte has developed. However, a simultaneous posterior stabilization procedure may be prudent if stability has been significantly threatened. Anterior revision of a midgraft fracture risks the problems inherent with postoperative scar formation.

The significance of pseudarthrosis, or more correctly, fibrous union, is as uncertain with strut grafts as it is with ventral discectomy and fusion. The incidence of this complication is less than 10% with autograft iliac crest, although it is reportedly as high as 30% with allograft fibula.[3] Hardware use may improve fusion rate. In one study late recurrent myelopathy in these patients could be attributed to a pseudarthrosis with hypertrophic changes, or new adjacent segment disease.[2]

When the neuroanatomic goals of corpectomy have been met and the patient made comfortable, the implications of a fibrous union at either end of the strut graft have received little critical discussion. Similarly, when decompression is achieved and good radiographic graft incorporation is documented, the significance of neck pain is not known. Because the incidence of radiographic pseudarthrosis is less than 10%, and that of postoperative neck pain even less, we have chosen to manage bony union issues as a neck pain problem. If positive radiographs are associated with neck discomfort, the patient is offered interspinous fusion. With inexplicable pain, the patient is

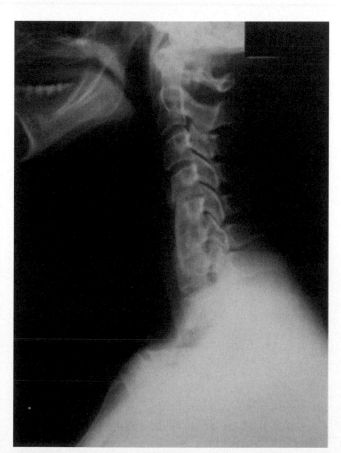

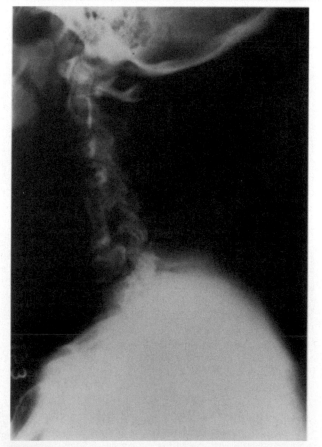

Figure 30.5 Lateral radiograph of a graft associated with kyphosis, without apparent clinical consequence. The authors have observed angulations as great as 20 degrees that have been effectively managed without revision.

Figure 30.6 Lateral radiograph showing hypertrophic changes and lucency at the caudal graft-vertebral body interface. This is consistent with pseudarthrosis. The patient was asymptomatic. Dynamic films demonstrated no motion.

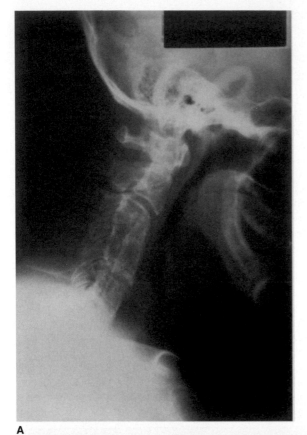

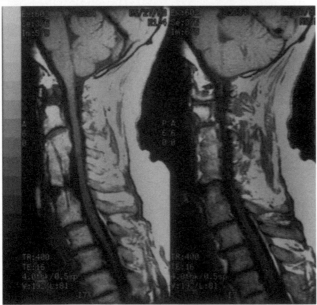

Figure 30.7 Lateral radiograph (**A**) and magnetic resonance imaging scan (**B**) are consistent with an old, healed midgraft fracture. The patient had no neck symptoms.

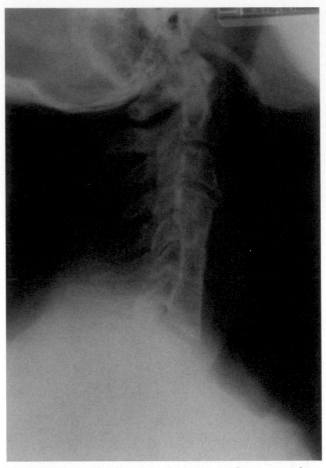

Figure 30.8 Lateral radiograph taken 5 years after strut grafting. Note continuity of cortical lines and complete absence of demarcation between vertebra and graft. Such a film excludes pseudarthrosis; dynamic films are unnecessary. Such maturity may require a year or more to achieve with iliac crest, and substantially longer with fibula.

offered posterior open assessment of segmental motion, and fusion is suggested if mobility is found. This latter strategy is plausible during the period of graft immaturity, 1 to 2 years postoperatively. Later the cortical lines are such that an absolute exclusion of nonunion by radiography alone is feasible (Figure 30.8). We have not performed explorations on a patient whose radiographs did not reveal anything. Patients with fibrous unions and late graft fractures are expected to be relieved of neck pain by successful posterior fusion and spinous process wiring.

Summary

Strut grafting after ventral cervical decompression ordinarily requires fastidious graft fit. If the graft cannot be displaced intraoperatively, it should remain in place. If, however, the spine is unstable, plating or extensive external bracing should be used.

REFERENCES

1. Awasthi D, Voorhies RM: Anterior cervical vertebrectomy and interbody fusion, technical note. *J Neurosurg* 76:159, 1992.
2. Emery SE, Bohlman HH, *et al*: Anterior cervical decompression and arthodesis for the treatment of cervical spondylotic myelopathy. *JBJS* 80A:941-951, July 1998.

3. Fernyhough JC, White JI, LaRocca HS: Fusion rates in multilevel cervical spondylosis comparing allograft fibula with autograft fibula. Presented at Cervical Spine Research Society, 18th annual meeting, San Antonio, November 28, 1990.

4. Herman JM, Sonntag VKH: Cervical corpectomy and plate fixation for postlaminectomy kyphoses. *J Neurosurg* 80:963, 1994.

5. Hughes SS, Pringle T, *et al*: Multilevel cervical corpectomy and fibular strut grafting: clinical and radiographic follow-up. Transactions of the 63rd Annual Meeting of the AAOS, Atlanta, GA, 1996.

6. Saunders RL: Anterior reconstructive procedures in cervical spondylotic myelopathy. *Clin Neurosurg* 37:682, 1991.

7. White AA, Panjabi MM: *Clinical Biomechanics of the Spine*, ed 2. Philadelphia, Lippincott-Raven, 1990, p 314.

CHAPTER 31

Interbody Cages

Donald A. Smith, D. Mark Melton, and David W. Cahill

Ventral cervical discectomy and cervical corpectomy for decompression of degenerative disease, trauma, tumor, and infection are among the most commonly performed spinal operations. Options for reconstruction of the anterior column include structural autografts and allografts, as well as an evolving genre of prosthetic devices. The objectives of reconstruction are to restore a stable load-bearing anterior column, to maintain intervertebral height, and to establish an anatomic cervical lordosis when possible. Ideally the construct will become biologically integrated into the native spine, with replacement by living bone over time. For simple discectomy and single-level corpectomy these endpoints are usually achievable with tricortical autografts harvested from the iliac crest. Complications such as graft collapse or extrusion are occasionally encountered, but the primary objection to the use of structural autografts relates to the relatively high rate of morbidity at the donor site. This may include chronic pain, numbness, infection, hematoma, and cosmetic deformity, and is reported to occur in the range of 10% to 25%.[6,10,24,25] A common observation among spine surgeons is that the morbidity associated with the bone graft harvest frequently exceeds the morbidity related to the primary procedure. This high rate of donor site morbidity has helped propel the search for alternative reconstructive possibilities. Structural allografts eliminate donor-site problems, but are associated with an increased risk of pseudarthrosis and graft resorption, especially in smokers. Although highly processed, lingering concerns remain about potential risk for disease transmission.

Reconstruction of a multilevel corpectomy bed poses yet a greater challenge. Iliac crest and fibula are the best autograft options available, but harvest of suitably long struts contributes significantly to patient morbidity. It can also be very difficult to match the graft to the cross-sectional and longitudinal geometry of the recipient site. These obstacles have prompted many surgeons to substitute fibular allograft as a simpler expedient. Fibular allografts are very straight and have a much smaller diameter than that of the cervical corpus. These features enable it to fit readily into the recipient bed, but may not indicate optimal load transfer characteristics. Fibular allograft is comprised almost exclusively of hard cortical bone. The mismatch in cross-sectional diameters and physical characteristics between the graft and recipient bone contributes to "pistoning" of the fibular strut through the adjacent central end-plates, a condition commonly observed as the reconstructed segment foreshortens during graft incorporation, with resultant loss of lordosis.[23] An additional concern is the heightened risk of nonunion that accompanies long segment allograft constructs.

Interbody Cages

A variety of prosthetic interbody cages are now available for use in the cervical spine, both for disc space arthrodesis and to bridge the larger voids created by single- or multilevel corpectomy. Current devices are fabricated, either from titanium alloy or polymer, and can be classified into screw-in, box-type, and cylindrical design categories.[15] Hydroxyapatite spacer-grafts, bioabsorbable implants, and artificial discs are also under investigation, but are not a primary focus of this chapter.

Interbody cages are intended to confer immediate structural integrity to the ventral spine. Although some surgeons have placed these as naked implants,[16] more typically, they are employed as carriers for osteoinductive or osteoconductive materials whose purpose is to secure long-term stability through biologic integration with the recipient spine. In the authors' experience, interbody cages are usually loaded with morselized autograft obtained from the cervical spine itself, or from cancellous harvest from the sternum or iliac crest at negligible added morbidity. Alternatives such as allograft bone, hydroxyapatite, and "biologics," including recombinant human bone morphogenetic protein (rhBMP), may even obviate this need.

Devices designed for disc space arthrodesis come prefabricated in a variety of sizes for direct implantation. Cages used for vertebral body replacement are provided as stock material, which can be rapidly modified on an individual basis to match the unique anatomic need. Many of these implants remain in development and are not released by the Food and Drug Administration (FDA) for clinical application in the United States at this time. The literature that bears on these devices includes animal-testing data,[29] biomechanical studies,[15,26,27] and clinical reports*; it is comparatively sparse and is devoid of any class 1 evidentiary material.

Screw-in Devices

The Bagby and Kuslich cervical cage (BAK/C, Sulzer Spine-Tech, Minneapolis) is the prototypic example of a "screw-in" design. The BAK/C cage is fundamentally an adaptation of a spinal instrumentation system already validated for disc-space arthrodesis in the lumbar spine. After successful completion of a prospective randomized multicenter trial, it has received FDA approval for use in the cervical spine.[11] Similar to the larger lumbar devices, a BAK/C implant consists of a hollow, threaded cage with multiple side-wall fenestrations. The cages are manufactured from a titanium alloy and are provided in a 12mm length, with a choice of 6, 8, 10, and 12mm diameters. Using a modification of the Cloward technique,[8] it is usually inserted as a single, midline cage after reaming and tapping of the adjacent central end-plates (Figure 31.1). Alternatively, two smaller (6 or 8mm) cages may be applied in a side-by-side fashion, although this necessarily limits the height of disc space

---

*References 1-3,5,7,9-14,16-22.

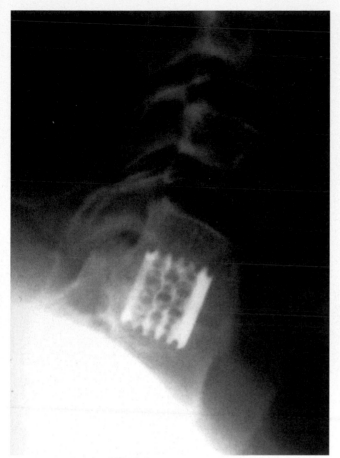

Figure 31.1 BAK/C cage.

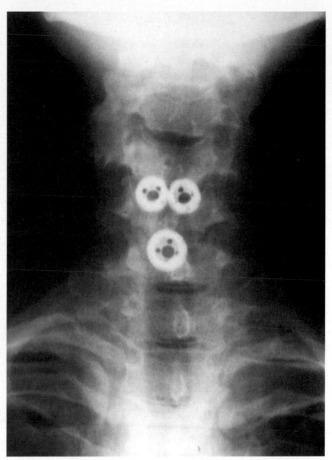

Figure 31.2 Side-by-side BAK cages with adjacent single-level cage.

distraction to be achieved (Figure 31.2). The cages are loaded with locally derived bone shavings, sometimes supplemented with allograft, according to volumetric needs. Sofamor Danek (Memphis) has recently released the Affinity cage in North America. This is similar in concept to the BAK/C, but has a conically tapered configuration whose purpose is to help establish cervical lordosis.

In the BAK/C study a single-level "fusion rate" of nearly 100% was reported. There were no device-related failures or complications, and other measures of clinical outcome appeared comparable to the noninstrumented ACDF "control" patients.[11] Furthermore these outcomes were achieved without the morbidity associated with iliac crest bone graft harvest observed in the control group. However, certain concerns linger about the consequences of violating the central vertebral end plates, as is required for insertion of this device. Hacker observed a 20% incidence of postoperative "sagittal alignment abnormalities" at follow-up. Lordotic reaming and tapping techniques and a tapered expansile cage (Varilift, Advanced Spine, Irvine, Calif.) have been developed in an effort to address this issue.

Because screw-in cages have a cylindrical cross section, the contact surface available for load transfer (and for fusion) is a comparatively narrow trough whose width is less than half of the cage diameter. This is mechanically disadvantageous in resisting lateral flexion, and the potential for subsidence of the implant with concomitant loss of cervical lordosis may be magnified if two or more adjacent

segments are instrumented. Disc-space restoration to an average height of 6 to 8mm requires implantation of 8 to 10mm diameter cages. When this is attempted at two or more adjacent levels the resultant encroachment into the intervening body can be substantial and may necessitate offset placement of the devices, and result in significant subsidence (Figure 31.3).

Box Cages

In Smith-Robinson type interbody fusions, the bony endplates are left intact, and a block-shaped structural graft with large, flat, superior and inferior contact surfaces is countersunk into the disc space.[28] From a biomechanical standpoint this construct is superior, because it retains the integrity of the end plates and provides a large surface area for load transfer and arthrodesis. Several box-type implant designs have been explored as alternatives to the more traditional tricortical autograft or structural allografts for Smith-Robinson fusion. These share a more or less rectangular configuration with a hollow core and fenestrations in their superior and inferior surfaces to allow the through-growth of bone. Both titanium and polymer cages have been produced. The Rabea cage (Signus Medizintechnik, Alzenau, Germany), the Syncage (Synthes, Davos, Switzerland), and the Tibon cage (Biomet-Merck, Berlin) are representative of titanium box designs.

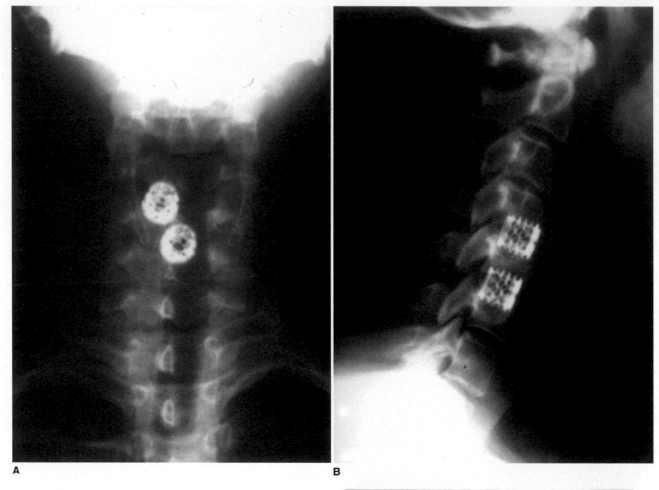

A

B

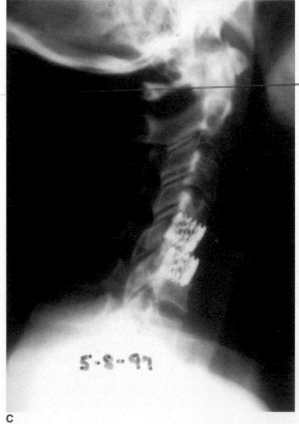

C

Figure 31.3 (**A**) Two-level BAK cages, anteroposteriorally. (**B**) Two-level BAK cages, lateral. (**C**) Same case, two-level BAK cages at 1-year follow-up showing subsidence.

With FDA approval, the Rabea cage is currently available as a "cement restrictor." It is made of forged titanium to ensure magnetic resonance imaging compatibility, and is prefabricated in a 12mm width, 12 and 14mm depths, and in heights ranging from 4 to 8mm (Figure 31.4). The Rabea is offered as a parallel end-plate design and as a "lordosed" version, with 5 degrees of divergence built in. The superior and inferior surfaces also bear retentive serrations to engage the end-plates and resist implant extrusion during neck flexion. Published experience with the Rabea cage is limited, but preliminary biomechanical studies and clinical reports are both favorable.[2,16,26] As with other metallic devices, it is hard to judge fusion, according to criteria of radiographically demonstrable bridging bone across the disc space and end-plates. Alternative criteria including less than 2 degrees of angulation in dynamic radiographs and absence of any peri-implant bony lucency are substituted.

Carbon fiber box cages have found favor as intervertebral implants in the lumbar spine.[4] These devices appear to be largely inert biologically; they exhibit good strength in all axes of applied stress, they are impact and fatigue resistant, their elastic modulus is purported to match well with that of the cortical bone of the recipient spine, and because they are radiolucent, they afford an opportunity for direct graft visualization and fusion assessment. Extending these advantages to a cervical interbody application, box-type polymer cages have been under active development abroad and are poised to enter the United States' market. Most designs have been fabricated from polyetheretherketone (PEEK), some also including a carbon fiber component (Cervical IF Cage, DePuy AcroMed, Raynham, MA). The Rabea device is now offered as a PEEK cage, again with approval in the United States for use as a cement restrictor. Other major vendors, including Stryker Instruments (Solis PEEK cage), Medtronic Sofamor Danek (CornerStone-SR), and Synthes (CR), have polymer cages already in place in overseas markets (Figure 31.5). Like the Rabea cage, they are offered in a variety of sizes and configurations, including parallel end-plates, lordotic, and superiorly convex designs to conform to individual disc space anatomic requirements. Shared features include a large central opening to contain graft material, ridged end plates to resist implant extrusion, and imbedded radio-opaque markers to allow x-ray visualization of the device.

Cho et al.[7] have recently reported on their preliminary experience with the Solis PEEK cage loaded with cancellous autograft in 40 patients undergoing mostly one- and two-level cervical discectomy and fusion.[7] Although the term of follow-up is unclear, the authors reported good functional outcomes, no device-related complications or failures, increased cervical lordosis, enlargement of neural foraminal cross-sectional area, and a 100% fusion rate. The complication rate was 2.5% in PEEK cage patients compared with a rate of 17.5% in a concurrent "control" group undergoing conventional discectomy and structural autografting in whom problems with graft collapse, dislodgement, and donor site morbidity were encountered. Radiolucent polymer cages are easily inserted; they appear to be biomechanically sound, and they hold much promise as interbody prostheses in the cervical spine, pending the outcome of more comprehensive clinical studies.

Cylindrical Mesh Cages

Vertically oriented cylindrical cages fabricated of titanium mesh are now gaining use in the cervical spine, both for disc-space arthrodesis and for segmental reconstruction after corpectomy. The Harms cage (DePuy AcroMed) is the primary example of this type of device; the SynMesh cage (Synthes, Davos, Switzerland) and Pyramesh cage (Sofamor Danek, Memphis, TN) are fundamentally similar designs. The FDA has granted approval for use of this instrumentation in the thoracic and lumbar spine. Published biomechanical data and clinical studies describing their use in the cervical spine are sparse. The senior author has now used these devices exclusively for postcorpectomy reconstruction for more than 5 years.

Similar to the box-cage designs, mesh cages are intended to interface with intact end-plates at the rostral and caudal ends of the construct. This increases the strength of the construct and reduces the risk for subsidence. Manufacturers provide stock material as sleeves of both circular and oval cross section, and in a variety of lengths and diameters. Cage diameters between 10 and 16mm are most suited for use in the cervical spine. In general the largest diameter that can be safely accommodated within the bed of the decompression is used, because the cage will then bear on the end plate perimeter, the

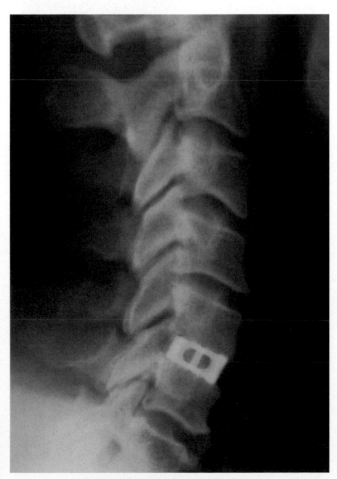

Figure 31.4 Single-level Rabea cage.

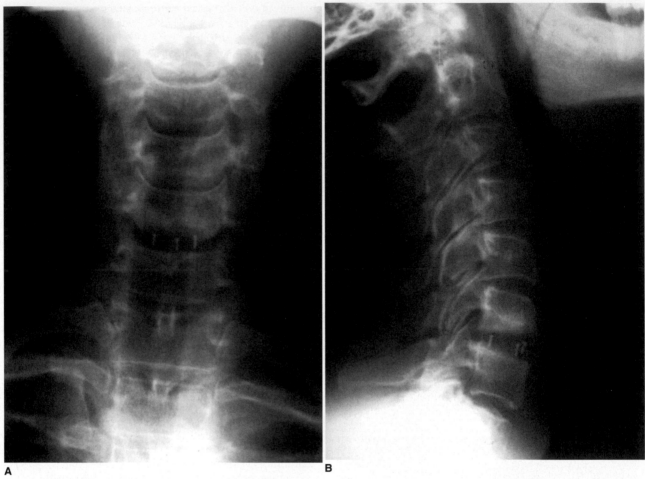

A

B

Figure 31.5 (**A**) Single-level Synthes CR cage, anterioposteriorally. (**B**) Single-level Synthes CR cage, lateral.

apophyseal ring, which is its strongest part. The mesh can be trimmed to any desired length and tailored to the particular reconstructive need if a stock length is not an exact match. All three systems can fit end caps to the top and bottom of the cylinder, thereby enlarging the metal-bone interface and lessening the risk of end plate perforation. Large central apertures within the end caps permit through-growth of bone. The palisading teeth of the cage ends project slightly above the plane of the end-caps, or the end caps themselves are serrated to grip the adjoining vertebral end plates and resist ventral cage extrusion. The Harms instrumentation provides a large selection of pre-cut straight and custom lordosed cages suitable as "off the shelf" implants for cervical disc-space arthrodesis. Cylindrical cages are usually loaded with densely packed autograft. As with other metallic devices, the radiographic evaluation of fusion status within mesh implants is indirect.

There is a paucity of literature pertaining to the use of mesh cages for cervical disc-space arthrodesis.[9,14] Our own experience with these devices in single- and multilevel discectomy operations suggests a significant potential for subsidence when these devices are used in a "stand-alone" mode. We attribute this to the relatively small contact area at the bone-implant interface in small-diameter disc-space

cages despite the use of end caps.[14] To retard subsidence we came to augment almost all ventral mesh cage reconstructions for degenerative disc disease with a dynamic anterior cervical plate. Although the addition of an anterior plate contributes only minimally to the duration and risk of operation, it does constitute a significant added expense. It is hoped that some of the newer box cage designs may yield satisfactory clinical results without a need for supplemental anterior fixation.

Mesh Cage Reconstruction of Corpectomy Defects

A more distinct advantage of using cylindrical mesh cage constructs is in the reconstruction of corpectomy defects. Indications for cervical corpectomy can include spondylosis, ossification of posterior longitudinal ligament, trauma, tumor, deformity correction, and occasional cases of infection. We and others have come to favor it in treatment of adjacent segment cervical disc disease as well.[12,17] Removal of a cervical corpus and the adjoining discs, and any associated osteophytes, can frequently be accomplished more expeditiously than two separate microdiscectomies (Figure 31.6). The quality of the decompression is unsurpassed, and ample bone is acquired from the corpectomy material to satisfy any need for graft.

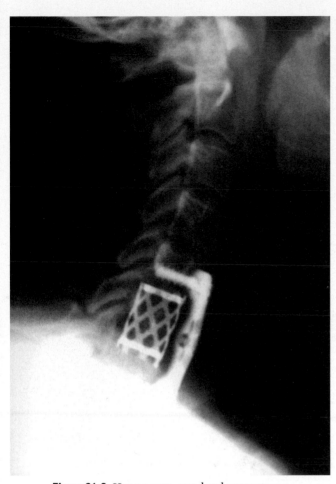

Figure 31.6 Harms cage, one-level corpectomy.

Except in cases of total spondylectomy for tumor, the central corpectomy bed is flanked on either side by a shell of lateral cortex and disc material. The method of decompression is addressed elsewhere in this volume. Ventral reconstruction seeks to restore the normal height of the vertebral column, which is frequently foreshortened with loss of cervical lordosis by the underlying conditions dictating the need for decompression. In the course of decompression axial distraction is routinely applied via halter or cranial tong traction, and a thin interscapular roll is placed to help establish slight neck extension. Screw-in posts are inserted into the ventral midbodies of the rostral and caudal vertebrae adjacent to the decompression. Powerful forces can then be applied using a rack and pinion distraction arm, which has the combined effect of lengthening the anterior column of the spine and restoring lordosis. In significantly kyphotic deformities, divergent distraction techniques may be advantageous. As a consequence of this maneuver, the planes of the recipient rostral and caudal end plates are brought more nearly to a parallel alignment. Some divergence will usually persist however, and this needs to be accounted for in the subsequent fashioning of the construct. Often there is a small ledge of osteophyte projecting caudally from the anteroinferior edge of the rostral vertebral body. This should be removed to create a relatively planar end plate surface that will allow unimpeded insertion of the construct. The car-

tilaginous end plates are scraped down with curettes, but every effort is made to leave the bony end plates inviolate.

Once the desired degree of distraction in the corpectomy bed has been obtained, calipers are used to measure the desired construct length at both its anterior and posterior limits. Because of the divergence of the end plates, the anterior height is often 1 to 2mm longer than the posterior measure. We are most experienced with the Harms system, which provides cages suitable for use in the cervical spine as straight cylindrical stock ranging from 12 to 16mm in diameter and from 30 to 50mm in length. Oval stock 15mm × 12mm is also available, as well as prelordosed tubular stock. We advise selecting the largest cage that can be safely accommodated within the corpectomy bed, without intruding on the ventral spinal canal. The cage is marked as to its desired anterior and posterior heights, according to caliper measurements, and is cut accordingly. For straight mesh stock spanning three or more levels, it may be advantageous to cut the lower end of the cage on a slight bias to optimally accommodate the divergence of the end plates to which they will be paired. Other systems offer end-fitted, lordotic end caps as an alternative to direct cage modification. Reference to intraoperative lateral fluoroscopy showing the rostral and caudal recipient end plates, with distraction applied, is helpful in forming a mental image of the desired cage geometry. Ideally there will be full cross-sectional contact between each end of the cage and the adjoining end plate.

An appropriately sized end-cap is fitted to one end of the cage. The bias cut is never so severe as to preclude a snug fit. The cage can then be loaded with morselized autologous bone obtained from the corpectomy bed itself, or elsewhere. This bone is repeatedly tamped down to create dense packing within the construct without any internal voids. Good packing of the construct is recognizable when graft material is seen extruding centrifugally through the interstices of the mesh. Only in cases of tumor and infection is locally derived graft material quantitatively or qualitatively insufficient. If necessary, it is easily supplemented by cancellous autograft obtained from the iliac crest or combined with allograft. The second end cap is seated, and a final bit of additional graft is packed into the central orifice of each end cap. Just before the cage is to be inserted, the distractor mechanism is opened to lengthen the corpectomy trough an additional 1 to 2mm. The cage is then seated in the corpectomy bed until a good friction fit is achieved. Small impactors are applied alternately over the rostral and caudal ends of the cage, tapping the cage deeper into the corpectomy trough until its presenting edge is recessed just below the ventral-most cortices of the adjacent vertebrae. At this point axial traction and distractive forces are removed to allow elastic recoil of the soft tissues to lock the construct in place. A nerve hook can be inserted behind the cage to assess the tightness of the fit and confirm the patency of the ventral spinal canal. Anteroposterior and lateral fluoroscopy are then used to control proper placement in coronal and sagittal planes, and any indicated adjustments are performed.

Reconstruction of one- and two-level corpectomies is generally straightforward. For degenerative conditions, we

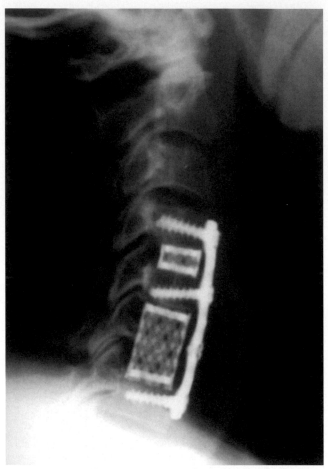

Figure 31.7 Harms cages, one-level corpectomy and adjacent disc-space arthrodesis.

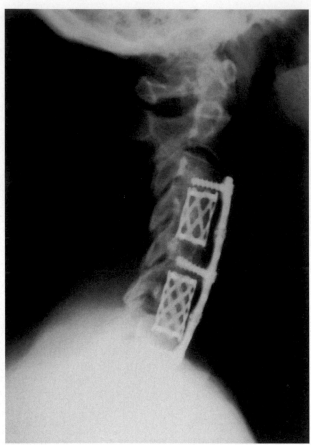

Figure 31.8 Harms cages, two-level discontinuous corpectomies.

secure the construct with a dynamic plate and screw system, which provides additional rigidity during neck extension and helps limit subsidence during healing. If bone quality and screw purchase are good, use of an external orthosis is optional in single-level corpectomy patients. In weakened osteoporotic bone, bicortical screw fixation of the anterior plate and an orthosis are used. Especially precarious constructs are supplemented with posterior instrumentation and fusion. For acute spinal traumas, a rigid plate and screw system is preferred because of the frequently associated soft-tissue injury and the heightened risk of instability. A minor degree of subsidence is routinely observed during healing, but graft or plate dislodgement or significant cervical straightening is distinctly unusual.

As an alternative to long-segment corpectomy or multi-level discectomy in patients with need for decompression/fusion at three or more motion segments, we have performed corpectomy plus adjacent level discectomy (three motion segments), or "discontinuous corpectomies" with retention of an intervening body (four motion segments). A ventral plate is thereby afforded at least two extra intermediary points of fixation (Figures 31.7 and 31.8). The advantage of this technique over multilevel discectomy is the speed and completeness of the decompression and the provision of locally derived autograft. We have experienced no instances of plate loosening or graft migration in this group of patients.

Reconstruction of three- and four-level corpectomies is more problematic. The potential for graft migration, plate loosening, and end-plate fracture is considerably greater. Frequently, such patients are being operated for correction of a kyphotic deformity and the bone quality can be suboptimal. Long-segment ventral plates fixated only at their rostral and caudal ends are very prone to failure. Failure typically occurs at the inferior end of the construct where the hardware either fractures or levers off of the caudal body (Figure 31.9). Simple "kick plates" fitted to the vertebral bodies at the rostral and caudal ends of the construct are worthy of consideration in this circumstance. They do not contribute to the inherent stability of the construct other than to prevent ventral extrusion of the implant. Immediate stability is secured by supplemental, instrumented posterior spinal fusion and/or halo immobilization (Figure 31.10).

Summary

Structural autografts and allografts have proved themselves generally satisfactory in single-level disc-space arthrodesis and in the reconstruction of single-level corpectomy defects. The risk of graft fracture, resorption, extrusion, and nonunion rises as fusion is extended over an increasing number of motion segments. A variety of interbody devices have been developed with shared advantages of strength,

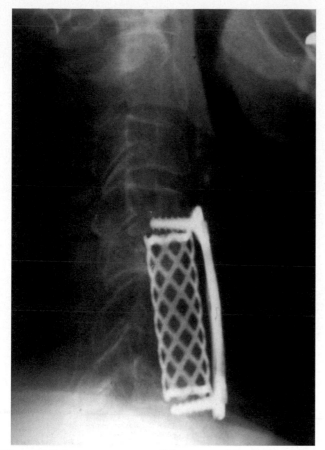

Figure 31.9 Long segment cage failure at caudal end of construct.

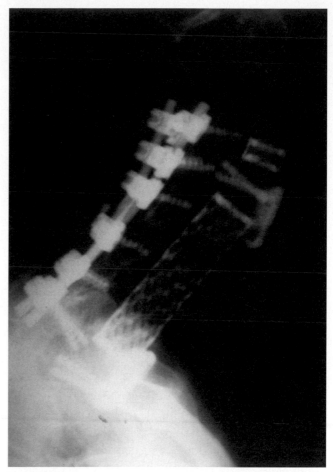

Figure 31.10 Long segment reconstruction with kick plate and posterior fixation.

resistance to collapse and extrusion, and an ability to function as carriers of bone graft "generators," while averting the morbidity associated with structural autograft harvest. Polymer cages have the additional benefits of radiolucency and a more physiologic elastic modulus.

Interbody cages have a mechanical function as spacer devices, restoring structural integrity to the load-bearing anterior column of the spine. The development of so-called biologics such as recombinant human bone morphogenetic protein (rhBMP) will begin to shift the focus from the mechanical properties of these devices to their biologic role as delivery systems for the mediators of bony fusion. Once fusion has been achieved, the function of the prosthesis itself has been supplanted. Bioabsorbable devices, which are "digested" after this function has been fulfilled, are therefore a logical next step in the future evolution of interbody device design. However, the ultimate role for interbody devices may be in the preservation or restoration of the physiologic motion segment rather than in its abolition. This seems to us to be the most auspicious direction for future pursuit in our own laboratory.

Disclosure Statement

Dr. Cahill received grant and research support from Medtronic Sofamor Danek and Synthes. Some of the devices described in this chapter have not received approval from the FDA for use as implants in the cervical spine. Please refer to product labeling information for approval status.

REFERENCES

1. Agrillo U, Mastronardi L, Puzzilli F: Anterior cervical fusion with carbon fiber cage containing coralline hydroxyapatite: preliminary observations in 45 consecutive cases of soft-disc herniations. *J Neurosurg* 96(3 Suppl): 273-276, 2002.

2. al-Hami S: Cervical monosegmental interbody fusion using titanium implants in degenerative, intervertebral disc disease. *Minim Invasive Neurosurg* 42:10-17, 1999.

3. Bartels RH, Donk R, van Azn RD: Height of cervical foramina after anterior discectomy and implantation of a carbon fiber cage. *J Neurosurg* 95(1Suppl):40-42, 2001.

4. Brantigan JW, Steffee AD, Geiger JM: A carbon fiber implant to aid interbody lumbar fusion. Mechanical testing. *Spine* 16(6 Suppl):S277-282, 1991.

5. Brooke NS, Rorke AW, King AT, Gullan RW: Preliminary experience of a carbon fibre cage prosthesis for treatment of cervical spine disorders. *Br J Neursurg* 11:221-227, 1997.

6. Castro FP, Holt RT, Majd M, Whitecloud TS III: A cost analysis of two anterior cervical fusion procedures. *J Spinal Disord* 13:511-514, 2000.

7. Cho D-Y, Liau W-R, Lee W-Y, *et al*: Preliminary experience using a polyetheretherketone (PEEK) cage in the treatment of cervical disc disease. *Neurosurgery* 51: 1343-1349, 2002.

8. Cloward RD: Treatment of acute fractures and fracture dislocations of the cervical spine by vertebral body fusion. *J Neurosurg* 18:205, 1961.

9. Das K, Couldwell WT, Sava G, Taddonio RF: Use of cylindrical titanium mesh and locking plates in anterior cervical fusion; technical note. *J Neurosurg* 94(1Suppl):174-178, 2001.

10. Hacker RJ: A randomized prospective study of an anterior cervical interbody fusion device with a minimum of 2 years of follow-up results. *J Neurosurg* 93(2Suppl):222-226, 2000.

11. Hacker RJ, Cauthen JC, Gilbert TJ, Griffith SL: A prospective randomized multicenter clinical evaluation of an anterior cervical fusion cage. *Spine* 25:2646-2655, 2000.

12. Hodges SD, Humphreys SC, Eck JC, et al: A modified technique for anterior multilevel cervical fusion. *J Orthop Sci* 7:313-316, 2002.

13. Kaden B, Schramm J, Fuhrmann G, Hoffmann CH: Titanium intervertebral disc and instrumentation for fusion in anterior cervical discectomy; technical note. *Neurosurg Rev* 18:25-29, 1995.

14. Kale S, Cahill DW: Current anterior techniques for single-level cervical disc disease. *Contemp Neurosurg* 24(6):1-8, 2002.

15. Kandziora F, Pflugmacher R, Schaefer J: Biomechanical comparison of cervical spine interbody fusion cages. *Spine* 26:1850-1857, 2001.

16. Lange M, Philipp A, Fink U, Oeckler R: Anterior cervical spine fusion using RABEA-Titan-Cages avoiding iliac crest spongiosa: first experiences and results. *Neurol Neurochir Pol* 34:64-69, 2000.

17. Majd ME, Vadhva M, Holt RT: Anterior cervical reconstruction using titanium cages with anterior plating. *Spine* 24:1604-1610, 1999.

18. Matge G: Anterior interbody fusion with the BAK-cage in cervical spondylosis. *Acta Neurochir* (Wien) 140:1-8, 1998.

19. Matge G, Leclercq TA: Rationale for interbody fusion with threaded titanium cages at cervical and lumbar levels. Results on 357 cases. *Acta Neurochir* (Wien) 142:425-433, 2000.

20. McAfee PC, Cunningham BW, Lee GA, et al: Revision strategies for salvaging or improving failed cylindrical cages. *Spine* 24:2147-2153, 1999.

21. Papavero L, Zwoenitzer R, Burkard I, et al: A composite bone graft substitute for anterior cervical fusion; Assessment of osseointegration by quantitative computed tomography. *Spine* 27:1037-1043, 2002.

22. Profeta G, de Falco R, Iannociello G, et al: Preliminary experience with anterior cervical microdiscectomy and interbody titanium cage fusion (Novus CT-Ti) in patients with cervical disc disease. *Surg Neurol* 53:417-426, 2000.

23. Saunders RL, Traynelis VC: Interbody strut techniques. In EC Benzel (ed): *Spine Surgery*. New York, Churchill-Livingstone, 1999, pp 241-248.

24. Savolainen S, Rinne J, Hernesniemi J: A prospective randomized study of anterior single-level cervical disc operations with long-term follow-up: surgical fusion is unnecessary. *Neurosurgery* 43:51-55, 1998.

25. Sawin PD, Traynelis VC, Menezes AH: A comparative analysis of fusion rates and donor-site morbidity for autogenic rib and iliac crest bone grafts in posterior cervical fusions. *J Neurosurg* 88:255-265, 1998.

26. Shimamoto N, Cunningham BW, Dmitriev AE, et al: Biomechanical evaluation of stand-alone interbody fusion cages in the cervical spine. *Spine* 26:E432-436, 2001.

27. Shono Y, McAfee PC, Cunningham BW, Brantigan JW: A biomechanical analysis of decompression and reconstruction methods in the cervical spine: emphasis on a carbon-fiber composite cage. *J Bone Joint Surg Am* 75A:1674-1684, 1993.

28. Smith GW, Robinson RA: Treatment of certain spine disorders by anterior removal of the intervertebral disc and interbody fusion. *J Bone Joint Surg Am* 40:607, 1958.

29. Zdeblick TA, Ghanayem AJ, Rapoff AJ, et al: Cervical interbody fusion cages: an animal model with and without bone morphogenetic protein. *Spine* 23:758-766, 1998.

CHAPTER 32

Cervical Laminotomy, Laminectomy, Laminoplasty, and Foraminotomy

Michael J. Ebersold and Richard B. Raynor

General Principles

Because there are multiple procedures that allow access to the spinal canal or neural foramina, each procedure has advantages and disadvantages. Ventral, dorsolateral (i.e., transpedicle and costotransversectomy), and dorsal options have been described.* The dorsal exposures have three advantages: (1) less surgical effort is required when exposing or decompressing multiple levels; (2) often, stability after the dorsal approach does not require the addition of instrumentation and/or fusion, and therefore may eliminate the need for immobilization and donor site morbidity; and (3) the procedure does not necessarily stiffen the motion segments, and therefore does not accelerate spondylotic degeneration at adjacent levels.

Severe spinal deformities, however, have resulted from inadequate consideration of overall spinal stability, especially the young patients and those with minimal degenerative changes who undergo laminectomy at multiple levels. Patients with extensive degenerative changes seem to have less overall spinal mobility, and the degenerative changes themselves can lend some additional stabilizing effect. Patients with neurologic disease such as intrinsic tumors or syrinxes, however, frequently seem to develop spinal deformity. This appears to be a result of compromised or asymmetric muscle tone, caused by altered neurologic input, in addition to the bone disruption from the surgery. Replacement of the dorsal elements may help to prevent spinal deformity in some cases.[23]

In other cases more extensive dorsal fusion, with or without instrumentation, may be required. In an effort to further minimize instability and abnormal spine biomechanics, various other modifications of the laminectomy have been developed. Partial hemilaminectomy, with or without foraminotomy, has become the standard dorsolateral exposure for the cervical and lumbar disc. An even more lateral exposure, using a transpedicular or costotransversectomy approach, is often used successfully for the more lateral thoracic disc because of the limited room

of the relatively smaller spinal canal. The standard laminectomy is not acceptable for the removal of the thoracic disc. The more broad-based central defects, especially those that extend into the spinal cord parenchyma itself, or those associated with a kyphotic deformity, are best approached through a more ventral approach.

Multiple-Level Laminectomies

The effects of multiple-level laminectomies on spinal stability have been of concern for some time. Tachdjian and Matson[31] reported a 40% incidence of cervical kyphosis in 115 children, whereas Dubousset et al.[5] reported the development of cervical deformity in 78% of 55 children undergoing laminectomy. Although not all of these deformities required further surgical treatment, improper spine mechanics (especially in the young and in the more mobile spine) can result in worrisome spinal deformity, musculoskeletal symptomatology, and deformity progression.

A recent review of problems associated with multiple-level lumbar laminectomy in 36 consecutive patients under age 30 also suggests a need for concern about the development of deformity. In this study 12 patients under age 17 and 24 patients between ages 18 and 30 were reviewed. Spinal deformity was diagnosed in five patients at 2 months to 7 years postoperatively. These patients were ages 16, 13, 17, 20, and 28 at the time of their initial operation. There was no obvious correlation among the incidence of the deformity, the number of lamina removed, and the neurologic condition after the laminectomy. A further review of these data suggests that it was extremely important to follow the patient (especially the young patient) who undergoes a lumbar laminectomy combined with unilateral total facetectomy.[24]

Laminoplasty

In an effort to further maintain the dorsal integrity of the spine, various additions and modifications of the laminectomy have been proposed. Various forms of laminoplasty that return the removed lamina to its original site have been developed. Some advocate total bilateral removal of the lamina. Others have suggested a modification of this removal; that is, the open-door laminoplasty, as initially described by Hirabayashi et al.[17] The open-door laminoplasty has recently been used in the treatment of cervical spondylotic myelopathy.[11,12,17,29] Reconstructing the spinal canal may, in fact, offer some benefits to the spinal cord function by creating a more natural environment. The effects of muscle scarring to the dura mater, rather than the normal spinal structures, would also seem to adversely affect mechanical aspects of the spine as a unit. In some cases it could result in additional postlaminectomy pain. Headaches and neck pain seem to be decreased in patients who undergo a posterior fossa craniectomy, if the craniectomy defect is covered by a cranioplasty. The explanation for this decrease in postoperative symptomatology is unclear, although one might postulate that the muscle-dural juncture can result in undesirable symptomatology. Care must be taken to not limit the decompression or increase the risks of surgery by doing the laminoplasty, because true instability or deformity development is rather

---

*References 1-17,26,30,32,34.

uncommon, especially when decompressing patients with degenerative disease free of any pre-existing instability.

Techniques

Intraoperative Patient Positioning and Monitoring

Most spine surgeons find the prone position quite acceptable for the dorsal approaches to the spine. Some, however, prefer the sitting position for surgery that involves the cervical level, and even the upper several thoracic levels. This is particularly so when instrumentation and fusion is not required. The problems associated with air embolism when using the sitting position are extremely infrequent, even though careful monitoring can detect air entering the venous system in nearly 7% of all cervical laminectomies in the sitting position.[16] However, the incidence of significant air embolism for operations at the upper cervical levels (i.e., a foramen magnum region procedure) is slightly more common. Routine monitoring methods include precordial Doppler and the measurement of end-expired carbon dioxide and nitrogen with a mass spectrometer. Esophageal echocardiography may be used in cases when the risk seems to be greater. When the sitting position is used, a venous catheter is generally placed with its tip in the upper-right atrium, so that any air that enters the venous system can be aspirated.

It is emphasized that air embolism can occur whenever a surgical procedure is done in which there are open veins in the surgical field at a height that is several centimeters above the heart. In such cases proper monitoring and therapeutic options should be used. When using the prone position, one is sometimes tempted to flex the neck to have better exposure to the foramen magnum region. This should generally be avoided, regardless of whether the prone or sitting position is used. This is especially so when there is a coexisting upper cervical instability.

As in any surgical case, care must be taken to properly position the patient to avoid undue pressure on nerves or bony prominences and to avoid brachial plexus or sciatic nerve stretch injuries.

Electrical monitoring for somatosensory evoked potentials and nerve root function should be considered, especially in cases that involve extensive spine surgery, long operative times, and significant potential for neurologic injury. Because of the extremely low likelihood of nerve root or spinal cord injury with cervical decompression, it is doubtful whether such monitoring is cost effective. Patients who undergo surgery involving extensive epidural dissections, instrumentation, and surgery for tumor removal, however, may be candidates for such monitoring. Another option is to do a "wake-up" test at various times in patients at significant risk.

Incisions and Spine Exposure

After the patient has been properly positioned, prepped, and draped, a vertical skin incision is made to expose only the dorsal elements that need to be addressed during the surgical procedure. Unnecessary dissection not only can cause increasing postoperative discomfort, but also can

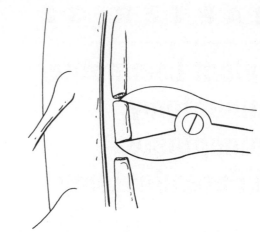

Figure 32.1 A rongeur can be used safely and efficiently, especially to begin the laminectomy if the jaws are biting parallel to the dura mater and do not compress the underlying dura or nerve elements. The tip of the rongeur must not be placed in a plane below the deepest extent of the lamina.

result in facet joint damage, unnecessary postoperative scarring, and soft-tissue injury, which can result in additional early, as well as possibly late, morbidity. In young children lamina exposure may result in undesired spontaneous dorsal element fusion. With such limited exposure, radiographs are usually needed to identify and confirm the appropriate level. A subperiosteal dissection is then carried out to free the muscle and soft tissue from the spinous process and lamina.

Dural Sac Decompression

Many dogmatic statements have been made concerning the technique used to remove the lamina. Suffice it to say that, whatever technique is used, great care must be taken not to compress the underlying dura or neural elements. Many spine surgeons use a high-speed drill to thin the lamina so that the very thin remaining lamina can be peeled from the dura with a curette, or possibly a very small angle Kerrison rongeur. Depending on the particular circumstances, however, even the 1mm foot plate of an angled Kerrison rongeur may not be appropriate to place between the dura and lamina if the canal is quite narrow.

Although much has been written about not using an Adson or Leksell rongeur to remove the lamina, these instruments can be used safely, if the jaws of the instruments are not placed beneath the lamina. If the instrument is used to thin the lamina, while avoiding the placement of the jaw beneath the lamina (Figure 32.1), the lamina can be very efficiently thinned, and in some cases removed without moving or compressing the underlying dura mater or elements. In the lumbar region, where there is somewhat more room because of the absence of the spinal cord and the more forgiving nature of the cauda equina, it is sometimes tempting to remove the lamina with an angled Kerrison rongeur (Figure 32.2). Once again, however, it should be remembered that the foot plate of an angled Kerrison rongeur can be placed in a manner to close it parallel to the dura rather than compressing the underlying dura. In the case of rather severe lumbar stenosis or a very large extruded disc, the

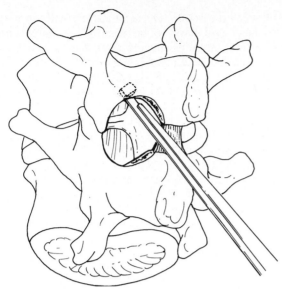

Figure 32.2 Great care must be used to not compress the underlying neural elements when placing the foot plate of an angled Kerrison rongeur under the lamina. In an already tight spinal canal, the aforementioned procedure is not acceptable. In the case of cervical foraminal stenosis the tight foramen may also not permit using even the smallest foot-plated Kerrison rongeur.

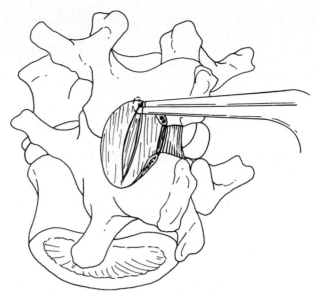

Figure 32.3 A curette or a very thin-footed Kerrison rongeur can be used to cut the ligamentous attachments to the lamina, after the desired amount of lamina has been removed.

nerve root or cauda may, in fact, be very compressed in the lateral recess, and the addition of the foot plate of the angled Kerrison rongeur in the lateral recess may result in neurologic injury. It is always important to remove bone in a way that does not result in any significant compression of the underlying dura mater or nerve root.

Many techniques have been used for removing the ligamentum flavum. However, one of the more common methods is to make a vertical incision parallel to the longitudinal axis of the spinal canal where the lamina meets the spinous process. After the dura mater can just be seen through this longitudinal cut, a blunt instrument such as the tip of a bayonet can be placed into this longitudinal division in the ligamentum flavum to further enlarge this opening in the direction of the fibers. The blunt tip of the bayonet would not be likely to go through the underlying dura mater, even when it is quite thin. After this vertical incision in the ligament has been made, a microangled Kerrison rongeur or curette can be used to cut the remaining ligament, as it attaches to the lamina above and below (Figure 32.3). By including a millimeter or so of bone in the jaw bite of the microangled rongeur, the ligament can be cut against the bone and maximize the dura exposure for the amount of bone removal. As previously stated, care should be taken not to remove more bone than is needed to deal with the pathology. Too small of a laminotomy or exposure, however, can require unnecessary nerve root or dural retraction, and certainly the removal of additional bone or ligament would be preferable to retraction of neural elements.

Nerve Root Decompression

The keyhole laminoforminotomy for cervical nerve root compression is generally quite safe and can provide ade-

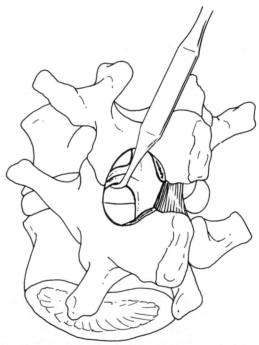

Figure 32.4 During a cervical discectomy, minimal upward retraction of the nerve root allows for exposure of the disc. Care must be taken to elevate both the sensory and the motor roots. Very minimal bone removal ("keyhole exposure") is acceptable, but not at the expense of inadequate exposure of the dura mater and nerve root, of excessive nerve root retraction, or of significantly increasing the risk of dural laceration.

quate exposure. It does not seem to add extra operative time or morbidity, and yet, preserves normal supportive anatomic structures (Figure 32.4). Enlarging the foramen can be accomplished without necessarily destroying the facet joint.[25] Facet joint destruction can result in decreased stability.[21] Raynor[28] demonstrated that more than 50% of bilateral facet removal significantly compromises sheer strength of the cervical spine. The entire length of the foramen can be enlarged safely with the use of curettes or a drill, with preservation of greater than 50% of the facet, by initially working parallel and just inferior to the nerve root and then, as room is gained, by removing the rim of foramen just dorsal to the nerve root (Figure 32.4).[23,28,33]

Surgery for Cervical Disc Herniation and Foraminal Stenosis

In the case of cervical disc disease or cervical nerve root compression caused by foraminal stenosis, the decompression is begun with a small partial hemilaminectomy above and below the site of expected pathology. Removing the inferior margin of the superior lamina laterally and the attached ligamentum flavum allows for identification of the lateral dural margin and the nerve root origin. The axilla is then easily exposed. Although the major exposure is inferior, it is desirable to also expose the superior border of the nerve root to allow for its complete identification and achieve some space for the minimal mobilization of the nerve root. This is required when the extruded disc is removed. Often there is a small amount of room inferior to the nerve root. This room can be enlarged with a curette or high-speed drill. Care must be taken to ensure one has enough of the nerve root axilla exposed so that the motor root is not confused with extruded disc material. Identification of the top of the pedicle is helpful in avoiding motor rootlet damage. Inadequate exposure within the axilla can result in the surgeon unknowingly separating the sensory and motor nerve roots, and assuming that one root is either fibrous tissue or disc material. After identifying the axilla and doing at least enough foraminotomy so that the surgeon is confident about the course of the nerve root, a blunt hook can be used to elevate the involved cervical nerve root slightly, so that the undersurface can be explored for the presence of a soft-disc extrusion (Figure 32.4).

If there is a soft-disc extrusion, the posterior longitudinal ligament (PLL) can be incised with a knife, and a small amount of pressure on the above PLL will sometimes cause the fragment to be milked outward beneath the slightly elevated root. A small forceps can then be used to remove this fragment. After removal, there is often some additional room so that the foramen can be better explored and enlarged, if necessary. If there is only a small, hard bony ridge beneath the nerve root, it is not necessary to remove this, because often simply decompressing the nerve root dorsally far out into the foramen provides adequate relief of symptoms. Nevertheless, it is sometimes desirable to remove a lateral osteophyte that rests ventral to the nerve root, if such seems to be significantly compressing the nerve root, even after the dorsal decompression. The PLL is opened below the axilla, and using the PLL to protect the nerve root and dura mater, a 2 to 3mm diamond burr can be inserted into the PLL opening, and the underlying bone and osteophyte can be drilled away. The thin, bony rim that remains can be fractured into the now underlying decompression site to decompress the cervical nerve root without undue

retraction of the root.[27] Occasionally a small amount of medial facet will have to be removed to satisfactorily visualize the course of the foramen, but in general the foramen can be enlarged while keeping the majority of the facet joint intact. This can be accomplished by restricting bone resection to the medial part of the facet.[23,28]

After an extruded cervical disc removal, it is not necessary or advisable to enter the cervical disc space to remove additional degenerated disc material from behind, since such manipulation can be dangerous. Usually, visualizing the interspace would require significant nerve root retraction, which in itself could result in nerve root injury. Fortunately, such additional disc material need not be removed, as suggested by the fact that the recurrence rate for a cervical disc without entering the disc space is less than 1% in most series.

Laminoplasty

Because of the high incidence of spinal cord compression secondary to ossification of the posterior longitudinal ligament (OPLL), (a condition prevalent in Japan), Japanese surgeons have been innovative in developing decompression procedures. The biomechanical effects of laminectomy have been under scrutiny, especially in extensive decompressions involving multiple levels. There have been reports of instability after laminectomy, but these cases appear to involve mainly children and younger individuals whose primary disease is neurologic or rarely, localized bone abnormalities. In our experience, standard decompressive laminectomy, including minimal facetectomy in the older patient with degenerative hyperostotic bone disease, does not significantly affect stability. Occasionally, adequate decompression does require partial facetectomy, and this can have a significant effect on spinal stability.[4,28]

The true biomechanical effect of laminoplasty on the cervical musculature has never been measured though computer simulations; however, attempts at biomechanical testing using devices such as weights and pulleys have been performed. Empirical evidence, as well as intuition, indicates that there is a strong anatomic reason for the multisegmental attachment of the dorsal musculature, an arrangement disturbed by laminectomy.

Quite often patients with cervical stenosis have three or more levels of significant spinal canal compromise. Ventral surgery eliminates motion at the operated segment. This results in additional stress in the remaining motion segments. The more segments fused the greater the incremental increase, especially in the immediately adjacent segments. Long-term follow-up on segmentally fused patients shows significant, often symptomatic, degenerative changes in the adjacent segment in about 8% of patients (personal data).

As the term implies, laminoplasty is a plastic procedure with most of the dorsal bony elements replaced after decompression. This permits the dorsal musculature that has been detached to reattach segmentally to bone. When necessary, a larger facetectomy can be performed on one or both sides, while stability is minimally affected. Cervical motion is slightly affected with the laminoplasty, but at

2 years there does appear to be a significant difference, when compared to ventral fusion over a similar number of levels.[10,18]

Laminoplasty, or laminectomy, is most appropriate when lordosis is present.[2] Reversal of the cervical lordosis (kyphosis) appears to be a contraindication to dorsal procedures, because the cord is unlikely to migrate dorsally after decompression. The straightened spine is a marginal situation. Flexion and extension radiographs may be helpful in the evaluation. Significant ventral compression is a relative contraindication to dorsal decompression, whereas dorsal compression favors the use of dorsal decompression. Although many laminoplasty variations have been described, there does not appear to be a significant difference in outcomes. The objective of a laminoplasty procedure is to decompress the neural elements, and to sustain the effects of this decompression. The technique described here is relatively simple and straightforward and accomplishes the desired objectives.

Technique

The early technique of laminoplasty is rarely done today. This technique involved dissecting the dorsal midline muscles free of their bony attachments, and then cutting the lamina free bilaterally at or near the facet joints. The lamina was then reattached by wires. This method is tedious, and it can be difficult to maintain the decompression space since these attachments do not provide a rigid fixation. The detached dorsal bony elements were often riding free and rarely underwent refusion to the lateral elements.

The Japanese have developed and popularized the technique of open-door laminoplasty. As the name implies, it is modeled after doors. There are basically two types of doors. The first type consists of a one-piece door hinged on one side, which swings open while attached to its hinges. The second type, a French door, consists of two half doors separated down the middle, with each half hinged along its lateral side and swinging open from the middle. There are a number of variations of open-door laminoplasty, but all fall into one of these two major categories.

Open-door laminoplasty

The earliest and probably most common technique is that of Hirabayashi,[14,16] which is described (with modifications) in the following paragraph.

The procedure may be performed in either the prone or sitting position, depending on the experience and preference of the surgeon. It is technically easier in the sitting position because of better operative exposure, but the possibility of air embolus requires experienced anesthesia and careful monitoring. It is emphasized that air can also enter veins when the patient is prone, if the surgical site is above the level of the heart. Rigid fixation of the head is advisable with either position. Some head-neck flexion without increasing spinal cord compression is the optimal position. It is generally advisable to decompress one level above and one level below the stenotic area. However, C2, with its profuse muscular attachments, should be left intact unless it is absolutely necessary to decompress at this level.

A midline skin incision is made over the area to be decompressed. This is extended down to the dorsal spines. Special care is taken to not damage the interspinous ligaments. Using the electrocautery and sharp periosteal elevators, the muscular attachments to the dorsal spines and lamina are dissected subperiosteally. Dissection is continued laterally to the facet margins, taking care to not damage the joint capsules. Appropriate retractors are then placed.

Open-door laminoplasty requires detaching one side of the lamina from its facet, while leaving the opposite side connected. The hinged side is generally on the opposite side of the predominant radicular symptoms.

The high-speed air drill with a small burr (preferably 2mm) is used to make a trough bilaterally in the laminae that are to be opened. This is performed at the lamina-facet junction (Figure 32.5). A trough several millimeters wide is thus created, extending the length of the decompression. This is performed bilaterally, leaving the hinged side with enough cortical bone for support, but thin enough to bend. On the opposite side the bone is burred to a thin layer, which is then resected with a fine Kerrison rongeur. There is usually a lateral extension of ligamentum flavum bridging the gap between the adjacent edges of the lamina. This must be carefully incised, using either a knife or scissors. It is advisable to use magnification to prevent injuring the underlying structures, since the tolerances are tight because of the degenerative changes.

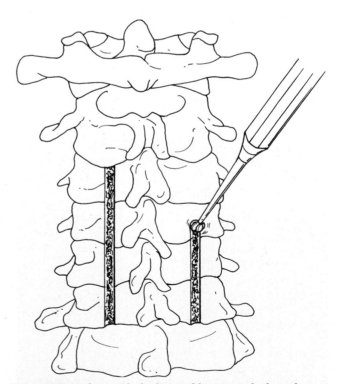

Figure 32.5 With use of a high-speed burr to make lateral cuts for a laminoplasty, the drill can be used to divide the lamina laterally. Fracturing the innermost 1mm of lamina with an osteotome, or completing this inner table bone division with a micro-Kerrison, eliminates the need to place any space-occupying instrument between the lamina and the underlying dura mater.

A "door" has now been formed. It is attached on one side by a thinned bridge of bone between the lamina and facet. The lamina is completely divided on the contralateral side (Figure 32.6).

At this point partial facetectomies and foraminotomies to decompress nerve roots can be performed. However, on the hinged side this is limited by the desirability of keeping a good hinge of bone intact. On the free side the decompression can be more extensive, though biomechanical considerations make it desirable to keep about two thirds of the facet joint intact.[28]

The door is now ready to be opened to provide the decompression of the spinal cord. A Kocher or similar clamp is placed on the intact dorsal spines. They are gently elevated and pulled toward the hinged side. If there is too much resistance, it may be necessary to further thin the bony hinges.

The opened side can also be levered up using the intact bone lateral to the trough as a fulcrum. This technique must be performed with care to prevent damage to the underlying neural structures. As the laminae are slowly and carefully elevated, the underlying soft tissues such as ligamentum flavum and adhesions become visible. These usually hinder the free elevation of the laminar door and must be carefully and sharply cut. The laminar door is elevated enough to give the surgeon a good view of the underlying structures. The dura mater should be cleared of any constricting bands, so that it can expand and freely migrate dorsally.

Once the door has been opened and the decompression achieved, it is necessary to stabilize this opening. Originally this was done by placing sutures between holes drilled in the lamina and the facet joint (Figures 32.7 and 32.8). The anchoring tissue was often sparse, and the sutures could pull out, allowing the door to partially close and diminish the effect of the decompression. Small metal plates are now generally used to maintain the desired lam-

inar elevation. Two or three of these plates, appropriately molded and placed, should stabilize the decompression and prevent the lamina from moving. The muscles are loosely sutured to the dorsal spines, and the wound is closed.

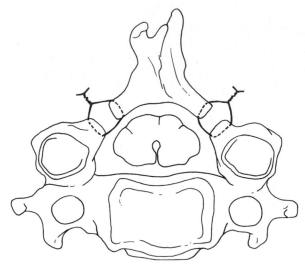

Figure 32.7 Laminoplasty. Cross section of vertebra showing placement of nonabsorbable suture in the distal lamina and medial facet, thus effectively holding the posterior elements up and away from the spinal canal. This effect moves the lamina about 3mm dorsal to its original location and enlarges the spinal canal slightly.

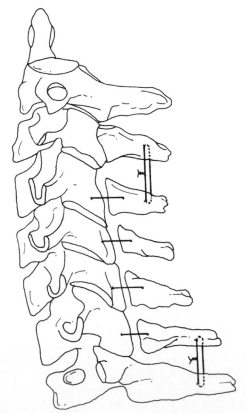

Figure 32.8 Laminoplasty. Lateral view of spine showing the appropriate wiring and suturing involved.

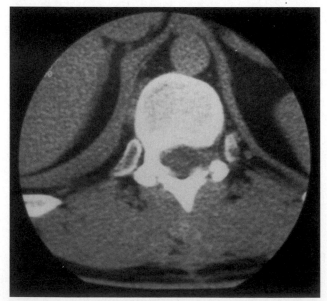

Figure 32.6 Open-door laminoplasty, accomplished by using the high-speed air drill to cut one side of lamina and then thin the opposite side, thus creating the door-like hinge.

French-door laminoplasty

The French-door variation requires splitting the lamina in the midline. The lamina-facet junction is thinned bilaterally, but left intact. Both hemilaminae are then opened, and a graft is placed between the separated medial edges of the lamina.

Comparison of Techniques

There is no difference in the results of the two methods. Open-door laminoplasty appears to be advantageous when decompressing more than two levels, especially in the younger patient prone to degenerative changes above and below a ventral fusion site.

Summary

The safety of the dorsal approaches to the spinal canal are increased by using proper surgical techniques and by being familiar with alternative approaches to the spinal canal. In general all intradural pathology is best approached from the dorsal, or possibly, dorsolateral, approach.

Laminoplasty has been advocated, especially for treating benign disease of the young patient. In older patients, extensive degenerative changes make instability or progressive deformity less of a concern. The risks of such additional surgery, and the associated increase in operative time, needs to be considered against the benefits to be achieved.

More bone removal is not necessarily better. The goal of the dorsal procedures is to achieve adequate visualization for decompression or pathology intervention, and to maintain or achieve spinal stability. Nevertheless, the removal of too little bone can increase the risk of dural tear, not adequately recognizing the nerve root, or missing a free fragment of disc or other pathology. Adding additional steps to any surgical procedure adds extra risk and surgical time. This cannot be defended unless there is a unique, expected benefit from this maneuver. The goal of any decompressive surgery of the cervical spinal cord and roots has to also include maintaining spinal stability without accelerating degenerative changes.

REFERENCES

1. Aldrich F: Posterolateral microdiscectomy for cervical monoradiculopathy caused by posterolateral soft cervical disc sequestration. *J Neurosurg* 72:370, 1990.
2. Benzel E: *Biomechanics of Spinal Stability*, ed 2. Rolling Meadows, IL, American Association of Neurological Surgeons, 2001.
3. Cochrane DD, Steinbok P: Laminotomy: a technical note. *Child's Nerv Syst* 8:226, 1992.
4. Cusick JF, Yoganandan N, Pintar F, *et al*: Biomechanics of cervical spine facetectomy and fixation techniques. *Spine* 13:808-812, 1988.
5. Dubousset J, Guillamant JI, Mechin J: Les compression medullaire non-traumatique de l'infant. *J Rougerie Massen*, Paris, 1973.
6. Ducker TB, Zeidman SM: The posterior operative approach for cervical radiculopathy. *Neurosurg Clin North Am* 4:61, 1993.
7. Fager CA: Management of cervical disc lesions and spondylosis by posterior approaches. *Clin Neurosurg* 24:488, 1977.
8. Fager CA: Posterior surgical tactics for the neurological symptoms of cervical disc and spondylotic lesions. *Clin Neurosurg* 25:218, 1978.
9. Henderson CM, Hennessy RG, Shuey HM, Shackelford EG: Posterior-lateral foraminotomy as an exclusive operative technique for cervical radiculopathy: a review of 846 consecutively operated cases. *Neurosurgery* 13:504, 1983.
10. Herkowitz HN: A comparison of anterior cervical fusion, cervical laminectomy, and cervical laminoplasty for the surgical management of multiple level spondylotic radiculopathy. *Spine* 13:774-780, 1988.
11. Herkowitz HN: Cervical laminoplasty: its role in the treatment of cervical radiculopathy. *J Spinal Disorders* 1:179, 1988.
12. Herkowitz HN: A comparison of anterior cervical fusion, cervical laminectomy, and cervical laminoplasty for the surgical management of multiple level spondylotic radiculopathy. *Spine* 13:774, 1988.
13. Herkowitz HN, Kurz LT, Overholt DP: Surgical management of cervical soft disc herniation: a comparison between the anterior and posterior approach. *Spine* 15:1026, 1990.
14. Herabayashi K: Expansive open-door laminoplasty for cervical spondylotic myelopathy. *Shujutsu* 32:1159-1163, 1978.
15. Hirabayashi K, Satomi K, Sasaki T: Ossification of the posterior longitudinal ligament in the cervical spine. In Sherk HH (ed): *The Cervical Spine*, ed 2. Philadelphia, Lippincott-Raven, 1989, pp 678-692.
16. Herabayashi K, Toyama Y, Cheba K: Expansive laminoplasty for myelopathy in ossification of the longitudinal ligament. *Clin Orthop Rel Res* 359:35-48, 1999.
17. Hirabayashi K, Watanabe K, Wakano K, *et al*: Expansive open-door laminoplasty for cervical spinal stenotic myelopathy. *Spine* 8:693, 1983.
18. Hosono N, Yonenobu K, Ono K: Neck and shoulder pain after laminoplasty: a noticeable complication. *Spine* 21:1969-1973, 1996.
19. Hunt WE, Miller CA: Management of cervical radiculopathy. *Clin Neurosurg* 33:485, 1986.
20. Klara PM, Foley K: Surgical treatment of osteophytes and calcified discs of the cervical spine. *Neurosurg Clin North Am* 4:53, 1993.
21. Krupp W, Schattke H, Muke R: Clinical results of the foraminotomy as described by Frykolm for the treatment of lateral cervical disc herniation. *Acta Neurochir* 107:22, 1990.
22. Losasso TJ, Muzzi DA, Dietz NM, *et al*: 50% nitrous oxide does not increase the risk of venous air embolism in neurosurgical patients operated upon in the sitting position. *Anesthesiology* 77:21, 1992.
23. Nowinski GP, Visarius H, Ing D, *et al*: A biomechanical comparison of cervical laminoplasty and cervical laminectomy with progressive facetectomy. *Spine* 18:1995, 1993.
24. Papagelopoulos P, Emmanuel R, Ebersold M, *et al*: Presented at the 62nd Annual Meeting of American Academy of Orthopedic Surgeons, Orlando, Feb. 16-21, 1995.

25. Raimondi AJ: *Pediatric Neurosurgery: Theoretical Principles, Art of Surgical Techniques*. New York, Springer, 1987, pp 98-105, 107-109.

26. Raynor RB: Anterior or posterior approach to the cervical spine: an anatomical and radiographic evaluation and comparison. *Neurosurgery* 12:7, 1983.

27. Raynor RB: Anterior and posterior approaches to the cervical spinal cord, discs, and roots: a comparison of exposures and decompressions. In Sherk HH (ed.): *The Cervical Spine*, ed 2. Philadelphia, Lippincott-Raven, 1989, pp 659-669.

28. Raynor RB, Pugh J, Shapiro I: Cervical facetectomy and its effect on spine strength. *J Neurosurg* 63:278, 1985.

29. Satomi K, Yukimi N, Kohno T, Hirabayashi K: Long-term follow-up studies of open-door expansive laminoplasty for cervical stenotic myelopathy. *Spine* 19:507, 1994.

30. Snow RB, Weiner H: Cervical laminectomy and foraminotomy as surgical treatment of cervical spondylosis: a follow-up study with analysis of failures. *J Spinal Disorders* 6:245, 1993.

31. Tachdjian MO, Matson DD: Orthopaedic aspects of intraspinal tumors in infants and children. *J Bone Joint Surg* 47A:223, 1965.

32. Yonenobu K, Hosono N, Iwakasi M, *et al*: Neurologic complications of surgery for cervical compression myelopathy. *Spine* 16:1277, 1991.

33. Zdeblick TA, Zou D, Warden KE, *et al*: Cervical stability after foraminotomy: a biochemical in vitro analysis. *J Bone Joint Surg* 74:22, 1992.

34. Zeidman SM, Ducker TB: Posterior cervical laminoforaminotomy for radioculopathy: review of 172 cases. *Neurosurgery* 33:356, 1993.

CHAPTER 33

Interspinous, Laminar, and Facet Fusion

Noel I. Perin and Joseph F. Cusick

Basic to the details of therapeutic intervention, either operative or nonoperative, is an understanding of the biomechanical principles of cervical spine function. These considerations permit the most effective planning of a specific treatment, especially the details of surgical intervention. Generally, in the cervical region the major mechanism of injury is transmission of force through the head. The corresponding changes are usually related to flexion, extension, or rotation, with associated axial compression or distraction. Clarification of these factors will assist the surgeon in designing the most appropriate procedure. A surgeon therefore desires to counteract the major force vectors responsible for the principal injury pattern. (One would not accentuate an extension-compression or extension-distraction injury by increasing extension forces with certain posterior fixation procedures.) The selected method of treatment should be based on the biomechanics of the injury and the experience and preference of the surgeon. This chapter covers the factors predisposing to instability in the subaxial (C3-7) cervical spine and the management of instability, using wire and cable techniques. Allen et al.[2] proposed a mechanistic classification based on biomechanical considerations of the injury vectors. Panjabi and White[25] proposed a working classification especially for acute instability, in which greater than 3.5mm of anterolisthesis, or more than 11 degrees of angulation, constitutes instability in the lower cervical spine, which may be helpful in evaluation. In awake patients who fail to demonstrate radiologic evidence of instability with routine cervical spine films, flexion-extension lateral radiographs should be obtained. Dynamic radiographs, however, should be approached with a level of caution. The situation is often best approached initially by computed tomography (CT), with sagittal reconstruction for full definition of the possible injury patterns. If instability is not demonstrated with the aforementioned studies, yet it is suspected from the increased prevertebral soft-tissue swelling and the severe neck pain, these patients should be placed in a firm cervical collar and the flexion-extension films repeated in 2 weeks. The elapsed time allows muscle spasm to abate and allows demonstration of ligamentous instability on the flexion-extension radiographs.

Initial Management

Accident victims with suspected cervical spine injury should have their head and neck immobilized in a firm cervical collar, or with sandbags, before being transported. In the emergency room, after stabilization of the respiratory and hemodynamic status, a rapid neurologic assessment is undertaken. Radiographs of the cervical spine are obtained, paying special attention to visualization of C7-T1 levels. Patients with evidence of instability on the initial evaluation are placed in traction using Gardner-Wells tongs or a halo ring. Traction is initiated with 10lb, with appropriate head and neck positioning dependent on the mechanism and radiologic appearance of the injury.

Muscle relaxation with agents such as diazepam (Valium) facilitates reduction of the subluxation and alignment of the spine. Weights are added in 5lb increments to a maximum of 35 to 40lb. Lateral cervical spine radiographs are obtained after each weight or position change to monitor cervical spine alignment. Patients who do not reduce on graded cervical traction, and those who cannot tolerate traction, are considered for early surgical reduction and stabilization. All patients with spinal cord injury with moderate to severe neurologic deficit are started on the Solu-Medrol protocol.[29]

Imaging Evaluation

After initial evaluation with plain radiographs, patients who are neurologically intact, and those with residual neurologic function below the level of the injury, should have a magnetic resonance imaging (MRI) scan or a myelogram with postmyelographic CT scan. These studies demonstrate the presence of any soft-tissue compression (disc herniation) on the neural elements. If an MRI scan is performed, a CT scan with bone windows should be obtained to assess the bony anatomy of the fracture. In patients without neurologic function below the level of the injury it may be sufficient to obtain CT images only to assess the anatomy of the fracture.

Timing of Surgery

Surgery for cervical spine instability may be performed ultra early (in less than 6 to 8 hours), early (in 24 to 72 hours), or late (several days to weeks later). The temporal course of events may be conditioned by the presence of other associated injuries, but generally most surgeons operate on these patients between 24 and 72 hours, unless during this period there is deterioration of the patient's neurologic status since admission. Deterioration of the neurologic status may suggest corresponding vertebral artery compromise or other events that may indicate consideration for emergent surgery. In patients with partial neurologic injury, and nonreduction of the subluxation, the ongoing bony or soft-tissue compression may suggest a theoretic advantage to early surgery in reducing secondary neurologic injury; the full validity of this concept has not been fully defined, however.[12] In neurologically intact patients, and patients with a complete neurologic deficit noted from the outset, timing is not as critical. However, early mobilization should minimize pulmonary and other complications.

Operative Techniques
Positioning, Intubation, and Monitoring

Patients in traction are brought to the operating room in their beds. Patients with normal neurologic function, and those with residual neurologic function below the level of the injury, are potential candidates for somatosensory-evoked potential (SSEP) monitoring. If this electrodiagnostic study is elected for use during the operative procedure, preoperative recordings should be obtained. Oral endotracheal intubation entails extension of the neck, which may be hazardous in patients with instability. In the presence of significant instability, after awake fiber-optic intubation the patient is turned to the prone position while awake, and a rapid neurologic examination is carried out before anesthesia is given.

The patient is turned to the prone position, in a firm cervical collar with manual traction applied to the head ring by the surgeon. The head is supported in a cerebellar head rest, and traction is re-established (Figure 33.1). Mayfield skull clamps can be used if alignment can be maintained without traction. The latter mode of fixation minimizes problems with pressure necrosis of the face and potentially disastrous ocular injury. A lateral cervical spine radiograph is obtained to check alignment after turning and positioning the patient.

Exposure

The neck (up to the occiput) and the area around the iliac crest and posterior superior iliac spine are routinely prepared and draped. A midline incision is made in the neck; the length of the incision depends on the number of segments to be addressed. It is critical to stay in the midline to avoid excessive bleeding. The paracervical muscles are stripped subperiosteally from the spine and laminae and retracted laterally. The possibility of pre-existing bony or ligamentous incompetence with associated instability or dural exposure cautions the surgeon to exercise care in the exposure of the posterior elements. Supported by preoperative imaging information, dissection is accomplished sharply; blunt dissection and monopolar cautery are avoided. The dissection is carried to the lateral edge of the facet joints. When possible the supraspinous and interspinous ligaments are preserved. Once the spine is exposed a lateral radiograph is obtained with a marker on the spinous process, to identify the levels to be fused.

Reduction of preoperatively unreduced, unilateral or bilateral locked ("jumped") facets should be attempted at this time. The tip of the superior facet is drilled. Using two straight curettes between the adjacent laminae in the "tire-lever" B-type maneuver and working medially to laterally toward the facet joint, the surgeon removes the superior facet ventral to the inferior facet (Figure 33.2). In cases in which there is a facet fracture with encroachment into the neural foramen this fragment of bone should be removed to relieve the pressure on the exiting nerve root. The surgeon should always be aware of the potential for a lateral mass fracture that mimics a unilateral facet displacement.

Wire and Cable Fixation

The dorsal anatomic configuration of the subaxial cervical spine favors the use of adjunctive wire and cable fixation techniques. Wire and cable can be passed through and around spinous processes, through facet joints, and underneath the laminae. Sublaminar passage of wire in the subaxial spine may injure the spinal cord. Thus most surgeons restrict the use of sublaminar cables and wires to the more

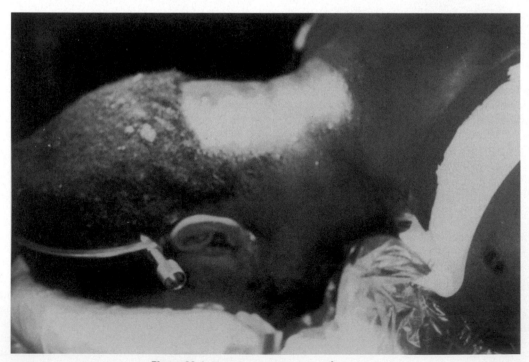

Figure 33.1 Patient prone in cervical traction.

capacious upper cervical spine only, avoiding the regions of cervical spinal cord enlargement. These wires and cables can also be used to hold the bone graft to spine, laminae, and facets.

For maximum efficiency the wire and cable should be strong, malleable, and MRI compatible. The cable systems on the market, in addition to fulfilling these criteria, are coupled with high-quality instrumentation and have generated a renewed interest in the use of wiring in the cervical spine.

Interspinous Wiring

The majority of patients with cervical spine instability can be treated with wiring. Since Rogers first reported a high success rate for cervical fusion with a single, interspinous wiring, numerous techniques of dorsal wiring have been defined. As previously noted, the availability of commercially prepared, braided-wire (cable) systems has improved the technical ease of applying some of these wiring methods. Basically the systems are 18 gauge (Songer) and 20 gauge (Codman), with varying characteristics that may offer improved usage in different constructs. Each system is available in stainless steel or titanium, with specific force application limits that are dependent on the specific type of metal. The braided character of the cables markedly improves strength and malleability. These characteristics are not meant to imply

a universal acceptance of the cable systems in creating dorsal constructs; some surgeons prefer the less malleable Luque wire, especially when applying compression techniques with spinous process wiring.

After exposure of the appropriate levels in the cervical spine and confirmation by radiography, the process of wiring has begun. A transverse hole is made at the junction of the spinous process and lamina of the most rostral level to be fused. This can be made using a power drill and can be completed with a large towel clip. Care should be taken not to angle the drill ventrally and enter the spinal canal. The use of a dental drill appliance permits a straight lateral drill path. The leader wire of the cable system is passed through the drill hole at the spinolaminar junction, and is then carried distally, parallel across the interspace, down to the next most rostral spinous process. The cable ends are then passed in opposite directions around the caudal aspect of that spinous process (Figure 33.3A,B). The cable is tightened with the Tensioner-Crimper, as defined by the recommendations of the system's manufacturer. The wire can also be looped around the rostral border of the spinolaminar junction of the upper level and then threaded in opposite directions through the drill hole at the spinolaminar junction, before being carried caudally.[21] Alternatively, the cable can be passed in the form of a loop through two drill holes at the base of the two spinous processes to be fused. In multilevel fusion each level is wired individually, beginning at the rostral end (Figure 33.4). This latter construct places the majority of the stress between the donor bone and wire, rather than between the spinous process and wire.

With dorsal cervical interspinous compression wiring in the subaxial spine,[3] the base of the most spinous process to be fused is cannulated. Double-stranded, 22-gauge, stainless-steel wire is passed through the hole in the upper spinous process and around the base of the lower spinous process. A single-stranded, 22-gauge wire (compression wire) is placed between the two spinous processes and underneath the twisted wire, and is used to secure the bone graft to the spinous processes. The two ends of the double-stranded cerclage wire are twisted together to achieve the required alignment of the cervical spine (Figure 33.5).

Triple-Wire Technique

Three wires are used in the triple-wire technique.[20] A drill hole is made at the spinolaminar junction, as described previously. Both levels to be fused have drill holes made at the spinolaminar junction. A single-stranded, 20-gauge wire is looped around the rostral border of the rostral process and then passed from opposite directions through the drill hole in that process. The wires are then passed

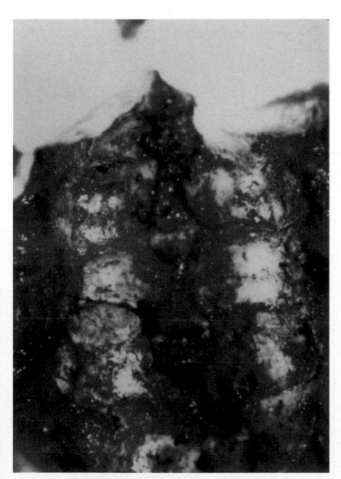

Figure 33.2 Reduction of jumped facet.

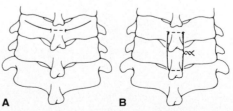

A   B

Figure 33.3 Interspinous wiring technique (single-level fusion).

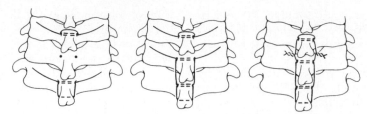

Figure 33.4 Interspinous wiring in multilevel fusion with equalization twists.

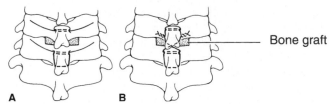

Bone graft

A   **B**

Figure 33.5 Compression wiring: two-wire crossover technique.

caudally, parallel across the interspace down to the drill hole in the lower process. One end of the wire is passed through the drill hole at the caudal process and then looped around the base of the spinous process at that level, before coming back through the same drill hole. It is torqued to the opposite end of the wire that is emerging from the rostral drill hole (Figure 33.6). This wiring arrangement is described as the tethering wire. Two separate 22-gauge wires are passed from either side through the same holes to secure the bone graft. After decortication the two corticocancellous strips of bone are wired down snugly. Biomechanical studies have verified the strength of this construct, and case reviews have described excellent union with this technique.[20]

Oblique Wiring

Most wiring techniques are effective in restricting flexion, but are less effective in limiting extension, especially rotation. Modification of wire fixation has been developed to aid in the treatment of rotational instability, especially as encountered with facet dislocation.[5] A standard dorsal midline incision is made in the neck, with the patient in the prone position. The segments to be fused are exposed, with care taken not to take down the supraspinous, interspinous, and capsular ligaments. After the segmental level is confirmed with lateral cervical radiographs the facet joint capsule at the level to be fused is taken down. If the facet dislocation is not reduced, this can be achieved manually, as described in the previous section. A small, angled curette is used to remove articular cartilage from within the facet joint to be fused. The facet joint is opened using

a Penfield, or periosteal, elevator, which is also used to protect the superior facet below during drilling. To open the facet joint and ease the wire passage, it is advisable to burr down the superior facet. Often the frustration of passing a facet wire is caused by the lack of a widely opened facet joint. A ^{3}/$_{32}$-inch drill, or burr, is used to make the hole in the inferior facet (Figure 33.7). The drill hole is made at the center of the inferior facet, angled slightly medially and caudally. A 22-gauge braided wire or cable is passed through the drill hole, with the facet joint kept open by the Penfield dissector. The end of the wire, or "leader" of the cable, is picked up within the joint with a curved hemostat. By a combination of pushing and feeding the wire from above, together with pulling from below, the wire is threaded. Vigorous pulling and pushing will produce a "Gigli saw" effect and cut through the inferior facet. The upper limb of the wire is passed through the interspinous ligament above the spinous process to be wired, and the lower limb of the wire is passed through the interspinous ligament below the spinous process to be wired (Figure 33.8). The wire is twisted, or the cable is torqued and crimped on the opposite side of the lower spinous process. The application, in a bilateral fashion, establishes both flexion and rotational stability.

If the inferior facet is fractured and cannot take a wire or cable, the wiring must skip to the next intact rostral inferior facet. The upper limb of the wire or cable, in this instance, instead of passing between the middle and caudal spinous processes, passes above the middle spinous process and then joins the caudal limb and passes below the caudal spinous process, as described previously.

Other variations on the technique depend on the injury and fracture pattern and will include unilateral and bilateral oblique wiring, with interspinous wiring and bone grafting.

Facet Wiring

The facet joints are major determinants of cervical motion. Numerous studies have demonstrated that facet joint instability occurs with both dorsal ligamentous and dorsal bony injuries. Functional unit studies have shown approximately a 30% decrease in stiffness to flexion-compression

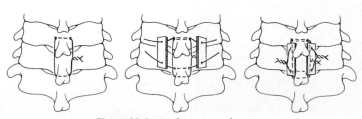

Figure 33.6 Triple-wire technique.

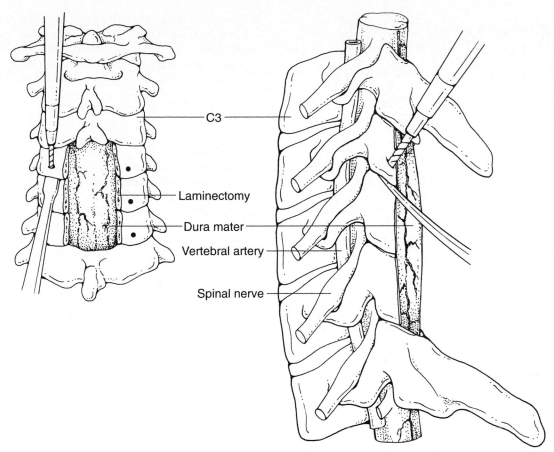

Figure 33.7 Drilling for facet fusion. The hole is being drilled through the inferior facet into the joint.

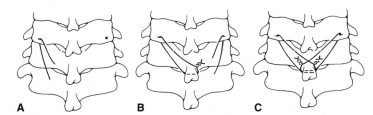

Figure 33.8 Oblique wiring technique: bilateral facet to spinous process wiring.

load with unilateral facetectomy and approximately a 50% decrease in stiffness with bilateral facetectomies. Facet-to-facet or facet-to-spinous process fixation resulted in significant restoration to intact levels, but demonstrated persistent interspinous motion.[11] This latter finding suggests that facet wiring techniques should be associated with spinous process wiring, if available. Other *in vitro* studies have verified the relative contribution of the facet joint to stability and the merits of fixation.[14,28]

The technique of wire placement is similar to oblique wiring. Again, the wide opening formed in the facet joint by drilling down the upper portion of the superior facet facilitates wire or cable passage. A bicortical, biconcave bone graft is laid over the decorticated facets to be fused, and the two limbs of the facet wires are brought around the bone graft and twisted (Figure 33.9).[6] This construct, however, may not provide adequate stiffening and is best considered primarily a method to secure the graft to the facets. A similar technique may also be used to wire down contoured rods and Luque rectangles, especially in post-

laminectomy patients. This latter form of stabilization will significantly decrease flexibility, offering a firmer construct with improved expectations for resistance to flexion, extension, and rotation.[19]

Often, securing the Luque rectangle, or similar metal construct, requires sublaminar and facet wiring, in conjunction with autologous bone grafting of the facets and facet joints. In the passage of sublaminar wires the operator must again consider the potential of compromising underlying neural structures, especially at the level of the cervical spinal cord enlargement. In this aspect preoperative MRI will assist in clarifying the epidural and subarachnoid space at the C2 and T1 levels. Some surgeons prefer Songer cables at the proximal and distal sublaminar points and soft-wire cables (Codman) for facet passage.

Fusion

Bone fusion should be performed in all patients who undergo dorsal subaxial wire or cable fixation. Autograft

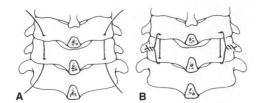

Figure 33.9 Interfacet wiring with ipsilateral wires.

should be used in all cases for best results. The iliac crest is the best source of bone for grafting. An incision is made over the posterior superior iliac spine and extended laterally over the dorsal iliac crest. The incision should not extend more than 6 to 7cm lateral to the posterior superior iliac spine. The cluneal nerves may be injured beyond this point. This can lead to postoperative gluteal numbness and painful neuralgias. The iliac crest is exposed subperiosteally, and the greater sciatic notch is palpated. The superior gluteal artery emerges from the greater sciatic notch and traverses between the gluteus medius and minimus muscles. Injury to the artery may be difficult to control, because the injured proximal stump of the vessel can retract into the pelvis, necessitating a pelvic exploration to control bleeding. Subperiosteal stripping of the gluteal muscles and avoiding the greater sciatic notch will prevent this complication. Strips of corticocancellous and cancellous bone are obtained for onlay grafting.

The dorsal elements of the subaxial spine to be fused are decorticated with a cutting burr. Roughening of the bone is usually sufficient in the cervical spine to facilitate onlay bone fusion. The facet joint to be fused is denuded of capsule, and a small, curved curette is used to remove the joint cartilage and roughen the opposing surfaces of the facet joint. Cancellous bone graft is interposed into the facet joint before the wire or cable is tightened. Further bone graft is laid around the wires over the decorticated spines and laminae. In the technique of facet wiring, bicortical bone graft, contoured in two planes, is laid over the decorticated lateral masses and facets to be fused and wired.

Summary

Injuries to the dorsal osseoligamentous complex are most suited for dorsal wire or cable techniques. The introduction of cable systems into the market has renewed an interest in wire fixation of the cervical spine. The particular technique chosen to stabilize an unstable cervical spine will depend on the injury pattern, the experience, and the preference of the surgeon.

REFERENCES

1. Alexander E: Decompression and fixation in cervical spine fractures: indications and techniques. *Clin Neurosurg* 27:401-413, 1980.
2. Allen BL, Ferguson RL, Lehman TR, *et al*: A mechanistic classification of closed, indirect fractures and dislocations of the lower cervical spine. *Spine* 7:1-27, 1982.
3. Benzel EC, Kesterson L: Posterior cervical interspinous compression wiring and fusion for mid to low cervical spinal injuries. *J Neurosurg* 70:893-899, 1989.
4. Braakman R: Some neurological and neurosurgical aspects of injuries to the lower cervical spine. *Acta Neurochir (Wien)* 22:245-260, 1970.
5. Cahill DW, Bellegarrigue R, Ducker TB: Bilateral facet to spinous process fusion: a new technique for posterior spinal fusion after trauma. *Neurosurgery* 13:1-4, 1983.
6. Callahan RA, Johnson RM, Margolis RH, *et al*: Cervical facet fusion for control of instability following laminectomy. *J Bone Joint Surg* 59A:991-1002, 1977.
7. Capen DA, Garland DE, Waters RL: Surgical stabilization of the cervical spine: a comparative analysis of anterior and posterior spine fusions. *Clin Orthop* 196:229-237, 1985.
8. Cheshire DJ: The stability of the cervical spine following the conservative treatment of fractures and fracture dislocations. *Paraplegia* 7:193-203, 1969.
9. Cooper PR: Operative management of cervical spine injuries. *Clin Neurosurg* 34:650-674, 1987.
10. Cooper PR, Cohen A, Rosiello A, Koslow M: Posterior stabilization of cervical spine fractures and subluxations using plates and screws. *Neurosurgery* 23:300-306, 1988.
11. Cusick JF, Yoganandan N, Pintar FA, Hussain H: Biomechanics of cervical spine facetectomy and fixation techniques. *Spine* 13:808-812, 1988.
12. Ducker TB, Bellegarrigue R, Scallion M, *et al*: Timing of operative care in cervical spinal cord injury. *Spine* 9:525-531, 1984.
13. Fielding W: Current concepts review: the status of arthrodesis of the cervical spine. *J Bone Joint Surg* 70A:1571-1574, 1988.
14. Goel VK, Clark CR, Harris KG, Schulte KR: Kinematics of the cervical spine: effects of multiple total laminectomy and facet wiring. *J Orthop Res* 6:611-619, 1988.
15. Larson SJ: Surgical treatment of cervical fractures. *Contemp Neurosurg* 6:1-4, 1984.
16. Maiman DJ, Barolat G, Larson SJ: Management of bilateral locked facets of the cervical spine. *Neurosurgery* 18:542-547, 1986.
17. Maravilla KR, Cooper PR, Sklar FH: The influence of thin section tomography in the treatment of cervical spine injuries. *Radiology* 126:131-139, 1978.
18. Marshall L, Knowlton S, Garfin SR, *et al*: Deterioration following spinal cord injury: a multicenter study. *J Neurosurg* 66:400-404, 1987.
19. Maurer PK, Ellenbogen RG, Ecklund J, *et al*: Cervical spondylotic myelopathy: treatment with posterior decompression and Luque rectangle bone fusion. *Neurosurgery* 28:680-684, 1991.
20. McAfee PC, Bohlman HH, Wilson WL: Triple wire technique for stabilization of acute cervical fracture dislocations. *Orthop Trans* 10:455-456, 1986.
21. Rogers WA: Treatment of fracture dislocations of the cervical spine *J Bone Joint Surg* 24:245-258, 1942.
22. Roy-Camille R, Saillant G, Berteaux D, *et al*: Early management of spinal injuries. In McKibbon B (ed): *Recent Advances in Orthopedics*. New York, Churchill Livingstone, 1979, pp 57-87.
23. Stauffer ES: Management of spine fractures C3-C7. *Orthop Clinic North Am* 17:45-53, 1986.

24. Wagner FC: Management of acute spinal cord injury. *Surg Neurol* 7:346-350, 1977.

25. White AA, Panjabi M: The role of stabilization in the treatment of cervical spine injuries. *Spine* 9:512-522, 1984.

26. White AA, Southwick WO, Panjabi MM: Clinical instability in the lower cervical spine. A review of past and current concepts. *Spine* 1:15-27, 1976.

27. Yashon D, Tyson G, Vise VM: Rapid closed reduction of cervical fracture dislocations. *Surg Neurol* 4:513-514, 1975.

28. Zdeblick TA, Zau DD, Warden KE, *et al*: Cervical stability after foraminotomy. *J Bone Joint Surg* 74A:22-29, 1992.

29. A randomized controlled trial of methylprednisolone or naloxone in the treatment of acute spinal cord injury: the 2nd National Acute Spinal Cord Injury Study. *New Engl J Med* 322:1405-1411, 1990.

CHAPTER 34

Combined Ventral-Dorsal Procedure

Jaime H. Nieto and Edward C. Benzel

The treatment of spinal disorders is constantly changing and the complexity of procedures continues to escalate. The growing knowledge and understanding of biomechanics, the development of new surgical techniques, and the qualitative improvement of spinal implants have made possible the treatment of much more complex pathology. Most cervical spine disorders that require surgical intervention can be treated with a single operative approach. However, in a very small percentage of patients, their pathology is much more complex, thus requiring a ventral and dorsal combined approach. In the past, such patients often underwent staged operations, subjecting them to repeated anesthesia, hospitalization between procedures, and a higher risk of infection.[9] This chapter addresses some of the common pathologies that require complex cervical spine operations, with emphasis on the combined ventral-dorsal surgical approach.

Trauma

Patients who are involved in motor vehicle accidents, falls, and sports injuries are at risk for cervical spinal cord injuries.[14] Most of these injuries are associated with cervical spine fractures. Of those patients needing surgery, the majority are treated with a single operation with either a ventral or dorsal approach. For complex acute traumatic lesions of the sub-axial cervical spine, a bidirectional (ventral and dorsal) approach may be required for about 1% to 5 % of patients.[5,17] The surgical treatment of cervical spine fractures has been in continuous evolution for the past three decades. The patients requiring a circumferential or combined approach were often initially treated by traction, realignment, and dorsal fusion. One week later, the patients would undergo a ventral decompression and fusion if there was an incomplete neurological recovery.[17,18] With an augmented knowledge of biomechanics and improved instrumentation, the procedure can be combined into a single-stage operation if the patient is medically stable. The benefits of the single ventral/dorsal approach include (1) single anesthetic session, (2) shorter hospital stay, (3) lower risk of infection,[9] (4) fewer airway complications,[19] and (5) preservation of alignment.[5]

Patient selection remains the most important factor relating to surgical success. The decision for surgery is based on the patient's neurologic status, co-morbidities, and presence of instability. There are a variety of methods for evaluating the stability of the spine. These include the three-column theory of Denis,[8] the two-column theory of Holdsworth,[11] the point classification of White and Panjabi,[22,33] and Allen's cervical spine fracture classification. Regardless of the classification system used, the surgeon must be aware of the extent of spinal instability in order to develop a treatment plan and avoid failure.[2,6,30,36] The patients at greatest risk for failure by a single approach are those in whom ligamentous injuries are missed and injuries that cause angulation and retrolisthesis, bilateral dislocation of the facets, and distraction of dorsal interspinous ligaments with or without vertebral dislocation.[2] The posterior longitudinal ligament is often injured by the angulation and retropulsion of bony fragments into the spinal canal.[2]

Imaging studies are of paramount importance. Most patients undergo radiographic or CT evaluation in the emergency department. MRI may be used to rule out occult ligamentous injuries and herniated discs. The best study for the bony anatomy remains the CT, particularly if done with 3-D reconstructions.

Once the patient is hemodynamically stable, the spine may be stabilized with axial traction. The patient may require vasopressors for blood pressure management. Controversy still exists regarding the timing of surgery. In general, if the patient is hemodynamically stable, with no significant co-morbidities, early surgery is facilitated.

In the operating room, traction is continued, and for incomplete or neurologically intact patients, neurophysiologic monitoring may be used. Turning the patient is usually safe once the initial decompression and arthrodesis is performed. In the past, surgeons have used the Stagnara wake-up test during the rotation from supine to prone position (or vice versa) if somatosensory-evoked potentials were not used.[1] Today, if the patient has retained neurologic function, motor- and sensory-evoked potentials are often used. The sequence of the operation components is usually ventral decompression and fusion, followed by dorsal arthrodesis and instrumentation.

Kyphotic Deformity

Rigid kyphotic deformity is a disabling condition and can be a source of pain. It impairs the ability to look forward and to open the mouth.[4,26] It is not only cosmetically unappealing, but it can be a functional handicap.

Kyphotic deformity can develop in patients after cervical spine trauma and after radiation therapy for malignancies in or around the spinal cord, as well as in patients who undergo wide laminectomies for stenosis or intramedullary tumors. With cervical spine trauma, the deformity can develop after the treatment of cervical spine fractures in which ligamentous injuries are missed.

Flexion-compression, flexion distraction, or burst fractures of the vertebral body, combined with dorsal disruption of the posterior longitudinal ligament, are injuries that are at risk of post-injury kyphosis if not treated appropriately.[18] Other conditions that increase the risk for development of kyphotic deformities are the treatment of cervical spinal cord tumors or degenerative spondylosis. Postlaminectomy kyphosis, or "swan neck" deformity, has been documented in as many as 50% of pediatric and 21% of adult patients undergoing bilateral laminectomy.[13,15,21,23,25] Kaptain et al.[13]

reported a 21% incidence of postlaminectomy kyphosis in their review of 46 patients treated with laminectomy for cervical spondylotic myelopathy. Individuals at higher risk are those who have a straightened spine on preoperative imaging studies.

Yeh *et al.*[35] reported the development of sagittal malalignment following laminectomy for intramedullary tumor in 12 out of 27 children. Long-term follow-up is necessary, since it can take several years for the deformity to develop. The population at highest risk is children undergoing bilateral laminectomy for intramedullary tumors, most commonly gliomas.[3]

Indications for surgery include progressive kyphosis of more than 40 degrees or fixed kyphosis of more than 40 degrees and an incomplete neurologic deficit.[18]

For posttraumatic or postlaminectomy kyphosis, the ventral approach with decompression and reconstruction alone has been associated with graft complications and instability.[23,34,37] McAfee *et al.*[18] recommend ventral release, with or without interbody grafting, combined with the dorsal arthrodesis and instrumentation. An illustrative case is depicted in Figure 34.1. It portrays the use of a "front-back-front" strategy, in which instrumentation was only used ventrally.

Neoplasms

Cervical spine involvement by primary bone tumors is 7% for benign primary bone tumors and 15% for malignant primary bone tumors.[7] The most common benign tumors in the cervical spine are osteoid osteoma, aneurysmal bone cyst, and osteoblastoma. In spite of their benign histologic character, they can behave aggressively by their rate of growth, infiltration, recurrence, and compression of neural elements. In these cases, tumor control requires aggressive surgical intervention.[20] The clinical presentation is usually that of a subacute onset and pain. Such initial symptoms are often more intense at night. In the case of osteoid osteoma, the pain is relieved by salicylates.

The cervical spine is affected by metastatic tumors, although much less so than the thoracic and lumbar spine.[31] The symptoms usually involve pain and radiculopathy, often with myelopathy. The common primary sites of origin are breast, lung, and prostate.[12,18] In most instances, steroids and radiation therapy is the primary mode of therapy. Surgical intervention is considered in those patients with progression of neurologic deficits, intractable pain, instability, and failure of conservative therapy. Occasionally, surgery is indicated as first line of treatment when there is a single metastatic radioresistant spine lesion in a patient who is medically fit for surgery.

The goals of surgery are to control pain, preserve neurologic function, and maintain stability with maximal local tumor control. The tumors that require a ventral and dorsal approach are those with extensive involvement of both ventral and dorsal elements or those that have a kyphotic deformity with compression of the spinal cord. In patients with a relatively good prognosis (expected survival greater than 6 months), surgery is indicated in order to achieve

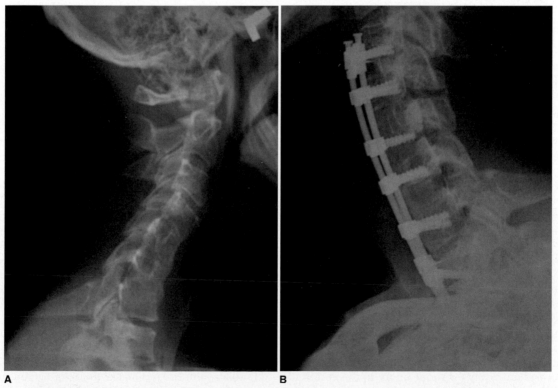

A   **B**

Figure 34.1 A 50-year-old male with prior ventral and dorsal procedures, resulting in significant neck pain and myelopathy. (**A**) A ventral "release" was performed at multiple levels via discectomies. This included the takedown of the old fusion at each segment. A dorsal release was then performed via facetectomies. (**B**) A ventral fusion and deformity correction with instrumentation at each segment level was thus facilitated.

optimal stability with decompression of neural elements. A dorsal decompression and fusion not only augments tumor control, but also provides for better reconstruction and prevention of postsurgical kyphosis. In McAfee's[18] series, ventral reconstruction following corpectomy was accomplished with polymethylmethacrylate with excellent results. One can now consider titanium mesh cages or expandable cages for ventral reconstruction.

Ankylosing Spondylitis

Patients with ankylosing spondylitis are susceptible to spinal injury. These fractures usually involve both the ventral and dorsal elements.[28] The severity of the trauma can be as mild as ground falls or minor motor vehicle accidents, but the effects can be devastating. When the alignment is normal or with minimal displacement, the fractures can be treated with dorsal lateral mass fusion and cervical spine orthosis only.[28] In cases with more than 11 degrees of angulation or more than 3mm of displacement, a ventral and dorsal surgical approach may be best.

Ankylosing spondylitis commonly results in severe kyphotic deformity. The lumbar and thoracic spine regions are affected more often than the cervical spine. Patients with severe deformities have difficulty looking ahead and eating because of difficulty opening the jaw. The deformity usually renders them unable to work, even in the presence of little or no neurologic deficits.

Smith-Petersen[27] first published reports of surgical correction of kyphotic deformity in 1945. Since then, many reports of kyphotic deformity correction by lumbar and thoracic osteotomies have been published.[24] The operation consists of single- or multiple-wedge osteotomies to reestablish the sagittal balance of the spine and for correction of the visual angle. Overcorrection of the sagittal balance can adversely affect the gaze angle.[24] Simmons et al.[26,29] reported their series of osteotomies for correction of cervical ankylosing spondylitis kyphosis using Urist method, with the patient in the sitting position and under local anesthesia. Today the principle remains the same. The osteotomy is performed at the cervico-thoracic junction C7-T1. This level is safe because the vertebral artery usually enters the foramen transversarium at C6. The lamina and spinous process of C7 is completely removed and partial C6 and T1 laminectomies are performed. Bilateral complete foraminotomies at C7-T1 are performed to expose the C8 nerve roots. The spine is then carefully fractured ventrally and the osteotomy gap closed. Today, the procedure is performed under general anesthesia. Internal fixation is used to avoid the plaster body jacket and the halo vest.[20] Duff et al.[10] reported a case of correction of the kyphotic deformity in a different manner. In their report, they performed a two-level wedge osteotomy at C3-4 and C4-5 with dorsal instrumentation, achieving excellent results without injury to the vertebral arteries. Bhojraj[4] reported the correction of kyphotic deformity secondary to Still's disease in a similar manner, but he added the ventral release via ventral discectomy as the first part of the procedure. The dorsal osteotomy and fusion was performed as described above.[4]

Multilevel Corpectomy

Cervical spondylotic myelopathy and ossification of the posterior longitudinal ligament often require multilevel corpectomies for their treatment. For one- and two-level involvement, corpectomies with autograft or allograft and ventral plating may suffice. For longer ventral decompressions, the risk of graft displacement and pseudoarthrosis increases significantly.[16,32] For multilevel corpectomies, the patients are usually placed in a halo vest postoperatively for up to 12 weeks if dorsal instrumentation is not performed. The placement of the halo vest is not only a physical handicap for the patient, but also has complications such as loosening, infection, and intracranial penetration of the skull pins. To avoid some of the inherent complications of the halo vest, immediate internal stabilization with a dorsal arthrodesis may be performed.

REFERENCES

1. Aebi M, Mohler J, Zach GA, Morscher E: Indication, surgical technique, and results of 100 surgically-treated fractures and fracture-dislocations of the cervical spine. *Clin Orthop* 203:244-257, 1986.
2. Allen BL, Ferguson RL, Lehmann TR: A mechanistic classification of closed, indirect fractures and dislocations of the lower cervical spine. *Spine* 7(1):1-28, 1982.
3. Alvisi C, Borromei A, Cerisoli M, Giulioni M: Long-term evaluation of cervical spine disorders following laminectomy. *J Neurosurg Sci* 32(3):109-112, 1988.
4. Bhojraj SY, Dasgupta D, Dewoolkar LV: One-stage "front" and "back" correction for rigid cervical kyphosis. A safer technique of correction for a rare case of adult-onset Still's disease. *Spine* 18(13):1904-1908, 1993.
5. Capen DA, Garland DE, Waters RL: Surgical stabilization of the cervical spine. A comparative analysis of anterior and posterior spine fusions. *Clin Orthop* 196:229-237, 1985.
6. Cybulski GR, Douglas RA, Meyer PR Jr, Rovin RA: Complications in three-column cervical spine injuries requiring anterior-posterior stabilization. *Spine* 17(3): 253-256, 1992.
7. Dahlin DC: *Bone Tumors: General Aspects and Data on 6221 Cases,* ed. 3. Charles C Thomas, Springfield, IL, 1978.
8. Denis F: Spinal instability as defined by the three-column spine concept in acute spinal trauma. *Clin Orthop* 189: 65-76, 1984.
9. Dick J, Boachie-Adjei O, Wilson M: One-stage versus two-stage anterior and posterior spinal reconstruction in adults. Comparison of outcomes including nutritional status, complications rates, hospital costs, and other factors. *Spine* 17(8 Suppl):S310-S316, 1992.
10. Duff SE, Grundy PL, Gill SS: New approach to cervical flexion deformity in ankylosing spondylitis. Case report. *J Neurosurg* 93(2 Suppl):283-286, 2000.
11. Holdsworth F: Fractures, dislocations, and fracture-dislocations of the spine. *J Bone Joint Surg Am* 52(8): 1534-1551, 1970.
12. Jonsson B, Jonsson H Jr, Karlstrom G, Sjostrom L: Surgery of cervical spine metastases: a retrospective study. *Eur Spine J* 3(2):76-83, 1994.

13. Kaptain GJ, Simmons NE, Replogle RE, Pobereskin L: Incidence and outcome of kyphotic deformity following laminectomy for cervical spondylotic myelopathy. *J Neurosurg* 93(2 Suppl):199-204, 2000.

14. Lasfargues JE, Custis D, Morrone F: A model for estimating spinal cord injury prevalence in the US. *Paraplegia* 33:62-68, 1995.

15. Lonstein JE: Post-laminectomy kyphosis. *Clin Orthop* 128:93-100, 1977.

16. Macdonald RL, Fehlings MG, Tator CH, *et al*: Multilevel anterior cervical corpectomy and fibular allograft fusion for cervical myelopathy. *J Neurosurg* 86(6):990-997, 1997.

17. McAfee PC, Bohlman HH: One-stage anterior cervical decompression and posterior stabilization with circumferential arthrodesis. A study of twenty-four patients who had a traumatic or a neoplastic lesion. *J Bone Joint Surg Am* 71(1):78-88, 1989.

18. McAfee PC, Bohlman HH, Ducker TB, *et al*: One-stage anterior cervical decompression and posterior stabilization. A study of one hundred patients with a minimum of two years of follow-up. *J Bone Joint Surg Am* 77(12):1791-1800, 1995.

19. McNamara MJ, Devito DP, Spengler DM: Circumferential fusion for the management of acute cervical spine trauma. *J Spinal Disord* 4(4):467-471, 1991.

20. Mehdian SM, Freeman BJ, Licina P: Cervical osteotomy for ankylosing spondylitis: an innovative variation on an existing technique. *Eur Spine J* 8(6):505-509, 1999.

21. Mikawa Y, Shikata J, Yamamuro T: Spinal deformity and instability after multilevel cervical laminectomy. *Spine* 12:6-11, 1987.

22. Panjabi MM, White AA 3rd: Basic biomechanics of the spine. *Neurosurgery* 7(1):76-93, 1980.

23. Schultz KD Jr, McLaughlin MR, Haid RW Jr, *et al*: Single-stage anterior-posterior decompression and stabilization for complex cervical spine disorders. *J Neurosurg* 93(2 Suppl):214-221, 2000.

24. Sengupta DK, Khazim R, Grevitt MP, Webb JK: Flexion osteotomy of the cervical spine: a new technique for correction of iatrogenic extension deformity in ankylosing spondylitis. *Spine* 26(9):1068-1072, 2001.

25. Sim FH, Svien HJ, Bickel WH, *et al*: Swan-neck deformity following extensive cervical laminectomy. A review of twenty-one cases. *J Bone Joint Surg (Am)* 56:564-580, 1974.

26. Simmons EH: The surgical correction of flexion deformity of the cervical spine in ankylosing spondylitis. *Clin Orthop* 86:132-143, 1972.

27. Smith-Petersen MN, Larson CB, Aufranc OE: Osteotomy or the spine for correction of flexion deformity in rheumatoid arthritis. *J Bone Joint Surg* 27:1-11, 1945.

28. Taggard DA, Traynelis VC: Management of cervical spinal fractures in ankylosing spondylitis with posterior fixation. *Spine* 25(16):2035-2039, 2000.

29. Urist MR. Osteotomy of the cervical spine: Report of a case of ankylosing rheumatoid spondylitis. *J Bone Joint Surg [Am]* 40:833, 1958.

30. Vaccaro AR, Cook CM, McCullen G, Garfin SR: Cervical trauma: rationale for selecting the appropriate fusion technique. *Orthop Clin North Am* 29(4):745-754, 1998.

31. Vieweg U, Meyer B, Schramm J: Tumour surgery of the upper cervical spine—a retrospective study of 13 cases. *Acta Neurochir (Wien)* 143(3):217-225, 2001.

32. Wang JC, Hart RA, Emery SE, Bohlman HH: Graft migration or displacement after multilevel cervical corpectomy and strut grafting. *Spine* 28(10):1016-1021, 2003.

33. White AA 3rd, Johnson RM, Panjabi MM, Southwick WO: Biomechanical analysis of clinical stability in the cervical spine. *Clin Orthop* 109:85-96, 1975.

34. Whitecloud T III, LaRocca H: Fibular strut graft in reconstructive surgery of the cervical spine. *Spine* 1:33-43, 1976.

35. Yeh JS, Sgouros S, Walsh AR, Hockley AD: Spinal sagittal malalignment following surgery for primary intramedullary tumours in children. *Pediatr Neurosurg* 35(6):318-324, 2001.

36. Zeidman SM, Ducker TB: Circumferential spinal fusion: cervical. In Schmidek HH (ed): *Schmidek and Sweet's Operative Neurosurgical Techniques*, ed 4. Philadelphia, WB Saunders, 2000.

37. Zdeblick TA, Bohlman HH: Cervical kyphosis and myelopathy. Treatment by anterior corpectomy and strut grafting. *J Bone Joint Surg (Am)* 71:170-182, 1989.

CHAPTER 35

Ventral and Ventrolateral Spine Decompression and Fusion

Eric M. Massicotte, Michael G. Fehlings, and Alexander R. Vaccaro

Ventral spinal decompression was described by Royle[66] as early as 1928. This approach remained unused until 1956 when Hodgson and Stock[31] reported the use of ventral spinal decompression in the treatment of tuberculous lesions. A progressive increase in the use of ventral and ventrolateral approaches for spinal decompression in treating various spinal lesions, such as tuberculosis, pyogenic osteomyelitis, kyphotic deformities, neoplasms (primary and metastatic), and burst fractures[9,29,67,68] has been observed. The types of ventral approaches used for different spinal levels are summarized in Table 35.1. Ventral and ventrolateral decompression principles for spinal tumors are discussed in depth. This is followed by the management of other types of spinal pathology that may be treated through a ventral decompression.

Spinal Tumors

Recently, the surgical management of patients with spinal tumors and associated spinal cord compression has shifted from a laminectomy approach to ventral approaches with ventral decompression.[9,18,28,72] Because most spinal tumors are located ventrally, a laminectomy can limit the degree of ventral resection and can exacerbate, or worsen, existing spinal instability associated with tumors that have destroyed spinal bony segments. Several authors[27,83] have reported that the results of ventral decompression of spinal tumors with spinal cord compression are significantly better in most cases when compared with radiation therapy (RT) alone or in conjunction with laminectomy. Dorsolateral approaches can also provide some degree of ventral spinal decompression, with the advantage that they allow for both ventral and dorsal decompression and dorsal stabilization with a single exposure. Because of the limited access of the contralateral ventral dural sac, however,

this exposure is more suitable in cases with unilateral spinal canal and vertebral involvement. The results of ventral decompression indicate that this is an effective method to preserve and improve neurologic function in patients with neural compromise from primary and metastatic tumors of the thoracic and lumbar spine.[9,29,38,73]

The principal indications for ventral decompressive surgery in patients with ventrally located spinal tumors are (1) progressive neurologic deficits, (2) pathologic fracture or impending spinal instability, and (3) mechanical or compressive pain. In rare circumstances, resection of a lesion to make the diagnosis is required when the computed tomography (CT) guided needle biopsy is nondiagnostic. The issue of pain can be controversial. If the etiology of the pain is from compression of the neural tissues or mechanical instability, justification for decompression and fixation can be made. The authors have intervened surgically on terminal patients with a life expectancy of 3 to 4 months, and for whom conservative measures have failed to provide sufficient pain relief.

The radiosensitivity of the tumor plays an important role in overall management. Radiosensitive tumors (e.g., lymphoma, myeloma, Ewing's sarcoma, or neuroblastoma) can be treated with radiation therapy initially, if the cord compression is the result of epidural tumor alone. Surgical decompression is the initial treatment when a significant degree of compression can be attributed to bony or ligamentous fragments or spinal deformity, as a result of destruction by tumor. In cases of failed radiation therapy with persistent or recurrent spinal cord compression, surgical intervention is also required. The increased complications associated with operating on a previously radiated site also favor surgery before radiation. Surgical decompression can be considered for radiation-resistant tumors, such as melanoma or renal cell carcinoma and intermediate radiosensitivity tumors like lung, breast, or prostate. The rate of clinical progression provides the surgeon with valuable information when deciding the optimal timing of intervention. Rapid progression of symptoms is best managed with surgery, since the effects of radiation can be initially associated with swelling. The medical status of the patient and ability to tolerate the surgery is also taken into consideration.

Preoperative Assessment

Initially, plain spine radiographs (anteroposterior and lateral) are used to determine the level and extent of tumor involvement. The spinal alignment can also be observed from these films. A CT scan with and without intravenous contrast at the appropriate spinal levels allows the degree of bony destruction of the spinal column to be defined. Although magnetic resonance imaging (MRI) is less precise than CT in outlining bony destruction, it provides the most precise means for illustrating the site and degree of cord compression by tumor or bone (Figure 35.1). Myelography and postmyelography CT scan can be used when MRI is contraindicated or is not available.

TABLE 35.1

TABLE 35.1

Classification of Ventral Surgical Approaches

Spinal Segment	Surgical Approach
Cervicothoracic C7-T2 (see Figure 35.11)	Extended ventral cervical (division of strap muscles) Transsternal Cervicosternotomy ("trapdoor" approach)
Upper thoracic T2-5 (see Figure 35.10)	High dorsolateral thoracotomy (third-rib approach with mobilization of scapula)
T6-12 (see Figures 35.2B, 35.7, 35.9)	Dorsolateral thoracotomy
Thoracolumbar T12-L2 (see Figures 35.1 and 35.8)	Transthoracic/retroperitoneal with 10th to 12th rib resection; division of diaphragm
Lumbar L2-5	Retroperitoneal/flank Transabdominal
Lumbosacral L5-sacrum	Ventral retroperitoneal ("pelvic brim" approach)

To avoid complications from intraoperative and postoperative instability of the spinal column, it is important to assess the spinal stability before performing a vertebral decompression. Stability can be considered in terms of the three-column theory, after the extent of bony destruction produced by tumor has been determined from imaging.[13,79] Single-column involvement can be considered relatively stable. The additive destabilizing effects of decompression, however, must factor into the decision-making process.

Anterior-column and middle-column involvement are the most common findings in symptomatic patients with spinal tumors and are frequently associated with some degree of vertebral body collapse and bony retropulsion into the spinal canal (Figure 35.1A). If these conditions are treated by corpectomy, with a strut graft used for fusion (Figure 35.1B,C), stability of the spinal column can be achieved.

Careful review of the degree of involvement of the dorsal elements is required. The need for augmentation of ventral fixation with dorsal instrumentation will be based on the integrity of the lamina, lateral masses, pars interarticularis, and facets. Corpectomy and vertebral replacement techniques can result in persistent dorsal element instability if overdistraction and opening of the facets is performed. This can prevent subsequent fusion and result in failure of the ventral fixation. The ease with which distraction can be obtained following decompression can also provide the surgeon with information regarding the degree of posterior instability. Intraoperative x-rays can be taken to ensure the proper amount of distraction. In cases when the posterior instability is deemed significant, posterior stabilization should be undertaken.

When planning surgery for spinal tumors, an assessment of stability must also take into account angulation and alignment.[79] Higher failure rates will be observed with a poorly aligned construct. It is also important to consider the nature of the tumor in terms of its capacity to infiltrate and destroy bony tissue and its response to RT or chemotherapy.

Preoperative Angiography and Embolization

Angiography, with a view to embolization, is recommended for patients with known vascular tumors (e.g., melanoma, renal cell carcinoma, metastatic thyroid tumor, or primary giant cell tumor) or in patients in whom imaging suggests a relatively vascular tumor. If these tumors are amenable to embolization, this should be performed no more than 48 hours prior to surgery. Waiting too long after embolization may result in recanalization. The expertise of the interventional neuroradiologist will influence greatly the success of the surgical intervention (Figure 35.1D-I).

Surgical Management

Intraoperative Monitoring and Anesthetic Management

The authors recommend electrophysiologic monitoring, if available, including somatosensory and motor evoked potentials, at all vertebral levels involving the spinal cord. Electromyography (EMG) monitoring is also useful in the lumbar region, if segmental pedicular fixation is contemplated. Monitoring setup time and cost are definite drawbacks to this type of technology, although its use is generally supported in the literature.[12,39,46,56,58] In approaches of the upper and middle thoracic spine, a double lumen endotracheal tube allows the lung in the operative field to be deflated, improving the surgical exposure. In lesions of the lower thoracic and thoracolumbar regions, the lung can be retracted easily. Invasive arterial pressure monitoring and central venous pressure (CVP) monitoring are recommended in any case in which more than minimal blood loss may occur.

Positioning

Patients are positioned in full lateral decubitus (Figure 35.2) with an axillary roll placed under the dependent axilla to prevent neurovascular compromise.

Incision and Exposure

The side of approach and the level of the spine that is involved are important factors in determining where to make the incision. To maximize resection, the decision to perform a right-sided or left-sided skin incision and approach should be determined by the side of the spine with greater tumor involvement. If neither side is predominantly involved by tumor, the spine is generally approached from the right side, at or above the T5 vertebral segment, to avoid the arch of the

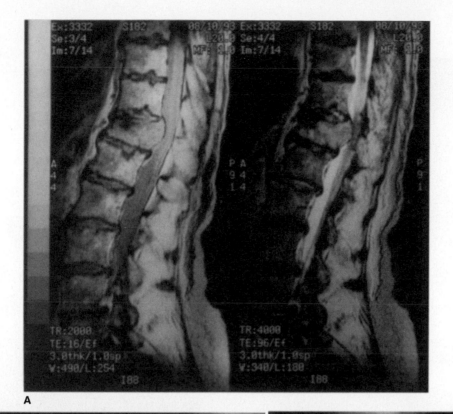

A

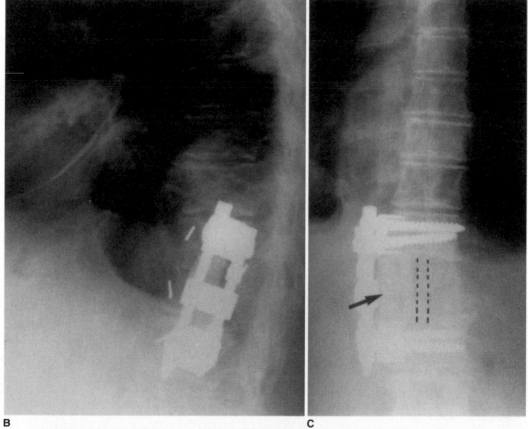

B   C

Figure 35.1 (**A**) Proton density and T_2-weighted sagittal MR image of metastatic carcinoma of the breast to the $T1_2$ vertebral body with angulation and severe spinal cord compression. (**B, C**) Postoperative lateral and anteroposterior radiographs after $T1_2$ vertebral body resection showing the placement of a rib bone graft, methylmethacrylate, and Kaneda instrumentation. Postoperatively, the patient recovered full neurologic function and was pain free. In view of the isolated vertebral body involvement, it was believed that good long-term survival was possible (thus the use of additional bone graft in the reconstruction). The patient, however, died of systemic metastatic cancer 8 months postoperatively.   *Continued*

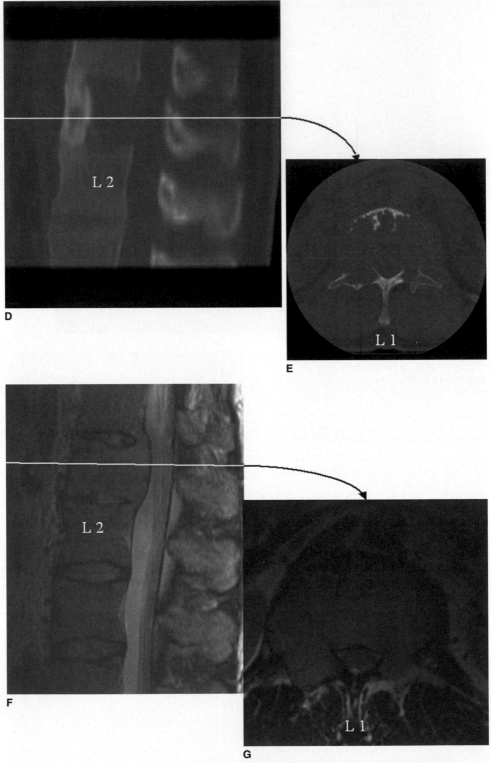

Figure 35.1 *cont'd* (**D**) Sagittal reconstruction CT scan and corresponding axial image of (**E**) a patient with plasmacytoma involving the L1 vertebral body. T$_2$-weighted magnetic resonance (MR) images in (**F**) sagittal and (**G**) axial of the same case. Images of the CT scan illustrate the bony destruction while the MR images show the spinal cord compression more accurately.

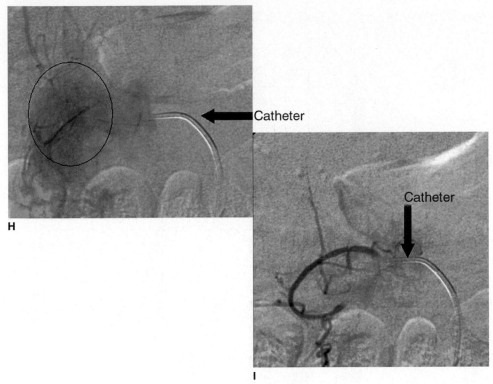

Catheter

Catheter

Figure 35.1 *cont'd* Preembolization angiogram showing (**H**) the vascular supply of the L1 lesion with a tumor blush *(circle)*. Postembolization angiogram with (**I**) a significant reduction in tumor blush in the same case.

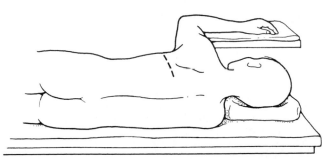

Figure 35.2 Patient is in the lateral position, and a dorsolateral thoracotomy skin incision is placed below the scapula.

aorta. Below T5, the spine is generally approached from the left side to minimize retraction on the liver.

Lesions involving the cervicothoracic (C7-T1), upper thoracic (T1-5), lower thoracic (T6-11), thoracolumbar (T12 and L1), and lumbar and sacral (L2 to sacrum) segments require specific approaches (Table 35.1) and considerations that have been described in other chapters.

Spinal Decompression

Spinal decompression requires a sequential approach that can be divided into four stages.

Exposure

The pleura is sharply incised and reflected. A rib head that overlies the level of the pathology in the midaxillary level is resected. The segmental vessels at the level of the

pathology and of the vertebral bodies above and below the lesion (Figure 35.3) are ligated and divided. Division of segmental vessels over the vertebral body in the middle of the body reduces the risk of vascular compromise of the spinal cord by taking advantage of collateral vessels from adjacent levels. The periosteum is reflected medially, and the anterior longitudinal ligament is identified.

Vertebral Body Decompression

The intervertebral discs above and below the involved vertebral body are identified and resected initially by sharp dissection (Figure 35.4). Disc material is cleared with curettes and pituitary rongeurs. Removing the rib head will allow identification of the ipsilateral pedicle and its continuation into the vertebral body. The pedicle is an important marker for the orientation and position of the spinal canal. Using sharp curettes, rongeurs, and a high-speed drill, the vertebral body is resected ventrally to dorsally, except for a rim of the ventral portion of the vertebral body. This protects the aorta and inferior vena cava from accidental trauma. Resection of the vertebral body can progress as far as the opposite pedicle (Figures 35.5 and 35.6), and the entire dorsal aspect of the vertebral body can be removed. Sufficient bone needs to be removed to clear the posterior longitudinal ligament of any compression of the dura. The dissection can also be continued dorsolaterally to allow decompression of the spinal nerve roots. The tumor involvement and the quality of the residual bone for instrumentation will determine the extent of bony removal. Techniques to augment the strength of the purchase into the bone are discussed in subsequent paragraphs.

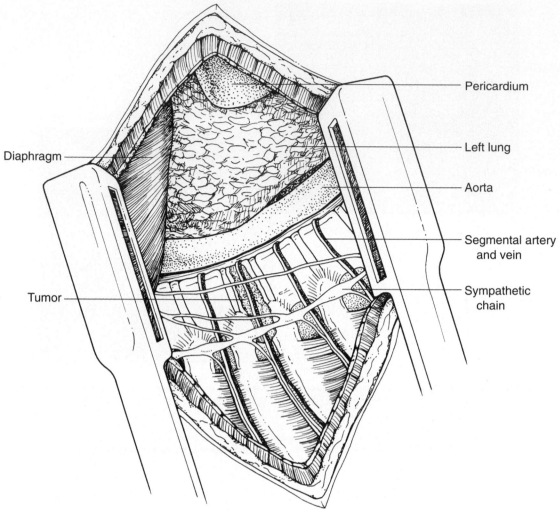

Figure 35.3 Exposure of the thoracic spine after entry into the thoracic cavity and placement of a self-retaining chest retractor. The parietal pleura has been separated from the ribs and spinal column with the segmental vessels along the side of the vertebrae identified.

Rostrocaudal Dissection

Special care is afforded to the cartilaginous end plates and the central regions of cancellous bone of vertebral bodies adjacent to the corpectomy site. Removal using a small high-speed burr or curettes (Figure 35.7) or osteotomes and rongeurs may be used, depending on the bony consistency. This allows troughs to be created in the vertebral bodies above and below the corpectomy site to allow subsequent reconstruction with a bone graft, implant, or acrylic. Preparing the end plates to accommodate the construct requires special attention. When the construct involves bone, either autograft or allograft, an eventual fusion will be desired. In this circumstance the end plates require adequate vascular supply for achieving fusion. Methylmethacrylate, on the other hand, will not fuse and the overall construct strength can be weakened by aggressive removal of the end plates. The risk of telescoping and the graph imploding into the vertebral body can also occur when the end plates are destroyed. The structural integrity of the graft can also fail if it is suboptimal or radiated.

Intraspinal Decompression

After adequate bony resection, decompression, and removal of all devitalized bone and tumor tissue, the posterior longitudinal ligament is resected to expose the dura mater that encloses the spinal cord and segmental nerve roots. Any tumor or bone impinging on the dural sac or nerve root is carefully removed to allow decompression of these structures. The goal of surgery should be radical tumor resection and decompression. In patients who have previously received RT, the posterior longitudinal ligament is frequently adherent to the dura mater and may be difficult to separate. In these cases, it may be advisable to leave it *in situ*.

Avoiding Complications During Spinal Decompression

Complications Related to the Approach

A thoracotomy carries pulmonary risks, such as atelectasis and pneumonia. The retroperitoneal exposure may injure

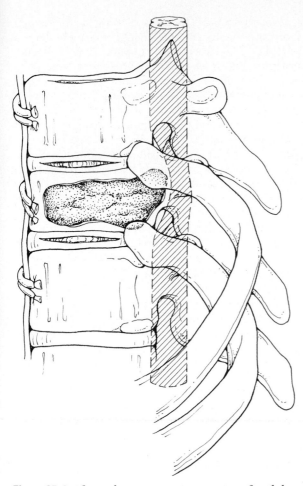

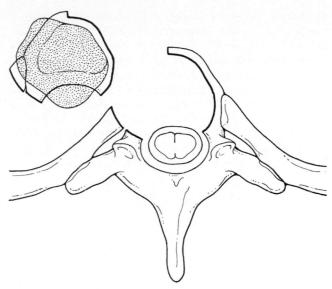

Figure 35.6 Remaining vertebra after bony decompression and tumor removal showing that the decompression extends from the ipsilateral pedicle to the contralateral pedicle.

Figure 35.4 After a thoracotomy via resection of a rib located one level rostrally, the pleura is reflected off the ventral spine. The segmental vascular bundles are isolated and ligated as shown. Vertebral decompression of the tumor begins by the excision of intervertebral discs above and below the involved vertebra. Following this, 1 to 2cm of the rib head is drilled down to expose the ipsilateral pedicle.

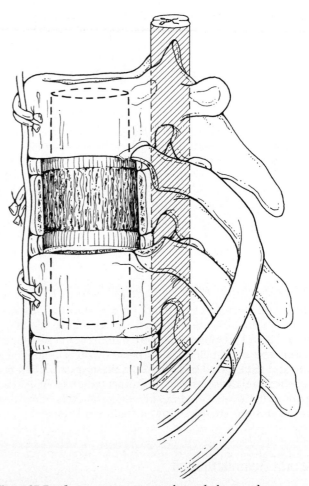

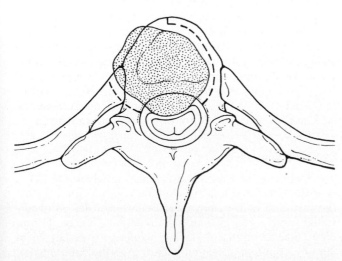

Figure 35.5 Axial section through vertebra involved with spinal tumor showing the extent of bony decompression necessary to allow adequate tumor resection.

Figure 35.7 After tumor resection, the end plates and cancellous bone of adjacent vertebral bodies are removed to the degree shown (*dotted line*) using an angled high-speed drill or angled curettes.

the spleen, kidney or ureter, and a prolonged postoperative ileus may occur. Any unrepaired defect in the abdominal wall or diaphragm may be the site of a later visceral herniation. Using vertebral body screws with manual confirmation of bicortical penetration requires considerable dissection of the contralateral aspect of the vertebral body, placing the aorta, inferior vena cava, and iliolumbar vessels at risk if this is not done meticulously. Injury to the lumbar hypogastric plexus at L5 in males may be complicated by retrograde ejaculation. Chyle leak from damage to the thoracic duct is best managed with immediate repair.

Inadequate Spinal Decompression

Inadequate decompression reduces the chance of adequate neurologic recovery and carries the risk of incomplete tumor resection. It is important that the decompression be performed to the contralateral pedicle.

Neurologic Injury

A careful, staged approach to spinal decompression with adequate exposure and identification of segmental vessels, nerve roots, and dural tube markedly reduces the risk of nerve root and spinal cord injury. Nuwer[56] concluded that intraoperative neurophysiologic monitoring is a cost-effective way of reducing the potential for a neurologic deficit. Intraoperative information is valuable not only to the prognosis but also by altering intraoperative and postoperative management. Hardware revision and removal during the operation may be performed, based on intraoperative neurophysiologic changes.

Dural Tears

Occasionally, a dural tear may occur while the tumor is being dissected from adjacent dura mater or because of erosion of the dura caused by the tumor. In these cases, the precise site of dural tear should be identified and the tear repaired with a nonabsorbable suture (e.g., 4-0 Neurolon [Ethicon]). In less discrete or poorly visualized dural tears, fibrin glue can be layered over the cerebrospinal fluid leakage site and allowed to adhere to underlying dura mater. A lumbar drain should be placed for 5 days postoperatively to facilitate dural closure.

Excessive Epidural Bleeding or Bleeding from Tumor

Preoperative angiography and embolization of vascular tumors reduce the risk of such intraoperative bleeding. After careful identification and mobilization, segmental vessels above and below the corpectomy site should be ligated and cut to avoid bleeding from these vessels when the vertebral bodies adjacent to the corpectomy site are spread apart. Other sites of epidural bleeding should be identified and hemostasis attained with bipolar coagulation.

Spinal Reconstruction

Graft Material

The appropriate type of material to use for spinal column reconstruction depends on the nature of the lesion and the patient's life expectancy. In cases of trauma, for benign lesions, or for patients with malignant tumors who have a relatively long life expectancy (greater than 2 years), reconstruction is best when using autogenous bone from the iliac crest or rib for single vertebral body defects. If two or more vertebral levels are involved with the neoplasm, an allograft (e.g., from the fibula or humerus) can be used. It is often useful to supplement the allograft strut with local autograft bone (Figure 35.8).

In patients with malignant disease and a short life expectancy, autogenous bone grafts have certain disadvantages: (1) if life expectancy is less than 1 year, solid bony fusion over the long-term is unnecessary, (2) the use of adjunctive radiation and chemotherapy will slow or prevent the bony fusion needed for stability, (3) any remaining local tumors may infiltrate the bone graft and weaken the construct, and (4) autogenous donor sites may not be suitable because of tumor involvement.

For patients with an expected survival of 18 months or less, a synthetic construct using polymethylmethacrylate (PMMA), with or without titanium cages, can be used. Expandable cages made of titanium can also be used to provide anterior support and reconstruction in difficult cases (Figure 35.8D,E). Biomechanical studies of intervertebral fixation have shown resistance of the implants to cyclic fatigue within typical normal physiologic loading and superior reduction of intervertebral motion and increased spinal stiffness.* The use of expandable vertebral prosthesis or cages has not received much attention in the literature. These expandable cages are usually complemented with dorsal fixation.

Reconstruction Technique

Reconstruction techniques aim to provide solid fixation to adjacent spinal segments. Failure of these constructs is usually the result of reconstruction material dislodging at proximal and/or distal ends at which it fits into adjacent spinal segments. Early spinal changes in the cancellous bone of adjacent vertebral segments, seen on postoperative MRI scans, can be an indication of potential failure of these regions to anchor the construct. Another important situation is one in which adjacent vertebral segments are involved with disease but are not collapsed and are not causing spinal cord compression. PMMA can be used to strengthen the adjacent bone. Alternatively, supplemental dorsal instrumentation may be required. The technique of vertebroplasty has grown significantly in popularity for osteopenic fractures in the elderly.[16,34,42,62,78] This technique can complement and add strength to an anterior or even posterior construct.

Synthetic Constructs

The technique of Errico and Cooper,[8] in which PMMA is pressure injected into a Silastic tube which is fitted against the vertebral bodies above and below, provides an ideally suited construct for patients with metastatic lesions (Figure 35.9). Silastic tubing of varying diameters (typically 15 to 20mm) is cut to a measured length (from the outer edge of the upper and lower troughs of adjacent vertebral segments

---

*References 6,35,47,49,50,53,77,84.

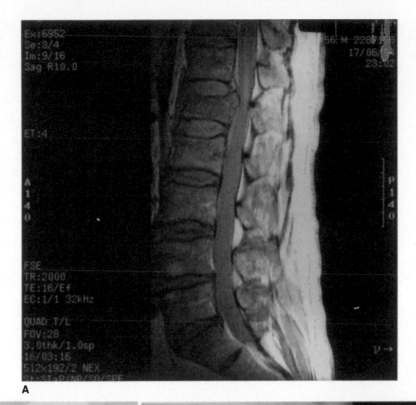

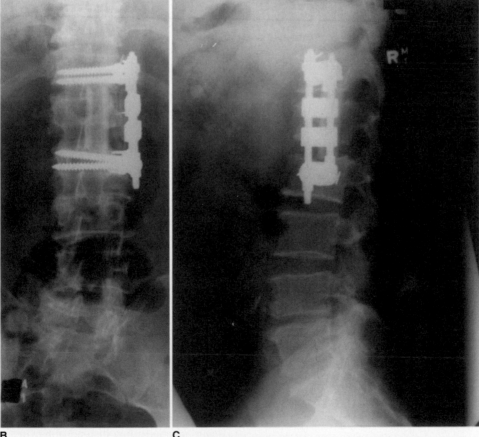

Figure 35.8 **(A)** Proton density sagittal MRI scan illustrating an L1 burst fracture with compression of the conus. **(B-C)** Postoperative anteroposterior and lateral radiographs after anterior decompression and stabilization using bone graft (combination of humeral allograft and rib autograft) and Kaneda instrumentation. *Continued*

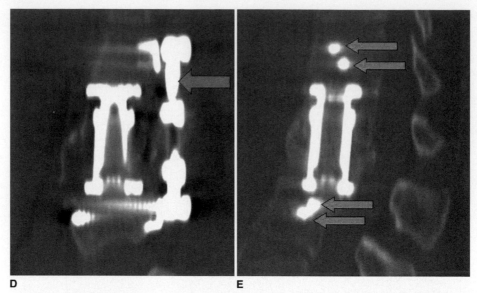

D   E

Figure 35.8 *cont'd* (**D**) Coronal and (**E**) sagittal CT scan images showing an expandable cage for the reconstruction of a two-level corpectomy. The Kaneda system is added to the construct for additional support to the anterior and middle column. The arrows in **E** identify the Kaneda screws into the body above and below the cage while the arrows in **D** show the connecting rods.

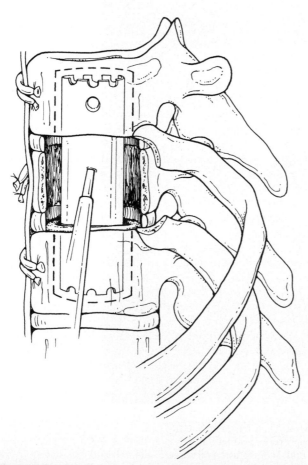

Figure 35.9 After the Silastic tubing is inserted into the spinal defect, a syringe is used to fill the tube with slow-curing, low-viscosity polymethylmethacrylate.

to the corpectomy site). One 6mm–diameter hole is made in the center of the tubing with a rongeur, and three small holes are made laterally, two at the rostral end and one at the caudal end. Small bites are also made at the ends of the tubing to allow extrusion of cement overflow. The three smaller lateral holes allow air bubbles and excess cement to flow out easily. The side of the Silastic tubing facing the spinal cord is free of the central and lateral holes to avoid cement extrusion into the spinal canal. The Silastic tubing is passed into the space between two adjacent vertebral bodies at the corpectomy site and positioned so that there is no bending of the tubing that could obstruct cement flow. Low-viscosity, slow-curing PMMA is prepared and is kept in a large 50ml syringe. When it has become semiliquid, the PMMA is injected through the center hole of the Silastic tubing, filling the tubing until PMMA can be seen passing out from the ends of the tube (see Figure 35.9). The tube must be observed carefully to avoid spilling the PMMA into the spinal canal. Curved Penfield dissectors can be used to protect the dural tube. As the PMMA in the Silastic tubing becomes harder, more PMMA is prepared and placed ventral and lateral to the Silastic tube until it is continuous with the borders of the upper and lower vertebrae. During polymerization and hardening of the PMMA, copious saline irrigation is used to help dissipate the heat. Hemostasis is attained with bipolar coagulation.

Using Silastic tubing instead of K-wires, in conjunction with PMMA, for reconstruction of the vertebral body defect, has certain advantages. First, the pliable Silastic tubing can be positioned with its ends sitting against the graft beds of the rostral and caudal adjacent vertebrae. This ensures the tubing is anchored against the adjacent vertebral bodies and does not remain unanchored in an open defect, thus reducing the risk of extrusion of the cement into the spinal canal and enhancing fixation to the adjacent vertebral column. Second, passing PMMA into the cancellous bone of adjacent vertebral segments further reinforces the vertebral bodies above and below the corpectomy site. Third, the pliable plastic filled with hardened PMMA becomes a long rigid construct that encompasses the length of the corpectomy site defect to facilitate anchorage into adjacent vertebrae. This reduces the risk of the construct dislodging from this position.

Degree of Vertebral Involvement

Most forms of metastatic spinal disease usually involve the vertebral body. When there is significant involvement of the dorsal elements, dorsal resection of the pathology can be performed by laminectomy. The decision to decompress using an anterior or posterior approach is based on the location of the pathology and the compression. Combined approaches are required when the destruction of the native spinal column is circumferential. Many surgeons prefer to proceed with anterior decompression initially, since this approach will more often provide a greater degree of decompression. Dorsal instrumentation will supplement the anterior construct and can be done either in combination with the initial operation or in a delayed fashion. Circumferential stabilization is recommended to prevent subsequent spinal instability, spinal deformity, or excessive spinal movement that may predispose to loosening and dislodgment of the spinal construct at the corpectomy site. The length of the posterior instrumentation will be based on the quality of the pedicular purchase and the overall alignment of the construct. Instrumentation will not be terminated in the midthoracic curve, minimizing the chance of pulling out the screws at the end of the instrumentation. Added consideration is given to the transition zones at the cervicothoracic and thoracolumbar levels. Bridging of these areas is often required to reduce the chance of failure of the spinal segment adjacent to the construct.

Bony Graft Fusion in Malignant and Nonmalignant Disease

In patients with nonmalignant disease, or with malignant disease with a relatively longer survival period (usually greater than 2 years), a bone graft is used to supplement the synthetic construct described above (see Figure 35.1).

Fusion

Distraction

After initial vertebral decompression, vertebral distraction is attained by using a vertebral distracter or by applying distraction after placing vertebral screws.

Graft Site Preparation

The end plates of vertebral bodies adjacent to the decompression site are prepared to accept a graft. The underlying cancellous bone should not be exposed by complete removal of the end plates. Destruction of the end plates will lead to reduction of the mechanical strength of the vertebral body and increase the risk of the graft telescoping into or penetrating the weakened vertebral bodies. The rostral and caudal end plates are of different shapes. This must be kept in mind and selective drilling used to ensure that the graft site has parallel surfaces with adequate cortical bone remaining to support the graft. One common mistake is the failure to remove sufficient ventral and dorsal end plate lip, resulting in a central gap between the bone graft and vertebral end plate. Another mistake that has more serious consequences is the "ramp effect" that occurs when excessive bone is removed from the ventral two thirds of the lower vertebral body. This results in a graft site that is longer ventrally than dorsally, predisposing to ventral dislocation of the graft.

Grafting

A firm, well-fitted graft is the result not only of a well-prepared graft site, but also of a well-proportioned, appropriately sized bone graft. A caliper and depth gauge should be used to measure the length and depth of the graft site accurately to determine the dimensions of the bone strut. The depth of the graft site is measured from the dorsal cortex to the ventral cortex along the midline of the vertebral body. The length of the graft site is measured with the vertebral bodies maximally distracted and is the distance between the end plates.

A tricortical iliac crest bone graft can be used up to a two-level corpectomy. More extensive decompressions may necessitate a humeral or fibular allograft. Such an allograft strut has greater biomechanical strength than an iliac crest, with a fusion rate similar to that of autologous bone. The high cortical bone content, however, means that it may take up to 1 year for the graft to incorporate.[5] A supplemental local autograft (e.g., from rib or vertebral body) enhances the rate of fusion when using allografts (Figure 35.8). If grafts are taken from the iliac crest, the osteotomies should be perpendicular to the surface of the iliac crest and parallel to each other. A double-bladed oscillatory saw is useful in obtaining parallel surfaces. When these grafts are to be used for subtotal or total vertebral body replacement, several extra millimeters should be taken to allow for further reshaping. In the midthoracic and upper thoracic spine, rib strut grafts taken at the time of the thoracotomy are usually adequate.

With the vertebral bodies distracted, the graft is gently placed into position and should fit without excessive force or hammering. Tactile inspection of the final position of the graft should be done using a blunt hook alongside the graft. Small pieces of cancellous bones can be gently impacted into the remaining gaps. However, care should be taken to avoid spinal canal compromise or compression of neural structures by these smaller pieces of bone. It is important to use a drill to remove any irregularities of the anterior surface of the vertebral bodies so the plate can sit flush against them. A greater plate-to-bone contact allows increased structural stability of this construct.

Avoiding Complications Related to Fusion

To reduce the morbidity that can be associated with this procedure, there are specific fusion-related complications that must be considered.

Hemorrhage

Although hemorrhage cannot be totally avoided, it is important to minimize the amount of blood loss during fusion by giving special consideration to the following three factors.

1. Careful positioning of the patient on the operating table will avoid unnecessary pressure on the abdomen. This is particularly relevant in the lateral and prone positions. Obstruction of the vena cava and collateral flow from the lower extremities into the paravertebral plexus will impact on the venous congestion of the epidural venous plexus and contribute to blood loss.
2. Timing of end plate preparation and decortication may be associated with additional blood loss; this should only be done after the bony exposure has been completed, soft tissue has been excised, and bone graft has been harvested. Bleeding from decortication sites should not be treated with bone wax because this reduces the capacity for osteogenesis.[25] Excessive bleeding usually settles after the graft is inserted and may be controlled with Gelfoam.
3. Avoiding inadvertent injury and excessive bleeding, the segmental vessels should be clearly identified and dissected so that they may be suture ligated and divided in a controlled, safe manner. In the lower thoracic and upper lumbar region, the artery of Adamkiewicz and other radicular arteries supplying the anterior and posterior spinal arteries can be identified by preoperative selective segmental vessel angiograms. This is recommended in instances in which there is a concern that these vessels may be at risk during the approach. The authors usually reserve preoperative spinal angiography for cases with a long-standing fixed kyphotic deformity in which the spinal cord blood supply may be tenuous or for cases in which preoperative embolization is desired.

Pseudarthrosis

Pseudarthrosis refers to a lack of bony union and may account for a poor clinical result. It is worth noting, however, that fibrous pseudarthrosis may limit spinal movement and allow a good clinical outcome with symptomatic relief. Moreover, even when bony fusion has occurred, patients can remain symptomatic. Meticulous attention to graft site preparation and use of autograft, where possible, enhances fusion rates. In cases of traumatic lesions, the supplementation of the fusion with a local vertebral body autograft that is osteoinductive may be appropriate.

Harvesting Autogenous Iliac Crest Bone

The iliac crest is the most common site from which bone grafts are taken. Consideration of the following complica-

tions during this procedure may help reduce the donor site morbidity associated with this procedure.[1,23,40,69] Donor site pain is common and can continue to be a problem in one out of five patients, lasting up to 2 years postsurgery.[51]

Cosmetic deformity can be a problem when full-thickness grafts are taken from the iliac crest. When larger grafts are taken and cosmetic deformity becomes a concern, three techniques are useful in preventing crest deformities: (1) the trapdoor method uses the crest as a hinge, (2) the subcrestal window avoids resection of the rostral margin of the crest,[4] and (3) oblique sectioning of the crest allows the crest to be reconstituted.[51,81] Reconstruction of the crest, using different techniques, has been described: rib,[11,30,75] bioactive apatite and wollastonite-containing glass ceramic,[3] or methylmethacrylate.[45] Although infection is not a major concern, it does occur occasionally. A deep wound infection at the iliac donor site is treated like other wound infections adjacent to bone. It will require drainage, irrigation, and appropriate antibiotic coverage. Hematoma is not uncommon at the wound site. Gelfoam or bone wax can be used, but microcrystalline collagen is best for reducing bleeding from cancellous bone.[7] Suction drainage may be used to reduce the incidence of wound hematomas, although not proven. Gait disturbance, with a limp or abductor lurch as a result of considerable stripping of the outer table muscles, can cause hip abductor weakness. With bone graft taken from the dorsal crest, patients may have difficulty with hip extension, which is evident when climbing stairs or rising from a chair.

Stress fractures can occur after full-thickness grafts are taken from the anterior iliac crest.[61] Stress fractures, as a result of the pull from the sartorius and rectus femoris muscles, can be avoided by harvesting the graft well away from the anterior superior iliac spine.[15] Moreover, taking long strips of bone along the iliac crest increases the risk of ilium fracture.

Perforation of the peritoneum can occur with a ventral approach to the inner table of the iliac crest because the peritoneum is closely related to the inner surface of the abdominal wall and iliacus muscles.[14] Herniation of abdominal contents can occur after removal of full thickness grafts that include the iliac crest.[57]

Placing the skin incision behind the anterior superior iliac spine can minimize injury to the lateral femoral cutaneous nerve. Anatomic variation of the lateral femoral cutaneous nerve places this nerve at risk in less than 10% when dissection is 3cm posterior to the anterior iliac spine.[54]

Instrumentation

The need for supplementary instrumentation depends on the spinal level involved and the degree of bony involvement.

T1 to T9

When the corpectomy involves only the thoracic spine, supplementary instrumentation is generally not necessary because the thoracic spine, unlike the lumbar spine, is supported by the rib cage. However, if there is three-column involvement, additional instrumentation will be necessary (Figure 35.10).[9] For the upper thoracic spine (T1-3), ventral cervical plates can be used (Figure 35.11).

T10 to L5

The T12 vertebral body and lumbar spine receive little or no additional support from the rib cage, and in this region there is a greater degree of extension of the spine with spinal motion. Ventral instrumentation is necessary to supplement the reconstruction and to prevent excessive extension that can lead to extrusion of the graft or synthetic construct.[36,38,48]

Supplemental Ventral Instrumentation

The rationale for using ventral instrumentation can be understood best by considering the biomechanics of the ventral fixation device. Shono et al.[70] and Gertzbein[26] have described the biomechanics of thoracolumbar ventral fixation devices when loss of anterior and middle

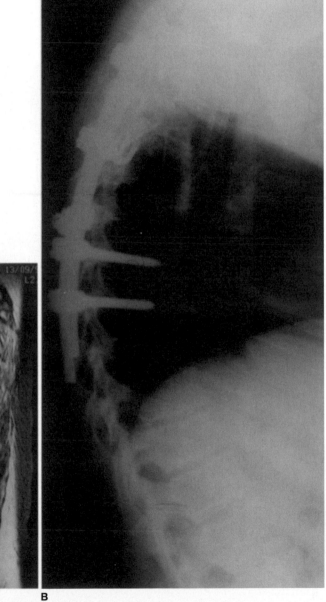

Figure 35.10 (A) Proton density and T_2-weighted sagittal MRI scan showing a T4-5 fracture dislocation with angulation and spinal cord compression in a 24-year-old woman with an incomplete spinal cord injury. A left third rib thoracotomy approach was used to perform a ventral decompression and reconstruction with rib autograft. In view of the three-column injury with associated rib fractures, posterior instrumentation (AO Universal Spine System) was performed. (B) Postoperative lateral radiographs show correction of the kyphotic deformity with posterior segmental stabilization.

column integrity is present. The Kaneda device,[36] which has two cross-fixed rods linked to four vertebral body screws (Figures 35.1 and 35.8), allows rigid stabilization against forces of axial compression, flexion, extension, and rotation. The quadrangular construct created by the two independent rods linked by the two cross-fixed bars provides greater resistance to flexion-extension and rotation than a single rod system, such as the Zielke system. The insertion of the vertebral body screws in nonparallel (triangular) alignment controls ventral and downward displacement. In the ventrally destabilized spine, the Kaneda construct provides superior fixation compared with dorsal instrumentation (such as a laminar hook or pedicle screw systems), especially against flexion and axial compression forces. If disruption of dorsal elements is present, ventral instrumentation alone is insufficient to

provide stability (Figure 35.10). Most important, regardless of the rigidity of instrumentation, the spinal construct will eventually fail unless solid bony fusion occurs. One of the key concepts of ventral fusion is that the bone graft should be placed under compression to allow greater graft stability and fusion to adjacent vertebral bodies.[81]

Instrumentation Technique

The basic principle entails inserting screws into the midpoint of the vertebral bodies above and below the corpectomy site and connecting these by a rod or plate. Initially, Kostuik-Harrington instrumentation was used. This has been supplanted by the Kaneda, CD Horizon® Anteres™ Spinal System and Z-plate systems. The Kaneda

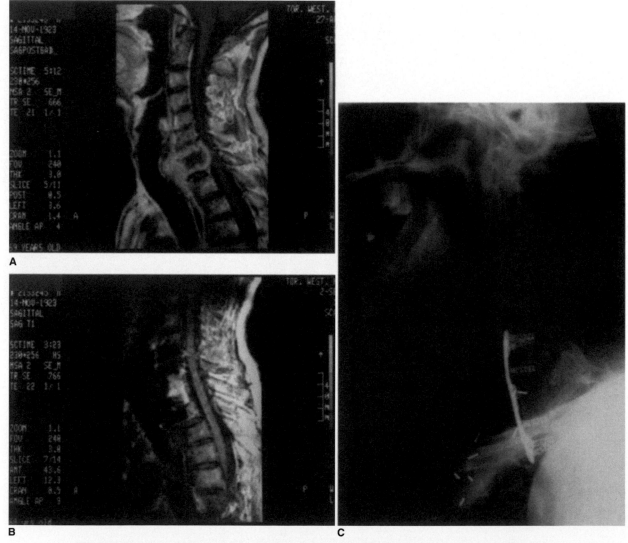

Figure 35.11 (A) Gadolinium-enhanced T_1-weighted sagittal MRI scan of a patient with tuberculosis of the cervicothoracic junction showing vertebral body involvement of T1 and extension into the spinal canal with severe spinal cord compression and paraspinal extension. Surgical exposure of this lesion was achieved via a right-sided cervicosternotomy approach. **(B-C)** Postoperative T_1-weighted sagittal MRI scan and lateral cervical spine radiograph after vertebral body resection and stabilization with an iliac crest bone graft and Synthes plate.

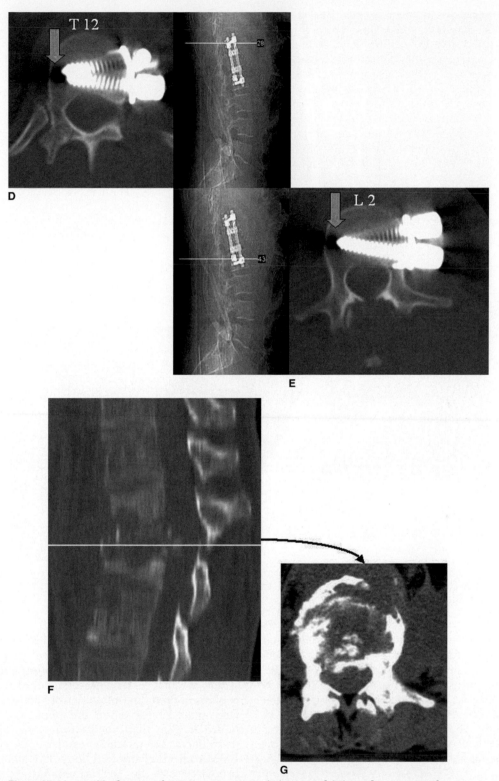

Figure 35.11 *cont'd* These axial CT scan images at **(D)** T12 and **(E)** L2 demonstrate the suboptimal screw placement (Kaneda system). The screws are convergent but do not engage the second cortex; the arrows show the gap. A case of Pott's disease at the T12 and L1 level. The CT scan images, **(F)** sagittal and **(G)** corresponding axial images show the bony destruction.

Continued

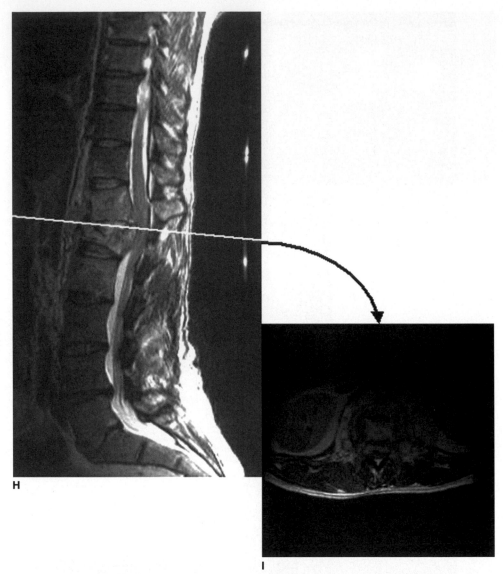

H

I

Figure 35.11 *cont'd* The MR images, (**H**) T$_2$-weighted sagittal and (**I**) corresponding axial image show the spinal cord compression.

and CD Horizon® Anteres™ Spinal systems are best used between T10 and L4. Above T10, the small size of the vertebral bodies may make screw placement difficult, although screws can usually be placed as high as T6 in select cases. Below L4, the iliac veins and origin of the inferior vena cava tend to impede the safe placement of the Kaneda system. The Z-plate system, which has a lower profile, has recently been modified to allow ventral instrumentation of the midthoracic and lower thoracic spine.

Avoiding Complications Related to Instrumentation

The role of instrumentation in the context of any spinal pathology is to provide stability either transiently, while fusion occurs, or permanently. Placement of instrumentation, however, carries risks and can cause complications. Direct trauma related to poorly positioned instruments is typically noted immediately. Erosion of screws into soft tissues can present in a delayed fashion. Poorly placed instruments can also fail to achieve the primary goal of providing stability. Patients will often complain of persistent mechanical pain. Assessment of the bone quality is often limited, and bone density studies can only provide limited information preoperatively. The interface between the instrumentation and the bone, also described as the purchase, can be improved by injecting PMMA into the vertebral body. The technique of vertebroplasty can be performed intraoperatively,[19,22,60] using radiopaque PMMA and injecting it while in liquid form under fluoroscopy to ensure safe distribution in the vertebral body and avoiding the spinal canal (Figure 35.11D,E).

Other Spinal Pathology

In addition to metastatic spinal disease, several other conditions require ventral spinal decompression and are dis-

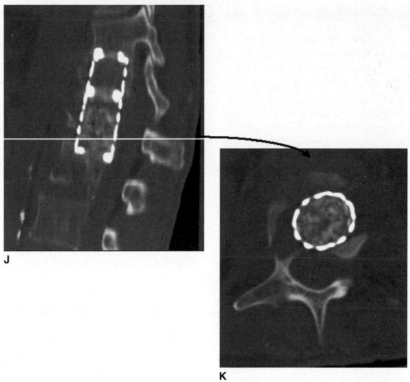

Figure 35.11 *cont'd* **(J-K)** A postoperative CT scan demonstrates the anterior reconstruction with a titanium cage filled with autologous bone graft. This construct was subsequently complemented with posterior instrumentation using pedicle screws above and below the cage (*not shown here*).

cussed below. Because the principles of ventral spinal decompression, fusion, and instrumentation are similar, only factors that are unique to these situations are outlined.

Osteomyelitis of the Spine

The most common infections of the spinal column are: (1) infections caused by pyogenic organisms (*Staphylococcus aureus* and *coliform bacilli* are the most common pyogenic bacteria found), (2) infections caused by fungi (actinomycetes and blastomycetes are the most common organisms), and (3) tuberculosis (Pott's disease) (Figure 35.11).

These organisms usually reach the spinal column by hematogenous spread. Infection becomes symptomatic as a result of neural compromise from an associated extradural abscess or a bony deformity from vertebral collapse with adjacent bone overgrowth that compromises the spinal canal (gibbus formation).

Identification of predisposing factors for infection following spinal surgery has been described by Wimmer *et al.*[81] Medical conditions, such as diabetes, obesity, corticosteroid therapy, chronic infection, and smoking were identified in patients with a higher rate of infection. Surgical variables, such as previous spinal surgery, extended preoperative hospitalization ($p<.04$), prolonged duration of operation ($p<.001$), and high blood loss ($p<.01$), were identified as risk factors. The role of prophylactic antibiotic administration has been demonstrated by Horwitz[32] to reduce wound infection with spinal surgery. Some institutions have adopted a prolonged duration

of antibiotic doses for patients at higher risk, using the above factors.

Patients with osteomyelitis usually have symptoms of back pain, local spinal tenderness, and paraspinal muscle spasm. Associated fever and leukocytosis is common. Erosion of several adjacent vertebral bodies with collapse and involvement of associated intervertebral disks is characteristic and an early radiographic finding on lateral and anteroposterior spine films. Bone scans are often positive at regions of vertebral infection, and the serum alkaline phosphatase level is often elevated.

In these infective cases, it is important to assess, using axial CT images, the degree of spinal canal narrowing from vertebral collapse or gibbus formation (Figure 35.11*F,G*). In the absence of spinal canal narrowing, an extradural abscess or granuloma is the likely cause of spinal symptoms. MRI or myelography to delineate neural (spinal cord or nerve root) compromise is also indicated for these patients before surgical decompression (Figure 35.11*H-K*).

Surgical decompression is indicated in patients with progressive symptoms of spinal cord compression. The thoracic region is the most common site of osteomyelitis, and dorsolateral spinal approaches (e.g., costotransversectomy) usually allow adequate spinal decompression. Occasionally, ventral decompressive procedures are necessary when there is (1) progressive spinal compression; (2) osteomyelitis of the cervical spine; (3) spinal infections with kyphotic angulation in the lower lumbar spine, in which a retroperitoneal approach with corpectomy can be performed; and (4) extensive involvement of the vertebral body that cannot be adequately decompressed by the dorsolateral approach (Figure 35.11).

The method of vertebral decompression and reconstruction is similar to that described earlier. The use of autogenous bone is favored in the setting of osteomyelitis. Internal fixation use is controversial. Some surgeons advocate its use in the setting of osteomyelitis provided that a good local débridement is achieved. For pyogenic infections, appropriate intravenous antibiotics are necessary for 4 to 6 weeks, followed by oral antibiotics, until the infection resolves both clinically and radiographically.

Some patients with tuberculosis of the spine and mild neurologic signs of spinal cord compression improve with antituberculous drugs, rest, and without requiring surgical decompression. However, close neurologic follow-up is required to ensure that symptoms are not progressive. It is important to remember that spinal infections can result in spinal cord symptoms without actual spinal cord compression. This occurs as a result of vascular thrombosis secondary to the inflammatory process. It is important, then, to confirm radiologically any evidence of spinal cord compression because these patients do not benefit from surgical decompression.

Kyphotic Deformities

Ventral corpectomy and fusion allow the correction of severe, symptomatic deformities. Surgical exposures are performed as described above, depending on the spinal level of the deformity. A ventral release with section of the anterior longitudinal ligament and discectomies is helpful for correcting the deformity. The adjacent discs involved in the kyphosis are identified and excised, and autologous bone (cortical iliac bone, section of rib, or fibula) is used for bone struts. This may be supplemented by ventral instrumentation to allow early ambulation of the patient. Most severe fixed kyphotic deformities require supplemental dorsal instrumentation and fusion.

Resection of Hemivertebra

A hemivertebra may become symptomatic and cause a severe, progressive deformity of the spine with neurologic compromise.[72] This usually occurs when the anomaly lies low in the lumbar spine and results in congenital scoliosis with the hemivertebra as the apical part of the curve. The hemivertebra is resected ventrally to dorsally, back to the level of the epidural space, with the base of the pedicle also resected. An autologous bony strut graft with ventral instrumentation can be used for stability. A second operation or, at the same setting, a dorsal approach is used to resect the dorsal elements of the hemivertebra.

Thoracic and Thoracolumbar Fractures

These fractures can be approached by a ventral, ventrolateral (Figures 35.8 and 35.10), dorsolateral or dorsal approach depending on certain features.[8,17,21,56] When lesions are ventral in the thoracic spine, available options for surgical exposure that allow decompression and stabilization include: costotransversectomy, a lateral extracavitary approach, a transthoracic extrapleural approach, or a

transthoracic transpleural approach. The authors favor the latter approach when neural decompression is an important goal, as in the patient with incomplete spinal cord injury (Figures 35.8 and 35.10). For burst fractures at the thoracolumbar junction, a transthoracic/retroperitoneal (10th rib approach) exposure is used to achieve ventral decompression and reconstruction (Figure 35.8). For midlumbar fractures (L2 or L3), a retroperitoneal approach is used. Low lumbar fractures (L4 or L5) are approached via a dorsolateral approach because the nerve roots may be retracted with greater facility, allowing easier decompression.

The transthoracic and retroperitoneal approaches allow a single staged procedure with decompression and removal of pathologic material ventral to the dura mater over several vertebral segments and reconstruction with bone graft and instrumentation. Three-column injuries necessitating the use of ventral decompression require supplemental dorsal instrumentation (Figure 35.10).

Decompression and Stabilization

Surgical exposures to other thoracic and lumbar levels (T1-3 and T3-L2) are described in other chapters. The fractured or retropulsed bony segment is identified under the microscope and removed, using curettes and a high-speed air drill. The intervertebral disks and end plates of adjacent vertebral bodies are removed to allow adequate fusion of the bony graft inserted between the intact adjacent vertebral bodies above and below the decompression. Certain important principles should be observed in spinal decompression associated with spinal trauma or fractures.

The decompression can often be performed without removing the entire vertebral body. The aim is to remove only the bony segment that is compromising the spinal canal. Using a high-speed burr, this can be performed by drilling away the bone ventral to the bony segment that protrudes into the spinal canal. This creates a vacant area ventral to the bony fragment impinging into the spinal canal. The retropulsed fragment can then be gently pushed away from the ventral aspect of the dura, using an angled curette, into the empty ventral space. This technique is similar to that used for the removal of a ruptured thoracic disc. For fracture decompressions, however, one-third to one-half of the vertebral body should be resected to allow adequate spinal decompression.

After a herniated disc or retropulsed bony fragment is removed, the spinal column needs to be stabilized. Rib struts, prepared from the resected rib, can be used for the bony graft in the upper thoracic and midthoracic spine. An iliac crest bone graft is used in the lower thoracic spine, thoracolumbar junction, or lumbar spine. Alternatively, allograft humerus or fibula supplemented with local autograft (rib or resected vertebral body) may be used. Subjacent intervertebral discs and cartilaginous end plates should be removed from vertebral bodies adjacent to the bony graft. Any spinal column deformity that is not fixed should be corrected using an appropriate distraction system. This is particularly useful in cases with significant kyphosis extending over several vertebral levels. Slots are drilled into vertebral bodies immediately above and below the decompression site to allow the bone grafts to be held in position. The decompressed vertebral segment is measured and a bone graft of appropriate size is prepared. The bone graft is gently tapped into the prepared interval between the two vertebral bodies using the bone set. A number of instrumentation systems are currently available for ventral instrumentation of the thoracolumbar spine, including the Kaneda device, Z-plate, CD Horizon® Anteres™ Spinal system and AO thoracolumbar locking plate.

Transthoracic Discectomy

Symptomatic thoracic intervertebral disc herniations are relatively uncommon with an incidence of 1 per million,[83] constituting approximately 0.25% to 0.75% of all symptomatic disc lesions. They usually occur between T4 and T12. Patients may appear with radicular symptoms or spinal cord compression, depending on whether the disc has herniated laterally or centrally. MR is the imaging technique of choice for the diagnosis (Figure 35.12). Initially, thoracic disc herniations were approached by laminectomy with poor results.* Although patients with lateral disc herniation fared better than those with central disc herniation, in both cases a number of patients failed to improve, continued to deteriorate, or had postoperative paraparesis as a complication.* In 1960, a lateral approach via a costotransversectomy was used with encouraging results.[34] Recently, a more direct ventral transpleural approach has provided further reduction in neurologic morbidity.[60,64]

Transthoracic (Transpleural) Discectomy

This approach allows direct exposure of the ventral and lateral regions of the intervertebral disc. If the surgeon is inexperienced in this approach, exposure should be performed by a thoracic surgeon. The patient's medical and pulmonary condition should be evaluated before surgery to ascertain the patient's ability to tolerate the procedure. A standard chest radiograph should be included as part of the pulmonary assessment and also to ensure the patient has 12 ribs. This anatomic detail is important when confirming the appropriate level intraoperatively.

The surgical approach to the appropriate vertebral level by thoracotomy is described in other chapters. The vertebral bodies above and below the herniated intervertebral disc are identified using the rib as a guide. The rib will articulate with the vertebral body above, therefore, the eighth rib head will point to the seventh and eighth disc space. Using x-ray to confirm the correct level is highly recommended.

An operating microscope may be used once the appropriate vertebral levels are identified. Dissection and proper visualization of the disc space, as previously described, is integral prior to proceeding with the discectomy. The amount of dissection is typically less extensive and limited to the rostral and caudal levels. The primary objective is to avoid retraction or manipulation of the dural sac at any time during the discectomy. To ensure adequate decompression and to allow smaller remnants of herniated disc to be removed, the floor of the spinal canal is palpated

---

* References 2,44,45,53,60,64,65,75,77.

gently with flat instruments, such as the Penfield dissector. These are then used to gently remove small, sequestered disc fragments. If the annulus fibrosus or posterior longitudinal ligaments are lax, or free, they can be pushed back into the intervertebral space and removed from this region. The operative site is then irrigated, and hemostasis is ensured once the spinal cord appears adequately decompressed.

Thoracic Endoscopic Surgery

Thoracic endoscopic surgery was first described for treatment of Pott's disease in 1951.[42] The expansion of video technology in the early 1990s impacted endoscopic capabilities, providing a better-quality image with smaller equipment.[24,66] Thoracoscopic approaches to the thoracic spine for sympathectomy, discectomy, and paraspinal neurogenic tumor with low morbidity and mortality have been described.[28] Thoracoscopic-assisted treatment of thoracic and lumbar fractures has been carried out on over 371 patients to date.[38] Expansion of these new minimally invasive techniques seems appealing when reported by a small number of authors.[20,28,38] Caution should be exercised when adopting these new surgical techniques since there is a significant learning curve. Certain pathologic entities still require open procedures to achieve adequate decompression and control bleeding.

Closure and Postoperative Care

Routine closure with approximation of all muscle layers in surgery involving the thoracic cavity is performed with one or two thoracostomy tubes, one passing to the apex and/or one to the dependent region of the chest cavity, connected to an underwater suction seal allowing drainage of air and blood. The drains are removed once the drainage is less than 100ml over a 12-hour period, which usually occurs by postoperative day 2 or 3. A major complication of both the transpleural and the ventrolateral approaches to the thoracolumbar spine is blood loss. This occurs during both the decompressive procedure and the fusion during which blood loss occurs from the cancellous surfaces of the bone graft and vertebral body sites. The blood lost should be estimated and should be replaced intraoperatively, and the hematocrit should be followed closely postoperatively. Pulmonary complications are low if relatively young, healthy patients are selected for these procedures.[10] Daily chest x-rays will help the physician monitor the pneumothorax and pleural effusions.

Patients who have undergone transthoracic surgery begin ambulation soon after removal of thoracostomy tubes. Sufficient analgesic must be given at all stages of postoperative care to reduce the postoperative pain that is associated with this type of surgery. Intercostal nerve blocks can be used before closure of the thoracotomy. Intrathoracic catheters for administration of narcotic analgesics are also helpful. Depending on neurologic recovery and capability for independence and support at home, the patient may return home or may require further rehabilitation at an appropriate facility.

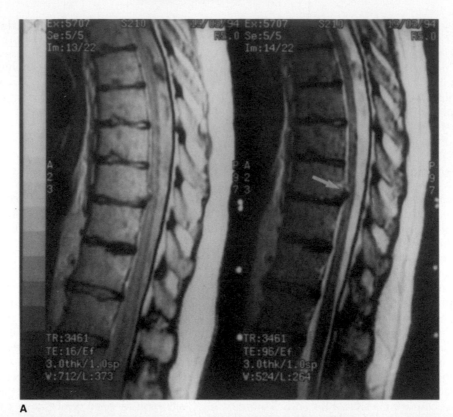

A

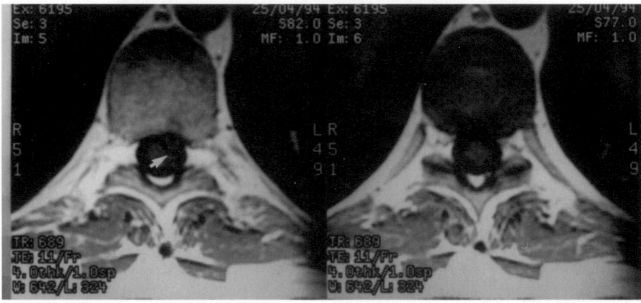

B

Figure 35.12 (**A**) Proton density and (**B**) T$_2$-weighted sagittal MR images of a patient with a T9-10 thoracic disc herniation with spinal cord compression.

Summary

Ventral and ventrolateral decompression, fusion, and instrumentation facilitate spinal canal and spinal cord decompression and provide stability in conditions with loss of anterior and middle column integrity, as what occurs in trauma (e.g., burst fracture), tumor, infection, degenerative disease, and congenital deformities. The techniques described allow decompression, correction of kyphosis, and stabilization to be performed as one-stage procedures and provide a stable construct with fixation involving the minimal number of segments. Postoperatively, excellent results for degree of decompression and rates of fusion have been obtained with minimal complications related to the surgical procedure.

REFERENCES

1. Arrington ED, Smith WJ, Chambers HG, et al: Complications of iliac crest bone graft harvesting. *Clin Orthop* Aug;300-309, 1996.

2. Arseni C, Nash F: Protrusion of thoracic intervertebral discs. *Acta Neurochir* (Wien) 11:418-430, 1963.

3. Asano S, Kaneda K, Satoh S, et al: Reconstruction of an iliac crest defect with a bioactive ceramic prosthesis. *Eur Spine J* 3:39-44, 1994.

4. Behairy YM, Al Sebai W: A modified technique for harvesting full-thickness iliac crest bone graft. *Spine* 26:695-697, 2001.

5. Bernard TN, Jr., Whitecloud TS III: Cervical spondylotic myelopathy and myeloradiculopathy: anterior decompression and stabilization with autogenous fibula strut graft. *Clin Orthop* Aug:149-160, 1987.

6. Burkus JK: Intervertebral fixation: clinical results with anterior cages. *Orthop Clin North Am* 33:349-357, 2002.

7. Cobden RH, Thrasher EL, Harris WH: Topical hemostatic agents to reduce bleeding from cancellous bone: a comparison of microcrystalline collagen, thrombin, and thrombin-soaked gelatin foam. *J Bone Joint Surg Am* 58:70-73, 1976.

8. Cook WA: Transthoracic vertebral surgery. *Ann Thorac Surg* 12:54-68, 1971.

9. Cooper PR, Errico TJ, Martin R, et al: A systematic approach to spinal reconstruction after anterior decompression for neoplastic disease of the thoracic and lumbar spine. *Neurosurgery* 32:1-8, 1993.

10. Dales RE, Dionne G, Leech JA, et al: Preoperative prediction of pulmonary complications following thoracic surgery. *Chest* 104:155-159, 1993.

11. Defino HL, Rodriguez-Fuentes AE: Reconstruction of anterior iliac crest bone graft donor sites: presentation of a surgical technique. *Eur Spine J* 8:491-494, 1999.

12. Deletis V, Sala F: The role of intraoperative neurophysiology in the protection or documentation of surgically induced injury to the spinal cord. *Ann N Y Acad Sci* 939:137-144, 2001.

13. Denis F: Spinal instability as defined by the three-column spine concept in acute spinal trauma. *Clin Orthop* Oct:65-76, 1984.

14. Dosoglu M, Orakdogen M, Tevruz M, et al: Enterocutaneous fistula: a complication of posterior iliac bone graft harvesting not previously described. *Acta Neurochir* (Wien) 140:1089-1092, 1998.

15. Ebraheim NA, Yang H, Lu J, et al: Anterior iliac crest bone graft: anatomic considerations. *Spine* 22:847-849, 1997.

16. Eck JC, Hodges SD, Humphreys SC: Vertebroplasty: a new treatment strategy for osteoporotic compression fractures. *Am J Orthop* 31:123-127, 2002.

17. Erickson DL, Leider LL, Browne W: One-stage decompression-stabilization for thoracolumbar fractures. *Spine* 2:143-153, 1977.

18. Errico TJ, Cooper PR: A new method of thoracic and lumbar body replacement for spinal tumors: technical note. *Neurosurgery* 32:678-680, 1993.

19. Evans AJ, Jensen ME, Kip KE, et al: Vertebral compression fractures: pain reduction and improvement in functional mobility after percutaneous polymethylmethacrylate vertebroplasty retrospective report of 245 cases. *Radiology* 226:366-372, 2003.

20. Fessler RG: Minimally invasive spine surgery. *Neurosurgery* 51:iii-iv, 2002.

21. Flesch JR, Leider LL, Erickson DL, et al: Harrington instrumentation and spine fusion for unstable fractures and fracture-dislocations of the thoracic and lumbar spine. *J Bone Joint Surg Am* 59:143-153, 1977.

22. Fourney DR, Schomer DF, Nader R, et al: Percutaneous vertebroplasty and kyphoplasty for painful vertebral body fractures in cancer patients. *J Neurosurg* 98:21-30, 2003.

23. Fowler BL, Dall BE, Rowe DE: Complications associated with harvesting autogenous iliac bone graft. *Am J Orthop* 24:895-903, 1995.

24. Friedel G, Linder A, Toomes H: Selective video-assisted thoracoscopic sympathectomy. *Thorac Cardiovasc Surg* 41:245-248, 1993.

25. Geary J, Frantz V: New absorbable bone wax: experimental and clinical studies. *Ann Surg* 132:1128, 1947.

26. Gertzbein SD, Offierski C: Complete fracture-dislocation of the thoracic spine without spinal cord injury: a case report. *J Bone Joint Surg Am* 61:449-451, 1979.

27. Hall AJ, Mackay NN: The results of laminectomy for compression of the cord or cauda equina by extradural malignant tumour. *J Bone Joint Surg Br* 55:497-505, 1973.

28. Han PP, Kenny K, Dickman CA: Thoracoscopic approaches to the thoracic spine: experience with 241 surgical procedures. *Neurosurgery* 51:88-95, 2002.

29. Harrington KD: Anterior cord decompression and spinal stabilization for patients with metastatic lesions of the spine. *J Neurosurg* 61:107-117, 1984.

30. Harris MB, Davis J, Gertzbein SD: Iliac crest reconstruction after tricortical graft harvesting. *J Spinal Disord Tech* 7:216-221, 1994.

31. Hodgson A, Stock F: Anterior spinal fusion: a preliminary communication on radical treatment of Pott's disease and Pott's paraplegia. *Br J Surg* 44:266, 1956.

32. Horwitz N, Curtin J: Prophylactic antibiotics and wound infections following laminectomy for lumbar disc herniation. *J Neurosurg* 43:727-731, 1975.

33. Hulme A: The surgical approach to thoracic intervertebral disc protrusions. *J Neurol Neurosurg Psychiatry* 23:133, 1960.

34. Jensen ME, Dion JE: Percutaneous vertebroplasty in the treatment of osteoporotic compression fractures. *Neuroimaging Clin N Am* 10:547-568, 2000.

35. Kanayama M, Cunningham BW, Haggerty CJ, et al: In vitro biomechanical investigation of the stability and stress-shielding effect of lumbar interbody fusion devices. *J Neurosurg* 93:259-265, 2000.

36. Kaneda K: *The Textbook of Spinal Surgery*. Philadelphia, Lippincott-Raven, 1991, p. 959.

37. Khoo LT, Beisse R, Potulski M: Thoracoscopic-assisted treatment of thoracic and lumbar fractures: a series of 371 consecutive cases. *Neurosurgery* 51:104-117, 2002.

38. Kostuik JP, Errico TJ, Gleason TF, et al: Spinal stabilization of vertebral column tumors. *Spine* 13:250-256, 1988.

39. Kothbauer K, Deletis V, Epstein FJ: Intraoperative spinal cord monitoring for intramedullary surgery: an essential adjunct. *Pediatr Neurosurg* 26:247-254, 1997.

40. Kurz LT, Garfin SR, Booth RE, Jr.: Harvesting autogenous iliac bone grafts: a review of complications and techniques. *Spine* 14:1324-1331, 1989.

41. Kux E: The endoscopic approach to the vegetative nervous system and its therapeutic possibilities. *Chest* 20:139-147, 1951.

42. Linville DA: Vertebroplasty and kyphoplasty. *South Med J* 95:583-587, 2002.

43. Logue V: Thoracic intervertebral disc prolapse with spinal cord compression. *J Neurol Neurosurg Psychiatry* 15:227, 1952.

44. Love J, Schorn V: Thoracic disc protrusion. *JAMA* 191:627, 1965.

45. Lubicky JP, DeWald RL: Methylmethacrylate reconstruction of large iliac crest bone graft donor sites. *Clin Orthop* Apr:252-256, 1982.

46. Luk KD, Hu Y, Wong YW, *et al:* Evaluation of various evoked potential techniques for spinal cord monitoring during scoliosis surgery. *Spine* 26:1772-1777, 2001.

47. Maciejczak A, Radek A: Lumbar interbody fusion: biomechanical significance for the spine. *Neurol Neurochir Pol* 32:1247-1259, 1998.

48. Manabe S, Tateishi A, Abe M, *et al:* Surgical treatment of metastatic tumors of the spine. *Spine* 14:41-47, 1989.

49. Matge G: Cervical cage fusion with 5 different implants: 250 cases. *Acta Neurochir (Wien)* 144:539-549, 2002.

50. Matge G, Leclercq TA: Rationale for interbody fusion with threaded titanium cages at cervical and lumbar levels: results on 357 cases. *Acta Neurochir (Wien)* 142:425-433, 2000.

51. Mirovsky Y, Neuwirth MG: Comparison between the outer table and intracortical methods of obtaining autogenous bone graft from the iliac crest. *Spine* 25:1722-1725, 2000.

52. Mueller R: Prolapse of thoracic intervertebral discs. *Acta Med Scand* 139:99, 1951.

53. Murakami H, Horton WC, Kawahara N, *et al:* Anterior lumbar interbody fusion using two standard cylindrical threaded cages, a single mega-cage, or dual nested cages: a biomechanical comparison. *J Orthop Sci* 6:343-348, 2001.

54. Murata Y, Takahashi K, Yamagata M, *et al:* Injury to the lateral femoral cutaneous nerve during harvest of iliac bone graft, with reference to the size of the graft. *J Bone Joint Surg Br* 84:798-801, 2002.

55. Norrell H: The treatment of unstable spinal fractures and dislocations. *Clin Neurosurg* 25:193-208, 1978.

56. Nuwer MR: Spinal cord monitoring. *Muscle Nerve* 22:1620-1630, 1999.

57. Ousmane ML, Herbecq P, Jasatis L, *et al:* Colon hernia through a defect in the iliac crest after bone graft harvesting. *Ann Fr Anesth Reanim* 19:749-750, 2000.

58. Owen JH: The application of intraoperative monitoring during surgery for spinal deformity. *Spine* 24:2649-2662, 1999.

59. Perot PL, Jr., Munro DD: Transthoracic removal of midline thoracic disc protrusions causing spinal cord compression. *J Neurosurg* 31:452-458, 1969.

60. Peters KR, Guiot BH, Martin PA, *et al:* Vertebroplasty for osteoporotic compression fractures: current practice and evolving techniques. *Neurosurgery* 51:96-103, 2002.

61. Porchet F, Jaques B: Unusual complications at iliac crest bone graft donor site: experience with two cases. *Neurosurgery* 39:856-859, 1996.

62. Predey TA, Sewall LE, Smith SJ: Percutaneous vertebroplasty: new treatment for vertebral compression fractures. *Am Fam Physician* 66:611-615, 2002.

63. Ransohoff J, Spencer F, Siew F, *et al:* Transthoracic removal of thoracic disc: report of three cases. *J Neurosurg* 31:459-461, 1969.

64. Reeves DL, Brown HA: Thoracic intervertebral disc protrusion with spinal cord compression. *J Neurosurg* 28:24-28, 1968.

65. Robertson DP, Simpson RK, Rose JE, *et al:* Video-assisted endoscopic thoracic ganglionectomy. *J Neurosurg* 79: 238-240, 1993.

66. Royle N: The operative removal of an accessory vertebra. *Med J Aust* 1:467, 1928.

67. Sacks S: Anterior interbody fusion of the lumbar spine. *J Bone Joint Surg* 47B:211, 1965.

68. Sacks S: Anterior interbody fusion of the lumbar spine: indications and results in 200 cases. *Clin Orthop* 44: 163-170, 1966.

69. Seiler JG III, Johnson J: Iliac crest autogenous bone grafting: donor site complications. *J South Orthop Assoc* 9:91-97, 2000.

70. Shono Y, Kaneda K, Yamamoto I: A biomechanical analysis of Zielke, Kaneda, and Cotrel-Dubousset instrumentations in thoracolumbar scoliosis: a calf spine model. *Spine* 16:1305-1311, 1991.

71. Slabaugh PB, Winter RB, Lonstein JE, *et al:* Lumbosacral hemivertebrae: a review of twenty-four patients, with excision in eight. *Spine* 5:234-244, 1980.

72. Sundaresan N, Galicich JH, Bains MS, *et al:* Vertebral body resection in the treatment of cancer involving the spine. *Cancer* 53:1393-1396, 1984.

73. Sundaresan N, Galicich JH, Lane JM, *et al:* Treatment of neoplastic epidural cord compression by vertebral body resection and stabilization. *J Neurosurg* 63:676-684, 1985.

74. Svein H, Karavitis A: Multiple protrusions of the intervertebral discs in the upper thoracic region: report of case. *Proc Staff Meet Mayo Clin* 29:375, 1954.

75. Torode IP: Pelvic reconstruction after bone-graft harvesting. *J Pediatr Orthop* 14:381-382, 1994.

76. Tovi D, Strang RR: Thoracic intervertebral disc protrusions. *Acta Chir Scand Suppl* 267:1-41, 1960.

77. Tsantrizos A, Baramki HG, Zeidman S, *et al:* Segmental stability and compressive strength of posterior lumbar interbody fusion implants. *Spine* 25:1899-1907, 2000.

78. Watts NB, Harris ST, Genant HK: Treatment of painful osteoporotic vertebral fractures with percutaneous vertebroplasty or kyphoplasty. *Osteoporos Int* 12:429-437, 2001.

79. White AA, III, Panjabi MM: *Clinical Biomechanics of the Spine.* Philadelphia, Lippincott-Raven, 1978.

80. Wimmer C, Gluch H, Franzreb M, *et al:* Predisposing factors for infection in spine surgery: a survey of 850 spinal procedures. *J Spinal Disord Tech* 11:124-128, 1998.

81. Wolfe SA, Kawamoto HK: Taking the iliac-bone graft. *J Bone Joint Surg Am* 60:411, 1978.

82. Wood KB, Blair JM, Aepple DM, *et al:* The natural history of asymptomatic thoracic disc herniations. *Spine* 22: 525-529, 1997.

83. Young RF, Post EM, King GA: Treatment of spinal epidural metastases: randomized prospective comparison of laminectomy and radiotherapy. *J Neurosurg* 53:741-748, 1980.

84. Zdeblick TA, Smith GR, Warden KE, *et al:* Two-point fixation of the lumbar spine: differential stability in rotation. *Spine* 16:S298-S301, 1991.

C H A P T E R   3 6

Lateral Extracavitary Decompression

**Dennis J. Maiman, Paul M. Arnold,
Dennis G. Vollmer, and Sanford J. Larson**

Indications

The lateral extracavitary approach (LECA) to the thoracic and lumbar spine[4,5] is a useful surgical procedure for approaching pathology located ventral and lateral to the spinal cord, as well as circumferential lesions. The LECA can be used effectively from T3 to S1 for the removal, under direct vision, of virtually any ventral extradural mass, including fractures,[4,5,10,13,14] tumors,[6,11,12] infection,[4,7] and herniated discs (Figures 36.1 to 36.4).[9] Bony interbody fusion and dorsal fixation are readily accomplished during a single procedure, through one incision, and in a logical sequence of decompression, stabilization, and fusion.[15,16] The LECA allows the surgeon to avoid the thoracic and abdominal cavities, while also avoiding associated complications. At the thoracolumbar junction, exposure of the T12 through L2 vertebral bodies is facilitated without takedown of the diaphragm.

Usually the procedure is performed from one side, but it can be carried out bilaterally to facilitate complete spondylectomy, including complete removal of the dorsal elements. Furthermore, contralateral transpedicular decompression, laminectomy, and dorsal instrumentation are facilitated through the same incision. If only a ventral/lateral exposure is requested, alternative incisions that minimize muscle dissection can be used; recently, we have employed minimally invasive techniques to the approach.

Surgical Preparation

A well-conceived, preoperative diagnostic work-up is essential for surgical planning. Imaging should include an assessment of bony integrity, as well as neural decompression. Magnetic resonance imaging (MRI) is ideal for the latter and provides critical information regarding ligament status. This is often important with respect to the decision-making process regarding dorsal fixation. Currently there is no conclusive evidence that early surgery for thoracolumbar trauma improves outcome; thus treatment of other traumatic lesions may take operative precedence.[5,7,8] Similarly, the decision to undertake a major spinal procedure in patients with known metastases requires knowledge of the primary tumor involvement and suspected outcomes. "Lesser" procedures may be appropriate in individuals with limited life expectancy; conversely, the LECA is ideal in patients who require decompression as well as fixation, recognizing that more traditional ventrolateral approaches are limited in terms of dorsal fixation.

Preoperative spinal angiography is sometimes useful in identifying the artery of Adamkiewicz for lesions between T7 and L2. This artery is located at the level of pathology in approximately 20% of the cases and may provide critical blood supply to the watershed zone in the lower thoracic spinal cord.[1] Although the popular consensus is that injury of this vessel does not produce neural injury, some studies, and the authors' anecdotal experience, suggest that it can. Hence caution is advised. When feasible, the authors recommend operating from the side opposite this vessel. Angiography for preoperative embolization is also quite valuable for many tumors. This should be performed within 24 to 36 hours of the surgery and may result in dramatically decreased blood loss.

Operative Technique
Surgical Preparation

Preoperative preparation is the same as for any major spinal procedure. Large-bore venous access, arterial pressure lines, Foley catheters, and antiembolism stockings are used. The authors usually perform this procedure on a Jackson frame, which decreases intraabdominal venous pressure, with careful attention paid to padding of pressure points. The Jackson frame allows the table to be rotated from the surgeon, often an advantage during decompression.

Balanced anesthesia, with a combination of inhalation agents and narcotics, is usually used. The authors do not recommend hemodilution or intentional hypotension during surgery. A cell-saver is used, except in cases of cancer or infection. The authors do not routinely use intraoperative sensory or motor evoked potential monitoring because thecal sac decompression is performed under direct vision, and the results and benefits of electrophysiologic monitoring have been inconsistent.[3,5-7] However, in cases of severe deformity it may be helpful.

Incision

Correct anatomic or radiographic localization is essential because the incision must be centered over the lesion. The skin incision should be marked after the patient is positioned. A metallic marker is placed over what is thought to be the level of pathology, and a radiograph is obtained. A curved, hockey stick-shaped incision is typically used (Figure 36.5). Although others have used an L-shaped incision, a devascularized corner can become necrotic. The hockey stick-shaped incision is typically made to the side of the worst pathology in the instance of fracture or tumor, unless precluded by the location of the artery of Adamkiewicz.[1,5,17] For disc herniation, if there is asymmetry, the authors prefer to operate from the side of the greatest spinal canal compromise.

If dorsal decompression or fixation is not to be performed, a linear paramedian incision over the lateral border of the paravertebral musculature should suffice. If the lesion is at T12 or below, the caudal aspect of the hockey-stick incision is situated over the iliac crest. In this case part of the iliac crest may be removed to facilitate

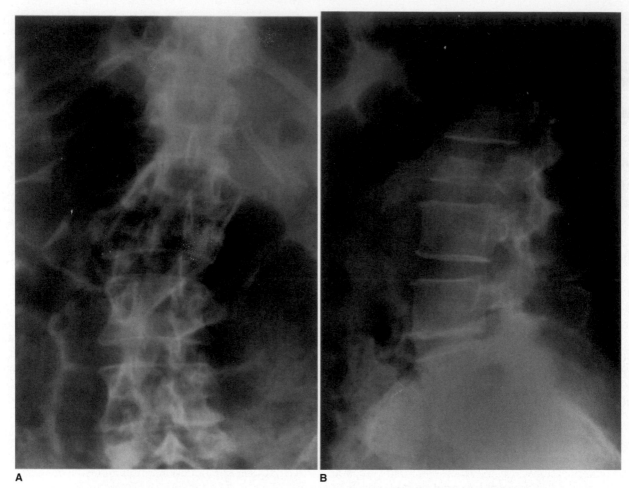

A   B

Figure 36.1 (A-B) Anteroposterior and lateral radiographs show L2 fracture secondary to
metastatic adenocarcinoma.

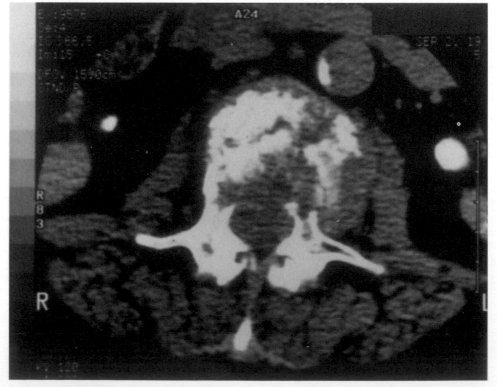

Figure 36.2 A CT scan shows destruction of vertebral body and left pedicle.

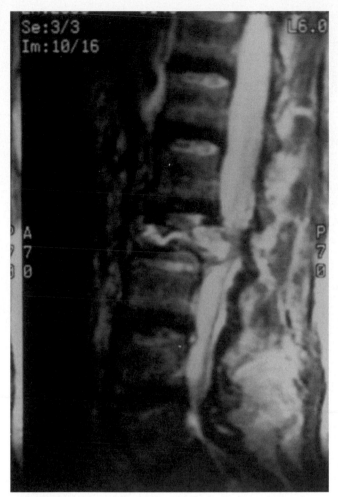

Figure 36.3 Sagittal T$_2$-weighted MRI image shows severe narrowing of spinal canal.

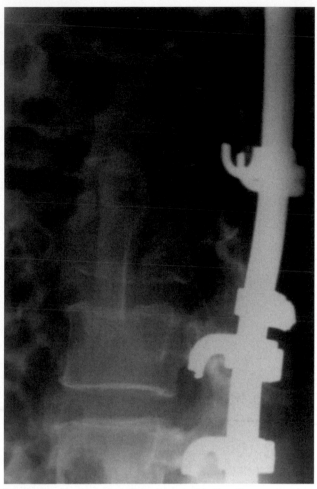

Figure 36.4 Postoperative film showing hook-rod construction (T10-L4) and interbody rib graft from L1 to L3.

exposure of the spinal canal. The iliac crest can then be used as grafting material. If the lesion is above L2, the ribs that are removed when approaching the spinal canal can be used for bone grafts.

Deep Dissection

After the skin incision is made, the subcutaneous tissue, fascia, and muscles are stripped from the spinous processes, lamina, and facet joints bilaterally, if dorsal instrumentation is to be used. A flap is developed, consisting of the thoracodorsal fascia (which has been elevated from the muscle) and subcutaneous tissue and skin, and retracted laterally. A plane is also developed, typically using blunt dissection, under the lateral aspect of the erector spinae muscle. These muscles are then retracted medially off the underlying ribs or transverse processes. A self-retaining retractor is used to hold the erector spinae muscle medially and the skin flap laterally. At this point the initial subperiosteal dissection from the midline structures is continuous with the just-completed dissection beneath the muscle bellies of the erector spinae muscle.[6,7]

Ribs must be dissected free from the underlying tissue before they can be removed. In general a single rib is removed for a single-level disc herniation; the proximal portions of two ribs are removed for fracture, tumor, or infection.

A Doyen instrument is used to free the soft tissue from the ventral side of the ribs. The rib is then disarticulated at the costovertebral joint with a periosteal elevator. Keep in mind that the underlying pleura can be torn. Rib disarticulation is facilitated by rongeuring back the transverse process. The rib is incised laterally with a rib cutter (about 8 to 10cm from the joint for tumor or trauma, and 3cm for disc) and saved for later use as bone graft. Often the twelfth rib must be removed for adequate exposure of L1 or L2. At levels below T12, the appropriate transverse processes are dissected and removed.[7]

For lesions of L3 or lower, portions of the iliac crest are removed with osteotomes after subperiosteal dissection of the overlying muscles. It is important to remove the medial aspect of the iliac crest to avoid neural injury and to avoid entering the sacroiliac joint. The bleeding cancellous bone is waxed as needed to prevent postoperative hematoma. The resected bone is saved for later use as a bone graft.

The exposed intercostal nerve is skeletonized with the use of blunt and sharp dissection to facilitate removal of the pedicle. The nerve is followed proximally to the neural

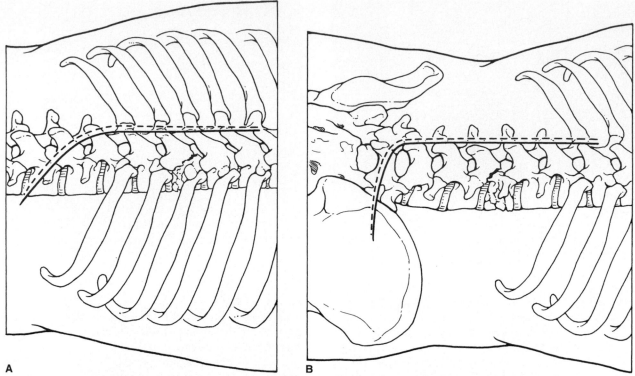

Figure 36.5 (**A**) Thoracic skin incision. Note that the incision extends three levels above and below lesion. The caudal portion is in a "hockey-stick," B-type curve. (**B**) Lumbar skin incision. Note that the caudal portion extends over the iliac crest. In both **A** and **B**, alternate incisions are also depicted.

foramen. At this point the table is rotated 20 degrees away from the surgeon, so that the ipsilateral side of the patient is higher, thus enabling the spine to be at an optimal angle for visualization by the surgeon. The venous plexus surrounding the nerve is coagulated at its junction with the dural sac, and the dura is freed from the bone. The foramen is enlarged circumferentially using a small 45-degree Kerrison rongeur and curettes, and continued dissection is performed with a nerve hook or dental tool. This is performed at levels rostral and caudal to the pathology before any effort to decompress the thecal sac is made. Thus in fractures and tumors, two intercostals are exposed.

The periosteum of the involved vertebrae is bluntly dissected away to identify disc spaces rostral and caudal to the pathology, and radiography is obtained to ensure that the surgery is at the appropriate level. Developing this plane helps to attain an unobstructed view of the entire lateral aspect of the spine. The pleura or peritoneum is retracted with a Dever or Thompson retractor. Occasionally, small pleural tears occur, either during the extracavitary dissection previously described or during rib removal. To prevent a pneumothorax or hemothorax, the pleura is oversewn, or in the case of a larger tear a thoracostomy tube is inserted and exteriorized to closed drainage through a separate incision.

Spinal Canal Decompression

The pedicle is now ready for removal. It can be thinned, although not removed, with a rongeur or high-speed drill. The excision is accomplished in a piecemeal fashion with a

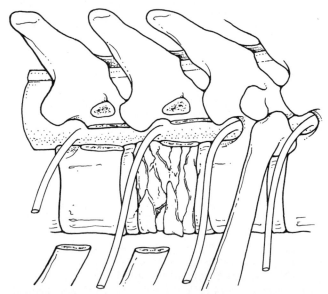

Figure 36.6 The pedicle has been removed after the intercostal nerve to the neuroforamen. The lesion and the compressed spinal cord are easily visualized.

Kerrison punch, while ensuring that there are no dural adhesions (which commonly occur in trauma). The entire pedicle and the lateral wall of the spinal canal should be completely removed above and below the lesion. Ideally, removal extends just beyond the end plate of the adjacent discs to afford direct visualization of the relationship between the dural sac and the pathology (Figure 36.6).

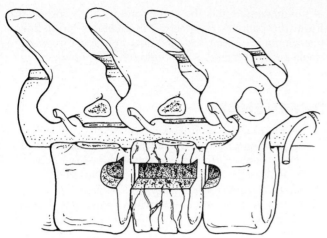

Figure 36.7 The disc spaces are drilled out with a Hudson brace after radiographic localization.

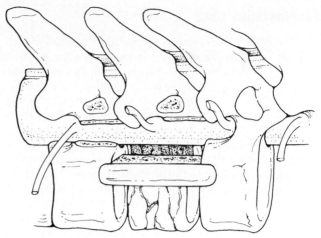

Figure 36.8 The bone graft is inserted after decompression and fixation have been completed

If the clinical pathology is a herniated disc and no vertebral resection is necessary, the disc is resected after removal of the pedicle. A no. 11 scalpel is used to incise the annulus about 1cm ventral to the spinal canal, and disc material is removed across the midline. Some use a Hudson brace and bit to drill out the hole. Down-biting curettes are then used to push the disc, compressing the spinal cord away until full decompression has been achieved. Decompression can be confirmed with dental mirrors or ultrasound. One or two small pieces of the previously resected ribs are cut to the appropriate size and used as an interbody graft, since instability is felt to be a prominent aspect of the pathogenesis of thoracic disc herniation.[18] If tumor, infection, or trauma is present, the vertebral body may require resection, along with the disc above and below. The discs are opened laterally. Generally, except for tumor in which more radical removal is needed, the disc is incised about 1 to 1.5cm ventral to the spinal canal (Figure 36.7). It is absolutely imperative that disc removal extend well across the spinal canal; the success of the vertebral decompression is dependent on this. Generally the authors employ a Hudson brace and bit to drill out the disc space, ensuring that the hole extends beyond the opposite side of the spinal canal.

After disc removal, attention can be turned to the vertebral body. The vertebral body is removed with a high-speed drill or a Leksell rongeur. Because this is done under direct vision, damage to the spinal cord can be averted. Care must be taken to avoid pushing a fractured piece of bone into the spinal canal.

The drill or Leksell rongeur is used to remove bone until a thin rim of bone (i.e., 2 to 3mm) is left dorsally, which is the floor of the canal. This thin rim, or "shelf" of the bone, is then removed in a downward (ventral) direction, ideally at the end-plates after the bone is dissected free from the dura mater. This can be accomplished with downward-angled curettes. Care must be taken to not damage the dural sac and contents with the "recoil" force resulting from the rebound of the dorsal bony fragments. Disc and bone removal should be accomplished well past the opposite lateral border of the spinal canal to ensure decompression of the entire thecal sac. Adequacy of resec-

tion can be confirmed by inspection with dental mirrors or intraoperative ultrasound to visualize the contralateral aspect of the dural sac. Significant epidural bleeding occasionally occurs during decompression, but can usually be controlled with topical hemostasis. Now that the thecal sac is decompressed, reduction, if indicated, and stabilization can be safely accomplished.

Spinal Instrumentation

The retractors are removed, the table is turned back prone, and attention is given to the previously accomplished subperiosteal dissection. Spinal instrumentation is usually required when the vertebral column is unstable.[2,3,7] The type and length of the construct depends on the surgeon's experience and the pathology. Adson-Beckman retractors are placed over the areas already dissected. Decortication and dorsal element and transverse process bone grafting can be performed at this time. The posterior muscle layer is closed after the instrumentation is completed, usually over a surgical drain.

Interbody Bone Graft Placement

Attention is now turned to the last portion of the procedure: placement of the interbody bone graft. Troughs are made with curettes in the vertebral bodies above and below the decompressed area. The previously resected ribs or iliac crest are cut to the appropriate length and then impacted into place. Two or three rib segments or one piece of tricortical iliac crest is optimal. If bone is structurally suboptimal, titanium mesh or other interbody devices can be employed. The grafts should be placed as far from the spinal cord as is technically feasible (Figure 36.8). If the grafts are slightly longer than the defect, impaction generally ensures solid placement.

Wound Closure

The wound is closed in layers, with a surgical drain placed adjacent to the operative site and kept in for 24 hours.

Postoperative Care

The postoperative care is generally straightforward. Patients occasionally require intensive care the night of surgery. Mobilization in an orthosis within 24 hours of surgery is desirable when systemically possible. Postoperative radiographs are obtained on the third postoperative day. The patient is usually ready for discharge on the fifth to seventh postoperative day, either to his or her home, or to a rehabilitation unit in cases of trauma or tumor. Patients being treated for thoracic disc herniation average 2.5 days of hospitalization. A postoperative orthosis is used depending on the pathology: although there is little evidence for this practice, the authors maintain the thoracolumbosacralorthosis (TLSO) for an average of 12 weeks in trauma or tumor, and 6 weeks for thoracic disc surgery.

Complications

Complications are those typical of major spine surgery, but are surprisingly uncommon. Infectious complications such as pneumonia or urinary tract infections are common in patients with paraplegia. Wound infections are relatively uncommon and are typically superficial. The authors have found that using a surgical drain and a hockey stick–shaped incision, as opposed to using an L-shaped incision, has diminished wound necrosis. The incidence of deep venous thrombosis is minimized with the use of pneumatic compression devices and stockings. Recently the authors have begun using low molecular weight heparin intraoperatively and postoperatively in selected patients, without evidence of increased blood loss. Hypovolemia and ileus may be problems in the early postoperative period but are usually self-limited. Interbody graft displacement is uncommon because the grafts are placed during the same procedure as the internal fixation, and repositioning is not required between stages as it is for an anteroposterior 360-degree fusion.

Historically, some surgeons have had problems with blood loss during this procedure. However, in recent years careful attention to hemostasis, especially during the initial dissection and removal of the pedicle, has dramatically decreased blood loss. Control of the arteries perforating the vertebral bodies ventrally is helpful as well.

Pulmonary complications such as hemothorax or pneumothorax are treated with thoracostomy, either intraoperatively or postoperatively. These complications are uncommon, however. Later complications include implant failure, nonunion, and excessive flexion deformity. These are uncommon as well, since both ventral and dorsal fusion have been performed. In an early series the authors had used single-level pedicle fixation for trauma. Although nonunion was infrequent, the loss of correction was unsatisfactory, and the technique is only rarely used. Indeed, in patients undergoing LECA with ventral iliac crest grafting and dorsal fixation with dorsal fusion for trauma, the nonunion rate is less than 3%.

Thus the LECA represents a rational approach to disorders of the spine that require vertebral resection and fusion, facilitating the employment of sound biomechanical principles and rational clinical decision-making. From a technical standpoint, good surgical technique and an understanding of the anatomy limits the complications of the procedure. From the patient's perspective, it facilitates the definitive management of complex problems in a single procedure, single anesthesia, and single postoperative period.

REFERENCES

1. Arnold PM, Hollowell JP, Bates SR, Mark LP: Role of spinal arteriography in the preoperative management of thoracolumbar pathology. Presented at the 62nd Annual Meeting of the American Association of Neurological Surgeons, April 1994, Chicago, IL.
2. Benzel EC: The lateral extracavitary approach to the spine using the three-quarter prone position. *J Neurosurg* 71:837, 1989.
3. Benzel EC, Larson SJ: Operative stabilization of the post-traumatic thoracic and lumbar spine: a comparative analysis of the Harrington rod and the modified Weiss spring. *Neurosurgery* 19:378, 1986.
4. Capener N: The evolution of lateral rhacotomy. *J Bone Joint Surg* 36B:173, 1954.
5. Larson SJ: Unstable thoracic fractures: treatment alternatives and the role of the neurosurgeon. *Clin Neurosurg* 27:624, 1980.
6. Larson SJ: Lateral extracavitary approach to the spine: indications and operative technique. *Contemp Neurosurg* 15:1-6, 1993.
7. Larson SJ, Holst RA, Hemmy DC, Sances A Jr: Lateral extracavitary approach to traumatic lesions of the thoracic and lumbar spine. *J Neurosurg* 45:628, 1976.
8. Larson SJ, Maiman DJ: Biomechanics of the spine: normal and pathologic. In *Surgery of the Lumbar Spine*. New York, Thieme, 1999, pp 13-34.
9. Larson SJ, Maiman DJ: Benign tumors of the spine. In *Surgery of the Lumbar Spine*. New York, Thieme, 1999, pp 183-200.
10. Larson SJ, Maiman DJ: Metabolic diseases of the bone. In *Surgery of the Lumbar Spine*. New York, Thieme, 1999, pp 51-78.
11. Larson SJ, Maiman DJ: Primary malignant tumors. In *Surgery of the Lumbar Spine*. New York, Thieme, 1999, pp 201-230.
12. Larson SJ, Maiman DJ: Metastatic tumors of the lumbar spine. In *Surgery of the Lumbar Spine*. New York, Thieme, 1999, pp 231-254.
13. Larson SJ, Maiman DJ: Bone grafts and orthoses In *Surgery of the Lumbar Spine*. New York, Thieme, 1999, pp 255-267.
14. Larson SJ, Maiman DJ: Trauma. In *Surgery of the Lumbar Spine*. New York, Thieme, 1999, pp 157-182.
15. Larson SJ, Maiman DJ: Surgical approaches. In *Surgery of the Lumbar Spine*. New York, Thieme, 1999, pp 267-325.
16. Maiman DJ, Larson SJ: Lateral extracavitary approach to the thoracic and lumbar spine. In Rengachary SS, Wilkins RM (eds): *Neurosurgical Operative Atlas*. Baltimore, Williams & Wilkins, 1992.
17. Maiman DJ, Larson SJ, Benzel EC: Neurologic improvement associated with late decompression of the thoracolumbar spinal cord. *Neurosurgery* 14:302, 1984.
18. Maiman DJ, Larson SJ, Luke E, El-Ghatit A: The lateral extracavitary approach to the spine for thoracic disc herniation: Report of 23 cases. *Neurosurgery* 14:178, 1984.

CHAPTER 37

Retropleural Approach to the Ventral Thoracic and Thoracolumbar Spine

Paul C. McCormick

Two of the most widely used approaches to the ventral thoracic and thoracolumbar spine are the transpleural thoracotomy and the lateral extracavitary approach.[1,5] Each approach has its advantages and disadvantages. The major advantage of the ventrolateral transpleural thoracotomy is that it provides unparalleled exposure of the ventral vertebral column over several segments. Nevertheless this exposure has several disadvantages. First, this approach is characterized by an extensive incision and soft-tissue dissection that are necessitated by a deep operative field. Secondly, because with this approach, the chest cavity is entered from the ventrolateral chest quadrant, significant retraction of the unprotected lung is required. Finally, identification and decompression of the ventral spinal canal is also problematic, because the rib head partially obscures the spinal canal and the epidural veins are difficult to control via this trajectory. The aforementioned factors can create a less secure operative environment, promote surgical morbidity, and hinder the attainment of the surgical objective(s).

The lateral extracavitary approach is particularly useful when circumferential spinal exposure is needed, but it is impractical for isolated ventral vertebral column exposure. Ventral vertebral exposure with this technique requires an extensive and often bloody paraspinal muscle and foraminal dissection. Intercostal nerves are sacrificed to optimize exposure. This may result in a painful neuroma or abdominal wall muscle weakness at lower thoracic and thoracolumbar levels. The foraminal dissection may inadvertently occlude a medullary vessel, which may risk spinal cord infarction. Finally, despite the extensive dissection, direct ventral spinal canal visualization extends only to the midline and provides insufficient exposure to place a lateral spinal implant.

A retropleural thoracotomy, ideally, is more suited for a ventral exposure of the thoracic and thoracolumbar spine.[3,4,6] Similar to ventrolateral thoracotomy, the line of vision provided with a retropleural thoracotomy is ventral to the ventral aspect of the spinal canal, but because the chest cavity is entered more dorsally, there is a significantly shorter distance to the ventral vertebral column and canal. The extrapleural nature of the dissection allows safer and more secure lung retraction and avoids postop-erative tube thoracostomy placement. This approach allows for earlier identification and entry into the lateral spinal canal, via a resected pedicle. It greatly facilitates ventral spinal canal decompression through the disc space and vertebral bodies. Unlike the lateral extracavitary approach, however, mobilization or sacrifice of the foraminal neurovascular structures is avoided. Thus retropleural thoracotomy represents a hybrid surgical approach, incorporating the advantages of both standard transpleural ventrolateral and dorsolateral extrapleural approaches, while avoiding their limitations.

Operative Planning

Retropleural thoracotomy is an appropriate approach for localized ventral thoracic and thoracolumbar vertebral lesions between T3 and L2. The side of the operative approach is determined primarily by the location of the lesion. Eccentric lesions are approached ipsilaterally. The choice of the approach for central lesions is determined by the proximity of the great vessels and viscera. For high thoracic lesions, the aortic loop favors a right-sided approach. Either side is appropriate at midthoracic levels, although an ectatic aorta in older patients may obscure the field with a left-sided approach. At thoracic and thoracolumbar levels a left-sided approach is preferred to avoid the vena cava and retraction of the liver.

Consistency must be ensured between the methods of preoperative and intraoperative determination of pathologic level to avoid a discrepancy. This is particularly likely to occur when the preoperative levels are determined by magnetic resonance imaging (MRI). MRI identifies levels according to an end-vertebrae reference point. For a lower thoracic lesion, for example, the pathologic level is numbered by counting up from the sacrum. This creates two areas of uncertainty. First, there may be transitional lumbosacral vertebrae. Second, MRI does not identify the number of ribs, size of the end rib, and number of non-rib lumbar vertebrae. From a surgical perspective, intraoperative localization is usually done according to a surgically verifiable landmark, such as the end rib. Therefore these two study methods must be consistent before surgery. If the location of the pathology has been identified with MRI, plain radiographs should be obtained to determine the size of the end rib and the number of nonribbed lumbar vertebrae.

Surgical Technique

After appropriate arterial and venous line access has been established induction and intubation is performed. A double lumen tube is used for lesions above the T6 vertebral level. An epidural catheter may be placed after intubation or at the conclusion of the procedure, for postoperative pain management. A broad-spectrum antibiotic is usually administered 30 minutes before the skin incision, and this may be continued for two postoperative doses. The patient is carefully turned into a lateral position on a beanbag chair, with a small, soft roll under the dependent axilla. The upper arm is supported on a pillow or sling. The lower leg is slightly flexed at the hip and knee to help secure the position. All bony prominences and subcutaneously coursing nerve trunks must be well padded. The ulnar nerve at the elbow and the peroneal nerve at the fibular neck are particularly vulnerable areas. Thoracolumbar lesions should be centered over the kidney break. The skin incision is planned according to the level of exposure. For midthoracic lesions (T5-9), a 14cm skin incision should extend from a point 4cm off the dorsal midline to the dorsal axillary line. Extension of the incision toward the midaxillary line expands ventral access and may be required in some cases (Figure 37.1, *center incision*). A curved incision that parallels the medial and inferior scapular border is used for upper (T3-4) thoracic lesions (see Figure 37.1, *rightmost incision*). For thoracolumbar exposure (T10-L2), the incision should parallel the rib one spinal segment above the pathologic level because of the more caudal inclination of the proximal portion of the lowest ribs (see Figure 37.1, *leftmost incision*). Therefore whereas the approach to a T7-8 disc is exposed through the T8 rib bed, a T12 lesion is approached through the bed of the T11 rib.

The skin incision is carried down to the rib (Figure 37.2). A 10 to 12cm rib segment, extending from the costotransverse ligament to the dorsal axillary line, is subpe-

riosteally exposed and removed with rib shears (Figure 37.3). The exposed bone surfaces are waxed. Note that the proximal 4cm of the rib, extending from the costotransverse articulation to the rib head, has yet to be removed. The bed of the resected rib is now inspected. Muscle fibers of an inconstant subcostal muscle may be seen. At thoracic levels above T10 the endothoracic fascia will be identified in the rib bed. The endothoracic fascia is analogous to the transversalis fascia of the abdominal cavity.[2] Both types of fascia line the walls of their respective visceral cavities and are reflected onto the surface of the diaphragm. The endothoracic fascia is tightly applied to or is continuous with the inner periosteum of the rib and vertebral bodies. The parietal pleuron maintains its attachment to the chest wall through a surface tension seal with the inner surface of the endothoracic fascia. The intercostal vessels, nerves, and sympathetic chain are contained within the endothoracic fascia. Although only a potential (subendothoracic) space exists between the endothoracic fascia and parietal pleura, a small amount of fluid and loose adipose tissue is occasionally identified, particularly dorsally near the rib head and vertebral bodies. Because the endothoracic fascia is continuous with the inner

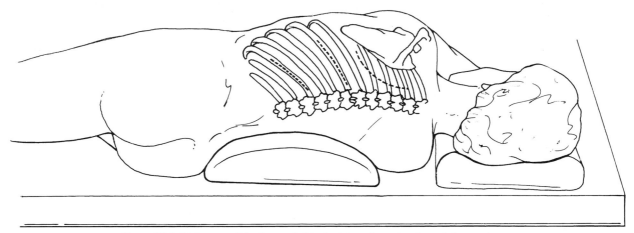

Figure 37.1 Patient positioning and skin incisions for retropleural thoracotomy.

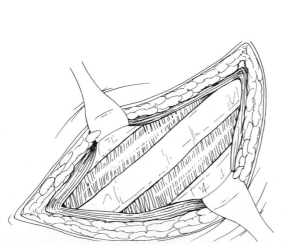

Figure 37.2 Skin incision is carried down to expose the rib to be resected.

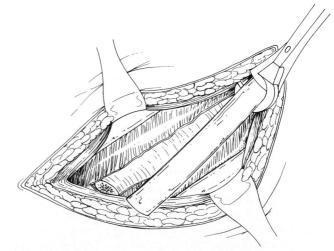

Figure 37.3 After a careful subperiosteal dissection, a 10 to 12cm rib segment is removed.

periosteum of the rib, it may be inadvertently torn during rib dissection and removal. This is common in older patients. If the endothoracic fascia is intact, it should be incised in line with the rib bed (Figure 37.4). The underlying parietal pleuron is bluntly and widely separated from the endothoracic fascia, either manually or with a Kittner (peanut) clamp (Figure 37.5). The endothoracic fascia incision is continued dorsally to the margin of the cut surface of the remaining proximal rib. Blunt dissection of the pleura off the proximal rib head extends dorsally to expose the vertebral bodies and disc space. When the ventral convex border of the vertebral body has been exposed, a self-retaining, table-mounted retractor maintains exposure of the vertebral column (Figure 37.6).

The endothoracic fascia incision is continued dorsally over the remaining proximal rib segment and onto the vertebral body with electrocautery. This divides the sympathetic chain that descends within the endothoracic fascia, just ventral to the rib head insertion on the surface of the vertebral column. The musculoligamentous attachments, including the costotransverse and stellate ligaments, are detached from the rib head segment, which is then removed. Removal of the rib head is critical because it allows identification of the pedicle (through which the lateral spinal canal entry will subsequently be accessed). For thoracic disc removal, the incised endothoracic fascia and vertebral body periosteum are elevated, in either direction from the disc space to the midvertebral body. The intercostal vessels, which run transversely at the midvertebral level, are preserved within the reflected tissue. The margins of the pedicle are defined with angled curettes and nerve hooks. The pedicle is resected with a high-speed drill, or Kerrison rongeurs. Removal of the pedicle provides lateral spinal canal identification and entrance. This lateral canal entrance, unlike the lateral extracavitary approach,

avoids a bloody foraminal dissection, as well as possible nerve root and radiculomedullary artery injury.

The lateral disc annulus fibrosus is sharply incised. The disc is evacuated with curettes and rongeurs. The adjacent end-plate and vertebral body margins are removed with a high-speed drill. The width and depth of the disc and adjacent vertebral body dissection must be adequate to ensure ventral spinal canal exposure and decompression. The depth should extend 3 to 3.5cm from the lateral body vertebral margin to reach the contralateral pedicle. The width should extend about 1cm on either side of the disc into the adjacent vertebral bodies (wider for larger calcified discs that have migrated, usually caudally, behind the vertebral body). The dissection is continued dorsally toward the spinal canal with disc curettage and a high-speed drill (Figure 37.7). Spinal canal identification through the disc space and adjacent vertebral bodies is readily achieved because of the previously exposed lateral spinal canal entrance through the resected pedicle bed. When the dissection is carried back to the dorsal cortical margin and dorsal annulus fibrosus, a sharp, reverse-angle curette is passed through the lateral spinal canal entrance to displace these structures away from the spinal canal and into the bed of the resected disc and adjacent vertebral bodies. This maneuver may precipitate epidural bleeding that can be effectively managed with bipolar cautery forceps, introduced through the lateral spinal canal margin or with small pieces of Surgicel. As in the ventral cervical region a thin dorsal layer of posterior longitudinal ligament (PLL) often remains after resection of the thicker ventral portion of the PLL (which is firmly attached to the dorsal disc annulus). Many calcified thoracic disc fragments are suspended within this thin dorsal PLL layer and are not located intradurally as often as the literature suggests. The ventral spinal canal should be probed with a microdissector and nerve hook for identification and delivery of these fragments that are suspended within this layer of ligament. The dura mater should be clearly identified before the decompression is considered complete. After adequate spinal canal decompression has been achieved, an interbody autologous rib graft is placed, although its efficacy after routine discectomy has as yet to be established (Figure 37.8).

A more extensive dissection is required for vertebral corpectomy, particularly if stabilization with a lateral metallic implant is planned. For a T8 corpectomy, after the initial exposure through the T8 rib bed, the T8 and T9 rib heads are removed to expose the T7-8 and T8-9 disc spaces. The segmental artery and vein at the T8 midvertebral body level are individually ligated and divided as ventrally as possible. After resection of the pedicle of the vertebral body to be resected, the discs above and below the vertebral body are incised and evacuated (Figure 37.9). Rongeurs and a high-speed drill are used to complete the corpectomy. Appropriate stabilization is then performed (Figure 37.10). If a lateral implant is planned, the lateral aspects of the instrumented segments must be well exposed. This includes subperiosteal reflection of the endothoracic fascia and suture ligation and division of the segmental vessels at the midvertebral body level. The rostral margin of the rib of the rostral instrumented vertebrae may also have to be removed to achieve adequate exposure for plate placement.

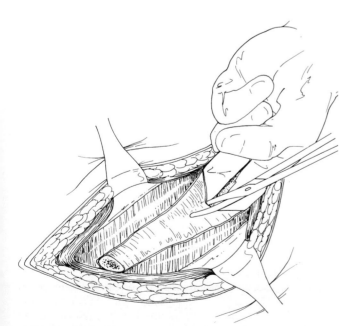

Figure 37.4 The endothoracic fascia is incised in line with the bed of the resected rib. Note that the underlying pleura are bluntly freed from the undersurface of the endothoracic fascia with gloved fingers.

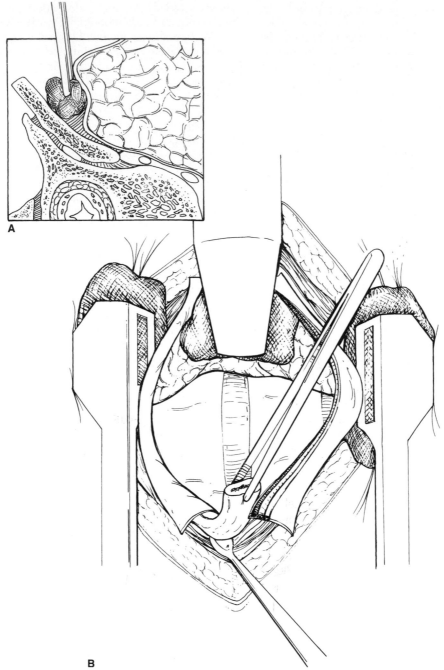

Figure 37.5 **(A)** The pleura are bluntly freed from the inner surface of the endothoracic fascia with Kittner clamps. **(B)** After a wide pleural dissection, the remaining endothoracic fascia overlying the remaining rib head and vertebral bodies is incised, and the rib head removed.

The retropleural approach is modified at the thoracolumbar junction (T10-L2), because of the caudal rib angulation and diaphragm attachments (Figure 37.11). At these levels the approach is through the rib, one level above the pathologic segment. When the initial rib segment is removed, the diaphragm, rather than the endothoracic fascia, remains in the bed of the rib at the lowest three rib levels. A Cobb elevator is used to detach the dorsal diaphragm margins from their attachment to the inner surfaces of the rib origins. This immediately unites the

retropleural and retroperitoneal compartments. The dissection continues dorsally to elevate the diaphragm from the dorsal abdominal wall attachments to the quadratus lumborum muscle (lateral arcuate ligament), the psoas muscle (medial arcuate ligament), and vertebral body (crus). The exposure is maintained with table-mounted retractors. Elevation of the psoas muscle with electrocautery is required at the L1 and L2 levels. Decompression and stabilization is then performed using the previously described techniques and principles. After decompression

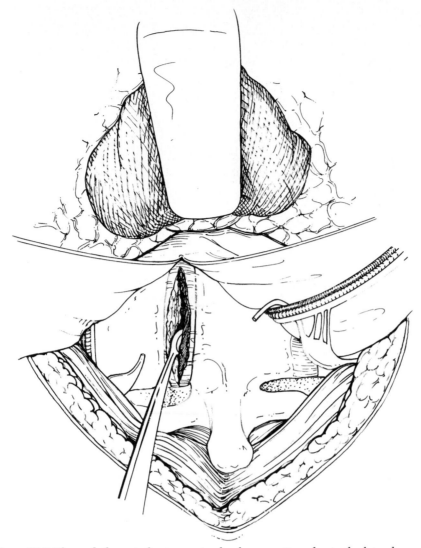

Figure 37.6 The endothoracic fascia opening has been continued onto the lateral aspect of the vertebral bodies. It is reflected away from the disc. The intercostal vessels remain within the reflected tissue. The thoracic sympathetic chain has been divided, and the disc has been incised.

and stabilization, the diaphragm is reattached to the psoas and quadratus muscles with suture.

The pleura are inspected before closure. Ideally, pleural tears should be repaired with sutures as soon as they occur. If the lung remains adherent to the parietal pleura at the conclusion of the procedure, no tube thoracostomy is placed, even if a prior pleural tear has been incurred. If separation between the lung and parietal pleura is present, indicating either an air leak (i.e., lung parenchymal entry) or a non-airtight pleural tear closure, a no. 32 tube thoracostomy is placed and brought out through a separate stab incision. It can usually be removed the next day. The remainder of the wound is closed carefully in layers with suture and skin staples.

Postoperative Care

Postoperative care is fairly standardized. If a tube thoracostomy has been placed, it can be removed on postoper-

ative day 1, unless an air leak or excessive drainage is present. The epidural catheter, through which a long-acting narcotic is instilled for perioperative pain relief, is removed 36 hours postoperatively. Ambulation or mobilization is encouraged on the first postoperative day. Ambulatory patients are usually discharged on postoperative day 3 or 4. Skin staples are removed on postoperative day 10.

Follow-up

The author's experience with this exposure includes 32 patients with a mean follow-up of 10 months. The morbidity and complications are less than the previous experience with the standard transpleural ventrolateral thoracotomy. Postoperative pain is similar to that encountered with dorsolateral approaches, which suggests that the pleural incision accounts for much of the postoperative intercostal neuralgia that has occurred in

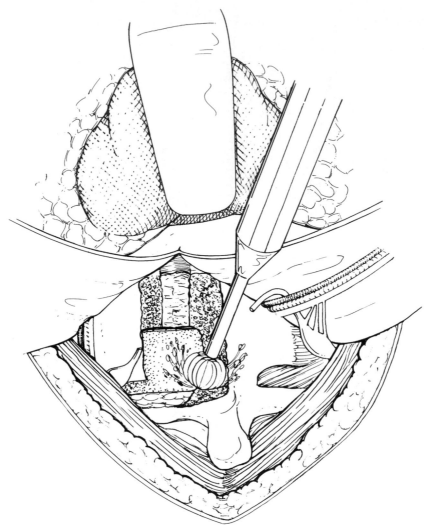

Figure 37.7 After disc curettage, the adjacent vertebral end-plates and pedicle are removed with a high-speed drill.

two out of the 32 patients (6%). In both patients (involvement of T11-12 disc space; L1 burst fracture) postoperative intercostal pain and dysesthesias eventually lessened and evolved into a mildly annoying numbness or hypersensitivity.

Summary

Retropleural thoracotomy has proved to be useful for ventral exposure of the thoracic and thoracolumbar spine. It incorporates the advantages of both the ventrolateral transpleural thoracotomy (i.e., direct ventral canal expo-

sure) and the lateral extracavitary approach (extrapleural dissection and initial lateral spinal canal entry via the pedicle or foramen), while avoiding the disadvantages of each approach, such as the extensive incision and soft-tissue dissection, deep operative field, and oblique spinal canal exposure of the transpleural thoracotomy and the bloody paraspinal and foraminal dissection, intercostal nerve sacrifice, and incomplete direct ventral spinal canal exposure associated with a lateral extracavitary approach. Retropleural thoracotomy should be considered when ventral exposure of up to three vertebral segments of the ventral thoracic and thoracolumbar spine is required.

(Continued on p. 446)

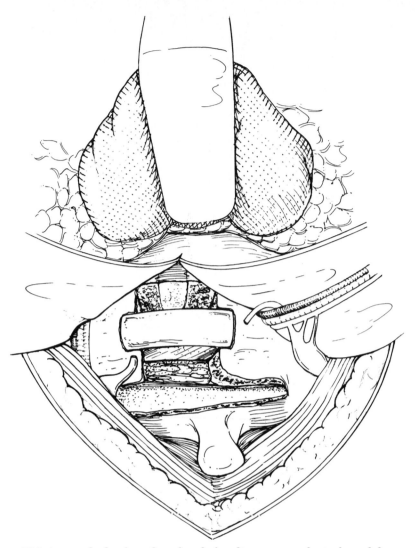

Figure 37.8 An interbody rib graft is placed after discectomy and spinal canal decompression.

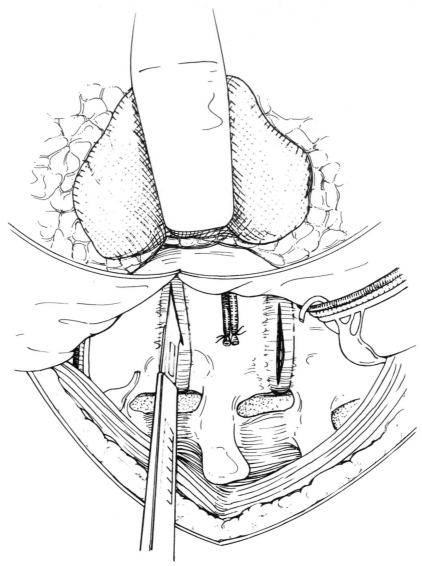

Figure 37.9 Adequate exposure for a corpectomy requires the additional removal of just the proximal rib head at the lower margin of the vertebral body to be resected. The segmental vessels are ligated and divided.

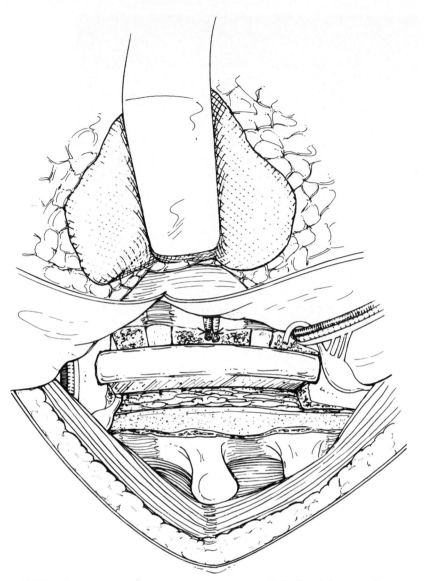

Figure 37.10 After corpectomy, reconstruction is accomplished with bone graft.

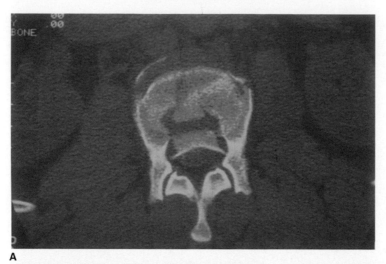

A

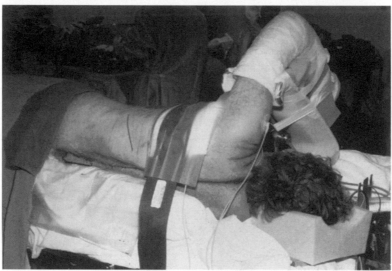

B

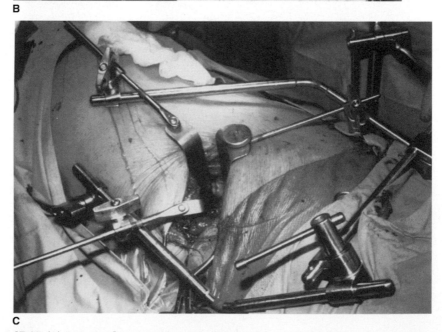

C

Figure 37.11 (**A**) Computed tomography scan of L1 burst fracture with large retropulsed fragment into the spinal canal. (**B**) Operative photograph demonstrating position and skin incision for a thoracolumbar approach for an L1 burst fracture. (**C**) After the initial dissection and exposure, an operative photograph demonstrates the table-mounted retractor that maintains retraction.

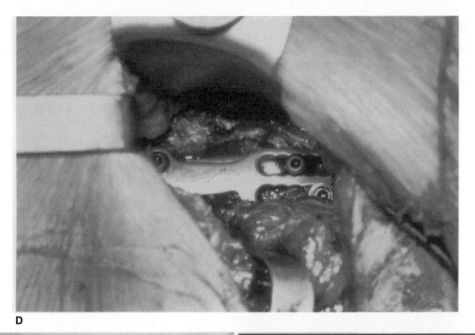

D

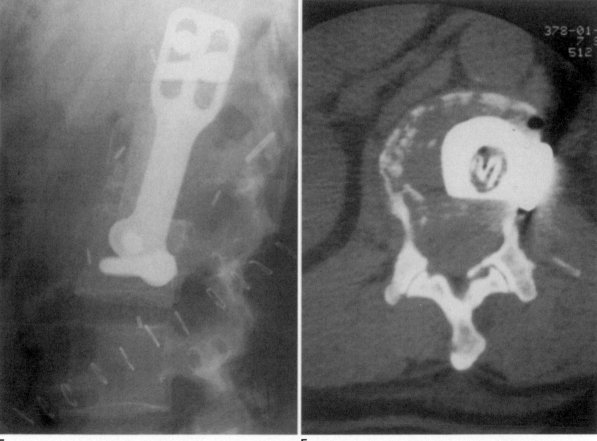

E

F

Figure 37.11 *cont'd* (**D**) After corpectomy, a reconstruction with interbody graft and a lateral plate has been accomplished. (**E**) Lateral radiograph after decompression and stabilization shows lateral plate and a large structural graft extending from T12 to L2. (**F**) Postoperative computed tomography scan demonstrates spinal canal reconstruction and placement of a large, structural femoral shaft allograft that has been filled with rib autograft. The lateral plate is in good position.

REFERENCES

1. Bohlman HH, Zdeblick TA: Anterior excision of herniated thoracic discs. *J Bone Joint Surg* 20A:1038-1047, 1988.

2. Hollinshead WH: *Textbook of Anatomy,* ed 3. Hagerstown, MD, Harper & Row, 1974, pp 496-501.

3. Louis R: *Surgery of the Spine.* New York, Springer-Verlag, 1983, pp 228-231.

4. McCormick PC: The lateral extracavitary approach to the thoracic and lumbar spine. In Holtzman RNN, McCormick PC, Farcy JPC (eds): *Spinal Instability.* New York, Springer-Verlag, 1993, pp 335-348.

5. McCormick PC: Retropleural approach to the thoracic and thoracolumbar spine. *Neurosurgery* 37:908-914, 1995.

6. Otani K, Yoshida M, Fujii E, *et al*: Thoracic disc herniation: surgical treatment in 23 patients. *Spine* 13:1262-1267, 1988.

CHAPTER 38

Laminotomy, Laminectomy, Laminoplasty, and Foraminotomy

Edward S. Connolly and Gordon R. Bell

Thoracic and lumbar laminotomies and laminectomies are two of the most commonly performed spinal procedures. They have remained basically unchanged since the 1930s, but have been refined with the advent of magnification and microtechnique, microinstrumentation, and power tools. These, along with use of perioperative antibiotics and better neurodiagnostic tests, have reduced the incidence of complications of these procedures.

The performance of thoracic and lumbar laminectomies, laminotomies, laminoplasties, and foraminotomies may be divided into five segments: (1) positioning, (2) exposure of the vertebral column, (3) bone removal, (4) wound closure, and (5) perioperative treatment.

Positioning

Positioning for thoracic and lumbar laminotomies, laminectomies, laminoplasties, and foraminotomies is dictated by the level of the vertebral column to be exposed. Exposure of the upper thoracic vertebral column requires the prone position—the patient has a moderately flexed neck, with the arms at their side, and their shoulders depressed. Middle and lower thoracic spine exposure requires the prone position, with the arms either at the side or abducted at the shoulders and flexed at the elbows. Lumbar exposure may be obtained in the prone position, knee-chest position, or in the lateral decubitus position. It is of prime importance to provide adequate visualization of the anatomy of the vertebral column that contains the pathology. The prone position allows complete exposure of the dorsal elements from the cranium to the sacrum. It allows an assistant to have an adequate view of the vertebral column and allows at least four hands to be available to help with the procedure. The disadvantages of the prone position are restriction of thoracic expansion, compression of the abdominal viscera (producing increased venous pressure in the epidural venous plexus), and the potential for ocular and peripheral nerve compression. It is important that these drawbacks be minimized to prevent pulmonary complications, bleeding complications, and neurologic complications.

To position for upper thoracic procedures (T1-5), the head is placed in three-point fixation, and the eyes are filled with ophthalmic ointment, taped shut, and covered with plastic goggles before the patient is turned to the prone position. Compression stockings and serial venous compression devices may be placed on the patient's legs to prevent phlebothrombosis and possible pulmonary embolization. When turning the patient to the prone position, care is taken to prevent twisting the neck. The patient is log-rolled onto soft bolsters that extend from the shoulders to the pelvis, allowing the weight to be carried at these four points and allowing expansion of the chest and freedom of the abdomen from compression. The skeletal head holder is positioned so that the cervical spine is mildly flexed. The elbows are surrounded with soft padding and the arms abducted at the shoulders and tucked to the side. Tape is used to depress the shoulders by extending it from the tip of one shoulder to the opposite side of the table in a criss-cross fashion, ensuring that the cross occurs at the thoracolumbar region and does not involve the upper thoracic region. The depression of the shoulders should not be so great as to stretch the brachial plexus, but should be sufficient to place the rhomboid muscles on slight tension. The operative table is then tilted in a mild, reverse Trendelenburg position to place the upper thoracic vertebrae parallel to the floor (Figure 38.1).

Positioning for exposure of the lower thoracic vertebrae requires the same eye protection and venous leg compression as the exposure for the upper thoracic vertebrae, but the head may either be turned to the side or placed in a sponge rubber cradle to help prevent ocular compression, if the neck is left in the neutral position. If the procedure is to be lengthy, the neutral position of the neck is preferred because turning the head to the side for prolonged periods may produce a postoperative torticollis, or neural or vascular compression. As the patient is log-rolled into the prone position on bolsters that extend from the shoulders to the pelvis, the arms are abducted 90 degrees at the shoulder, the elbows are flexed 90 degrees, with the forearms resting on padded arm boards, and the axillae and elbows are padded (Figure 38.2).

Positioning for exposure of the lumbar vertebrae may be accomplished in the prone position, lateral decubitus position, or knee-chest position. One author prefers placing the patient in the knee-chest position on an Andrews operating table for lumbar exposures. This provides the least abdominal and thoracic compression. This position is limited, however, to patients who weigh less than 300lb and are between 54 and 80 inches in height. It also is limited to patients who are able to bend both hips and knees 90 degrees. For most adults this is an excellent method of positioning for lumbar exposures. The authors have used this position without difficulty for many patients in the late stages of pregnancy. If a patient weighs more than 300lb or is extremely tall, a special frame may be required.

If the Andrews table is used, it is important to measure the chest-to-knee distance accurately before turning the patient to the prone position. As with all face-down positioning, eye protection is necessary and venous compression stockings and alternating leg compression devices are important. The patient is carefully log-rolled onto the Andrews operating table, with the neck held carefully in the neutral position and with the head in a sponge cradle. If the patient has a catheter, it is important that the catheter or the catheter drainage tube not be caught in the table

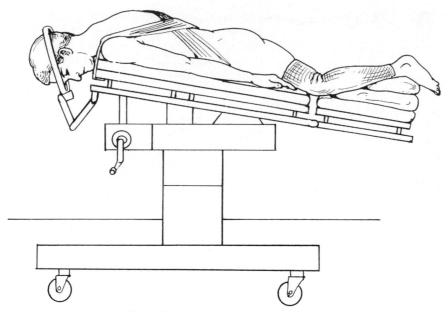

Figure 38.1 Prone position for upper thoracic laminectomy.

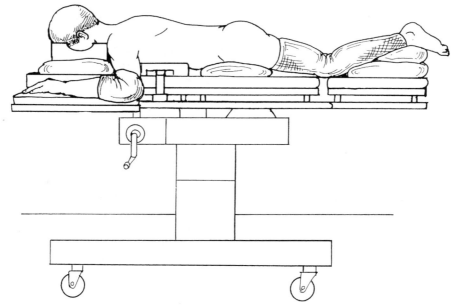

Figure 38.2 Prone position for middle and lower thoracic laminectomy.

mechanism. The patient's feet should be padded before they are placed in the stirrups. As the patient is being slid into the knee-chest position it is important to keep sliding until the thighs are flexed 90 to 95 degrees. The butt board should be placed high on the buttocks so that it does not compress the sciatic nerves in the upper thigh and does not compress the scrotum in males. Arms are abducted 90 degrees at the shoulders, and the elbows are flexed 90 degrees, with the padding of the axilla and the elbow to prevent peripheral nerve compression. If a Bovie unit is to be used, it is essential after positioning the patient that no skin is touching any metal portion of the operative table. Also, proper grounds should be checked before skin preparation and draping are started (Figure 38.3).

Exposure of the Vertebral Column

Exposure of the vertebral column usually requires radiographic confirmation of the levels to be exposed; one cannot always rely on external or bony landmarks. It is also important to have the neuroradiologic studies that demonstrate the pathology on view in the operating room before an incision is made. These diagnostic studies should also show the exact vertebral levels involved. This is particularly true in the thoracic region, in which magnetic resonance imaging (MRI) often demonstrates the pathology but is insufficient to precisely define the vertebral level.

Before the skin is prepared, the chart should be checked in regard to allergies. The skin preparation should

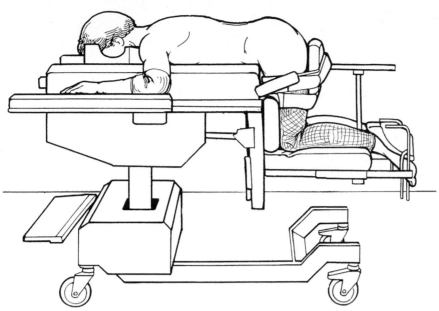

Figure 38.3 Knee-chest position on an Andrews operating table for lumbar laminectomy.

be much larger than the area that is to be exposed, so that if (during the procedure) unforeseen greater exposure is necessary, the wound could be extended without entering an unprepared area. After the skin has been prepared, an incision is made that is long enough to adequately expose the involved vertebrae. Hemostasis may be improved by injecting 0.5% Xylocaine with epinephrine 1:200,000 along the incision line. If the patient is not allergic to iodine, the authors prefer an iodinated adhesive drape over the skin incision. The incision is carried down to the deep fascia. The subcutaneous fat is reflected off the deep fascia with a periosteum elevator. Small perforating vessels are coagulated and divided as they penetrate the thoracolumbar fascia. This allows a good view of the thoracolumbar fascia for precise fascial closure at the conclusion of the procedure. If a unilateral exposure of the vertebral column is used, as in the case of a unilateral laminotomy or foraminotomy, the deep fascia is incised just lateral to the spinous process, leaving enough attached to the bone for closure. The Bovie unit is used to dissect the paraspinous muscles from the spine and lamina in a subperiosteal manner. Care is taken not to injure the facet capsules as the muscles are retracted laterally. A long muscle release allows less retraction on the muscles. The exposure should be extensive enough so that all of the bony structures overlying the pathology are exposed. The muscles may be held by various self-retaining retractors. Care should be taken to not damage the facet capsules. Soft-tissue hemostasis should be complete, and the interspace should be cleaned of soft tissue before bone work is performed. All soft-tissue hemostasis should be completed before bone removal. It is also essential that radiographs be taken intraoperatively.

Bone Removal

Bone may be removed with a high-speed drill or with bone-biting instruments. Both hands should be used to hold a high-speed drill while the assistant irrigates and provides suction. Instruments will "jump," even in expert hands. Using two hands may prevent dural or neural injury. It is important that instruments not be passed over the exposed wound, because a dropped instrument, particularly on an exposed thoracic spinal cord, could produce significant spinal cord injury. In the thoracic spine it is important to thin the lamina with a high-speed drill to permit decompression of the bony structures without placing large instruments within the spinal canal, which could cause further spinal cord compression (Figure 38.4). The use of a high-speed drill allows one to remove the dorsal arch intact so that it may be replaced as a laminoplasty. This is particularly important in the young growing spine to prevent a delayed spinal deformity. As much bone work as possible should be accomplished before removing the ligamentum flavum, because it adds another protective layer. The ligamentum flavum is opened over an instrument or cotton pad to prevent a dural injury (Figure 38.5). The ligamentum flavum is removed after it is freed from the underlying dura mater with sharp dissection. It is essential that the ligament be completely freed before it is removed. In cases of long-standing spinal stenosis in which the ligamentum flavum and the dura mater are tightly adherent, and also in cases in which a synovial cyst is compressing the dural sac, dural tears are more likely to occur. Often there are severe adhesions among the ligamentum flavum, the synovial cyst, and the dura mater. Great care and gentle dissection are required to free these adhesions before removing the ligament. The laminectomy or foraminotomy may be widened by undercutting the facet joints, using a high-speed drill or a sharp chisel. If a high-speed drill is used to undercut the facet joint, a malleable retractor, rubber strip, or cottonoid pad needs to be placed over the dura for protection (Figure 38.6). Large bites with an angled punch should not be used because it is easy to crack or fracture the facet joint or the pars interarticularis with this maneuver. A high-speed drill

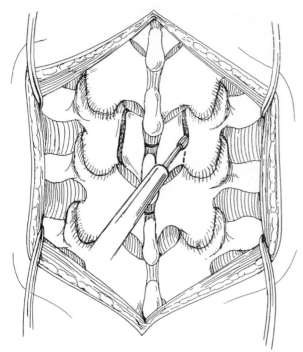

Figure 38.4 Laminectomy with high-speed drills prevents the need for placing instruments into the spinal cord and allows replacement of the posterior arch (laminoplasty).

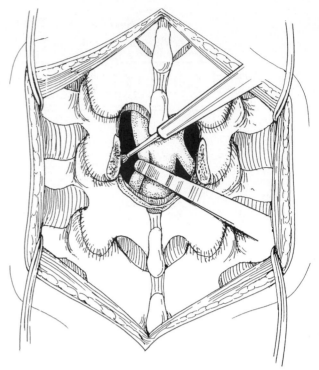

Figure 38.6 The dura mater and nerve root should be protected by a malleable retractor when a medial facetectomy is performed with a high-speed drill.

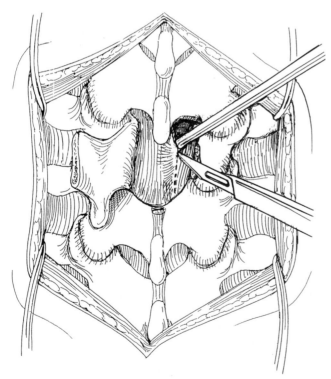

Figure 38.5 Ligamentum flavum is opened over another instrument or cotton pad to prevent injuring the dura mater.

may be used to drill down to an eggshell thickness, so that a small punch may be used to remove the last little pieces of bone without injury to the joint itself. This can also be done by using a sharp chisel to loosen the bone and then removing it with a small angled punch. Epidural venous

bleeders should be controlled with bipolar coagulation and divided. Bone bleeding can be controlled with bone wax. If a facet is inadvertently fractured, it may be prudent to remove the fractured fragments in the lumbar region.

It is important to repair any dural tears that may occur. If direct suturing is not possible because of the location of the tear, a piece of fascia and fibrin glue may be used.

If a laminoplasty is to be performed, the use of miniplates and screws is an effective and safe method of reapplying the dorsal arches (Figure 38.7). The plate is placed on the laminar side bilaterally and screwed in place. The facet side screw is placed last. Using the miniplates reduces the risk of drilling holes through the facet and passing wire or suture material. Miniplates also provide a more stable fixation than suture material.

Unilateral laminotomy for discectomy is tailored by the amount of interlaminar space available. Usually no more lamina needs to be removed than the insertion of the ligamentum flavum (Figure 38.8).

Wound Closure

The most important aspect of closure of thoracic and lumbar laminectomies and laminotomies is the closure of the deep thoracolumbar fascia. This provides the major strength of the closure. The deep thoracolumbar fascia should be closed with interrupted sutures. Dexon, or an equivalent absorbable suture, is appropriate. Absorbable sutures are less likely to cause stitch abscesses and spitting of foreign material from the wound. If a dural tear occurs during the procedure, even though the dura mater has been repaired, a running, locking suture of the deep fascia

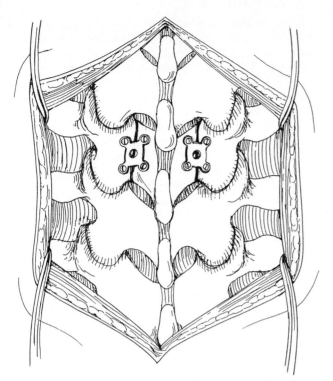

Figure 38.7 The use of miniplates and screws to replace the dural laminar arch in a laminoplasty.

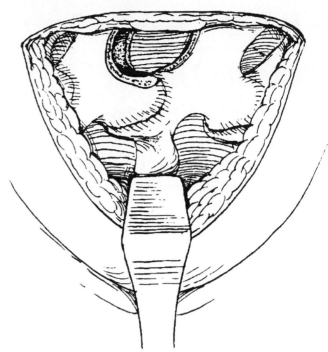

Figure 38.8 Laminotomy. Usually bone removal should not be required above the insertion of the ligamentum flavum.

may be prudent after the interrupted sutures are placed in the deep fascia layer. The subcutaneous tissues are then closed with an interrupted inverted layer of absorbable suture material. In the upper thoracic region in which there is tension from the pectoral girdle muscles, it may be prudent to close the skin with interrupted mattress sutures or staples and with deep retention sutures over bolsters to prevent separation of the wound. Patients may be placed in a figure-eight dressing to keep the shoulders back and help ensure that they do not use the arms to pull during the immediate postoperative period. The sutures are normally kept in place in the upper thoracic area for at least 2 weeks. Wounds are then covered with a light, dry, sterile dressing.

Perioperative Treatment

Administration of prophylactic antibiotics before the induction of anesthesia is an important adjunct to reducing the complication of infection. The use of compressive stockings and early ambulation both play a role in reducing the chances of phlebothrombosis and pulmonary embolization. Adequate pain management is necessary to assist with early ambulation. If Ketorolac Tromethamine is used, Cytotec should be given for protection against gastric ulcers. As soon as wounds are well healed, a progressive stretching program is begun to prevent muscle shortening and chronic mechanical discomfort.

CHAPTER 39

Posterior Lumbar Interbody Fusion

Diana Barrett Wiseman, Christopher I. Shaffrey, and Giuseppe Lanzino

Posterior Lumbar Interbody Fusion

Posterior lumbar interbody fusion (PLIF) is a procedure that has enjoyed variable popularity over the past 40 years. Although the procedure meets most of the criteria of an "ideal" fusion procedure it has always been technically demanding and associated with the risk of significant complications. Recent advances in spinal instrumentation and minimal assess techniques have revitalized the interest in PLIF. PLIF is closely linked with Ralph Cloward, who pioneered and popularized the procedure.[25-31] Cloward first performed this operation in 1940, facing formidable technical challenges. Only 4 years before Cloward's first PLIF, Mercer, after reviewing the pertinent literature, stated that "the ideal operation for fusing the spine would be an interbody fusion" but that "the surgical difficulties encountered in performing such a feat would make the operation technically impossible."[71]

Cloward's first patient was a schoolteacher with acute sciatica. "After removing a large intraspinal disc fragment, there was a big hole left in the disc space, and it occurred to me that I might be able to obtain some stability of the spine by putting a bone graft into this hole. Accordingly, I cut off the spinous process, shaped it with a rongeur and pounded it into the interspace."[28] Because of the death of this patient secondary to a pulmonary embolus, Cloward abandoned the procedure until 1943 when the operation developed as a wartime necessity.

Cloward was the only neurosurgeon available for duty in the Pacific theater during the early phases of World War II. The physical effort required to build defense structures resulted in many low back injuries. The traditional operation (laminectomy) developed for sciatica was effective in relieving the radicular pain, but many laborers were unable to return to work because of residual low back pain. By October 1947 Cloward had treated 100 patients and had presented his results to the Harvey Cushing Society. He recalled that the manuscript was received "with anything but enthusiasm." Eighty-two of the 100 patients returned to manual labor, and Cloward concluded, "If my colleagues did not like the operation, my patients did, so I continued to treat all of my lumbar cases in this manner." Since then PLIF has gradually become more widely accepted and numerous variations of the original procedure have been developed. The indications for PLIF and variants of it, such as transforaminal interbody lumbar fusion (TLIF) have expanded and include numerous pathologic conditions other than sciatica. Currently PLIF is routinely performed for spondylolisthesis, degenerative scoliosis, degenerative disc disease, and recurrent disc herniations.

Proponents of PLIF claim it has several distinct advantages over other lumbar fusion techniques. Unlike the ventral approach, a dorsal route permits better exposure, decompression, and inspection of the neural structures by laminotomy, medial facetectomy, foraminotomy, and discectomy.[85,107] When compared with the outcome of a dorsal or dorsolateral (intertransverse) fusion, the theoretic advantages of the bone fusion obtained with PLIF include the following: fusion occurs at approximately the center of the axis of rotation; the graft is subjected to compressive rather than tensile forces; a wide area of bone surface is involved; and an excellent source of blood supply is obtained through the cancellous portion of the vertebral body when the cortical end-plates have been partially or totally removed.[22,61,63] Placement of the bone graft or fusion device maintains the interbody height, preserves patency of the lateral spinal canal, improves anatomic relationships among different vertebral elements, and following successful fusion, limits mechanical traction on the nerve root from the surrounding scar tissue.[62] A successful fusion also arrests microinstability and hypertrophic degenerative changes, thus removing the impetus for progressive tropism and stenosis.[107] Excision of the entire disc prevents recurrent disc herniation and may reduce the rate of additional surgery.[85]

A successful PLIF or TLIF therefore maintains disc height, protects nerve roots, immobilizes the unstable degenerated disc area, restores weight-bearing to ventral structures, and places the annulus under tension.[17] Despite numerous reports of outstanding clinical outcomes and fusion rates, the procedure is technically demanding, with a very steep learning curve.[*] The indications for PLIF, the specific surgical technique, the need for interbody or pedicle screw instrumentation, the type of bone graft (i.e., local autograft, iliac crest autograft, allograft or bone morphogenic protein [BMP]), the clinical outcome, as well as the fusion rates when compared with those for ventral interbody and intertransverse fusion techniques are all controversial elements.

The "classic" PLIF operation described by Cloward consisted of subtotal disc removal with decompression of the neural elements, followed by interbody fusion of the vertebral bodies. The operation has been modified because of new technical adjuncts, failures of the original technique, and availability of sophisticated materials for fixation and bone grafting. Modifications of the operation that limit thecal sac and nerve root retraction, including unilateral or bilateral complete facetectomies to approach the disc space through the "triangular working zone," are gaining in popularity.

The distinction between the approach to the disc space in PLIF and TLIF procedures is beginning to blur by working in the space between the thecal sac and the nerve root. The TLIF procedure was originally described by Dr. Harms. The procedure involves a unilateral hemifacetectomy of the superior and inferior facets of the level to

---

[*]References 11,12,44,64,68,85,90,92.

452

be fused. The pars interarticularis is removed, which allows access to the lateral aspect of the disc. A near-complete discectomy is performed from this far lateral approach, often with less retraction of the dural sac and nerve roots than required for a standard PLIF. Bone graft and cages are then placed unilaterally and "rolled" across to the opposite side. The advantages of the TLIF procedure are a unilateral approach versus a bilateral approach typically required for the PLIF procedure with less required retraction on the nerve roots or the dural sac for exposure. The classic PLIF technique must often be limited to L3-S1 levels because of the required retraction of the dural sac, whereas the TLIF procedure may be performed higher.

Patient Selection

Patient selection remains the most critical factor for surgical success.[39,66] Although there is some debate regarding surgical indications, all patients should meet established criteria for decompression and fusion. Numerous publications have demonstrated the efficacy of the PLIF technique for degenerative conditions, spondylolisthesis, and discogenic back pain. Accurate diagnosis and appropriate surgical indications are crucial for the efficacy of the procedure. Careful history and physical examination, and appropriate radiologic evaluation including dynamic radiographs, are required to make the correct diagnosis. Psychologic assessment and treatment of depression are also important, as is awareness of compensation and litigation, because these factors have a significant impact on patient outcomes after surgery.[38]

The biologic rationale for justifying PLIF is that interbody fusion eliminates the instability that can be the principal cause of pain. The definition of "instability," however, continues to be debated. Gross instability can be measured radiographically and can result from previous lumbar spine surgical procedures (wide laminectomy, facetectomy, failed lumbar fusion), congenital or acquired spondylolisthesis, or other degenerative conditions. At times, however, vertebrae are subjected to forces that exceed normal physiologic parameters, and "microinstability" may develop. Microinstability is related to intervertebral disc and facet degeneration. It presents radiographically with narrowing of the joint space, subarticular sclerosis and cyst formation, osteophyte formation, facet hypertrophy, and signal intensity changes on magnetic resonance imaging (MRI). Although degenerative changes in the lumbar spine are almost universally apparent by the age of 60, the incidence of symptomatic individuals is low.[35]

Unless a focal neurologic deficit is present, a vigorous trial of nonoperative therapy is essential in every patient before surgery is considered. This trial should be extended over many months. Only those patients who still have persistent, disabling pain after such a trial should be considered for surgical treatment. It is critical to select patients who have few, if any, negative variables, such as chronic pain syndrome, psychosocial disorders, or potential secondary gains. Screening studies should include spine radiography (including flexion-extension lateral radiography) and a structural imaging technique, such as computed

tomography (CT), CT-myelography, or MRI. CT-myelography still plays a critical role in the evaluation of patients with disabling low back and radicular pain in the elderly because it identifies other pathologic entities such as lumbar and foraminal stenosis that are often associated with degenerative disc disease. Because the correlation between structural changes and symptoms can be minimal and misleading, several other ancillary tests have been devised to attempt to correlate lumbar pain and clinicoradiographic signs of degenerative disc disease that can be improved with interbody fusion. These methods include provocative discography,[33,87] response to rigid bracing, and intradiscal steroid injection. These methods, however, lack scientific confirmation of their efficacy in diagnosing symptomatic instability or discogenic pain.

Theoretically, PLIF fulfills the criteria required of an ideal surgical procedure designed for the correction of recurrent disc herniations, most lumbar degenerative conditions, and spondylolisthesis, whether congenital, degenerative, or iatrogenic (postsurgical).[29,88] It permits decompression of the neural elements, distracts and aligns the vertebral bodies, and stabilizes the motion segment.[61] A range of indications for PLIF has been reported in the literature. Cloward was the strongest proponent of the procedure and believed that all lumbar disc operations should be accompanied by a PLIF.[30] Others have suggested that this procedure can be a valid therapeutic option in those patients with chronic low back pain secondary to disc derangements. Lee et al.[58] have reported encouraging results in 62 patients with chronic disabling low back pain who were unresponsive to aggressive conservative management and in whom provocative discography pointed to the intervertebral disc as the source of the unremitting pain. Other indications described in the literature include recurrent disc herniation, persistent pain after chemonucleolysis,[62,89] treatment of lateral disc herniations in obese patients (in these cases it is speculated that discectomy with PLIF may prevent the rapid postoperative settlement of the disc space),[68] spondylolisthesis, symptomatic spinal stenosis with or without degenerative scoliosis or spondylolisthesis,[45] iatrogenic lumbar spinal instability, and failed back syndrome.

Contraindications to the use of PLIF include severe symptomatic adhesive arachnoiditis, severe osteoporosis, recent discitis, and severe subchondral sclerosis with no viable bone marrow tissue seen on MRI scans.[65] The authors believe that the operation is indicated in selected cases of spondylolisthesis, with or without sciatica, and in patients who complain of persistent back pain after traditional discectomy. Certain selected patients with discogenic low back pain, diagnosed by MRI and with concordant findings on provocative discography, with one or two levels of involvement, may also be surgical candidates.

Surgical Technique
Positioning

The patient is placed very carefully in the prone position to lessen its adverse effects.[1] The optimal position for spinal surgery is one that facilitates exposure, minimizes bleeding and the likelihood of violation of vital structures in the operative field, and permits proper ventilation. Care must be taken not to allow pressure on the abdomen, because this may cause venous engorgement, stasis, and increased bleeding from the epidural veins. To prevent compression of the ventral abdominal wall, two firm rolls support the iliac crest, lateral rib cage, and clavicle. Alternatively, an operative spinal frame or table can be used. The use of a Jackson spinal table that keeps the abdomen free, resulting in decreased epidural bleeding, but keeps the hips extended to maximize lumbar lordosis during the fusion procedure, has been a useful adjunct in PLIF surgery. An additional benefit of the Jackson spinal table is the ability to perform a 360-degree radiographic evaluation, a distinct advantage aiding in the placement of spinal instrumentation. A Foley catheter is inserted before surgery to ensure that bladder distension does not increase intraabdominal pressure during the procedure.

Exposure

The classic Cloward PLIF consists of three steps: (1) laminectomy or laminotomy, (2) removal of the intervertebral disc, and (3) spinal fusion.[25,27,28,30] After administration of perioperative antibiotics and infiltration of the skin and paraspinal muscles with 1% bupivacaine (Marcaine), a midline skin incision of approximately 10cm is made slightly rostral to the pathologic disc space. Dissection is carried down to the level of the lumbosacral fascia, which is opened along the midline. The spinous processes and the laminae of the vertebrae above and below the level of the pathology are exposed and cleaned of all soft tissues. Only a deep notch is made in the laminae of interest. Complete laminectomies are not performed. Preservation of the dorsal portion of the motion segment prevents slippage of the adjacent vertebral bodies in case fusion does not occur, allows for reattachment of the muscle to the motion segment enhancing the stability of the grafts in the disc space, and serves as a rigid mechanical barrier that protects the neural structures during intradiscal instrumentation (if used). Special instruments devised for this purpose, such as the vertebrae spreader,[26,31] a self-retaining retractor inserted between the spinous processes in the midline, allow excellent exposure of the intervertebral space with a minimal amount of bone removal. By the use of this instrument, the interspace can be distracted to nearly twice its normal height and held in position throughout the procedure.

Removal of the lower third of the inferior facet and the medial two thirds of the superior facet widens the exposure of the spinal canal and allows visualization of the lateral half of the intervertebral disc and provides adequate exposure of the nerve roots above and below the disc space. In cases in which transpedicular instrumentation is used, a complete facetectomy permits complete neural decompression and a direct approach to the disc space with minimal neural retraction. Preparation of the disc space for PLIF requires sufficient release of possible scar tissue and adhesions to allow sufficient mobilization of the thecal sac for safe access. After the dural sac and superior and inferior nerve roots are gently retracted, they must be protected during the exposure and procedure in the disc space; self-retaining nerve root retractors specifically designed for this purpose can be used in this stage of the operation.[31] Great care must be taken to avoid overdistraction and traction of the neural structures during any of these steps. Typically the nerve root exiting below the superior pedicle is at the greatest risk for injury, especially with the placement of intervertebral instrumentation. Injury to the dorsal root ganglion in this area may result in permanent neuropathic pain that is very resistant to all treatment modalities. Temporary distraction moves the nerve root at risk superiorly, making access less problematic. The epidural venous plexus over the dorsal annulus must be meticulously cauterized to maintain a dry field, reduce intraoperative blood loss, and keep good visualization of the dorsal annulus and the floor of the spinal canal.

Discectomy and Preparation of the Graft Site

The disc space is entered, and a 7mm intradiscal shaver (Figure 39.1A) is inserted on one side, parallel to the end plates, and rotated a number of times. These shavers have side-cutting flutes so that disc material and end plate are removed. By alternating sides in 2mm increments, the shavers also result in distraction of the disc space. This also leads to the disc space being aggressively cleaned of disc material bilaterally. In PLIF, 80% to 90% of the dorsal disc material should be removed, because a large area of bone contact between the grafts and the vertebral bodies improves the chance of a successful interbody fusion.

Adequate preparation of the host graft site and removal of the cartilaginous end-plates are important steps to ensure successful fusion. The lumbar cortical end plates are thinner in young patients; therefore when a young patient undergoes PLIF, curetting to the level of oozing cortical bone is often sufficient to ensure adequate vascularization

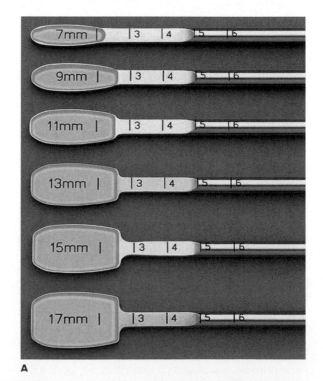

A

Figure 39.1 (A) Intervertebral Disc Shavers. Allow breakdown of nucleus pulposus to facilitate removal while also removing cartilaginous tissue from the end plate.

of the grafts. In older patients with matured cortical end plates; however, it is suggested that many islands of decortication to the cancellous bone are created. Because blood is supplied to the end plate by end arteries, the removal of a thin layer of cortical bone sufficient to change the color from white (cortical end plate) to a brownish shade (subcortical cancellous bone) is sufficient to ensure an adequate blood supply.[65] Because the bone texture is more porous in the central portion of the vertebral body, partial decortica-

tion prevents the graft from settling into the softer cancellous bone.[65] Total decortication down to the anterior longitudinal ligament, as advocated by Cloward,[27] should be avoided unless excellent visualization is achieved because it carries with it the risk of vascular injury.

The danger of injuring the ventral vascular structures was one of the main factors that discouraged surgeons from attempting PLIF.[66] Because the average depth of the disc space ranges from 25mm under the facet to 35mm in the center of the interspace, Lin suggested the use of instruments with a 3cm marker so that their exact depth in the disc space can be judged readily at any time during the procedure, thus minimizing the risk of injuring ventral vascular structures.[66] Instruments specifically designed for the preparation of the host site are now commercially available (see Figure 39.1). Sagittal, axial, and operative views of the exposure are presented in Figure 39.2.

Grafting

Once the disc space has been adequately cleaned, the graft material is inserted. Before the routine use of transpedicular instrumentation, the grafts are held in the interspace mainly by axial intervertebral forces. Therefore it was crucial that the disc space be maximally distracted (with care taken to avoid a reversal of the physiologic lordotic curve, the so-called "flat back") before the grafts are inserted. The interbody grafts were relatively fixed by the combination of the recoil force of the annulus, gravity, and effect of muscle pull. Although there are numerous reports of excellent clinical and radiographic outcomes of "stand-alone" PLIF procedures, most surgeons currently use transpedicular instrumentation to reduce the incidence of graft displacement, loss of disc space height, pseudarthrosis, and progressive kyphosis.[21,77,78]

Autologous cancellous bone interbody graft, alone, is of inadequate mechanical strength to resist the forceful recoil against the graft, even with transpedicular instrumentation. Some form of vertical column support can be provided either by hard cortical bone in a corticocancellous graft or by an intervertebral fusion device that maintains disc space height as the graft heals. In addition, a tight, close fit is critical to grafting, because bone is less successful in bridging a gap greater than about 200μm.[14,80,81]

Since the early 1950s several methods of support and several graft substitutes have been developed to reduce the problems associated with donor bone grafts (Box 39.1).* Tricortical grafts, as originally described by Cloward (Figure 39.3), provide soft cancellous bone, as well as rigid support to the column, but the cortical portions integrate with the fusion very slowly, and the precise cutting of rectangular tricortical grafts that match the recipient holes requires special skills and instruments. Rectangular grafts also have sharp lateral corners that may potentially injure a nerve root, ganglion, or the dura mater during insertion. Simmons has recommended the use of local bone (laminae, spinous processes, facets) packed tightly into the disc space,[90] whereas Branch and

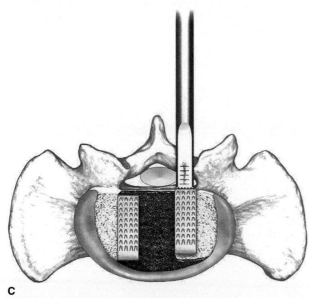

B

C

Figure 39.1 *cont'd* (B) Intervertebral Disc Excisors. These facilitate removal of disc material while preparing the end plates without damaging the subchondral bone. **(C)** An example of two PLIF Spacers within the disc space. The spacers are contoured, wedge-shaped cortical allograft. *(From Synthes, with permission.)*

---

*References 2,7-15,17,32,33,44,45,47,53,56,59,62,64,65,68,72,73,75, 80-84,102,104.

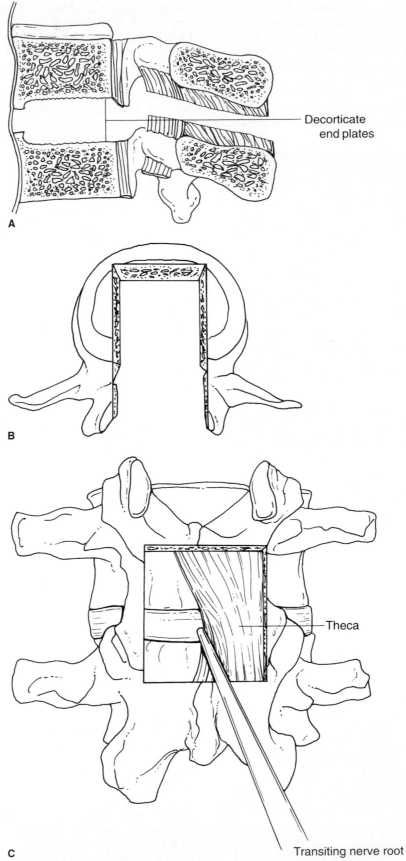

Figure 39.2 Sagittal (**A**), axial (**B**), and operative (**C**) views of the exposure.

39.1

Methods for posterior lumbar interbody fusion

1. Tricortical grafts (Cloward, Lin, Ma)
2. Rectangular grafts (Ma, Collis, Branch)
3. Bone dowels (Wiltberger, Blume, Ray)
4. Loose PLIF chips (Simmons)
5. Threaded bone dowel (Otero-Vich)
6. Tubular container, autologous bone (Bagby)
7. Threaded tubular container (Ray, Kuslich, Michelson)
8. Knurled, toothed container/spacer (Herman, Stryker, Biomat, others)
9. Open "box" support (Brantigan)
10. Cancellous metal block (Krüger-Henssge, Waisbrod) Titanium mesh block (Leong)
11. PLIF Spacers—Contoured wedge-shaped cortical allograft (Synthes)

Modified from Ray CD: Spinal interbody fusions: a review, featuring new generation techniques. *Neurosurg Quart* 7:135-156, 1997.

Branch[11,12] have reported the use of vertical support columns cut from spinous processes inserted into the disc space successively filled with cancellous bone chips. To solve the problem associated with the cutting of precise rectangular inserts, Wiltberger[104] in 1953 and others thereafter have recommended the use of round bone dowels (Figure 39.4). Using these dowels, the round inserts and recipient holes were much easier to cut precisely; however, these grafts were still associated with problems, such as extrusion and collapse.

In 1986 Bagby[2] first described a threaded steel basket filled with autologous bone that he used for fusion of the cervical spine in horses. Brantigan and colleagues[13,14,17] developed a carbon fiber reinforced polymer implant to aid interbody fusion (Figure 39.5). This implant has ridges or teeth to resist retropulsion, struts to use for support, and a hollow area to allow packing of autologous bone graft.[17] The carbon fiber cages have the advantage of being radiolucent and having a modulus of elasticity similar to cortical bone.[24] In 1988 Ray[79-84] used a threaded, perforated titanium alloy cage into which autologous cancellous bone was packed (Figures 39.6 to 39.8).

Cages similar to the Ray cages have also been described by Michelson[72] and Kuslich.[56] BAK cages have been extensively used and studied. Goh *et al.*[42] have shown that progressive size increase in BAK cages provides increasing stability in facetectomized human cadaver models. Of note this study is performed with bilateral facetectomies and insertion of two BAK cages without additional internal fixation. Small BAK cages (13mm) returned extension stiffness to that of the intact functional unit. Medium cages (15mm) restored extension and lateral bending stiffness to baseline level. Large cages (17mm) returned extension, lateral bending, and torsional stiffness to baseline measurements. Of note, the discectomy required for insertion of the cages significantly decreased flexion stiffness. This was not significant improved with the placement of the cages. Pitzen *et al.*[77] found that BAK cages in a human cadaver PLIF model without instrumentation had a range

of motion of 10.6 degrees in torsion. No comment on the size of the BAK cage used is made; however, this degree of motion can lead to a pseudarthrosis. In contrast, Lund *et al.*[49] found in a human cadaver model, that cages of various manufacturers, Ray, Brantigan, and Stratec significantly stabilized the spine in flexion and lateral bending. No effect on stability was noted with lateral bending or axial rotation. Cage type also did not significantly affect stability. The use of threaded cortical bone dowels (TCBDs) has been shown to be effective at bony fusion. Under static loading, biomechanic studies have shown they can bear an average compressive load of 25kN, more than two times higher than the physiologic loads experienced when lifting heavy objects. TCBD can be removed in a piecemeal fashion, if required. Cagli *et al.*[21] found that threaded cages versus threaded bone dowels in cadaver models biomechanically performed similarly. Both constructs alone, though, were less stable than those constructs augmented with posterior instrumentation.

Cylindric fusion devices inherently require more thecal sac and nerve root retraction compared with rectangular interbody fusion devices to achieve the same amount of intervertebral distraction. Barnes *et al.*[4] retrospectively evaluated TCBDs versus Allograft-impacted wedges in PLIF supplemented with posterior segmental instrumentation. A minimum of a 1-year follow-up was evaluated for 49 patients; 27 who underwent PLIF with wedges and 22 who underwent PLIF with TCBD. Permanent nerve root injury was noted in 13.6% of TCBDs versus a 0% rate among impacted wedges. Fusion rates were 95.4% and 88.9% respectively, whereas satisfactory outcome rate was 72.7% and 85.1% respectively. The difference in fusion rates was not statistically significant; however, the difference in outcomes was significant.

On completion of graft insertion, the distracting instruments are removed to allow the fused segment to compress to prevent graft extrusion. With the use of transpedicular instrumentation, active compression is performed to accentuate lumbar lordosis and optimize graft compression. In stand-alone applications, care must be taken to develop an undercut in the graft bed, both ventrally and dorsally, to avoid retropulsion or anteropulsion of the graft material. The dorsal surface of the graft should be curvilinear to adapt to the shape of the vertebral body, and the grafts should be countersunk so that they lie 2 to 3mm below the surface of the adjacent vertebral bodies.

New advances in interbody devices include the resorbable interbody cage, 70/30 poly (L-lactide-co-D, L-lactide). These constructs have been evaluated in a ventral interbody animal model and have been found to be a viable alternative to metals.[97] Future clinical trials will bear out their efficacy compared to other implants as an interbody fusion device.

The long-standing controversy on whether to use autografts or allografts remains unresolved. Although some authors have noted no differences in the fusion rates between patients with autologous or homologous (tissue bank) grafts,[85,107] others[16,17] have observed better results and fusion rates with autologous bone. Although allografts have the advantage of allowing previous modeling of the graft to fit the interspace, most surgeons prefer autologous graft material, especially cancellous bone, with its intrinsic

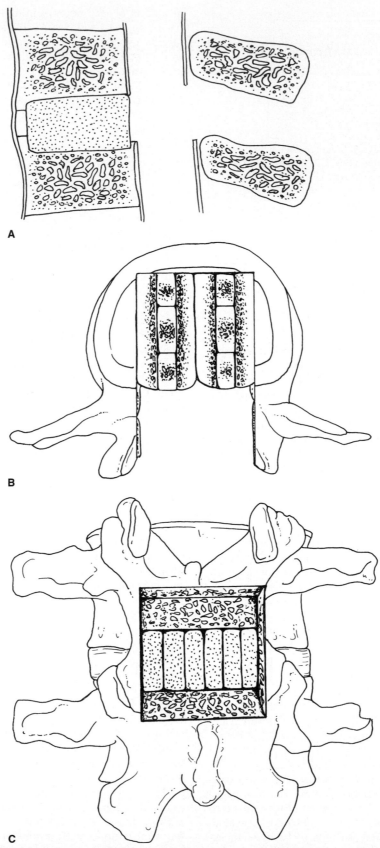

A

B

C

Figure 39.3 Sagittal (**A**), axial (**B**), and operative (**C**) views using Cloward's rectangular tricortical graft technique.

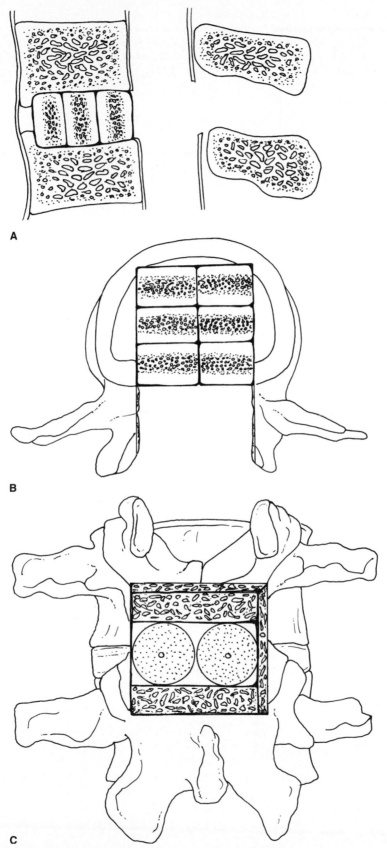

Figure 39.4 Sagittal (**A**), axial (**B**), and operative (**C**) views using bone dowels (rectangular [*A* and *B*] and cylindrical *[C]*).

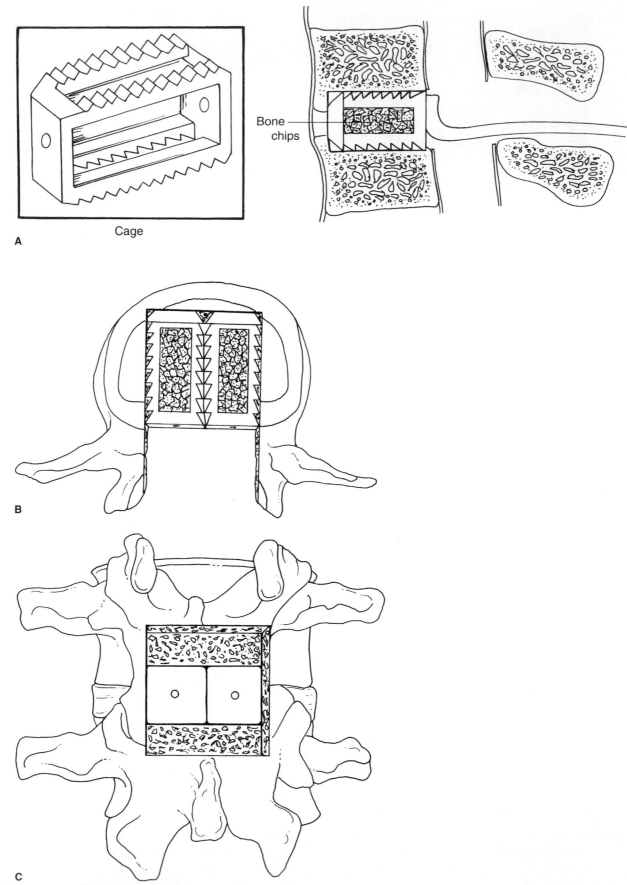

Cage

Bone
chips

A

B

C

Figure 39.5 Sagittal (**A**), axial (**B**), and operative (**C**) views using Brantigan's carbon-fiber fusion cage.

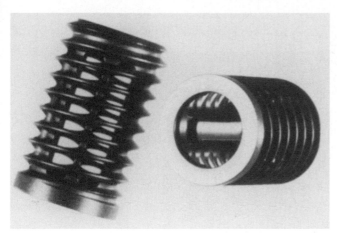

Figure 39.6 Lateral and end views of a Ray threaded fusion cage.

growth factors and natural compatibility. However, this bone is too soft to support intervertebral forces, and the harvesting of autologous grafts is cumbersome, with its own set of delayed and immediate complications. Therefore sterile, prepared bank bone, such as homologous, freeze-dried bone dowels or tricortical grafts, is often used. Rish *et al.*,[85] in one comparative study of autologous and homologous (tissue bank) grafts, showed no significant differences in the observed fusion rates, 84% for autograft versus 86% for allograft. Other authors, however, have reported lower fusion rates with allografts compared with autografts.[16,17]

Interbody graft substances may ultimately be radically changed by the recent approval of rhBMP-2 for interbody fusion. Currently rhBMP-2 is only approved for anterior interbody fusion. Studies have shown that rhBMP-2 collagen-soaked sponges placed within an anterior interbody cage provides a fusion rate of 100% without the need for autologous bone graft. The use of rhBMP-2 has not been approved for posterior use, secondary to the theoretic concern that bony overgrowth into the spinal canal through the disrupted posterior longitudinal ligament may occur. A recent animal model, though using OP-1 (BMP-7) with a hydroxyapatite spacer found a significantly increased fusion rate compared to autograft via a TLIF approach supplemented with posterior instrumentation.[6] No complications were noted with the OP-1/HA group. Further studies are needed to assess the full safety of BMPs used in posterior interbody fusions.

Uninstrumented "Stand-Alone" PLIF (PLIF Without the Addition of Posterior Segmental Instrumentation)

The classic PLIF technique involves grafting of the lumbar interbody space without the addition of posterior segmental instrumentation. The concern for this technique is that the interbody graft alone may not provide enough stability to allow adequate healing and thus eventual bony fusion. Several authors have evaluated their experience with PLIF using various interbody grafts. Since the 1980s there have been several reports on large series of patients undergoing PLIF. Because of variations in technique in each series, it is difficult to accurately judge the procedure

in general.[107] This confusion and the impossibility of exact statistical comparisons are increased because selection criteria and patient populations vary greatly. Results of PLIF are usually assessed by evaluating the rate of clinical success and the rate of fusion.[16,17] In 1985 Cloward reported a clinical success rate of 87% to 92% and a fusion success rate of 92% in his 40-year experience with the operation.[31] These results have been confirmed in large series by others who applied minor modifications to the procedure.[40]

A stand-alone fusion device depends on the strength of the end-plate to totally resist all compressive loads. Even with added transpedicular instrumentation, patients with osteoporosis are at risk for cage subsidence. Lund *et al.*[67] evaluated the effect of bone mineral density on stability. They found, in a human cadaver model, increasing bone density improved stabilization provided by cages without supplemental instrumentation. As bone mineral density increased, stabilization was improved in regard to flexion, extension, and lateral bending. Axial rotation, however, was not significantly affected.

Using their "keystone technique," Branch and Branch obtained "satisfactory results" in 129 of 172 patients (75%).[11,12] Among workers' compensation cases, the result was satisfactory in 61% of patients, in contrast to an 89% rate among non-workers' compensation patients.[11] Patients previously operated on or those with failed backs achieved a 70% satisfactory result overall; a 60% satisfactory result was reported if patients had undergone more than one previous surgical procedure.

In 1997 Ray[82] published the results of 236 patients undergoing a PLIF with the Ray-TFC (Surgical Dynamics, Norwalk, Conn.). Of note no posterior lateral segmental instrumentation was placed. Five hundred eighty-seven cages were implanted with average follow-up of 32 months. Disc space settling was no more than 1.5mm, with approximately all disc spaces settling 1mm. Intraoperative complications included 13 dural tears. Postoperatively, no cage displaced or dislodged. Temporary foot weakness or numbness occurred in 10% of cases but resolved by the week 6 of the follow-up period in all cases except two. Seven wound infections occurred—five superficial and two deep. Of those patients who had completed 2-year follow-ups, 208 (96%) had radiographic evidence of fusion. Prolo scale outcomes found 40% excellent, 25% good, and 21% fair outcomes.

Chitnavis *et al.*[23] demonstrated a 95% fusion rate using carbon fiber cages. A very small percentage of their patients had supplemental instrumentation that is not delineated in the fusion rate numbers. All patients but one were single-level procedures. One pair of cages was found to have fractured; however, the patient went on to a solid fusion with good clinical result. Sixty-six percent of patients had a good to excellent outcome by Prolo assessment.

Kuslich *et al.*[54] reviewed their results in a prospective multicenter study using BAK cages (Spine-Tech Inc., Minneapolis). The devices were used alone without supplemental fixation. Stability and fusion were assessed using flexion-extension lateral lumbar radiographs. PLIF procedures were performed in 356 cases with 272 of these being one level and 84 being two levels. Spondylolisthesis was minimal. Fusion rates at 12 and 24 months were 85.3% and 90.6% respectively. Fusion success was affected by

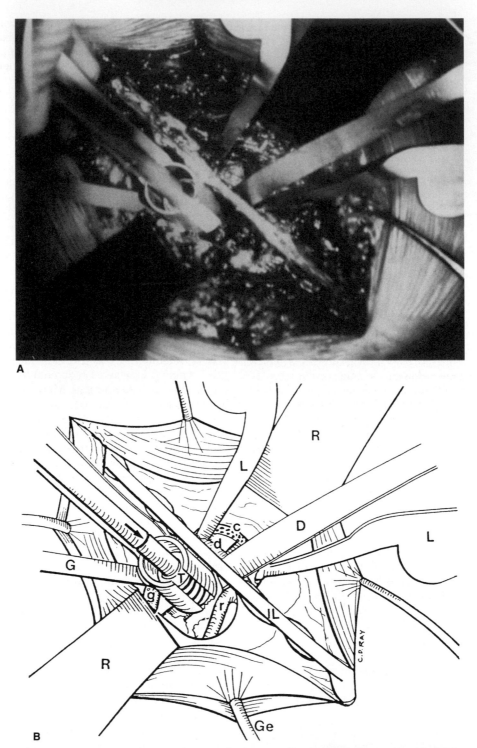

Figure 39.7 Intraoperative photograph (**A**) and schematic drawing (**B**) of a Ray threaded fusion cage implantation showing the bilateral wide black retractors (*R*), a narrow ganglion-protecting retractor (*G*), a Cloward lamina spreader (*L*), a dural retractor (*D*) passed from the opposite side beneath the interspinal ligament and the protective C retractor (*C*). The shaft of the spiral tap (*T*) drives the tap as it enters the circular hole drilled between the vertebral bodies. Note the protection provided to the nerve by the C retractor. Note also the intact interspinous ligament (*IL*). Further note the depth markings, engraved bands around the shaft of the tap, just distal to the reference letter "T." (*From Ray CD: Spinal interbody fusions: a review, featuring new generation techniques.* Neurosurg Quart *7:135-156, 1997, with permission.*)

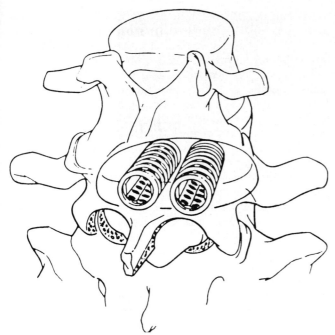

Figure 39.8 Schematic drawing of a pair of Ray threaded fusion cages placed at the L5-S1 space. Note the correct position of the perforations and lateral ribs within the disc. Also note the circular laminotomies bilaterally cut using a circular lamina cutter guided by a centering rod placed within the disc space bilaterally. *(From Ray CD: Spinal interbody fusions: a review, featuring new generation techniques. Neurosurg Q 7:135-156, 1997, with permission.)*

level, L4-5 had a slightly lower fusion rate at 12 and 24 months postprocedure. Patients who received a single implant/level had a lower fusion rate at 12 months; however, the fusion rate was comparable to two implants/level by 24 months. The study is limited in regard to outcome measures for PLIF because it combines both PLIF and ALIF data. Of both surgical types 85% of patients experienced pain relief at 24 months postoperatively.

In a follow-up study, Kuslish et al.[55] reported their 4-year results of the aforementioned patients. For PLIF data, 68 patients were available, 50 of these were one level and 18 were two levels. Fusion rates were 100% and 94.4% for the one and two levels respectively.

Unilateral and Instrumented PLIF

Most of the variations of the original PLIF technique involve grafting of the interspace and the use of different implants. These techniques have been substantiated by the excellent results reported by authors using their own innovations. Two other modifications to the classic Cloward technique that do not involve grafting the interspace are the unilateral PLIF, as advocated by Blume,* and the instrumented PLIF.

Because radicular symptoms and signs are often unilateral, Blume[7-10] proposed a unilateral PLIF. Compared with the bilateral fusion, the unilateral procedure causes

less morbidity because the contralateral, asymptomatic side remains untouched. After the unilateral procedure, postoperative conventional radiographs in his series showed a delay in consolidation; this delay, however, did not seem to have any untoward effect on clinical outcome. For his unilateral fusions, Blume used multiple cylindric autologous bone grafts obtained from the patient's ileum.

Although adequate recipient bed preparation and graft placement are critical requirements for a successful fusion, it has become clear that the success of the PLIF operation is dependent on many factors, with restraint of motion during fusion growth being one of the most important. The failures encountered with classic, uninstrumented PLIF, and the availability of new spinal instrumentation systems to stabilize and immobilize the spine while bone fusion occurs, have prompted several authors to suggest the use of implanted instrumentation in combination with the interbody fusion.[93,94] At one extreme, Wiltse[105] has stated that donor bone PLIF without instrumentation routinely fails. In 1982 Steffee[93,94] developed the so-called variable screw placement system of segmental spine plates with transpedicular screw fixation in conjunction with PLIF to align and stabilize the spine. Constant pressure is applied on the graft, and thus osteosynthesis is accelerated. Moreover, he suggested that by providing significant rigidity, the variable screw placement system prevents future spondylotic slippage and allows for early postoperative mobilization.

The use of an additional internal fixation device is especially indicated when the dorsal portion of the motion segment is incompetent, as in all forms of spondylolisthesis or in postlaminectomy instability associated with facet disruption. The concurrent use of instrumentation enhances the fusion rates by increasing rigidity at the fusion site.[51,52] In a cadaver model Goel[41] has demonstrated a 70% decrease in flexion and extension, a 65% decrease in lateral bend, and a 65% decrease in axial motion with bilateral segmental pedicle plate fixation. Lund et al.[67] demonstrated in a human cadaver model that dorsal instrumentation significantly improved stabilization of dorsally inserted interbody cages. This was regardless of the three cage designs tested (Ray, Brantigan, and Stratec). The addition of cross-bracing to the dorsal instrumentation had a small significant positive effect on axial rotation without significantly affecting flexion, extension, or lateral bending. Klemme et al.[50] evaluated the effect threaded cages alone versus vertical cages supplemented with compressive dorsal transpedicular instrumentation had on segmental lumbar lordosis. On average, patients receiving threaded cages had a mean lordotic loss of 3 degrees, whereas patients with instrumentation and vertical cages had a mean lordotic gain of 5 degrees per segment. Additional instrumentation and stabilization are especially recommended in patients with multilevel disease and spondylolisthesis who seem to have unsatisfactory results with classic PLIF.[85]

Many authors have reviewed their experiences with PLIF, plus dorsal segmental instrumentation. In 1993 Gill and Blumenthal,[40] after a 2-year follow-up, reported their results in 238 patients who had undergone PLIF and instrumentation with the Wiltse pedicle screw fixation

---

*References 7-10,16,40,93-95.

system. A solid fusion (determined by routine anteroposterior and lateral radiographs) occurred in 92% of the cases; after 2 years, 21% of the patients experienced complete recovery without recurrences; 40% had no pain but had experienced one or more recurrences of sciatica or low back pain during the follow-up period; 26% had a mild or moderate level of pain but were able to perform all activities; and the remaining 13% had a mild to moderate level of persistent pain.

Steffee and Brantigan[94] reviewed 169 patients treated with PLIF and instrumentation using the variable screw placement system. Results were satisfactory in 86% of patients with spondylolisthesis, in 80% of patients with postsurgical failed back syndrome, and in 78% of patients presenting with spinal stenosis. Fusion rates were 91.5%, 92%, and 97%, respectively. In 1994 Brantigan[16] reported on 25 patients treated with PLIF and Steffee plates. The PLIF and posterolateral fusion was performed with allograft bone and autograft, respectively. A fusion rate of only 56% was found.

Barnes et al.[3] reviewed their experience with TCBDs used in PLIF, plus instrumented posterior fixation without fusion in 23 patients with mechanical low back pain secondary to degenerative disc disease. In these patients, 70% satisfactory outcome with fusion in 95% of patients was noted. Postoperative complications included one nerve root injury and two wound infections. Brantigan et al.[15] found a 100% fusion rate using the carbon cages supplemented with posterior instrumentation. Tullberg et al.[98] showed that PLIF using carbon cages supplemented with instrumentation had an 86% fusion rate.

Leufven and Nordwall[60] reported their experience of PLIF augmented with posterolateral fusion and instrumentation on chronic disabling low back pain. Twenty-nine patients were evaluated, of which nine had isthmic spondylolisthesis. All patients had pain exceeding 2 years' duration and had failed conservative management. Disc herniations and spinal stenosis were excluded. Patients had positive findings on discography. Patient follow-up was at least 2 years postoperatively. Back pain on average was reduced approximately 50%. No back pain was reported in 38%, improved back pain was reported in 31%, and unchanged and worsened back pain was reported in 17% and 14%, respectively. Leg pain on average was reduced approximately 50%. Thirty-two percent of patients returned to full working ability and 27% could perform light duty, while 7% had mild restrictions. Fusion rate was 93%.

Circumferential PLIF vs. Posterolateral Fusion (PLF) with Instrumentation

PLIF with posterolateral fusion provides for a 360-degree spinal fusion and restoration of anterior column height at the level fused. It is not clear that combining PLIF with posterolateral fusion provides any better outcomes than posterolateral fusion alone. Typically, more muscular dissection and retraction is required for a posterolateral fusion, compared with a PLIF plus segmental posterior instrumentation without PLF. This additional dissection must be balanced with the increased surface area available for bony fusion.

Madan and Boeree,[69] in a retrospective study, compared patients with symptomatic isthmic spondylolisthesis (Grade I or II) who were treated with either instrumented posterolateral fusion or PLIF with instrumented posterolateral fusion. Twenty-one patients were in the posterolateral group and 23 patients were in the PLIF group. By Oswestry index, satisfactory outcome was 81% for posterolateral fusion and 69% for the PLIF group. Degree of correction and maintenance of this was better with PLIF versus posterolateral fusion; however, this was not a statistically significant difference. Two nonunions occurred in the posterolateral group. Results did not separate out back pain and leg pain symptom improvement. Madan et al.[70] then went on to perform a similar study comparing instrumented posterolateral fusion alone to instrumented posterolateral fusion plus PLIF for lumbar disc disease. No significant difference in outcome as evaluated by the Oswestry disability index was noted for either procedure, 63.9% rate of satisfaction versus 80% for PLF versus PLIF, respectively. Two patients in the PLF were noted to have a nonunion, whereas none in the PLIF group were found.

Suk et al.[96] evaluated 2-year outcomes of how adding PLIF to posterolateral fusion and instrumentation for spondylolytic spondylolisthesis would affect fusion rates. Forty patients had a posterolateral fusion with pedicle screw instrumentation, whereas 36 patients had the PLIF procedure (using autogenous tricortical iliac bone block, in addition to the aforementioned posterolateral fusion. None of the PLIF plus instrument patients developed a pseudarthrosis, whereas 7.5% of the others did. Reduction of listhesis was significantly greater for PLIF patients versus posterolateral instrumented fusion, 41.6% versus 28.3%, respectively. In regard to preoperative symptoms of neurogenic claudication, both groups had satisfactory results in approximately 90% of patients. In contrast, those patients who underwent PLIF had a 75% excellent outcome in regard to back pain, whereas only 45% had excellent results in the posterolateral fusion group.

Rompe et al.[86] evaluated the effect of posterolateral fusion and instrumentation with and without PLIF for degenerative lumbar spine disease. They found no significant difference between the two procedures. In their analysis of patients with fair to poor outcomes they noted a preoperative greater degree of lumbar kyphosis, motor weakness, and a significantly larger number of previous lumbar spine procedures.

PLIF vs. ALIF

Anterior lumbar interbody fusion, with or without posterior instrumentation, is another method to achieve interbody fusion. Anterior fusion is performed through either an endoscopic or open laparotomy. Secondary to vascular anatomy the disc spaces amenable to this procedure are largely limited to L4-5 and L5-S1 levels. Risks include vascular injury and significant hemorrhage, bowel injury, and sympathetic plexus injury that is associated with retrograde ejaculation in males. Advantages of the procedure are the ability to easily excise the disc and place large interbody devices without any retraction of the nerve roots. Controversy exists about the use of stand-alone ALIF versus ALIF with supplemental posterior instrumentation. In addition the decision to perform an ALIF versus PLIF in the future may be swayed by the recent Food and Drug Administration (FDA) approval of rhBMP-2 for ALIF only.

Both biomechanical and clinical studies comparing ALIF with PLIF have been performed. Voor et al.[101] performed a cadaver study comparing ALIF and PLIF with posterior instrumentation. ALIF was noted to be slightly superior to PLIF, particularly in regard to left torsion. Anterior cages alone have been noted to stabilize better in axial rotation and lateral bending than posteriorly inserted cages.[76] Barnes et al.,[3] in a retrospective series, evaluated the effect of stand-lone ALIF versus PLIF with supplemental instrumentation in the treatment of mechanical discogenic low back pain. Of the 28 patients available for outcome analysis, eight ALIF and 20 PLIF/PSIF, a 70% satisfactory outcome was noted in PLIF patients and 38% in ALIF patients.

PLIF vs. TLIF

The transforaminal lumbar interbody fusion procedure was originally described by Dr. Harms (Figure 39.9). The procedure involves a unilateral hemifacetectomy of the superior and inferior facets of the level to be fused. The pars interarticularis is removed, allowing access to the lateral aspect of the disc. A near-complete discectomy is performed from this far lateral approach, often with less retraction of the dural sac and nerve roots than required for a standard PLIF. In previously operated levels, this often facilitates removal of bone lateral to the previous surgery site and thus provides for a fresh working channel. Bone graft and cages are then placed unilateral and "rolled" across to the opposite side. The advantages of the TLIF procedure are a unilateral approach versus a bilateral approach required for the PLIF procedure with less required retraction on nerve roots or the dural sac for exposure. The unilateral approach also reduces the chance of injury to the opposite nerve root, which remains untouched. The PLIF technique must often be limited to L3-S1 levels because of the required retraction, whereas the TLIF may be performed higher.

On review of the literature one study performs a comparison of the two techniques. Humphreys et al.[43] performed a nonrandomized comparison of 34 patients who received PLIF versus 40 patients who underwent TLIF procedures. The procedures were performed for degenerative disc disease, grades I and II spondylolisthesis, and central disc herniations. No complications occurred in the TLIF group, whereas 10 of the 34 PLIF patients had complications. Blood loss was significantly less for the two-level TLIF procedures versus the two-level PLIF procedures.

As the TLIF technique becomes more widely used, further studies may elucidate further the advantages and disadvantages of the procedure in comparison to the PLIF.

Complications and Complication Avoidance

PLIF is a technically demanding procedure; several serious complications can occur if it is attempted by an

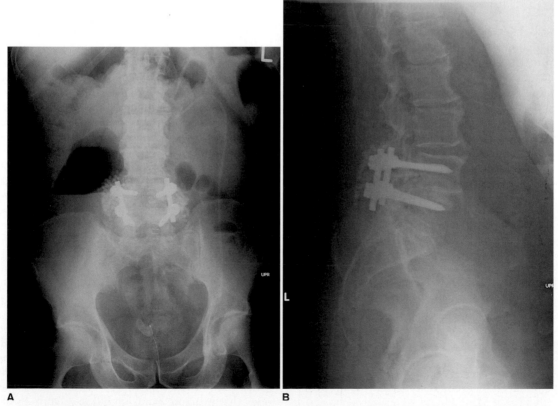

Figure 39.9 (A) AP and **(B)** lateral example of an instrumented posterior transforaminal lumbar interbody fusion.

inexperienced spinal surgeon. Some of the complications encountered during and after PLIF are common to other surgical procedures that involve a dorsal approach to the lumbar spine and the neural structures, whereas other complications are specific to the PLIF operation. PLIF-related complications seem to follow a precise timetable: those caused by technical errors and trauma become clinically evident immediately or within the first 3 months; problems related to instability and strain, such as listhesis, become apparent by 6 months; tropism secondary to unsuccessful fusion and degenerative changes, or actual sequestra of pseudarthrotic bone plugs are usually encountered after the first year.[85] Table 39.1 summarizes complications of the PLIF operation and possible measures to avoid them.

Identification of the Correct Level

Adequate identification of the correct level is of utmost importance. Patients with transitional vertebral segments that may confuse proper localization need special attention. Comparison of plain radiographs with contrast studies is helpful. Accuracy can be increased by intraoperative manual palpation of the sacrum. To adequately localize the correct level, however, there is no substitute for the intraoperative radiograph. After incising the ligamentum flavum with a no. 11 blade, a no. 4 dissector is inserted through the opening. The correct position of the probe for intraoperative localization is within the disc space. The probe can cause an inadvertent durotomy, especially in patients with associated lumbar stenosis, so care must be exercised during this maneuver.

Injury of the Neural Elements

Recognizing anatomic factors and variations is a critical step in the prevention of injury to neural structures. Such variations include enlargement in size of the nerve root, tumors that can mimic disc pathology, and variations of bone structure. MRI enhances the accuracy of preoperative planning and facilitates the preoperative recognition of some of these variations that in the past were often missed by traditional contrast studies.

New or increased neurologic deficits occur postoperatively in 0.5% to 4% of the patients after PLIF.* Undue traction on the nerve roots to gain exposure during the procedure must be carefully avoided (especially on the nerve root passing around the pedicle below the level of the fusion). The nerve root exiting the foramen above this interspace is also at risk from friction during the insertion of the fusion plugs. The upper exiting nerve root, in fact, traverses the interspace just out of direct view in the lateral recess and can be damaged when grafts are inserted into the disc space. Retraction of the sacral nerve roots during the operation can result in postoperative transient urinary retention.[31,40] Neural injury reported in earlier series was, in part, related to the limitations of working space while trying to preserve the facet joints.[107] This complication is minimized by preliminary wide decompressive

laminectomy and variable facetectomy. Positioning the patient is extremely important for minimizing the chances of possible nerve injuries; flexing the hips and knees as much as possible relaxes the nerves and permits their displacement to the midline.[45]

PLIF augmented with transpedicular instrumentation allows the surgeon to remove a greater degree of bone, while maintaining posterior stabilization, and thus obtain better exposure for the subsequent discectomy and cage placement. Distraction across the disc space either with an intralaminar spreader or across the pedicle screws allows the disc space to be opened up and moves the superior nerve root farther cephalad from the working channel. As noted earlier, Barnes et al.[4] found that the choice of implant could affect incidence of nerve root injury. Cylindric cages had a higher rate of nerve root injury compared to allograft wedges.

Increased Tropism at Adjacent Levels

One of the possible disadvantages of the PLIF technique is that a single-level fusion adjacent to a segment already showing degenerative changes may precipitate the disease at the adjacent level.[57] This problem was reported by Rish in 3 out of 250 patients who had undergone PLIF.[85] A two-level fusion procedure or a standard procedure without fusion is recommended in these cases. Discs at levels adjacent to the fused segment frequently show signs of degeneration and collapse, a consequence of making a segment rigid and the entire spine less flexible. Increased flexion of segments adjacent to a fusion can also be observed.[34,36,37,103] In addition, the dorsal elements are rendered more flexible as a result of the surgery, which may influence the behavior of adjacent segments. The neural arch, in fact, is normally restrained in flexion by the dorsal ligaments (tension band). If some of these ligaments are disrupted by surgery, an imbalance of forces can cause the dorsal elements to bend (flex) excessively.[36,37]

The motion segment adjacent to the fused spine may undergo accelerated degeneration because of the increased stress that occurs at the segment next to a fusion. Lee reported 18 patients who developed new symptoms from the segment adjacent to a fusion after an average symptom-free interval of 8.5 years.[57] The most common pathologic conditions at the adjacent segments were hypertrophic facet joints and disc degeneration. Spondylosis and spondylolisthesis are also reported after lumbar fusion.[20]

Graft Retropulsion

Postoperative graft retropulsion with possible catastrophic neurologic sequelae is a serious complication of the PLIF operation. Graft displacement is reported to occur in 0.3% to 2.4% of patients undergoing this procedure.[66] Surgeons who have performed more than 60 PLIF operations report an incidence of graft retropulsion of 1.6%, whereas the incidence of graft displacement increases to 9% for surgeons with less experience.[66] As Lin indicated, conditions that promote graft migration include the following: (1) inadequate design construction, (2) mobility of the grafts within the disc space, (3) delayed fusion, (4) improper size

---

*References 7,33,40,45,58,65,68,85.

TABLE 39.1

Complications of Posterior Lumbar Interbody Fusion and Possible Solutions

Complication	Solution
Blood loss	Perform layer by layer hemostasis
	Use autologous blood
	Use recycling unit
Epidural bleeding	Position patient properly
	Use bipolar cautery
	Use thrombin-Gelfoam packing
End-plate bleeding	Perform good decortication but minimize depth
	Use well-packed bone graft
Nerve root injury	Perform careful decompression
	Perform judicious nerve root retraction
	Perform lateral disc exposure
	Perform ample facetectomy/foraminotomy
	Visualize and protect adjacent nerve root at time of graft impaction
Intraabdominal vessel injury	Directly visualize anterior annulus
	Obtain palpable "feel" while evacuating disc (instrument on bone)
Graft retropulsion	Shape end plate appropriately
	Accurately size the graft
	Place graft 2-4mm below posterior vertebral margin
	Maintain segmental stability
	Provide appropriate internal fixation
	Provide postoperative bracing
Pseudarthrosis	Perform end plate decortication
	Completely remove disc and annulus
	Completely pack disc space
	Maintain stability
	Use high quality and low antigenicity allograft, autograft, or composite bone
	Use pulsing electromagnetic fields
Instability	Maintain two thirds of facet joint
	Maintain supraspinous ligaments
	Maintain graft stability
	Provide appropriate internal fixation
	Completely fill disc space
Graft resorption	Use allograft of low antigenicity
	Use composite graft
	Avoid overcompression
	Maintain stability
Infection	Use preoperative antibiotics (for gram-positive and gram-negative organisms)
	Use frequent antibiotic irrigation
	Use closed drainage postoperatively
	Close dead space
	Debride nonviable muscle
Epidural scar	Perform hemostasis
	Use gentle retraction
	Use delicate dissection
	Use fat graft
	Perform stabilization
	Perform appropriate internal fixation
Arachnoiditis	Use same measures as for epidural scar
Dural tears	Perform careful dissection
	Perform adequate repair

Modified from Simmons JW: Posterior lumbar interbody fusion. In Frymoyer JW (ed): *The Adult Spine: Principles and Practice*. Philadelphia, Lippincott-Raven, 1991, with permission.

and shape of the graft, and (5) instability of the motion segment.[66]

Preparation of the host site and graft is a vital step for the success of PLIF and ensures optimal conditions for fusion. If the cartilage prevents the graft from obtaining adequate blood supply from the vertebral body, the graft will absorb, decrease in size, and move with movements of the spine.[31] Decortication is therefore recommended to allow incorporation of the graft. Total decortication, however, is not necessary, because partial decortication to oozing bone layer on all exposed cortical end plates is sufficient.[66] Good compressive strength can be achieved if the force is uniformly distributed across a large area of the bone graft. To carry body weight safely without crushing bone tissue, the graft must cover approximately two thirds of the area of the end-plate.[61]

The crush resistance of the cancellous bone of the vertebral bodies is markedly site dependent; the more central the location, the weaker the resistance. Grafts should be positioned as peripherally as possible, extending across the entire surface of the body. Additionally, the cancellous bone is strongest beneath the end-plates and weakest at mid-body. Thus in preparing the body for grafting, the amount of bone removed should be the minimum that is commensurate with providing a flat, bleeding surface.[36,37] Total end-plate removal should also be avoided because this can induce the graft to collapse into the vertebral body. The countersunk position also traps bone plugs and prevents normal fusion hyperostosis from compromising the spinal canal or foraminal exit route.[85] The graft should be larger than the opening to the disc space, and once in the disc space, it should be locked and kept in place by the physiologic lumbar lordosis.

Avoiding trauma around the operated interspace in the immediate postoperative period is crucial. Patients should be advised against flexion-extension exercises, torsion, vertical impact, trauma, and Valsalva maneuvers until the process of osteosynthesis is complete.[85] Unless the grafts are impacted tightly, even a small flexion-extension movement of the graft after surgery tends to decrease the rate of fusion and promotes graft migration.[66] Rish reported 5 patients out of 250 (2%) who required subsequent surgery after trauma during the first 3 months after PLIF.[85] Three of these patients had falls and retropulsed a bone plug, which caused compressive radiculopathy. In two cases a plug was extruded after a Valsalva maneuver. One patient had a flulike syndrome with severe stretching during her third postoperative week. She noted the immediate recurrence of sciatica pain and had a retropulsed bone plug in the canal. Another patient, a smoker with chronic bronchitis, had a coughing spasm in the postoperative night and had recurrent symptoms secondary to plug extrusion.

As stressed by Hutter,[45] positioning of the patient is a critical factor. The use of knee-chest frames to free the abdomen from pressure creates an accentuation of the lumbar lordosis. The increase of this lordosis shapes the disc space in a way that favors graft extrusion. Therefore lumbar lordosis should be controlled.[107] Instrumentation systems stabilize and immobilize the spine while fusion occurs.[46] With immediate stabilization, the patient may be mobilized much sooner in the postoperative course. In addition, the risk of graft migration is eliminated in part by the enhanced rigidity afforded by the segmental fixation.

Although the use of dorsal fixation as an adjunct to PLIF reduces the probability of graft displacement, neurologic injury, and nonunion,[95] the advantages gained by the use of these techniques have to be weighed against the additional complications. These complications include extensive exposure and dissection, increased blood loss and infection rate, and spinal canal and neural foramen compromise by the hardware, causing neurologic injury. In addition, radiologic imaging studies performed to assess the results of the fusion are difficult to interpret in the presence of hardware required for the fixation.

The development and commercial availability of fusion cages represent a significant improvement over more traditional means of grafting. These systems provide structural support to the graft while fusion occurs, and they contain the graft material preventing problems associated with graft extrusion. In the multicenter FDA study evaluating the use of the Ray threaded fusion cage, no cases of graft extrusion or migration were reported.[81-84] Disc space preparation and assuring a proper fitting cage are critical to the success of the interbody fusion.

Hemorrhage

Copious bleeding from epidural veins is frequently encountered but rarely represents a clinically significant problem. Knowledge of the anatomy of the blood supply of the spine is important to obtain adequate hemostasis. The arterial blood supply is fairly constant, and coagulation of arteries before they start to bleed can greatly reduce blood loss. Coagulation of the epidural veins as they are encountered also greatly decreases the chance that excessive bleeding can be a problem. The importance of adequate and careful positioning in preventing unnecessary bleeding that results from increased intraabdominal pressure has already been stressed. Hypotensive anesthesia to the level of 80 to 90mmHg systolic may be used to decrease the amount of bleeding.[45,107]

Blood loss is also related to the number of levels fused. In a study of 238 patients Gill and Blumenthal reported an average blood loss of 180ml for single-level fusion, 350ml for two-level fusion, and 500ml for three-level fusion.[40] In a multilevel procedure a blood product recycling unit such as a CellSaver-4 (Haemonetics Corp., Braintree, Mass.) can help contain blood loss.[11] Epidural drains for 24[100] or 48 hours[11] are used by some surgeons to prevent development of postoperative hematomas. Humphreys *et al.,* in an analysis of PLIF versus TLIF, noted that for a single-level procedure blood loss was approximately equal, but for two-level procedures PLIF had a higher blood loss than TLIF.[43] Brantigan reviewed his experience with PLIF using a carbon fiber cage and transpedicular instrumentation. Blood loss averaged 1066, 1843, and 2561ml for one-, two-, and three-level PLIF, respectively. One death occurred in his series secondary to blood loss.[18]

Complications Related to Graft Harvesting

The use of autologous bone does not expose the patient to the risk of transmissible disease or to an inflammatory response related to banked bone, but carries with it the additional morbidity and postoperative pain related to iliac bone harvesting. In a metaanalysis of published studies on lumbar fusion,[99] donor site complications were reported in 10.85% of the patients. These included donor site infection (1.5%), donor site chronic pain (8.7%), and donor site pelvic instability (1.9%).

The most common and readily available source for bone grafting is the iliac crest. Great care must be taken to prevent injury to the sacroiliac joint by overzealous harvesting of graft material and, deep in the wound, injury to the vessels coursing through the greater sciatic notch (superior gluteal artery, vein, or branches).[106] Cluneal neuritis has been reported in 4% of the patients who undergo iliac crest graft harvesting.[44] All of these patients required re-exploration and sectioning of the nerve.

To obviate the need for banked bone or the harvest of autogenous iliac bone, Branch and Branch[11,12] described a keystone graft technique in which the confluence of the lamina and the spinous process is removed en bloc during the exposure and is afterward contoured into three keystone plugs. The ventral third of the disc space is packed with bone fragments, and the keystone plugs are tapped in dorsal to the bone fragments and locked into place. Excess bone fragments are laid over the facet joints bilaterally and over the transverse processes, if necessary, to fuse the facet joints and create a dorsal fusion. Using this technique, Branch and Branch have obtained good to excellent results in 75% of their patients.[11]

Postoperative Scar Tissue Formation

Epidural fibrosis is a postoperative phenomenon in which adhesive constrictions can form around the neural structures and result in their compression. Epidural scar tissue can result in postoperative pain, although its occurrence is usually asymptomatic. Recurrent disc herniations or postoperative epidural scar formation must be suspected in patients with delayed postoperative recurrent pain. Because scar tissue enhances and disc material does not, these two entities are best differentiated with gadolinium-enhanced MRI. In reviewing 12 patients with failed PLIF, Wetzel and LaRocca identified excessive epidural scar formation as a problem in 11 patients in whom the canal was re-explored.[103]

It is conceivable that the extensive epidural manipulation of the neural elements required during the PLIF procedure to allow adequate exposure of the disc space may increase the likelihood of postoperative scar formation. To avoid violation of a virgin asymptomatic side and to prevent diffuse epidural scarring, some authors advocate a unilateral approach to the disc space, except in those cases in which clinical reasons dictate bilateral surgical access.[85] Prevention of scar tissue formation is primarily related to meticulous hemostasis and gentle surgical manipulation of neural structures; interposition of physical barriers, such as a fat graft obtained from subcutaneous tissue, or artificial material, such as absorbable gelatin sponge (Gelfoam), helps preserve a plane between the scar and neural structures and prevents traction of the neural elements after scar retraction. Large fat grafts should be avoided because they can cause compressive symptoms secondary to nerve root compression, requiring re-exploration and removal in some cases.[85]

Infection

The overall infection rate after PLIF ranges from 0.2% to 7%.[11,33,40,44,87] Postoperative infections are differentiated into two types—superficial wound infections and deep wound infections. Although treatment of these two types is eventually the same, the different degree of involvement of the tissue dictates the length of the appropriate antibiotic treatment.[5] In addition, the long-term outcome is different between the two types of infections.[5] Superficial wound infections are defined as those occurring above the thoracolumbar fascia. These infections are clinically characterized by tenderness and local erythema. Systemic signs and symptoms are usually absent, although patients at times can be febrile. The peripheral white blood cell count and differential count are usually within normal limits, but erythrocyte sedimentation rate and C reactive protein levels are elevated.[5]

Unlike superficial wound infections, deep infections are more difficult to diagnose. Deep infections must be suspected in patients with persistent pain that occurs after a pain-free postoperative period. Generalized malaise and low-grade fever may be present. Radicular pain is reported, especially if an epidural abscess has formed. Levels of acute phase reactants are usually elevated, whereas white blood cell counts can be normal. MRI can confirm the diagnosis. Confirmatory diagnosis can be obtained through fine-needle aspiration of the material. This procedure also helps in choosing the appropriate antibiotic treatment on the basis of culture results. Surgical treatment consists of aggressive débridement of all tissues involved, until normal bleeding healthy tissues are visualized.

All the authors' patients receive cefazolin 30 minutes before the skin incision is made. In patients with penicillin allergy, vancomycin is used because of the risk of cross reaction with cephalosporin. Rigorous adherence to aseptic principles and use of careful surgical technique that minimizes tissue damage are the most important factors in preventing wound infections. Careful soft-tissue hemostasis is also crucial because postoperative hematomas and fluid collections represent favorable culture media for bacterial growth.

Dural Tears

Perforations of the dura mater are more common in reoperations than in primary surgery. Inadvertent damage to the dural membrane can be incurred with sharp instruments, such as the Kerrison rongeur, during dissection of hypertrophic ligament adherent to the sac in patients with severe lumbar stenosis, or during attempts to free the neural elements from epidural scars in patients who have undergone previous spinal surgery. PLIF requires displacement of the dura mater to near the midline and use of sharp instruments in the spinal canal. The occurrence of an inadvertent durotomy is usually recognized immediately because cerebrospinal fluid (CSF) suddenly flows through the defect and appears in the field. Gentle handling of the dural sac and perhaps the use of the surgical microscope during the initial decompression may reduce the incidence of this complication.

Once recognized, these defects should be repaired primarily because they predispose to CSF leakage and formation of pseudomeningocele. In addition, persistent drainage of CSF through the defect may cause tedious postoperative spinal headache. Closure is achieved in a watertight manner with 5-0 or 6-0 silk or nylon suture. If the defect is large, repair with a dural substitute may be considered. If it is in a location such as the ventral surface of the thecal sac, in which tight closure presents a technical problem, a fat or muscle graft and use of fibrin glue can enhance the chance of successful closure. Extreme care must be exercised, because nerve roots can often herniate through the defect and can be easily damaged during further dissection or repair of the tear. Using the operative microscope for dural repair may reduce the risk of nerve entrapment or laceration. If nerve root herniation has occurred through the defect, the nerve root must be gently pushed through the hole with the help of a small pattie.

In patients with a recognized or suspected dural tear the fascia layer must be closed in a watertight fashion using several interrupted nylon sutures. Careful attention must be given to the closure of the rostral and caudal limits of the fascial opening. These extremes are often undermined under the skin, making adequate closure difficult. In such cases it can be helpful to extend the rostral and caudal limits of the skin incision to allow more room for fascial closure. Patients who have suffered an intraoperative dural tear are confined to flat bed rest for at least 24 hours. If a CSF leak occurs through the wound, a lumbar drain is inserted and kept in place for 72 hours, in addition to the bedrest restriction.

Pseudarthrodesis

In general there is an overall positive relationship in lumbar fusion between percentage of patients with solid arthrodesis and satisfactory outcome.[99] The incidence of nonfusion varies according to its definition.[19] Rish reported the rate of radiologic fusion, evaluated independently by a radiologist and a neurosurgeon, in 250 patients undergoing PLIF.[85] Positive signs for fusion included homogeneous assimilation of the vertebral and graft interfaces, trabeculation of the graft, block configuration of the two vertebrae, and stability on motion studies. Halo formation along a graft surface, resorption of the graft plug, retropulsion of the graft, and sequestration of a bone wedge were definitive signs of nonunion.[85] Using these criteria, Rish reported a radiologic fusion rate of 85.6%. In his series, nonunion did not universally result in a clinical failure; 50% of the patients with nonunion were considered clinical failures, compared with only 8% of patients with evidence of radiologic fusion.[85]

Although proper recipient bed preparation and graft material placement are essential, it has become clear that the greatest successes are related to a variety of factors. Two of the most important are structural support for the graft and restraint of motion while fusion occurs. Fusion cages provide adequate mechanical strength during fusion maturation and enhance the fusion rates. Brantigan and Steffee reported their results using a carbon fiber cagelike implant; using radiographic criteria they obtained 100% fusion in a 2-year follow-up period.[15] In the multicenter FDA Ray[81-84] threaded fusion cage study, the fusion rate was 82% at 6 months and 96% after 1 year. Although external restriction of motion by external bracing has been found to clearly increase the success rate, this method is poorly tolerated and causes significant discomfort to the patient. Internal fixation of the motion segment by implanted instrumentation is the best method of restraining the motion segment while fusion takes place. As previously indicated, different fixation systems are often used in combination with the interbody fusion. They enhance immobilization and facilitate fusion, although their efficacy

has to be weighed against the additional morbidity associated with their use. As mentioned previously in this chapter, biomechanical studies have shown that stand-alone PLIF constructs tend to have more motion than PLIF augmented with transpedicular instrumentation. This trend toward increased motion can lead to pseudarthrosis.

Several adjuncts have been suggested for increasing fusion rates. Simmons recommended the use of pulsed electromagnetic fields to salvage failed arthrodesis.[91] Mooney reported that the use of pulsed electromagnetic fields in interbody fusion achieved a 92% fusion rate compared with a 65% fusion rate without pulsed electromagnetic fields.[74] If pseudarthrosis occurs, a trial of pulsed electromagnetic fields can be tried. For definite pseudarthrosis, dorsolateral fusion with instrumentation or revision of the PLIF should be considered.

Failed PLIF

A failed PLIF has a worse outcome than failure of any other fusion procedure.[15] Careful patient selection is required for the success of any surgical procedure, and this applies particularly to the PLIF procedure because its failure is accompanied by disastrous clinical outcomes. Wetzel and LaRocca[103] evaluated the problems presented by 12 patients with failed PLIF who underwent a total of 37 procedures. Chronic radiculopathy was present in all individuals, as detected with electromyography or nerve conduction velocity examination. In the 11 patients in whom the spinal canal was re-explored, all had extensive epidural fibrosis. Four patients had evidence of motion dysfunction at nearby levels; two patients had positive discograms adjacent to the PLIFs; one patient had developed a facet syndrome at L5-S1, caudal to an L4-5 PLIF; and one patient demonstrated frank segmental instability at L2-3 rostral to a previous PLIF at L3-4. These authors concluded that they were unable to recommend any successful salvage for the failed PLIF. They recommend an instrumented PLIF as a possible solution in patients with failed primarily noninstrumented PLIF. In patients with a failed instrumented PLIF a ventral interbody fusion may be considered to avoid excessive scar resulting from the original operation.

Future Directions

Minimally invasive spine surgery is rapidly becoming a more widely studied and practiced form of spine surgery. Minimally invasive posterior interbody fusions have been described. Khoo et al. published their results with this procedure augmented by minimally invasive posterior segmental instrumented fusion in three patients.[48] Their average operative time was 3.5 hours per level with estimated blood loss of 185ml, and average inpatient stay was 2.8 days. With these encouraging early results minimally invasive fusions may play an increasingly larger role in the treatment of spondylolisthesis. Future studies will be needed to compare the results of these procedures with open treatment.

Summary

Excellent results have been reported by several authors. However, PLIF has not yet gained wide acceptance because of the technical difficulties of the procedure. When these difficulties occur, complications can be catastrophic, and revision of a failed PLIF is usually unsuccessful. In experienced hands, however, the procedure leads to excellent clinical and radiologic results in selected patients with a variety of lumbar spine pathologies.

REFERENCES

1. Amudson G, Garfin SR: Minimizing blood loss during spine surgery. In Garfin S (ed): *Complications of Spine Surgery.* Baltimore, Williams & Wilkins, 1989, pp 29-52.

2. Bagby G: Stainless steel implants for intervertebral body fusions. In Proceedings of the Annual Meeting of the North American Spine Society, Banff, Alberta, Canada, 1987.

3. Barnes B, *et al*: Threaded cortical bone dowels for lumbar interbody fusion: over 1-year mean follow up in 28 patients. *J Neurosurg* 95(1 Suppl):1-4, 2001.

4. Barnes B, *et al*: Allograft implants for posterior lumbar interbody fusion: results comparing cylindrical dowels and impacted wedges. *Neurosurgery* 51(5):1191-1198, 2002; discussion 1198.

5. Bell GW: Complications of lumbar spine surgery. In *The International Society for the Study of the Lumbar Spine: The Lumbar Spine.* Philadelphia, WB Saunders, 1996, pp 945-968.

6. Blattert TR, *et al*: Successful transpedicular lumbar interbody fusion by means of a composite of osteogenic protein-1 (rhBMP-7) and hydroxyapatite carrier: a comparison with autograft and hydroxyapatite in the sheep spine. *Spine* 27(23):2697-2705, 2002.

7. Blume HG: Unilateral posterior lumbar interbody fusion: simplified dowel technique. *Clin Orthop* (193):75-84, 1985.

8. Blume HG: Unilateral posterior lumbar interbody fusion: simplified dowel technique. In Gill K, Lin P, (eds): *Lumbar Interbody Fusion.* Rockville, MD, Aspen Publishers, 1989, pp 201-209.

9. Blume HG, Rojas CH: Unilateral lumbar interbody fusion (posterior approach) utilizing dowel grafts: experience in over 200 patients. *J Neurol Orthop Surg* 2:171-178, 1981.

10. Blume HG, Rojas CH: Unilateral lumbar interbody fusion by posterior approach with dowel grafts. In Lin PM (ed): *Posterior Lumbar Interbody Fusion.* Springfield, IL, Charles C. Thomas, 1982, pp 252-275.

11. Branch CL, Branch CL Jr: Posterior lumbar interbody fusion with the keystone graft: technique and results. *Surg Neurol* 27(5):449-454, 1987.

12. Branch CL Branch CL Jr: Posterior lumbar interbody fusion: the keystone technique. In Gill K, Lin PM (eds): *Lumbar Interbody Fusion.* Rockville, MD, Aspen Publishers, 1989.

13. Brantigan JW, Steffee AD, Geiger JM: A carbon fiber implant to aid interbody lumbar fusion. Mechanical testing. *Spine* 16(6Suppl):S277-S282, 1991.

14. Brantigan JW, *et al*: Compression strength of donor bone for posterior lumbar interbody fusion. *Spine* 18(9): 1213-1221, 1993.

15. Brantigan JW, Steffee AD: A carbon fiber implant to aid interbody lumbar fusion. Two-year clinical results in the first 26 patients. *Spine* 18(14):2106-2107, 1993.

16. Brantigan JW: Pseudarthrosis rate after allograft posterior lumbar interbody fusion with pedicle screw and plate fixation. *Spine* 19(11):1271-1279, 1994; discussion 1280.

17. Brantigan JW, *et al*: Interbody lumbar fusion using a carbon fiber cage implant versus allograft bone. An investigational study in the Spanish goat. *Spine* 19(13): 1436-1444, 1994.

18. Brantigan JW, *et al*: Lumbar interbody fusion using the Brantigan I/F cage for posterior lumbar interbody fusion and the variable pedicle screw placement system: two-year results from a Food and Drug Administration investigational device exemption clinical trial. *Spine* 25(11):1437-1446, 2000.

19. Brodsky AE, Kovalsky ES, Khalil MA: Correlation of radiologic assessment of lumbar spine fusions with surgical exploration. *Spine* 16(6Suppl):S261-S265.

20. Brunet JA Wiley JJ: Acquired spondylolysis after spinal fusion. *J Bone Joint Surg Br* 66(5):720-724, 1984.

21. Cagli S, *et al*: Biomechanics of grade I degenerative lumbar spondylolisthesis. Part 2: treatment with threaded interbody cages/dowels and pedicle screws. *J Neurosurg* 94(1Suppl):51-60, 2001.

22. Cautilli R: Theoretical superiority of posterior lumbar interbody fusion. In Thomas CC, Lin PM (eds): *Posterior Lumbar Interbody Fusion.* Springfield, IL, Charles C. Thomas, 1982, pp 82-93.

23. Chitnavis B, *et al*: Posterior lumbar interbody fusion for revision disc surgery: review of 50 cases in which carbon fiber cages were implanted. *J Neurosurg* 95(2Suppl): 190-195, 2001.

24. Christel P: The applications of carbon fiber-reinforced carbon composites (CRFC) in orthopaedic surgery. *CRC Crit Rev Biocompatibility* 2:189-218, 1986.

25. Cloward R: The treatment of ruptured lumbar intervertebral disc by vertebral body fusion. II. Method of use of banked bone. *Ann Surg* 136:987-992, 1952.

26. Cloward R: Lumbar intervertebral disc surgery. Description of a new instruments, the vertebral spreader. *Surgery* 32:852-857, 1952.

27. Cloward R: The treatment of ruptured lumbar intervertebral disc vertebral fusion. Indications, operative technique, aftercare. *J Neurosurg* 10:154-166, 1953.

28. Cloward R: History of PLIF. Forty years of personal experience. In Thomas CC, Lin PM (eds): *Posterior Lumbar Interbody Fusion.* Springfield, IL, Charles C. Thomas, 1982.

29. Cloward RB: Spondylolisthesis: treatment by laminectomy and posterior interbody fusion. *Clin Orthop* (154):74-82, 1981.

30. Cloward RB: The treatment of ruptured lumbar intervertebral discs by vertebral body fusion. *Clin Orthop* 193:5-15, 1985.

31. Cloward RB: Posterior lumbar interbody fusion updated. *Clin Orthop* (193):16-9, 1985.

32. Collins JS: The technique of total disc replacement: a modified posterior lumbar interbody fusion. In Gill K, Lin PM (eds): *Lumbar Interbody Fusion.* Rockville, MD, Aspen Publishers, 1989, pp 221-232.

33. Collins JS: Total disc replacement: a modified posterior lumbar interbody fusion. Report of 750 cases. *Clin Orthop* (193):64-67, 1985.

34. Dekutoski MB, *et al*: Comparison of in vivo and in vitro adjacent segment motion after lumbar fusion. *Spine* 19(15):1745-1751, 1994.

35. Eisenstein S: The trefoil configuration of the lumbar vertebral canal. A study of South African skeletal material. *J Bone Joint Surg Br* 62-B(1):73-77, 1980.

36. Evans JH: Biomechanics of lumbar fusion. *Clin Orthop* (193):38-46, 1985.

37. Evans JH: Biomechanics of lumbar fusion. In Gill K, Lin PM (eds): *Lumbar Interbody Fusion*. Rockville, MD, Aspen Publishers, 1989, pp 9-15.

38. Fager CA, Freidberg SR: Analysis of failures and poor results of lumbar spine surgery. *Spine* 5(1):87-94, 1980.

39. Gill K: Clinical indications for lumbar interbody fusion. In Gill K, Lin PM (eds): *Lumbar Interbody Fusion*. Rockville, MD, Aspen Publishers, 1989, pp 35-53.

40. Gill K, Blumenthal SL: Posterior lumbar interbody fusion. A 2-year follow-up of 238 patients. *Acta Orthop Scand Suppl* 251:108-110, 1993.

41. Goel VK, *et al*: Effects of rigidity of an internal fixation device. A comprehensive biomechanical investigation. *Spine* 16(3Suppl):S155-S161, 1991.

42. Goh JC, *et al*: Influence of PLIF cage size on lumbar spine stability. *Spine* 25(1):35-39, 2000; discussion 40.

43. Humphreys SC, *et al*: Comparison of posterior and transforaminal approaches to lumbar interbody fusion. *Spine* 26(5):567-571, 2001.

44. Hutter CG: Posterior intervertebral body fusion. A 25-year study. *Clin Orthop* (179):86-96, 1983.

45. Hutter CG: Spinal stenosis and posterior lumbar interbody fusion. *Clin Orthop* (193):103-114, 1985.

46. Jackson JD: Posterior lumbar interbody fusion utilizing power instrumentation and posterior wire stabilization. In Gill K, Lin PM (eds): *Lumbar Interbody Fusion*. Rockville, MD, Aspen Publishers, 1989, pp 233-241.

47. Jaslow IA: Intercorporeal bone graft in spinal fusion after disc removal. *Surg Gynecol Obstet*, 82:215-220, 1946.

48. Khoo LT, Palmer S, Laich DT, Fessler RG: Minimally invasive percutaneous posterior lumbar interbody fusion. *Neurosurgery*, 51(5Suppl):166-171, 2002.

49. Kitchel. In Proceeding of the Annual Meeting of the North American Spine Society, San Francisco, 1997.

50. Klemme WR, *et al*: Lumbar sagittal contour after posterior interbody fusion: threaded devices alone versus vertical cages plus posterior instrumentation. *Spine* 26(5):534-537, 2001.

51. Krag MH: Fixation of the lumbosacral spine: experience with the Vermont spinal fixator. In Gill K, Lin PM (eds): *Lumbar Interbody Fusion*. Rockville, MD, Aspen Publishers, 1989, pp 251-260.

52. Krag MH: Overview of options and posterior internal fixation devices. In Frymoyer JW (ed): *The Adult Spine: Principles and Practice*. Philadelphia, Lippincott-Raven, 1991.

53. Kruger M, Henssge EJ, Sellin D: [Cast metal spongioid bone implants in animal experiments.] *Z Orthop Ihre Grenzgeb*, 123(6):962-965, 1985.

54. Kuslich SD, *et al*: The Bagby and Kuslich method of lumbar interbody fusion. History, techniques, and 2-year follow-up results of a United States prospective, multicenter trial. *Spine* 23(11):1267-1278, 1998; discussion 1279.

55. Kuslich SD, *et al*: Four-year follow-up results of lumbar spine arthrodesis using the Bagby and Kuslich lumbar fusion cage. *Spine* 25(20):2656-2662, 2000.

56. Kuslish SD, Oxland TR, Jansen RC, Ulstrom CL: The BAK interbody fusion system: early clinical results of treatment for chronic low back pain. In Proceedings of the Annual Meeting of the North American Spine Society, San Diego, 1993.

57. Lee CK: Accelerated degeneration of the segment adjacent to a lumbar fusion. *Spine* 13(3):375-377, 1988.

58. Lee CK, Vessa P, Lee JK: Chronic disabling low back pain syndrome caused by internal disc derangements. The results of disc excision and posterior lumbar interbody fusion. *Spine* 20(3):356-361, 1995.

59. Leong JC, Chow SP, Yau AC: Titanium-mesh block replacement of the intervertebral disc. *Clin Orthop* (300):52-63, 1994.

60. Leufven C, Nordwall A: Management of chronic disabling low back pain with 360 degrees fusion. Results from pain provocation test and concurrent posterior lumbar interbody fusion, posterolateral fusion, and pedicle screw instrumentation in patients with chronic disabling low back pain. *Spine* 24(19):2042-2045, 1999.

61. Lin P: Introduction to PLIF, biomechanical principles and indications. In Thomas CC, Lin M (eds): *Posterior Lumbar Interbody Fusion*. Springfield, IL, Clarence C. Thomas, 1982, pp 3-57.

62. Lin P: Editorial comment. *Clin Orthop* 193:2-4, 1985.

63. Lin P: Posterior lumbar interbody fusion. In Cauthen J (ed); *Lumbar Spine Surgery. Indications, Techniques, Failures and Alternatives*. Baltimore, Williams & Wilkins, 1988, pp 228-247.

64. Lin PM, Cautilli RA, Joyce MF: Posterior lumbar interbody fusion. *Clin Orthop* (180):154-168, 1983.

65. Lin PM: Posterior lumbar interbody fusion technique: complications and pitfalls. *Clin Orthop* (193): 90-102, 1985.

66. Lin PM: Technique and complications of posterior lumbar interbody fusion. In Gill K, Lin PM (eds): *Lumbar Interbody Fusion*. Rockville, MD, Aspen Publishers, 1989, pp 171-199.

67. Lund T, *et al*: Interbody cage stabilisation in the lumbar spine: biomechanical evaluation of cage design, posterior instrumentation and bone density. *J Bone Joint Surg Br* 80(2):351-359, 1998.

68. Ma GW: Posterior lumbar interbody fusion with specialized instruments. *Clin Orthop* (193):57-63, 1985.

69. Madan S, Boeree NR: Outcome of posterior lumbar interbody fusion versus posterolateral fusion for spondylolytic spondylolisthesis. *Spine* 27(14):1536-1542, 2002.

70. Madan SS, Harley JM, Boeree NR: Circumferential and posterolateral fusion for lumbar disc disease. *Clin Orthop* (409):114-123, 2003.

71. Mercer W: Spondylolisthesis with a description of a new method of operative treatment and notes of ten cases. *Ed Med J Neurosurg* 43:545, 1936.

72. Michelson GK: Threaded spinal implant. U.S. Patent 5,015,247, May 14, 1991.

73. Mitsunaga MM, Chong G, Maes KE: Microscopically assisted posterior lumbar interbody fusion. *Clin Orthop* (263):121-127, 1991.

74. Mooney V: A randomized double-blind prospective study of the efficacy of pulsed electromagnetic fields for interbody lumbar fusions. *Spine* 15(7):708-712, 1990.

75. Otero Vich JM: Anterior cervical interbody fusion with threaded cylindrical bone. *J Neurosurg* 63(5):750-753, 1985.

76. Oxland TR, Lund T: Biomechanics of stand-alone cages and cages in combination with posterior fixation: a literature review. *Eur Spine J* 9(Suppl1):S95-101, 2000.

77. Pitzen T, *et al*: Motion of threaded cages in posterior lumbar interbody fusion. *Eur Spine J* 9(6):571-576, 2000.

78. Pitzen T Matthis D, Steudel WI: The effect of posterior instrumentation following PLIF with BAK cages is most pronounced in weak bone. *Acta Neurochir (Wien)* 144(2):121-128, 2002; discussion 128.

79. Ray CD: Transfacet decompression with dowel fixation: a new technique for lumbar lateral spinal stenosis. *Acta Neurochir Suppl (Wien)* 43:48-54, 1988.

80. Ray CD: Lumbar interbody threaded prostheses. In Brock M, Mayer HM, Weigel K (eds): *The Artificial Disc*. Berlin, Springer-Verlag, 1991, pp 53-67.

81. Ray CD: Posterior lumbar interbody fusions by implanted threaded titanium cages. In White A, Schoffermann JA (eds): *Spine Care*. St. Louis, CV Mosby, 1995, pp 1223-1232.

82. Ray CD: Threaded titanium cages for lumbar interbody fusions. *Spine* 22(6):667-679, 1997; discussion 679-680.

83. Ray CD: Threaded fusion cages for lumbar interbody fusions. An economic comparison with 360 degrees fusions. *Spine* 22(6):681-685, 1997.

84. Ray CD: Spinal interbody fusions: a review featuring new generation techniques. *Neurosurg Quart* 7:135-156, 1997.

85. Rish BL: A critique of posterior lumbar interbody fusion: 12 years' experience with 250 patients. *Surg Neurol* 31(4):281-289, 1989.

86. Rompe JD, Eysel P, Hopf C: Clinical efficacy of pedicle instrumentation and posterolateral fusion in the symptomatic degenerative lumbar spine. *Eur Spine J* 4(4):231-237, 1995.

87. Schechter NA, France MP, Lee CK: Painful internal disc derangements of the lumbosacral spine: discographic diagnosis and treatment by posterior lumbar interbody fusion. *Orthopedics* 14(4):447-451, 1991.

88. Schlegel KF, Pon A: The biomechanics of posterior lumbar interbody fusion (PLIF) in spondylolisthesis. *Clin Orthop* (193):115-119, 1985.

89. Sepulveda R, Kant AP: Chemonucleolysis failures treated by PLIF. *Clin Orthop* (193):68-74, 1985.

90. Simmons JW: Posterior lumbar interbody fusion with posterior elements as chip grafts. *Clin Orthop* (193):85-89, 1985.

91. Simmons JW: Treatment of failed posterior lumbar interbody fusion (PLIF) of the spine with pulsing electromagnetic fields. *Clin Orthop* (193):127-132, 1985.

92. Simmons JW: Posterior lumbar interbody fusion. In White A, Rothman RH, Ray, CD (eds): *Lumbar Spine Surgery. Techniques and Complications*. St. Louis, CV Mosby, 1987.

93. Steffee AD: The variable screw placement system with posterior lumbar interbody fusion. In Lin P, Gill K (eds): *Lumbar Interbody Fusion*. Rockville, MD, Aspen Publishers, 1989, pp 81-93.

94. Steffee AD, Brantigan WJ: The VSP spinal fixation system. Report of a prospective study of 250 patients enrolled in FDA clinical trials. In Proceedings of the North American Spine Society, Boston, 1992.

95. Stonecipher T, Wright S: Posterior lumbar interbody fusion with facet-screw fixation. *Spine* 14(4):468-471, 1989.

96. Suk SI, *et al*: Adding posterior lumbar interbody fusion to pedicle screw fixation and posterolateral fusion after decompression in spondylolytic spondylolisthesis. *Spine* 22(2):210-219, 1997; discussion 219-220.

97. Toth JM, *et al*: Evaluation of 70/30 poly (L-lactide-co-D, L-lactide) for use as a resorbable interbody fusion cage. *J Neurosurg* 97(4Suppl):423-432, 2002.

98. Tullberg T, *et al*: Fusion rate after posterior lumbar interbody fusion with carbon fiber implant: 1-year follow-up of 51 patients. *Eur Spine J* 5(3):178-182, 1996.

99. Turner JA, *et al*: Patient outcomes after lumbar spinal fusions. *JAMA* 268(7):907-911, 1992.

100. Verlooy J De Smedt K, Selosse P: Failure of a modified posterior lumbar interbody fusion technique to produce adequate pain relief in isthmic spondylolytic grade 1 spondylolisthesis patients. A prospective study of 20 patients. *Spine* 18(11):1491-1495, 1993.

101. Voor M.J, *et al*: Biomechanical evaluation of posterior and anterior lumbar interbody fusion techniques. *J Spinal Disord* 11(4):328-334, 1998.

102. Waisbrod H: Treatment of metastatic disease of the spine with anterior resection and stabilization by means of a new cancellous metal construct. A preliminary report. *Arch Orthop Trauma Surg* 107(4):222-225, 1988.

103. Wetzel FT, LaRocca H: The failed posterior lumbar interbody fusion. *Spine* 16(7):839-845, 1991.

104. Wiltberger BR: The prefit dowel intervertebral body fusions used in lumbar disc therapy. *Am J Surg* 86: 723-734, 1953.

105. Wiltse LL: Surgery for intervertebral disc disease of the lumbar spine. *Clin Orthop* (129):22-45, 1977.

106. Zindrick MR, Selby D: Lumbar spine fusion: different types and indications. In *The International Society for the Study of the Lumbar Spine: The Lumbar Spine*. Philadelphia, WB Saunders, 1996.

107. Zuckerman JF, Selby D, DeLong WB: Failed posterior lumbar interbody fusion. In White A, Rothman RH, Ray CD (eds): *Lumbar Spine Surgery. Techniques and Complications.*. St. Louis, CV Mosby, 1987.

CHAPTER 40

Anterior Lumbar Interbody Fusion

Robert F. Heary, Edward C. Benzel, and Ceslovas Vaicys

Anterior lumbar interbody fusion (ALIF) reconstructs the anterior column of the lumbar spine, improving sagittal plane alignment. It also facilitates restoration, or at least improvement, of normal lumbar lordosis. In addition, the neural foramina are enlarged secondary to the distractive effect produced by the "spacer" that replaces the degenerative disc. It has become increasingly popular, mainly because of improved understanding of the biomechanics of the spine.

Dorsal decompression, without fusion, has suffered from difficulties that involve the development of chronic low back pain. Posterior lumbar interbody fusion (PLIF) has had unacceptably high complication rates, as well as inferior fusion rates, when compared with ALIF. The biomechanically superior construct that results from ALIF has further led to its increased popularity.

Possibly more than any other spinal surgical procedure, a careful consideration of the indications for ALIF is essential for a good surgical outcome. Chronic low back pain is the principal indication for ALIF.[*] ALIFs are not used to decompress the neural elements because of inadequate visualization. Therefore safe ventral decompression cannot be performed.[9,27,64]

ALIF is associated with a low complication rate. Complications include difficulties with respect to the approach, the discectomy, the donor site, and the fusion, and can be divided into preoperative, intraoperative, and postoperative components.

History

ALIF has evolved considerably over the past century. Ventral approaches to the lumbar spine were first reported for the treatment of tuberculosis. In 1892 Vincent[88] described a costotransversectomy that was used to treat tuberculosis of the ventral lumbar spine. In 1906 Muller[61] described a transperitoneal decompressive operation for the lumbar spine. Ito et al.,[38] in 1932, described a transperitoneal approach to the lumbar spine that incorporated fusion.

Spondylolisthesis has been treated with ventral lumbar surgery since 1933. At that time Burns described a transperitoneal approach using a tibial graft for fusion of the L5-S1 interspace.[5] Numerous other investigators have

followed with modifications of ventral lumbar surgery for spondylolisthesis.[*] The retroperitoneal approach to the lumbar spine was first reported by Iwahara[39] in 1944. In 1948, Lane and Moore[49] described a series of patients with isolated lumbar disc pathology who were treated with ALIF.

The ventral approach to interbody lumbar fusion avoids the neural elements. As such, most early experiences with this surgical procedure were those of orthopedic surgeons. Over the past two decades the increased experience with this technique has been shared by both orthopedic and neurologic surgeons. Although modifications to the standard technique have been devised, the basic tenets of the operation continue to be removal of the disc via a ventral approach, followed by placement of a spacer to maintain disc height, provide anterior column stability, and facilitate bony fusion.

Preoperative Considerations

Proper patient selection is vital to the success of an ALIF procedure[64] and is the best predictor of a good surgical outcome. Operative indications for ALIF include degenerative disc disease with back pain.[†] Degenerative spondylolisthesis with back pain often accompanies degenerative disc disease.[‡] A failure of prior dorsal surgery may be an indication for ALIF.[§] Most important, the symptoms must have persisted for a prolonged period. In general, symptoms are present for 6 months or more before a patient undergoes an ALIF procedure. Likewise, a prolonged trial of conservative therapy should have been attempted and failed before planning an ALIF procedure.[8,50,52,80]

Contraindications for ALIF are absolute or relative. The only true absolute contraindication is advanced osteoporosis that prevents the vertebral bodies from maintaining a bone graft.[9] Relative contraindications occur in varying degrees. Neural compression as a result of either disc pathology or stenosis is a relative contraindication. If neural compression is present, it is most safely and thoroughly approached from dorsally. Other relative contraindications to ALIF include prior retroperitoneal surgery, severe peripheral vascular disease,[9,14,22,90] an active disc space infection, a neoplasm,[90] an infrarenal aortic aneurysm, an anomalous genitourinary system[89] with only a single ureter, and systemic medical illness that precludes the surgery. As a general rule, an ALIF procedure is associated with less blood loss and is better tolerated than the majority of dorsal lumbar surgical procedures.[30,47,75]

A trial of nonoperative therapy is mandatory before undergoing ALIF.[1,8,50,52,80] Mainstays of nonoperative treatment include optimizing body weight, which as a general rule consists of weight loss in most patients; cessation of smoking is also important. In addition, an exercise program that includes back and abdominal muscle strengthening and stretching exercises should be instituted. Consultation with a pain management specialist,[53] as well

---

[*]References 9,11,13,19,47,50,53,75,83,89.

[*]References 20,24,31,36,41,58,59,68,82,94.
[†]References 8,11,50,76,83,89.
[‡]References 17,19,23,25,40,70,76,79.
[§]References 9,11,17,23,25,27,47,53,64,75,80,83.

as a psychological evaluation,[*] are useful adjuncts in determining the optimal candidates for this procedure. Chronic pain may cause varying degrees of depression, anxiety, and aggression, and these behavioral changes can be reversed if the cause of pain is discovered and corrected.[10,81] The efficacy of other conservative therapies such as epidural steroid injections, acupuncture, chiropractic, biofeedback, and modalities is debatable. A preoperative trial of bracing is often recommended, and advocates of preoperative bracing believe that surgical results are superior if there is a good response to use of an external orthosis preoperatively.[60,72,93]

It is important to assess the patient's level of function before surgery, and it should also be determined whether the patient is able to maintain employment and enjoy recreational activities. In addition, simple parameters such as walking distances in a pain-free state, as well as total walking distance, should be assessed. If the preoperative level of function is equivalent to the level that a good surgical result would yield, ALIF should not be performed. Back pain of a magnitude sufficient to consider a fusion procedure should substantially limit a patient's level of function.

It is essential for both the surgeon and the patient to have realistic expectations of the surgical outcome, and this is the reason for a long, conservative trial. Surgical success should be evaluated by a return to the activities of daily living rather than by the hope for a return to high-level athletic activities. Surgical success cannot be fully evaluated until a minimum of 6 to 12 months after the operation.[†] In general, it is not until fusion has been completed that surgical success can be fully evaluated.

Well-known negative prognostic indicators include involvement in workers' compensation or litigation cases,[‡] because these patients are known to have suboptimal long-term clinical results. This is particularly worrisome because the operative indications for ALIF are subjective (low back pain) rather than objective (neurologic deficit).

Before considering an ALIF procedure, a detailed radiographic imaging work-up is required. The initial work-up includes a plain film radiographic series, with flexion and extension lateral views.[30] Flexion and extension radiographs may not reveal segmental instability because most painful motion segments are probably caused by rotational destabilization.[16] These radiographs are used to evaluate spinal stability as well as to confirm the number of true lumbar vertebrae. In preoperative planning, these images are correlated with advanced radiographic imaging studies, such as magnetic resonance imaging (MRI), computed tomographic (CT) scans, and CT myelography. It is important to evaluate lumbar interspaces beyond the zone of the previous spinal surgery to identify additional sources of pain.

A myelogram with a postmyelogram CT scan is considered by some to be the gold standard to rule out neural compression.[8,30,36,47,53] A myelogram and a CT scan are particularly useful in cases of lateral recess stenosis. In addition, CT is an excellent tool for evaluating bony pathology and recording measurements of the cross-sectional diameters of the vertebral bodies on the axial views.

MRI is extremely useful in defining soft-tissue pathology. In particular, T_2-weighted sagittal images are valuable in determining disc dehydration as evidenced by decreased signal intensity.[77,89] In addition, MRI can evaluate adjacent motion segments, neural compression secondary to a herniated lumbar disc, and central stenosis. Furthermore, axial measurements to be used in preoperative planning can be accurately obtained from MRIs.

Discography is a more controversial preoperative radiographic imaging technique. Some advocates of discography promote the use of a provocative discogram to evaluate patients who are considering lumbar interbody fusion.[*] With a provocative discogram, the patient's typical pain pattern must be reproduced at the involved level in an awake, nonsedated state. In addition, injection at other levels of the lumbar spine must not reproduce the patient's typical low back pain pattern. Discography should be used only to confirm MRI findings. It can be most effective in determining the number of levels to be fused in cases of multilevel pathology. In patients who show discrepancies between the results of discography and MRI, consideration should be given to delaying surgical therapy and pursuing other conservative treatments. In other words, diagnostic imaging techniques should be used to decrease, *not increase*, the percentage of surgical candidates.

The number of levels to be fused is an important yet controversial topic. Many studies have clearly demonstrated that pseudarthrosis rates are increased with each increased level of fusion.[†] In addition, clinical success rates are lessened with each additional fused level.[25] Furthermore, there is an increased chance of adjacent motion segment degeneration with longer fusions, which is particularly problematic at the level immediately rostral to a lumbar interbody fusion.[6,8] The number of levels fused is most frequently determined by a review of the radiographic imaging studies. Typically, plain flexion and extension radiographs that demonstrate pathologic motion at the proposed fusion site are helpful.[30,91] In addition, MRI scans, especially T_2-weighted sagittal images, which demonstrate loss of signal consistent with disc dehydration, may help to define the involved segments.[77,89] Finally, it is the opinion of some authors that a provocative discogram confirming the results of the MRI and/or the flexion and extension radiographs may be useful in determining the number of levels to be fused.[‡]

Before undergoing ALIF, a detailed general medical evaluation should be completed. Smoking is known to decrease fusion rates in spinal surgical procedures,[3,44,52] and as a general guideline, patients are requested to quit smoking a minimum of 8 weeks before surgery and to continue to not smoke until radiographic fusion has been confirmed. Additional factors known to detrimentally affect both clinical and radiographic fusion rates include diabetes mellitus, an immunocompromised state, and chronic corticosteroid use.

ALIF is performed for chronic low back pain. As such, patients who have experienced prolonged courses of narcotic analgesics use have a poorer clinical outcome with

[*]References 1,10,17,25,26,37,53,70,80,88,89.
[†]References 8,10,17,23,25,47,50,80,83.
[‡]References 1,17,26,30,52,75,83.

[*]References 8,21,30,37,44,47,52,64,75.
[†]References 22,25,37,47,52,83.
[‡]References 7,8,9,17,19,21,25,30,37,44,47,50,52,64,75,77.

respect to overall pain control than patients who have not used narcotics preoperatively.[10,80] It is unclear whether the worsened clinical outcome in patients requiring narcotic analgesics preoperatively is a result of more severe pathology, to a changing of the pain receptor mechanisms, or to psychologic factors.

The use of oral contraceptives or any drugs containing estrogens is known to increase the incidence of deep vein thromboses during the postoperative period.[12] As a result, these drugs should be discontinued preoperatively for a minimum of 3 months. If there is any chance that an ongoing spinal infection or neoplastic process is present, it should be thoroughly evaluated before considering surgery.[89] The presence of peripheral vascular disease should also be investigated preoperatively with a detailed evaluation by physical examination of the aorta and lower extremities.[9,22,91] Likewise, if there are genitourinary abnormalities, imaging studies should be performed to confirm the presence of two functioning kidneys and two functioning ureters. Abnormalities of the reproductive system, particularly evidence for ejaculatory dysfunction in a male, should be evaluated preoperatively. The presence of osteoporosis should be evaluated with a bone scan and bone mineral density testing before any consideration of surgery.[90]

The decision to undergo ALIF may include a bowel preparation the night before surgery. A bowel preparation makes retraction of the intraperitoneal structures easier and increases safety by decreasing the possibility of an iatrogenic bowel injury.[22,50,75] In addition, routine preoperative antibiotic coverage directed at *Staphylococcus* spp. and *Streptococcus* spp. should be administered. This is usually accomplished with a first-generation cephalosporin antibiotic.

Intraoperative Considerations

Most complications of ALIF can be avoided by following strict preoperative indications, careful preoperative planning, and meticulous intraoperative technique. When complications do occur intraoperatively, most can be managed immediately during the surgical procedure. Some complications are not detectable until the postoperative period. In the following discussion the operation is broken down into each of its components, which are considered separately.

Positioning

Operative positioning depends on the level to be operated on. Most ALIFs are performed at the two most caudal motion segments of the spine.*

General principles of spine surgery should be followed for operative positioning. As a rule, all bony prominences must be padded, with particular attention paid to protection of the ulnar nerve at the elbow[80] and the peroneal nerve at the fibular head.[44] In addition, antiembolic stockings and sequential compression devices are useful intraoperative adjuncts. Because no neural decompression is performed during an ALIF procedure, there is no need for evoked potential monitoring or the use of electromyo-

graphy intraoperatively. The operating table must allow for both anterior/posterior and for lateral fluoroscopy, because this feature is essential for accurate placement of a bone graft and/or an intervertebral cage.

The best operative positioning is obtained by placing the lumbar spine in a position of lordosis. This position is achieved by reversing the flex on the table and placing a roll or bump under the low back region. These maneuvers help open the interspace ventrally, improve the sagittal plane alignment, and facilitate discectomy. In addition, the left iliac crest should be prepared and draped and included in the operative field if a separate incision is necessary for harvesting iliac crest autograft.

When possible, it is best to keep the patient in a true supine position. This is ordinarily achievable without difficulty at the L4-5 and L5-S1 levels. At progressively rostral levels it may be necessary to position the patient slightly in a right lateral decubitus position. Lateral positioning may be necessary to aid in retraction of the intraperitoneal contents during retroperitoneal exposure. Any lateral positioning leads to increased difficulty in maintaining orientation to the true bony midline. As a general rule, thin patients can be maintained in a true neutral supine position, whereas more obese patients require some lateral rotation on the operating table to allow gravity to assist with retraction.

Incision

In any surgical procedure a properly placed skin incision is essential for achieving optimal exposure. The usual approach for an ALIF procedure is via retroperitoneal exposure from the patient's left side. The left side is considerably safer than the right because it allows the great vessels to be approached from the side of the aorta. It is substantially safer to retract the infrarenal aorta from left to right than to retract the inferior vena cava from the patient's right side. A left-sided retroperitoneal approach minimizes the need for any retraction of the inferior vena cava and thus decreases the possibility of injuring[2,48] or thrombosing[88] this structure.

The nerves, muscles, and ureters that surround the lumbar spine are ordinarily symmetric. Only vessel asymmetry determines the need for a left-sided incision. Occasionally, prior abdominal or retroperitoneal surgery may determine the need to perform ALIF from the patient's right side.

Incisions vary based on the level of surgery. Single-level ALIF at either the L4-5 or L5-S1 interspace is performed using a right-angled incision. The standard retroperitoneal incision includes a horizontal limb extending from the midline to the linea semilunaris (lateral border of the rectus abdominis muscle). This horizontal limb is located at a point between the umbilicus and the pubic tubercle. The vertical limb of the incision extends up the linea semilunaris for a variable length, depending on the number of levels to be fused. For a single-level ALIF, the vertical limb is approximately the same length as the horizontal limb (Figure 40.1). When multiple levels are to be fused, the vertical limb extends a longer distance than the horizontal limb. At progressively higher levels, it is necessary to orient the incision in an oblique fashion, extending

---

*References 8,9,19,34,37,44,50,52,75,82.

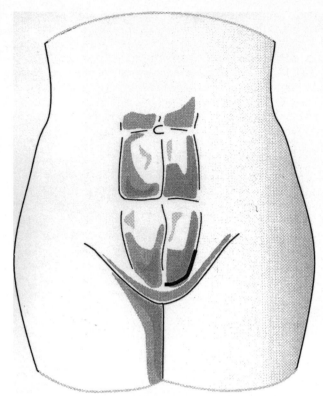

Figure 40.1 Incision for an L5-S1 or L4-5 anterior lumbar interbody fusion. (*Copyright University of New Mexico, Division of Neurosurgery, with permission.*)

toward the tip of the left twelfth rib. This oblique incision may be necessary to gain access to the retroperitoneal space of the L1-2 and L2-3 interspaces. At more rostral levels care must be taken to avoid retraction on the spleen, which is susceptible to minor blunt trauma from the retractors.[33]

Exposure

ALIF can be approached by a variety of exposures. The most commonly used technique is left-sided retroperitoneal dissection. Other methods include a transperitoneal open procedure, as well as a laparoscopic approach.* The difficulties with transperitoneal surgery include prolonged postoperative ileus, as well as problems with fluid management and "third spacing" secondary to fluid shifts from an edematous bowel. As such, the open transperitoneal approach has been essentially abandoned in favor of retroperitoneal exposure. Laparoscopic techniques are discussed elsewhere; however, they do not as yet have long-term follow-up data that support their use.

It is mandatory that a surgeon who is comfortable with the surgical approach provide the exposure. This procedure can be performed by a general surgeon or a vascular surgeon familiar with the retroperitoneal region, as well as management of the potential complications that may occur during the operation. Proper techniques of vessel ligation are vital to successful exposure of the disc spaces.[11] With a left retroperitoneal approach, the intraperitoneal contents are dissected away from the retroperitoneal space from the

left side toward the midline. The ureter must be identified and protected. During the exposure, it is best to avoid cutting longitudinally oriented structures.[89,90] The dissection must be performed ventral to the psoas muscle. In thin patients it is possible to dissect into the retropsoas space, which can result in excessive postoperative fluid collection, blood loss, and the possibility of injury to the genitofemoral and ilioinguinal nerves.

In patients who have not undergone prior retroperitoneal surgery, gentle blunt dissection is the safest, quickest, and easiest technique. If the peritoneum is violated during the retroperitoneal approach, it should be immediately closed to prevent development of a postoperative hernia.[81] This is accomplished by isolating the edges of the peritoneum and using an absorbable suture with a continuous stitch. An unrecognized peritoneal violation can result in a postoperative hernia and subsequent bowel obstruction. If the bowel proper is violated during retroperitoneal exposure, it should be treated with immediate irrigation, followed by layered closure, with the mucosal and serosal layers repaired separately, and abortion of the ALIF procedure. In addition, broad-spectrum antibiotics with anaerobic coverage should be instituted immediately. In spite of the excellent bony and vascular anatomic landmarks present in the ventral lumbar spine, radiographic confirmation of the correct level is mandatory before performing ALIF. Intraoperative radiographs should be compared to preoperative plain radiographs to confirm the appropriate level.[12,34,91] Surgery at the incorrect level has been previously reported.[83]

Each level of the lumbar spine has distinct anatomic structures that must be addressed during a retroperitoneal approach. In general, lumbar segmental arteries should be preserved unless specific damage has occurred to one of them. There is no need to routinely ligate these vessels, which are involved in supplying blood to the vertebral body proper.[12]

At the L5-S1 interspace, there is no need to mobilize the iliac vessels. This interspace is routinely located between the right and left common iliac vessels, and is easily visualized without vessel dissection. Important structures at the L5-S1 level include the autonomic nerves that traverse the prevertebral space at this level. These nerves may be damaged by a monopolar electrocautery, and this can lead to autonomic dysfunction. In males, this is manifested as retrograde ejaculation. To avoid this complication a monopolar electrocautery should not be used in the prevertebral space.* In addition, a vertical opening of the midline prevertebral space should be used with gentle blunt dissection laterally to free all overlying soft tissues, and in the process, to gently dissect the hypogastric plexus away from the ventral disc space at the L5-S1 level (Figure 40.2).[89,91]

At the L4-5 interspace the left common iliac vessels routinely traverse the prevertebral space and thus prevent direct access to the space. These vessels must therefore be mobilized from left to right to expose the bony midline. Before mobilizing the iliac vessels, however, vessel loops should be passed proximally and distally to obtain vascular control of both the left common iliac artery and the common iliac vein. In addition, the left iliolumbar vein

---

*References 3,6,55,56,65-67,73,74,95.

*References 11,12,25,42,75,89,90.

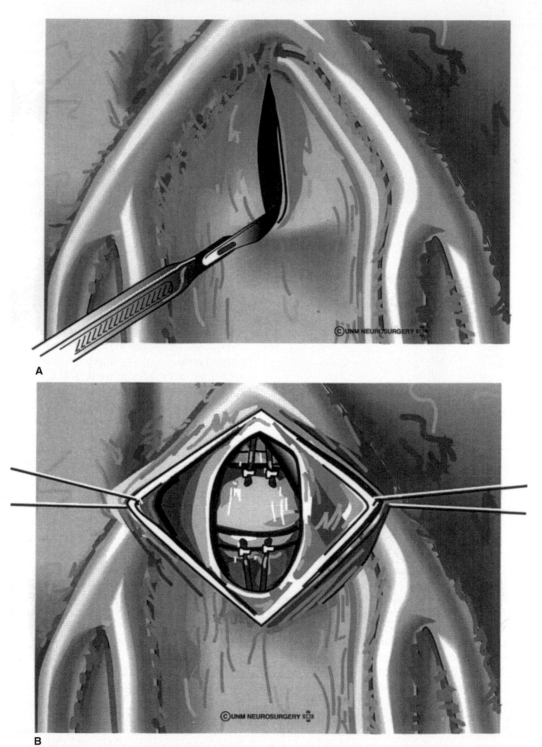

Figure 40.2 After retraction of the retroperitoneal and abdominal structures, a vertical incision is made in the prevertebral space. **(A)** Gentle retraction laterally gains access to the L5-S1 and, occasionally, the L4-5 disc interspace. Vessels are ligated and clipped, or tied **(B)**. *(Copyright University of New Mexico, Division of Neurosurgery, with permission.)*

routinely enters the left common iliac vein laterally at a variable distance caudal to the inferior vena cava. It is necessary to locate and ligate the left iliolumbar vein before medially mobilizing the left common iliac vein. If the common iliac vein is mobilized without ligation of the iliolumbar vein, extensive hemorrhaging can occur secondary to avulsion of this vessel (Figure 40.3A).[2,48] If an iliac vein is damaged, direct pressure should be applied and proximal and distal vascular control obtained. Fine, nonabsorbable suture is used to primarily close the venous defect with a continuous suturing technique. Common iliac vein injuries have been described in 2% to 4.5% of cases.[46,69,70,81] Although they have been reported, injuries of the common iliac artery[69] and inferior vena cava[2,48] are very rare.

At the L3-4 disc space the iliac vessels must be mobilized medially. In addition, a minimal amount of mobilization of the distal aorta from left to right is necessary (Figure 40.3B). There is no need to mobilize the inferior vena cava during a left-sided approach to the lumbar spine at any level. If surgery is necessary at the L1-2 levels, the aorta will need to be mobilized from left to right to gain exposure to the true bony midline. In addition, care must be exerted at the L1-2 level to avoid iatrogenic injury to the left renal artery if overly vigorous medial displacement of the aorta is performed.

Retraction

After exposure of the retroperitoneal space, a table-mounted self-retaining retraction system is useful; it should have malleable, broad-bladed retractors to evenly disperse pressure. Laparotomy pads are used to cover the retractor blades to protect the sensitive intraperitoneal structures. After the self-retaining retractor system is positioned and the correct level identified, a lateral fluoroscopic image can confirm the appropriate level.[12,34,89,91] An anteroposterior (AP) fluoroscopic image is necessary to mark the true bony midline with an indelible marking pen or methylene blue dye. Maintaining orientation to the bony anatomic midline is critical to the safe performance of an ALIF procedure.

Excessive retraction can lead to injuries to the peritoneum, the intraperitoneal structures, or the major blood vessels. The intraperitoneal contents are best retracted using the self-retaining retractor system; however, the iliac vessels and the aorta should not be retracted by this method. The use of self-retaining retractors on these vessels can be associated with an increased risk of vascular injury and an increased risk of thrombosis of either the artery or the vein.[9,12,34] The major vessels are best retracted by hand-held instruments manipulated by a surgical assistant under direct vision. Thus pressure on the vessels can be frequently released, which helps to prevent development of an intramural thrombus. If one of the iliac vessels or the aorta is injured, the umbilical tapes, which provide distal and proximal vascular control, are used to halt the bleeding. This is followed by primary vessel repair using nonabsorbable sutures. This repair is ordinarily performed by either a general or vascular surgeon. Iliac artery thrombosis can be detected by carefully monitoring peripheral pulses and skin color in the lower extremities. If a thrombus is detected or strongly suspected, an intraoperative angiogram should be obtained immediately.

Thrombectomy is often the treatment for a positive angiogram.[22] Additionally, if the ureter is injured during the retraction or exposure, placement of a ureteral stent is ordinarily performed by a general or urologic surgeon.[57]

Discectomy

After the correct level has been confirmed with lateral fluoroscopy, and an AP fluoroscopic image has confirmed the midline, the midline is marked on the vertebral bodies above and below the disc space to help maintain orientation. At this stage in the operation, long instruments are very useful. Commercially available curettes and rongeurs 13 to 15 inches long facilitate performance of the discectomy. To determine the depth of the discectomy, confirmation should be made based on the preoperative MRI study and/or CT scan. Particularly at the L5-S1 interspace, it is important to confirm that all tissue overlying the disc space has been gently and bluntly swept laterally before incising the ventral annulus fibrosus. Once again, avoidance of monopolar electrocautery diminishes the incidence of autonomic dysfunction postoperatively.*

A symmetric window is cut into the ventral annulus fibrosus, taking care to preserve the lateral aspects of the disc bilaterally (Figure 40.4). It is essential to maintain orientation to the midline and stay within the annulus fibrosus, with care being taken not to violate the annulus laterally or dorsally. The nucleus pulposus is removed entirely, up to the dorsal annulus fibrosus. Calibrated tips on the instruments are useful at this stage. With use of some of the newer cage and bone dowel techniques, a predetermined cylinder of disc and bone material is removed. In a standard lumbar interbody fusion, all articular cartilage is removed from the bony end plates above and below the disc space, with care taken to preserve the subchondral bone of the end-plates. As a general rule, disc material is removed 25 to 30mm in depth and 30 to 35mm in width, centered at the bony midline. These measurements are quite consistent for the lower lumbar motion segments. Variations exist in the anteroposterior dimensions of the vertebral bodies. The oval shape of the lumbar vertebrae accounts for a larger depth in the midline than in the lateral portions of the vertebra.[11] It is important to avoid use of bone wax for bleeding cancellous bone because foreign bodies may decrease the fusion rates postoperatively.

Excessive depth of the discectomy can be catastrophic. The dorsal annulus fibrosus is not well visualized from an ALIF approach, and if it is violated, epidural bleeding or a dural injury can occur. These are usually not controllable by using a limited exposure and are best avoided. If the dorsal annulus fibrosus is violated, the disc space must be observed for bleeding or a cerebrospinal fluid (CSF) leak. Bleeding is best controlled with copious amounts of irrigation, as well as with the use of thrombin-soaked Gelfoam. Patience is the key, because access in this area is extremely poor. It is unrealistic to attempt bipolar cautery on a bleeding epidural vessel unless it is directly visualized, because it is not usually possible. Monopolar electrocautery must be avoided at all times in the epidural space. If a CSF leak occurs, free muscle and fascia grafts, with or without fibrin

---

*References 11,12,25,42,75,89.

COMMON ILIAC VEIN
COMMON ILIAC ARTERY   ILIO-LUMBAR VEIN, DIVIDED
PSOAS MUSCLE

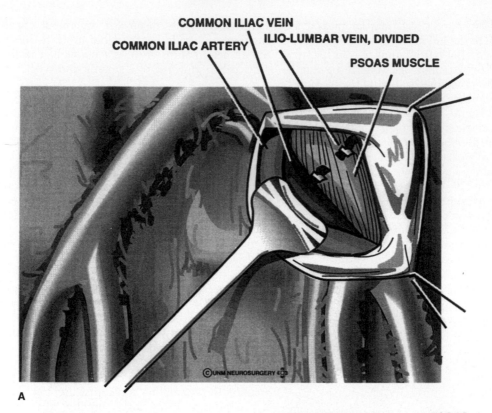

A

ILIO-LUMBAR VEIN,
DIVIDED   PSOAS
MUSCLE

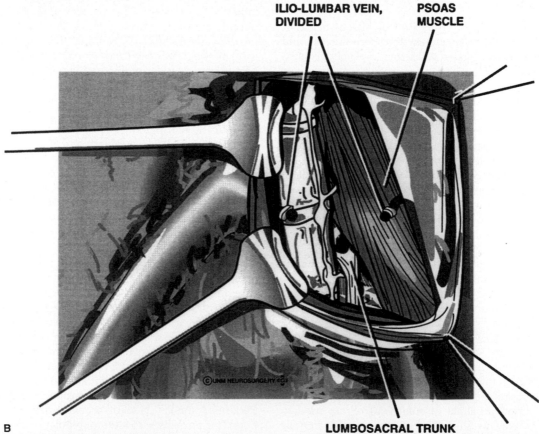

B

LUMBOSACRAL TRUNK

Figure 40.3 At the L4-5 interspace, lateral retraction initially exposes the left common iliac vein beneath the left common iliac artery (**A**). The iliolumbar vein is then clipped, ligated, or tied. After this, further retraction gains access to the ventral L4-5 and L3-4 disc interspaces (**B**). (*Copyright University of New Mexico, Division of Neurosurgery, with permission.*)

glue, are used to attempt to control the egress of spinal fluid. Consideration should be given to placement of a lumbar subarachnoid drain to divert CSF during the immediate postoperative period.[54] Safe and reliable decompression of the thecal sac or nerve roots is not realistic from an ALIF approach, and if neural decompression is necessary, it should be performed using a dorsal procedure or as part of a combined procedure.

Distraction

Several commercially available systems have been developed for ALIF. These systems have disc space distractors with calibrated tips to prevent excessively deep disc space distraction (Figure 40.5). Improved distraction can also be obtained by proper patient positioning. This helps to maintain lumbar lordosis and in the process opens up the ventral aspect of the interspace. Particularly in larger

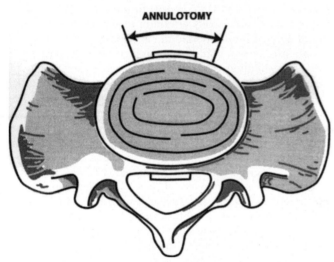

Figure 40.4 An annulotomy, taking great care to not proceed too far excessively laterally is performed, as depicted. (*Copyright University of New Mexico, Division of Neurosurgery, with permission.*)

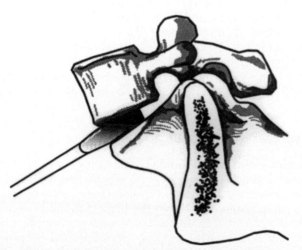

Figure 40.5 An interbody strut, several types of which are available, can be used to increase disc interspace height, as depicted. (*Copyright University of New Mexico, Division of Neurosurgery, with permission.*)

patients, the operating surgeon should wear a headlamp to improve visualization to perform the discectomy safely.

The interspace can be distracted with either a system developed specifically for ALIF or with a laminar spreader, a straight osteotome, or a Cobb periosteal elevator. The danger of excessively deep placement of a distractor is violation of the dorsal annulus fibrosus, with subsequent entrance into the epidural space. This can be associated with epidural bleeding, which may be difficult to control, or neurologic injury or durotomy, which cannot be adequately visualized and repaired.

Bone Graft Harvest

The highest fusion rates in lumbar surgery are obtained when autograft bone is used as a fusion substrate. This bone can be used alone, in combination with allograft bone, or with a cage. If the iliac crest is within 5cm of the retroperitoneal skin incision, dissection through the same skin incision allows access to the iliac crest for harvesting bone graft. If more than 6cm separates the skin incision from the iliac crest, a separate skin incision will be necessary to harvest the bone graft.

When harvesting iliac crest autograft, the medial-most aspect of the skin incision should be at least 2cm lateral to the anterior superior iliac spine (ASIS). The lateral femoral cutaneous nerve is subcutaneous in this location and typically runs within 2cm of the ASIS. If this nerve is transected, permanent anesthesia of the ventrolateral skin of the thigh results.[53,54] If it is compressed, a temporary sensory deficit, caused by neurapraxic injury, results. When ALIF is performed using iliac crest autograft as the sole graft source, the medial and lateral aspects of the crest need to be exposed and an oscillating saw used to harvest tricortical strut grafts. Osteotomes can also be used; however, they have been shown to be associated with an increased incidence of microfractures of the tricortical bone graft.[43] If the iliac crest autograft is being used to augment allograft bone or a cage, then a small cortical window can be opened on either the medial or lateral surface of the iliac crest and, with the use of curettes and gouges, cancellous bone removed from the iliac crest. In extremely thin patients the medial crest is favored for its cosmetic advantages, and in heavier patients, the lateral crest is more easily accessible. Ordinarily harvesting iliac crest autograft does not result in cosmetic deformity.

Excessive exposure of the medial iliac crest can lead to a hernia through the transversalis fascia. If the transversalis fascia is violated, it should be repaired immediately to prevent development of a postoperative hernia. After removal of the iliac autograft, the wound should be copiously irrigated and packed with thrombin-soaked gauze. Bone wax should be avoided because it is associated with an increased incidence of wound infections. After removal of all packing and copious irrigation, hemostasis is obtained. A drain should also be considered.

Complications associated with iliac crest autograft harvesting include lateral femoral cutaneous nerve (LFCN) palsies that result from medial placement of the skin incision. A postoperative hematoma may develop if inadequate hemostasis has occurred.[75] This complication can be avoided by paying attention to hemostasis, and perhaps with the use of a drain. Postoperative wound infections and subsequent pain may also occur,[8,47,69] and are avoided by use of generous quantities of irrigation, drainage of the wound, use of prophylactic antibiotics, and consideration of pulse lavage following graft harvest.

Fusion

ALIF is performed for low back pain, and long-term bony fusion is necessary for the best postoperative results.[25,34,83] Fusion can be judged both clinically, as evidenced by the relief of back pain, and radiographically, as evidenced by radiographic incorporation of the graft. The meticulous performance of ALIF is critical.

After the discectomy is completed, a spacer must be placed in the involved interspace. A variety of materials have been employed to function as spacers. Iliac crest autograft can be used to function as a spacer, in which case two tricortical grafts are typically placed side by side. Allograft bone can also be used. The different forms of allografts used in ALIF procedures include femoral ring, tibia, humerus, and iliac crest. Of all of these femoral ring is the best choice because it can be sculpted to anatomically fit the defect and then be packed with cancellous autograft bone. The use of iliac crest allograft is a poor choice because this bone does not have the same structural strength as comparable autografts. Recently, threaded dowels of bone derived from femoral allograft have been developed. They are placed in predetermined channels, a method similar to the Cloward technique used for the cervical spine. Likewise, cages have become increasingly popular[3,15,51] and can be made of either titanium or carbon fibers. The Food and Drug Administration (FDA) has approved titanium cages, which are threaded cages that lie flat within the interspace side by side and are filled with autograft iliac crest cancellous bone. Additionally, a titanium cage can be used that stands upright as a single trapezoidal cage within the interspace. Typically, carbon fiber cages are placed as two cages lying flat within the interspace side by side.

Spacers are used to maintain disc height after a discectomy and to facilitate bony fusion. Ideally a spacer is slightly larger than the disc height as measured by preoperative sagittal plane imaging studies. Likewise, an optimal spacer has a slightly trapezoidal configuration, with the larger end placed ventrally to increase lumbar lordosis. The depth of the spacer is determined by careful examination of the preoperative axial images from either CT or MRI. Spacers perform a variety of functions, including restoration of lumbar lordosis and improvement of sagittal plane alignment of the lumbar spine. In addition, a spacer serves to improve disc height, and in so doing, increases the size of the corresponding neural foramina.

Two principles of bony fusion are applicable to ALIF: (1) the need for compression, and (2) the need for immobilization to increase the chances of acquiring stable bony fusion. Unlike dorsal fusion, with ventral fusion the graft can be maintained in a position of compression.* Compression is best achieved by distracting the interspace and placing a slightly oversized spacer in this disc space.

Compressive forces felt by a spacer in the intervertebral space are many times greater in magnitude than any compression achieved by an onlay graft dorsally. Immobilization is obtained by firmly fitting a spacer into the intervertebral disc space. In addition, an external orthosis may be used to diminish motion at the lower lumbar spine. There is no need for internal instrumentation with ALIF.

The grafting technique itself involves removal of all articular cartilage overlying the surfaces to be grafted. The interspace is distracted, and a slightly oversized spacer is selected. A portion of cancellous bone from the vertebral body immediately above and below the interspace is exposed using a drill, curette, or gouge. The exposed cancellous bone of the vertebral body should be aligned with the exposed cancellous portion of the bone graft, which allows for optimal fusion, as well as provides immediate hemostasis. The ventral-most aspect of the spacer should be slightly countersunk beneath the ventral-most surface of the vertebral bodies above and below. Bone wax should be avoided because it decreases fusion rates. When placing a spacer, meticulous attention to maintenance of the orientation of the bony midline is important. If two spacers are used, they should be symmetrically placed on each side of the midline, and if a single spacer is used, it should be centered on the midline. After placement of the spacer, AP and lateral fluoroscopic confirmation should be obtained immediately.[12,34,90,92] If any modification of the positioning of the spacer is necessary, it should be addressed immediately. A particular concern regarding the placement of two spacers side by side is assurance that when the second spacer is positioned, it does not cause loosening of the first spacer. This must be confirmed after placement of the second spacer, and if the initial spacer has been loosened, modification must be made before wound closure. Strict adherence to symmetric placement of the spacers with respect to the midline helps avoid this problem.

In situations in which circumferential instability is present, anterior/posterior circumferential fusion should be considered. This procedure involves a significantly larger operation, more operative time, and greater operative blood loss. If neural compression is present, requiring a dorsal operation, and there is a need for anterior column restoration, then both a ventral and dorsal operation may be preferable. In addition, ventrodorsal fusions may be indicated in conditions with known diminished fusion rates. This involves smokers, diabetics, immunocompromised patients, and patients on chronic corticosteroid use.

Postoperative Complications

Postoperative complications related to ALIF can be divided into four categories: (1) complications related to the operative approach, (2) neurologic complications, (3) complications related to the bone graft, and (4) complications related to the fusion. Neurologic complications are quite unusual in properly performed ALIF procedures. They tend to appear in the first 2 days after the operation and require prompt diagnosis and intervention. Complications related to the operative approach and those related to the iliac crest donor site both occur between

---

*References 11,12,34,50,80,91.

3 and 14 days after surgery. Complications related to the fusion proper tend to consist of the development of chronic pain syndromes. Fusion problems are usually not detectable until 6 to 12 months postoperatively.[*]

Operative Approach

After ALIF, it is possible to develop a postoperative hernia,[37,69,76] which may lead to bowel obstruction[9,35,36] and possible bowel infarction. Violation of the peritoneum during ALIF with the retroperitoneal approach, or violation of the transversalis fascia during iliac bone graft harvest, can lead to the development of both internal hernias and subsequent bowel obstruction. When the peritoneum or the transversalis fascia is violated, postoperative hernias are best prevented by immediate operative repair of the defects during the index surgical procedure.[81] If these structures are violated and are inadequately repaired or not appreciated, a hernia may result.

An injury to the bowel may occur during retroperitoneal exposure, and this extremely rare complication requires immediate detection and treatment. The treatment is aggressive irrigation followed by direct repair of the bowel, with separate, layered closures of the mucosal and serosal layers. Prophylactic antibiotics are administered, and the ALIF procedure is aborted at this point. If not already present during the surgery, a general surgeon should perform or assist in the bowel repair. Bowel injuries are best avoided by using a preoperative bowel preparation, including an enema to help decompress the loops of bowel, as well as placement of a nasogastric tube before the retroperitoneal procedure is performed.[22,50,75]

Major blood vessel injuries are rare during operative exposure. Injuries to the iliac arteries or veins, the inferior vena cava, and the aorta occur in 2% to 4% of ALIF operations.[†] To avoid vessel injuries, a self-retaining retractor should not be used on the vessels during the exposure portion of the operation.[9] In addition, before mobilizing the iliac vessels or the aorta, proximal and distal control should be obtained with vessel loops, which are used when a major vessel is injured. Should this type of injury occur, a vascular surgeon should perform or assist in vessel repair. Major vessel injuries are repaired primarily using nonabsorbable sutures. Sometimes smaller vessels are injured. The left iliolumbar vein can be avulsed if not ligated before mobilizing the left common iliac vein.[2,48] This vessel is safely ligated at any time and should be ligated before common iliac vein mobilization. Likewise, lumbar segmental arteries can be ligated safely at any level; however, these vessels ordinarily are spared during the surgical procedure.

Retrograde ejaculation is a serious complication that may occur in male patients after ALIF.[22,25,42,75] It occurs when the autonomic nerves are injured, usually at the L5-S1 level. The hypogastric plexus is a continuation of the preaortic sympathetic chain that extends down from the thoracic region ventral to the aorta and lumbar vertebrae in the retroperitoneal space.[42,89,90] As stated, the use of a monopolar electrocautery overlying the L5-S1 interspace

has been associated with an increased incidence of retrograde ejaculation and should be avoided.[*] This problem occurs in 0.5% to 2% of all ALIF procedures performed on males.[8,18,52,83] The mechanism of retrograde ejaculation involves the presence of dry ejaculate secondary to relaxation of the internal bladder sphincter, with retrograde flow of ejaculate into the bladder.[42,90] There is no surgical management for this complication, and it becomes prograde in 25% to 33% of patients by the end of the second year.[18,35]

Thrombosis of either venous or arterial structures may occur after ALIF. Venous thrombosis has been reported in 1% to 11% of all ALIF procedures, but arterial thrombosis is extremely rare.[†] To avoid these thromboses, retraction should not be prolonged, and self-retaining retractors should not be used on major vessels. If thrombosis is suspected, an immediate angiogram or venogram should be obtained. The treatment is open surgical thrombectomy.[22] Likewise, an embolus in the arterial vascular tree in the lower extremities can occur on rare occasions and is particularly likely if the patient is elderly. To avoid arterial embolization, retraction should not be prolonged and care should be taken not to use self-retaining retractors on blood vessels. An arterial embolus is detected in the perioperative period by loss of distal pulses and a cool extremity and is best treated by immediate vascular surgical removal.

General systemic medical problems may arise during the postoperative period. Urinary retention occurs in 5% to 27% of cases and is usually temporary.[‡] It may be related to the use of perioperative narcotic analgesics. If urinary retention occurs, it is important to rule out an injury to the ureter or cauda equina syndrome. If urinary tract dysfunction occurs in the late postoperative period, obstruction of the distal ureter from retroperitoneal scarring must be ruled out.[57] Postoperative ileus is also common during the postoperative period and usually resolves less than 1 week after the operation. Prolonged postoperative ileus has been reported in 1% to 8% of all ALIF procedures[§] and also may be related to the use of perioperative narcotic analgesics. An internal hernia that causes bowel obstruction secondary to violation of the peritoneum or transversalis fascia must be ruled out in cases of prolonged postoperative ileus. Serious general medical problems that have been reported include both fatal[11,87] and nonfatal[19,83] cardiac arrest, fatal[19,80] and nonfatal[||] pulmonary embolus, and aortic aneurysm rupture.[69]

Neurologic Complications

Neurologic complications are quite rare after ALIF because the epidural space ordinarily is not entered, and no attempt is made to decompress the neural elements during this procedure. Most neurologic complications are related to injuries to the nervous structures during the operative procedure. If neurologic deterioration occurs during the postoperative period, immediate neuroimaging with either MRI or CT myelography should be performed.

If an epidural hematoma that causes neurologic dysfunction is detected, the patient should be immediately returned to the operating room. Epidural hematomas are best treated using a dorsal approach that provides the safest and easiest access to the thecal sac and nerve roots to decompress the hematoma. An incomplete neurologic deficit requires that imaging studies be promptly performed. The surgeon's judgment determines whether repeat surgery or expectant observation is the solution. Cauda equina syndrome must be ruled out and, if detected, treated with laminectomy. The decision to observe or explore a patient for postoperative bowel and bladder dysfunction is based on postoperative neuroradiographic imaging studies.

Specific nerve root syndromes are manifested as radiculopathies and should be worked up immediately with neuroimaging studies. Based on the results of these studies, either expectant observation or dorsal exploration should be undertaken. Injuries to the genitofemoral or ilioinguinal nerves may occur after an ALIF procedure.[8,22,50] These injuries are characterized postoperatively by numbness in the groin and/or the medial thigh region. They are most common in patients who undergo ALIF procedures at the upper lumbar levels. Palsies in these nerves usually resolve spontaneously and are usually treated by observation alone.

Compression of the thecal sac during the postoperative period secondary to hematoma, infection, or retropulsed disc material is best treated with dorsal exploration.[50,78] A dural tear is ordinarily detectable intraoperatively. However, it is usually not adequately treated via an ALIF approach. Placement of a lumbar subarachnoid drain to divert the spinal fluid during the first week after surgery is the usual treatment for an intraoperative dural tear that results from an ALIF procedure.[54] Injury to the sympathetic nerves on the side ipsilateral to the retroperitoneal approach may occur. Usually, partial sympathectomy occurs and is manifested by vasodilatation of blood vessels in the ipsilateral foot.[8,28,52] The usual patient complaint is a cold feeling in the contralateral foot.[22,90] Sympathectomy symptoms usually resolve spontaneously in the first 3 to 6 months following surgery. Discitis[34,84] and osteomyelitis[21,86] each occur in approximately 1% of all ALIF procedures. These infections are a result of the operative technique and may occur in a variable time frame. Their treatment involves reexploration for a confirmed abscess, using either a ventral or a dorsal approach, and wound culture and drainage of the abscess. If infection is present, in the absence of an abscess, treatment with prolonged antibiotics and immobilization can be used. Surgical exploration may also be necessary in such cases.

Bone Graft Harvest

Postoperative infections of the iliac crest donor site wound occur in 1% to 9% of all ALIF procedures[8,47,69] and are usually detected secondary to pain, which is followed by eventual purulent discharge from the wound. Iliac wound infections are best prevented by avoiding the use of foreign material in the wound (e.g., bone wax), use of prophylactic antibiotics perioperatively, copious irrigation, and meticulous intraoperative hemostasis. The use of large-bore drains in iliac wounds may prevent accumulation of a hematoma and decrease wound infection rates; however, they lead to an egress of organisms through and around the drain. When iliac crest wound infection occurs, treatment requires surgical re-exploration of the wound, cultures, and drainage.

Postoperative iliac crest wound hematomas usually are manifested as pain in the iliac crest region, which may radiate toward the groin.[75] These hematomas are best avoided by meticulous hemostasis and generous intraoperative wound irrigation. The use of a postoperative large-bore drain may diminish the incidence of postoperative hematomas. Most of these hematomas resolve spontaneously and can be managed by observation. Based on the surgeon's preference, it may be necessary to drain them if they become large or painful.

Fusion

Complications related to the bony fusion portion of the operation are the most common complications of ALIF. Persistent low back pain is the most frequent complication and is usually the result of pseudarthrosis, or nonunion, of the fusion. This complication is reported at extremely variable rates, ranging from 3% to 58%.[*] It is not possible to diagnose lumbar pseudarthrosis secondary to an ALIF procedure until 6 to 12 months after surgery.[†] The workup includes plain radiographs to detect evidence of a persistent lucent line between the graft and the vertebral body. In addition, tomograms and CT scans with sagittal re-formations may be useful for detecting this lucent line.[71] Flexion and extension lateral radiographs can detect persistent motion consistent with pseudarthrosis.[52] MRI is difficult to interpret after ALIF and is not particularly useful in revealing postoperative pseudarthrosis.

The treatment of symptomatic pseudarthrosis secondary to ALIF is prolonged immobilization of the patient, which can be accomplished with a thoracolumbosacral orthosis (TLSO) or with a body cast. It may also be helpful to consider electrical stimulation. In addition, reoperation using an anterior or posterior approach may be necessary. Rarely, a ventrodorsal combined procedure is necessary for treatment of pseudarthrosis. Several authors have stated that there is no correlation between radiographic pseudarthrosis rates and clinical outcome results.[‡] No treatment is required for asymptomatic pseudarthrosis, and the patient should be observed with serial radiographs.

Collapse of the spacer is ordinarily the result of suboptimal technique. Graft collapse occurs in 1% to 2% of all ALIF procedures,[9,32,52,92] and ordinarily results from excessive removal of subchondral bone from the vertebral body bony end plate.[47] A kyphotic deformity may develop. The treatment is surgical re-exploration via an anterior approach. Graft resorption may occur and is particularly likely in patients who are smokers,[4,44,52] diabetic, or immunosuppressed. Graft dislodgment occurs in 1% of all

---

ALIF procedures, and the treatment is reoperation using an anterior approach.[22,52,83]

After a successful ALIF procedure, the motion segments immediately adjacent to the fusion are exposed to increased stress. Months to years after a successful procedure, adjacent-level disc herniation or degeneration may occur and is particularly likely to take place at the motion segment cephalad to the ALIF.[6,8] Detection of adjacent-level disc problems is best accomplished with good long-term follow-up.

Multilevel ALIF

Complication rates increase when multiple motion segments are fused. Several investigators have noted a direct correlation between the number of levels fused and postoperative pseudarthrosis rates. With each additional level fused, the pseudarthrosis rate increases.[*] Likewise, clinical success rates decrease for each additional level fused.[25] In addition, because of the longer lever arms that result from multilevel ALIF, adjacent-segment disc problems increase after multilevel procedures. Complications related to the retroperitoneal approach also increase because of the larger surgical exposure. Furthermore, systemic medical problems secondary to the longer duration of surgery with increased blood loss are also more common in multilevel procedures. Finally, iliac donor site problems are increased when additional bone is necessary to fuse multiple levels.

New Horizons

Following the lead developed by gynecologic and general surgeons, clinicians have developed laparoscopic approaches to the lumbar spine for ALIF procedures, and they are particularly useful at the L5-S1 level.[†] In this region the iliac vessels are located lateral to the L5-S1 space, providing direct access for an ALIF procedure to be safely performed laparoscopically. Once again, it is essential to avoid using a monopolar electrocautery over the L5-S1 disc, since this may result in higher rates of retrograde ejaculation in males.[‡] The laparoscopic approach provides good visualization but makes hemostasis difficult. Likewise, maintaining orientation to the true bony midline may be more difficult laparoscopically. AP and lateral fluoroscopy are essential to the laparoscopic approach. Because of the need to mobilize the large blood vessels at levels rostral to the L5-S1 interspace (iliac artery and vein, inferior vena cava, aorta), laparoscopic methods are more dangerous at these levels.[95] There are no long-term data available on the success rates of laparoscopic ALIF.

Recently, the use of cages to function as spacers in ALIF procedures has gained popularity.[3,15,51] These cages first received FDA approval in 1996 and are available in many forms. Both threaded titanium cages and carbon fiber cages can be obtained. These cages are routinely packed with iliac crest cancellous autograft bone. In addition, threaded bone dowels from allograft femur have also been used as spacers. Current long-term follow-up data are not available; however, short-term follow-up results have been promising.

Summary

In properly selected patients, the results of ALIF in treating patients with chronic low back pain secondary to degenerative disc disease have been encouraging. ALIF offers the advantages of immediate immobilization of the motion segment, a larger fusion area than is achievable with dorsal or dorsolateral techniques, a fusion construct under compression, improved sagittal plane alignment that restores lumbar lordosis, restoration of intervertebral disc height, and an increase in the height of the neural foramina. In addition, the spinal canal is avoided, as well as many of the difficulties related to scarring that commonly occur with dorsal approaches.[8,27] ALIF is generally well tolerated and is associated with less operative blood loss compared with equivalent dorsal procedures.[30,47,75]

The end result of an ALIF procedure should be a biomechanically strong construct, compared with its dorsal counterparts. Long-term follow-up is necessary until both clinical and radiographic fusion are demonstrated. Complication rates are reasonable, and many problems can be treated intraoperatively. Complications are (1) related to the operative approach, (2) neurologic, (3) related to the iliac donor site, and (4) directly related to the fusion proper. Fusion complications are the most common. It is the adequacy of the long-term bony arthrodesis that provides long-term pain relief in patients undergoing ALIF procedures, and long-term results are promising.[*] Continued modifications, including the use of laparoscopic approaches and cages, must undergo long-term scrutiny to determine their efficacy.

REFERENCES

1. An HS, Booth RE, Rothman RH: Complications in lumbar disc disease and spinal stenosis surgery. In Balderston R, An HS (eds): *Spinal Surgery*. Philadelphia, WB Saunders, 1991, pp 61-78.
2. Baker JK, Reardon PR, Reardon MJ, Heggeness MH: Vascular injury in anterior lumbar surgery. *Spine* 18:2227-2230, 1993.
3. Brantingan JW, Steffee AD: A carbon fiber implant to aid interbody lumbar fusion: two year clinical results in the first 26 patients. *Spine* 18:2106-2117, 1993.
4. Brown CW, Orme TJ, Richardson HD: The rate of pseudoarthrosis (surgical nonunion) in patients who are smokers and patients who are nonsmokers: a comparison study. *Spine* 11:942-943, 1986.
5. Burns BH: An operation for spondylolisthesis. *Lancet* 224:1233, 1933.
6. Calandruccio RA, Benton BF: Anterior lumbar fusion. *Clin Orthop* 35:63-68, 1964.

---

*References 8,22,25,37,47,52,83.
†References 55,56,63,66,67,73,74.
‡References 11,12,25,42,75,89,90.

---

*References 8,9,19,29,50,64,70,75.

7. Calhoun E, McCall IW, Williams L: Provocation discography as a guide to planning operations of the spine. *J Bone Joint Surg Br* 70B:267-271, 1988.

8. Chow SP, Leong JCY, Ma A, Yau AC: Anterior spinal fusion for deranged lumbar intervertebral disc: a review of 97 cases. *Spine* 5:452-458, 1980.

9. Collis JS, Rojas C, Janack M: Anterior total disc replacement: a modified anterior lumbar interbody fusion. In Lin P, Gill K (eds): *Lumbar Interbody Fusion*. Rockville, MD, Aspen Publishers, 1989, pp 149-152.

10. Crock HV: Observations on the management of failed spinal operations. *J Bone Joint Surg Br* 58B:193-199, 1976.

11. Crock HV: Anterior lumbar interbody fusion: indications for its use and notes on surgical technique. *Clin Orthop* 165:157-163, 1982.

12. Crock HV: Lumbar vertebral interbody fusion. In Lin P, Gill K (eds): *Lumbar Interbody Fusion*. Rockville, MD, Aspen Publishers, 1989, pp 115-125.

13. Dennis S, Watkins RG, Landaker S, *et al*: Comparison of disc space heights after anterior lumbar interbody fusion. *Spine* 14:876-878, 1989.

14. Dodge LD, Bohlman HH, Rhodes RS: Concurrent lumbar spinal stenosis and peripheral vascular disease: a report of nine patients. *Clin Orthop* 230:141-148, 1988.

15. Enker P, Steffee AD: Interbody fusion and instrumentation. *Clin Orthop* 300:90-101, 1994.

16. Farfan HF: *Mechanical Disorders of the Low Back*. Philadelphia, Lea & Febiger, 1973.

17. Flynn JC, Hogue A: Anterior fusion of the lumbar spine: end result with long-term follow-up. *J Bone Joint Surg Am* 61A:1143-1150, 1979.

18. Flynn JC, Price CT: Sexual complications of anterior fusion of the lumbar spine. *Spine* 9:489-492, 1984.

19. Freebody D, Bendall R, Taylor RD: Anterior transperitoneal lumbar fusion. *J Bone Joint Surg Br* 53B:617-629, 1971.

20. Friberg S: Studies on spondylolisthesis. *Acta Chir Scand* 55:7-134, 1939.

21. Fujimaki A, Crock HV, Bedbrook GM: The results of 150 anterior lumbar fusion operations performed by two surgeons in Australia. *Clin Orthop* 165:164-167, 1982.

22. Gill K: Technique and complications of anterior lumbar interbody fusion. In Lin P, Gill K (eds): *Lumbar Interbody Fusion*. Rockville, MD, Aspen Publishers, 1989, pp 95-106.

23. Gill K, O'Brien JP: Observations of resorption of the posterior lateral bone graft in combined anterior and posterior lumbar fusion. *Spine* 18:1885-1889, 1993.

24. Gjessing MH: Osteoplastic anterior fusion of the lower lumbar spine. *Acta Orthop Scand* 20:200-213, 1951.

25. Goldner JL, Urbaniak JR, McCollum DE: Anterior disc excision and interbody spinal fusion for chronic low back pain. *Orthop Clin North Am* 2:543-568, 1971.

26. Greenough CG, Taylor LJ, Frazer RD: Anterior lumbar fusion: a comparison of non-compensation patients with compensation patients. *Clin Orthop* 300:30-37, 1994.

27. Hammerberg KW: Anterior lumbar interbody fusion. In Margulies JY, Floman Y, Farcy JP, Neuwirth MG (eds): *Lumbosacral and Spinopelvic Fixation*. New York, Lippincott-Raven, 1996, pp 495-505.

28. Harmon PH: Anterior disc excision and fusion of the lumbar vertebral bodies: a review of diagnostic level testing with operative results in more than seven hundred cases. *J Int Coll Surg* 40:572-586, 1963.

29. Harmon PH: Anterior excision and vertebral body fusion for intervertebral disc syndromes of the lower lumbar spine: three to five year results in 244 cases. *Clin Orthop* 26:107-127, 1963.

30. Harmon PH: Anterior lumbar disc excision and fusion: operative technique including observations upon variations in the left common iliac veins and their connections. *Clin Orthop* 18:185-198, 1960.

31. Henschen C: Operation der spondylolisthesis durch transabdominelle lumbosacrale verschraubung und zusatzliche transplantative spanversteifung. *Helv Med Acta* 9:25-28, 1942.

32. Hirabayashi K: Anterior lumbar spinal body fusion with the addition of A-O screwing and wiring. In Lin P, Gill K (eds): *Lumbar Interbody Fusion*. Rockville, MD, Aspen Publishers, 1989, pp 127-131.

33. Hodge AW, DeWald RL: Splenic injury complicating anterior thoracolumbar surgical approach for scoliosis. *J Bone Joint Surg Am* 65A:396-397, 1983.

34. Hodgson AR, Wong SK: A description of a technique and evaluation of results in anterior spinal fusion for deranged intervertebral disc and spondylolisthesis. *Clin Orthop* 56:133-162, 1968.

35. Humphries AW, Hawk WA, Berndt AL: Anterior fusion of lumbar vertebrae: a surgical technique. *Surg Clin North Am* 41:1685-1700, 1961.

36. Ingerbrigtsen R: Indications for anterior transperitoneal fusion in the treatment of spondylolisthesis. *Acta Chir Scand* 105:172-181, 1953.

37. Inoue SJ, Watanabe T, Hirose A, *et al*: Anterior discectomy and interbody fusion for lumbar disc herniation: a review of 350 cases. *Clin Orthop* 183:22-31, 1984.

38. Ito H, Tsuchiya J, Asami G: A new radical operation for Pott's disease. *J Bone Joint Surg* 16B:499-515, 1934.

39. Iwahara T: A new method of vertebral body fusion. *Surgery* (Japan) 8:271, 1944.

40. Iwahara T, Ikeda K, Hirabayashi K: Results of anterior spine fusion by extraperitoneal approach for spondylosis and spondylolisthesis. *J Jpn Orthop Assoc* 36:1049-1067, 1963.

41. Jenkins JA: Spondylolisthesis. *Br J Surg* 24:80-85, 1936.

42. Johnson RM, McGuire EJ: Urogenital complications of anterior approaches to the lumbar spine. *Clin Orthop* 154:114-118, 1981.

43. Jones AA, Dougherty PJ, Sharkey NA, Benson DR: Iliac crest bone graft: osteotome versus saw. *Spine* 18:2048-2052, 1993.

44. Knox BD, Chapman TM: Anterior lumbar interbody fusion for discogram concordant pain. *J Spine Disord* 6:242-244, 1993.

45. Kostuik JP: Anterior spinal cord decompression for lesions of the thoracic and lumbar spine: techniques, new methods of internal fixation, results. *Spine* 8:512-531, 1983.

46. Kostuik JP: Anterior fixation for burst fractures of the thoracic and lumbar spine with or without neurologic involvement. *Spine* 13:286-293, 1988.

47. Kozak JA, O'Brien JP: Simultaneous combined anterior and posterior fusion: an independent analysis of a

treatment for the disabled low-back pain patient. *Spine* 15:322-328, 1990.

48. Kozak JA, Heilman AE, O'Brien JP: Anterior lumbar fusion options. *Clin Orthop* 300:45-51, 1994.

49. Lane JD, Moore ES: Transperitoneal approach to intervertebral disc in lumbar area. *Ann Surg* 127:537-551, 1948.

50. Leong JCY: Anterior interbody fusion. In Lin P, Gill K (eds): *Lumbar Interbody Fusion*. Rockville, MD, Aspen Publishers, 1989, pp 133-148.

51. Leong JCY, Chow MS, Yan ACH: Titanium-mesh block replacement of the intervertebral disc. *Clin Orthop* 300: 52-63, 1994.

52. Loguidice VA, Johnson RG, Guyer RD, *et al*: Anterior interbody fusion. *Spine* 13:366-369, 1988.

53. Long DM, Filtzer DL, BenDebba M, Hendler NH: Clinical features of the failed-back syndrome. *J Neurosurg* 69:61-71, 1988.

54. Marshall LF: Cerebrospinal fluid leaks: etiology and repair. In Rothman RS, Simeone FA (eds): *The Spine*. Philadelphia, WB Saunders, 1992, pp 1892-1898.

55. Mathews HH, Evans MT, Kyles MK: Laparoscopic discectomy with fusion. Proceedings of the Ninth Annual Meeting of the North American Spine Society, Minneapolis, October 1991, p 63.

56. McAfee PC: Laparoscopic fusion and BAK stabilization of the lumbar spine. In Regan JJ, McAfee PC, Mack MJ (eds): *Atlas of Endoscopic Spine Surgery*. St. Louis, Quality Medical Publishing, 1995, pp 306-320.

57. McMaster WC, Silber J: A urological complication of Dwyer instrumentation. *J Bone Joint Surg Am* 57A: 710-711, 1975.

58. Mercer W: Spondylolisthesis with a description of a new method of operative treatment and notes of ten cases. *Edinburgh Med J* 43:545-572, 1936.

59. Merle d'Aubigne R, Cauchoix J, Faulong M: L'arthrodese par voie anterieure transperitoneale dans la cure du spondylolisthesis. *Rev Orthop* 36:490-494, 1950.

60. Morris JM: Low back bracing. *Clin Orthop* 103:120-132, 1974.

61. Muller W: Transperitoneale freilegung der wirbelsaule bei tuberkuloser spondylitis. *Dtsch Z Chir* 85:128, 1906.

62. Nisbet NW, James A: Results of intervertebral bony fusion. *J Bone Joint Surg Br* 38B:952-953, 1956.

63. Novotney SR, Guyer RD, Regan JJ: Laparoscopic assisted anterior lumbar interbody fusion. Proceedings of the Ninth Annual Meeting of the North American Spine Society. Minneapolis, October 1991, pp 61-62.

64. O'Brien JP, Dawson MHO, Heard CW, *et al*: Simultaneous combined anterior and posterior fusion: a surgical solution for failed spinal surgery with a brief review of the first 150 patients. *Clin Orthop* 203:191-195, 1986.

65. Obenchain TG: Laparoscopic lumbar discectomy: case report. *J Laparoendosc Surg* 1:145-149, 1991.

66. Obenchain TG, Cloyd D: Outpatient lumbar discectomy: description of technique and review of first twenty-one cases. *Surg Tech Int* 2:415-418, 1994.

67. Obenchain TG, Cloyd DW: Laparoscopic lumbar retroperitoneal and transperitoneal discectomy. In Regan JJ, McAfee PC, Mack MJ (eds): *Atlas of Endoscopic Spine*

Surgery. St. Louis, Quality Medical Publishing, 1995, pp 243-254.

68. Ramser R: Transabdominelle operation der nichttraumatischen spondylolisthesis. *Helv Med Acta* 10:365-375, 1942.

69. Raney FL, Adams JE: Anterior lumbar disc excision and interbody fusion used as a salvage procedure. *J Bone Joint Surg Am* 45A:667-668, 1963.

70. Raugstad TS, Harbo K, Skeie S: Anterior interbody fusion of the lumbar spine. *Acta Orthop Scand* 53:561-565, 1982.

71. Rothman SLG, Glenn WV Jr: CT evaluation of interbody fusion. *Clin Orthop* 193:47-56, 1985.

72. Saal JA, Saal SS: Physical rehabilitation of lower back pain. In Frymoyer JW (ed): *The Adult Spine*. New York, Lippincott-Raven, 1997, pp 1805-1819.

73. Sacks BL, Scwaitzberg SD: Laparoscopic lumbosacral discectomy and interbody fusion technique: early clinical experience. Proceedings of the Ninth Annual Meeting of the North American Spine Society, Minneapolis, October 1991, p 67.

74. Sacks BL, Scwaitzberg SD: Lumbosacral (L5-S1) discectomy and interbody fusion technique. In Regan JJ, McAfee PC, Mack MJ (eds): *Atlas of Endoscopic Spine Surgery*. St. Louis, Quality Medical Publishing, 1995, pp 275-292.

75. Sacks S: Anterior interbody fusion of the lumbar spine. *J Bone Joint Surg Br* 47B:211-223, 1965.

76. Sacks S: Anterior interbody fusion of the lumbar spine: indications and results in 200 cases. *Clin Orthop* 44: 163-170, 1966.

77. Schneiderman G, Flannigan B, Kingston S, *et al*: Magnetic resonance imaging in the diagnosis of disc degeneration: correlation with discography. *Spine* 12: 276-281, 1987.

78. Sicard A: Remarks in discussion. *Mem Acad Chir* 78:216, 1952.

79. Sijbrandij S: The value of anterior interbody vertebral fusion in the treatment of lumbosacral insufficiency with special reference to spondylolisthesis. *Arch Chir Neerl* 14:37, 1962.

80. Sorenson KH: Anterior interbody spine fusion for incapacitating disc degeneration and spondylolisthesis. *Acta Orthop Scand* 49:269-277, 1978.

81. Southwick WO, Robinson RA: Surgical approaches to the vertebral bodies in the cervical and lumbar regions. *J Bone Joint Surg Am* 39A:631-644, 1957.

82. Speed K: Spondylolisthesis: treatment by anterior bone graft. *Arch Surg* 37:175-189, 1938.

83. Stauffer RN, Coventry MB: Anterior interbody lumbar spine fusion. *J Bone Joint Surg Am* 54A:756-768, 1972.

84. Stein SC: Laparoscopic lumbar discectomy. Proceedings of the Ninth Annual Meeting of the North American Spine Society, Minneapolis, October 1991, p 61.

85. Storen H: Remarks in discussion of spondylolisthesis. *Nord Med* 44:1802, 1950.

86. Stray K: Remarks in discussion of spondylitis. *Nord Med* 44:1802, 1950.

87. Taylor TKE: Anterior interbody fusion in the management of disorders of the lumbar spine. *J Bone Joint Surg Br* 52B:784, 1970.

88. Vincent E: Contribution a la chirurgie rachidienne du drainage vertebrale dans la mal du Pott. *Rev Chir Orthop* 12:273, 1892.

89. Watkins RG: Assessment of results and complications of anterior lumbar fusion. In Lin P, Gill K (eds): *Lumbar Interbody Fusion*. Rockville, MD, Aspen Publishers, 1989, pp 153-169.

90. Watkins RG: Anterior approaches to the lumbar spine. In Torrens MJ, Dickson RA (eds): *Operative Spinal Surgery*. New York, Churchill Livingstone, 1991, pp 161-171.

91. Watkins RG: Anterior lumbar interbody fusion—surgical complications. *Clin Orthop* 284:47-53, 1992.

92. Whitecloud TS, Butler JL: Anterior lumbar fusion utilizing transvertebral fibular graft. *Spine* 13:370-373, 1988.

93. Willner S: Effect of a rigid brace on back pain. *Acta Orthop Scand* 56:40-42, 1985.

94. Zaaijer JH: Transabdominale behandlung van spondylolisthesis. *Neder T Gen* 96:518-520, 1952.

95. Zuckerman JF, Hsu K, Implacito D: Instrumented transperitoneal laparoscopic fusion. In Margulies JY, Floman Y, Farcy JP, Neuwirth MG (eds): *Lumbosacral and Spinopelvic Fixation*. New York, Lippincott-Raven, 1996, pp 579-585.

CHAPTER 41

Lumbar Interbody Cages

**Branko Prpa, Melvin D. Whitfield,
and Isador H. Lieberman**

Interbody fusion procedures are increasingly used in the treatment of a variety of disorders. It is estimated that every month in the United States alone, more than 5000 interbody fusion procedures are performed.[46] The majority of interbody fusion procedures are completed at the L4-5 or L5-S1 vertebral segments. The current interest in performing lumbar arthrodesis with cages is attributable to three factors: (1) the high rate of pseudarthrosis associated with use of interbody bone graft alone[3,15,16]; (2) the risk associated with use of dorsal pedicle-screw instrumentation[29,59]; (3) and the initial success associated with use of stand-alone interbody fusion cages and autogenous bone graft, thus obviating the need to perform a 360-degree lumbar arthrodesis with dorsal instrumentation.[12]

Background

Early techniques of lumbar arthrodesis with use of autograft and allograft were associated with a high failure rate. Stauffer and Coventry[58] reported on 83 patients who had an anterior interbody arthrodesis between 1959 and 1967. Of 77 patients who were followed for an average of 3.75 years after the procedure, 28 (36%) had good (76% to 100%) relief, 15 (19%) had fair (26% to 75%) relief, and 34 (44%) had poor (0% to 25%) relief. Thirty (44%) of 68 patients who were evaluated radiographically at a minimum of 18 months postoperatively had a pseudarthrosis. They defined radiographic fusion as a "pattern of continuous trabeculae traversing the grafted region and the adjacent vertebral bodies, with no evidence of motion when the patient was bending." These results, and the equally unfavorable results reported by other investigators,[15,16,24] prompted investigation into alternative devices to improve the long-term outcome of spinal arthrodesis.

History

Bagby[3] was the first to work on the early development of the lumbar interbody fusion cage. Working with Grant (a veterinarian) and a series of thoroughbred horses that had wobbler syndrome (a form of spondylotic myelopathy that leads to ataxia), he found that the Cloward technique,[15] which requires obtaining bone from the iliac crest, resulted in unacceptable morbidity. Bagby then proceeded to develop the first interbody stainless-steel basket, the Bagby basket, which was 30mm long and 25mm in diameter, and had 2mm fenestrations in its walls to allow ingrowth. Subsequent studies demonstrated that the horses treated with the Bagby basket had improved neu-

rologic outcomes; some not only survived for years but several also won races. Several other investigators began making modifications on his technique, including adding external threads to the basket,[50,66] adaptation of the cage for use in dorsal interbody fusion, and improving in the inherent compressive strength.[50] DeBowes et al.,[19] in another study of horses, compared the results of arthrodesis using bovine xenograft with those of arthrodesis with the use of autogenous graft inside a Bagby basket; they found that the rate of fusion was better when the Bagby basket had been used and that the device did not collapse. After the arthrodesis, the gross appearance of the bovine xenograft was pale, and seven of eight sites that were examined demonstrated fibrous tissue. The autogenous graft and the Bagby basket contained little or no fibrous tissue.

Types of Fusion Cages

A number of cages are currently available, each with its own indications, advantages, and disadvantages. This chapter focuses on five devices: (1) the Bagby-and-Kuslich device[39] (BAK; Sulzer Spine-Tech, Minneapolis) (Figure 41.1); (2) the threaded interbody fusion device, or Inter Fix (TIBFD; Medtronic Sofamor-Danek Group, Memphis) (Figure 41.2); (3) the Ray cage (U.S. Surgical, Norwalk, Conn.) (Figure 41.3); (4) the Harms titanium-mesh cage (DePuy-Acromed, Raynham, Mass.); and (5) the Brantigan rectangular and rounded cages (DePuy-Acromed) (Figure 41.4).

Mechanical and Physiologic Roles of Fusion Cages

Kanayama et al.[35] performed mechanical tests to assess different types of fusion cages in 60 calf-spine units, each consisting of one vertebral disc space and the adjacent vertebrae. There were six specimens in each group. The devices tested included two BAK cages, two BAK proximity cages, two Ray cages, two TIBFDs, one Harms cage, two Harms vertical cages, two Brantigan cages, one femoral ring allograft, and two bone dowel allografts. Intracage pressures were then tested with a pressure needle transducer throughout various loading conditions after silicone elastomer gel had been injected. No significant differences were detected among the 10 cage constructs with regard to construct stiffness ($p > .05$).

Chen et al.,[13] in a study of nine fresh-frozen lumbar spines with foraminal stenosis, constructed silicone molds of the neuroforamina. After the application of cages, the neuroforaminal volume increased by 23% at the fourth and fifth lumbar levels and by 22% at the fifth lumbar and first sacral level. The dorsal disc height increased by 37% at the fourth and fifth lumbar level and by 45% at the fifth lumbar and first sacral level ($p < .001$).

Several authors have demonstrated that interbody cages do not augment segmental biomechanic stability.[17,21,27,43,63] Lund et al.[43] performed a biomechanic study on human cadaver spines to determine the effect of three different cage designs, with and without dorsal instrumentation, on the three-dimensional flexibility of the spine. They studied the Brantigan cage, the Ray cage, and the porous titanium

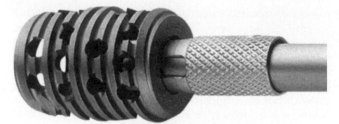

Figure 41.1 BAK cage.

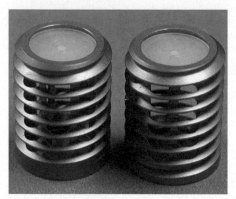

Figure 41.2 Threaded Interbody Fusion Device.

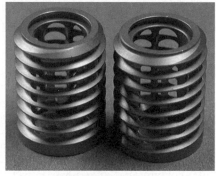

Figure 41.3 Ray cage.

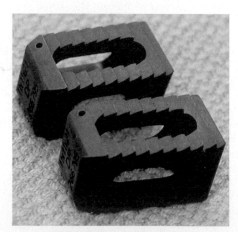

Figure 41.4 Brantigan cage.

cage (Stratec). Six lumbar functional spinal segments for each cage were subjected to multidirectional flexibility testing. No significant difference in the stabilizing potential of the three cage designs was found. The cages used alone significantly decreased the intervertebral movement in flexion and lateral bending, but no stabilization was achieved in *extension* or axial rotation. For all types of cages, the greatest stabilization in flexion and extension and lateral bending was achieved by the addition of dorsal instrumentation.

Sagittal balance is very important in the overall stability of spinal constructs.[28,36,48] Klemme[36] compared the alterations in lumbar sagittal balance after dorsal lumbar fusion using threaded interbody devices alone versus vertical cages combined with dorsal instrumentation. The radiographs of 30 patients were compared. Results demonstrated that threaded fusion devices placed under distraction with the end plates parallel failed to preserve or reestablish segmental lordosis. Cages, when combined with dorsal instrumentation, maintained both segmental lordosis and correct sagittal plane deformity.

Goals of Lumbar Fusion

The primary goal of lumbar surgery in the degenerative setting is the relief of the patient's pain with improvement in overall functional status. It has long been thought that this would be best achieved by correction of existing mechanical deformation to its anatomic baseline and by minimizing abnormal pain-producing motions. In theory lumbar interbody fusion has been the preferred surgical technique to achieve these goals.

As a result, interbody cages have been developed with the aim of overcoming these problems. They strive to:

1. Correct the existing mechanical deformation.
2. Provide stability to the segment until arthrodesis is obtained.
3. Provide the best possible environment for successful arthrodesis.
4. Achieve fusion with limited morbidity associated with their use.
5. Serve as a delivery mechanism for osteogenic, osteoinductive, and/or osteoconductive material (i.e., osteoprogenitor cells, bone morphogenic proteins [BMPs]).

Correction of Existing Mechanical Deformation

An interbody cage should restore disc height, restore annular fibers to "normal" tension, recreate lordosis through the lumbar segment, reduce subluxed facet joints, enlarge the neuroforaminal space, and restore to normal the proportion of weight bearing through the anterior column. To date there are no controlled studies that demonstrate symptom relief with correction of mechanical deformation with interbody cages.

Provision of Mechanical Stability

An interbody cage device should provide immediate stiffness to the segment, be able to withstand applied vertical loads, and provide adequate resistance to translational and rotational forces in all directions. Threaded cages often provide significant fixation of the lumbar motion segment to promote interbody fusion without supplemental dorsal stabilization in all degrees of freedom except extension. How much extension stability is needed still has to be investigated.

Provision of Optimal Environment for Arthrodesis

An optimal environment for interbody fusion consists of six criteria: (1) complete discectomy so that no soft tissue obstructs the fusion beds; (2) complete excision of the cartilaginous end plate to bleeding compacted cancellous bone; (3) preservation of the bony end-plate to maintain structural integrity and prevent subsidence; (4) use of smallest cage volume (as cage volume increases, graft volume decreases[46]); (5) optimal amounts of graft—preferably autogenous—with the widest possible interface with the fusion beds; and (6) maintenance of compression across anterior load-bearing portion of vertebral body.

Limit Morbidity

An ideal cage provides all of the preceding surgical goals while not adding any subsequent morbidities. Cage insertion should also minimize operative time and blood loss. Surgeon preference, reproducibility, and ease of insertion also play largely into its application.

Delivery Mechanisms for Osteogenic and/or Osteoinductive Materials

The use of a cage as a delivery and/or containment device is of theoretic advantage. This is discussed in detail in the last section of this chapter.

Selection of Patients for Arthrodesis

Ray[53] selected patients for insertion of a lumbar interbody fusion cage with the use of six criteria: (1) severe, disabling, intractable pain; (2) degenerated disc spaces with resultant pain; (3) an absence of disc space or systemic infection; (4) no previous interbody arthrodesis at the target levels; (5) an absence of degeneration at adjacent disc spaces, whether or not they were painful; and (6) no Meyerding grade-I spondylolisthesis. The disabling pain had to have been present for 1 year and refractory to nonoperative care. Patients who had a disc height of more than 12mm were also excluded.

Over the past several years, cages have been used for patients who have general disc pain or disc spaces that appear desiccated on magnetic resonance imaging (MRI) studies (so-called *black disc disease*). In general a more conservative approach is preferred. Cages should be limited to selected patients who have postlaminectomy syndrome or disc-space collapse with foraminal narrowing. Cages should not be the first line of treatment for patients who simply have black disc disease or who have a positive discogram. Patients should have at least a 3- to 6-month trial of nonoperative treatment before arthrodesis is considered. Cages should not be used for those with involve-

ment of more than two levels. If associated instability is present at more than two levels, then posterior augmentation with a pedicle screw construct should be planned. (Figure 41.5).

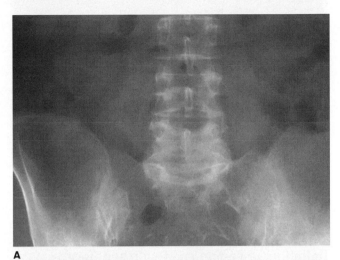

A

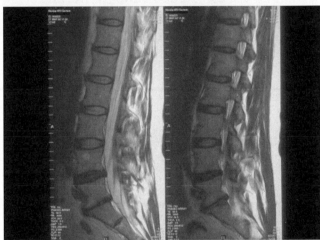

B

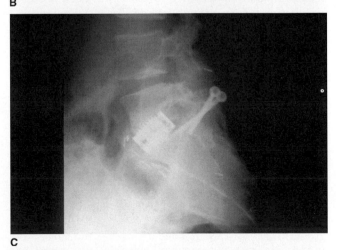

C

Figure 41.5 A 42-year-old female with 1-year history of severe low back pain that has failed multiple attempts at nonoperative treatment. **(A)** Anteroposterior lumbar spine. **(B)** T_2-weighted sagittal MRI demonstrating loss of L5-S1 disc space height. **(C)** and **(D)** Anteroposterior/lateral after laparoscopic anterior cage placement followed by translaminar facet screw fixation.

Continued

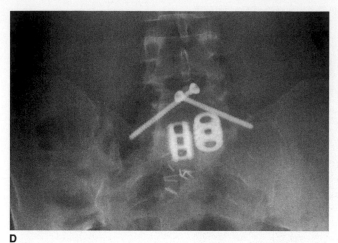

D

Figure 41.5 *cont'd*

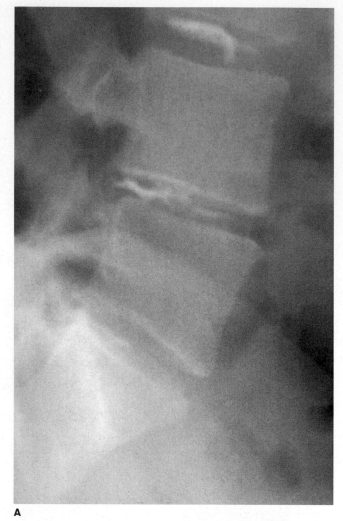

A

Figure 41.6 A 41-year-old male with progressive deterioration of L4-5, L5-S1. **(A)** Discogram with extravasation at L4-5 and concordant pain.

Definition of Fusion and Published Results

By virtue of the fact that there is no single definition of fusion in the literature, it is difficult to compare the results of different studies. The rates of fusion are approximately 20% higher when the sole criterion is loss of motion rather than continuous trabeculae across the graft and vertebral interfaces.[4,12,60] The criteria for successful fusion in patients managed with a cage are often different from those used in previous reports. Kumar et al.[38] looked at 32 patients and found that 21 (66%) had radiographic union and stability on flexion and extension. Four (13%) had nonunion and instability. For the remaining seven patients (22%) the results were ambiguous. They coined the term "functional arthrodesis," which indicates less than 2 degrees of motion on flexion and extension radiographs with bridging bone either anterior or posterior, although the fusion was less than complete.

Stauffer and Coventry[58] defined fusion as bridging and no motion. Many authors have thought that more than 5 degrees of motion as seen on lateral flexion and extension radiographs indicates a failure of fusion.[9,11] Yet others have defined fusion with use of stricter criteria (2 to 3 degrees of motion).[25,42] Hacker[30] states that nonunion is present when radiolucent areas that are wider than 2mm and that extend along at least 50% of bone adjacent to the implant are indicative of failure.

Attempting to decide whether a fusion is present on flexion and extension radiographs is difficult for many reasons. The difference in asymptomatic individuals can range anywhere from 7 to 14 degrees.[11] Second, measurement in patients with pedicle screw constructs may be unreliable because motion may be restricted in a pseudarthrosis, thus giving a false-positive finding of fusion. And finally, the radiographs may not accurately demonstrate a patient's range of motion secondary to pain and splinting.

In a prospective, multicenter clinical trial, Yuan et al.[66] used the following definition of fusion to study the BAK cage. The fusion was considered solid if there were no dramatically obvious radiolucencies and there was less than 5 degrees of vertebral motion in the sagittal plane, as assessed with digitization methods. An independent radiologist evaluated all radiographs that demonstrated between 3 and 7 degrees of sagittal motion. Patients with a two-level procedure were considered fused if both levels exhibited no motion (Figure 41.6).

Ray[12] defined fusion according to six criteria: (1) lack of dark halo around implant; (2) lack of any visible motion, or less than 3 degrees of intersegmental change, as seen on flexion and extension radiographs; (3) minimum loss of disc-space height, indicating a resistance to collapse of the cancellous vertebral bone; (4) lack of substantial sclerotic changes in the recipient bone bed; (5) lack of visible fracture of the device, graft, or vertebrae; and (6) visible bone within the hollow Ray titanium cage, as seen on multiple radiographic views. If the radiologist determined that the vertebral bodies were fused but the surgeon thought they were not, fusion was considered not to have occurred.

Diedrich et al.[20] looked at 64 patients who had a PLIF performed with cages. Conventional radiographs were obtained at 6 weeks, 3 and 6 months, and then yearly. Radiographic evaluation was performed using the fusion

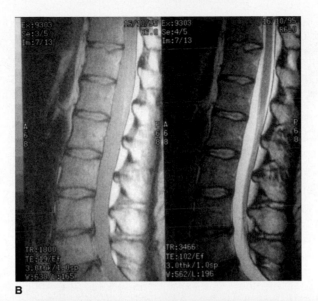

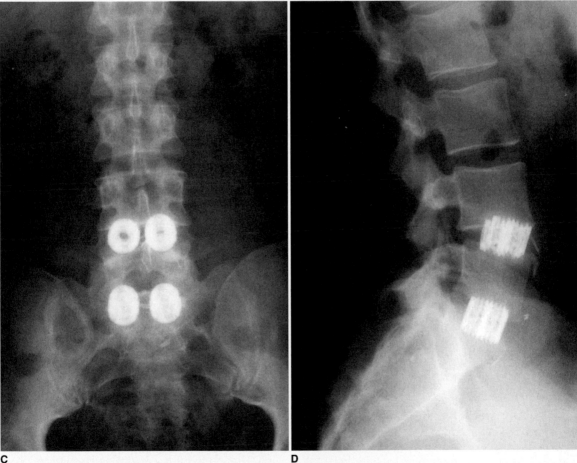

Figure 41.6 *cont'd* **(B)** An MRI demonstrating L4-5 and L5-1 disc space narrowing.
(C) Anteroposterior radiograph following cage placement. **(D)** Lateral postoperative radiograph.

criteria described by Brantigan and Steffee.[11] A fusion rate of 51.5% after 12 months, 61.4% after 24 months, 66.7% after 36, and 77.8% after 48 months postoperatively was found. There was evidence that radiographic fusion criteria occurred in a specific chronological order.

Fusion rates are also affected by technical aspects. McAfee *et al.*[45] in 1994 evaluated the role of a complete discectomy versus a partial discectomy in fusion rates. One hundred consecutive patients were involved and divided equally into two groups. At 2 or more years of follow-up, all patients who had a complete discectomy achieved solid fusion. There were no revisions. In the partial discectomy group, seven patients had pseudarthrosis and eight required revision. An overall pseudarthrosis rate of 14% was present in the partial discectomy group.

Biologic Cages

O'Brien[33] described a biologic fusion cage consisting of a femoral cortical allograft ring packed with autogenous cancellous bone graft. Thirty-two patients had posterior instrumentation and eight did not. The reported fusion rate was 70 (96%) of 73 levels. The average interbody disc height returned to preoperative levels at an average of 1.4 years (range, 1 to 2.4 years).

Kozak et al.[37] looked at 45 patients in whom two 6.5mm cancellous bone screws with washers were used to prevent anterior femoral allograft dislodgement. Twenty-one patients were treated for disc-disruption syndrome, 12 patients for postlaminectomy syndrome, and 11 patients for failed posterolateral fusion and pseudarthrosis. Thirty-eight patients (84%) had no motion as seen on flexion and extension radiographs 2 years postoperatively. Six (13%) had a radiolucent line on one or both sides of the femoral allograft; however, fusion was suggested by bridging the bone either anteriorly or posteriorly to the allograft. Overall fusion rate was 97% (44 of 45 patients).

Clinical Series Results
BAK Cage

Yuan et al.,[66] Kuslich et al.,[39] and Alpert[2] reported on 947 patients in a prospective, multicenter trial of the BAK device. A total of 591 patients had a ventral approach (62%), and 356 patients (38%) had a dorsal approach. Spondylolisthesis was observed in 114 patients (12%). The average duration of symptoms was 5.5 years before operation; 767 patients (81%) had the symptoms for more than 1 year. Two hundred and forty-six patients (26%) were smokers, and 341 (36%) had a previous spinal procedure.

Functional outcome was evaluated with the use of a numeric scale, according to seven parameters: the ability to walk, sit, stand, squat, put on socks and shoes, the level of recreational activity; and the level of work. The best possible score (lowest) was 7 points, and the worst was 32 points. The average functional score was 20.9 preoperatively, 15.2 points at 12 months, and 14.4 points at 24 months.

Yuan et al.[66] also followed the patients with their ability to return to work. A total of 843 patients were considered to be ineligible for work or had been receiving disability compensation before the operation. Five hundred and seventy-three (68%) of these patients returned to work at 12 months, and 658 (78%) returned at 24 months. Fusion rate was determined to be 91% in 283 patients (defined as absence of radiolucencies and less than 5 degrees of vertebral motion).

Ray Titanium Cage

The study[54] consisted of 211 patients who were followed for 24 months postoperatively. The indications for the procedure were severe disabling pain in 203 patients (96%);

annular degeneration in 156 patients (74%); disc herniation in 120 patients (57%); a decrease in the disc space height of more than 10% (91 patients, 43%); and formation of osteophytes (44 patients, 21%). Previous operations were performed in 95 patients (45%). At follow-up, 203 patients (96%) had radiographic evidence of fusion, defined as absence of motion on flexion and extension radiographs with use of radiographic overlay technique,[31] absence of dark halo, and continued presence of visible bone within cage, as seen on Ferguson view. The clinical outcome according to the Prolo et al.[52] scale was excellent for 48 patients (40%), good for 53 (25%), fair for 44 (21%), and poor for 30 (14%).

Brantigan Cage

Excellent fusion rates (>90%)[1,8,10,14] have been reported with the insertion of Brantigan cages. Brantigan cages filled with autogenous bone, in combination with pedicle screw instrumentation, were compared to those of a control group that had been managed with ethylene-oxide–sterilized allograft bone blocks and pedicle screw fixation.[10] Clinical success was derived from the scale of Prolo et al.[52] The scores for pain, function, work status, and use of medication were combined. Scores ranging from 4 to 20 were possible. A score of 17 to 20 indicated an excellent result; 13 to 16, a good result; 9 to 12, a fair result; and 4 to 8, a poor result. A clinical success was defined as a 2-year rating of excellent or good. A successful fusion was achieved in 262 (97%) of 271 patients who had been treated with the Brantigan cage compared with 59 (79%) of 75 who had been managed with an allograft. A successful clinical result was achieved in 248 (87%) of 285 patients who had been managed with Brantigan cage and 65 (80%) of 81 who had been managed with an allograft.

Brantigan et al.[8] examined the efficacy of the carbon cage with pedicle screw fixation. The clinical study consisted of 221 patients at six centers. Fusion success was achieved in 176 (98.9%) of 178 patients. In the management of degenerative disc disease in patients with prior failed discectomy surgery, clinical success was achieved in 79 (86%) of 92 patients, and radiographic arthrodesis in 91 (100%) of 91 patients. Fusion success was not diminished over multiple levels.

Harms Cage

The vertical upright titanium-mesh cage was developed by Harms et al. in 1991.[31] The Harms cage differs from horizontal cages because it needs to be cut for appropriate sizing. The device was created as an anterior load-sharing support for defects created after a ventral corpectomy for treatment of fractures and tumors. Harms used an anterior interbody approach, combined with a posterior approach, in 21 patients with a grade I or II spondylolisthesis. In the 83 patients who had a higher-grade slip (grade III or IV), Harms et al. performed a posterior lumbar interbody arthrodesis and insertion of cage packed with autogenous bone chips. The edges of the cage are designed to dig into the vertebral end plates and prevent dislodgement. To date there have been no widespread multicenter studies.

Eck *et al.*,[22] in a study of 66 consecutive patients (ages 20 to 81), examined the outcomes of titanium mesh cages implanted into the ventral column. Average follow-up was 2 years (range 24 to 62 months). No cage failure or extrusion was observed. Seventy-eight percent of the cages were judged to be fused by observers examining plain radiographs. The outcome at follow-up for patients with suspected pseudarthrosis was similar to the group of patients with fusions rated as solid.

Complications of ALIF

Penta *et al.*[51] studied 52 patients, using MRI 10 years after an anterior lumbar interbody fusion (ALIF) that had not included the insertion of a fusion cage to determine if the arthrodesis increased the rate of adjacent level disc disease. They found normal adjacent discs associated with a solid fusion to the sacrum in 67% (35) of the patients and concluded that the procedure does not cause adjacent level disc disease. Wetzel studied 12 patients who had failure of a previous posterior lumbar interbody fusion (PLIF). All 12 patients had chronic radiculopathy caused by extensive perineural fibrosis as a result of epidural manipulation that was required during the procedure. Adjacent unfused segments became symptomatic in four cases, which suggested a mechanical problem inherent in the procedure.

Glassman[26] reported complications were more likely to occur when the cage was inserted through an anterior approach. Titanium cages (trapezoidal) inserted through a dorsal approach retropulsed into the spinal canal, causing neurologic involvement. Subsequently, these patients underwent cage removal and placement of a femoral ring packed with autogenous cancellous bone graft.

Ray and BAK Device

There have been no reported cases of fracture of titanium cages, whereas a fairly substantial rate of pedicle screw breakage (range, 0.9% to 27%) has been reported.[40,41] Kuslich *et al.*[39] reported the reoperation rate for patients who had a fusion cage to be 4% (42 of 947), and reoperation was most common in the first 100 days because of migration of the cage. Dural tears have a reported prevalence of 10.1% in 356 patients, and exclusively occur during the posterior approach.[66] Retrograde ejaculation (1.9%), major vessel damage (1.7%), urologic complications (1.4%), and postoperative ileus (2.2%) have been associated with the anterior retroperitoneal approach (in 591 patients).[66]

Elias *et al.*[23] examined the complication rate in 67 patients who underwent interbody fusion with a threaded interbody cage. A total of 15% (10) were complicated by a dural tear. In three cases bilateral cages could not be placed. Twenty-eight patients (42%) experienced significant low-back pain at 3 months, and in 10 (15%) of these cases it persisted beyond 1 year. In 10 patients postoperative radiculopathy was demonstrated. One patient incurred a permanent motor deficit with sexual dysfunction. Pseudarthrosis was suggested with evidence of motion on flexion and extension films (10 cases), lucencies around the implants (7 cases), and dorsal migration of the cage (2 cases) Fourteen patients required additional surgery for signs of spinal instability.

Brantigan Cage

Most complications in the Investigational Device Exemption study were not caused by the cage but rather to the pedicle screw system.[11] Seventy-eight (36%) of 219 patients had removal of pedicle screws, 30 (14%) had device-related complications, and 18 (8%) had a revision operation.

Anterior Open and Anterior Laparoscopic Cage Insertion

Regan *et al.*[55,56] looked at 250 consecutive patients who had a laparoscopic arthrodesis at the fourth and fifth lumbar and first sacral vertebrae with insertion of a BAK cage. The control group consisted of 591 patients who had an open anterior arthrodesis with insertion of a BAK device by 42 surgeons at 19 medical centers. Forty percent of patients had a previous laminectomy. The patients who had a laparoscopic procedure at the fourth and fifth lumbar levels had a significantly longer operative time ($p < .001$), but significantly less blood loss ($p = .023$) and a significantly shorter hospital stay ($p = .003$). Six instances of iatrogenic disc herniation as a result of lateral placement of taps, reamers, and cages were noted, leading to nerve root compression in the laparoscopic group. Regan stated that the learning curve was steep and became as safe and effective as the open procedure after the first five to ten procedures[55,56] (Figure 41.7).

McAfee[44] reported one instance of emergent conversion from a laparoscopic to open procedure for a laceration of left common iliac vein (in 100 patients). Other studies[45,47] indicate that the most important operative devices in a laparoscopy are the retractors and vascular clamps needed to convert the procedure to a standard open laparotomy. In an effort to avoid vascular complications, some authors[49,55] recommend performing the operation in the lateral decubitus position and that the cage be inserted in a transverse direction. This approach can be used from the first to the fifth lumbar levels, but should be avoided at the first sacral level. McAfee *et al.*[49] performed arthrodesis at the first through fifth lumbar levels with the use of a minimally invasive anterior retroperitoneal approach and insertion of a BAK device in a transverse direction. The average hospital stay was 2.9 days. No patient had migration or pseudarthrosis at 24.3 months (range 12 to 40 months) postoperatively. With this technique of lateral insertion, mobilization of the vessels is usually not necessary. Dorsal instrumentation was not used.

Fusion Cages and Osteoinductive Materials

Cunningham *et al.*[18] performed an endoscopic study in the thoracic spine in sheep to compare the use of a BAK cage filled with osteogenic protein-1 with a BAK cage filled with autogenous iliac-crest bone graft. Solid fusion was defined as bridging of the trabecular network from end plate to end plate, as seen in the cage on midsagittal microradiographs. The authors evaluated the biomechanic, computed tomography (CT), microradiography, and quantitative histomorphometric measurements.

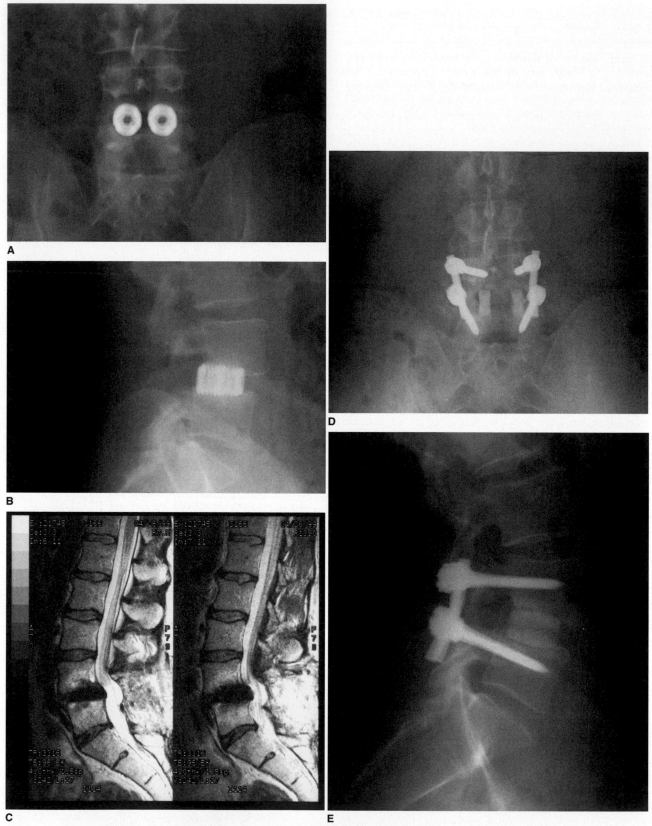

Figure 41.7 A 45-year-old man 2 years status post previous anterior cage insertion presents with worsening back pain and bilateral lower extremity paresthesias that have failed nonoperative intervention. (**A**) Preoperative anteroposterior radiograph (status post L4-5 cage insertion). (**B**) Preoperative lateral radiograph. (**C**) Sagittal MRI with thecal sac displacement. (**D**) Anteroposterior radiograph following cage removal and femoral allograft insertion with pedicle screw fixation. (**E**) Lateral postoperative radiograph.

Multilevel thoracic decompression was performed in 12 sheep through a thoracoscopic approach. Three non-contiguous sites (the fifth and sixth, seventh and eighth, and ninth and tenth thoracic vertebral levels) were randomly treated with one of five protocols. Group 1 (six specimens) was treated with destabilization only; Group 2, with an empty BAK cage; Group 3, autogenous graft only; Group 4, BAK device with autogenous graft; Group 5, BAK device with osteogenic protein-1. Four months after the operation, groups 3, 4, and 5 had significantly higher levels of segmental stiffness ($p < .05$) than did the control groups as demonstrated with three of the five testing modalities. Significantly more trabecular bone was present in the treatment groups ($p < .05$). The authors concluded that the arthrodesis with use of osteogenic protein-1 was biomechanically and histomorphometrically equivalent to that of arthrodesis with use of autogenous iliac-crest graft.

Boden[6] described his findings in five adult rhesus monkeys that had laparoscopic exposure of the lumbrosacral spine, followed by insertion of a hollow titanium cylindrical cage filled with bone morphogenic protein-2. All five monkeys had solid fusion as determined by manual palpation. CT scans demonstrated fusion with trabecular bone growth through the cage.

Osteoinductive Growth Factors

Urist[61] was the first to discover the osteoinductive capacity of bone. Demineralized bone matrix, when placed in the muscle pouches of rats, induced ingrowth of connective tissue cells and differentiation of cartilage and bone. Studies and advances in protein isolation technology subsequently yielded evidence of a series of soluble, low molecular weight glycoproteins, identified as BMPs. Because BMPs make up 1% of all bone protein, large volumes of allograft are required to extract small amounts of osteoinductive factors. In the 1980s Wosney[65] identified several BMP molecules, of which all but one belong to the TGF-B family of proteins. Several recombinant BMP molecules have been produced as singular molecular species in virtually unlimited quantities using genetically modified cell lines. In 1990 Wang et al.[62] described osteoconductivity of rhBMP-2 in a rat ectopic assay system. This activity was also shown for rhBMP-4 and for rhBMP-7 (OP-1). Since 1993 the efficacy of rhBMP-2 has been shown in spinal fusion models in rabbits, dogs, sheep, goats, and rhesus monkeys.[5,32]

The use of rhBMP-2 in cylindric fusion devices was first studied in animal models. Sandu[57] in 1996 reported that successful anterior lumbar fusion had occurred in sheep after implantation of cylindric titanium cages filled with rhBMP-2 soaked collagen sponges. Although only 33% of cages filled with autograft were associated with fusion in this model, all animals with rhBMP-2 filled cages had successful fusion and excellent bony consolidation. In another study cylindric freeze-dried allograft bone dowels were filled with either rhBMP-2 or autogenous bone graft from the iliac crest and implanted into rhesus monkeys.[32] At 3 months there was radiographic evidence of fusion in the sites that were implanted with rhBMP-2. By 6 months, there was both radiographic and histologic evidence of solid fusion in all sites implanted with rhBMP-2.

The first clinical demonstration of clinical efficacy of rhBMP-2 for spinal fusion was a multicenter trial involving 14 patients.[7] All patients had single-level lumbar disease. They were randomized to either tapered Ti fusion cages that contained an rhBMP-2 (1.5mg/ml) soaked bovine collagen sponge or morselized autogenous bone graft from the iliac crest. Of the patients who received rhBMP-2, 10 of 11 achieved fusion by 3 months, and all had fusion by 6 months. Only one of the three controls achieved fusion by 12 months.

At this time data-exploring alternative osteoinductive materials are promising but sparse. Although the optimal graft substitute and delivery system for lumbar intervertebral fusion has not been established, the preliminary data from trials incorporating rhBMP-2 has been favorable. Whether to use threaded interbody implants, or traditional femoral ring allografts will depend on further clinical research and outcome analysis.

Summary

The key question to answer when considering the effectiveness of cages is to determine whether fusion has taken place. The use of titanium and tantalum cages makes routine assessment of fusion even more difficult because of artifacts on CT and MRI scans.[40] The main criteria for determining successful fusion are different for each of the different types of fusion devices. The Brantigan[11] cage is radiolucent and allows direct visualization of graft within the cage. The success of the Ray[54] cage was evaluated with

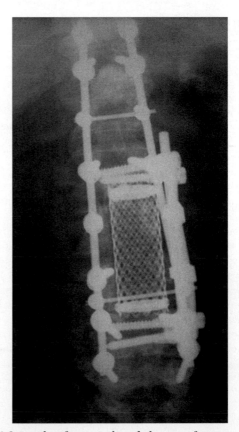

Figure 41.8 Lumbar fusion with pedicle screw fixation and Harm's cage with anterior instrumentation.

the use of radiographic overlay method of Hutter.[34] When superimposed flexion and extensions views were compared, fusion was present when no motion was evident. The BAK device was evaluated on the basis of decreased motion on lateral flexion and extension radiographs, with the use of 3 degrees[39] or 5 degrees[2] as the essential value (Figure 41.8).

Questions relating to the success of an arthrodesis cannot be adequately addressed unless standard criteria are used. Assessment of fusion should be based on increased density of the graft within the disc space, bridging trabecular bone, and continuous intervertebral cortical bridges from the dorsal border of one vertebral body joining the cortex of the caudad vertebral body. Researchers should use conventional criteria for determining fusion, such as bridging trabecular bone in continuity with two adjacent end-plates. Investigators performing prospective, randomized trials should use the same radiographic criteria for both the control group as for the cage group. If CT images do not demonstrate trabecular bone, then the fusion mass is indeterminate. A lack of motion of flexion and extension lateral radiographs should not be equated with successful fusion. The determination of duration and follow-up necessary to adequately identify a fusion mass is, to date, unknown.

The rates of fusion after interbody fusion have improved, from 66%[58] to 2-year rates of 91%[39] with the use of the BAK titanium device, and 96% with the use of the Ray titanium device.[54] However, one must keep in mind that longer clinical and radiographic follow-up is necessary before the actual effectiveness (period free of revision) and true fusion rates are known.

REFERENCES

1. Agazzi S, Reverdin A, May D: Posterior lumbar interbody fusion with cages: an independent review of 71 cases. *J Neurosurg* 91:186-192, 1999.
2. Alpert S: Summary of effectiveness and safety—BAK interbody fusion system—PMA P950002, PMA Document Mail Center (HFZ-401), Center for Disease and Radiological Health. Washington D.C., Food and Drug Administration, Sept 20, 1996.
3. Bagby GW: Arthrodesis by the distraction-compression method using a stainless steel implant. *Orthopedics* 11: 931-934, 1988.
4. Blumenthal SL, Gill K: Can lumbar spine radiographs accurately determine fusion in postoperative patients? Correlation of routine radiographs with a second surgical look at lumbar fusions. *Spine* 18:1186-1189, 1993.
5. Boden SD, Horton WC, Martin G: Laparoscopic anterior spinal arthrodesis with rhBMP-2 in a titanium interbody threaded cage. *J Spinal Disord* 11:95-101, 1998.
6. Boden SD, Schimandle JH, Hutton WC: The use of osteoinductive growth factor for lumbar spine fusion. *Spine* 20:2633-2644, 1995.
7. Boden SD, Zdeblick TA, Sandu HS, Heim SE: The use of BMP-2 in interbody fusion cages: Definitive evidence of osteoinduction in humans. *Trans Am Acad Orthop Surg*, 1999.
8. Brantigan J, Steffee A, Lewis M, *et al*: Lumbar interbody fusion using Brantigan I/F cage for posterior lumbar

interbody fusion and the variable pedicle screw placement system. *Spine* 25:1437-1446, 2000.
9. Brantigan JW: Pseudoarthrosis rate after allograft posterior lumbar interbody fusion with pedicle screw and plate fixation. *Spine* 19:1271-1280, 1994.
10. Brantigan JW, McAfee PC, Cunningham BW, *et al*: Interbody lumbar fusion using a carbon fiber cage implant versus allograft bone. An investigational study in the Spanish goat. *Spine* 19:1436-1444, 1994.
11. Brantigan JW, Steffee AD, Lewis ML, *et al*: Lumbar interbody fusion using the Brantigan I/F cage for PLIF and the VSP pedicle screw system: two-year results of a Food and Drug Administration IDE clinical trial. In Husson JL, Le Heuc JC (eds): *Intersomatique du Rachis Lumbaire*. Montpelier, France, Sauramps Medical, 1996.
12. Brodsky AE, Kovalsky ES, Khalil MA: Correlation of radiologic assessment of lumbar spine fusions with surgical exploration. *Spine* 16:261-265, 1991.
13. Chen D, Fay LA, Lok J, *et al*: Increasing neuroforaminal volume by anterior interbody distraction in degenerative lumbar spine. *Spine* 20:74-79, 1995.
14. Chitnavis B, Barbagallo G, Selway R: Posterior lumbar interbody fusion for revision disc surgery: review of 50 cases in which carbon fiber cages were implanted. *J Neurosurg* 95:190-195, 2001.
15. Cloward RB: The treatment of ruptured lumbar intervertebral discs by vertebral body fusion. I. Indications, operative technique, after care. *J Neurosurg* 10:154-168, 1953.
16. Crock HV: Observations on the management of failed spinal operations. *J Bone Joint Surg* 58B:193-199, 1976.
17. Cunningham BW, Haggerty CJ, McAfee PC: A quantitative densitometric study investigating the stress-shielding effects of interbody spinal fusion devices—emphasis on long term fusions in thoroughbred racehorses. Read at the Annual Meeting of the Orthopedic Research Society, New Orleans, March 9, 1998.
18. Cunningham BW, Kanayama M, Parker LM, *et al*: Osteogenic protein (rhOP-1) versus autologous fusion in sheep thoracic spine. *Spine* 24:509-518, 1999.
19. DeBowes RM, Gant BD, Bagby GW, *et al*: Cervical vertebral interbody fusion in the horse: a comparative study of bovine xenografts and autografts supported by stainless steel baskets. *Am J Veter Res* 45:191-199, 1984.
20. Diedrich O, Perlick L, Schmitt O, Kraft C: Radiographic characteristics on conventional radiographs after posterior lumbar interbody fusion: comparative study between radiolucent and radiopaque cages. *J Spinal Disord* 14: 522-532, 2001.
21. Dimar J, Beck D, Glassman S, *et al*: Posterior lumbar interbody cages do not augment segmental biomechanical stability. *Am J Orthop* 636-639, August 2001.
22. Eck K, Bridwell K, Ungacta F, *et al*: Analysis of titanium mesh cages in adults with minimum of two-year follow-up. *Spine* 18:2407-2415, 2000.
23. Elias W, Simmons N, Kaptain G, *et al*: Complications of posterior lumbar interbody fusion when using a titanium threaded cage device. *J Neurosurg* 93:45-52, 2000.
24. Fraser RD: Interbody, posterior, and combined lumbar fusions. *Spine* 20:167-177, 1995.

25. Frymoyer JW, Hanley EN, Howe J, Kuhlman D: A comparison of radiographic findings in fusion and non fusion patients ten or more years following lumbar disc surgery. *Spine* 4:435-440, 1979.

26. Glassman S, Johnson JB, Raque G, et al: Management of iatrogenic spinal stenosis complicating placement of a fusion cage. A case report. *Spine* 21:2383-2386, 1996.

27. Glazer PA, Colliou O, Lotz JC, Bradford DS: Biomechanical analysis of lumbrosacral fixation. *Spine* 21:1211-1222, 1996.

28. Goldstein J, Macenski M, Griffith S, McAfee P: Lumbar sagittal alignment after fusion with a threaded interbody cage. *Spine* 26:1137-1142, 2001.

29. Grubb SA, Lipscomb HJ: Results of lumbrosacral fusion for degenerative disc disease with and without instrumentation. Two to five year follow-up. *Spine* 17: 349-355, 1992.

30. Hacker RJ: Comparison of interbody fusion approaches for disabling back pain. *Spine* 22:660-666, 1997.

31. Harms J: Screw-threaded rod system in spinal fusion surgery. *Spine* 6:541-575, 1992.

32. Hecht BP, Fischgrund JS, Herkowitz HN: The use of recombinant human bone morphogenetic protein 2 (rhBMP-2) to promote spinal fusion in a non-human primate anterior interbody fusion model. *Spine* 24:629-636, 1999.

33. Holte DC, O'Brien JP, Renton P: Anterior lumbar fusion using a hybrid interbody graft. *European Spine J* 3:32-38, 1994.

34. Hutter CG: Posterior intervertebral body fusion. A 25-year study. *Clin Orthop* 179:86-96, 1983.

35. Kanayama M, Haggerty CJ, Cunningham BW, et al: The biomechanical stability and stress-shielding of lumbar interbody fusion implants: an in-vitro comparative study. Read at the Annual Meeting of the Orthopedic Research Society, New Orleans, March 17, 1998.

36. Klemme W, Owens B, Dhawan A, et al: Lumbar sagittal contour after posterior interbody fusion. *Spine* 26:534-537, 2001.

37. Kozak JA, Heilman AE, O'Brien JP: Anterior lumbar fusion options. Technique and graft materials. *Clin Orthop* 300:45-51, 1994.

38. Kumar A, Kozak JA, Doherty BJ, Dickson JH: Interspace distraction and graft subsidence after anterior lumbar interbody fusion with femoral strut allograft. *Spine* 18:2393-2400, 1993.

39. Kuslich SD, Ulstrom CL, Griffith SL, et al: The Bagby and Kuslich method of lumbar interbody fusion. History, techniques, and 2-year follow-up results of a United States prospective, multicenter trial. *Spine* 23:1267-1279, 1998.

40. Larsen JM, Rimoldi RL, Capen DA: Assessment of pseudoarthrosis in pedicle screw fixation: a prospective study comparing pain radiographs, flexion/extension radiographs, CT scanning, and bone scintigraphy with operative findings. *J Spinal Disord* 9:117-120, 1996.

41. Lehman TR, Spratt KF, Tozzi JE: Long-term follow-up of lower lumbar fusion patients. *Spine* 12:97-104, 1987.

42. Lin PM: Posterior lumbar interbody fusion technique: complications and pitfalls. *Clin Orthop* 193:90-102, 1985.

43. Lund T, Oxland R, Jost B, et al: Interbody cage stabilization in the lumbar spine. *J Bone Joint Surg Br* 80:351-359, 1998.

44. McAfee P: Current concepts review: Interbody fusion cages in reconstructive operations on the spine. *J Bone Joint Surg Am* 81:859-879, 1999.

45. McAfee PC: Complications of anterior approaches to the thoracolumbar spine. Emphasis on Kaneda Instrumentation. *Clin Orthop* 306:110-119, 1994.

46. McAfee PC: Interbody fusion cages in reconstructive operations in the spine. *J Bone Joint Surg Am* 81:859-889, 1999.

47. McAfee PC, Farey ID, Sutterlin CE: Device-related osteoporosis with spinal instrumentation. *Spine* 14:919-926, 1989.

48. McAfee P, Lee G, Fedder I, Cunningham B: Anterior BAK instrumentation and fusion: Complete versus partial discectomy. *Clin Ortho Rel Research* 394:55-63, 2002.

49. McAfee PC, Regan JJ, Geis WP, Fedder IL: Minimally invasive anterior retroperitoneal approach to the lumbar spine. *Spine* 23:1476-1484, 1998.

50. Otero Vich JM: Anterior cervical interbody fusion with threaded cylindrical bone. *J Neurosurg* 63:750-753, 1985.

51. Penta M, Sandhu A: Magnetic resonance imaging assessment of disc degeneration 10 years after anterior lumbar interbody fusion. *Spine* 20:743-747, 1995.

52. Prolo DJ, Oklund SA, Butcher M: Toward uniformity in evaluating results of lumbar spine operations. A paradigm applied to posterior lumbar interbody fusions. *Spine* 11:601-606, 1986.

53. Ray CD: Threaded fusion cages for lumbar interbody fusions. An economic comparison with 360 degrees fusion. *Spine* 22:681-685, 1997.

54. Ray CD: Threaded titanium cages for lumbar interbody fusion. *Spine* 22:667-680, 1997.

55. Regan JJ, McAfee PC, Guyer RD, Aronoff RJ: Laparoscopic fusion of the lumbar spine in a multicenter series of the first 34 consecutive patients. *Surg Laparscop Endosc* 6:459-468, 1996.

56. Regan JJ, McAfee PC, Mack MJ: *Atlas of Endoscopic Spine Surgery.* St. Louis, Quality Medical, 1995.

57. Sandu HS, Kabo JM, Turner AS: Augmentation of titanium fusion cages for experimental anterior lumbar fusion. *Orthopedic Transactions* 21:92, 1997.

58. Stauffer RN, Coventry MB: Anterior interbody lumbar spine fusion. Analysis of Mayo Clinic Series. *J Bone Joint Surg* 54A:756-768, 1972.

59. Steffee AD, Sitkowski DJ: Posterior lumbar interbody fusion and plates. *Clin Orthop* 227:99-102, 1988.

60. Togawa D, Bauer T, Brantigan J, Lowery G: Bone graft incorporation in radiographically successful human intervertebral body fusion cages. *Spine* 26:2744-2750, 2001.

61. Urist MR: Bone formation by autoinduction. *Science* 150:893-899, 1965.

62. Wang EA, Rosen V, D'Alessandro JS: Recombinant human bone morphogenetic protein induces bone formation. *Proc Natl Acad Sci USA* 87:2220-2224, 1990.

63. Weiner BK, Fraser RD: Spine update: lumbar interbody cages. *Spine* 23:634-640, 1998.

64. Wetzel FT, LaRocca H: The failed posterior lumbar interbody fusion. *Spine* 16:839-845, 1991.

65. Wosney JM: The bone morphogenetic family and osteogenesis. *Mol Reprod Dev* 32:160-167, 1992.

66. Yuan H, Kuslich SD, Dowdle JA, et al: Prospective multicenter clinical trial of the BAK interbody fusion system. Read at the Annual Meeting of the NASS, New York, Oct. 22, 1997.

CHAPTER 42

Dorsal and Lateral Thoracic and Lumbar Fusion

George J. Kaptain, Christopher I. Shaffrey,
Andrea L. Halliday, Michael Schneier,
and John A. Jane

Historic Perspective

In 1911 Albee[3] and Hibbs[40] independently described two methods of arthrodesis to treat patients with thoracolumbar deformities secondary to Pott's disease. With both techniques greenstick fractures of the spinous process were used to expose fresh cortical surfaces to facilitate fusion. Albee augmented the fusion with tibial autograft. Realizing the potential applications offered by spinal fusion, researchers applied the technique to patients with scoliosis,[41] spondylolisthesis,[43] and fracture dislocations. MacKenzie-Forbes[53] and Hibbs[41] described techniques of laminar decortication that extended the fusion bed laterally. In 1924 Hibbs denuded the cartilaginous articulation of the facet joints to enhance fusion in his series of scoliosis patients.[41] Howorth,[43] McBride,[60] and Moe[62] further modified facet joint preparations. Hall and Goldstein devised modifications of dorsal element decortication in the treatment of scoliosis.[8,31]

In 1936 Mathieu and Demirleau[57] introduced transverse process fusion as an alternative to dorsal fusions. Adkins[2] applied this technique to spondylolisthesis to improve on the results of interlaminar fusions. These techniques were especially valuable in the lumbar spine in cases in which laminectomy precluded dorsal fusion. Watkins[86] devised a paramedian approach to the dorsal aspect of the lumbar spine by exposing the transverse processes lateral to the paraspinous musculature. This technique retained the advantage of permitting access to the lateral aspect of the spine without disturbing the spinous process and interspinous ligament. Wiltse and colleagues[87,88] were able to gain access to more medial structures through a paramedian approach, splitting the fascial plane between the multifidus and longissimus divisions of the paraspinous musculature, rather than dissecting lateral to the entire muscle group. Recently the application of internal fixation has improved the capability to correct spinal deformity and reduce the incidence of pseudarthrosis after thoracolumbar fusion procedures.[33,74,89,94] These devices temporarily immobilize the spine and permit the synthesis of an osseous rather than a fibrous union.

Bone Anatomy and Physiology

Bone is specialized connective tissue composed of a calcified matrix that contains osteocytes, osteoblasts, and osteoclasts. Osteoblasts synthesize bone matrix, which is composed of hydroxyapatite crystals, organic collagen fibrils, and an amorphous ground substance. The ground substance, composed of glycosaminoglycans, stimulates the calcification of the matrix. Once osteoblasts are surrounded by a completely calcified matrix, they become osteocytes.

The secondary structure of bone matures as it is exposed to compressive or tensile forces. Primary bone appears initially in embryonic development, but also occurs in maturing fracture sites. Woven bone is a type of primary bone found at fracture sites during rapid osseous formation and is characterized by a random deposition of fine collagen fibrils that contain a dense population of osteocytes. Because of the disorderly arrangement of these structures, this construct is relatively weak. Primary bone, however, reorganizes to gain a secondary structure more capable of bearing force.

Cortical and cancellous bone are both forms of secondary bone and are found in the mature human skeleton. The osteon is the primary structural unit of cortical bone and is characterized by a concentric array of parallel collagen fibers situated around a central or Haversian canal that brings nutrients to compact bone. The Haversian canals communicate with the marrow cavity, the periosteum, and with each other via transverse or oblique Volkmann canals. Cancellous or spongy bone is located deep in cortical bone and contains marrow elements. The beams and struts of cortical bone are covered by a fine endosteum, which is a source of osteoprogenitor cells. Intersecting osseous bars called trabeculae are present in cancellous bone. There are both horizontal and vertical components that are oriented in response to stress and lend strength and support to the bone.[58]

Biology of Bone Grafting

Unlike other tissue, bone heals by regeneration with complete restoration of tissue integrity. The components and organization essential to fracture healing are also central to bone synthesis incurred by surgical fusion procedures. A rich vascular network delivers oxygen to the graft site, as well as to a population of inflammatory cells that accumulates in the wound hematoma within hours after surgery.[75] Macrophages congregate in the graft bed and remove necrotic debris while secreting growth factors that stimulate the migration of other inflammatory cells.[70] Platelets secrete platelet-derived growth factor and other substances that are chemotactic for fibroblasts and other mesenchymal cells necessary for fracture healing.[73]

Inflammatory cells and platelets that congregate at the surgical or fracture site recruit a population of primitive mesenchymal cells that are stimulated first to proliferate and then to transform to an osseous or chondroid lineage.[19] These mesenchymal cells are found in the bone marrow, the endosteum, the cambial or inner layer of the periosteum, and the perivascular spaces.[67] Transformation of this pool of undifferentiated cells is induced by bone morphogenic protein (BMP), the final factor essential for bone synthesis.[69,90,91]

This regenerative process may be divided into three stages: (1) inflammation, (2) repair, and (3) remodeling.[75] In the first phase of healing the inflammatory signals summon cells that either participate in the deposition of bone or remodel and ingest necrotic debris. During repair, macrophages remove blood clots, damaged bone matrix, and injured cells. Osteoclasts at the fracture site resorb dead bone and remove mineralized matrix while new blood vessels grow into the graft or fracture site. Cartilaginous matrix or osteoid is deposited by pre-existing osteoblasts, chondroblasts, or cells derived from converted mesenchymal cells. Primary and woven bone are then formed as the osteoid or cartilaginous callus is mineralized. If ossification is incomplete, a fibrous nonunion or pseudarthrosis occurs. As mechanical stress is placed on the construct, remodeling restores the bone to its original shape, structure, and mechanical strength.[48]

Although both fracture healing and surgical arthrodesis use identical cellular and molecular cascades to effect regeneration, the central challenge of surgical arthrodesis is to incorporate transplanted graft to create a modified osseous structure. Optimum surgical fusion relies not only on the properties of the fusion bed but also on the nature of the graft. Graft material may manifest osteogenic, osteoinductive, or osteoconductive properties together or in isolation. Osteogenesis refers to the ability of the bone graft to transmit viable osteoblasts to the fusion site. Osteogenic grafts are favorable because they supply a population of osteoprogenitor cells independent of the nature of the fusion site. Vascularized autografts contain the highest number of viable osteoprogenitor cells. Autogenous cancellous material also contains large numbers of cells, but few survive transplantation.[49] Osteoinduction induces undifferentiated mesenchymal cells to divide and then transform into osseous or chondroid phenotypes.[69] BMP, which has been defined and purified by recombinant techniques, is found within the bone matrix and induces the transformation of the undifferentiated cells into those required for fracture healing or arthrodesis.[90,91] Osteoconductive grafts supply a scaffolding to support the ingrowth of sprouting capillaries and osteoprogenitor cells from the recipient host bed into the structure of an implant or graft.[66] This property is characteristic of autograft, allograft, and bone matrix substitutes.

Bone grafts are incorporated by a process known as "creeping substitution" mediated by osteoclasts, in which the resorbed bone graft is replaced with new bone.[18] As osteoclasts resorb grafted material, blood vessels invade the implant. The net result is an increase in porosity of the bone graft with a weakening of its initial mechanical strength. As the bulk of the graft is replaced by regenerated bone, the density and strength of the construct increase.[66]

Graft Selection for Dorsal and Lateral Thoracolumbar Fusions

Successful arthrodesis depends on the biologic vitality of both the implant and the fusion bed. An ideal graft contains independently functional vascular channels, a supply of viable osteoprogenitor cells, and a source of BMPs; it is also antigenically compatible to the host tissue.[79] An adequately prepared fusion site should offer these elements and, to maximize the area of osseous contact, should also be free of soft-tissue or necrotic debris. Stabilization of the fusion bed also promotes graft incorporation.[71]

Vascularized autologous bone is the most biologically active graft. Bone implanted with a vascular pedicle is more rapidly incorporated than is nonvascularized material, although the use of this material is rarely practical for most thoracolumbar fusions.[72] Cortical and cancellous autograft and allograft are used for the vast majority of thoracolumbar fusions. Cancellous graft differs from cortical bone grafts in the rate and completeness of repair. Autogenous cancellous bone is a better graft material than cortical bone for thoracolumbar fusion applications, because it is more rapidly revascularized and is more osteoinductive.[1,80,91] The initial mechanical strength of cortical bone as a grafting material is useful in procedures that require graft rigidity, such as ventral thoracolumbar fusions. Cortical bone grafts, however, become progressively weaker as graft material is resorbed during the incorporation process.

Allografts also have osteoinductive and osteoconductive properties, but they are inferior to autogenous substances because they incur immunologic responses from the host.[37,72] Allografts are useful in patients with a limited bone supply who require a large quantity of graft material.[16] Although autogenous materials are more biologically active than allografts, their procurement can result in a significant number of complications.[47,50,81,92] Despite the apparent biologic disparity of these two substances, equivalent clinical outcomes and fusion rates have been reported in a series that compares the use of allograft and autograft in certain patient populations undergoing dorsal thoracolumbar fusions. In a series of pediatric patients with scoliosis, Montgomery et al.[63] treated 18 patients with autografts and 12 with allografts. Solid fusion was identified in 94.5% of the autograft group and in 100% of the allograft group. A compilation of the results from this and several other series indicates that similar fusion rates can be achieved through the use of allografts, in conjunction with segmental instrumentation in young patients with thoracolumbar scoliosis.[6,12,26,27] The efficacy of allograft in these procedures may be related to the restricted range of motion in the thoracic spine and a conductive environment for fusion in pediatric patients.

In contrast, the results of autografting are far superior to those of allografting in adults undergoing lumbar intertransverse fusions. An et al.[4] conducted a prospective study that evaluated the efficacy of autografts versus allografts in 20 patients who had undergone instrumented interlaminar and intertransverse fusions. In each patient they applied an autograft on one side and an allograft on the other. They found 80% and 35% fusion rates in the autografted and allografted sides, respectively. Other studies also demonstrate higher pseudarthrosis rates with the use of allograft, compared to autograft in intertransverse and interlaminar fusions of the lumbar spine.[21,39,44,64] The greater degree of mobility in the lumbar spine may account for the failure of allograft in these cases.

Indications

Spinal fusion is used to maximize the weight-bearing capacity of the spine while limiting pathologic motion across joint complexes. The objectives of this procedure include the relief of pain, preservation of neurologic function, and maintenance of spinal alignment. Currently, dorsal and dorsolateral fusion techniques are used to manage spinal instability or deformity that result from congenital or idiopathic scoliosis, isthmic spondylolisthesis, spinal fractures, primary and metastatic tumors, and spinal infections, as well as an assortment of degenerative conditions. Absolute indications for fusion include conditions that compromise the structural integrity of the spine that could result in neural injury (Table 42.1). Spinal fusion has also been shown to arrest the progression of deformity in congenital and idiopathic scoliosis[24] and in patients with spondylolisthesis. In his review of the treatment of spondylolisthesis Hanley concluded that fusion is indicated in patients who suffer from a documented progression of spondylolisthesis, in children who present with a symptomatic grade III or IV slip, or in those with a low-grade slip if symptoms persist despite conservative therapy.[34]

Degenerative abnormalities of the lumbar spine may result in symptoms from either compression of neural structures or from abnormal mechanical stress placed on the facet-intervertebral disc joint complex. Alterations in the mechanical properties of the spine are multifactorial but probably begin with desiccation of the intervertebral disc. Although disc desiccation occurs with aging, in certain persons this process is followed by bulging of the annulus fibrosus, hypertrophy of facet joints and the ligamentum flavum, and the eventual development of spinal stenosis. Lumbar stenosis is characterized by constriction of the vertebral canal, resulting in compression of neural elements, which causes neurogenic claudication, low back pain, radicular symptoms, or even incontinence (rarely). Although these spondylotic changes may restrict the mobility of the lumbar spine, most symptoms result from compression of the neural elements and are relieved by spinal decompression. The benefit of adding a fusion after decompressions is therefore controversial. Spondylotic changes associated with lumbar stenosis, on occasion, result in unstable conditions or deformities, such as degenerative spondylolisthesis or scoliosis; these changes may further restrict the area of the vertebral canal. The use of spinal arthrodesis for either the treatment of degenerative disc disease or lumbar disc herniation continues to be an area of debate, and no definitive benefit has been proven.[76,84] However, fusion has been shown to be effective in treating instability (spondylolisthesis) or deformity (scoliosis) resulting from degenerative disc disease.

Lumbar stenosis in association with degenerative spondylolisthesis has been studied prospectively by Herkowitz and Kurz,[38] who randomized 50 patients according to decompression alone versus decompression in conjunction with a noninstrumented fusion. They found good to excellent outcomes in 24 out of 25 patients treated with decompression and fusion, whereas only 11 out of 25 patients treated with decompression alone experienced good or excellent results. Criteria for instability may be evaluated radiographically by the presence of traction spurs[55] or by abnormal angular or translational motion on lateral flexion-extension radiographs. Reported results of fusion for patients who present with localized back pain with these radiographic abnormalities has varied widely with success rates ranging from 30% to 90%.[34] Intraoperative assessment of stability is another factor that influences the decision to augment lumbar decompression with fusion. Fox et al.[28] demonstrated that patients who undergo multiple-level decompressions are more likely to suffer from postoperative instability and slip progression. The lateral extent of the decompression, which is essential for the relief of radicular symptoms, also impacts on postoperative stability. Lombardi et al.[52] compared three groups of patients. The first group had total laminectomies with preservation of the facet joints. The second group had laminectomies, as well as bilateral facetectomies. The third group had laminectomies, partial facetectomies, and intertransverse fusions. Worse outcomes and a higher incidence of slip progression were noted in the group that received facetectomy without fusion.[52]

Internal fixation should also be considered for patients who are candidates for spine fusion. Before the advent of fixation systems, failure rates of noninstrumented fusions for scoliosis ranged from 20% to 40%, with a 35% incidence of loss in correction. Adding segmental fixation has decreased the failure rate to 10%.[85] Instrumentation has also improved fusion rates and clinical outcomes in patients with degenerative disease of the lumbar spine.[30,85,93] Zdeblick described a series of 124 patients who underwent lumbar or lumbosacral fusion. He noted a fusion rate of 65% in patients who were treated without instrumentation. In the remaining two patient groups semirigid instrumentation resulted in a 77% fusion rate, whereas rigid instrumentation resulted in successful arthrodesis in 95% of cases. Clinical outcomes paralleled the rate of successful fusion.[94]

TABLE 42.1

Indications for Spinal Fusion

Recommended	Relative	Rare
Two-third column injury	Degenerative spondylolisthesis	Routine discectomy
Trauma	Abnormal movement on dynamic	Stable spinal stenosis
Tumor	films with appropriate pain	
Infection	or neurologic deficit	
Iatrogenic instability		
Isthmic instability		

Modified from Sonntag VKH, Marciano FF: *Spine* 20:138S-142S, 1995, with permission.

Surgical Technique
Positioning

After the patient is intubated, compressive devices are placed on the lower extremities. Bladder catheterization should be considered for lengthy procedures or when significant blood loss is expected. All dorsal approaches to the lumbar spine are performed with the patient in the prone position, with limited hip flexion for lumbosacral fusion and moderate hip flexion for thoracic fusions. With procedures involving the lower thoracic and lumbar spine, the patient's arms are abducted and the elbows are flexed. The upper extremities are adequately padded, particularly at the elbow to avoid ulnar nerve injury; the arm is not abducted beyond 80 degrees to avoid brachial plexus injury. With dissections involving the upper or midthoracic spine, or in patients with arthritis of the shoulder or elbow, the arms should be padded and fixed in the anatomic position. With concerns about arm position affecting the performance of radiographs, a preoperative study should be performed, and positioning should be adjusted before beginning surgery.

Prevention of epidermal, appendicular, and ocular compressive injuries should be ensured during patient positioning by proper padding over all pressure points. Before transfer, all electrocardiogram leads and wires should be removed from the chest and abdomen to avoid skin breakdown. Chest rolls or frames are used so that the abdomen hangs freely to avoid excessive intraabdominal pressure. The anterior superior iliac spine (ASIS) and knees are padded, and a pillow is placed under the legs so that the toes hang freely. The dorsalis pedis pulse is palpated to guard against femoral artery compression. Urinary catheters should be free of tension, and if chest rolls are used, the breasts should be displaced medially. Finally, goggles should be placed over the eyes to prevent pressure injury to the globes.

Soft-Tissue Approaches
Median Approach to the Thoracic and Lumbar Spine

The median approach to the thoracolumbar spine permits bilateral exposure of the dorsal elements and vertebral canal through one fascial incision. The spinous processes are palpated, and a longitudinal incision is directed through the epidermis, dermis, and superficial fascia to expose the deep thoracolumbar fascia. Self-retaining retractors are then placed, and the fascia is incised with either a monopolar cautery or a scalpel. Once the tips of the spinous processes are visualized, a periosteum or Cobb elevator is used to maintain lateral traction on the paraspinous musculature to facilitate visualization of muscular insertions into the spinous process and medial lamina. Optimal hemostasis is maintained only if these structures are sharply severed directly at their insertion, using either a second Cobb elevator, electrocautery, or curved Mayo scissors. The detachment of these structures facilitates a subperiosteal dissection of the soft tissue from the spinous process, lamina, and the medial portion of the facet joint. The structure of the thoracic vertebrae affords an exposure of the transverse process at this point. Gauze sponges are inserted into the dissection plane, using periosteum elevators to improve exposure and hemostasis. After this is completed, self-retaining retractors can be advanced deep into the superficial fascia. The insertions of the rotares muscle group can be separated at the point at which they insert into the caudal tip of each lamina.

The transverse process of the lumbar vertebrae is located in a deeper sagittal plane relative to the facet joint and pars interarticularis. The terminal branches of the segmental lumbar artery are located rostral, caudal, and lateral to the facet joints (Figures 42.1 and 42.2). Identification and coagulation of these vessels during the course of dissection will reduce bleeding. Arterial bleeding from these

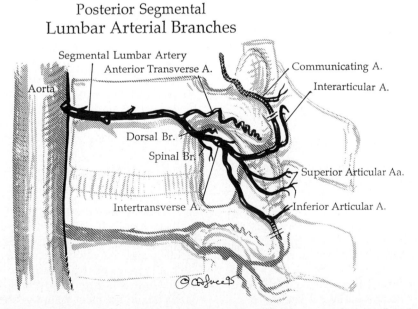

Posterior Segmental Lumbar Arterial Branches

Figure 42.1 Lateral view of the lumbar segmental artery as branches course proximal to the neural foramina before becoming apparent dorsal to the intertransverse ligament.

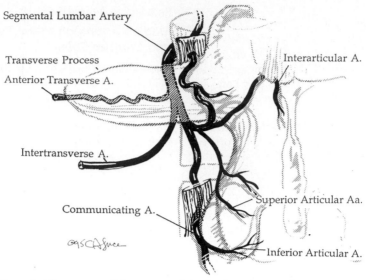

Figure 42.2 Dorsal oblique view of the course of the lumbar segmental artery as it pierces the intertransverse ligament.

vessels should be controlled with bipolar electrocautery to avoid transmission of thermal damage to nerve roots exiting the nearby neural foramina. Fracture of the transverse process should be avoided while performing a periosteal dissection lateral to the zygapophyseal joints. Exposure of the ventral face of the transverse process is hazardous because this area houses both the anterior transverse artery and the exiting nerve root. Advancement of self-retaining retractors permits visualization of the dorsal aspect of the dorsal elements. Care should be taken to periodically release self-retaining retractors so soft-tissue trauma is reduced. Exposure of the L5 transverse process and the ala of the sacrum is complicated by multifidus and sacrospinalis muscle origins that are firmly attached at the sacral ala and dorsal sacrum. The lateral aspect of the superior facet of the sacrum and sacral ala should be periosteally exposed and decorticated to the depth of the L5 transverse process for lumbosacral fusions.

Large, crank-type retractors that can produce excessive force on paraspinal musculature should be avoided when attempting to expose transverse processes. Hand-held retractors provide sufficient exposure of the facet joints and transverse processes to permit decortication and pedicle screw placement, while limiting the possibility of muscle necrosis.

Paramedian Approach to the Lumbar Spine

A median incision is made, as described previously, and the thoracolumbar fascia is widely exposed.[88] A longitudinal incision is made in the deep fascia (bilaterally, if necessary) two finger widths lateral to the spinous process. The fascial plane that separates the multifidus from the longissimus muscles is defined, and a finger is inserted into this avascular plane until a facet joint is palpated. Self-retaining retractors are then placed deep into the lumbodorsal fascia, and a subperiosteal dissection of the musculature is performed over the transverse process, facet joint, and lateral lamina (if indicated). Knowledge of the anatomy of the terminal branches of the segmental artery is necessary to control arterial bleed-

ing. Exposure at the L5-S1 level may be complicated by the laterally projecting fibers of the multifidus as they sweep toward their sacral insertion. These muscles should be detached subperiosteally from their attachments on the sacral ala to permit decortication for lumbosacral fusion.

Bone Dissection
Interlaminar and Intertransverse Fusion

Any remaining soft tissue is removed, and the dorsal aspect of the lamina or transverse process is decorticated with rongeurs, gouges, or osteotomes; the bone chips are set aside to be used with other graft materials. Decortication of the lateral aspect of the superior facet, the region of the mamillary and accessory processes, and the transverse processes should proceed medially to laterally. This decortication should not extend further than the dorsal surface of the transverse process. The intertransversarii muscles and the intertransverse ligament should not be detached to avoid damage to the contents of the neural foramen. In lumbosacral fusions it is essential to decorticate the superior articular facet of the sacrum, as well as the ala of the sacrum to prevent pseudarthrosis. To avoid postoperative degenerative change or spondylolisthesis, the facet joint immediately above or below the fusion mass must not be violated. Onlay graft material is then placed over the decorticated area (Figures 42.3 and 42.4).

Facet Joint Preparation

In the thoracic spine en bloc removal of the superior facet can be accomplished with a straight osteotome, using Hall's method (Figure 42.5).[8] An initial cut is made at the level of the caudal border of the transverse process and is extended medially and caudally. The cartilage and synovium of the joint are removed to expose the underlying cancellous bone. Graft is inserted into this space to facilitate fusion. Moe's method of facet stripping uses a curette or gouge to first reflect the osteocartilaginous rind of the superior facet joint.[62] This flap is left connected to the caudal border of

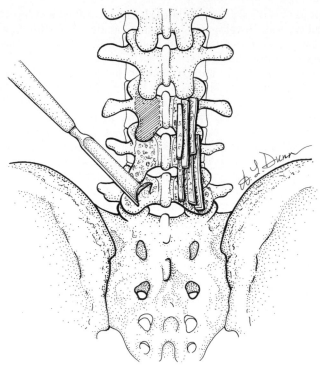

Figure 42.3 Dorsal view of an interlaminar fusion demonstrating the decortication of the lamina and facet joint surfaces with the placement of bone graft contralaterally. Note that the facet joint of the rostral border of the fusion site should not be disturbed to guard against postoperative instability.

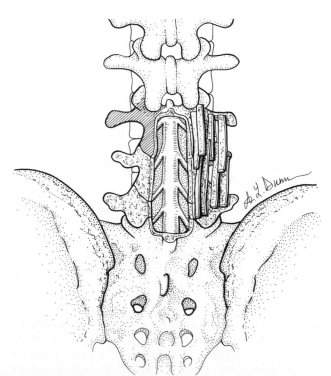

Figure 42.4 Dorsal view of a dorsolateral fusion after total laminectomy. Fusion bed involves the dorsal aspect of the transverse process, the facet joint, and the pars interarticularis.

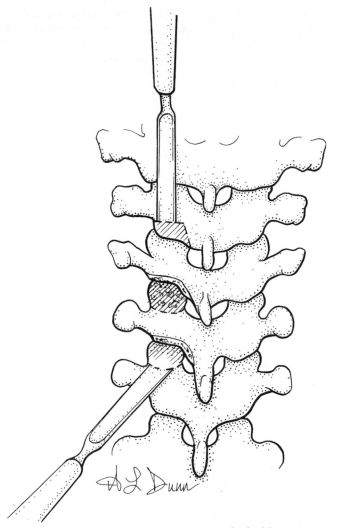

Figure 42.5 Dorsal view demonstrating a method of facet joint preparation in the thoracic spine.

the rostral transverse process and is reflected caudally. The same procedure is used to denude the caudal facet of the motion segment. This flap is reflected rostrally and left attached to the rostral margin of the transverse process. Soft tissue or cartilage is removed from the fusion site and grafting material is added to the site.

In the lumbar spine osteocartilaginous plates may be removed using osteotomes. Initial cuts should be oriented parallel to the axis of the joint space. Osteocartilaginous plates of bone are removed from the superior and inferior joint surface. These pieces are morcellized or cut into strips and may be used as graft material.

The importance of complete soft-tissue removal in the areas lateral to the facet joint and overlying transverse process during intertransverse fusion cannot be overemphasized.

Complications and Avoidance
Positioning
Hemorrhage

Intraoperative venous hemorrhage can be greatly reduced if the abdomen is properly placed during positioning.

Hemodynamic pressure in the epidural and paravertebral venous plexus is greatly increased by the functional obstruction of the caval system through an increase in intraabdominal pressure.[7] Venous hypertension is reduced if the abdomen hangs freely during the procedure. The knee-chest, kneeling, and prone positions on a spinal frame maintain abdominal decompression while permitting access to the dorsal aspect of the spine.

Loss of Lumbar Lordosis

Loss of lumbar lordosis ("flat back" syndrome) has been associated with pain and gait abnormalities in patients who have undergone thoracolumbar fusion for scoliosis.[36] Tan et al.[82] compared the degree of lumbar lordosis in patients placed in various positions for dorsal thoracolumbar surgery and found that the closest approximation to normal lumbar lordosis is obtained by placing the patient in the prone position with extended lower extremities.

Compression and Traction Injuries

Neural, ocular, and epidermal structures may be damaged by compression and traction during positioning. These injuries are minimized by proper padding of pressure points, such as the knees and the region of the lateral femoral cutaneous nerves, and by avoiding stretching of the brachial plexus by positioning the arms at an 80-degree angle or less to the body.

Surgical
Pseudarthrosis

The success of fusion is determined clinically by amelioration of symptoms and, anatomically, by evidence of bridging trabecular bone on radiographs. Pseudarthrosis after spinal fusion is defined by the incomplete development of a rigid osseous construct, thus permitting motion across a joint complex. The diagnosis of pseudarthrosis is determined with plain radiographs, flexion and extension views, plain tomography, and computed tomography (CT). These images may demonstrate the absence of osseous material at the graft site or movement at the joint with flexion-extension images. These studies are not as sensitive or as specific for determining the status of a fused segment when compared with intraoperative observations during a "second look" surgery.[9,14,45] The difficulty in radiographically characterizing a fusion mass is further complicated in the thoracic spine in which motion is limited, and in instrumented fusions in which artifact obscures imaging. Failure to achieve a solid fusion has been associated with increased morbidity in a variety of pathologic conditions. Pseudarthrosis is known to allow the progression of deformity in scoliosis,[24,32,59,62,63] as well as a recurrence of symptoms in spondylolisthesis.[5,35] The significance of pseudarthrosis as a complication of surgery, however, is not always straightforward. DePalma and Rothman[22] and Frymoyer et al.[29] have all demonstrated that solid arthrodesis does not correlate with patient satisfaction, alleviation of pain, or disability.

The treatment of pseudarthrosis depends on the recognition of its varied clinical presentation. Pseudarthrosis after spinal surgery for scoliosis or spondylolisthesis may present with a progression of deformity, radiologic instability, pain, myelopathy, or radiculopathy. Reexploration may be required to establish a definitive diagnosis and repair of pseudarthrosis.

The diagnosis and treatment of pseudarthrosis in patients with persistent low back pain or neurologic symptoms after lumbosacral fusion is a more difficult issue. The "failed back" syndrome includes individuals with persistent symptoms after surgical treatment of a variety of conditions, such as lumbar stenosis, lumbar disc herniation, spondylolisthesis, or degenerative disc disease. In the absence of infection, hardware failure, or new neurologic deficit, it is essential to avoid reexploration until a sufficient interval has elapsed to allow for maturation of the fusion mass. At the conclusion of this interval radiologic evaluation may or may not demonstrate a pseudarthrosis. Other sources of persistent pain or neurologic deficit include disc herniation, painful degenerative changes at adjacent levels, and residual spinal or foraminal stenosis. Magnetic resonance imaging (MRI), CT, and myelography are helpful to delineate the presence of these conditions. Reexploration of the surgical site should proceed only in patients who do not respond to conservative therapy.

Treatment of nonunion should begin with an identification of factors that inhibit bone healing. The distribution of forces within the graft site influences the effectiveness of healing. In patients with scoliosis, pseudarthrosis varies with the degree of correction, as well as with the expanse of curvature.[59] Pseudarthrosis is also more commonly a problem in patients with spondylolisthesis, especially in those individuals with a higher grade of subluxation.[11] In both scoliosis and spondylolisthesis normal spinal biomechanics are altered so that large tensile forces are imposed on the graft site, limiting the capacity of fusion.

Motion across the fusion site is also associated with pseudarthrosis. The pseudarthrosis rate increases with an increasing number of spinal segments because of a longer fusion mass and more total motion across the area.[22,74] Spinal instrumentation reduces pseudarthrosis rates by limiting motion across the area.[74,89,93,94] Schwab and colleagues[85] reported significantly improved union rates in patients with lumbar spondylosis. In cases of fusion for degenerative disc disease, noninstrumented fusions have pseudarthrosis rates ranging from 20% to 40%, whereas the addition of pedicle screw fixation decreases the rate to 5%. Although it is generally accepted that instrumentation facilitates fusions, some authors report no difference in rates of arthrodesis using internal fixation.[61] The decision to use instrumentation must be tempered with the understanding that intraoperative device-related complication rates have been reported to be approximately 5% to 10%, although the majority of these occurrences do not result in permanent sequelae.[30] Additionally, although hardware improves fusion rates in most instances, up to 20% of instrumented patients require reoperation for the removal of hardware.[10,74] These rates, however, are comparable to the incidence of revision surgery for the repair of pseudarthrosis in noninstrumented fusions.[30]

Methods of pseudarthrosis repair in patients with scoliosis are related to the degree of deformity. A one-stage repair of pseudarthrosis is possible if the patient has maintained an appropriate spinal contour. Under these conditions the fusion mass is exposed, the instrumentation is removed, the bone is decorticated, and large quantities of autologous cancellous bone are applied. Internal fixation is then reapplied and compressive forces are placed across the area of nonunion. A two-stage procedure is advocated in persons who develop significant scoliosis as a result of pseudarthrosis. In these patients the fusion mass is exposed, the hardware is removed, and multiple osteotomies are performed in an effort to realign the spine. The deformity is reduced during a course of halo-femoral traction after which the patient undergoes bone grafting and reinstrumentation.[20,78] Ventral discectomy and bone grafting followed by dorsal instrumentation and fusion have also been recommended.

Repair of lumbosacral dorsal and lateral fusions can be approached by a re-exploration of the fusion mass, with decortication and application of additional bone graft. Fusion rates in patients undergoing pseudarthrosis repair are significantly improved by the application of dorsal segmental instrumentation.[74,94] Interbody fusion has also been advocated as an alternative in patients with pseudarthrosis and persistent low back pain.[77] Although successful fusion has been reported in 81% of patients, the approach is not familiar to many spine surgeons and is associated with complications, including hemorrhage resulting from great vessel injury, unintentional sympathectomy, and retrograde ejaculation in males.[83]

The general medical condition of the patient also influences fusion and fracture healing. Smoking has been associated with an increased incidence of pseudarthrosis.[15,17] Partial oxygen arterial pressures were significantly reduced in the population of smokers, reinforcing the concept that oxygen delivery is an essential component in bone deposition.[15] Osseous healing is also facilitated by immunologically mediated messages between cells. If possible, glucocorticoid administration should be tapered before surgery to increase the possibility of engraftment. Nutritional status is also an essential preoperative consideration in patients undergoing elective arthrodesis; malnourished patients may benefit from dietary supplementation before their surgery.[12,49]

Hemorrhage

Significant blood loss from thoracolumbar fusions may be the result of perforation of the terminal branches of lumbar and thoracic segmental arteries.[54] These vessels are encountered while exposing the transverse processes in the vicinity of the facet joint and the proximal portion of the transverse process. They lie deep in the intermediate fascia of the paraspinal musculature; the rostral and caudal articular arteries lie superior and inferior to the facet joint, the communicating artery travels lateral to the joint on the dorsal surface of the transverse process, and the interarticular artery courses medially (Figures 42.1 and 42.2). Identification and coagulation of these vessels before dissection will avoid hemorrhage and excessive use of cautery.

Venous bleeding can be the result of increased intraabdominal pressure with a resultant increase in flow through Batson's plexus. Bleeding can be avoided by careful posi-

tioning, as outlined in the previous section. Venous bleeding from the decorticated segment of bone at the graft site may also occur. Although some degree of hemorrhage is preferable to a dry fusion bed, excessive intraoperative bleeding is avoidable if decortication follows all other portions of the procedure.

Autologous blood banking should be offered as an alternative to patients when operative blood loss may require blood transfusion. This option is essential in scoliosis surgery in which exposures are expansive and blood loss may be significant. Oga et al.[65] outlined an algorithm using a cell saver and autologous blood banking. In their system harvested autologous blood and cell savers were used in patients in whom operative blood loss was expected to exceed 1000ml. The cell saver alone was used in procedures in which blood loss of less than 1000ml was expected. Blood loss in their series ranged from 2000 to 3000ml. Homologous transfusion was required in only 10% of their patients.[65]

Infection

Infection rates in spinal surgery vary with the complexity and duration of the procedure. Whereas 2% to 4% of non-instrumented fusions become complicated by infection, procedures that involve the placement of internal fixators result in rates between 6% and 11%.[56] *Staphylococcus aureus* is the most common pathogen isolated from deep wound infections. Streptococcal species and a variety of gram-negative enteric organisms have also been identified as pathogens. Seeding may occur intraoperatively by direct inoculation of the organism; therefore adherence to strict sterile technique minimizes risk. Familiarity with decortication, harvesting, and instrumentation techniques shortens operative time and therefore minimizes the possibility of wound colonization. The use of allograft and other implants has also been associated with an increased risk of infection. The possibility that these materials will transmit microbes is minimized if sterile packaging is opened at the last possible moment to prevent contamination.[63]

Hematogenous seeding of wound infections is also possible during and after surgery. The recognition and treatment of remote infections minimize the possibility of colonization from this source. Urinary catheters should be removed soon after completion of the procedure to prevent the possibility of urinary tract infections. Patient mobilization, pain control, and spirometry should be encouraged to prevent atelectasis and pneumonia.

Perioperative antibiotics and intraoperative wound irrigation are effective adjuncts that should minimize infection rates.[42] A first- or second-generation cephalosporin sufficiently covers the most common pathogens encountered in this population of patients. Preservation of the viability of tissues within the wound is of paramount importance; self-retaining retractors should be repositioned often to reduce tissue damage, and monopolar electrocautery should be used sparingly. If placed, drains should be directed away from the perineum and should be removed by the second postoperative day.[56]

Re-exploration of wound infections is indicated not only to obtain diagnosis but also to débride infected and necrotic material. A complete exposure of the fusion mass should include the removal of unincorporated bone graft and necrotic material. After the wound is thoroughly irrigated, washed bone graft material may be replaced. Levi et al.[51] have demonstrated that deep, instrumented wound infections should be treated without the removal of hardware. They were able to eradicate 16 of 17 deep wound infections by using a combination of débridement and systemic and local antibiotic administration.[51]

Postfusion Spondylosis

Interlaminar fusion has been associated with vertebral canal stenosis, as well as with acquired pars defects. Maturation of the fusion mass may result in the inward protrusion of the lamina to obstruct the vertebral canal. These complications usually occur at the cranial edge of the fusion site and may be associated with hypertrophy of the ligamentum flavum.[13,46,54] Postfusion stenosis is accentuated in persons with associated disc bulges or congenital stenosis; this complication may be avoided through careful patient selection. Alternative treatments that overcome this phenomenon include intertransverse fusion, as well as a procedure, as described by DiPierro et al., to decompress nerve roots and stabilize the lumbar spine in patients with lumbar stenosis, and involve unilateral decompressive hemilaminectomy (Figure 42.6).[25] The contralateral lamina and facet are decorticated and packed with autograft. The impact of laminar hypertrophy in dorsal fusions may be minimized by this unilateral decompression.

General Medical Complications

Lumbar fusion is commonly used in patients with degenerative spinal conditions. The utility of spinal arthrodesis in several forms of degenerative disease, however, is speculative. In an effort to clarify the risk imposed by spinal fusion in comparison with spine surgery without fusion, Deyo et al.[23] compared the cost, complications, and reoperation rates in elderly patients on Medicare. Patient selection was based on the diagnosis as defined by International Classification of Diseases, Ninth Revision Clinical Modification. These investigators found that mortality, the rate of nursing home hospitalization, and the duration of hospitalization were significantly increased in patients who required a concomitant fusion for a given diagnosis. Outcome, as measured by the incidence of reoperation 4-year follow-up, was no different in both groups.[23]

In a separate review of 1000 patients who underwent spinal fusion, Prothero et al.[68] found that urinary retention and paralytic ileus were the most common medical complications. Deep venous thrombosis occurred in 4.2% of patients. The risk of acquiring thrombotic complications, however, was significantly reduced by a factor of 2 when the duration of postoperative bed rest was decreased.[68]

Conclusion

Dorsal and dorsolateral spine fusion are currently used for a variety of traumatic, neoplastic, congenital, and degenerative conditions. The development of segmental instrumentation systems has permitted correction of spinal deformity and reduced pseudarthrosis rates at the price of a slightly increased operative complication rate. Spinal instrumentation will fail with time unless adequate bony fusion occurs. Meticulous preparation of the fusion bed and adequate quantities of bone graft are key factors in obtaining a solid fusion. Complications are reduced by a thorough understanding of operative anatomy and proper preoperative, intraoperative, and postoperative care.

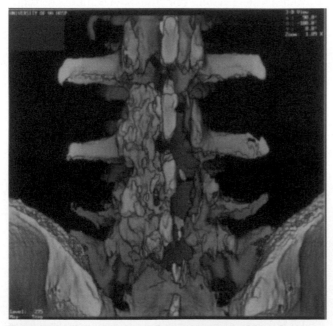

Figure 42.6 Three-dimensional reconstruction of fine-slice computed tomography data showing a unilateral dorsal decompression with contralateral interlaminar fusion. (*From DiPierro CG, Helm GA, Shaffrey CI, et al: J Neurosurg 84: 166-173, 1996, with permission.*)

REFERENCES

1. Abbot LC, Schottstaedt ER, Saunders JB, Bost FC: The evaluation of cortical and cancellous bone as grafting material: a clinical and experimental study. *J Bone Joint Surg* 29:381-414, 1947.
2. Adkins EWO: Lumbo-sacral arthrodesis after laminectomy. *J Bone Joint Surg* 37B:208-233, 1955.
3. Albee FH: Transplantation of portions of the tibia into the spine for Pott's disease. *JAMA* 57:885-886, 1911.
4. An HS, Lynch K, Toth J: Prospective comparison of autograft vs. allograft of adult posterolateral lumbar spine fusion: differences among freeze dried, frozen, mixed grafts. *J Spine Disord* 8:131-135, 1995.
5. Apel DM, Lorenz MA, Zindrick MR: Symptomatic spondylolisthesis in adults: four decades later. *Spine* 14: 345-348, 1989.
6. Aurori BF, Weierman RJ, Lowell HA, *et al*: Pseudarthrosis after spinal fusion for scoliosis. A comparison of autogenic and allogeneic bone grafts. *Clin Orthop* 199: 153-158, 1985.

7. Batson OV: The function of the vertebral veins and their role in the spread of metastases. *Ann Surg* 112:138-149, 1940.

8. Bernardi R, Mueller W: Thoracic fusion techniques using bone. In Menezes AH, Sonntag VKH (eds): *Principles of Spine Surgery.* New York, McGraw-Hill, 1996, pp 1173-1183.

9. Blumenthal SL, Gill K: Can lumbar spine radiographs accurately determine fusion in postoperative patients? Correlation of routine radiographs with a surgical second look at lumbar fusion. *Spine* 18:1186-1189, 1993.

10. Blumenthal SL, Gill K: Complications of the Wiltse pedicle screw fixation system. *Spine* 18:1867-1871, 1993.

11. Boxall D, Bradford DS, Winter RB: Management of severe spondylolisthesis in children and adolescents. *J Bone Joint Surg* 61A:479-486, 1979.

12. Bridwell KH, O'Brien MF, Lenke LG, *et al*: Posterior spinal fusion supplemented with only allograft bone in paralytic scoliosis. Does it work? *Spine* 19:2658-2666, 1994.

13. Brodsky AE: Post-laminectomy and post-fusion stenosis of the lumbar spine. *Clin Orthop* 115:130-139, 1976.

14. Brodsky AE, Kovalsky ES, Khalil MA: Correlation of radiologic assessment of lumbar spine fusions with surgical exploration. *Spine* 16:S261-S265, 1991.

15. Brown CW, Orme TJ, Richardson HD: The rate of pseudarthrosis (surgical nonunion) in patients who are smokers and patients who are nonsmokers: a comparison study. *Spine* 11:942-943, 1986.

16. Butterman GR, Glazer PA, Bradford DS: The use of allografts in the spine. *Clin Orthop* 324:75-85, 1996.

17. Carpenter CT, Dietz JW, Leung KYK, *et al*: Repair of a pseudarthrosis of the lumbar spine. *J Bone Joint Surg* 78A:712-720, 1996.

18. Chase CW, Herndon CH: The fate of autogenous and homogenous bone grafts. A historical review. *J Bone Joint Surg* 37A:809-841, 1955.

19. Cook SD, Rueger DC: Osteogenic protein. I. Biology and applications. *Clin Orthop* 324:29-38, 1996.

20. Cummine JL, Lonstein JE, Moe JH: Reconstructive surgery in the adult for failed scoliosis fusion. *J Bone Joint Surg* 61A:1151-1161, 1979.

21. Dawson EG, Lotysch M, Urist MR: Intertransverse process lumbar arthrodesis with autogenous bone grafts. *Clin Orthop* 154:90-96, 1981.

22. DePalma AF, Rothman RH: The nature of pseudarthrosis. *Clin Orthop* 59:113-118, 1968.

23. Deyo RA, Ciol MA, Cherkin DC, *et al*: Lumbar spine fusion. A cohort study of complications, re-operations, and resource use in the Medicare population. *Spine* 18: 1463-1470, 1993.

24. Dickson JH, Erwin WD, Rossi D: Harrington instrumentation and arthrodesis for idiopathic scoliosis: a twenty-one year follow up. *J Bone Joint Surg* 72A: 678-683, 1990.

25. DiPierro CG, Helm GA, Shaffrey CI, *et al*: Treatment of lumbar stenosis by extensive unilateral decompression and contralateral autologous bone fusion: operative technique and results. *J Neurosurg* 84:166-173, 1996.

26. Dodd CAF, Fergusson CM, Freedman L, *et al*: Allograft versus autograft bone in scoliosis surgery. *J Bone Joint Surg* 70B:431-434, 1988.

27. Fabry G: Allograft versus autograft in idiopathic scoliosis surgery: a multivariate statistical analysis. *J Pediatr Orthop* 11:465-468, 1991.

28. Fox MW, Onofrio BM, Hanssen AD: Clinical outcomes and radiological instability following decompressive lumbar laminectomy for degenerative spinal stenosis: a comparison of patients undergoing concomitant arthrodesis versus decompression alone. *J Neurosurg* 85:793-802, 1996.

29. Frymoyer JW, Hanley EN, Howe J, *et al*: A comparison of radiographic findings in fusion and nonfusion patients ten or more years following lumbar surgery. *Spine* 4:435-440, 1979.

30. Garfin SR: Summation. *Spine* 19:2300S-2305S, 1994.

31. Goldstein LA: Results in the treatment of scoliosis with turnbuckle plaster cast correction and fusion. *J Bone Joint Surg* 41A:321-335, 1959.

32. Graham JJ: Pseudarthrosis in scoliosis: routine exploration of forty-five operative cases. *J Bone Joint Surg* 50A:850, 1968.

33. Grubb SA, Lipscomb HJ: Results of lumbosacral fusion for degenerative disc disease with and without instrumentation. Two and five year follow up. *Spine* 17: 349-355, 1992.

34. Hanley EN: The indications for spinal fusion with and without instrumentation. *Spine* 20:143S-153S, 1995.

35. Hanley EN, Levy JA: Surgical treatment of isthmic lumbosacral spondylolisthesis. Analysis of variables influencing results. *Spine* 14:48-50, 1989.

36. Hasday CA, Passoff TL, Perry JP: Gait abnormalities arising from iatrogenic loss of lumbar lordosis secondary to Harrington rod instrumentation in lumbar fractures. *Spine* 8:501-511, 1983.

37. Heiple KG, Chase SW, Herndon CH: A comparative study of the healing process following different types of bone transplantation. *J Bone Joint Surg* 45A:1593-1616, 1963.

38. Herkowitz HN, Kurz LT: Degenerative lumbar spondylolisthesis with spinal stenosis. A prospective study comparing decompression with decompression and intertransverse process arthrodesis. *J Bone Joint Surg* 73A:802-808, 1991.

39. Herron LD, Newman MH: The failure of ethylene oxide gas-sterilized freeze-dried bone graft for thoracic and lumbar spine fusion. *Spine* 14:496-500, 1989.

40. Hibbs RH: An operation for progressive spinal deformities. *NY J Med* 93:1013-1016, 1911.

41. Hibbs RA: A report of fifty-nine cases of scoliosis treated by the fusion operation. *J Bone Joint Surg* 6A:3-37, 1924.

42. Horwitz NH, Curtin JA: Prophylactic antibiotics and wound infection following lumbar disc surgery: a retrospective study. *J Neurosurg* 43:727-731, 1975.

43. Howorth MB: Evolution of spinal fusion. *Ann Surg* 117:278-289, 1943.

44. Jorgenson SS, Lowe TG, France J, Sabin J: A prospective analysis of autograft versus allograft in posterolateral lumbar fusion in the same patient. A minimum of 1 year follow up in 144 patients. *Spine* 19:2048-2053, 1994

45. Kant AP, Daum WJ, Dean MS: Evaluation of lumbar spine fusion. Plain radiographs versus direct surgical exploration and observation. *Spine* 20:2313-2317, 1995.

46. Kestler OC: Overgrowth (hypertrophy) of lumbosacral grafts causing complete block. *Bull Hosp Jt Dis Orthop Inst* 27:51-57, 1966.

47. Kurz LT, Garfin SR, Booth RE: Harvesting autogenous iliac crest bone grafts: a review of complications and techniques. *Spine* 14:1324-1331, 1989.

48. Kushner A: Evaluation of Wolff's law in bone formation. *J Bone Joint Surg* 22A:589-596, 1940.

49. Lane JM, Muschler GF: Principles of bone fusion. In Rothman RH, Simeone FA (eds): *The Spine*, ed 3. Philadelphia, WB Saunders, 1992, pp 1739-1755.

50. Laurie SWS, Kaban LB, Mulliken JB, Murray JE: Donor site morbidity after harvesting rib and iliac bone. *Plast Reconstr Surg* 73:933-938, 1984.

51. Levi ADO, Dickman CA, Sonntag VKH: The management of postoperative infections after spinal instrumentation. *J Neurosurg* 86:975-980, 1997.

52. Lombardi JS, Wiltse LL, Reynolds J, *et al*: Treatment of degenerative spondylolisthesis. *Spine* 10:821-827, 1985.

53. MacKenzie-Forbes A: Technique of an operation for spinal fusion as practiced in Montreal. *J Orthop Surg* 2B:509-514, 1920.

54. MacNab I: The blood supply of the lumbar spine and its application to the technique of intertransverse lumbar fusion. *J Bone Joint Surg* 53B:628-638, 1971.

55. MacNab I: The traction spur. An indicator of segmental instability. *J Bone Joint Surg* 53A:663-670, 1971.

56. Massie JB, Heller JG, Abitbol JJ, *et al*: Postoperative posterior spinal wound infections. *Clin Orthop* 284:99-108, 1992.

57. Mathieu P, Demirleau P: Traitement chirurgical du spondylolisthesis douloureaux. *Rev Orthop* 23:352, 1936.

58. Matthews JL: Bone structure and ultrastructure.. In Urist MR (ed): *Fundamental and Clinical Bone Physiology*. Philadelphia, Lippincott-Raven, 1980, pp 4-44.

59. May VR, Mauck WR: Exploration of the spine for pseudarthrosis following spinal fusion in the treatment of scoliosis. *Clin Orthop* 53:115-122, 1967.

60. McBride ED: A mortised transfacet bone block for lumbosacral fusion. *J Bone Joint Surg* 31A:385-393, 1949.

61. McGuire RA, Amundson GM: The use of primary internal fixation in spondylolisthesis. *Spine* 18:1662-1672, 1993.

62. Moe JH: A critical analysis of methods of fusion for scoliosis. An evaluation in two hundred and sixty six patients. *J Bone Joint Surg* 40A:529-554, 1958.

63. Montgomery DM, Aronson DD, Lee CI, Lamont RL: Posterior spine fusion: allograft versus autograft bone. *J Spinal Disord* 3:370-375, 1990.

64. Nugent JP, Dawson EG: Intertransverse process lumbar arthrodesis with allogenic fresh-frozen bone graft. *Clin Orthop* 287:107-111, 1991.

65. Oga M, Ikuta H, Sugioka Y: The use of autologous blood in the surgical treatment of spinal disorders. *Spine* 17:1381-1385, 1992.

66. Prolo DJ: Morphology and metabolism of fusion of the lumbar spine. In Youmans JR (ed): *Neurological Surgery*, ed 4. Philadelphia, WB Saunders, 1996, pp 2449-2460.

67. Prolo DJ, Rodrigo JJ: Contemporary bone graft physiology and surgery. *Clin Orthop* 200:322-342, 1985.

68. Prothero SR, Parkes JC, Stinchfield FE: Complications after low-back fusion in 1000 patients: a comparison of two series one decade apart. *Clin Orthop* 306:5-11, 1994.

69. Reddi AH, Weintroub S, Muthukumaran N: Biologic principles of bone induction. *Orthop Clin North Am* 18:207-212, 1987.

70. Rifas L, Shen V, Mitchell K, Peck WA: Macrophage-derived growth factor for osteoblast-like cells and chondrocytes. *Proc Natl Acad Sci USA* 81:4558-4562, 1984.

71. Sauer HD, Schoettle H: The stability of osteosynthesis bridging defects. *Arch Orthop Trauma Surg* 95:27-30, 1979.

72. Schaffer JW, Field GA, Goldberg VM: Fate of vascularized and nonvascularized autografts. *Clin Orthop* 197:32-43, 1985.

73. Scher CD, Shepard RC, Antoniades HN, Stiles CD: Platelet-derived growth factor and the regulation of the mammalian fibroblast cell cycle. *Biochim Biophys Acta* 560:217-241, 1979.

74. Schwab FJ, Nazarian DG, Mahmud F, Michelsen CB: Effects of spinal instrumentation on fusion of the lumbosacral spine. *Spine* 20:2023-2028, 1995.

75. Simmons DJ: Fracture healing perspectives. *Clin Orthop* 200:100-112, 1985.

76. Sonntag VKH, Marciano FF: Is fusion indicated for lumbar spinal disorders? *Spine* 20:138S-142S, 1995.

77. Stauffer RN, Coventry MD: Anterior interbody lumbar spine fusion. *J Bone Joint Surg* 54A:756-768, 1972.

78. Steinmann JC, Herkowitz HN: Pseudarthrosis of the spine. *Clin Orthop* 284:80-90, 1992.

79. Stevenson S, Emery SE, Goldberg VM: Factors affecting bone graft incorporation. *Clin Orthop* 323: 66-74, 1996.

80. Stringa G: Studies of the vascularization of bone grafts. *J Bone Joint Surg* 39B:395-420, 1957.

81. Summers BN, Einstein SM: Donor site pain from the ilium. *J Bone Joint Surg* 71B:677-680, 1989.

82. Tan SB, Kozak JA, Dickson JH, Nalty TJ: Effect of operative position on sagittal alignment of the lumbar spine. *Spine* 19:314-318, 1994.

83. Tiusanen H, Seitsalo S, Osterman K, Soini J: Anterior interbody lumbar fusion in severe low back pain. *Clin Orthop* 324:153-163, 1996.

84. Turner JA, Ersek M, Herron L, *et al*: Patient outcomes after lumbar spine fusion. *JAMA* 268:907-911, 1992.

85. Vaccaro AR, Garfin SR: Internal fixation (pedicle screw fixation) for fusions of the lumbar spine. *Spine* 20: 157S-165S, 1995.

86. Watkins MB: Posterolateral fusion of the lumbar and lumbosacral spine. *J Bone Joint Surg* 35A:1014, 1953.

87. Wiltse LL, Spencer CW: New uses and refinements of the paraspinal approach to the lumbar spine. *Spine* 13:696-706, 1988.

88. Wiltse LL, Bateman JG, Hutchinson RH: The paraspinal sacrospinalis splitting approach to the lumbar spine. *J Bone Joint Surg* 50A:919-926, 1968.

89. Wood GW, Boyd RJ, Carothers TA, *et al*: The effect of pedicle screw/plate fixation on lumbar/lumbosacral

autogenous bone graft fusions in patients with degenerative disc disease. *Spine* 20:819-830, 1995.

90. Urist MR: Bone: formation and autoinduction. *Science* 150:893-899, 1965.

91. Urist MR, Hay PH, Dubuc F, Buring K: Osteogenic competence. *Clin Orthop* 64:194-220, 1969.

92. Younger EM, Chapman MW: Morbidity at bone graft donor sites. *J Orthop Trauma* 3:192-195, 1989.

93. Yuan HA, Garfin SR, Dickman CA, Mardjetko SM: A historical study of pedicle screw fixation in thoracic, lumbar and sacral spinal fusions. *Spine* 19:2279S-2296S, 1994.

94. Zdeblick TA: A prospective, randomized study of lumbar fusion: preliminary results. *Spine* 18:983-991, 1993.

CHAPTER 43

Trauma Surgery: Occipitocervical Junction

Curtis A. Dickman, Tanvir F. Choudhri, and Jürgen Harms

The occipitocervical junction includes the skull base at the foramen magnum, C1, C2, and the associated ligamentous, neural, and vascular structures. Because of the important neural and vascular structures in the region, occipitocervical junction injuries have the potential to cause significant neurologic morbidity or mortality. Therefore, careful recognition, diagnosis, and management of these injuries are essential. The association with high-impact trauma and occipitocervical junction injuries is well recognized. However, the potential for injuries even with relatively minor trauma should be remembered, especially with abnormal bone (e.g., osteoporosis) and/or ligaments (e.g., rheumatoid arthritis).

Occipitocervical junction injuries can be classified in several ways (Box 43.1). One useful system describes occipitocervical junction injuries as isolated ligamentous injuries, isolated fractures, or mixed ligamentous and bony injuries. Occipitocervical junction trauma can also be described by the site and/or level(s) of injury. At most sites, classification systems have been developed for specific injury patterns (e.g., C2 odontoid fractures). Finally, occipitocervical junction injuries can be described based on their stability. Stability is generally determined with clinical and radiographic assessment, sometimes using dynamic flexion/extension radiographs. A stable injury does not demonstrate significant radiographic deformity, pain, or neurological dysfunction with normal physiological loads and movement. An example of a stable injury would be an isolated C2 spinous process fracture, which meets the above criteria. Some injuries are clearly unstable, such as occipitocervical dislocations. Other injuries may initially appear stable but have a reasonable chance of developing delayed instability with time, gravity, movement, and/or relaxation of paraspinal muscle spasm. This category reflects the reality that clinical and radiographic assessment of long-term stability may be indeterminate.

The above classification systems are helpful in injury assessment and planning management. However, the management of a patient with occipitocervical junction trauma is best determined by considering the nature of the injury (including associated injuries), the patient characteristics (e.g., age, medical risk factors, bone quality, desire/ability to tolerate use of a halo orthosis), and the physician's experience. Although much less common, penetrating trauma to the occipitocervical junction presents unique issues that relate to the specific location and trauma modality (bullet, knife, etc.). This class of injuries will not be specifically discussed in this chapter but is addressed in the chapter on Penetrating Spinal Cord Injuries. Although most of the principles from blunt trauma are applicable to penetrating trauma, it is important to point out some important differences. Compared with blunt trauma, penetrating trauma typically results in less ligamentous injury and therefore for a similar fracture may be more stable. However, penetrating trauma more commonly result in trauma to vascular or other important regional structures.

General Principles

The initial management of occipitocervical junction injuries is focused on basic trauma management principles including establishment and maintenance of airway, breathing, and circulation; careful immobilization and transportation; and recognition and management of any associated injuries. These principles have evolved over time and have been published in numerous settings.[28,29]

Occipitocervical junction injuries are frequently recognized on routine cervical spine imaging. However, these injuries may be difficult to detect on initial diagnostic studies. Clinical suspicion based on history and physical exam can aid recognition. Routine radiographs and clinical assessment are often inadequate to fully characterize the injury, and more specialized imaging is usually indicated. Coronal, curved coronal, sagittal, and/or 3-D CT reconstruction views can be extremely helpful in characterizing the presence and nature of injury. MRI imaging may be difficult or impossible to obtain acutely but can often provide essential information on spinal canal compromise and may suggest the presence and degree of ligamentous injury. Dynamic imaging with plain x-rays, CT, and/or MRI can be valuable in assessing stability but should be performed carefully. Occasionally, stability is checked with real-time fluoroscopy during careful flexion and extension controlled by a qualified examiner. For example, fluoroscopic flexion/extension imaging may be helpful when there is urgent need to assess the stability of the cervical spine in an unresponsive patient.

Once occipitocervical junction injuries are diagnosed, management decisions are based on several factors, including the extent and stability of injury, the presence or progression of neurological deficits, and patient-specific factors that influence the risks with different treatments. Nonoperative management typically includes some type of rigid (halo) or semirigid (collar) orthosis. Operative management is generally indicated for injuries that are unstable, have significant potential for delayed instability, have

43.1

Occipitocervical junction injury classification systems

A. Location of bone or ligamentous injury
Pure ligamentous injuries
Occipitoatlantal dislocations
Transverse ligament injuries
Rotatory C1-2 dislocations

Isolated fractures
Occipital condyle fractures
C1 (lateral mass, ring)
C2 (odontoid, body, hangman, posterior element)

Mixed ligamentous and bony injuries

B. Site/Level of Injury
Occipital bone (C0)	(e.g., condyle fracture)
C0-1 ligaments	(e.g., occipitoatlantal dislocation)
C1	(e.g., lateral mass, ring fractures)
C1-2 ligaments	(e.g., transverse ligament injuries)
C2	(odontoid, body, hangman, posterior element fractures)

C. Degree of stability
Stable
Low probability of delayed instability
High probability of delayed instability
Unstable

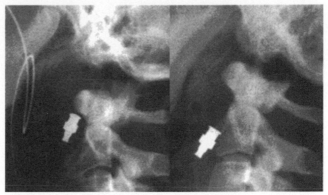

Figure 43.1 Lateral cervical x-rays demonstrating occipitocervical dislocation. The craniovertebral instability is apparent in the two images. (*From Dickman CA, Spetzler RA, Sonntag, VKH [eds]: Surgery of the Craniovertebral Junction. New York, Thieme, 1998.*)

progressive neurological deficits, and/or cause significant deficits or symptoms that are not controlled with nonoperative measures. Operative planning may include obtaining additional imaging (e.g., dedicated studies for image-guidance), ensuring the availability of appropriate instrumentation, and arranging neurophysiologic monitoring where appropriate.

Diagnosis and Management
Occipitocervical Dislocations

Occipitocervical dislocations are relatively uncommon ligamentous injuries that usually result from hyperflexion and distraction during high-impact blunt trauma.[1,36] These injuries are highly unstable, frequently fatal, and usually result in significant neurologic injury from stretching, compression, and/or distortion of the spinal cord, brainstem, and cranial nerves.[8] In addition, significant morbidity and mortality can result from vertebral artery injury. Recognition and rapid management of these injuries may limit further injury, but even with appropriate care, neurologic deficits can progress. Although initially felt to be rare, several series of trauma fatalities have revealed an incidence between 8% and 19%.[1]

Lateral cervical spine radiographs may recognize occipitocervical dislocations (sensitivity 0.57), especially in severe injuries. However, these injuries can be difficult to diagnose with plain radiographs alone, especially with less-severe dislocations. In addition, the frequent presence of coexisting significant head trauma can delay recognition of spinal injury. Diagnostic clues include prevertebral soft-tissue swelling, an increase in the dens-basion distance, and separation of the occipital condyles and C1 lateral masses (Figure 43.1). CT imaging with reconstruction

views (sensitivity 0.84) usually provides a better assessment of fractures and alignment than plain x-rays. The presence of subarachnoid hemorrhage supports but does not confirm the diagnosis. MRI imaging can be helpful for diagnosis (sensitivity 0.86), to assess the extent of spinal cord compression and injury, and to demonstrate compressive hematoma lesions.[29]

Based on the injury pattern, occipitoatlantal dislocations have been classified by Traynelis[44] into four types: type I (anterior), type II (longitudinal), type III (posterior), and "other" (complex). A number of diagnostic radiographic criteria have been described that assess the relationship between the skull base and cervical spine (Figure 43.2). Although developed for lateral plain x-rays, these criteria can also be used on sagittal-reconstruction CT views provided there are no significant artifactual distortions. Wackenheim's clival line extends along the posterior surface of the clivus and should be tangential to the tip of the dens.[45] Ventral or dorsal translation of the skull in relation to the dens will shift the clival line to either intersect or run posterior to the dens, respectively. Power's ratio is based on the relationship of the B-C line (from the basion to the C1 posterior arch) and the O-A line (between the opisthion and the C1 anterior arch).[39] Normal BC/OA ratios average 0.77, while pathologic ratios (greater than 1.0) typically represent occipitocervical dislocations. However, false-negatives can occur with longitudinal or posterior dislocations. The Wholey dens-basion technique assesses the distance from the basion to the dens tip.[46] Although variability is common, in adults the average distance is about 9 mm and pathological distances are greater than 15mm.[12] Dublin's method, the least reliable method, measures the distance from the mandible (posterior ramus) to the anterior part of C1 (normally 2 to 5mm) and C2 (normally 9 to 12mm).[15]

Initial management of these injuries focuses on immobilization, almost always with a halo orthosis. Cervical collars are potentially dangerous because they may produce distraction and thereby promote further injury. Similarly, traction can cause neurologic worsening (2 of 21 patients) and should be avoided or used with extreme caution.[28,29] Nonoperative management does not provide definitive treatment of these injuries because of the significant liga-

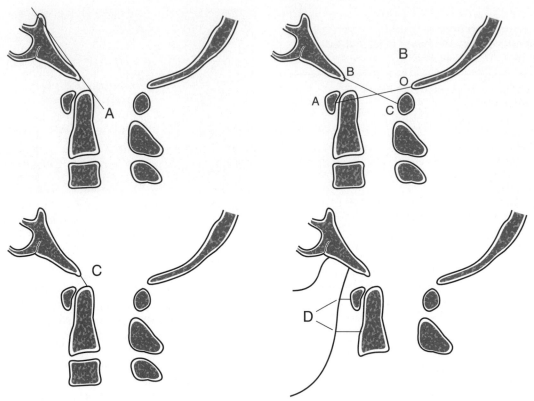

Figure 43.2 Four radiographic methods for assessing occipitocervical dislocation:
(A) Wackenheim's clival line; **(B)** Power's ratio (BC/OA); **(C)** Wholey dens-basion technique;
and **(D)** Dublin's method. See text for details. *(From Barrow Neurologic Institute, with permission.)*

mentous disruption that cannot be expected to heal even
with prolonged rigid (halo) external immobilization (11 of
40 patients had a nonunion and/or neurologic deterioration).[29] Operative stabilization consists of an occipitocervical arthrodesis with rigid internal fixation (discussed below
and in the chapter on High Cervical and Occipitocervical
Plate, Rod, Wire, and Bone Techniques). Decompression
and restoration of alignment may also be necessary to maximize neurologic recovery.

Transverse Ligament Injuries

Isolated traumatic transverse ligament injuries are unstable injuries that can result in significant upper cervical
spinal cord injury either during the initial trauma or after-
wards. These injuries are more common in hyperflexion
injuries. Because transverse ligament injuries may be difficult to recognize on initial (neutral) plain x-rays, an elevated index of suspicion is required in some settings—for
example, high-impact trauma.

Transverse ligament injuries are suggested or diagnosed with radiographic imaging. A widened atlantodental
interval (ADI) on flexion lateral cervical radiographs
(greater than 3mm in adults, greater than 5mm in children) suggests transverse ligament insufficiency. Thin-cut
CT imaging with reconstruction views may suggest the
diagnosis by demonstrating a C1 lateral mass avulsion fracture at the ligamentous insertion. Thin-cut MRI with
attention to the transverse ligament when using gradient

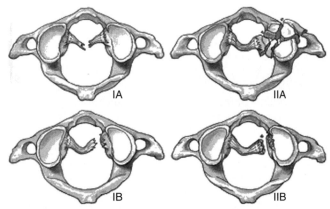

Figure 43.3 Classification of transverse ligament injuries. Type I
injuries are disruptions of the transverse ligament in its
midportion (IA) or periosteal insertion laterally (IB). Type II
injuries lead to transverse ligament insufficiency through
fractures that disconnect the C1 lateral mass tubercle (insertion
of the transverse ligament) via a comminuted fracture (IIA) or
an avulsion fracture (IIB). *(From Barrow Neurologic Institute,
with permission.)*

echo sequences can directly demonstrate a transverse ligament injury.[13] If the diagnosis is uncertain, dynamic (flex-
ion/extension) imaging is appropriate for cooperative
patients. Based on CT and MRI traumatic transverse ligament injuries can be classified into two categories (Figure
43.3). Type I injuries involve disruptions of the midportion

(IA) or periosteal insertion laterally (IB). Type II injuries involve fractures that disconnect the C1 lateral mass tubercle for insertion of the transverse ligament via a comminuted fracture (IIA) or an avulsion fracture (IIB).[11]

The management of transverse ligament injuries is based on the type of injury. Type I injuries are pure ligamentous injuries that cannot be expected to heal with nonoperative external fixation. Therefore, operative stabilization with a posterior C1-2 arthrodesis and fixation is indicated. The surgical options include C1-2 posterior wiring, C1-2 Halifax clamps, C1-2 transarticular screws, and/or C1-2 segmental screw fixation (see later section and Chapter 111). Type II injuries have a much higher chance of healing with halo immobilization (up to 74%).[11] If a nonunion is still present after a prolonged period of immobilization (greater than 3 months) then operative stabilization is generally appropriate.

Rotatory C1-2 Subluxations

Rotatory C1-2 subluxations are ligamentous injuries that are more common in children and adolescents. These injuries typically present with neck pain and a fixed, rotated "cocked-robin" head position. Open mouth x-rays may demonstrate an asymmetry of the C1 and C2 lateral masses. CT imaging can confirm the rotatory subluxation diagnosis and demonstrate coexisting fractures. C1-2 axial rotation greater than 47 degrees confirms the diagnosis. Three-view CT imaging (15 degrees to left, neutral, and 15 degrees to right) can also be helpful in establishing the diagnosis.[16,17] MRI imaging may detect a coexistent transverse ligament injury.

The treatment of C1-2 rotatory subluxations is generally nonoperative. Axial traction with a halter device or Gardner-Wells tongs can usually achieve reduction of the injury. Prolonged traction and/or the use of muscle relaxants may be needed. Periodic imaging may help to assess progress but clinical improvement in the alignment and symptoms often provides confirmation of a successful reduction. Operative reduction and fixation are reserved for irreducible injuries, recurrent subluxations, and transverse ligament injuries.

Occipital Condyle Fractures

Occipital condyle fractures generally occur with axial trauma and are almost always unilateral (greater than 90%). These injuries are classified into three types according to Anderson and Montesano.[3] Type I injuries are comminuted fractures that result from axial trauma. Type II fractures are extensions of linear basilar skull fractures. Type III injuries, the most common, are avulsion fractures of the condyle that can result from a variety of mechanisms. The incidence of occipital condyle fractures has been estimated to be between 1% and 3% of blunt craniocervical trauma cases.[33] Although plain radiographs (usually open mouth x-rays) may occasionally identify the injury, they have an unacceptably low sensitivity (estimated 3.2%) and should not be relied on when the diagnosis is suspected. CT imaging with reconstruction views provides the best assessment of fracture pattern and alignment.[33, 37]

Occipital condyle fractures are generally stable and therefore are typically managed with an external nonrigid orthosis (collar) until the fracture heals (often 12 weeks). Type III fractures are felt to be more prone to instability and, when significant displacement or clinical concern exists, halo immobilization may be appropriate. Operative stabilization with an occipitocervical fusion is generally reserved for situations when there are associated cervical fractures or significant ligamentous injuries.

C1 Fractures

Isolated C1 fractures comprise approximately 5% of cervical spine fractures. These injuries occur with axial trauma with or without lateral bending.[27] Open mouth x-rays may suggest the injury, but CT imaging with reconstruction views provides the best assessment of fracture pattern and alignment. Fractures can include almost any part of the ring or lateral masses of C1. Aside from unilateral lateral mass fractures, the fractures usually occur at multiple sites (Figure 43.4). Jefferson fractures are four-part fractures with bilateral ventral and dorsal ring fractures. The assessment of these injuries is focused on evaluating the integrity of the transverse ligament and on recognizing any additional fractures.

The management of C1 fractures is based on the integrity of the transverse ligament that can be assessed indirectly with several radiographic criteria such as a widened atlantodental interval (ADI, greater than 3mm) and increased spread of the lateral masses of C1 over C2 (greater than 6.9mm, Rule of Spence)[42] or directly through high-resolution MRI (Figure 43.5). If the transverse ligament is intact, isolated C1 fractures are generally stable and can be treated with an external orthosis (e.g., SOMI) primarily for symptom control until the fracture heals. With transverse ligament insufficiency, operative stabilization is indicated by using a C1-2 fusion technique such as dorsal C1-2 wiring techniques, C1-2 transarticular screws, C1 lateral mass-C2 pars/pedicle screws, or ventral C1-2 screw fixation (see chapter on High Cervical and Occipitocervical Plate, Rod, Wire, and Bone Techniques). The surgical choice is primarily based on patient anatomy and fracture pattern as well as surgeon experience/preference. Postoperatively, most operations employing rigid internal fixation can be managed with a non-rigid external orthosis (e.g., collar or SOMI) but C1-2 dorsal wiring without additional instrumentation generally warrants the use of a halo.[41]

C2 Fractures

C2 fractures comprise about 20% of all cervical spine fractures and are classified as either odontoid, body, or other fractures (e.g., hangman, laminar, or spinous process).

Odontoid Fractures

C2 odontoid fractures can occur from a number of mechanisms but most often are caused by hyperextension injuries. Although lateral cervical spine x-rays may demonstrate some fractures, especially those with displacement,

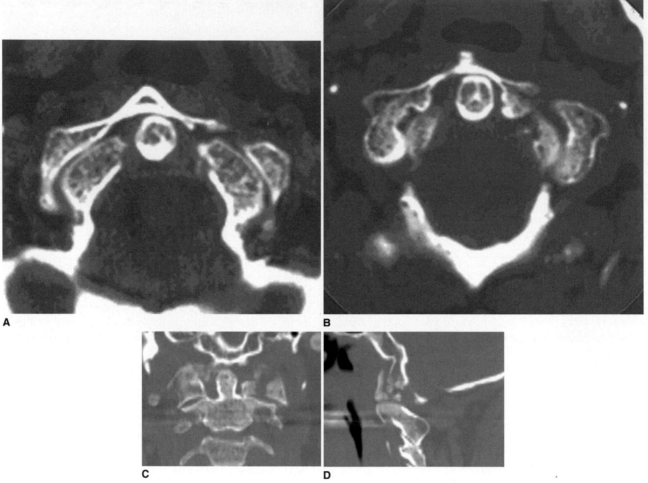

Figure 43.4 C1 lateral mass fracture. Axial CT images **(A-B)** and coronal **(C)** and sagittal **(D)** CT reconstruction views of right C1 lateral mass fracture from high-speed MVA. The fracture healed with 3 months' external immobilization.

this technique can easily miss fractures, especially those with degenerative changes or minimal displacement. Open-mouth radiographs are very helpful to diagnose most odontoid fractures, but these also may be inconclusive. Thin-cut CT images with sagittal and coronal view reconstruction views are the best way to diagnose and characterize odontoid fractures as well as to find associated fractures and plan treatment.[23, 26]

Anderson and D'Alonzo classified odontoid fractures into three types based on the location of the fracture line through the odontoid tip (type I), odontoid base (type II), or C2 body (type III)[2] (Figure 43.6). Type I fractures are essentially avulsion fractures of the odontoid tip and are rare, generally stable, and usually managed with an external semirigid (collar) or rigid (halo) orthosis. Type II fractures are the most common type of odontoid fracture. These fractures are unstable and prone to nonunion because they occur in an area of relatively reduced osseous vascularity. Therefore, rigid halo immobilization or surgical stabilization is often necessary. Hadley *et al.* described Type IIA fractures that are comminuted fractures at the base of the dens with associated free fragments.[25] These fractures are considered particularly unstable and surgical stabilization is advisable, usually with a posterior C1-2

fusion. Type III fractures involve the vertebral body and are discussed below.

C2 Body Fractures

The C2 body can be defined as the C2 bone mass caudal to the dens and ventral to the pars interarticularis bilaterally. Benzel *et al.*[6] have classified C2 body fractures based on the orientation of the fracture line: coronal, sagittal, or transverse (a.k.a. horizontal rostral). The transverse type of C2 body fracture is a more appropriate description of type III odontoid fractures. The coronal and sagittal types represent "vertical" fractures. Of the vertical fractures, the coronal type was much more common (4:1) and resulted from multiple (four) different mechanisms. Sagittal type C2 body fractures were caused by axial loading trauma. Figure 43.7 shows an example of C2 body fracture.

Although standard cervical radiographs will often recognize the fracture, the injury is best characterized with high-resolution CT scanning with multiplanar reconstruction views. It is important to look for radiographic evidence of involvement of the foramen transversarium and clinical signs of vertebral artery injury. If there is a significant degree of suspicion, an assessment of the vertebral

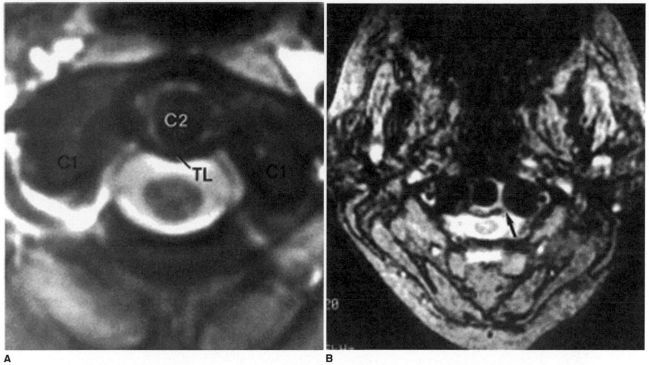

A   **B**

Figure 43.5 Axial MRI images demonstrating an intact (**A**) and ruptured (**B**) transverse ligament. (*From Dickman CA, Spetzler RA, Sonntag, VKH [eds]:* Surgery of the Craniovertebral Junction. *New York, Thieme, 1998.*)

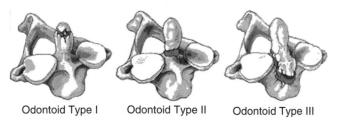

Odontoid Type I   Odontoid Type II   Odontoid Type III

Figure 43.6 C2 odontoid fractures as described by Anderson and D'Alonzo. Type II fractures are better described as C2 body fractures as discussed later. (*From Barrow Neurologic Institute, with permission.*)

artery with CT, MR, or transfemoral catheter angiography should be obtained. The stability of C2 body fractures can be assessed either with fracture characteristics (displacement, etc.) or with careful dynamic (flexion/extension) imaging when stability appears likely.

A majority of C2 body fractures can be managed nonoperatively. Depending on the alignment, degree of displacement, and fracture location either a collar or halo may be advisable. Occasionally, surgical intervention with a posterior C1-2 fusion is indicated, particularly for highly unstable fractures and in patients prone to nonunion.

Other C2 Fractures

Traumatic spondylolisthesis fractures of the axis (a.k.a. hangman fractures) are characterized by bilateral fractures through the C2 pars/pedicle (Figure 43.8). Although these fractures may be unstable, they do not generally cause sig-

nificant compromise of the spinal canal or neurologic injury. Effendi and colleagues[18] have classified these injuries into three groups based on mechanism. Type I fractures occur with axial loading and hyperextension. Type II fractures are hyperextension injuries with rebound hyperflexion. Type III fractures are primarily flexion injuries with rebound extension. Levine and Edwards[34] modified the system by adding a Type IIA, which represents flexion-distraction injuries. Type I and II injuries are generally stable and can usually be managed in a collar. With significant displacement (greater than 4 to 6 mm) halo immobilization may be advisable. Type IIA injuries are more likely to be unstable, especially with displacement greater than 4 to 6mm or angulation more than 11 degrees. If one or both of these findings are present, surgical stabilization may be necessary. Type III injuries are unstable and typically require surgical stabilization. Isolated C2 laminar or spinous process fractures are stable and therefore are usually managed with an orthosis (e.g., collar).

Combination Occipitocervical Junction Injuries

Combination occipitocervical junction fractures involve bony and ligamentous injuries of the foramen magnum (e.g., occipital condyles), C1, and/or C2. These injuries are usually unstable, occur with high-impact trauma, and frequently result in death or major neurologic injury. Management of these injuries is similar to that of occipitocervical dislocations. Initial management involves airway management, craniovertebral immobilization, and medical stabilization. Patients who are medically stable are consid-

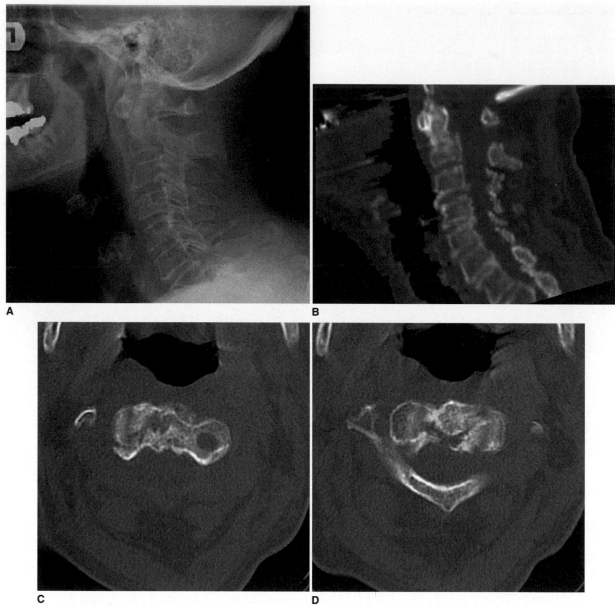

Figure 43.7 C2 body fracture. An 80-year-old woman presented with neck pain after a fall. A lateral cervical radiograph (**A**) suggests C1-2 instability from a C2 fracture. A sagittal CT reconstruction image (**B**) suggests a C2 body fracture with a transverse fracture line (also described as type III odontoid fracture) and a vertical (coronal) fracture line in addition. Axial CT images (**C-D**) confirm the C2 vertical fracture component.

ered for more prolonged stabilization with rigid external halo immobilization and/or surgical stabilization. For incomplete spinal cord injuries, decompression of any compressive bony or hematoma lesions may also be necessary and are performed when the patient is medically stable. With complete spinal cord injuries, the timing of surgical stabilization and/or decompression is less urgent.

Combined C1-2 fractures occur with axial trauma with or without lateral bending. Although plain x-rays may indicate a combined fracture, a CT with multiplanar reconstruction views is usually necessary to fully characterize the fractures and alignment and to plan treatment.

Compared with isolated C1 and C2 fractures, combined C1-2 fractures are typically associated with a higher rate of instability, nonunion and neurologic injury. Treatment of these injuries is based on the degree and location of bony and ligamentous injuries. Because of the instability, rigid external (halo) and/or internal fixation are usually required. Standard surgical procedures (e.g., posterior C1-2 interspinous fusion) may not be possible because of the extensive fractures. Advances in instrumentation and surgical technique have allowed the development and increased use of newer types of surgical stabilization such as C1-2 transarticular screws or C1-2 segmental fixation.[30,40]

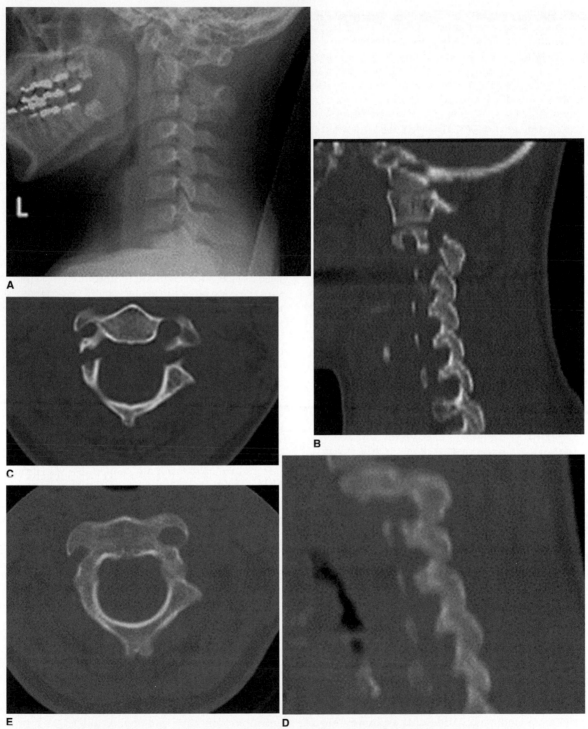

Figure 43.8 C2 hangman fracture. A 21-year-old woman presented with neck pain after a motor vehicle accident. Initial studies with a lateral cervical radiograph (**A**), sagittal CT reconstruction image (**B**), and axial CT image (**C**) demonstrate the fracture through the C2 pars/pedicle with moderate displacement. The fracture healed with 3 months' external immobilization as evidenced by the delayed sagittal CT reconstruction (**D**) and axial CT (**E**) images.

Surgical Procedures
General Principles
Preoperative

There are multiple indications for surgical intervention with occipitocervical trauma. Decompression may be necessary to relieve compromise of the spinal canal or neural foramina from bone or soft tissue (e.g., hematoma) lesions. Internal stabilization may be necessary to treat acute or impending instability, to promote fracture healing, and to improve and/or correct alignment.

Preoperative care is focused on optimizing medical stability; obtaining the necessary imaging to assess the injury location, alignment, and stability; and determining the nature and timing of any needed intervention. The timing of surgery is based on the patient's medical stability, the degree of spinal compression, the presence or progression of neurologic deficits, and the availability of optimal operating room equipment and personnel. When appropriate likelihood of benefit exists, incomplete spinal cord injuries with compressive lesions warrant surgical intervention as soon as possible. This is particularly true when there are progressive neurologic deficits. However, it is important to note that neurologic deterioration may be related to the natural history of the neurologic injury and/or medical deterioration (such as hypoxia, hypotension, and/or fever) that would not necessarily be assisted with surgical intervention. Rather, it is possible that the patient would have a better chance of tolerating, and hopefully benefiting from, the procedure by delaying surgery until the medical issues have been optimized. Where possible, early surgical intervention is desirable to promote early mobilization and transfer to rehabilitation.

Preoperative planning includes selection of a primary surgical plan, as well as backup plans, which may become necessary. When needed, specialized equipment (image-guidance, instrumentation, etc.) and/or neurophysiologic monitoring should be reserved or arranged in advance. When possible, preoperative studies should be loaded onto image-guidance equipment (if used) in advance to permit preoperative surgical planning.

Intraoperative

The intraoperative setup and positioning are directed by the nature of the injury and surgical approach. In general, occipitocervical junction trauma procedures use a midline dorsal approach in the prone position with cranial fixation or a high ventral cervical approach in the supine position. Transoral, transfacial, and far lateral skull base approaches are not commonly used in the trauma setting. When there is sufficient neurologic function and degree of potential new or exacerbated neurologic injury, spinal monitoring (sensory and/or motor evoked potentials) may prove useful for determining whether the final surgical positioning is satisfactory.

Exposure of the occipitocervical junction for trauma may require special considerations. For example, throughout the case, careful attention is advised to maintain appropriate alignment and minimize/avoid pressure on unstable or compressed neurologic structures. Traumatic injuries to the subcutaneous and paraspinal soft tissues can distort and obscure anatomic landmarks. Additional exposure (length of incision, number of levels, etc.) may aid recognition and management of the abnormal anatomy because of increased exposure of adjacent normal anatomy.

Decompression and stabilization are two primary objectives of surgery. Decompression of neurologic structures may be accomplished by correcting alignment or removing compressive bone, ligaments, or other space-occupying lesions such as hematomas. The goals of stabilization are to achieve stability and, where appropriate and possible, to maintain/improve alignment, maximize neurologic function, and improve symptoms. Achieving bony

fusion is the best way to achieve long-term stability. At surgery, the standard principles of arthrodesis should be followed with careful attention to the exposure and preparation of bone fusion surfaces and the choice of structural or morselized bone graft material. For the majority of cases, internal fixation with instrumentation is utilized to maintain alignment and promote osseous union. Nonrigid external orthoses (e.g., collar, SOMI) do not provide substantial immobilization of the occipitocervical junction. Therefore, instrumentation should be optimized with some (or all) of the following strategies: including all segments involved in the construct, using larger diameter or length screws as possible, and achieving bicortical purchase where advisable.

Occipitocervical junction trauma operations may require special closure considerations. For example, these cases may have an increased risk of postoperative infection as the incision typically extends beyond the suboccipital hairline. Copious irrigation is therefore advised before closure. Leaving one or more Jackson Pratt or Hemovac drains may reduce the incidence of postoperative hematoma or seroma collections. However, these drains should be used cautiously if the dura was compromised from the trauma or during the procedure. In the event of dural compromise, primary closure and/or augmentation (patch, fibrin glue product, etc.) and extra attention to fascial closure are often used. A running locked suture may be used for the skin closure. For cases with significant dural compromise that is not possible to repair, several days of postoperative spinal drainage via local (through or near incision) or distal (typically lumbar) placement of an intrathecal catheter may reduce chances of a postoperative spinal fluid collection or leak.

Postoperative

Postoperatively, a rigid external orthosis (halo) is used if instrumentation is not used or if concern exists regarding the instrumentation or bone quality. Otherwise, some type of nonrigid orthosis is advisable in most cases. Because standard cervical collars do not immobilize the occipitocervical junction well, special orthoses are often used (e.g., SOMI braces). Although not officially studied or approved for cervical spine application, use of an external spinal stimulator may improve the fusion rate. Stimulators may be used as a primary adjunct in patients prone to nonunion (e.g., smokers) or in an attempt to salvage a nonunion. Patients with spinal cord injury require special attention to nutrition, skin care, pulmonary toilet, DVT prophylaxis, and often psychiatric support. Patients with poor nutrition are prone to wound healing problems and sutures may need to be left for a prolonged period (2 to 3 weeks or more).

Postoperative imaging with plain x-rays and/or CT imaging is generally obtained when possible to assess final anatomy and alignment, extent of decompression, and position of instrumentation. Interval imaging is followed as needed to assess bony fusion. When sufficient stability is achieved either from the internal fixation and/or bone fusion, the orthosis can be weaned. Dynamic imaging with flexion/extension views can provide an assessment of stability and bony fusion.

Occipitocervical Junction Fusions

Occipitocervical junction fusions are performed through a posterior midline approach. Ventral occipitocervical junction fusions may be technically possible, but the transoral approach for trauma is prone to infection and may be difficult to expose because of the altered anatomy and difficult to close because of the instrumentation. Finally, the ventral approach is not ideal for placement of instrumentation because the surgeon is limited in the extent of rostrocaudal exposure.

At surgery, careful transfer to the prone position is required. The patient's head is fixed with a Mayfield head clamp unless the patient is already in a halo ring/vest. In this case, it is possible to turn the patient in the halo ring/vest. After locking the halo ring to the operating table with a Mayfield halo adapter, the posterior part of the halo vest and connecting bars are disassembled to permit adequate exposure. As much as possible, the head should be positioned in an appropriate alignment such that the patient will naturally look forward (i.e., avoid hyperflexed or hyperextended positioning to maximize patient visualization and comfort). The iliac crest region is prepped to harvest bone graft. The exposure should extend from the inion down to C3 at least, with the ability to continue further caudally as necessary. Decompression of the foramen magnum should be performed if necessary, but the ability to achieve a midline fusion and take advantage of the thicker midline bone is limited by an extensive midline suboccipital decompression.

Structural unicortical strips are harvested from the iliac crest along with cancellous bone. Local autograft from the cranium or posterior spinal elements is significantly less effective in achieving fusion. Allograft is least likely to achieve fusion and generally should not be relied on. Instrumentation options include inverted U rods with wiring, inverted-Y plate/screw constructions, and specialized cranial plate attachments for polyaxial cervical screws.[5,31] The midline bone is thickest and allows placement of longer screws with better purchase. The construct should be extended to at least C2 and sometimes lower to achieve optimal fixation. However, advances in instrumentation have made the longer constructs to the lower cervical spine or cervicothoracic junction uncommon unless additional subaxial cervical spine injuries exist. Dorsal C0-1 transarticular screw fixation has recently been described by Grob[24] and by Gonzales *et al.*[22] The utility of this procedure is still evolving. The instrumentation options and techniques are discussed further in Chapter 111. Postoperatively, a collar or SOMI brace is used until bony fusion occurs (usually 12 weeks). Halo immobilization is used when the bone quality or fixation is suboptimal.

Dorsal C1-2 Fixation

Dorsal C1-2 fusions are indicated for unstable C1 and/or C2 fractures and are performed through a dorsal midline approach. C1-2 fusion requires sacrifice of the movement at C1-2 (primarily rotation); therefore, for appropriate fractures with an intact transverse ligament, odontoid screw fixation may be preferable.

At surgery, the positioning is similar to that used in occipitocervical junction fusions. However, if transarticular screw placement is planned, then the head should be flexed as possible to facilitate screw placement. The exposure should extend from the foramen magnum through C3. If the dorsal elements of C1 and C2 are intact and do not need to be decompressed, then structural autograft from the iliac crest is harvested for placement between or along the posterior elements of C1 and C2. Careful exposure, preparation, and decortication of the fusion surfaces are important to maximize the chances of achieving fusion. The caudal edge of C1 is a common site for nonunion and deserves special attention.

Instrumentation options include C1-2 wiring alone or with additional screw instrumentation, C1-2 Halifax clamp fixation, C1-2 transarticular screw fixation, and C1-2 segmental screw fixation.[30,40] The wiring options include the Brooks, Gallie, and Sonntag interspinous fusion operations.[*] The relative advantages and disadvantages of the various options are listed in Box 43.2. Postoperatively, a collar or SOMI brace is used until bony fusion occurs (usually 12 weeks). Halo immobilization is used when the bone quality or fixation is suboptimal.

Odontoid Screw Fixation

Ventral odontoid screw fixation is appropriate for many unstable C2 odontoid fractures that require operative fixation. The main advantages of odontoid screw fixation are the preservation of C1-2 mobility and the relatively

---

[*]References 7,9,14,20,21,35,38.

BOX 43.2

Advantages and disadvantages of dorsal C1-2 fusion operation

C1-2 Wiring (Brooks, gallie, sonntag)
Advantages: Familiar technique, avoids screw
Disadvantages: Least rigid, requires more external fixation, higher nonunion rate

C1-2 Transarticular screw fixation
Advantages: Most rigid
Disadvantages: Potential for vertebral artery injury

C1-2 Segmental fixation
Advantages: Familiar technique, avoids screw, very rigid
Disadvantages: Venous plexus bleeding, potential vertebral artery injury

C1-2 Sublaminar hooks (Halifax clamps)
Advantages: Avoids screw placement risks
Disadvantages: Less rigid than screws, weak in extension, may narrow canal

short and well-tolerated nature of the procedure. However, the procedure is not possible for many patients and fractures because of anatomic limitations. For example, patients with short necks, barrel chests, inability to tolerate cervical extension, insufficient transverse ligaments, oblique fracture lines and/or significantly comminuted fractures are poor candidates for this procedure. For these patients, a posterior C1-2 fusion is typically chosen.

At surgery, the patient is positioned supine with the head extended, usually in a fixed position with a Mayfield head holder. Biplanar fluoroscopy is generally used. Using a lower cervical incision about at C5-6, a standard high ventral cervical approach is followed to the C2-3 region. A variety of standard or specialized retractors can be used to maintain exposure. Using a Kerrison rongeur or high-speed drill, a midline trough is made in the anterior-superior C3 vertebral body. Next, by using the trough, a power drill with a 2mm bit is used to drill a pilot hole from the anterior inferior border of C2, across the fracture line, and to the tip of the odontoid process. The appropriate length screw is determined by preoperative x-ray or CT measurements, intraoperative fluoroscopy, and/or by measuring the length of drill bit. If reduction of the fracture is needed, then a lag screw of an appropriately shorter length should be selected. Even without significant fracture displacement, lag screws can promote fusion by providing a compressive force across the fracture line. The screw is threaded into the pilot hole in the same trajectory. One or two screws may be placed,

but one is typically used because the outcomes appear similar.[32,43] Several odontoid screw systems exist with specialized instrumentation and screws.[4] One system includes cannulated screws that can be placed over a threaded drill bit (Figure 43.9).[10] See Chapter 111 for additional details on the instrumentation.

Patients are managed with a postoperative external orthosis (collar) until the fracture heals (usually 10 to 12 weeks). Success rates are high, with fusion rates between 81% and 96%.[32,43] In the event of a nonunion, a posterior C1-2 technique can be used.

Ventral C1-2 Fixation

Ventral C1-2 transarticular fixation can be used if an odontoid screw fixation is not successful during an anterior approach. In addition, the approach may be used if a posterior approach is not feasible for some reason or a posterior C1-2 fusion has failed. The technique involves bilateral screws through the lateral vertebral body of C2 into the lateral mass of C1. Careful preoperative assessment of the course of the vertebral artery is essential to determine whether the procedure is feasible.

At surgery, the positioning, approach, and exposure are similar to odontoid screw placement. An entry point is marked with a pilot hole at the groove between the C2 body and superior articular facet. This point is just medial to the vertebral artery. The screw trajectory is about 20 degrees lateral and rostral as needed to

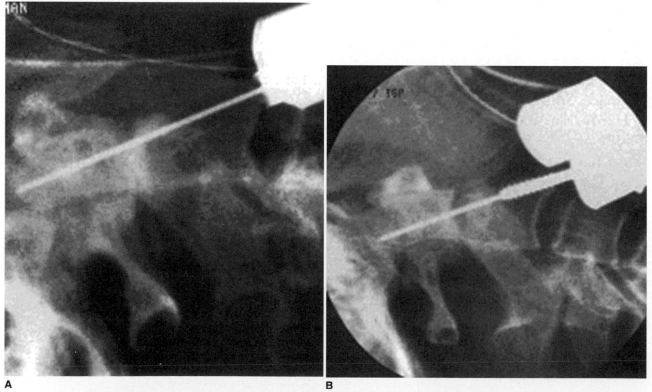

A   **B**

Figure 43.9 C2 odontoid screw placement with a cannulated screw system. Initially a K-wire drill bit is placed (**A**). Next, the screw is carefully threaded over the drill bit under fluoroscopic guidance (**B-C**). (*From Dickman CA, Spetzler RA, Sonntag, VKH [eds]: Surgery of the Craniovertebral Junction. New York, Thieme, 1998.*)   *Continued*

engage the C1 lateral mass securely. The screws are placed with fluoroscopic guidance (ideally biplanar) (Figure 43.10). Although placing onlay bone graft may be possible, the technique does not allow direct placement of bone between C1 and C2 and aims to have fusion occur at the articulation between the C1 and C2 lateral masses. Therefore the C1-2 facet should be scraped with a small curette as possible to promote arthrodesis. Postoperatively, a collar or SOMI brace is used until bony fusion occurs (usually 12 weeks). Halo immobilization is used when the bone quality or fixation is suboptimal.

Ventral C2-3 Fixation

Ventral C2-3 discectomy and fusion are used for some traumatic C2 hangman fractures that demonstrate suffi-

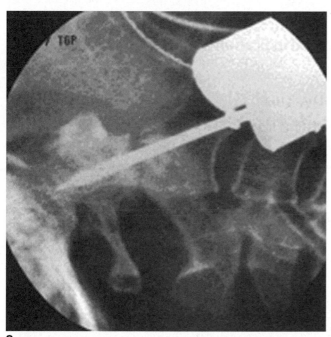

C

Figure 43.9 *cont'd*

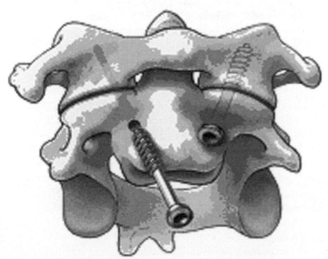

Figure 43.10 Anterior C1-2 transarticular instrumentation. *(From Barrow Neurological Institute, with permission.)*

cient instability to warrant operative fixation.[19] By using a high cervical incision, a standard high anterior cervical approach and limited C2-3 discectomy is performed. If there is canal compromise from osteophytes or a herniated disc, then a more extensive dorsal osteophytectomy and/or discectomy is performed. The alignment, if abnormal, is optimized as much as possible. After preparing the end plates, a C2-3 arthrodesis is performed with structural iliac crest autograft or allograft. Then C2-3 ventral cervical plating is performed (see the chapter on High Cervical and Occipitocervical Plate, Rod, Wire, and Bone Techniques and the chapter on Ventral Subaxial Cervical Fixation Techniques). Extra attention is required for the C2 screws because of the unique anatomy. A narrow low-profile plate is preferred to facilitate placement. The patient is managed with a postoperative external orthosis (collar) for 6 or more weeks depending on the degree of preoperative instability.

Dorsal C2-3 fixation does not adequately treat these fractures unless direct dorsal C2 screw placement across the fracture is used. C1-3 dorsal segmental instrumentation with intervening screw or sublaminar wiring at C2 is another alternative procedure.

Summary

Occipitocervical junction trauma can result in a variety of injury patterns involving the regional bony, ligamentous, neurologic, and vascular structures. Because of the vital nature of these threatened structures, accurate diagnosis and careful management are required. In particular, careful attention is directed to achieving and maintaining an appropriate alignment from the onset of trauma. After initial airway management and medical stabilization, relevant diagnostic imaging should be obtained. Although many of the injuries are able to be recognized on plain radiographs, high-resolution CT scanning with multiplanar reconstruction views generally provides the most useful information. MR imaging may be difficult to obtain but is usually best to assess any spinal canal compromise and the integrity of important ligaments. Flexion/extension imaging is most useful for cooperative patients who do not have significant spinal canal compromise.

The primary focus of the imaging is to identify and characterize injuries and to guide management. If instability is documented or presumed based on imaging, then some combination of external and/or internal stabilization is necessary to protect neurologic function and permit mobilization. If malalignment is present, correction with an orthosis, traction, and/or operation is considered depending on the degree of deformity and its relation to current or potential neurologic injury. When needed, traction should be performed cautiously and only with a solid understanding of the injury, as distraction can exacerbate certain injuries (e.g., occipitoatlantal dissociation).

Operative procedures generally require rigid intraoperative fixation via a halo ring/adaptor or Mayfield head clamp. Surgical intervention is focused on decompressing significant compressive lesions (bone, hematoma, etc.), restoring alignment, and achieving stabilization with arthrodesis and usually internal fixation. Advances in instrumentation and surgical technique (e.g., image guidance, surgical innovation) have led to the development of better, stronger internal fixation constructs that can spare motion (e.g., odontoid screw fixation), reduce the number of levels to be fused, and avoid or minimize use of uncomfortable orthoses such as halos, which have inherent risks themselves (pulmonary compromise, skull pin site complications, etc.). These instrumentation techniques are discussed further in the chapter on High Cervical and Occipitocervical Plate, Rod, Wire, and Bone Techniques. Achieving bony fusion is an important goal of stabilization, and careful attention to technique is required. Although many trauma patients are good fusion candidates (young, healthy patients), liberal use of autograft is advised in most cases, because many patients may be or become critically ill and malnourished because of spinal or systemic injuries. Furthermore, nonunions can be difficult to manage and may require more substantial operative intervention. Overall, the treatment of occipitocervical injuries must be individualized on the basis of patient/injury characteristics and surgeon experience.

REFERENCES

1. Alker AJ, Oh YS, Leslie EV: High cervical spine and craniocervical junction injuries in fatal traffic accidents: a radiological study. *Ortho Clin North Am* 9:1003-1010, 1978.
2. Anderson LD, D'Alonzo RT: Fractures of the odontoid process of the axis. *J Bone Joint Surg Am* 56:1663-74, 1974.
3. Anderson PA, Montesano PX: Morphology and treatment of occipital condyle fractures. *Spine* 13:731-6, 1988.
4. Apfelbaum RI, Lonser RR, Veres R, Casey A: Direct anterior screw fixation for recent and remote odontoid fractures. *J Neurosurg* 93(2 Suppl):227-36, 2000.
5. Apostolides PJ, Dickman CA, Golfinos JG, Papadopoulos SM, Sonntag VK: Threaded Steinmann pin fusion of the craniovertebral junction. *Spine* 21:1630-7, 1996.
6. Benzel EC, Hart BL, Ball PA, Baldwin NG, Orrison WW, Espinosa M: Fractures of the C-2 vertebral body. *J Neurosurg* 81:206-12, 1994.
7. Brooks AL, Jenkins EB: Atlanto-axial arthrodesis by the wedge compression method. *J Bone Joint Surg Am* 60: 279-284, 1978.
8. Bucholz RW, Burkhead WF: The pathological anatomy of fatal atlanto-occipital dislocations. *J Bone Joint Surg Am* 61A:248-250, 1979.
9. Dickman CA, Crawford NR, Paramore CG: Biomechanical characteristics of C1-2 cable fixations. *J Neurosurg* 85: 316-22, 1996.
10. Dickman CA, Foley KT, Sonntag VK, Smith MM: Cannulated screws for odontoid screw fixation and atlantoaxial transarticular screw fixation. Technical note. *J Neurosurg* 83:1095-100, 1995.
11. Dickman CA, Greene KA, Sonntag VKH: Injuries involving the transverse atlantal ligament: classification and treatment guidelines based upon experience with 39 injuries. *Neurosurgery* 38:44-50, 1996.
12. Dickman CA, Greene KA, Sonntag VKH: Traumatic injuries of the craniovertebral junction. In Dickman CA, Spetzler RA, Sonntag, VKH (eds): *Surgery of the Craniovertebral Junction*. New York, Thieme, 1998, 175-196.
13. Dickman CA, Mamourian A, Sonntag VK, Drayer BP: Magnetic resonance imaging of the transverse atlantal ligament for the evaluation of atlantoaxial instability. *J Neurosurg* 75:221-7, 1991.
14. Dickman CA, Sonntag VK, Papadopoulos SM, Hadley MN: The interspinous method of posterior atlantoaxial arthrodesis. *J Neurosurg* 74:190-8, 1991.
15. Dublin AB, Marks WM, Weinstock D, Newton TH: Traumatic dislocation of the atlanto-occipital articulation (AOA) with short-term survival: With a radiographic method of measuring the AOA. *J Neurosurg* 52:541-546, 1980.
16. Dvorak J, Hayek J, Zehnder R: CT-functional diagnostics of the rotatory instability of the upper cervical spine. Part 2. An evaluation on healthy adults and patients with suspected instability. *Spine* 12:726-31, 1987.
17. Dvorak J, Panjabi MM, Hayek J: Diagnosis of hyper- and hypomotility of the upper cervical spine using functional computerized tomography. *Orthopade* 16:13-9, 1987.
18. Effendi B, Roy D, Cornish B, Dussault RG, Laurin CA: Fractures of the ring of the axis. A classification based on the analysis of 131 cases. *J Bone Joint Surg Br* 63:319-27, 1981.
19. Francis WR, Fielding JW, Hawkins RJ, Pepin J, Hensinger R: Traumatic spondylolisthesis of the axis. *J Bone Joint Surg Br* 63:313-8, 1981.
20. Gallie WE: Skeletal traction in treatment of fractures and dislocations of the cervical spine. *Ann Surg* 106:770-776, 1937.
21. Gallie WE: Fractures and dislocations of the cervical spine. *Am J Surg* 46:495-499, 1939.
22. Gonzalez LF, Crawford NR, Chamberlain RH, Perez Garza LE, Preul MC, Sonntag VK, Dickman CA: Craniovertebral junction fixation with transarticular screws: biomechanical analysis of a novel technique. *J Neurosurg* 98:202-9, 2003.
23. Greene KA, Dickman CA, Marciano FF, Drabier JB, Hadley MN, Sonntag VK: Acute axis fractures. Analysis of management and outcome in 340 consecutive cases. *Spine* 22:1843-52, 1997.
24. Grob D: Transarticular screw fixation for atlanto-occipital dislocation. *Spine* 26:703-7, 2001.
25. Hadley MN, Browner CM, Liu SS, Sonntag VK: New subtype of acute odontoid fractures (type IIA). *Neurosurgery* 22:67-71, 1988.
26. Hadley MN, Dickman CA, Browner CM, Sonntag VK: Acute axis fractures: a review of 229 cases. *J Neurosurg* 71:642-7, 1989.
27. Hadley MN, Dickman CA, Browner CM, Sonntag VK: Acute traumatic atlas fractures: management and long-term outcome. *Neurosurgery* 23:31-5, 1988.
28. Hadley MN, Walters BC, Grabb PA, Oyesiku NM, Przybylski GJ, Resnick DK, Ryken TC, Mielke DH: Guidelines for the management of acute cervical spine and spinal cord injuries. *Clin Neurosurg* 49:407-98, 2002.
29. Hadley MN, Walters BC, Grabb PA, Oyesiku NM, Przybylski GJ, Resnick DK, Ryken TC, Mielke DH: Management of acute central cervical spinal cord injuries. *Neurosurgery* 50:S166-72, 2002.
30. Harms J, Melcher RP: Posterior C1-C2 fusion with polyaxial screw and rod fixation. *Spine* 26:2467-71, 2001.

31. Hurlbert RJ, Crawford NR, Choi WG, Dickman CA: A biomechanical evaluation of occipitocervical instrumentation: screw compared with wire fixation. *J Neurosurg* 90:S84-90, 1999.

32. Jenkins JD, Coric D, Branch CL Jr: A clinical comparison of one- and two-screw odontoid fixation. *J Neurosurg* 89:366-70, 1998.

33. Leone A, Cerase A, Colosimo C, *et al.*: Occipital condylar fractures: A review. *Radiology* 216:635-44, 2000.

34. Levine AM, Edwards CC: The management of traumatic spondylolisthesis of the axis. *J Bone Joint Surg Am* 67: 217-26, 1985.

35. Melcher RP, Puttlitz CM, Kleinstueck FS, Lotz, JC, Harms J, Bradford DS: Biomechanical testing of posterior atlantoaxial fixation techniques. *Spine* 27:2435-2440, 2002.

36. Muhonen MG, Menezes AH: Weaver syndrome and instability of the upper cervical spine. *J Pediatr* 116:596-9, 1990.

37. Mody BS, Morris EW: Fracture of the occipital condyle: case report and review of the world literature. *Injury* 23:350-2, 1992.

38. Naderi S, Crawford NR, Song GS, Sonntag VK, Dickman CA: Biomechanical comparison of C1-C2 posterior fixations. Cable, graft, and screw combinations. *Spine* 23:1946-55, 1998.

39. Powers B, Miller MD, Kramer RS, Martinez S, Gehweiler JA Jr: Traumatic anterior atlanto-occipital dislocation. *Neurosurgery* 4:12-17, 1979.

40. Resnick DK, Benzel EC: C1-C2 pedicle screw fixation with rigid cantilever beam construct: case report and technical note. *Neurosurgery* 50:426-8, 2002.

41. Sonntag VK, Hadley MN, Dickman CA, Browner CM: Atlas fractures: treatment and long-term results. *Acta Neurochir Suppl (Wien)* 43:63-8, 1988.

42. Spence KF Jr, Decker S, Sell KW: Bursting atlantal fracture associated with rupture of the transverse ligament. *J Bone Joint Surg Am* 52:543-9, 1970.

43. Subach BR, Morone MA, Haid RW Jr, *et al.*: Management of acute odontoid fractures with single-screw anterior fixation. *Neurosurgery* 45:812-9,1999.

44. Traynelis VC, Marano GD, Dunker RO, Kaufman HH: Traumatic atlanto-occipital dislocation: Case Report. *J Neurosurg* 65:863-870, 1986.

45. Wackenheim A: *Roentgen Diagnosis of the CrANIOVERtebral Region.* New York, Springer-Verlag, 1974.

46. Wholey MH, Bruwer AJ, Baker HL: The lateral roentgenogram of the neck (with comments on the atlanto-odontoid-basion relationship). *Radiology* 71: 350-356, 1958.

CHAPTER 44

Trauma Surgery: Cervical Spine

Scott D. Daffner, Alexander R. Vaccaro, Charles Stillerman, and L. Erik Westerlund

Injury to the cervical spine should be suspected in any patient complaining of neck pain after trauma. Initial management of the multiply injured patient will be dictated by established advanced trauma life support (ATLS) protocols, with priority directed to management of airway, breathing, and circulatory compromise. The "chin lift and jaw thrust" method of securing an airway may decrease the space available for the spinal cord (beyond that seen with nasal or oral intubation) and should be avoided in the patient with a known or suspected cervical spine injury. Spinal precautions (to include cervical spine immobilization) should be maintained throughout the early stages of evaluation and resuscitation of the multi-trauma patient.[3] The most common causes of injury to the neck are motor vehicle accidents (MVAs), diving into shallow water, and sporting-related activities. A thorough history of a given accident may further influence clinical suspicion for the presence of a cervical spine injury. Did the patient strike his or her head? Was there evidence of cranial impact to the windshield from inside the vehicle? Was the patient ejected? Was there any indication of weakness or paralysis noted at the accident scene? Was the patient neurologically intact at the scene with later deterioration in neurologic function? Information gathered through such questioning will guide clinical suspicion for neck injury and may provide important prognostic information when neurologic compromise is present. Obtaining information regarding prior history of injury, underlying preexisting cervical spine disease, or systemic conditions (such as ankylosing spondylitis) is important as well.

The physical examination of the patient with known or suspected cervical spine injury begins at the patient's head and progresses distally. It is complete only after a thorough evaluation of the entire musculoskeletal system has been performed.[5] Abrasions or lacerations about the scalp, face, or neck provide mechanistic clues, alerting the examining physician to the potential for underlying spine trauma. The posterior cervical spine should be palpated carefully to evaluate for focal tenderness, step-off, or hematoma. Range of motion should be prohibited until the radiographic evaluation of the neck has been completed. All voluntary motion of the arms, hands, fingers, legs, feet, and toes should be observed, graded, and recorded, along with any noted sensory or deep tendon reflex compromise. Incomplete spinal cord lesions are described by a constellation of characteristic neurologic findings determined by the anatomic location of an injury. Examples include Brown-Sequard syndrome, central cord syndrome,[13] anterior cord syndrome, and posterior cord syndrome (Table 44.1). A rectal examination is essential (particularly in the neurologically injured patient in order to document any degree of sacral sparing) and should be accompanied by bulbocavernosus reflex testing to assess for spinal shock. Spinal shock is the transient loss of all motor, sensory, and reflex function distal to the level of an acute spinal cord injury. The classification of a neurologic deficit as complete or incomplete cannot be determined until spinal shock has resolved.

The radiographic evaluation often begins with the ATLS screening series that includes a cross-table lateral view of the cervical spine from the occiput to C7/T1. Care should be taken that the lower part of the cervical spine is completely visualized; superimposition of the shoulders may be overcome with caudally directed manual traction on the patient's arms. Experience at multiple centers has demonstrated that most missed cervical fractures and subluxations are those present at the lower aspect of the cervical spine.[8,14] A swimmer's view often proves useful for complete visualization of the cervicothoracic junction.[4] An open-mouth odontoid view, an anteroposterior (AP) and lateral plain radiograph of the entire spine should be obtained if a fracture is found resulting from the frequent occurrence of noncontiguous spinal injuries. Radiographic findings suggestive of cervical instability are summarized in Table 44.2.

Segmental injuries are common and the presence of injury at one level should prompt a careful search for subtle injuries elsewhere in the spine.[14] Computed tomography (CT) should be routinely used to provide a more accurate delineation of osseous injuries.[1,2] Sagittally reconstructed images are helpful in illustrating the sagittal alignment of the spine as well as injuries at the cervicothoracic junction. It is often helpful in demonstrating those fracture lines passing in the plane of the transaxial CT cuts. Magnetic resonance imaging (MRI) is used to further evaluate the nature and extent of neural and connective soft tissue injury. As such, MRI may be used to identify intracanilicular associated disc herniations, spinal cord contusions and often ligamentous disruption, and occult fractures.[5,6] Flexion and extension dynamic radiography is frequently used in the awake neurologically intact patient with isolated neck pain and normal plain radiographs. These films are often repeated in patients with persistent neck pain to minimize masked instability secondary to acute muscle spasm.

Soft-Tissue Neck Injuries

Isolated soft tissue injury is a common occurrence that has been variably described as whiplash, cervical sprain, cervical strain, acceleration injury, and hyperextension injury.[8,19,21,24,25] Each of these is nearly always the result of an excessive acceleration force acting to violently extend the neck beyond normal restraints. The overwhelming majority of these injuries occur as the result of MVAs.[23]

Symptoms may include nonfocal neck pain with or without accompanying radicular symptoms, isolated cervical

TABLE 44.1

Incomplete Spinal Cord Injury Syndromes

Central cord syndrome		The central cord syndrome is the most commonly encountered of all incomplete spinal cord injuries. Its presence is characterized by upper extremity motor weakness with relative sparing of the lower extremities. Expected neurologic recovery is fair to poor.
Anterior cord syndrome		Anterior cord syndrome results from damage to the interior two - thirds of the spinal cord with sparing of the posterior third. There is loss of motor function and pain and temperature sensation. There is preservation of vibration and position sense. Potential for recovery is variable.
Posterior cord syndrome		The posterior cord syndrome is the least common. Injury to the posterior columns results in loss of vibration and position sense. There may be sparing of crude touch. Potential for functional recovery is fair.
Brown-Sequard syndrome		Brown-Sequard syndrome is an uncommon injury pattern that is secondary to injury to half of the spinal cord. This is characterized by ipsilateral motor weakness and loss of proprioception, and contralateral loss of light touch, pain, and temperature sensation. Prognosis for ambulation is excellent in this setting.

TABLE 44.2

Radiographic Findings Suggestive of Cervical Instability

Direct Evidence of Instability	Indirect Evidence of Instability
Angulation > 11 degrees between adjacent segments[16] Anteroposterior translation > 3.5 mm[16] Segmental spinous process widening on lateral view[18] Facet joint widening[17] Malalignment of spinous processes on AP view Rotation of facets on lateral view[12] Lateral tilt of vertebral body on AP view[12]	Increased retropharyngeal soft-tissue margin[5] Avulsion fractures at or near spinal ligament insertions Minimal compression fractures of the anterior vertebral bodies[7,10,11,15] Nondisplaced fracture lines through the posterior elements or vertebral body[9]

radiculopathy, cervical myelopathy, and various related lumbar pain syndromes. Closed head injuries may be associated with these injuries. Intracranial manifestations include chronic headache, concussion, extra axial/intracranial bleeding, and sympathetic dysfunction. Additionally, psychiatric changes, including sleep disturbance, depression, mood changes or frank personality changes, may occur.[19]

The most common radiographic finding is the loss of normal cervical lordosis as seen on a lateral plain radi-

ograph.[18] Delayed flexion and extension radiographs are again obtained 2 weeks after resolution of acute muscle spasm to evaluate for evidence of potential destabilizing soft tissue disruption.[20] Bone scan has a limited role in screening for occult fractures in selected patients with atypical chronic pain.[19] If positive, a CT scan may then be performed for further evaluation.

Early intervention and treatment is based on the presenting injury subtype, including its pathomechanics, severity, and the overall medical status of the patient.[22] In the setting of a whiplash-type injury, initial use of a soft collar will improve comfort in many patients, although use should be limited to a 2- to 4-week period to minimize dependence, muscle atrophy, and decreased neck range of motion.[23] Isometric exercises and gentle, supervised range of motion should be initiated as soon as symptoms permit (or within 2 weeks of injury). The regimen should be performed several times a day and should include neck flexion/extension, rotation, and lateral flexion. Enlisting the assistance of a physical therapist may be beneficial, particularly in the early phases of recovery.

Transient Quadraplegia

A neurapraxia-type injury to the cervical spinal cord resulting in transient quadriplegics is most commonly seen in athletes participating in contact sports. The incidence among collegiate football players is 7.3 per 10,000 athletes. Plain radiographs are normal in this setting. The mechanism of injury is most often axial compression combined with hyperflexion or hyperextension. Sensory and motor neurologic deficits are bilateral and usually persist from several minutes to 48 hours following trauma. There is an association with developmental cervical stenosis, although effective guidelines for identification of predisposed athletes have been difficult to establish. Efforts to establish sensitive and specific screening methods to reliably identify "at-risk" athletes are under way.

Injuries to the Occipitocervical Articulation

Injuries to the occipitocervical junction are being recognized with increasing frequency while patient mortality rates are declining. Improved outcomes are likely a direct benefit of present trauma protocols that begin at the scene of an injury, supporting those who would not have previously survived. Heightened suspicion and early detection (with current imaging techniques) have further contributed to the above-noted trends.

The occipital condyles are paired, semi-lunar-shaped projections from the inferior aspect of the occiput that articulate with the atlantal lateral masses.[26] This articulation bears lit-tle intrinsic osseous stability, depending instead on the external and internal craniocervical ligaments for constraint. The internal craniocervical ligaments (tectorial membrane, cruciate ligament, and paired alar and apical ligaments) provide the predominance of the intrinsic occipito-atlantal stability. Injury to the craniocervical junction commonly occurs by three primary forces: distraction, compression, and lateral rotation.[39] Injuries may be mild and stable or life threatening (with complete osteoligamentous disruption).[33]

Occipital Condyle Fractures

Occipital condyle fractures are most often identified incidentally on head CT in the unconscious patient, though awake patients with complaints of deep suboccipital pain or occipital headache should be suspected of having sustained an injury to the occipital cervical junction.[26,37] The neurologic examination in survivors is often normal, although mild cord injury and cranial nerve injury has been reported. Classification of occipital condyle fractures is based on CT morphology (Figure 44.1).[26,38] A type I fracture is a comminuted fracture of the condyle resulting from impaction of the condyle by the lateral mass of C1. The mechanism is often a direct blow to the head. A type II injury is characterized by the presence of a related basilar skull fracture. Type III injuries are avulsion fractures occurring at the attachment site of the alar ligaments. They may be bilateral in up to 50% of cases and, in this circumstance, are associated with an atlanto-occipital dislocation. Treatment of stable type I and II injuries is cervical immobilization in a hard collar, cervicothoracic brace, or halovest for 6 to 8 weeks. Type II fractures demonstrating separation of the occipital condyle from the occiput may have inadequate lateral column support, thus requiring 8 to 12 weeks of halovest immobilization. Instability is commonly noted in type III injuries and is demonstrated by occipito-atlantal anterior-posterior displacement, longitudinal diastasis, or joint incongruity. Injuries identified as unstable are best managed with a posterior occipital-cervical arthrodesis.

Occipitocervical Dislocation/Dissociation

Until recently, few cases of patients surviving this entity had been reported.[28-32,40] Occipitocervical dislocation or dissociation often results from high-energy trauma, is

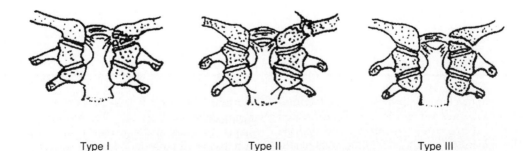

Type I　　　　Type II　　　　Type III

Figure 44.1 Occipital condyle fracture classification. A type I fracture is a comminuted fracture of the condyle resulting from the impaction of the condyle by the lateral mass of C1. The mechanism is often a direct blow to the head. A type II injury is characterized by the presence of a related basilar skull fracture. A type III injury is an avulsion-type fracture occurring at the attachment site of the alar ligaments.

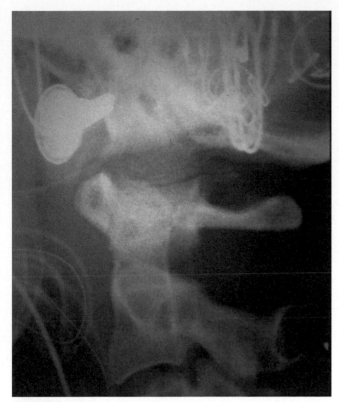

Figure 44.2 A lateral plain radiograph revealing longitudinal diastasis of the occipital-C1 articulation.

highly unstable, and is frequently fatal (Figure 44.2). High-resolution CT (with or without MRI) is often required to evaluate these injuries because they may be difficult to appreciate on plain radiographs unless significant displacement is present (Figure 44.3A). Occipitocervical instability (subluxation and dislocation) is classified according to the direction of displacement of the occiput.[27,34,36] Type I injuries are anterior subluxations of the occipital condyle relative to the atlantal lateral masses. These represent the most commonly observed injury pattern. Type II injuries are vertical displacements of the occipital condyles greater than 2mm beyond normal. C1-2 distraction injuries are included in this category. Type III injuries are posterior occipital dislocations and are exceedingly rare. In evaluating these injuries, more than 2mm of subluxation at the atlanto-occipital articulation indicates a functional loss of integrity of the major occipital-cervical stabilizers such as the alar ligaments and the tectorial membrane.[33,39] Treatment of occipitocervical instability is through closed or open reduction and surgical stabilization.[35] Traction is to be avoided in these injuries (Figure 44.3B,C).

Injuries to the First Cervical Vertebra

Traumatic Transverse Atlantal Ligament Insufficiency

Insufficiency or disruption of the transverse atlantal ligament (TAL) may occur following a violent flexion force to the upper cervical spine. Associated head injuries are common. Although survival after acute traumatic rupture had previously been thought unusual, it is now being reported

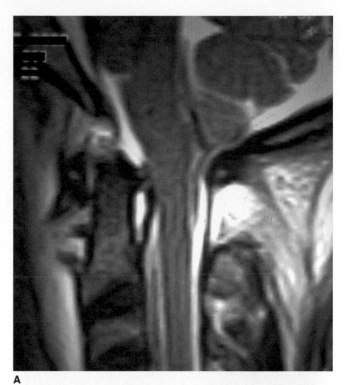

A

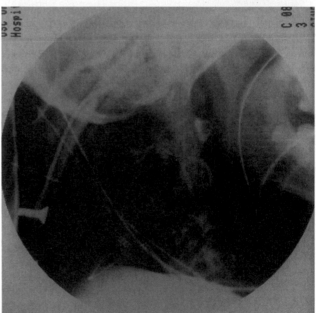

B

Figure 44.3 A, A sagittal MRI revealing longitudinal diastasis of the occipital C1 and C1-2 articulation. **B,** Lateral x-ray film of type IIB occipital-atlantal-axial dislocation. Note that in addition to the longitudinal distraction of the occiput relative to the atlas, a distractive injury also exists at the atlantoaxial segment. *Continued*

with increasing frequency.[43,52,67] Findings range from normal to transient quadriparesis. Permanent quadriparesis is rare given the fatal sequelae that typically follow complete injury at this level.[46,52,60] Associated clinical signs include cardiac and respiratory changes secondary to brain stem compromise, or dizziness, syncope, and/or blurred vision as a result of vertebral artery disruption. Symptoms may be exacerbated by neck flexion. A lateral plain radiograph often demonstrates abnormal translation (greater than 5mm) at the atlanto-dens interval (ADI).

Nonoperative treatment strategies have generally failed to provide satisfactory results, and the treatment of choice in most patients is a C1/C2 arthrodesis.

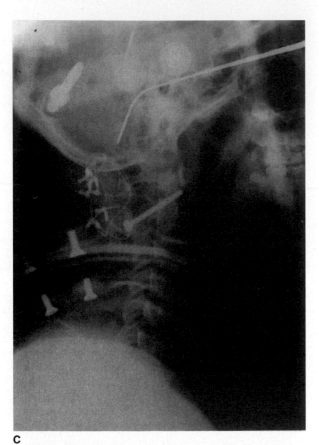

C

Figure 44.3 *cont'd* C, Postoperative lateral x-ray film demonstrates the screw-cable-rib construct used to stabilize this occipital-atlantal-axial instability. Posterior C1-2 transarticular screw fixation was used to provide rigid fixation across the atlantoaxial level, thereby blocking rotational movement at this level. Multiple titanium cables were also placed to achieve occiput to C2 fixation. Rib was used because it conforms to the occipital-atlantal-axial contour. (**B** and **C,** from Stillerman CB, Ranjan SR, Weiss MH: Cervical spine injuries: diagnosis and management. In Wilkins RH, Rengachary SS. *Neurosurgery,* ed 2, vol II. New York, McGraw-Hill Medical Publishing, 1995, p 2883.)

Acute disruption of the TAL may also be noted in association with a Jefferson-type burst fracture of C1.[56,59,65] Treatment in this circumstance should consist of cervical immobilization for 10 to 12 weeks awaiting union of the C1 arch. Persistent instability after completion of cervical immobilization may then be addressed with a C1/C2 fusion.[47,56]

Traumatic Rotatory Subluxation

Acute trauma is an unusual cause of acute C1-2 rotatory subluxation. The clinical presentation of C1-2 rotatory subluxation is the complaint of neck pain with findings of torticollis, and it is more commonly seen in children than adults. Four types of C1-2 rotatory injuries have been described (Figures 44-4 and 44-5).[45] Type I injuries involve poor rotational changes without associated subluxation. In the type II pattern there are 3 to 5mm of displacement of C1 on C2 (with one lateral mass acting as a pivot while the other rotates anteriorly). Type III injuries have more than 5mm of forward displacement of both lateral masses. Type II and III injuries are both associated with TAL incompetence, and neurologic involvement is common. Treatment is with halo or Gardner-Wells traction-reduction, followed by external immobilization for 2 to 3 months. Delayed instability is managed with a posterior stabilization procedure. Fixed or irreducible deformities as well as delayed presentation of this condition are again best managed with surgical stabilization.

Fractures of the First Cervical Vertebra

Fractures of C1 occur either as an isolated injury or often in combination with a fracture to the C2 vertebrae. The most common associated cervical spine injuries are a type II odontoid fracture and spondylolisthetic fracture of C2.[44,53-56,63] Fractures of C1 comprise up to 10% of all spine injuries and are thus encountered with relative frequency.[55] Neurologic injury is unusual.[41,42,54,63]

Fractures of C1 are classified generally into three categories. This classification scheme has proven useful in determining treatment options, expected clinical course, and prognosis (Figure 44.6). Type I fractures are limited to involvement of the dorsal arch, are often bilateral, and will typically occur at the junction of the lateral masses and posterior arch. This is the most common pattern of C1

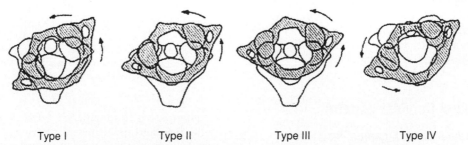

| Type I | Type II | Type III | Type IV |

Figure 44.4 Classification of rotatory subluxation. Type I, simple rotatory displacement without anterior shift. The odontoid acts as a pivot point. Type II, rotatory displacement with anterior displacement of 3 to 5mm. The lateral articular process is the pivot point. Type III, rotatory displacement with anterior displacement of more than 5mm. Type IV, rotatory displacement with posterior translation. (*From Fielding JW, Hawkins RJ Jr.: Atlanto-axial rotatory fixation [fixed rotatory subluxation of the atlanto-axial joint].* J Bone Joint Surg 59A:37-44, 1977.)

fracture and likely occurs secondary to hyperextension in conjunction with an axial load. A type II atlas fracture is a unilateral lateral mass injury that occurs as the result of an asymmetrically applied axial load. Intraarticular extension is not common but is reported.[50] A type III (or Jefferson) fracture is a burst-type fracture that involves three or more fractures through the anterior and posterior aspects of the C1 ring. The mechanism of this second most common pattern is that of a pure axially applied load.

Plain radiographs are useful in the evaluation of these injuries and will often demonstrate widening of the retropharyngeal soft tissue shadow from C1 to C3 (though these changes may take 6 or more hours to develop).[61,66] The open-mouth odontoid view will show lateral displacement of the lateral masses in a Jefferson-type fracture and may appear normal with the more common Type I posterior arch fracture. If total combined lateral displacement of the C1 lateral masses over C2 is greater than 6.9mm,[42,63,66] the transverse atlantal ligament has been disrupted, resulting in an unstable injury.[48,53,56,65] Type II fractures appear radiographically as unilateral displacement of the affected lateral mass on an open-mouth odon-

toid radiograph. Improvements in technique and image quality have made CT in the plane of the C1 ring helpful in fully defining these injuries.

The most important factor governing treatment and outcome is the occurrence of other simultaneous occurring injuries.[44,53,56] Treatment of isolated C1 fractures has traditionally been nonoperative, although some European centers have reported the successful surgical reduction and stabilization of markedly displaced Jefferson burst fractures.

Results with nonoperative treatment have been good,[50,64] although mild neck pain is a chronic sequelae in up to 80% of these patients.[54] There has been no reported correlation between fracture union/nonunion and functional outcome.*

Fractures of the Second Cervical Vertebra

Fractures of the Odontoid Process

Fractures of the odontoid process of the axis are relatively common among injuries of the upper cervical spine, although the exact prevalence is not well established. Odontoid fractures in young adults are most often secondary to high-energy trauma, such as MVAs or violent blows to the head (57% to 81%).[69,72,76,83] Those sustained by the elderly or very young are more commonly due to lower-energy falls.[74,86,89] As with other upper cervical injuries, the importance of clinical suspicion is critical to early recognition, since several studies have reported a high incidence of missed injuries, especially in patients with depressed mental status. The degree of neurologic involvement is widely variable; however, the majority of patients have a normal neurologic examination. Odontoid fractures are best visualized on lateral and open-mouth AP plain radiographs, as well as on reformatted sagittal CT images (because routine axial imaging may miss the fracture).

The most widely adopted classification system is that proposed by Anderson and D'Alonzo[69] following their experience with 60 patients with odontoid fractures treated over an 8-year period. This classification identifies three fracture types based on the anatomic location of the fracture line (Figure 44.7). Type I fractures are the least common and are described as an oblique fracture involving the

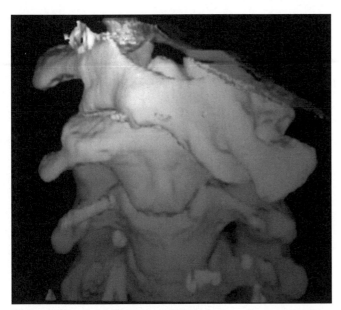

Figure 44.5 A three-dimensional CT scan revealing a traumatic rotatory dislocation of C1-2.

*References 49,51,54,57,58,62.

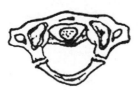 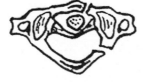 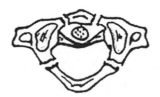

Type I   Type II   Type III

Figure 44.6 Classification of fractures of C1. Type I fractures are limited to involvement of the posterior arch, are often bilateral, and will typically occur at the junction of the lateral masses and posterior arch. A type II atlas fracture is usually a unilateral injury defined by involvement of the lateral mass (with fracture lines passing both anteriorly and posteriorly) as the result of an asymmetrically applied axial load. A type III (or Jefferson) fracture is a burst-type fracture that involves three or more fractures through the anterior and posterior aspect of the C1 ring.

superior tip of the dens. Type II odontoid fractures occur at the junction of the base of the dens and the body of the axis. This is the most common of the three types and the most controversial when discussing treatment.[72,75] Type II fractures have the highest rate of nonunion when treated nonoperatively, especially in the elderly. In type III fractures, the fracture line occurs in the body of the axis (primarily involving cancellous bone).

Isolated type I odontoid fractures are considered stable (unless they are associated with instability involving the occipital-cervical junction) and may be treated with a Philadelphia collar or similar orthosis. Type III fractures are often successfully managed with collar or halo immobilization. Type II fractures, however, lack both periosteum and cancellous bone at the fracture site, increasing the propensity for non-union.[68] Fractures that are significantly displaced may be realigned with traction reduction and immobilized with a halo vest until definitive treatment measures are selected. Factors considered to be associated with non-healing of Type II fractures include the degree of displacement, angulation, age of patient, loss of fracture reduction, and medical co-morbidities. Surgical stabilization, when chosen, may proceed through an anterior or posterior approach, depending on patient variables and fracture subtype.[70,77]

Traumatic Spondylolisthesis of the Axis

Traumatic spondylolisthesis of the axis is a bipedicular fracture of the second vertebrae that has been of interest for decades given its unique distinction as the "hangman's fracture.[71,82,84,85,88] The lesion encountered today, fre-

quently a result of an MVA, is similar in terms of location to the originally described hangman's fracture, but from a mechanistic standpoint bears little resemblance to the fracture subtype characteristic of judicial hanging.[79,80] The majority of these injuries are the result of motor-vehicle trauma and are infrequently associated with injury to the spinal cord (6.5%).[73] The basic mechanism of injury is that of rapid deceleration with forward flexion, axial impaction of the head on the windshield, followed by hyperextension after impact.[79,80] Each of the three primary fracture types[77-79] (Figure 44.8) are characterized further by variations of this mechanism. Dynamic radiography may be required to differentiate injury types.

Type I fractures occur through the neural arch in the region just posterior to the vertebral body. There is less than 3mm of translation and no angulation at the fracture site. This fracture subtype is the result of hyperextension and axial load. These may be treated with immobilization in a cervical orthosis for 3 months.

Type II fractures are divided further into type II and type IIA injuries. Type II fractures have greater than 3mm of displacement and significant angulation. The mechanism of injury is a combined force comprised of hyperex-

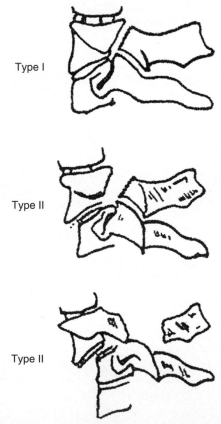

Figure 44.8 Classification of traumatic spondylolisthesis of the axis. Type I fractures occur through the neural arch in the region just posterior to the vertebral body. There is less than 3mm of translation and no angulation at the fracture site. Type II fractures have greater than 3mm of displacement and significant angulation. Type III fractures describe a type I (pars) fracture with an associated bilateral facet dislocation at C2-3. The critical feature is the classic presence of a free-floating posterior arch of C2.

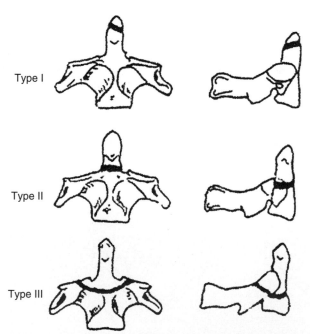

Figure 44.7 Classification of odontoid fractures. Type I fractures are the least common and are described as an oblique fracture involving the superior tip of the dens. Type II odontoid fractures occur at the junction of the base of the dens and the body of the axis. This is the most common type. Type III odontoid fractures are characterized by the fracture line passing through the cancellous bone of the vertebral body.

tension and axial loading (extension immediately followed by flexion). Fracture reduction may be achieved with skeletal traction in extension with immediate or delayed conversion to halo-vest immobilization. Surgical stabilization is infrequently necessary, although several surgical options exist in patients in whom a reduction cannot be maintained or in those unable to tolerate prolonged halo traction or halo-vest immobilization. In reducible fractures a primary pedicle screw osteosynthesis of C2 is possible. In fractures that are not anatomically reducible, or in cases of displaced nonunion, an anterior C2-3 arthrodesis is a viable treatment option (Figure 44.9).

Type IIA fractures are distinguished by an oblique fracture line often running from posterior-superior to anterior-inferior along the length of the pars. The mechanism is a flexion-distraction force. This fracture subtype is seen less than 10% of hangman's fractures. Reduction is by extension and slight axial loading; axial traction will accentuate the deformity. Reduction should be followed by immobilization in a halo-vest for 3 months.

Type III fractures describe a type I (pars) fracture with an associated bilateral facet dislocation at C2-3. The critical feature is the classic presence of a free-floating posterior arch of C2. These are unstable and irreducible by closed means, requiring surgical intervention.

An additional group of injuries may also be described as traumatic spondylolisthesis of C2-3 with either bilateral laminar fractures (Type IV) or bilateral facet fractures of the inferior articular processes of C2 (Type V). The mechanism of both types is flexion or shear, producing a highly unstable pattern.[78-81,87]

Injuries to the Lower Cervical Spine

The C3 through C7 vertebrae are similar in anatomy, biomechanics, and generally incur fracture patterns that are similar. However, the C7 vertebrae is exposed to greater axial compression and flexion load because of its location at the junction of the cervical and thoracic spine. Closed indirect injuries to the head and neck often produce patterns of injury that are therefore characteristic to the lower cervical vertebral column. The most severe neurologic sequelae arise as a result of a translational deformity, establishing ligamentous integrity as critically important to stability and treatment.

Both two- and three-column models are presently used in discussing traumatic pathoanatomy of the lower cervical spine. The three-column model was originally described in 1984 with specific reference to thoracolumbar injuries[93] but has since been modified to address cervical spine stability. It may be of greater utility to discuss the cervical spine as a two-column entity composed of an anterior and posterior column.[90,96,97,102] In the two-column model, the anterior spine consists of the posterior longitudinal ligament (PLL) and all remaining ventral structures, while the posterior column is comprised of all structures dorsal to the PLL (Table 44.3). The anterior and posterior columns are then reciprocally affected by flexion and extension moments.[96]

A mechanistic classification of subaxial cervical spine injuries was described by Allen et al.[90] in 1982. This classification divides mid- and low-cervical fractures into six groups based on force vector (initial dominant force) and subsequent incremental tissue failure (based on the attitude of the spine at failure). Abnormal relationships between adjacent vertebrae imply ligamentous failure, suggesting a shear force mechanism (since ligaments do not fail in compression). The three most common injury groups are compressive flexion, compressive extension, and distractive flexion. Vertical compression injuries occur with intermediate frequency, whereas distractive extension and lateral flexion injuries occur the least.[90] The presence of neurologic injury has not been strongly associated with any individual group within the classification, although it is

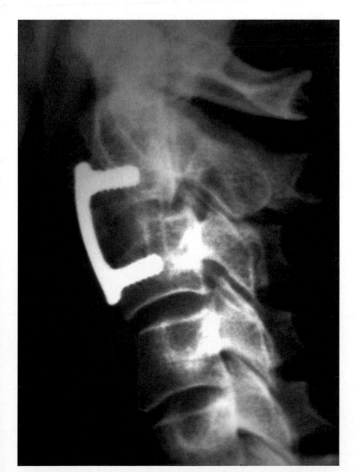

Figure 44.9 A lateral plain radiograph following an anterior C2-3 fusion for late instability of a type II hangman's fracture.

TABLE 44.3

The Two-Column Model of the Lower Cervical Spine

Anterior Column Components	Posterior Colum Components
Anterior longitudinal ligament	Pedicles and posterior vertebral arch
Intervetebral disc & anulus fibrosus	Posterior interspinous ligament complex
Vertebral body	
Posterior longitudinal ligament	

related to progressive osteoligamentous disruption or the severity of injury within a particular subgrouping.

Injuries as identified on plain radiographs should undergo further evaluation with CT scanning and possibly MRI. Assessment of plain radiographic, CT, and MRI findings assist in the evaluation of spinal stability.

Compressive Flexion

Compressive flexion injuries are caused by a ventral and axially directed load of increasing intensity. Compressive fractures without facet fracture or subluxation are usually stable injuries. Higher stages of injury involve increased ventral osseous and dorsal ligamentous injury and may be unstable (Figures 44-10 and 44-11). Treatment is tailored accordingly, although a frequent complication is late instability with conservative management.*

Surgical intervention often involves a cervical corpectomy and instrumented fusion with a structural graft. Adjunctive dorsal stabilization may be necessary in highly unstable advanced-stage lesions.

Compressive Extension

Compressive extension injuries result in a spectrum of pathology ranging from unilateral vertebral arch fractures to bilateral laminar fractures and finally to vertebral arch fractures with full ventral displacement of the vertebral body (Figure 44.12). Management is tailored based on injury severity and instability. An initial dorsal reduction

*References 91,92,94,95,99-101,103.

and stabilization procedure is often required, followed by adjunctive ventral stabilization if necessary.

Distractive Flexion

Distractive flexion injuries are also known as the flexion dislocation injuries. There is typically little osseous injury except for minor compression failure of the caudal vertebral segment. However, there is severe ligamentous damage involving the dorsal facet capsule complex, ligamentum flavum, and interspinous ligaments, and (depending on the presence of a unilateral or bilateral dislocation) injury to the posterior longitudinal ligament and intervertebral disc (Figures 44-13 and 44-14). A significant number of patients with this injury have also had an associated closed head injury.[98] Radiographic changes may be minimal in the early stages (*flexion sprain*) of this injury subtype. MRI is often useful to delineate the full extent of soft tissue disruption (including injury to the disc), although obtaining this study in an awake, alert, and cooperative patient should not delay traction reduction when plain radiographs demonstrate a translational displacement. Some physicians recommend a prereduction MRI prior to closed or open reduction of this injury subtype. All injuries in this family should be considered at risk for further displacement, making surgical stabilization the primary mode of treatment. Following a successful closed reduction, MRI should be obtained to evaluate for the presence of a herniated disc (Figure 44.15). If present, a ventral decompression and stabilization is the preferred surgical approach. If a closed reduction is not feasible, the surgical approach is predicated on the presence of an

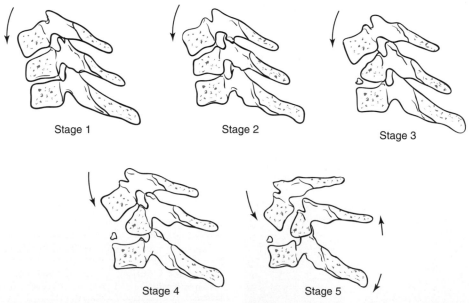

Stage 1   Stage 2   Stage 3

Stage 4   Stage 5

Figure 44.10 Compression flexion injury. Stage 1: Blunting and rounding-off of anterosuperior vertebral margin. Stage 2: Loss of anterior vertebral height with anteroinferior beaking. Stage 3: Fracture line extending from anterior surface of vertebral body extending obliquely through the subchondral plate (fractured beak). Stage 4: Less than 3mm of the posteroinferior vertebral margin into the neural canal. Stage 5: Greater than 3mm of displacement of the posterior aspect of the vertebral body with complete disruption of the posterior ligamentous complex. The vertebral arch is intact. (*From Rizzolo SJ, Cotler JM: Unstable cervical spine injuries:specific treatment approaches.* J Am Acad Orthop Surg 1:57-66, 1993.)

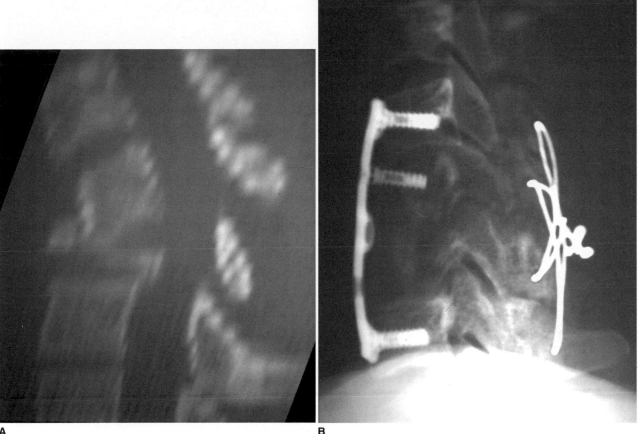

A

B

Figure 44.11 (**A**) A sagittal CT reconstruction revealing an advanced stage flexion compression cervical spinal injury. (**B**) A plain radiograph following an anterioposterior cervical decompression and stabilization procedure.

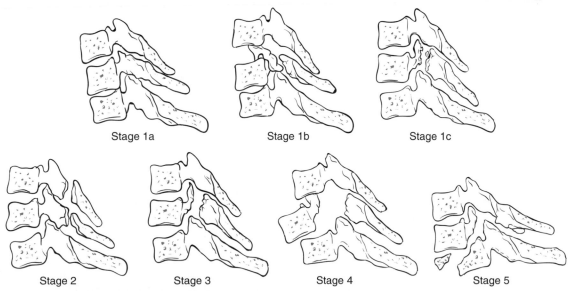

Stage 1a

Stage 1b

Stage 1c

Stage 2

Stage 3

Stage 4

Stage 5

Figure 44.12 Compression extension injury. Stage 1: Unilateral vertebral arch fracture through the articular process (stage 1a), the pedicle (stage 1b), or lamina (stage 1c), either with or without a rotary spondylolisthesis of the centrum. Stage 2: Bilaminar fracture at one or more levels. Stage 3: Bilateral fractures of the vertebral arch with partial-width anterior vertebral body displacement. State 4: Partial-width anterior vertebral body displacement. Stage 5: Complete anterior vertebral body displacement. (*From Rizzolo SJ, Cotler JM: Unstable cervical spine injuries: specific treatment approaches.* J Am Acad Orthop Surg 1:57-66, 1993.)

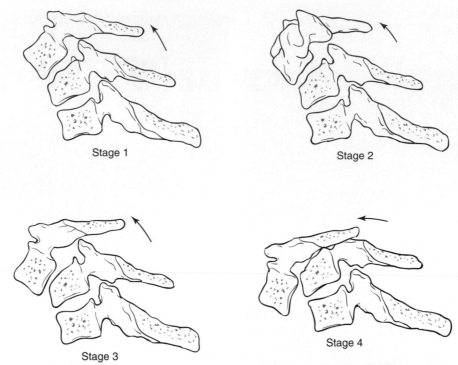

Stage 1

Stage 2

Stage 3

Stage 4

Figure 44.13 Distractive flexion. Stage 1: Flexion sprain injury with facet subluxation in flexion and divergence of spinous processes. There may be some blunting of the anterosuperior vertebral margin (similar to stage 1 compression-flexion injury). Stage 2: Unilateral facet dislocation with or without rotary spondylolisthesis. Stage 3: Bilateral facet dislocation with up to 50% vertebral body displacement. Stage 4: Completely unstable motion segment with full-width vertebral body displacement. *(From Rizzolo SJ, Cotler JM: Unstable cervical spine injuries: specific treatment approaches.* J Am Acad Orthop Surg *1:57-66, 1993.)*

extruded disc fragment. If present, a ventral decompression is required with or without an attempted ventral open reduction followed by a stabilization procedure. In the absence of an extruded disc fragment, a dorsal open reduction and stabilization procedure is often sufficient to obtain adequate spinal stability.

Vertical Compression

A vertical compression fracture is described as a cervical burst fracture caused by an axial-loading mechanism. Osseous failure is considered more significant by far than injury to the ligamentous structures in this injury (Figure 44.16). Treatment with halo immobilization is usually sufficient, although injuries at the cervical thoracic junction (C7) have a tendency to settle into kyphosis, which may require surgical intervention.[95] Ventral surgical decompression and stabilization is often necessary in patients with an incomplete neurologic deficit.

Distractive Extension

Distractive extension injuries are usually caused by forces acting to place the anterior elements under tension (Figures 44-17 to 44-20). Ventral disc space widening is the characteristic radiographic finding, although failure

may occur in a ventral-to-dorsal direction through the vertebral body. Less severe injuries may have little displacement, making radiographic detection difficult.[90,99] The presence of a ventral avulsion fracture resulting from an avulsion of the anterior longitudinal ligament may provide a clue to this injury type. This injury is especially unstable in a patient with ankylosing spondylitis or diffuse idiopathic skeletal hyperostosis (DISH) where there exist two rigid moment arms joined at an unstable junction. Distraction extension injuries are commonly associated with neurologic impairment. Patients frequently present with neurologic evidence of a central cord syndrome with significant weakness involving the upper extremities and relative sparing of the lower extremities. Spontaneous recovery is common.[90] Most distractive extension injuries without disc space disruption are stable and may be treated nonoperatively with late flexion-extension radiographs to confirm stability. Unstable injuries benefit from a ventral reconstructive procedure with ventral plate fixation acting as a ventral tension band.

Lateral Flexion

Lateral flexion injuries are secondary to asymmetric compressive loading resulting in unilateral vertebral body compression failure and ipsilateral posterior arch fracture

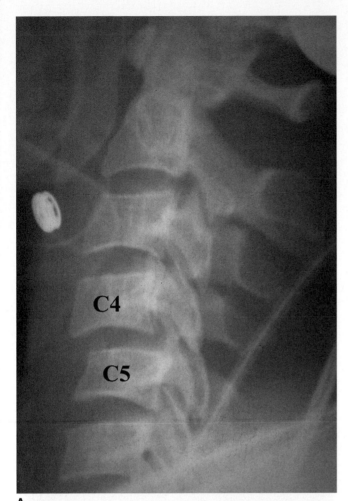

A

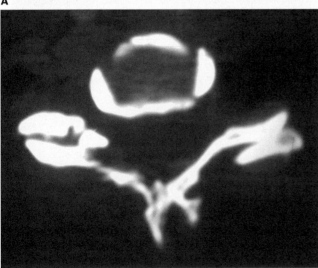

B

Figure 44.14 (A) A lateral plain radiograph revealing evidence of a C4-5 unilateral facet dislocation (type II distractive flexion injury). Note the 25% anterior subluxation of C4 on C5. (B) A transaxial CT scan revealing a left-sided unilateral facet dislocation. Note that the left C4 inferior articular process is anterior to the left C5 superior articular process.

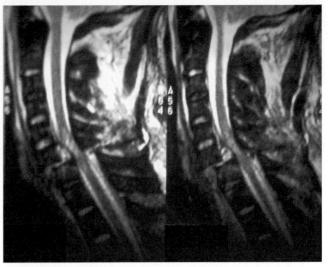

Figure 44.15 A sagittal MRI revealing significant cord edema and hemorrhage at the level of a C6-7 bilateral facet dislocation (type IV distractive flexion injury). Note the soft tissue density behind the body of C6, which may represent an extruded disc fragment.

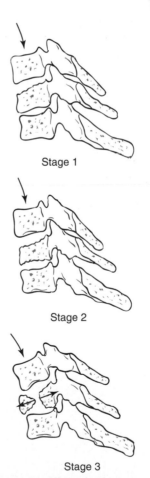

Stage 1

Stage 2

Stage 3

Figure 44.16 Vertical compression injury. Stage 1: Central "cupping fracture" of the superior or inferior vertebral end plate. Stage 2: Fracture of both superior and inferior end plates. Stage 3: Displacement and fragmentation of the vertebral body. (*From Rizzolo SJ, Cotler JM: Unstable cervical spine injuries: specific treatment approaches.* J Am Acad Orthop Surg *1:57-66, 1993.*)

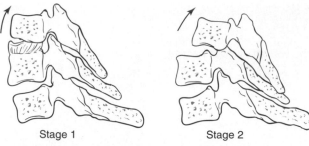

Stage 1   Stage 2

Figure 44.17 Distractive extension injury. Stage 1: Failure of anterior ligamentous complex, which may present as a widening of the disc space or a nondeforming transverse fracture through the centrum. Stage 2: Injury may be identified radiographically by an anterior marginal avulsion fracture of the centrum. Posterior ligamentous disruption may be identified by posterior displacement of the superior vertebra. *(From Rizzolo SJ, Cotler JM: Unstable cervical spine injuries: specific treatment approaches. J Am Acad Orthop Surg 1:57-66, 1993.)*

(Figure 44.21). As noted previously, this is the least common pattern of lower cervical spine disruption and is often stable, requiring cervical immobilization for 6 to 12 weeks.

Summary

Over half of the reported 50,000 annual new spinal cord injuries seen in the United States each year occur in the cervical spine. Of these, 11,000 have some degree of permanent deficit. Further advancement and implementation of advanced trauma life support (ATLS) protocols may be expected to continue producing increases in the incidence of multi-trauma survivors with proportional increases in the incidence of cervical spine trauma presenting in our emergency departments. These trends and statistics underscore the socioeconomic importance of cervical spine trauma, and they add greater emphasis to the critical nature of early injury recognition, evaluation, and proper treatment.

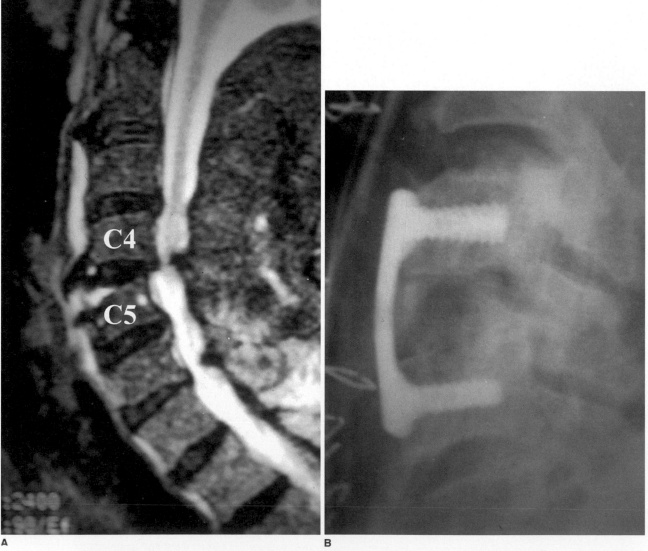

A   B

Figure 44.18 **(A)** A sagittal MRI revealing a distraction extension injury at the C4-5 level with retrolisthesis of C4 on C5. **(B)** A plain lateral radiograph following an anterior tension band (instrumented fusion) reconstruction of this injury.

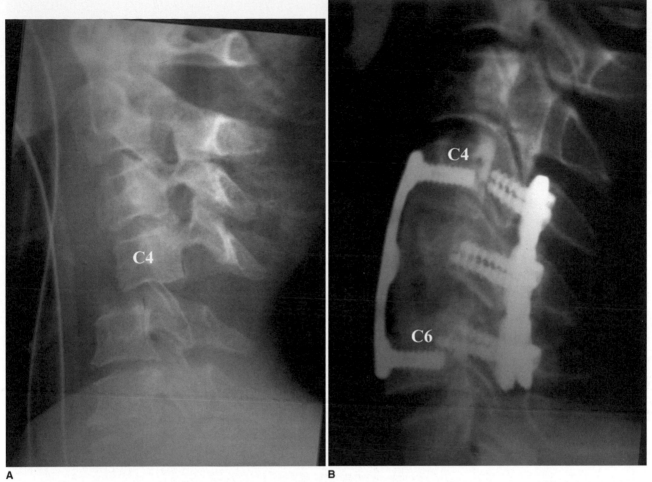

Figure 44.19 **(A)** A lateral plain x-ray revealing a high-grade distraction extension cervical injury at the C4-5 level. **(B)** A lateral plain x-ray following a posterior-anterior reconstruction procedure to obtain adequate spinal stability.

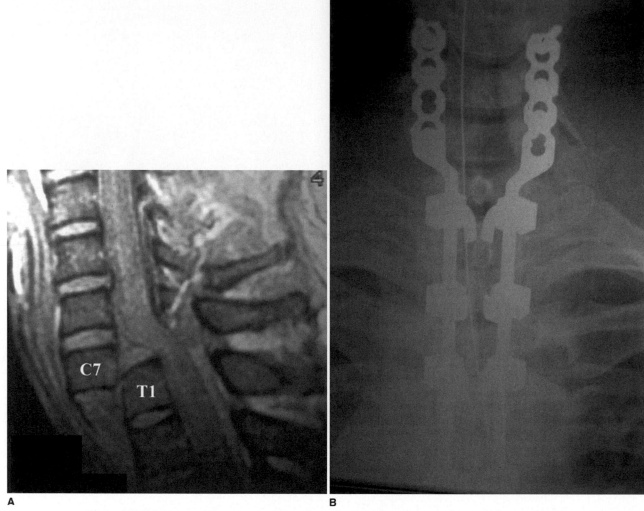

A

B

Figure 44.20 **(A)** A sagittal MRI revealing a high-grade distraction extension injury at the C7-T1 level. **(B)** The patient underwent a posterior open reduction and stabilization procedure using a cervicothoracic plate rod implant to obtain adequate spinal stability.

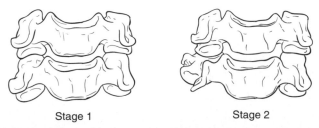

Stage 1   Stage 2

Figure 44.21 Lateral flexion. Stage 1: Asymmetric compression fracture of the centrum with associated ipsilateral vertebral arch fracture seen on lateral radiograph; no displacement is noted on the anteroposterior (AP) view. Stage 2: Displacement is evident on the AP as well as the lateral radiograph. There may also be tension failure of the contralateral ligaments and facet joint. *(From Rizzolo SJ, Cotler JM: Unstable cervical spine injuries: specific treatment approaches.* J Am Acad Orthop Surg *1:57-66, 1993.)*

REFERENCES

1. Alker G: *Computed Tomography With and Without Myelography.* Philadelphia, JB Lippincott, 1989.
2. Allen BL, Ferguson RL, Lehman TR, Obrien RP: A mechanistic classification of closed indirect fractures and dislocations of the lower cervical spine. *Spine* 7:1-27, 1982.
3. American College of Surgeons: *Advanced Trauma Life Support Manual.* Chicago, American College of Surgeons, 1984.
4. Clark CR, Ingram CM, El Khoury GY, Ehara S: Radiographic evaluation of cervical spine injuries. *Spine* 13:742-747, 1988.
5. Dunn EJ, Blazer S: Soft tissue injuries to the lower cervical spine. *Instr Course Lect* 36:499-512, 1987.
6. Goldberg AL, Rothfus WE, Deeb ZL: The impact of magnetic resonance on the diagnostic evaluation of acute cervicothoracic spinal trauma. *Skeletal Radiol* 17:89-95, 1988.
7. Herkowitz HN, Rothman RH: Subacute instability of the cervical spine. *Spine* 9:348-357, 1984.
8. Kirshenbaum KJ, Nadimpalli SR, Fantus R, Cavallino RP: Unsuspected cervical spine fractures associated with significant head trauma: the role of CT. *J Emerg Med* 8:183-198, 1990.
9. Lee C, Kim KS, Rogers LF: Sagittal fractures of the cervical vertebral body. *AJR* 139:55-60, 1982.
10. Mazur JM, Stauffer ES: Unrecognized spinal instability associated with seemingly simple cervical compression fractures. *Spine* 8:687-692, 1983.
11. Mori S, Nobuhiro O, Ojima T, *et al:* Observation of "tear drop" fracture-dislocation of the cervical spine by CT. *J Jpn Orthop Assoc* 57:373-378, 1983.
12. Scher AT: Unilateral locked facet in cervical spine injuries. *AJR* 129:45-48, 1977.
13. Schneider RC, Thompson JM, Bebin J. The syndrome of acute central cervical spinal cord injury. *J Neuro Neurosurg Psych* 21:216-227, 1958.
14. Vaccaro AR, An HS, Lin S, *et al:* Non-contiguous injuries to the spine. *J Spine Disord* 5:320-329, 1992.
15. Webb JH: Hidden flexion injury of the cervical spine. *J Bone Joint Surg* 55B:322-327, 1976.
16. White AA, Punjabi MM: Update on the evaluation of instability of the lower cervical spine. *Instr Course Lect* 36:499-520, 1987.
17. Woodring JH, Goldstein SJ: Fractures of the articular process of the spine. *Am J Radiol* 139:341-344, 1982.

Soft-Tissue Neck Injuries

18. Daffner RH: Evaluation of cervical cerebral injuries. *Semin Roentgenol* 27:239-253, 1992.
19. Gay Jr, Abbott KH: Common whiplash injuries of the neck. *JAMA* 152:1968-2704, 1953.
20. Herkowitz HN, Rothman RH: Subacute instability of the cervical spine. *Spine* 9:348-357, 1984.
21. Hohl M: Soft tissue injuries of the neck in automobile accidents: factors influencing prognosis. *J Bone Joint Surg (Am)* 56:1675-1682, 1974.
22. Joliffe VM: Soft tissue injury of the cervical spine: consider the nature of the accident. *BMJ* 307:439-440, 1993.
23. LaRocca HL. Cervical spine syndrome: diagnosis, treatment and long term outcome. In Frymoyer JW, Ducker TB, Hadler NM, *et al.* (eds): *The Adult Spine.* New York, Raven Press, 1991, pp 1051-1062.
24. McNab I: Acceleration injuries of the cervical spine. *J Bone Joint Surg (Am)* 46:1797-1799, 1964.
25. Wickstrom JK, Martinez JL, Rodriguez RPO, Haines DM: Hyperextension and hyperflexion injuries to the head and neck of primates. In *Neckache and Backache,* Springfield Press, 1970, pp 108-117.

Injuries to the Occipitocervical Articulation

26. Anderson PA, Montesano PX: Morphology and treatment of occipital condyle fractures. *Spine* 13:731-736, 1988.
27. Anderson PA, Montesano PX: Traumatic Injuries of the Occipito-Cervical Articulation. In Camins, O'Leary (eds): *Disorders of the Cervical Spine.* Baltimore, Williams & Wilkins, 1992.
28. DeBeer JDV, Thomas M, Walters J, Anderson P. Traumatic atlanto-axial subluxation. *J Bone Joint Surg (Br)* 70B:652-655, 1988.
29. Dibenedetto T, Lee CK: Traumatic atlanto-occipital instability: a case report with follow-up and a new diagnostic technique. *Spine* 15:595-597, 1990.
30. Eismont FJ, Bohlman HH: Posterior atlanto-occipital dislocation with fractures of the atlas an odontoid process: report of a case with survival. *J Bone Joint Surg (Am)* 60:397-399, 1978.
31. Evarts CM: Traumatic occipito-atlantal dislocation: report of a case with survival. *J Bone Joint Surg (Am)* 52:1653-1660, 1970.
32. Gabrielsen TO, Maxwell JA: Traumatic atlanto-occipital dislocation. *AJR* 97:624-629, 1966.
33. Harris JR Jr, Carson GC, Wagner LK, Kerr N: Radiographic diagnosis of traumatic occipitovertebral dissociation: comparison of three methods of detecting occipitovertebral relationships on lateral radiographs of supine subjects. *AJR.* 162:887-892, 1994.
34. Jevitch V: Traumatic lateral atlanto-occipital dislocation with spontaneous bony fusion: a case report. *J Spinal Disord* 4:251-263, 1991.
35. Koop SE, Winter RB, Lonstein JE: The surgical treatment of instability of the upper part of the spine in children and adolescents. *J Bone Joint Surg (Am)* 66:403-411, 1984.
36. Montane I, Eismont FJ, Green BA: Traumatic occiptoatlantal dislocation. *Spine* 16:112-116, 1991.
37. Stroobants J, Fidlers L, Storms JL, *et al:* High cervical pain and impairment of skull mobility as the only symptoms of an occipital condyle fracture: a case report. *J Neurosurg* 81:137-138, 1994.
38. Wackenheim A: *Roentgen Diagnosis of the Craniovertebral Region.* Berlin, Springer-Verlag, 1974.
39. White AA, Panjabi MM: Kinematics of the spine. In *Clinical Biomechanics of the Spine (ed 2).* Philadelphia, JB Lippincott, 1990, pp 92-97.
40. Zigler JE, Waters RL, Nelson RW, *et al:* Occipito-cervico-thoracic spine fusion in a patient with occipito-cervical dislocation and survival. *Spine* 11:645-646, 1986.

Injuries to the First Cervical Vertebra

41. Alker G, Oh Y, Leslie E, *et al:* Post mortem radiology of head and neck injuries in fatal traffic accidents. *Radiology* 114: 611-617, 1975.

42. Bucholz R, Burkhead W: The pathological anatomy of fatal atlanto-occipital dislocations. *J Bone Joint Surg (Am)* 61:248-250, 1979.

43. Dunbar HS, Ray BS: Chronic atlanto-axial dislocations with late neurologic manifestations. *Surg Gyncol Obstet* 113:747, 1961.

44. Esses S, Langer F, Gross A: Fracture of the atlas associated with fracture of the odontoid process. *Injury* 12:310-312, 1981.

45. Fielding JW, Hawkins RJ, Hensinger RN, *et al:* Atlantoaxial rotary deformities. *Orthop Clin North Am* 9: 955-967, 1978.

46. Gonzalez TA, Vance M, Helper M: *Legal Medicine: Pathology and Toxicology.* New York, Appleton Century, 1940, p 312,.

47. Hamilton AR. Injuries of the atlanto-axial joint. *J Bone Joint Surg (Br)* 33:434-435, 1951.

48. Hatchette S. Isolated fracture of the atlas. *Radiology* 36:233-235, 1941.

49. Highland T, Salciccioli G: Is immobilization adequate treatment of unstable burst fractures of the atlas? A case report with long-term follow-up evaluation. *Clin Orthop* 201:196-200, 1985.

50. Hinchey J, Bickel W: Fractures of the atlas: review and presentation of data on eight cases. *Ann Surg* 121: 826-832, 1945.

51. Jefferson G: Remarks on fractures of the first cervical vertebra. *Br Med J* 2:153-157, 1927.

52. Krantz P: Isolated disruption of the transverse ligament of the atlas: an injury easily overlooked at post-mortem examination. *Injury* 12:168-170, 1980.

53. Levine A: Avulsion of the transverse ligament associated with a fracture of the atlas: a case report. *Orthopaedics* 6:1467-1471, 1983.

54. Levine A, Edwards C: Fractures of the atlas. *J Bone Joint Surg (Am)* 73:680-691, 1991.

55. Levine A, Edwards C: Treatment of injuries in the C1/C2 complex. *Orthop Clin North Am* 17:31-44, 1986.

56. Lipson SJ: Fractures of the atlas associated with fractures of the odontoid process and transverse ligament ruptures. *J Bone Joint Surg (Am)* 59:940-943, 1977.

57. Marlin A, Williams G, Lee J: Jefferson fractures in children. *J Neurosurg* 58:277-279, 1983.

58. Milward F: An unusual case of fractures of the atlas. *BMJ* 1:458, 1933.

59. O'Brien JJ, Butterfield WL, Gossling HR: Jefferson fracture with disruption of the transverse ligament. *Clin Orthop* 126:135-138, 1977.

60. Pennecot GF, Leonard P, DesGachons SP, *et al:* Traumatic ligamentios instability of the cervical spine in children. *J Pediatr Orthop* 4:339-345, 1984.

61. Penning L: Paravertebral hematoma in cervical spine injury: incidence and etiologic significance. *AJR* 136: 553-561, 1981.

62. Plaut H: Fracture of the atlas resulting from automobile accidents: a survey of the literature and a report of 6 cases. *AJR* 40:867-890, 1938.

63. Segal L, Grimm J, Stauffer E: Non-union of fractures of the atlas. *J Bone Joint Surg (Am)* 69:1423-1434, 1987.

64. Sherk H, Nicholson J: Fractures of the atlas. *J Bone Joint Surg (Am)* 52:1017-1024, 1970.

65. Spence KF, Decker S, Sell KW: Bursting atlantal fracture associated with rupture of the transverse ligament. *J Bone Joint Surg (Am)* 52:543-549, 1970.

66. Templeton P, Youhg J, Mirvis S, *et al:* The value of retropharyngeal soft tissue measurements in trauma of the adult cervical spine: cervical spine soft tissue measurements. *Skel Radiol* 16:98-104, 1987.

67. Wigren A, Anici F: Traumatic atlanto-axial dislocation without neurologic disorder, *J Bone Joint Surg (Am)* 55:642, 1973.

Fractures of the Second Cervical Vertebrae

68. Amling M, Hahn M, Wening VJ, *et al:* The microarchitecture of the axis as the predisposing factor for fracture of the base of the odontoid process. *J Bone Joint Surg (Am)* 76:1840-1846, 1994.

69. Anderson LD, D'Alonzo RT: Fractures of the odontoid process of the axis. *J Bone Joint Surg (Am)* 56:1663-1674, 1974.

70. Bohler J: Anterior stabilization for acute fractures and nonunions of the dens. *J Bone Joint Surg (Am)* 64:18-27, 1982.

71. Bucholz RW: Unstable hangman's fractures. *Clin Orthop* 154:119-124, 1981.

72. Clark CR, White AA III: Fractures of the dens: a multicenter study. *J Bone Joint Surg (Am)* 67:1340-1348, 1985.

73. Francis WR, Fielding JW, Hawkins RJ, *et al:* Traumatic spondylolisthesis of the axis. *J Bone Joint Surg (Br)* 63:313-318, 1981.

74. Hanigan WC, Powell FC, Elwood PW, Henderson JP: Odontoid fractures in elderly patients. *J Neurosurg* 78: 32-35, 1993.

75. Holsbeeck EV, Stoffelen D, Fabry G: Fractures of the odontoid process: conservative and operative treatment, prognostic factors. *Acta Orthop Belg* 59:17-21, 1993.

76. Husby J, Sorensen KH: Fractures of the odontoid process of the axis. *Acta Orthop Scand* 45:182-192, 1974.

77. Jeanneret B, Vernet O, Frei S, Magerl F: Atlantoaxial mobility after screw fixation of the odontoid: a computed tomographic study. *J Spinal Disord* 4:203-211, 1991.

78. Levine AM, Edward CC: The management of traumatic spondylolisthesis of the axis. *J Bone Joint Surg (Am)* 67:217-226, 1985.

79. Levine AM, Edwards CC: Treatment of injuries in the C1/C2 complex. *Orthop Clin North Am* 17:31-44, 1986.

80. Levine AM, Edwards CC: Traumatic lesions of the occipitoatlantoaxial complex. *Clin Orthop* 239:53-68, 1989.

81. Levine Am, Rhyne Al: Traumatic spondylolisthesis of the axis. *Semin Spine Surg* 3:47-60, 1991.

82. Mollan RAB: Hangman's fracture: injury. *Br J Accident Surg* 14(3):265-267, 1982.

83. Osgood RB, Lund CC: Fractures of the odontoid process. *N Engl J Med* 198:61-72, 1928.

84. Pepin JW, Hawkins RJ: Traumatic spondylolisthesis of the axis: hangman's fracture. *Clin Orthop* 157:133-138, 1981.

85. Schneider RC, Livingston KE, Cave AJE, *et al:* "Hangman's fracture" of the cervical spine. *J Neurosurg* 22:141-154, 1965.

86. Seimon LP: Fracture of the odontoid process in young children. *J Bone Joint Surg (Am)* 59:943-947, 1977.

87. Starr JK, Eismont FJ: Atypical hangman's fracture. *Spine* 18:1954-1957, 1993.

88. Termansen NB: Hangman's fracture. *Acta Orthop Scand* 45:529-539, 1974.

89. Wisoff HS: Fracture of the dens in the aged. *Surg Neurol* 22:547-555, 1984.

Injuries to the Lower Cervical Spine

90. Allen BL, Ferguson RL, Lehman TR, Obrien RP: A mechanistic classification of closed, indirect fractures and dislocations of the lower cervical spine. *Spine* 7:1-27, 1982.

91. Capen DA, Nelson RW, Zigler J, et al: Surgical stabilization of the cervical spine: a comparative analysis of anterior and posterior spine fusions. *Paraplegia* 25:111-119, 1987.

92. Capen DA, Zigler J, Garland DE: Surgical stabilization in cervical spine trauma. *Contemp Orthop* 14:25-32, 1987.

93. Denis F: Spinal instability as defined by the three column spine concept in acute spinal trauma. *Clin Orthop* 189:65-76, 1983.

94. Evans DK: Dislocations of the cervicothoracic junction. *J Bone Joint Surg (Br).* 65:124-127, 1983.

95. Grady MS, Howard MR, Jane JA, Persing JA: Use of the Philadelphia collar as an alternative to the halo vest in patients with C2-C3 fractures. *Neurosurgery* 18:151-156, 1985.

96. Harris JH: Radiographic evaluation of spinal trauma. *Orthop Clin North Am* 17:75-86, 1986.

97. Panjabi MM, White AA III, Johnson RM: Cervical spine mechanics as a function of ligament transection. *J Bone Joint Surg (Am)* 57:582, 1975.

98. Rorabeck CH, Rock MG, Hawkins AJ, Bourne RB: Unilateral facet dislocation of the cervical spine: an analysis of the results of treatment in 26 patients. *Spine* 12:23-27, 1987.

99. Stauffer ES: Management of spine fractures C3-C7. *Orthop Clin North Am* 17:45-53, 1986.

100. Stauffer ES, Kelly EG: fracture dislocations of the cervical spine: instability and recurrent deformity following treatment by anterior interbody fusion. *J Bone Joint Surg (Am)* 59:45-48, 1977.

101. Van Peteghem PK, Schweigel JF: The fractured cervical spine rendered unstable by anterior cervical fusion. *J Trauma* 19:110-114, 1979.

102. White AA III, Southwick WO, Panjabi MM: Clinical stability in the lower cervical spine: a review of past and current concepts. *Spine* 1:15-27, 1976.

103. Zigler J, Rockowitz N, Capen D, et al: Posterior cervical fusion with local anesthesia: the awake patient as the ultimate spinal cord monitor. *Spine* 12:206-208, 1987.

CHAPTER 45

Trauma Surgery: Thoracic and Thoracolumbar Spine

James S. Harrop, Alexander R. Vaccaro, Kevin T. Foley, and Iain Kalfas

In the United States approximately 160,000 patients a year incur traumatic spinal column injuries, with 10% to 30% of them having a concurrent spinal cord injury.[31,51] Cervical and lumbar (L3-5) spine fractures comprise the majority of these vertebral column injuries. However, between 15% and 20% of traumatic fractures occur at the thoracolumbar junction (T11-L2), whereas 9% to 16% occur in the thoracic spine (T1-10).[29,39] Thoracic and thoracolumbar fractures are associated with a high incidence of neurologic injuries because of the significant kinetic energy required to create these lesions and the relatively small size of the spinal canal in the thoracic region.[51] These patients are typically younger males who were involved in high-speed motor vehicle accidents. The transfer of axial loads through the transition from the rigid thoracic kyphosis to the mobile lumbar region results in a high incidence of thoracolumbar junction fractures.

Trauma to the thoracic spine and thoracolumbar junction, as a result of its anatomy, and biomechanical characteristics, is efficiently classified according to its radiographic presentation, biomechanical deficiencies, and clinical presentation of the patient. A thorough understanding of the principles of trauma care and an awareness of the unique biomechanic properties of the thoracic spine afford the treating physician a knowledge base that facilitates the effective management of these patients, both nonoperatively and operatively.

Anatomy

The vertebral column provides humans with the ability to maintain an upright posture, protects the neural and visceral organs (i.e., heart, lungs, abdominal contents), and aids with motility. It consists of 29 vertebrae arranged in four major curves, two primary curves (thoracic and sacral), and two compensatory or secondary curves (cervical and lumbar).[41] The vertebral column also provides a protective environment for the spinal cord and neural elements. The vertebral body, pedicles, and dorsal elements surround the spinal cord, allowing the spinal nerves to exit through the paired neural foramina The laminae are formed as a dorsal-medial extension of the pedicles and fuse in the midline to create the spinous processes (Figure 45.1).

The thoracic spine typically consists of 12 vertebrae (T1-12) and is the longest segment of the spinal column. However, in this chapter the thoracic spine is considered from level one to ten (T1-10). It is the thoracolumbar junction from thoracic vertebrae 11 to the second lumbar vertebrae (T11-L2).

The primary spinal curves are present at birth, are maintained through life, and are relatively rigid or stiff. The secondary curves are more flexible and are the result of development or adaptation. The cervical lordosis is created first, at approximately 3 to 9 months of age, when the infant begins supporting his or her head and sitting upright. The lumbar lordosis develops later (between 12 and 18 months), as the child begins to ambulate and assumes and upright posture.[41] A thorough knowledge of the thoracic spine and thoracolumbar junction anatomy facilitates a greater understanding of the biomechanical, radiographic, and surgical techniques that are used to surgically treat spinal fractures.

Thoracic Spine

The thoracic spine differs from the cervical and lumbosacral spines because of its articulation with the rib cage (T1-12) through an extensive ligamentous support network, its coronal facet joint orientation, and its small spinal canal to neural element ratio (Figure 45.2). There is significant variability in what is considered the "normal" sagittal curvature of the thoracic spine. This value has been reported to be between 20 and 45 degrees,[34,85,97] with each individual vertebral body contributing approximately 3.8 to 3.9 degrees of kyphosis through its wedged-shaped angulation.[85] This variability is further influenced by age (increases with aging) and gender; females have a greater degree of kyphosis than males.[34,97] There is also a significant degree of variability on a segmental basis, particularly at the transitional regions with the lordotic cervical and lumbar spine.[11,13,94]

The apex of thoracic kyphosis is at the seventh thoracic vertebrae. The thoracic spine typically has a mild, right-sided lateral curvature.[41,97] The causes of the right-sided lateral curve is debated but is believed to be either the result of hand dominance (right-hand majority) or created by pulsations of the thoracic aorta.[41] The thoracic vertebrae increase in size (height, width, and depth) as the spine is descended.[7,11,85,105,108] These bodies differ from the other vertebral bodies in that the ventral portion is shorter than the dorsal portion, which contributes to the thoracic kyphosis. In the transverse plane the thoracic vertebrae have a triangular configuration and appear heart shaped. The diameter of the thoracolumbar pedicles also increases in size as the spine is descended and have an oval configuration, with a greater height (mean 15 to 16mm) than width (mean 8 to 9mm).[105]

The thoracic pedicles are situated toward the rostral portion of the vertebral body in close proximity to the superior disc space (Figure 45.3). The pedicle location on the vertebral body progressively migrates as the spine is descended in a caudal direction. In the rostral thoracic spine, the pedicles have a greater angle of insertion into the vertebral body (approximately 15 degrees for T1).

This lessens to approximately 10 degrees at T3-11, and finally to 5 degrees at T12.[7,76,97] The medial pedicle cortical wall is approximately two to three times thicker than the lateral wall.[61] Clinically, this is manifested by a greater incidence of lateral compared to medial breeches during the insertion of thoracic pedicle screws. This protects the medially located neural elements.

The thoracic transverse processes project laterally from the dorsal articular pillars and decrease in length caudally.[29] However, unlike the lumbar spine the relationship between the transverse process and the midpoint of the pedicle is not as clearly defined. McCormick *et al.*[70] showed that there is a significant degree in the variability of the transverse process to pedicle relationship. The mid-

point of the T1 transverse process is approximately 5mm rostral to the center of the pedicle, whereas at T12 the transverse process to pedicle relationship changes to approximately 6mm caudal.[70] This distance difference is greater than 1cm between T1-12, and is approximately 0 at the T6-7 level.[70]

The thoracic spine facet articulations are considered apophyseal joints and are composed of a ligamentous capsule with a synovial lining. The ligament is thicker than their cervical counterpart's lining. The joints are located at the rostral and caudal borders of the lamina and situated medial to the transverse processes (Figure 45.3). The inferior facet's ventral surface articulates with the superior facet's dorsal surface. Thoracic facet joints are oriented in a coronal plane and therefore limit the degree of flexion and extension of the thoracic spine.[28]

The ribs articulate with the thoracic vertebrae at two locations. The rib tubercle articulates with the transverse process of the vertebral body at the costotransverse articulation, except at T1, T11, and T12. This articulation is supported with a large superior costotransverse ligament, which connects the rostral rib segment to the caudal transverse process (Figure 45.2). The second rib articulation is the rib head with the same numbered vertebral body and the rostral disc space through the two costal demifacets (T2-10). The strong ligamentous structures that compose the costovertebral joint make the thoracic disc the strongest of all the vertebral discs.[1a] The superior demifacet (rostral on the vertebral body and caudal to the rib) is located over the pedicle, such that the sixth rib articulates with the fifth and sixth vertebral bodies and overlies the sixth vertebral pedicle. Because of the rostral location of the thoracic pedicle on the vertebral body, the sixth rib overlies the T5-6 disc space. Understanding the anatomic

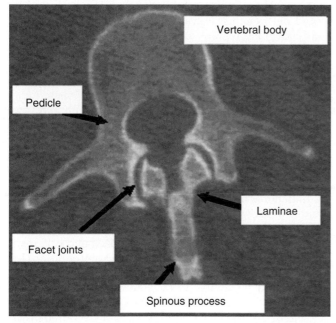

Figure 45.1 Axial CT image of L2 vertebral body identifying the dorsal elements.

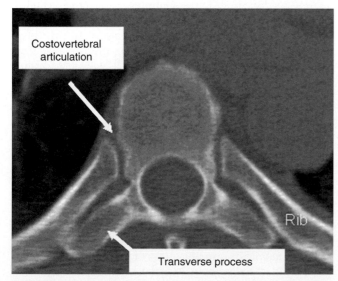

Figure 45.2 Axial CT image of T6 vertebral body identifying the relationship between the vertebral body and the rib head's articulations.

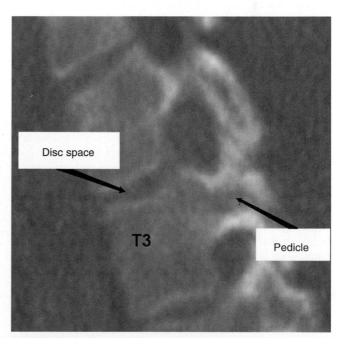

Figure 45.3 Sagittal CT reformatted image of T2-3 vertebral bodies illustrating the relationship of the pedicle to the intervertebral disc space in the thoracic spine.

relationship of the rib head to the pedicle allows the surgeon to remove the rib-head and identify the neurovascular bundle, along with the neural foramina and thecal sac at that level.

In the thoracic spine the laminae are short and broad, which prevents hyperextension.[35] The volume of the spinal canal varies throughout the vertebral column, and is the narrowest in the midthoracic region (T3-9).[7,85,95] The transverse spinal canal diameter decreases from T1-3 and then increases caudally into the lumbar region. The anteroposterior diameter, however, is more varied.[85,95] Therefore, in the thoracic region a minor degree of canal encroachment may compromise the narrow canal and may result in neurologic compromise.[9,10] The thoracic spinal cord has the most tenuous blood supply.[85] The small canal size, limited blood supply, and high degree of energy required to create a thoracic fracture results in a 90% incidence of neurologic deficit in patients who sustain a thoracic fracture.[74]

Thoracolumbar Junction

The transition from a relatively rigid thoracic kyphosis to a mobile lumbar spine occurs at the thoracolumbar junction. This transition generally occurs at T11-12, although in elderly female patients the thoracolumbar inflexion point migrates caudally, as a result of their increased degree of thoracic kyphosis.[11,94,97]

The lowest thoracic ribs (T11 and T12) afford less stability at the thoracolumbar junction region compared to the rostral thoracic region, because they do not connect to the sternum and are free floating. Only a single rib articulation is present on the eleventh and twelfth vertebral bodies, and there are no accessory ligamentous attachments, such as the rib's tubercle to the vertebral body via the costotransverse ligament, or the ligamentous attachment to the transverse process.[41] Conversely, the surrounding thoracolumbar ligaments, such as the interspinous and thoracolumbar fascia, which provide a significant amount of stability, are the strongest caudally.[105]

The thoracolumbar junction facet joints are again of the apophyseal type and are composed of a ligamentous capsule with a synovial lining. As mentioned previously, the joints of the midthoracic region are oriented in the coronal plane, limiting flexion and extension while providing substantial resistance to anteroposterior translation.[29] In the lumbosacral region the facet joints are oriented in a more sagittal alignment, which increases the degree of potential flexion and extension at the expense of limiting lateral bending and rotation. Therefore in the region of the thoracolumbar junction there is a gradual change in facet orientation to a more oblique orientation in the upper lumbar spine. Depending on the spatial orientation of the spinal column (i.e., flexion or extension), the facet joints may support a third of the axial load. These joints, however, provide substantial support and resistance to approximately 35% to 45% of the torsional and shear forces experienced in this region.[27,39]

During infancy the spinal cord terminates at the end of the vertebral column or lumbosacral junction. However, the location of the terminal end of the spinal cord or conus medullaris varies as the infant develops.[68] In neonates the spinal cord terminates between the first and third lumbar vertebrae, whereas in adults it is positioned between the twelfth thoracic vertebrae and the second lumbar vertebrae.[68]

Imaging

Plain radiographic studies are often difficult to interpret because of surrounding soft tissue and bony overlap. Patients with spinal fractures often sustain concurrent life-threatening injuries and may be obtunded or sedated and require emergent resuscitation. Therefore it is not uncommon in these clinically unstable trauma patients for fractures to not be identified early in the resuscitative period. It has been reported that between 5% and 15% of multisystem trauma patients have occult fractures not diagnosed on their initial evaluation.[17,30,63] Although thoracic vertebral fractures are only a minor proportion of traumatic fractures, they are extremely difficult to visualize compared to other vertebral or appendicular fractures. Approximately 20% to 50% of superior thoracic spinal fractures are not diagnosed by admission plain radiographs.[29,99,103] Therefore, all suspected spinal trauma admissions should be immobilized until a thorough and detailed spinal evaluation can be performed. If appropriate stabilization precautions are not taken in this patient population, unforeseen neurologic compromise may result.[40]

Initial imaging studies performed on all thoracolumbar trauma patients should consist of standard anteroposterior (AP) and lateral plain radiographs. These initial radiographs should be reviewed in an organized and systematic manner. On the AP view the pedicles, vertebral bodies, disc spaces and spinous processes, and soft tissue relationships should be examined in detail. The vertebral body heights, disc space relations, vertebral body alignment, and paraspinal swelling should be carefully assessed on the lateral view. These plain radiographs are particularly useful to assess overall sagittal and coronal balance. If a deformity exists, a useful radiographic measurement of the degree of deformity is the Cobb measurement, which is the subtended angle measured between a perpendicular line drawn from the superior end-plate of the vertebral body above the injured body and the inferior end-plate one level below the injured vertebral body (see Figure 45.20). This method of measuring spinal sagittal angulation has been shown to have the highest degree of intraobserver and interobserver reliability.[62]

In the presence of a vertebral injury the entire spine should be imaged in an orthogonal manner, because of the high incidence (5% to 20%) of noncontiguous spinal fractures.[16,87,92] The rostral thoracic spine can be difficult to visualize on lateral plain radiographs because of the patient's shoulders and body habitus, and a swimmer's view may allow better visualization of the cervicothoracic junction down to the third thoracic vertebral body.[22] Radiographically, a typical superior end-plate thoracic fracture manifests visually as loss of vertebrae height, with or without malalignment, a widened paraspinal line, and possibly, a widened mediastinum.[103] Because of difficulties in imaging the upper thoracic region, a high index of suspicion is required by the physician to avoid missing injuries at this level. The physician perhaps should have a low threshold for ordering supplemental imaging modalities to assist in the diagnosis, such as computed tomography and magnetic resonance imaging.

Computed tomography (CT) provides a fast and accurate imaging assessment of the vertebral column. This imaging modality has been very useful in the classification and understanding of these fractures.[26,49,69] CT is more sensitive in detecting fractures than plain radiographs in the thoracic spine. It is also useful in defining the three-dimensional anatomy of complex fractures through reformation in the sagittal and coronal planes. CT imaging permits a more detailed and precise assessment of fracture configuration by its ability to remove extraneous artifacts, such as the ribs and soft tissue structures. This facilitates the quantification of the degree of spinal canal encroachment by retropulsed middle column bone and the presence of a nondisplaced laminae fracture on transaxial imaging, all not possible with standard plain radiography (Figure 45.4). Serial CT has confirmed the spontaneous remodeling and bone reabsorption of retropulsed bone fragments in the spinal canal at the time of long-term follow-up of traumatic burst fractures.[8,23,60]

CT image reconstruction is also invaluable at the cervicothoracic junction because of the overlay of the scapula, shoulders, and surrounding tissues. In the obtunded patient this technique has been reported to identify more than 10% of fractures not visualized on plain radiographs.[55] CT, however, has a limited capacity to visualize disc herniations, epidural or subdural hematomas, ligamentous disruption, or spinal cord parenchymal changes.[33]

Magnetic resonance imaging (MRI) has further improved the ability to visualize and comprehend the pathoanatomy of the soft-tissue, ligamentous, intervertebral disc and the neural element disruption that occurs after spinal injury. Unfortunately MRI is not always available because of its expense, takes a longer time to implement, and cannot be performed on patients with specific ferromagnetic implants. Today it has supplanted CT myelography as the imaging tool of choice of the neuroaxis, because it is faster, noninvasive, and allows improved visualization of the spinal cord parenchyma.[57] MRI provides the physician the ability to identify edema and/or hemorrhage of the spinal cord[57] (Figure 45.5). These images have been correlated with neurologic outcomes, where the presence of hemorrhage in the spinal cord parenchyma is associated with minimal neurologic recovery.[93]

MRI evaluation is especially useful at the thoracolumbar junction because of the variable location of the cauda equina and conus medullaris in the adult population at this level. A neurologic examination can be difficult to interpret at the conus/cauda equina transition level, as a result of the presence of lumbar spinal nerve sparing, the presence of concurrent injuries, sedation, in-dwelling catheters, and delayed reflex recovery (Figure 45.6). Accurate neural visualization may help in clarifying the pathoanatomy in this clinical situation.

Biomechanics

The thoracic spine assumes a relatively rigid kyphotic posture between the flexible lordotic cervical and lumbar segments, with the thoracolumbar junction providing the transition between the thoracic and the lumbar spine. The spinal column provides humans with the ability to maintain an upright position by balancing all applied forces that affect the spine while keeping the head centered over the pelvis. The vertebral body is the primary load-bearing structure of the spine, with the intervertebral disc transferring all forces applied to the adjacent

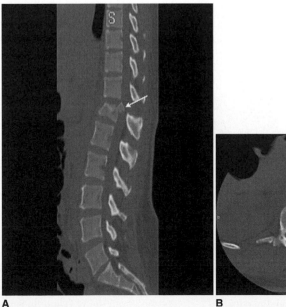

A   B

Figure 45.4 T12 burst fracture sustained after an MVA. (**A**) Note the high definition of the posterior displaced fragment (*arrow*), along with the vertebral body sagittal fracture (**B**, *arrow*) and the associated laminae fracture.

vertebral bodies.[39,86] The annulus fibrosus of the intervertebral disc supports a significant portion of all applied axial and lateral loads and resists tension and shearing.[67]

The spinal ligamentous structures are essential in maintaining overall sagittal balance. The posterior longitudinal

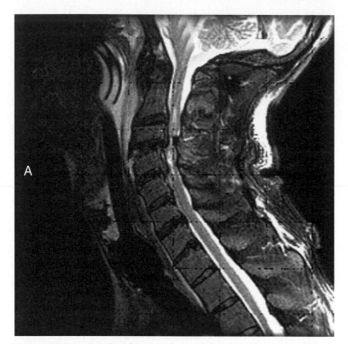

Figure 45.5 T_2-weighted MRI of cervical spine of C5 ASIA A spinal cord injured patient after an automobile crash. The images illustrate severe intraparenchymal edema, along with hemorrhage in the spinal cord.

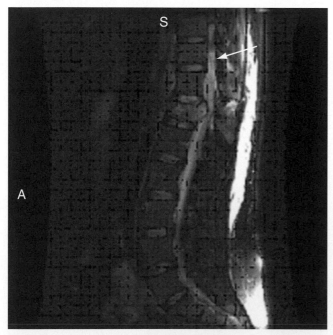

Figure 45.6 T12 burst fracture with retropulsion of fragment into canal. Note that the fragment is compressing the conus medullaris and there is resulting spinal cord edema. Clinically the patient has a severe lower-extremity paresis and loss of bowel and bladder function.

ligament (PLL) is a relatively weak ligament that provides some restriction to hyperflexion, along with the ligamentum flavum. The thick anterior longitudinal ligament (ALL) functions in resisting spinal hyperextension and distraction.[82] This thick ligament has fatigue loading values that are approximately double any other spinal ligaments,[67,82,86] and its strength increases caudally from C3 to the sacrum.[82] The intrinsic strength of the spinal ligaments is only an isolated factor in the overall stability of the spinal column. The lever arm by which these ligaments act on the spine also significantly affects the overall stability of the vertebral column (Figure 45.7). For example, the facet capsules are very strong ligaments and act with a short lever arm by their relationship to the instantaneous axis of rotation (IAR), whereas the intraspinous ligaments are relatively weak but act with a great lever arm because of their increased distance from the IAR. Based on the ligaments' relative strengths, it would seem that the intraspinous ligaments are not important, but both ligaments significantly affect the strength and structure of the spine.

The thoracic spine differs from the remainder of the spinal column because it is supported and maintains articulations with the ribs (Figure 45.2). The intact rib cage increases the axial load-resisting capacity of the thoracic spine by a magnitude of four. The rib cage and facet articulations limit rotation, and therefore most thoracic spine fractures occur from a flexion or axial compression force vector.[47] The majority of stability in flexion is provided by the costovertebral articulations.[42] A significant factor in the degree and extent of fracture character is the rate of force impact loading.[102]

The IAR is defined as the axis where all forces and moments are balanced on a specific motion segment.[43] This axis is a geometric concept and does not apply to a specific anatomic location.[44] However, in the normal thoracic and thoracolumbar spine the IAR is located in the ventral vertebral body.

The IAR is analogous to a fulcrum, where during flexion the structures anterior to this axis will come under compression, whereas structures dorsal to this axis are exposed to tensile forces. The bending moment or arm is defined as the product of the lever arm (distance at right angle to the point of force application) and the magnitude

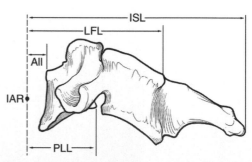

Figure 45.7 The lever arm of the ligaments to the instantaneous axis of rotation (*IAR*) greatly influences the stability of the spine. The weaker interspinous ligaments work at the greatest distance from the IAR and therefore provide significant resistance to gravitational influences. *ALL*, Anterior longitudinal ligament; *Cap*, capsular ligaments; *IS*, interspinous ligaments; *PLL*, posterior longitudinal ligament.

of force transmitted on the object. Therefore forces or loads that are applied to the IAR at a greater distance are at a biomechanic advantage as a result of their greater moment arm.

Gravitational forces exert a significant axial load on the vertebral column in the standing adult human. The center of gravity of the body, located where all forces are counterbalanced such that there is no net movement when positioned through this point, is approximately 4cm anterior to the first sacral vertebra.[105] This results in a ventral bending (angular) vector acting on the spinal column. This bending force draws or attracts the ventral spinal column closer to the center of gravity such that a lower energy state may be achieved by the paraspinous musculature. The dorsal ligamentous complex and dorsal paraspinal musculature, acting as a dorsal tension band, counteracts these forces, such that the net sum of the vectors acting on the spine equals zero. Therefore the dorsal ligamentous, osseous, and musculature components are essential for overall support of the spine to prevent a change in the spine's sagittal alignment. Trauma resulting in disruption of the spinal ligaments or osseous structures may change the net vector sum from zero, resulting in the potential for spinal imbalance. These new vectors acting on the spine, if not corrected, may result in a gradual spinal deformity associated with or without pain or neurologic deterioration. Whiteside used the analogy of a construction crane to illustrate this mechanical principle (Figure 45.8).[106] In this analogy the weight to be lifted is anterior to the crane where the boom (anterior vertebral column) is under compressive forces and the guide wires (posterior columns) are under tension. Failure of either supporting structure independent of the other will result in mechanical failure or collapse.

The thoracic and thoracolumbar vertebrae are at an increased risk for developing compression fractures after trauma as a consequence of axial loads resulting from the natural kyphotic curvature of the thoracic spine.[45] The kyphotic posture results in the placement of axial forces on the ventral portion of the vertebral body. An axial load causes all points that are ventral to the IAR of the spine to come closer together while simultaneously all points that are dorsal are spread apart. Therefore if the strength of the ventral vertebral body is exceeded, a fracture of the vertebral body occurs, resulting in a vertebral compression fracture (VCF). The traumatic forces may also exceed the strength of the dorsal vertebral body and ligamentous elements, resulting in disruption of the dorsal tension band. The destruction of the ventral vertebral stabilizing elements (vertebral body, disc, ligaments, annulus) causes the IAR to migrate dorsally to the region with intact supporting structures.[45,46] The dorsal migration of the IAR causes the previous mechanical advantage of a longer level arm from which the dorsal ligaments and muscles acted to be shortened. This migration of the IAR simultaneously increases the distance of the center of gravity to the IAR, thereby placing further distraction on the dorsal spinal column and compression on the ventral spinal column (Figure 45.7).[45,46] The shortened dorsal lever arm and potentially disrupted dorsal tension band, along with a greater ventral bending moment arm, creates a viscous cycle that places the vertebral bodies at a greater risk for further compression fractures and subsequent deformity progression.

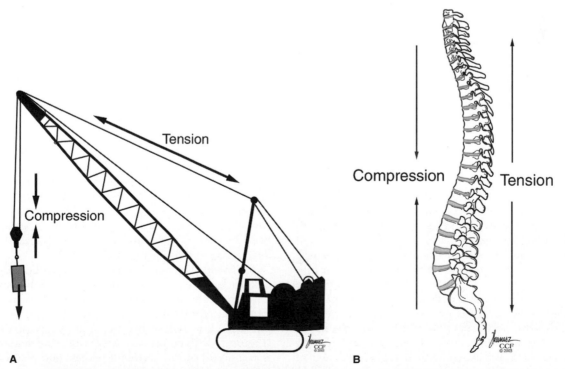

A　　**B**

Figure 45.8 (**A** and **B**) Whiteside's analog of the spine illustrates the delicate equilibrium of the anterior compression vectors against the posterior tension vectors. (*Copyright Cleveland Clinic Foundation, 2003.*)

Concurrent Injuries

Thoracic Spine Fractures

The osseous structures, ligaments, rib cage, and the anatomy of the thoracic spine's structural integrity provide more resilience to sustaining fractures then the remaining vertebral column. Therefore when a fracture occurs over this region, the physician must be aware that a high degree of energy was required to produce this lesion. These forces on impact are dispersed and transmitted to the soft tissue and viscous elements contained within and around the thoracic cavity, resulting in a high incidence of concurrent injuries. The incidence of concurrent injuries is reported to be greater than 80%, and involves the thorax, appendicular skeleton, and abdominal region.[84,92,103] These high-energy impacts also affect remote areas from the trauma, such as the cranial vault. Petitjean et al.[84] reported a 65% incidence of head injuries after high-velocity impacts, which resulted in incomplete thoracic spinal cord injury with 12% of these injuries classified as severe (Glasgow Coma Scale [GCS] score less than 8).[84]

The thoracic cavity consists of the heart, lung, trachea, esophagus, and great vessels. Any of these structures may be injured as a result of blunt trauma and manifest as hemodynamic instability. Tearing or rupture of the aorta has been associated with thoracic vertebral fractures.[101] Hemodynamic instability may result from injury to any vascular structure, or even from blood loss secondary to a thoracic vertebral fracture.[24,104] Hemothorax has also been reported to occur between 24% and 32% of patients with thoracic fractures.[2,37] Pulmonary injuries have been reported in 85% of patients and typically consist of pulmonary contusions.[84] Infrequently, perforation of the esophagus and tracheal injuries have also been associated with thoracic fractures.[20,79,100] The mechanism of perforation is believed to be caused by ischemia of the esophageal tissue after becoming devascularized as a result of a deceleration-traction injury.[20,100]

Thoracolumbar Junction Fractures

The thoracolumbar region is more vulnerable to concurrent injuries than the thoracic region because it is not provided the protection of the thoracic rib cage. Petitjean[84] reported a 71% incidence of associated blunt abdominal injuries after thoracolumbar fractures. Typically these consist of hollow viscous injuries, such as intestinal perforations, mesenteric avulsions, or solid organ injuries.[4,84,88]

The most common mechanism of abdominal injuries is distraction or seat-belt injuries.[4,52,84,88] Blunt abdominal aortic dissections are associated with distraction-rotational injuries of the thoracolumbar region.[52] These aortic injuries can range from an intimal tear to a full-thickness laceration. CT provides accurate imaging of this injury in the stable and asymptomatic patient. A large degree of energy is involved in this distraction-type mechanism, accounting for the large number of associated injuries. Multiple-level thoracic and lumbar fractures are also associated with a high incidence of abdominal injuries.[52,88]

Axial load injuries, particularly in patients that have jumped or fallen and landed on their feet, may manifest as

both thoracolumbar fractures and also calcaneal fractures. Isolated transverse process fractures of the lumber spine should not be overlooked as a minor injury. Miller reported a 48% incidence of concurrent abdominal injuries associated with transverse process fractures.[76] Therefore a physician treating vertebral column injuries must not only be aware of the presence of spinal fractures, but also the possibility of concurrent, nonspinal, soft tissue and bony injuries.

Classification

Fracture classification schemes provide physicians with the ability to organize and treat fractures through predetermined protocols to maximize patient outcomes. A classification scheme must therefore be simple to understand, easy to apply, and have consistent outcomes with the application of the same treatment algorithm. Unfortunately, the thoracic spine does not have a uniformly agreed upon classification scheme, and the systems available for the thoracolumbar junction injuries are inconsistently used because of their complexity, difficulty in application, and clinical irrelevance.*

Nicholl[83] developed the first detailed thoracic and thoracolumbar spinal fracture classification scheme and attempted to define unstable versus stable fractures after trauma in a series of flexion and flexion rotation injuries. This classification system was originally intended to guide the treatment and work status of injured miners. Nichol emphasized the importance of the dorsal interspinous ligament in spinal stability.[83] Later, Holdsworth,[50] after clinical failures in immobilizing pure flexion fractures per the recommendations of Watson, Jones, and Davis, further studied the importance of the spinal ligamentous complexes after thoracolumbar junction injuries. He classified fractures, according to their mechanism of injury, into four main types: flexion, flexion and rotation, extension, and compression. Holdsworth[50] further classified these fractures as unstable if the posterior ligamentous complex, consisting of the intervertebral disc, spinous ligaments, facet capsules, and the ligamentum flavum, was disrupted. He noted that in compression, flexion, and extension injuries, the dorsal ligamentous complex is typically not ruptured and these fractures were therefore considered stable. However, he reported that flexion and rotational injuries were at a much greater risk for disruption of the dorsal ligamentous complex and subsequent instability. Rennie and Mitchell[89] added a fifth category of thoracolumbar junction fractures consisting of flexion distraction fractures or seat-belt injuries, based on the description and reporting of Chance.[18]

Kelly and Whiteside[59] reported that without dislocation of the dorsal elements of the spinal column neurologic injuries rarely occur. They classified fractures based on structural criteria and considered the spine to consist of not one, but rather two separate supportive columns (Figure 45.9). The primary weight-bearing ventral column is composed of the vertebral bodies, and a second structural column consists of the posterior neural arches and

---

*References 25,26,32,50,59,65,66,72,83.

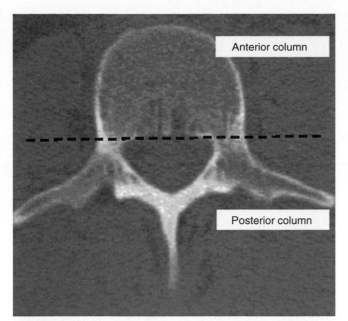

Figure 45.9 Axial CT of lumbar vertebral body illustrating Kelly and Whiteside's two-column theory of spine stability, which classifies the spine into two equal columns of support consisting of equal anterior and posterior columns.

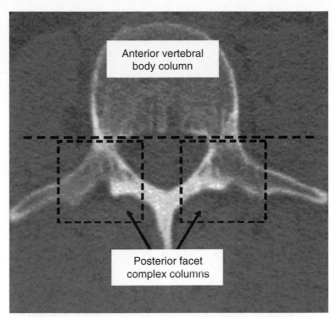

Figure 45.10 Axial CT of lumbar vertebral body illustrating Louis' three-column figure theory of spine structure. This classification system divides the spine into an anterior column consisting of the vertebral body and two equal posterior columns consisting of the facet complexes.

ligaments. The structural classification scheme provided surgeons the ability to predict the degree of instability of the spine based on the degree of resulting structural damage after trauma. Based on this assessment, treatments were devised to enhance neurologic and spinal stability. Later, Louis[65] further modified this structural classification scheme by proposing a third column. Louis' three-column concept consisted of one ventral column, the vertebral bodies, and two dorsal columns involving each facet articulation (Figure 45.10).

Technological advancements in the form of superior imaging studies have allowed a greater understanding of the pathoanatomy of spinal trauma. Several biomechanic studies have documented that an isolated rupture of the posterior spinal ligamentous complex is insufficient to create instability.[5,6,85,91] However, if the PLL, along with the posterior annulus fibrosis, is also disrupted, then the vertebral column will become unstable, particularly in flexion. Denis used the enhanced imaging techniques CT, along with *in vitro* biomechanic data to further modify the spinal column theories into a different three-column classification scheme (Figure 45.11). In this classification the ventral column consists of the ventral longitudinal ligament (VLL), the anterior annulus fibrosis, and the anterior half of the vertebral bodies. The middle column consists of the PLL, the dorsal annulus fibrosis and the dorsal half of the vertebral bodies. Lastly, the posterior column, analogous to what Holdworth defined as the dorsal ligamentous complex, consists of the bony neural arch, posterior spinous ligaments, and ligamentum flavum, as well as the facet joints. According to the Denis classification scheme, rupture of the dorsal ligamentous complex only creates instability if and when there is concurrent disruption of at least the PLL and dorsal annulus.

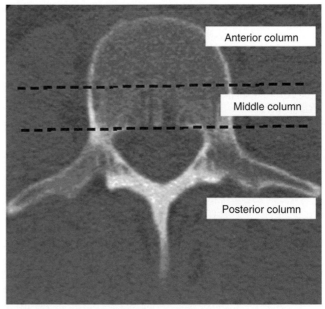

Figure 45.11 Axial CT of lumbar vertebral body illustrating Denis' three-column classification scheme of spine stability. This classification system divides the spine into an anterior column consisting not only of the anterior half of the vertebral body, but also the anterior longitudinal ligament. The middle column consists of the posterior half of the vertebral body and the posterior longitudinal ligament. The posterior column consists of the facets, laminae, and ligamentous complex.

Denis defined failure of the anterior column alone under compression (compression fracture) with an intact posterior column as a stable fracture (Figure 45.12). Burst fractures were defined as being generated through an axial compressive load, and involved failure of the anterior and

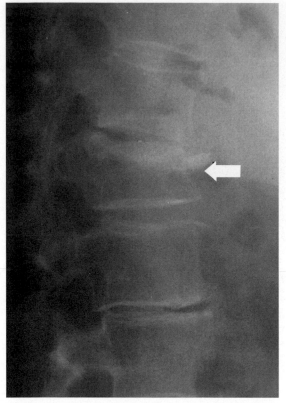

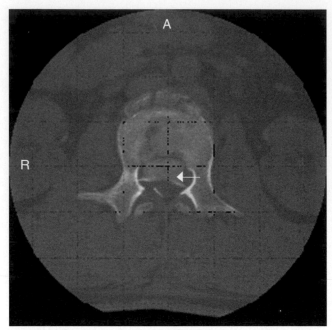

Figure 45.13 An 18-year-old male who sustained a 25-foot fall. Axial CT image of L2 burst fracture detailing the canal encroachment of the retropulsed fracture *(arrow)*. Note the disruption of the posterior vertebral wall and the splaying of the pedicles.

Figure 45.12 L1 vertebral compression fracture *(arrow)*. Note the posterior vertebral body's height is maintained, and in the Denis classification only the anterior column is disrupted.

middle columns (Figure 45.13). Severe tensile injuries resulted in seat-belt fracture or flexion distraction injuries, which involve a disruption of the posterior and middle columns with an intact anterior column that serves as a fulcrum or hinge (Figure 45.14). The last category in Denis' scheme is fracture dislocations, which are defined as a mechanical failure of all three columns, which makes them extremely unstable injuries (Figure 45.15).

Denis organized instability into three categories: mechanical, neurologic or both mechanical and neurologic. Mechanical instability may result in a late kyphotic deformity. For example, a seat belt or severe compression fracture with compromise to the dorsal ligamentous complex may result in the spinal column falling into kyphosis, rotating around the intact middle column because of the deficient dorsal tension band. External immobilization, and when appropriate, operative reduction and stabilization, may prevent this deformity progression. Neurologic instability may occur after a severe burst fracture in which the middle column has ruptured under axial loads. This disruption and retropulsion of bone fragments into the spinal canal predisposes these patients to an increased risk for neurologic injury, especially with increased spinal motion. Denis reported that 20% of patients with severe burst fractures and dorsal ligamentous injuries that were treated nonoperatively with external immobilization, developed a subsequent neurologic deficit. Neurologic and mechanical instability may develop after a burst fracture or fracture/dislocation, with or without an initial neurologic deficit. These are very unstable

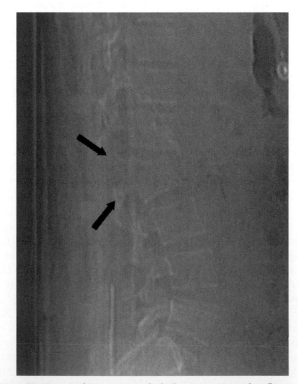

Figure 45.14 L2 Chance or seatbelt fracture. Note this flexion distraction injury splits the pedicle and facets *(arrows)*, leaving the anterior column intact.

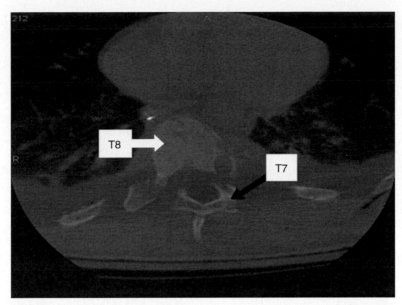

Figure 45.15 A 38-year-old male driven over by a truck presented with thoracic T7-8 dislocation and complete loss of motor and sensation below the injury. The spine was fractured and dislocated, therefore separating all three columns of stability as detailed in the Denis classification.

injuries and according to Denis' analysis require decompression and internal stabilization.

Magerl developed a comprehensive classification scheme based on pathomorphologic criteria. This system is modeled after the AO long bone fracture classification (Miller) and consists of a grid with three major fracture types, subdivided into three more groups, which are further subgrouped into three more categories.[75] The main categories include: (A) compression injuries of the vertebral bodies, (B) distraction injuries that affect the anterior and posterior elements, and (C) axial torque or multidirectional injuries with translation that also affects the anterior and posterior elements. The severity of the fractures is inherent with this scheme as one progresses from type A to C. Although this classification system is extremely organized and comprehensive, it is underused clinically because of its complexity.

McCormack[72] created a classification system based on a load-sharing principle that uses a graded point system based on the integrity of the vertebral bodies or anterior and middle column. Points are based on the amount of vertebral body comminution, spread of fragments at the fracture site, and the amount of corrected traumatic kyphosis (Figure 45.16). Traumas with the highest degree of energy cause bone fragments to be greatly dispersed such that they are displaced further and not in continuity with the other fragments. This classification can be applied preoperatively to quantitatively estimate the extent of disruption of the anterior and middle columns. The patients with increased point values (greater than six) have a large void or gap, resulting in the least supportive anterior and middle columns. The fractures with the greatest dispersion of fragments and least bone contact create the highest degree of cantilever bending loads on the pedicle screw implants and predisposes the posterior instrumentation to failure.[73,107] This classification scheme assists the surgeon in deciding if ventral spinal support is necessary after dorsal instrumentation, based on the

premise that inadequate anterior column support will result in excessive loads being transferred to the dorsal elements (and instrumentation), thus increasing the risk for failure.

Treatment Options and Strategies

There is a significant amount of controversy regarding not only the need for surgical versus nonsurgical management of thoracolumbar injuries, but also the approach and type of surgery if operative intervention is chosen. No definitive treatment algorithm has been universally accepted for this spinal disorder, despite the numerous classification systems that exist. Stability of the vertebral column over the thoracic and thoracolumbar region, like the remainder of the spine, is dependent on the integrity of the osseous and ligamentous components. Once these structures are disrupted the stability of the vertebral column can become compromised, resulting in an unstable spine. One difficulty in treating these fractures is that the definition of instability of the spine is difficult to assess, based on clinical and radiographic findings. White and Panjabi have the most detailed description of instability: "the loss of the ability of the spine under physiological loads to maintain relationships between vertebrae in such a way that there is either damage or subsequent irritation to the spinal cord or nerve roots, and in addition, there is development of incapacitating deformity or pain due to structural changes."[105] However, even this definition leaves a large degree of ambiguity because of the large spectrum of spinal disorders.

Treatment algorithms are based on maximizing neurologic recovery and prevention of neurologic decline and deformities, while maximizing pain relief. This is accomplished by identifying fractures that are "unstable" such that their structural support can be augmented to maximize clinical outcomes. Each patient and management strategy must be individualized depending on the type of

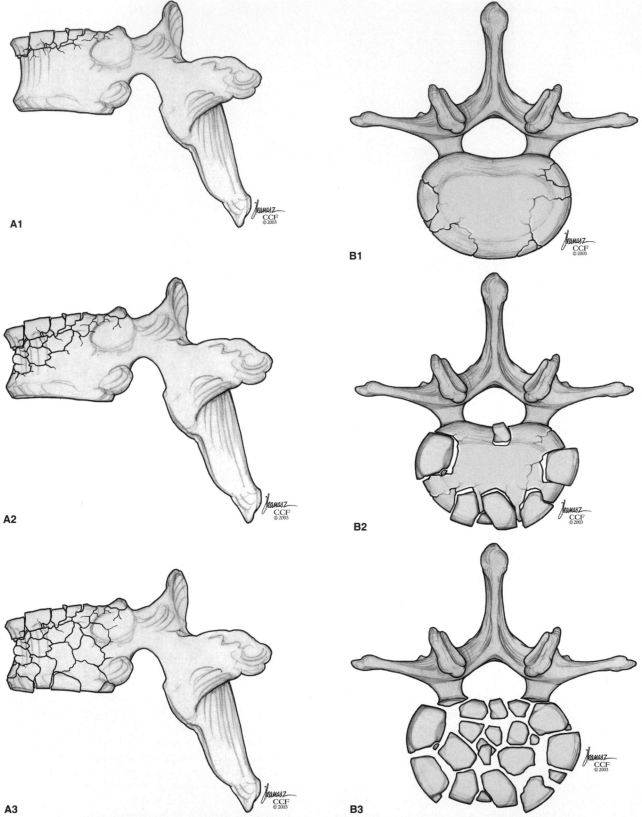

A1

B1

A2

B2

A3

B3

Figure 45.16 McCormick grading scheme or load-sharing classification. Communition of fragments based on a sagittal CT reformat as either **(A1)** little (<30%), one point; **(A2)** moderate (30% to 60%), two points; or **(A3)** gross (>60%), three points. Apposition of fragments based on an axial CT image as either **(B1)** minimal one point, **(B2)** spread defined as greater than 2mm in less *than* 50% of the body two points, or **(B3)** wide, 2mm in greater than 50% of the body three points.

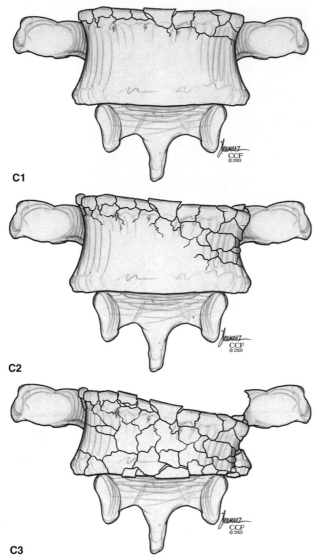

C1

C2

C3

Figure 45.16 *cont'd* Kyphosis correction on plain radiographs (**C1**) <3 degrees, one point, (**C2**) 4 to 9 degrees, two points, or (**C3**) >10 degrees, three points. (*Copyright Cleveland Clinic Foundation, 2003.*)

fracture, location, other traumatic comorbidities, neurologic outcomes, and medical comorbidities.

Nonoperative Strategies

The majority of fractures in the thoracic and thoracolumbar regions consist of compression, stable burst, and isolated dorsal column fractures. These fractures are generally classified as stable because there is little risk of neurologic compromise from osseous compression or deformity progression. The acquired stability of the preserved ligaments and osseous structures usually prevent acute instability; however, a low potential for chronic or glacial instability still remains. Glacial instability usually presents as mechanical pain, but could also present as a neurologic deficit. VCFs, as defined by the Denis' three-column scheme, consist of a loss of anterior column or ventral vertebral body height as a result of axial compression (Figure 45.12). These fractures are considered stable anatomically, if the dorsal ligamentous complex, along with the dorsal verte-

bral body, is not disrupted. The intact dorsal ligaments and dorsal elements provide a significant tension band. Further stability is also provided by the remaining intact anterior and middle columns. Neurologic function should not be impaired as a result of these fractures, because the dorsal cortex of the vertebral body is not violated and because there is no encroachment of fracture fragments on or into the spinal canal.

In approximately a third of patients these vertebral compression fractures unfortunately are persistently painful and can require bracing, prolonged bed rest, and narcotic therapy. Such VCFs may be satisfactorily treated nonoperatively with a hyperextension brace or corsette. This bracing technique maintains alignment through three-point bending principles and results in axial loads being displaced through the dorsal vertebral body and fracture. The redirection of axial loads through the dorsal portion of the fracture may impede the degree of anterior column subsidence and therefore minimize the extent of eventual thoracic kyphosis. In the elderly, symptomatic compression fractures associated with severe pain and functional morbidity, which have not responded to a minimum of 6 weeks of conservative management, have been treated with polymethylmethacrylate (PMMA) augmentation, either via vertebroplasty or via a cavitation and endplate elevation procedure (Figure 45.17). These techniques have been associated with a significant improvement in patient function and pain relief.[3,64]

Burst fractures, as defined by Denis, are vertebral body fractures involving the anterior and middle columns, such that the ALL and vertebral body, including the dorsal vertebral body cortex, are disrupted (Figures 45.4, 45.6, 45.11, and 45.13). A burst fracture in a neurologically intact patient without posterior ligamentous or dorsal element fractures is usually considered a stable injury. James *et al.*[54] confirmed this clinically in his reported series of patients with burst-type fractures with an intact dorsal bony architecture, all of whom became stable with a bracing regimen. Thoracic burst fractures (T1-10) comprise a minor subset of burst injuries, representing approximately 5% to 10% of the total number of burst fractures. These burst fractures are inherently more stable because of the presence of the costovertebral ligamentous complex, along with the support of the rib cage.[15] Therefore, like VCFs, conservative therapy has been the mainstay of treatment through bracing and postural reduction.[5,6,36,81]

The incidence and degree of kyphosis and neurologic deterioration after a thoracic and thoracolumbar burst fracture are not known. In the neurologically intact patient with a mild kyphotic deformity (<15 degrees) and minimal dorsal ligamentous disruption, a bracing strategy may be appropriate (Figure 45.18). However, significant divergent splaying of the spinous processes on lateral plain radiographs, which implies dorsal ligamentous complex disruption, often implies the potential for progressive instability. Therefore surgical intervention should be considered. Brown *et al.*[15] advocated nonoperative treatment of burst fractures with less than 50% of vertebral body collapse, less than 30 degrees of kyphotic deformity, and no more than 3cm of offset from the standard sagittal vertical angle on lateral scoliosis films. These recommendations are

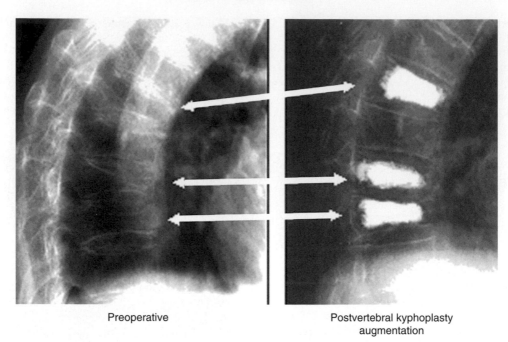

Preoperative   Postvertebral kyphoplasty
                                                        augmentation

Figure 45.17 Three levels of kyphoplasty vertebral augmentation with PMMA.

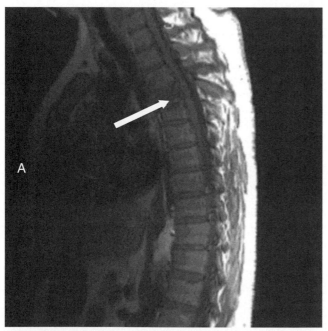

Figure 45.18 A 35-year-old male sustained a T4 burst fracture (*arrow*) with minimal retropulsion and normal strength and examination. Treated in thoracic brace with cervical extension and has had no neurologic decline of progression of kyphosis.

supported by the findings of Cantor and associates,[16] where evidence of dorsal ligamentous complex disruption was present if there was greater than 30 degrees of kyphosis, greater than 50% loss of ventral vertebral body height, splaying of the spinous processes, facet fracture or subluxation, and pars interarticularis fractures. Brown's management protocol recommended immediate casting of the hemodynamically stable patient in a hyperextension body cast, followed by serial radiographs. Casts were maintained for 6 to 12 weeks, followed by a Jewett orthosis and then serial radiographs every 4 weeks. This management strategy facilitated early mobilization, reduced hospital stays and costs, and if successful, avoided the risks of surgical therapy. Nonoperative management therefore may be used in the neurologically intact patient, even with a large degree of spinal canal stenosis from retropulsed bone fragments, as long as there is no significant kyphosis representing significant disruption of the dorsal osteoligamentous complex. CT has confirmed the spontaneous remodeling through bone reabsorption of retropulsed bone fragments in the spinal canal in patients immobilized nonoperatively.[8,23,60] However, if there is a decline in the patient's neurologic status during nonoperative treatment, operative intervention is indicated in the presence of documented instability or neural compression.[81]

Operative Strategies

After assessing the patient with a thoracic or thoracolumbar junction fracture, the surgeon must examine the fracture in relation to neurologic impairment and spinal structural integrity. Optimal imaging studies are important to clearly define the extent of the injury and degree of osseous and ligamentous disruption. The two main goals of spinal surgery after traumatic fractures are to adequately decompress the spinal canal to maximize neurologic recovery and the creation of spinal stability so that a painful deformity and potential future neurologic decline is prevented. Surgical reconstruction provides immediate stabilization and allows earlier mobilization than nonoperative and therefore can prevent or minimize the sequelae of prolonged bed rest, such as pulmonary dysfunction, urinary tract infection, deep vein thrombosis, and cutaneous decubiti.

During the past several decades there has been a rapid progression in the development and advancement of surgical treatments, particularly in the realm of spinal implants. Although internal fixation devices have greatly facilitated the management of thoracic and thoracolumbar injuries, the ultimate outcome is dependent on the attainment of a solid fusion or arthrodesis. If a bone fusion is not achieved, the instrumentation usually will eventually fatigue and fail.

Neurologic Decompression for Incomplete Injuries

Neurologic injuries are present in 42% of patients with thoracolumbar junction fractures.[39] Approximately 90% of patients with a thoracic fracture, excluding a VCF, have a concurrent neurologic injury, with 63% having a complete neurologic deficit.[74] The compression of the spinal cord after thoracic or thoracolumbar trauma is typically caused by a ventral retropulsed bone fragment from the vertebral body. Complete loss of neurologic function below the level of the injury usually occurs at the moment of trauma, and therefore removing the presence of retropulsed bone in the setting of a complete neurologic injury (ASIA A) rarely, if ever, enhances neurologic recovery.[8] However, in the presence of an incomplete neurologic deficit with persistent compression of the neural elements, a decompressive procedure may maximize the potential for neurologic recovery.[19] Boerger[8] performed a metaanalysis of the world literature to analyze surgical outcome after decompression of the spinal cord after thoracolumbar burst fractures. Patients with an incomplete neurologic deficit who underwent an operative decompression and stabilization procedure were shown to have an enhanced neurologic recovery compared to nonoperatively treated patients.[8,10,12,56] Operative therapy has also been shown to decrease pain, reduce periods of postural reduction or bedrest, and improve sagittal alignment.[38] Presently, surgical decompression in patients with a complete neurologic injury has not demonstrated true benefit in terms of overall neurologic improvement.[9]

A ventral or dorsolateral approach may effectively decompress the neural elements in the setting of spinal cord compression. The ventral approach is particularly useful for decompressing midline ventral lesions and correcting severe kyphotic deformities.[9,10] Bohlman[9] reported superior neurologic outcomes after a ventral, compared to a dorsal, decompressive procedure in the setting of an incomplete thoracic spinal cord injury. The major limitation of a ventral exposure is the potential surgical violation of the pleural and/or peritoneal cavities. McCormick[71] reported the effective use of an extrapleural technique for the exposure of the ventral thoracic and thoracolumbar spine, thus avoiding violation of the pleural cavity.

Biomechanically, ventral reconstruction and instrumentation provides superior mechanical stability over an equal number of spinal segments to compressive loads than do dorsal instrumentation strategies.[96] A patient with midline ventral spinal cord compression, an incomplete neurologic injury, and an unstable thoracic or thoracolum-

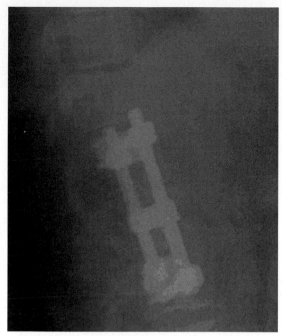

Figure 45.19 Anterior corpectomy and decompression after a burst fracture, followed with an anterior iliac crest bone graft fusion with a Kaneda device.

bar junction burst fracture is most effectively treated with a ventral decompression and reconstruction procedure (Figure 45.19). A variety of ventral instrumentation systems are now available that may be applied to the ventral spinal elements after an adequate decompression and fusion procedure. Biomechanically, ventral bicortical screws purchase provides a 25% to 50% increase in screw purchase strength, compared to unilateral screw purchase.[14]

Dorsal decompression via laminectomy after thoracic and thoracolumbar injuries has been shown to be ineffective and should not be performed as an isolated treatment strategy.[9,80] The surgical removal or destruction of the dorsal ligamentous complex, along with the dorsal osseous elements, may permit temporary neurologic recovery. However, the vertebral column may not be able to maintain its alignment with the loss of the dorsal tension band and instability, along with the potential progression of a kyphotic deformity, may ensue (Figure 45.20). The immediate result of removing the dorsal osseous components is dorsal migration of the spinal cord if the spine has a lordotic alignment. However, the normal untraumatized spinal column at the thoracolumbar junction maintains a slightly kyphotic posture. Spinal trauma typically results in an increase in the kyphotic deformity or angulation. Therefore removing the dorsal tension band after trauma in the setting of ventral compression from bone fragments may result in further neurologic compromise, caused by tethering of the neural elements (bowstring effect) over ventral bony elements.

An axial compression fracture subjected to surgical intervention requires the application of a distractive force to realign the spinal column. This can be accomplished either with ventral distraction (ventral to the IAR) through a ventral approach or through dorsal distraction, fracture reduction, and realignment via ligamentotaxis. Ligamentotaxis requires a partially intact PLL, as well as Sharpey fibers, in order for the applied distraction force to tension (tighten) these ligamentous fibers and therefore reduce the retropulsed bone fragments ventrally and out of the spinal canal. Overdistraction may result in neurologic worsening or progression of the kyphotic deformity, especially if applied to a flexion-distraction injury.

Harrington rods were the first spinal implants widely used for the treatment of vertebral fractures. The dorsal spinal elements are distracted to reduce and realign the vertebral column via ligamentotaxis.[48] Unfortunately, this artificially applied distraction force can result in the loss of the normal spinal curvature (loss of lordosis or exaggeration of kyphosis), resulting in muscles and ligaments working at a biomechanical disadvantage. As a result of the ensuing sagittal imbalance (or the creation of a flat back deformity), the patient's muscles may fatigue over time, as they strain to maintain an upright position. This can result in significant pain and disability.[53] Rod and proximal and distal hook dorsal internal fixation strategies that rely on distraction and ligamentotaxis require the spanning of multiple spinal segments in order to achieve biomechanical efficacy. This, along with their inability to efficiently control sagittal alignment, has given way to other more biomechanically friendly devices (multiple segmental hook/rod or pedicle screw based systems) that facilitate better control of the sagittal and coronal curvatures of the spine.

An advantage of a dorsal approach is that it provides excellent visualization and access to the dorsal thecal sac. This is useful in certain fracture types, since the reported incidence of thecal sac lacerations (with a potential for nerve root incarceration) after traumatic thoracic and thoracolumbar burst fractures is 7% to 16%.[58,98] The lumbar nerve roots are prone to entrapment through these lacerations. A ventral approach will not provide access to repair this deficiency.[77] The presence of a central split or greenstick fracture of the spinous process on preoperative transaxial CT imaging studies may be an indicator of a dural laceration, depending on its size and displacement during impact.[78]

Additional Operative Considerations

Fracture-dislocations are the most unstable of traumatic vertebral column injuries. The fractures are created by significant high-energy loads that result in a complete dissociation of the osseous structures and ligamentous complexes. Typically, these have a complete loss of neurologic function.[21,26] (Figure 45.15). Flexion-distraction-dislocation injuries have a significant distraction component and differ from seat-belt type injuries in that there is a large rotatory or torque component that causes a disruption of all three spinal columns.[25] An injury of this type in the thoracic region almost always results in a complete spinal cord injury. This is so because the spinal canal is smaller at this level, there is a diminished vascular supply to the thoracic spinal cord, and a significant amount of energy is required to cause such an injury. Such injuries are associated with the highest incidence of concurrent neurologic injuries.[25,50,66] Denis reported that over 50% of patients with this fracture subtype had a complete paraplegia.

Patients with a complete neurologic injury involving the thoracic spine may frequently benefit from surgical

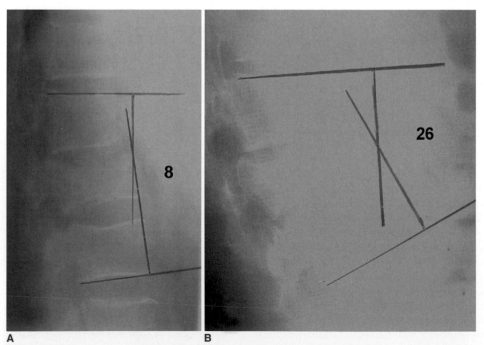

A   **B**

Figure 45.20 A 50-year-old male with L2 burst fracture after a fall. **(A)** Plain sagittal radiograph illustrating 8 degrees of kyphosis. **(B)** Treated in a body cast and then braced but had progressive back pain, and follow-up radiographs illustrate progression of the kyphosis to 26 degrees.

intervention to realign a deformity, provide immediate stability, and prevent further or future neurologic injury. Postural reduction and bed rest mandate at least 6 to 12 weeks of prolonged immobilization before the spine heals enough to attain any degree of intrinsic stability.[21]

The immediate stability provided to the vertebral column by spinal instrumentation provides an environment conducive to soft tissue healing and bone graft maturation. The use of screws placed through the pedicles permits immobilization of all three spinal columns and is quite effective in injuries involving the thoracolumbar junction. This form of instrumentation provides substantial load-sharing capabilities. However, without adequate anterior column support, pseudarthrosis may ensue with possible fatiguing of the instrumentation. McCormack *et al.*[72] illustrated the need to assess the structural stability of the anterior column with a load-sharing classification. The ability of the anterior column to support axial loads can be assessed through examination of the kyphotic angulation, the number and comminution of the fracture fragments, and the dispersion or space between fragments. If the anterior column does not remodel and form a solid column that supports axial loads, dorsal instrumentation constructs are at risk for eventual failure.

Indirect augmentation of the anterior column via a dorsal transpedicular approach, without removal or replacement of the contiguous intervertebral discs, does not appear to provide sufficient anterior column support. Alanay *et al.*[1] demonstrated that short segment transpedicular screw fixation, with and without transpedicular bone graft augmentation, via a dorsal approach failed equally (approximately 50%). The lateral extracavitary approach provides access to both the ventral and dorsal portion of the vertebral column through a single dorsal incision. However, this approach has limited usefulness in thoracic and lumbar trauma because of its high incidence of associated morbidities. Resnick and Benzel[90] reviewed their series of 33 trauma patients treated with this approach and reported a 55% incidence of morbidity.

Fracture dislocations are extremely unstable and early surgery with instrumentation provides immediate spinal stability and facilitates early entry into the rehabilitation process. The surgeon must carefully assess the structural integrity of the anterior column when planning an operative procedure. If the anterior column is intact or only minimally damaged, dorsal reduction and instrumentation with bone grafting may be appropriate, without the need for an additional ventral procedure. However, if there is a large degree of anterior column compromise, a ventral reconstruction may prevent late progression of spinal deformity and instrumentation failure.

Summary

Neurologically intact patients with compression fractures or stable burst fractures may be managed successfully with conservative external orthosis. Patients with an incomplete neurologic injury may benefit from an operative decompression and stabilization procedure to maximize the potential for neurologic recovery. It is clear that fracture dislocation injuries are unstable and require operative stabilization to restore sagittal alignment and prevent posttraumatic deformities. However, injuries that are without obvious kyphotic misalignment on presenting plain radiographs, but with clear disruption of the dorsal osteoligamentous complex on advanced imaging studies, may require surgical intervention. It is generally agreed that injuries involving destruction of the dorsal osteoligamentous complex manifested as splaying of the spinous processes or severe kyphotic deformities (greater than 30 degrees) are considered unstable, often benefiting from surgical intervention.

Flexion-distraction or bony Chance fractures are also potentially unstable injuries. These injuries are created through large-energy force vectors that involve both a distraction and a flexion component, resulting in both middle and posterior column disruption.[25] The vertebral body is stronger in tension than compression, and therefore distraction injuries usually result in failure at the disc-end-plate interface. Compressive forces typically disrupt the vertebral body.[67] In these Chance or seat-belt type injuries, the anterior column may be compressed if the IAR involves the anterior of the middle spinal column. These injuries are characterized by horizontal fractures through the posterior and middle column osseous structures, but variants involve tissue disruption that may involve the contiguous soft tissue structures. These injuries may be difficult to visualize on CT, because the fracture lines may be horizontally oriented and in the line of gantry of the CT image acquisition.

Patients who do not have an obvious unstable injury on initial presentation may still have occult instability that may manifest late as mechanical pain or a progressive neurologic deficit if not followed on a routine basis.

REFERENCES

1. Alanay A, Emre A, Muharrem Y, *et al:* Short-segment pedicle instrumentation of thoracolumbar burst fractures: Does transpedicular intracorporeal grafting prevent early failure? *Spine* 26(2):213-217, 2001.
1a. Andriacchi TP, Schultz AB: A model for the studies of mechanical interactions between the human spine and rib cage. *J Biomech* 7:497-507, 1974.
2. Argenson C, Bouleau P, de Peretti F, Lovett J: Les fractures du rachis thoracique (T1-10). A propos de 105 cas. *Rev Chir Orthop* 75(6):370-386, 1989.
3. Barr JD, Barr MS, Lemley TJ, McCann RM: Percutaneous vertebroplasty for pain relief and spinal stabilization. *Spine* 25(8):923-928, 2000.
4. Beaunoyer M, St-Vil D, Lallier M, Blanchard H Abdominal injuries associated with thoraco-lumbar fractures after motor vehicle collision. *J Ped Surg* 36(5):760-762, 2001.
5. Bedbrook GM: Stability of spinal fractures and fracture dislocations. *Paraplegia* 9:23-32, 1971.
6. Bedbrook GM: Treatment of thoracolumbar dislocation and fracture with paraplegia. *Clin Orthop* 112:267-284, 1979.
7. Berry JL, Moran JM, Berg WS, Steffee AD: A morphological study of human lumbar and selected thoracic vertebrae. *Spine* 12:362-366, 1987.

8. Boerger TO, Limb D, Dickson RA: Does 'canal clearance' affect neurological outcome after thoracolumbar burst fractures? *J Bone Joint Surg* 82B:629-635, 2000.

9. Bohlman HH: Traumatic fractures of the upper thoracic spine with paralysis. *J Bone Joint Surg [Am]* 56:1299, 1974.

10. Bohlman HH, Freehafer A, Dejak J: The results of treatment of acute injuries of the upper thoracic spine with paralysis. *J Bone Joint Surg [Am]* 67:360-369, 1985.

11. Boyle JJ, Singer KP, Milne N: Morphological survey of the cervicothoracic junctional region. *Spine* 21(5): 544-548,1996.

12. Bradford DS, Akbarnia BA, Winter RB: Surgical stabilization of fractures and fracture dislocations of the thoracic spine. *Spine* 2:185-196, 1977.

13. Breathnach AS: *Fraser's Anatomy of the Human Skeleton*, ed 5. London: J&A Churchill, Ltd, 1958.

14. Breeze SW, Doherty BJ, Noble PS, *et al*: A biomechanical study of anterior thoracolumbar screw fixation. *Spine* 23(17):1829-1831, 1998.

15. Brown CW, Gorup JM, Chow GH: Nonsurgical treatment of thoracic burst fractures in controversies In Zdeblick TA, Benzel EC,Anderson PA, Stillerman CB (eds): *Spine Surgery*, St. Louis, Quality Medical Publishing, 1999, pp 86-96.

16. Cantor JB, Lebwohl NH, Garvey T, Eismont FJ: Non-operative management of stable thoracolumbar burst fractures with early ambulation and bracing. *Spine* 19:1731-1740, 1993.

17. Chan RNW, Ainscow D, Sikorski JM: Diagnostic failures in the multiple injured. *J Trauma* 20:684-687, 1980.

18. Chance CQ. Note on a type of flexion fracture of the spine. *Br J Radiol* 21:452, 1948.

19. Chapman JR, Anderson PA: Thoracolumbar spine fractures and neurologic deficits (review). *Orthop Clin North Am* 25:595-612, 1994.

20. Chiliimindris CP: Rupture of the thoracic esophagus from blunt trauma. *J Trauma* 17:968-971, 1977.

21. Convery FR, Minteer MA, Smith RW, Emerson SM: Fracture-dislocation of the dorsal-lumbar spine: Acute operative stabilization by Harrington instrumentation. *Spine* 3:160, 1978.

22. Daffner RH, Deeb ZL, Rothfus WE: Thoracic fractures and dislocations in motorcyclists. *Skeletal Radiol* 16: 280-284, 1987.

23. Dai LY: Remodeling of the spinal canal after thoracolumbar burst fractures *Clin Ortho Rel Res* 382:119-123, 2001.

24. Dalvie SS, Burwell M, Noordeen MHH: Haemothorax and thoracic spinal fracture: a case for early stabilization. *Injury* 31:269-270, 2000.

25. Denis F: The three column spine and its significance in the classification of acute thoracolumbar spinal injuries. *Spine* 8(8):817-831, 1983.

26. Denis F, Burkus JK: Shear fracture dislocations of the thoracic and lumbar spine associated with forceful hyperextension (lumberjack paraplegia). *Spine* 17:152, 1992.

27. Dickman CA, Fessler RG, MacMillan M, Haid RW: Transpedicular screw-rod fixation of the lumbar spine: operative technique and outcome in 104 cases. *J Neurosurg* 77:860-870, 1992.

28. Ebraheim NA, Xu R, Ahmad M, Yeasting RA: Projection of the thoracic pedicle and its morphometric analysis. *Spine* 22:233-238, 1997.

29. El-Khoury GY, Whitten CG: Trauma to the upper thoracic spine: anatomy, biomechanics and unique imaging features. *AJR* 160:95-102, 1993.

30. Enderson BL, Reath DB, Meadows J: The tertiary trauma survey: a prospective study of missed injury. *J Trauma* 30:666-669, 1990.

31. Evans L: Risk of fatality from physical trauma versus sex and age. *J Trauma* 28:368-378, 1988.

32. Ferguson RL, Allen BL Jr: A mechanistic classification of thoracolumbar spine fractures. *Clin Orthop* 189:817-831, 1983.

33. Flanders AE: Thoracolumbar trauma imaging overview. *Instructional Course Lectures* 48:429-431, 1999.

34. Fon G, Pitt MJ, Thies AC: Thoracic kyphosis: range in normal subjects. *Am J Roentgenol* 134:979-983, 1980.

35. Fessler RG, Greenwald D, Peace D: Surgical exposures of the cervicothoracic and upper thoracic spine. In Benzel EC, Stillerman CB (eds): *The Thoracic Spine*. St Louis, Quality Medical Publishing, 1999, pp 197-207.

36. Frankel HL, Hancock DO, Hyslop G: The value of postural reduction in the initial management of closed injuries of the spine with paraplegia and tetraplegia. *Paraplegia* 7:179-92, 1969.

37. Freysz M, Adamon O, Wilkening M, Sautreaux JL: Hemothorax et fractures de la colonne dorsale. *Sem-Hop* 59(32):2229-2231, 1983.

38. Gertzbein SD: Scoliosis Research Society: Multicenter spine fracture study. *Spine* 17:528-540, 1992.

39. Gertzbein SD: *Fractures of the Thoracic and Lumbar Spine*. Baltimore: Williams & Wilkins, 1992.

40. Gertzbein SD: Neurologic deterioration in patients with thoracic and lumbar fractures after admission to the hospital. *Spine* 19:1723-1725, 1994.

41. Gray H: Anatomy, descriptive and surgical. In Pick TP, Howden R (eds): *Revised American Edition from the Fifteenth English Edition*. New York, Bounty Books, 1977.

42. Haber TR, Filmy WT, O'Brien M: Thoracic and lumbar fractures: diagnosis and management. In Bridwell KH, DeWald PR (eds): *The Textbook of Spinal Surgery*. Philadelphia, Lippincott, 1991, pp 857-910.

43. Haher TR, O'Brien M, Felmly WT, *et al*: Instantaneous axis of rotation as a function of the three columns of the spine. *Spine* 17(6 Suppl):S149-S154, 1992.

44. Haher TR, Bergman M, O'Brien M, *et al*: The effect of the three columns of the spine on the instantaneous axis of rotation in flexion and extension. *Spine* 16(8 Suppl): S312-S318, 1991.

45. Haher TR, Tozzi JM, Lospinuso MF, *et al*: The contribution of the three columns of the spine to spinal stability: a biomechanical model. *Paraplegia* 27(6): 432-439, 1989.

46. Haher TR, Felmy W, Baruch H, *et al*: The contribution of the three columns of the spine to rotational stability. A biomechanical model. *Spine* 14(7):663-669, 1989.

47. Hanley EN, Eskay ML: Thoracic spine fractures. *Orthopedics* 12:689-696, 1989.

48. Harrington RM, Budorick T, Hoyt J, *et al*: Biomechanics of indirect reduction of bone retropulsed into the canal in vertebral fracture. *Spine* 18:692-699, 1993.

CHAPTER 46

Trauma Surgery: Fractures of the Lumbar and Sacral Spine

Paul Santiago and Richard G. Fessler

Patients with isolated fractures of the lumbar and sacral spine represent a small subset of the more than 150,000 individuals in the United States who sustain vertebral column injuries annually. The majority of lumbar fractures occur in combination with fractures of the lower thoracic spine at the thoracolumbar junction. The anatomy and physiology of the lumbar and sacral spine make these regions more resistant to injury than the thoracic spine. Therefore, it is not uncommon for patients with lumbar and sacral fractures to have significant closed head, pulmonary, intraabdominal, and extremity injuries. A thorough understanding of the pathophysiology of these fractures is required to appreciate which fractures must be stabilized in the context of significant comorbidity.

Initial Management

All patients involved in major trauma should be treated as having a potential spinal injury until proven otherwise. Initial management in the field should follow an advanced life support protocol. A stable airway, adequate ventilation, and hemodynamic stability should be established. Once a patient is stabilized, a neurologic examination should be performed, keeping in mind that concomitant head injury, intoxication, or extremity injury may make a thorough examination difficult or impossible.[4] A "normal" neurologic examination in the field does not rule out a spinal injury. The majority of spinal fractures occur in the absence of neurologic deficit. For this reason, patients should be transferred from the field to a hospital, using full spinal precautions. This includes multiperson patient transfer, log rolling, and the use of a cervical orthosis and backboard. Every attempt should be made to maintain the spinal column in as near neutral alignment as possible. Of spinal cord injury (SCI) patients, 1.8% to 10% have been reported to experience deterioration in their neurologic function after admission to hospital.* A significant number of these patients suffered secondary injuries that could have been prevented. Finally, certain injury mechanisms should raise the suspicion of associated spinal fractures. Patients jumping or falling from heights with significant lower-extremity injury, calcaneal injuries in particular, are at high risk for accompanying lumbar and thoracolumbar spine injuries. Patients involved in motor vehicle accidents

and wearing lap belts only are at risk for flexion distraction injuries. These injuries can sometimes be difficult to identify on plain films and axial CT.

Because of the magnitude of the forces required to cause fractures in the lumbar and sacral spine, these injuries have been associated with significant comorbidity. Head and extremity injuries are common.[4] Lumbar fractures have been associated with abdominal and urologic trauma, particularly in cases of lap belt injuries.[38] Sacral fractures are often associated with pelvic injury. An indication of the severity of these injuries is the 10% to 20% mortality that has been reported in closed pelvic trauma.[54]

Upon the patient's arrival to the hospital from the field, airway, pulmonary, and cardiovascular status should be reassessed. In patients with hemodynamic instability, diagnostic peritoneal lavage, CT of the chest and abdomen, and/or diagnostic ultrasound is indicated. Workup of altered mental status should include a head CT. During the initial workup, a lateral C-spine, anteroposterior (AP) chest and AP pelvis radiographs are obtained. Among the many injuries that can be detected with these screening tools are gross malalignment of the spine and pelvis.

A detailed spinal examination may commence once immediate life-threatening injury has been ruled out. Care should be taken to inspect the patient's skin and posture. Bruising of the abdomen may be a sign of an underlying lap belt type injury. An abnormal posture may be indicative of muscle spasm and associated spinal injury. Using full spinal precautions, the patient should be log rolled and the skin and contour of the neck and back examined. Bruising, step-off, deviation from the normal spinal curvature, or pain with dorsal midline palpation may be indicative of an underlying bony and ligamentous injury.

Neurologic examination should be carried out in a systematic and standardized fashion. Results should be communicated using the accepted standard. This facilitates communication between treating specialties. Progressive neurologic deterioration is a widely accepted indication for acute intervention. It is, therefore, imperative that an accurate assessment of baseline neurologic function be established. The ASIA/IMSOP scale is the currently accepted standard. This scoring system is described elsewhere and is summarized in Figure 46.1 and Table 46.1.

Diagnostic Imaging

Radiologic workup of a patient with a presumed spinal injury begins with plain radiographs of the spine. In compliant patients with unaltered metal status, no distracting injuries, and lack of midline spinal tenderness, the patient's spine can be cleared without obtaining screening plain radiographs.[52] However, if the patient does not meet any of the above criteria, a "complete spine series" is mandatory. One should bear in mind that between 5% and 20% of all spine fractures are multiple and 5% occur at noncontiguous levels.[9] The "complete spine series" includes, at a minimum: AP and lateral views of the cervical, thoracic, lumbar and sacral spine, and open mouth odontoid view. These can be supplemented with swimmer's views to define the cervicothoracic junction and oblique views to assess the facet complex and pars interarticularis. Flexion/extension studies are generally avoided

---

*References 1,8,10,13,22,25,29,44,50,61.

in the workup of acute fractures. Spinal alignment should be assessed in both planes. The margins of the vertebral bodies, the spinolaminar line, facets, the interspinous and interpedicular distance, and the position of the transverse process should be studied. Acute kyphotic angulation or loss of lordosis may be indicative of an acute bony or ligamentous injury. Loss of disk height at the level above a vertebral body fracture is often observed in acute flexion injuries, but it may also be seen in cases of degenerative disk disease. Bare or "naked" facets may be indicative of posterior ligamentous injury as a result of a distraction type injury. Abnormalities of the soft tissues, such as a paraspinal mass or loss of the psoas stripe can help identify areas of adjacent bony injury.

Poorly visualized segments or pathologic segments should be examined with fine cut CT (minimum 3mm slices), extending from one level above to one level below the region of interest. Coronal and sagittal reformations may prove helpful in the diagnosis of axially oriented injuries, such as Chance fractures. CT myelography can be useful in the study of nerve root injury above the sacral spine, since the thecal sac ends at S2 in most patients. MRI can be useful in the study of patients with neurologic deficit to determine the extent of compression on the

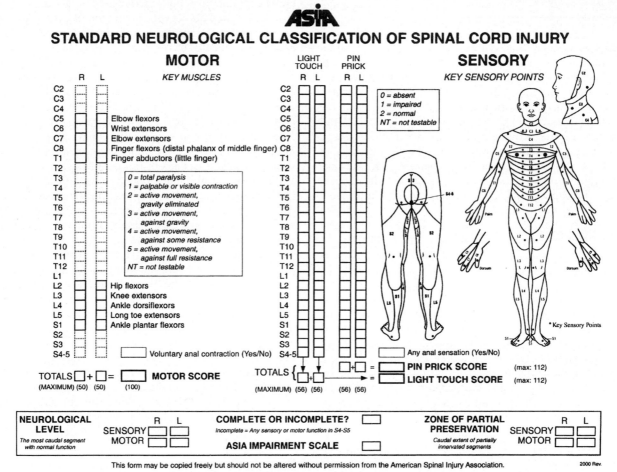

Figure 46.1 Summary of the spinal component of the neurologic examination as endorsed by the American Spinal Injury Association.

TABLE 46.1	
ASIA Impairment Scale	
A.	Complete: No motor or sensory function is preserved in the sacral segments S4-S5.
B.	Incomplete: Sensory but no motor function is preserved below the neurologic level and includes the sacral segments S4-S5.
C.	Incomplete: Motor function is preserved below the neurologic level, and more than half of key muscles below the neurologic level have a muscle grade less than 3/5.
D.	Incomplete: Motor function is preserved below the neurologic level, and at least half of key muscles below the neurologic level have a muscle grade of 3/5 or more.
E.	Normal: Motor and sensory functions are normal.

Courtesy of American Spinal Injury Association.

neural elements. Although current MRI techniques are in many ways more sensitive than CT in detecting areas of acute injury, they do not provide the bony detail provided by conventional CT. Increased signal on T_2-weighted imaging may be used to detect fractures not well visualized on plain radiographs or CT. Short tau inversion recovery (STIR) sequences are quite sensitive for the detection of ligamentous and intervertebral disk injury not otherwise detected by plain radiographs or CT.

In one series, 49% of sacral fractures were missed on initial hospital presentation and included 24% with "unexplained" neurologic deficit, later explained by the presence of a fracture.[23] The sacrum is poorly visualized on standard AP views of the pelvis, so the treating physician must rely on other cues to prompt a more detailed survey of this region. A history of direct trauma, fracture of a lower lumbar transverse process, ventral pelvic ring fracture without an identifiable dorsal pelvic ring fracture, asymmetry of the sacral notch, clouding of the trabecular pattern in the lateral sacral mass, or irregularity of the arcuate lines of the upper three sacral neural foramina on AP pelvic radiographs should prompt more detailed studies. These studies should include a Ferguson's view (true AP of the sacrum with the beam directed 30 degrees rostrally) and a lateral sacral film including the coccyx. CT with coronal and axial reformations is the most sensitive modality for defining complex pelvic and sacral fractures.

Neurologic Injury

Injury to adjacent spinal cord segments and nerve roots is of great concern in acute spinal injury. The pattern of neurologic injury observed is dependent on the location of spinal injury. In the majority of patients, the conus medullaris lies directly opposite the L1 vertebral body. The conus medullaris contains the anterior horn cells of the L5 through S5 nerves. Additionally, all exiting lumbar roots pass behind the L1 vertebral body. Injuries to the L1 vertebral body, such as burst fractures, can lead to significant neurologic deficit. Both upper motor neuron (conus injury) and lower motor neuron (cauda equina) injury can occur.[32,34] The injury pattern runs the spectrum from a complete injury below L1 to incomplete syndromes resulting in partial motor and sensory preservation with sacral dysfunction. The sacral nerve roots are the most sensitive to injury and the least likely to improve after injury. Injury to the sacral spinal cord and nerve roots can result in loss of bowel and bladder function; sexual function is often less severely affected. Injuries from L2-5 can result in isolated root injuries or cauda equina syndrome. Root injuries can appear as monoradiculopathy or polyradiculopathy. Cauda equina syndrome appears as a variable sensory, motor, bowel, and bladder dysfunction. Sensory and motor loss tends to be asymmetric. This is in contradistinction to the conus medullaris syndrome where deficits are usually more symmetrical. Sphincteric dysfunction is common and is often permanent.

Denis et al.[18] reported a 21% incidence of nerve injury with sacral fractures. Injury to the sacral ala (Zone I) was associated with 5.9% rate of injury to the L5 nerve root and presented with symptoms of a sciatica-type syndrome.

Of fractures through the sacral foramina (Zone II), 28.4% were associated with unilateral L5-S2 injuries. Finally, more than half (56.7%) of fractures through the sacral canal (Zone III) were associated with sphincteric dysfunction and saddle anesthesia.

Anatomic Considerations

Anatomic differences have a significant effect on the types of fractures encountered along the lumbar and sacral spine.[48,59] For the purposes of this discussion, the upper lumbar spine L1-2 should be considered as part of the thoracolumbar junction (T11-L2). The upper thoracic spine is relatively rigid, and the lumbar spine is relatively mobile. Biomechanically, this difference results in a region of high stress at the interface between these two segments. Second, the thoracic spine deforms in kyphosis and the lumbar spine deforms in lordosis, resulting in nearly pure compressive forces at the thoracolumbar junction. Third, the thoracic spine is highly resistant to rotational forces because of the stabilizing effect of the rib cage.[2] The inwardly directed facets of the lower lumbar spine help resist rotational forces. The thoracolumbar spine lacks attachments to the rib cage and has a transitional facet structure that is unable to resist rotational forces. As a result, 60% of all spinal fractures occur between T12 and L2 and 90% occur between T11 and L4.[36,46,51] Fractures of the lower lumbar spine (L3-5) account for approximately 4% of all spinal fractures because of their relatively large size, significant muscular attachments, and the stability of their inwardly directed facets.[41,42]

The sacrum with its intimate attachments to the pelvis is an incredibly stable structure.[49] The relatively immobile sacroiliac joint and strong ventral and dorsal ligamentous attachments between the sacrum and pelvis account for this stability. The sacrum lies at a 40-degree incline from horizontal at the lumbosacral junction. Axial loads, therefore, result in rotational forces. These rotational forces are resisted by the strength of the sacrotuberous and sacrospinous ligaments, which attach opposite the S4 neural foramina. The sacrum forms a portion of the dorsal pelvic arch and, as a result, 90% of reported sacral fractures occur in conjunction with pelvic fractures.[6] Removal of the sacrum distal to the S1-2 interspace weakens the pelvic ring by 30% and resection up to S1, thereby removing half of the sacroiliac joint, which weakens the pelvic ring by 50%.[27] Thus any discussion of stability of the sacrum must also include a discussion of pelvic stability.

Fracture Classification

Several classification systems have been developed to describe fractures of the thoracic and lumbar spine. Since most spinal fractures occur in the thoracolumbar junction region (classically defined as extending from T11-L2), these systems are most suited to describing pathology in this region.[16,46] Over time, however, these systems have been applied to the remainder of the thoracic spine and to the subaxial cervical spine. Holdsworth[33] first proposed a two-column concept of the cervical spine in the early 1960s. He described a two-column model, with a ventral, weight-bearing vertebral body and a dorsal ligamentous

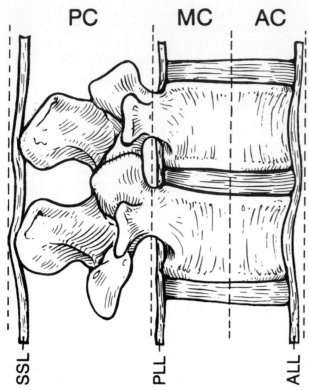

Figure 46.2 Three columns of the spine: anterior column (*AC*), middle column (*MC*), and posterior column (*PC*). *ALL,* Anterior longitudinal ligament; *PLL,* posterior longitudinal ligament; *SSL,* supraspinous ligament. (*From Haber TR, Felmly WT, O'Brien M: Thoracic and lumbar fractures: diagnosis and management. In Bridwell KH, DeWald RL [eds]:* Textbook of Spinal Surgery, *vol 2. Philadelphia, JB Lippincott, 1991, pp 857-910.*)

complex. Instability was defined as failure of the dorsal ligamentous complex. Later, biomechanical and clinical data did not support this model.[16,46,59] In 1983 both Denis and McAfee[16,46] independently published three-column models that have become widely accepted (Figure 46.2). More recently, Magerl *et al.*[43] proposed a system based upon the three basic forces (compression, distraction, and rotation). The utility of this model has yet to be established.

The three-column models of Denis and McAfee are very similar but do have some fundamental differences (Table 46.2). Each model divides the vertebra into three columns: anterior column (anterior longitudinal ligament, ventral one half of the vertebral body, and ventral one half of the annulus fibrosus), middle column (posterior longitudinal ligament, dorsal one half of the vertebral body, and dorsal one half of the annulus fibrosus), and posterior column (supraspinous and infraspinous ligaments, ligamentum flavum, articular processes, joint capsules, spinous processes, and laminae). In Denis's model, instability requires injury to at least two columns with an emphasis on preservation of the middle column for the maintenance of stability. Fractures are divided into four groups: wedge compression, lap belt-type injury, burst fracture, and fracture dislocation. Instability varies in magnitude: first degree (mechanical), second degree (neurologic), and third degree (mechanical and neurologic). McAfee's system places more emphasis on preservation of the posterior column for the maintenance of stability and defines six fracture patterns: wedge compres-

sion, Chance fracture, flexion-distraction injury, stable burst, unstable burst, and translational injury.

Wedge Compression Fractures

Wedge compression fractures are common injuries, accounting for 58% of all spinal fractures. They result from isolated failure of the anterior column, which fails in flexion and compression (Figure 46.2). Severe cases may result in partial failure of the posterior column "tension band." By definition the middle column is preserved. Minimal and moderate wedge compression fractures are stable. Multilevel fractures may progress to kyphosis and may require treatment in an orthosis. Severe wedge compression fractures with failure of the posterior column may progress to mechanical instability and should be treated as unstable. Neurologic deficit is rare.

Burst Fractures

Burst fractures comprise 17% of all spinal fractures. Burst fractures occur as a result of failure of the anterior and middle columns under axial compression. In severe burst fractures, the posterior elements may also be injured (Figure 46.3). However, injury to the dorsal elements is not universal and, for this reason, McAfee distinguishes between stable and unstable burst fractures, that is, two-column versus three-column injury, respectively. Additionally, isolated horizontal laminar fractures do not impact upon the stability of the posterior column and should not be counted as part of a three-column injury. Bony fragments may be retropulsed into the spinal canal and can result in significant neurologic deficit. The extent of neurologic deficit is highly dependent on the level of injury. Injuries at the conus level and above (above L1-2) can result in a complete SCI or anterior cord syndrome. Symptoms of spinal stenosis may develop in a delayed fashion in initially asymptomatic patients with high degrees of spinal canal compromise treated without surgical decompression. So-called "stable" burst fractures are most often treated with an orthosis and serial imaging. Indications for surgical decompression and stabilization are highly controversial. The literature does not support surgical decompression for patients with incomplete injuries lasting more than 48 hours.[5] In general, incomplete spinal cord and cauda equina injuries with greater than 40% spinal canal compromise, greater than 50% loss of vertebral body height (compared to average height of the vertebral bodies above and below the level of injury), or greater than 20 degrees of segmental kyphosis have been treated with surgical intervention.[*] The correlation between the extent of canal compromise and neurologic dysfunction remains controversial.[†] Timing of surgery in incomplete lesions remains controversial.[‡] A benefit to early surgical decompression has not been consistently demonstrated with respect to improvement in neurologic function. Early intervention allows for early mobilization and rehabilitation.[§] Early intervention has also been shown to decrease complications such

---

[*]References 3,5,21,26,45,47.
[†]References 12,14,16,24,30,31,39,40,46,47,56,58.
[‡]References 3,12,20,21,37,45,53.
[§]References 7,15,19,21,28,34,35,47.

TABLE 46.2

Comparison of Three-Column Classification Schemes

Fracture type		Spinal column failure			Assessment of stability	
Denis	McAfee	Anterior	Middle	Posterior	Denis	McAfee
Wedge compression	Wedge compression	X			Stable*	Generally stable†
Lap belt type injury	Chance fracture		X	X	Unstable‡	Generally stable§
	Flexion distraction	X	X	X		Generally unstable
Burst fracture	Stable burst	X	X		Unstable‖	Stable
	Unstable burst	X	X	X		Unstable
Fracture dislocation	Translational injury	X	X	X	Unstable¶	Unstable

*Severe wedge compression fractures may result in progressive kyphosis over time.
†Multilevel wedge compression fractures may require surgical therapy.
‡Potential mechanical instability.
§Unstable if there is facet dislocation, subluxation, or facet fracture.
‖Burst fractures are either neurologically unstable, or both mechanically and neurologically unstable.
¶Fracture dislocations are both mechanically and neurologically unstable.
Modified from McCormack B, MacMillan M, Fessler RG: Management of thoracic, lumbar and sacral injuries. In Tindall GT, Cooper PR, Barrow D (eds): *The Practice of Neurosurgery*, vol II. Baltimore, Williams & Wilkins, 1996, pp 1721-1740.

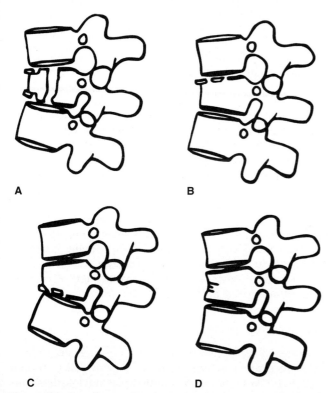

Figure 46.3 Four types of compression fractures, as described by Denis: (**A**) Compression of fracture detaching anterior vertebral body from posterior vertebral body. (**B**) Failure of superior end plate. (**C**) Failure of inferior end plate. (**D**) Failure of superior and inferior end plates. (*From Denis F: The three column spine and its significance in the classification of acute thoracolumbar spinal injuries.* Spine 8:817-831, 1983.)

as decubitus ulcer formation, deep vein thrombosis, and pneumonia. Finally, the benefit of dorsal decompression in neurologically intact patients is also controversial. Some centers adopt the approach of a limited dorsal stabilization in the acute period, followed by a staged ventral decompression and fusion.

Lap Belt Type Injuries

Lap belt type fractures were first described by Chance[11,16] in 1948 and comprise 6% of all spinal injuries. In Chance fractures, the fulcrum is moved to the anterior abdominal wall by the lap belt, as opposed to anterior wedge compression fractures, where the fulcrum of flexion is in the anterior column. Therefore, the middle and posterior columns fail in flexion and distraction (Figure 46.4). Injury may extend into the anterior column, but the anterior longitudinal ligament is usually preserved along with enough of the remainder of the anterior column to preserve alignment. Neurologic injury usually does not occur. These injuries are quite painful and often result in significant soft tissues disruption. Bruising and widening of the interspinous space is often detected on physical examination. Several variants exist involving one or two levels and may be purely bony, purely ligamentous, or combined. The classic Chance fracture is a pure bony injury and is defined as a horizontal fracture through the dorsal arch and pedicles, extending into the dorsal aspect of the vertebral body. "Bony" Chance fractures can be treated in an orthosis or Risser cast with serial imaging. MRI is useful in these cases to document preservation of the disk and ligamentous structures. Injuries involving the ligamentous structures and disk are usually treated with surgical stabilization. Untreated patients tend to fail in flexion over time, hinging on the preserved anterior column.

Fracture Dislocation

Fracture dislocations represent 19% of all spinal fractures.[16] By definition, these fractures involve all three columns and result in displacement of one vertebral body with respect to the others. Three subtypes are defined according to the mechanism of injury: flexion-rotation, flexion-distraction, and shear or hyperextension (Figure 46.5). Shear injuries are very rare and occur in accidents where the victim is struck by a large object across the mid-back.[17] As the spine fails in extension, surgical stabilization should be performed with the patient positioned

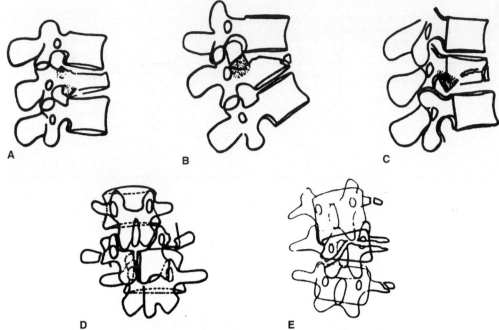

Figure 46.4 Classification of burst fractures (by Denis). **(A)** Fracture of both end plates. **(B)** Fracture of the superior end plate. **(C)** Fracture of the inferior end plate. **(D)** Burst rotation. **(E)** Burst lateral flexion. *(From Denis F: The three column spine and its significance in the classification of acute thoracolumbar spinal injuries. Spine 8:817-831, 1983.)*

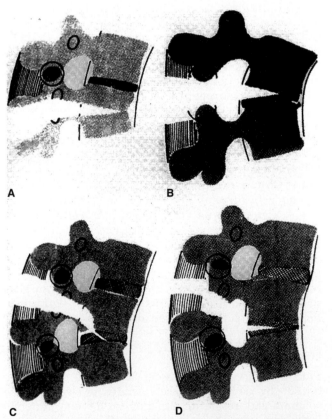

Figure 46.5 **(A)** One-level lap belt type injury through the bone (Chance fracture). **(B)** One-level lap belt type injury through the ligament. **(C-D)** Variants of two-level lap belt type injuries: **(C)** two-level lap belt type injury through the bone; **(D)** two-level lap belt type injury through the ligaments. *(From Denis F: The three column spine and its significance in the classification of acute thoracolumbar spinal injuries. Spine 8:817-831, 1983.)*

in flexion (e.g., positioned prone on a Wilson frame). This injury type results in disruption of all ligamentous and supporting structures of the spine. In many flexion-distraction and flexion-rotation injuries the anterior longitudinal ligament is preserved. Because of this, spinal alignment is often maintained in the supine position, and these fractures are erroneously classified as burst or lap belt type injuries. These fractures are unstable and may require treatment with surgical stabilization. Neurologic deficit is observed in 75% of patients, with 50% being complete SCIs.[16] Dural lacerations, with associated nerve root injury, are common. Figure 46.6 shows classification of fracture dislocation types, according to Denis.

Miscellaneous Fractures

Fractures of the transverse and spinous processes, isolated facet fractures, fractures caused by penetrating trauma (e.g., bullet wounds), and traumatic spondylolisthesis are classified as minor fractures and are often treated with serial imaging only. With the exception of penetrating trauma, they are rarely associated with neurologic deficit and are considered stable fractures. Exceptions to this are bilateral pars interarticularis fractures and pedicle fractures, which can lead to progressive deformity. A more extensive discussion of these injuries can be found in the discussion of spondylolisthesis.

Sacral Fractures

Bonnin[6] was the first to attempt a systematic classification of sacral fractures. He classified these fractures into six types: juxtailiac-marginal fractures; fractures involving the S1 or S2 foramen with upward displacement of the lateral

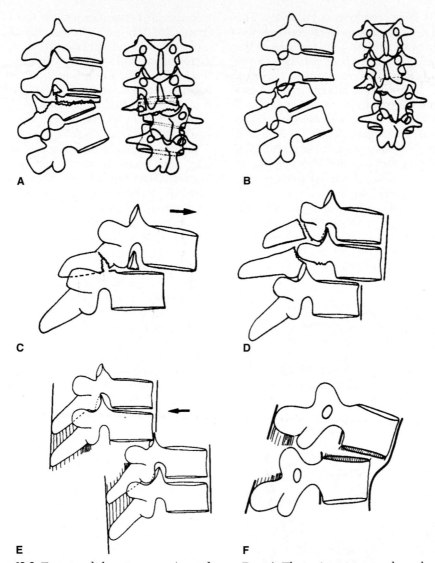

Figure 46.6 Fracture dislocation types (according to Denis). Flexion/rotation type through (**A**) the bone (**B**) and disc. Note the difference in rotation between both spinal segments. (**C**) Shear (posteroanterior) subtype; the segment above is sheared off forward on the top of the segment below. This may leave (**D**) a floating dorsal arch. A dural tear and complete paraplegia are very common with this type of fracture. (**E**) Shear (anteroposterior subtype). (**F**) Flexion/distraction type resembles a lap belt type fracture but, in addition, there is stripping of the anterior longitudinal ligament during subluxation or dislocation. (*From Denis F: The three column spine and its significance in the classification of acute thoracolumbar spinal injuries. Spine 8:817-831, 1983.*)

mass; fractures through the neural foramina, separating the lateral mass from the body of the sacrum; comminuted fractures of the upper sacrum; avulsion fractures of the attachment of the sacrotuberous ligament; and transverse fractures of the sacrum. This system describes commonly seen fracture types but does not correlate with mechanism of injury and does not aid in the clinical evaluation or prognostication process. In 1984, Schmidek *et al.*[55] proposed a system of dividing fractures into those caused by direct injury to the sacrum and those arising from forces indirectly applied to the sacrum. If the sacroiliac joints above the S1 neural foramina are intact, fractures resulting from direct injury to the sacrum are stable and do not require stabilization. This includes transverse fractures of the

sacrum, most common through the neural foramina of S4, which can be caused by a hard fall onto the buttocks. The distal fragment is displaced ventrally and, in severe cases, may perforate the rectum. The indirect mechanism of injury to the sacrum involves concomitant injury to the lumbar spine and/or pelvic ring. The sacrum fails in flexion, often as a result of an injury involving hip flexion with knee extension. This can result in a traumatic spondylolisthesis through the neural foramina of S1 or S2, with forward displacement of the spine above the fracture. One quarter of transverse sacral fractures incurred after falls have been associated with thoracolumbar burst fractures.

Additionally, lumbosacral fracture-dislocations also have a high coincidence of concomitant transverse sacral fractures and can involve the S1 facet, resulting in instability. The majority of sacral fractures caused by indirect forces are vertical fractures, observed in conjunction with fractures of the pelvis. Schmidek described four fracture patterns: lateral mass fractures, juxta-articular fractures, cleaving fractures, and avulsion fractures along the attachments of the sacrotuberous and sacrospinous ligaments. In 1988, Denis et al.[18] published a simplified scheme that divides the sacrum into three anatomic regions: alar region (Zone I), foraminal region (Zone II), and region of the central sacral canal (Zone III) (Figure 46.7). Zone II fractures include combination fractures of Zones I and II, and a Zone III fracture may include a fracture extending into Zones I and II.

Zone I fractures are usually the result of lateral compression of the pelvis with preservation of the sacroiliac ligaments. Vertical shear injuries of the pelvis may result in upward displacement of the sacral ala after a Zone I injury. If severe enough, the upwardly displaced fragment may

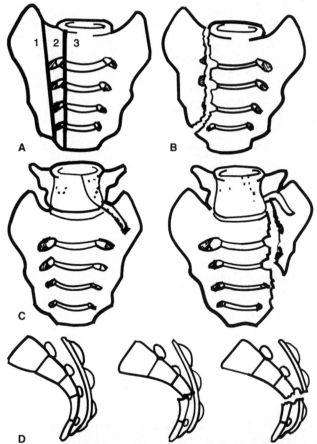

Figure 46.7 (**A**) Classification of sacral fractures into Zone I, region of the ala; Zone II, region of the sacral foramina; and Zone III, region of the central sacral canal. (**B**) Zone II fracture. (**C**) Mechanism of L5 nerve root damage or entrapment in the traumatic "far out" syndrome. The L5 root is caught between the sacral ala and the transverse process of L5 as the fragment migrates superiorly and posteriorly. (**D**) Sagittal view of Zone III fractures: (*left*) normal sacrum; (*middle*) sacral burst fracture with a high potential for sacral root compression; and (*right*) sacral fracture dislocation with a higher potential for sacral root disruption. (*From Denis F, Davis S, Comfort T: Sacral fractures: an important problem. Retrospective analysis of 236 cases. Clin Orthop 227:67-81, 1988.*)

trap the L5 nerve root against the L5 transverse process (traumatic "far-out" syndrome).[60] Zone I fractures also include avulsion fractures at the insertion of the sacrospinous and sacrotuberous ligaments at the level of the S4 foramen. Little injury occurs to the sacrum itself because of the extensive ligamentous injury, and the pelvis is often left unstable.

Zone II injuries comprise fractures extending through one or more sacral foramina but lateral to the sacral canal. These fractures are often seen in shear type injuries but may also occur as the result of lateral compression. Vertical shear injuries are the result of significant force transmission to the sacrum and pelvis and usually result in concomitant injury to the sacroiliac joint. As a result, they are unstable. Nerve root injury has been reported in 28% to 54% of Zone II injuries.[18,55]

Zone III fractures include vertical shear injuries, high and low transverse fractures, and traumatic spondylolisthesis of L5 on S1 (highly unstable in flexion). Transverse sacral fractures are commonly seen after falls from large heights. These fractures usually cross the S2-3 level below the level of the sacroiliac joints with ventral and caudal displacement of the spine above the fracture. Zone III fractures have a high incidence of bilateral nerve root injury and cauda equina dysfunction. In addition to the features mentioned above, the following are also associated with a risk of instability: high transverse, bilateral sacral fractures, and vertical shear fractures.

The management of sacral fractures remains controversial. Early management is often complicated by significant comorbidity. Damage to the internal iliac vessels and presacral venous plexus can be associated with significant hemorrhage and is a contraindication to anterior approaches to the sacrum. Most sacral fractures can be treated with bed rest and pelvic immobilization. In the acute setting, application of an external fixator may help to tamponade life-threatening bleeding. However, this may not be enough to stabilize the pelvis long-term. Stability with respect to the sacrum is defined as the ability to bear physiologic loads without further displacement. Reduction of an alar or Zone I fracture may be necessary to decompress an L5 nerve root injury.[61] In some cases, stabilization of the pelvis along with bed rest will suffice, particularly in cases where the dorsal ligamentous complex of the pelvis is intact. Dorsal fixation of the sacrum can be performed by dorsal fixation of the pelvis, using plates and threaded rods. Zone II injuries causing radiculopathy are best treated by bed rest. Residual symptoms despite conservative therapy can be treated by sacral laminectomy and foraminotomy as needed. Weakness from S1 nerve root entrapment may require early decompression. Transverse Zone III fractures are usually not associated with pelvic instability. High transverse fractures are the exception and may require instrumentation and surgical decompression of the neural elements. Transverse fractures may also lead to compression of the cauda equina. Early decompression is advocated in an attempt to restore bowel, bladder, and sexual function.[49]

Summary

Due to a better understanding of the fracture pathophysiology and improved technology, a variety of surgical approaches exist for arthrodesis and instrumentation for those fractures not amenable to bracing. Surgical approaches for the management of lumbar and sacral fractures are discussed at length elsewhere in this text.

REFERENCES

1. Aito S, El Masry WS, Gerner HJ, *et al:* Ascending myelopathy in the early stage of spinal cord injury. *Spinal Cord* 37(9):617-623, 1999.

2. Andriacchi T, Schultz A, Belytschko T, Galante J: A model for studies of mechanical interactions between the human spine and rib cage. *J Biomech* 7(6):497-507, 1974.

3. Benzel EC, Larson SJ: Functional recovery after decompressive operation for thoracic and lumbar spine fractures. *Neurosurgery* 19(5):772-778, 1986.

4. Bohlman H: The neck. In D'Ambrosia R (ed): *Musculoskeletal Disorders, Regional Examination Differential Diagnosis.* Philadelphia, JB Lippincott, 1985, pp 219-286.

5. Bohlman HH: Treatment of fractures and dislocations of the thoracic and lumbar spine. *J Bone Joint Surg Am* 67(1):165-169, 1985.

6. Bonnin J: Sacral fractures and injury to the cauda equina. *J Bone Joint Surg Am* 27:113-127, 1945.

7. Bradford DS, McBride GG: Surgical management of thoracolumbar spine fractures with incomplete neurologic deficits. *Clin Orthop* (218):201-216, 1987.

8. Burke DC, Berryman D: The place of closed manipulation in the management of flexion-rotation dislocations of the cervical spine. *J Bone Joint Surg Br* 53(2):165-182, 1971.

9. Calenoff L, Chessare JW, Rogers LF, *et al:* Multiple level spinal injuries: importance of early recognition. *Am J Roentgenol* 130(4):665-669, 1978.

10. Castillo M, Quencer RM, Green BA, Labus JB: Acute, ascending cord ischaemia after mobilisation of a stable quadriplegic patient. *Lancet* 1(8588):759-760, 1988.

11. Chance G: Note on a type of flexion fracture of the spine. *Br J Radiol* 21:452, 1948.

12. Clohisy JC, Akbarnia BA, Bucholz RD, *et al:* Neurologic recovery associated with anterior decompression of spine fractures at the thoracolumbar junction (T12-L1). *Spine* 17(8 Suppl):S325-S330, 1992.

13. Colterjohn NR, Bednar DA: Identifiable risk factors for secondary neurologic deterioration in the cervical spine-injured patient. *Spine* 20(21):2293-2297, 1995.

14. Dall BE, Stauffer ES: Neurologic injury and recovery patterns in burst fractures at the T12 or L1 motion segment. *Clin Orthop* Aug:171-176, 1988.

15. Davies WE, Morris JH, Hill V: An analysis of conservative (non-surgical) management of thoracolumbar fractures and fracture-dislocations with neural damage. *J Bone Joint Surg Am* 62(8):1324-1328, 1980.

16. Denis F: The three-column spine and its significance in the classification of acute thoracolumbar spinal injuries. *Spine* 8(8):817-831, 1983.

17. Denis F, Burkus JK: Shear fracture-dislocations of the thoracic and lumbar spine associated with forceful hyperextension (lumberjack paraplegia). *Spine* 17(2):156-161, 1992.

18. Denis F, Davis S, Comfort T: Sacral fractures: an important problem. Retrospective analysis of 236 cases. *Clin Orthop* 227:67-81, 1988.

19. Dickson JH, Harrington PR, Erwin WD: Results of reduction and stabilization of the severely fractured thoracic and lumbar spine. *J Bone Joint Surg Am* 60(6):799-805, 1978.

20. Dolan EJ, Tator CH, Endrenyi L: The value of decompression for acute experimental spinal cord compression injury. *J Neurosurg* 53(6):749-755, 1980.

21. Dunn HK: Anterior spine stabilization and decompression for thoracolumbar injuries. *Orthop Clin North Am* 17(1):113-119, 1986.

22. Farmer J, Vaccaro A, Albert TJ, *et al:* Neurologic deterioration after cervical spinal cord injury. *J Spinal Disord* 11(3):192-196, 1998.

23. Fishman EK, Magid D, Brooker AF, Siegelman SS: Fractures of the sacrum and sacroiliac joint: evaluation by computerized tomography with multiplanar reconstruction. *South Med J* 81(2):171-177, 1988.

24. Fontijne WP, de Klerk LW, Braakman R, *et al:* CT scan prediction of neurological deficit in thoracolumbar burst fractures. *J Bone Joint Surg Br* 74(5):683-685, 1992.

25. Frankel HL, Hancock DO, Hyslop G, *et al:* The value of postural reduction in the initial management of closed injuries of the spine with paraplegia and tetraplegia. Part I. *Paraplegia* 7(3):179-192, 1969.

26. Gertzbein SD, Court-Brown CM, Marks P, *et al:* The neurological outcome following surgery for spinal fractures. *Spine* 13(6):641-644, 1988.

27. Gunterberg B: Effects of major resection of the sacrum: clinical studies on urogenital and anorectal function and a biomechanical study on pelvic strength. *Acta Orthop Scand Suppl* 162:1-38, 1976.

28. Hanley EN, Jr., Eskay ML: Thoracic spine fractures. *Orthopedics* 12(5):689-696, 1989.

29. Harrop JS, Sharan AD, Vaccaro AR, Przybylski GJ: The cause of neurologic deterioration after acute cervical spinal cord injury. *Spine* 26(4):340-346, 2001.

30. Hashimoto T, Kaneda K, Abumi K: Relationship between traumatic spinal canal stenosis and neurologic deficits in thoracolumbar burst fractures. *Spine* 13(11):1268-1272, 1988.

31. Herndon WA, Galloway D: Neurologic return versus cross-sectional canal area in incomplete thoracolumbar spinal cord injuries. *J Trauma* 28(5):680-683, 1988.

32. Holdsworth F: Fractures, dislocations, and fracture-dislocations of the spine. *J Bone Joint Surg Am* 52(8):1534-1551, 1970.

33. Holdsworth FW: Fractures, dislocations and fracture-dislocations of the spine. *J Bone Joint Surg Am* 45B:6-20, 1963.

34. Holdsworth FW, Hardy A: Early treatment of paraplegia from fractures of the thoracolumbar spine. *J Bone Joint Surg Br* 35:512-531, 1953.

35. Jacobs RR, Casey MP: Surgical management of thoracolumbar spinal injuries: general principles and controversial considerations. *Clin Orthop* (189):22-35, 1984.

36. Jefferson G: Discussion on spinal injuries. *Proc R Soc Med* 8:625-648, 1927.

37. Kaneda K, Abumi K, Fujiya M: Burst fractures with neurologic deficits of the thoracolumbar-lumbar spine: results of anterior decompression and stabilization with anterior instrumentation. *Spine* 9(8):788-795, 1984.

38. Kauffler S, Hayes JT: Lumbar fracture dislocations: a study of twenty-one cases. *J Bone Joint Surg Am* 48:788-795, 1966.

39. Keene JS, Fischer SP, Vanderby R Jr, *et al:* Significance of acute posttraumatic bony encroachment of the neural canal. *Spine* 14(8):799-802, 1989.

40. Lemons VR, Wagner FC, Jr., Montesano PX: Management of thoracolumbar fractures with accompanying neurological injury. *Neurosurgery* 30(5):667-671, 1992.

41. Levine AM: The surgical treatment of low lumbar fractures. *Semin Spine Surg* 2:41-53, 1990.

42. Levine AM, Edwards CC: Low lumbar burst fractures: reduction and stabilization using the modular spine fixation system. *Orthopedics* 11(10):1427-1432, 1988.

43. Magerl F, Aebi M, Gertzbein SD, *et al:* A comprehensive classification of thoracic and lumbar injuries. *Eur Spine J* 3(4):184-201, 1994.

44. Marshall LF, Knowlton S, Garfin SR, *et al:* Deterioration following spinal cord injury. A multicenter study. *J Neurosurg* 66(3):400-404, 1987.

45. McAfee PC, Bohlman HH, Yuan HA: Anterior decompression of traumatic thoracolumbar fractures with incomplete neurological deficit using a retroperitoneal approach. *J Bone Joint Surg Am* 67(1):89-104, 1985.

46. McAfee PC, Yuan HA, Fredrickson BE, Lubicky JP: The value of computed tomography in thoracolumbar fractures: an analysis of one hundred consecutive cases and a new classification. *J Bone Joint Surg Am* 65(4):461-473, 1983.

47. McAfee PC, Yuan HA, Lasda NA: The unstable burst fracture. *Spine* 7(4):365-373, 1982.

48. Panjabi MM, Goel V, Oxland T, *et al:* Human lumbar vertebrae: quantitative three-dimensional anatomy. *Spine* 17(3):299-306, 1992.

49. Perin NI, Stanley MI: Sacral fractures. In Youmans JR (ed): *Neurological Surgery*. Philadelphia, WB Saunders, 1996, pp. 2097-2102.

50. Poonnoose PM, Ravichandran G, McClelland MR: Missed and mismanaged injuries of the spinal cord. *J Trauma* 53(2):314-320, 2002.

51. Post MJD: *Radiographic Evaluation of the Spine: Current Advances with Emphasis on Computed Tomography*. New York, Masson, 1980.

52. Radiographic assessment of the cervical spine in asymptomatic trauma patients. *Neurosurgery* 50(3 Suppl):S30-S35, 2002.

53. Rivlin AS, Tator CH: Effect of duration of acute spinal cord compression in a new acute cord injury model in the rat. *Surg Neurol* 10(1):38-43, 1978.

54. Rubash HE, Mears DC: External fixation of the pelvis. *Instr Course Lect* 32:329-348, 1983.

55. Schmidek HH, Smith DA, Kristiansen TK: Sacral fractures. *Neurosurgery* 15(5):735-746, 1984.

56. Starr JK, Hanley EN, Jr.: Junctional burst fractures. *Spine* 17(5):551-557, 1992.

57. Tator CH, Duncan EG, Edmonds VE, *et al:* Comparison of surgical and conservative management in 208 patients with acute spinal cord injury. *Can J Neurol Sci* 14(1):60-69, 1987.

58. Trafton PG, Boyd CA, Jr.: Computed tomography of thoracic and lumbar spine injuries. *J Trauma* 24(6):506-515, 1984.

59. White AA, Panjabi MM: *Clinical Biomechanics of the Spine*. Philadelphia, JB Lippincott, 1978.

60. Wiltse LL, Guyer RD, Spencer CW, *et al:* Alar transverse process impingement of the L5 spinal nerve: the far-out syndrome. *Spine* 9(1):31-41, 1984.

61. Yablon IG, Ordia J, Mortara R, *et al:* Acute ascending myelopathy of the spine. *Spine* 14(10):1084-1089, 1989.

CHAPTER 47

Cervical Discectomy

Richard L. Saunders and Richard B. Raynor

Surgery of the cervical disc is a gratifying challenge from several perspectives. It involves a readily defined pathologic process, elementary clinical neurology if lesions are radicular (potentially confounding when myelopathic), management judgments that are often important to outcome, surgical strategies ranging from simple to complex, and a potential for substantial complications.

Pathology

The essential feature of degenerative disc disease is disc desiccation. This process, associated with annular fissures, creates the setting for the acute sequestered disc syndrome, whereas consequential disc space narrowing impacts the facet joint, alters the lordotic curve, and probably instigates the formation of marginal osteophytes. Disc changes influence, and are influenced by, coincidental features of the cervical spine, such as congenital spinal canal narrowing and segmental anomalies. These factors are a critical consideration in management algorithms. For example, by imaging studies, a simple disc sequestrum may appear to be an elementary challenge, but in the presence of congenital spinal stenosis, there is little latitude for technical error. Management decisions are multifactorial but are based predominantly on the clinical syndrome. Informed management couples specifics of the clinical syndrome and its course with modern imaging. The trap of the asymptomatic disc protrusion has been appreciated since the report by Hitselberger and Witten[5] and has been reemphasized since the advent of magnetic resonance imaging (MRI) studies. In formulating the approach to a particular patient, the imaging is but one factor to be considered with the history and examination.

Perineural Fibrosis

Whereas disc disease associated with congenital spinal stenosis is so commonplace that management decisions are elementary, the pathology of perineural fibrosis is not frequently discussed. Frykholm[3] first described this process and its increased prevalence with age. Perineural fibrosis may be an important consideration during surgical planning for a chronic or subacute radiculitis because it

requires a strategy wherein the nerve root can be fully visualized and neurolysis can be carried out (extradurally, not intradurally, as recommended by Frykholm).

In a typical fibrosis case, a severe radiculitis fails to fully resolve and surgical intervention is undertaken 6 months or more after onset. Imaging may not be impressive. The pathology is a constricting broad band that fixes the nerve root to the ventral aspect of the neuroforamen. Bony decompression alone may fail. Elimination of movement by ventral fusion may ameliorate brachialgia but is unpredictable. Perineural fibrosis may be the explanation for surgical failures for radiculitis, in spite of appropriate indications and patient selection. This is especially true with ventral surgical strategies. A dorsal approach with wide exposure and visualization of the nerve root should be considered in this group of patients.

Osteophytic Disease

The spondylotic spur impacting the spinal cord or nerve root may commonly become symptomatic with or without soft disc changes. These changes are clearly demonstrated by MRI, in which the signal from the disc protrusion and the reactive posterior longitudinal ligament contrast with that from the osteophyte. Inflammatory products from the disc may incite neurologic symptoms, which resolve with time, despite the persisting osteophytic process.

In patients whose symptoms fail to resolve with time, both the osteophyte and the disc should be considered as targets for surgical intervention. The surgical strategy for a symptomatic level may require treating apparent asymptomatic disease to avoid surgical morbidity. For example, a ventral procedure may be more prudent than a simple foraminotomy for a C6 radiculitis associated with asymptomatic but significant spinal cord compression from spondylosis. Surgical alteration of the motion patterns by interbody fusion may hasten degenerative change at adjacent spondylotic segments. This may result in symptomatic disc pathology at a later date. The frequency of this detrimental adjacent segment effect increases with time and recurrent clinical problems are not uncommon.

Significant degenerative disc disease is usually associated with cervical spine straightening and, not infrequently, kyphosis. The biomechanical alterations associated with these changes in spinal configuration are occasionally important in the tailoring of strategies for soft disc disease management. For example, a sequestrum at a hypermobile segment may occur adjacent to an autofused spondylotic segment. Strategies taken in such a case must address the need to stabilize as well as decompress.

Clinical Syndromes

The basic nature of nerve root compression syndromes warrants little comment. Most disc protrusion syndromes are not those of spinal cord compression because of the propensity for the soft disc to be dorsolateral. In the unusual myelopathic presentation from disc sequestra the surgeon's challenge is primarily imaging interpretation. The indications for surgery in situations other than those of neural compression are tenuous, such as for the entity of the so-called painful disc. This is controversial at best and will not be further considered here. Similarly, disc surgery for neck ache or headache primarily should be cautiously considered, even though such symptoms may accompany the typical nerve root compression presentation.

The C5 Nerve Root Syndrome

The so-called shoulder girdle disc, or C5 nerve root compression syndrome, is occasionally confused with rotator cuff disease and other shoulder derangements. Most radiculitis patients, however, have some element of pain radiation and radial paresthesiae. Motor impairment may be missed if the arm is tested only in abduction: The disc patient who cannot reach above his or her head because of shoulder pain will not experience pain when the arm is passively elevated; the shoulder derangement will be painful with active or passive elevation. In nerve root syndromes, symptom relief by arm abduction and elevation is almost diagnostic. Conversely, patients whose symptoms are aggravated by reaching above the head usually do not have nerve root compression.

The C5 nerve root, for unclear reasons, is unpredictable in cervical surgery.[9] If the root is in the area of a surgical decompression (i.e., C4-5 discectomy, laminectomy, or corpectomy), the patient should be made aware of the potential for symptoms of a complicating radiculitis postoperatively. Symptoms may be delayed in onset, often occurring a day or two after surgery. They are often painful and do not necessarily reflect undue nerve root manipulation or inadequate decompression. This is rarely an indication for further surgery, and the patient usually recovers, although occasionally some deficit persists indefinitely.

The C8 Nerve Root Syndrome

Another area fraught with potential confusion is the C8 nerve root syndrome. Reflexes are normal, and the motor findings are restricted to the intrinsic muscles of the hand. No proximal motor findings are present, despite the complaint of dorsolateral arm pain. The sensory complaints are suggestive of an ulnar neuropathy. However, the nature of the pain should separate an entrapment from a radiculitis syndrome. Careful preoperative assessment of the intrinsic musculature of the hand is of critical importance. Informed consent includes the major impact that motor worsening could have on hand use. For example, a weak thumb from surgery would disable a surgeon.

In the evaluation of possible C7-T1 disc symptoms, the workup should not stop at cervical MRI since the C8 syndrome may be the first manifestation of an apical lung lesion.

Spinal Reflexes

Reflexes related to the C6 and C7 nerve roots are usually depressed or unobtainable in patients with significant related nerve root compression syndromes. This is particularly true in acute situations. However, in the more chronic condition, the reflexes may not be so predictable. Accordingly, surgical intervention is not necessarily contraindicated by intact reflexes, but the history, imaging, and overall picture must be clear and consistent. Similarly, although patients may commonly describe sensory symptoms with nerve root compression, there may be no objective sensory findings.

The Surgery of Cervical Discs
An Overview

Ordinarily, cervical radiculitis not responding to expectant treatment will be relieved by ventral or dorsal surgery. The appropriateness of a given approach in a specific clinical situation is based on the surgeon's preferences.

As a general rule, ventral strategies are preferable for their stiffening effect in situations in which marked osteophytic disease coexists or the disc protrusion is central or paracentral. On the other hand, dorsal approaches for the removal of soft lateral sequestra have low morbidity and no motion segment impact.[4]

Although ventral strategies can be technically easier to master than microsurgical facetectomy, their morbidity is greater. Disproportionate local mobility or frank instability associated with a nerve root syndrome is eliminated incidental to a ventral approach. In such cases, surgical planning must include a means to protect, or secure, the bone graft. In recent years, there has been increasing use of plates with allograft intervertebral spacer, even for single-level discectomy, rationalized on the basis of the advantage of "internal" orthosis and enhanced graft incorporation. These arguments have been shown to be compelling[8] but continue to be controversial. Nevertheless, plating should be considered a surgical option, but not mandatory. It is emphasized that good clinical results with well-executed ventral surgery have been achieved without hardware for 50 years.

Indications

The natural history of nerve root compression syndromes is that of pain resolving within a few weeks of onset. The surgical case is the exception. Marked motor deficit or agonizing intractable radicular pain in the face of appropriate disc imaging is the principal indication for expedient intervention in root syndromes. Additionally, a myelopathic picture from soft central disc sequestra is ordinarily reason for prompt surgery. For the less compelling "root" picture, 3 to 6 weeks of anti-inflammatory drugs, inactivity, and analgesics are prescribed. Traction, if comforting, is frequently used but is not critical to outcome. A cervical orthotic may help by reducing neck movement. Chronic persistent brachialgia with nerve root symptoms appropriate to imaging findings ultimately warrants the offering of surgical treatment. In an otherwise surgical case, delaying surgery for its own sake longer than 6 weeks may increase the chance of a suboptimal outcome.

Ventral Surgery with Interbody Fusion

The principal advantage of ventral approaches is their simplicity: simple access, minimal local postoperative symptoms, and the benefits of coincidental fusion. Despite such elegance, attempts at further simplification have made ventral discectomy one of the most litigated of procedures. Tight, tiny keyhole exposure leading to undue soft-tissue tension and compromised exposure can ruin the best of surgeries. It is likely that vocal cord paralysis, swallowing dysfunction, esophageal tears, and stridor are not always the consequence of dissection but tissue ischemia from sustained forceful retraction. During the wide soft-tissue exposure required for a multilevel corpectomy, for example, soft-tissue morbidity may be reduced to less than 2%, simply by wide prevertebral dissection and intermittent relaxation of retraction. Consistent with this observation has been the beneficial effect on postoperative hoarseness by deflation of the endotracheal tube balloon cuff after applying retractors.

The use of the operating microscope for ventral disc surgery has been of particular value. Far from being the gimmick that its early detractors envisioned, it has become an important surgical adjunct. In this era of increasing endoscopic applications, it is more than likely that such technology will bring further refinement to surgery of the cervical disc. In particular, the transdiscal removal of a soft lateral disc without interbody fusion may essentially yield to a percutaneous endoscopic method.

Side of Approach

The side of approach has been given excessive emphasis. This has occurred because postoperative hoarseness has been misconstrued as the consequence of dissection. This presumption has been overemphasized. It should be remembered that as high as 5% incidence of hoarseness is observed after noncervical exposures. More practical concerns should dictate the side of the incision (e.g., previous surgery and the side of radicular symptoms). Of even more importance is the side from which the surgeon is most comfortable or familiar.

There is the potential for subclinical damage to the recurrent laryngeal nerve (RLN) from prior neck or chest surgery. Accordingly, with such prior history, preoperative vocal cord examination is prudent. Alternatively, the anticipated procedure could be performed on the same side as the prior surgery. Should subclinical vocal cord weakness be compounded by that surgery from the opposite side, respiratory distress and a permanent tracheotomy are possible.

If the aforementioned concern does not apply, there may be an advantage in approaching the ventral spine from the side opposite the nerve root compression since the obliquity of the surgeon's perspective facilitates the view of the opposite side of the interspace (Figure 47.1).

Indications for Ventral Surgery

The ventral approach to the cervical spine is particularly suited to disc fragments situated ventral to the spinal cord, especially central and paracentral discs. Lesions in the neural foramen are generally best approached by medial microsurgical facetectomy, especially in the absence of substantial spondylosis. Discs at the cord-root junction are amenable to either a ventral or a dorsal approach, depending on whether a fusion is desirable, the presence of bony osteophyte, and the surgeon's experience and preference.[6]

Ventral Technique*
Positioning

Careful attention paid to the initial positioning of the patient obviates orientation problems during surgery. The patient is placed supine with a roll placed behind the shoulders. This tends to extend the neck slightly, thus aiding the surgical exposure. The head may be placed in a halter and carefully positioned straight up. Five-pound weights are attached to the halter to stabilize the head position.

During graft insertion, the weight is increased to 15 lb or more to distract the interspace. A 5-lb sandbag is placed under the hip to be used for graft harvest. Bandage rolls are placed around both wrists and the ends loosely secured to the foot of the operating table. These are used to pull the shoulders down when radiography is performed for localization because the shoulders usually interfere with the visualization of the cervical spine below C5, especially in patients with short necks.

Skin Incision

For a one- or two-level exploration, the incision is transverse, following a normal neck crease. It is approximately 5 to 6cm in length and carried through the subcutaneous tissues up to, but not including, the platysma muscle. It may be made on either side of the neck according to the surgeon's preference. It begins close to the midline and overlaps the leading edge of the sternomastoid muscle, extending laterally 1 to 2cm, depending on the level of the interspaces to be approached. The higher the interspace, the less the overlap because the sternomastoid muscle moves dorsally and laterally as it approaches its insertion on the mastoid bone. The platysma muscle is split longitudinally along the ventral edge of the sternomastoid muscle. It is usually necessary to separate the platysma from the overlying subcutaneous tissues for about 2cm above and below the incision.

Soft-Tissue Dissection

When the ventral border of the sternomastoid muscle has been identified, dissection is both blunt and sharp. There is a natural plane between the great vessels laterally and the visceral fascia about the tracheoesophageal complex medially. Remaining in this plane may lessen the risk of damage to the recurrent nerve. A finger is used to gently define the plane. Structures, such as vessels, crossing this plane are divided. Depending on the spinal level, the superior thyroid artery and the omohyoid muscle may be encountered. Both of these may be divided, but the muscle ends should be tagged and reapproximated at the end of the procedure.

Dissection is continued to the ventral aspect of the spine and the appropriate disc identified by radiograph. Frequently, the midline of the vertebral body can be identified by the presence of a small bony spine near the disc. If degenerative disease is present, the local anatomy and landmarks may be distorted, making the midline more

---

*Per R.B.R.

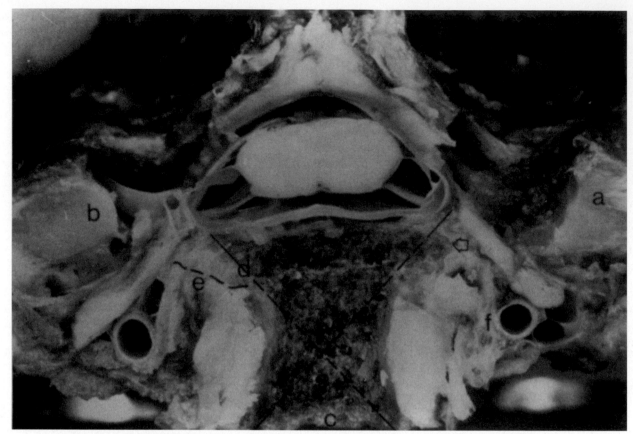

Figure 47.1 The C4-5 interspace has been disarticulated and the viewer is looking rostrally at the undersurface of C4. **(A)** One-half of the facet joint has been removed on the right to expose 4mm of nerve root. **(B)** On the left one-quarter of the facet joint has been resected and 5mm of the nerve root has been exposed. **(C)** A Cloward procedure has been done. **(D)** The line of vision from the right side of the specimen to the left nerve root has been drawn. Note that neither the dural edge nor the nerve root can be seen. On the opposite side, the line of maximal lateral visualization is also drawn. The bone of the uncovertebral joint has been resected for several millimeters laterally *(open arrow)* beyond the limits of visualization. The dural edge and the nerve root would be seen if the posterior longitudinal ligament and its lateral expansion were removed. **(E)** On the left, the resection of the uncovertebral joint was similarly performed. Radiographs taken with markers verified that the extent of the lateral nerve root exposure achieved was the same anteriorly and posteriorly. Note **(F)** the vertebral artery position, in relation to the depth of the vertebral body.

difficult to locate. The medial borders of the longus colli muscles are identified and then stripped laterally until the lateral mass of the involved upper vertebrae is identified. This usually necessitates dissecting the muscles from most of the vertebral body of the upper vertebrae and half the body of the lower vertebrae. The midline bulge of the midsections of the upper vertebral body should now be visible, and these aid in confirming midline orientation. Dissection of the medial borders of the longus colli muscles to expose the lateral masses of the vertebral bodies facilitates the use of self-retaining retractors. The toothed blades of self-retaining retractors, such as the Caspar or Cloward retractors, are anchored into the medial borders of the longus colli muscles. Anchoring into the medial muscle border minimizes medial pressure against the tracheoesophageal complex and the possible adverse consequences of such pressure. The medial blade of the retractor system has a tendency to ride up and pull out of the muscle. A bandage roll looped around the medial retractor arm and attached to a 5-lb weight prevents this and prevents the blade from dislodging. Blunt blades are used to aid rostral-caudal retraction and visualization. The periosteum is split in the midline and flapped back, the disc is incised, and easily mobilized material is removed. At this point, the use of magnification is considered. Loupes with a magnification of 3.5 are desirable, although the use of the microscope may be more desirable in certain circumstances.

Neural Decompression

Findings of preoperative imaging studies determine the size of the decompression needed to remove the disc and its fragments. The minimum transverse distance necessary to decompress the dural sac appears to be 15mm. The vertical extent of the decompression depends on whether and how far disc material has migrated behind a vertebral body. If the herniated disc material is confined to the interspace, the cortical end plates are at least thinned and perforated in several places to expose cancellous bone. It is usually desirable to remove the end plates because cancellous bone provides a better graft bed. The dissection is done with a high-speed air drill, initially using a burr and then switching to a diamond tip as the dorsal margin of the body is approached. More disc material is removed as the dissection proceeds more deeply until the posterior longitudinal ligament is exposed. If the ligament appears hypertrophied and a possible cause of dural compression, or if a hidden disc fragment is suspected, the ligament is carefully incised and removed, either with a fine Kerrison rongeur or by sharp dissection; otherwise, it is left intact.

The nerve root and its neuroforamen of exit frequently lie several millimeters rostral to the disc space and lateral to the usual operative exposure and, therefore, are not under direct vision (Figure 47.1).[6] Small upcutting curettes are used to clean these lateral recesses, affording an extra 3 to 5mm of decompression. The instrument is swept from the medial portion toward the interspace. If the vertebral body is divided into quarters (depthwise, ventrally to dorsally), dissection is confined to the deepest quarter because the vertebral artery lies approximately at midlevel, depthwise. Staying deep prevents arterial injury during this blind dissection. A fine, small-angled punch may also be used to remove bone, again confining removal to the deepest portion. An intact posterior longitudinal ligament offers protection to the nerve root because the ligament fans out laterally from the vertebral body to cover the medial aspect of the neuroforamen. If the posterior longitudinal ligament has been removed, the curette is a safer instrument to use for this additional lateral decompression. It also tends to catch any small hidden disc fragments as it is swept beneath the vertebral body. The dorsal edges of both vertebral bodies bordering the interspace area are also undercut using up-angled curettes and a fine Kerrison punch, again affording a few extra millimeters of decompression. Ultrasonography can be used intraoperatively to visualize the nerve roots laterally and the spinal cord pulsations longitudinally in instances in which there are far-lateral disc fragments or in which fragments have migrated behind a vertebral body for any significant distance.[7] In a number of instances, missed disc fragments or osteophytes have been identified and removed after what was considered to be an adequate decompression. Bleeding is controlled with bipolar cautery, bone dust, and Gelfoam.

Fusion and Closure

A tricortical bone graft, at least 2mm greater in length than the cervical decompression, is taken from the iliac crest. This larger size ensures a secure countersinking of the bone graft into mortise. The harvest site should be at least 1cm away from the anterior superior iliac spine to prevent its fracture (which increases patient pain and morbidity). The graft is trimmed and shortened to fit the bed, weight is added to the cervical traction, and the graft is gently tapped into place, countersinking it slightly. The periosteum is smoothed back over the vertebral bodies. The platysma edges are reapproximated, and a subcuticular layer of absorbable sutures is used to close the skin.

A ¼-inch drain may be brought out through the incision and left in place for 24 hours, with one suture to be tied when the drain is removed. The patient is placed in a collar and ambulated the day of surgery.

Ventral Technique*

The overall method is very similar to that described above. Minor differences are the transection of the platysma rather than splitting and ignoring repair of the transected omohyoid muscle. In moving the longus colli muscles laterally, the stripping is largely by monopolar cautery primarily on the side ipsilateral to the surgeon. The uncinate processes facilitate orientation in the interspace. The method of retraction is important. Longus colli impaling instruments, such as the Cloward or Caspar systems, are inherently dangerous regarding their potential for slipping into the great vessels or esophagus. A table-fixed system with toothless blunt blades provides an appealing alternative. The relaxation of retraction periodically during lengthy procedures is important and simpler with such a system. A fivefold decrease in the incidence of stridor and swallowing obstruction in the immediate postoperative period after establishing the routine of timed retraction was also observed. However, no change in the incidence of vocal cord paralysis (3%) was observed (Saunders, unpublished data).

No special attention is paid to preservation of the end plates during the decompression. Bone impeding access to adequate visualization of the posterior longitudinal ligament (PLL) is aggressively removed. An air-driven burr may be used for much of the bone removal, especially in the deep midline dorsally, to avoid inadvertent spinal cord impact with Kerrisons and curettes. The PLL is more often opened than not to exclude significant ligament thickening and the epidural sequestra. If a major sequestrum is evident behind an involved vertebra, the procedure should be modified to that of a corpectomy.

After placing the bone graft the neck is flexed and extended under direct visualization in an attempt to actually displace the graft. When unchanged by this effort, the graft rarely moves in convalescence.

Ventrolateral Foraminotomy

Described by Verbiest and Paz-geuze[11] this approach should have anatomic appeal for surgeons. However, for reasons that are uncertain, it has not been widely embraced. With this exposure, the uncinate process is removed after a deliberate exposure and retraction of the vertebral artery, and the nerve root is followed down to the thecal sac (Figure 47.2). The elegance of such an approach resides in two facts: the nerve root is completely skeletonized while minimizing the removal of intervertebral disc, and a fusion or spacer is not even a consideration, much less a necessity. A practical concern, at least for the novice, is the potential for vertebral artery or carotid sheath injury, as well as the almost expected Horner's syndrome from this more lateral approach.

---

*Per R.L.S.

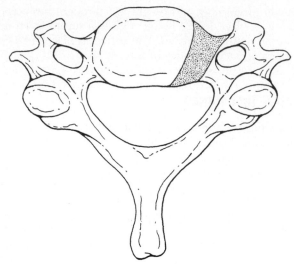

Figure 47.2 Axial view of an uncinate process resection for decompression of the cervical nerve root. Note proximity of the vertebral artery and the potential avenue for decompression of the ventral spinal cord.

Dorsal Technique
Medial Facetectomy

One of the few refinements of laminectomy, an old and perhaps crude procedure, is that of nerve root decompression by partial medial resection of the facet joint.[4] The fundamental attractiveness of this operation is the degree to which the nerve root is visualized in comparison with ventral procedures. The problem affecting the nerve root can be identified, whether it is an osteophyte, a soft sequestrum, or a perineural fibrosis. The two principal disadvantages of facetectomy are postoperative neck pain from the requirement for retraction of a major muscle mass and the potential for nerve root injury by excessive manipulation.

The use of the operating microscope is critical to the elegance of facetectomy. The two disadvantages are thus ameliorated by precise nerve root exploration with limited muscular trauma through smaller exposures.

Operative adjuncts include prophylactic antibiotics, optional steroids, and positioning. Three-point head fixation with a neutral to slightly flexed neck position is ideal. In the sitting position this is easily realized. In the so-called "Concord" prone position the cervical curve should follow that of the thoracic kyphosis to maintain a neutral position. Neck positioning is particularly important if spinal canal caliber is marginal, regardless of the presence or absence of spinal cord symptoms. In spite of controversy as to the hazard of air embolism in the sitting position, this remains legitimate, especially for the obese or pulmonary patient. The position requires careful attention to maintenance of mean arterial blood pressure especially in the elderly or myelopathic. Whether or not a central venous catheter adds to the overall safety of the sitting position is unsettled.

Skin Incision and Soft-Tissue Dissection

The incision measures 4 to 5cm and is positioned according to the spinous processes, if palpable, correlated with prior radiographs. Allowing for spinous process inclination, the caudal end of the skin incision is not beyond lower process of the level of interest so as to place that facet joint in the middle of the deep exposure. Paralytic anesthesia is allowed to wear off as the skin incision is deepened. This permits the detection of a motor response if the surgery about the nerve root is unduly rough. The lateral fascial attachments at the tips of the two exposed spinous processes are cut only on the side to be exposed. A sharp narrow periosteal elevator is passed along each lamina to the level of the facet joint, in a deliberate attempt to peel off the periosteum. This is the first step in minimizing muscle injury, bleeding, and postoperative pain. The soft tissue separating these two periosteal tunnels is then divided with monopolar cutting current, fully exposing the facet joint. A lateral radiograph with a marker in place should absolutely confirm the level of surgery.

Retractors are placed only after the entire facet joint is visualized. Regardless of the retractor type used, the nuchal ligament should be protected. One means is by use of a table-fixed narrow retractor blade whereby there is no need for medial counter-traction. Another method places the medial point of the Williams self-retaining retractor against the spinous process. A refinement of the Williams retractor system is the Ducker retractor, which broadens the medial retractor component. At this point, the operating microscope may replace loupe magnification.

Decompression

The keyhole facetectomy begins at the interlaminar space, medial to the estimated pedicle position along the caudal edge of the rostral lamina. The interlaminar ligamentum flavum is usually thin and requires no dissection from either lamina. Having removed about 1cm² of upper lamina, the 1-mm Kerrison rongeur is turned caudally and forced through the thin ligamentum flavum and into the lower lamina to take the upper 2 to 3mm of edge. This caudal laminotomy accesses the epidural space superficial to the venous plexus overlying the lateral gutter and nerve root. Bony removal at the caudal lamina then proceeds laterally to the inferior pedicle. The pedicle is the key landmark for cervical nerve root decompression and exploration. The nerve root axilla lies at and above this landmark and is the principal avenue through which the disc sequestrum or osteophyte is found. Bony removal proceeds rostrally and laterally to the line of the inferior pedicle. The foramen is thus entered. About half of the facet width is taken as the decompression approaches the rostral pedicle (Figures 47.1, 47.3, and 47.4). The nerve root may yet to be visualized, and fat may be present in spite of significant foraminal pathology.

Epidural bleeding, especially if surgery is performed in the prone position, is troubling as one proceeds laterally with the facetectomy. Bleeding is stemmed by placing 2mm pieces of thrombin-soaked Gelfoam ahead of the Kerrison rongeur. One avoids cottonoid patties by using a vented suction tip.

When bony decompression is complete, the epidural venous layer can be defined and coagulated at its medial edge over the thecal sac with a blunt micro-dissector, hook, or Penfield dissector. The tips of the bipolar forceps,

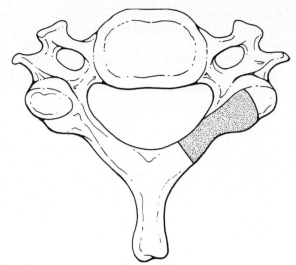

Figure 47.3 Axial view of a medial facetectomy. Note that the pedicle landmark lies well medial to the lateral extent of facet joint resection.

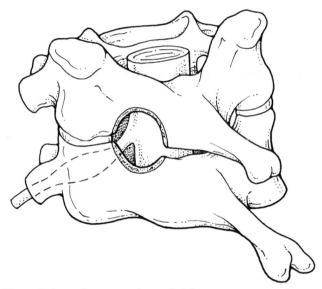

Figure 47.4 En face view of a medial facetectomy. Note the extent of lamina removal required to expose the nerve root axilla.

one superficial and the other deep to this layer, effectively coagulate the full thickness of the plexus medially to laterally, parallel with the course of the nerve root. This is followed by cutting the plexus superficial to and along the axis of the nerve root. The nerve root is thus fully exposed. There may be a scarifying layer beneath the venous layer that should also be sharply freed from the nerve root, which allows the flattened root to reexpand.

Exploration of the root axilla is the final and critical aspect of nerve root exploration. Rarely is exploration over the nerve root shoulder revealing. It may be fairly bloody here as well. The ventral spinal canal below the nerve root next to the pedicle is now visualized with minimal thecal sac retraction. A blunt nerve hook here is then swept medially, rostrally, and then laterally under the dural sac/nerve

root, respectively. A sequestrum often presents itself after the application of pressure against the annulus in this maneuver. The nerve root should not be substantially retracted during such a search. At this point, one should be cautious not to mistake the often separate motor component of the proximal root for the disc fragment. Frequently, it will be necessary to incise the PLL in the axilla to allow extrusion of a disc sequestrum retained by the ligament. The disc space is never entered with a rongeur, as one would in lumbar surgery. Not only is disc space evacuation unnecessary, but one can unknowingly traverse the interspace into unforgiving ventral neck anatomy.

Lastly, the lateral adequacy of bony decompression is checked with a Penfield dissector. The decompression is extended as far as necessary, even if total facetectomy is required for complete decompression. It should be recognized that, if more than one-half of the facet joint is taken, there is a significant impact on that segment's stability. No effort is ordinarily made to actually remove the incidental osteophyte. An air-driven burr rather than a Kerrison may be preferred for the bony decompression, especially if the foramen is particularly tight.

Closure

Soft-tissue closure is performed only after absolute hemostasis is obtained. Twenty-four hours of suction drainage should be considered for persistent oozing. A soft collar can be comforting but is not required.

Avoiding Complications
General Concepts

General problems associated with cervical discectomy include pain control, complicating medical illness, and those problems consequent to surgery, such as pneumonia, pulmonary embolism, and myocardial infarction. Adequacy of pain control may actually dictate surgical timing. When a surgical lesion is present, early surgery is preferable to protracted and ineffective narcotic management. In general, no patient should be allowed to become bedridden and frightened by pain either preoperatively or postoperatively.

The simplicity and thus the attractiveness of ventral discectomy and fusion may be undermined by the postoperative pain resulting from autogenous bone harvest. Because the iliac crest donor site is often the most significant postoperative source of pain, several techniques have been developed to avoid this problem. These include omission of an interbody spacer entirely or the use of spacers of allograft fibula, methylmethacrylate, or hydroxyapatite. All these approaches have associated disadvantages that must be compared with the donor site morbidity. Because failure of complete interbody bony bridging is not necessarily harmful or the equivalent of poor outcome, the surgeon's judgment must guide the choice and use of spacers.

Soft-Tissue Complications

Soft-tissue complications are diverse with ventral cervical spine surgery. In Flynn's[2] monumental survey of more than

80,000 ventral disc procedures, there were only four presumably symptomatic epidural hematomas (Table 47.1). These were not associated with soft-tissue hematomas.

Infection after ventral cervical spine surgery is rare. Indeed this event should raise the question of esophageal injury. Wound problems after dorsal surgery are more frequent and often stem from inadequate hemostasis and/or wound care.

Vascular and visceral injuries following ventral surgery are rare. Carelessly placed sharp-toothed retractors and scars from previous surgery are usually the culprits. Damage to the esophagus and recurrent laryngeal nerve is a particular concern. Vertebral artery injury occurs when the surgeon is anatomically lost or is too aggressive with attempts at lateral decompression. Anteroposterior radiographs with metal interspace markers, respect for the uncinate process as a lateral landmark, and conservative lateral decompression should minimize vascular complications, except perhaps for those arising from a medial loop anomaly of the vertebral artery. The latter anomaly can be suspected from preoperative CT scans and occurs in approximately 3% of cadavers.[1]

Bone Graft Complications

There is a potential for interbody bone graft collapse and displacement. The incidence of bone graft collapse with allograft can be minimized by using fibula rather than iliac crest. Nonosteopenic autogenous tricortical iliac crest rarely collapses and has the advantage of rapid incorporation in comparison with fibula. Interspace collapse is not often of immediate clinical importance representing only a radiographic disappointment. If such collapse results in a kyphotic angulation, there may be future symptoms, cervical imbalance, and consequent degenerative changes at cephalad motion segments. Ventral displacement of the interbody spacer is usually inconsequential, but interspace collapse may narrow the foramen to the degree that there is recurrent root pain or neck pain from loading the facet complex. Significant dysphagia can also occur with complete displacement of a large graft.

Pseudarthrosis is the persistence of motion at an operated motion segment and not, actually, a false joint. Without evidence of instability, such persistence is of uncertain clinical significance. Substantial mobility results in progressive osteophyte formation, with the potential for recurrent neural compression, but it more practically can be the source of persistent neck pain. Nevertheless, good clinical results are commonly achieved in the face of radiographic nonunion.

Neck pain, in the presence of a stable, but failed fusion, may prompt tenuous cause-and-effect assumptions. It is naive to indict this radiographic finding after ventral disc surgery as the cause of poor outcome, pejoratively called *symptomatic pseudarthrosis*. There is no clear consensus on whether or not the clinical result in ventral disc surgery relates to the success or failure or interbody fusion. Indeed, with corpectomy, there was no absolute correlation between success or failure of solid bony union and neck comfort in more than 350 cases (R.L.S., unpublished data). The substantial avoidance of nonunion by the use of ventral plates should clarify, ultimately, the impact of radiographic findings on overall outcome. Salvage surgery for ventral discectomy ordinarily is best rationalized for neurologic indications and instability—that for axial pain only with stable nonunion is tenuous and requires clear preoperative consent.

Failure of bony union, in the absence of instability, should simply be referred to as a persistent motion segment. The surgical intent, when neural structures are compressed in the otherwise stable spine, should be neural decompression and the maintenance of a nonpathologic relationship between the spinal column and neural elements. This focus should, perhaps, induce more precise decompressive efforts and, if used, fastidious spacer placement.

Neurologic Complications of Disc Surgery

The neurologic complications of disc surgery include: (1) worsened radiculitis (see earlier comments on the C5 root), (2) cerebrospinal fluid (CSF) leak, and (3) myelopathy.

Radicular worsening after ventral surgery is unusual and probably warrants immediate postoperative imaging. These studies should be interpreted with caution in light of often obscuring surgical artifacts (especially those from metal debris on MRI resulting from the use of burrs in decompression). Radicular worsening after facetectomy is usually due to excessive root manipulation; persistent or recurrent radicular pain probably warrants a ventral procedure after reimaging. Recurrent sequestrum does occur, but very rarely, after dorsal surgery and would be the primary indication for facetectomy revision.

A CSF fistula, or pseudomeningocele, can develop after inadvertent dural opening. Nerve root sleeve tears are not likely to be consequential but thecal sac tears, unless suture repair is water-tight, warrant consideration of a lumbar drain for several days. Pseudomeningocele after ventral surgery usually resolves if left untreated, although this may take months. Persistent CSF problems suggest unappreciated elevated CSF pressure.

Myelopathic complications after cervical disc surgery are rare (see Table 41.1). They should prompt reassessment of the surgical strategy used, principally as it relates to the adequacy of decompression and the overall caliber of the spinal canal. U and Wilson[10] reported that epidural hematomas complicating ventral discectomy were of arterial origin and were marked by

TABLE 47.1

Etiology of Operative Myelopathy

Etiology of Deficit	Immediate	Delayed	Total
No etiology given	7	1	8
No etiology apparent	7	9	16
Intraoperative trauma	36	2	38
Epidural hematoma	2	2	4
Infection	0	3	3
Other	1	0	1

From Flynn TB: Neurologic complications of anterior interbody fusion. *Spine* 7:536, 1982.

catastrophic immediate progressive postoperative quadriplegia. Nevertheless, such hematomas must be very rare indeed. Flynn[2] suggested that few postoperative myelopathies had a clear explanation, and those handled expectantly did as well as, or better than, those that were treated by reoperation.

Summary

Cervical disc prolapse management has been refined through advances in technique and imaging, and it has long been a gratifying aspect of spine surgery. Attention to detail is critical to the outcome, from indications for surgery to adequacy of neural decompression. No single approach is necessarily all-encompassing, and the complete surgeon should be proficient in both ventral and dorsal strategies.

REFERENCES

1. Curylo L, Mason H, Bohlman H, Yoo J: Anomalous vertebral artery: a cadaveric and clinical case study. *Spine* 25:2860, 2000.
2. Flynn TB: Neurologic complications of anterior interbody fusion. *Spine* 7:536, 1982.
3. Frykholm R: Lower cervical nerve roots and their investments. *Acta Chir Scand* 101:457, 1951.
4. Henderson CM, Hennessy RG, Shuey HM, *et al:* Posterolateral foraminotomy as an exclusive operative technique for cervical radiculopathy: a review of 846 consecutively operated cases. *Neurosurgery* 13:504, 1983.
5. Hitselberger WE, Witten RM: Abnormal myelograms in asymptomatic patients. *J Neurosurg* 28:204, 1968.
6. Raynor R: Anterior or posterior approach to the cervical spine: an anatomical and radiographic evaluation and comparison. *Neurosurgery* 12:7, 1983.
7. Raynor R: Intraoperative ultrasound for immediate evaluation of anterior cervical decompression and discectomy. *Spine* 22:389-395, 1997.
8. Shapiro S: Banked fibula and the locking anterior cervical plate in anterior cervical fusions following cervical discectomy. *J Neurosurg* 84:161, 1996.
9. Saunders R: On the pathogenesis of the radiculopathy complicating multilevel corpectomy. *Neurosurgery* 37:408, 1995.
10. U HS, Wilson CB: Postoperative epidural hematoma as a complication of anterior cervical discectomy. *J Neurosurg* 49:288, 1978.
11. Verbiest H, Paz-geuze HD: Antero-lateral surgery for cervical spondylosis in cases of myelopathy or nerve compression. *J Neurosurg* 25:611, 1966.

CHAPTER 48

Thoracic Discectomy

Charles B. Stillerman, Paul C. McCormick, and Edward C. Benzel

It has been estimated that up to 20% of the population has a thoracic disc herniation on magnetic resonance imaging (MRI).[3,4] However, the need for discectomy is relatively rare. Surgery for removal of thoracic disc herniations is thought to comprise less than 4% of all disc operations.[29,30,32] Historically, these operations have been associated with suboptimal outcomes. The reason for this is multifactorial and, in part, related to diagnostic delays. These delays are a result of the rarity of symptomatic thoracic discs and the lack of a characteristic presentation pattern. It is hoped that a growing awareness of this disorder will lead to better outcomes as a result of earlier treatment. Additionally, there is uncertainty about the natural history of this disease. There is no consensus regarding the indications for disc removal. Most surgeons generally avoid prophylactic surgery for disc herniation; however, this practice has not been based on prospective studies. Generally, surgery is reserved for patients with severe, intractable radicular pain or for those with myelopathy, especially when progressive or severe. Finally, there are numerous operations for the removal of these lesions. Regrettably, there are no universally accepted selection criteria to help determine the best operation for each individual situation. Recently, surgical selection guidelines were proposed that were based on a large series of ventrolateral and lateral operations, the well-documented success of groups using the transpedicular approach, and preliminary experience with newer procedures, including transthoracic thoracoscopy, retropleural thoracotomy, and transfacet pedicle-sparing approaches (Table 48.1).[29-31]

Until the 1950s, laminectomy, with or without disc removal, was the treatment of choice for the surgical management of this disorder. Logue's[17] historical review in 1952 revealed the poor results achieved using laminectomy.[32,34] Consequently, other methods of performing discectomy were developed. These operations were intended to improve the exposure to the ventral spinal canal throughout the thoracic spine. Although these approaches were successful at improving access to the disc space, they were technically formidable and associated with considerable morbidity. Each of these approaches has a unique set of potential complications. These complications are necessary to appreciate so that they can be avoided. This chapter emphasizes these techniques and focuses on the advantages and disadvantages of each procedure. Fourteen contemporary thoracic disc series are summarized, with special attention given to the reported complications.[29] In closing, a new management paradigm for the treatment of symptomatic thoracic discs is presented.[29]

Surgical Approaches for Thoracic Discectomy
Dorsal Approaches
Laminectomy

The initial approach used for thoracic disc herniation was laminectomy, either with or without disc removal. In 1952, Logue[17] reviewed the thoracic discectomy literature and found that the results were poor. A significant percentage of patients were left paraplegic. Although the precise reasons for these results were not known, it was postulated that laminectomy alone did not significantly reduce the ventral forces created by a thoracic disc herniation acting on the spinal cord.[33] Additionally, when discectomy was performed, spinal cord manipulation was generally not well-tolerated. The limited space available for the spinal cord, as well as the comparatively tenuous blood supply, was thought to increase the susceptibility of the thoracic spinal cord, to injury during disc removal (Figure 48.1).

Advantages and Disadvantages. Although laminectomy is technically the simplest decompressive spinal operation, the only indication for its use in thoracic disc disease may be in the treatment of thoracic spondylosis.[32]

Dorsolateral Approaches
Transpedicular Approach

Patterson and Arbit[23] first reported the transpedicular approach in 1978. It was initially performed on three patients with thoracic disc herniations. Two of the patients had complete resolution of their symptoms, and the third was markedly improved. Subsequently, several other series have also reported excellent results (Figure 48.2).*

Technique. The patient is placed in the prone position and taped to the table to facilitate rolling away from the surgeon during the disc removal. The spinous process, lamina, and facet joints are exposed using a linear midline incision. Most of the facet joint is removed, as is the pedicle caudal to the disc space. The pedicle is drilled out flush with the vertebral body. A small cavity measuring 1.5 to 2.0cm in depth is created in the vertebral body to enable depressing the overlying disc away from the ventral dura mater. Additionally, whenever necessary, hemilaminotomies are performed to visualize the dorsolateral dura mater.[6,16,22,32-34]

Advantages. This approach is considerably less invasive than most other operations for thoracic disc removal, particularly the transthoracic (TT) and the lateral extracavitary approaches (LECA). This is thought to lessen perioperative pain, shorten hospital stays, and enable earlier return to premorbid activity.[16,21,22,29-31] The surgery avoids problems associated with thoracotomy, rib resection, and extensive muscle dissection. Operating time and blood loss also appear to be less than with other surgeries.

---

*References 6,16,21,24,30,31.

Disadvantages. Critics of this procedure point out the limited ability to visualize across the spinal canal, making decompression of central and contralateral portions of disc a relatively blind procedure. Sometimes, difficulty is encountered in managing calcified and intradural disc fragments. The authors[16,21,30] believe that safety is enhanced by

using specially designed thoracic microdiscectomy instrumentation (Figure 48.3) and endoscopic techniques.[16,29,30] Although there have been reports of removal of intradural fragments and central, densely calcified discs using the dorsolateral techniques,[16,21,24,29,31] the authors[29,31] have not had success with these entities. Dense calcifications involving the dorsal margin of the disc space tend to be strongly adherent to the ventral dura mater.[29,31] The possibility of significant dural adherence may lead one to use one of the ventrolateral or lateral procedures in those situations.[29,31]

The final disadvantage of this procedure relates to the removal of the facet-pedicle complex, without the ability to place an interbody graft. It has been reported that patients operated on using the transpedicular approach have somewhat disappointing results from the standpoint of localized back pain.[16,21,24,30,31] The desire to improve these results led to the development of the transfacet pedicle-sparing approach.[29-31] It was postulated that the avoidance of pedicle removal should minimize postoperative back pain. The preliminary experience has suggested that this, in fact, may be the case.[29-31]

Transfacet Pedicle-Sparing Approach

The transfacet pedicle-sparing approach was developed as a simpler alternative to the formidable ventrolateral and lateral operations for the treatment of thoracic disc disease.[29,30] Initially, morphometric studies were carried out and improved the authors' orientation to the disc space and ventral spinal canal, thereby aiding discectomy. Cadaveric studies demonstrated that a keyhole facetectomy alone, without associated pedicle or lamina removal, did not sacrifice the exposure achieved with the transpedicular approach.[29,30] Although the safety and overall effectiveness of the transpedicular approach has been well-documented,[16,17,21,24] it was hoped that avoidance of

TABLE 48.1

Surgical Approaches for Herniated Thoracic Discs

Surgical Approach	General Indications
Ventral	
Trans-sternal	Upper thoracic spine
	Densely calcified centrolateral
Ventrolateral	
Transthoracic/ Thoracoscopic	Densely calcified centrolateral
	Selected mildly calcified centrolateral
Retropleural	Selected high medical risk static severe myelopathy
Lateral	
A. Extracavitary/	
B. Costotransversectomy	A and B, Selected densely calcified centrolateral
	Mildly calcified centrolateral
C. Parascapular	C, Upper thoracic spine Calcified centrolateral
Dorsolateral	
Transfacet pedicle-sparing/	All soft herniated discs Calcified lateral
Transpedicular	Mildly calcified centrolateral All high medical risk except densely calcified centrolateral

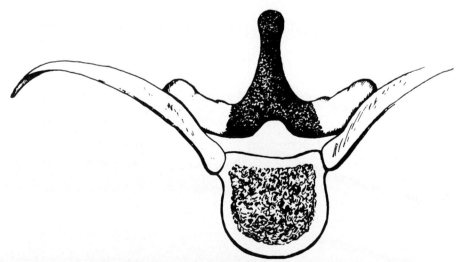

Figure 48.1 Laminectomy approach. The lamina and spinous process is removed, often extending above and below the level of disc herniation. This approach has been associated with suboptimal outcomes. It may be used for the management of thoracic spondylosis. (*From Stillerman CB, Weiss MH: Principles of surgical approaches to the thoracic spine. In Tarlov EC [ed]: Neurosurgical Topics: Neurosurgical Treatment of Disorders of the Thoracic Spine. Park Ridge, IL, AANS, 1991, pp 1-19.*)

pedicle removal and limiting the amount of facet resected would improve localized back pain results.[30,31]

Technique. The operation is performed with the patient in the prone position on a radiolucent frame and spinal table. The arms are placed at the sides, and the patient is taped to the table. Anteroposterior (AP) fluoroscopic

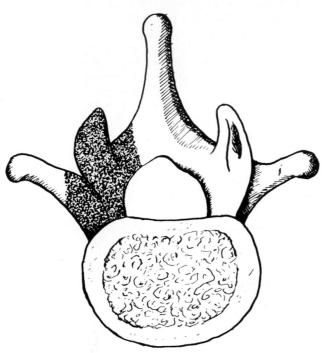

Figure 48.2 Transpedicular approach. On the side ipsilateral to the herniation, the facet joint and pedicle flush to the vertebral body and are generally removed. A hemilaminectomy may also be performed. (*From Stillerman CB, Weiss MH: Management of thoracic disc disease.* Clin Neurosurg 38:325-352, 1992.)

imaging is used to identify the appropriate disc space. A 4-cm linear skin incision is centered over the disc space. The paraspinal muscles are subperiosteally reflected laterally, exposing the ipsilateral spinous process, lamina, facet joint, and transverse processes above and below the disc space. A small, self-retaining retractor is placed, and the fluoroscope is introduced to verify the correct level and the precise location of the underlying disc relative to the facet joint. Once this relationship is ascertained, a high-speed drill is used to facilitate a partial facetectomy (Figure 48.4*A*). Care is taken to preserve the lateral margin of the inferior and superior articular processes of the facet joint and the entire pedicle directly caudal to the disc. When the partial facetectomy is completed, the underlying neuroforaminal fat is coagulated with bipolar cautery. The nerve root, which exits the spinal canal under the more rostral pedicle, is rarely encountered, except in the upper thoracic spine (Figure 48.4*B*). The underlying annulus is coagulated and incised. The disc herniation is removed using conventional microdiscectomy techniques (Figure 48.4*C*). As with the transpedicular approach, no fusion is required.[30]

Advantages. Advantages of the transfacet pedicle-sparing approach may include diminished operating time, decreased blood loss, and limited bone and soft tissue removal. Like the transpedicular approach, perioperative pain, hospital stay, and return to premorbid activity appear to compare favorably with the more formidable ventrolateral and lateral approaches.[29-31] When necessary, multiple disc herniations may be treated.[9] The exposure is identical to that provided by the transpedicular approach. Preservation of the pedicle may improve long-term localized back pain results.[29-31]

Disadvantages. The disadvantages are the same as for the transpedicular approach.[31-33] Specially designed thoracic

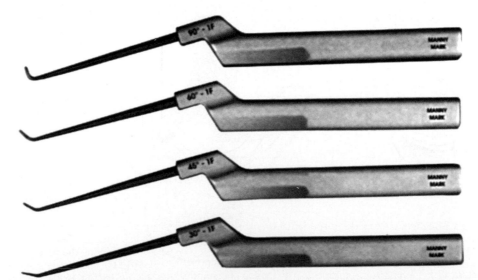

Figure 48.3 Photograph of a portion of the Manny-Mark Stillerman thoracic microdiscectomy instruments. These were developed to facilitate disc removal during a dorsolateral approach without damaging the medially situated spinal cord. (*From Stillerman CB, Chen TC, Day JD, et al: The transfacet pedicle-sparing approach for thoracic disc removal: cadaveric morphometric analysis and preliminary clinical experience.* J Neurosurg 83:971-976, 1995.)

microdiscectomy instrumentation[30] and, on occasion, open endoscopic visualization of the disc and ventral dural mater have been helpful in enhancing safety during the disc removal.[16,29,30]

Lateral Approaches
Lateral Extracavitary Approach

Lateral extracavitary approach (LECA) was developed and refined by Larson.[15] It was first performed for the management of Pott's disease. It provides the best exposure to the ventral spinal canal of all lateral operations. Large thoracic discectomy series have documented its safety and efficacy (Figure 48.5).[20,33]

Technique. The procedure is performed with the patient prone and taped to the table with arms at the side. The skin incision consists of a hockey stick-shaped incision, with the vertical portion centered over the area of pathology (Figure 48.5A).[15,20,32,34] Caudally, the incision is gently curved off the midline for 8 to 12cm, enabling the skin, subcutaneous tissue, and fascial flap to be rotated far laterally. Alternatively, a paramedian lunar-shaped incision may be used. The erector spinae muscles are subperiosteally dissected off the dorsal ribs and transverse processes and flapped medially.[11] The erector spinae muscle complex may be wrapped in a moistened laparotomy pad and gently retracted medially. Intraoperative imaging helps ensure removal of the rib that articulates with the correct disc space (Figure 48.5B). Once the proximal 8 to 12cm of rib is resected, the underlying intercostal nerve is identified

and traced into the neural foramen (Figure 48.5C). The pedicle caudal to the disc is identified and removed. This exposes the lateral aspect of the dura mater (Figure 48.5D). At this point, the dorsal third of the disc space is removed. Care is taken to leave intact the dorsal most margin of disc and the posterior longitudinal ligament (Figure 48.5E). The dorsal-caudal quarter of the rostral vertebra is drilled out, as is the dorsal-rostral quarter of the caudal vertebra. This creates a cavity so that the remaining dorsal disc and posterior longitudinal ligament can be gently depressed away from the spinal cord (Figure 48.5F). The ventral dura mater can then be inspected either directly, with small dental mirrors, or with an endoscope. The rib, which was resected to facilitate exposure of the disc space, is then fashioned into strut grafts and then carefully impacted across the cavity (Figure 48.5G). The ventral dura mater and spinal canal are then inspected again to ensure that there is no encroachment by the bone grafts.

Advantages. One major advantage of this procedure is the enhanced safety during the disc removal because of direct visualization of the dura mater before and during the decompression.[15,20,32-34] The removal of the pedicle helps facilitate this. Additionally, because of the extensive amount of rib removed compared with the other lateral procedures, the exposure to the ventral spinal canal is improved. Surgeon orientation is almost truly lateral. By remaining extrapleural, the procedure avoids the complications observed with intrathoracic surgery.[33] These include the need to place a thoracostomy tube and various pulmonary complications (cerebrospinal fluid-pleural

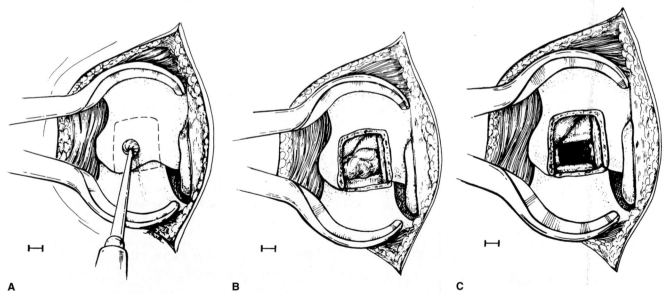

A　　　　　　　　**B**　　　　　　　　**C**

Figure 48.4 Transfacet pedicle-sparing approach. Diagrams illustrating surgical sequence. Bar scale represents 0.8cm = 1cm. A mesial facetectomy is centered over the disc herniation. **(A)** Fluoroscopy is used to limit the amount of bone removed. Upon completing the partial facetectomy, **(B)** the foraminal fat is coagulated and the disc is exposed. **(C)** The disc herniation is removed using conventional microdiscectomy techniques. Specially designed thoracic microdiscectomy instruments are helpful to facilitate safety during discectomy. Additionally, open endoscopy can be used to improve visualization of the central and contralateral spinal canal during disc removal. *(From Stillerman CB, Chen TC, Day JD, et al: The transfacet pedicle-sparing approach for thoracic disc removal: cadaveric morphometric analysis and preliminary clinical experience.* J Neurosurg 83:971-976, 1995.)

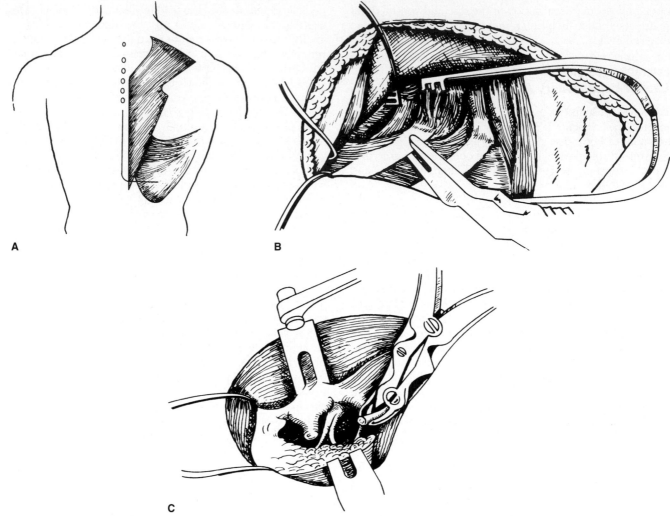

Figure 48.5 Lateral extracavitary approach. A *hockey stick*-shaped incision centered over the level of disc herniation is generally used. **(A)** Caudally, the incision is curved off the midline to maximize the amount of rib that can be exposed and removed. Shorter portions of rib resections create a more dorsolateral orientation to the disc space. Conversely, extensive removal of rib will facilitate a more lateral approach to the disc space. The skin, subcutaneous tissue, and fascia are rotated laterally. **(B)** The erector spinae muscles are then flapped medially, exposing the underlying rib(s), which are then resected flush with the vertebral body. **(C)** Removal of the proximal rib head, transverse process, and pedicle directly caudal to the disc space enables exposure of the neural foramen and lateral dura mater.   *Continued*

fistula, pneumonia, and complications related to the need to take down the diaphragm at the thoracolumbar junction). A ventral strut graft can be placed with relative ease. Finally, in the rare instance of multiple symptomatic discs,[9,29] multiple levels can be exposed.[20,33]

Disadvantages. The major disadvantage of LECA is that it is a formidable operation with a potential for significant perioperative pain.[29-31] Additionally, there is a potential for prolonged operating time and considerable blood loss, especially early on in a surgeon's series. In experienced hands, however, these parameters appear to be comparable to the ventrolateral approaches.[15,20] Densely calcified central discs, intradural fragments, ventral dural tears, or discs that are completely enveloped by the dura mater may be difficult to remove without the need to elevate the dura mater.[29] These situations may be better treated using

a ventrolateral approach. Finally, as is the case with ventrolateral surgeries, LECA is generally not recommended by the authors in the medically high-risk patient.[29]

Lateral Parascapular Extrapleural Approach

Fessler, Dietze, MacMillan, *et al*[12] developed a modification of LECA called the lateral parascapular extrapleural approach (LPEA). This operation simplifies removal of a thoracic disc herniation in the upper thoracic spine.

Technique. Patients are placed prone and taped to the table so they can be rotated 15 to 20 degrees away from the surgeon during the decompression. The arms are kept at the sides. A midline incision extends two spinous processes above and below the disc to be removed. Caudally, the incision is gently curved laterally to the

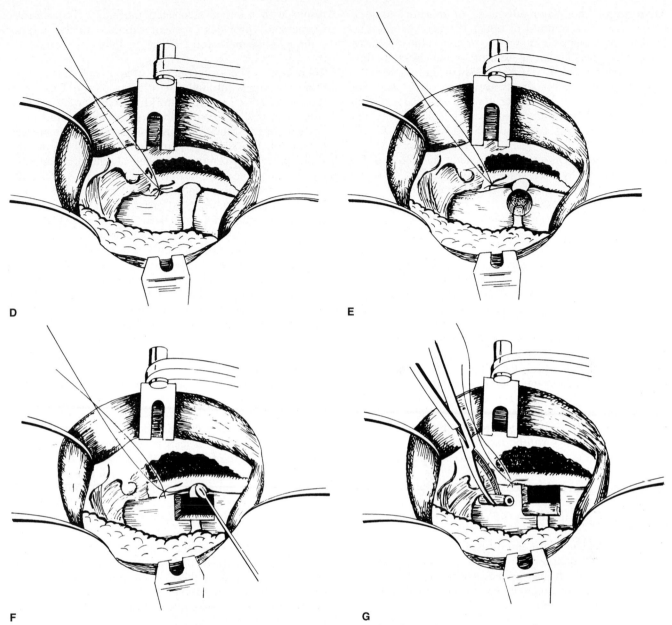

Figure 48.5 *cont'd* (**D**) The intercostal nerve is identified and traced into its respective foramen. This is tagged and cut. Care must be taken to avoid traction on this nerve. (**E**) The lateral annulus is incised and a portion of nucleus is removed enabling drilling through the disc to the contralateral side. The dorsal portion of the disc, posterior longitudinal ligament, and disc herniation are left intact. A cavity is created by removal of a portion of the rostral and caudal vertebral bodies. (**F**) The remaining disc and posterior longitudinal ligament are then depressed into this cavity. Once the ventral dura and spinal canal are directly inspected for retained fragments, (**G**) the rib that was removed during the exposure is fashioned into struts and gently impacted across the defect. *(From Stillerman CB, Weiss MH: Management of thoracic disc disease. Clin Neurosurg 38:325-352, 1992.)*

scapular line on the side of pathology. To minimize postoperative seroma formation, the incision is carried down to the deep fascia, with only minimal subcutaneous undermining. The rhomboid and trapezius muscles are then dissected off the spinous processes. A myocutaneous flap is rotated toward the medial scapular border. The caudal fibers of the trapezius muscle are transected to reflect the flap. It is important to protect the rostral latissimus dorsi fibers while cutting the inferior portion of the trapezius muscle. The musculocutaneous flap is limited by the skin incision and the medial scapula. The scapula rotates laterally as the trapezius and rhomboid muscles are mobilized. This increases the exposure of the ribs laterally for better orientation to the ventral spinal cord and central disc space.[11,12]

Most of the advantages and disadvantages of LECA are identical to its LPEA modification. The following emphasizes points that are specific to the LPEA surgery.

Advantage. The major advantage of this technique is that it simplifies removal of upper thoracic disc herniations by providing a far lateral orientation to the disc space at this level. This far lateral exposure enhances safety during decompression by improving visualization across the ventral spinal canal. There is avoidance of the superior mediastinal structures, which may be traumatized with other approaches to the upper thoracic spine. Recurrent laryngeal nerve palsies are also avoided.[12]

Disadvantages. Disadvantages include the potential for shoulder morbidity from scapular mobilization, T1 nerve injury, Horner's syndrome, sympathectomy, and intercostal neuralgia.

Costotransversectomy

The costotransversectomy approach was initially reported by Ménard[7,32,33] for the treatment of Pott's disease. The orientation to the disc space is more dorsal than with either LECA or LPEA. This is the result of a more limited rib resection.

Technique. Different costotransversectomy techniques have been proposed. Patient positioning options vary from prone to modified lateral decubitus.[7] Skin incisions likewise vary and include the paramedian incision along the lateral border of the erector spinae muscles, and a semilunar incision. A skin, subcutaneous tissue, and fascial flap may be rotated medially toward the spinous process. The trapezius muscle can be incised in line with the skin incision and retracted medially. The erector spinae muscles are then dissected from their attachments and can be reflected medially. Some surgeons prefer to cut this muscle complex and reapproximate it at the time of closure. From this point, surgical decompression is the same as for LECA.

Advantages. The skin and muscle manipulation and amount of rib resected is somewhat less than with LECA or LPEA. This offers the theoretical advantage of comparatively diminished perioperative pain and may shorten the length of hospitalization.

Disadvantages. This is a more dorsal approach than that provided by the other two lateral surgeries. Consequently, the visualization of the central spinal canal is not as good as with those approaches.

Ventrolateral Approaches
Transthoracic Thoracotomy

The transthoracic thoracotomy approach was first reported independently in 1969 by Perot and Munro[24] and Ransohoff et al.[25] These two groups reported on a combined number of five patients. Despite the limited number of patients initially undergoing this approach, it has developed into one of the surgical cornerstones for the management of symptomatic thoracic disc herniations.[29,31] Two large series of thoracic discectomy patients were compared in 1992.[33] One group primarily used the transthoracic thoracotomy approach and the other group exclusively used the lateral extracavitary approach. It was determined that these two formidable procedures provided very good

results with minimal associated morbidity. Transthoracic thoracotomy provides excellent exposure to the anterior column between T3 and L1 (Figure 48.6).

Technique. The preferred side of approach in the upper thoracic spine is through a right thoracotomy. This avoids the heart as well as the carotid and subclavian arteries. When the disc herniation involves the middle and lower portions of the thoracic spine, most spinal surgeons perform a left thoracotomy. Approaching the disc from this side avoids manipulation of the delicate inferior vena cava, which may prove difficult to repair if injured. Additionally, at the thoracolumbar junction the liver is avoided. A double lumen endotracheal tube may be used to facilitate single lung ventilation (particularly in the upper thoracic spine). Care is taken to place the patient in a true lateral decubitus position. A bean bag and tape are used to maintain this position so that the patient may be rolled during the decompression. When possible, the area of pathology is centered over the break in the table. All pressure points are padded. A tangential incision is made over the rib to be resected. This enables the removal of additional ribs when necessary. The skin and subcutaneous tissue are incised from the lateral border of the paraspinal muscles to the sternocostal junction (Figure 48.6A). The thoracic muscular layers are then incised and a rib retractor is introduced. It is helpful to verify that the proper rib is being resected by intraoperative AP fluoroscopy. The periosteum of the rib is then incised and exposed using subperiosteal dissection. A Doyen elevator is used to strip the periosteum from the ventral surface of the rib without violating the underlying endothoracic fascia and pleura. Small defects in these layers should be closed primarily; the rib is then resected. Bone edges of the rib are waxed and the resected portion of rib is saved so that it can be used to form an interbody bone graft upon completion of the discectomy. The parietal pleura is then incised along the line of the rib bed and the wound is held open by introducing a rib spreader (Figure 48.6C). The lung is covered with a moistened laparotomy pad and can be gently retracted medially and ventrally. It may be selectively collapsed to facilitate additional exposure of the spinal column. The parietal pleura, which covers the vertebral bodies, are incised. A Cobb elevator can be used to prepare the vertebral bodies. This dissection must avoid injury to the segmental vessels, as well as the sympathetic chain that crosses the middle portion of each vertebral body (Figure 48.6D). It may be necessary to ligate or clip these vessels. To expose the dorsolateral disc space, ventral spinal canal, and entire neuroforamen, it is necessary to incise the radiate ligament and to drill off the head of the overlying rib. The overlying transverse process, neurovascular foramen, and the rostral and caudal boundaries of the pedicle that is directly caudal to the appropriate disc space are palpated with a small nerve hook. The pedicle can be removed. This exposes the lateral dura mater. When necessary, additional exposure of the neuroforamen can be facilitated by sectioning the intercostal nerve proximal to the dorsal root ganglia. At this point, the surgeon should have precise orientation regarding the location of the ventral floor of the spinal canal. The dorsal portion of the annulus is incised and the discectomy is carried across the vertebral body approaching the other side. Care is taken to leave intact the most dorsal margin of disc and the posterior longitudinal ligament. A high-speed drill is used to create a small cavity in the dorsal-caudal quadrant of the rostral vertebral body and the dorsal-rostral portion of the caudal vertebral body. Once this cavity has been created, the overlying dorsal disc margin and posterior longitudinal ligament can be incised and gently depressed into the cavity, away from the ventral dura mater. A reverse angled curette may aid the decompression without manipulating the spinal cord (Figure 48.6*E*). The ventral spinal canal and dura mater should be directly inspected subsequent to placement of bone grafts to ensure that there is no encroachment of the spinal canal. The lung is then expanded under direct visualization. The parietal pleura are closed over a thoracostomy tube.

Advantages. The main advantage of the transthoracic thoracotomy relates to the ventrolateral exposure of the disc space and the ventral spinal canal. This orientation enables improved exposure for the removal of midline densely calcified discs and intradural fragments. Repair of ventral dural tears is also simplified as is interbody bone graft placement. Finally, it is possible to remove more than one disc in the rare situation of multiple symptomatic herniations.*

Disadvantages. The main disadvantage is similar to that of the more extensive lateral exposures; this is a formidable operation with significant potential for considerable

---

*References 9,24,25,29,31,33.

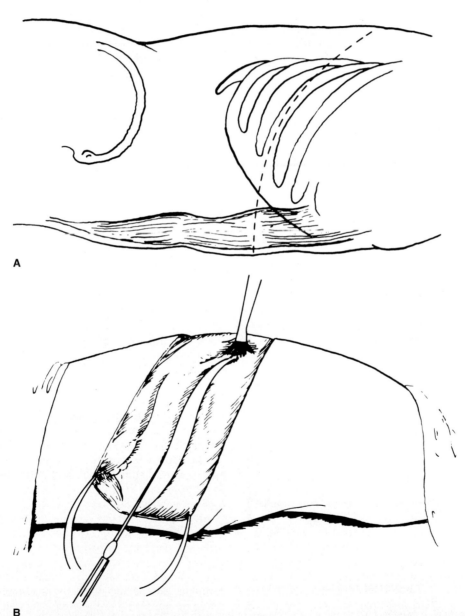

A

B

Figure 48.6 Transthoracic thoracotomy approach. The patient is placed in the lateral decubitus position. **(A)** The incision extends from the border of the paraspinal muscles to the sternocostal junction. The rib is exposed and resected flush with the lateral spinal column. **(B)** Removal of the rib head exposes the appropriate disc space and neural foramen.

postoperative pain.[29,31] Because of the visceral exposure, several unique risks are possible. These include cerebrospinal fluid-pleural fistulas and pulmonary complications secondary to lung collapse. Additionally, closed chest drainage is required in the postoperative period. Disc herniations that occur at the thoracolumbar junction may require at least partial takedown of the diaphragm. Finally, the operation is technically demanding and may require collaboration with a thoracic surgeon.

Transthoracic Thoracoscopy

The use of thoracoscopy for the treatment of thoracic disc herniations was reported as early as 1994.[13,27] Subsequently, growing enthusiasm for this procedure has developed with several surgeons demonstrating proficiency.[10,14,18,26] The technique as described by Rosenthal et al.[27] uses a right-sided approach. Four small incisions are made along the midaxillary line so that four trocars may be inserted in a triangular fashion along this line

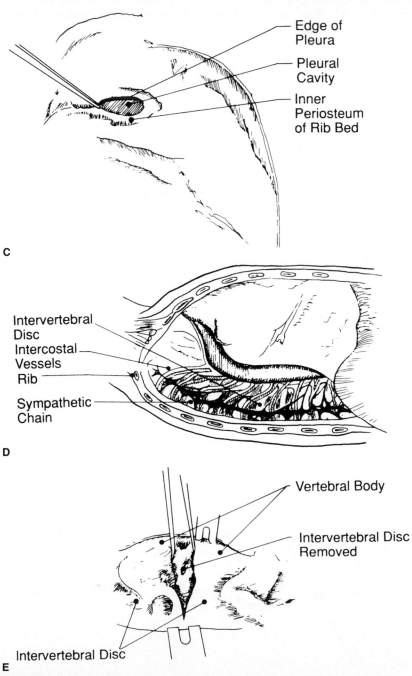

Figure 48.6 *cont'd* (**C**) The pleura are opened in line with the rib bed. The lung is gently retracted and the parietal pleura overlying the spinal column is incised and carefully reflected. It is often necessary to ligate the intercostal vessels. (**D**) The sympathetic chain must be left intact. (**E**) The disc space is exposed and the disc herniation can now be removed. *(From Stillerman CB, Weiss MH: Management of thoracic disc disease. Clin Neurosurg 38:325-352, 1992.)*

converging on the disc space. An endoscope with a 30-degree angled lens is introduced through one of the trocars, leaving the other three as working ports. Specially designed long instruments are introduced through the working ports. At this point, the discectomy proceeds similarly to an open thoracotomy.

Advantages. Proponents of this approach believe that compared with transthoracic thoracotomy, transthoracic thoracoscopy allows for complete disc removal with a reduction in surgical trauma. Thus it is thought to be associated with significantly less pain and morbidity and enables faster recovery time.[10,27]

Disadvantages. In its present form, there are several limitations to this technique. This includes the need for pleural entry with all the attendant risks of intrathoracic surgery, including the need for a postoperative thoracostomy tube. A steep learning curve exists because of the need to develop techniques requiring new hand-eye coordination skills, limited tactile feedback during the surgery, and difficulties with the three-dimensional visualization during disc removal. Additionally, in an era when growing cost constraints are impacting on surgical methodology, the cost effectiveness of this procedure will need to be evaluated from the standpoint of duration of hospitalization, length of surgery, and cost of the instrumentation required to perform this technique. Finally, despite being touted by some as a *minimally invasive* technique for thoracic disc removal, it is important to keep in mind that this operation currently requires multiple stab incisions for the insertion of the camera, two working ports, and on occasion, a retractor for the diaphragm, or an incompletely collapsed lung. In its present form, this procedure is perhaps more invasive than other techniques.[31] The exposure that this technique provides is identical to thoracotomy.[29,31] If this procedure is proven clinically safe and effective over long-term follow-up, it would appear to be best suited as an alternative to open thoracotomy in distinction to being a substitute for the dorsolateral, lateral, and retropleural operations.[31]

Retropleural Thoracotomy Approach

Retropleural thoracotomy was recently refined and popularized by McCormick.[19] This operation provides an exciting option in the management of ventral spinal pathology by providing orientation that is similar to the other ventrolateral approaches and avoids key complications (Figure 48.7).

Technique. Like the transthoracic procedures, the side of the approach is determined by the location of the pathology. The patient is placed in the lateral decubitus position on a bean bag with a small roll under the dependent axilla. Lesions that occur at the thoracolumbar junction should be centered over the break in the table. Between T5 and T10, a 12-cm skin incision is made, extending from the posterior axillary line to a point 4cm lateral to the dorsal midline over the rib at the level of pathology. For upper thoracic spine lesions, a *hockey stick* incision that parallels the medial and caudal scapular border, is performed (Figure 48.7A). The incision is then carried through the scapular muscles (trapezius and rhomboids) to the ribs. The scapula is then rotated rostrally to expose the appropriate rib. After the appropriate level is identified, a subperiosteal detachment of intercostal muscles is performed over 8 to 10cm of rib. The rib is then resected and removed (Figure 48.7B). The most proximal 4cm of rib that has attachments to the vertebral body and transverse process remains intact. Once the rib resection is completed, a well-defined layer of tissue is identified in the rib bed. This layer is the endothoracic fascia. It is analogous to the transversalis fascia in the abdomen.

The endothoracic fascia lines the entire chest cavity. The underlying parietal pleura maintains an attachment to the inner chest wall through this layer. There is a potential space between the endothoracic fascia and parietal pleura that may contain loose areolar tissue. The endothoracic fascia is continuous with the inner periosteum of the rib and the thoracic vertebral body. It is important to remember that the thoracic sympathetic chain, the intercostal neurovascular elements, the thoracic duct, and the azygous veins are contained against the thoracic wall and the vertebral bodies within this fascial layer. Once identified, the fascia is incised in line with the rib bed (Figure 48.7C). The underlying parietal pleural is bluntly dissected from the undersurface of the endothoracic fascia, in much the same way that the peritoneum is freed from the transversalis fascia. Proximally, the pleura are dissected from the vertebral column. At this point, a table-mounted malleable retractor maintains retraction of a laparotomy pad-covered lung (Figure 48.7D). The opening can be further widened by placement of a rib retractor.

The endothoracic fascia should be opened over the remaining 4cm of proximal rib. The costotransverse ligaments are divided and the rib head is removed. The fascia and periosteum over the vertebral body are elevated away from the disc space. The intercostal vessels that cross the midvertebral body transversely may be preserved. Once the rib head is resected, the boundaries of the neuroforamen and pedicle are identified and the rostral portion of the pedicle directly caudal to the disc space may be resected. From this point on, the decompression is identical to the other ventrolateral approaches (Figures 48.7E and 48.7F). At the thoracolumbar junction, because of the diaphragm and the greater angulation of the ribs, the procedure is modified. A 12- to 14-cm skin incision is generally made over the 10th rib that extends from the posterior axillary line to 4cm off the midline (Figure 48.7A). A 10-cm portion of rib is then exposed and resected. The pleural surface of the diaphragm is then identified. It should be noted that the endothoracic fascia is reflected over the diaphragm and tightly applied to its surface.

The initial exposure may be somewhat cramped because of the diaphragm's attachment to the ribs. If the endothoracic fascia is present in the rib bed, it is opened. Caudally, the pleural surface of the diaphragm is depressed and detached from the ventral surface of the T11 and T12 ribs with Cobb elevators. Once this is completed, there is a communication between the retropleural and retroperitoneal space. Medially, the detachment is continued so that the arcuate ligaments are elevated off the quadratus lumborum and psoas muscles. Division

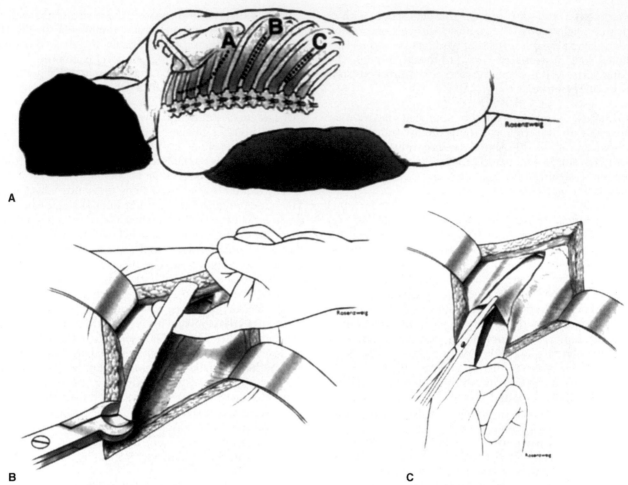

Figure 48.7 Retropleural thoracotomy approach. (**A**) The patient is placed in the lateral decubitus position. Incision *A* is used for upper thoracic spine disc herniations. Incision *B* is used for herniations between T5 and T10. Incision *C* is used for thoracolumbar herniated discs. The skin incision is extended through the muscle layers and the rib is exposed. (**B**) All but the most proximal 4cm of rib is removed. After rib removal, the well-defined endothoracic fascia is identified within the rib bed. (**C**) This is then opened in line with the rib bed. The pleura are then swept away from the undersurface of the endothoracic fascia.   *Continued*

of the crus of the diaphragm completes the mobilization of the diaphragm. At this point, table-mounted malleable retractors are inserted as rib spreaders. The proximal 4cm of rib are then removed. The decompression at this point continues as described above.[19]

Advantages. This operation provides exposure to the ventral spinal canal and dura mater that is identical to the intrathoracic operations discussed above. However, it avoids pleural entry. Thus many of the significant complications that may arise from these procedures are avoided.

Also important is that the retropleural thoracotomy approach provides the shortest direct surgical route to the ventral thoracic and thoracolumbar spine. This may enhance safety during the decompression, as well as enable the surgery to be performed using smaller incisions with less soft-tissue dissection. This should lessen perioperative pain and diminish the length of hospitalization. In contrast to the ventrolateral approaches, the diaphragm can be

mobilized quite easily at the thoracolumbar junction without its incision. Additionally, the exposure rendered is less obscured by the aorta and vena cava. In contrast to the lateral approaches, exposure to the lateral spinal canal is achieved without dissection or sacrifice of the intercostal nerve or potentially occluding the intraforaminal radicular medullary artery. Overall, this procedure appears to offer advantages over the other ventrolateral surgeries (both closed and open), and lateral approaches.[19]

Disadvantages. When compared with the dorsolateral operations (transfacet and transpedicular), the orientation to the disc space and ventral spinal canal is more direct.[19] This must be weighed against the more extensive muscle and bone manipulation required by this surgery. If safety and efficacy are demonstrated clinically, the retropleural thoracotomy approach may be ideally suited for disc herniations that cannot be reliably treated using one of the less invasive dorsolateral techniques.

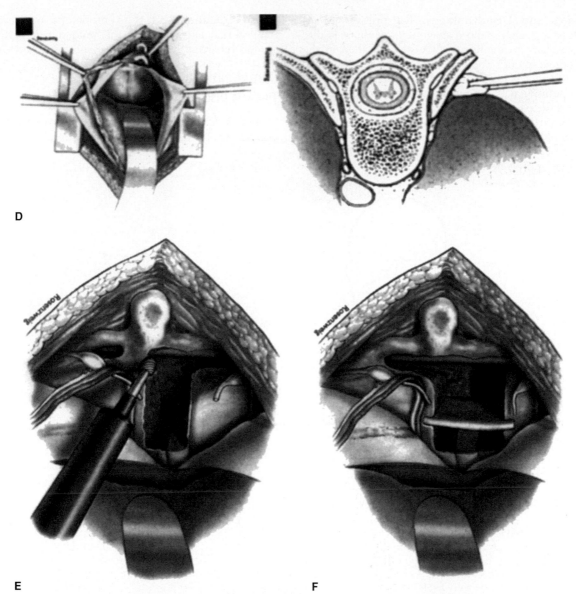

Figure 48.7 *cont'd* (**D**) Proximally, the pleura are dissected off the spinal column. The rib head is removed along with the rostral portion of the pedicle directly caudal to the disc space. (**E**) The overlying transverse process can also be removed. This exposes the neural foramen and the lateral dura. (**F**) The disc is then removed, the spinal canal and ventral dura are directly examined, and the rib that was removed can be fashioned into strut grafts and impacted across the defect. (*From McCormick PC: Retropleural approach to the thoracic and thoracolumbar spine.* Neurosurgery 37:1-7, 1995.)

Ventral Approaches
Trans-sternal Approach

The trans-sternal approach may be an option for the management of midline densely calcified herniations between T2 and T5 (Figure 48.8).[32-34] When the surgery requires access to the T4-5 levels, preoperative imaging must define the relationship between the aortic arch and the ventral spinal column.

Technique. This operation is generally performed through a T-shaped skin incision that has its vertical limb extending from the lower cervical skin crease to a few centimeters below the xiphoid process (Figure 48.8A). The strap muscles are then divided, and the precervical fascia and pretracheal fascia incised at the level of the sternal notch. The sternum is then split and retracted laterally. After the exposure of the pericardium and thymus, the thymus is retracted to the right, exposing the left innominate vein, which can be sacrificed. The working space is between the left common carotid artery and the innominate artery, the trachea, esophagus, and thyroid. Gentle retraction of these structures exposes the ventral region of the spinal column (Figure 48.8B). Once the ventral spine is exposed, the disc is removed using standard microdiscectomy techniques that are used during ventral cervical microdiscectomy.[32-34]

Advantages and Disadvantages. The primary advantage of this approach is the management of thoracic disc herniations that are midline and densely calcified in the upper thoracic spine.[29] The other advantages are similar to those for the ventrolateral approaches. This is clearly a formidable operation with the potential for significant physiologic cost to the patient. Fortunately, disc herniations in the upper thoracic spine are quite rare, constituting just a fraction of symptomatic disc herniations.[29] Most of these herniations can be treated successfully using one of the other less invasive approaches. In addition to all the disadvantages encountered with the ventrolateral approaches, the trans-sternal approach has the unique risk of injury to the left recurrent laryngeal nerve and the thoracic duct.[33]

Complications
Thoracic Disc Series

Several independently reported reviews of thoracic disc herniations have appeared in the literature.° Many of

°References 1-3,5,8,17,24,28.

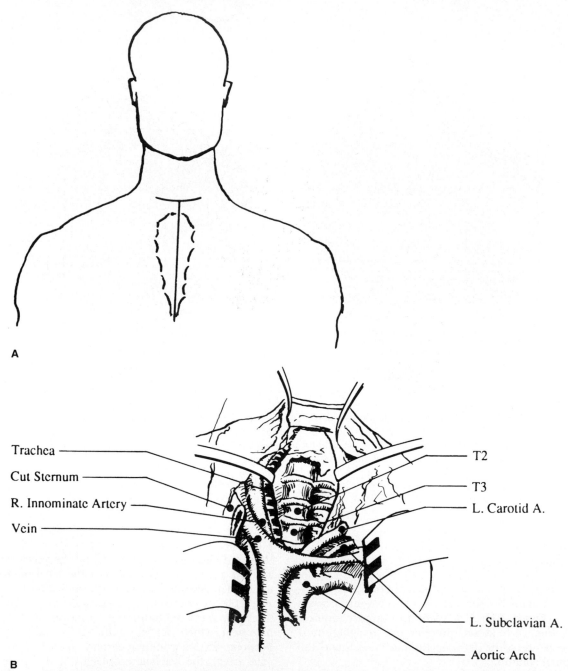

A

Trachea
Cut Sternum
R. Innominate Artery
Vein

T2
T3
L. Carotid A.

L. Subclavian A.
Aortic Arch

B

Figure 48.8 Transsternal approach. **(A)** T-shaped incision with the transverse limb along the lower cervical skin crease and the vertical limb extending along the midline to below the xiphoid process. **(B)** The vertebral column is exposed following sternal splitting, dissection, and retraction of the intervening structures. (*From Stillerman CB, Weiss MH: Management of thoracic disc disease. Clin Neurosurg 38:325-352, 1992.*)

these reports provide excellent historic perspectives that include surgeries performed before the 1930s. For a better understanding of the overall effectiveness of modern thoracic disc herniation management, a focused review of several large series performed during the past decade is presented (Table 48.2).[29] Recently, Stillerman et al.[29] reported their experience with the operative management of 82 symptomatic herniated thoracic discs. In this series the overall complication rate was 12/82 (14.6%).

There were three major complications (3.6%) consisting of one perioperative death from cardiopulmonary complications in a high medical risk patient, spinal instability requiring further surgery, and an increase in the severity of a preoperative paraparesis. There were 9/82 (11%) minor complications, which consisted of one transient paraparesis that completely resolved after 48 hours, one compression fracture treated with 3 months of bracing, three superficial wound infections, three pneumonias, and one postoperative seizure. All of the minor complications were treated medically with no sequela (Table 48.3).[29] Results of the Stillerman et al.[29] and the 13 other contemporary series were then compared (Table 48.4). The review group reported a 6.1% major complication rate (16/263) compared to a 3.6% rate (3/82) in the Stillerman series. This difference was not found to be statistically significant (chi-square test). Although several deaths have been reported in earlier series[2,5,6,17,24] there were none in the 13 contemporary

TABLE 48.2

Thoracic Disc Series 1986–1997[29]

| Name | Year | Surgical Approach | PTS/DISCS | Pain | | Motor Deficit Pre/Post | Bowel/Dysfunction Pre/Post | Complications Bladder |
				Back Pre/Post	Radicular Pre/Post			
Lesoin et al.	1986	Lam 3 MTP 16 TT 2	21/22	NR	5/5	16/10	NR	Major 1 (4.5%) Paraparesis permanent Minor 1 (4.5%) Paraparesis transient Total (9%)
Bohlman and Zdeblick	1988	Costo 11 TT 8	19/22	13/10	4/1 + NR	14/12	8/2 + NR	Major 2 (9%) 1 paraparesis permanent 1 wrong lev. ⇒ redo surgery Minor 1 (4.5%) Paraparesis transient Total (13.6%)
Blumenkopf	1988	TT 4 TP 3	9/#7	7/7	4/4	3/2	1/1	NR
Otani et al.	1988	MCos 23	23/23	NR	NR	23/23	23/18	NR
El-Kalliny et al.	1991	TP 8 TT 8 Costo 5	21/23	15/11	13/11	10/8	6/NR	Major 3 (13%) 1 Paraparesis permanent – TT 1 Pleural effusion ⇒ Surgery for CSF Leak ⇒ TT 1 CVA Minor 1 (4.3%) Pleural effusion Total (17.4%)
Singounas et al.	1992	Costo 14 MCos 4	14/14	NR	NR	NR	NR	Major 3 (21.4%) 1 paraparesis 1 discitis 1 comp. fx. from discitis
Le Roux et al.	1993	TP 20	20/23	17/14	17/16	3/3	1/1	NR
Fessler	1993	LEC 17	17/22	15/10	7/5	8/8		Minor 2 (9%) 1 anesthesia dolorosa 1 pneumonia

Continued

review series. The minor complications reported in the review group were composed of 8.7% (23/263), compared to 11% (9/82) in the Stillerman series. The total complication rate reported was 14.8% (39/263) in the review group and 14.6% (12/82) in the Stillerman series. Like the case with major complications, there was no sig-

nificant difference in either the total complication rate or minor complications.

Based on experience gained with the ventrolateral and lateral surgeries during the course of the series of 82 thoracic discectomies, the well-documented success by others using the dorsolateral transpedicular approach, the preliminary

TABLE 48.2

Thoracic Disc Series 1986–1997[29] *cont'd*

Name	Year	Surgical Approach	PTS/DISCS	Pain		Motor Deficit Pre/Post	Bowel/ Dysfunction Pre/Post	Complications Bladder
				Back Pre/Post	Radicular Pre/Post			
Ridenour *et al.*	1993	Lam 4 Costo 15 TP 12	31/3311/7	12/5	18/9	13/8		Major 3 (9%) 1 increased myelopathy 1 Wrong level additional surgery 1 Incomplete disc Removal redo surgery Minor 3 (9%) 3 Superficial wound infection Total (18.2%)
Simpson *et al.*	1993	MCos 16	21/23	19/19	6/4	4/3	NR	
Oppenheim *et al.*	1993	Costo 8	12/8	7/6	NR	1/1		Major 1 (12.5%) 1 Wrong diagnosis progressive weakness. Avm found 3 levels Caudal operated level
Currier *et al.*	1994	TT19	19/22	15/10	11/7	6/NR		Major 3 (13.6%) 1 Nonfatal PE 1 Intraop hemodynamic Instability v. tack. + hypotension 1 Spinal instability kyphosis after lam+TT Minor 9 (41%) 1 Incisional hernia 1 Dural tear intraop repair + drain 2 transient urinary retention 2 UTIs 4 chronic thoracotomy pain Total (54.5%)

TABLE 48.2

Thoracic Disc Series 1986–1997[29] cont'd

Name	Year	Surgical Approach	PTS/DISCS	Pain Back Pre/Post	Pain Radicular Pre/Post	Motor Deficit Pre/Post	Bowel/ Dysfunction Pre/Post	Complications Bladder
Bilsky and Patterson	1997	TP20	20/20	7/5 MCos 4	6/4	11/11	6/5	Minor 3 (15%)1 Pseudomeningitis 1 Deep wound infection 1 Transient increase in myelopathy

From Stillerman CB, Chen TC, Couldwell WT, *et al:* Surgical experience in the operative management of 82 symptomatic herniated thoracic discs and review of the literature. *J Neurosurg* 88:623-633, 1998.
Pre/post, Preoperative signs + symptoms/postoperative patients with resolution or improvement; *NR,* not reported; *Lam,* laminectomy; *TP,* transpedicular; *Costo,* costotransversectomy; *TT,* transthoracic; *MTP,* modified transpedicular; MCos = modified costotransversectomy; *LEC,* lateral extracavitary; *#7,* 7 discs operated (2 treated conservatively); *#8,* 8 discs operated (4 treated conservatively).

TABLE 48.3

Surgical Complications in 82 Thoracic Microdiscectomies

Complication Type	Number of Complications
Death	1 (1.2%)
Loss of spinal integrity Stable compression	
Fx: braced	1 (1.2%)
Fx with kyphosis: surgery	1 (1.2%)
Increased weakness	
Transient (resolved 48 h)	1 (1.2%)
Permanent mild residual deficit	1 (1.2%)
Superficial wound infection	3 (3.7%)
Pneumonia	3 (3.7%)
Seizure	1 (1.2%)
Total	12 (14.6%)

From Stillerman CB, Chen TC, Couldwell WT, *et al:* Surgical experience in the operative management of 82 symptomatic herniated thoracic discs and review of the literature. *J Neurosurg* 88:623-633, 1998.

experience reported with the transthoracic thoracoscopy, retropleural thoracotomy, and transfacet pedicle-sparing approaches, guidelines for selections for surgical approaches have been developed (see Table 48.1).[29]

Special Considerations

Localization

Care must be exercised when attempting to localize a lesion totally on the basis of an MRI scan. For example, the MRI may count the level of the lesion according to counting from an end vertebrae (i.e., the sacrum or C2). At operation, it is often not possible to count from the end vertebrae, but one must count from the rib. In a small but not insignificant percentage of the population, there may be variations in the number of non-rib-bearing lumbar vertebrae or even in the size of the 12th lumbar rib. Therefore, it might be important to reconcile the MRI level with plain films to know the number of non-rib lum-

bar vertebrae and the size of the 12th rib. Other measures, such as preoperative marking with fluoroscopy, may provide useful information about the level of the herniation.

Failure to Achieve Objective

A thorough review of preoperative studies to determine the size and location of the disc herniation within the spinal canal (i.e., centrolateral vs. lateral, extradural vs. intradural, migration away from the disc space) helps the surgeon determine whether the disc herniation has been completely removed. Examination of the ventral spinal canal with dental mirror, or through endoscopy, or perhaps the appreciation of the restoration of dural pulsations following the removal of the disc are all means of gaining information on the extent of disc herniation that has been removed. It is important to realize that there is often a very thin layer of posterior longitudinal ligament that remains after the standard removal of the disc. This layer must be fenestrated so that the actual dura is identified to minimize the possibility of a retained disc fragment.

Management of Dural Openings

A CSF leak is not nearly as problematic for the posterolateral extrapleural approaches as it is for the transthoracic approaches. A CSF pleural fistula may be difficult to treat. When a dural opening is made during transthoracic surgery, an attempt to achieve a water-tight dural closure either primarily or with use of a graft should be made. A small pleural flap may be utilized. Additionally, fibrin glue to reinforce the suture line may be helpful. The utilization of a chest tube with water seal in instituting spinal drainage are two other techniques to circumvent CSF pleural fistula.

New Paradigm for Thoracic Disc Herniations

Based on an evaluation of the aforementioned contemporary series, a management paradigm was developed for treating this disorder (Figure 48.9).[29] Patients with symptoms of

TABLE 48.4

Thoracic Disc Series Comparison

	13 Contemporary Series 1986–1997	Stillerman *et al.*
Demographics and disc characteristics		
Patients/discs	247/263	71/82
Sex (f/m)	112/95 (1.18:1) 37/34 (1.09:1)	
Age	18–79	19–75
Trauma	37% (59/161)	37% (26/71)
Levels	T1–L1 (total 244)	T4–L1 (total 82)
Frequency	T8–9: 17% (41)	T9–10: 26% (21)
	T11–12: 16% (39)	T8–9: 23% (19)
	T10–11: 11% (26)	T10–11: 17% (14)
Calcified	22% (33/151)	65% (53/82)
Intradural	6% (5/90)	7% (6/82)
Canal location		
Central/centrolateral	77% (113/146)	94% (77/82)
Lateral	23% (33/146)	6% (5/82)
Multiple discs	8% (20/242)	14% (10/71)
Presenting signs and symptoms		
Localized/axial pain	56% (111/199)	61% (43/71)
Radicular pain	51% (94/185)	16% (11/71)
Sensory deficit	64% (145/226)	61% (43/71)
Bowel/bladder deficit	35% (72/208)	24% (17/71)
Motor impairment	55% (114/208)	61% (43/71)
Results (no. resolved or improved/total no. of patients in groups reporting this result)		
Pain: total	76% (106/140)	87% (47/54)
localized/axial	80% (39/49)	86% (37/43)
radicular	74% (29/39)	91% (10/11)
Sensory deficit	NR	84% (36/43)
Bowel/bladder deficit	80% (47/59)	77% (13/17)
Motor impairment	69% (65/94)	58% (25/43)

From Stillerman CB, Chen TC, Couldwell WT, *et al:* Surgical experience in the operative management of 82 symptomatic herniated thoracic discs and review of the literature. *J Neurosurg* 88:623-633, 1998.

thoracic disc herniations are placed into one of three groups: localized/axial pain, radicular pain, or myelopathy.

Localized/Axial Pain

Patients with back pain alone who do not have myelopathy or severe unrelenting radicular pain are a difficult management problem because of the nonspecific nature of their pain syndrome. Surgery has a high failure rate in these patients and has to be individualized.

Radiculopathy

Patients who are experiencing severe radiculopathy that is refractory to aggressive nonoperative management are evaluated for surgery. This generally consists of a dorsolateral approach for decompression because radiculopathy alone is generally associated with a far lateral disc or an osteophyte.

Myelopathy

Patients with myelopathy who are shown to have a disc herniation are treated based on the status of their neurologic deficit. The following is intended to serve as suggested considerations; the ultimate choice of procedure must be influenced by the surgeon's familiarity and skill

with the different approaches. Patients who have a nonsevere static deficit without functional impairment and whose pain is tolerable, are managed nonoperatively. Patients who are improving from the standpoint of their myelopathy are likewise treated conservatively. When the myelopathy is either severe and nonprogressive or progressing, the patients are entered into either a high medical risk or a low medical risk group. In the low medical risk group, the parameters influencing the selection of a particular approach include the position of the disc in the spinal canal (i.e., centrolateral vs. lateral herniation) and the consistency of the disc (soft vs. mildly calcified vs. densely calcified). Additionally, the location of the calcium in the disc (i.e., ventral vs. dorsal) is important in ascertaining the likelihood of significant dural adherence by the disc material. High medical risk patients with severe (static or progressive) myelopathy should undergo dorsolateral decompression unless their disc is midline or central-lateral, large, and densely calcified. Patients with these types of discs are operated on, using either a transthoracic thoracoscopy or retropleural approach, or on occasion, a transthoracic thoracotomy. The high medical risk patients with densely calcified central-lateral discs and static myelopathies are initially treated conservatively. However, if their symptoms prove to be refractory they are operated on with the same surgical approaches that

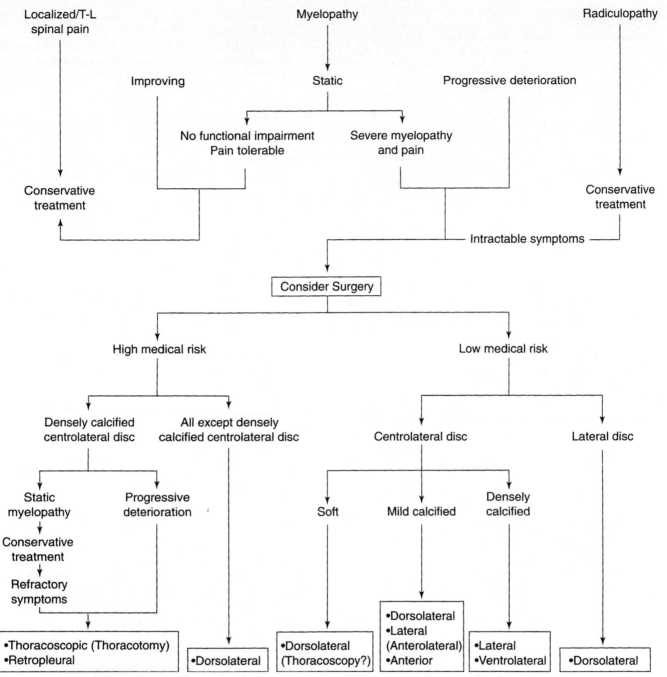

Figure 48.9 Management scheme for treating symptomatic thoracic disc herniations. *(From Stillerman CB, Chen TC, Couldwell WT, et al: Surgical experience in the operative management of 82 symptomatic herniated thoracic discs and review of the literature.* J Neurosurg 88:623-633, 1998.)

are used for patients found to have progressive deterioration in their myelopathy.

Summary

The review of contemporary thoracic disc herniation management has illustrated that its treatment still poses a significant problem. Patient outcome has improved considerably from earlier series. Further refinement of management, however, is necessary. The optimal treatment strategy must be designed based on the patient presentation, medical condition, disc characteristics, and familiarity of the surgeon with each approach. Because all of the surgical cornerstones for the treatment of symptoms of thoracic disc herniations have the potential for significant morbidity, there needs to be continued effort in the improvement of *minimally invasive* techniques. It is unlikely that one particular operation will become a panacea for all situations. Therefore, it is important that treating clinicians maintain proficiency in multiple surgical options.

REFERENCES

1. Arce CA, Dohrmann GJ: Thoracic disc herniation: improved diagnosis with computed tomographic scanning and a review of the literature. *Surg Neurol* 23:356-361, 1985.

2. Arce CA, Dohrmann GJ: Herniated thoracic discs: symposium on neurosurgery. *Neurol Clin* 3:383-392, 1985.

3. Arseni C, Nash F: Thoracic intervertebral disc protrusion: a clinical study. *J Neurosurg* 17:418-430, 1960.

4. Awad EE, Martin DS, Smith KR, Jr., *et al:* Asymptomatic versus symptomatic herniated thoracic discs: their frequency and characteristics as detected by computed tomography after myelography. *Neurosurgery* 28:180-186, 1991.

5. Benjamin V: Diagnosis and management of thoracic disc disease. *Clin Neurosurg* 30:577-605, 1983.

6. Bilsky MH, Patterson RH: The transpedicular approach for thoracic disc herniations. In Benzel EC, Stillerman CB (eds): *The Thoracic Spine.* St Louis, Quality Medical Publishing, 1998.

7. Borges LF: Thoracic disc disease and spondylosis. In Tindall GT, Cooper PR, Barrow DL (eds): *The Practice of Neurosurgery.* Baltimore, Williams & Wilkins, 1996, 2461-2471.

8. Brown CW, Deffer PA, Akmakjian J, *et al:* The natural history of thoracic disc herniation. *Spine* 17:S97-S102, 1992.

9. Chin LS, Black KL, Hoff JT: Multiple thoracic disc herniations: case report. *J Neurosurg* 66:290-292, 1987.

10. Dickman CA, Rosenthal D, Karahalios DG, *et al:* Thoracic vertebrectomy and reconstruction using a microsurgical thoracoscopic approach. *Neurosurgery* 38:201-219, 1996.

11. Dietze DD, Jr., Fessler RG: Thoracic disc herniations. *Neurosurg Clin North Am* 4:75-90, 1993.

12. Fessler RG, Dietze DD, Jr., MacMillan M, *et al:* Lateral parascapular extrapleural approach to the upper thoracic spine. *J Neurosurg* 75:349-355, 1991.

13. Horwitz MB, Moossy JJ, Julian T, *et al:* Thoracic discectomy using video assisted thoracoscopy. *Spine* 9:1082-1086, 1994.

14. Krasna MJ, Mack MJ: *Atlas of Thoracoscopic Surgery.* St Louis, Quality Medical Publishing, 1994, pp 206-211.

15. Larson SJ, Holst RA, Hemmy DC, *et al:* Lateral extracavitary approach to traumatic lesions of the thoracic and lumbar spine. *J Neurosurg* 45:628-637, 1976.

16. Le Roux PD, Haglund MM, Harris AB: Thoracic disc disease: experience with the transpedicular approach in twenty consecutive patients. *Neurosurgery* 33:58-66, 1993.

17. Logue V: Thoracic intervertebral disc prolapse with spinal cord compression. *J Neurol Neurosurg Psychiatry* 15:227-241, 1952.

18. McAfee PC, Regan JR, Zdeblick T, *et al:* The incidence of complications in endoscopic anterior thoracolumbar spinal reconstructive surgery. *Spine* 20:1624-1632, 1995.

19. McCormick PC: Retropleural approach to the thoracic and thoracolumbar spine. *Neurosurgery* 37:1-7, 1995.

20. Maiman DJ, Larson SJ, Luck E, *et al:* Lateral extracavitary approach to the spine for thoracic disc herniation: report of 23 cases. *Neurosurgery* 14:178-182, 1984.

21. Patterson RH: Thoracic disc herniation: operative approaches and results. *Neurosurgery* 12:305, 1983.

22. Patterson RH: Thoracic disc disease: experience with the transpedicular approach in twenty consecutive patients. *Neurosurgery* 33:66, 1993.

23. Patterson RH, Jr., Arbit E: A surgical approach through the pedicle to protruded thoracic discs. *J Neurosurg* 48:768-772, 1978.

24. Perot PL, Munro DD: Transthoracic removal of midline thoracic disc protrusions causing spinal cord compression. *J Neurosurg* 31:452-458, 1969.

25. Ransohoff J, Spencer F, Siew F, *et al:* Transthoracic removal of thoracic disc: report of three cases. *J Neurosurg* 31:459-461, 1969.

26. Regan JJ, Mack MJ, Picetti GD: A technical report on video-assisted thoracoscopy in thoracic spinal surgery. *Spine* 20:831-837, 1995.

27. Rosenthal D, Rosenthal R, De Simone A: Removal of a protruded thoracic disc using microsurgical endoscopy: a new technique. *Spine* 19:1087-1091, 1994.

28. Russell T: Thoracic intervertebral disc protrusion: experience of 67 cases and review of the literature. *Br J Neurosurg* 3:153-160, 1989.

29. Stillerman CB, Chen TC, Couldwell WT, *et al:* Surgical experience in the operative management of 82 symptomatic herniated thoracic discs and review of the literature. *J Neurosurg* 88:623-633, 1998.

30. Stillerman CB, Chen TC, Day JD, *et al:* The transfacet pedicle-sparing approach for thoracic disc removal: cadaveric morphometric analysis and preliminary clinical experience. *J Neurosurg* 83:971-976, 1995.

31. Stillerman CB, Couldwell WT, Chen TC, *et al:* Thoracic disc (invited response) neurosurgical forum. *J Neurosurg* 85:187-190, 1996.

32. Stillerman CB, Weiss MH: Principles of surgical approaches to the thoracic spine. In Tarlov EC (ed): *Neurosurgical Topics: Neurosurgical Treatment of Disorders of the Thoracic Spine.* Park Ridge, IL, AANS, 1991, pp 1-19.

33. Stillerman CB, Weiss MH: Management of thoracic disc disease. *Clin Neurosurg* 38:325-352, 1992.

34. Stillerman CB, Weiss MH: Surgical management of thoracic disc herniation and spondylosis. In Menezes AH, Sonntag VKH (eds): *Principles of Spinal Surgery.* New York, McGraw-Hill, 1996, pp 581-601.

CHAPTER 49

Lumbar Discectomy

Bruce L. Ehni, Edward C. Benzel, and Robert S. Biscup

Lumbar laminectomy for disc hernia or annular prolapse is one of the most common operations performed by North American spine surgeons and remains one of the most successful operations. To the casual observer, it can appear to be simple and unchallenging. It is not without pitfalls, however. In fact, they are numerous: in the form of patient selection, neuroimaging, timing of surgery, technical nuances in the performance of the surgery, and in subsequent patient follow-up to ensure that success has been achieved with a minimal complication rate. There can hardly be a more unhappy patient than one who has experienced a poor outcome from lumbar discectomy. Short-term outcomes are widely accepted as excellent, but the focus needs to be applied to the long-term outcome as well. Complications remain a significant problem despite the adherence to well-developed precepts.

Outcomes

Relief of radiculopathic leg pain can be expected in 85% to 90% of patients appropriately selected for lumbar discectomy.* The problem that has long faced successful performance of this usually straightforward procedure is that one of the most common causes for poor outcome is the poor definition of selection criteria for surgery.[22,71] The procedure can be expected, with a high degree of certainty to relieve radiculopathic leg pain, but relief of back pain cannot be predicted.[129,130,136] Recurrent radiculopathy occurs in 5% to 10% of patients,[136] which approaches the lifetime incidence of disc surgery.[22] Less likely causes for failure include perineurial fibrosis and arachnoiditis.

The long-term outcomes of surgery and conservative treatment are similar, but in the short-term, surgery provides the prospect of quicker relief.[10,55,129,130] Quicker relief with surgery may translate into reduced economic cost.[124] There are wide regional and interregional variations in the rates at which surgery is offered and performed.[10]

It is difficult to define preoperative findings that are predictive of success or failure, even in the largest series of patients. Part of the problem arises from the fluctuation of results over time, with as much as 40% of patients crossing over from the favorable to unfavorable postoperative groups and vice versa.[135] Nevertheless, risk factors associated with poor outcome include female gender, downtime off work in excess of 3 months, psychosocial problems, and plain radiographic changes. Factors predictive of a good

outcome include absence of back pain, absence of work-related injury, presence of radicular pain to the foot, positive straight-leg raise, and reflex asymmetry.[3] Obesity, although complicating anesthesia and convalescence, does not of itself adversely affect outcome.[3,7] Smoking is an indicator of risk for chronic low back pain.[38,75] Perhaps because of the location of the dorsal root ganglion and because of the difficulty associated with surgical approaching lateral hernias, the outcome for extraforaminal hernias is not as good as that for paramedian hernia.[85,90] The outcome for the cauda equina syndrome is better if there is unilateral sciatic pain and worse if there is bilateral sciatica; it is very poor if there is saddle hypesthesia. Patients with complete perineal anesthesia are at risk for permanent sphincter dysfunction. The mode of onset of symptoms may also be important, with the acute onset of symptoms over hours thought to be a prognosticator of poorer outcome, particularly bladder function, than a more insidious onset over days or weeks.[69]

History

A condition recognized as sciatica, although not associated with spinal abnormality, was described before the time of Alexander the Great.[27] In 1779, Pott[96] was able to associate deformity of the spinal column with sciatic pain, but it remained for Lane[69a] to describe sciatic pain and its origin in a living patient in 1893 and for Bailey and Casamajor,[11] in 1911, to describe a small series, complete with radiographic studies. Also in 1911, Goldthwait,[46] who thought herniations of the disc were capable of producing sciatic and low back pain, presented a patient with lumbosacral disc hernia and paraplegia. In 1916, Elsberg[28] (who operated on the patients of Bailey and Casamajor and often noted relief after apparently no more than decompressive laminectomy) described it as attributable to a condition of cauda equina radiculitis, Parker and Adson[94] in 1925, Putti[99] in 1927, Dandy[21] in 1929, Mauric[84] in 1933, and others attributed sciatic pain to nerve root involvement within the spinal canal and believed that adjacent vertebral structures were responsible. In 1934, Mixter and Barr[86] published their milestone paper on the pathology and surgical findings associated with a ruptured nucleus pulposus, not only in the lumbar canal but also in the cervical and thoracic canals, complete with their diagnoses of the condition preoperatively.

The surgical procedure of choice for many of these pioneering surgeons was complete laminectomy, and it was used to good advantage often providing significant relief. Mixter and Barr favored a hemilaminectomy approach, as did Love,[78] for the cases of simple herniated disc that were amenable to preoperative localization. As experience accumulated, it became apparent that dural incision was unnecessary in most cases.

The complicating effect that developmental lumbar stenosis had on the pathology of disc diseases was appreciated in Verbiest's[122,123] reports from 1949 through 1955. It remains true more than 40 years later that some of the more serious complications of surgery for lumbar disc hernia can be attributed to lack of preoperative appreciation of this anatomic variation and failure to tailor the procedure accordingly.

---

*References 3,22,23,85,88,93,115.

Working only with myelography and the power of clinical preoperative and subsequent intraoperative observation, the early surgeons were able to learn much and to steadily improve upon the surgical approach to lumbar disc disease. Currently, with the advantages of improved neurodiagnostic modalities, there is no longer much occasion for "surgical exploration," and it should not be common to find an intraoperative surprise. There is no place in the modern era for a therapeutic trial of back surgery. Surgeons should be capable not only of making the preoperative diagnosis but also of adhering to a secure surgical plan, one that should accomplish the goal of radicular or cauda decompression with minimal risk of complication or injury.

Indications for Discectomy

Patient selection is so integral regarding good patient outcomes in lumbar microdiscectomy that it can be said that for success, technique may not be as important as patient selection. The patient selection pitfalls to be encountered, recognized, and avoided in lumbar discectomy surgery are numerous. One of the most common errors is the misinterpretation of leg pain of some other origin for radiculopathy, and to then correlate it with an unrelated neuroimaging finding. The most important determinant in favor of proceeding to surgery should be strict correlation between the distribution of the radiculopathic leg pain and the nerve root compression seen on preoperative imaging studies. Performed carefully and correctly, clinical examination can predict findings of neuroimaging and subsequent surgery approximately 70% to 80% of the time.[4,116,126,127]

In practice, and as a prerequisite for successful surgery, there should be a strong correlation between the pain, neurologic deficit, and the preoperative imaging findings. This rule should be inflexible.

Back Pain

Low back pain is a poor indicator for discectomy surgery. An anatomic cause is impossible to establish despite modern neuroimaging. In western medicine, plain radiographs are, despite a widely known lack of correlation with back pain, expected and pressed for by the patient.[65,104] They will often lead to more sensitive imaging studies such as MRI. MRI, in turn, is so sensitive and generally readily accessible that these virtues in a certain way can be looked upon as drawbacks. It is a rare scan that is read as normal or even normal for age, yet it is well known that sizable protrusions and extrusions exist commonly in asymptomatic patients.[58] Therefore, interpretation of the neuroimaging studies by the operating surgeon must be made in the context of clinical correlation rather than in the absence of reasonably detailed clinical description. There is "an increasing realization that information about morphology alone is not enough to make a definitive diagnosis."[58] It is difficult for the backache patient (and perhaps even the referring doctor) to conceive that radiographs and MRI or CT-myelogram that show pathology, have no relationship to the pain. In fact, just the knowledge of pathology can adversely affect outcome.[65] If pres-

ent at multiple levels, the presence of a "dark nucleus" on MRI begins to predict a likelihood of back pain, but the pain generator still remains unknown, whether it is the annulus, the vertebrae, ligaments, fascia, muscles, or facets.[79] The advantage of such sensitivity, of course, is that modern neuroimaging, particularly MRI, has eliminated the need for surgical exploration in many cases.

As mentioned, back surgery as described in this chapter, may do little for back pain itself.[31] The presence or absence of back pain should have little bearing on the patient's selection for surgery, with a couple of exceptions. If a large hernia appears to be responsible for radiographically visible elevation of the posterior longitudinal ligament off the vertebral bodies, particularly in midline,[85] discectomy and the resultant relaxation of the tension on the ligament may well result in relief of the resultant back pain. If the hernia is large and midline, or if the lumbar spinal canal is shallow and, as a result, central stenosis of the lumbar canal is caused by disc herniation, the patient develops a reflexive posture of lumbar flexion (the shopping cart position). This results in lumbar fatigue and pain. The symptoms can often be relieved by surgical decompression of the involved motion segment. However, it should be made clear to the patient without mechanical instability facing the prospect of simple one-level surgery for degenerative disc disease that surgery may have no impact on the lumbar pain. Lumbar pain is manageable by other interventions outside the scope of this chapter, such as exercises and other conservative measures, injection treatments, and surgical fusion.[14]

Radicular Symptoms

Assessment of the depth of the spinal canal by preoperative imaging is an integral part of the decision to operate. Central spinal canal capacity and the presence or absence of lateral recess stenosis has significant bearing on the presence of nerve root compression and the patient's amenability to surgery. A small bulge or prolapse in one patient with developmental or acquired stenosis can be more damaging to the traversing nerve root or roots than a large extrusion in another patient with capacious canal.

Straight leg raise and elicitation with Valsalva maneuver is more likely to be positive in herniations of L4-5 and L5-S1, where the compression and irritation are more likely to be at the axilla of the nerve root. The femoral stretch test is more likely to be positive at higher lumbar levels.[125] Monoradiculopathic leg pain, or sciatica, is the most useful clinical correlate. It is superior to straight leg raising, scoliosis, and sensorimotor deficits.[4] Leg pain is often more severe in extraforaminal hernia than intraforaminal or paramedian hernia, perhaps resulting from the location of the dorsal root ganglion and its direct compression by the hernia.[90]

Leg pain is perhaps the most common indicator for discectomy, and the best indicator. Conservative measures should be applied for a period of several weeks or longer from onset, if at all possible, prior to consideration for surgery, since long-term outcomes (4 years and more) are similar for both conservative and operative care.[55,129,130] In practice, however, the time required for spontaneous resolution of radiculopathy to occur may be more than some patients can bear, so pain becomes an important determinant for surgery. It is commonly accepted that the longer pain and numbness exist prior to decompression, the longer they will last following decompression. Furthermore, there is a legitimate fear that even permanent deafferentation pain can result from untreated compression.[31,87] Inflammation from the disc hernia can adversely affect the nerve root over time, and thus affect prognosis.[135] Chronic pathologic changes can occur in the nerve root from prolonged compression, and over time (estimated at 3 to 6 months), there may be irreversible neuropathic changes.[31,55,85] Literature review and common clinical experience dictates that there is, however, no consensus on what constitutes an appropriate conservative trial, and there is no consensus on what constitutes the factors leading to irreversible nerve root damage. Solid evidence for the hypothesis that delayed surgery impairs results is lacking.[32]

The patient's economic imperatives become an important and valid factor in the selection of surgery in the presence of work disability and the requirement for rapid return to work. Surgery provides more rapid relief than conservative measures.[10] Also, long-term conservative care may ultimately be more expensive than surgery (in properly selected surgical candidates).[124]

Motor and sensory deficits are surgical indicators. It is practical to observe mild motor weakness and to follow for a period of time if stable. Motor deficit that is not improving, however, may be considered a surgical indicator,[31] as should progressively worsening motor deficit,[85] and, of course, severe motor deficit.[32]

Spontaneous resorption of disc material undeniably occurs and should be allowed to progress given the absence of severe motor deficit and the patient's ability to comply. It is, almost paradoxically, a phenomenon likely to be more satisfactory and complete in larger hernias, when there is true extrusion, rather than simple contained annular prolapse. Extrusion past the annulus marshals the processes of inflammation and phagocytosis of the mass.[49,55,56,81,92]

In summary, the ideal patient for discectomy is one in severe, disabling unilateral radiculopathic leg pain without severe sensorimotor loss, for whom conservative measures over a period of a few weeks to 2 months have yielded little.[31] A poorer recovery can be expected in the presence of severe persistent sensorimotor loss, once pain has remitted or has acquired the burning deafferentation quality suggestive of nerve root damage. Changes induced in the course of back pain through discectomy are unpredictable. The relatively soft and poorly defined nature of these indication guidelines has resulted in widely variable rates of surgery, as much as a threefold difference between surgeons and between countries.[63]

Cauda Equina Syndrome

A somewhat separate issue is the cauda equina syndrome. Bladder and bowel sphincter dysfunction and bilateral neurologic deficits are the strongest indicators for surgery. Cauda equina compression often exists in the sensitizing presence of developmental lumbar stenosis. Unlike with the lesser indications discussed above, compression of the cauda equina constitutes a medical emergency or urgency and should be relieved as soon as possible after diagnosis.[14,69] If the onset of symptoms is abrupt, the symptoms and prognosis for full recovery are worse than if the symptoms are slower in onset[69] and by inference the urgency for decompression greater. Other poor prognostic signs for the recovery of sphincter control in cases of cauda equina compression include saddle hypesthesia and bilateral radiculopathic leg pain.

Technique

There are only a few basic tenets of disc surgery. The object of the surgery is to decompress the nerve root and to leave it freely relaxed and untraumatized, not necessarily to manipulate the disc. The presence of annular prolapse should be differentiated from true hernia; not all abnormal annuli require enucleation, not all bulges are true hernias, and not all nerve root compressions are caused by a true hernia. An injection of irrigant into the disc, as is described below, can be done if there is any doubt that the annulus is torn and there is a true hernia in contrast to a bulging but competent annulus. If the disc is merely bulging, it is meddlesome to incise its annulus and to enucleate its contents. The object of the surgery is to remove the compression in a conservative fashion, leaving behind as little encouragement for scar formation as possible. The removal of some bone is necessary in most cases, but overly aggressive or misplaced bone removal can result in subsequent fracture (of the pars) and resultant chronic microinstability, or even the risk of overt instability and the necessity of fusion. Patients are rarely symptomatic from multiple levels and, therefore, multilevel discectomy should be exceptionally rare and the indications for it very strong (if performed).

The preoperative surgical plan should include an appraisal of the presence or absence of stenosis. In the case of concomitant spinal stenosis, either acquired through spondylosis or congenital stenosis, radiculopathic pain and neurologic deficit may be worse than in a deeper canal, given a similar-sized herniation mass within the canal. Since crowding of the cauda equina already exists and there is an intolerance to further incursion into the canal during the surgery, it is prudent in the course of the operation and in the presence of stenosis to decompress widely prior to manipulating the dural sac to facilitate discectomy.

Conventional laminectomy and discectomy work as well as microdiscectomy. The advantage to microdiscectomy is the smaller and more comfortable incision and the shortened hospital stay and diminished trauma to the adjacent motion segments and paraspinous musculature. Microdiscectomy requires the use of magnification. The choice of loupes and headlight or microscope is moot. Results from surgery are the same with both techniques.[3,85] Loupes, with the use of a coaxial or near coaxial headlight, offers the same or nearly the same magnification and the same or nearly the same size incision in the case of microdissection as does the operating microscope. The advantage of the microscope lies in its use by an observer or assistant, the disadvantage being some additional encumbrance and perhaps expense to the patient.

The following discussion assumes that discectomy is the planned end result of the surgery, not to be followed by fusion, in which case restrictions on bone removal would not be as significant.[20]

Operative Positioning and Patient Preparation

The disc space is avascular and, as a result, less resistant to infection. There is evidence that the risk of disc space infection may be reduced through the use of perioperative antibiotics.[48]

The preoperative placement of elastic stockings to prevent thromboembolism is recommended.[36] A urinary catheter is usually unnecessary, unless the procedure is expected to take more than 2 hours.

For most surgeons, the prone position on a frame works well. Often, such devices are inadequate for preventing increased intraabdominal pressure (and thus increased ventilatory, venous, and cerebrospinal fluid pressures) in obese patients. Obese patients are better positioned in such a manner that the abdominal panniculus hangs unimpeded, without bearing any of the patient's weight (e.g., the knee-chest position). The eyes and facial prominences should be well padded and inspected after turning the patient to the prone position because ocular pressure, or a combination of pressure and hypotension, can lead to blindness.[62] The arms, if held abducted on armboards, must be well padded over bony prominences and over the ulnar nerves.[95] To prevent costoclavicular compression of the brachial plexus, care should be taken to avoid hyperabduction over 90 degrees at the shoulders and shoulder hyperextension. The radial pulse on each side should be felt. Women should bear the weight of the chest on the ventrolateral rib cage (not on the breasts, which should be moved medially). All skin in contact with the frame or with pads on the frame should be protected with a layer of linens; skin should not be allowed to touch the bare occlusive surface of vinyl or silicone rubber cushions. The urinary catheter (if placed) is inspected after the patient is turned. Male genitalia must not be subject to compression between the approximated thighs. All bony prominences of the legs must be padded, and in particular, the toes must bear no weight of the foot. A diminished or absent pedal pulse may indicate femoral artery compression. This can be encountered on a conventional frame, as well as in the knee-chest position.[9] The patient, when positioned, should be stable so that vigorous intraoperative manipulation will not cause movement. Hardware in the room, such as IV stands, light sources, carts, tables, and anesthetic equipment should be arranged to allow easy access for both radiograph equipment and film cassette holders.

Lateral decubitus positioning is occasionally used in obese patients because the intraabdominal pressure can be kept low, and thus, epidural venous bleeding at a minimum. It may be the favored position if a patient has significant respiratory compromise. The surgeon may have a personal preference for the lateral decubitus position because it can allow greater lumbar flexion than does the prone position, and it allows blood from the wound to drain away from the operative field (rather than aspirated). Those who favor the lateral decubitus position generally prefer to have the symptomatic side up, because a little table flexion immediately beneath the operated lumbar segment can help with interlaminar distraction, and the position also helps with visualization. As with the prone position, the patient requires adequate padding and intraoperative support. This may be enhanced in the lateral decubitus position by a beanbag pad.

After the patient is positioned, a standard scrub is applied, and the patient is draped for surgery in a sterile fashion. A radiograph may be taken at this point, using a radiopaque localizer. If the planned incision is likely to be longer, as in conventional laminectomy, the radiograph can be delayed until an instrument can be applied to one of the exposed spinous processes. In any case, obtaining an intraoperative radiograph is recommended to avoid erroneous interpretation of the level or levels exposed. The point verified by the radiopaque marker should then be visibly marked in the operative exposure before removal of the marker. Palpation of the iliac crests as a landmark for the L4-5 interspace, percussion of the sacrum to elicit its characteristic sound, and counting interspinous spaces from the desired level to that of the myelogram injection point can all be relied upon to localize the incision. However, these serve only as guides, particularly because skin traction and patient positioning can alter these critical relationships. Microdissection and either the use of the headlight and loupes or of the operating microscope demands accurate placement of the initial skin incision and of all subsequent dissection therefrom.

Before the skin incision is made, the surgeon should have taken the opportunity to become familiarized with the patient's particular anatomy and pathology, and the operation should have been planned. Ideally, the interpretation of the preoperative studies, how they relate to the patient, and the intraoperative plan in brief terms should be committed to the chart. Thus, in the event of the images being unavailable at the time of surgery, the surgeon can proceed unimpaired and prepared for anatomic variation. For example, the surgeon should know whether the patient has L5 or S1 spina bifida occulta.

Developmental spinal stenosis, if present, is a flag of caution, and its presence must be acknowledged with a variation of the standard techniques than would otherwise be used. The removal of herniated L5-S1 nucleus pulposus that is concurrent with an L5 spondylolysis may not adequately decompress the nerve root if hypertrophic fibrocartilaginous material is responsible for the patient's symptoms.

Conventional Laminotomy (Laminectomy) and Standard Techniques

Although the term *conventional laminotomy* may imply the absence of visual magnification, some form of magnification is often used. The skin incision for laminotomy for disc herniation is conventionally about three spinous processes in length, 10 to 12 cm for a one-level operation. When performed in this manner, conventional laminotomy has the advantage of facilitating surgical assistance.

Furthermore, illumination is not quite as problematic as with shorter incisions, and the longer incisions have been suggested to be less traumatic to the paraspinous musculature than shorter incisions (that require greater retractor pressure). After the incision is made, hemostasis is obtained and retractors are placed. As with any incision, tension on the skin retractor should be inspected intermittently throughout the operation because pressure necrosis of the skin edge is a significant source of infectious wound complications. After the skin has been incised, the subcutaneous tissue is divided. This can be accomplished without bleeding or trauma with blunt dissection. The lumbodorsal fascia is then exposed, and for ease of subsequent closure, it is prudent to sweep the subcutaneous fat off a short distance laterally. The fascia is then incised, just lateral to the spinous process, rather than in the midline. This allows preservation of interspinous ligaments. If the laminotomy is to be performed bilaterally, as in cases of developmental stenosis with superimposed disc hernia, a fascial incision on both sides of the spinous processes results in a saved strip, the width of the spinous processes, in the midline, complete with the interspinous ligament.

The paraspinous musculature is then taken down, off the spinous processes and out the laminae above and below, with a sharp periosteum elevator. To do this as atraumatically as possible requires division of the tendinous attachments to the caudal lip of the lamina as lateral dissection proceeds.

With the field prepared for bone work, the overhanging caudal lip of the rostral lamina can be partially removed, allowing for further exposure of the interlaminar ligamentum flavum. The amount of bone removal is at the surgeon's discretion. The hernia and the annulus can be accessed with little or no removal of bone, if one is comfortable with the amount of force necessary to retract the nerve root medially.[85,113,131,132] Wider exposure via laminotomy and medial facetectomy, flush with the medial surface of the caudal pedicle, minimizes the need to mobilize the nerve root aggressively. Paramedian discs at higher lumbar levels represent a slightly greater challenge than those at L4-5 and L5-S1 because of the lamina and facet structure. The spinal canal is smaller in caliber, the lamina and facets descend more caudally, the facets are positioned more medially, and the facet clefts are more sagittally oriented than more caudal segments. Each of these features makes it necessary not only to remove more bone, but also makes progressive removal more risky to the integrity of the pars and the facet. This anatomy becomes particularly important when addressing intraforaminal disc hernia by the midline approach (see below).

Using a cutting burr or a Leksell rongeur, a small amount of bone is removed from the medial caudal edge of the rostral hemilamina, just below the spinous process. Here the spinal canal should be at its deepest, and the potential for anatomic confusion and for injury to the spinal canal contents the least. The ligamentum flavum attaches to the caudal lip of the rostral lamina and to its inner surface, so that the drill or rongeur meets the ligamentum flavum before endangering the dural sac. The ligamentum is then exposed rostrally. It can then be deliberately violated. An incision is made with a sharp knife through its superficial fibers and is completed with a dull instrument, such as a blunt hook or Freer instrument. The blunt dissector is then used to gently palpate within the central canal or lateral recess of the spinal canal, feeling for available room. This is an important step, for if a simple blunt hook will not fit into a pathologically narrowed lateral recess, it is certain that the foot of a large punch will not fit without damaging the underlying nerve root. With the large instrument, the surgeon loses tactile sensitivity and may not appreciate the compression. The laminar bone is further removed with a series of punches (of increasingly larger size), removing with it the attached ligamentum flavum. As bone removal proceeds rostrally, the lateral margin of the removal must migrate medially toward the midline, in a fashion that makes the defect appear triangular or lung shaped so that the structural integrity of the pars interarticularis is not compromised. Compromise of the pars by an overly aggressive bone removal can result in a pars interarticularis fracture, either during the course of surgery or during convalescence. More than half the bone of the pars, in its lateral dimension, should be left to avoid fracture (Figure 49.1).[105] As mentioned above, this is particularly important at midlumbar segments, where the pars is narrower and the facet cleft more sagittally oriented than at lower motion segments. Pars fracture isolates the facet, functionally resulting in complete facetectomy, which increases the failure rate due to back pain and instability.[3]

Alternatively, a minimalist approach can be taken to bone and ligamentum removal as described by Williams.[132] This does have the disadvantage of reduced visualization and increased traction upon the nerve root during its medial mobilization. While the amount of bone removal is discretionary, as a rule, decompressive removal should be more generous in the case of concomitant developmental stenosis. At times, it can be minimal when the interlaminar space is large.

Perineurial scar has been blamed for postsurgical failure to relieve sciatica. There are many means of dealing with its development. The ligamentum flavum is one such potential source of fibrosis if left in large shreds beneath the lamina. The ligamentum is therefore reasonably dealt with in one of two ways: (1) with minimal fenestration of the ligament, leaving its slick inner surface approximated to the nerve root as a natural barrier,[85,113,131] or (2) with its complete removal from the lateral recess. Because of impaired visualization and mobility of the underlying thecal sac and nerve root sleeve during the surgery and the variable ability to access the lateral recess and its contents with a minimal approach (dependent on the level operated and concomitant spondylotic enlargement of the facet and lateral recess stenosis), complete flavectomy is usually preferred. With angled curettes, removal from the undersurface of the remaining rostral lamina should be thorough. Its raw surface may lead to a significant postoperative fibroblastic response and scar formation. Its continuation with the medial facet capsule contributes to lateral recess and foraminal stenosis.

After partial removal of the rostral lamina and ligamentum in this manner, attention is turned to the caudal lamina. The thin rostral lip is removed medially to laterally, along with the remaining ligamentum flavum. Care must be taken to avoid compression of the underlying neural elements.

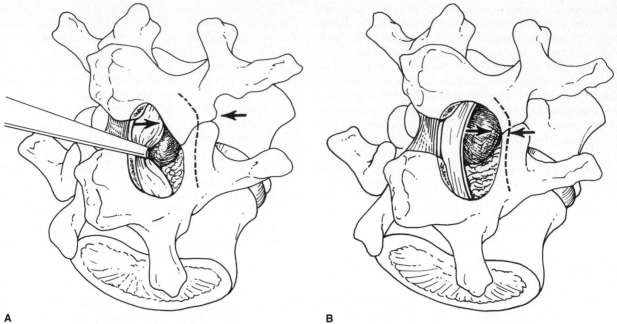

Figure 49.1 **(A)** Inadequate bone removal results in necessary excessive nerve root and dural sac retraction. **(B)** More generous bone removal reduces the likelihood of nerve root injury. Maintaining pars interarticularis integrity is emphasized. In this regard, bone removal should not extend past the *dotted lines*.

Removal of bone in the caudal direction does not need to be as extensive as the rostral removal. It must, however, be extended enough laterally to be flush with the medial side of the pedicle of the caudal vertebra, and enough caudally to allow ensuing visualization of the disc space, usually a 3- or 4-mm distance from the rostral edge. During the course of bone removal, the underlying epidural fat is protected.

The decompressive approach as described here could be described as semihemilaminectomy, medial facetectomy, and hemiflavectomy. Performed as described, it would typically span a distance of 20 to 25mm longitudinally and 10 to 15mm laterally. It provides adequate room for nerve root and lateral thecal sac visualization and safe mobilization, yet does not weaken the motion segment. The amount of bone removed is variable and depends on the motion segment involved, the amount of lumbar flexion afforded during positioning, the amount of spondylotic change present, and the patient's developmental anatomy. Often, little work is required on the bone at the lumbosacral interspace. During the course of bone removal, there is no occasion for blind removal. With strong illumination and adequate exposure and hemostasis, visualization should not present a problem.

The location of the foot of the punch or the edge of the curette and the location of the nerve root sleeve should be well perceived by the operating surgeon. It is worth noting that a risk of dural tear is present in every case. If a scar is present, adhering the dura mater to overlying bone, the risk of a dural tear is increased. The chance of tear is also increased in the elderly (particularly elderly women) in whom the dura mater is thin and in whom a noncompliant scar may be present, even in the absence of prior surgery. An inflammatory response to the hernia itself is often present.[49,56,92] The geometry of the instrumentation involved is

crucial because the dura mater can fold over the foot of a punch or the edge of the curette that is not applied closely to the underside of the bone. This is a blunder that can be worsened if the dura mater is distended under increased intrathecal pressure; like epidural venous bleeding, its risk can be reduced by careful positioning, with attention paid to intraabdominal pressure reduction. Piecemeal bone removal is not slowed by cautious inspection. Caution simply requires keeping the eyes on the target, letting the assistant clean the punch, and judiciously appreciating the tactile input.

A dural tear is a significant problem only if it is not cared for properly. In some cases, dural tears are almost unavoidable, and their occurrence even predictable. It is a problem encountered by the best of surgeons. The risk of a tear is high in the elderly, but it is also a risk if the herniated disc fragment has been present long enough to result in dural adhesions. A mistake is to be cavalier about the occurrence of a CSF leak and not to repair the leak properly. If the tear is dorsal or lateral, it will be problematic for the remainder of the case if not attended to. The defect should be protected from further tearing or from aspiration of nerve roots by the placement of Gelfoam and a cottonoid beneath the suction tip over the tear. It should be exposed, with further bone removal, and repaired in a watertight fashion (preferably immediately after its occurrence). Repair can be tedious and time-consuming at a point in the operation at which much remains to be done. The temptation to delay it until later is most often best resisted. Attention may not be paid to the details of adequately repairing the leak after an unusually lengthy procedure, if the repair is one of the last tasks. If the arachnoid is also involved and spinal fluid is being lost, thecal sac collapse occurs, and epidural venous bleeding intensifies because of decreased tamponade. This obscures visualization, and blood can enter the thecal sac and can result in arachnoidal adhesions. Other possible results of unrepaired dural tear include radiculopathic pain and deficit secondary to herniation of nerve roots through the dural defect, of symptomatic pseudomeningocele, the possibility of meningitis, and persistent orthostatic headache complaints.[76,89,121,128] Repaired primarily, CSF leaks incurred intraoperatively have no impact on ultimate surgical outcome.[128] On occasion, the tear may be located on the ventral aspect of the nerve root sleeve or thecal sac, in which case, while it may be impossible to repair without marked difficulty, it nevertheless does not risk the problems of a dorsal tear and will more than likely tamponade itself.

Preservation of the epidural fat is a worthwhile goal during the development of the interlaminar exposure. Some cases of considerable residual postoperative radiculopathic pain are attributable to epineurial scar formation and the resultant tethering of the nerve root to the adjacent bone and annulus fibrosus. As with hemostasis, attention must be paid to the epidural fat to ensure an optimal outcome. Epidural fat, however, should not be allowed to obscure the field to the detriment of the outcome. It is crucial that the nerve root sleeve and the ventral disc space be fully visualized. If necessary, the fat can be pulled off the dorsum of the nerve root sleeve and moved medially, divided gently with the bipolar tips, or rubbed aside and protected with a cotton stamp. When the nerve root and disc pathology is definitively addressed, the fat can be moved back into a protective position.

With the medial aspect of the facet joint and capsule partially removed so that the medial surface of the caudal pedicle can be observed and felt, the need for medial retraction on the nerve root to allow visualization of the disc space should be minimized (see Figure 48.1B). Before retraction instruments are inserted, room ventral to the nerve root and dural sac must be assessed (Figure 49.2). With a small-caliber aspiration tip (5 or 7 Fr.), blunt hook, or ball-ended dissector, the nerve root can be mobilized medially, and while doing so, the amount of ventral fibrosis or compression can be determined. This palpation should be gentle, and if resistance to mobilization in this manner is met, the surgeon must determine the cause, as well as a solution to the problem of mobilization. The axilla of the nerve root may straddle a sharp focal prominence of annulus fibrosus. Forcing the nerve root up and over it may invite neural injury. In such a case, the prominence can be trimmed or impacted down, medial to the nerve root in the axilla, following which the nerve root can be mobilized medially and the disc pathology better addressed. Poor ability to mobilize may reflect a nerve root anomaly such as low origin.

Conjoined nerve roots, low root origins, and interradicular anastomoses often affect the lower lumbar levels and represent something of a surgical challenge for a number of reasons. They can confuse the surgical anatomy, and if the conjoined root is large and pulled or pushed tightly into the lateral recess by the disc pathology, they can be mistaken for the hernia itself.[97] If a low origin from the dura results in a lateral course over the disc space, they can be impossible to safely mobilize to access the disc. Therefore, a thorough decompression of the nerve root

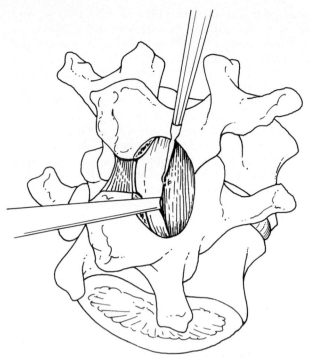

Figure 49.2 Adequacy of room is assessed before inserting any retraction device capable of excessive compression of underlying structures.

may be very difficult to achieve. The presence of a conjoined root should be readily anticipated from modern neuroimaging, however.

Often, the herniated nucleus pulposus is sequestered beneath the posterior longitudinal ligament, rather than being free in the spinal canal or lateral recess. A simple poke with the bipolar tips through the ligament may be all that is necessary to initiate its delivery. Perhaps the most atraumatic method of removing the hernia is to grasp a small slip of the fragment with a pituitary instrument and deliver it slowly up through the ligamentous tear, serially repositioning the instrument to catch more of its bulk while doing so. The residual ligament protects the adjacent nerve root from traction.

Occasionally, the hernia represents a complete nuclear extrusion, and its attempted removal in one piece may force the nerve root medially to such an extent that injury results. It is, therefore, often optimal to remove it piecemeal. When the prominence has been reduced by removal of some of the herniated disc material, the nerve root is more relaxed and more room is available for exploration with blunt angled dissecting instruments, such as a ball-ended dissector. The ventral epidural space is thoroughly palpated for any residual fragments by sweeping the dissector over the disc space. The subligamentous space is similarly palpated, as is the neural foramen rostral and lateral to the pedicle. The intervertebral disc space is then thoroughly explored and emptied of nucleus, using a combination of straight and angled pituitary rongeurs. It is often necessary to enlarge the annular tear to permit entrance of the rongeurs into the disc interspace. It is recommended that this be accomplished sharply and generously with a no. 15 or 11 blade on a long handle, fashioning a rectangular window through the annulus fibrosus. After discectomy, the annulus, if otherwise left in the lateral recess, may prolapse or adhere to the nerve root and produce recurrent symptoms.

To reduce the chances of recurrent disc hernia, all loose nucleus material should be removed. It is neither possible nor desirable to remove all disc material. Overly aggressive curettage with removal of end plate cartilage and excessive removal of interspace volume can result in a patulous annulus, poor mechanical support of the motion segment, and therefore potential foraminal stenosis or instability. Removal should be limited to loose fragments within reach of the annular opening.

With the annulus and the cartilaginous end plates being retained, the surgeon must stay focused on an envisioned estimate of the anatomy of the intervertebral space because this is a blind procedure. The majority of vascular and visceral injuries that result from perforation of the ventral annulus occur at L4-5 and L5-S1, although injury can occur at other levels as well.* The firm ventral and lateral annular margins can usually be palpated with the rongeurs, and the depth of penetration can be controlled. It is possible, however, as a result of ventral annular tears,[33,47,74,109] that the annulus fibrosus does not adequately restrain the instruments to blind palpation. Tarlov[119] suggests penetrating the annular space to no more than a depth of 1.125 inches and marking the operative instruments at this depth.

Shevlin[110] reported a case in which atraumatic passage of a rongeur to an unusual depth was followed by the observation that irrigating fluid then emptied out the ventral annulus, and suggests this as a sign of potential problems, as what occurred with his case. During discectomy and shortly thereafter, any sudden vagal or hypovolemic response should be seriously regarded as indicating possible vascular, ureteral, or intestinal injury. Most often, bleeding from the annular space is not noted in major vascular injuries.

Catastrophic problems occurring as a result of perforation through the ventral annulus are possible, even with skilled surgeons. There is an incidence of 1.6 to 17 per 10,000 cases of ventral perforation with vascular or visceral injury.[47,91,100,119] Body habitus, the operating surgeon's experience, patient positioning, and the type of surgical instrumentation used (including the microscope) do not appear to influence the risk. Good outcome is entirely dependent on early recognition and swift appropriate action. However, mortality may still reach 47% with vascular injury.

If the annulus fibrosus is simply bulging over a broad area or is partially dislodged from its attachment to the vertebral lip rostral or caudal to it and does not appear to be torn (permitting expression of the nucleus), it is best left intact. Nerve root decompression can be achieved by removal of overlying bone and ligamentum flavum, allowing the preservation of the motion segment. The decision to violate the posterior longitudinal ligament and annulus can be made by some surgeons with greater assurance by using an intradiscal injection of saline. A small amount of indigo carmine dye, just enough to color the irrigant, and 5ml of saline are drawn up in a 6 or 10ml syringe, a

22-gauge spinal needle is fitted, and the nuclear space is injected through the annulus. If the irrigant can be observed readily extravasating from the disc space, it can be assumed that the annulus is incompetent and that its contents should, perhaps, be emptied. If the disc accepts only a few milliliters of fluid, and no extravasation is observed, the annulus can be assumed to be competent, despite its bulge, and is best left undisturbed.

Intervertebral disc hernia may be encountered at unusual locations within the canal on occasion. Immediately upon entering the canal, just under the ligamentum, the surgeon might be met with a dorsally migrated epidural fragment of disc material.[102] It is an interesting and occasionally unexpected finding but should not be difficult to remove and trace to its source. More difficult to manage are the rare intradural and intraradicular hernias. Because of adhesion of the dura to the annulus, a hernia may rarely perforate the dura mater and be located within the thecal sac or within the nerve root itself.[106,118]

Adhesion is a consequence of prior surgery, or it is the result of inflammatory changes incurred by the hernia itself, or perhaps congenital adhesion is already present. To find the pathology in these cases requires the surgeon to be vigilant for any discrepancies between what is observed in the field and what was observed on the neuroimaging studies, and to simply be aware that such conditions exist. It has been postulated that some cases of failure may indeed be due to such pathology that has been overlooked.[118]

When the ligamentum flavum is aggressively removed, the nerve root decompressed, the fat replaced, and hemostasis obtained, the wound is closed. Irrigating solution is used to flood the wound. A secure, but nonstrangulating, absorbable suture reapproximates the muscle to the midline to eliminate dead space. The fascia is closed in a watertight fashion, and the subcutaneous fat and skin are closed. The surgeon can elect to place a Depo-Medrol-soaked Gelfoam pledget or morphine (Duramorph) over the nerve root before closure or to infiltrate the paraspinous muscle with bupivicaine before closure of the skin.[45]

Microlaminotomy

The term *microlaminotomy* denotes the use of a short skin and fascial incision and, by necessity of the short incision, visual magnification of some sort. To accomplish the task accurately and effectively through a microlaminotomy incision, loupes with a magnification with a strong headlight, with the beam coaxial with the line of sight, or the binocular operating microscope are required. As with the use of loupes, the use of the microscope has certain advantages and disadvantages.

Properly fitted loupes and a coaxial headlight can be worn comfortably for an extended period of time. With loupes, there is no impediment to the surgeon's mobility in the field or in the room. The line of sight can be adjusted to refocus attention to other details in the field without hesitation and without removing hands or instruments from their position or task. Intraoperative radiographs may be obtained with minimum movement of equipment. The disadvantage of loupes is the poor view afforded to surgical assistants.

The most significant advantage of the microscope is the ability of the surgical assistant to obtain a view that is

---

*References 12,15,24,109,111,112,119.

the same as the surgeon's. It is also possible to use a much higher magnification, although for laminotomy this is not usually necessary. The disadvantage of use of the microscope is the encumbrance of the device.

Microlaminotomy has the theoretical advantage (supported by 25 years of experience since Williams first described the technique) of decreased postoperative pain. As a result, the complications of postoperative atelectasis and postoperative temperature elevation may be reduced.[18,64] The high magnification used in its completion encourages gentle tissue handling.

Positioning and preparation are unchanged from conventional laminotomy, except that some form of radiographic localization is absolutely required. A spinal needle introduced into the interspinous ligament makes an excellent marker, and when the radiograph returns, it can be used to estimate the optimum trajectory to the disc space. The incision can be centered on or placed somewhat above or below the puncture. In slender adults, a 2 to 3cm incision is more than adequate, although if necessary, there should be no hesitation to lengthen it. The fascia to the side of the hernia is incised cleanly along the spinous process the same length as the skin incision, and the muscle is stripped subperiosteally, as accomplished with conventional laminotomy. For wound retraction, there is a choice of instruments, although most surgeons favor Williams or Caspar retractors.

There is no subsequent difference in technique between conventional and microlaminotomy for the remainder of the surgery, other than the use of magnification. It is possible to perform disc surgery using the operating microscope without removing much, if any, bone and little ligamentum flavum. In fact, when microlaminotomy was first described by Williams,[133] this was recommended. The focus of the operation, however, should be thorough nerve root decompression and the minimization of the chance for recurrent symptoms, rather than an exercise in leaving the least trace. Without a more or less conventional amount of bone removal, the chances of overlooked pathology and a compromised outcome are increased. It is strongly advised, therefore, that microlaminotomy be performed in the same fashion as one would a conventional laminectomy. Results from both conventional laminectomy and microlaminectomy are similar.[22,43] The theoretical benefit of microdiscectomy is its applicability to outpatient usage.[6,13,120]

Complete Laminectomy

Once a popular method of exposure for all disc surgery, complete laminectomy with bilateral removal of the medial facets and laminae and of the spinous process has fallen into disfavor because of its inherently destructive nature. In severe developmental stenosis with superimposed disc hernia or large central adherent disc hernia, however, it may be advisable to perform an aggressive exposure such as this before discectomy to avert compressive nerve root or cauda equina injury during the discectomy. In some cases of hernia, the nuclear fragment can tear and enter the thecal sac and requires dural incision and repair for its treatment. This is facilitated by complete laminectomy. This is more common with postoperative recurrent hernia than in de novo cases because of epidural fibrosis with tethering of the dura mater. High lumbar disc hernia (at L1-2 or L2-3) may be at the level of the conus medullaris, a structure that is intolerant of retraction and compression. Some consideration may be given to complete laminectomy in the upper lumbar spinal canal if this is thought to be a risk. Finally, in some cases of significant vertebral subluxation complicating disc hernia, a complete laminectomy with discectomy may be required for bilateral decompression before fusion, particularly if reduction cannot be obtained.

Complete laminectomy deprives the multifidus, rotators, interspinalis, and spinalis muscles of origin and insertion. Some degree of mechanical dysfunction and pain will naturally result. Therefore, complete laminectomy for discectomy should be avoided, if possible.

The Lateral and Far Lateral Hernia

Far lateral disc hernia, with resulting compression of the nerve root in, or lateral to, the intervertebral neuroforamen is an unusual variant of annular prolapse or disc.* It is estimated that about 10% of all symptomatic disc hernias are of the far lateral variety. Most commonly, far lateral disc herniation occurs at L3-4, L4-5, or higher levels. They occur in an older patient population than do the more common dorsolateral hernias.[29,30,70,125] As a corollary to its frequency at midlumbar and higher lumbar levels, there is some likelihood that patients with ventral thigh pain and sensory deficit, quadriceps weakness, a positive femoral stretch test, and reduced patellar reflex, harbor a far lateral hernia. Recognition of this has been facilitated by use of myelography and postmyelographic CT.[68] MRI, particularly the sagittal images, may best demonstrate the pathology.[59,60] Pain may be more severe than that incurred in paramedian disc hernia because of the location of the sensory root ganglion.[90]

It facilitates preoperative planning to conceive of the hernia location to be in one of three areas and its accessibility by one of several options. First, the lateral hernia may lie within the proximal foramen just at the medial aspect of the pedicle, and in this case, can be approached through a modification of the paramedian laminotomy. Second, it may lie in the lateral foramen and must then be approached by means of a lateral facetectomy. Third, it may lie in an extraforaminal location in which case an extraforaminal or parasagittal approach would be necessary to avoid complete facetectomy. It may be necessary, in a patient with developmental stenosis and therefore unusually large, medially located and coronal facets, to opt for one of the lateral approaches over a more conventional medial facetectomy. Although complete facetectomy has been historically reported to be relatively benign, perhaps more benign at the caudal two levels,[29] facetectomy should be avoided, if possible. Facetectomy results in delayed instability and failure due to chronic back pain.[3]

Despite its recognition, it is still difficult to effectively treat a far lateral hernia. The variety of surgical trajectories is illustrated in Figure 49.3. The most popular approach is a standard midline incision and interlaminar exposure

---

*References 1,2,26,29,42,50,54,57,77,83,107.

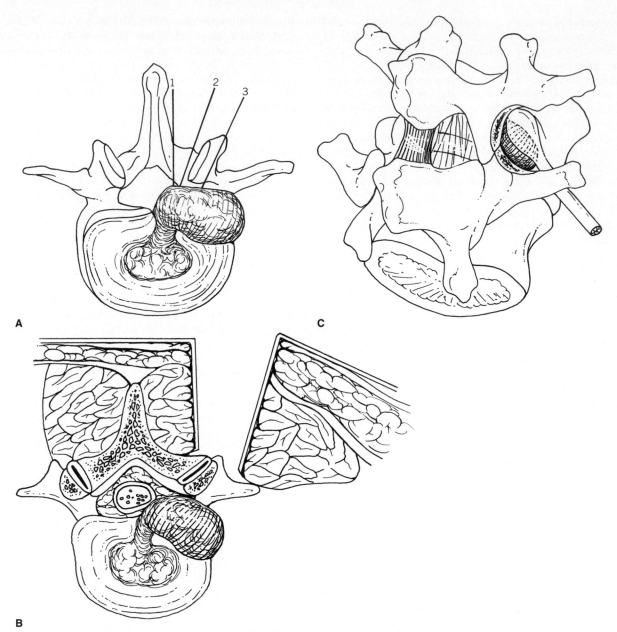

Figure 49.3 (**A**) Trajectories achieved by the varieties of exposure for lateral disc hernia. *1*, midline; *2*, interlaminar and extralaminar approach; *3*, paramedian muscle splitting. (**B**) Paramedian muscle splitting approach achieves an optimal angle of exposure to discs situated beyond the pedicle. (**C**) For most approaches to a lateral disc hernia, a modest lateral facetectomy is performed, thus providing direct access to the hernia.

with medial facetectomy.[1,2,29,30,77] This approach has the advantages of greater familiarity of the surgeon with surgical anatomy, absence of bleeding, early exposure of the affected nerve root, and the ability to perform discectomy to preclude recurrence. It is most appropriate for hernia within the proximal foramen. Often, the amount of bone that must be removed to gain exposure to the neuroforamen is greater than in simple dorsolateral hernias. It helps visualization considerably to tilt the table toward the operator. It may even require complete facetectomy.[29,30,42] It has been suggested that complete facetectomy is tolerated well, with little likelihood of instability,[29,30,42,50] particularly at the lowest two lumbar motion segments.[29,50] It must be recognized, however, that delayed spinal instability and chronic pain can

potentially result.[3,105] Therefore, complete facetectomy is not recommended in most cases.[70] Intervertebral foraminotomy, with some form of partial facetectomy, is still the most popular surgical option, despite the inherent disadvantage of aggressive bone removal.

Using a modification of the midline approach to address hernia within the lateral foramen, a combined interlaminar and extralaminar exposure has been described by Hood[54] in which the muscle is not dissected off the spinous processes but rather 1 cm lateral to the midline. The facet joint is exposed. A drill and punch are used to produce a partial lateral facetectomy, through which the rostral and caudal pedicles can be palpated. The nerve root, forced dorsally by the pathologic hernia, lies deep to the facet capsule and ligamentum flavum. It can be mobilized and retracted to address the disc hernia. If necessary, the lateral recess and retained disc material within the spinal canal can then be approached through a standard interlaminar route with a minimum of bone removal, thus maintaining the integrity of the facet joint.

In another modification of the midline approach, the interlaminar exposure of the proximal neuroforamen and affected nerve root is performed first at the level of hernia. The volume of bone removed is minimized by the addition of an extralaminar procedure similar to that of Hood's.[57]

Di Lorenzo et al.[25] have recently reported on a novel approach to intraforaminal disc hernia, producing a small ovoid window through the pars, sparing an isthmus of bone on both its medial and lateral aspects, leaving the inferior facet connected to the pedicle and lamina. This approach may have limited applicability. The pars must be intrinsically generously wide enough to permit fenestration without compromising its integrity. The foramen must be large enough, uninvolved by stenosis, to permit manipulation of the root as well as the hernia. The approach is limited only to intraforaminal hernia and does not permit enucleation of the disc space. It cannot be modified with the addition of laminectomy to address pathology more medial to its exposure.

In another modification of the midline approach, the intention is to improve visibility of the nerve root in the foramen. A safe and standard exposure of the affected root through a routine interlaminar midline approach is performed, one level rostral to the neural foramen (e.g., the L4 nerve root compressed in the L4-5 foramen is exposed at L3-4 through a routine interlaminar approach). The nerve root is then followed a short distance with a small amount of bone removal from the rostral edge of the caudal lamina and facet at this level. The extralaminar approach is then used to deal with the nerve root, now identified and protected under a dissector in the neuroforamen.[26]

In the foregoing procedures, the paraspinous musculature is removed from the spinous processes or is dissected using the column approach, 1cm lateral to the paraspinal musculature. Exposure of the neuroforamen is via a trajectory that is almost directly dorsal. This hampers efforts to preserve the facet joint. In this regard, manipulation within the neuroforamen can be performed from a more lateral trajectory.

The paramedian, muscle-splitting approach[34,83,107,134] has the advantage of sparing the patient the loss of bone and of providing a somewhat more oblique view of the neuroforamen. It is most useful for hernias within the lateral foramen or which are extraforaminal. A paramedian skin and fascial incision, about 3cm from the midline (or further lateral at lower levels), is made just over the natural plane groove between the multifidus and longissimus muscles. Descending through the paraspinous musculature between the transverse processes onto the neuroforamen from a lateral orientation, the surgeon is able to locate the lateral facet and its capsule and perhaps be able to remove only a small amount of lateral facet, if necessary (Figure 49.3). The medial transverse processes are exposed, the multifidus muscular attachments to the facet are incised, and the intertransverse muscle and ligament are incised. It is then

possible to expose the affected nerve root in the neuroforamen, retract it aside, and address the disc hernia. This is not too dissimilar to the lateral extracavitary approach described by Larson et al.[72] It finds its greatest usefulness at the lower levels, L4-4 and L5-S1, where the lateral hernia is more likely to lie outside the access provided by a midline approach.[70,101] Although the major advantage is the preservation of the pars interarticularis and the facet joint, it has the disadvantages of surgical unfamiliarity, deeper dissection, possibly poorer visualization, difficulty enucleating the disc space, potential injury to the nerve root within the neuroforamen, and dealing with sequestered fragments beneath the posterior longitudinal ligament.[29,30] The exposure at the lower levels gained by the muscle-splitting approach can be more difficult to achieve than at higher levels because of the gradually decreasing room available between the confines of the transverse and accessory processes and the sacral ala.[44,101]

Although most intraforaminal disc hernias can be cared for from the midline approach, the surgeon should be familiar with the paramedian approach and should be capable of opting for it when the nerve root is compressed lateral to the neuroforamen[77] or when a lateral disc at L4-5 or L5-S1 is encountered. With the availability of these options, there should be little reason to sacrifice the entire facet joint.

Other approaches, such as the ventrolateral retroperitoneal approach and osteoplastic removal and replacement of the pars interarticularis and facet, have been advocated, but they appear to be more complex than warranted, especially with the availability of simpler procedures. Limited experience has been gained with augmentation of midline approaches using endoscopy to access the foramen.[40] No matter which surgical approach is taken, it is wise to not displace the nerve root within the foramen aggressively because the dorsal root ganglion within it is sensitive and its manipulation may worsen the symptoms.[59]

The historically reported results of treatment for lateral disc hernia are similar to those of more classical dorsolateral hernias* in patients of the same age group. However, more recent reports suggest a lower response rate than that of paramedian disc.[85,90]

Prevention of Perineurial Scar Formation

Throughout the history of lumbar disc surgery, failure has been attributed to scar formation around the nerve root and, therefore, the interest in scar formation prevention has been high. Scar formation tethers the root within the otherwise slick interfaces of the lateral recess and sensitizes it to compression, tension, and ischemia, that would otherwise theoretically be asymptomatic. In the circumstance of recurrent hernia following discectomy, fibrosis around the root certainly impacts symptoms and reoperation rate. Fibrosis results in unusual anatomic problems, including intraradicular and intradural herniations.[106,118] Because of fibrosis and tethering of the dura mater, the

---

*References 2,26,29,30,42,83.

presentation of recurrent hernia or prolapse may be polyradicular rather than monoradicular.

Determinants of scar formation include soft tissue traumatization and blood left behind in the operative field. Therefore, surgical minimization and cleanliness can be expected to improve outcomes if indeed scar lends itself to failure, and these are reasonable and naturally accepted tenets. Gelatin sponge has been reported to increase scar formation. Therefore, the manufacturer recommends its removal from the field after hemostasis is achieved. Urokinase has been used in an animal model to break down the small amount of blood that invariably remains or accumulates after surgery. This has reduced scar formation and lends credence to the theory of blood products being at least partially responsible.[19] A number of substances have been proposed to reduce scar formation in addition to clean technique.

One of the most popular measures is the use of epidural steroids, in use for the last 20 years or so, yet without supportive clinical data. The use of epidural methylprednisolone or dexamethasone, however, is in common use and has been shown in animal models to reduce the epidural scar.[39,45,53]

Free fat grafts taken from the subcutaneous space or paraspinous tissue have also been used for the last 20 years. Fat grafts can be placed in the interlaminar defect dorsally and may prevent the formation of a dorsal scar or "laminectomy membrane," but cannot be placed circumferentially around the nerve root, including its ventral surface. Support in the literature for this practice is variable,[80,114] but there can be little downside to the application of a small pledget of fat into the interlaminar defect.

Carbohydrate polymer in gelatin, Adcon-L, has proven efficacy in the reduction of scar formation around the nerve root, by both animal histologic and human radiographic studies, when placed around the root following discectomy.[16,37,103] In fact, it is evidently so effective that there may be an increased incidence of postoperative cerebrospinal fluid leakage.[52,73] Hyaluronic acid has also been used in animal trial[114] and is used in other surgical fields for the purpose of discouraging scar formation, though it has not been used clinically in laminectomy patients. Both agents inhibit the initial influx of inflammatory cells and the ingrowth of fibroblasts, and both agents are biodegradable. Clinical efficacy has not been demonstrated.

The interposition of bone wax, silastic or Dacron sheeting, and fascial graft has been used. However, none can be recommended. Common to the use of these materials is a lack of proven efficacy in the prevention of postoperative residual radiculopathy in large trials.[43] Outside of the connection between postoperative adhesions and the odd intradural or intraradicular recurrent hernia, the relationship between scar and failure is one in theory only.[37]

Management of Complications

In either the prone or the lateral decubitus position, air embolism can occur, though in neither position is it considered to be enough of a risk to warrant invasive line placement. If, however, a Doppler monitor is placed, it provides the earliest diagnosis. With paradoxical embolism across a patent foramen ovale, a decrease in arterial carbon dioxide pressure, a decrease in end-tidal carbon dioxide pressure, an increase in arterial carbon dioxide pressure, and subsequent hypotension and tachycardia may all be observed. Proper management consists of ceasing nitrous oxide administration, flooding the field with saline, waxing the bony surfaces, and repositioning the patient quickly to lower the field in relation to the heart.[5]

The hazard of a dural tear lies not with the meningeal injury sustained, recognized, and repaired adequately at the time of surgery, but rather with injury that is not recognized at surgery or is acquired postoperatively. Dural tear can result in subsequent delayed wound dehiscence and CSF leakage or in symptomatic pseudomeningocele.[76,89,121] Pseudomeningocele can cause recurrent back and leg pain, the latter being the result of nerve root herniation into the dural sac.[89] Treatment, if the patient is symptomatic, requires reoperation. Good results, with resolution of symptoms by primary closure of the dural defect, can be expected.

Injury of abdominal organs or viscera occurs in 1.6 to 17 per 10,000 cases.[47] Effective management of visceral or vascular injury requires prompt recognition of its occurrence. Mortality, in cases of untreated vascular or visceral injuries, approaches 100%.[47] In some reported cases of bowel and ureteral injury, visceral tissue was found in the disc specimen submitted for examination. As mentioned in the above section on technique, injury may be suspected intraoperatively because of hypotension, the unexplained egress of irrigation fluid through the annulus and out of the field, or persistent bleeding up through the annulus not explained by bone or epidural bleeding. There appears to be no common risk factors predisposing patients to this type of hazard, apart from ventral annular tear. A sound knowledge of retroperitoneal anatomy is useful (Figure 49.4). Even with treatment, mortality of these injuries is high, at nearly 50%, and therefore if suspected the injury demands immediate attention.[47] Unfortunately, the initial lack of clinical signs of injury usually accounts for any delay encountered, and in a majority of cases, the surgeon fails to recognize perforation of the annulus or ligament and intraabdominal injury. In convalescence, persistent flank or abdominal pain, ileus, hypotension, and fever may all signal intraabdominal injury and should be investigated. Plain abdominal radiographs, CT, IVP, angiography, and abdominal ultrasound may all be necessary.

A patient may be sensitized to major vascular injury through one of two or three anatomic variations. Since the anterior longitudinal ligament provides a barrier to the passage of an instrument through the annulus into the retroperitoneum, a high aortic bifurcation results in the iliac vessel lying lateral to the protection of the ligament. A spondylotic ridge may result in attenuation of the ligament.[33] Also, peridiscal inflammation, resulting in fibrosis, can result in adhesion of a large vessel to the annulus. Of injured named vessels, the left iliac artery is the most common. Arterial injury is at times large enough and hypotension is rapid enough that there may not be time for angiography or scanning. In such cases, immediate laparotomy is indicated. If the vessel is small, hemorrhage from

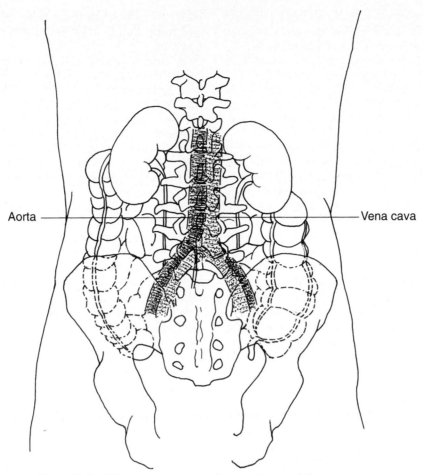

Figure 49.4 Abdominal viscera at risk through ventral disc penetration.

the disc space notable, and the patient stable, angiography is useful in determining its location prior to laparotomy.[67] There may be an initial lack of clinical signs of vascular injury until significant blood loss has occurred and the patients are in danger of vascular collapse, particularly in healthy young patients with significant cardiovascular reserve (if a small vessel such as a medial sacral vessel has been injured).

Bowel motility is slowed by the use of general anesthesia, but it can also result from the surgery itself, and ileus can affect both the large and small bowel. Usually, it is not a significant problem, but it can last several days and can require nasogastric suction.[98] A more severe form of impaired bowel motility, pseudo-obstruction of the colon, or Ogilvie's syndrome, is a life-threatening complication characterized by massive cecal distention that can lead to perforation. Bowel sounds are present from areas of active motility, but cecal distention and tenderness are also present. Decompression by colonoscopy is the treatment of choice unless rupture has already occurred.[35]

Infections can be categorized as those involving the bone or the disc interspace and simple wound infections. The risk of wound infection is about 0.5%. A frank wound infection that does not involve the disc space or bone can be managed with drainage and a brief 1- or 2-week course of appropriate antibiotics. Surveillance measures should be taken to rule out a deepening process. Nearly 80% of infections in discectomy patients appear in the first postoperative

month. Diabetic, elderly, alcoholic, and immunocompromised patients are at greatest risk. Excessive use of monopolar cautery and excessive tissue trauma and tissue retraction predispose to infectious complication. If extending to the surface, an infected wound may be probed to determine its depth and to drain the purulent material. If probing or scanning demonstrates a wound separation down to the bone, the likelihood of disc interspace involvement is higher.

If disc interspace infection is present, the superficial wound is often well healed, with the nidus of infection contained in the disc space. Marked persistent spastic back pain, marked sedimentation rate elevation, and elevated C-reactive protein are clinical and laboratory indicators of disc interspace infection. In these cases, discitis should be assumed until it has been ruled out.[108] The presence of unusually severe pain in the postoperative period, even if the wound is well healed, should prompt a workup for disc interspace infection because superficial evidence of wound infection is unusual. MRI is a very sensitive indicator and can show evidence of infection early in its course. Patients with sedimentation rates of over 45mm/min and C-reactive protein levels higher than 2.5mg/L on the fifth or sixth postoperative day are suspected of having disc interspace infections. Although the temperature and peripheral white blood cell count may be elevated, this is not always the case. If disc interspace infection is present, antibiotics should be appropriate for the infectious agent as proven by open or CT-guided biopsy or by peripheral blood culture (which is positive in 25% of cases). Intravenous antibiotics should be administered for a period of 6 weeks. If there is reason to suspect involvement of adjacent vertebral bone, by MRI or CT or by progressive deformity, intravenous antibiotics should be continued for 6 to 8 weeks, followed by oral antibiotics for another 8 weeks. Immobilization is generally recommended.

The radiographic changes of disc interspace infection are often delayed. Optimally, the presence of infection should be recognized before its radiographic appearance. Plain radiographs do not show a change until 6 weeks after the onset of infection, until there is erosion of the subchondral cortical bone. The most sensitive radiographic study early in the course of infection is the MRI scan, which shows: (1) a diffuse decrease in the T1 signal from vertebral body bone adjacent to the disc as a result of edema fluid in the marrow; (2) blurring of the margins between vertebral bone, cartilaginous end plates, and disc; and (3) an increased T2 signal in the area of inflammation, particularly in the disc. There may be swelling of paravertebral soft tissues and, with gadolinium infusion, epidural contrast enhancement. Bone scanning and indium labeled leukocyte scanning are also quite sensitive and positive relatively early in the course of infection.

Staphylococcus aureus can produce, in addition to abscess formation and recurrent neurologic deficit on the basis of space-occupying mass effect, exotoxins with local and distant effects. Toxic shock syndrome is attributable to this, with vascular collapse and encephalopathy. Reportedly, local staphylococcal wound infection after lumbar laminectomy can even result in a cauda equina syndrome, without a compressive mass effect.[8]

Recurrent radiculopathic pain may be due to traction injury of a root fixed in perineurial or arachnoidal scar, or it may be due to recurrent or residual disc hernia or prolapsed annulus. Recurrent radiculopathy (as a result of recurrent hernia or secondary degenerative change and stenosis) resulting in reoperation occurs in from about 5% to 20% of patients in long-term studies.[23,66,82,136] Higher figures in long-term studies may also include the risk of acquiring radiculopathy unrelated to surgery. When radiculopathic leg pain reappears or does not remit, repeat neuroimaging is indicated. Optimally, this would be a high-quality MRI without and with gadolinium enhancement. The finding of perineurial scar only is neither a surgical complication nor an indication for revision surgery. However, lateral recess stenosis, annular prolapse, foraminal stenosis, and recurrent or residual disc herniation are all to some extent, secondary complications that can be responsible for symptoms and indicate revision surgery. The management of repeat or incompletely treated nerve root compression is similar to that of an otherwise untreated hernia, with the exception that there is a variable amount of scar around the nerve root. The fibrosis can make anatomic planes difficult to discern and dissect and can result in unusual anatomic problems, such as intraradicular and intradural herniations, as mentioned in the section on technique. Also, because of fibrosis and tethering of the dura mater, the presentation may be polyradicular rather than monoradicular. The anatomy is easier to understand if the bony exposure is made wider and fresh dura is identified around the periphery of the exposure.

A time-honored belief was that recurrent hernia required fusion. There is, however, little reason to proceed with fusion unless the motion segment is demonstrably unstable. Of course, the addition of fusion increases the likelihood of its own complications and reoperation rate.[82] Therefore, an initial recurrent disc hernia or secondary stenosis can be treated with conventional or microlaminotomy, with good results.[17,51,117] In the case of multiple recurrences, because of the implication of the role of instability, repetitive revision may indicate the need for thorough decompression and fusion.[41] With the need for repetitive revisions, poorer results are encountered.[66]

Recurrent symptoms may result from, or be exacerbated by, poor bone and ligamentous healing. Bone healing may not be as important to outcome in discectomy as it would be in attempted fusion, but it is nevertheless significant in bone remodeling postoperatively. Good bone remodeling is important for the reacquisition of normal pars strength, and therefore to long-term results and return to preoperative activities. Systemic factors demonstrated to inhibit bone healing and likely to interfere with optimum outcome include smoking, malnutrition, diabetes, rheumatologic conditions, and osteoporosis. Additionally, to be avoided are courses of steroid and nonsteroidal medications and cytotoxic medications in the perioperative period, particularly the first 2 postoperative weeks.[61] It is suggested that postoperative patients engage in and maintain daily reconditioning, including low impact aerobic exercises, such as walking and swimming and active range of motion exercises.

REFERENCES

1. Abdullah AF, Ditto EW, III, Byrd EB, *et al:* Extreme-lateral lumbar disc herniations: clinical syndrome and special problems of diagnosis. *J Neurosurg* 41:229-234, 1974.
2. Abdullah AF, Wolber PG, Warfield JR, *et al:* Surgical management of extreme lateral lumbar disc herniations: review of 138 cases. *Neurosurgery* 22:648-653, 1988.
3. Abramovitz JN, Neff SR: Lumbar disc surgery: results of the Prospective Lumbar Discectomy Study of the Joint Section on Disorders of the Spine and Peripheral Nerves of the American Association of Neurological Surgeons and the Congress of Neurological Surgeons. *Neurosurgery* 29: 301-307; discussion 307-308, 1991.
4. Albeck MJ: A critical assessment of clinical diagnosis of disc herniation in patients with monoradicular sciatica. *Acta Neurochir (Wien)* 138:40-44, 1996.
5. Albin MS, Ritter RR, Pruett CE, *et al:* Venous air embolism during lumbar laminectomy in the prone position: report of three cases. *Anesth Analg* 73:346-349, 1991.
6. An HS, Simpson JM, Stein R: Outpatient laminotomy and discectomy. *J Spinal Disord Tech* 12:192-196, 1999.
7. Andreshak TG, An HS, Hall J, *et al:* Lumbar spine surgery in the obese patient. *J Spinal Disord Tech* 10:376-379, 1997.

8. Arend SM, Steenmeyer AV, Mosmans PC, *et al:* Postoperative cauda syndrome caused by *Staphylococcus aureus. Infection* 21:248-250, 1993.

9. Aschoff A, Steiner-Milz H, Steiner HH: Lower limb compartment syndrome following lumbar discectomy in the knee-chest position. *Neurosurg Rev* 13:155-159, 1990.

10. Atlas SJ, Deyo RA, Keller RB, *et al:* The Main Lumbar Spine Study, Part II: 1-year outcomes of surgical and nonsurgical management of sciatica. *Spine* 21:1777-1786, 1996.

11. Bailey PaC, L: Osteo-arthritis of the spine as a cause of compression of the spinal cord and its roots: with reports of five cases. *J Nerv Ment Dis* 38:588-609, 1911.

12. Bashkoff E, Gadaleta D, Moccio C: Postlaminectomy aortic pseudoaneurysm. *J Spinal Disord Tech* 5:219-221, 1992.

13. Bookwalter JW, III, Busch MD, Nicely D: Ambulatory surgery is safe and effective in radicular disc disease. *Spine* 19:526-530, 1994.

14. Borenstein DG: Epidemiology, etiology, diagnostic evaluation, and treatment of low back pain. *Curr Opin Rheumatol* 13:128-134, 2001.

15. Brewster DC, May AR, Darling RC, *et al:* Variable manifestations of vascular injury during lumbar disc surgery. *Arch Surg* 114:1026-1030, 1979.

16. Brotchi J, Pirotte B, De Witte O, *et al:* Prevention of epidural fibrosis in a prospective series of 100 primary lumbo-sacral discectomy patients: follow-up and assessment at re-operation. *Neurol Res* 21(suppl 1): S47-S50, 1999.

17. Carroll SE, Wiesel SW: Neurologic complications and lumbar laminectomy: a standardized approach to the multiply-operated lumbar spine. *Clin Orthop:*14-23, 1992.

18. Caspar W, Campbell B, Barbier DD, *et al:* The Caspar microsurgical discectomy and comparison with a conventional standard lumbar disc procedure. *Neurosurgery* 28:78-86; discussion 86-77, 1991.

19. Ceviz A, Arslan A, Ak HE, *et al:* The effect of urokinase in preventing the formation of epidural fibrosis and/or leptomeningeal arachnoiditis. *Surg Neurol* 47:124-127, 1997.

20. Chhabra MS, Hussein AA, Eisenstein SM: Should fusion accompany lumbar discectomy? A medium-term answer. *Clin Orthop* Apr:177-180, 1994.

21. Dandy W: Loose cartilage from intervertebral disc simulating tumor of the spinal cord. *Arch Surg* 19: 660-672, 1929.

22. Daneyemez M, Sali A, Kahraman S, *et al:* Outcome analyses in 1072 surgically treated lumbar disc herniations. *Minim Invasive Neurosurg* 42:63-68, 1999.

23. Davis RA: A long-term outcome analysis of 984 surgically treated herniated lumbar discs. *J Neurosurg* 80:415-421, 1994.

24. De Saussure R: Vascular injury coincident to disc surgery. *J Neurosurg* 16:222-229, 1959.

25. Di Lorenzo N, Porta F, Onnis G, *et al:* Pars interarticularis fenestration in the treatment of foraminal lumbar disc herniation: a further surgical approach. *Neurosurgery* 42:87-89; discussion 89-90, 1998.

26. Donaldson WF, III, Star MJ, Thorne RP: Surgical treatment for the far lateral herniated lumbar disc. *Spine* 18:1263-1267, 1993.

27. Ehni GJ: Effects of certain degenerative diseases of the spine, especially spondylosis and disc protrusion, on the neural contents, particularly in the lumbar region: historical account. *Mayo Clinic Proc* 50:327-338, 1975.

28. Elsberg CA: *Diagnosis and Treatment of Surgical Diseases of the Spinal Cord and Its Membranes.* Philadelphia, WB Saunders, 1916.

29. Epstein NE: Evaluation of varied surgical approaches used in the management of 170 far-lateral lumbar disc herniations: indications and results. *J Neurosurg* 83: 648-656, 1995.

30. Epstein NE, Epstein JA, Carras R, *et al:* Far lateral lumbar disc herniations and associated structural abnormalities: an evaluation in 60 patients of the comparative value of CT, MRI, and myelo-CT in diagnosis and management. *Spine* 15:534-539, 1990.

31. Errico TJ, Fardon DF, Lowell TD: Open discectomy as treatment for herniated nucleus pulposus of the lumbar spine. *Spine* 20:1829-1833, 1995.

32. Eysel P, Rompe JD, Hopf C: Prognostic criteria of discogenic paresis. *Eur Spine J* 3:214-218, 1994.

33. Ezra E, Richenberg JL, Smellie WA: Major vascular injury during lumbar laminectomy. *J R Soc Med* 89:108P-109P, 1996.

34. Faust SE, Ducker TB, VanHassent JA: Lateral lumbar disc herniations. *J Spinal Disord Tech* 5:97-103, 1992.

35. Feldman RA, Karl RC: Diagnosis and treatment of Ogilvie's syndrome after lumbar spinal surgery: report of three cases. *J Neurosurg* 76:1012-1016, 1992.

36. Ferree BA: Deep venous thrombosis following lumbar laminotomy and laminectomy. *Orthopedics* 17:35-38, 1994.

37. Fischgrund JS: Perspectives on modern orthopaedics: use of Adcon-L for epidural scar prevention. *J Am Acad Orthop Surg* 8:339-343, 2000.

38. Fogelholm RR, Alho AV: Smoking and intervertebral disc degeneration. *Med Hypotheses* 56:537-539, 2001.

39. Foulkes GD, Robinson JS, Jr.: Intraoperative dexamethasone irrigation in lumbar microdiscectomy. *Clin Orthop* Dec:224-228, 1990.

40. Frank E: Removal of a lateral disc herniation with malleable endoscopic forceps: technical note. *Neurosurgery* 41:311-312; discussion 312-313, 1997.

41. Fritsch EW, Heisel J, Rupp S: The failed back surgery syndrome: reasons, intraoperative findings, and long-term results: a report of 182 operative treatments. *Spine* 21:626-633, 1996.

42. Garrido E, Connaughton PN: Unilateral facetectomy approach for lateral lumbar disc herniation. *J Neurosurg* 74:754-756, 1991.

43. Gibson JN, Grant IC, Waddell G: The Cochrane review of surgery for lumbar disc prolapse and degenerative lumbar spondylosis. *Spine* 24:1820-1832, 1999.

44. Gioia G, Mandelli D, Capaccioni B, *et al:* Surgical treatment of far lateral lumbar disc herniation: identification of compressed root and discectomy by lateral approach. *Spine* 24:1952-1957, 1999.

45. Glasser RS, Knego RS, Delashaw JB, *et al:* The perioperative use of corticosteroids and bupivacaine in the management of lumbar disc disease. *J Neurosurg* 78: 383-387, 1993.

46. Goldthwait J: The lumbo-sacral articulation: an explanation of many cases of "lumbago," "sciatica," and paraplegia. *Boston Med Surg J* 164:365-372, 1911.

47. Goodkin R, Laska LL: Vascular and visceral injuries associated with lumbar disc surgery: medicolegal implications. *Surg Neurol* 49:358-370; discussion 370-372, 1998.

48. Haines SJ: Systemic antibiotic prophylaxis in neurological surgery. *Neurosurgery* 6:355-361, 1980.

49. Hall H: Surgery: indications and options. *Neurol Clin* 17:113-130, 1999.

50. Hazlett JW, Kinnard P: Lumbar apophyseal process excision and spinal instability. *Spine* 7:171-176, 1982.

51. Herron L: Recurrent lumbar disc herniation: results of repeat laminectomy and discectomy. *J Spinal Disord Tech* 7:161-166, 1994.

52. Hieb LD, Stevens DL: Spontaneous postoperative cerebrospinal fluid leaks following application of anti-adhesion barrier gel: case report and review of the literature. *Spine* 26:748-751, 2001.

53. Hinton JL, Jr., Warejcka DJ, Mei Y, *et al:* Inhibition of epidural scar formation after lumbar laminectomy in the rat. *Spine* 20:564-570; discussion 579-580, 1995.

54. Hood RS: Far lateral lumbar disc herniations. *Neurosurg Clin N Am* 4:117-124, 1993.

55. Ito T, Takano Y, Yuasa N: Types of lumbar herniated disc and clinical course. *Spine* 26:648-651, 2001.

56. Ito T, Yamada M, Ikuta F, *et al:* Histologic evidence of absorption of sequestration-type herniated disc. *Spine* 21:230-234, 1996.

57. Jane JA, Haworth CS, Broaddus WC, *et al:* A neurosurgical approach to far-lateral disc herniation: technical note. *J Neurosurg* 72:143-144, 1990.

58. Jarvik JG, Deyo RA: Imaging of lumbar intervertebral disc degeneration and aging, excluding disc herniations. *Radiol Clin North Am* 38:1255-1266, vi, 2000.

59. Jenis LG, An HS: Spine update: lumbar foraminal stenosis. *Spine* 25:389-394, 2000.

60. Jenis LG, An HS, Gordin R: Foraminal stenosis of the lumbar spine: a review of 65 surgical cases. *Am J Orthop* 30:205-211, 2001.

61. Kalfas IH: Principles of bone healing. *Neurosurg Focus* 10:1-4, 2001.

62. Katz DM, Trobe JD, Cornblath WT, *et al:* Ischemic optic neuropathy after lumbar spine surgery. *Arch Ophthalmol* 112:925-931, 1994.

63. Keller RB, Atlas SJ, Singer DE, *et al:* The Maine Lumbar Spine Study, Part I: background and concepts. *Spine* 21:1769-1776, 1996.

64. Kelly RE, Dinner MH, Lavyne MH, *et al:* The effect of lumbar disc surgery on postoperative pulmonary function and temperature: a comparison study of microsurgical lumbar discectomy with standard lumbar discectomy. *Spine* 18:287-290, 1993.

65. Kendrick D, Fielding K, Bentley E, *et al:* Radiography of the lumbar spine in primary care patients with low back pain: randomised controlled trial. *BMJ* 322:400-405, 2001.

66. Keskimaki I, Seitsalo S, Osterman H, *et al:* Reoperations after lumbar disc surgery: a population-based study of regional and interspecialty variations. *Spine* 25:1500-1508, 2000.

67. Kiev J, Dupont JR, Kerstein MD: Injury of a medial sacral vessel during lumbar laminectomy. *Ann Vasc Surg* 10:63-65, 1996.

68. Kornberg M: Extreme lateral lumbar disc herniations: clinical syndrome and computed tomography recognition. *Spine* 12:586-589, 1987.

69. Kostuik JP, Harrington I, Alexander D, *et al:* Cauda equina syndrome and lumbar disc herniation. *J Bone Joint Surg Am* 68:386-391, 1986.

69a. Lane WA: Spondylolisthesis associated with progressive paraplegia: Laminectomy. *Lancet* 1:991, 1893.

70. Lanzino G, Shaffrey CI, Jane JA: Surgical treatment of lateral lumbar herniated discs. In Rengachary SS, Wilkins RH (eds): *Neurosurgical Operative Atlas*, vol 8. Park Ridge, IL, American Association of Neurological Surgeons, pp 243-251.

71. Larequi-Lauber T, Vader JP, Burnand B, *et al:* Appropriateness of indications for surgery of lumbar disc hernia and spinal stenosis. *Spine* 22:203-209, 1997.

72. Larson SJ, Holst RA, Hemmy DC, *et al:* Lateral extracavitary approach to traumatic lesions of the thoracic and lumbar spine. *J Neurosurg* 45:628-637, 1976.

73. Le AX, Rogers DE, Dawson EG, *et al:* Unrecognized durotomy after lumbar discectomy: a report of four cases associated with the use of ADCON-L. *Spine* 26:115-117; discussion 118, 2001.

74. Leavens ME BF: Ruptured intervertebral disc: report of a case with a defect in the anterior annulus fibrosus. *J Neurosurg* 10:544-546, 1953.

75. Leboeuf-Yde C: Smoking and low back pain: a systematic literature review of 41 journal articles reporting 47 epidemiologic studies. *Spine* 24:1463-1470, 1999.

76. Lee KS, Hardy IM, II: Postlaminectomy lumbar pseudomeningocele: report of four cases. *Neurosurgery* 30:111-114, 1992.

77. Lejeune JP, Hladky JP, Cotten A, *et al:* Foraminal lumbar disc herniation: experience with 83 patients. *Spine* 19:1905-1908, 1994.

78. Love J: Removal of protruded intervertebral discs without laminectomy. *Proc Staff Meet Mayo Clin* 14:800, 1939.

79. Luoma K, Riihimaki H, Luukkonen R, *et al:* Low back pain in relation to lumbar disc degeneration. *Spine* 25:487-492, 2000.

80. MacKay MA, Fischgrund JS, Herkowitz HN, *et al:* The effect of interposition membrane on the outcome of lumbar laminectomy and discectomy. *Spine* 20:1793-1796, 1995.

81. Maigne JY, Rime B, Deligne B: Computed tomographic follow-up study of forty-eight cases of nonoperatively treated lumbar intervertebral disc herniation. *Spine* 17:1071-1074, 1992.

82. Malter AD, McNeney B, Loeser JD, *et al:* 5-year reoperation rates after different types of lumbar spine surgery. *Spine* 23:814-820, 1998.

83. Maroon JC, Kopitnik TA, Schulhof LA, *et al:* Diagnosis and microsurgical approach to far-lateral disc herniation in the lumbar spine. *J Neurosurg* 72:378-382, 1990.

84. Mauric G: *Le disque intervertébral: physiologie, pathologie, et indications thérapeutiques.* Paris, Masson & Cie, 1933.

85. McCulloch JA: Focus issue on lumbar disc herniation: macro- and microdiscectomy. *Spine* 21:45S-56S, 1996.

86. Mixter W, Barr, JS: Rupture of the intervertebral disc with involvement of the spinal canal. *N Engl J Med* 211, 1934.

87. Nachemson AL: Advances in low-back pain. *Clin Orthop* Nov:266-278, 1985.

88. Nashold BS HZ: *Lumbar Disc Disease: A Twenty Year Followup Study.* St. Louis, CV Mosby, 1971.

89. Nishi S, Hashimoto N, Takagi Y, *et al:* Herniation and entrapment of a nerve root secondary to an unrepaired small dural laceration at lumbar hemilaminectomies. *Spine* 20:2576-2579, 1995.

90. Ohmori K, Kanamori M, Kawaguchi Y, *et al:* Clinical features of extraforaminal lumbar disc herniation based on the radiographic location of the dorsal root ganglion. *Spine* 26:662-666, 2001.

91. Oppel F SA, Schirmer M, *et al:* Results and complicated course after surgery for lumbar disc herniation. In Wullenweber R BM, Hamer J, *et al* (eds): *Advances in Neurosurgery,* vol 4. New York, Springer-Verlag, 1977, p 36.

92. Ozaki S, Muro T, Ito S, *et al:* Neovascularization of the outermost area of herniated lumbar intervertebral discs. *J Orthop Sci* 4:286-292, 1999.

93. Pappas CT, Harrington T, Sonntag VK: Outcome analysis in 654 surgically treated lumbar disc herniations. *Neurosurgery* 30:862-866, 1992.

94. Parker HL AA: Compression of the spinal cord and its roots by hypertrophic osteo-arthritis. *Surg Gynecol Obstet* 41:1-14, 1925.

95. Parks BJ: Postoperative peripheral neuropathies. *Surgery* 74:348-357, 1973.

96. Pott P: Remarks on that kind of palsy of the lower limbs which is frequently found to accompany a curvature of the spine, and is supposed to be caused by it, together with its method of cure. *Med Classics* 1:281-297, 1936.

97. Prestar FJ: Anomalies and malformations of lumbar spinal nerve roots. *Minim Invasive Neurosurg* 39:133-137, 1996.

98. Price SJ, Buxton N: A dynamic ileus complicating lumbar laminectomy: a report of two cases. *Br J Neurosurg* 12: 162-164, 1998.

99. Putti V: New conceptions in the pathogenesis of sciatic pain. *Lancet* 2:53-60, 1927.

100. Ramirez LF, Thisted R: Complications and demographic characteristics of patients undergoing lumbar discectomy in community hospitals. *Neurosurgery* 25:226-230; discussion 230-231, 1989.

101. Reulen HJ, Muller A, Ebeling U: Microsurgical anatomy of the lateral approach to extraforaminal lumbar disc herniations. *Neurosurgery* 39:345-350; discussion 350-351, 1996.

102. Robe P, Martin D, Lenelle J, *et al:* Posterior epidural migration of sequestered lumbar disc fragments: report of two cases. *J Neurosurg* 90:264-266, 1999.

103. Robertson JT, Maier K, Anderson RW, *et al:* Prevention of epidural fibrosis with ADCON-L in presence of a durotomy during lumbar disc surgery: experiences with a pre-clinical model. *Neurol Res* 21(suppl 1):S61-S66, 1999.

104. Roland M, van Tulder M: Should radiologists change the way they report plain radiography of the spine? *Lancet* 352:229-230, 1998.

105. Rosen C, Rothman S, Zigler J, *et al:* Lumbar facet fracture as a possible source of pain after lumbar laminectomy. *Spine* 16:S234-S238, 1991.

106. Schisano G, Franco A, Nina P: Intraradicular and intradural lumbar disc herniation: experiences with nine cases. *Surg Neurol* 44:536-543, 1995.

107. Schlesinger SM, Fankhauser H, de Tribolet N: Microsurgical anatomy and operative technique for extreme lateral lumbar disc herniations. *Acta Neurochir (Wien)* 118:117-129, 1992.

108. Schulitz KP, Assheuer J: Discitis after procedures on the intervertebral disc. *Spine* 19:1172-1177, 1994.

109. Shaw ED, Scarborough JT, Beals RK: Bowel injury as a complication of lumbar discectomy: a case report and review of the literature. *J Bone Joint Surg Am* 63:478-480, 1981.

110. Shevlin WA, Luessenhop AJ, Fox JL, *et al:* Perforation of the anterior annulus during lumbar discectomy: case report. *J Neurosurg* 38:514-515, 1973.

111. Smith DW, Lawrence BD: Vascular complications of lumbar decompression laminectomy and foraminotomy: a unique case and review of the literature. *Spine* 16: 387-390, 1991.

112. Smith EB, DeBord JR, Hanigan WC: Intestinal injury after lumbar discectomy. *Surg Gynecol Obstet* 173:22-24, 1991.

113. Song J, Park Y: Ligament-sparing lumbar microdiscectomy: technical note. *Surg Neurol* 53:592-596; discussion 596-597, 2000.

114. Songer MN, Rauschning W, Carson EW, *et al:* Analysis of peridural scar formation and its prevention after lumbar laminotomy and discectomy in dogs. *Spine* 20:571-580; discussion 579-580, 1995.

115. Spurling RG GE: The end-results of surgery for ruptured intervertebral discs: a follow-up study of 327 cases. *J Neurosurg* 6:57-64, 1949.

116. Stankovic R, Johnell O, Maly P, *et al:* Use of lumbar extension, slump test, physical and neurological examination in the evaluation of patients with suspected herniated nucleus pulposus: a prospective clinical study. *Man Ther* 4:25-32, 1999.

117. Suk KS, Lee HM, Moon SH, *et al:* Recurrent lumbar disc herniation: results of operative management. *Spine* 26: 672-676, 2001.

118. Suzer T, Tahta K, Coskun E: Intraradicular lumbar disc herniation: case report and review of the literature. *Neurosurgery* 41:956-958; discussion 958-959, 1997.

119. Tarlov EC: Major vascular injury secondary to spine surgery. In Tarlov EC (ed): *Complications of Spinal Surgery.* Park Ridge, IL, American Association of Neurological Surgeons, 1991.

120. Tomaras CR, Blacklock JB, Parker WD, *et al:* Outpatient surgical treatment of cervical radiculopathy. *J Neurosurg* 87:41-43, 1997.

121. Tsuji H, Handa N, Handa O, *et al:* Postlaminectomy ossified extradural pseudocyst: case report. *J Neurosurg* 73:785-787, 1990.

122. Verbiest H: Further experiences on the pathological influence of a developmental narrowness of the bony canal. *J Bone Joint Surg* 37B:576-583, 1955.

123. Verbiest H: A radicular syndrome from developmental narrowing of the lumbar vertebral canal. *J Bone Joint Surg* 36B:230-237, 1954.

124. Vroomen PC, de Krom MC, Knottnerus JA: When does the patient with a disc herniation undergo lumbosacral discectomy? *J Neurol Neurosurg Psychiatry* 68:75-79, 2000.

125. Vroomen PC, de Krom MC, Wilmink JT: Pathoanatomy of clinical findings in patients with sciatica: a magnetic resonance imaging study. *J Neurosurg* 92:135-141, 2000.

126. Vucetic N, de Bri E, Svensson O: Clinical history in lumbar disc herniation: a prospective study in 160 patients. *Acta Orthop Scand* 68:116-120, 1997.

127. Vucetic N, Svensson O: Physical signs in lumbar disc hernia. *Clin Orthop* Dec:192-201, 1996.

128. Wang JC, Bohlman HH, Riew KD: Dural tears secondary to operations on the lumbar spine: management and results after a two-year-minimum follow-up of eighty-eight patients. *J Bone Joint Surg Am* 80:1728-1732, 1998.

129. Weber H: Lumbar disc herniation: a controlled, prospective study with ten years of observation. *Spine* 8:131-140, 1983.

130. Weber H: The natural history of disc herniation and the influence of intervention. *Spine* 19:2234-2238; discussion 2233, 1994.

131. Wenger M, Mariani L, Kalbarczyk A, *et al:* Long-term outcome of 104 patients after lumbar sequestrectomy according to Williams. *Neurosurgery* 49:329-334; discussion 334-335, 2001.

132. Williams R: Microlumbar discectomy: a conservative surgical approach to the virgin herniated lumbar disc. *Spine* 3:175-182, 1978.

133. Wiltse LL BJ, Hutchinson RH, Nelson WE: The paraspinal sacrospinalis-splitting approach to the lumbar spine. *J Bone Joint Surg* 50A:919, 1960.

134. Woertgen C, Rothoerl RD, Brawanski A: Influence of macrophage infiltration of herniated lumbar disc tissue on outcome after lumbar disc surgery. *Spine* 25:871-875, 2000.

135. Woertgen C, Rothoerl RD, Breme K, *et al:* Variability of outcome after lumbar disc surgery. *Spine* 24:807-811, 1999.

136. Yorimitsu E, Chiba K, Toyama Y, *et al:* Long-term outcomes of standard discectomy for lumbar disc herniation: a follow-up study of more than 10 years. *Spine* 26:652-657, 2001.

CHAPTER 50

Percutaneous Approaches to Lumbar Discectomy

Maurice M. Smith, Joseph Watson, and Joseph C. Maroon

Technical and research developments have provided new treatment modalities for the patient with spinal disc disease since its description by Mixter and Barr[30] in 1934. Percutaneous techniques derive their origins and continued success from these medical advances and the patients' desire for a less invasive yet effective therapy for this common ailment. Advances in percutaneous techniques and endoscopy have allowed for an explosion of interest and work in the field of minimally invasive discectomy that complements the current popularity of outpatient surgery.

Percutaneous techniques include chemonucleolysis, manual and automated discectomy, and endoscopic-assisted discectomy. These approaches, although diverse in their methodology, share some common, desirable qualities. They may be performed under local anesthesia, afford a minimal amount of soft-tissue dissection, and do not preclude the use of open surgery in the future.

The lumbar spine has been the target of most of the percutaneous approaches to the disc. Access to the cervical and thoracic disc spaces is also possible. Many of the principles presented here apply to these regions as well. They are not, however, the focus of this chapter. Experience with percutaneous needle access to the nucleus pulposus provided the impetus for percutaneous discectomy. The dorsolateral approach is common to the percutaneous techniques. Other less often used approaches, such as transperitoneal and direct endoscopic dorsal approaches, are discussed.

Needle Placement

Accurate and safe needle placement is critically important for complication avoidance with the dorsolateral percutaneous procedures. High-quality fluoroscopy is a prerequisite for the safe execution of these procedures, as is a fluorocompatible operating table. Anatomic variations of retroperitoneal structures should be ruled out by preoperative imaging studies. For all procedures, prophylactic intravenous antibiotics, administered at least 15 minutes before skin puncture, is recommended. The authors[2,45] prefer to use cefazolin (2g rather than 1g because the higher dose provides detectable intradiscal antibiotic levels). In a patient with a penicillin allergy, vancomycin may be substituted for cefazolin. The patient may be positioned prone or, if a biportal technique is not required, in the lateral decubitus position with the symptomatic side up. When the prone position is used, the authors prefer to place the patient on a Wilson type frame with the back slightly flexed and the abdomen free. After positioning, the patient's back is carefully prepared and draped. The fluoroscopy machine is also draped so that it may be moved from anteroposterior (AP) to lateral projections without contamination of the field.

The approach for needle placement was originally described for the purpose of percutaneous spinal biopsy in 1948. It has withstood the test of time regarding safety.[48] The technique requires a dorsolateral entry point, 8 to 10cm from the midline. With a uniportal technique, if the pathology is lateralized, entry is on the symptomatic side. Local anesthesia is used to numb the skin and subcutaneous tissue. Deep infiltration is not necessary initially but is added if severe discomfort is encountered around the facet joint. Care is taken to not anesthetize the nerve root so that accurate patient feedback is attained regarding nerve root irritation.

Before needle entry, identification of the appropriate disc space with fluoroscopy is mandatory. Any patient rotation is corrected by repositioning the patient and/or the fluoroscopy unit because rotation will alter the essential landmarks.

The skin entry point is located approximately 8 to 10cm lateral to midline. The appropriate sagittal orientation is determined by choosing an entry point that is directly in line with the mid-portion of the disc space on the lateral fluoroscopic view. In this manner, the needle enters the disc space parallel to the end plates, allowing for the maximum degrees of freedom for working within the disc space.

The target for the needle is the triangular working zone. This zone is defined anatomically, rostrally, and ventrally by the exiting nerve root, dorsally by the superior articular process, caudally by the lower vertebral body and pedicle, and medially by the traversing nerve root and dura mater. The initial needle angle should be directed about 45 degrees medially toward the lateral facet. The needle should pass just lateral to the facet and parallel to the vertebral body end plates, entering the disc in its midposition. Once the needle has reached the annulus, its position should be confirmed by both AP and lateral fluoroscopy. On the lateral view, the tip of the needle should be at the dorsal vertebral body line, and on the AP view, within the interpedicular lines. In most cases, the initial positioning is suboptimal, requiring repositioning. It is better for an initial approach to be too medial and risk colliding with the facet and lamina, than to be too lateral and entering the abdomen. It is perfectly acceptable and safe to initially dock on the lateral aspect of the facet and then reposition the needle into the triangular working zone. Once docked on the lateral aspect of the facet, the needle is withdrawn 2 to 3cm and then redirected with a more acute angle to bypass the facet and fall into the triangular working zone. When the needle is repositioned, confirmation of placement with both AP and lateral fluoroscopy is mandatory. When satisfactory needle placement is confirmed, the needle is advanced into the disc space until the center of the disc is reached. If a biportal technique is used, the same approach is used on the other side with the goal of having the needles parallel to each other and meeting at the post-central portion of the disc. From this point, one may proceed with the desired technique for disc removal.

Needle placement at L5-S1 can be difficult secondary to the disc's location low within the pelvis. The iliac crest prevents a direct parallel approach, so a slightly more rostral entry is required at this level. In general, the same skin entry point for L4-5 is appropriate for L5-S1. Because of the rostral entry required at L5-S1, biportal needles may not meet in the center of the disc space. The needle passes obliquely through the disc in a rostral to caudal direction toward the sacrum, making the biportal approach difficult and sometimes impossible at L5-S1.

Percutaneous Techniques

Chemonucleolysis

Intravenous papain injection in rabbits was found to result in floppy ears from a transient loss of cartilage. This discovery was cleverly applied to disc disease and found to dissolve the nucleus in humans. The initial experience was presented in 1964.[50] Its use has been the subject of much controversy in the subsequent years.

Technique

Immediate preprocedural preparation includes the administration of prophylactic antibiotics and prophylactic histamine blockade (both H1 and H2). The technique involves unilateral needle placement, as described above, under local anesthesia into the disc space via the dorsolateral approach and fluoroscopic guidance. Discography with water-soluble contrast, such as Omnipaque 1ml, is advocated to further confirm needle placement and to rule out an intrathecal communication. Then 1 to 1.5ml of the enzyme (300 to 1500 units) is injected into the disc space over several minutes. The wide range of dosage used reflects the debate over the minimal effective dose. The needle is left in for another 3 to 5 minutes to keep the enzyme from escaping from the needle tract, and then it is withdrawn.

Treatment of sciatica with chymopapain had been shown to be effective compared with placebo, in three randomized, blinded trials, in giving relief of symptoms at 6 to 12 months in 70% to 80% of patients.[6,12,19] A previous randomized blinded study had failed to demonstrate a statistical improvement over placebo, giving rise to some initial skepticism regarding the technique.[26]

Chemonucleolysis compares favorably to automated percutaneous discectomy. A randomized study of 141 patients comparing the two techniques found a significant difference in reported patient outcome in patients with sciatica, with 66% good outcome in the chymopapain group versus only 37% in the automated percutaneous discectomy group.[44] Chemonucleolysis has also been compared to open surgery in patients with radiculopathy. In a prospective, randomized study of chymopapain versus open discectomy, no statistical differences in outcome were observed at 1 and 4 years.[17] Another randomized, prospective trial did not support the efficacy of chemonucleolysis compared with open surgery for a contained disc rupture with radiculopathy. This was because of a high initial failure rate within the chymopapain group who then underwent open surgery.[32]

Complications

Despite studies demonstrating the efficacy of chemonucleolysis, its side effect profile has limited its continued widespread use in many countries. The complications, the actual numbers of which are small, may be quite serious. These include urticaria, anaphylaxis, arachnoiditis, transverse myelitis, and central nervous system hemorrhage.[6,33,51] Occasionally, back stiffness and muscle spasm are observed that may require intravenous pain control for several days. This, however, dissipates in 90% of patients at 6 months.[18] The risk of anaphylaxis may be reduced by avoiding patients with a history of papaya ingestion and specific antigen testing to papaya. Advocates of the procedure maintain that the complications, other than allergic reactions, are preventable with accurate needle placement and the avoidance of an intrathecal injection. Egress of spinal fluid from the needle, or the visualization of discography dye in the thecal sac, is a contraindication to the chymopapain injection. Should intrathecal injection occur, usually manifesting as abrupt hypertension and headache, immediate lumbar tap and drainage of spinal fluid is indicated. This maneuver may be lifesaving.[51] Discitis after chemonucleolysis is a potential risk (about 0.25%).[1,7,22,33]

It is clear from the literature that complications from chemonucleolysis are small.[1,22,32] The soiled reputation of chymopapain, however, may be unrecoverable.

Percutaneous Nucleotomy

The first report of percutaneous discectomy was in 1975, using a unilateral dorsolateral approach to the disc.[16] Although the dorsolateral approach was the most widely used, a more lateral, retroperitoneal approach was proposed.[10] This was not widely accepted because of the risk of damage to retroperitoneal structures.

The next significant improvement in the technique came in the 1980s with the use of an automated disc extractor, giving rise to the automated percutaneous lumbar discectomy.[26,37] The automated discector is a suction shaver that can perform controlled removal of disc material. The laser has been applied with some success using this approach.[4,5,35,42,45] Although most of the experience has been in the lumbar spine, series of cervical cases have been reported but are not the focus of this chapter.[17,53]

Controversy and criticism surround the large reports concerning the percutaneous nucleotomies. These techniques may all be considered indirect techniques because they remove the central disc but do not directly address the offending pathology of nerve root compression. Central disc removal reduces the pressure within the disc space, an effect casually known as *popping the balloon*. Furthermore, it creates a defect in the annulus fibrosus through which disc material may herniate in the future. This herniation is directed away from the nerve root. Also, with an indirect approach to the pathology, epidural scar formation is eschewed. The crux of the debate is over the indications and patient selection. This fact makes patient selection crucial because patients with a diffuse bulge may be expected to derive more benefit from nucleotomy than a patient with focal root compression. Most authors agree that removal of the nucleus alone will not be effective in the case of a sequestered disc fragment.

In carefully selected patients, the reported efficacy of percutaneous discectomy by various techniques (the manual technique, the automated technique, the biportal discoscopic technique, and the laser technique) is 70% to 80%.[5,26,31,39,48] In some hands, however, the results have been poor, on the order of 50% improvement.[20] None of these series, however, were randomized controlled trials. When the percutaneous technique was subjected to the standards of a randomized, controlled trial, the results were not promising. One trial was terminated prematurely because of the apparent inefficacy at interval analysis of automated percutaneous discectomy, and the other failed to show efficacy.[3,44]

Technique

The nucleotomies are typically performed with the patient prone, but may be done laterally if a uniportal technique is used. Local anesthesia with intravenous sedation is the preferred anesthetic technique. General or regional anesthesia is contraindicated because an important factor in avoiding root injury is feedback from the awake patient during instrument positioning. Prophylaxis against discitis should be used as a one-time preincisional intravenous dosing. A guidewire is inserted via a dorsolateral approach. A needle may also serve as the guidewire, especially if discography is also desired. With a safe pathway to the disc established, a dilator is inserted over the guidewire to dock on the annulus. A working cannula is then inserted over the dilator, and its position is confirmed with fluoroscopy. The dilator is then removed, establishing a small tubular corridor to the triangular working zone. Instruments, such as elongated rongeurs, an automated discector, or a laser, may be passed into the disc space for the removal of the central nucleus pulposus.

Because the discectomy is performed without visualization, a technical challenge is to know how much disc to remove. With the standard instruments and the automated disc extractor, an estimate of disc removal can be made from the tissue recovered. Objective estimates are not possible with the laser techniques because the laser vaporizes the disc in situ. Estimates of removal are based on the amount of time the laser is activated within the disc space. This uncertainty over the exact extent of disc removal is another criticism of the blind percutaneous techniques.

Complications

Experience with the percutaneous techniques has proven them to be safe. As with chemonucleolysis, the most important step in avoiding complications is accurate needle placement. Reported complications include discitis in less than 1%, anecdotal cases of psoas hematoma, and nerve root injury.* Two cases of a cauda equina syndrome have been reported from injury by the nucleotome.[8,38] In at least one of these cases, improper instrument place-

ment resulted in the described injury. The patient also reported an excruciating headache when the nucleotome was activated, which was a warning of dural breech.[38] The potential exists for intraabdominal or vascular injury. A contralateral injury to the ureter has been described.[9]

Despite the lack of reports of intraabdominal injury, there is nothing inherently safer about this procedure than an open discectomy regarding these complications. The procedure is designed to work within the confines of the disc space, and only careful technique and evaluation of instrument position with fluoroscopy will prevent breech of the annulus fibrosus and inadvertent injury to the surrounding structures. Once the cannula has docked on the disc space, within the triangular working zone, it cannot be allowed to migrate. The cannula itself serves as a protective conduit to the disc. By allowing the cannula to come off the annulus, surrounding structures may be injured. A retroperitoneal colon may predispose a patient to an inadvertent bowel injury with the dorsolateral approach. The actual incidence of a retrorenal colon by prone computed tomography (CT) scan is less than 1 in 1000.[15] It still behooves the operating physician to carefully study the preoperative CT or magnetic resonance imaging (MRI) to rule out variations in anatomy, which may place the patient at risk.

Safety regarding the approach and needle/instrument placement may be increased by incorporating imaging techniques. CT-guided stereotaxis for percutaneous uniportal discectomy has been reported in more than 250 patients, without any complications from instrument positioning.[14,23] Frameless image-guided technology is ideally suited for the percutaneous techniques. Constraints with accurate frameless registration in the unopened spine have not yet been worked out, and therefore this technology is not currently available.

Injury to the exiting roots or the lumbar plexus during instrument insertion is avoided with the use of local anesthesia rather than general, epidural, or spinal anesthesia. If the patient complains of nerve root stimulation, the instrument should be repositioned. Therefore, local anesthesia of the nerve root should be avoided. Additionally, excessive intravenous sedation should be avoided because it is essential that the patient be able to answer specific questions regarding painful stimuli. Specifically, the patient must be able to distinguish pain caused by annular fiber stimulation (hip and back pain), from that caused by nerve root stimulation. Use of the endoscope after needle placement, but before insertion of working instruments into the disc space, has been advocated as a method to ensure further that the nerve root is away from the operative portal.[21]

Although there is a role for these indirect percutaneous techniques, it is clear from the literature that strict exclusion criteria must be used to maximize results. Patients with a suspected free fragment disc rupture, spinal stenosis, lateral recess stenosis, or severe neurologic signs such as a cauda equina syndrome, are generally excluded in favor of other treatments. These exclusion criteria eliminate a large percentage of surgical patients.

Endoscopic Discectomy

The marriage of the endoscope with the percutaneous technique was a logical progression. Percutaneous evalua-

---

*References 8,11,38,39,46,47.

tion of the spinal canal, and the endoscopic description of disc pathology were described in 1938.[40,41] Endoscopy was used to improve on the blind technique of percutaneous nucleotomy, by allowing the surgeon to confirm instrument placement and to observe the disc removal from within the disc space.[48,49] The next limitation of the percutaneous procedures to overcome was the inability to remove directly the disc under the nerve root in the spinal canal. Intradiscal approaches could only indirectly remove herniated disc material by pulling it down into the disc space. Endoscopic approaches with a working channel scope were developed to visualize directly (rather than indirectly) and address the pathology at the nerve root level.

Technique

The discoscopic approach brought the endoscope to percutaneous discectomy. This modification was designed to view the dorsal portion of the nucleus pulposus, in an attempt to identify and remove the offending disc material and, at least theoretically, to make the procedure safer and more effective.[48] The procedure uses a biportal approach, with working instruments on one side and an endoscope on the other side. Two operators are required. One removes the disc and the other follows with the endoscope. The initial discectomy is performed in a blind manner. This creates a working space within the disc. Now with the endoscope in the disc space, working instruments are used on the contralateral side to remove disc until the resection cavities meet in the central portion of the disc space. The endoscope is then used to view disc removal. The endoscope and working instruments are commonly changed from side to side to obtain a more comprehensive visualization within the disc space. It is essential to use endoscopes angled off-axis to improve visualization of the dorsal portion of the disc space. With such an angled scope, annular tears may occasionally be identified from within the disc space, and attempted reduction and removal of the nucleus pulposus may be performed. The use of the endoscope changes a blind procedure into a visually directed one. However, limited ability to directly address the herniation with this technique does not allow for effective treatment of sequestered fragments. Therefore, it did not greatly expand the indications for the procedure.

Another focus has been on using the endoscope to modify the traditional procedure by directing attention even more dorsally, in the region of the annular tear.[13,21,29,47] With the trajectory provided by the dorsolateral approach, the end of the cannula is pointed away from the dorsal portion of the disc space and toward the central portion of the disc, instead of toward the herniation. Upbiting flexible instruments and more accurately angled endoscopes provide access and visualization of the dorsal annulus fibrosus that had not been possible with the dorsolateral approach. Visual guidance allows this to be performed with minimal fear of nerve root injury. A randomized study comparing this percutaneous endoscopic technique with open microdiscectomy for contained disc rupture proved it to be as effective at 2 years post-procedure.[29]

Direct Endoscopic Approaches

The desire to expand the patient pool for endoscopic techniques led to the direct endoscopic approaches. With direct approaches, disc material in the spinal canal could be accessed regardless of its relationship to the central disc. The endoscopic transforaminal approach (the foraminoscopic approach) was the first percutaneous approach to visualize directly the pathology of nerve root compression. The epidural space, and any pathology involving either the exiting or traversing nerve root, can be seen through the neural foramen.[28] A uniportal approach, with a small fiberoptic scope and 6-mm working channel, is performed. With the foraminoscopic approach, a more lateral skin entry point for the needle placement, 10 to 12cm from midline, allows for a flatter trajectory, and facilitates visualization of the neuroforamen. Continuous saline irrigation is used to clear the field of frequently encountered venous bleeding. The technique seems particularly well suited for the treatment of far lateral disc herniation, although this represents less than 10% of symptomatic disc rupture. Initial experience with this transforaminal approach is good, but the indications are still limited. Specifically, the small size of the scope and foramen limit size of working instruments and the ability to remove large fragments of disc.

The primary goal of lumbar disc surgery is to decompress the affected nerve root. This may require extensive bony decompression, nerve root manipulation, and/or disc removal. All of the previously mentioned minimally invasive techniques, despite their popularity, have not been able to reproducibly achieve this goal. Therefore, open surgery remains the gold standard.

Microendoscopic Discectomy

The Microendoscopic Discectomy (MED) System was designed to decompress the nerve root by applying standard open surgical techniques through a tubular retractor under direct endoscopic vision. A laminotomy, medial facetectomy, foraminotomy, nerve root retraction, and discectomy are performed in a minimally invasive fashion under direct endoscopic vision. The MED System allows for nerve root decompression using similar instruments and techniques to open surgery, while preserving the advantages of a percutaneous approach. In so doing, the reliability of conventional open surgery has been combined with the benefits of a minimally invasive approach.

Microendoscopic discectomy can be performed under local, regional, or general anesthesia. Patient feedback is not necessary because the nerve root is directly visualized, as with open surgery. The patient is positioned prone. The entry point is approximately one fingerbreadth (1.5cm) off the midline on the symptomatic side, directly over the appropriate disc level. Under lateral fluoroscopy, the guidewire is advanced to the caudal edge of the rostral lamina. The skin incision is extended for a total length of 16mm. Sequential dilators are inserted over the guidewire and each other. The tubular retractor is passed over the largest dilator, down to the lamina. The dilators are removed, establishing an operative corridor. The endoscope is inserted into the tubular retractor. The remaining portion of the case is performed under direct endoscopic vision. Soft tissue overlying the lamina and interlaminar space is removed with a pituitary rongeur. The laminar edge is identified using a curette. If bony work is necessary, a laminotomy and medial facetectomy can be performed with a Kerrison punch or high-speed drill. The ligamentum flavum is opened using a curved curette and Kerrison punch. The nerve root is identified, retracted medially, and the volar epidural space explored. The offending pathology, whether it be a free fragment or a contained herniation, can then be identified and removed. Intradiscal and extradiscal work can be carried out as one would normally perform during a standard open microdiscectomy. The perineural space is explored to ensure adequate decompression. The tubular retractor is removed and the wound closed in a standard fashion.

Laparoscopic Techniques

With the popularity of laparoscopic techniques in abdominal and thoracic surgery, reports of discectomy of the lumbar spine have appeared.[34,36,43] The approach in these cases often involves the general surgeons because complications of the approach require their specific expertise. However, despite improved visual access to the disc, the neural elements cannot be easily visualized. General anesthesia is used for these techniques, which separates them from the other approaches discussed in this chapter. The ventral approach is primarily limited to the L4-5 and L5-S1 disc spaces because of the relation of the aorta and vena cava to the spine.

Complications

The risks with the endoscopic procedures are essentially the same as with the percutaneous procedures, although direct surgical vision should provide a safety factor. For the biportal endoscopic technique, discitis appears to be the most common complication, occurring in 1% to 2% of cases. An arterial injury to a small sigmoid colon branch has been reported because of a bent needle guide.[48] This underscores the importance of accurate needle placement for these techniques.

Currently, the experience with the transforaminal approach and the microendoscopic approach is too limited to have firm data on complications. In a series of 18 patients treated with the transforaminal approach for far-lateral disc herniation, there were no complications encountered.[52] Epidural scar formation is avoided, but scar in the dorsolateral safe zone may occur. It is of unknown significance. Only one complication, an incidental durotomy, was encountered in the initial results with 41 patients using the microendoscopic approach. Epidural cicatrization with this technique is expected to be equal to that of an open approach.

For the lumbar laparoscopic technique, the common complication of transient adynamic ileus can be averted with the use of the retroperitoneal approach, instead of the transperitoneal approach. Discitis and an incisional hernia have been reported.[34] Sexual dysfunction and retrograde ejaculation, as a result of injury to the sacral autonomic plexus, is a risk with closed or open ventral approaches.[24] The advantage of the decreased risk of local versus general anesthesia is lost with this approach. It is

the risk of injury to the great vessels and to the retroperitoneal structures that will likely prevent this technique from achieving preference over an open technique for simple discectomy.

Summary

The percutaneous discectomy techniques are generally safe and well tolerated. Their usefulness is determined by their comparison to the standard treatment of focal disc rupture, open discectomy. Open discectomy and microdiscectomy are accepted as highly effective and well tolerated. With respect to safety and complications, the percutaneous techniques compare favorably to open discectomy. Most percutaneous techniques provide some advantage over an open exposure, such as avoidance of epidural cicatrice formation. Convincing efficacy data, especially compared with open discectomy, are lacking. The indirect techniques do not provide direct access to the offending pathology. Therefore, the number of patients in whom an indirect technique will work is limited and is the subject of much speculation. A direct approach (e.g., the microendoscopic discectomy approach) provides the familiarity and reliability of an open procedure, while maintaining the advantages of a percutaneous one, such as a smaller incision and minimal muscle dissection. However, comparison data for the direct techniques are not available.

Technologic advances, such as three-dimensional endoscopy, heat-free lasers, and frameless stereotaxy, should continue to fuel advances in minimally invasive disc surgery. Patients seek out these techniques for their reputation of less pain and shorter recovery. It behooves the health care provider to be familiar with these treatment modalities. The data clearly show that there are certain patients in whom the procedures are quite effective. The art of surgery will be in understanding the individual patient well enough to provide the best treatment.

REFERENCES

1. Agre K, Wilson RR, Brim M, McDermott DJ: Chymodiactin postmarketing surveillance. *Spine* 9:479, 1984.
2. Boscardin JB, Ringus JC, Feingold DJ, Ruda SC: Human intradiscal levels with cefazolin. *Spine* 17:S145, 1992.
3. Chatterjee S, Foy PM, Findlay GF: Report of a controlled clinical trial comparing automated percutaneous lumbar discectomy and microdiscectomy in the treatment of contained lumbar disc disease. *Spine* 20:734, 1995.
4. Choy DS, Ascher PW, Saddekni S, *et al*: Percutaneous laser disc decompression. *Spine* 17:949, 1992.
5. Choy DSJ, Case RB, Fielding W, *et al*: Percutaneous laser nucleolysis of lumbar discs. *N Engl J Med* 317:771, 1987.
6. Dabezies EJ, Langford K, Morris J, *et al*: Safety and efficacy of chymopapain (Discase) in the treatment of sciatica due to a herniated nucleus pulposus: results of a randomized, double-blind study. *Spine* 13:561, 1988.
7. Eggen PJ, ter Bruggen JP, Wein BB, Tonino AJ: Aseptic spondylodiscitis: a complication of chemonucleolysis? A case report. *Spine* 18:2358-2361, 1993.

8. Epstein NE: Surgically confirmed cauda equina and nerve root injury following percutaneous discectomy at an outside institution: a case report. *J Spinal Disord Tech* 3:380, 1990.

9. Flam TA, Spitzenpfeil E, Steg A, Debre B: Complete ureteral transection associated with percutaneous lumbar disc nucleotomy. *J Urol* 148:1249, 1992.

10. Friedman WA: Percutaneous discectomy: an alternative to chemonucleolysis? *Neurosurgery* 13:542, 1983.

11. Gill K: Retroperitoneal bleeding after automated percutaneous discectomy of the lumbar spine: case report. *Spine* 15:1376, 1990.

12. Gogan WJ, Fraser RD: Chymopapain: a ten year, double-blind study. *Spine* 17:388, 1992.

13. Guyer RD, Kambin P: Arthroscopic microdiscectomy: posterolateral approach. In Regan JJ, McAfee PC, Mack MJ (eds): *Atlas of Endoscopic Spine Surgery.* St Louis, Quality Medical Publishing, 1995, p 257.

14. Heikkinen ER: "Whole body" stereotaxy: application of stereotactic endoscopy to operations of herniated lumbar discs. *Acta Neurochir* 54(suppl):89, 1992.

15. Helms CA, Munk PL, Witt WS, *et al:* Retrorenal colon: implications for percutaneous discectomy. *Radiology* 171:864, 1989.

16. Hijikata S, Yamgishi M, Nakayama T, Oomori K: Percutaneous discectomy: a new treatment method for lumbar disc herniation. *J Toden Hosp* 5:5, 1975.

17. Hoogland T, Scheckenbach C: Low-dose chemonucleolysis combined with percutaneous nucleotomy in herniated cervical discs. *J Spinal Disord Tech* 8:228, 1995.

18. Javid M: A 1- to 4-year follow-up review of treatment of sciatica using chemonucleolysis or laminectomy. *J Neurosurg* 76:184, 1992.

19. Javid MJ, Nordby EJ, Ford LT, *et al:* Safety and efficacy of chymopapain (Chymodiactin) in herniated nucleus pulposus with sciatica: results of a randomized, double-blind study. *JAMA* 249:2489, 1983.

20. Kahanovitz N, Viola K, Goldstein T, Dawson E: A multicenter analysis of percutaneous discectomy. *Spine* 15:713, 1990.

21. Kambin P: Posterolateral percutaneous lumbar discectomy and decompression: arthroscopic microdiscectomy. In Kambin P (ed): *Arthroscopic Microdiscectomy: Minimal Intervention in Spinal Surgery.* Baltimore, Urban & Schwarzenberg, 1991, p 67.

22. Kitchel SH, Brown MD: Complications of chemonucleolysis. *Clin Orthop* 284:63, 1992.

23. Koutrouvelis PG, Lang E: Stereotactic lumbar microdiscectomy. *Neurosurg Clin N Am* 7:49, 1996.

24. Kuslich SD, McAfee PC, Regan JJ: Spinal instrumentation. In Regan JJ, McAfee PC, Mack MJ (eds): *Atlas of Endoscopic Spine Surgery.* St Louis, Quality Medical Publishing, 1995, p 293.

25. Maroon JC, Allen RC: A retrospective study of 1,054 APLD cases: a twenty-month clinical follow-up at 35 U.S. centers. *J Neurol Orthop Med Surg* 10:335, 1989.

26. Maroon JC, Onik G: Percutaneous automated discectomy: a new method for lumbar disc removal. *J Neurosurg* 66:143, 1987.

27. Martins AN, Ramirez A, Johnston J, Schwetschenau PR: Double-blind evaluation of chemonucleolysis for herniated lumbar discs: late results. *J Neurosurg* 49:816, 1978.

28. Mathews HH: Transforaminal endoscopic microdiscectomy. *Neurosurg Clin N Am* 7:59, 1996.

29. Mayer HM, Brock M: Percutaneous endoscopic discectomy: surgical technique and preliminary results compared to microsurgical discectomy. *J Neurosurg* 78:216, 1993.

30. Mixter WJ, Barr JS: Rupture of intervertebral disc with involvement of the spinal canal. *N Engl J Med* 211:201, 1934.

31. Mochida J, Arima T: Percutaneous nucleotomy in lumbar disc herniation: a prospective study. *Spine* 18:2063, 1993.

32. Muralikuttan KP, Hamilton A, Kernohan WG, *et al:* A prospective randomized trial of chemonucleolysis and conventional disc surgery in single level lumbar disc herniation. *Spine* 17:381, 1992.

33. Nordby EJ, Wright PH, Schofield SR: Safety of chemonucleolysis: adverse effects reported in the United States, 1982–1991. *Clin Orthop* 293:122, 1993.

34. Obenchain TG, Cloyd D: Laparoscopic lumbar discectomy: description of transperitoneal and retroperitoneal techniques. *Neurosurg Clin N Am* 7:77, 1996.

35. Ohnmeiss DD, Guyer RD, Hochschuler SH: Laser disc decompression: the importance of proper patient selection. *Spine* 19:2054, 1994.

36. Ominus M, Papin P, Gangloff S: Extraperitoneal approach to the lumbar spine with video assistance. *Spine* 21:2491, 1996.

37. Onik G, Helms CA, Ginsberg L, *et al:* Percutaneous lumbar discectomy using a new aspiration probe. *AJR* 144:1137, 1985.

38. Onik G, Maroon JC, Jackson R: Cauda equina syndrome secondary to an improperly placed nucleotome probe. *Neurosurgery* 30:412, 1992.

39. Onik G, Mooney V, Maroon JC, *et al:* Automated percutaneous discectomy: a prospective multi-institutional study. *Neurosurgery* 26:228, 1990.

40. Pool JL: Direct visualization of dorsal nerve roots of the cauda equina by means of a myeloscope. *Arch Neurol Psych* 39:1308, 1938.

41. Pool JL: Myeloscopy: intraspinal endoscopy. *Surgery* 11:169, 1942.

42. Quigley MR, Maroon JC: Laser discectomy: a review. *Spine* 19:53, 1994.

43. Regan JJ: Percutaneous endoscopic thoracic discectomy. *Neurosurg Clin N Am* 7:87, 1996.

44. Revel M, Payan C, Vallee C, *et al:* Automated percutaneous lumbar discectomy versus chemonucleolysis in the treatment of sciatica. *Spine* 18:1, 1993.

45. Rhoten RL, Murphy MA, Kalfas IH, *et al:* Antibiotic penetration into cervical discs. *Neurosurgery* 37:418, 1995.

46. Savitz MH: Same-day microsurgical arthroscopic lateral-approach laser-assisted (SMALL) fluoroscopic discectomy. *J Neurosurg* 80:1039, 1994.

47. Schaffer JL, Kambin P: Percutaneous posterolateral lumbar discectomy and decompression with a 6.9 millimeter cannula: analysis of operative failures and complications. *J Bone Joint Surg* 73:822, 1991.

48. Schreiber A, Leu H: Percutaneous nucleotomy: technique with discoscopy. *Orthopedics* 14:439, 1991.

49. Schreiber A, Suezawa Y: Transdiscoscopic percutaneous nucleotomy in disc herniation. *Orthop Rev* 15:75, 1986.

50. Smith L: Enzyme dissolution of the nucleus pulposus in humans. *JAMA* 265:137, 1964.
51. Smith L: Chemonucleolysis: personal history, trials, and tribulations. *Clin Orthop* 287:117, 1991.
52. Smith MM, Foley KT, Ondra SL: Endoscopic working channel discectomy for far lateral disk herniation. Presented at the CNS Annual Meeting, San Francisco, CA, October 1995 (Abstract).
53. Zhou YC, Zhou YQ, Wang CY: Percutaneous cervical discectomy for treating cervical disc herniation: a report of 12 cases. *J Tongji Med Univ* 14:110, 1994.

CHAPTER 51

The Black Disc

Kenneth S. Yonemura and Hansen A. Yuan

The importance of degenerative processes involved with the development of magnetic resonance imaging (MRI) findings referred to as "black disc disease" should not be overlooked. Unfortunately, the common use of the MRI description of the intervertebral disc does not by itself indicate pathology that consistently results in clinical symptoms. Nevertheless, there are distinct situations in which significant clinical symptoms can occur and, with appropriate screening, surgical intervention may be beneficial.

In the simplest form, the degenerative process of disc dehydration resulting in the "black disc," is common to all disc spaces in the body and is the earliest sign of normal osteoarthritis of the spine. Thus, a method to distinguish between symptomatic versus asymptomatic degeneration of the disc space has been developed. A common sequela of disc degeneration was discussed in the prior chapter and involves herniation of disc material into the spinal canal with nerve root or spinal cord compression. The symptomatic "black disc," however, refers to intrinsic changes in the disc that can result in primary joint pain without compression of the traversing spinal nerve roots or spinal cord.

An alternative term for this process, *internal disc disruption*, was initially described by Crock[8] in 1970 and further presented in his presidential address to the International Society for the Study of the Lumbar Spine (ISSLS). More recently, the term *internal annular tear* has been used based on subtle findings on high-resolution MRI and lumbar discography; this also would be synonymous with a symptomatic annular tear. The pain provocative aspect of discography has also led to the use of the term *discogenic pain* which can be seen in cases of annular degeneration without a discrete tear. For consistency in this chapter, the terms *annular tear* and *annular degeneration* are used in reference to discogenic pain. Less specific terms such as *black disc disease*, *dark disc disease*, *post-laminectomy syndrome*, and *failed back syndrome* should be avoided in favor of more specific terminology.

Historically, a distinction has not been made between studies examining the cause and treatment of radicular leg pain, as compared to axial back pain. Though radicular pain may be associated with axial back pain, it is also recognized that axial back pain may occur independently. Thus, it is difficult to obtain accurate or reasonable epidemiologic estimates for the incidence, prevalence, or natural history of discogenic pain, as compared to radiculopathy with axial back pain.

Prior to the advent of axial tomography and MRI, myelography was used extensively to localize spinal canal pathology resulting in nerve root compression. Discography was introduced by Lindblom[19] to evaluate the disc anatomy, and it was Hirsh[13] who first described the provocation and localization of axial back pain despite a normal myelographic study. As is discussed later, the use of discography is imperative for the diagnosis of discogenic pain.

Etiology of Pain

The development of intractable axial back pain in the face of "normal" degenerative changes in the lumbar discs has definitely created some controversy. Although the most common sources for midline axial back pain remain muscular or ligamentous injuries, chronic pain with specific postural changes has been attributed to the facet joints or intervertebral discs. This is the focus of this chapter. The natural history with progressive disc collapse and loss of mobility of the functional spine unit should lead to gradual resolution. However, the time course can vary widely. The dilemma, therefore, lies in the lack of understanding why intervertebral discs with nearly identical morphology should behave differently, with some chronically painful and others asymptomatic.[19]

The lumbar disc is supplied with pain fibers from the sympathetic chain via the sinuvertebral nerve[9] that innervates the outer six layers of the annulus fibrosus.[11] Stimulation of these pain fibers can occur from noxious breakdown products of the nucleus pulposis or from mechanical stimulation. Following injury to the annulus fibrosus, sprouting of pain fibers into the site of injury has been observed and may also be a factor in the formation of a symptomatic annular tear.[7] Pressure within the disc space has been shown to be greatest in the sitting position and, therefore, the association of sitting intolerance and resolution with recumbency fit well for a mechanical basis of pain. An annular tear may allow disc material to extend into the outer region of the disc with mechanical stimulation of the c-fibers mediating pain.

A wide variety of putative inflammatory agents have been reported to occur in the nucleus pulposus as part of the degenerative process and are listed in Figure 51.1. Of potential putative agents, phospholipase A2 has received significant attention.[22] Other agents may ultimately be shown to be of greater importance.[10,15] Leakage of these substances into the outer annulus may be one mechanism of pain generation, and exposure of the dorsal root ganglion has also been shown to result in histologic damage to the myelin sheaths and ganglion.[6,16] This inflammatory process may be the basis of neuropathic pain, which may also accompany discogenic pain.

Clinical Presentation

Frequently, low back pain and radicular leg pain are felt to have a common etiology: nerve root compression. In a majority of cases, this assumption is true. However, the art of the practice of spine surgery lies in the desire and ability to detect subtle patterns of pain that are atypical for classic radiculopathy. The presence of atypical pain should prompt the collection of additional data and the inclusion of further testing based on a larger differential diagnosis.

626

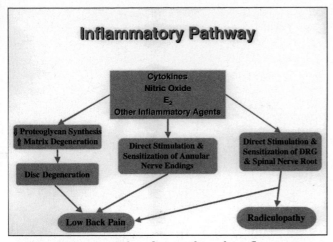

Figure 51.1 Potential mediators of annular inflammation.

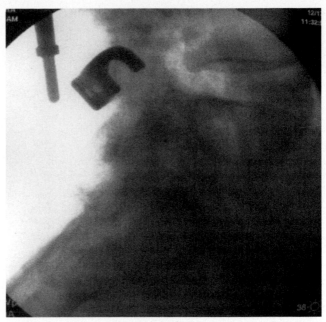

Figure 51.2 A 35-year-old female with scoliosis treated with a T6-L4 Harrington rod fusion 20 years earlier has symptoms of primary right-sided lumbosacral back pain without radiculopathy. Hook dislodgment at L4 with L3-4 pseudoarthrosis noted on plain films.

Not uncommonly, lumbar disc herniations have a history of acute back pain at onset, prior to the development of radicular leg pain. On further questioning, some of these patients acknowledge the complete resolution of their original back pain with a delayed but acute onset of radicular leg pain. Though cause and effect are difficult to prove, it is not inconceivable that the initial symptoms of a symptomatic annular tear resolved as internal pressure on the annular pain fibers decreased with herniation of nuclear material into the spinal canal.

A hallmark of a symptomatic annular tear is a pattern of activity-related back pain that is characterized by sitting intolerance and relief with recumbency. The lumbosacral back pain is usually described as a deep midline aching discomfort, which frequently extends into the gluteal region and occasionally radiates into the lower extremities. The leg pain that arises from a symptomatic annular tear may be mistaken for true radiculopathy but typically extends into the dorsal thigh. It rarely extends below the knee. Occasionally, pain can be described as extending distally into the foot but in the absence of nerve root compression on MRI. This may be best described as pseudoradiculitis. The treatment of discogenic pain should be reserved for patients resistant to conservative management because a majority of patients note slow resolution over 3 to 6 months.

Despite the description of significant pain, the physical examination is usually normal. On close observation, there may be a tendency for frequent changes in position and a relative intolerance to sitting, especially forward flexion. The absence of physical findings may prompt the diagnosis of malingering or psychogenic pain. Formal psychometric testing should be used liberally to rule out potential psychosocial issues and to quantify the effect of longstanding pain on coping mechanisms. Many of these factors, as well as the presence of active litigation have been shown to be predictive of a poor outcome with surgical treatment.[4] Close observation of the patient by the surgeon at the time of discography can be helpful and a formal psychometric evaluation can be invaluable.[2]

In addition to pain of discogenic origin, there are alternative sources of activity-related back pain. Facet pain has frequently been implicated, based on facet arthropathy and relief with facet injections or rhizolysis procedures. Tumors may occasionally be associated with vague back pain symptoms but are rarely missed with current MRI scan technology. Osteoporotic or pathologic fractures frequently present with isolated back pain but are easily recognized with standard radiographs and acutely with MRI. Isthmic spondylolisthesis is also commonly felt to result in chronic back pain but may be asymptomatic, except acutely in the adolescent or with radiculopathy in the adult. An incomplete transitional vertebra syndrome with unilateral or bilateral pseudojoint formation can also be a potential source. This can be easily missed without an angled anteroposterior (Ferguson's) view of the lumbosacral junction (Figures 51.2 and 51.3).

Diagnostic Testing

Without specialized testing, discogenic pain is not adequately assessed by conventional radiographs, CT, and MRI. Standard spine radiographs are warranted to rule out vertebral instability, but otherwise are not helpful in the diagnosis of a symptomatic annular tear. Osteophyte formation and foraminal narrowing may also be observed, but the absence of true radicular pain makes these findings relevant only if there is concomitant spinal stenosis with a history of claudication.

A unique MRI finding in the dorsal annulus fibrosus, referred to as a high-intensity zone (HIZ) lesion, has been described.[26] This finding, consisting of a discrete bright zone within the dorsal annulus, has been felt to represent either disc material visualized within an annular tear or edema fluid located within the dorsal annulus (Figures 51.4 and 51.5). This finding may be helpful in localizing

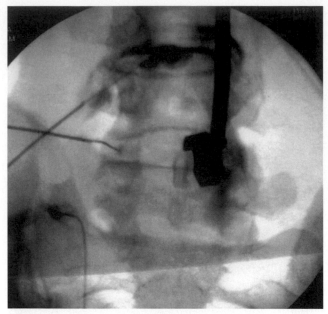

Figure 51.3 Anteroposterior fluoroscopic images show needle placement with injection of the L3-4 disc and right L5-S1 pseudojoint formation. Unilateral enlargement of the right L5 transverse process with articulation with the sacrum and pelvis is noted. Injection of the pseudojoint as demonstrated resulted in concordant pain reproduction.

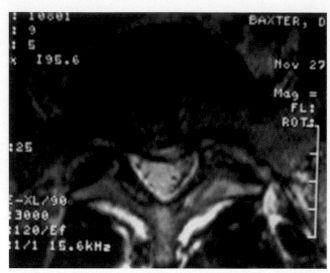

Figure 51.5 The axial T2 MRI demonstrates the L5-S1 high intensity zone lesion without significant central or lateral recess stenosis.

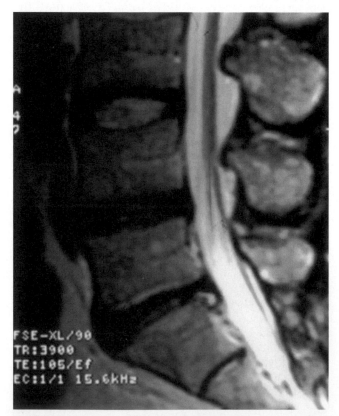

Figure 51.4 A 53-year-old male with chronic intractable axial back pain and sitting intolerance. Sagittal T2 MRI demonstrates the L5-S1 high intensity zone lesion.

the site of pain. However, it may also be asymptomatic.[5,14] Additional findings have been characterized by Modic that describe changes in the vertebral bodies adjacent to the affected disc space.

Recently, studies have indicated the association of Modic[3] type 1 findings with discogenic pain. However, the sensitivity of this finding has been questioned.

Clearly the MRI findings are not independently diagnostic, and clinical correlation can only be obtained with provocative testing of the disc space via discography,[12] if at all. Lumbar discography was initially described by Lindblom[19] in 1948 for evaluation of disc herniations, but with the advent of water-soluble contrast agents and MRI, discography has been used primarily for the evaluation of discogenic pain with chronic axial back pain.

Discography involves the injection of water-soluble iodine contrast into the disc with the observation of the contrast pattern, volume of injection, effect of pressure, and, most importantly, the patient's pain response (Figures 51.6 and 51.7). If there are lateralizing symptoms, the reproduction of the pain at the time of discography may be helpful to determine the level of concordance based on the development of the patient's typical referred pain. This should not be confused with true radiculopathy. Though the development of concordant pain is key, equally important is the absence of significant pain from a control level.

Discography requires the use of fluoroscopy for localization but does not necessarily require a biplane facility. Coaxial placement of a 6-inch, 22-gauge spinal needle through a standard length 18-gauge spinal needle minimizes the potential for iatrogenic discitis. The trajectory is usually paramedian. Typically, the entry point is 8 to 10cm from the midline. At L5-S1, disc entry can be difficult because of the limitation of the iliac crests, combined with large facet joints. However, entry into the disc space can usually be attained by placing a gentle curve in the tip of the 22-gauge needle. Occasionally, a midline transdural approach may be required at L5-S1.

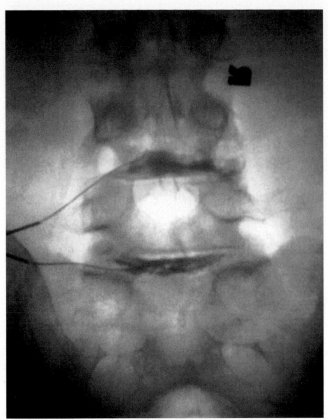

Figure 51.6 The anteroposterior fluoroscopic image demonstrated needle position and contrast pattern following L4-5 and L5-S1 contrast injection.

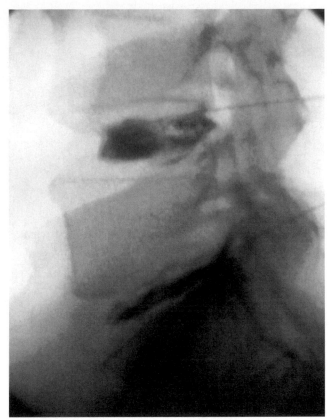

Figure 51.7 The lateral fluoroscopic image shows nonspecific degenerative findings at both L4-5 and L5-S1. Concordant pain was noted at L5-S1 and no significant pain was noted at L4-5.

Injection of contrast media should be to a firm endpoint and the volume injected should be recorded. The use of manometry may help standardize the injection process. Close observation and recording of the pattern and intensity of the pain response must be made. The reliability of this information is intimately related to accurate communication between the patient and physician. Therefore, sedation during the test should be minimized and avoided if possible. A discogram should not be considered positive or concordant without exact reproduction of the patient's typical pain. Based on the need for clinical correlation, the operating surgeon may be in the best position to assess the validity of the test, whether through the direct performance of the procedure or by review of a video recording of the procedure.

The various radiographic appearances of the disc space containing contrast material has been described and grading systems have been devised. The observed contrast patterns have not, however, been shown to be associated with clinical symptoms (Figure 51.8). Computed tomographic images are usually obtained immediately after the injection and may help with operative planning, especially for percutaneous treatment strategies that involve direct treatment of a demonstrated annular tear.

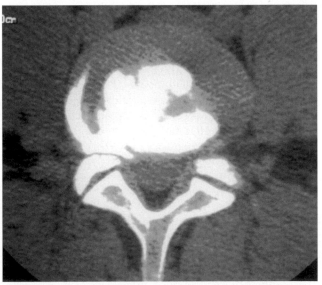

Figure 51.8 The axial CT following disc injection shows an asymptomatic L4-5 annular tear.

Percutaneous treatments are highly desirable from a patient standpoint but appear to have a more limited application at the early stages of the degenerative cascade. During the early stages, the lack of advanced disc space collapse provides an environment that facilitates the manipulation of catheters, electrodes, and endoscopic instruments within the disc space (Figures 51.9 to 51.11).

Treatment

Various treatment strategies are currently available for discogenic pain with widely differing levels of complexity.

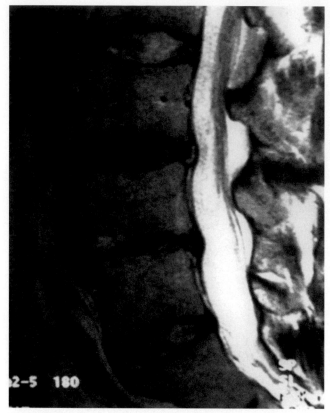

Figure 51.9 A 45-year-old female with intractable back lumbar back pain. The T$_2$-weighted MRI scan demonstrates a high intensity zone lesion at L3-4. Discography was concordant solely at L3-4.

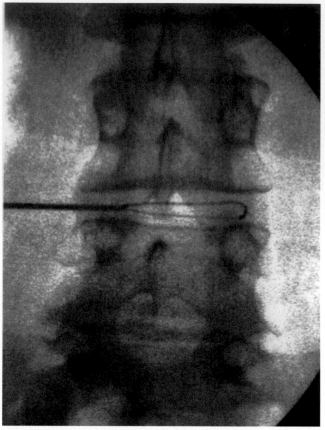

Figure 51.10 An anteroposterior fluoroscopic image showing the intradiscal electrothermal therapy catheter positioned within the L3-4 disc space.

The potential for direct treatment of an internal annular tear has prompted the development of two disparate forms of treatment. The first involves the placement of a resistive heating coil catheter into the dorsal annulus, intradiscal electrothermal therapy (IDET).[23-25] With heating of the coil to 90°C, the temperature of the surrounding annular tissue is elevated. Denervation occurs at greater than 45°C and denaturation of collagen fibers above 65°C. The denaturation, through cross-link disruption, results in contraction of collagen fibers and may promote healing of annular tears. The acute effects of IDET have been questioned,[17] but the long-term effects are of greater importance. A recent prospective randomized of the IDET procedure has shown significant differences between controls and treated patients at 6 months.[21]

A second form of direct treatment involves the intradiscal treatment of annular tears with the use of endoscopy and laser annuloplasty. Recent reports from Yeung[27] indicate the effectiveness of this treatment, but it remains to be seen if the technique can be standardized and replicated.

In cases of advanced disc space collapse or with failure of percutaneous treatment, surgical fusion of the affected disc space can also be offered. The relative merits of ventral versus dorsal procedures will be discussed in other chapters. As a basic rule, the presence of significant intracanal pathology usually indicates the need for a dorsal approach for spinal canal decompression and may be combined with a ventral interbody or dorsal fusion, based on surgeon preference. Although caution regarding surgical treatment of internal disc disruption has been advocated,[28] there have been some published series with exceptional results.[18] Ultimately, the permanent changes in spinal biomechanics and morbidity of fusion procedures may be counterproductive in the long run.

More recently, the potential for joint reconstruction has prompted several clinical trials involving either the use of a prosthetic nucleus pulposus or total disc replacement. The prosthetic nucleus has concentrated on the use of hydrogel polymers that rely on the natural bone end plates for support, versus disc replacement strategies that use paired metallic end plates and core substance, usually ultra high molecular weight polyethylene (Figure 51.12). Both forms of disc replacement have been used clinically for many years in Europe, and clinical trials in the United States are currently under way.

One form of total disc replacement, PRODISC®, was implanted in 64 patients in Europe by two surgeons from 1990 through 1993. Minimum follow-up of 7 years was obtained in 61 patients, of whom 33% underwent 2 level implantation. There was no evidence of implant subsidence or implant failure, and none of the implants required removal. Severe back pain was noted in 77.8% of the patients prior to implantation and this decreased to 9.3% following PRODISC® insertion with 56.4% with only mild or no reported pain. Overall, 92.7% of the

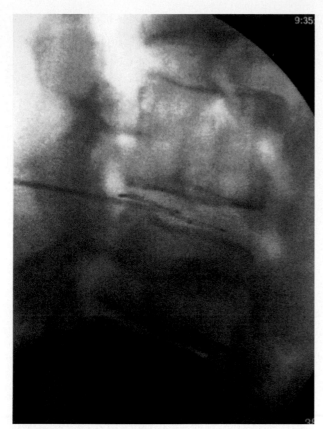

Figure 51.11 A lateral fluoroscopic image shows the intradiscal electrothermal therapy catheter located correctly in the posterior annulus at the site of the high intensity zone lesion.

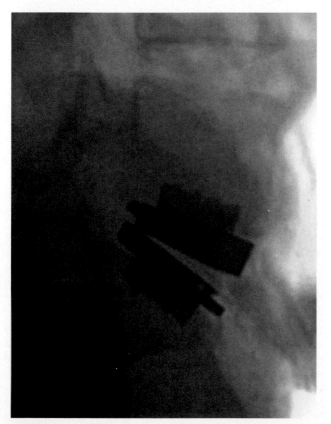

Figure 51.12 A lateral fluoroscopic image showing implantation of a PRODISC® at L5-S1.

patients were satisfied with the results of the surgery. Bertagnoli,[1] who found similar results in 108 patients with 90.8% excellent results and no associated implant failures or complications, has now replicated this initial pilot study.

Summary

Literature and experience over the past 25 years has substantiated the existence of discogenic pain, whether associated with discrete annular tears or diffuse annular degeneration. This literature supports the premise that there may be both mechanical and biochemical factors involved in the genesis of discogenic pain. Standard diagnostic tests alone are not sufficient to make the diagnosis, and close observation with provocative testing is mandatory. Ultimately, the restoration of biomechanical function, elimination the painful spinal motion segment, and avoidance of fusion morbidity should be the goals of future treatment strategies.

REFERENCES

1. Bertagnoli R, Kumar S: Indications for full prosthetic disc arthroplasty: a correlation of clinical outcome against a variety of indications. *Eur Spine J* 11(suppl 2):S131-S136, 2002.
2. Block AR, Vanharanta H, Ohnmeiss DD, Guyer RD: Discographic pain report: influence of psychological factors. *Spine* 21(3):334-338, 1996.
3. Braithwaite I, White J, Saifuddin A, *et al:* Vertebral end-plate (Modic) changes on lumbar spine MRI: correlation with pain reproduction at lumbar discography. *Eur Spine J* 7(5):363-368, 1998.
4. Carragee EJ: Is lumbar discography a determinate of discogenic low back pain: provocative discography reconsidered. *Curr Rev Pain* 4(4):301-308, 2000.
5. Carragee EJ, Paragioudakis SJ, Khurana S: 2000 Volvo Award winner in clinical studies: lumbar high-intensity zone and discography in subjects without low back problems. *Spine* 25(23):2987-2992, 2000.
6. Chen C, Cavanaugh JM, Ozaktay AC, *et al:* Effects of phospholipase A_2 on lumbar nerve root structure and function. *Spine* 22(10):1057-1064, 1997.
7. Coppes MH, Marani E, Thomeer RT, Groen GJ: Innervation of "painful" lumbar discs. *Spine* 22(20): 2342-2349; discussion 2349-2350, 1997.
8. Crock HV: The presidential address: ISSLS, internal disc disruption, a challenge to disc prolapse fifty years on. *Spine* 11: 650-653, 1986.
9. Edgar MA, Ghadially JA: Innervation of the lumbar spine. *Clin Orthop* (115):35-41, 1976.
10. Gronblad M, Virri J, Ronkko S, *et al:* A controlled biochemical and immunohistochemical study of human synovial-type (group II) phospholipase A2 and inflammatory cells in macroscopically normal, degenerated, and herniated human lumbar disc tissues. *Spine* 21(22):2531-2538, 1996.
11. Gronblad M, Weinstein JN, Santavirta S: Immunohistochemical observations on spinal tissue innervation: a review of hypothetical mechanisms of back pain. *Acta Orthop Scand* 62(6):614-622, 1991.

12. Guyer RD, Ohnmeiss DD: Lumbar discography. Position statement from the North American Spine Society Diagnostic and Therapeutic Committee [see comments]. *Spine* 20(18):2048-2059, 1995.

13. Hirsh C, Schazowicz F: Studies on structural changes in the lumbar annulus fibrosus. *Acta Orthop Scand* 22:184-223, 1952.

14. Ito M, Incorvaia KM, Yu SF, *et al:* Predictive signs of discogenic lumbar pain on magnetic resonance imaging with discography correlation. *Spine* 23(11):1252-1258; discussion 1259-1260, 1998.

15. Kang JD, Stefanovic-Racic M, McIntyre LA, *et al:* Toward a biochemical understanding of human intervertebral disc degeneration and herniation. *Spine* 22(10):1065-1073, 1997.

16. Kawakami M, Tamaki T, Hashizume H, *et al:* The role of phospholipase A_2 and nitric oxide in pain-related behavior produced by an allograft of intervertebral disc material to the sciatic nerve of the rat. *Spine* 22(10):1074-1079, 1997.

17. Kleinstueck FS, Diederich CJ, Nau WH, *et al:* Acute biomechanical and histological effects of intradiscal electrothermal therapy on human lumbar discs. *Spine* 26(20):2198-2207, 2001.

18. Lee CK, Vessa P, Lee JK: Chronic disabling low back pain syndrome caused by internal disc derangements. *Spine* 20(3):356-361, 1995.

19. Lindblom K: Diagnostic puncture of intervertebral discs in sciatica. *Acta Orthop Scand* 17:231-239, 1948.

20. Nachemson A, Zdeblick TA, O'Brien JP: Lumbar disc disease with discogenic pain. What surgical treatment is most effective? *Spine* 21(15):1835-1838, 1996.

21. Pauza K, *et al:* A randomized, double-blind, placebo controlled trial evaluating the efficacy of intradiscal electrothermal annuloplasty (IDET™) for the treatment of chronic discogenic low back pain: 6-month outcomes. In *International Spinal Injection Society*. Austin, TX, 2002.

22. Saal JS, Franson RC, Dobrow R, *et al:* High levels of inflammatory phospholipase A_2 activity in lumbar disc herniations. *Spine* 15:674-678, 1990.

23. Saal JA, Saal JS: Intradiscal electrothermal treatment for chronic discogenic low back pain: a prospective outcome study with minimum 1-year follow-up. *Spine* 25(20): 2622-2627, 2000.

24. Saal JA, Saal JS: Intradiscal electrothermal treatment for chronic discogenic low back pain: prospective outcome study with a minimum 2-year follow-up. *Spine* 27(9):966-973; discussion 973-974, 2002.

25. Saal JS, Saal JA: Management of chronic discogenic low back pain with a thermal intradiscal catheter: a preliminary report. *Spine* 25(3):382-388, 2000.

26. Schellhas KP, Pollei SR, Gundry CR, Heithoff KB: Lumbar disc high-intensity zone: correlation of magnetic resonance imaging and discography. *Spine* 21(1):79-86, 1996.

27. Yeung AT, Tsou PM: Posterolateral endoscopic excision for lumbar disc herniation: Surgical technique, outcome, and complications in 307 consecutive cases. *Spine* 27(7): 722-731, 2002.

28. Zdeblick TA: The treatment of degenerative lumbar disorders: a critical review of the literature. *Spine* 20 (24 suppl):126S-137S, 1995.

CHAPTER 52

Cervical Spondylosis

Richard L. Saunders, Edward C. Benzel, and Henry Bohlman

Background

In the closing years of the nineteenth century, a time of increasing scientific medicine, the understanding of spinal disease was confounded by a lack of imaging, the prevalence of tuberculous spinal "caries," and the terms *protruded disc* for osteophyte, and *enchondroma* for disc fragment. There was a nihilistic perception that the osteophytes so commonly found at autopsy were inconsequential because in life they were not ordinarily associated with a crippling impairment. The term *spondylitis* was and is often still used interchangeably for spondylosis. Clinical neurologists resorted to fanciful descriptive diagnoses for neurologic problems that were likely the complications of spondylosis. Rail travel ultimately would prove important in recognizing the potential clinical importance of cervical spondylosis. A near epidemic of railcar collisions and their attendant liability would lead to the concept of acceleration injuries. Accident claims described subjective complaints with features suspiciously similar to those we now recognize as the central cord syndrome, for which the diagnoses spinal cord "congestion" or "anemia" were coined.

Other markers of the unfolding story of cervical spondylosis were the long uncertainty of the cause of soft disc fragments and the beginnings of surgery of the spinal nervous system. Early pathologic confusion of disc sequestra with cartilaginous tumors would persist until the 1930s.[17] A pioneer of neurologic surgery, Sir Victor Horsley would be credited with the first procedure for the clinical diagnosis of symptomatic cervical disc. His operative note suggests that the operation involved the decompression of an osteophyte. That compressive osteophytes had the "potential" for neurologic impairment had been appreciated a century earlier. Whether or not Horsley's osteophyte was, in fact, the clinical culprit remains doubtful in that his quadriplegic patient also had signs of optic neuritis before complete recovery with Sir Victor's surgery. Another 60 years would pass before the landmark paper of Russell Brain appeared in *Brain*, characterizing the neurologic consequences of spondylosis.[3]

Pathology of Spondylosis

Cervical spondylosis is a ubiquitous degenerative disease that affects primarily the intervertebral disc, the facet joint, and related ligaments. It worsens with age and inordinate stress (e.g., trauma, ongoing or in the past). These changes take on clinical significance in the presence of congenital spinal canal narrowing and/or consequential segmental derangements, such as kyphosis and instability.

The basic aging process of spondylosis involves the desiccation of the nucleus pulposis with resulting disc space narrowing. These changes are related to decreases in disc proteoglycans, substances that are critical to water transfer and nucleus health.[4] There probably is a familial propensity to spinal aging. Cigarette smoking potentiates the process by an adverse affect on chondrocytes, in particular. Curiously, however, fibrous tissue metaplasia to chondrocytes and, in turn, cartilage ossification, are pathologic changes seen in spondylosis

Both major trauma and relatively minor trauma such as acceleration injury can set the stage for subsequent spondylotic changes. Injury to the annulus fibrosus initiates a repair process that often includes the formation of osteophytes at and around the insertion of the annular ligament. Injury to the disc may lead to internal fragmentation of the nucleus. Trauma leads to minor tears of the facet joint cartilage. This may result in a reparative process that includes arthritic lipping. The role of injury to the dorsal ligaments, in particular the interspinous ligaments, is often overlooked. These structures are particularly vulnerable in flexion injuries of the cervical spine. Excessive stretch of these ligaments, with very small tears, may never allow return to the premorbid length and elasticity, thus permitting secondary changes to take place. Ligamentous laxity may have a detrimental effect on the lordotic curve. Subclinical trauma is inherent to many occupations (e.g., hod carriers, dentists, violinists). Older swimmers may be subject to accelerated cervical spine degeneration. Chronic vibration has been shown to have a deleterious effect on lumbar discs.[26]

Whereas the aforementioned spinal pathologies are the essential changes of spondylosis, it is the spine's consequential architectural changes that have clinical relevance. Among these are foraminal and canal stenosis, alteration of the cervical lordosis, and changes in cervical mobility (Figure 52.1). Narrowing of the neuroforamina is primarily the result of facet joint degenerative disease and hypertrophy, but is also related to loss of disc height.

Spinal narrowing is caused by osteophyte formation at the disc margin ventrally and shingling dorsally. Shingling can be thought of as the combined result of loss of disc height, facet joint narrowing, and postural lordosis or hyperlordosis. The spinal canal can also be narrowed because of infolding of the ligamentum flavum as the cervical spine is telescoped from the degenerative disc changes. The normal, slightly lordotic posture is usually altered to a straightened curve. Kyphosis, and the less common hyperlordosis, are the extreme forms of postural change.

Mobility of the cervical spine is often altered in spondylosis. Not infrequently, mobility is reduced with disc hardening and osteophyte formation. Facet joint

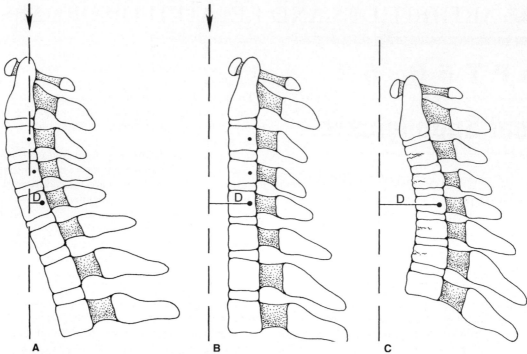

Figure 52.1 **(A)** In the normal spine the dorsal vertebral body height is less than the ventral height. As the degenerative process proceeds, ventral disc height is lost and the spine "straightens." **(B)** A moment arm *(D)* is thus created. This predisposes to further deformation after the application of axial loads. **(C)** A kyphosis results.

degenerative changes add to this general reduction in mobility. Severe changes may result in almost total resorption of the disc and segmental autofusion at one or more levels. In other patients, facet joint degeneration, perhaps with laxity of capsular ligaments, results in segmental hypermobility and olisthesis. Excessive segmental translation at upper cervical interspaces in association with lower cervical immobility is a relatively common finding in the elderly patient presenting with clumsy hand myelopathy (Table 52.1).

Neuropathology Associated with Spondylosis

Permanent changes in the spinal cord and nerve roots, as well as their coverings, represent the most serious problems complicating spondylosis. Nerve root sleeve fibrosis and intradural fibrosis have been appreciated since the work of Frykholm in 1951.[11] Adherence of the richly innervated dura mater to the surrounding bony and cartilaginous structures in the neuroforamen may be a source of pain.

Chronic changes in the spinal cord may take the form of spinal cord atrophy and, in fact, have the histologic appearance of infarction. The latter is recognized as a bright signal change observed on T_2-weighted magnetic resonance imaging (MRI). The role of dural adhesions, spinal cord tethering by arachnoid scar, and microvascular changes in spondylotic myelopathy are not well understood. Dentate ligaments, once believed to play a prominent role in the pathophysiology of cervical spondylotic myelopathy, probably have some minor importance in the tethering of the spinal cord against a rough osteophytic ridge in the presence of a kyphotic deformity of the cervical spine.[15]

Clinical Correlates of Spondylosis

Cervical spondylosis generally presents with one or more of the following signs: axial pain, arm pain, and myelopathy. Consequent symptoms may occur alone or in combination, although it is recognized that often even severe myelopathy is not associated with neck pain.

Axial Pain

Axial or neck pain may be caused by facet joint inflammation from loading, ligamentous stretching, postural strain, or spinal cord impingement. It may also result from input from the dorsal primary division(s) of a compressed and irritated cervical nerve root or annular pain fibers. The management of neck pain is more difficult and less rewarding than dealing with other clinical problems related to cervical spondylosis. The challenge is at least twofold: (1) defining the source of pain and (2) identifying a specific therapeutic maneuver to deal with the pain. Muscles, particularly the dorsal paraspinous muscles, may be a source of pain (myofascial pain). One should also consider the viscera and vessels of the neck as a possible source of pain in rare cases.

Arm Pain

Arm pain, usually in a dermatomal distribution, results from compression of the corresponding cervical nerve root or roots and ganglia. More severe nerve root compression may result in muscle weakness and atrophy, and sensory symptoms of tingling or numbness.

TABLE 52.1

Pathology and Clinical Status Assessment

	Plain Radiography Including Flexion Extension Views	Magnetic Resonance Imaging	Myelography	Computed Tomography	Injection of Local Anesthetic	Electro Diagnostics
Disc degeneration	X	X		X	X°	
Canal narrowing or shingling	X	X	X			
Alteration in curvature	X	X	X			
Alteration in mobility and facet joint disease	X				X†	
Neuroforaminal narrowing	X	X	X	X	X‡	X
Spinal canal narrowing	X	X	X	X		

°Injected into a disc suspected of being a source of pain
†Injected into a facet joint suspected of being a source of pain.
‡Injected at the level of a neuroforamen to identify the particular nerve root or roots associated with the patient's pain.

Myelopathy

Myelopathy can result from spinal canal narrowing from disc protrusion, ventral spinal canal osteophytes, laminar shingling, ligamentous infolding, and microvasculature changes. Usually these architectural changes take on myelopathic significance only in the face of congenital stenosis of the spinal canal.[16] It is, however, not uncommon to see asymptomatic patients whose MRI scans show variably severe osteophytic indentation of the spinal cord or nerve root sleeves.[25] If such patients have no abnormal findings on neurologic examination, they should be followed indefinitely, because they will not infrequently develop correlative signs and symptoms and benefit from early diagnosis and treatment.

Cooper's group[5] has analyzed the pattern of myelopathic deficit in a surgical cohort. An impairment of hand function was present in 75% of their patients, and the most common motor finding was weakness of hand intrinsics. Gait difficulties and upper extremity sensory symptoms were the most frequent complaints (greater than 80%). Proximal weakness and spasticity characterized the gait dysfunction. Bladder dysfunction was reported in 10% of cases. Bilateral hand impairment can be almost entirely subjective and commonly has been diagnosed and treated as carpal tunnel syndrome. Even in the face of finger astereognosis and prehension loss, there may be no gait findings, spasticity, or Babinski sign. This potentially confounding picture for the generalist has been referred to as the "clumsy hand syndrome."

Medical Management

A trial of nonoperative therapy is the rule, ordinarily, for patients who have only neck or arm pain or whose symptoms of paresthesias are of nerve root rather than cord origin. Treatment modalities include rest, traction, analgesics, antiinflammatory agents, and drugs for muscle spasm.

Depending on the severity of symptoms, bed rest with the head and neck in a nonweight-bearing position may be necessary. In less severe pain syndromes, local immobilization with a firm neck support may provide symptomatic relief. Large pillow use, a propensity of the elderly, should be eliminated. There is often an association of symptom escalation from sustained automobile travel.

Sometimes traction is helpful to reduce pressure against a nerve root. To be most effective, it should be applied several times a day. Most patients tolerate 10 to 12 lb of traction for 15 minutes. It is vital that patients maintain their head and neck in a neutral position throughout the period of traction. Neck extension, in particular, is to be avoided. A few degrees of flexion are usually well tolerated. If, however, patients report that traction increases their pain, this form of treatment should be discontinued, as long as it has been established that the patient had been applying it correctly.

Analgesics should be provided as indicated. Allowing the patient to remain in severe pain sometimes causes an awkward compensatory position, itself a source of new pain. Acetaminophen (without or with codeine), propoxyphene, hydrocodone, or oxycodone may all be used sparingly in appropriate dosages. Stronger narcotic medication is rarely necessary.

Antiinflammatory medication may be very helpful. A large number of such medications are now available. Occasionally it is beneficial to administer short courses of oral steroids (methylprednisolone or dexamethasone). Prepackaged formulations with a "programmed" dosage taper facilitates dosage. Because some patients exhibit gastrointestinal irritation from these medications, it is helpful to provide a histamine H_2-receptor antagonist (cimetidine), gastric secretion inhibitor (omeprazole), or an antacid together with antiinflammatory medication.

Antispasm medication is occasionally helpful when neck muscle spasm is a significant feature of the clinical presentation. Methocarbamol, cyclobenzaprine, and diazepam (occasionally for severe muscle spasm) should all be considered.

Surgical Management: The Fundamentals
Relative Contraindications

Although advanced age alone does not represent a contraindication to surgery, age-related factors such as osteoporosis must be considered in planning a particular surgical approach. There are few situations in which some type of appropriate decompressive surgery cannot be undertaken, particularly when spinal cord compression is the issue. Laminectomies and foraminotomies have been performed in the elderly with very good outcomes.

In almost every patient, cardiac, pulmonary, and neural problems can be managed adequately to meet the needs of general anesthesia and surgery. However, the conduct of surgery/anesthesia must be impeccable: blood loss must be minimized and hypotension must be avoided. Occasionally the patient with borderline pulmonary function should remain intubated until the postoperative depression of consciousness is absolutely dissipated. Some have suggested such extremes should be taken after protracted ventral procedures in the severely impaired to avoid complications of secondary airway obstruction. Emery *et al.* reported on seven patients who had upper airway obstruction after multilevel cervical corpectomies for severe myelopathy. Early compromise of airway was believed to be secondary to edema, and not hematoma.[7]

Occasionally a severely myelopathic patient has an imaging study that shows such severe spinal cord atrophy that the osteophytes, although sizable, do not appear to make contact with the spinal cord. Such cases raise questions regarding diagnosis. Before determining that such atrophy mitigates against surgery, an MRI scan obtained in neck flexion and extension should be performed. Similarly, myelography with computed tomography (CT-myelography), still complementary with MRI, can be very revealing when diagnosis is not entirely certain on initial imaging. The presence of a thin line of circumferential dye on axial images is to be expected even in severe spinal cord compression. On the other hand, a wide halo of dye about a crenulated cord is the picture of major atrophy.

Surgical Indications

Although most surgery for cervical spondylosis is elective in nature, it is still possible to distinguish relative degrees of necessity for surgical intervention. Even pain that is without associated impairment and that is unresponsive to conservative management, depending on its characteristics and severity, may be an indication for surgical intervention. Unequivocal anatomic correlation between the pain and a defined structural abnormality must be present in such instances and is critical to surgical planning. For example, Lhermitte's sign may be terribly disquieting, and although not necessarily associated with significant signs, usually responds quite nicely to an appropriate decompression. Similarly, chronic axial pain from a dorsal ligamentous injury that is aggravated by movement, a purely subjective problem, will respond to a single-level posterior fusion (Figure 52.2).

Intractable radiculitis pain with associated sensory and motor signs that shows no trend to improvement with conservative methods represents a clear indication for surgical

therapy. This is particularly true in older patients and in the presence of muscle atrophy, when recovery of muscle strength is even more problematic and less likely to be complete. The resulting disability can be quite severe if definitive treatment is delayed unduly.

Symptomatic spinal cord compression is a surgical indication until proven otherwise by co-morbidities and/or an inconsequential course. Since neurologic recovery after spinal cord compression can be unpredictable and problematic, prompt intervention is not radical. Delay in treatment and severity of impairment are the critical factors in outcome. Impairment of sphincter control or hand dexterity may be devastatingly persistent after surgery if their cause has not been expediently defined and promptly managed. Even spasticity, hand dysfunction, and sensory loss from spinal cord compression, if not neglected, can improve with proper surgery. In Cooper's series[5] about 80% improved, but gait impairment, usually from spastic-

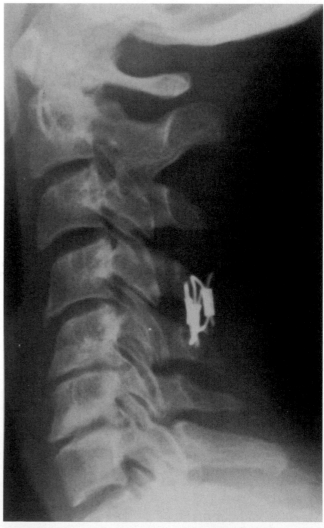

Figure 52.2 Cervical spine radiograph of a 36-year-old woman who underwent posterior cervical fusion with bone graft and cable for segmental instability at C4-5. The patient had sustained a cervical flexion injury in a motor vehicle accident 3 years earlier and had persistent neck pain, which was relieved by local anesthetic injection into the C4-5 interspinous ligament. Fusion relieved her neck pain.

ity, persisted in half of the cases.[5] Emery *et al.*[6] reviewed 108 patients with myelopathy, followed for 2 to 17 years after ventral decompression and fusion. The Nurick functional grade improved from 2.4 preoperatively to 1.2 postoperatively. Of 82 patients with gait abnormalities, 38 became normal, 33 improved, and 6 had no change.

Problems
Axial Pain

There are few unequivocal and isolated facet joint problems that correlate well with a clinical state. Arthrosis of the C1-2 facet joint is an exception. Typically these patients present with pain in the mastoid region or angle of the jaw or with suboccipital headache on the affected side; pain is aggravated by neck rotation. The diagnosis is supported by C1-2 joint sclerosis on open-mouth plain films of the cervical spine (Figure 52.3) and is confirmed by a radiographically controlled block procedure. It is effectively treated by dorsal C1-2 fusion using bone graft and wire cables. Ghanayem *et al.*[13] reported long-term follow-up of 15 patients treated by posterior arthrodesis with excellent results for relieving pain. There is also a group of patients with similar stories but without radiographic arthrosis findings in whom pain relief by a CT-guided C2 root block is diagnostic. There is almost always a history of neck trauma. This group often responds to C2 rhizotomy or neurolysis without fusion.[22]

Other painful facet joints can often be identified by palpation, but the level of the involved facet joint has to be confirmed fluoroscopically. It is then advisable to determine whether instilling local anesthetic, or local anesthetic with steroid medication into the joint in question, will relieve the patient's pain. With such block effect, dorsal cervical fusion at the level of a diseased and painful facet joint is an option, even when there are no neurologic symptoms or signs.

A cervical intervertebral disc suspected as being the source of neck pain can be injected with a contrast agent, local anesthetic, or a combination of these, but the validity of these tests and their interpretation remain controversial.[23] Reliance is placed on reproducing the specific pain complaint at hand ("concordance") with acute distention of the cervical disc, but overlapping patterns of pain make this a less than totally reliable diagnostic test.

Radiographically controlled diagnostic blocks also can be helpful in identifying the interspinous ligament as a source of pain.[16] Often such blocks should be confirmed on one or more occasions, because this is the only screening tool for an otherwise subjective problem, and the only definitive treatment is a dorsal interspinous fusion (Figure 52.2). In general, diagnostic blocks performed in attempts to define the pain generator in axial syndromes should be repeated several times, preferably with different agents, including short-acting and long-acting local anesthetics and even saline to identify patients with other than classical pain syndromes. Currently there is no simple treatment for neck pain associated with a kyphotic curvature without associated neurologic features. The extensive realignment of the spine and fusion necessary to correct the deformity is, in most cases, excessive surgery for a largely subjective problem (Figure 52.4). However, if the patient with kyphosis has loss of cervical muscle control, or has associated spondylotic neural compression (even without neural deficit), then correction of the deformity with stabilization will often relieve the pain.

Nerve Root Syndromes

Patients presenting with shoulder and arm pain presumed to be caused by nerve root compression should be evaluated most carefully when pain is the only symptom, in the

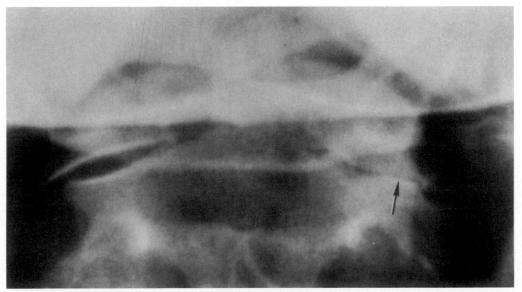

Figure 52.3 Open-mouth ventrodorsal radiograph of C1-2 articulation (*arrow*) shows severe degenerative changes in 74-year-old woman who presented with symptoms of left-sided neck pain exacerbated by neck rotation, earache, and suboccipital pain and tenderness even to pillow contact. The patient underwent a C1-2 dorsal fusion with iliac crest bone, reinforced with cable fixation. Pain relief was complete after her fusion.

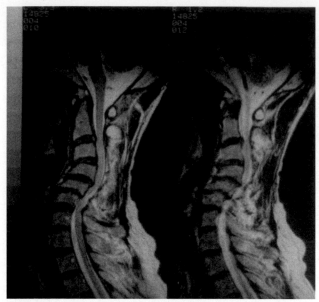

Figure 52.4 MRI of 44-year-old male patient who complained of neck pain. Note S-shaped curve, congenital stenosis typically opening to normal caliber at C2 and C7, and the fact that the magnitude of the surgical correction challenge is disproportionate to the subjective problem.

absence of motor or sensory features. Thus the differential diagnosis is diligently pursued and should include shoulder impingement syndromes, thoracic outlet and superior (pulmonary) sulcus syndromes, suprascapular, cubital tunnel, and carpal tunnel entrapment neuropathies, and peripheral neuropathies. Rarely, autonomically mediated pain syndromes are a consideration.

Specific diagnosis and directed surgical therapy is also of concern in elderly patients where imaging studies often reveal multiple levels of potential nerve root compression. Whereas the pattern of pain may be characteristic of a particular dermatome, there is enough dermatome overlap that some would feel it best to define, by fluoroscopically controlled nerve blocks, which, if not both, of two adjacent nerve roots is symptomatic. This approach, it is argued, allows the most limited surgical strategy. Others would see this as contrived self-deception. At the very least one must be circumspect in interpreting the effects of diagnostic injections, although at times they may be therapeutic in themselves.

The classical nerve root-specific syndromes of radicular pain, motor and sensory impairment, and corresponding reflex changes usually do not present significant diagnostic challenges. Good clinical/imaging correlation is essential before proposing surgical intervention. In the absence of complicating factors the usual initial approach is simple root decompression by medial facetectomy. It is, of course, well established that an osteophyte compressing a nerve root may extend medially and compress the spinal cord as well. Thus the syndrome of myeloradiculopathy, in theory, should exist. In fact, simultaneous symptoms from both the nerve root and spinal cord are observed infrequently. The majority of patients present with either nerve root or myelopathic symptoms, and the essential issue is not the presentation, but the most prudent surgical strategy.

Myelopathic Syndromes

The choice of the optimal surgical approach for myelopathy must take several factors into account: (1) whether the lordotic curve is preserved, (2) the overall spinal canal caliber, (3) cervical mobility, and (4) the number of compressing segments. When surgical fusion is integral to a surgical option, the age and general health of the patient, smoking history, osteopenia, and anticipated orthosis compliance are of particular importance. Multilevel osteophytic disease, involving three or more spinal levels, may pose greater challenges. Ventral decompressive techniques prescribed for the straight or kyphotic spine often involve central trough corpectomies, and the placement of a single longitudinal graft. Alternatively, multilevel discectomies and interbody fusion have their advocates, especially since the advent of ventral plates and multiple-level vertebral body fixation.

Hypermobility of the spine in the presence of spondylotic myelopathy requires stabilization. Indeed, decreasing mobility, even if not excessive, may be ameliorating to a myelopathy. When a ventral procedure is performed, elimination of the hypermobile segment is integral to the procedure. Plate and screw fixation may be prudent here if segmental stability is substantially compromised. When laminectomy is performed for decompression of multilevel spondylosis, the use of lateral mass plates have been found to lessen postoperative pain and possibly improve outcome over that of the unplated.[15] In some cases there may be a similar advantage from the stiffening after laminoplasty.[18] This factor in laminoplasty remains uncertain, however.

Surgery of Spondylosis: The Strategies

The technique, details, and nuances of specific procedures in cervical spine surgery are elaborated elsewhere in this text. Accordingly, the comments that follow are essentially the authors' editorial "bites" on the several strategies used in the surgery of spondylosis.

Foraminotomy

For uncomplicated nerve root compression at one or more levels, enlargement of the root foramen via a microsurgical medial facetectomy is likely preferable to ventral interbody osteophytectomy by virtue of its simplicity. Such foraminotomies, ordinarily, do not involve an attempt at removing the offending ventral osteophyte. They only provide room for the nerve root to back away from the bony ridge. It has been amply demonstrated that this relieves symptoms for most patients. A few will require a subsequent ventral osteophyte resection and fusion for persisting root complaints. Another potential complication of medial facetectomy is segmental destabilizing when more than half of the facet must be resected for adequate decompression.

Microsurgical medial facetectomy has the advantage of sparing the motion segment, a particularly important consideration in the spondylotic patient who is more likely to have some early changes at adjacent levels, even though these are not the cause of symptoms. Other advantages of medial facetectomy are the fact that no postoperative immobilization is necessary and the risks to cervical vessels and viscera of ventral surgery are avoided.

Laminectomy

Because laminectomy only decompresses the spinal cord dorsally, the logic of this procedure is predicated on the presence of some lordotic curvature (Figure 52.4).[1] The practical dilemma is that the majority of aged spines are straightened, or have reversal of the lordotic curve, thus eliminating laminectomy as an attractive decompression strategy. Laminectomy may be effective when the cervical spine is straightened, but the decompression may have to extend into C2, and even C1 to permit dorsal migration of the dural tube sufficient to allow the spinal cord to move away from offending ventral osteophytes. Laminectomy is ineffective for spinal cord compression when there is kyphotic angulation wherein ventral decompression is the preferred procedure.[27]

Laminectomy or laminoplasty may be recommended for spinal cord decompression in congenital canal stenosis because of the longitudinal extent of the problem; however, since the narrowing usually begins subaxially and opens to normal at C7, a long, ventral decompressing corpectomy is feasible.[24] In patients with multilevel spondylosis with only minor degrees of kyphosis, particularly if the patient can extend the spine, fusion and instrumentation (lateral mass screw fixation) may be prudently employed. In all such patients a postoperative magnetic resonance study may be performed to ensure that the intended decompression was achieved. Long-term follow-up is often indicated in light of the expected progression of disease at the remaining motion segments.

Hyperlordosis of the cervical spine may be the result of compounding cervical degenerative changes by the postural stress of accommodating a significant thoracic kyphosis.[8] When spinal cord compression occurs in this situation, laminectomy, although the principal approach, poses some unique problems. The inherent dorsal migration of the spinal cord after laminectomy may be so extreme that ventrally fixed nerve roots are excessively angulated or stretched. The complication may be a severe and untreatable radiculopathy. However, a ventral procedure in the hyperlordotic spine is not usually an effective strategy. A judiciously planned limited laminectomy, with geometric factors taken into account remains the preferred approach.

Ventral Strategies

When a single ventral osteophyte is the principal pathology impacting the spinal cord, bone resection with interbody fusion is preferable to dorsal decompression, even with a preserved lordotic curve. It has been argued that osteophytic resection, without placement of a bone graft, provides an equivalent form of surgical therapy. Spontaneous fusion will usually occur in most of these patients, even in the absence of a bone graft. There is, however, a risk of symptomatic foraminal narrowing, as well as segmental kyphotic angulation when a bone graft is omitted.

When there is incontrovertible imaging evidence of coexisting asymptomatic spinal cord compression (not merely indentation of the subarachnoid space) and a nerve root syndrome, a ventral cervical disc and osteophyte resection with interbody fusion is also preferred. The nerve root, as well as the spinal cord, can be adequately decompressed and the foraminal decompression maintained by the distraction of the interbody graft.

When more than one or two levels of ventral spinal cord compression are present, there is a persisting debate as to the approach in the absence of a kyphotic curve. The more extensive ventral surgery can take the form of multilevel discectomies, spacers, and plating, or with more global canal compromise, as in ossification of posterior longitudinal ligament (OPLL) or congenital stenosis, multilevel corpectomy with interbody strut fusion are surgery options.

If a disadvantage of ventral surgery lies in problems with and consequences of fusion,[9] this may be answered by the optional strategy of the so-called oblique corpectomy. George described an approach apparently as effective as conventional multilevel corpectomy wherein the bony boundaries of ventral spinal canal are drilled away from a far lateral access, which spares the anterior column.[12] Enough structural spinal support is thereby retained that no subsequent strut graft is necessary. Provisos are that the disc spaces should be narrowed, and there should be no hypermobile segments involved. In effect, the neck should be nearly autofused.

Ventral Hardware

Ventral plate and screw fixation with multilevel corpectomies, as well as with most other ventral surgery, are now probably the rule rather than the exception.[19] Instrumentation for the otherwise uncomplicated ventral fusion can be rationalized for a number of reasons, some solid and some tentative. Clearly, ventral hardware utilization, simply to forgive poor patient selection or surgical technique, is to be discouraged. For example, graft displacement without hardware almost always occurs in the first few days of surgery and never if the graft cannot be dislodged by intraoperative flexion and extension of the neck. Displacement is therefore more than likely the result of an error in securing the graft, by either excessive graft impaction against the lateral trough wall or inadequate mortising. Accordingly, hardware should not be primarily used for the prevention of graft displacement. Further, it is naïve to rationalize the use of hardware because it replaces the requirement of learning to perform solid and secure strut grafting technique. Plating clearly diminishes the risk of pseudarthrosis. However, this is an infrequent clinical problem, although it is arguably a common radiographic disappointment.

On the other hand the problems of kyphosis and instability[20,27] are compelling reasons to use ventral plates and screws. Importantly, the internal orthosis of instrumentation obviates the use of uncertain conventional orthotics and diminishes the impact of poor patient compliance.

The appeal of plating an extra long ventral graft lies in the concern for the lever-arm stress placed on the caudal mortise, usually at C7, the site of most graft displacements. Actually, ventral plates do not effectively diminish this risk, whereas dorsal instrumentation does.[10]

The reader should remember that the "attractive nuisance" of reports on novel technology having near zero morbidity and great benefit are often from centers with vast experience, and as such can be a dangerous trap for the average practitioner. The potential danger of plates and screws must forever be weighed against their practical benefit. The noninstrumented construct is still legitimate (Figure 52.5).

Summary

Whereas cervical spondylosis is usually without surgical consequence, there exists a significant number of patients, especially myelopaths, that suffer complications of this ubiquitous consequence of aging. Improvements in imaging detail, pathophysiologic insight, and surgical strategies allow the thoughtful spine surgeon reason for confident optimism in managing a condition that was associated with substantial nihilism in the not too remote past.

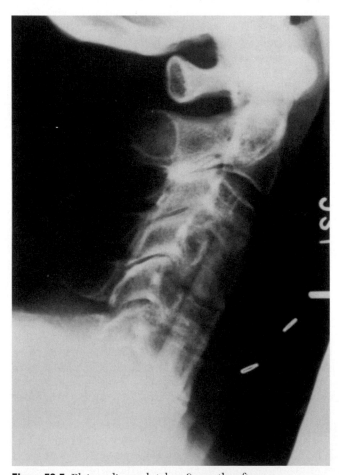

Figure 52.5 Plain radiograph taken 8 months after an uninstrumented three-level corpectomy for spondylotic myelopathy in a 55-year-old male. Preoperative studies showed mild reversal of the lordotic curve. Note that the rostral placement of the graft is into the ventral cortex secured in a dove-tail construct to support the anterior column, addressing the moment arm on the instantaneous axis of rotation, lengthened by the spondylotic process.

REFERENCES

1. Batzdorf U, Batzdorff A: Analysis of cervical spine curvature in patients with cervical spondylosis. *Neurosurgery* 22:827, 1988.
2. Benzel EC: Degenerative and inflammatory diseases of the spine. In Benzel EC (ed): *Biomechanics of Spine Stabilization: A Clinical Approach.* New York, McGraw-Hill, 1998.
3. Brain WR, Northfield D, Wilkinson M: The neurological manifestations of cervical spondylosis. *Brain* 75[Part II]:187, 1952.
4. Brodin H: Paths of nutrition in articular cartilage and intervertebral discs. *Acta Orthop Scand* 24:171, 1955.
5. Chiles BW III, Leonard MA, Choudhri HF, Cooper PR: Cervical spondylotic myelopathy: patterns of neurological deficit and recovery after anterior cervical decompression. *Neurosurgery* 44:762-769, 1999.
6. Emory SE, Bohlman HH, Bolesta MJ, Jones PK: Anterior cervical decompression and arthrodesis for the treatment of cervical spondylotic myelopathy. *J Bone Joint Surg,* 80A(7):941-951, July 1998.
7. Emory SE, Smith MD, Bohlman HH: Upper-airway obstruction after multilevel cervical corpectomy for myelopathy. *J Bone Joint Surg* 73A(4), 544-551, April 1991.
8. Epstein JA, Carras R, Epstein BS, *et al*: Myelopathy in cervical spondylosis with vertebral subluxation and hyperlordosis. *J Neurosurg* 32:421, 1970.
9. Fernyhough J, White J, LaRocca H: Fusion rates in multilevel cervical spondylosis comparing allograft fibula with autograft fibula in 126 patients. *Spine* 16:S562, 1991.
10. Foley K: Personal communication, 2001.
11. Frykholm R: Cervical nerve root compression resulting from disc degeneration and root sleeve fibrosis: a clinical investigation. *Acta Chir Scand* (Suppl 160):1-149, 1951.
12. George B, Gauthier N, Guillaume L: Multisegmental cervical spondylotic myelopathy and radiculopathy treated by multilevel oblique corpectomies with fusion. *Acta Neurochir (Wein)* 121:187, 1993.
13. Ghanayem AJ, Leventhal M, Bohlman HH: Osteoarthrosis of the atlanto-axial joints. *J Bone Joint Surg* 78-A(9), 1300-1307, Sept 1996.
14. Green JD, Harle TS, Harris JH Jr: Anterior subluxation of the cervical spine: hyperflexion sprain. *AJNR* 2:243,1981.
15. Kahn EA: The role of the dentate ligaments in spinal cord compression and the syndrome of lateral sclerosis. *J Neurosurg* 4:191, 1947.
16. Kessler JT: Congenital narrowing of the cervical spinal canal. *J Neural Neurosurg Psychiatry* 38:1218, 1975.
17. Keyes DC, Compere EL: The normal and pathological physiology of the nucleus pulposus of the intervertebral disc: an anatomical, clinical, and experimental study. *J Bone Joint Surg* 14:897, 1932.
18. Kumar V, Rea G, Mervis L, McGregor J: Cervical spondylotic myelopathy: functional and radiographic long-term outcome after laminectomy and posterior fusion. *Neurosurgery* 44:771, 1999.
19. Mayr MT, Subach BR, Comey CH, *et al*: Cervical spinal stenosis: outcome after anterior corpectomy, allograft

reconstruction, and instrumentation. *J Neurosurg (Spine 1)* 96:10, 2002.

20. Miyazaki K, Tada K, Matsuda Y, *et al*: Posterior extensive simultaneous multisegment decompression with posterolateral fusion for cervical myelopathy with cervical instability and kyphotic and/or S-shaped deformities. *Spine* 14:1160, 1989.

21. Ohmori K, Ishida Y, Suzuki K: Suspension laminotomy: a new surgical technique for compression myelopathy. *Neurosurgery* 21:950, 1987.

22. Pikus H, Phillips J: Characteristics of patients successfully treated for cervicogenic headache by surgical decompression of the second cervical root. *Headache* 35:621, 1995.

23. Roth DA: Cervical analgesic discography: a new test for the definitive diagnosis of the painful-disc syndrome. *JAMA* 235:1713, 1976.

24. Saunders R, Pikus H, Ball P: Four level cervical corpectomy. *Spine* 23:2455, 1999.

25. Teresi LM, Lufkin RB, Reicher MA, *et al*: Asymptomatic degenerative disc disease and spondylosis of the cervical spine: MR imaging. *Radiology* 164:83,1987.

26. Wilder DG, Woodworth BB, Frymoyer JW, *et al*: Vibration and the human spine. *Spine* 7:243, 1982.

27. Zdeblick TA, Bohlman HH: Cervical kyphosis and myelopathy: treatment by anterior corpectomy and strut-grafting. *J Bone Joint Surg* 71A:170, 1989.

CHAPTER 53

Thoracic and Lumbar Spondylosis

Christopher B. Shields, Carole A. Miller, and Stewart B. Dunsker

The spectrum of *spondylosis* encompasses degenerative disc disease with its associated vertebral osteophytosis, ligamentous disease, facet joint disease, and neurologic complications. To some extent the condition usually begins by age 45,[40] and is found on plain radiographs in 95% of men and 80% of women older than 65 years.[38] Using magnetic resonance imaging (MRI) scans, Powell *et al.*[55] found that the prevalence of degenerative disc disease is greater than 33% in 20-year-old women, and that it increases to 95% in women older than 70 years. It is one of the main causes of work loss, particularly among heavy manual laborers. Spondylosis occurs in all spinal segments but is most often present in the cervical and lumbar segments, which are the most mobile segments of the spine; intervertebral disc disease is not as prevalent in the thoracic region of the spine. The normal kyphosis of the thoracic spine, however, may cause the ventral edges of the vertebral bodies to compress disc tissue so that the anterior portion of the disc is subject to increased degeneration.

Lumbar spondylosis, more common in males,[47] is more prominent in the caudal segments, the same segments that are affected by degenerative disc disease.[69] It is one of the most frequent causes of low back and leg pain. Spondylosis is the primary cause of lumbar spinal stenosis, and it is responsible for most of the clinical syndromes that require surgical intervention.

Historic Background

In 1893 W.A. Lane of Guys Hospital in London described spondylosis with stenosis and its surgical treatment.[68] The patient had cauda equina syndrome and complained of "weakness of her back and insecurity of her legs." Lane was able to diagnose the presence of spondylolisthesis at operation.

Neurogenic claudication and its relief by forward flexion were described in 1889 and 1911. Hypertrophic changes in the lumbar spine were stressed in early reports. The concept of "congenital stricture of the spinal canal" was later proposed by Sarpyener.[59] Verbiest[67] discussed the contribution of congenital narrowing of the spinal canal and implicated a hypertrophied ligamentum flavum. Verbiest also defined the clinical syndrome with myelography and demonstrated the spinal obstruction. MacNab drew attention to spondylolisthesis with an intact neural arch.[43] Kirkaldy-Willis *et al.*[35] conducted a thorough review of lumbar spinal stenosis in 1974. Currently the relative roles of congenital narrowing versus hypertrophic changes are debated. Undoubtedly both play a role in producing the clinical syndrome.

In 1921 Sicard and Forestier found that a herniated disc with nerve root compression could give rise to sciatica, and they confirmed the presence and site of the disc rupture by myelography.[61] In 1927 Putti described an emerging nerve root entrapment in the subarticular gutter that was caused by superior articular facet hypertrophy.[56] In 1934 Mixter and Barr wrote their well-known article confirming that a herniated disc could indeed compress an emerging nerve root and cause sciatic pain.[48]

Sarpyener,[59] however, recognized that bony compression of a nerve root could also give rise to radicular pain. The diagnosis of spinal stenosis was then indiscriminately applied to all cases with sciatic pain not resulting from herniated nucleus pulposus. In fact, many patients have multisegmental spondylosis and stenosis with no symptoms whatsoever. Jensen *et al.*[25] observed that in 98 individuals without back pain, annular defects of the outer fibrous ring of the disc occurred in 14% of patients, and facet arthropathy in 8% of patients. The mere radiographic demonstration of a lateral recess stenosis does not mean that the cause and site of the neurologic condition have been identified. Although a patient may have a lateral recess stenosis that involves both sides at several levels, the symptoms may be unilateral or monoradicular. MacNab[43] reviewed 432 patients with sciatica associated with radiologic demonstration of bilateral recess stenosis, with 403 of these patients presenting with unilateral monoradicular sciatica.

Spinal stenosis may be: (1) lateral spinal canal stenosis (caused by hypertrophic apophyseal joints that may compress the emerging nerve root[s]); (2) central spinal canal stenosis (caused by a thickened laminar arch), which threatens the cauda equina; or (3) a combination of both lateral and central stenoses. Lateral bony compression of the nerve roots can arise as a result of subarticular entrapment, pedicular kinking, or foraminal impingement caused by posterior joint subluxation.[66] The term *spinal stenosis* refers to an anatomic abnormality. It is not a clinical diagnosis.

Anatomic Diagnosis

There are no universally accepted diagnostic criteria for lumbar spinal stenosis. Most authors have described a set of stereotypical symptoms in patients with associated radiographic findings. Most would also agree with Epstein and Epstein that there is "an incongruity between the capacity and the contents of the lumbar spinal canal that may give rise to compression of the roots of the cauda equina."[15] The anteroposterior (AP) diameter of the spinal canal varies in symptomatic patients from 10 to 15 mm; these measurements overlap widely in asymptomatic persons. Thus there can be no definition of spinal stenosis based solely on measurements of canal diameters.

Intervertebral disc degeneration most likely plays a major role in causing spinal canal stenosis.[69] However, its importance is suspect. Lumbar facet joint arthritis rarely occurs without radiologic evidence of disc space degeneration or disc protrusion.[6] Congenital stenosis of the spinal canal is an important factor in the development of symptomatic spinal stenosis. Developmentally, the lumbar spinal canal reaches its full internal diameter in childhood. The AP and lateral diameters are smallest at the level of L3 and L4, and indeed, stenosis is most common at this level.[21] Before computed tomography (CT) was available the normal AP diameter of the lumbar spinal canal was generally considered to be 12 to 15mm when measured radiographically or intraoperatively. Using dynamic CT-myelographic techniques, Penning and Wilmink[53] evaluated the internal diameter and cross-sectional area of the dural sac myelographically in proven cases of lumbar stenosis, as well as in controls. All measurements were taken in flexion and extension and were corrected for radiographic enlargement. They found no significant difference between bony sagittal or interpedicular diameters between the two groups. However, there was a significant discrepancy in the size of the cross-sectional area of the dural sac at the L4-5 disc level: a mean of 105mm^2 (range: 70 to 138mm^2) in patients with clinical stenosis versus a mean of 145mm^2 (range: 86 to 230mm^2) in the controls. The key to stenosis is the enlarging apophyseal joints. The cross-sectional area of the canal enlarges in flexion and is reduced in extension, thus explaining the usual symptomatic relief that is reported on flexion.[72]

The nerve root courses downward and outward, passing beneath the medial border of the inferior articular facet before passing close to the caudal surface of the pedicle and emerging through the foramen. Hypertrophy of the superior articular facet, particularly its medial border, may compress the nerve root against the dorsal surface of the vertebral body.

When advanced intervertebral disc degeneration is associated with marked narrowing of the disc, the adjacent vertebral bodies approach one another. As the upper vertebral body descends, the caudal surface of the pedicle may kink the exiting nerve root, particularly if asymmetric collapse of the disc has occurred. Often this is observed with degenerative scoliosis (Figure 53.1) in which the nerve root is compressed in a gutter formed by osteophytes from the collapsed disc and the pedicle above. Pedicular kinking of the nerve root at L5 is common in spondylolisthesis.[70]

As the nerve root exits through the foramen, it lies rostral to the tip of the superior articular facet of the vertebra below. When the intervertebral disc narrows, the superior (anterior) articular process slides further rostrally into the foramen and the exiting nerve root may be compressed, another example of the *syndrome of the superior facet* (Figure 53.2).

Three different types of nerve root compression may occur as the nerve passes through the foramen: (1) compression by the tip of the subluxing inferior articular facet, (2) compression between the superior articular facet and the caudal surface of the pedicle above, and (3) compression between an osteophyte arising from the superior

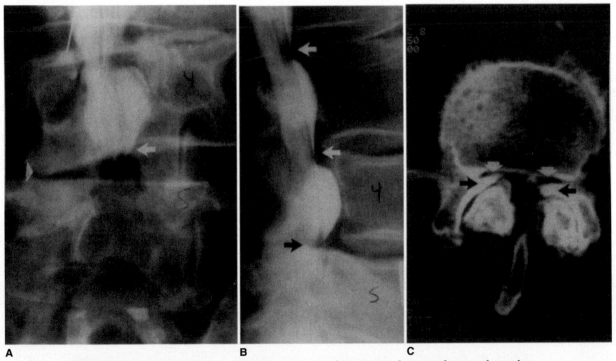

A   B   C

Figure 53.1 Lumbar myelogram showing severe spinal stenosis with a complete myelographic block at L4-5. **(A)** AP view. Note the lateral olisthesis and retrolisthesis, hypertrophic facet on the right side, unilateral narrowing of the L4-5 discspace (*arrowhead*), and total myelographic block (*arrow*). **(B)** The lateral view shows a diffuse annular bulge at the L2-3 and L3-4 levels (*white arrows*) and grade I spondylolisthesis with a complete block at L4-5 (*black arrow*). **(C)** Axial CT scan at L4-5 showing severe hypertrophic facet disease of both the superior (*black arrows*) and inferior facets with marked lateral recess stenosis (*white arrows*). Minimal contrast agent is noted in the subarachnoid space.

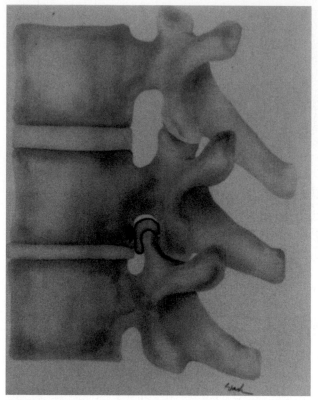

Figure 53.2 Severe discspace narrowing is associated with marked upward migration of the superior articular process of the lower vertebrae and severe compression on the exiting nerve root *(arrow)*. The intervertebral disc also narrows the foramen anteriorly.

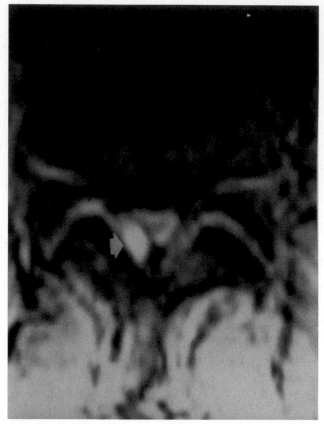

Figure 53.3 MRI scan demonstrating a high signal synovial cyst *(arrow)* in the epidural space arising from the medial aspect of the right L4-5 facet joint.

articular facet and the posterior surface of the adjacent vertebral body.[65] Occasionally, ganglion-like, intraspinal synovial cysts (another cause of spinal stenosis) arise from the apophyseal joints. Synovial cysts are usually seen in patients older than 50 years. They often arise from the apophyseal joints from L3 to L5, and particularly from L4 and L5. Synovial cysts extend from the anteromedial margin of the apophyseal joint and compress the dural sac or the descending or exiting nerve root. They are usually less than 1cm in diameter and may be filled with fluid, fat, or gas. This condition is diagnosed most readily by CT or MRI scans (Figure 53.3).

Central spinal stenosis may also follow degenerative disc disease when, with narrowing of the intervertebral disc space, the spinal canal is constricted by a diffuse annular bulge, anterior buckling of the ligamentum flavum, and shingling of the laminar arch. This situation may then be further aggravated by hypertrophic changes in the arthritic posterior joints, and the development of spondylotic spurs from the margins of the vertebral bodies, thereby encroaching on the midline. These bony changes may cause symptoms in elderly patients and even in middle-aged patients, if there is concomitant congenital spinal stenosis.[34,36]

Also, forward displacement of the lamina (as in degenerative spondylolisthesis) can produce central stenosis, as can degenerative retrolisthesis. Hypertrophy of the superior articular facet of the subjacent vertebrae adds subar-

ticular stenosis to the problem (Figure 53.4). Thickening of the lamina in certain pathologic states, such as fluorosis and Paget's disease, may also cause posterior encroachment on the spinal canal. Furthermore, any method of spinal fusion that involves decortication of the lamina with the addition of a bone graft may result in overgrowth of the posterior elements and cause constriction of the spinal canal. Postfusion spinal stenosis is especially likely to occur if the patient is already suffering from either congenital stenosis of the spinal canal or narrowing of the canal produced by degenerative changes.

Chen *et al.*[8] evaluated 48 patients who underwent dorsal decompressive surgery for lumbar spinal stenosis without fusion. Their findings were as follows: no significant bone regrowth (regrowth of 10% or less) in 6% of the patients; mild regrowth (regrowth of 11% to 40%) in 50%; moderate regrowth (regrowth of 41% to 70%) in 29%; and marked regrowth (regrowth of 71% to 100%) in 15%. The factors associated with a moderate to marked bony regrowth are a total block of contrast agent as observed on the preoperative myelogram, a follow-up period of greater than 5 years, decompression at more than three spinal levels, and patients younger than 60 years. They also noted that bone regrowth was greater in the presence of postoperative spinal instability. Postacchini and Cinotti[54] performed a similar study in 40 patients. Their results showed no bone regrowth in 12%, mild regrowth in 48%, moderate regrowth in 28%, and marked regrowth in 12% of patients.

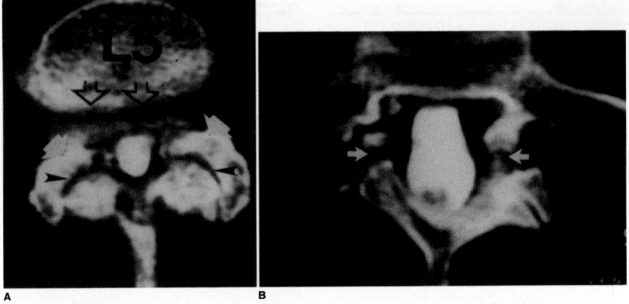

Figure 53.4 (A) Markedly hypertrophic facets *(white arrows)* and irregular facet surfaces at L4-5 *(black arrowheads)*. The space between the posterior aspect of L4-5 vertebral bodies is seen as well *(black open arrows)*. **(B)** Bilateral pars interarticularis defects *(white arrows)* are seen as well as the characteristic oblong appearance of the dural tube at the level of the pars defect.

Some authors have reported that the ligamentum flavum may be 7 to 8mm thick instead of the usual 4mm or less, but ligament thickness may not be real because of the volume redistribution in the shortened interlaminar space.

Any or all combinations of central and lateral compressions can occur. Two adjacent roots may be entrapped by different mechanisms. For example, because of its obliquity, the fifth lumbar nerve root may be compressed as it courses under the inferior articular facet at L5, and it may also be compressed in its foramen by the tip of the articular facet of S1.[31] Although laminar compression may occur by itself, it is often associated with lateral or apophyseal root entrapment at the same or at different segments.

Severe degenerative disc disease will result in diffuse annular bulging, buckling of the ligamentum flavum, and retrolisthesis caused by subluxation of the articular facets, resulting in shingling of the lamina and further encroachment on the spinal canal.

Central compression may occur as much as two levels higher than the segments at which the lateral stenosis is present. In such instances the central compression is readily apparent on myelography, but if surgical intervention is confined to decompressing the pathology in the midline, the patient may have persistent symptoms arising from lateral stenosis. Paradoxically, the myelogram will be normal.

In degenerative joint disease the characteristic findings on CT include hypertrophy of the articular processes (especially the superior process); osteophyte formation of the joint margins; narrowing and irregularity of the joint spaces; juxtaarticular calcification in the joint capsule or in the ligamentum flavum; and, occasionally, gas in the facet joint.[64]

Symptomatic stenosis attributed to developmental changes is often superimposed on congenital spinal stenosis, neither of which alone would have been symptomatic. There have been no definitive studies regarding whether patients with congenitally shallow spinal canals have more extensive osteoarthritis.

The pathology of spinal stenosis thus is thickened laminae, thickened ligamentum flavum, facet hypertrophy, and synovial cysts arising from apophyseal joint capsules. Sometimes the whole situation is worsened by forward or backward slipping of one vertebra on an adjacent vertebra. All of the aforementioned factors may cause severe spinal stenosis as seen on imaging studies, but there are few if any clinical symptoms.

These variables make the performance of the appropriate diagnostic studies critical, but before embarking on any surgical intervention, these studies must be scrupulously correlated with clinical findings. Correcting demonstrable anatomic abnormalities that may be entirely asymptomatic is inappropriate.

Clinical Diagnosis

Patients with lumbar spinal stenosis may present with low back pain, sciatica, or a combination of both.[51] The cardinal symptom of lumbar stenosis is neurogenic intermittent claudication (Table 53.1).[2,51]

Neurogenic claudication is precipitated and gradually intensified by walking and standing. It differs from the claudication of vascular insufficiency because it is first felt proximally and is not relieved just by the cessation of activity.[52] Clinical evaluation of patients with spinal stenosis supports the thesis that the complaint of radicular pain implies lateral or apophyseal stenosis, now commonly referred to as lateral recess stenosis.

Lumbar spinal stenosis occurs primarily in elderly men; however, women are more likely to develop degenerative spondylolisthesis ("pseudospondylolisthesis"), particularly

TABLE 53.1

Frequency of Signs and Symptoms in 145 Patients with Lumbar Spinal Stenosis

Symptoms/Signs	Frequency (%)
Pain on motion	100
Neurogenic claudication	100
Restriction of extension	77
Dermatomal sensory impairment	47
Reflex deficit	40
Motor deficit	29
Limited straight leg raising	23

at L4-5. The symptoms are difficult to correlate with a single nerve-root entrapment, and abnormal signs on physical examination are scarce or absent, which frequently leads to misdiagnosis. Individuals with spinal stenosis are often misdiagnosed as having osteoarthritis of the hip or trochanteric bursitis, with the converse also occurring, which leads to inappropriate therapy being administered before the correct diagnosis is made.

The cardinal symptoms of lumbar spinal stenosis are bilateral neurogenic claudication (pseudoclaudication) and absence of pain when seated.[32] Patients complain of pain or weakness in the muscles of the thighs and calves, provoked by both standing and walking, and relieved within minutes by sitting, bending forward, or lying in the fetal position.[2] Patients often report numbness that may be described as a "rubbery" or a pins-and-needles sensation. Sparing of the sacral roots occurs because of their central protected position in the stenotic lumbar spinal canal. They may at times be involved, however, and male patients complain of having to sit down to void. Voiding dysfunction was noted preoperatively by 12 of 18 (65%) male and female patients with lumbar spinal stenosis.[20] However, urodynamic studies were abnormal in only two patients (one showed detrusor hyperreflexia; the other, urethral obstruction).

If patients continue to walk, their legs weaken and they may fall. Low back and lower extremity discomfort is exacerbated by lumbar extension. Symptoms decrease or resolve when the patients adopt a flexed position of the lumbar spine.[31] They can achieve this position by leaning forward on shopping carts, church pews, lawn mowers, etc. These patients avoid lines in supermarkets or shopping in malls, and when forced to stand for long, will shift weight from one foot to the other. In advanced cases patients adopt a simian posture and, even in recumbency, will assume a flexed or fetal position. Flexion-extension studies have shown the highly significant increased area of the dural sac in flexion. This also includes an increase in the sagittal diameter of the dural sac and increase in the length of the spinal canal in flexion.[10]

With vascular claudication, muscle pain is experienced as cramping without a paresthetic quality, which is provoked by walking and relieved by standing. Although cycling exacerbates the symptoms of vascular claudication, cycling is often well tolerated when lumbar spinal stenosis is present because the spine is not weight bearing and is flexed. It is much easier for patients with lumbar spinal stenosis to go upstairs than down for the same reasons.

When asked to show where the pain is, a standing patient will describe its distribution with a sweeping downward movement of both hands, from the buttocks to the heels. The Valsalva maneuver does not produce symptoms, whereas in discogenic sciatica, it often does. Low back pain, when present in spinal stenosis, has a mechanical quality.

The diagnosis of neurogenic intermittent claudication caused by lumbar spinal stenosis is usually made from the patient's history. There may be few physical signs. Decreased range of lumbar motion, although usually reported, is of little value in making the diagnosis. Forward flexion may be normal; in fact, patients may be able to touch their toes. The straight-leg raising test of Lasègue is usually negative. Weakness is usually mild, is either unilateral or bilateral, and is usually found in muscles innervated by the L5 and the S1 roots. This weakness can be evoked by asking patients to walk on their heels or toes and is manifested as a wide-based gait and positive Romberg's test.[32] When patients stand up for a few minutes they seek a flexed posture and lean on the examining table. Walking nonstop for a few minutes will induce symptoms. At times the deep tendon reflexes may disappear or be reduced when checked after exertion.[30] Patients with lumbar spinal stenosis experience thigh pain and neuromuscular defects after 30 seconds of lumbar extension.[32] Another fundamental test was described as a screening procedure in patients with neurogenic intermittent claudication: downhill walking. A positive test consisted of discomfort (positive predictive value of 86%) and changes in the neurologic status (predictive value of 89%).[26]

Bony compression of an emerging nerve root does not invariably give rise to claudication pain. It may simply present as sciatica, being aggravated by general and specific activities. The clinical picture of bony nerve root entrapment differs in several aspects from the syndrome of ruptured disc. Disc ruptures are by far the most common cause of radicular pain in patients younger than age 40. In patients between 40 and 50 years of age, bony nerve root entrapment and a herniated disc occur with equal frequency, but in those older than age 65, bony nerve root entrapment syndromes are the most common source of root irritation.[30] Pain at rest, at night, and on coughing are as common with lateral spinal stenosis as with disc herniation. Individuals with disc herniations are more likely to require increased analgesic medication.[30]

Patients with bony nerve root entrapment usually have a history of long-standing backache and recent onset of sciatica. On examination one remarkable finding is that straight-leg raising test is rarely limited significantly in central spinal stenosis, despite severe sciatic pain. However, the straight-leg raising test pulls the nerve root over the herniated disc. In lateral recess or foraminal stenosis the nerve root is firmly caught at the point of bone entrapment and the nerve root moves very little on raising the straight leg. This causes severe pain on the straight-leg raising test, but not as severe as with a herniated disc.[30]

A disc herniation rarely occurs at more than one segment. Lateral recess or foraminal stenosis, however, frequently involves several spinal levels. A large central disc may involve more than one root. When there is clinical evidence of multiple root involvement, the probability is much greater that root entrapment is caused by stenosis of arthritic origin at several levels.

What causes the radicular pain? Ischemia of the nerve roots has been proposed.[4] Mechanical compression prevents the nerve roots from receiving the necessary blood supply. This is why the characteristic leg pain is similar to the symptoms of claudication observed with peripheral vascular disease.[4]

In elderly patients the main psychologic factor that should not be overlooked is depression. Disincentives to improvement, such as wage-replacement benefits and litigation, must be considered, but these factors seldom apply to patients older than 65 years of age. Primary depression, which is not uncommon in this age group can, however, result in a confusing differential diagnosis. Most patients who have true depression have some somatic complaints, and prompt recognition and early treatment of the underlying depression may result in marked diminution of such symptoms.

Diagnostic Tests

Electromyography

Electromyographic and neurographic studies may be performed on the lower extremities. The incidence of bilateral neurogenic changes was 87.5% in total spinal occlusion, and in severe lumbar spinal stenosis (with no occlusion) 81%; multisegmental electromyographic abnormalities were present in 94% of patients with total spinal occlusion and in 75% of patients with severe lumbar spinal stenosis (with no occlusion). For patients with a normal myelogram, the rates of abnormal test findings were 29% and 21%, respectively.[28] Thus electromyography is somewhat helpful, but it has a fairly high rate of false-negative and false-positive results.

Somatosensory evoked potentials can be of diagnostic value when performed before and after a walking stress test. When tested preoperatively, 31 of 37 patients exhibited the onset of an abnormality of stress-induced stress somatosensory evoked potentials immediately after walking. When tested postoperatively, the somatosensory evoked potentials returned to normal after stress-induced testing. This test may help differentiate vascular from neurogenic intermittent claudication.[37]

Plain Lumbar Spine Radiographs

Imaging studies are the key to the confirmation of the diagnosis of lumbar stenosis (see Chapter 131). Plain radiographs of the lumbar spine are necessary to exclude other pathologic processes. Although the diagnosis of lumbar spinal stenosis can be suspected on the basis of plain radiographs, additional studies are mandatory before surgical intervention. Because most patients with degenerative stenosis are elderly, there is a higher likelihood of neoplasm. Consequently, a bone scan is another important diagnostic test that should be performed.

Radiographs in lumbar spondylosis and spinal stenosis have several characteristics. Frequently, the bony nerve root entrapment syndromes are associated with subluxation of the facet joints. On a lateral view the joint-body line (a line

drawn along the caudal border of the vertebral body and extended dorsally) should pass above the tip of the apophyseal joint (Figure 53.5). With subluxation secondary to degenerative disc disease, it passes through the middle aspect of the joint. With chronic subluxations, especially with lordosis, the inferior articular facet impinges on the lamina. A reactive ridge of bone is often formed and is recognizable as a white crescent on the oblique view. In severe degrees of subluxation the tip of the superior articular facet may impinge against the pedicle above. Narrowing of the interlaminar space, noted on the AP view of the spine, is also characteristic of lateral spinal stenosis. The interlaminar space may be encroached on by overgrowth of the facets, by an abnormal configuration of the lamina, by subluxation of the facet joints, or by osteoarthritis of the facet joints.[41]

Radiographs of the lumbar spine show degenerative disc disease in 78% of the elderly (older than 65 years) patient population[38] and osteoarthritis of the facet joints in 62%. When AP radiographs of the lumbar spine show apophyseal joint hypertrophic changes, it is suggestive of stenosis because it indicates that the spinal canal is severely narrowed. Degenerative spondylolisthesis, usually grade 1, is observed most often at L4-5 and usually occurs late in the development of osteoarthritis of the facet joints.

Plain radiographs are ideally suited to demonstrate degenerative scoliosis, as scoliotic curves (up to 30 degrees),

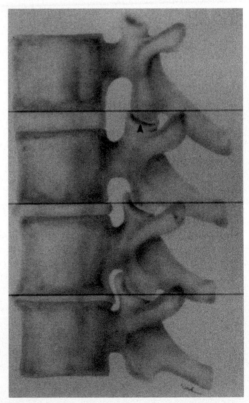

Figure 53.5 A lateral lumbar spine with a line drawn along the inferior surface of the vertebral body and continued posteriorly through the posterior articular joint. In a normal disc (*upper*) the posterior line passes above the articular joint (*arrowhead*). In moderately degenerative discdisease (*middle*) the line passes through the articular joint. If severe degenerative disease exists (*lower*) the line passes through the lower aspect of the articular joint.

disc space narrowing, and lateral olisthesis facet hypertrophy are all clearly depicted on these films (Figure 53.6).

Myelographic Findings

The myelogram may not show a discrete myelographic defect. However, there may be a nerve root sleeve cutoff, either unilaterally or bilaterally. Degenerative spinal stenosis is frequently associated with multilevel diffuse annular bulges. The dorsal hump produced by the annular bulge is associated with narrowing of the dye column, producing an hourglass constriction (Figure 53.7).

If the bony constriction is confined to the lateral recess, the myelogram usually shows only root sleeve cutoff. When lateral encroachment is combined with central constriction of the spinal canal, with or without a diffuse bulge of the annulus, there may be a complete cutoff of the flow of contrast medium. The paintbrush or rat tail appearance at the end of the contrast column distinguishes this myelographic (extradural) defect from that produced by an intradural tumor, with its characteristic meniscus.

Preoperative myelography is of value in predicting the results of adequately performed decompressive lumbar surgery. Herno et al.[22] reported that good-to-excellent outcomes were observed in 76% of the block stenosis group (complete or subtotal block); in 61% of the relative stenosis group (AP diameter of 10 to 12mm); and in 56% of the absolute stenosis group (AP diameter less than 10mm).

CT and CT-Myelography

CT scans are commonly overinterpreted as demonstrating evidence of lumbar spinal stenosis. CT scans are most helpful when performed with intrathecal contrast metrizamide in the spinal canal. CT alone is inferior to CT with intrathecal contrast and myelography.[21]

Lumbar myelography followed by CT (CT-myelography) allows one to make an accurate diagnosis of spinal stenosis and also provides critical information necessary for effective preoperative planning.[3,19,60] This combination allows for the precise measurement of the diameter and cross-sectional area of the dural sac. The extent of the decompression that is necessary can also be determined by studying the CT-myelograms. When there is a complete block or a high-grade stenosis, the CT scans must be studied distal to the block to determine the length of surgical decompression that will be necessary, because the contrast agent will not ascend above the block. The contrast agent used during myelography should be run up to the midthoracic level to identify any lesions present at these higher levels.[46]

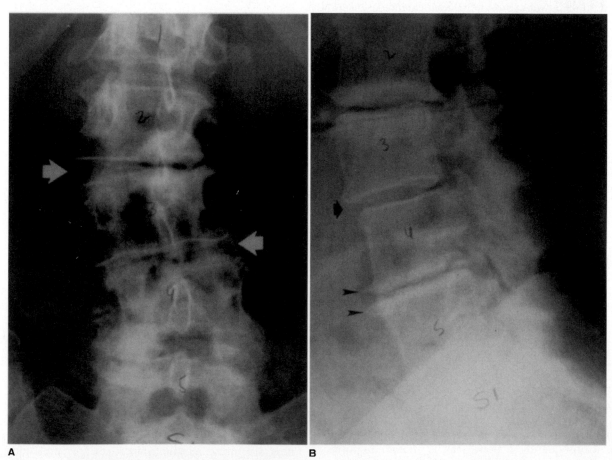

A   **B**

Figure 53.6 (**A**) AP view of a thoracolumbar spine that shows a marked degree of degenerative scoliosis of 25 degrees. This deformity resulted from degenerative discdisease and hypertrophic facets, as well as from distress at L2-3 and L3-4 (*arrows*). (**B**) Lateral view of lumbar spine showing narrow L2-3 and L4-5 discspaces. Also note traction spurs at L4 and L5 (*arrowheads*) and grade I spondylolisthesis at L3-4 (*arrow*).

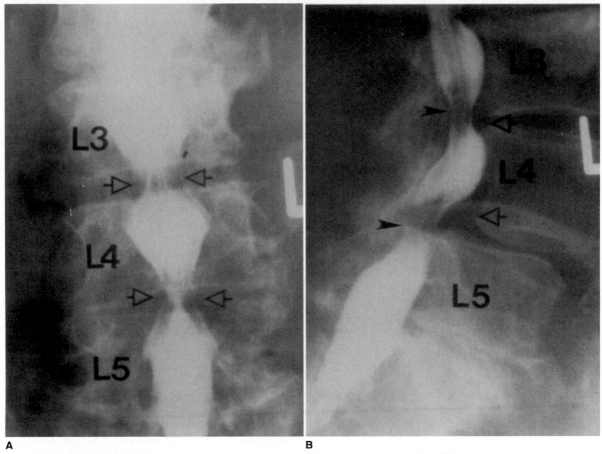

A   **B**

Figure 53.7 **(A)** AP myelogram demonstrates spinal stenosis at L3-4 and L4-5 *(open arrows)*. **(B)** Concentric narrowing at both L3-4 and L4-5 on the lateral view, caused by hypertrophic facet disease located posteriorly *(arrowheads)* and the annular bulge anteriorly *(open arrows)*.

Flexion and extension films can allow one to further evaluate the lumbar canal under stress.[71] Functional (flexion-extension) myelography is of value in preoperative evaluation of segmental spinal instability. If instability is present preoperatively, it is predictive of a poor prognosis after surgery without fusion (p <.01), particularly in women. Postoperative slipping was noted in 26 of 61 patients (42%), especially in those patients who experienced an unsatisfactory outcome (p <.001).[29] Fox *et al.*[17] pointed out that predictors of postoperative subluxation included instability on flexion-extension studies, particularly if preoperative spondylolisthesis was present. These authors stressed that radiologic progression of the slippage postoperatively does not necessarily correlate with a poor clinical outcome.

Magnetic Resonance Imaging

MRI is used more frequently for assessing patients with spinal disorders,[14,60] although currently the authors prefer the combination of myelography followed by CT scan.

Gadolinium DTPAB–enhanced MRI of the lumbar spinal canal in patients with neurogenic intermittent claudication often reveals abnormal intrathecal enhancement at the level of severe lumbar spinal stenosis, which may extend cranially or caudally. The enhancement pattern is

linear, curvilinear, punctate, or diffuse in configuration. This is thought to be caused by enhancement of dilated veins that drain the cauda equina, or it may be evidence of blood-nerve barrier breakdown associated with mechanical injury, inflammatory response, and wallerian degeneration and regeneration of compressed nerve roots.[27]

Surgical Indications

Symptomatic degenerative lumbar spinal stenosis occurs mainly in the over age 65 population. Age alone does not represent a contraindication to surgery. The critical indicator for surgery revolves around the patients' perception of their quality of life and the status of their medical health. These variables vary among individuals, but they form a major criterion when considering surgical intervention.[42,73]

Absolute indications for surgical decompression are: (1) actual or impending cauda equina syndrome; (2) increasing neurologic abnormality of the legs, such as weakness and numbness; and (3) increasing or unrelenting pain.

Surgery should be considered for patients with severe lumbar spinal stenosis when the pain is intractable or when appropriate nonoperative treatment has failed and other causes of pain have been ruled out. Psychologic evaluation should be considered for patients whose report of pain is disproportionate to the apparent disease process.

Lumbar spinal stenosis commonly presents with symptoms of monoradiculopathy. In such cases, if the involved nerve root can be determined correctly, limited decompression of the root alone is all that is necessary.[7]

Lumbar retrolisthesis is occasionally observed in lumbar spinal stenosis. Of men with low back pain, 30% have retrolisthesis on spinal extension. In later stages, degeneration of the facet joints may lead to symptoms of lateral recess stenosis and foraminal encroachment. This usually requires lumbar decompression.

Bridwell et al.[5] studied the effect of fusion in 44 patients who had degenerative spondylolisthesis with lumbar spinal stenosis. They noted that patients who underwent decompression and fusion with instrumentation and autogenous bone grafts had a more successful outcome than those patients who had decompression without fusion or with noninstrumented autogenous iliac crest bone grafts ($p = .001$). Without an instrumented spine fusion there was a significant progression of spondylolisthesis.

Degenerative scoliosis is a late development of degenerative disc disease and facet disease of the lumbar spine. Lateral olisthesis of the lumbar spine is often associated with significant rotational deformities. Symptoms of central and lateral recess spinal stenosis or back pain are common indicators for spinal surgery. Recent reviews suggest that decompression alone is insufficient treatment for many patients with degenerative scoliosis or lumbar spinal stenosis, and they often require concomitant instrumentation with bony fusion.[24,44,49,62]

Attempts at surgical correction of the aging, degenerating spine should be approached with caution. Patients and their families must be fully aware of the chances of failure or of worsening of the condition.[58] After extensive spinal decompression without fusion, worsening of preexistent deformity is occasionally observed.[24] Furthermore, accentuation of the deformity is often asymptomatic. Predisposition to postoperative deformities includes: (1) a large disc space height at the time of decompression, (2) the presence of traction spurs extending from the margins of the vertebral bodies, (3) radical removal of the disc facets at the time of decompression, (4) age younger than 50, (5) obesity, (6) scoliosis, and (7) asymmetric, narrowed discs.[24] The presence of these predictive factors has been used as an indication of fusion at the time of decompression.[17,24,49]

Nonsurgical Treatment

If the patient's symptoms of lumbar spinal stenosis become intractable, the prognosis for relief by prolonged bed rest is not as good as that of the patient with a disc herniation. This is understandable when one considers the following: a disc herniation gradually recedes into the disc space after 5 to 7 days of bed rest. Bed rest for a patient who is suffering from the syndrome of lumbar spinal stenosis from bony entrapment may result in a decrease in the inflammatory reaction of the affected nerve roots. As edema diminishes, there may be enough room for the neural elements, despite the existing narrowing of the canal. Nonoperative therapy includes the use of nonsteroidal antiinflammatory and analgesic medications. If these fail to produce significant improvements, steroids may be administered into the epidural space. However, epidural steroid injections provide only limited benefit. Rosen et al.[57] reported that approximately 50% of patients with radicular symptoms received temporary relief, but less than 25% experienced benefit at follow-up 8 months after epidural injections.[57] Physical therapy (infrared heat, ultrasound, diathermy, and active lumbar exercises) may provide temporary relief of symptoms arising from muscle spasms. Salmon calcitonin has been recommended for the treatment of pain and neurogenic intermittent claudication in lumbar spinal stenosis, but the results are conflicting.[16,51]

Surgical Technique

General Considerations

Preoperative planning for surgery should include evaluation of the patient's general medical condition and treatment of comorbidities.[9,63]

Surgery for lumbar spinal stenosis consists of spinal decompression to remove the bone and soft tissues that are compressing the dural sac and nerve roots. The extent of the decompression depends on the case-specific anatomy. The most frequent error is either too little decompression (with residual stenosis) or excessive decompression (causing segmental spinal instability).

Infrequently, spinal fusion is indicated at the same time as decompression, but in some cases it is necessary.[24,49,62] The need for fusion can often be predicted preoperatively. An extensive decompression may destabilize the spine (segmental spinal instability), necessitating concomitant spinal fusion.

After induction of anesthesia and the administration of intravenous antibiotics, the patient is placed prone on an appropriate frame. Care must be taken to avoid external pressure on the eyes. The abdomen should hang free, the hips should be flexed, and the lumbar spine should be flattened. If spinal fusion is planned, appropriate adjustment of the frame will preserve the normal lumbar lordosis. The placement of a urinary catheter is recommended if the surgery is expected to be lengthy or if the patient's medical condition requires it.

Although the use of evoked potential monitoring may help determine whether an adequate decompression has been accomplished, its use is controversial in lumbar spinal stenosis. The surgeon cannot rely on somatosensory evoked potentials alone to evaluate the completeness of the decompression.

After the skin incision is made, dissection proceeds to the lumbodorsal fascia, at which self-restraining retractors are placed. Spinous processes are identified, and an incision is made directly over the middle of each spinous process. A subperiosteal dissection of muscle from the spinous processes and laminae is performed to minimize bleeding. An attempt is made to preserve the muscle's pseudocapsule. Dissection is continued laterally along the laminar arches as far as the apophyseal joints. If a dorsolateral intertransverse fusion is planned, the dissection is carried over the apophyseal joints to a point lateral to the tips of the transverse processes. Muscle must be assiduously stripped from the bone to increase the success of the fusion. The white inter-transverse ligament should be clearly exposed after removal of overlying muscle to improve the rate of fusion. Successful fusion, occurring in approximately 90% of these cases, is dependent on technique.

When this phase of the dissection has been completed, large, self-retaining Scoville retractors are positioned. At this point a lateral intraoperative radiograph is taken with an instrument placed at the base of a spinous process or through the interlaminar space to confirm that one is at the correct level. The precise determination of level may be uncertain in obese patients. Once the approach phase is completed, decompression of the central or lateral elements can commence.

Central Stenosis

Of the various types of stenotic spinal syndromes, central canal stenosis is the most easily treated. For example, if the major stenotic segment is at the L4-5 interspace, the caudal portion of the L4 spinous process, the rostral portion of the L5 spinous process, and the adjacent portions of the laminar arches and medial third of the facets are removed. Lateral decompression should extend at least to the medial surface of the pedicles. The thickened ligamentum flavum is opened in the midline with Kerrison rongeurs or a scalpel. The midline is chosen for opening the ligamentum flavum because the dorsal epidural fat pad often lies between the dura and ligamentum flavum, serving as a protective barrier.

A no. 4 Penfield dissector or equivalent is then used to separate the ligamentum flavum from the dura mater laterally. Cottonoid patties are placed beneath the ligamentum flavum to facilitate its excision and protect the dura from damage, which may be caused by the Kerrison rongeur.

When the laminotomies have been performed above and below the hypertrophic apophyseal joint, dissection proceeds in a rostral to caudal direction, toward the region of maximum stenosis (which is approached last). The lamina and medial facets are then thinned with a high-speed drill, and the laminectomy is completed by chipping out the thin, residual laminar bone with curettes or small Kerrison punches. Care must be taken to preserve the pars interarticularis to prevent postoperative fracture of the pars. An intact pars will also increase the available surface area for lateral mass fusion if a fusion is to be performed.

In patients with spinal stenosis the dura mater is often adherent to the undersurface of the lamina and ligamentum flavum. This is particularly true in the region of the lateral recess. Upbiting rongeurs are used to remove the anterior surface of the thickened lamina, thereby remodeling the shape of the spinal canal. A central, midline decompression is thus created from L4 to L5, which provides excellent release of the dural tube in the central portion of the spinal canal. There is little advantage in removing the entire lamina of L4 and L5, because the stenosis can nearly always be relieved by limiting the structures removed to those causing the central canal stenosis; that is, the hypertrophic infolded ligamentum flavum, the caudal half of the lamina of L4, and the rostral third of the lamina of L5.

When the midline dura mater has been exposed in its entirety, the surgeon proceeds to clear the lateral gutters, including a medial facetectomy, working from the opposite side of the table with 45-degree–angled Kerrison rongeurs or a high-speed drill. Hemostasis is obtained with Gelfoam. Epidural veins located in the lateral recesses are thrombosed with bipolar coagulation in order to avoid spread of thermal injury to the adjacent nerves, which may be caused by monopolar coagulation.

At this point the sizes of the neuroforamina are evaluated, using blunt probes of varying lengths and sizes. Usually, at the site of compression there is very little or no epidural fat.

Often the dura mater is adherent to the undersurface of the lamina and to the undersurface of the ligamentum flavum, especially in the lateral recess. Dural tears occur in approximately 5% of patients with spinal stenosis who have not had a previous operation. They occur more often in reoperations as a result of severe epidural fibrosis and the absence of a clearly defined plane between the dura and epidural scar. If possible, these tears should be repaired immediately with absorbable sutures.

Lateral Stenosis

Foraminotomy, if necessary, may be accomplished using a variety of methods, depending on the degree of spinal stenosis. If the stenosis is mild, a simple undercutting of the superior articular facet with a 45-degree–angled punch may be adequate. If the stenosis is severe, it may be necessary to remove most or all of the pars interarticularis. If the latter procedure is performed, particularly bilaterally, a fusion must be performed. If the patient already has degenerative spondylolisthesis, the consideration of a fusion with instrumentation becomes even more relevant.

If the pedicle is a major source of neural compression, resulting in kinking of the exiting nerve root, the use of an osteotome or high-speed drill to remove the caudal aspect of the pedicle, where the nerve root rounds it, may help to decrease the angular deformity of the nerve root. Osteotomes and gouges are ideally suited for shaving the offending pedicle. The fragment of pedicle to be removed must not be turned into the nerve root, and meticulous attention must be paid to removing all bone fragments from the foramen. When using a chisel, bone must be removed with great precision and control while the exiting nerve root is continually kept under direct visualization. Decompression of the lateral recess and foraminotomy includes the removal of the joint capsular ligament, osteophytes, superior and inferior articular processes, and occasionally part of the pedicle and reduction of disc margin osteophytes. A small 45-degree–angled Kerrison rongeur can be used to remove the ventral portion or tip of the superior articular process, which is narrowing the foramen. Because of marked osteophytic overgrowth of the articular process, a significant amount of bone can be removed without entry into the joint itself or weakening of the articulation.

If the foramen is markedly stenotic because of a hypertrophic superior articular facet, it may be necessary to decompress the entire foramen. Bone is removed along the base of the superior articular process using the surface of the caudal pedicle as a landmark. The superior articular process can often be removed in a single piece if bony removal is carried laterally far enough. It is important to remember that the foramen has a width of approximately 1cm, and a hypertrophic superior articular process may extend along its entire width, causing nerve root compression along the entire length of the tip of the superior articular process. Removal of the medial portion of the superior articular facet (window foraminotomy) will fail to provide adequate decompression of the foramen.

A foraminotomy can also be accomplished with small chisels, because they are easy to use with precision. With sharp osteotomes and gouges ranging from a few millimeters to 1.5cm in width, driven with a light awl, small shavings of the bony margins of the foramen can be removed, with the foramen being sculpted to its new dimension. If a fusion is not planned, it is important not to remove more bone than necessary, to avoid destabilization. However, it is desirable to overdecompress the foramen and spinal canal, as well as the lateral recesses, to ensure for adequate decompression, even if this results in spinal instability. Such iatrogenically induced instability can be readily and easily corrected by a spinal fusion during the same operation, with or without instrumentation.

It may be necessary to remove the medial half of the superior facet of the caudal vertebra. With a lateral recess stenosis the overhanging superior facet may often need to be undercut or removed. This is easily accomplished with a small, sharp osteotome, breaking away the bone without fully penetrating the process. The bone chips are removed with a forceps. If the bony and ligamentous removal is adequate, the dura mater should be pulsatile, the nerve roots should be free and mobile, and a 2 to 4mm probe should pass easily along the root sleeve into the foramen. Up to 50% of the facet joint may be removed without a loss of spinal stability.

The disc space should be inspected. A bilateral disc ectomy may be performed if a disc herniation is present. Hemostasis is obtained, and a piece of autogenous fat laid in the epidural space may minimize periradicular scarring.

Isolated Unilateral Recess Stenosis

When the pathology is confined to a unilateral recess, a midline incision is made, and only the laminae on the involved side are exposed. The lateral recess is divided into three zones: entrance, midzone, and exit. If only the entrance zone is stenotic, a medial facetectomy provides adequate decompression. The midzone is bounded ventrally by the vertebral body, dorsally by the pars interarticularis, and laterally by the pedicle and foramen. The dorsal root ganglion, which has the largest diameter of any portion of the nerve root, usually lies in this zone and can be easily compressed there. Stenosis in this region may also be caused by the abundant, hypertrophic, capsular ligament associated with spondylosis. The exit zone contains the ventral ramus, and can only be decompressed by a far lateral foraminotomy.

Complications of Decompression

Complications of decompression include segmental spinal instability, dural tears, arachnoiditis, infection, nerve injury, and epidural fibrosis. Sophisticated biomechanical analysis has shown that sacrifice of more than 50% of both facets or the sacrifice of one entire facet may produce a significant loss of mechanical integrity.[23] This research tends to confirm the clinical experience of others. Radiologic evidence of postoperative instability, however, is not always associated with clinical symptoms. In many studies progressive symptoms are found in up to 19% of patients. It is also probable that slowly progressing deformity can occur even after carefully obtained radiographs fail to show increased mobility at the time of surgery.[34]

Clinical experience indicates that other factors may influence the long-term result. Advanced age, marked disc space narrowing, and osteophytes are generally thought to reduce the need for fusion because of the additional stiffness in the motion segment. By contrast, operations on a younger patient, particularly when radical facet resections are performed, can lead to a spine that is unstable. If disc excision is performed in conjunction with facetectomies, the degree of instability is increased.[33,39,50]

Dural tears occur in 0.3% to 13% of previously unoperated patients with lumbar spinal stenosis. The incidence of dural tears increases to 17.6% in previously operated patients. These tears should be repaired immediately.[18]

Results

Deen et al.[12] used the exercise tolerance test on the treadmill to measure the effectiveness of lumbar decompressive laminectomy in 20 patients with neurogenic intermittent claudication from lumbar spinal stenosis. Following a specific protocol, they noted that the mean time to first symptoms was 2.68 minutes (median time, 1.31 minutes) and the mean time to severe symptoms was 5.47 minutes (median time, 3.42 minutes) preoperatively. In the postoperative trial at the same speed, the mean time to first symptoms was 11.2 minutes (median time, 15 minutes) and the mean time to severe symptoms was 11.81 minutes (median time, 15 minutes). This is a safe, easily administered, and quantifiable method for assessing the outcome following laminectomy in patients with symptomatic lumbar spinal stenosis, which measures the real value of decompression.

Deen et al.[13] analyzed 45 patients who had no improvement after lumbar decompression for lumbar spinal stenosis. They reported that only 23 patients (51%) had the clinical syndrome of neurogenic intermittent claudication preoperatively, 15 patients (33%) had midline low back pain without a radicular component, three patients had peripheral neuropathy, and three patients had atypical leg pain. Only 10 out of the 45 patients had radiographic evidence of severe spinal stenosis. In an additional 10 patients the surgical decompression was inadequate. They concluded that the surgical outcome can be improved by a more careful selection of patients and by performing adequate surgical decompression.

Bladder function is expected to improve after lumbar decompression for spinal stenosis.[11] Of 20 patients in that series who had some degree of bladder dysfunction preoperatively, 12 patients (60%) noted subjective improvement in bladder function postoperatively; in eight patients the bladder function was unchanged and no patient demonstrated worsening function. Both postvoiding residual urine volume and urine flow rates showed improvement, but cystometrography, electromyography, urine flow pattern, and bladder capacity remained unchanged.

Airaksinen *et al.*[1] retrospectively reviewed 439 patients who had undergone decompressive laminectomy for lumbar spinal stenosis. They concluded that a good outcome could be predicted by several variables. The ability to return to work postoperatively depended on the patient's ability to work before surgery. Age younger than 50 years at the time of the operation and absence of prior back surgery were also positive predictors of being able to return to work. Men had a lower incidence of reoperation for recurrent stenosis or instability (6%) than did women (28%).[45]

Summary

Clinical awareness of spinal stenosis, thoughtfully performed diagnostic imaging procedures, sophisticated understanding of the pathophysiology of lumbar spinal stenosis and neurogenic intermittent claudication, and appropriate surgical treatment are important for the successful treatment of this condition. Failure in any one of these features will result in failure to relieve the patient's disabling symptoms. Poorly planned and unjustified surgery may actually worsen the patient's symptoms because of epidural fibrosis, arachnoiditis, or spinal instability.

REFERENCES

1. Airaksinen O, Herno A, Saari T: Surgical treatment of lumbar spinal stenosis: patients' postoperative disability and working capacity. *Eur Spine J* 3:261, 1994.
2. Amundsen T, Weber H, Lilleas F, *et al*: Lumbar spinal stenosis: clinical and radiologic features. *Spine* 20:1178, 1995.
3. Bolender NF, Schonstrom NSR, Spengler DM: Role of computed tomography and myelography in the diagnosis of central spinal stenosis. *J Bone Joint Surg* 67A:240, 1985.
4. Bridwell KH: Lumbar spinal stenosis: diagnosis, management, treatment. *Clin Geriatr Med* 10:677, 1994.
5. Bridwell KH, Sedgewick TA, O'Brien MF, *et al*: The role of fusion and instrumentation in the treatment of degenerative spondylolisthesis with spinal stenosis. *J Spinal Dis* 6:461, 1993.
6. Butler D, Trafimow JH, Andersson GBJ, *et al*: Disc s degenerate before facets. *Spine* 15:111, 1990.
7. Caspar W, Papavero L, Sayler MK, Harkey HL: Precise and limited decompression for lumbar spinal stenosis. *Acta Neurochir (Wien)* 131:130, 1994.
8. Chen Q, Baba H, Kamitani K, *et al*: Postoperative bone regrowth in lumbar spinal stenosis: a multivariate analysis of 48 patients. *Spine* 19:2144, 1994.
9. Ciol MA, Deyo RA, Howell E, Kreif S: An assessment of surgery for spinal stenosis: time trends, geographic variations, complications, and reoperations. *J Am Geriatr Soc* 44:285, 1996.
10. Dai LY, Xu YK, Zhang WM, Zhou ZH: The effect of flexion-extension motion of the lumbar spine on the capacity of the spinal canal: an experimental study. *Spine* 14:523, 1989.
11. Deen HG Jr, Zimmerman RS, Swanson SK, Larson TR: Assessment of bladder function after lumbar decompressive laminectomy for spinal stenosis: a prospective study. *J Neurosurg* 80:971, 1994.
12. Deen HG Jr, Zimmerman RS, Lyons MK, *et al*: Measurement of exercise tolerance on the treadmill in patients with symptomatic lumbar spinal stenosis: a useful indicator of functional status and surgical outcome. *J Neurosurg* 83:27, 1995.
13. Deen HG Jr, Zimmerman RS, Lyons MK, *et al*: Analysis of early failures after lumbar decompressive laminectomy for spinal stenosis. *Mayo Clin Proc* 70:33, 1995.
14. el Gammal T, Brooks BS, Freedy RM, Crews CE: MR myelography: imaging findings. *Am J Roentgenol* 164:173, 1995.
15. Epstein NE, Epstein JA: Individual and coexistent lumbar and cervical spinal stenosis. In Hopp E (ed): *Spine: State of the Art Reviews*, vol 1. Philadelphia, Hanley & Belfus, 1987, p 401.
16. Eskola A, Pohjolainen T, Alaranta H, *et al*: Calcitonin treatment in lumbar spinal stenosis: a randomized, placebo-controlled, double-blind, cross-over study with one-year follow-up. *Calcif Tissue Int* 50:400, 1992.
17. Fox WM, Onofrio BM, Hanssen AD: Clinical outcomes and radiological instability following decompressive lumbar laminectomy for degenerative spinal stenosis: a comparison of patients undergoing concomitant arthrodesis versus decompression alone. *J Neurosurg* 85:793, 1996.
18. Goodkin R, Laska LL: Unintended "incidental" durotomy during surgery of the lumbar spine: medicolegal implications. *Surg Neurol* 43:4, 1995.
19. Gundry CR, Heithoff KB: Imaging evaluation of patients with spinal deformity. *Orthop Clin North Am* 25:247, 1994.
20. Hellstrom PA, Tammela TL, Niinimaki TJ: Voiding dysfunction and urodynamic findings in patients with lumbar spinal stenosis and the effect of decompressive laminectomy. *Scand J Urol Nephrol* 29:167, 1995.
21. Helms CA, Vogler JB III, Hardy DC: CT of the lumbar spine: normal variants and pitfalls. *Radiographics* 7:447, 1987.
22. Herno A, Airaksinen O, Saari T, Miettinen H: The predictive value of preoperative myelography in lumbar spinal stenosis. *Spine* 19:1335, 1994.
23. Herron LD, Trippi AC: L4-5 degenerative spondylolisthesis. The results of treatment by decompressive laminectomy without fusion. *Spine* 14:534, 1989.
24. Hopp E, Tsou PM: Postdecompression lumbar instability. *Clin Orthop* 227:143, 1988.
25. Jensen MC, Brant-Zawadzki MN, Obuchowski N, *et al*: Magnetic resonance imaging of the lumbar spine in people without back pain. *N Engl J Med* 331:69, 1994.
26. Jensen OH, Schmidt-Olsen S: A new functional test in the diagnostic evaluation of neurogenic intermittent claudication. *Clin Rheumatol* 8:363, 1989.
27. Jinkins JR: Gd-DTPA enhanced MR of the lumbar spinal canal in patients with claudication. *J Comput Assist Tomogr* 17:555, 1993.
28. Johnsson KE, Rosen I, Uden A: Neurophysiologic investigation of patients with spinal stenosis. *Spine* 12:483, 1987.

29. Johnsson KE, Redlund-Johnell I, Uden A, Willner S: Preoperative and postoperative instability in lumbar spinal stenosis. *Spine* 14:591, 1989.

30. Jonsson B, Stromqvist B: Symptoms and signs in degeneration of the lumbar spine. A prospective, consecutive study of 300 operated patients. *J Bone Joint Surg* 75B:381, 1993.

31. Katz JN, Dalgas M, Stucki G, Lipson SJ: Diagnosis of lumbar spinal stenosis. *Rheum Dis Clin North Am* 20:471, 1994.

32. Katz JN, Dalgas M, Stucki G, *et al*: Degenerative lumbar spinal stenosis. Diagnostic value of the history and physical examination. *Arthritis Rheum* 38:1236, 1995.

33. Kawai S, Hattori S, Oda H, *et al*: Enlargement of the lumbar vertebral canal in lumbar canal stenosis. *Spine* 6:381, 1981.

34. Kirkaldy-Willis WH, Farfan HF: Instability of the lumbar spine. *Clin Orthop* 165:110, 1982.

35. Kirkaldy-Willis WH, Paine KW, Cauchoix J, McIvor G: Lumbar spinal stenosis. *Clin Orthop* 99:30, 1974.

36. Knutsson F: The instability associated with disc degeneration in the lumbar spine. *Acta Radiol* 25:593, 1944.

37. Kondo M, Matsuda H, Kureya S, Shimazu A: Electrophysiological studies at intermittent claudication in lumbar stenosis. *Spine* 14:862, 1989.

38. Lawrence JS: disc degeneration. Its frequency and relationship to symptoms. *Ann Rheum Dis* 28:121, 1969.

39. Lee CK: Lumbar spinal instability (olisthesis) after extensive posterior spinal decompression. *Spine* 8:429, 1983.

40. Lewin T: Osteoarthritis in lumbar synovial joints. *Acta Orthop Scand* 73(Suppl):1, 1964.

41. Lipson S: Radiologic imaging for spinal stenosis. *Semin Spine Surg* 1:145, 1989.

42. Lombardi JS, Wiltse LL, Reynolds J, *et al*: Treatment of degenerative spondylolisthesis. *Spine* 10:821, 1985.

43. MacNab I: Spondylolisthesis with an intact neural arch: the so-called pseudo-spondylolisthesis. *J Bone Joint Surg* 32B:325, 1950.

44. Markwalder TM: Surgical management of neurogenic claudication in 100 patients with lumbar spinal stenosis due to degenerative spondylolisthesis. *Acta Neurochir* 120:136, 1993.

45. McCullen GM, Bernini PM, Bernstein SH, Tosteson TD: Clinical and roentgenographic results of decompression for lumbar spinal stenosis. *J Spinal Disord* 7:380, 1994.

46. McGuire RA, Brown MD, Green BA: Intradural spinal tumors and spinal stenosis. Report of two cases. *Spine* 12:1062, 1987.

47. Miller JA, Schmatz C, Schultz AB: Lumbar disc degeneration: correlation with age, sex, and spine level in 600 autopsy specimens. *Spine* 13:173, 1988.

48. Mixter WJ, Barr JS: Rupture of the intervertebral disc with involvement of the spinal canal. *N Engl J Med* 211:210, 1934.

49. Nasca RJ: Rationale for spinal fusion in lumbar spinal stenosis. *Spine* 14:451, 1989.

50. Natelson SE: The injudicious laminectomy. *Spine* 11:966, 1986.

51. Onel D, Sari H, Donmez C: Lumbar spinal stenosis: clinical/radiologic therapeutic evaluation in 145 patients.

52. Paine KW: Clinical features of lumbar spinal stenosis. *Clin Orthop* 115:77, 1976.

53. Penning L, Wilmink JT: Posture-dependent bilateral compression of L4 or L5 nerve roots in facet hypertrophy. A dynamic CT-myelographic study. *Spine* 12:48, 1987.

54. Postacchini F, Cinotti G: Bone regrowth after surgical decompression for lumbar spinal stenosis. *J Bone Joint Surg* 74B:862, 1992.

55. Powell MC, Wilsonn M, Szypryt P, *et al*: Prevalence of lumbar disc degeneration observed by magnetic resonance in symptomless women. *Lancet* 2:1366, 1986.

56. Putti V: New conceptions in the pathogenesis of sciatic pain. *Lancet* 2:53, 1927.

57. Rosen CD, Kahanovitz N, Bernstein R, Viola K: A retrospective analysis of the efficacy of epidural steroid injections. *Clin Orthop* 228:270, 1988.

58. Sanderson PL, Wood PL: Surgery for lumbar spinal stenosis in old people. *J Bone Joint Surg* 75B:393, 1993.

59. Sarpyener MA: Congenital stricture of the spinal canal. *J Bone Joint Surg* 27B:70, 1945.

60. Schnebel B, Kingston S, Watkins R, Dillin W: Comparison of MRI to contrast CT in the diagnosis of spinal stenosis. *Spine* 14:332, 1989.

61. Sicard JA, Forestier J: Methode radiographique d'exploration de la cavite epidural par le lipiodol. *Rev Neurol* 37:1264, 1921

62. Simmons ED Jr, Simmons EH: Spinal stenosis with scoliosis. *Spine* 17 (Suppl 6):S117, 1992.

63. Simpson JM, Silveri CP, Balderston RA, *et al*: The results of operations on the lumbar spine in patients who have diabetes mellitus. *J Bone Joint Surg* 75A:1823, 1993.

64. Teplick JG: *Lumbar Spine CT and MRI*. Philadelphia: JB Lippincott, 1992, p 353.

65. Tsuji H, Tamaki T, Itoh T, *et al*: Redundant nerve roots in patients with degenerative lumbar spinal stenosis. *Spine* 10:72, 1985.

66. Verbiest H: A radicular syndrome from developmental narrowing of the lumbar vertebral canal. *J Bone Joint Surg* 36B:230, 1954.

67. Verbiest H: Pathomorphologic aspects of developmental lumbar stenosis. *Orthop Clin North Am* 6:177, 1975.

68. Verbiest H: Introduction. In Hopp E (ed): *Spine: State of the Art Reviews*, vol 1. Philadelphia, Hanley & Belfus, 1987, p 366.

69. Vernon-Roberts B, Pirie CJ: Degenerative changes in the intervertebral disc s of the lumbar spine and their sequelae. *Rheumatol Rehabil* 16:13, 1977.

70. Wiesel SW, Bernini P, Rothman RH: Developmental anatomy and pathophysiology of lumbar disc disease. In *The Aging Lumbar Spine*. Philadelphia, WB Saunders, 1982, p 20.

71. Wiesel SW, Tsourmas N, Feffer HL, *et al*: A study of computer-assisted tomography. I. The incidence of positive CAT scans in an asymptomatic group of patients. *Spine* 9:549, 1984.

72. Wiltse LL, Rothman SL: Spondylolisthesis: classifications, diagnosis and natural history. *Semin Spinal Surg* 1:78, 1989.

73. Wiltse LL, Kirkaldy-Willis WH, McIvor GW: The treatment of spinal stenosis. *Clin Orthop* 115:83, 1976.

Conservative treatment or surgical intervention? *Spine* 18:291, 1993.

CHAPTER 54

Spondylolisthesis: Sagittal Plane Lumbar Spine Deformity Correction

Nevan G. Baldwin, Shunji Matsunaga, and Bruce L. Ehni

The first description of a spondylolisthesis is credited to Herbiniaux, a Belgian obstetrician who diagnosed the condition by pelvic examination and noted that a lumbar vertebra ventral to the sacrum was an obstruction to labor.[92] The name of the condition arises from the Greek words *spondylous*, meaning spine, and *olisthesis*, which refers to slipping.[88] The first use of the term *spondylolisthesis* is credited to Kilian, who believed the problem was caused by subluxation of the facet joints.[84]

Since the initial description, spondylolisthesis has been classified in a number of ways, usually being grouped according to anatomic and etiologic subtypes. The most widely accepted classification scheme in current clinical use is probably the one described by Wiltse, Newman, and MacNab in 1976.[156] Similar to its predecessors, this scheme is based on etiologic and anatomic features. The importance of classifying the condition is that both treatment and prognostic factors are related to the type of underlying defect. The following categories comprise the Wiltse-Newman-MacNab classification: dysplastic, isthmic, degenerative, traumatic, and pathologic types (Box 54.1). Some authors consider the postsurgical occurrence of a spondylolisthesis to be a separate (iatrogenic) type.[2,154] In their original article, Wiltse *et al.*[156] included it as a subtype of the pathologic form and called it spondylolisthesis acquisita. It is probably more reasonable, however, to give this type its own category because the treatment is more straightforward and the prognosis is better for this type than for most of the other conditions in the pathologic subtype.

A number of other terms are used frequently in association with spondylolisthesis. The ventral displacement of one vertebra in relation to the adjacent caudal vertebra is referred to as olisthesis, olisthetic defect, or slip. Spondylolysis refers to the presence of a defect in the pars interarticularis that is not associated with an olisthesis. The defect in spondylolysis is bilateral in the majority of cases.[39,58] A severe spondylolisthesis, in which there is complete or near-complete subluxation of one vertebral body over another, is called spondyloptosis. Spondyloptosis occurs most commonly at the lumbosacral junction.

The most widely used clinical method to describe a spondylolisthesis is that described by Meyerding.[85] This method involves dividing the rostral surface of the lower vertebral body into fourths and expressing the slip in terms of the number of fourths that the subluxation encompasses. For example, a displacement of up to 25% is referred to as a grade I slip; a displacement of 25% to 50% is called a grade II slip, and so forth (Figure 54.1). Because spondylolistheses are often associated with significant deformities of the vertebral body end plates, precise definition of the degree of slip can be quite difficult. A number of other methods to define the slip and associated features, such as angles of articulation, have been described.[*] These methods may be of some use to researchers in this area, but for clinical use, Meyerding's method is a simple and practical tool that is without equal.

Anatomy of Spondylolisthesis

An understanding of the anatomic features of each type of spondylolisthesis is important because these play a role in presentation, prognosis, evaluation, and treatment selection.

Dysplastic Spondylolisthesis

Dysplastic spondylolisthesis occurs almost exclusively at the lumbosacral junction. Occasionally it will occur one level higher in the presence of a transitional vertebra. Abnormalities of the upper sacral surface or the neural arch of the last mobile lumbar vertebra (e.g., malformed inferior facets) permit the olisthesis to occur.[70] Spina bifida is a commonly associated component of neural arch anomalies. Abnormalities of the facet joints, most commonly a reduction in the transverse articular dimension, provide insufficient stabilization and ultimately allow subluxation by failure of the bony hook of the dorsal elements (Figure 54.2).[46] As this type of slip progresses, it can lead to elongation of the pars, with eventual development of a pars defect. It is still, however, identifiable as a separate entity by the presence of facet joint subluxation. The neural arch is usually intact (with the exception of a possible gap of spina bifida) in this type, and unless the pars elongates, the slip cannot exceed about 35% of the width of the sacral end-plate without producing symptoms of severe cauda equina compression.[158] Therefore the intact neural arch results in a greater frequency of neurologic deficits in this type of spondylolisthesis than with the isthmic type.[149]

Isthmic Spondylolisthesis

Isthmic spondylolisthesis is the result of abnormalities of the pars interarticularis, and it is the most common variety.[94] Changes at the pars interarticularis occur over time and give rise to a spectrum of appearances for this disorder. The changes are postulated to be a result of repeated fractures of the pars with healing and remodeling.[88,151,153] The different appearances of the pars give rise to three subtypes of isthmic spondylolisthesis. Subtype A has complete separation of the components of the pars, whereas subtype B has elongation of the pars without separation. Repeated

---

*References 13,37,68,84,143,155.

BOX

54.1

Wiltse-Newman-MacNab classification of spondylolisthesis

Dysplastic: Spondylolisthesis caused by abnormalities of the upper sacrum or the neural arch of the last mobile lumbar vertebra, which permit the olisthesis to occur.

Isthmic: Spondylolisthesis caused by a lesion in the pars interarticularis. There are three subtypes.

Degenerative: Spondylolisthesis caused by long-standing intersegmental instability and the changes resulting from abnormal motion in the unstable segments.

Traumatic: Spondylolisthesis caused by fractures in portions of the "bony hook" other than the pars. The bony hook consists of the pedicles, the pars, and the superior and inferior articular processes.

Pathologic: Spondylolisthesis caused by changes in the bone as a result of either localized or generalized disease. Cases of iatrogenic or postsurgical spondylolisthesis are also included in this category.

From Wiltse LL, Newman PH, MacNab I: Classification of spondylolysis and spondylolisthesis. *Clin Orthop* 117:23-29, 1976.

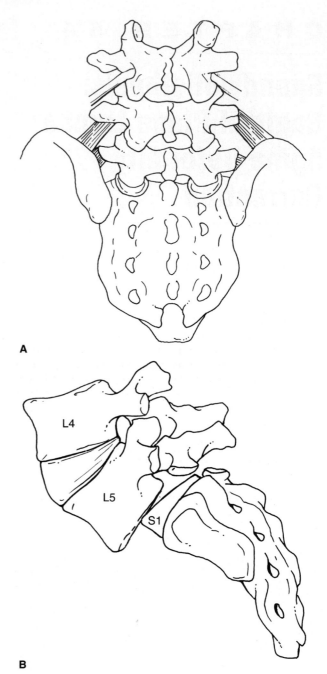

A

B

Figure 54.2 (A-B) Dysplastic spondylolisthesis. Note the axially oriented facets.

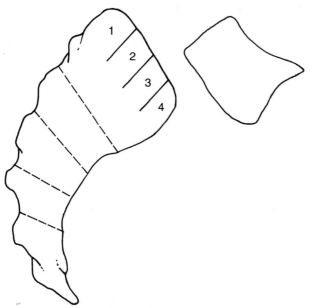

Figure 54.1 The Meyerding method for grading spondylolisthesis describes the slip as the amount of displacement of the upper vertebra relative to the width of the upper end-plate of the lower vertebrae. The categories are as follows: grade I—0% to 25%; grade IIC—25% to 50%; grade III—50% to 75%; and grade IV—more than 75%.

microfracture of the pars leads to a progressively more abnormal appearance and may eventually result in a fracture that does not heal, changing the condition to subtype A. The facet joints remain intact. In subtype C there is an acute pars fracture (Figure 54.3). Usually there is only spondylolysis in this condition, but it can, however, progress over time to include an olisthetic component. Most patients with spondylolysis will progress to some degree of olisthesis, but the slip is usually low grade and the patients are most commonly asymptomatic.[39,153] Pars defects are common in the general population (prevalence

of approximately 4% to 6%).[39,118,157] Therefore it may be difficult to determine the acuteness of the lesion in an accident victim. Radioisotope bone scans and single photon emission tomography can be used to distinguish between the acute and chronic lesions, as will be discussed later in this chapter.[6,73,107,121] If no increased uptake of the isotope is seen at the site, a chronic defect can be assumed. If, however, increased uptake is present, the distinction between an acute lesion and inflammatory changes resulting from trauma at the site of a preexisting lesion may not be made with certainty. Plain radiographs can also help in

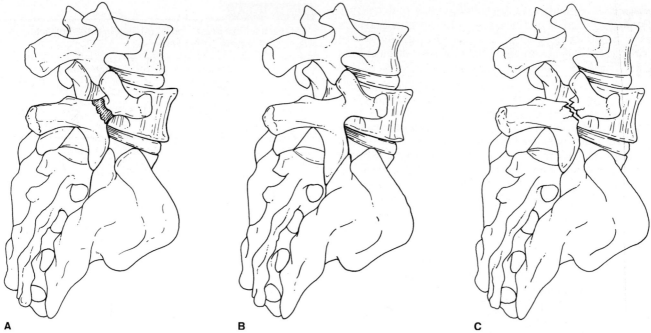

Figure 54.3 **(A)** Isthmic subtype A spondylolisthesis has a pars interarticularis defect that is filled with fibrous tissue. **(B)** Isthmic subtype B spondylolisthesis has elongation of the pars in association with subluxation of the vertebral body. **(C)** Isthmic subtype C spondylolisthesis arises from an acute fracture of the pars *(jagged line)* with subsequent subluxation of the vertebral body.

demonstrating sclerotic margins in the defect that clearly define the lesion to be preexisting.

Degenerative Spondylolisthesis

Degenerative spondylolisthesis is essentially a lesion of the facet joints.[45,46] It does not involve abnormalities of the pars interarticularis, nor is it associated with spina bifida.[91,116] With aging and the development of any abnormal motion at the facet joints, there is ongoing remodeling of the articular processes in the joints.[56] Over time the orientation of the facets becomes more sagittal, which allows progression of the spondylolisthesis.[45,46,56]

The slip in degenerative spondylolisthesis usually does not exceed approximately 30% of the width of the subjacent vertebral body.[91,116] The subluxation of the upper vertebral level is halted when its isthmus or inferior articular processes abut the upper margin of the superior articular processes or the dorsal margin of the body of the lower vertebrae (Figure 54.4).[1,84,116] Therefore acute, severe neurologic deficits are uncommon in patients with degenerative spondylolisthesis. The degenerative type of slip is found most often at the L4-5 level, about six times more often than either the L3-4 or the L5-S1 subluxations.[116] It is often associated with sacralization of the last lumbar vertebra and diminished lumbar lordosis.[116,117]

Degenerative spondylolisthesis is encountered in routine clinical practice. Many reports are available concerning operative treatment of this condition.* Spinal fusion for degenerative spondylolisthesis is controversial.[34,36,52,53] The radiographic diagnosis of degenerative spondylolisthesis is

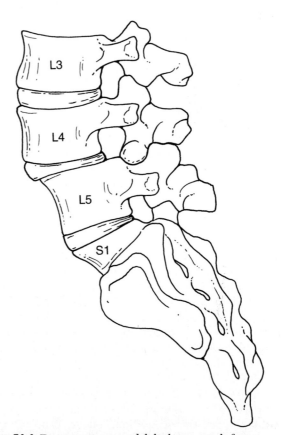

Figure 54.4 Degenerative spondylolistheses result from subluxation of a degenerated facet joint that allows the vertebral body to slip ventrally. In this example the inferior facet of L4 has abutted the dorsal aspect of the L5 body, thereby preventing further subluxation.

*References 14,19,20,34,38,52.

not difficult. Patients with this condition may undergo surgery for lumbago or neurologic symptoms without conservative treatment. Few studies have documented the clinical course of nonoperated patients with degenerative spondylolisthesis. Such information should be useful for determining indications for surgery and the choice of surgical procedures. A prospective study with more than 10 years follow-up on the nonoperated patients was performed to determine the progression of slippage, changes in clinical symptoms, and final functional status.[80] A total of 203 patients underwent conservative treatment because they had no clear neurologic deficits, except lumbago or pain in the lower extremities at the time of the initial examination. The conservative treatment of these patients consisted of bracing, the use of antiinflammatory agents, or lumbago exercises. Forty of 203 patients who underwent conservative treatment dropped out of this study during follow-up. A total of 53 of the remaining 163 patients underwent surgery because of the presence of neurologic compromise during follow-up. The development of a neurologic deficit did not correlate with progression of slippage. Finally, 145 unoperated patients (36 men and 109 women), who were followed up over more than 10 years, were the subjects of this study. They included 110 patients with conservative treatment and 35 of those who refused surgery. Of these patients, 47 were heavy workers, such as farmers or fishermen, 41 were desk workers, and 57 were housekeepers. A total of 46 of the 145 patients followed to the end of their life. The average age at the time of initial examination was 58.6 years. The period of observation was 10 to 18 years (average 15.8 years), and their ages at the end of the survey ranged from 69 to 85 years (average age 76 years). The percent slippage at initial examination was 7% to 20% (average 13.6%), and the site of slippage was the third lumbar vertebral body in five cases, the fourth lumbar vertebral body in 125, and the fifth lumbar vertebral body in 27. Twelve patients had two lesions.

With the assumption that an increase in slippage of 5% or more constitutes progression of slippage, progression was found in 49 cases (34%). The final percent slippage averaged 15.6% (7% to 29%). Percent slippage of 25% or more was observed in 10 cases. The patients who already had decreased intervertebral disc space height to half of normal exhibited no subsequent progression of slippage. In contrast, 49 (96%) of 51 patients who had no decrease in intervertebral disc space height exhibited progression of slippage. The extent of intervertebral disc space height was significantly larger in the nonprogressive group than in the progressive slip group (Table 54.1). Angular displacement of slipped segments was calculated with lateral radiographs in the ventral flexion position. With the assumption that an angular displacement of 9 degrees or more constitutes instability according to Posner's criteria,[109] 76 patients exhibited such instability at the time of the first visit. However, this instability decreased over the follow-up periods (Figure 54.5).

A total of 110 patients had lumbago, with or without pain, in the lower extremities at initial examination. The pain in the lower extremities was transitory and was considered to be radicular in nature. The duration of lumbago averaged 3.2 months (1.5 to 6.8 months) and the frequency of episodes of lumbago decreased with time.

TABLE 54.1

Decrease in Size of Intervertebral Space of the Segment with Spondylolisthesis During Follow-Up

Slippage	Progression (n = 49)	Not Progression (n = 96)	P Value
mean ± SD (mm)	1.5 ± 0.8	7.9 ± 1.6	<.005

Figures show the decrease in intervertebral space in both groups.

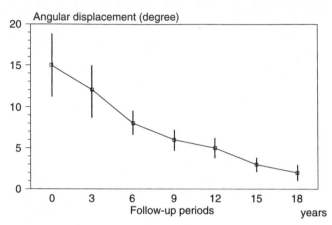

Figure 54.5 Change in angular displacement of the slipped segments in 76 patients with abnormal angular displacement at the first visit. Values are mean ± SD. (*From Matsunaga S, Ijir S, Hayashi K: Nonsurgically managed patients with degenerative spondylolisthesis: a 10- to 18-year follow-up study.* J Neurosurg 93:194-198, 2000.)

A total of 85 (77%) of the 110 patients exhibited improvement of lumbago during follow-up. All 25 patients who had no change in lumbago were heavy laborers. Finally, 84 of the 110 patients who had no neurologic deficits at initial examination remained free of neurologic deficits such as sensory disturbance, muscle weakness, and cauda equina symptoms after 10 years' follow-up. The remaining 26 patients had minor neurologic deficits such as numbness, but did not require surgery. A total of 48 (86%) of 56 patients who had pain in the lower extremities exhibited improvement of pain with conservative treatment, but these symptoms recurred in 37% of them. A total of 29 (83%) of the 35 patients who had neurologic symptoms such as those of intermittent claudication or vesicorectal disorder as a result of cauda equina pathology at initial examination and refused surgery, had deterioration of these symptoms. Development of neurologic deficits was not correlated with progression of slippage. The only symptom that changed when a radiographic decrease in intervertebral disc space height developed was lumbago. A total of 85 (90%) of 94 patients who had decreases in intervertebral disc space height exhibited improvement of lumbago (Figure 54.6).

Degenerative spondylolisthesis develops as a result of degeneration of the lumbar spine.[8,94] It is characterized in most patients by hypertrophy of the facet joint, resulting in segmental instability, predominantly in the sagittal plane.[94]

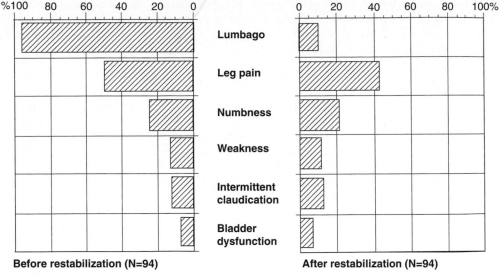

Figure 54.6 Changes in symptoms after the onset of decrease in intervertebral space size. *(From Matsunaga S, Ijir S, Hayashi K: Nonsurgically managed patients with degenerative spondylolisthesis: a 10- to 18-year follow-up study.* J Neurosurg 93:194-198, 2000.)

Disc degeneration is associated with degenerative spondylolisthesis to a varying degree. Decreases in intervertebral disc space height, osteophyte formation, ossification of spinal ligaments, and degeneration of the facet joint were proposed as radiographic findings of restabilization by Kirkaldy-Willis.[66] Patients who already had a decrease in intervertebral disc space height have been observed to exhibit no subsequent progression of slippage.[80] This suggests that restabilization occurred over the natural course of degenerative spondylolisthesis. The decrease in range of motion of the slipped segment in the long-term study of Matsunaga *et al.*[80] supports the development of clinically significant restabilization.

Whether spinal fusion should be performed for the treatment of degenerative spondylolisthesis is controversial. In the opinion of some authors, good results can be obtained by decompression alone[34,53,129]; opposing opinions, however, are also found.* Whether fusion is required, based on the observation of the natural course of this condition, has not been determined. Lumbago, the major symptom of patients with degenerative spondylolisthesis, improved after spontaneous restabilization. Patients who had a decreased intervertebral disc space height exhibited improvement of lumbago. Moreover, spinal instability, a major pathophysiologic component of this condition, disappeared without fusion as a result of spontaneous restabilization. Spinal fusion for instability associated with this condition should perhaps not be performed if the patient exhibits lumbago alone. An exception may be a selected few heavy workers. When spinal fusion is considered for this condition, the natural course of this condition should also be considered; that is, if restabilization has already been functioning in the natural course, spinal fusion is not required. An exception may be a destabilized spine after laminectomy. Fusion for spondylolisthesis can occasionally

be necessitated by the iatrogenic destabilization caused by decompression surgery. Less invasive surgery for decompression that does not cause instability should be attempted. When spontaneous restabilization is not present, the need for spinal fusion should be dictated in part by the age and daily life activities of the patient. Sanderson and Wood[123] recommended the performance of decompressive surgery alone for elderly patients. An evidence-based approach is required to clarify indications.

The mechanism of the development of clinical symptoms in degenerative spondylolisthesis is very complicated, and intervertebral disc degeneration, facet joint degeneration, spinal instability, compression of nerve tissues by herniated intervertebral disc and other factors are intimately involved in the process.[7,45,56,87] Particularly in the case of spinal instability, no clear conclusion has been reached concerning the extent of instability that is clinically relevant. A better definition of clinically relevant instability is required to determine the indication for spinal fusion.

Traumatic Spondylolisthesis

Traumatic spondylolisthesis results from a fracture along the bony hook of the dorsal elements that does not involve the pars. The spondylolisthesis occurs over weeks or months after injury.[154] If a slip is present acutely, the injury is categorized as a fracture dislocation. If the pars is involved in the fracture, the lesion is classified as isthmic subtype C. Simple immobilization will lead to healing in most cases of traumatic spondylolisthesis. If failure of healing occurs in a symptomatic patient, or if progression of the slip is documented, surgical stabilization should be performed.

Pathologic Spondylolisthesis

Alterations of the bone tissue of the spine result in loss of the ability of the bony hook to maintain spinal alignment,

---

*References 4,5,14,19,20,52.

leading to the pathologic type of spondylolisthesis. There are two subtypes, generalized and local. In the generalized subtype, widespread changes such as those of Paget's disease, hyperthyroidism, osteopetrosis, and syphilitic disease are present.[32,154] In the localized subtype, tumor, localized infection, or other destructive processes result in failure of the bony hook to maintain spinal alignment.

The pathologic type of spondylolisthesis is perhaps the most difficult of all the types to treat. Therapies directed at the underlying cause are naturally the most effective avenues to prevent progression and perhaps avoid the need for surgery. With surgical intervention, it is often difficult to obtain adequate fixation to maintain spinal stability, and impaired bone healing may make it difficult to obtain a solid arthrodesis.

Postsurgical spondylolisthesis is included in the category of pathologic spondylolisthesis, but these patients do not have bone tissue problems that adversely affect the healing of a fusion. During the era of dorsal lumbar fusions, because the pars interarticularis is the weakest part of the neural arch, repeated loading often led to stress fractures ventral to the fusion mass (through the pars), and the occurrence of a spondylolisthesis was therefore a common postoperative complication (Figure 54.7).[114] Dorsal fusion has been largely abandoned in favor of dorsolateral fusion or other techniques, and postsurgical spondylolisthesis is therefore less common. The prognosis for patients with postsurgical spondylolisthesis is more favorable than for patients with most other subgroups of pathologic spondylolisthesis, because these patients respond well to reoperation and fusion. It is therefore reasonable to categorize postsurgical spondylolisthesis as a separate type.

Clinical Presentation

The most common presenting symptom of spondylolisthesis, regardless of the type, is pain. In children and young adults, isthmic and dysplastic slips constitute the most common cause of clinically significant low back pain.[68] The degenerative type is found more commonly in patients over age 50. The pain of spondylolisthesis is typically a steady ache and is usually related to the position or posture, suggesting a mechanical component in the cause of the pain. Other factors postulated as causes of the pain include ligamentous strain and osteoarthritis arising from instability, chronic nerve root irritation and traction, and degeneration of the involved intervertebral disc.[101,112] More significant symptoms may arise with the development of spinal stenosis. Symptoms of the lower extremities (including pain, numbness, or weakness) that are exacerbated by walking and relieved by rest and postural change may be the predominant reason for a patient to seek evaluation. This symptom complex, neurogenic claudication, is particularly common in patients with degenerative slips. In patients without spondylolisthesis, neurogenic claudication is usually relieved by bending forward. In the presence of a spondylolisthesis, the best posture for relief may be extension, because extending the spine reduces the degree of slip if any instability is present.

The incidence of isthmic defects in women is approximately half of that found in men. Women, however, are more likely to become symptomatic, and they account for about half of all symptomatic spondylolisthesis cases.[39,101,102] Also, women are five times more likely to develop degenerative spondylolisthesis than men.[44,53,138]

The neurologic examination is usually normal in spondylolisthesis patients. In patients with dysplastic or isthmic slips, there is often a palpable "step-off" of the lumbar spinous processes, and the waistline does not have its usual taper above the iliac crests. In older patients examination for signs of peripheral vascular disease and degenerative or inflammatory disease of the hips should be performed, because these can mimic the symptoms of degenerative spondylolisthesis.[91]

The tight hamstring syndrome is a characteristic presentation in younger spondylolisthesis patients. This syndrome produces a stooped posture with flexion at the hips and knees and is accompanied by a waddling gait.[93] This may be a result of postural exaggeration to compensate for changes in the lumbar lordotic curve. In patients with isthmic or dysplastic spondylolisthesis, the lumbar lordosis is most commonly exaggerated. The tight hamstring syndrome may simply represent a flexed posture that patients assume in order to reposition their center of gravity and maintain balance. With chronic flexion, mild tendon contractures may result in the fixed deformity of tight hamstring syndrome.

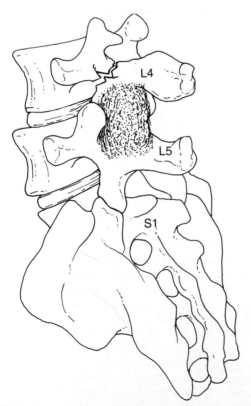

Figure 54.7 After interlaminar fusion (*shaded area at L4-5*), a stress fracture (*jagged line through the pars interarticularis of L4*) may occur at the pars of the uppermost vertebra in the fusion mass with resulting spondylolisthesis. In this example, L4 has subluxed ventrally on L5.

Diagnostic Work-Up

Spondylolisthesis is diagnosed readily on plain radiographs. Spondylolysis, on the other hand, may be somewhat more difficult to diagnose. In the presence of exaggerated lordosis, oblique views may not readily display the pars interarticularis at the lumbosacral junction, and defects of the pars can be obscured by overlying bone. The facet joints are frequently sclerotic in spondylolisthesis patients, and this can also obscure an adjacent defect in the pars interarticularis.

On computed tomography (CT) scans, spondylolysis can be diagnosed by the "incomplete ring" sign. Langston and Gavant[67] described this sign based on the premise that a continuous ring of cortical bone surrounding the spinal canal should be visible on at least one axial CT image in the normal vertebrae with an intact neural arch. If such a complete ring is not observed on a CT scan, using thin-section images, the presence of a pars defect can be assumed (Figure 54.8). Evaluation by CT has also been reported to be the best radiographic technique to demonstrate a pseudarthrosis in patients with a suspected failed fusion.[15]

Magnetic resonance imaging (MRI) plays an increasingly important role in evaluation of spondylolisthesis. This modality offers superior imaging of the soft tissues of the spine, and its multiplanar views allow evaluation of the pars interarticularis in the sagittal plane that will readily demonstrate many pars defects.[58,59] If surgery is planned, MRI is also an incomparable technique for ascertaining whether the discs at adjacent levels are responsible for the patient's symptoms.[44,58,142] With video motion MRI scanning also available, dynamic flexion-extension images can be added. Sagittal view MRI is particularly valuable for assessing neuroforamina. Detailed MRI evaluation of the neuroforamina is an invaluable tool for surgical planning in the proposed treatment for spondylolisthesis with radiculopathy.

Myelography and postmyelogram CT scanning are useful tools for evaluating spondylolisthesis patients, and sagittal reconstruction images have also been advocated. Definition of the bony anatomy is better with these studies than with MRI. Also, patients may tolerate myelography better than they do MRI because a high-quality diagnostic study requires less time, with the patient remaining in one position. Good quality dynamic flexion and extension images can be obtained during the myelogram with conventional hardware. These images may demonstrate pathology that is not seen with other modalities.

Radioisotope scanning is, in selected cases, a sensitive and useful addition to the diagnostic work-up. Bone scanning may be positive for pars injury that is otherwise radiographically inapparent. A positive scan results from active bone turnover. The implication of a positive scan is that repair of injury is occurring. This may be a radiographic reflection of the symptoms of either local back pain or of referred pain of facet joint origin.[6,73,107,122]

Diagnosing true symptomatic instability may be more problematic than diagnosing the radiographic abnormalities of spondylolysis or spondylolisthesis. Flexion-extension lateral radiography is a simple and time-honored method but is associated with a significant incidence of false-negative results. Other radiographic means of diagnosing

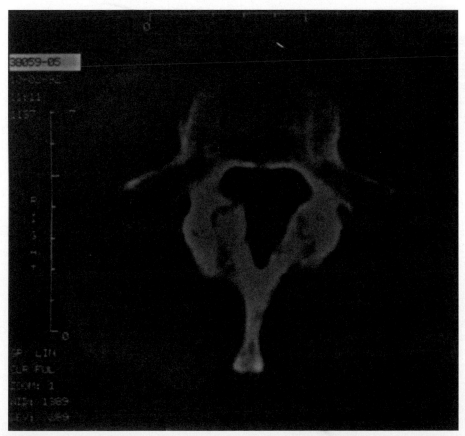

Figure 54.8 A defect in the pars interarticularis causes the "incomplete ring sign" on a CT scan. With such defects, none of the tomographic slices will contain a complete ring of bone surrounding the spinal canal because of the defect in the bony neural arch.

instability include placing a standardized load or traction, obtaining radiographs in the standing and recumbent positions, and assessing motion stereographically.[41,74,139]

More invasive means of diagnosis have also been used to verify instability in spondylolisthesis patients. In selected patients with severe, longstanding pain, Olerud has used percutaneously placed external spinal fixation, similar to a brace, to evoke clinical improvement as a predictor of benefit with fusion in cases of questionable instability.[99] Pope et al[108] have used percutaneously placed strain gauges and LED devices to aid in the quantitation of instability. Although this is obviously a highly invasive technique, it may be a more refined way to determine whether simpler techniques are giving false-negative results in difficult cases.

Treatment

The mainstay of therapy for spondylolisthesis and spondylolysis patients remains, even in the era of modern spine surgery and instrumentation, the conservative nonoperative approach. Among symptomatic patients, Rombold[115] reported that 22% eventually required surgery. In patients with symptomatic spondylolisthesis, only 10% to 15% fail conservative therapy and require surgical intervention.[95,116,153,154]

Nonoperative Therapy

A trial of nonoperative therapy is indicated for any spondylolysis or spondylolisthesis patient who presents with no neurologic compromise or with a chronic stable deficit. Therapies are generally aimed at relief of symptoms in the short term, because the symptoms themselves tend to run a course of acute exacerbation followed by remission. The two most important concepts in conservative therapy for these patients are the following: (1) the treatment should be of sufficient duration (usually at least several months) to convince the prudent clinician that it is not succeeding in providing relief, and (2) the patient must understand that to a large measure, improvement results from the patient's efforts to comply with treatment. The initial plan for nonoperative therapy should also address associated components of the symptomatology, such as fear of disability, narcotic addiction, litigation or potential secondary gains through pain behavior, and any other psychosocial concerns. The clinician who addresses these issues early and directly will more readily earn the trust of the patient, motivate the patient, and predispose the situation to a better outcome.

The best treatment for spondylolisthesis and spondylolysis patients is usually a multimodality approach. The use of medication, usually nonsteroidal antiinflammatory drugs or muscle relaxants, should be coupled with an exercise program that includes stretching and strengthening components and with specific educational components tailored to the needs of the patient, where applicable. For example, a patient who is a heavy laborer may require training in proper lifting techniques or retraining for another career, if practical. The patient who is an office worker may benefit more from abdominal muscle strengthening or the use of an orthotic device to improve posture.[77,135] Stretching may be of greater benefit than strengthening exercises, and

such patients may benefit from such simple measures as referral for yoga instruction. Evaluation by a physical therapist adds a considerable number of options, such as ultrasound, massage, whirlpool, traction, and other modalities. Their efficacy, however, remains unproven.

For the obese patient, weight loss is clearly the first goal in treating a lumbar spine disorder. Abdominal mass hanging over the belt ventrally places an excessive force on the lower back because of the lever arm arising from the ventrally displaced mass (Figure 54.9). It should be stressed that the best means of avoiding surgical complications in spondylolisthesis patients is to manage these individuals nonoperatively.

A trial period of external spinal immobilization has long been considered a screening test for evaluating patients preoperatively for the potential benefits of surgical fusion. Various orthotic devices and body casts, as well as percutaneously placed external fixator devices, have been employed for this purpose. Long-term follow-up evaluations have shown that such data do not reliably predict outcome after surgical fusion.[100] Bracing, even with the use of a thoracolumbosacral orthosis with unilateral thigh extension (hip immobilization), does not provide a consistent or significant immobilizing effect on spinal translational movements.[5,136]

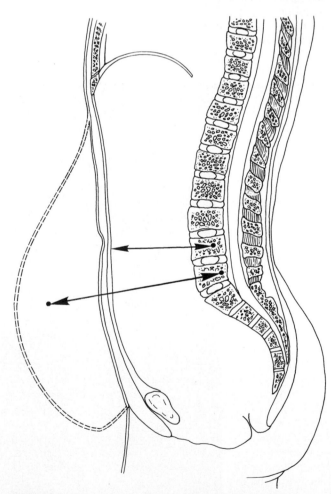

Figure 54.9 The presence of a pendulous abdomen places an excessive load on the ventral aspect of the lumbar spine. A well-toned flat abdomen will have substantially lessened ventral load forces.

The improvement that is frequently observed in patients treated with orthotic devices may be largely a result of the postural changes invoked by such treatments.[136]

Corticosteroids and long-acting local anesthetic agents are of some temporizing value when injected into the facet joints or epidural space. Injection directly into the pars defect, when present, may be of value in predicting the response to surgical fusion.[141]

The use of narcotics plays a limited role in the treatment of spondylolisthesis patients. The symptoms of an acute exacerbation may sometimes be managed appropriately with these drugs, but their use should only be short term. Narcotics have no place in therapy for chronic low back pain, because long-term use of these drugs will simply add the component of addiction to a problem that is complex from the start.

Eventually, having failed conservative treatment, 10% to 20% of patients will require surgical treatment for relief of radiculopathy and back pain.[44,138] The results of fusion for back pain caused by instability in spondylolisthesis are better than the results obtained from fusion for degenerative disease and prior discectomy, or for failed back syndrome.[57]

Indications for Surgical Treatment

Because all surgical procedures for treatment of spondylolysis and spondylolisthesis are major operations, the indications for surgery in every patient must be carefully considered. If symptoms of pain or neurologic deficit significantly disrupt lifestyle and do not improve with conservative management, surgical intervention should be considered. The general indications for surgery include the following: failure of an adequate trial of conservative therapy, radiographic instability with symptoms, documented progression of the slip to greater than grade II, symptomatic grade III slip, grade IV slip, or spondyloptosis.* An adequate trial of conservative therapy includes a multimodality approach, consideration and addressing of psychosocial concerns, a duration of the treatment of at least 3 to 4 months, and adequate patient compliance. The patient who is motivated and interested in improving can be expected to lose weight, exercise, stretch, and follow other prescribed tasks. Motivation is called into question when patients fail to comply and instead offer excuses for the lack of completion of their portion of the conservative therapy. Relative contraindications to surgery (particularly to fusion) include multilevel disease, poor patient motivation or compliance, very low activity level, osteoporosis, and habitual tobacco abuse.[35,48]

Patients presenting with bowel or bladder dysfunction attributable to spondylolisthesis should undergo more urgent surgical intervention. If any neurologic deficit attributable to a spondylolisthesis occurs acutely, urgent or emergent operative decompression is indicated. Decisions regarding inclusion of fusion and instrumentation should be made by the same criteria for these operations, regardless of whether they are performed as emergencies or as elective operations.

Patients with low-grade slips (grade I or II) seldom require surgery. Most of these patients are asymptomatic, and the likelihood of progression is low—approximately 10%.[50,89,153] One study has even suggested that the occurrence of significant or disabling low back pain in middle-aged patients with isthmic spondylolisthesis is not more likely than in the normal population.[147] In terms of patient satisfaction, surgery for low-grade spondylolistheses produces no improvement compared to conservative therapy alone, and the results are considerably worse than those after surgery for more severe (higher grade) spondylolistheses.[40]

Surgical Options

After the decision for surgical intervention is made, the selection of an appropriate operation for the patient is the next crucial step. The major decision points are the operative approach, the number of levels to be involved, whether to perform decompression, whether to perform fusion, and whether to include internal fixation.

The choice of operative approach is usually straightforward. The majority of these operations are performed through a dorsal midline incision. This is the approach with which spine surgeons are invariably the most familiar, and it is therefore the simplest approach. Unless significant advantages are foreseen by the use of an alternative approach, the dorsal method should generally be the technique of choice.

Ventral Approach

A ventral approach is sometimes a useful alternative technique. If a ventral approach is chosen, arthrodesis is recommended in all instances. The quantity of disc material removed in this approach can reach almost 100%. Without fusion, the patient who already has a spondylolisthesis will be left with a spine that is further destabilized by disruption of the intervertebral disc and the anterior longitudinal ligament (ALL). Therefore instrumentation is also a useful adjunct if interbody fusion is used.[128] A number of devices are manufactured specifically for instrumentation of the ventral spine.[132]

The ventral approach offers some advantages and may be particularly useful for the patient with a previously failed fusion. Interbody fusion gives the largest amount of bony surface for arthrodesis. Placement of grafts in the interspace maintains the height of the interspace and therapy preserves the size of the neuroforamen. These advantages must be weighed against the disadvantages of limited visualization of the nerve roots and the possibility of complications, such as impotence, ureteral injury, and vascular injury.[95] High rates of nonunion have also been reported for ventral interbody fusion.[65,124,144]

Because of the lordotic curve of the lumbar region, the lowest lumbar interspace and the lumbosacral interspace are tilted downward out of the line of sight of the surgeon using the ventral approach. In isthmic spondylolistheses the lumbar lordotic curvature is usually increased, thereby exaggerating this tilt.[71] Therefore visualization of the interspace can be difficult with the ventral approach, especially if there is a high-grade slip at the L5-S1 level.

---

*References 29,37,42,88,138,153.

Dorsal Operations

In cases of isthmic spondylolisthesis it is usually only necessary to operate from a dorsal approach at the L5-S1 level. The only exception to this may be the occasional patient who presents with a symptomatic disc herniation at the next rostral level. However, in degenerative spondylolisthesis, the slip is most common at the L4-5 level.[116] In these patients, if fusion is planned, the decision must also include consideration of whether to fuse only the involved level or to include the lumbosacral junction as well. Some surgeons consider arthrodesis at L4-5 alone to be a "floating fusion" that results in increased stress and accelerated degeneration of the lumbosacral junction. On the other hand, fusion of longer spinal segments simply amplifies the stress that will be transmitted to the remaining nonfused or noninstrumented levels.[90,104] Therefore it seems to be a sounder approach to include only the level(s) of demonstrated instability or other surgical pathology for most patients. Such a strategy preserves maximum lumbar spinal motion. If, however, significant degenerative changes are present in the disc or facet joints at the lumbosacral junction, fusion to the sacrum may be justified.

Fusion Without Decompression

Some series of spondylolisthesis patients undergoing arthrodesis have suggested that fusion alone, without decompression, relieves symptoms and leads to resolution of some neurologic deficits.[102,126] Relief of radicular symptoms by arthrodesis suggests that the neurologic symptoms in these patients were caused by nerve root traction or intermittent compression that arose from abnormal segmental motion. Common sites of nerve root compression include the spinal canal, lateral recess, and neuroforamen.[30,58] In patients undergoing surgery for refractory back pain or for demonstrated instability with no radicular symptoms or neurologic deficit, this is often a satisfactory approach. Fusion without decompression substantially reduces operative time, thereby lessening blood loss, infection risk, and other risk factors for intraoperative complications. For patients with radicular symptoms, decompression relieves nerve root symptoms with greater certainty than does fusion alone.

Decompression

In patients with degenerative spondylolisthesis the radicular symptoms may be associated with anatomic derangements other than the slip itself. Hypertrophic facet joints with thickened capsules, synovial cysts, osteophyte formation, and ligamentous thickening can all contribute to nerve root compression, in either the lateral recess or the neuroforamen. In cases of isthmic spondylolisthesis, nerve root compression is more likely to involve the L5 root in the L5-S1 neuroforamen than the S1 root in the lateral recess. The mechanism of compression is often multifactorial. The reparative process present in the pars defect causes pars enlargement that is often covered by fibrocartilaginous overgrowth. Other associated factors may be involved simultaneously, such as bulging of the disc, hypertrophy of the ligamentum flavum, and hypertrophy of the facet.[17,33,113]

The symptoms of many spondylolisthesis patients result from spinal stenosis, as well as from individual nerve root compression. It is often difficult to make clear and precise distinctions between the symptoms caused by these two causes. Therefore it is recommended that decompression be performed with most surgical treatments for spondylolisthesis. Radical dorsal decompression procedures, such as complete laminectomy, are best avoided in cases of significant instability if no fusion is planned, because they are likely to aggravate slip. Similarly, aggressive bone removal, when addressing the facet joints, is to be avoided, even if fusion is planned.[72] The integrity of the disc should not be violated if it is not frankly herniated, because damage to the intervertebral discs may also adversely affect long-term stability.[39,53] For spondylolisthesis patients with a low-grade slip, in whom the only symptom is back pain of a mechanical nature with no radicular component and in whom there is no radiographic suggestion of stenosis, arthrodesis without decompression is probably a good choice.

Fusion and Instrumentation

The dorsal approach is the method of choice for surgical treatment of spondylolisthesis and spondylolysis in the majority of cases. For patients with degenerative spondylolisthesis in the absence of gross instability, decompression alone may be adequate. For young patients with isthmic spondylolistheses, persistent localized back pain or radiculopathy considered to be the result of spondylolisthesis are indications for surgery if conservative therapy fails. If surgery is performed in such patients, arthrodesis should be included in the procedure. Some recent studies have demonstrated better outcomes for arthrodesis procedures when instrumentation is included, compared to those performed without internal fixation.[152,160] Instrumentation provides for preservation of lumbar lordosis and a high fusion rate, even in the presence of a previously failed fusion attempt.[28] In patients at risk for pseudarthrosis, such as those who are tobacco users, internal fixation is even more useful as an adjunctive measure because the rate of successful fusion in this group is considerably lower.[16,138,160] Although a large amount of clinical data on the use of an implantable electrical stimulator to enhance bone growth is unavailable, this technique may also be of benefit in this group.[64]

Ventral-Dorsal Approach

For patients with a high-grade spondylolisthesis, or for patients with a previous failed fusion, some authors have advocated surgery from both the ventral and the dorsal approach. This circumferential operation, dubbed the "360" approach, may be of benefit to a select group of patients. The potential benefits must, however, be weighed against the risks of this large surgical undertaking. The additive potential for complications with two approaches, additional blood loss, and longer operative times must be taken into account. Since the fusion rates for single approach procedures, either ventral or dorsal, commonly exceed 80%, the need for this additional surgery is questioned. Reasonable indications for the 360 approach are revision surgery in high-grade slips and spondyloptosis in patients in whom previous procedures have failed.[146]

Internal fixation is commonly used in spinal surgery. The growth of this practice has been aided by newer, more rigid implant techniques and instrument systems that are more user friendly. External bracing, one of the mainstays of therapy, does not provide rigid fixation and has not been demonstrated to provide any significant lasting benefit,[86,136] although it has some advocates.[6,134,137] In one study, external bracing was even shown to aggravate instability in some patients.[86] However, bracing remains a reasonable temporary therapeutic method, an element in the decision process of whether or not to fuse. Bracing is often used postoperatively as an adjunct to internal fixation. Since the introduction of rigid internal fixation systems that are easy to use and widely available, bracing alone has little place as a primary treatment for spondylolisthesis. It is, however, an option for patients who decline surgery or for those who are considered to be poor surgical risks.

Complications: Avoidance and Management

Patient Selection

One of the reasons for poor surgical outcome in spondylolisthesis patients is poor patient selection. Inadequate trials of conservative therapy may precede surgery for patients who would otherwise have benefitted from a more intensive effort at nonsurgical treatment. Another source of patient selection errors is symptoms that arise from other courses, such as disc degeneration or herniation at an adjacent level.

Any operative therapy for spondylolisthesis is a major surgical undertaking, and these operations are, with rare exception, elective in nature. Therefore only patients who are suitable candidates for major elective surgery should be considered. The usual considerations of cardiopulmonary health, age, and other associated risk factors are important, as are the issues of bone quality and patient motivation and compliance. Multilevel degenerative disease, particularly at levels rostral to the spondylolisthesis, may be a relative contraindication to arthrodesis. Fusion places additional stress on adjacent levels during volitional motion, and accelerated degenerative changes at these sites may lead to a poor long-term result.[139]

It is important that before surgery, patients be given a realistic description of the results of surgery and of their period of recovery. Convalescence after major spinal operations is seldom simple, the pain is substantial, and it sometimes results in continued symptoms, even though the severity may be markedly lessened. For patients who expect a perfect result, even a little residual back pain can be a disappointment.

Technical Factors and Outcome

Inadequate surgery is a potential pitfall in surgery for spondylolisthesis and spondylolysis patients. Potential sources of surgical error include inadequacy of exposure, decompression of the involved neural structures, preparation of graft site, and installment of implants. The spinal subluxation of spondylolisthesis results in an abnormal neuroforamen in which the roots can be compressed.[30] A thick, fibrous band of connective tissue that usually spans the defect is present at the level of the slip.[12,75] Microscopically this resembles normal ligamentous tissue. It will often cross directly over the nerve root and may contribute to compression, particularly if significant spinal instability exists. To adequately decompress the nerve roots, these bands should be divided over the root or resected completely. Nerve root distortion or compression at the margins of the vertebral body should be relieved by retracting the root and contouring the bone by curettage.

When arthrodesis is part of the planned treatment for spondylolisthesis or spondylolysis, strict attention should be paid to technical features of the procedure. The subluxation of a vertebral body, particularly if it happens to be at the L5-S1 level, leads to spinal geometry that can be confusing to identify anatomically. The transverse processes of the ventrally displaced vertebral body are more difficult to expose, and juxtaposition of the iliac bones obscures the view. Removal of the soft tissues overlying the transverse processes, critical for optimal fusion results, can therefore be tedious. A thorough knowledge of the anatomy of the superior, interarticular, and inferior articular arteries and muscular branches of the lumbar arteries can make the dissection relatively bloodless.[76]

In cases of high-grade spondylolisthesis, the subluxation can result in a near-horizontal orientation of the fusion mass that is biomechanically suboptimal for axial weight bearing (Figure 54.10). In these cases inclusion of another level into the fusion provides a more vertically oriented fusion mass with better load-bearing capability.[23,68,88] The orientation of the fusion mass may also be improved by reduction of the slip.

Definite morbidity is associated with the use of spinal implants. Therefore the use of internal stabilization should be included only when the potential benefits outweigh the risks.[133,150] In patients with degenerative spondylolisthesis, there is often no overt instability. For these patients, if symptoms of neural compression predominate (either radiculopathy or symptomatic stenosis), decompression without fusion may be the optimal surgical procedure.[1,53,61,62] However, with such decompressions, caution should be exercised to remove no more than a third to a half of the medial aspect of the facet joints to avoid progressive instability.* A trend toward increased slip has been noted after laminectomy without fusion in degenerative spondylolisthesis patients.[51,55,69] This does not, however, appear to adversely affect outcome.[35,61,63,127] In fact, there may be no correlation between progression of the slip and clinical symptoms in degenerative spondylolisthesis patients.[81]

Gill Procedure

Laminectomy with removal of the loose dorsal elements in patients with lytic lumbar spondylolisthesis was reported by Gill and colleagues[43] in 1955. This operation is simple to perform, avoids the risks of arthrodesis, and in multiple series, it has been shown to be an effective treatment.[3,21,25,101]

---

*References 42,53,63,69,117,140.

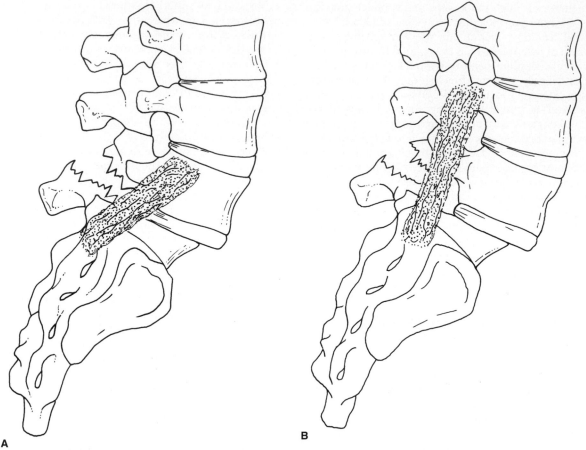

Figure 54.10 In high-grade spondylolistheses, an intertransverse fusion mass may have a near-horizontal spatial orientation, as shown by shaded area (**A**). Inclusion of an additional level in the fusion will alter the orientation of the fusion mass to a more vertical position that is better suited to spinal load bearing as shown by shaded area (**B**).

The Gill procedure is contraindicated in adolescents or adults younger than age 30.[101]

Direct Pars Repair

Direct repair of the pars interarticularis is another surgical option for isthmic spondylolisthesis patients. This can be achieved by screw fixation of the lamina to the pedicle or by tension-band wiring of the lamina to the transverse processes.* Another recently described technique involves placement of pedicle screws, followed by compression wiring of the lamina to the screws.[122] The success of these techniques is critically dependent on the anatomic defect being the source of the patient's pain. Infiltration of the pars defect can be performed as a functional test to evaluate the source of pain.[35,141] Because these techniques are difficult to perform in severe slips, and because disc degeneration and ligamentous changes invariably accompany severe slips in adults, pars repair is contraindicated in patients older than age 30 and in patients with slips exceeding 3 to 4mm.[9,98,112,138,141]

Reduction of Spondylolistheses

The principal feature of a spondylolisthesis is malalignment of the spine. Therefore the option to reduce the subluxation during operative intervention is appealing, and a number of techniques for performing reduction of a spondylolisthesis have been described. The earliest methods involved traction and casting, but these techniques often failed, and if reduction was successful, recurrence of the slip was also common.[93] Intraoperative reduction without decompression has been reported to carry significant risk of neurologic injury.* In trauma patients, attention to possible disc injury is also essential to prevent cauda equina or nerve root compression after reduction and fixation of the dislocation.[24] Reduction of a spondylolisthesis after neural element decompression is a somewhat different issue.

Placement of bone screws into the pedicles of the vertebrae has given a new degree of control and rigidity in spinal fixation. Bone screws can be rigidly affixed to a longitudinal member (usually a rod or plate), allowing force to

---

*References 9,18,47,60,96,98,105,141.

*References 28,35,40,106,110,138.

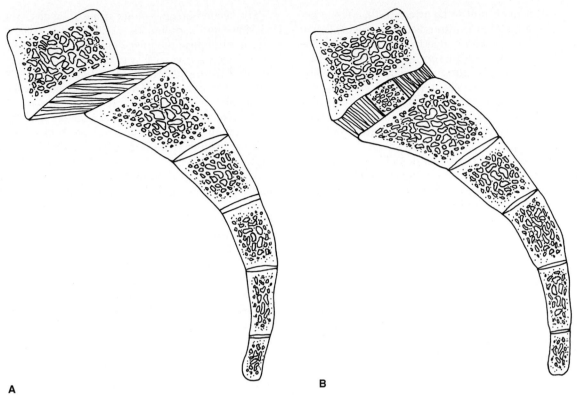

A   B

Figure 54.11 (**A**) Fibers of the annulus fibrosus, at the level of a spondylolisthesis, are oriented in the direction of the slip. (**B**) Placement of an interbody graft restores the intervertebral height and a tension band is created by the fibers of the annulus.

be applied to the vertebra with much greater control than was possible with conventional hook devices. Although the hook systems are actually tension-band fixators, screws attached rigidly to a rod provide rigid fixation in three dimensions. Therefore reduction with screws after neural element decompression is a different procedure than what is discussed in much of the literature on the topic of spondylolisthesis reduction. With decompression via wide laminectomies, the spinal canal and neuroforamina are easily visualized, and reduction with instrument systems using bone screws can be accomplished in a more judicious manner than was possible historically. Excellent results from surgical reduction of spondylolisthesis after decompression have been reported with instrumentation of the pedicles with bone screws.[54,78,79] Significant complications, however, are still associated with these operations, and improvement over the results of nonreductive procedures remains unproved.[4,54,110] Reduction of a spondylolisthesis, however, increases the amount of bony surface available for interbody fusion. It has long been recognized that the risk of a failed fusion, or pseudarthrosis, can be reduced by increasing the area of the fusion mass.[14,27]

Reduction of a spondylolisthesis can be performed in different degrees. A common practice is to use a spinal surgery frame that maintains the natural lumbar lordosis. In patients without gross spinal instability, positioning to preserve lordosis gives a natural postural reduction with no more force exerted on the spine than the amount the patient may apply in performing routine daily activities. Therefore ligamentous tension is within the physiologic range, and the facet joints are held at positions within their

usual range of motion. The application of force to the spine for reduction, usually by distraction, places additional stress on the implants and has been associated with loss of reduction in the postoperative period.[4,10] In patients with severe slips or spondyloptosis, reduction may be indicated to enhance approximation of bony surfaces for fusion, improve biomechanical load-bearing capacity, and relieve neural compression.[10,97] If applied-force reduction is performed, interbody fusion should also be considered because this may decrease the incidence of loss of reduction (Figure 54.11).[4,10,97]

Some degree of scoliosis is frequently present in spondylolisthesis patients, and it is present in 5% to 7% of patients with spondylolisthesis and spondylolysis.[2] In their series of 91 patients undergoing surgery, Laurent and Osterman[68] observed scoliosis in 44 patients (48%). This was most commonly postural scoliosis, but structural scoliosis was observed as well. In patients with degenerative spondylolisthesis and scoliosis, reduction of the curvature may be warranted if surgical treatment is undertaken. Because acceleration of degenerative changes is sometimes observed at the level immediately above a fusion, reducing scoliotic angulation below the fusion can restore a more physiologic pattern of load bearing and, in theory, may reduce the rate of degeneration at adjacent levels.

The angular orientation of the facet joints forces rotation to occur if lateral bending takes place. This is the biomechanic principle of coupling of segmental spinal motion. A scoliotic curve in the lumbar spine will result in rotation of the vertebral bodies such that the transverse processes are displaced ventrally on the concave side of the curve.[103] It is important to be aware of this phenomenon because rotation of the vertebra can cause a change in the position of nerve roots relative to the transverse processes. For example, the L2 root typically courses ventral to the L3 transverse process and remains in the plane ventral to the intertransversarius muscles. With ventral transverse process displacement, the nerve root may bulge slightly dorsal to the transverse process in the intertransverse space. If the plane of the intertransversarius muscles is then violated, injury to the root can occur.

Reduction of degenerative scoliotic deformities is usually simple and does not require complex preplanning or derotation maneuvers. By compressing on the convex side and distracting on the concave side, the coronal plane deformity is easily reduced. The rotational component that is invariably present because of the coupling phenomenon is simultaneously reduced.

Misplacement of Implants

A dreaded complication of spinal instrumentation is misplacement of implants. Although it is theoretically possible to instrument the spine properly every time, this complication is not rare.[130] Almost all spine surgeons who perform a substantial number of spinal instrumentation surgeries will encounter this problem. In a normal spine, proper identification of implant placement sites and orientation of screw insertion angles are quite simple. Spines that require instrumentation, however, are frequently grossly abnormal anatomically. Landmark distortion by degenerative changes, trauma, congenital deformity, scoliosis, and alignment changes because of spondylolisthesis are some of the commonly encountered alterations that dramatically increase both the difficulty and the risk in hardware placement.

A number of techniques can help reduce the risks of hardware placement. One of the simplest of these is fluoroscopy. The fluoroscope identifies the pedicles and confirms the correct identification of spinal levels. It should be borne in mind, however, that the two-dimensional view obtained by fluoroscopy does not provide a clear appreciation of any rotational component that may be present. Coronal plane deformity can also cause the pedicles of a given vertebra to be misaligned. In the lateral fluoroscopic projection, this can lead to misidentification of the position of a pedicle. The preoperative CT scan can be useful for identifying positional changes caused by scoliotic deformities. Viewing by fluoroscopy in two planes can be helpful, but changing the position of the equipment intraoperatively can be cumbersome. Fluoroscopy also requires the use of a radiolucent operating table if anteroposterior (AP) views are needed.

The use of image guided surgery technology has become increasingly popular as a tool to avoid hardware misplacement. These devices take two general approaches. The first is to incorporate images obtained preoperatively and to then register these into a defined stereotactic space intraoperatively. This allows manipulation of instruments and implants within this space intraoperatively. Typically this technique is used with either CT or MRI images. The advantages of this method include the ability to use multiplanar views and three-dimensional reconstructed image technology.

The second image-guided strategy involves the use of a reference grid applied to an imaging device, such as a C-arm, to acquire the image data intraoperatively. A reference device is placed in the operative field and securely attached to the patient. It is critical with this technique that no movement of that device (relative to the patient) occurs after registration. The images are then acquired and stereotactic space is thereby defined. The image guidance system can then track the position of implants or instruments in the defined space and display them on the acquired images.

As is the case with any technology, errors can occur in the use of image guided methods. Movement of the reference grid or the in-field reference device, obliquity of images, and field distortions that naturally occur at the periphery of acquired images can all result in loss of accuracy and subsequent surgical misadventure. Anatomic abnormalities may not be easily seen on intraoperative images. Another potential source of error is to rely too heavily on a single registration. Frequent checking of accuracy against known landmarks in the surgical field can help to reduce these errors in long procedures. When numerous spinal levels are involved, multiple registrations are usually recommended to lessen the risk of misguidance. Despite the high level of technologic advancement represented by the image-guidance systems, the surgeon's most important asset in the prevention of errors when using them is a high index of suspicion for misguidance and frequent accuracy checks.

A certain way to identify the vertebral pedicles is by direct visualization of the structures. Simply by wide decompression, the pedicles can be observed, and screw placement becomes more certain. This technique is particularly valuable if rotational deformities are present. Exposure of both pedicles at a given level gives the surgeon an excellent appreciation of the degree of asymmetry resulting from rotation and coronal plane changes in pedicle alignment. The nerve root adjacent to the pedicle can also be retracted by the assistant during screw placement, so that if the medial margin of the pedicle is violated inadvertently, no significant complication will result; the implant is simply redirected and installed.

Another measure of avoiding hardware misplacement is to carefully sound the pedicle after placing the probe. This helps ascertain that there is bone surrounding the entire length of the tract and that the ventral cortex of the vertebral body has not been violated. Placing Kirschner wires into the pedicles and obtaining AP and lateral view radiographs before screw insertion also helps prevent improper placement of implants.

If misplacement of implants is diagnosed intraoperatively, the faulty piece(s) can be repositioned or removed and replaced. More commonly, however, the diagnosis of misplaced hardware is made by postoperative radiographs. The occurrence of misplaced hardware often relates to difficulties in obtaining adequate intraoperative films of fluoroscopy. Problems arising from patient obesity, osteopenia, and spinal deformities may all contribute to deterioration of the technical quality of radiographs. In the absence of good quality radiographic data, the risk of malpositioned implants rises considerably.

The decision to reoperate for misplaced spinal instrumentation is usually a difficult one. If there is a reasonable expectation that no serious adverse sequelae will arise from the misplacement, reoperation should not be undertaken. The potential adverse effects of misplacement include insufficient stabilization, neurologic injury, and visceral or vascular injury. For example, stabilization may be perfectly adequate with a misplaced pedicle screw, if good thread purchase is achieved with all of the other screws. However, in a patient with significant osteopenia, stabilization may be inadequate with a misplaced screw, and further instrumentation may be necessary. Such a patient should be followed closely and if there is any evidence of loosening hardware, reoperation should be performed, provided that the patient is symptomatic. If the patient is asymptomatic, solid arthrodesis may eventually occur despite a small amount of segmental movement, or an asymptomatic pseudarthrosis may result and no therapy will be needed.

Malpositioned spinal instrumentation can lead to injury of vascular or neural structures. Probably the most common of these serious soft-tissue injuries is spinal cord or nerve root compression or transection. If the spinal cord is compromised by an instrument pressing into the canal, reoperation should be performed immediately to relieve the compression, unless there is a complete myelopathy. In the patient with a complete myelopathy, reoperation should also be considered, particularly if the compression involves the level of the conus medullaris. Reoperation for conus compression may lead to substantial recovery. If a complete myelopathy is caused by compression of the thoracic spinal cord, there is little hope for meaningful functional recovery. If a complete myelopathy existed preoperatively, malpositioned instrumentation may have no ill consequences as long as the spine is adequately stabilized.

If a nerve root is transected, the only action regarding the root is to check for the leakage of cerebrospinal fluid (CSF). The instrument in question, however, is likely to be in poor position, and it may not provide adequate stabilization. If the nerve root is partially intact, repositioning of the hardware may prevent tethering and chronic irritation of the functional portion of the root.

Other soft-tissue structures at risk from misplaced instrumentation include blood vessels, ureters, and intestines. These injuries typically arise from penetration by the screw of the anterior bony cortex of the vertebrae. Penetrating screws often simply protrude into the psoas muscle, and no further treatment should be entertained. Ventral penetration may result in screws abutting large arteries, particularly the iliac arteries at the L5 level. If the postoperative radiographs suggest ventral penetration, a CT scan should be obtained. If a screw is shown to impinge on a large artery, it should be replaced with a shorter implant. Injury to the bowel and ureters has also been reported from screw penetration of the ventral cortex of the sacrum. Treatment and repair of these injuries should be undertaken with the assistance of urologists, general surgeons, or other consultants as appropriate.

Infection and Blood Loss

Infection represents another common complication in surgery for spondylolisthesis. Because these cases most commonly involve foreign body implants, infection can be especially problematic. The management of this complication is, however, not specific to the spondylolisthesis patient, and it should be treated in essentially the same manner as for any surgical spinal infection.

Another major complication of spondylolisthesis surgery is large-volume blood loss. The use of a spinal surgery frame that allows the abdomen to hang freely, typically a knee-chest position frame, will reduce venous congestion in the epidural space and will reduce blood loss. During the dissection, exposure up to only the facet joints allows decompression, while preventing the oozing of blood in the lateral gutters that will occur after the transverse processes are exposed. The transverse processes are then exposed after the decompression and immediately before instrumentation. Other measures to deal with blood loss include preoperative autologous blood donation by the patient and the use of a Cell Saver for reinfusion of blood lost during surgery. Early intraoperative hemodilution, removal of a unit of blood by the anesthesiologist at the beginning of surgery, and replacement with crystalloid will also allow for less loss of erythrocyte mass in a given volume of blood. The withdrawn blood is reinfused at the completion of the operation.

CSF Leakage

A further complication of spondylolisthesis surgery is the possibility of a CSF leak. Leakage of CSF can be stopped by suturing the dura, if possible, or by placing some Gelfoam over the leak. Fibrin tissue sealant is also a useful adjunct for this purpose. The intraoperative repair should be tested by having the anesthesiologist induce a Valsalva maneuver. If the adequacy of the repair remains in question or if the leak is not diagnosed until the postoperative period, a lumbar CSF drain may be inserted and left in place for 3 to 5 days.

Implant Failure and Pseudarthrosis

Failure of spinal instrumentation and failure to obtain solid arthrodesis are two more complications found in the surgical treatment of spondylolisthesis and spondylolysis. Historically, it had been thought that fusion failures were as likely to be asymptomatic as symptomatic.[11,27,148] In the postfusion patient with ongoing symptoms, fusion failure remains the likely source of difficulty.

Pseudarthrosis rates are increased in certain individuals at risk, including those with anemia, postmenopausal osteoporosis, malabsorption syndromes, vitamin D derangements, and antacid use with phosphate depletion.[111] It has long been recognized that tobacco abuse contributes to fusion failure, perhaps because of its effect on blood supply to the graft.[22] Alcohol abuse is also thought to predispose to failed fusion.

Apart from the host conditions, fusion may also be at risk because of particular technical factors. Coronal orientation of the facets or their operative modification can yield greater stresses on the fusion mass.[44] Likewise, a more horizontally oriented fusion mass faces higher shear forces and may be at risk from resulting vertical motion. Intertransverse fusion has been reported to result in lower rates of nonunion than interbody fusion (7% versus 30%).[76,125] An overall failure rate of about 13% is standard.[57]

With the engineering refinements of the current generation of spinal instrumentation systems, actual breakage of the implants is far less common than with earlier systems. However, implant fractures do occur in 10% or more of cases, and the risk of this complication can be substantially reduced with some simple precautions.[82,104,133,136,159] Ascertaining that an adequate length of rod protrudes beyond the screws or hooks at the ends of the construct and that locking washers are properly tightened and not cross threaded is among the easiest ways to avoid major complications.[31] Instrument breakage typically occurs from an inordinate amount of stress at a single point that produces metal fatigue and eventual breakage. Such stress risers can be avoided by carefully contouring the longitudinal members (rods or plates) to allow easy attachment of the segmental fixation devices (hooks, screws, wires, or cables) with minimal stress. Bends in the longitudinal members should be gentle arcs, and point bending should be avoided if possible, because the resulting angle will have a stress riser at the apex. Overbending the member and then reducing the bend should be strictly avoided, especially with titanium implants, because this back-and-forth bending causes low-cycle metal fatigue. Because of its brittle nature, titanium is extremely susceptible to low-cycle fatigue. Caution should also be taken to ensure that the junctions at which the longitudinal and segmental members are joined are as flush as possible because any mismatch at the junction will also produce a stress riser or a poor fit, either of which can cause failure.

Postoperatively, spondylolysis and spondylolisthesis patients may continue to experience substantial symptoms. Initially, unless new neurologic findings are present, the only work-up indicated is plain roentgenography for detecting misplaced implants or worsening spinal alignment. If symptoms suggesting nerve root compression persist for more than 2 to 3 months, work-up to rule out continued compression should be considered. As fusion progresses, symptoms may resolve, even in the presence of continued nerve root compression. The work-up, if instrumentation was included at surgery, may have to include myelography, because myelogram images are less affected by the presence of implants than are CT and MRI. If the implants are made of titanium, MRI can be performed because image quality is not significantly degraded by titanium devices.[120]

Persistence of symptoms for more than 1 year after surgery or the appearance of new symptoms several months after surgery may suggest pseudarthrosis formation. This diagnosis can sometimes be confirmed with conventional radiographs. If alignment changes or further degenerative changes such as the formation of or enlargement of traction spurs are observed, a pseudarthrosis is likely. Signs of loosening implants, such as a halo appearance around screws, are also suggestive of pseudarthrosis.

The diagnosis of pseudarthrosis can be difficult to make with certainty.[15,133] The most certain method to prove solid bony fusion is operative exploration.[119] Evaluation by CT scan has been reported to be the best radiographic technique to evaluate failed fusions.[15]

Bone scintigraphy can also help determine the solidity of a fusion in some cases.[49,83,131,145] The limiting factor with this technique is that there is a time window for its use. At 4 to 6 months postoperatively, the bone scan shows increased uptake in the region of a fusion that is progressing well.[26] Long after surgery, a well-established pseudarthrosis may not demonstrate any increased uptake in the adjacent bone.[49] If a bone scan demonstrates increased uptake in a patient more than 1 year after surgery, an ongoing inflammatory, neoplastic, or remodeling process can be assumed. In the appropriate clinical setting this strongly suggests a pseudarthrosis. An additional advantage of bone scintigraphy is that it is less affected by the presence of spinal implants than are other radiographic techniques.

Summary

The potential complications occurring with surgical treatment of spondylolysis and spondylolisthesis are numerous and sometimes severe. Avoidance of surgical complications is most easily achieved by the use of nonoperative treatment, which is the appropriate management for the majority of these patients. Surgical interventions are, however, indicated in many cases, and with an appropriate operative procedure, the results are usually gratifying.

REFERENCES

1. Alexander E Jr, Kelly DL Jr, Davis CH Jr, et al: Intact arch spondylolisthesis. A review of 50 cases and description of surgical treatment. J Neurosurg 63:840-844, 1985.
2. Amundson G, Edwards CC, Garfin SR: Spondylolisthesis. In Rothman RH, Simeone FA (eds): The Spine. Philadelphia, WB Saunders, 1992, pp 913-969.
3. Amuso SJ, Neff RS, Coulson DB, et al: The surgical treatment of spondylolisthesis by posterior element resection. J Bone Joint Surg 52A:529-536, 1970.
4. Ani N, Keppler L, Biscup RS, et al: Reduction of high-grade slips (grades III-V) with VSP instrumentation. Report of a series of 41 cases. Spine 16:S302-S310, 1991.
5. Axelsson P, Johnsson R, Stromqvist B: Lumbar orthosis with unilateral hip immobilization. Effect on intervertebral mobility determined by roentgen stereophotogrammetric analysis. Spine 18:876-879, 1993.
6. Blanda J, Bethem D, Moats W, et al: Defects of pars interarticularis in athletes: a protocol for nonoperative treatment. J Spinal Disord 6:406-411, 1993.
7. Boden SD, Riew KD, Yamaguchi K, et al: Orientation of the lumbar facet joint: association with degenerative disc disease. J Bone Joint Surg [Am] 78: 403-411, 1996.
8. Bolesta MJ, Bohlman HH: Degenerative spondylolisthesis. Instr Course Lec 38:157-165, 1986.
9. Bonnici AV, Koka SR, Richards DJ: Results of Buck screw fusion in grade I spondylolisthesis. J R Soc Med 84: 270-273, 1991.
10. Boos N, Marchesi D, Zuber K, et al: Treatment of severe spondylolisthesis by reduction and pedicular fixation. A 4-6-year follow-up study. Spine 18:1655-1661, 1993.

11. Bosworth DM: Technique of spinal fusion: pseudarthrosis and method of repair. In Blount WP, Banks SW (eds): *American Academy of Orthopedic Surgery Instructional Course Lectures*. St Louis, CV Mosby, 1948, pp 295-313.

12. Bosworth DM, Fielding JW, Demarest L, *et al:* Spondylolisthesis: a critical review of a consecutive series of cases treated by arthrodesis. *J Bone Joint Surg* 37A: 767-786, 1955.

13. Boxall D, Bradford DS, Winter RB, *et al:* Management of severe spondylolisthesis in children and adolescents. *J Bone Joint Surg* 61A:479-495, 1979.

14. Bridwell KH, Sedgewick TA, O'Brien MF, *et al:* The role of fusion and instrumentation in the treatment of degenerative spondylolisthesis with spinal stenosis. *J Spinal Disord* 6:461-472, 1993.

15. Brodsky AE, Kovalsky ES, Khalil MA: Correlation of radiologic assessment of lumbar spine fusions with surgical exploration. *Spine* 16:S261-S265, 1991.

16. Brown CW, Orme TJ, Richardson HD: The rate of pseudarthrosis (surgical nonunion) in patients who are smokers and patients who are nonsmokers: a comparison study. *Spine* 11:942-943, 1986.

17. Brown M, Lockwood J: Degenerative spondylolisthesis. In Blount WP, Banks SW (eds): *American Academy of Orthopedic Surgery Instructional Course Lectures*. St Louis, CV Mosby, 1983, pp 162-169.

18. Buck JE: Direct repair of the defect in spondylolisthesis. Preliminary report. *J Bone Joint Surg* 52B:432-437, 1970.

19. Caputy A, Luessenhop A: Long-term evaluation of decompressive surgery for degenerative lumbar stenosis. *J Neurosurg* 77:669-676, 1992.

20. Cauchoix J, Benoist M, Chassaing V: Degenerative spondylolisthesis. *Clin Orthop* 115:123-129, 1976.

21. Cedell CA, Wiberg G: Long-term results of laminectomy in spondylolisthesis. *Acta Orthop Scand* 40:773-776, 1969.

22. Daftari TK, Whitesides TE, Jr., Heller JG, *et al:* Effect of nicotine on the revascularization of bone graft. An experimental study in rabbits. *Spine* 19:904-911, 1994.

23. Dandy DJ, Shannon MJ: Lumbo-sacral subluxation (Group 1 spondylolisthesis). *J Bone Joint Surg* 53B: 578-595, 1971.

24. Davis AA, Carragee EJ: Bilateral facet dislocation at the lumbosacral joint. A report of a case and review of literature. *Spine* 18:2540-2544, 1993.

25. Davis IS, Bailey RW: Spondylolisthesis. Long-term follow-up study of treatment with total laminectomy. *Clin Orthop* 88:46-49, 1972.

26. Dawson EG, Clader TJ, Bassett LW: A comparison of different methods used to diagnose pseudarthrosis following posterior spinal fusion for scoliosis. *J Bone Joint Surg* 67A:1153-1159, 1985.

27. DePalma AF, Rothman RH: The nature of pseudarthrosis. *Clin Orthop* 59:113-118, 1968.

28. Dickman CA, Fessler RG, MacMillan M, *et al:* Transpedicular screw-rod fixation of the lumbar spine: operative technique and outcome in 104 cases [see comments]. *J Neurosurg* 77:860-870, 1992.

29. Dupuis PR, Yong-Hing K, Cassidy JD, *et al:* Radiologic diagnosis of degenerative lumbar spinal instability. *Spine* 10:262-276, 1985.

30. Edelson JG, Nathan H: Nerve root compression in spondylolysis and spondylolisthesis. *J Bone Joint Surg* 68B:596-599, 1986.

31. Edmunds I, Cummine J, Fearnside M: Prevention of dislodgement of Cotrel-Dubousset rods from tulip screws. *Spine* 18:2325-2326, 1993.

32. Elghazawi AK: Clinical syndromes and differential diagnosis of spinal disorders. *Radiol Clin North Am* 29: 651-663, 1991.

33. Epstein J, Epstein B, Lavine L: Nerve root compression associated with narrowing of the lumbar spinal canal. *J Neurol Neurosurg Psychiatry* 25:165-176, 1962.

34. Epstein NE: Decompression in the surgical management of degenerative spondylolisthesis: advantages of a conservative approach in 290 patients. *J Spinal Disord* 11:116-122, 1998.

35. Esses SI, Huler RJ: Indications for lumbar spine fusion in the adult. *Clin Orthop* 279:87-100, 1992.

36. Feffer H, Weisel S, Cuckler J, *et al:* Degenerative spondylolisthesis: To fuse or not to fuse. *Spine* 10: 286-289,1985.

37. Fischgrund J, Kurz LT: The radiographic assessment of spondylolisthesis. *Semin Spine Surg* 5:301-307, 1993.

38. Fischgrund JS, Mackay M, Herkowitz HN, *et al:* Degenerative lumbar spondylolisthesis with spinal stenosis: a prospective, randomized study comparing decompressive laminectomy and arthrodesis with and without spinal instrumentation. *Spine* 22:2807-2812, 1997.

39. Fredrickson BE, Baker D, McHolick WJ, *et al:* The natural history of spondylolysis and spondylolisthesis. *J Bone Joint Surg* 66A:699-707, 1984.

40. Frennered AK, Danielson BI, Nachemson AL, *et al:* Midterm follow-up of young patients fused in situ for spondylolisthesis. *Spine* 16:409-416, 1991.

41. Friberg O: Lumbar instability: a dynamic approach by traction-compression radiography. *Spine* 12:119-129, 1987.

42. Frymoyer JW, Selby DK: Segmental instability. Rationale for treatment. *Spine* 10:280-286, 1985.

43. Gill GG, Manning JG, White HL: Surgical treatment of spondylolisthesis without spine fusion. *J Bone Joint Surg* 37A:493-520, 1955.

44. Grobler L, Wiltse L: Classification, non-operative, and operative treatment of spondylolisthesis. In Frymoyer JW (ed): *The Adult Spine: Principles and Practice*. Philadelphia, J.B. Lippincott, 1991, pp 1655-1704.

45. Grobler LJ, Robertson PA, Novotny JE, *et al:* Decompression for degenerative spondylolisthesis and spinal stenosis at L4-5. The effects on facet joint morphology. *Spine* 18:1475-1482, 1993.

46. Grobler LJ, Robertson PA, Novotny JE, *et al:* Etiology of spondylolisthesis. Assessment of the role played by lumbar facet joint morphology. *Spine* 18:80-91, 1993.

47. Hambly M, Lee CK, Gutteling E, *et al:* Tension band wiring-bone grafting for spondylolysis and spondylolisthesis. A clinical and biomechanical study. *Spine* 14:455-460, 1989.

48. Hanley EN Jr, Levy JA: Surgical treatment of isthmic lumbosacral spondylolisthesis. Analysis of variables influencing results. *Spine* 14:48-50, 1989.

49. Hannon KM, Wetta WJ: Failure of technetium bone scanning to detect pseudarthroses in spinal fusion for scoliosis. *Clin Orthop* 123:42-44, 1977.

50. Harrington PR, Tullos HS: Spondylolisthesis in children. Observations and surgical treatment. *Clin Orthop* 79:75-84, 1971.

51. Hazlett JW, Kinnard P: Lumbar apophyseal process excision and spinal instability. *Spine* 7:171-176, 1982.

52. Herkowitz HN, Kurz LT: Degenerative lumbar spondylolisthesis with spinal stenosis. *J Bone Joint Surg [Am]* 73:802-807, 1991.

53. Herron LD, Trippi AC: L4-5 degenerative spondylolisthesis. The results of treatment by decompressive laminectomy without fusion. *Spine* 14:534-538, 1989.

54. Hirabayashi S, Kumano K, Kuroki T: Cotrel-Dubousset pedicle screw system for various spinal disorders. Merits and problems. *Spine* 16:1298-1304, 1991.

55. Iida Y, Kataoka O, Sho T, et al: Postoperative lumbar spinal instability occurring or progressing secondary to laminectomy. *Spine* 15:1186-1189, 1990.

56. Inoue S, Watanabe T, Goto S, et al: Degenerative spondylolisthesis. Pathophysiology and results of anterior interbody fusion. *Clin Orthop* 227:90-98, 1988.

57. Jackson RK, Boston DA, Edge AJ: Lateral mass fusion. A prospective study of a consecutive series with long-term follow-up. *Spine* 10:828-832, 1985.

58. Jinkins JR, Matthes JC, Sener RN, et al: Spondylolysis, spondylolisthesis, and associated nerve root entrapment in the lumbosacral spine: MR evaluation. *AJR Am J Roentgenol* 159:799-803, 1992.

59. Johnson DW, Farnum GN, Latchaw RE, et al: MR imaging of the pars interarticularis. *AJR Am J Roentgenol* 152:327-332, 1989.

60. Johnson GV, Thompson AG: The Scott wiring technique for direct repair of lumbar spondylolysis. *J Bone Joint Surg* 74B:426-430, 1992.

61. Johnsson KE, Redlund-Johnell I, Udén A, et al: Preoperative and postoperative instability in lumbar spinal stenosis. *Spine* 14:591-593, 1989.

62. Johnsson KE, Willner S, Johnsson K: Postoperative instability after decompression for lumbar spinal stenosis. *Spine* 11:107-110, 1986.

63. Jonsson B: Vertebral slipping after decompression for spinal stenosis. *Acta Orthop Scand Suppl* 251:76-77, 1993.

64. Kahanovitz N, Arnoczky SP: The efficacy of direct current electrical stimulation to enhance canine spinal fusions. *Clin Orthop* 251:295-299, 1990.

65. Kim NH, Kim HK, Suh JS: A computed tomographic analysis of changes in the spinal canal after anterior lumbar interbody fusion. *Clin Orthop* 286:180-191, 1993.

66. Kirkaldy-Willis WH, Farfan HF: Instability of the lumbar spine. *Clin Orthop* 165:110-123, 1982.

67. Langston JW, Gavant ML: "Incomplete ring" sign: a simple method for CT detection of spondylolysis. *J Comput Assist Tomogr* 9:728-729, 1985.

68. Laurent LE, Osterman K: Operative treatment of spondylolisthesis in young patients. *Clin Orthop* 117:85-91, 1976.

69. Lee CK: Lumbar spinal instability (olisthesis) after extensive posterior spinal decompression. *Spine* 8:429-433, 1983.

70. Lim TH, Goel VK: Biomechanical aspects of spondylolisthesis. *Semin Spine Surg* 5:288-296, 1993.

71. Lindholm TS, Ragni P, Ylikoski M, et al: Lumbar isthmic spondylolisthesis in children and adolescents. Radiologic evaluation and results of operative treatment. *Spine* 15:1350-1355, 1990.

72. Lombardi JS, Wiltse LL, Reynolds J, et al: Treatment of degenerative spondylolisthesis. *Spine* 10:821-827, 1985.

73. Lowe J, Schachner E, Hirschberg E, et al: Significance of bone scintigraphy in symptomatic spondylolysis. *Spine* 9:653-655, 1984.

74. Lowe RW, Hayes TD, Kaye J, et al: Standing roentgenograms in spondylolisthesis. *Clin Orthop* 117:80-84, 1976.

75. Lusskin R: Pain patterns in spondylolisthesis. A correlation of symptoms, local pathology and therapy. *Clin Orthop* 40:123-136, 1965.

76. MacNab I, Dall D: The blood supply of the lumbar spine and its application to the technique of intertransverse lumbar fusion. *J Bone Joint Surg* 53B:628-638, 1971.

77. Magora A: Conservative treatment in spondylolisthesis. *Clin Orthop* 117:74-79, 1976.

78. Markwalder TM: Surgical management of neurogenic claudication in 100 patients with lumbar spinal stenosis due to degenerative spondylolisthesis. *Acta Neurochir (Wien)* 120:136-142, 1993.

79. Markwalder TM, Saager C, Reulen HJ: Isthmic spondylolisthesis: an analysis of the clinical and radiological presentation in relation to intraoperative findings and surgical results in 72 consecutive cases. *Acta Neurochir (Wien)* 110:154-159, 1991.

80. Matsunaga S, Ijir S, Hayashi K: Nonsurgically managed patients with degenerative spondylolisthesis: a 10- to 18-year follow-up study. *J Neurosurg* 93:194-198, 2000.

81. Matsunaga S, Sakou T, Morizono Y, et al: Natural history of degenerative spondylolisthesis: pathogenesis and natural course of slippage. *Spine* 15:1204-1210, 1990.

82. McAfee PC, Weiland DJ, Carlow JJ: Survivorship analysis of pedicle spinal instrumentation. *Spine* 16:S422-S427, 1991.

83. McMaster MJ, Merrick MV: The scintigraphic assessment of the scoliotic spine after fusion. *J Bone Joint Surg* 62B:65-72, 1980.

84. McPhee B: Spondylolisthesis and spondylolysis. In Youmans JR (ed): *Neurological Surgery*. Philadelphia, WB Saunders, 1990, pp 2749-2784.

85. Meyerding HW: Spondylolisthesis. *Surg Gynecol Obstet* 54:371-377, 1932.

86. Miller RA, Hardcastle P, Renwick SE: Lower spinal mobility and external immobilization in the normal and pathologic condition. *Orthop Rev* 21:753-757, 1992.

87. Morgan FP, King T: Primary instability of lumbar vertebrae as a common cause of low back pain. *J Bone Joint Surg [Br]* 38: 6-21, 1957.

88. Nachemson A, Wiltse LL: Spondylolisthesis, editorial. *Clin Orthop* 117:2-3, 1976.

89. Nachemson AL: Newest knowledge of low back pain. A critical look. *Clin Orthop* 279:8-20, 1992.

90. Nagata H, Schendel MJ, Transfeldt EE, et al: The effects of immobilization of long segments of the spine on the adjacent and distal facet force and lumbosacral motion. *Spine* 18:2471-2479, 1993.

91. Nelson PB: Degenerative lumbar spondylolisthesis. *Contemp Neurosurg* 14:1-5, 1992.

92. Neugebauer FI: The classic: a new contribution to the history and etiology of spondylolisthesis. *Clin Orthop* 117: 4-22, 1976.

93. Newman PH: A clinical syndrome associated with severe lumbo-sacral subluxation. *J Bone Joint Surg* 47B:472B481, 1965

94. Newman PH: Stenosis of the lumbar spine in spondylolisthesis. *Clin Orthop* 115:116-121, 1976.

95. Newman PH: Surgical treatment for spondylolisthesis in the adult. *Clin Orthop* 117:106-111, 1976.

96. Nicol RO, Scott JH: Lytic spondylolysis. Repair by wiring. *Spine* 11:1027-1030, 1986.

97. O'Brien JP, Mehdian H, Jaffray D: Reduction of severe lumbosacral spondylolisthesis. A report of 22 cases with a ten-year follow-up period. *Clin Orthop* 300:64-69, 1994.

98. Ohmori K, Suzuki K, Ishida Y: Translamino-pedicular screw fixation with bone grafting for symptomatic isthmic lumbar spondylolysis. *Neurosurgery* 30:379-384, 1992.

99. Olerud S, Sjostrom L, Karlstrom G, *et al:* Spontaneous effect of increased stability of the lower lumbar spine in cases of severe chronic back pain. The answer of an external transpeduncular fixation test. *Clin Orthop* 203:67-74, 1986.

100. Ordeberg G, Enskog J, Sjostrom L: Diagnostic external fixation of the lumbar spine. *Acta Orthop Scand Suppl* 251:94-96, 1993.

101. Osterman K, Lindholm TS, Laurent LE: Late results of removal of the loose posterior element (Gill's operation) in the treatment of lytic lumbar spondylolisthesis. *Clin Orthop* 117:121-128, 1976.

102. Osterman K, Schlenzka D, Poussa M, *et al:* Isthmic spondylolisthesis in symptomatic and asymptomatic subjects, epidemiology, and natural history with special reference to disc abnormality and mode of treatment. *Clin Orthop* 297:65-70, 1993.

103. Panjabi MM, Oxland TR, Yamamoto I, *et al:* Mechanical behavior of the human lumbar and lumbosacral spine as shown by three-dimensional load-displacement curves. *J Bone Joint Surg* 76A:413-424, 1994.

104. Pashman RS, Hu SS, Schendel MJ, *et al:* Sacral screw loads in lumbosacral fixation for spinal deformity. *Spine* 18:2465-2470, 1993.

105. Pedersen AK, Hagen R: Spondylolysis and spondylolisthesis. Treatment by internal fixation and bone-grafting of the defect. *J Bone Joint Surg* 70A:15-24, 1988.

106. Peek RD, Wiltse LL, Reynolds JB, *et al:* In situ arthrodesis without decompression for Grade-III or IV isthmic spondylolisthesis in adults who have severe sciatica. *J Bone Joint Surg* 71A:62-68, 1989.

107. Pennell RG, Maurer AH, Bonakdarpour A: Stress injuries of the pars interarticularis: radiologic classification and indications for scintigraphy. *AJR Am J Roentgenol* 145: 763-766, 1985.

108. Pope MH, Frymoyer JW, Krag MH: Diagnosing instability. *Clin Orthop* 279:60-67, 1992.

109. Posner L, White AA, Edward WT, *et al:* A biomechanical analysis of the clinical stability of lumbar and lumbosacral spine. *Spine* 7:374-389, 1982.

110. Poussa M, Schlenzka D, Seitsalo S, *et al:* Surgical treatment of severe isthmic spondylolisthesis in

111. adolescents. Reduction or fusion in situ. *Spine* 18:894-901, 1993.

111. Raney FL, Kolb FD: The effect of metabolic bone disease on spinal fusion. In Rothman RH, White AH, Ray DC (eds): *Lumbar Spine Surgery.* St Louis, CV Mosby, 1987, pp 246-249.

112. Rauschning W: Pathoanatomy of lumbar disc degeneration and stenosis. *Acta Orthop Scand Suppl* 251:3-12, 1993.

113. Rissanen PM: Comparison of pathological changes in intervertebral disc and interspinous ligaments of the lower part of the lumbar spine in the light of autopsy findings. *Acta Orthop Scand* 34:54-65, 1964.

114. Robertson PA, Grobler LJ: Stress fracture of the pedicle: a late complication of posterolateral lumbar fusion. *Spine* 18:930-932, 1993.

115. Rombold C: Treatment of spondylolisthesis by posterolateral fusion, resection of the pars interarticularis, and prompt mobilization of the patient. An end-result study of seventy-three patients. *J Bone Joint Surg* 48A:1282-1300, 1966.

116. Rosenberg NJ: Degenerative spondylolisthesis. Predisposing factors. *J Bone Joint Surg* 57A:467-474, 1975.

117. Rosenberg NJ: Degenerative spondylolisthesis: surgical treatment. *Clin Orthop* 117:112-120, 1976.

118. Rosenberg NJ, Bargar WL, Friedman B: The incidence of spondylolysis and spondylolisthesis in nonambulatory patients. *Spine* 6:35-38, 1981.

119. Roy-Camille R, Benazet JP, Desauge JP, *et al:* Lumbosacral fusion with pedicular screw plating instrumentation. A 10-year follow-up. *Acta Orthop Scand Suppl* 251:100-104, 1993.

120. Rupp R, Ebraheim NA, Savolaine ER, *et al:* Magnetic resonance imaging evaluation of the spine with metal implants. General safety and superior imaging with titanium. *Spine* 18:379-385, 1993.

121. Ryan PJ, Fogelman I: The role of nuclear medicine in orthopaedics [see comments]. *Nucl Med Commun* 15: 341-360, 1994.

122. Salib RM, Pettine KA: Modified repair of a defect in spondylolysis or minimal spondylolisthesis by pedicle screw, segmental wire fixation, and bone grafting. *Spine* 18:440-443, 1993.

123. Sanderson PL, Wood PL: Surgery for lumbar spinal stenosis in old people. *J Bone Joint Surg [Br]* 75:393-7, 1993.

124. Saraste H: Spondylolysis and spondylolisthesis. *Acta Orthop Scand Suppl* 251:84-86, 1993

125. Selby DK, Henderson RJ, Blumenthal S, *et al:* Anterior lumbar fusion. In Rothman RH, White AH, Ray DC (eds): *Lumbar Spine Surgery.* St Louis, CV Mosby, 1987, pp 383-402.

126. Shelokov A, Haideri N, Roach J: Residual gait abnormalities in surgically treated spondylolisthesis. *Spine* 18:2201-2205, 1993.

127. Shenkin HA, Hash CJ: Spondylolisthesis after multiple bilateral laminectomies and facetectomies for lumbar spondylosis. Follow-up review. *J Neurosurg* 50:45-47, 1979.

128. Shirado O, Zdeblick TA, McAfee PC, *et al:* Biomechanical evaluation of methods of posterior stabilization of the spine and posterior lumbar interbody arthrodesis for lumbosacral isthmic spondylolisthesis. A calf-spine model. *J Bone Joint Surg* 73A:518-526, 1991.

129. Silvers HR, Lewis PJ, Asch HL: Decompressive lumbar laminectomy for spinal stenosis. *J Neurosurgery* 78: 695-701,1993.

130. Sim E: Location of transpedicular screws for fixation of the lower thoracic and lumbar spine. Computed tomography of 45 fracture cases. *Acta Orthop Scand* 64: 28-32, 1993.

131. Slizofski WJ, Collier BD, Flatley TJ, *et al:* Painful pseudarthrosis following lumbar spinal fusion: detection by combined SPECT and planar bone scintigraphy. *Skeletal Radiol* 16:136-141, 1987.

132. Slone RM, MacMillan M, Montgomery WJ, *et al:* Spinal fixation. Part 2. Fixation techniques and hardware for the thoracic and lumbosacral spine. *Radiographics* 13: 521-543, 1993.

133. Soini J, Laine T, Pohjolainen T, *et al:* Spondylodesis augmented by transpedicular fixation in the treatment of olisthetic and degenerative conditions of the lumbar spine. *Clin Orthop* 297:111-116, 1993.

134. Soren A, Waugh TR: Spondylolisthesis and related disorders. A correlative study of 105 patients. *Clin Orthop* 193:171-177, 1985.

135. Spratt KF, Weinstein JN, Lehmann TR, *et al:* Efficacy of flexion and extension treatments incorporating braces for low-back pain patients with retrodisplacement, spondylolisthesis, or normal sagittal translation. *Spine* 18:1839-1849, 1993.

136. Steffee AD, Brantigan JW: The variable screw placement spinal fixation system. Report of a prospective study of 250 patients enrolled in Food and Drug Administration clinical trials. *Spine* 18:1160-1172, 1993.

137. Steiner ME, Micheli LJ: Treatment of symptomatic spondylolysis and spondylolisthesis with the modified Boston brace. *Spine* 10:937-943, 1985.

138. Stillerman CB, Schneider JH, Gruen JP: Evaluation and management of spondylolysis and spondylolisthesis. *Clin Neurosurg* 40:384-415, 1993.

139. Stokes IA, Wilder DG, Frymoyer JW, *et al:* 1980 Volvo award in clinical sciences. Assessment of patients with low-back pain by biplanar radiographic measurement of intervertebral motion. *Spine* 6:233-240, 1981.

140. Stromqvist B: Postlaminectomy problems with reference to spinal fusion. *Acta Orthop Scand Suppl* 251:87-89, 1993.

141. Suh PB, Esses SI, Kostuik JP: Repair of pars interarticularis defect. The prognostic value of pars infiltration. *Spine* 16:S445-S448, 1991.

142. Szypryt EP, Twining P, Mulholland RC, *et al:* The prevalence of disc degeneration associated with neural arch defects of the lumbar spine assessed by magnetic resonance imaging. *Spine* 14:977-981, 1989.

143. Taillard WF: Etiology of spondylolisthesis. *Clin Orthop* 117:30-39, 1976.

144. Turner JA, Ersek M, Herron L, *et al:* Patient outcomes after lumbar spinal fusions. *JAMA* 268:907-911, 1992.

145. Valdez DC, Johnson RG: Role of technetium-99m planar bone scanning in the evaluation of low back pain. *Skeletal Radiol* 23:91-97, 1994.

146. Verbiest H: The treatment of lumbar spondyloptosis or impending lumbar spondyloptosis accompanied by neurologic deficit and/or neurogenic intermittent claudication. *Spine* 4:68-77, 1979.

147. Virta L, Ronnemaa T: The association of mild-moderate isthmic lumbar spondylolisthesis and low back pain in middle-aged patients is weak and it only occurs in women. *Spine* 18:1496-1503, 1993.

148. Watkins MB, Bragg C: Lumbosacral fusion: results with early ambulation. *Surg Gynecol Obstet* 102:604-608, 1956.

149. Wenger DR, Lee CS: Spondylolisthesis in children and adolescents. *Semin Spine Surg* 5:308-319, 1993.

150. West JL, Ogilvie JW, Bradford DS: Complications of the variable screw plate pedicle screw fixation. *Spine* 16: 576-579, 1991.

151. White AAI, Panjabi MM: *Clinical Biomechanics of the Spine*. Philadelphia, JB Lippincott, 1990.

152. Whitecloud TS, Butler JC, Cohen JL, *et al:* Complications with the variable spinal plating system. *Spine* 14:472-476, 1989.

153. Wiltse LL, Jackson DW: Treatment of spondylolisthesis and spondylolysis in children. *Clin Orthop* 117:92-100, 1976.

154. Wiltse LL, Rothman SLG: Spondylolisthesis: classification, diagnosis, and natural history. *Semin Spine Surg* 5: 264-280, 1993.

155. Wiltse LL, Winter RB: Terminology and measurement of spondylolisthesis. *J Bone Joint Surg* 65A:768-772, 1983.

156. Wiltse LL, Newman PH, MacNab I: Classification of spondylolysis and spondylolisthesis. *Clin Orthop* 117: 23-29, 1976.

157. Wiltse LL, Widell EH Jr, Jackson DW: Fatigue fracture: the basic lesion is isthmic spondylolisthesis. *J Bone Joint Surg* 57A:17-22, 1975.

158. Wynne-Davies R, Scott JHS: Inheritance and spondylolisthesis: a radiographic family survey. *J Bone Joint Surg* 61B:301-305, 1979.

159. Yashiro K, Homma T, Hokari Y, *et al:* The Steffee variable screw placement system using different methods of bone grafting. *Spine* 16:1329-1334, 1991.

160. Zdeblick TA: A prospective randomized study of lumbar fusion: preliminary results. *Spine* 18:983-991, 1993.

CHAPTER 55

Degenerative Rotatory Scoliosis: Coronal Plane Lumbar Spine Deformity Correction

Edward C. Benzel and Russ P. Nockels

Degenerative lumbar rotatory scoliosis is a manifestation of accelerated degenerative disease of the lumbar spine. Its extent, as illustrated by imaging studies, does not necessarily correlate with symptoms or neurologic deficits, a fact that presents a significant dilemma to the treating physician. Management options are complicated by the wide variety of treatment choices.

When surgery is considered, its rationale must be clearly delineated. Surgery is indicated in lumbar degenerative rotatory scoliosis for one of two reasons: (1) instability or (2) neural compression.

Instability can take many forms, ranging from the instability associated with mechanical low back pain to overt deformity progression or frank instability. Instability usually manifests itself by pain of a mechanical nature (pain that is deep and agonizing in nature that is worsened by activity [loading] and improved by rest [unloading]).

The treatment for neural compression is often surgical decompression, and the treatment for instability is joint immobilization. Surgery is a common option for the latter. Neurogenic claudication (a neurologic syndrome) does not respond to spinal fusion. Conversely, mechanical low back pain *uncommonly* responds to laminectomy. One must separate these clinical manifestations carefully so that surgical management can be specifically tailored to the patient's complaints and to the structural pathology.

As we age our spines "loosen" somewhat until midlife. Then, at about the age of 55, the degenerative process begins to accelerate and spinal stiffening occurs (i.e., spinal restabilization). This stiffening process, although associated with spinal degeneration and spinal deformation, leads to a progressively more stable spine in most cases. Therefore this scenario, which is the rule rather than the exception, should mandate a surgically conservative approach in the majority of patients. For example, even with significant spinal deformation, a patient with neurogenic claudication may be best managed by a carefully performed decompression procedure—not a radical decompression, deformity reduction, fusion, and instrumentation procedure.

Finally, methods of deformity reduction and maintenance are described in this chapter. Adjuncts to this aspect of the management of degenerative rotatory scoliosis, such as ventral "release" procedures or orthotic management, are not. In the clinical scenarios presented in this chapter, it is assumed that the patient has a symptomatic and mechanically unstable spine and that adjuncts to the surgical scheme under discussion are also undertaken when appropriate.

Pathophysiology of Disc Degeneration and the Spondylotic Process

Lumbar spondylosis is not a pathologic process. It is but a manifestation of the wear-and-tear phenomenon that is associated with aging. It is defined as vertebral osteophytosis secondary to degenerative disc disease[12] and is not an inflammatory process. Noninfectious inflammatory processes are grouped together as arthritides and are excluded from this discussion.

Spondylosis and associated osteophytosis is universally accompanied by degeneration of the intervertebral disc. The intervertebral disc is an amphiarthrodial joint (no synovial membrane) with particular traits that result in a characteristic degeneration pattern. Conversely, arthritides classically involve the synovial membranes of diarthrodial joints (joints lined with synovium and lubricated with synovial fluid [e.g., facet joints]). Facet joints, however, are also affected by the spondylotic process.[5,10]

The degenerative process primarily involves the disc interspace and alters intradiscal dynamics that result in spinal deformation. The resultant excessive motion and stresses cause extradiscal soft-tissue proliferation. Finally, spinal deformation predisposes to further deformation (see "Osteoporosis" section). Osteoporosis contributes to the latter process, with a resultant asymmetric vertebral body collapse.

Intradiscal Dynamics

Chronically elevated intradiscal pressure causes disc interspace narrowing (collapse), distorting the annulus fibrosus and the facet joint capsule. This in turn accelerates the degenerative process.

The water content of the disc interspace gradually decreases throughout life, which contributes to alterations in the chemical and anatomic makeup of the disc. Fibroblasts become defective, and the desiccated disc is less effective as a cushion. Fissures then develop in the cartilaginous end-plates. Schmorl's nodes are manifestations of this pathologic process. Gas may accumulate in the disc (the vacuum phenomenon). An ingrowth of fibrocartilage (mucoid degeneration) with obliteration of the nucleus fibrosus ensues. Relative incompetence of the disc itself and relative instability result, and annulus fibrosus bulging and tension occur as a result of this process.[5]

Disc Deformation

Bulging of the annulus fibrosus results in periosteal elevation and subperiosteal bone formation. Spondylotic ridges (osteophytes) are laid down, and this can result in spinal canal encroachment. These ridges occur most commonly on the concave side of a curvature. Therefore natural cervical and lumbar lordosis predisposes the spine to osteophyte formation toward the spinal canal, causing spinal canal encroachment. The thoracic region, by virtue of its intrinsic kyphotic posture, is relatively spared this process.

Although osteophyte formation occurs predominantly on the concave side of a scoliotic curvature (where annulus fibrosus bulging is most significant), disc herniation occurs commonly on the convex side of a spinal bend. The thin dorsal annulus fibrosus and relatively weak lateral aspect of the posterior longitudinal ligament (PLL) combine with the migratory tendencies of the nucleus pulposus to encourage dorsolateral disc herniation.[5]

In the laboratory, (1) flexion (causing dorsal nucleus pulposus migration), (2) lateral bending away from the side of disc herniation (causing lateral nucleus pulposus migration), and (3) application of an axial load (causing an increase in intradiscal pressure) are required for the creation of a herniated lumbar disc. A degenerated disc is also necessary as a predisposing factor.[1] This complex loading pattern results in the application of tension on the weakest portion of the annulus fibrosus (the dorsolateral position, the location of the herniation), migration of the nucleus pulposus toward this position, and an asymmetric increase in intradiscal pressure. The age-related increased frequency of annulus fibrosus tears and a peaking of nucleus fibrosus pressures in people 35 to 55 years of age[10] also predisposed to an increased incidence of disc herniation.

Asymmetric collapse of the disc interspace is often a result of the disc degeneration process and places asymmetric focal stresses on portions of the spine.

Extradiscal Soft-Tissue Involvement

Hypertrophy and buckling of the ligamentum flavum, as well as other soft tissue proliferative processes, can result in spinal canal encroachment. Excessive pathologic segmental motion predisposes to this process and is a major factor related to the development of spinal stenosis.

Osteoporosis

Osteoporosis leads to a decrease in bony integrity, and this in turn leads to vertebral body collapse. The presence of thoracic kyphosis predisposes the thoracic spine to ventral vertebral body collapse, whereas asymmetric disc interspace collapse (which is commonly associated with degenerative disc disease) predisposes to lateral vertebral body collapse. The latter is a major predisposing factor related to the development of scoliotic deformations; that is, deformity begets deformity (deformity progression). Deformity and deformity progression ensue because of the application of loads (usually axial loads) to progressively longer and longer moment arms. This creates a "vicious cycle" that perpetuates the process.

Spinal Configuration

The configuration of the spine should be considered carefully before determining the surgical approach (which includes application of a spinal implant) for a spinal disorder. The thoracic and lumbar regions are affected differently in this regard. Thoracic spine disc interspace height loss occurs predominantly in the ventral aspect of the disc. This results in progression of the natural kyphotic defor-

mity as the degenerative process ensues, thus exaggerating deformity progression propensities. The rib cage, however, substantially stabilizes the thoracic spine.

The coupling phenomenon (whereby one movement of the spine about or along an axis obligates another movement about or along another axis)[5] plays a significant role in the development of degenerative spinal deformations in the lumbar region (whereas it is of minimal significance regarding degenerative deformities in the thoracic region). This is because thoracic degenerative deformities are often orientated in the sagittal plane, whereas degenerative lumbar deformities are usually orientated in the coronal plane (excluding degenerative lumbar spondylolisthesis). The absence of uncovertebral joints (in contrast to the cervical region) and the sagittal orientation of the facet joints (in contrast to the cervical and thoracic regions) creates a situation that causes obligatory rotation of the spine in response to lateral bending (coupling). The progression of lateral bending deformities in the lumbar spine (scoliosis) thus predisposes to rotation of the spine (Figure 55.1).

Furthermore, lateral bending deformation predisposes to lateral bending deformity progression in the lumbar spine, as the presence of kyphotic deformation predisposes to the progression of kyphotic deformation in the thoracic spine. An asymmetric loss of height of the lumbar intervertebral disc may progress to an asymmetric collapse of the vertebral body, as described previously in this chap-

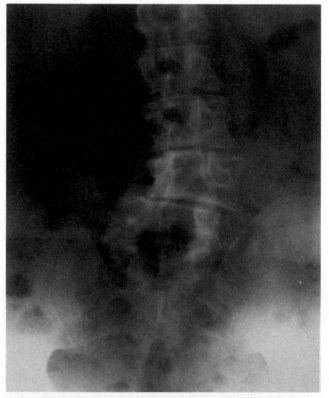

Figure 55.1 Radiograph of the lumbar spine of a patient with degenerative rotatory scoliosis. This illustrates that, via the coupling phenomenon, the scoliosis is obligatorily associated with a rotatory deformation of the spine. Note that the spinous processes are rotated toward the concave side of the curvature, which is in contradistinction to the situation in the cervical spine where the coupling phenomenon results in an obligatory rotation of the spinous processes toward the convex side of the curvature.

ter. As this scoliotic deformity progresses, it is obligatorily associated with rotation of the spine, with the spinous processes rotating toward the concave side of the curve (coupling).[5] Of note is that because of the aforementioned osteophyte development propensities, osteophytes occur predominantly on the concave side of the curvature.

The obligatory association of rotation with lateral bending (coupling) complicates lumbar spinal instrumentation surgery. Transverse process exposure and dissection can cause injury to underlying nerve roots because of the relative dorsal migration of the root with respect to the transverse processes. Furthermore, deformity correction via distraction of the concave side of the curvature may result in excessive stretching of foreshortened and tethered nerve root(s). The nerve roots become foreshortened because of their shorter course on the concave side of the curve. Therefore care must be taken both during surgical exposure of the lumbar transverse processes and during deformity reduction (concave-side distraction).

Deformity Correction

A variety of techniques can be used to correct lumbar spinal deformities. Deformity correction is accomplished via the application of rotatory or translational forces to the spine along one or a combination of the three axes of the Cartesian coordinate system.[5] Distraction can be used to reduce compression deformations, as well as coronally and sagittally oriented translational deformations. Compression can be employed for the latter as well. Similarly, three- or four-point bending forces can be applied. Finally, bending moments can be applied in either the coronal or sagittal planes to correct spinal curvatures. Complex bending moment forces are often applied.

Methods of deformity reduction and deformity reduction maintenance are discussed in this chapter. When indicated, ventral release procedures can provide the "relaxation" necessary to achieve the desired reduction. Conversely, excessive deformity reduction for degenerative lumbar rotatory scoliosis is seldom necessary. Alleviation of symptoms (both for the short and long term), not necessarily the attainment of a perfectly reduced spinal deformity, is the goal of any surgical management scheme.

Distraction and Compression

Distraction can be applied to the spine to reduce coronal and sagittal plane deformations. Ligamentous or other soft tissue integrity is mandatory for this type of force application to be effective in these circumstances. Distraction via this ligamentotaxis mechanism can be effective as an isolated mechanism of deformity correction.

Distraction force application on the concave side of the curve and compression force application on the convex side of the curve can be used to correct coronal plane deformities. This force couple[5] applies a coronal plane bending moment.

Three- and Four-Point Bending Fixation

Three- and four-point bending of the spine, as defined by White and Panjabi,[13] involves the loading of a long structure (i.e., the spine) with one or two transverse forces on one side and two on the other.[13] In a four-point bending construct, the bending moment is constant between the two intermediate points of force application if all forces are equal. In a three-point bending construct the bending moment peaks at the intermediate point of force application.

The crossed-rod technique is a complex variant of three- or four-point bending fixation. It is a traditional and common method of thoracic and lumbar kyphotic deformity correction and was first used with Harrington distraction rods. Subsequently, it involved the Luque multisegmental sublaminar wiring technique.[4] Most recently, it has been employed with the sequential hook insertion (SHI) technique with universal spinal instrumentation constructs.[6] Regardless of the specific method used, the crossed-rod technique involves sequential and gradual application of kyphosis reduction forces to the spine via moment arms through longitudinal members.

Applied Moment Arm Cantilever Beam Force Application

Applied moment arm cantilever beam constructs are most appropriate in situations in which short-segment constructs are particularly desirable.[5] This type of construct mandates that a significant force be applied by the implant to the spine. Although this type of construct is most often applied for sagittal plane deformities, it can also be used (although uncommonly) for coronal plane deformity correction.

These are constructs frequently applied as either flexion or extension bending moments via pedicle screws.[9] They can be used with distraction, compression, or coronal plane bending moment force application, and can also be applied with an accompanying ventral dural sac decompression and interbody bone graft placement. Furthermore, they can be applied so that deformity is reduced and compression of the bone graft is achieved. This technique of (1) sequential application of distraction (load bearing), (2) decompression of the dural sac, (3) interbody fusion placement, and (4) compression of the construct to share the load with the ventral spinal elements is termed *load-bearing to load-sharing force application*. It provides biomechanical advantages (load sharing), as well as clinical advantages.[5]

Short-Segment Parallelogram Deformity Reduction

Short-segment parallelogram deformity reduction is a rigid cantilever beam pedicle fixation technique that applies bending moments for the reduction of lateral translational deformations.[5] This technique is most useful when short-segment fixation is deemed optimal. It involves (1) placement of pedicle screws, (2) appropriate dural sac decompression, (3) attachment of the longitudinal members to the screws (rods), (4) application of a rotatory and distraction force to the rods, (5) maintenance of the achieved spinal reduction via rigid cross-fixation, (6) placement of a fusion (interbody and/or lateral), and finally, (7) compression of the screws so that load sharing is achieved and the interbody bone graft is secured in its acceptance bed.[5] It applies load-bearing to load-sharing forces (Figure 55.2).

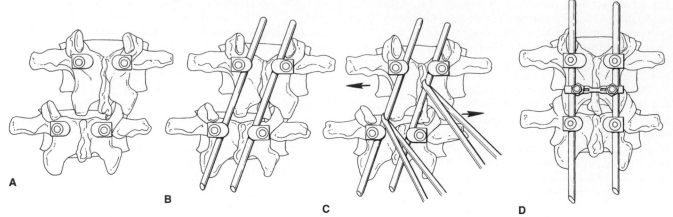

Figure 55.2 Short-segment parallelogram deformity reduction. A lateral translational deformity is reduced by first inserting pedicle screws into each of the pedicles (**A**). Next, rods are attached to each of the screws (**B**). Bending moments are then simultaneously applied to each of the rods by rod grippers (**C**). A rigid cross-member is then used for deformity reduction maintenance and stability augmentation purposes (**D**).

In Vivo Implant Contouring

Segmental relationships can be altered by rod or plate contouring. Employment of *in vivo* implant contouring for segmental relationship alteration is an effective method of deformity reduction. A multisegmental fixation system can be inserted in such a manner that it conforms to a spinal deformity, such as scoliosis. After insertion, rod contouring can be used to "straighten" the spine. Adequate implant-bone juncture security is mandatory. Implant contouring alters the forces applied by the implant to the spine at each segmental level. For example, hooks can overtighten or loosen, infringe on the spinal canal, or migrate laterally or medially.[5]

Intrinsic Implant Bending Moment Application about the Long Axis of the Spine: The Derotation Maneuver

As discussed in the chapter, an obligatory rotatory component coexists with scoliotic deformities (coupling). This phenomenon can be used to an advantage by applying the spinal derotation maneuver. Spinal derotation involves conversion of a scoliotic curvature to a kyphotic curvature.[8] The resultant kyphotic curvature can be reduced, if appropriate, via rod contouring. The derotation maneuver is accomplished by first inserting the rods via hooks, screws, or wires, which are relatively loosely attached to the rod (with friction-glide tightness), so that rotation of the rod can occur at its juncture with the hooks, screws, or wires. The attachment should not be so tight as to allow dislodgment (friction–glide tight or "just right tight" is preferable). This allows the hooks, screws, or wires to maintain their relationship with the spinal attachment site. The rods are then simultaneously rotated 90 degrees, which converts a scoliotic deformity to a kyphotic deformity. The rods can be contoured to eliminate an excessive kyphotic curvature. The junctures are then tightened and secured, and cross-fixation is employed to maintain the reduction (Figure 55.3A).

These maneuvers should be used in a gradual manner so that continuous assessment and reassessment of the implant-spine relationships can be made. For example, a hook may not rotate on the rod during the derotation maneuver, thus placing significant stress on the hook-bone attachment (Figure 55.3B).

Intrinsic Implant Bending Moment Application about the Axial Axes of the Spine

Intrinsic implant bending moment can be applied in either the sagittal or coronal plane. One or two segment lumbar scoliotic deformations can be partially or completely corrected by this technique. In applying this procedure pedicle screws are inserted and the rods are attached to the screws. The screws on the concave side of the curvature are then distracted (usually 1 to 2cm), whereas the screws on the convex side of the curvature are compressed. Cross-fixation to maintain the correction is then used (Figure 55.4A and B). A similar technique can be employed to correct sagittal plane deformities by using rod or plate-screw systems on the lateral aspect of the spine.

One should be cognizant of the type of screw-rod juncture (i.e., variable angle versus fixed angle). The application of distraction forces to a variable-angle screw that is *not* tightened to a friction-glide extent may result in screw flexion at the screw-rod juncture, which can cause application of an untoward bending moment to the spine. This can be prevented by tightening the screw carefully to friction-glide tightness before applying distraction forces.

Maintenance of Correction

Cross-Fixation

Cross-fixation is the connection of bilaterally placed constructs to each other and can result in a substantial increase in the integrity of the construct. In general, cross-fixation of

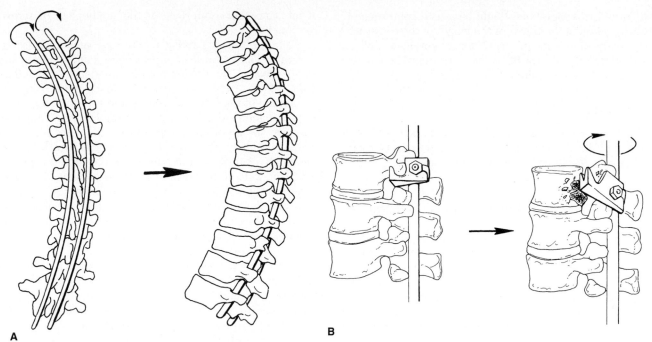

A   **B**

Figure 55.3 The derotation maneuver. A scoliotic curvature can be reduced by first attaching contoured rods (contoured to the shape of the deformity) to the affected portion of the spine at multiple attachment sites. Each rod is then rotated gradually and carefully by 90 degrees *(curved arrows)* (**A**). The resultant kyphotic deformity can then be reduced by *in situ* rod bending techniques. Care must be taken not to overtighten the hook-rod juncture. If this juncture is overtightened, rotation of the rod may result in hook cutout (**B**).

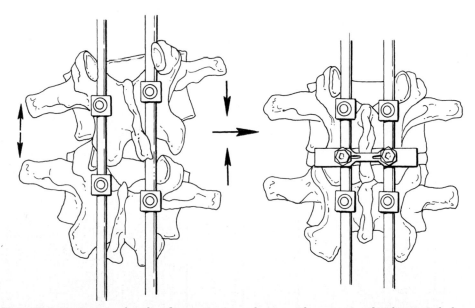

Figure 55.4 Intrinsic implant bending moment application. The concave side of a coronal plane curvature is distracted, and the concave side of the curvature compressed (each no more than 2cm). A rigid cross-member is used to assist in reduction maintenance. A similar technique can be used to correct sagittal plane deformities.

short constructs is of no significant benefit. However, in selected cases it can be used to maintain deformity reduction. In such situations very rigid cross-members should be used because substantial bending moments are applied (resisted) at the cross-member-rod juncture.

With longer constructs, cross-fixation provides a quadrilateral, framelike construct. This in turn results in rotatory stability and implant-bone juncture integrity augmentation. With long constructs, two cross-members are better than one; however, more than two add very little to construct integrity.[5] Cross-members should be placed approximately at the junction of the thirds of the length of the construct.[5]

Cross-fixation can be used for maintenance of an appropriate interrod width so that hook migration, screw dislodgment from the ilium, can be prevented.

Screw Toe-In

Screw toe-in can play an important role in lateral translational deformity prevention. It can be used with cross-fixation to achieve maintenance of deformity reduction.[5]

Low Lumbar and Lumbosacropelvic Techniques

Surgical management of lumbosacral deformities is fraught with complications. Therefore it should be considered only if there is a neurologic deficit in the presence of spinal canal compromise and/or instability.[5] If, indeed, surgery is indicated, multiple options are available.

The lumbosacral region presents many anatomic and biomechanical challenges. If adequate axial load-supporting capacity exists or has been attained surgically by a ventral interbody operative procedure, the stabilization process (via a spinal implant) is simplified or rendered unnecessary.

Conversely, if axial load-supporting capacity is not adequate or was not achieved surgically, acquisition of a stable spine will indeed be complex and difficult. Surgical alternatives include pedicle fixation, complex lumbosacroiliac fixation techniques, and combination multisegmental fixation techniques.

Pedicle fixation construct application in the absence of adequate axial load-supporting capacity places excessive stresses on the implant and the implant-bone juncture. Repetitive loading of such a construct may produce failure

at the screw-bone interface or the screw-plate or screw-rod juncture.[5]

Complex lumbosacroiliac techniques, such as the slingshot and Galveston techniques,[2] are cumbersome and involve fixation to predominantly low-density medullary bone. Thus they may provide inadequate fixation. Prevention of lumbosacral fixation and extension therefore may be inadequate because of poor implant-bone juncture integrity (as mentioned previously) and because of an inability to apply an adequate moment arm. Furthermore, the ability of these techniques to effectively reduce coronal plane deformities is poor because of their rigid one-piece design. Iliac screw fixation techniques using bicortical ilial fixation (BIF) are applicable as viable alternatives to these techniques.[3] They allow the surgeon to use a tripodlike implant geometry for buttressing the sacroiliac segment (Figure 55.5).[3,5]

A ventromedial orientation of sacral screws is, in general, superior to a ventrolateral (alar) orientation. Greater bone density, and hence provision of a stronger implant-bone juncture, can be achieved in the region of the midline sacral promontory or the L5-S1 disc interspace.[5,7] Additional implant-sacrum junctures can be used to prevent lumbosacral flexion and extension, including the first sacral lamina (for sublaminar wire fixation), the second dorsal sacral neuroforamina (for hook fixation), and the dorsum of the sacrum itself (via a buttressing effect) (Figure 55.6).

Combination multisegmental lumbosacral fixation techniques provide the ability to distract the lumbosacral spine, restore height to collapsed vertebral segments, allow two or more points of sacral fixation, and permit use of the sacrum as a buttress for axial load support of the torso. This allows the use of multiple fixation modalities (Figure 55.7).[5]

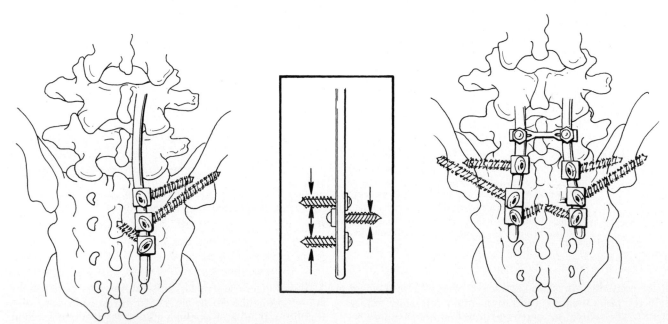

Figure 55.5 BIF achieves a tripodlike geometry. Rigid cross-fixation can be used to augment the fixation by enhancing the tripod effect. *BIF,* Bicortical ilial fixation.

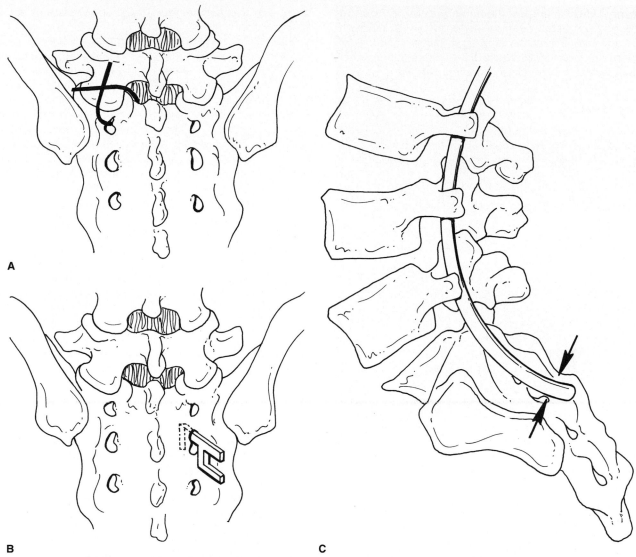

Figure 55.6 Additional sacrum fixation techniques. These involve the first sacral lamina for sublaminar wire fixation (**A**), the second dorsal sacral neuroforamina for hook fixation (**B**), and the dorsum of the sacrum itself for buttressing the rod (**C**).

Lumbosacroiliac fixation techniques should be used with the lumbosacral pivot point in mind. This is defined as the point of intersection of the middle osteoligamentous column (a region of the PLL) in the sagittal plane and the L5-S1 intervertebral disc (Figure 55.8). Constructs that employ lumbosacroiliac fixation via bone screws are most effective in resisting flexion and extension deformation if the ventral extent of the screws extends ventrally to this point (Figure 55.7).[11]

Clinical Applications

Clinical application of some of the techniques described in this chapter may indeed be difficult and dangerous. Therefore management options should be carefully considered and individualized. Reduction, fusion, and stabilization procedures are often not indicated despite the presence of a significantly degenerated and deformed spine. In fact, as we age (past approximately 55 years), a spinal restabilization process ensues (as a result of osteophyte formation, disc interspace collapse, and calcification). Deformity progression, which has been relentless before this, may slow down or cease. Therefore attempts at reduction and fusion in this patient population may be ill-advised.

Even when indicated, the universal application of a single surgical technique to all clinical situations is imprudent. For example, although pedicle fixation is, in general, a useful and efficacious technique, its universal application is inappropriate. For instance, it should not be applied over an unstable segment if ventral axial load-supporting ability is inadequate. Longer techniques, or the use of ilial fixation augmentation, may be beneficial (Figure 55.7).

Similarly, several options are available to correct scoliotic deformities. These include distraction, short-segment parallelogram deformity reduction techniques

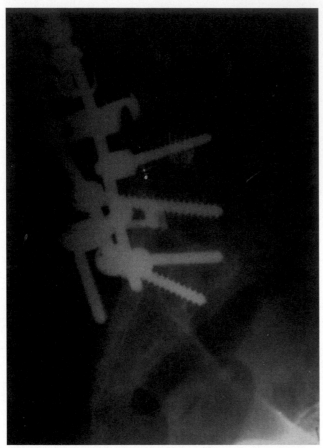

Figure 55.7 Use of multiple fixation techniques. Bicortical iliac fixation, laminar fixation, and sacral screw fixation are depicted in a single case.

(Figure 55.2), the derotation maneuver (Figure. 55.3), and intrinsic implant bending moment application (Figure 55.4). Each procedure is indicated in specific circumstances; however, these indications are currently poorly defined.

REFERENCES

1. Adams MA, Huton WC: Prolapsed intervertebral disc: a hyperflexion injury. *Spine* 7:184-191, 1982.
2. Allen BL, Ferguson RL: The Galveston technique for L-rod instrumentation of the scoliotic spine. *Spine* 7: 276-284, 1982.
3. Baldwin NG, Benzel EC: Sacral fixation using iliac instrumentation and a variable-angle screw device. *J Neurosurg* 81:313-316, 1994.
4. Benzel EC: Luque rod segmental spinal instrumentation. In Rengachary SS, Wilkins RH (eds): *Neurosurgical Operative Atlas*. Park Ridge, IL: American Association of Neurological Surgeons, 1992, pp 433-438.
5. Benzel EC (ed): *Biomechanics of Spine Stabilization: Principles and Clinical Practice*. New York, McGraw-Hill, 1995, pp 101-278.

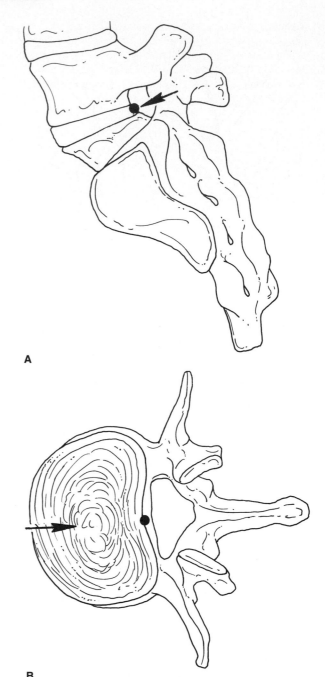

A

B

Figure 55.8 The lumbosacral pivot point is essentially the dorsal aspect of the intervertebral disc (**A-B**). Note that the ilial and sacral screw tips depicted in Figure 55.7 are positioned ventral to the lumbosacral pivot point.

6. Benzel EC, Ball PA, Baldwin NG, Marchand EP: The sequential hook insertion technique for universal spinal instrumentation application. *J Neurosurg* 79:608-611, 1993.
7. Carlson GD, Abitbol JJ, Anderson DR, *et al*: Screw fixation in the human sacrum. *Spine* 17:S196-S203, 1992.
8. Cotrel Y, Dubousset J, Guillaumat M: New universal instrumentation in spinal surgery. *Clin Orthop* 227:10-23, 1988.
9. Dick W: The "fixatuer interne" as a versatile implant for spine surgery. *Spine* 12:882-900, 1987.

10. Kramer J: *Intervertebral Disc Disease: Causes, Diagnosis, Treatment, and Prophylaxis*, ed 2. New York, Thieme, 1990.

11. McCord DH, Cunningham BW, Shono Y, *et al*: Biomechanical analysis of lumbosacral fixation. *Spine* 17:S235-S243, 1992.

12. Weinstein PR, Ehni G, Wilson CB: *Lumbar Spondylosis: Diagnosis, Management and Surgical Treatment*. Chicago, Year Book Medical Publishers, 1977.

13. White AA, Panjabi MM: *Clinical Biomechanics of the Spine*, ed 2. Philadelphia, JB Lippincott, 1990.

CHAPTER 56

Rheumatoid Arthritis

Robert F. Heary, Frederick A. Simeone, and H. Alan Crockard

Rheumatoid arthritis is a systemic disease of unknown cause that primarily involves small blood vessels and synovium. It is a chronic disease that is generally more common in females. Rheumatoid arthritis is characterized by polyarticular symmetric involvement of the smaller joints of the appendicular skeleton. It destroys the articular joint surfaces and the joint capsules and the ancillary ligaments that support the joints.[36] In addition, rheumatoid arthritis can be associated with osteoporosis and erosion and cyst formation in the bone.[46] The extent of myelopathy in patients with rheumatoid arthritis is difficult to evaluate because their disease may be complicated by peripheral joint destruction, peripheral neuropathies, nerve entrapments, and rheumatoid myopathy.[75]

The most common skeletal manifestation of rheumatoid arthritis is the involvement of the metatarsophalangeal joints of the feet. This is followed in frequency by rheumatoid involvement of the cervical spine and the metacarpophalangeal joints of the hands.[6] Cervical spine involvement is very common, and symptoms do not necessarily accompany extensive bony changes of the spine.[7] Rheumatoid involvement of the cervical spine may be present with minimal or no clinical or radiologic expression elsewhere in the body.[6] The major clinical problems in the spine result from erosive changes in the cervical spine that lead to pathologic subluxation or dislocation.[78] Although much less common, the thoracic and lumbar regions may also be involved.

The three most common lesions that cause neurologic involvement and intractable pain are atlantoaxial subluxation, subaxial subluxation, and vertical subluxation of the odontoid process.[66] The onset of cervical spine instability is often insidious. It may be masked by weakness and loss of function associated with peripheral joint disease.[85] Although any synovial joint in the spine may be involved, the earliest changes are usually observed at the occipitocervical junction.[75] Rheumatoid involvement of the cervical spine appears to begin early and progress in relationship to peripheral joint involvement. The cervical spine abnormalities are the result of destruction in the joints, ligaments, and bone by synovitis.[46]

Atlantoaxial subluxation represents the most common and significant manifestation of rheumatoid involvement of the cervical spine.[78] The degree of neurologic deficit does not correlate with the degree of subluxation observed on lateral radiographs. This discrepancy may be the result of the formation of pannus between the dens and the dura mater. This may contribute to spinal cord compression but cannot be visualized on plain radiographs. In 1830, Sir Charles Bell[4] reported the first case of an atlantoaxial subluxation resulting in an inflammatory process. Incompetence of the transverse ligament was demonstrated pathologically.

The rate of development of neurologic signs and symptoms is usually slow. Numerous large surgical and nonsurgical series of patients with rheumatoid arthritis have demonstrated that the average duration of disease before surgery is 15 to 20 years.[*] Although life expectancy in patients with moderate or severe rheumatoid arthritis is less than that of the general population, cervical subluxation does not influence life expectancy.[79]

The most common clinical finding in rheumatoid involvement of the cervical spine is severe and persistent pain. Typically, this pain is located in the occipital region[6,37,54,55] or in the neck[64] or it may radiate toward the vertex of the skull.[54] Typically, this pain is exacerbated by neck motion.[6,7,58] Tears in the transverse and alar ligaments and in the atlantooccipital membrane may give rise to retro-orbital or temporal pain.[58] Pain in the arms is typically absent. This type of pain helps to distinguish these disorders from cervical spondylosis.[61] Neurologic signs and symptoms that are useful for detection of the onset of myelopathy in rheumatoid arthritis patients include neck pain, occipital neuralgia, L'hermitte's sign (electric-like shocks produced with neck flexion), and the patient's account of diminished motor ability or a documented worsening in the motor examination from the previous neurologic examination.[18]

Myelopathy may develop from spinal cord compression. This usually occurs in late middle age after many years of disability.[61] Because of the frequent, severe deforming effects of rheumatoid arthritis in the extremities, long tract signs may be useful in detecting myelopathy. These include hyperreflexia and extensor plantar responses.[55,61] The myelopathy that occurs in rheumatoid arthritis is most likely caused by the effects of compression, stretch, and movement, not by ischemia.[33]

Because of patient selection and referral patterns, there is a marked discrepancy between the incidence of neurologic involvement of rheumatoid disease of the cervical spine in surgical and nonsurgical series. In two large nonsurgical series of more than 2000 patients with rheumatoid arthritis reported by Smith et al.[79] and Nakano et al.,[61] the incidence of cervical myelopathy was less than 3% in each series. Interosseous erosive disease of the peripheral joints is correlated to the severity of involvement of the cervical spine.[29,64]

The executive committee of the American Rheumatism Association has established criteria for rheumatoid arthritis that must be applied only to patients with a clear-cut diagnosis. In addition, this committee has adopted a classification of functional capacity that is used in rheumatologic studies.[83]

Ranawat et al.[66] developed a classification based on signs and symptoms. In this surgical series, neurologic deficits were divided into three classes:

I. No neurologic deficits
II. Subjective weakness, hyperreflexia, dysesthesias

---

*References 37,41,61,66,76,79,85,88.

III. Objective weakness, long tract signs
  A. Ambulatory
  B. Quadriparetic, not ambulatory

This classification scheme is widely used in most surgical series. The strength of the Ranawat classification system is that it measures a functional, rather than a neurologic, capacity. The ideal classification system has not been developed for rheumatoid arthritis patients. In an ideal system, an objective functional score should produce consistent, reliable interobserver and intraobserver results that can be compared between different studies.

Vertebral artery compression leading to vertebrobasilar insufficiency may occur in rheumatoid arthritis. The three possible sites for mechanical compression of the vertebral artery include the foramen transversarium, the atlantoaxial joint, and the occipitoatlantal joint. Vertebral artery insufficiency may be the result of kinking of the vertebral artery at one of these locations or the involvement of the brain stem by upward migration of the dens.[29] Symptoms that have been attributed to vertebral artery insufficiency secondary to rheumatoid disease of the cervical spine include dizziness, tinnitus, vertigo, diplopia, suboccipital headache, dysphasia, blurring of vision, cortical blindness, nystagmus, transient blackout spells, confusion, and dysarthria.[29,55,70,81] The frequency with which vertebral artery symptoms may occur is poorly documented. Henderson et al.[33] published nine autopsy cases of severe end-stage rheumatoid arthritis with vertical subluxation of the dens that showed the vertebral artery to be patent in all specimens.

The pathologic changes in rheumatoid arthritis of the cervical spine are predominantly secondary to synovitis. Synovitic proliferation destroys the facet joints, erodes and deforms the dens, and weakens the ligamentous attachments.[29] A characteristic pannus forms between the odontoid peg and the ventral dura mater that can compress the spinal cord. This pannus is usually firm, gray-pink tissue that shows end-stage chronic inflammation of synovial tissue.[18] In addition to this proliferation of the synovial tissue, osteoporosis and destruction of cartilage and subchondral bone can occur.[6,83] Localized bone loss around the inflamed joints is the result of prostaglandin and cytokine synthesis during the inflammatory process, which increases bone resorption.[86] Inflammatory destruction of the lateral atlantoaxial joints can lead to vertical translocation of the dens.[29] When the odontoid process herniates through the foramen magnum, it can cause flattening, softening, and atrophy of the medulla.[11]

The specific mechanism by which ischemia causes damage to the spinal cord is unclear. Two separate studies have postulated that intermittent compression of the ventral spinal artery was responsible for the spinal cord injury.[36,61] However, in a necropsy study of nine patients, Henderson et al.[33] demonstrated that the histopathologic changes were localized principally to the dorsal white matter of the spinal cord. The territory of the ventral spinal artery was spared. Most recently, O'Brien et al.[62] performed a histologic study of specimens removed during ventral decompressions of the cervicomedullary junction. They determined that repetitive mechanical damage caused by instability at the atlantoaxial joint, rather than an acute compressive effect from an inflammatory pannus, is the cause of spinal cord compression and subsequent axonal injury. In addition, Crockard and Grob[18] have stated that there is no evidence that avascular necrosis or vasculitis is involved in the inflammatory process of rheumatoid arthritis involvement of the spine. They believe that it is the repetitive movement of the unstable atlantoaxial joint against the neuraxis that causes a mechanical "wear-and-tear" phenomenon that leads to the development of a myelopathy.

In rheumatoid arthritis, osteophytes do not form because of deficient osteogenesis.[6,36,54] This may be contrasted to osteoarthritis that is characterized by the development of osteophytic spurs that have a stabilizing effect.[36,54,58]

Operative Indications

The presence of myelopathy or a progressive neurologic deficit is generally agreed upon as a good indication for surgery.[*] Likewise, intractable pain is an indication for operative intervention.[†] A much more controversial topic is whether a patient with markedly abnormal radiographs in the absence of pain or progressive neurologic deficit should undergo surgery. Numerous authors[33,63,65,66] believe that radiologic evidence of an impending neurologic deficit is an indication for surgery. Pellicci et al.[64] believe that radiographic evidence of disease progresses to a greater degree than does neural involvement. As such, they believe that no fusion should be recommended on the basis of a radiographic abnormality or radiographic deterioration alone. Others[8,46,58,76] have supported this more conservative viewpoint. In an intermediate position, Boden et al.[8] stated that only patients with a neurologic deficit underwent surgery in their series. However, they recommended surgery for patients with or without a neurologic deficit, if certain radiographic criteria are met.

Recently, the third author (H.A.C.) reviewed his results with 55 severe end-stage rheumatoid arthritis patients (Ranawat grade IIIB). He found that those patients who are bed-bound for more than 3 months fare extremely poorly, regardless of whether surgical intervention is undertaken. In addition, with these Ranawat grade IIIB patients, mortality rates are unacceptably high in many cases. Therefore, one must question the previously held view that the presence of a myelopathy in a long-term, bed-bound Ranawat grade IIIB patient is an absolute indication for surgery.

Radiographic Imaging Studies

A variety of radiographic imaging modalities are used to image the spine in rheumatoid arthritis. These modalities include plain radiography, computed tomography (CT), myelography, a combination of CT and myelography,

---

*References 8,25,29,33,40,41,46,58,63-66,75,78.
†References 25,29,40,41,46,64,75,78.

magnetic resonance imaging (MRI), and tomography. In addition, flexion and extension views may be used to augment the information provided by any of these studies. Because the occiput-C1-2 complex is the most frequently involved region of the spine in rheumatoid arthritis, the majority of imaging studies focus attention on this area. When clinically indicated, imaging studies of the subaxial cervical spine and of the thoracic and lumbar spines should also be performed.

On plain radiographs, small or absent osteophytes, osteoporotic vertebrae, and eroded vertebral end plates characterize rheumatoid arthritis.[6] In the absence of rheumatoid arthritis, degenerative changes are more marked in the lower cervical spine with advancing age. Radiographic changes at the C1-2 level are not present unless a specific process, such as rheumatoid arthritis, is affecting this region. These changes are independent of age.[69] Bland et al.[7] found 86% of patients with classic or definite rheumatoid arthritis to have evidence of cervical spine involvement on plain radiographs. These changes may frequently be asymptomatic and may not be associated with any neurologic deficit. In patients with severe polyarticular rheumatoid arthritis for more than 20 years, Santavirta et al.[76] found radiographic subluxation of the cervical spine in more than 80% of patients.

The most common radiologic abnormality in rheumatoid arthritis is ventral subluxation of the atlas. The atlantodens interval (ADI) measures the distance between the ventral dens and the dorsal ring of the atlas. In normal patients, this distance is less than 3mm.[91] An ADI of between 3 and 5mm in an adult is abnormal and indicates a tear or insufficiency of the transverse ligament. A separation of greater than 5mm indicates rupture or attenuation of the alar ligaments in addition to the transverse ligament.[54] Many studies have shown a poor correlation between abnormalities of the ADI and neurologic deficits. In an innovative study, Boden et al.[8] defined the dorsal atlanto-odontoid interval (AOI) as the distance between the dorsal surface of the dens and the ventral edge of the dorsal ring of the atlas measured along the transverse axis of the ring of the atlas. They demonstrated an excellent correlation between the dorsal AOI and the severity of the neurologic deficit. A dorsal AOI of less than 14mm correlated significantly with the presence and severity of a neurologic deficit. This dorsal AOI was also found to be a good predictor of neurologic recovery postoperatively. These authors stated that the weak correlation of the ventral ADI with a neurologic deficit may be due to variations in the diameter of the atlas as well as the presence of a pannus behind the odontoid process. Weissman et al.[88] studied 109 patients with rheumatoid arthritis and atlantoaxial subluxations for 5 years. They found that the ADI increased by greater than 2mm in 41% remained unchanged in 40% and decreased by more than 2mm in 19%. Of the patients whose ADI decreased, more than half had developed vertical subluxation of the odontoid process. Henderson et al.[33] have stated that vertical subluxation may cause a pseudofixation of the atlantodens interval. Interpretation of the ADI must therefore be made in conjunction with measurement of the vertical axial subluxation.

Vertical subluxation of the dens is an upward migration of the dens into the foramen magnum (Figure 56.1). In this

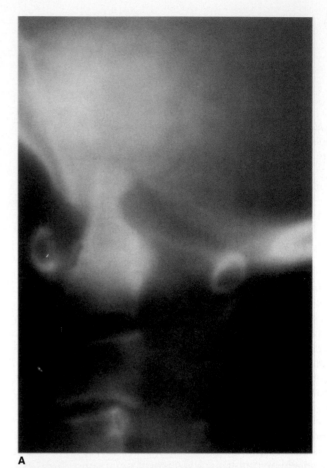

A

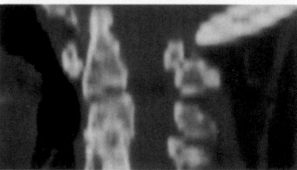

B

Figure 56.1 (**A**) Plain tomogram, lateral view. Vertical subluxation of the odontoid process is clearly demonstrated. The tip of the odontoid is seen posterior to the clivus in an intracranial position. The arch of the atlas has telescoped down the body of C2. This level of severe bony deterioration can cause the atlantodental interval to actually decrease. (**B**) Sagittal reformation of a CT scan (same patient as in **A**). Bony detail and intracranial location of the odontoid are well visualized. The anterior translation of the atlas is more apparent in this view.

location, the dens competes for space with the spinal cord and the brain stem. Vertical subluxation requires the lateral facet joints to be destroyed.[61] Vertical subluxation is the second most common upper cervical spine abnormality in rheumatoid arthritis after atlantoaxial subluxation and frequently accompanies ventral atlantoaxial subluxation. An increase in the vertical subluxation may actually produce a decrease in the measured ventral atlantoaxial subluxation.[88] In vertical subluxation, the presence of a rheumatoid

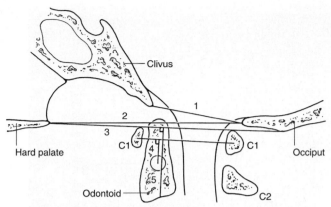

Figure 56.2 Common craniometry lines. *1,* McRae's line; *2,* Chamberlain's line; *3,* McGregor's line; *4,* Ranawat's line; *5,* Jones's level.

pannus together with the invaginated dens may produce ventral compression of the cervicomedullary junction.[55]

In an attempt to quantify vertical subluxation of the dens, numerous lines and indices have been proposed (Figure 56.2). These lines are characteristically drawn between bony landmarks that are identifiable on a lateral cervical spine radiograph. The tip of the dens is then measured with respect to the various lines. McGregor's line is drawn from the hard palate to the occiput, and it is probably the most traditional measure.[46] A shortcoming of these lines is that the hard palate, the dorsal edge of the foramen magnum, and the tip of the dens are not always visualized on routine lateral cervical spine radiographs in a patient with vertical subluxation of the odontoid. To avoid these difficulties, Ranawat *et al.*[66] developed an index that measures the distance between the diameter of the ring of the first cervical vertebra to the center of the pedicle of the second cervical vertebra. In men and women with normal cervical spines, this distance measured 17mm in men and 15mm in women. No normal patients had an interval of less than 15mm.

The cervical myelogram provides an indirect visualization of the spinal cord and adjacent structures silhouetted by contrast media in the subarachnoid space.[9] The information obtained by myelography may be augmented by a postmyelogram CT. Computerized myelotomography with multiplanar reconstruction can clearly demonstrate the important contribution of proliferative rheumatoid pannus behind the odontoid peg to ventral cervicomedullary compression. In addition, bone windows on the CT scan can demonstrate bony abnormalities well.

Currently, MRI is considered the ideal study to demonstrate the level and extent of spinal cord compression.[9,80] The advantages of MRI include direct imaging of the entire length of the spinal cord and the cervicomedullary junction, direct imaging in multiple planes, superior demonstration of soft-tissue structures, and the lack of image degradation by bone artifact at the cervicomedullary junction (Figure 56.3). In addition, MRI is noninvasive (no intrathecal contrast is needed), it can be performed on an outpatient basis, it does not expose the patient to the dangers of ionizing radiation, and it is generally well tolerated.[5,9,80] A limitation of MRI is that it does not image compact bone as accurately as CT.[80]

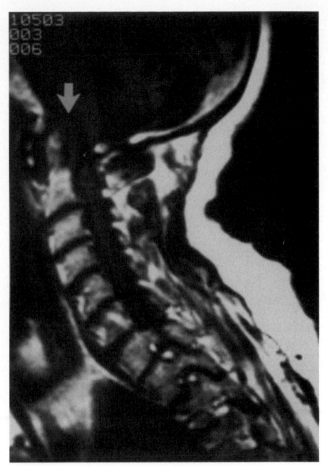

Figure 56.3 Sagittal T_1-weighted (TR 500/TE 11) MRI image of ventral compression from a large inflammatory pannus (*white arrow*). The cervicomedullary junction is deformed and attenuated by this soft-tissue mass.

Furthermore, Dickman *et al.*[21] have shown that the transverse atlantal ligament can be consistently and clearly visualized with MRI. This determination of a loss of anatomic continuity of the transverse ligament is useful for operative planning. For patients who are unable to undergo MRI, CT with multiplanar reconstructions provides better information than polytomography. It is important to visualize the neuraxis before surgery; therefore, a few milliliters of water-soluble contrast injected into the lumbar subarachnoid space will provide a CT scan and myelogram.

Dynamic views of the cervical spine in flexion and extension provide useful information about the degree of instability of the occiput-C1-2 complex (Figure 56.4). These flexion and extension views can be obtained on plain films, tomograms, computerized myelotomography scans, and MRI scans. Dickman *et al.*[20] recommend routine lateral cervical radiographs in flexion and extension for all patients undergoing transoral surgery. Furthermore, Sharp and Purser[77] recommend lateral flexion and extension radiographs in any patient with severe rheumatoid arthritis undergoing general anesthesia for any surgical procedure. Bell and Stearns[5] have found MRI in flexion and extension to be very useful for demonstrating dynamic changes in spinal cord configuration. They

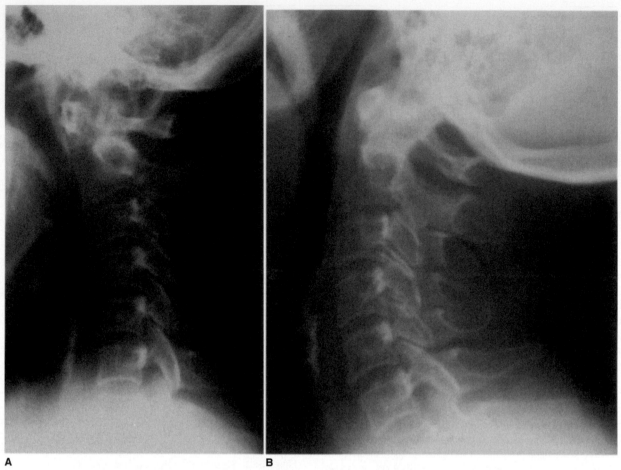

A   **B**

Figure 56.4 **(A)** Plain radiograph, lateral flexion view. Significant widening of the atlantodental interval with flexion is demonstrated. The occiput-C1 complex translates forward over the C2 vertebra. **(B)** Plain radiograph, lateral extension view (same patient as in **A**). The odontoid process is well reduced in extension with an atlantodental interval within normal limits (less than 3mm).

have used this information to determine the proximal extent of fusion required and have stated that it provides an accurate and dynamic study of the relationship between the spinal cord and the surrounding bony and soft-tissue structures.

Specific Regions of the Spine
Upper Cervical Spine

To fully understand the complex pathologic changes that occur in the occiput-C1-2 region, a thorough understanding of the biomechanics of this region is necessary. The majority of axial rotation occurs in the upper cervical spine. Approximately 60% of the axial rotation of the entire cervical spine and occiput is found in the upper region (occiput-C1-2) and 40% is found in the lower region (below C2). There is no axial rotation between the occiput and C1 unless there has been an occipitoatlantal disruption.[28] An extensive amount of axial rotation, 47 degrees, occurs at the C1-2 level.[90] White and Panjabi[91] have identified two distinct reasons why this increased motion can occur at the C1-2 level. First, the articular surfaces of the lateral masses of both C1 and C2

have a convex orientation in the sagittal plane that allows for considerable mobility. Second, a taut yellow ligament is not present between the dorsal elements of C1 and C2. Instead, a loose readily mobile atlantoaxial membrane connects the dorsal elements of C1 and C2, thereby enhancing the motion capacity of this region. Craniovertebral junction instability in rheumatoid arthritis patients occurs from a combination of bone softening, ligamentous destruction, and inflammatory pannus formation.[20] Unlike the lower cervical spine, the upper cervical spine cannot clearly be divided into ventral and dorsal elements with corresponding mechanical properties.[30] White and Panjabi[90] have defined clinical instability as "loss of the capacity of the spine under physiologic loads to maintain relationships between vertebrae so that no spinal cord or nerve root damage occurs and no incapacitating deformity or pain develops." This definition has led to certain anatomic measurements from plain film radiographs that can lead to a suspicion of clinical instability. In adults, a ventral ADI of greater than 3mm on a lateral radiograph is regarded as potentially unstable. Although less widely used, a dorsal AOI of less than 14mm is also suspicious for clinical instability.[8] With this basic understanding of the biomechanical relationships of the upper cervical spine, the two most common abnormalities in this region are ventral atlantoaxial subluxation, caused by incompetent ligaments, and vertical subluxation of the odontoid process that occurs because of lateral mass erosion.

Atlantoaxial Subluxation

Ventral atlantoaxial subluxation is the most common abnormality of the spine in rheumatoid arthritis. Classically, atlantoaxial subluxation is considered present if the ADI is greater than 3mm in an adult or greater than 4mm in a child.[29] Owing to selection biases between surgical and nonsurgical studies of patients with rheumatoid arthritis, there are marked discrepancies in the frequency with which atlantoaxial subluxation occurs. In a large study in the rheumatologic literature on the prevalence of atlantoaxial subluxation in rheumatoid arthritis patients, the authors found that an atlantoaxial subluxation was present in 1 out of 30 patients with any evidence of rheumatoid arthritis, in 1 out of 15 patients with clinical evidence of the disease, and in 1 out of 5 patients with rheumatoid arthritis admitted to the hospital.[77] This last group of patients are those most likely to be seen by a spine surgeon. Indeed, in the study by Weissman et al.,[88] ventral atlantoaxial subluxation was found to occur in one fourth to one third of patients with rheumatoid arthritis. Disruption of the transverse ligament of the atlas is the most important pathologic abnormality responsible for atlantoaxial instability.[21]

The degree of atlantoaxial subluxation is poorly correlated with clinical evidence of a compressive myelopathy.[9] Similarly, no correlation between the magnitude of an atlantoaxial subluxation and mortality was found in a 10-year follow-up study.[76] In a large review of 189 rheumatoid arthritis patients with atlantoaxial subluxations, Weissman et al.[88] found the incidence of spinal cord compression to be 11%. These findings underscore the necessity of an accurate history and physical examination to determine which patients with atlantoaxial subluxations are demonstrating evidence of neurologic abnormalities related to this radiographic abnormality. A characteristic clinical finding of ventral atlantoaxial subluxation is difficulty in raising the head to the neutral position following downward gaze. This sensation of the head "falling forward" has been referred to as the Sharp-Purser sign.[77]

An extremely rare abnormality is dorsal atlantoaxial subluxation. For a dorsal atlantoaxial subluxation to occur, the dens must be destroyed, fractured, or congenitally absent; or the ventral arch of the atlas must be destroyed or congenitally absent.[27,38,88,91] Vertical subluxation of the dens can occur simultaneously with a ventral atlantoaxial subluxation. When this occurs, the ADI can appear to actually decrease in size.[52] Isolated ventral subluxation is more common than either vertical subluxation or a combination of ventral subluxation and vertical subluxation. Kraus et al.[41] studied 55 patients with atlantoaxial subluxations who received dorsal fusion and found that none developed subsequent vertical subluxations. They believed that the dorsal fusion operation may have a protective effect in preventing vertical subluxation. This protective effect of dorsal fusion has not been demonstrated in a prospective study.

Vertical Subluxation of the Odontoid

Vertical subluxation of the dens is referred to by a variety of terms, including *atlantoaxial impaction, cranial settling, upward migration of the odontoid, pseudobasilar invagination, translocation of the dens, superior migration of the odontoid, basilar invagination, and vertical settling.* These terms have been used interchangeably in the medical literature. Vertical subluxation occurs as a consequence of loss of substance of the lateral masses, usually the atlas. However, the lateral masses of the axis and, less commonly, the occipital condyles may also be involved.[33] In vertical subluxation, the ventral arch of C1 gradually articulates with caudal portions of C2, first via the base of the dens and then with the body of C2.[88] If there is more than 18mm of translocation, the ring of the atlas is usually broken and the base of the axis has migrated within the disrupted ring. Significant vertical subluxation of the dens is generally agreed to be an indication for a fusion operation.*

Neurologic abnormalities are far more common with vertical subluxation of the dens than with atlantoaxial subluxation. The abnormal neurologic symptoms are the result of compression of the brain stem or upper cervical spinal cord. Neurologic abnormalities detected in vertical subluxation of the dens include hyperreflexia, extensor plantar reflexes, limb paresthesias, progressive difficulty with ambulation, a central cordlike syndrome, neurogenic bladder, and lower cranial nerve palsies.[55] Rheumatoid arthritis patients with vertical subluxation are more likely to be symptomatic from spinal cord compression.[8,53,55,76,88]

Lower Cervical Spine

As with abnormalities of the upper cervical spine, the presence of subaxial subluxations of the lower cervical spine vary greatly in reported series. Subaxial subluxation is a gradual process in which there is a forward displacement of one or more vertebral bodies on the vertebral body immediately below (Figure 56.5). The rheumatoid process attacks the apophyseal and uncovertebral joints, weakens the supporting ligaments, and erodes the intervertebral discs. These effects loosen the various intervertebral fixations and permit luxation between adjacent vertebral bodies.[36] Subaxial subluxations are usually reducible by traction; however, the reduction is difficult to maintain.[40] Classically, subaxial subluxation is a translation of one vertebra in relation to an adjacent vertebra of greater than 3.5mm on a lateral cervical spine radiograph.[91] Boden et al.[8] found that the diameter of the subaxial sagittal, spinal canal reflected the presence and degree of a neurologic deficit, more often than did the percentage of vertebral body slip. In addition to the bony luxations, compression from epidural rheumatoid granulations have been reported.[6,46,75]

Subaxial subluxations are usually late developments in the aggressive forms of rheumatoid arthritis.[6,76] The severity of these subaxial subluxations is also closely related to

---

*References 8,53-55,64-66,76,88.

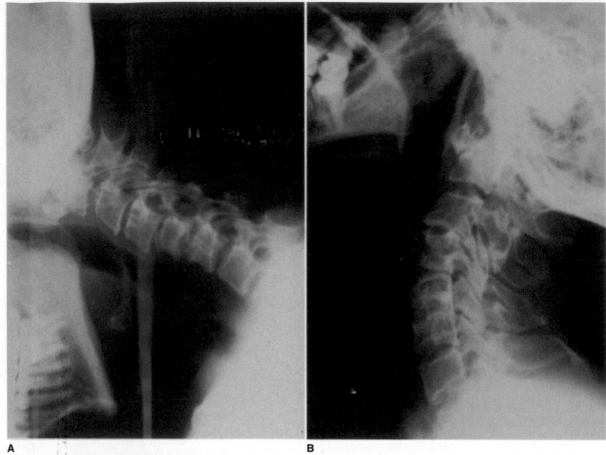

Figure 56.5 (A) Plain radiograph, lateral flexion view. Multiple subaxial subluxations are seen with neck flexion producing a "staircase" effect. The vertebral body translates forward with respect to the immediate subjacent vertebral body. Vertical subluxation of the odontoid process is also seen in this view. (B) Plain radiograph, lateral extension view (same patient as in **A**). Neck extension causes a marked correction in the degree of subaxial subluxations. There is no change in the relationship between the atlas and the axis with neck motion.

the duration of rheumatoid disease.[6,79] When compared with patients with atlantoaxial subluxations, the incidence of neurologic deficits is higher in patients with subaxial subluxation, and the final results are poorer.[85]

Typically, subaxial subluxations show a "staircase" appearance with multiple subluxations observed sequentially in the cervical spine.[46,61,78] Subaxial subluxations may result in nerve root impingement from foraminal narrowing or possibly from myelopathic changes.[78] The presence of a subaxial subluxation should be suspected when bizarre weakness of the hands is observed in a patient with rheumatoid arthritis. This may be difficult in patients with long-standing disease who already have crippling deformity of the hands.[3] This subaxial spinal cord involvement may cause myelopathy and may explain why some patients do not respond to surgical decompression at the craniocervical junction.[33] The most common site for subaxial subluxation is at the C3-4 level; however, it often occurs at multiple levels, and these typically lack osteophytes.[12,46,75]

Subaxial subluxations may be present at the time of surgery for an upper cervical instability. The caudal extent of the instrumentation and fusion must, therefore, be carefully selected to incorporate any segments with a significant subaxial subluxation.[17,24] In an autopsy study of nine patients with severe end-stage rheumatoid arthritis, Henderson *et al.*[33] found subaxial compression in eight of the nine patients. More commonly, subaxial subluxations may occur after fusion operations in the upper cervical spine.[12,41,75,78] As a result, it is essential that patients who undergo upper cervical fusions be followed up closely with lateral cervical spine radiographs both for evidence of a good osseous fusion and for the development of subaxial subluxations. Kraus *et al.*[41] found a much higher incidence of subaxial subluxations in patients whose upper cervical fusion incorporated the occiput. They postulated that this was perhaps because of a longer lever arm that results in higher forces generated at the lower cervical levels and that leads to a subaxial subluxation. Subaxial cervical subluxations in patients with rheumatoid arthritis have been associated with quadriplegia, sudden death, and other neurologic complications resulting from damage of the spinal cord or from interference with the flow of the vertebral arteries.[23]

The most accurate radiographic imaging study currently available to detect the site and type of spinal cord compression in subaxial subluxation of the rheumatoid spine is MRI.[76] All patients with subaxial subluxations and atlantoaxial subluxations with neurologic deficits or vertical subluxations of the dens should have an MRI scan, if possible.[85]

Thoracic and Lumbar Spines

Involvement of the thoracic and lumbar spines in patients with rheumatoid arthritis is rare. Heywood and Meyers[34] have stated that subcervical rheumatoid spondylitis is more common than is generally believed and have found an incidence of 0.9% in their clinic. Most other series of rheumatoid arthritis patients do not even address the topic of the thoracic and lumbar spine. In a study by Redlund-Johnell and Larsson,[68] of 100 patients with severe rheumatoid arthritis who had previously undergone occipitocervical fusion, four patients with subluxation of the upper thoracic spine were found. These changes in the upper thoracic spine were radiologically similar to the destructive type of subaxial subluxation typically observed in the cervical spine. The authors believed that this upper thoracic subluxation may have been caused by increased motion as compensation for decreased mobility in the cervical spine. The pathogenesis of rheumatoid spondylitis in the thoracic and lumbar spines is believed to be the result of a facet joint synovitis that leads to instability. In addition, involved costovertebral joints can spread their involvement to the disc space, causing a discitis between the disc and the vertebral end plates that can lead to further instability.[34] Rheumatoid granulation tissue causing compression of the thoracic spine has been reported.[2,6,87] In addition, an extensive inflammatory synovitis of the costovertebral and costotransverse joints can occur in the thorax.[14]

Rheumatoid involvement of the lumbar spine is rarely recognized as a cause of nerve root or cauda equina compression. Intraspinal rheumatoid granulomatous nodules can lead to nerve root compression, causing back and leg pain.[2,26] In addition, rheumatoid granulation tissue can develop in the lumbar facet joints and spread to the periarticular structures to contribute to cauda equina compression.[45,49]

The plain radiographic features of subcervical rheumatoid spondylitis include an ill-defined, blurred, and eroded margin to the vertebral end plates and an ill-defined, eroded facet joint complex.[34] If not specifically sought, these radiographic abnormalities may be easily overlooked. Frequently, patients with rheumatoid arthritis have stiff, high-positioned shoulders that may conceal the cervicothoracic junction on conventional radiographs. If clinically indicated, an MRI allows for better visualization of the cervicothoracic junction and the remainder of the thoracic and lumbar spines.[68]

Surgical Management of the Rheumatoid Spine

Many different operations have been recommended for patients with rheumatoid arthritis of the spine (Figure 56.6). The various options include a dorsal cervical fusion of C1-2, an occipitocervical fusion, a transoral approach, ventral and dorsal approaches to the subaxial cervical spine, and various combinations of these approaches. With the advent of spinal instrumentation techniques, surgeons have a wealth of different treatment options available to treat patients with rheumatoid arthritis. In addition, nonoperative modalities including traction, halo vest immobilization, and adjuvant medical therapies such as steroids, nonsteroidal anti-inflammatory agents, penicillamine, and methotrexate enter into the decision-making process.

The majority of patients with rheumatoid arthritis never develop spinal instability and never require spine surgery. As previously described, large studies of patients from rheumatology clinics have demonstrated that the clinical course of rheumatoid arthritis is usually benign. However, the natural history of the disease is that a certain proportion of patients with rheumatoid arthritis eventually require surgery. Pellicci et al.[64] followed 106 patients for more than 5 years and found that diligent use of a supportive collar will not alter the natural history of the disease. Similarly, More and Sen[58] have stated that the realistic treatment goals achieved by conservative measures are pain abatement and reduction of inflammation. The natural history of the disease is not altered. Pellicci's study also documented that rheumatoid involvement of the cervical spine does not appear to shorten life expectancy.[64] These findings are most likely a result of the small number of rheumatoid arthritis patients who develop cervical myelopathy. When cervical myelopathy is established, the natural history without surgical intervention is grave.[46] In addition, the development of a subaxial subluxation or a vertical subluxation in a patient with a preexisting atlantoaxial subluxation was found to be a poor prognostic sign.[64] The factors that influence the treatment of upper cervical lesions in rheumatoid arthritis are reducibility of the abnormality with traction, the type of compressive lesion (whether of a bony or a soft-tissue component), and the direction and mechanics of the spinal cord or brain stem compression.[53]

There is a general agreement among the majority of neurologic and orthopedic surgeons that intractable pain, progressive neurologic deficit, and the presence of myelopathy are indications for surgical intervention. On the other hand, there is considerable disagreement over surgery for the "risk of instability," which is usually construed by a variety of criteria analyzing radiographic imaging studies of the upper cervical spine.

With appropriate operative indications, the treatment of an isolated atlantoaxial subluxation is a dorsal C1-2 fusion. In these cases, the occiput should not be incorporated into the fusion because the higher complication rate, lower fusion rate, and morbidity associated with the decreased range of neck motion all mitigate against this procedure.

If vertical subluxation of the dens is present, or a combination of a vertical subluxation with an atlantoaxial subluxation is present, an occipitocervical fusion may be required. To determine whether an occipitocervical fusion alone is adequate, or a ventral decompression is necessary, cervical traction, in addition to the dorsal stabilization, may be used to determine whether the subluxation is reducible.[20,55,88] Transoral decompression may also be deemed necessary if significant soft-tissue rheumatoid granulation—that is, a rheumatoid pannus—is responsible for compression of the spinal cord.[16]

Viewpoints in the management of vertical subluxation of the dens are divergent, as has been shown in numerous studies published by Menezes et al.[53-55] and Crockard et al.[17,18,60] Menezes et al. maintains that it is the reducibility of a vertical subluxation that is the primary determinant

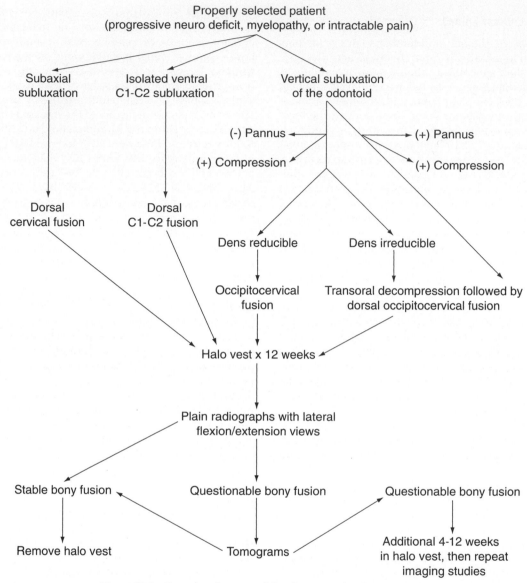

Figure 56.6 Algorithm for care of the rheumatoid arthritis patient.

of whether a transoral decompression is necessary. They determined that in 80% of their patients, an adequate reduction of the vertical subluxation could be achieved with traction and therefore, only a dorsal occipital cervical fusion was necessary. Despite the reducibility, all 45 patients in this series were symptomatic because of compression of the cervicomedullary junction. Menezes et al.[55] have stated that decompression of the cervicomedullary junction via a transoral approach is necessary for irreducible lesions. They found that all patients with greater than 20mm of penetration of the dens through the foramen magnum were unable to have their deformity reduced with cervical traction and required a transoral decompression. Dickman et al.[20] have also recommended a transoral decompressive procedure for irreducible craniovertebral junction compression. Both Menezes et al. and Dickman et al. recommend that the ventral decompressive surgery should be performed first and subsequent dorsal internal fixation later.[20,55] Transoral surgery involves the

resection of the dens, the ventral arch of the atlas, the ventral longitudinal ligament, the apical ligament, the alar ligament, the transverse ligament, and the tectorial membrane.[20] As such, the spine is destabilized after this procedure, necessitating a dorsal fusion. The advantages of the transoral approach to irreducible craniovertebral junction pathology have been described by Menezes and van Gilder. These include performing surgery in an avascular midline plane, accessibility to both bony and soft-tissue pathology, and performing surgery with the patient's head in an extended position (which decreases brain stem angulation and compression during the surgery). This approach allows for exposure from the lower half of the clivus to the C2-3 interspace. These authors strongly emphasize the need for a tracheotomy in all transoral surgeries.[53]

Crockard has stressed the contribution of a ventral compressive agent, the rheumatoid pannus, to be as important as any bony deformity in the development of spinal cord compression.[17] He has stated that the overall results of dorsal cervical surgery alone for patients with cervical myelopathy have been unsatisfactory with excessively high morbidity and mortality rates.[18] For patients with an established myelopathy in whom the pannus has been demonstrated to contribute to the cervicomedullary junction compression, Crockard performs a transoral decompression with a dorsal occipitocervical fusion in a single one-stage operation with the patient in the lateral position. Traditional skull traction is not used at any stage, but the head is held in the Mayfield retractor with a tilt table, which, in effect, functions like skull traction. In his experience, this one-stage procedure has led to fewer complications and better long-term results than either a two-stage operation or a dorsal fixation procedure alone.[17] Performing both operations at a single sitting avoids the discomfort of prolonged bed rest and the complications associated with prolonged immobilization. In most patients, Crockard has not found it necessary to perform a tracheotomy.[17,18,60]

As with the operative approaches to vertical subluxations, treatment of subaxial subluxations of the cervical spine is varied. Simpson et al.[78] have stated that surgery for subaxial subluxations involves a dorsal fusion and that the role of ventral surgery is unclear in this condition. Santavirta et al.[75] have indicated that reduction of the bony subluxation with a fusion is not adequate in patients with spinal cord compression from subaxial subluxation because rheumatoid granulation tissue in the sublaminar space may continue to compress the neural elements. Therefore, they recommend laminectomy in addition to this fusion procedure. King[40] has stated that a dorsal decompression may relieve the spinal cord compression. It may also, however, worsen spinal instability. At present, the optimal surgical treatment for subaxial subluxation of the rheumatoid cervical spine is unclear. Further experience with the various ventral and dorsal techniques will be necessary to clearly delineate which procedure is most advantageous.

Surgical Techniques

Once it has been determined that a patient with rheumatoid arthritis will require a surgical procedure, the correct operation must be chosen. The most frequent problem in this regard is deciding whether to incorporate the occiput into an upper cervical fusion. Including the occiput into an upper cervical fusion leads to a lower fusion rate and increased morbidity with respect to neck motion. However, it is frequently necessary to arrest the progression of a vertical subluxation of the odontoid. Other operative considerations that are less frequently problematic include the decision of whether to extend the fusion into the subaxial cervical spine when subluxations are present in that region.

It must be remembered that rheumatoid arthritis is a benign disease. As such, a stable arthrodesis is necessary for long-term success in the patient with rheumatoid arthritis. All instrumentation constructs fatigue with time and only a stable bony fusion will provide satisfactory long-term results.

Recently, the need for bone grafting in all patients has been challenged. Although it is uniformly agreed that young patients and patients with a reasonable prospect for long-term survival require grafting, Crockard et al.[17,18] and Moskovich et al.[60] contend that the results of arthrodesis in end-stage rheumatoid arthritis patients are very poor. Therefore, they evaluate each case on an individual basis, and in selected situations, perform a fixation procedure without a supplemental bony fusion.

C1-2 Stabilization

C1-2 stabilization and fusion procedures have been performed since the early twentieth century. Techniques have been established and many modifications of these techniques have been proposed. As new techniques are developed, they must be compared to time-honored, successful procedures that are currently in use. In addition, improved fusion rates and acceptably low complication rates are necessary before a new surgical procedure can be advocated.

In 1910, Mixter and Osgood[57] described a patient with atlantoaxial instability secondary to a nonunion of an odontoid fracture. They successfully treated this fracture by fixing the dorsal arch of the atlas to the spinous process of the axis using a stout, braided silk thread that had been soaked in tincture of benzoin. This case report represented the first documented C1-2 stabilization procedure. Although not mentioned in the report by Mixter and Osgood, use of bone graft materials to promote a long-term stable bony fusion of the axis and the atlas was soon recognized to be a necessary portion of any upper cervical spine stabilization procedure.

Axial rotation is the major motion that occurs at the C1-2 level. Although this motion is a movement that is clinically important to control,[90] translation is the main pathologic movement at the C1-2 level. Gallie,[28] in 1939, described a method to prevent the recurrence of cervical subluxation at the C1-2 level. He fastened the two vertebrae together with a fine steel wire passed beneath the dorsal arch of the atlas and around the spinous process of the axis. He stated that the risk of a late recurrence could be eliminated if bone grafts were applied to the construct. Gallie used a tricortical bone graft in an onlay fashion. Dickman et al.[22] have described a modification of a Gallie-type C1-2 fusion. In their modification, they interpose a bicortical iliac graft between the dorsal arch of C1 and the lamina of C2. This construct attempts to compress the bone graft between the two bony surfaces of the dorsal elements in an attempt to increase the fusion rate (Figure 56.7).

The next major modification to the Gallie-type C1-2 fusion procedure was proposed by Brooks and Jenkins[10] in 1978. They described a wedge compression arthrodesis of the atlantoaxial joint that was performed by placing sublaminar wires beneath the lamina of C2 and the dorsal arch of C1 bilaterally. Separate bone grafts were placed on each side of the midline and were secured separately. The authors stated that the procedure was rarely indicated in patients with long-standing rheumatoid arthritis or in patients with severe osteopenia. Despite this warning, Brooks-type fusions have been performed frequently for rheumatoid arthritis.

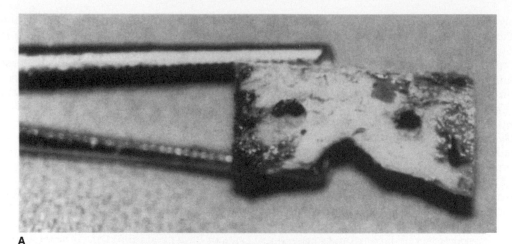

A

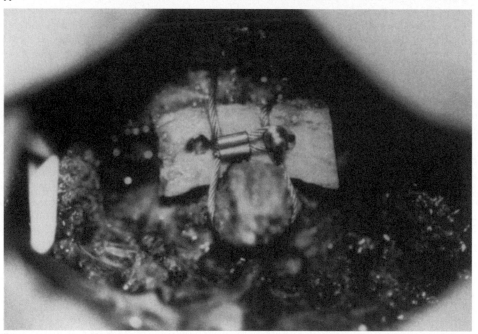

B

Figure 56.7 (**A**) Bicortical bone graft harvested from the iliac crest to be interposed between the arch of the atlas and the spinous process of the axis. Holes in the graft allow for the cables to pass through and add further stability to the construct. (**B**) A modified Gallie construct using an autogenous bicortical iliac crest graft that is compressed between the posterior elements of the atlas and the axis with a Songer cable. The free ends of the cable exit the construct through the holes in the graft where they are secured.

The dangers inherent in both the Brooks-type and the Gallie-type fusions are the necessity to pass the wire beneath the dorsal elements of the upper cervical spine. In doing so, compression from a ventrally located pannus can actually be increased and can lead to neurologic worsening. In an attempt to avoid this complication, techniques were developed that attempted to avoid the need to pass a sublaminar wire. In 1984, Holness et al.[35] reported the use of an interlaminar clamp. This device was originally developed in Halifax, Nova Scotia, Canada, and is commonly referred to as the Halifax clamp. The Halifax clamp involves the bilateral placement of hooks over the dorsal arch of C1 and under the lamina of C2, which are held together by a screw. In their original description, Holness et al.[1,59] did not advocate routine bone grafting.

They did, however, endorse bone grafting in rheumatoid arthritis patients. The Halifax clamp provided numerous advantages, including a decreased risk of dural penetration, a decreased risk of neurologic injury, ease of use, elimination of wire cutout in osteoporotic bone, and more recently, the development of MRI-compatible clamps to allow for better postoperative imaging. The motion for which the Halifax clamp is particularly suited is the resistance of flexion. This is the pathologic movement for which a C1-2 fusion is usually performed.[59] Rotational instability can occur and this can lead to failure.[1,59]

The optimal mechanical construct to provide internal fixation of the C1-2 segment should consist of a three-point fixation.[18,30] In an innovative attempt to achieve three-point fixation, Magerl and Seeman[48] devised a technique using transarticular screw fixation of the lateral facet joints of the atlas and the axis. Placement of a bone graft dorsally between the arch of C1 and the spinous process of C2 allows for a true three-point fixation. Recent studies by Marcotte et al.[50] and Stillerman and Wilson[84] have also provided an optimistic outlook for this procedure. The advantages of the C1-2 transarticular facet screws include improved fusion rates, ease of placement, improved mechanical strength, and overall patient safety.[84] Postoperative bracing in a halo vest apparatus may not be necessary when using this technique.[50,84] Jeanneret and Magerl[39] have recommended the use of transarticular screw fixation rather than a Brooks-type or Gallie-type fusion whenever a dorsal C1-2 fusion is indicated. As a result of potential technical difficulties, this technique has not yet gained widespread acceptance. As with any new technical modification, long-term follow-up results will be necessary to prove the efficacy and safety of this approach.

Grob et al.[30] performed a biomechanical evaluation of four different cervical fixation techniques. In their study, the techniques tested were the Gallie fusion, the Brooks fusion, the Halifax interlaminar clamp, and the transarticular screw fixation of Magerl. They determined that the Gallie-type fixation was the least stable and allowed a significantly greater range of motion in all directions than did the other three constructs. They determined that the transarticular screw fixation technique provided a true three-point fixation when a bone graft was placed dorsally. This construct was the most stable for lateral bending and axial rotation. The overall result of the cadaver study by Grob et al. was that the immediate three-dimensional stabilizing capability of the Brooks fusion, the Halifax interlaminar clamp, and the transarticular screw fixation technique of Magerl provided similar biomechanical results.

Additional modifications to C1-2 stabilization techniques include the use of multistranded cables, rather than twisted wires. These cables are easier to pass, are stronger than the twisted wires, and are available in titanium, which improves postoperative imaging. Polymethylmethacrylate (PMMA) is a synthetic cement compound that has been used in lieu of bone to augment instrumentation constructs. Polymethylmethacrylate has been associated with significant wound complications, interference with bony arthrodesis, and less than optimal rigid fixation.[24] It is therefore not advisable to use this material in C1-2 fusion operations for rheumatoid arthritis. Although the majority of C1-2 fusions have used iliac crest as the donor site of bone grafts, Sagher et al.[73] have described a technique that uses the occipital bone as the donor site for atlantoaxial fusions. Although their mean follow-up time was less than 1 year, all patients in their study proceeded to develop solid bony fusions. This interesting technique allows only a single incision to be made in the skin.

Occipitocervical Fusion

When vertical subluxation of the dens is present, with or without a concurrent atlantoaxial subluxation, an atlantoaxial fusion is not adequate treatment. In these cases, it is necessary to extend the fusion to include the occiput. Inclusion of the occiput in the fusion mass will significantly decrease head and neck motion, and as a result, it should not be performed in cases with an isolated ventral atlantoaxial subluxation.

In 1987, Wertheim and Bohlman[89] described a technique for occipitocervical fusion using rigid wiring of the occiput through the external occipital protuberance to the cervical spine by use of large iliac crest bone grafts. This technique avoided the need to penetrate both tables of the skull, allowed for immediate rigid internal fixation, permitted early patient mobilization, and resulted in a successful fusion in all 13 patients in their study. Of note, eight of these patients had rheumatoid arthritis. Modifications of the technique of Wertheim and Bohlman include placement of occipital burr holes to secure the occipital portion of the fusion.[13] In addition, Stambough et al.[82] described a technique for occipitocervical fusion in osteopenic rheumatoid arthritis patients using bone in combination with PMMA. The authors believed that this technique provided immediate stability and optimized the chances for long-term bony stability. Fusion constructs using PMMA for benign disease will, however, be prone to failure.

In 1986, Ransford et al.[67] described a method of occipitocervical stabilization with an anatomically contoured steel loop secured by occipital and sublaminar wires. This rigid dorsal internal fixation system provides immediate stabilization at the craniocervical junction. The authors stated that the loop system provided the necessary stability to allow the patient to mobilize without major external support. The use of this system was originally described in patients after transoral decompressive surgeries. It has, however, been subsequently widely used for primary occipitocervical surgical stabilizations. A similar modification of this technique incorporates a malleable rod and segmental wiring. This technique, described by Fehlings et al.[24] also provides immediate rigid stabilization, and the authors have stated that it avoids the need for an external orthosis.

Rogers et al.[71] have recently described a useful clinical tool to help determine which surgical techniques are safest. They have stated that although motor examination may be difficult in patients with severe rheumatoid arthritis, testing of sensation remains relatively straightforward. A loss of proprioception suggests a severe dorsal compressive component, usually at the occipitocervical junction, and passage of sublaminar wires in these cases may be hazardous and may result in neurologic morbidity. Grob et al.[31] described a technique for occipitocervical plating that uses screws into the occiput and the lateral masses in the cervical spine, obviating the need for sublaminar wires. This technique also provides immediate rigid internal fixation and good rotational stability.

Each of these newer techniques for occipitocervical fusion must be compared with the highly successful technique of Wertheim and Bohlman[89] in long-term follow-up studies. It should be noted that there is not adequate inherent stability in any bone-wire or bone-cable constructs, and as a result, external immobilization is mandatory whenever these techniques are used. Constructs that incorporate plates and screws or rectangles and cable or wire have greater inherent stability and may diminish the requirements for postoperative external immobilization.

Patients with rheumatoid arthritis and vertical subluxation of the dens, as a general rule, have had long-standing disease and are frequently osteopenic. Thus, it is necessary to evaluate these patients over time to determine the optimal method of fusion and the need for postoperative external support.

Transoral Surgery

In the transoral approach to the odontoid, a midline dorsal pharyngeal incision is made. This allows for exposure of the lower clivus to the level of the C2-3 junction. Depending on the preference of the operating surgeon, splitting the soft palate, performing a tracheotomy, using cervical traction, and using a halo vest postoperatively are all considerations with this surgery. In addition, the transoral decompression can be combined simultaneously with a dorsal cervical stabilization procedure to allow for immediate mobilization of the patient postoperatively.[60] On the other hand, the dorsal stabilization can be performed separately later.[20,55]

Menezes has stated that if the vertical subluxation has caused the dens to penetrate the foramen magnum by greater than 20mm, an acceptable reduction with prolonged traction cannot be achieved. These patients may require a transoral resection of the dens.[54] In 14 rheumatoid arthritis patients with irreducible vertical subluxation, Menezes and van Gilder[53] found a sequestered odontoid process protruding into the pons intradurally in four of the cases.

The specific aspects of the surgical procedure are open to debate. However, there appears to be uniform agreement among investigators experienced in this technique that the ventral transoral decompression should precede the dorsal cervical stabilization.[20,55]

Subaxial Cervical, Thoracic, and Lumbar Surgery

In cases of subaxial subluxations of the cervical spine, there is not adequate proof that a ventral, dorsal, or combined ventral and dorsal approach is the optimal treatment. Likewise, lesions affecting the thoracic or lumbar spine are so rare that specific treatments must be individualized on a case-by-case basis. Thus, no attempt will be made in this section to analyze the limited information available on these lesions.

Postoperative External Orthoses

There is no consensus in the orthopedic and neurosurgical literature regarding the optimal type of external orthosis to be used after an upper cervical stabilization procedure. Opinion ranges from the need for postoperative halo vest immobilization for a minimum of 12 weeks, followed by 4 to 8 weeks' additional time, if flexion-extension views do not show a stable fusion[63] to no need for any external orthosis postoperatively.[67] The majority of opinions fall into three categories: routine use of the halo vest postoperatively; routine use of an external orthosis other than the

halo vest such as a Minerva jacket, Philadelphia collar, or a SOMI brace; and use of a halo vest when fixation is deemed tenuous, with a lesser device used when the fixation is considered more secure.

Halo vests are used routinely by numerous authors* for 6 to 12 weeks postoperatively in all patients having upper cervical fusions. Others† prefer a Philadelphia collar, a SOMI brace, or a two- or four-post rigid orthosis postoperatively and do not recommend a halo vest. A compromise is made by some who believe that when the fixation is tenuous, a halo vest should be used; however, when the fixation is deemed more secure, a less rigid external orthosis can be applied.*

This lack of agreement regarding the use of external orthoses postoperatively may be the result of varied new surgical procedures currently being developed. In the Magerl[48] transarticular screw fixation of C1-2, if a bone graft is incorporated dorsally, a true three-point fixation can be achieved. Similarly, some occipitocervical fusion techniques also allow for a three-point fixation and thus may eliminate the need for a halo vest.[32,60,67] Long-term follow-up results will be needed to determine whether the benefit of improved patient comfort postoperatively in a lesser orthosis will outweigh the risk of an inferior fusion rate if the external support is inadequate. The need for the rigid support of a halo vest orthosis may be unnecessary in patients who are able to have a true three-point fixation internally.

Postoperative Results

Surgery on the rheumatoid cervical spine is indicated for intractable pain, myelopathy, or progressive neurologic deficit. The postoperative results can thus be categorized into neurologic results and bony fusion results. A solid bony arthrodesis is necessary for relief of intractable pain present preoperatively. Likewise, an adequate decompression is necessary for stabilization or improvement of neurologic status postoperatively. Finally, because much of the surgery for rheumatoid arthritis is performed at the occipitocervical junction, postoperative morbidity from systemic problems and postoperative mortality rates must be measured.

Neurologic Outcome

Boden et al.[8] found that the severity of the neurologic deficit present preoperatively was an accurate predictor of the postoperative neurologic status. They also stated that the duration of the neurologic deficit preoperatively did not affect the prognosis for neurologic recovery after the operation. Hultquist et al.[37] found that most of their patients had relief of their pain and amelioration of their neurologic symptoms; however, there was little evidence of improved overall functional capacity. In spite of this, most of their patients expressed great satisfaction in being pain-free postoperatively.

Once again, there is considerable discrepancy in the results of neurologic outcome among reported series. In the review by Menezes et al.[55] all 45 patients with vertical

---

subluxation of the odontoid had an improvement in their functional neurologic grade and amelioration of their neurologic dysfunction. On the other hand, Chan et al.[12] found that no patient with a preoperative myelopathy improved neurologically in the postoperative period.

The lack of improvement in some published series once a myelopathy has been established has led some investigators to recommend that early operative stabilization be considered before the onset of neurologic deficit, when radiographic instability is present. Although all patients in their series had evidence of a neurologic deficit before surgery, Boden et al.[8] have recommended that surgery be performed in neurologically intact patients who have a vertical subluxation of the dens compounding a marked atlantoaxial subluxation. In pain-free neurologically intact patients with a severe radiographic abnormality, the decision to intervene will depend on both accurate serial neurologic examinations and accurate serial radiographic imaging studies.

Fusion Outcome

A surgical success with a dorsal cervical fusion operation requires that a stable bony arthrodesis be achieved. A nonunion, also termed *pseudarthrosis,* is more likely to occur in patients with rheumatoid arthritis because of the well-documented problems of osteoporosis or osteopenia that occur in rheumatoid arthritis patients. In addition, many of these patients have been on long-term corticosteroid therapy that is also known to inhibit fusion rates.

Moskovich and Crockard[59] have defined the requirements for considering a solid dorsal atlantoaxial fusion a success: lateral flexion and extension radiographs that show no motion and evidence of trabecular bone in continuity between the dorsal elements and the graft. In cases of doubt, plain tomograms are excellent for determining continuity of the fusion. Chan et al.[12] agreed with this definition, and in addition, they defined a fibrous union as the presence of less than 2mm of motion on flexion-extension radiographs. Dickman et al.[22] have stressed that patients with fibrous unions must be followed closely for the signs of delayed instability or wire breakage.

In patients with rheumatoid arthritis, radiographic determination of an occipitocervical fusion may be difficult. Recently, Moskovich et al.[60] have reviewed a series of 152 rheumatoid arthritis patients who underwent occipitocervical stabilization procedures. In 80% of their patients, no bone grafting was used to augment the stabilization procedure with a contoured steel loop. To evaluate the occipitocervical complex for postoperative stability, these authors measured the angle between the occiput and the upper cervical vertebrae. The difference in the angle between flexion and extension radiographs provides an indication of stability. This method allows one to determine postoperative stability regardless of whether a bone graft is used to supplement the stabilization procedure.

Variability in the reporting of fusion rates postoperatively in patients with rheumatoid arthritis may be a result of discrepancies about whether a given author classifies patients with fibrous union along with the successful bony fusion patients or whether patients with fibrous union are classified along with the nonunion, or pseudarthrosis, patients. When pseudarthrosis occurs after atlantoaxial fusions, it is most common between the dorsal bone graft and the ring of C1.[59,78] The reasons for nonunion at this location include the high cortex-to-medulla ratio of the dorsal ring of C1, which is relatively sclerotic,[59] and frequent erosion of the dorsal arch of C1 in patients with rheumatoid arthritis.[78] In subaxial subluxations, failure of a ventral fusion may be a result of angulation, pseudarthrosis, or collapse of the graft in the bone graft bed.[66] Santavirta et al.[76] believed that ventral procedures for subaxial subluxation often fail because of vertebral body osteoporosis, and they stated that acrylic cement and metal rods are of little use as stabilizers in rheumatoid cervical spines.

Fusion rates vary between 50% to 100% in reported series of atlantoaxial fusions and occipitocervical fusions. Menezes et al.[55] have stated that a stable bony fusion occurred in 100% of their 45 patients with fusion for vertical subluxation of the odontoid. Similarly, all seven rheumatoid arthritis patients of Dickman et al.[22] developed stable osseous unions with a bicortical iliac bone graft in a modified Gallie-type fusion. Tricortical iliac crest bone grafts in dorsal atlantoaxial fusions are associated with a higher rate of fibrous union.[22,43] Fusion rates from 75% to 90% have been reported with Halifax interlaminar clamps,[1,59] a modified Gallie approach,[22,63] and the transarticular screw fixation technique of Magerl.[72,84] Fusion rates between 50% and 75% have been reported with traditional Gallie fusions[76] and after combined transoral and dorsal fusion operations for vertical subluxation of the odontoid.[20]

Many series of upper cervical fusions include rheumatoid patients along with young, healthy trauma patients. As a general rule, victims of trauma will have better bone stock and better fusion rates postoperatively when compared with patients with rheumatoid arthritis. As previously stated, different external orthoses were used to supplement the internal stabilization procedures in these series, and this can also affect fusion rates.

Mortality

Mortality in patients with rheumatoid arthritis varies greatly in reported series. Surgical series must be compared to the natural history of rheumatoid arthritis in patients never subjected to surgical procedures. In a 15-year prospective follow-up study of patients with new-onset rheumatoid arthritis, Corbett et al.[15] found only a small increase in mortality in rheumatoid arthritis patients compared with the general population over the same 15-year period.[42] They found an increased mortality at 15 years in rheumatoid arthritis patients with concurrent heart disease. Males were over-represented in this study.[15]

Davis and Markley[19] reported the first case of an autopsy-proven death in a rheumatoid arthritis patient secondary to compression of the medulla by herniation of the odontoid process through the foramen magnum. This was followed by two separate case reports by Martel and Abell[51] of autopsy-proven sudden death secondary to atlantoaxial subluxation. As the danger of sudden death was more widely reported, it became apparent that spinal cord damage may not always have been recognized as a cause of death in rheumatoid arthritis patient fatalities in the past. Smith et al.[79] stated that spinal cord involvement may have been responsible for more deaths than had previously been apparent.

Reported mortality in the first month postoperatively have varied between 4% and 10%.[12,41,53,60] Many deaths have been attributed to postoperative myocardial infarction; however, it is possible that spinal cord compression may contribute to these deaths. Santavirta et al.,[76] while operating on patients with severe rheumatoid arthritis, found that 50% of these patients died over a 10-year follow-up period postoperatively. These authors estimated that the average age of death of these patients was approximately the same as that of other patients with equally severe rheumatoid arthritis.[76] Like the nonsurgical long-term follow-up study of Corbett et al.,[15] Santavirta et al.[76] reported a significantly increased rate of death postoperatively when cardiac disease was also present.

The natural history of rheumatoid arthritis has demonstrated that the disease will be present for 15 to 20 years before the need for surgical correction of the abnormalities in the cervical spine. At the time of surgery, these patients are often severely debilitated from the general disease process. Therefore, long-term postoperative mortality must be compared with the mortality of patients with equally severe rheumatoid arthritis who do not require cervical spine operations. The definitive comparative analysis has yet to be completed.

Medical Adjuncts

Patients with long-standing rheumatoid arthritis requiring surgery on the cervical spine have often been treated with glucocorticoid medications for many years. These medications are well known to exert deleterious effects on bone. Skeletal damage resulting from long-term treatment with supraphysiologic doses of glucocorticoids occur in four ways: inhibition of bone growth, delayed union of fractures, osteoporosis, and osteonecrosis.[56]

Corbett et al.[15] in a 15-year prospective follow-up study of patients with new-onset rheumatoid arthritis, found that long-term use of steroids in rheumatoid arthritis was associated with higher mortality. In addition, Hall et al.[32] have stated that the cumulative dose of steroid is more important with respect to this negative effect than is the daily dose. Santavirta et al.[76] found that patients who had received steroid treatments for greater than 4 years had more fibrous unions and more pseudarthroses in a 10-year follow-up study. Laan et al.[43] found that low-dose prednisone therapy had a deleterious effect on the bone mineral density of postmenopausal women. These postmenopausal patients are at an increased risk for developing axial osteopenia and vertebral fractures. A similar bone density loss in men was not demonstrable. In patients with active rheumatoid arthritis, low doses of glucocorticoid can cause marked vertebral trabecular bone loss in the initial month of therapy.[43,55] After cessation of steroid therapy, this bone loss may be partially reversible.[32,44] Papadopoulos et al.[63] found that radiologic

progression of atlantoaxial subluxation occurs more rapidly in patients with systemic disease severe enough to require maintenance steroid therapy.

In an attempt to counteract these deleterious effects of glucocorticoids on bone in rheumatoid arthritis patients, new prednisone derivatives have been developed. Deflazacort, an oxazolone derivative of prednisone, has been developed and used to reduce the incidence of the catabolic glucocorticoid actions of prednisone and still maintain its beneficial actions. In a randomized double-blind study, deflazacort was found to decrease the amount of corticosteroid-induced osteoporosis.[56]

Another medical adjunct that may be of use in the future is estrogen replacement. In postmenopausal women with rheumatoid arthritis, estrogen replacement is protective with regard to the risk of spinal osteoporosis. Sambrook et al.[74] concluded that estrogen therapy should be considered in postmenopausal women with rheumatoid arthritis who are at risk for osteoporosis.

Additional research is necessary to develop medications that can provide the patient the symptomatic relief of prednisone while eliminating or reducing its harmful side effects on bone in rheumatoid arthritis patients who are predisposed to osteoarthritis by the disease process itself. Recent trends among rheumatologists to use less steroid medications have led to increased use of nonsteroidal anti-inflammatory agents, penicillamine, and methotrexate as additional treatment alternatives in patients with long-standing disease.

Summary

Because the majority of operative interventions on the spine in patients with rheumatoid arthritis occur at the C1-2 level, complications must be avoided because there is no effective management for them. Complication avoidance begins with proper patient selection for operative intervention. The authors recommend performing surgery for intractable pain, myelopathy, or progressive neurologic deficit. In the isolated case of an end-stage rheumatoid arthritis patient who has been bed-bound for more than 3 months, consideration may be given to a nonoperative treatment regimen. However, even with these patients, occasional rewarding results have been achieved surgically. An accurate and thorough history and physical examination, a detailed review of all radiologic imaging studies, and an understanding of the natural history of rheumatoid arthritis of the cervical spine are all necessary. A knowledge of past successes and failures can help optimize the results.

Patients with abnormal radiographs in the absence of pain or an abnormal neurologic exam should be followed closely with serial neurologic exams and serial radiographic imaging studies. Numerous rheumatologic studies have demonstrated clearly that many of these patients will never require operative intervention and that they may have a life expectancy similar to that of rheumatoid arthritis patients with an equivalent extent of disease with the exception of the spinal involvement.

The radiographic imaging workup can be very extensive. Although it is not cost-effective, each of the different imaging modalities provides useful information, both for preoperative planning and for following patients nonoperatively. In a patient with rheumatoid arthritis who is suspected of having spinal involvement, the authors routinely obtain plain radiographs, a CT scan, and an MRI scan. The plain radiographs allow calculation of the ventral ADI and the dorsal AOI and assessment for any evidence of vertical subluxation of the odontoid. In addition, the subaxial cervical spine can be imaged to look for subluxations. CT of the upper cervical spine provides the most accurate bony detail of this region. Identification of the foramen transversaria is best obtained on a CT scan, and this is mandatory if a transarticular C1-2 screw fixation is contemplated. MRI helps determine the extent of ventral soft-tissue pathology, (i.e., rheumatoid pannus) and the extent of spinal cord compression from both the ventral and dorsal directions. MRI is also excellent for screening for abnormalities of the subaxial cervical spine and, if necessary, of the thoracic and lumbar spines also. In cases where MRI cannot be performed, CT and myelography should be performed.

A detailed medical evaluation is required for any patient before undergoing surgery. This is best done in conjunction with a rheumatology consultant. When possible, steroids should be tapered or discontinued. This may not be possible in the severely debilitated end-stage rheumatoid arthritis patient with polyarticular disease. In all circumstances, smokers should be strongly advised to quit smoking. Because surgical procedures are routinely performed on an elective basis, baseline somatosensory-evoked potentials should be obtained, and arrangements should be made for donation of autologous blood before surgery.

Intraoperative considerations include the routine use of somatosensory-evoked potentials as well as fiberoptic intubation. Traction via a halo ring that can later be converted to a halo vest is preferable to Gardner-Wells traction. Whenever possible, autograft iliac crest is the preferred donor site for fusion operations. In patients with an osteoporotic pelvis who are unable to provide autograft, allograft bone may be used. This may be supplemented with a bone morphogenic protein preparation. Occasionally, one may also consider fixation without a concurrent fusion. It must be remembered that unlike ventral fusion operations in which the bone graft is under compression, dorsal onlay fusions are not under compression. Therefore, the need for long-term rigid immobilization to obtain a stable bony fusion is essential for any dorsal fusion operation. Because these patients are suffering from a benign disease with a potential for long life, PMMA should not be used on rheumatoid arthritis patients.

Following strict operative indications, the operative techniques that the authors recommend are as follows. For an isolated ventral C1-2 subluxation, a modified Gallie operation using bicortical iliac crest graft, advocated by Sonntag and others,[22,63] is used. The numerous other stabilization techniques for isolated C1-2 instability are generally acceptable. An important consideration is that incorporation of the occiput into the fusion construct may increase the risk of a poor result, and this should only be done if clearly indicated. When a vertical subluxation of the dens is present, an occipitocervical fusion with lateral plates (or a bent rod) that extends from the occiput to the cervical spine is ideal. These plates can be extended caudally in cases of subaxial subluxation. If the vertical subluxation is irreducible, or if significant ventral pathology causing compression is present, a transoral decompression is necessary. This transoral decompression should usually be performed before any dorsal surgery. Depending on the patient's physical condition, the ventral surgery may be followed by the dorsal operation in the same sitting, or the dorsal surgery can be performed later. The majority of subaxial subluxations of the cervical spine are best treated with lateral mass plating. Because thoracic and lumbar spine involvement in rheumatoid arthritis is very rare, the surgical management of these cases must be individualized on a case-by-case basis. As a general rule, ventral pathology should be decompressed and stabilized ventrally and dorsal pathology should be decompressed and stabilized dorsally. The authors routinely use cables over wire or twisted wire constructs. In addition, titanium cables and plates may be used. It should be recognized, however, that titanium implants are more difficult to work with and fail more easily than traditional steel; also, postoperative neuroimaging studies show significant erosion in the immediate regions of the implant. In addition, bending of the titanium plates or rods at the occipitocervical junction may cause them to weaken.

Postoperatively, the authors recommend using a halo vest for a minimum of 12 weeks. The reasons for halo immobilization include the historically poor fusion results of dorsal cervical fusions in rheumatoid arthritis patients, the osteopenia frequently observed in these patients, and the inability to place the grafts under adequate compressive forces. Therefore, immobilization is the key to obtaining a good bony fusion. After 12 weeks in the halo, plain radiographs are obtained to document a stable osseous arthrodesis. If any question exists, flexion and extension views should be obtained. Plain tomograms should be used in cases in which plain radiographs are not able to demonstrate a fusion definitively. If a stable fusion has not been obtained at 12 weeks, the halo should be continued for 4 to 12 additional weeks. Some of the newer techniques such as transarticular C1-2 screw fixation and occipitocervical plating may provide adequate three-point fixation to allow for long-term internal immobilization and thus allow for postoperative external immobilization in a lesser device than a halo.

A nonunion or a pseudarthrosis may require revision surgery. If the initial surgical indication was intractable pain, a postoperative pseudarthrosis may be painful and may require a revision surgery. If surgery was performed for a neurologic deficit, and this has improved, revision surgery may not be necessary. These patients must be followed closely, particularly patients with an asymptomatic fibrous union because some of them will develop a delayed bony union. It is preferable to continue using the halo for up to 24 weeks before determining that a nonunion has occurred. In patients with evidence of a successful bony fusion, the external orthosis is removed. It is mandatory to continue to watch these patients closely for development of delayed subaxial subluxations. These subluxations below the level of an upper cervical fusion are common.

Finally, the majority of surgical procedures on patients with rheumatoid arthritis of the spine are performed in the upper cervical region. Most of the complications arise from difficulties with fusion or instrumentation; these problems are much more common than a worsened neurologic deficit. Several pitfalls can be avoided by operating only when absolutely necessary on patients with intractable pain or a neurologic deficit. In addition, careful preoperative planning allows for use of the appropriate operative procedure that will give optimal results.

REFERENCES

1. Aldrich EF, Weber PB, Crow WN: Halifax interlaminar clamp for posterior cervical fusion: a long-term follow-up review. *J Neurosurg* 78:702-708, 1983.

2. Baggenstoss AH, Bickel WH, Ward LE: Rheumatoid granulomatous nodules as destructive lesions of vertebrae. *J Bone Joint Surg* 34A:601-609, 1952.

3. Bailey RW: Rheumatoid arthritis and other noninfectious inflammatory diseases. In The Cervical Spine Research Society: *The Cervical Spine*. Philadelphia, Lippincott-Raven, 1983.

4. Bell C: *The nervous system of the human body. Embracing the papers delivered to the Royal Society on the subject of the nerves*. London, Longman, Rees, Orme, Brown, and Green, 1830.

5. Bell GR, Stearns KL: Flexion-extension MRI of the upper rheumatoid cervical spine. *Orthopedics* 14:969-974, 1991.

6. Bland JH: Rheumatoid arthritis of the cervical spine. *J Rheumatol* 1:319-342, 1974.

7. Bland JH, Davis PH, London MG, *et al:* Rheumatoid arthritis of the cervical spine. *Arch Intern Med* 112:892-898, 1963.

8. Boden SD, Dodge LD, Bohlman HH, Rechtine GR: Rheumatoid arthritis of the cervical spine. *J Bone Joint Surg* 75A:1282-1297, 1993.

9. Breedveld FC, Algra PR, Vielvoye CJ, Cats A: Magnetic resonance imaging in the evaluation of patients with rheumatoid arthritis and subluxations of the cervical spine. *Arthritis Rheum* 30:624-629, 1987.

10. Brooks AL, Jenkins EB: Atlanto-axial arthrodesis by the wedge compression method. *J Bone Joint Surg* 60A:279-284, 1978.

11. Chamberlain WE: Basilar impression (platybasia): a bizarre developmental anomaly of the occipital bone and upper cervical spine with striking and misleading neurological manifestations. *Yale J Biol Med* 11:487-496, 1938; 1939.

12. Chan DPK, Ngian KS, Cohen L: Posterior upper cervical fusion in rheumatoid arthritis. *Spine* 17:268-272, 1992.

13. Clark CR: Occipitocervical fusion for the unstable rheumatoid neck. *Orthopedics* 12:469-473, 1989.

14. Cohen MJ, Ezekiel J, Persellin RH: Costovertebral and costotransverse joint involvement in rheumatoid arthritis. *Ann Rheum Dis* 37:473-475, 1978.

15. Corbett M, Dalton S, Young A, *et al:* Factors predicting death, survival and functional outcome in a prospective study of early rheumatoid disease over fifteen years. *Br J Rheumatol* 32:717-723, 1993.

16. Crockard HA: The transoral approach to the base of the brain and upper cervical cord. *Ann R Coll Surg Engl* 67:321-325, 1985.

17. Crockard HA, Calder I, Ransford AO: One-stage decompression and posterior fixation in rheumatoid atlanto-axial subluxation. *J Bone Joint Surg* 72B:682-685, 1990.

18. Crockard HA, Grob D: Rheumatoid arthritis: upper cervical involvement. In Clark CR (ed): *The Cervical Spine*. Philadelphia, Lippincott-Raven, 1995.

19. Davis FW, Jr., Markley HE: Rheumatoid arthritis with death from medullary compression. *Ann Int Med* 35:451-454, 1951.

20. Dickman CA, Locantro J, Fessler RG: The influence of transoral odontoid resection on stability of the craniovertebral junction. *J Neurosurg* 77:525-530, 1992.

21. Dickman CA, Mamourian A, Sonntag VKH, Drayer BP: Magnetic resonance imaging of the transverse atlantal ligament for the evaluation of atlantoaxial stability. *J Neurosurg* 75:221-227, 1991.

22. Dickman CA, Sonntag VKH, Papadopoulos SM, Hadley MN: The interspinous method of posterior atlantoaxial arthrodesis. *J Neurosurg* 74:190-198, 1991.

23. Fam AG, Cruickshank B: Subaxial cervical subluxation and cord compression in psoriatic spondylitis. *Arthritis Rheum* 25:101-106, 1982.

24. Fehlings MG, Errico T, Cooper P, *et al:* Occipitocervical fusion with a five-millimeter malleable rod and segmental fixation. *Neurosurgery* 32:198-208, 1993.

25. Ferlic DC, Clayton ML, Leidholt JD, Gamble WE: Surgical treatment of the symptomatic unstable cervical spine in rheumatoid arthritis. *J Bone Joint Surg* 57A:349-354, 1975.

26. Friedman H: Intraspinal rheumatoid nodule causing nerve root compression. *J Neurosurg* 32:689-691, 1970.

27. Frigaard E: Posterior atlanto-axial subluxation in rheumatoid arthritis. *Scand J Rheumatol* 7:65-68, 1978.

28. Gallie WE: Fractures and dislocations of the cervical spine. *Am J Surg* 46:495-499, 1939.

29. Grantham SA: Rheumatoid arthritis and other noninfectious inflammatory diseases: atlantoaxial instability. In The Cervical Spine Research Society: *The Cervical Spine*. Philadelphia, Lippincott-Raven, 1983.

30. Grob D, Crisco JJ, III, Panjabi MM, *et al:* Biomechanical evaluation of four different posterior atlantoaxial fixation techniques. *Spine* 17:480-490, 1992.

31. Grob D, Dvorak J, Panjabi M, *et al:* Posterior occipitocervical fusion: a preliminary report of a new technique. *Spine* 16(suppl 3):S17-S23, 1991.

32. Hall GM, Spector TD, Griffin AJ, *et al:* The effect of rheumatoid arthritis and steroid therapy on bone density in post menopausal women. *Arthritis Rheum* 36:1510-1516, 1993.

33. Henderson FC, Geddes JF, Crockard HA: Neuropathology of the brainstem and spinal cord in end stage rheumatoid arthritis: implications for treatment. *Ann Rheum Dis* 52:629-637, 1993.

34. Heywood AWB, Meyers OL: Rheumatoid arthritis of the thoracic and lumbar spine. *J Bone Joint Surg* 68B:362-368, 1986.

35. Holness RO, Huestis WS, Howes WJ: Posterior stabilization with an interlaminar clamp in cervical injuries:

technical note and review of the long term experience with the method. *Neurosurgery* 14:318-322, 1984.

36. Hughes JT: Spinal cord involvement by C4-C5 vertebral subluxation in rheumatoid arthritis: a description of 2 cases examined at necropsy. *Ann Neurol* 1:575-582, 1977.

37. Hultquist R, Zygmunt S, Saveland H, *et al:* Characterization and functional assessment of patients subjected to occipito-cervical fusion for rheumatoid atlanto-axial dislocation. *Scand J Rheumatol* 22:20-24, 1993.

38. Isdale IC, Corrigan AB: Backward luxation of the atlas: two cases of an uncommon condition. *Ann Rheum Dis* 29:6-9, 1970.

39. Jeanneret B, Magerl F: Primary posterior fusion C1/2 in odontoid fractures: indications, technique, and results of transarticular screw fixation. *J Spinal Disord Tech* 4: 464-475, 1992.

40. King TT: Rheumatoid subluxations of the cervical spine, editorial. *Ann Rheum Dis* 44:807-808, 1985.

41. Kraus DR, Peppelman WC, Agarwal AK, *et al:* Incidence of subaxial subluxation in patients with generalized rheumatoid arthritis who have had previous occipital cervical fusions. *Spine* 16(suppl):S486-S489, 1991.

42. Laan RFJM, Buijs WCAM, Verbeek ALM, *et al:* Bone mineral density in patients with recent onset rheumatoid arthritis: influence of disease activity and functional capacity. *Ann Rheum Dis* 52:21-26, 1993.

43. Laan RFJM, van Riel PLCM, van Erning LJTO, *et al:* Vertebral osteoporosis in rheumatoid arthritis patients: effect of low dose prednisone therapy. *Br J Rheumatol* 31:91-96, 1992.

44. Laan RFJM, van Riel PLCM, van de Putte LBA, *et al:* Low-dose prednisone induces rapid reversible axial bone loss in patients with rheumatoid arthritis: a randomized, controlled study. *Ann Intern Med* 119:963-968, 1993.

45. Linquist PR, McDonnell DE: Rheumatoid cyst causing extradural compression. *J Bone Joint Surg* 52A:1235-1240, 1970.

46. Lipson, SJ: Rheumatoid arthritis in the cervical spine. *Clin Orthop* 239:121-127, 1989.

47. MacKenzie AI, Uttley D, Marsh HT, Bell BA: Craniocervical stabilization using Luque/Hartshill rectangles. *Neurosurgery* 26:32-36, 1990.

48. Magerl F, Seeman PS: Stable posterior fusion of the atlas and axis by transarticular screw fixation. In Kehr P, Weidner A (eds): *The Cervical Spine,* vol 1. New York, Springer-Verlag, 1987, pp 322-327.

49. Magnaes B, Hauge T: Rheumatoid arthritis contributing to lumbar spinal stenosis. *Scand J Rheumatol* 7:215-218, 1978.

50. Marcotte P, Dickman CA, Sonntag VKH, *et al:* Posterior atlantoaxial facet screw fixation. *J Neurosurg* 79:234-237, 1993.

51. Martel W, Abell MR: Fatal atlanto-axial luxation in rheumatoid arthritis. *Arthritis Rheum* 6:224-231, 1963.

52. Mathews JA: Atlanto-axial subluxation in rheumatoid arthritis: a 5-year follow-up study. *Ann Rheum Dis* 33: 526-531, 1974.

53. Menezes AH, van Gilder JC: Transoral-transpharyngeal approach to the anterior craniocervical junction: ten-year experience with 72 patients. *J Neurosurg* 69:895-903, 1988.

54. Menezes AH, van Gilder JC: Anomalies of the craniovertebral junction. In Youmans JR (ed): *Neurological Surgery.* Philadelphia, WB Saunders, 1990, pp 1394-1400.

55. Menezes AH, van Gilder JC, Clark CR, El-Khoury G: Odontoid upward migration in rheumatoid arthritis. *J Neurosurg* 63:500-509, 1985.

56. Messina OD, Barreira JC, Zanchetta JR, *et al:* Effect of low doses of deflazacort vs. prednisone on bone mineral content in premenopausal rheumatoid arthritis. *J Rheumatol* 19:1520-1526, 1992.

57. Mixter SJ, Osgood RB: Traumatic lesions of the atlas and axis. *Ann Surg* 51:193-207, 1910.

58. More J, Sen C: Neurosurgical management of the rheumatoid cervical spine. *Mt Sinai J Med* 61:257-264, 1994.

59. Moskovich R, Crockard HA: Atlantoaxial arthrodesis using interlaminar clamps. *Spine* 17:261-267, 1992.

60. Moskovich R, Crockard HA, Shott S, Ransford AO: Occipitocervical stabilization for myelopathy in patients with rheumatoid arthritis. Implications of not bone-grafting. *J Bone Joint Surg [Am]* 82(3):349-365, 2000.

61. Nakano KK, Schoene WC, Baker RA, Dawson DM: The cervical myelopathy associated with rheumatoid arthritis: analysis of 32 patients, with 2 postmortem cases. *Ann Neurol* 3:144-151, 1978.

62. O'Brien MF, Casey ATH, Crockard HA, *et al:* Histology of the rheumatoid atlantoaxial joints: a clinico-pathologic analysis of 33 operative cases. In Abstracts of the *22nd Annual Meeting of the Cervical Spine Research Society,* Baltimore, 1994, pp 83-84.

63. Papadopoulos SM, Dickman CA, Sonntag VKH: Atlantoaxial stabilization in rheumatoid arthritis. *J Neurosurg* 74:1-7, 1991.

64. Pellicci PM, Ranawat CS, Tsairis P, Bryan WJ: A prospective study of the progression of rheumatoid arthritis of the cervical spine. *J Bone Joint Surg* 63A:342-350, 1981.

65. Peppelman WC, Kraus DR, Donaldson WF III, Agarwal A: Cervical spine surgery in rheumatoid arthritis: improvement of neurologic deficit after cervical spine fusion. *Spine* 18:2375-2379, 1993.

66. Ranawat CS, O'Leary P, Pellicci P, *et al:* Cervical spine fusion in rheumatoid arthritis. *J Bone Joint Surg* 61A: 1003-1010, 1979.

67. Ransford AO, Crockard HA, Pozo JL, *et al:* Craniocervical instability treated by contoured loop fixation. *J Bone Joint Surg* 68B:173-177, 1986.

68. Redlund-Johnell I, Larsson EM: Subluxation of the upper thoracic spine in rheumatoid arthritis. *Skeletal Radiol* 22:105-108, 1993.

69. Redlund-Johnell I, Pettersson H: Radiographic measurements of the cranio-vertebral region. Designed for evaluation of abnormalities in rheumatoid arthritis. *Acta Radiol [Diagn]* 25:23-28, 1984.

70. Robinson BP, Seeger JF, Zak SM: Rheumatoid arthritis and positional vertebrobasilar insufficiency. *J Neurosurg* 65: 111-114, 1986.

71. Rogers MA, Crockard HA, Moskovich R, *et al:* Nystagmus and joint position sensation: their importance in posterior occipitocervical fusion in rheumatoid arthritis. *Spine* 19: 16-20, 1994.

72. Ronderos J, Knightly JJ, Levy DI, *et al:* Stabilization of atlantoaxial instability in rheumatoid arthritis. Published abstract from *62nd Annual Meeting of the American Association of Neurological Surgeons,* San Diego, CA, 1994.

73. Sagher O, Malik JM, Lee JH, *et al:* Fusion with occipital bone for atlantoaxial instability: technical note. *Neurosurgery* 33:926-929, 1993.

74. Sambrook P, Birmingham J, Champion D, *et al:* Postmenopausal bone loss in rheumatoid arthritis: effect of estrogens and androgens. *J Rheumatol* 19:357-361, 1992.

75. Santavirta S, Konttinen YT, Sandelin J, Slatis P: Operations for the unstable cervical spine in rheumatoid arthritis. *Acta Orthop Scand* 61:106-110, 1990.

76. Santavirta S, Konttinen YT, Laasonen E, *et al:* Ten-year results of operations for rheumatoid cervical spine disorders. *J Bone Joint Surg* 73B:116-120, 1991.

77. Sharp J, Purser DW: Spontaneous atlanto-axial dislocation in ankylosing spondylitis and rheumatoid arthritis. *Ann Rheum Dis* 20:47-77, 1961.

78. Simpson JM, An HS, Balderston RA: Complications of surgery of the spine in rheumatoid arthritis and ankylosing spondylitis. In Balderston RA, An HS (eds): *Complications in Spinal Surgery.* Philadelphia, WB Saunders, 1991, pp 169-175.

79. Smith PH, Benn RT, Sharp J: Natural history of rheumatoid cervical luxations. *Ann Rheum Dis* 31:431-439, 1972.

80. Smoker WRK, Keyes WD, Dunn VD, Menezes AH: MRI versus conventional radiologic examinations in the evaluation of the craniovertebral and cervicomedullary junction. *Radiographics* 6:953-994, 1986.

81. Snelling JP, Pickard J, Wood SK, Prouse PJ: Reversible cortical blindness as a complication of rheumatoid arthritis of the cervical spine. *Br J Rheumatol* 29:228-230, 1990.

82. Stambough JL, Balderston RA, Grey S: Technique for occipito-cervical fusion in osteopenic patients. *J Spinal Dis* 3:404-407, 1990.

83. Steinbrocker O, Traeger CH, Batterman RC: Therapeutic criteria in rheumatoid arthritis. *JAMA* 140:659-662, 1949.

84. Stillerman CB, Wilson JA: Atlanto-axial stabilization with posterior transarticular screw fixation: technical description and report of 22 cases. *Neurosurgery* 32:948-955, 1993.

85. Stirrat AN, Fyfe IS: Surgery of the rheumatoid cervical spine. *Clin Orthop* 293:135-143, 1993.

86. van den Brink HR, Lems WF, van Everdingen AA, Bijlsma JWJ: Adjuvant oestrogen treatment increases bone mineral density in postmenopausal women with rheumatoid arthritis. *Ann Rheum Dis* 52:302-305, 1993.

87. van der Horst-Bruinsma IE, Markusse HM, Macfarlane JD, Vielvoye CJ: Rheumatoid discitis with cord compression at the thoracic level. *Br J Rheumatol* 29:65-68, 1990.

88. Weissman BNW, Aliabadi P, Weinfeld MS, *et al:* Prognostic features of atlantoaxial subluxation in rheumatoid arthritis patients. *Radiology* 144:745-751, 1982.

89. Wertheim SB, Bohlman HH: Occipitocervical fusion. *J Bone Joint Surg* 69A:833-836, 1987.

90. White AA, III, Panjabi MM: The clinical biomechanics of the occipitoatlantoaxial complex. *Orthop Clin North Am* 9:867-878, 1978.

91. White AA III, Panjabi MM: *Clinical Biomechanics of the Spine.* Philadelphia, Lippincott-Raven, 1990, pp 92-97, 296.

CHAPTER 57

Ankylosing Spondylitis and Related Disorders

John K. Webb, Patrick W. Hitchon, and Dilip K. Sengupta

Ankylosing spondylitis is a chronic inflammatory disease that affects the axial skeleton, causing pain and progressive stiffness and deformity. Strumpell[84] in 1897, and Marie[57] in 1898, first described the rheumatologic entity now known as ankylosing spondylitis. In the past ankylosing spondylitis has been referred to as von Bechterew's arthritis, rheumatoid spondylitis, pelvospondylitis ossificans, and spondylitis ankylopoietica. Rheumatologists in the United States officially adopted the term "ankylosing spondylitis" in 1963.[10]

Ankylosing spondylitis is a member of seronegative spondyloarthropathies. In the 1970s, a group of British authors from Leeds suggested that some of the diseases considered seronegative "variants of classic rheumatoid arthritis" are so closely interrelated that they may be included in a single group: the seronegative spondyloarthritidis.[65] All the members of this group of diseases are closely related to ankylosing spondylitis and include Reiter's syndrome and reactive arthritis, psoriatic arthritis, arthritis associated with inflammatory bowel disease, plus other undifferentiated forms that do not meet the criteria for definitive category. The common features of seronegative spondyloarthropathies include negative tests for rheumatoid factors, absence of subcutaneous (rheumatoid) nodules, radiologic sacroiliitis with or without spondylitis (often asymmetrical), peripheral inflammatory arthritis, evidence of clinical "overlap" between group members, and tendency to familial aggregation.[69] A detailed classification criteria for the entire group of the seronegative spondyloarthropathy has been described by Amor et al.,[2] and by the European Spondylarthropathy Study Group (ESSG).[23]

Prevalence of seronegative spondyloarthropathies, including ankylosing spondylitis, are directly correlated with prevalence of HLA-B27 in the population.[47] Ankylosing spondylitis is virtually nonexistent in African blacks who do not possess the B27 antigen. In contrast, highest prevalence of the disease (4.5%) is found in Canadian Haida Indians whose 50% population is B27 positive. Among the Europeans, the prevalence of B27 antigen in the general population ranges between 3% and 13%, and the prevalence of ankylosing spondylitis is estimated at 0.1% to 0.23%.[69]

Over 90% of patients with ankylosing spondylitis are HLA-B27 positive. The risk of an antigen-positive individual developing ankylosing spondylitis is under 2%.[15] However, if a patient is antigen-positive and also has a family history of ankylosing spondylitis, the likelihood of developing the clinical syndrome is 20%.[51,92]

Pathogenesis

The discovery that HLA-B27 is linked to ankylosing spondylitis (AS) and other seronegative spondyloarthropathies has provided new approaches to the study of the possible causation of these diseases. Experimental evidence suggests that HLA-B27 is itself involved in the pathogenesis of seronegative spondyloarthropathies. Population and peptide-specificity analysis of HLA-B27 suggest it has a pathogenic function related to antigen presentation.[56] Several theories have been proposed to explain these associations but only one, namely molecular mimicry, has provided a specific etiological agent for these diseases. *Klebsiella pneumoniae* shares a sequence of six consecutive amino acids with the HLA-B27 antigen. Elevated immune responses to *Klebsiella* microbes have been demonstrated in AS patients from 10 different countries. This wide geographic distribution suggests that the same etiological agent is probably related in producing this condition.[24] The HLA-B27 antigen may distinguish a group of people whose immune response to such an infectious agent predisposes them to develop spondyloarthropathy through the phenomenon of molecular mimicry.

Whether ankylosing spondylitis is caused by these bacteria can only be resolved by tissue typing all the patients early in the course of their disease and then assessing their response to antibiotic chemotherapy in longitudinal studies involving double-blind crossover trials. It is possible that in the future, the course of AS could be modified by adequate antibiotic chemotherapy or even diets that affect the substrates on which these bacteria grow.[24]

Pathology

The earliest lesion in AS is at the sacroiliac joint[11] (Figure 57.1). The lumbar spine is usually involved progressively upward. Skip lesions may occur, especially in women.[59] Hips and shoulders are affected frequently, but peripheral joints are rarely involved.

Although the synovium is the primary site of joint disease in rheumatoid arthritis, the primary site in the spondyloarthropathy is less well-defined.[6] Ball[4] claimed that enthesitis (inflammation at sites where ligaments, tendons, or joint capsules are attached to bone) is the hallmark of ankylosing spondylitis and other spondyloarthropathies. Synovitis is secondary to liberation of proinflammatory mediators from the enthesis.[58] Francois et al.[31] believe that the course of events is more complex than earlier claimed, and may be a combination of enthesitis, synovitis, and subchondral marrow changes, followed by fibrosis, cartilage metaplasia and ossification; none can thus far be distinguished as a unique hallmark.

In the early stages, chronic inflammatory cells localize to the subchondral bone at the sites of ligament attachment in the sacroiliac joints and discovertebral joints, resulting in periarticular osteopenia. Enthesitis at the insertion of the annulus fibrosus on the vertebral bodies in the erosive phase result in square appearance of the vertebra on lateral radiographs (Figure 57.2) As the disease progresses, articular cartilage is destroyed by osteoclasts and replaced by granulation tissue, which in radiograph show extensive erosion and destruction of the joint space.

In the late stage, granulation tissues are replaced with fibrous tissue that undergoes ossification and completely obliterates the joint, leading to "bamboo," or "poker," spine[21] (Figure 57.3). Surprisingly, the anterior longitudinal ligament remains free from ossification.

The sequence of events in the synovial joints between the facets, caudal part of the sacroiliac joints, and the peripheral joints resembles rheumatoid arthritis, although the exact target of inflammatory changes and the nature of

cellular exudates may differ.[31] Proliferation of synovial tissue and accumulation of plasma cells and lymphocytes at the joint margin lead to formation of pannus, which infiltrates and destroys the articular cartilage and the subchondral bone. This is followed by fibrosis and later, bony ankylosis in the reparative phase.

Extraskeletal involvement is seen in the iris, myocardium and aorta, lungs, and kidneys.[35,74] Fibrosis of the septum and the atrioventricular bundle may cause conduction defects. Focal necrosis at the root of the aorta often leads to dilatation of the aortic ring, causing aortic incompetence.

Clinical Manifestations

Seronegative spondyloarthropathies have common clinical and radiologic signs that are sacroiliitis, inflammatory spinal pain, peripheral arthritis and enthesitis, dactylitis, chest wall pain, aortic incompetence together with conduction disturbances, conjunctivitis, uveitis, and lesions of the lung apices. All of these may also occur in isolation.[69]

Ankylosing spondylitis often occurs in young adults between ages 17 and 35. Although usually thought to be more common in men, the disease also frequently affects women but with less severe involvement.[15] The juvenile-onset ankylosing spondylitis, with the onset of symptoms earlier than 16 years, has a higher incidence of hip disease. Patients with hip joint involvement show a faster progression of the spinal disease. In absence of hip disease, there is little difference between juvenile-onset and adult-onset ankylosing spondylitis in severity of spinal and extraskeletal manifestations.[14]

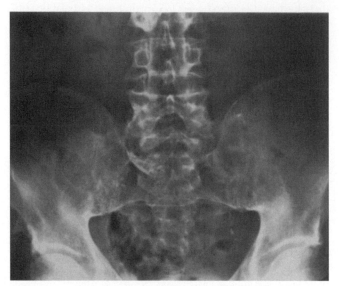

Figure 57.1 Early changes in ankylosing spondylitis with obliteration of the sacroiliac joints with maintenance of the vertebral end plates.

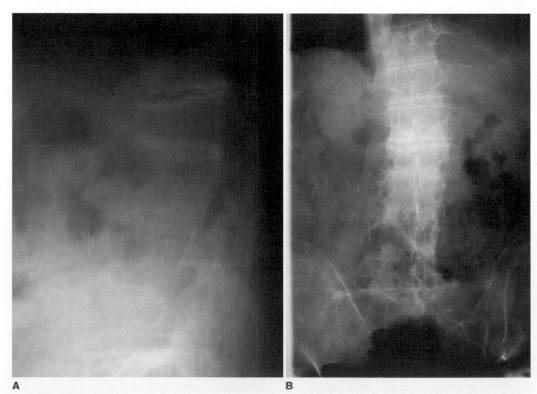

A   **B**

Figure 57.2 (A,B) Advanced changes in ankylosing spondylitis with vertebral osteoporosis, squaring of vertebral bodies, and Andersson lesion (spondylodiscitis).

Inflammatory back pain distinguishes itself from mechanical back pain by insidious onset before age 40, pain persisting for at least 3 months, morning stiffness, and improvement with exercise. Buttock pain typically alternates from side to side. Pain and stiffness in the cervical spine generally starts at a later stage.[16]

Incidence of peripheral joint involvement is 20% to 40%. Peripheral arthritis in spondyloarthritis is oligoarticular, asymmetric, and often affects hips or shoulders. Temporomandibular joint pain and stiffness occur in about 10% of patients. Less frequently involved joints include knees, ankles, elbows, and wrists. Involvement of hip joint is more important from the clinical viewpoint, since hip disease is far more disabling than spinal rigidity.[69]

Painful peripheral enthesitis often involve heel insertion of the Achilles tendon and plantar fascia. Other sites of enthesitis include superior and inferior poles of patella, tibial tubercle, pubic attachment of adductor longus, femoral trochanters, humeral epicondyles, and nuchal crests.

With the progress of the disease the spine is gradually ankylosed with a generalized kyphotic deformity. To maintain upright posture the patient hyperextends the hips and flexes the knees. Involvement of the hip joints seriously compromises the compensatory postures. Hyperextension of the cervical spine helps in maintaining the forward gaze. In advanced cases, when cervical spine becomes ankylosed in flexion, forward gaze and jaw opening are affected.

As the disease process immobilizes the spine, the majority of painful symptoms resolve. The inflammatory process tends to become inactive as bony ankylosis sets in, in the late fourth or fifth decade.[18]

Rarely, patients with ankylosing spondylitis develop cauda equina syndrome. One large study demonstrated neurologic symptoms only in 2.1% of 290 patients.[25] Unlike in lumbar disc herniation, the cauda equina syndrome in ankylosing spondylitis develops insidiously, and a high index of suspicion is necessary to make the diagnosis. In a meta-analysis of 52 papers reporting 86 patients of ankylosing spondylitis with cauda equina syndrome, Ahn et al.[1] found that only 22% complained of radicular symptoms and only 10% complained of back pain, and as many as 30% of the male patients had undergone prostate surgery before the realization that the cause of incontinence was not secondary to prostate but rather to the condition of the cauda equina. The polyradiculopathy or cauda equina syndrome may not be a result of skeletal changes but are associated with dilatation of the dural sac and the formation of thecal diverticula. There may be large arachnoid cysts that have eroded through the lamina and even into the spinous processes. The pathogenesis is not well understood.[76]

Radiologic Features

Radiographic changes are minimal in the early stages. Technetium 99m bone scan may demonstrate the sacroiliitis before radiographic changes.[75] Symmetric bilateral patchy areas of osteoporosis along the ill-defined sacroiliac joint are often suggestive of early disease. Later, subchondral erosions followed by patchy areas of ossifications develop that eventually lead to obliteration of the sacroiliac joint.

An early radiologic feature is squaring of the anterior corners of the thoracic and lumbar vertebrae due to osteopenia at the attachment of the anterior annulus. Vertebral osteopenia also accompanies the loss of normal concavity of the end plates.[37] Ossification extends within the substance of the annulus forming syndesmophytes, which bridges the adjacent vertebral bodies and develops into the bamboo spine in late stages[5] (Figure 57.3). Posterior vertebral structures are also ossified. These include the capsule of the facet joints, supraspinous and interspinous ligaments, and ligamentum flavum.

In the subaxial cervical spine, extensive ankylosis with varying degrees of kyphosis is seen in the advanced stages. In contrast, the upper cervical spine may demonstrate hypermobility resulting from atlantoaxial instability.[7]

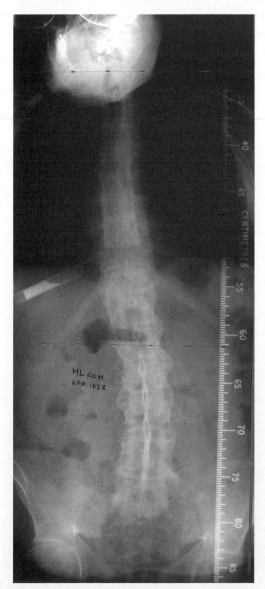

Figure 57.3 Advanced changes in ankylosing spondylitis with appearance of "bamboo spine" and obliteration of the sacroiliac joint.

Surgical Conditions Involving the Spine

The natural history of ankylosing spondylitis is benign in many cases. In a group of patients followed over a 35-year period, 92% remained functionally active, 68% had lifelong back problems, and only 41% of patients were affected by some degree of spinal immobility.[18] Most patients with ankylosing spondylitis do not require surgical intervention.

In a review of 33 patients with ankylosing spondylitis who required surgery at the Mayo Clinic, spinal fractures (traumatic or pseudarthrosis), progressive spinal deformity, rotary instability secondary to atlantooccipital or atlantoaxial subluxation, and spinal stenosis with associated neurologic deficit, pain, or spinal instability were the most common indications for surgery. In this series of 41 operations performed, 17 were of the cervical spine, 14 of the thoracic spine, and 10 of the lumbar spine.[30] Rarely, development of cauda equina syndrome may indicate surgical intervention.

Spinal Fractures

Spinal fractures in ankylosing spondylitis are pathologic fractures and differ from fractures in normal spine in many aspects. These fractures (1) often result after trivial trauma, (2) are usually highly unstable and displace more frequently, (3) almost always involve all three columns, (4) are more often associated with neurologic complications, and (5) are associated with epidural bleeding.[9]

Patients with ankylosing spondylitis are more prone to developing spinal fractures[20,34,43,68] secondary to osteoporosis and altered biomechanics. Generalized osteoporosis weakens the spine. The ankylosis makes it less resilient to absorb energy efficiently after an injury. The apex of normal thoracic kyphosis is usually at T7. The apex shifts distally, close to the thoracolumbar junction as a result of global kyphotic deformity in ankylosing spondylitis, rendering the junction more susceptible to fracture after an injury.

The spine in ankylosing spondylitis is stiff, brittle, and deformed in kyphosis. Because of ossification of all the ligaments and discs in advanced stage, the spine resembles the diaphysis of a long bone. When it fractures, everything fractures; there is no soft tissue left to support the spine, leaving the fracture highly unstable (Figure 57.4). The fracture classification systems developed for normal spines are therefore not applicable.[68] The fracture opens up in extension or flexion, depending on the position of the patient.

Neurologic deficit is frequent. Many reports suggest that it could be as high as 75%.[34,43] In a review of 31 consecutive patients with fractures in ankylosing spondylitis, Olerud et al.[68] reported immediate neurologic impairment

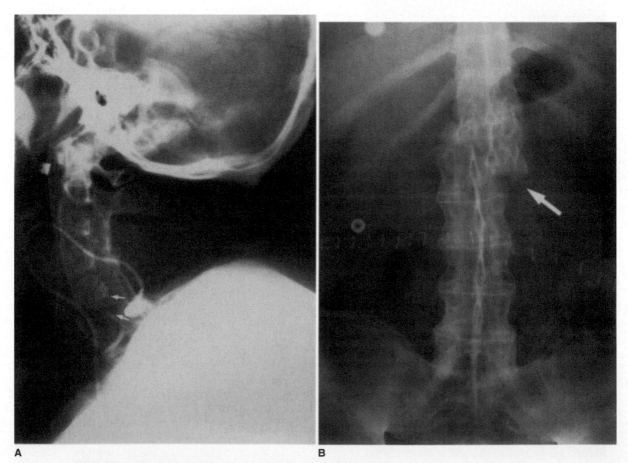

A   **B**

Figure 57.4 This 52-year-old patient showed symptoms of shock secondary to intraabdominal infection. Emergency attempt to intubate and give cardiopulmonary resuscitation resulted in both (**A**) cervical and (**B**) thoracic fractures.

in one third of patients and a further one third developed neurologic impairment subsequently. The secondary neurologic deterioration could be a result of epidural bleeding,[9,68] but more commonly result from displacement of the fracture. Displacement in hyperextension is considered to be most dangerous for neurologic impairment.[9,68,85] Because of the kyphotic deformity, the spine tends to displace in hyperextension when the patient lies in a supine position.[68]

The mean age of spinal fractures in ankylosing spondylitis patients is around the sixth decade.[30,68] The mid-cervical spine is the most frequent site of fracture, followed by the thoracolumbar junction.[43,68,96] Radiologic demonstration of the fractures may be difficult because of osteopenia and associated deformities.[66,96] Patients with a history of back or neck pain after trivial trauma or sudden progression of deformity should undergo a thorough radiologic evaluation including CT scan, and the clinician should have a very high index of suspicion for occult fracture (Figure 57.5). Multiple fractures are a strong consideration in patients with ankylosing spondylitis, and the coexistence of cervical and thoracic fractures has been demonstrated clearly in this patient population[30,68] (Figure 57.4).

Complications are frequent following spinal fracture. Most reports in the literature[86,98] suggest associated morbidity rate around 50% and mortality rate around 20% to 30%[68,86,98] after spinal fracture. Pulmonary involvement is particularly high among medical complications and often needs ventilatory support with or without tracheostomy. Vascular injuries such as aortic rupture have been reported in fractures resulting from higher-energy trauma.[77,78,88] Aortic root disease and connective tissue inelasticity predisposes to vascular injury. Even low-energy trauma may lead to significant paraspinal hemorrhage, hemothorax,[44] or epidural hematoma.[13,29,42,91,101]

Cervical Spine Fractures

Minimally displaced cervical spine fractures may be treated conservatively. Satisfactory results have been reported with prolonged bed rest either in traction or in a cervical collar[3,34,43] or early mobilization in a halo vest if the fracture segment remains stable.[67,98] It is important to follow up periodically with radiograph to recognize persistent movement or progressive subluxation, which indicate surgical stabilization. Many authors have found that nonoperative immobilization alone is difficult and frequently inadequate because of marked instability. Neurologic deterioration may result from distraction,[73] with simple maneuvers like transfer to a stretcher[98] or during halo-vest application.[30,98]

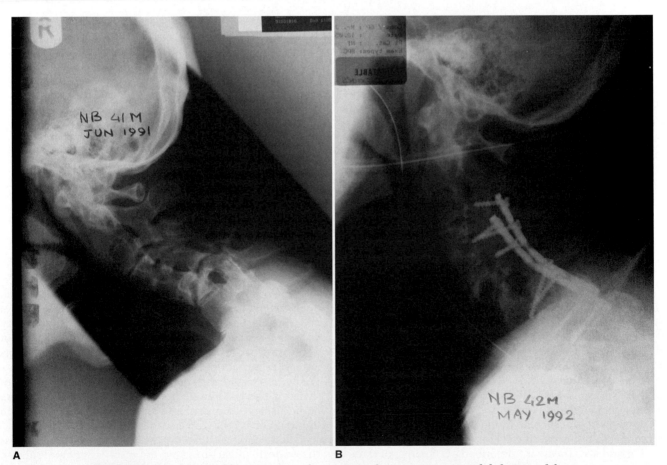

A **B**

Figure 57.5 This 41-year-old patient showed symptoms of progressive pain and deformity of the cervical spine with no history of trauma. (**A**) X-ray showed a fracture at the lower cervical spine. (**B**) Initial posterior fixation alone failed.

Continued

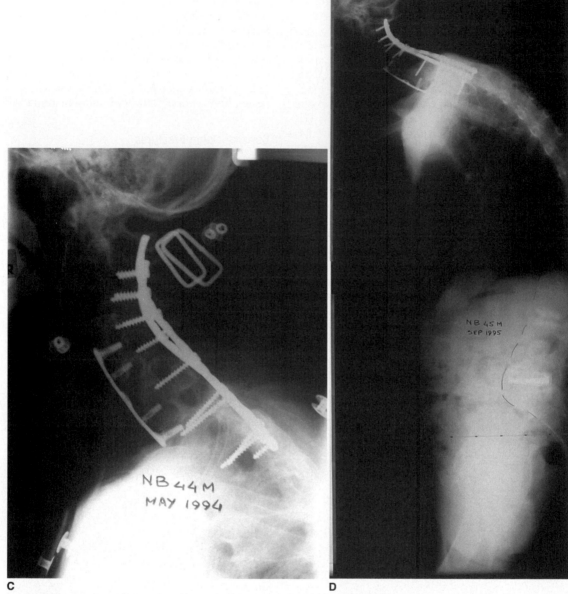

C   D

Figure 57.5 *cont'd* (C) The fracture healed only after subsequent anterior fixation and bone
grafting, revision of the posterior fixation, and additional external support for 3 months. A year
later he returned with increasing back pain and progressive kyphotic deformity.

Because of frequent incidence of neurologic deterioration, failure of union, or inadequate immobilization at the
fracture site with conservative treatment, many authors°
support surgical stabilization as the treatment of choice. For
the minimally displaced fractures in the Mayo Clinic series,
Fox *et al.*[30] recommended posterior spinous process wiring
with bone graft onlay followed by 3 to 6 months of external
immobilization. Most authors[22,30] recommend additional
external immobilization using halo or cervicothoracic brace
following posterior surgery. Immobilization in a cervical collar may result in failed surgical fusion.[98]

Taggard and Traynelis[86] described a technique of three-
point internal fixation combining lateral mass plate and

interspinous wiring, spanning at least two levels above and
below the fracture. Postoperatively they used only cervical
collar support and could avoid the need for a halo vest.
Lateral mass screw placement is difficult in this patient
population because the usual landmarks of the facet joints
are lost as a result of bony ankylosis. Extrapolation from a
recognizable landmark may be necessary to find the point
of screw entry. As an additional measure of safety, these
authors suggested use of screws 14mm or shorter in length
to avoid nerve root damage.

Dorsal stabilization alone may not be adequate unless
the anterior load-bearing column is competent. In
ankylosing spondylitis the disc is usually calcified, and
additional anterior stabilization or bone grafting is not
necessary. However, in the patient who has had a

°References 8,9,22,30,68,86.

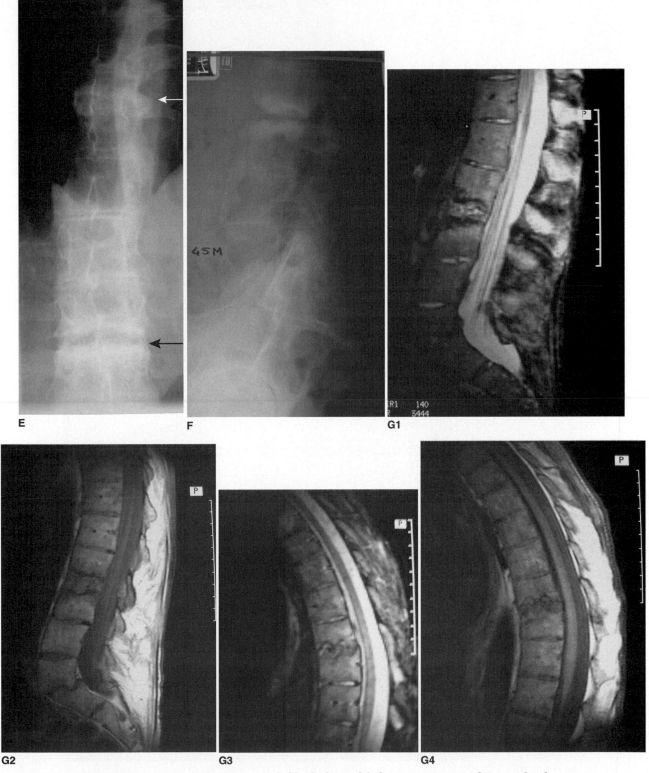

Figure 57.5 *cont'd* (D,E,F) X-rays revealed he had spondylodiscitis at T10-11 and at L2-3 levels.
(G1-G4) MRI scans more clearly diagnose these lesions and may also help to rule out any cord
compression, which is common.   *Continued*

subacute or chronic fracture with instability and
pseudarthrosis formation, it may be appropriate to
remove this granulation tissue and replace it with the
patient's own bone.[86] Anterior stabilization in the cervical
spine may be difficult in the presence of flexion deformity at the cervicothoracic junction.

Loss of fixation is a major concern in this patient group
because of osteopenia. In a review of 31 cases Olerud
et al.[68] reported three cases of loss of fixation out of 10
with "one side only" (anterior or posterior) approach. In
contrast, they found no loss of fixation in seven cases with
combined anterior and posterior stabilization. A combined

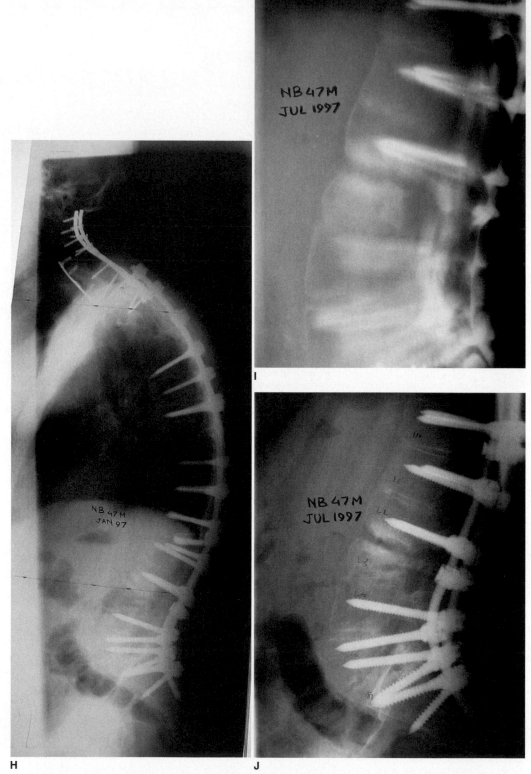

H   J

Figure 57.5 *cont'd* (H) Initial treatment was posterior stabilization of the whole spine, with correction of the deformity by compression at the spondylodiscitis levels and additional posterior polysegmental closing wedge osteotomies at the thoracic spine. Two years follow-up showed nonunion **(I,J)**.

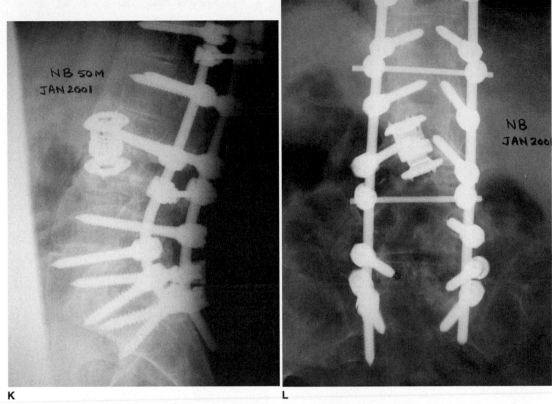

Figure 57.5 *cont'd* (**K,L**) Revision anterior surgery with excision of the pseudoarthritic tissue, and reconstruction of the anterior column with Synex Cage® and autogenous bone graft achieved union despite cage migration into the osteoporotic vertebral body.

Continued

approach has also been recommended by others in the recent literature.[26,95]

Upper Cervical Spine Fractures

Although the mid-cervical spine is the commonest site of fracture in ankylosing spondylitis, less commonly the proximal cervical spine may be involved. This may be in the form of acute fracture through the dens or chronic subluxation or ankylosis of the atlantoaxial joint or atlantooccipital joint resulting from erosive changes. Bony ankylosis of the atlantooccipital joint or the lower cervical spine may make the odontoid susceptible to fracture after minor trauma.[64,70] Spontaneous fracture of the odontoid without history of trauma may occur only after severe neurologic deficit.[48] Most of these injuries may be treated by halo-jacket immobilization alone[46] or in combination with posterior occipitocervical fusion.[48,70]

Thoracic and Lumbar Spine Fractures

Fractures in the thoracic and lumbar spine involve all three columns and are inherently unstable with a high possibility of secondary neurologic deterioration. Displacements are common, particularly toward hyperextension when the patient is positioned supine.[68,89] Surgical stabilization is therefore mandatory.

Trent *et al.*[89] suggested that reduction of the displacement and stabilization is best achieved with a Luque rectangular rod system, and laminectomy is not indicated.

Compression across the fracture site is desirable for union, and it is difficult to achieve by Luque system. A pedicle screw/hook and rod system like Cotrel-Dubousset instrumentation or Universal Spinal System may provide more stable posterior fixation. Reduction of the fracture may be achieved by positioning the patient on the table. Fracture site may be used at surgery to correct the kyphotic deformity, with caution, when it occurs below the level of the spinal cord. Hyperextension must be avoided; possible neurologic damage after anesthesia and positioning on the operation table has been reported.[68] Simmons[82] indicated that if the weight bearing can be shifted to posterior to the fracture site, uncomplicated healing should be expected.

In a retrospective review of 266 cases at the University of Iowa by one of the authors (PH), 11 cases of fractures (six thoracic and five lumbar) were identified. All the fractures were unstable involving three columns, and all but one resulted from trivial injuries like ground level falls or during patient transfers from bed to trolley. Nine cases developed hyperextension deformity and six cases had neurologic deficit on admission. Nine cases were treated by surgical stabilization using hooks and/or pedicle screws (Figure 57.6), and two of them had an additional anterior stabilization. Only two cases were treated conservatively. All cases had external orthosis for an average of 5 months. Neurologic deficit improved in three cases by at least one Frankel grade and remained unchanged in the other three. Correction of kyphotic deformity could be achieved in seven of the nine operated cases with an average 12 ± 10 degrees (SD).

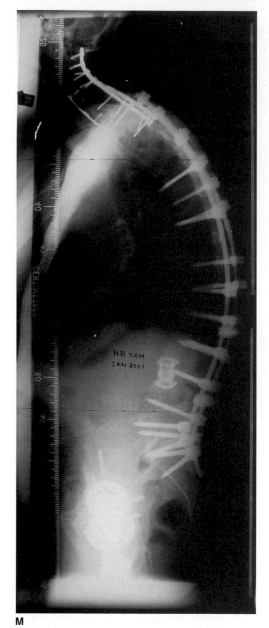

Figure 57.5 *cont'd* (**M**) End result was satisfactory.

Unrecognized or untreated fractures may contribute to the development of the typical flexion deformity or pseudarthrosis. In the presence of an anterior column defect or pseudarthrosis, strong consideration has to be given to operating both ventrally (to remove the granulation tissue and bone grafting) and dorsally (to stabilize with wires or instrumentation and again add additional bone). Even after a combined ventral and dorsal procedure, further immobilization of the patient with a body cast or TLSO should be considered.

Spinal Deformity

A progressive generalized kyphotic deformity is typical in ankylosing spondylitis. Osteopenia and fractures further worsen the kyphosis. Flexion deformity results in loss of sagittal balance and difficulty in forward gaze. In the early

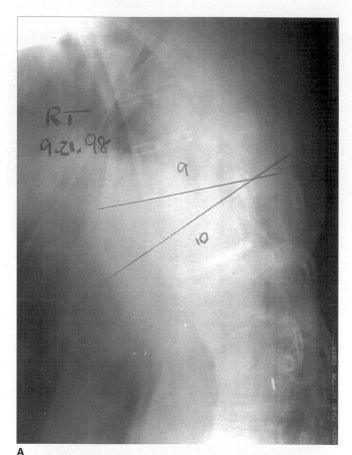

A

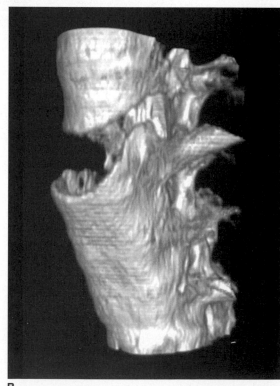

B

Figure 57.6 (**A**) Lateral radiograph reveals an extension fracture at T9-10 in a 44-year-old man with paraparesis involved in a car accident. He also sustained an unstable extension fracture at C6-7 necessitating anteroposterior cervical spine instrumentation. (**B**) Three-dimensional CT scan shows the three-column extension fracture across the caudal end of T9 and facets with posterior dislocation of T9 relative to T10.

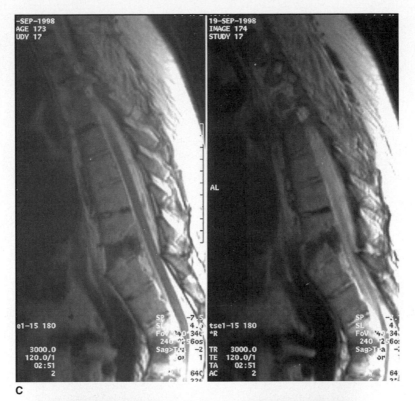

C

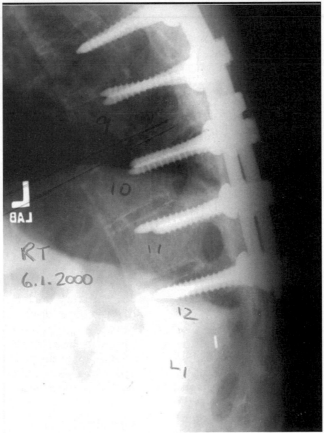

D

Figure 57.6 *cont'd* (**C**) Sagittal T2-weighted MRI shows the posterior compression of the spinal cord by the T10 lamina. (**D**) Postoperative lateral radiograph at 2-years' follow-up shows posterior fixation with pedicle screws and rods from T8-10.

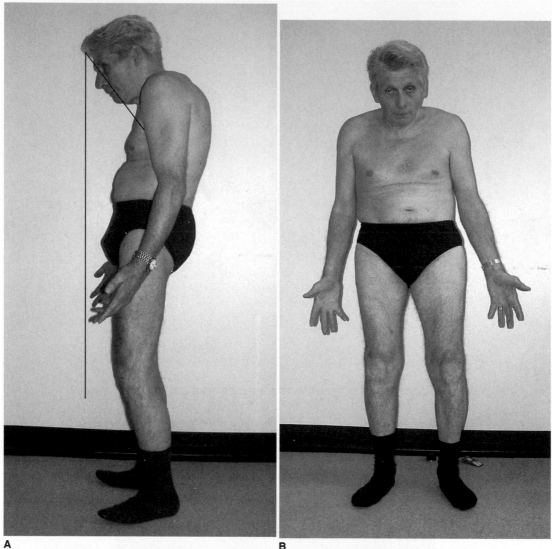

A   **B**

Figure 57.7 In the presence of global kyphosis, patients tend to lean backward, with flexion of the knees and hyperextension of the hips to regain the sagittal balance and achieve forward gaze. Gaze angle is measured as (**A**) chin-brow to vertical angle. (**B**) The eyeball rolls upward to further compensate for the forward gaze. The compensatory mechanisms should be taken care of before deformity planning. The gaze angle correction and posterior shift of the plumb line should be estimated from a lateral radiograph taken when the patient stands with relaxed hips, extended knees, and looks forward with eyeballs in the middle.

phase of the disease, patients try to compensate their sagittal balance by hyperextension of the hips and flexion of the knees. Hyperextension of the cervical spine helps to maintain forward gaze. When hips are involved with the disease, fixed flexion deformity develops and further interferes with the sagittal balance. In advanced stages of the disease the cervical spine is ankylosed, resulting in a global kyphotic deformity, interfering severely with compensation of the gaze angle. Severe kyphotic deformities may produce compression of the abdominal viscera and limitation of the pulmonary function by restriction of the diaphragmatic excursion.

Indications for Deformity Correction

Surgical intervention is indicated when kyphosis is decompensated. This means the patient cannot maintain a horizontal gaze when the hips and knees are extended and eyeballs are in the neutral position[32] (Figure 57.7). In practice, however, the general condition of the patient, the feasibility of correction and perhaps above all else, the morale and earnest desire of the patient to accept the risks and rehabilitative measures required for correction become more important decisive factors before considering surgery.

Preoperative Planning

Perhaps the most important step before surgical correction of deformity is planning of surgery. The goals are (1) restoration of sagittal balance, (2) correction of gaze angle, and (3) the safety of the procedure.

The level of osteotomy to correct a global kyphotic deformity has a disparate effect on gaze angle and sagittal balance (Figure 57.8). Sagittal balance is restored by redirecting the

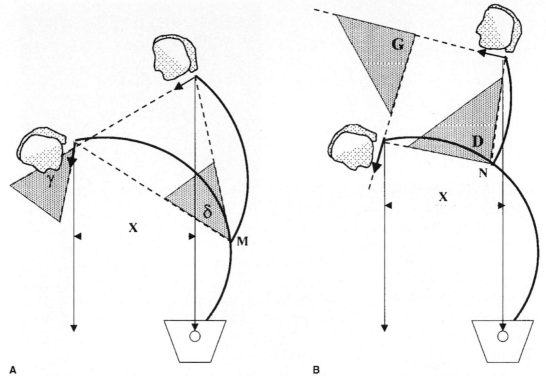

A   B

Figure 57.8 Level of osteotomy has a disparate effect on sagittal balance and gaze angle. Restoration of sagittal balance is achieved by posterior shift of the plumb line (X). The correction of the gaze angle (γ and G) is always the same as the corresponding osteotomy angle (δ and D), respectively. $\delta = \gamma$ and D=G. **(M)** When osteotomy is performed at a lower level, **(A)** an osteotomy angle δ is needed for restoration of the sagittal balance (X). When osteotomy is performed at a higher level (N), **(B)** a larger osteotomy angle (D) is needed (D> δ) for the same degree of sagittal balance restoration. Because osteotomy angle is always same as the gaze angle correction (D=G), the correction of the gaze angle will be larger (G> γ) with a higher level of osteotomy. This may lead to overcorrection of the gaze angle upward. *(From Sengupta DK, Khazim R, Grevitt MP, Webb JK: Flexion osteotomy of the cervical spine: a new technique for correction of iatrogenic extension deformity in ankylosing spondylitis. Spine 26:1068-1072, 2001.)*

spine posteriorly at the level of osteotomy so that the head lies vertically above the pelvis. The angle by which the spine is redirected at the osteotomy site (the osteotomy angle) for full restoration of the sagittal balance depends on the level of osteotomy. When the osteotomy is performed at a higher level, the osteotomy angle must be greater than that required for osteotomy at a lower level in the spine to achieve the same degree of correction in the sagittal balance.[52,80] In contrast, the visual angle (by which the gaze is redirected forward) will always be the same as the osteotomy angle, irrespective of the level of the osteotomy.

As mentioned earlier, in presence of global kyphosis in ankylosis spondylitis, patients try to extend their hips and flex their knees as much as possible to correct the sagittal balance and also to achieve a forward gaze. An estimate of gaze angle and sagittal balance correction from the lateral radiograph taken in this posture will underestimate both these parameters (Figure 57.7). The simple way to resolve this problem is to take the lateral radiograph when the patient stands with relaxed hips, without making an effort to correct the spinal balance or forward gaze. The degree of gaze angle correction needed is determined by the Chin-brow to vertical angle.[81] This is an angle between the

line drawn from the chin to the brow and a vertical line (Figure 57.7A). The sagittal balance correction is estimated from the degree of posterior shift of the plumb line required to bring it back to the sacrum.

Van Royen *et al.*[94] described a precise method for planning deformity correction, which involves the use of mathematical analysis with trigonometric equations, to construct a nomogram for individual patient. However, practical application of such an accurate estimate of the angle of osteotomy would require "a more exact and controllable surgical procedure," and special measurement device like "a customized mechanical or computer-assisted goniometer to measure the closing wedge osteotomy" during surgery. None of these is currently available.

The authors estimate the angle of osteotomy needed for a given level of osteotomy, usually at L2-3 level, to achieve posterior shift of the plumb line over the sacrum, from a cut-out of a transparent paper tracing over the full-length lateral radiograph (Figure 57.9). If this angle appears to be smaller than the estimated gaze angle correction, additional smaller osteotomies are planned at a higher level, which has a greater effect on the shift of the

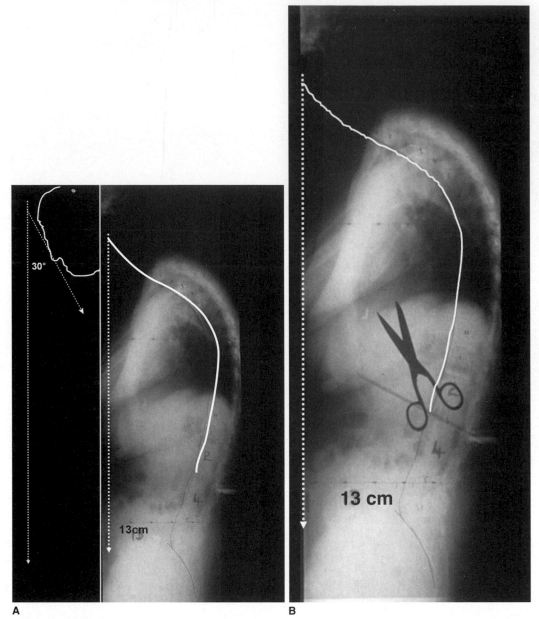

A   **B**

Figure 57.9 Preoperative planning for deformity correction. Chin-brow to vertical angle in this case measures 30 degrees. **(A)** The sagittal vertical axis drops 13cm in front of the S-1. **(B)** A silhouette of the spine is drawn on a tracing paper, and the level of the osteotomy is marked at L3 vertebra.

gaze angle than the shift of the plumb line. This usually involves a cervicothoracic osteotomy at a later date. On the other hand, when the estimated osteotomy angle appears to be too large to be obtained from a single level of osteotomy, a multisegmental osteotomy is planned. The largest osteotomy angle is planned at the lumbar level, and smaller angles at one or more thoracic levels; the sum total angular correction should match the estimated gaze angle correction.

Presence of hip flexion deformity severely affects both the sagittal balance and the gaze angle, and this must be corrected by total hip replacement before spinal osteotomy is undertaken.

When both lumbar and cervical osteotomy is needed, we perform the lumbar osteotomy in the first stage, achieving maximum correction of the sagittal balance. Cervical osteotomy is performed subsequently for fine-tuning the sagittal balance and gaze angle correction.

Lumbar Osteotomy—Historical Aspects and Types of Osteotomy

The different techniques of osteotomy described in the lumbar spine may be classified in three basic types:

A. *Ventral monosegmental open wedge osteotomy* (Figure 57.10). In this technique a large wedge of bone is

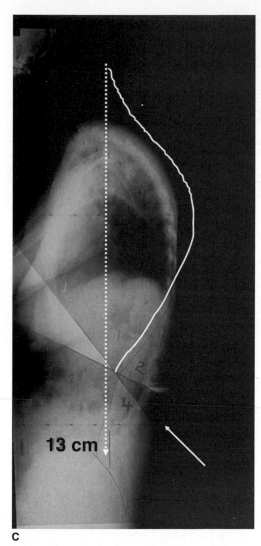

C

Figure 57.9 *cont'd* (C) The tracing paper is now cut at the level of osteotomy and rotated backward, centering the anterior border of the L3 vertebra, until the projected plumb line drops over the sacrum. The angle of rotation gives an estimate of the angle of osteotomy needed to restore the sagittal balance, which is 28 degrees in this case. This osteotomy will also correct the gaze angle by 28 degrees, which is close to full correction of the chin-brow to vertical angle in this case. If larger gaze angle correction would be required, additional cervical osteotomy or polysegmental thoracic osteotomy might be planned instead. The arrow indicates the amount of bone to be resected from the posterior elements of the spine, which on closure after osteoclasis at the anterior border of L3 will reproduce the effect of the osteotomy as planned.

resected from the posterior elements including the lamina and the facet joints and pedicle in the lumbar spine, usually at L2 level, just below the level of the spinal cord. The wedge is then closed by hyperextension of the spine with manual pressure. This manipulation causes disruption of the anterior longitudinal ligament and opens up a large gap in the anterior aspect of the vertebral column. This was the earliest technique described by Smith-Petersen *et al.*[83] in 1945 in six patients. They performed two- or three-level osteotomies through the facet joints at L1-3 levels, and closed the gap by osteoclasis of the vertebral body. Le

Chapple[53] described a similar technique in two stages; laminectomy at L2 under local anesthesia followed by anterior open-wedge osteotomy at L2-3 and bone grafting 2 weeks later. Many modifications of anterior open wedge osteotomy has been described since that time.* The main disadvantage of this technique was serious vascular and neurologic complications resulting from sudden elongation of the anterior column during closed osteoclasis maneuver and a large anterior opening of a monosegmental procedure.[17,41,49,54,97] The mortality rates up to 12% and complication rates up to 50% are not unusual.[32] The angular correction achieved by monosegmental wedge correction is around 40 degrees.[93]

B. *Polysegmental wedge osteotomy* (Figure 57.11). In this technique multiple posterior lumbar wedge osteotomies are made through the facet joints. Closing these wedges by osteoclasis gives a more gradual correction and creates only small bony defects anteriorly, thus avoiding the serious vascular and neurologic complications.

Wilson and Turkell[99] first reported polysegmental osteotomy in one patient in 1949. Zielke[36,38,71] described polysegmental osteotomies, usually four to six levels between T12-L1 and L4-5, using instrumentation, initially with Harrington and later with pedicle screws. The mortality rates as low as 4% and complication rates of about 27% have been reported.[32] The total degree of correction achieved may be the same as with open wedge osteotomy, which corresponds to about 10 degrees per level of osteotomy.

C. *Lumbar closing wedge osteotomy* (Figure 57.12). In this technique the posterior element of one vertebra including the lamina, facet joints, pedicles, and the posterior wedge of the vertebral body are resected by transpedicular decancellation procedure. The wedge is closed by hyperextension of the lumbar spine, hinging on the anterior cortex of the vertebral body.

Since there is no elongation of the anterior column, and correction is slow, serious complications are rare. The consolidation at the osteotomy site is rapid. However, the degree of angular correction achieved is less compared to the previous two techniques. This technique was initially described by Scudese *et al,*[79] but later popularized by Thomasen[87] in 1985. This technique is particularly beneficial in patients with advanced sclerosis of the large vessels.

Ideally, kyphotic deformity is best corrected when the osteotomy is placed at the site of maximum deformity. In practice, however, thoracic osteotomy is not preferred even when the maximum deformity is in the thoracic spine, since the rigid thorax limits correction, and the greater risk of spinal cord damage. Pelvic osteotomy to achieve sagittal balance of the trunk has been reported but has never been popular.[100] The most preferred site for osteotomy is below the level of the spinal cord in the lumbar spine to avoid serious neurologic complication, irrespective of the location of maximum kyphosis.

Zielke[32] emphasized that polysegmental osteotomy, besides minimizing vascular and neurologic complications, achieves a harmonious correction that satisfactorily corrects the thoracic hyperkyphosis. Using relatively weak

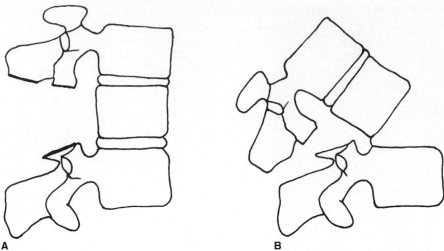

Figure 57.10 Diagrams of the opening wedge osteotomy. **(A)** Lateral view outlining the bone block to be resected. **(B)** Postoperative lateral view showing how correction is achieved by closure of the posterior elements and creating an open wedge of the anterior column. *(From Van Royen BJ, De Gast A: Lumbar osteotomy for correction of thoracolumbar kyphotic deformity in ankylosing spondylitis: a structured review of three methods of treatment.* Ann Rheum Dis *58:399-406, 1999.)*

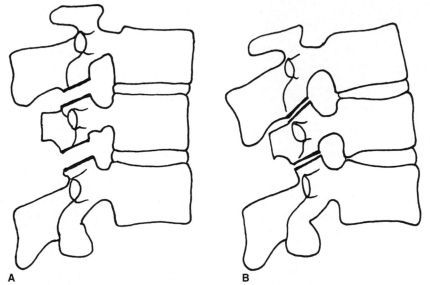

Figure 57.11 Diagrams of the polysegmental wedge osteotomies. **(A)** Lateral view outlining the bone blocks to be resected through the original facet joints in the direction of the interspinal foramen. **(B)** Postoperative lateral view showing how correction is achieved by closure of the posterior osteotomies. *(From Van Royen BJ, De Gast A: Lumbar osteotomy for correction of thoracolumbar kyphotic deformity in ankylosing spondylitis: a structured review of three methods of treatment.* Ann Rheum Dis *58:399-406, 1999.)*

Harrington compression instrumentation, which produces an uneven distribution of segmental compression forces, he could achieve harmonious correction in only 44% of cases. Later he used transpedicular fixation and described harmonious lordosis in 73% of cases in a large series of 177 cases.[39] In the remaining 27% of cases, the majority of correction still occurred at one or two levels. A similar result was also experienced by McMaster,[62] who found that despite multilevel osteotomies, the majority of correction often occurred at one level.

Surgical Technique

The authors prefer to do monosegmental lumbar closing wedge osteotomy below the level of conus, usually at L2 or L3 level, when the total angular correction is estimated around 40 degrees. When larger correction is required, we perform additional osteotomies at one or two levels in the thoracic spine, where smaller angular correction is achieved, averaging 10 to 20 degrees at each level.

The patient is positioned prone on rolls, with the table broken down like a jackknife. Usually, three levels are

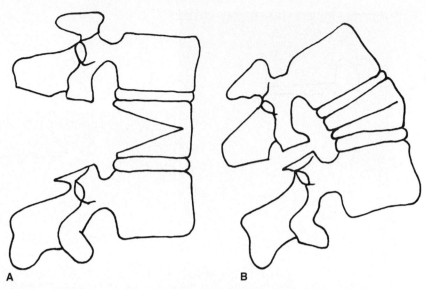

Figure 57.12 Diagrams of the closing wedge osteotomy. (**A**) Lateral view outlining the bone block to be resected. (**B**) Postoperative lateral view showing how correction is achieved by closure of the intravertebral osteotomy. *(From Van Royen BJ, De Gast A: Lumbar osteotomy for correction of thoracolumbar kyphotic deformity in ankylosing spondylitis: a structured review of three methods of treatment.* Ann Rheum Dis 58:399-406, 1999.*)*

instrumented on either side of the osteotomy levels. We use Universal Spinal System with side-opening pedicle screws. Once the screws are inserted, the osteotomy is performed. The apex of the osteotomy is usually placed at the anterior aspect of the vertebral body at the selected level. The amount of bone to be removed from the posterior element is determined from the cutout on the tracing paper at the time of the preoperative planning (Figure 57.9). Usually around 3cm of bone needs to be removed from the lamina and the facet joints. The lamina must be undercut to prevent impingement on the cauda equina as the osteotomy is closed. The pedicle of the vertebra at the level of osteotomy is removed (pedicle subtraction); this ensures adequate space for the exiting nerve roots and prevents entrapment. The dorsal part of the vertebral body is removed by transpedicular decancellation.

The precontoured rods are inserted into the proximal segment. Additional supralaminar hooks making a claw-construct with the proximal end screws provide protection to the proximal fixation. The two rods are connected with a cross-link proximal to the osteotomy, providing additional support to the proximal instrumentation. Before the osteotomy is completed it is important to temporarily secure the proximal and distal segment, to prevent sudden displacement which increases the risk of neurologic complications. Sticks are connected to the screw-heads both on the proximal and distal segments, and they are loosely connected to straight rods. The osteotomy is then gradually completed and the wedge is closed by firm manual pressure and straightening the operation table; the osteoclasis of the anterior vertebral wall feels like a snap as if breaking a green tree. The extension sticks slide along the loosely connected straight rod, thus permitting closure of the osteotomy wedge but prevents any anteroposterior displacement. The con-

toured rods are then reduced to the screw heads at the distal fragments and instruments are completed. The whole procedure is performed under spinal cord monitoring and wake-up tests are done in case of loss of monitoring signals (Figure 57.13).

Additional osteotomies are performed at one or two thoracic levels when indicated after preoperative planning. Generous chevron osteotomies are done through the facet joints and these are closed by applying compression with the instrumentation. The instrumentation is extended to the upper thoracic spine in such cases (Figure 57.13).

Postoperatively, molded thoracic lumbar sacral orthosis (TLSO) is used for mobilization out of bed until the osteotomy is consolidated.

Results and Complications

Van Royen and Gast[93] made a structured review of the three methods of lumbar osteotomy. From 856 cases reported in 41 articles published between 1945 and 1998, they selected 523 cases that met the inclusion criteria for analysis of outcome data. They found that average correction ranged between 37 and 40 degrees. Closing wedge osteotomy achieved 3.8 degrees less correction than the other two methods. In contrast, loss of correction was common with open wedge and polysegmental osteotomies but least with closing wedge osteotomy. Rupture of the aorta or its branches was reported only after open wedge osteotomy and the incidence was 0.9% (4 of 451 cases). Vascular injuries occurred when osteotomy was performed at L1-2 or L2-3 level. No vascular injury was reported with osteotomy below L3 level. Neurologic complications were often related to the displacement at the level of osteotomy. This was reported in 2.7% after open wedge procedure and 2% after closing wedge procedure. Perioperative mortality was

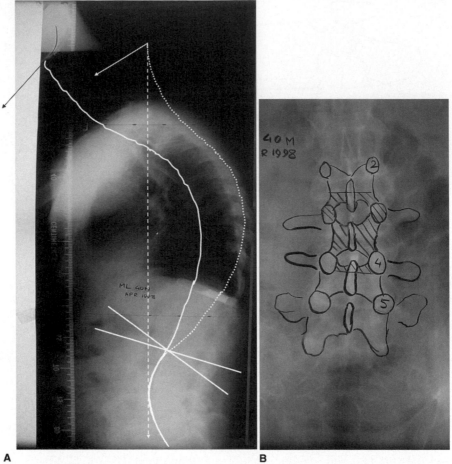

A   **B**

Figure 57.13 (**A**) Preoperative planning indicated that only 30 degrees of corrective osteotomy at L3 level would adequately restore the sagittal balance but not the gaze angle, which needed around 50 degrees of correction. (**B**) A 20-degree osteotomy is therefore planned at the L3 level and the amount of bone to be resected is marked out. Posterior closing wedge osteotomy performed with subtraction of the L3 pedicle.

reported in 5.8% with open wedge osteotomy, 2.4% with polysegmental osteotomy, and only 1.3% with closing wedge osteotomy. The data were not suitable for any statistical analysis. They concluded that although there was a trend that closing wedge osteotomy causes fewer complications and better results, the data were not adequate to make a decision as to which surgical procedure is preferable.

Cervical Osteotomy

Severe flexion deformity in the cervicothoracic region in ankylosing spondylitis may lead to characteristic "chin on chest" posture, which causes severe restriction of the forward gaze and interferes with jaw opening. Cervicothoracic deformity itself does not produce significant problems with the sagittal balance in absence of thoracolumbar kyphotic deformity. The corrective osteotomy therefore should be planned at the cervicothoracic junction.

The preferred site of cervical osteotomy is C7-T1 level. The vertebral artery and vein pass in front of the transverse process of C7 and enters the cervical through the transverse foramen at the C6 vertebra and is less likely to kink when the neck is extended. In addition, the spinal canal is relatively wide at this level, and C8 nerve root injury is less detrimental to hand function than damage to the other cervical nerve roots.

Urist[90] first described a case of cervical osteotomy under local anesthesia with the patient in sitting position in 1953. Law described cervical osteotomy under general anesthesia in 10 patients in 1962 with one death.[50] Since then there have been few reports of this hazardous procedure in more than a few patients. The only large series was reported by Simmons[82] on 42 cases, under local anesthesia, using a technique described by Urist, except the deformity was corrected by manipulation at operation, followed by postoperative immobilization in a halo jacket. In 1997 McMaster[60] described internal fixation with Luque wire in three of his 15 cases to prevent subluxation at the osteotomy site. The only case of a flexion osteotomy to correct iatrogenic extension osteotomy was reported by Sengupta et al.[80]

Surgical Technique

The authors operate with the patient under general anesthesia and in the prone position, which is more comfortable to the surgeon and the patient compared to operation with

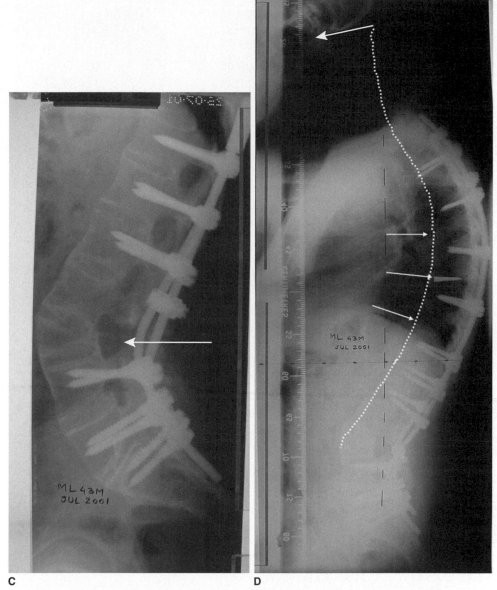

Figure 57.13 *cont'd* **(C,D)** Three more polysegmental osteotomies were performed in the thoracic spine, with around 10 degrees of correction at each level, to compensate for the deliberate undercorrection at the lumbar spine. The net effect was total visual angle correction by 50 degrees and, at the same time, adequate correction of the sagittal balance.

Continued

the patient in the sitting position and under local anesthesia. Spinal cord monitoring is routinely used. Intubation may be particularly difficult and use of fiber optic flexible laryngoscope and awake intubation under local anesthetic may be helpful adjuncts. The caveat in cervical osteotomy is to prevent translation at the site of osteotomy during surgery, before the instrumentation stabilizes the spine. To prevent this we use preoperative halo application, which helps to control head position on the table after osteotomy, and transparent drapes that help to ascertain the desired position of the head after osteotomy, before the spine is fixed in that position.

The spine is exposed through a dorsal midline approach from C3 to T5 inclusive. Drill holes are made in the lateral mass in the C4, C5, C6 and pedicle screws in T2, T3, and T4. A dorsal based wedge is resected. This includes the whole of the lamina of C7 and caudal and rostral part of the laminae of C6 and T1, respectively. Superficial layers of the bone may be removed using a burr, but the deeper layers should be removed using an up-cutting Kerrison rongeur, to prevent dural tear, which is often adherent. Dura is exposed and protected with neuro-patties. The osteotomy is extended laterally to decompress the C8 nerve roots thoroughly. The fused C7-T1 facet joints and the C7 and T1 pedicles are removed with the drills, and the margins of the C6 and T1 laminae are undercut, to prevent impingement of the C8 nerve roots when the osteotomy is closed (Figure 57.14).

The authors stabilize with AO Cervifix® 3.5mm rods and clamps both above and below the osteotomy. The rod is contoured to the anticipated degree of correction and fixed above the osteotomy level on one side only. Clamps should

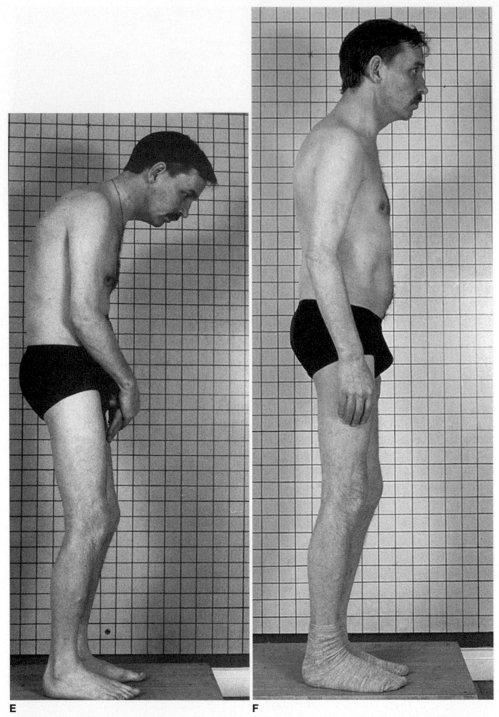

E   F

Figure 57.13 *cont'd* (E,F) Preoperative and postoperative clinical photographs show satisfactory correction of both the sagittal balance and visual angle.

be kept loose on the rod. The distal set of clamps are threaded to the rod but not fixed to the thoracic vertebra. As the osteotomy is completed by careful, controlled manipulation, correcting the deformity, the distal part of the rod will approach the thoracic vertebra. These clamps are then fixed to the predrilled holes in the pedicles of the thoracic vertebra. The other side is then fixed (Figure 57.14).

Mehdian *et al.*[63] described an alternate technique. A malleable rod (usually the template used to measure the rod length) may be used to temporarily hold the spine both above and below the osteotomy level until the osteotomy is made. When the osteotomy is completed the flexible rod allows bending the spine to correct the deformity but prevents the sudden translation. The other side is fixed with a regular implant. The malleable rod is then replaced with a regular Titanium rod (Mehdian technique[1]).

Often the cervicothoracic osteotomy needs to be performed as a secondary procedure after previous thoracic or lumbar osteotomy, in which case 6mm Titanium rods will already be in place, almost up to T2 vertebrae, from previ-

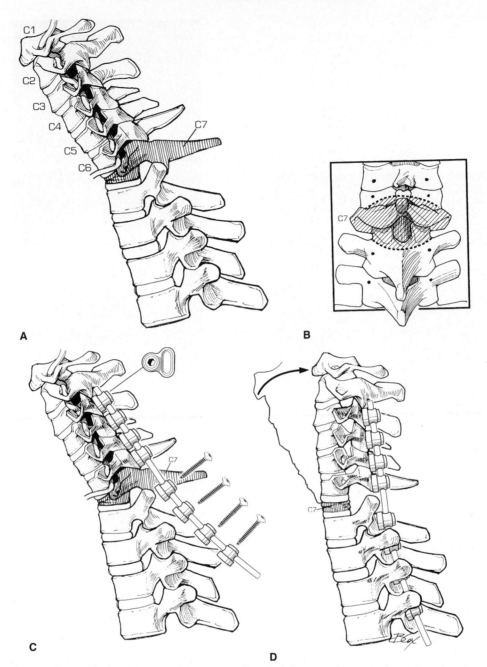

Figure 57.14 **(A)** Cervical osteotomy to correct flexion deformity. The inset shows the area of bone to be removed from C7. The margins of the C6 and T1 lamina should be undercut to prevent impingement on closure of the osteotomy. **(B)** C8 nerve root should be thoroughly decompressed. **(C)** The proximal segment of the spine is instrumented and drills are prepared in the distal segment before completion of the osteotomy to prevent translation. As soon as the osteotomy is completed, the spine should be stabilized immediately. *(From Webb JK, Sengupta DK: Posterior cervicothoracic osteotomy. In Vaccaro AR, Albert TJ [eds]:* Tricks of the Trade of Spine Surgery. *New York, Thieme, 2002.)*

ous surgery. In these situations a combination of 6mm Titanium rod for the thoracic spine below the osteotomy level, and 3.5mm CerviFix rod for cervical spine above the osteotomy level, connected together with a step-down connecting bar would be the ideal implant (Figure 57.14).

A ventral CSLP plate fixation of the osteotomy site ensures against postoperative translation. Postoperatively halo-jacket immobilization is used for additional support for 6 to 8 weeks followed by a period of molded collar until the osteotomy is consolidated.

Figure 57.15 summarizes the effect of osteotomy at the lumbar, thoracic, and cervical spine in a case of global kyphotic deformity because of ankylosing spondylitis, and explains well the need for proper deformity planning.

Spondylodiscitis

The prevalence of spondylodiscitis in ankylosing spondylitis is reported between 5% to 8%.[27,45,55] Most lesions are

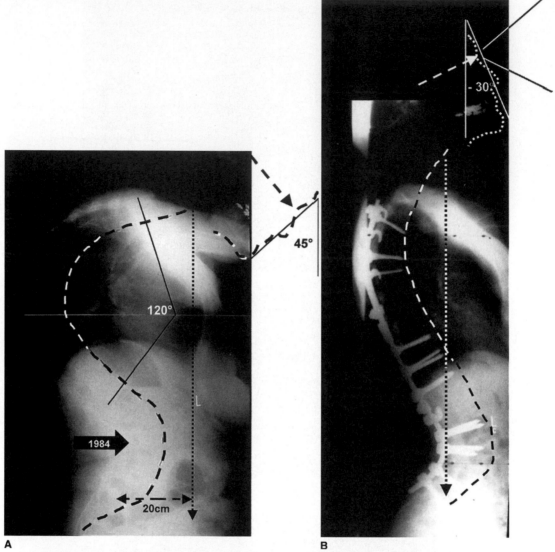

Figure 57.15 (**A**) Lateral radiograph of a 40-year-old woman with global kyphotic deformity from ankylosing spondylitis who underwent corrective osteotomy of the lumbar spine in 1984. Ten years later she presented with recurrence of kyphotic deformity measuring 120 degrees, predominantly in the thoracic spine. The plumb line from odontoid was 20cm in front of S1. The chin-brow angle measured 45 degrees, limiting the field of vision to within 2.5m of her feet. (**B**) She was treated with multiple osteotomies at T6 and at T8, with posterior stabilization from T2 to L5. The sagittal balance was well corrected, but the gaze angle was deviated upward. The chin-brow angle measured −30 degrees, and the patient could not see anything within 3m of her feet.

asymptomatic.[45] In half the cases the lesion may be multiple. The commonest location is in the lower thoracic and upper lumbar region, but the cervicothoracic junction may also be involved.

Neither trauma nor infection has been found to be involved in most cases.[45,72] However, due to similar distribution as thoracolumbar fracture, many believe that these lesions represent pseudarthrosis resulting from the instability of a chronic nonunion.[19] Histologic studies also support the view that these lesions are compatible with pseudarthrosis.[28] Radiologically, these lesions often appear like disc space infection and are referred to as Andersson lesions[72] (Figure 57.2). Spondylodiscitis may cause localized stenosis at the site of the pseudarthrosis and result in

neurologic symptoms. An MRI evaluation is therefore indicated in such cases.

Good results after conservative treatment with NSAID, rest, and physiotherapy have been reported, particularly when symptoms are minimal.[72] For established cases with persistent symptoms, principles of management of pseudarthrosis need to be followed. These lesions may be treated by posterior surgery alone if sagittal balance can be restored with a shift of the plumb line behind the vertebral body and compression applied with the instrumentation.[38] When spinal stenosis results with neurologic symptoms, an anterior approach with excision of the pseudarthrosis tissue, bone grafting, and instrumentation may be recommended[27] (Figure 57.5).

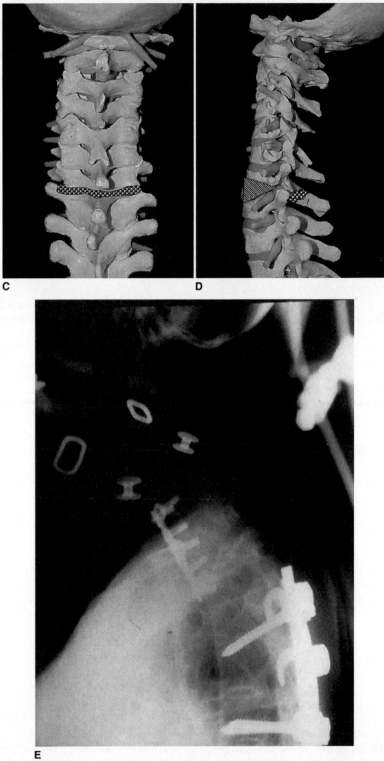

C   D

E

Figure 57.15 *cont'd* (**C,D**) A flexion osteotomy was performed at the level of C7, as shown in a spine model. Posterior transverse osteotomy was made through the lamina of C7-T1 followed by an anterior closing wedge osteotomy at C7 and plate fixation. (**E**) Postoperative lateral radiograph shows the corrected position immobilized in a halo. *(From Sengupta DK, Khazim R, Grevitt MP, Webb JK: Flexion osteotomy of the cervical spine: a new technique for correction of iatrogenic extension deformity in ankylosing spondylitis. Spine 26:1068-1072, 2001.)*

REFERENCES

1. Ahn NU, Ahn UM, Nallamshetty L, *et al:* Cauda equina syndrome in ankylosing spondylitis (the CES-AS syndrome): meta-analysis of outcomes after medical and surgical treatments. *J Spinal Disord Tech* 14:427-433, 2001.

2. Amor B, Dougados M, Mijiyawa M: Criteria of the classification of spondylarthropathies. *Rev Rhum Mal Osteoartic* 57:85-89, 1990.

3. Apple DF, Jr., Anson C: Spinal cord injury occurring in patients with ankylosing spondylitis: a multicenter study. *Orthopedics* 18:1005-1011, 1995.

4. Ball J: Enthesopathy of rheumatoid and ankylosing spondylitis. *Ann Rheum Dis* 30:213-223, 1971.

5. Barozzi L, Olivieri I, De Matteis M, *et al:* Seronegative spondylarthropathies: imaging of spondylitis, enthesitis and dactylitis. *Eur J Radiol* 27(suppl 1):S12-S17, 1998.

6. Benjamin M, McGonagle D: The anatomical basis for disease localisation in seronegative spondyloarthropathy at entheses and related sites. *J Anat* 199:503-526, 2001.

7. Berens DL: Roentgen features of ankylosing spondylitis. *Clin Orthop* 74:20-33, 1971.

8. Bohler J, Gaudernak T: Anterior plate stabilization for fracture-dislocations of the lower cervical spine. *J Trauma* 20:203-205, 1980.

9. Bohlman HH: Acute fractures and dislocations of the cervical spine: an analysis of three hundred hospitalized patients and review of the literature. *J Bone Joint Surg Am* 61:1119-1142, 1979.

10. Boland FW: Ankylosing spondylitis. In Hollander JL (ed): *Arthritis and Allied Conditions: A Textbook of Rheumatology*, ed 7. Philadelphia, Lea & Febiger, 1966, p 633.

11. Braun J, Sieper J: The sacroiliac joint in the spondyloarthropathies. *Curr Opin Rheumatol* 8:275-287, 1996.

12. Briggs H, Keats S, Schlesinger PT: Wedge osteotomy of spine with bilateral intervertebral foraminotomy: correction of flexion deformity in five cases of ankylosing arthritis of the spine. *J Bone Joint Surg Br* 29:1075, 1947.

13. Broom MJ, Raycroft JF: Complications of fractures of the cervical spine in ankylosing spondylitis. *Spine* 13:763-766, 1988.

14. Brophy S, Calin A: Ankylosing spondylitis: interaction between genes, joints, age at onset, and disease expression. *J Rheumatol* 28:2283-2288, 2001.

15. Calin A, Fries JF: Striking prevalence of ankylosing spondylitis in "healthy" with 27 positive males and females. *N Engl J Med* 293:835-839, 1975.

16. Calin A, Porta J, Fries JF, Schurman DJ: Clinical history as a screening test for ankylosing spondylitis. *JAMA* 237:2613-2614, 1977.

17. Camargo FP, Cordeiro EN, Napoli MM: Corrective osteotomy of the spine in ankylosing spondylitis: experience with 66 cases. *Clin Orthop* Jul:157-167, 1986.

18. Carette S, Graham D, Little H, *et al:* The natural disease course of ankylosing spondylitis. *Arthritis Rheum* 26: 186-190, 1983.

19. Chan FL, Ho EK, Fang D, *et al:* Spinal pseudarthrosis in ankylosing spondylitis. *Acta Radiol* 28:383-388, 1987.

20. Cooper C, Carbone L, Michet CJ, *et al:* Fracture risk in patients with ankylosing spondylitis: a population-based study. *J Rheumatol* 21:1877-1882, 1994.

21. Cruickshank B: Pathology of ankylosing spondylitis. *Clin Orthop* 10:393, 1971.

22. Detwiler KN, Loftus CM, Godersky JC, Menezes AH: Management of cervical spine injuries in patients with ankylosing spondylitis. *J Neurosurg* 72:210-215, 1990.

23. Dougados M, van der Linden S, Juhlin R, *et al:* The European spondylarthropathy study group preliminary criteria for the classification of spondylarthropathy. *Arthritis Rheum* 34:1218-1227, 1991.

24. Ebringer A, Ahmadi K, Fielder M, *et al:* Molecular mimicry: the geographical distribution of immune responses to Klebsiella in ankylosing spondylitis and its relevance to therapy. *Clin Rheumatol* 15(suppl 1):57-61, 1996.

25. Edgar MA: Letter: nervous system involvement in ankylosing spondylitis. *Br Med J* 1:394, 1974.

26. Einsiedel T, Kleimann M, Nothofer W, Neugebauer R: Special considerations in therapy of injuries of the cervical spine in ankylosing spondylitis (Bechterew disease). *Unfallchirurg* 104:1129-1133, 2001.

27. Escosa Bage M, Garcia Navarrete E, Pascual Garvi JM, Sola RG: Surgical treatment of spondylodiscitis in ankylosing spondylitis: two cases report. *Rev Neurol* 33:964-966, 2001.

28. Fang D, Leong JC, Ho EK, *et al:* Spinal pseudarthrosis in ankylosing spondylitis: clinicopathological correlation and the results of anterior spinal fusion. *J Bone Joint Surg Br* 70:443-447, 1988.

29. Fitt G, Hennessy O, Thomas D: Case report 709: transverse fracture with epidural and small paravertebral hematomata, in a patient with ankylosing spondylitis. *Skeletal Radiol* 21:61-63, 1992.

30. Fox MW, Onofrio BM, Kilgore JE: Neurological complications of ankylosing spondylitis. *J Neurosurg* 78:871-878, 1993.

31. Francois RJ, Braun J, Khan MA: Entheses and enthesitis: a histopathologic review and relevance to spondyloarthritides. *Curr Opin Rheumatol* 13:255-264, 2001.

32. Giehl JP, Hehne HJ, Zielke K: Kyphosis correction in ankylosing spondylitis using transpedicular instrumentation. In Bridwell KH, DeWald RL (eds): *The Textbook of Spinal Surgery*. Philadelphia, Lippincott-Raven, 1997, pp 1159-1167.

33. Goel MK: Vertebral osteotomy for correction of fixed flexion deformity of the spine. *J Bone Joint Surg Am* 50:287-294, 1968.

34. Graham B, Van Peteghem PK: Fractures of the spine in ankylosing spondylitis: diagnosis, treatment, and complications. *Spine* 14:803-807, 1989.

35. Gran JT, Husby G: Clinical, epidemiologic, and therapeutic aspects of ankylosing spondylitis. *Curr Opin Rheumatol* 10:292-298, 1998.

36. Halm H, Metz-Stavenhagen P, Schmitt A, Zielke K: Surgical treatment of kyphotic spinal deformities in ankylosing spondylitis using the Harrington compression system: long-term results based on the MOPO scales in the framework of a retrospective questionnaire. *Z Orthop Ihre Grenzgeb* 133:141-147, 1995.

37. Hanson CA, Shagrin JW, Duncan H: Vertebral osteoporosis in ankylosing spondylitis. *Clin Orthop* 74: 59-64, 1971.

38. Hehne HJ, Becker HJ, Zielke K: Spondylodiscitis in kyphotic deformity of ankylosing spondylitis and its healing affected by dorsal correction osteotomies: report of 33 patients. *Z Orthop Ihre Grenzgeb* 128:494-502, 1990.

39. Hehne HJ, Zielke K, Bohm H: Polysegmental lumbar osteotomies and transpedicled fixation for correction of long-curved kyphotic deformities in ankylosing spondylitis: report on 177 cases. *Clin Orthop* Sep:49-55, 1990.

40. Herbert JJ: Vertebral osteotomy: technique, indications and results. *J Bone Joint Surg Am* 30:680-689, 1948.

41. Herbert JJ: Vertebral ostetomy for kyphosis, especially in Marie-Strumpell Arthritis. *J Bone Joint Surg Am* 41: 291-302, 1959.

42. Hissa E, Boumphrey F, Bay J: Spinal epidural hematoma and ankylosing spondylitis. *Clin Orthop* Jul:225-227, 1986.

43. Hunter T, Dubo H: Spinal fractures complicating ankylosing spondylitis. *Ann Intern Med* 88:546-549, 1978.

44. Juric G, Coumas JM, Giansiracusa DF, Irwin RS: Hemothorax: an unusual presentation of spinal fracture in ankylosing spondylitis. *J Rheumatol* 17:263-266, 1990.

45. Kabasakal Y, Garrett SL, Calin A: The epidemiology of spondylodiscitis in ankylosing spondylitis: a controlled study. *Br J Rheumatol* 35:660-663, 1996.

46. Kaplan SL, Tun CG, Sarkarati M: Odontoid fracture complicating ankylosing spondylitis: a case report and review of the literature. *Spine* 15:607-610, 1990.

47. Khan MA, van der Linden SM: Ankylosing spondylitis and other spondyloarthropathies. *Rheum Dis Clin North Am* 16:551-579, 1990.

48. Kremer P, Despaux J, Benmansour A, Wendling D: Spontaneous fracture of the odontoid process in a patient with ankylosing spondylitis. Nonunion responsible for compression of the upper cervical cord. *Rev Rhum Engl Ed* 62:455-458, 1995.

49. Law WA: Osteotomy of the spine. *Clin Orthop* 66:70-76, 1969.

50. Law WA: Osteotomy of the spine. *J Bone Joint Surg Am* 44:1199-1206, 1962.

51. Lawrence JS: The prevalence of arthritis. *Br J Clin Pract* 17:699, 1963.

52. Lazennec JY, Saillant G, Saidi K, *et al:* Surgery of the deformities in ankylosing spondylitis: our experience of lumbar osteotomies in 31 patients. *Eur Spine J* 6:222-232, 1997.

53. Le Chapelle EH: Osteotomy of the lumbar spine for correction of kyphosis in a case of ankylosing spondyloarthritis. *J Bone Joint Surg* 28:851-858, 1946.

54. Lichtblau PO, Wilson P: Possible mechanism of aorta rupture in orthopaedic correction of rheumatoid spondylitis. *J Bone Joint Surg Am* 38:123-127, 1956.

55. Little H, Urowitz MB, Smythe HA, Rosen PS: Asymptomatic spondylodiscitis: an unusual feature of ankylosing spondylitis. *Arthritis Rheum* 17:487-493, 1974.

56. Lopez-Larrea C, Gonzalez S, Martinez-Borra J: The role of HLA-B27 polymorphism and molecular mimicry in spondylarthropathy. *Mol Med Today* 4:540-549, 1998.

57. Marie P: Sur la spondylose rhizomelique. *Rev Med* 18:285, 1898.

58. McGonagle D, Gibbon W, Emery P: Classification of inflammatory arthritis by enthesitis. *Lancet* 352: 1137-1140, 1998.

59. McGonagle D, Khan MA, Marzo-Ortega H, *et al:* Enthesitis in spondyloarthropathy. *Curr Opin Rheumatol* 11:244-250, 1999.

60. McMaster MJ: Osteotomy of the cervical spine in ankylosing spondylitis. *J Bone Joint Surg Br* 79:197-203, 1997.

61. McMaster MJ, Coventry MB: Spinal osteotomy in akylosing spondylitis: technique, complications, and long-term results. *Mayo Clin Proc* 48:476-486, 1973.

62. McMaster PE: Osteotomy of the spine for fixed flexion deformity. *J Bone Joint Surg Am* 44:1207, 1962.

63. Mehdian SM, Freeman BJ, Licina P: Cervical osteotomy for ankylosing spondylitis: an innovative variation on an existing technique. *Eur Spine J* 8:505-509, 1999.

64. Miller FH, Rogers LF: Fractures of the dens complicating ankylosing spondylitis with atlantooccipital fusion. *J Rheumatol* 18:771-774, 1991.

65. Moll JM, Haslock I, Macrae IF, Wright V: Associations between ankylosing spondylitis, psoriatic arthritis, Reiter's disease, the intestinal arthropathies, and Behcet's syndrome. *Medicine (Baltimore)* 53:343-364, 1974.

66. Moussellard H, Pointillart V, Mangione P, *et al:* Spontaneous vertebral pseudarthrosis in ankylosing spondylitis: apropos of 3 cases. *Rev Chir Orthop Reparatrice Appar Mot* 82:453-457, 1996.

67. Murray GC, Persellin RH: Cervical fracture complicating ankylosing spondylitis: a report of eight cases and review of the literature. *Am J Med* 70:1033-1041, 1981.

68. Olerud C, Frost A, Bring J: Spinal fractures in patients with ankylosing spondylitis. *Eur Spine J* 5:51-55, 1996.

69. Olivieri I, Barozzi L, Padula A, *et al:* Clinical manifestations of seronegative spondyloarthropathies. *Eur J Radiol* 27(suppl 1):S3-S6, 1998.

70. Peh WC, Ho EK: Fracture of the odontoid peg in ankylosing spondylitis: case report. *J Trauma* 38:361-363, 1995.

71. Puschel J, Zielke K: Corrective surgery for kyphosis in Bekhterev's disease: indication, technique, results (transl). *Z Orthop Ihre Grenzgeb* 120:338-342, 1982.

72. Rasker JJ, Prevo RL, Lanting PJ: Spondylodiscitis in ankylosing spondylitis, inflammation or trauma? A description of six cases. *Scand J Rheumatol* 25:52-57, 1996.

73. Rowed DW: Management of cervical spinal cord injury in ankylosing spondylitis: the intervertebral disc as a cause of cord compression. *J Neurosurg* 77:241-246, 1992.

74. Rumancik WM, Firooznia H, Davis MS, Jr., *et al:* Fibrobullous disease of the upper lobes: an extraskeletal manifestation of ankylosing spondylitis. *J Comput Tomogr* 8:225-229, 1984.

75. Russell AS, Lentle BC, Percy JS: Investigation of sacroiliac disease: comparative evaluation of radiological and radionuclide techniques. *J Rheumatol* 2:45-51, 1975.

76. Russell ML, Gordon DA, Ogryzlo MA, McPhedran RS: The cauda equina syndrome of ankylosing spondylitis. *Ann Intern Med* 78:551-554, 1973.

77. Savolaine ER, Ebraheim NA, Stitgen S, Jackson WT: Aortic rupture complicating a fracture of an ankylosed

thoracic spine: a case report. *Clin Orthop* Nov:136-140, 1991.

78. Schaberg FJ, Jr.: Aortic injury occurring after minor trauma in ankylosing spondylitis. *J Vasc Surg* 4:410-411, 1986.

79. Scudese VA, Calabro JJ: Vertebral wedge osteotomy: correction of rheumatoid (ankylosing) spondylitis. *JAMA* 186:627-631, 1963.

80. Sengupta DK, Khazim R, Grevitt MP, Webb JK: Flexion osteotomy of the cervical spine: a new technique for correction of iatrogenic extension deformity in ankylosing spondylitis. *Spine* 26:1068-1072, 2001.

81. Simmons EH: Ankylosing spondylitis: surgical considerations. In Rothman RH, Simeone FA (eds): *The Spine*, ed 3. Philadelphia, WB Saunders, 1992, pp 1447-1511.

82. Simmons EH: Kyphotic deformity of the spine in ankylosing spondylitis. *Clin Orthop* 128:65-77, 1977.

83. Smith-Petersen MN, Larson CB, Aufranc OE: Osteotomy of the spine for correction of flexion deformity in rheumatoid arthritis. *J Bone Joint Surg* 27:1-11, 1945.

84. Strumpell A: Bemerkiing uber die chronische ankylosirende Entzundung der Wirbelsaule und der Huftgelenke. *Dtsch Z Nervenheilkd* 11:338, 1897.

85. Surin VV: Fractures of the cervical spine in patients with ankylosing spondylitis. *Acta Orthop Scand* 51:79-84, 1980.

86. Taggard DA, Traynelis VC: Management of cervical spinal fractures in ankylosing spondylitis with posterior fixation. *Spine* 25:2035-2039, 2000.

87. Thomasen E: Vertebral osteotomy for correction of kyphosis in ankylosing spondylitis. *Clin Orthop* 194:142-152, 1985.

88. Tiesenhausen K, Thalhammer M, Koch G, Schleifer P: Traumatic aortic rupture in ankylosing spondylitis: a fatal complication. *Unfallchirurg* 104:1101-1103, 2001.

89. Trent G, Armstrong GW, O'Neil J: Thoracolumbar fractures in ankylosing spondylitis: high-risk injuries. *Clin Orthop* 227:61-66, 1988.

90. Urist MR: Osteotomy of the cervical spine: report of a case of ankylosing rheumatoid spondylitis. *J Bone Joint Surg Am* 40:833-843, 1958.

91. Van de Straete S, Demaerel P, Stockx L, Nuttin B: Spinal epidural hematoma and ankylosing spondylitis. *J Belge Radiol* 80:109-110, 1997.

92. van der Linden S, Valkenburg H, Cats A: The risk of developing ankylosing spondylitis in HLA-B27 positive individuals: a family and population study. *Br J Rheumatol* 22:18-19, 1983.

93. Van Royen BJ, De Gast A: Lumbar osteotomy for correction of thoracolumbar kyphotic deformity in ankylosing spondylitis: a structured review of three methods of treatment. *Ann Rheum Dis* 58:399-406, 1999.

94. Van Royen BJ, De Gast A, Smit TH: Deformity planning for sagittal plane corrective osteotomies of the spine in ankylosing spondylitis. *Eur Spine J* 9:492-498, 2000.

95. Vaverka M, Hrabalek L: Injuries of the cervical spine in patients with ankylosing spondylitis. *Rozhl Chir* 80:5-8, 2001.

96. Wade W, Saltzstein R, Maiman D: Spinal fractures complicating ankylosing spondylitis. *Arch Phys Med Rehabil* 70:398-401, 1989.

97. Weatherley C, Jaffray D, Terry A: Vascular complications associated with osteotomy in ankylosing spondylitis: a report of two cases. *Spine* 13:43-46, 1988.

98. Weinstein PR, Karpman RR, Gall EP, Pitt M: Spinal cord injury, spinal fracture, and spinal stenosis in ankylosing spondylitis. *J Neurosurg* 57:609-616, 1982.

99. Wilson MJ, Turkell JH: Multiple spinal wedge osteotomy: its use in a case of Marie Strumpell spondylitis. *Am J Surg* 77:777-782, 1949.

100. Wilson PD, Jr., Levine DB: Compensatory pelvic osteotomy for ankylosing spondylitis: a case report. *J Bone Joint Surg Am* 51:142-148, 1969.

101. Wu CT, Lee ST: Spinal epidural hematoma and ankylosing spondylitis: case report and review of the literature. *J Trauma* 44:558-561, 1998.

CHAPTER 58

Ossification of the Posterior Longitudinal Ligament

Nancy E. Epstein and Kazuo Yonenobu

Cervical myelopathy is often attributed to ossification of the posterior longitudinal ligament (OPLL).[1,2] OPLL appears in males twice as frequently as in females. It begins as an initial hypertrophy of the posterior longitudinal ligament with accompanying punctate ossification centers (early OPLL).[1] With progressive coalescence of these centers, frank ossification of the ligament emerges.[2] Patients with early OPLL become symptomatic in their mid-40s, and those with classic OPLL are typically in their mid to late 50s. Both anterior surgery, consisting of single to multilevel corpectomies with fusion with or without posterior instrumentation, and posterior procedures, including laminectomy with fusion or laminoplasty, may be used to treat the myelopathy related to cervical OPLL.

Prevalence of OPLL

OPLL may be encountered on plain radiographs in 0.12% of North Americans but in a higher 2.2% of Japanese patients without symptoms of myelopathy. However, where myeloradiculopathy is present, OPLL may be defined using CT/MR in 25% of patients in the United States and in 27% of patients in Japan.[3-6] Seventy percent of OPLL occurring in the cervical spine involves 2.7 to 4.0 levels and progresses in a caudal-rostral fashion. The remaining 30% is evenly divided between the proximal thoracic (T1-4) and proximal lumbar regions (L1-3).

Genetics

Studying 91 sibling pairs of patients with OPLL within 53 Japanese families, a likely genetic locus for OPLL was found near the human leukocyte antigen (HLA) site on chromosome 6-p.[7,8] Patients with diffuse idiopathic skeletal hyperostosis (DISH), 50% of whom have concurrent OPLL, test positive for HLA.[9] Evidence of OPLL is found in 26.15% of parents and 28.89% of siblings of patients with OPLL; an autosomal dominant mode of inheritance is therefore inferred.[10] A 53% expression rate of OPLL in patients with two concurrent HLA strands compared with 24% with one concurrent strand supported this hypothesis.[11] Alternatively, an autosomal recessive mode of inheritance was suggested when radiographically 56% of patient's siblings with both HLA haplotypes were sympto-matic with OPLL and those with only one HLA haplotype were not.[12]

Genetically modulated factors, like increased concentrations of growth hormone (GH) receptors and activins, contribute to the expression of OPLL.[13,14] A heightened potential for osteogenesis, attributed to elevated concentrations of bone morphogenetic proteins (BMPRs) in nonossified ligaments of OPLL patients, was identified in 347 families of patients with OPLL, including 1030 relatives of probands.[14] Koga et al.[7,8] identified two unique genetic factors in 18 patients with OPLL compared with 51 age-matched controls without OPLL; these included BamHI 10.0/10.0kb and HindIII 19.0/19.0/kb genotypes.

Anatomy

Posterior Longitudinal Ligament

The posterior longitudinal ligament (PLL) is comprised of collagen fibers with elastin densely concentrated at its center. It originates at the base of the clivus and ends at the sacrum. The PLL attaches to each disc annulus where it is widest and to each mid-vertebra, where it is narrowest. The ligament, 1 to 2mm thick centrally, thins out laterally.

Hypertrophy of the PLL is attributed to fibroblastic hyperplasia followed by increased collagen deposition. Progressive mineralization and cartilaginous ingrowth lead to ossification centers which later coalesce, eventually producing mature Haversian canals actively engaged in bone marrow production. OPLL enlarges an average of 0.4mm per year in its anterior-posterior dimension, while longitudinal expansion occurs at a rate of 0.67mm per year.

In Vitro Characteristics of Cultured PLL in North American Patients with OPLL

The PLL is osteogenic in patients with OPLL both in Japan and in the United States.[7,8,11,13,14] Immunohistochemical evaluation of PLL cells for patients undergoing anterior cervical decompression for cervical disease revealed "up-regulation of proliferating cell nuclear antigen" in patients with OPLL.[15] Epstein et al.[16] also evaluated the osteogenicity of the PLL in myelopathic North American patients with radiographically proven OPLL. Osteocalcin synthesis, reflecting the osteoblastic phenotype of the cells, was studied by collecting supernatants of PLL obtained from patients with OPLL and comparing them with PLL from others with spondylosis alone as controls. The quantity of osteocalcin induced was determined by incubating these PLL cells with $1,25(OH)_2$ Vitamin D3 at 10E-8M for 72 hours in serum free medium.[17] Cell lines from patients with OPLL grew to confluence and those with spondylosis did not respond to Vitamin D3 priming. This supported the osteogenicity of the PLL in non-Asian, North American patients with OPLL.

Mechanisms of Neural Injury in OPLL

Two major mechanisms contribute to neural injury in patients with OPLL: ischemic injury and direct mechanical compression. Direct ventral compression of the spinal cord produces a greater functional loss in the anterior (spinothalamic, motor) and anterolateral (corticospinal) tracts, while ischemia results in a disproportionate loss of the posterolateral tracts. Neural injury may begin with edema but is rapidly succeeded by progressive demyelination, myelomalacia, and atrophy.

Classification of OPLL

Early OPLL

OPLL represents a continuum of maturation, which starts with hypertrophy of the PLL and ends with ossification.[1,3,4] Early OPLL usually originates opposite multiple interspaces in patients in their mid-40s (Figures 58.1 and 58.2). Unlike routine disc herniations, it begins with retrovertebral extension seen on enhanced MR studies performed with GD-DTPA and punctate ossification demonstrated on CT examinations.

Classic OPLL

There are four classic types of mature OPLL.[18] The segmental variant (39%) located behind the vertebral bodies does not cross the intervening disc spaces. The continuous type (27%) extends from vertebra to vertebra, traversing the disc spaces. The mixed form (29%) simultaneously includes both continuous and segmental elements with "skip" areas, and the "other" form (5%) is localized to the disc spaces with limited degrees of rostral and caudal retrovertebral extension.

Myelopathy Scales

Two major myelopathy scales are used worldwide: the Nurick scale and the Japanese Orthopedic Association scale.

Nurick Scale 0-V

The Nurick Myelopathy scale offers six grades of neurologic classification: Grade 0: intact, mild radiculopathy without myelopathy; Grade I: mild myelopathy; Grade II: mild to moderate myelopathy; Grade III: moderate myelopathy; Grade IV: moderate to severe myelopathy; and Grade V: severe myelopathy, quadriplegic.[3,4]

JOA Scale

The Japanese Orthopedic Association scale (JOA) categorizes the severity of myelopathy using a 17-point scale.[19,20] Yononbu et al.[21] recently confirmed the reliability of the JOA score system.

Clinical Presentation of OPLL

Patients with early OPLL become symptomatic in their mid-40s. Symptoms typically include mild radiculopathy and/or myelopathy. Alternatively, those with classic (mature) OPLL are in their mid-50s and show symptoms with moderate to severe myelopathic syndromes character-

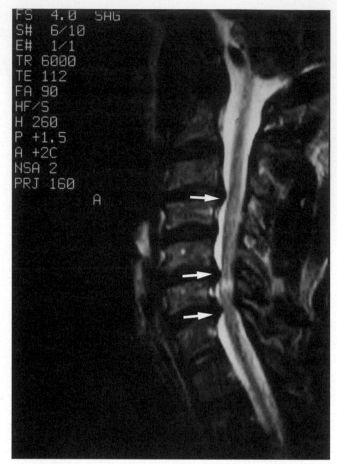

Figure 58.1 On this midline sagittal T_2-weighted MR image, early OPLL impinges ventrally on the thecal sac and cord at the C3-4, C5-6, and C6-7 levels *(white arrows)*. Differentiating early OPLL from disc disease is difficult, the multiplicity of levels involved, and the degree of retrovertebral extension signaling the presence of PLL ligamentous hypertrophy. Observe the high intrinsic signal in the cord opposite the C5-6 level.

ized by increased difficulty in the activities of daily living. Males are affected twice as frequently as females. Most patients develop symptoms in a subacute fashion over a 12-month period, but 10% present with acute deterioration associated with trauma (hyperextension injury).

Minor trauma may precipitate acute irreversible neurologic deterioration in patients with severe OPLL. When Katoh et al.[22] evaluated 27 OPLL patients with minor trauma out of a series of 118 patients, 13 newly developed myelopathy, 7 demonstrated further deterioration of preexisting myelopathy, and 7 remained unchanged. Furthermore, 18 of 19 patients with the narrowest cervical canals were most adversely affected. In Fujimura's et al.[23] series, 26 out of 91 patients operated on for OPLL had sustained minor trauma preoperatively and postoperatively were left with more major myelopathic deficits. Patients with more mobile spines associated with segmental, mixed, and other OPLL exhibited poorer outcomes when compared to those with more rigid spines attributed to continuous OPLL. Typical complaints included neck and arm pain or dysesthesias in over half of the patients, and neurologic signs included arm or leg weakness in one quarter of the patients who also demonstrated spasticity and ataxia.

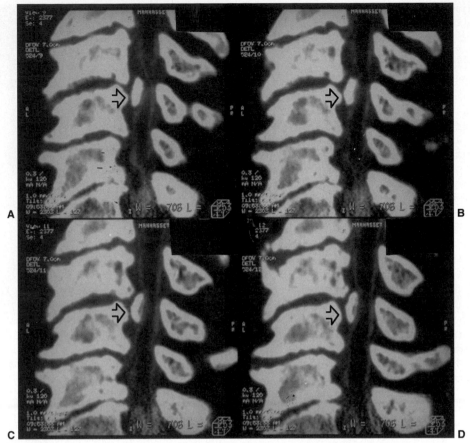

Figure 58.2 Hypertrophied PLL, on these sagittal and parasagittal Myelo-CT images, separates the vertebrae ventrally from a markedly compressed cord dorsally between the C2-6 levels. At the C3-4 level *(arrow)* a large "pearl of ossification" located within the hypertrophied PLL, contributed to marked cord compromise.

Associated Conditions

Patients with OPLL may frequently be diabetic or have coexisting hypoparathyroidism, acromegaly, vitamin D–resistant rickets, spondyloepiphyseal dysplasia, and myotonic muscular dystrophy.

Neurodiagnostic Studies

Radiographs

Based on lateral plain x-rays obtained 6 feet from the patient or tomography, the normal AP dimension of the cervical spinal canal measures an average of 17mm between the C3-7 levels. With absolute stenosis the canal is narrowed to 10mm or less, and those with relative stenosis have canals measuring from 10 to 13mm. The extent of OPLL is readily described by the occupancy ratio, a ratio determined by dividing the thickness of the measured ossified lesion by the anterior/posterior developmental canal diameter. If the ratio is greater than 40%, the risk of myelopathy increases.[2]

Magnetic Resonance Imaging (MRI)

T_1- and T_2-weighted MR studies and MR examinations, performed without and with contrast (Gadolinium-DTPA) are capable of demonstrating the spinal column, spinal cord, and nerve roots, intrinsic cord disease, and extrinsic cord compression from the occiput through the cervicothoracic junction in three planes: transaxial, coronal, and sagittal. On non-contrast MR studies, hypertrophied PLL often appears opposite multiple disc spaces, demonstrates accompanying retrovertebral extension, is slightly hyperintense (see Figure 58.1), and enhances with Gadolinium DTPA. Classical OPLL is readily identified on T_1-weighted MR studies in 50% of patients by a hyperintense signal reflecting the presence of fat within mature Haversian canals actively engaged in bone marrow production. Otherwise, the ossified portion of OPLL appears hypointense. MR examinations also help identify disc herniations (hypointense masses) at maximum compression levels of OPLL approximately 60% of the time and disc protrusions being found in conjunction with segmental OPLL in 81% of cases.[24]

Intrinsic cord swelling, myelomalacia, or irreversible myelomalacia or gliosis may produce hyperintense signals on T_2-weighted images. These findings constitute a poorer prognostic sign for patients with cervical spondylotic myelopathy (CSM) as compared with OPLL, where symptoms and findings are more frequently irreversible.[24,25] Despite the 43% incidence of increased preoperative cord signals on MR studies that failed to resolve postoperatively, OPLL patients exhibited better outcomes compared with those with CSM. Dynamic MR studies may also prove useful in demonstrating "dynamic" compression preoperatively and residual cord compromise postoperatively.

Magnetic Resonance Angiography (MRA)

Measurement of the interpedicular distance on preoperative CT scans typically dictates the medial/lateral dimension of the surgical trough to be created and may therefore vary from an average of 14mm in the Japanese population to 18 to 20mm in the North American population. Therefore, selected patients undergoing multilevel ACF may benefit from preoperative MRA studies if the vertebral artery appears to be following an unusually tortuous course. Occasional arterial loops may appear superficially, lateral to the anterior vertebral body margin, extending ventrally as it courses between the individual foramen transversarium. Alternatively, loops may be aberrantly medially located lateral to the spinal canal.

Management of vertebral arterial injuries is controversial. Direct surgical repair of the injured vessel is often difficult and carries substantial risks. The advent of interventional neuroradiology provides a preferred "endovascular" solution. For injuries less than 6 hours old, transient vessel tamponade may be immediately followed by acute stent placement. On the other hand, those injuries over 6 hours old, endovascular trapping with coils may be performed. Both endovascular alternatives avoid the risk of delayed reopening of the vessel, prevent pseudoaneurysm formation, and limit the potential for cephalad clot propagation and cranial embolization.

Computed Tomography Scan (CT)

CT-based examinations, including the non-contrast CT, intravenous enhanced contrast CT, 2D, and 3D reconstructed CT, and Myelo-CT studies, directly demonstrate punctate ossification characteristic of early OPLL or frank ossification typical of classical OPLL (Figures 58.3 and 58.4; see also Figure 58.2). CT studies also demonstrate degenerative changes adjacent to levels of prior surgery.[25] Where non-contrast CT studies fail to demonstrate lateral or foraminal root pathology, double-dose intravenous contrast-enhanced CT images may increase resolution, while differentiating postoperative scar (enhances) from new disc pathology (nonenhancing). Two-dimensional and 3D non-contrast CT reconstructed images provide a sagittal overview of the extent of cord compression without incurring the risk associated with Myelo-CT studies. In particular, younger patients with normal-sized spinal cords are at greater risk for acute deterioration following myelography compared to older individuals with significant underlying cord atrophy.

Where feasible, Myelo-CT studies contribute to a detailed "overview" of the extent of spinal cord and nerve root compression attributed to OPLL. Dorsally, Myelo-CT studies may show shingling of the lamina accenting significant congenital stenosis, along with infolding of the yellow ligament or ossified yellow ligaments (OYL). Ossification of the anterior longitudinal ligament, OPLL, spondylosis and disc pathology may also be readily identified. Furthermore, flexion and extension myelograms and Myelo-CT studies demonstrate cord compression not as readily viewed on static studies.

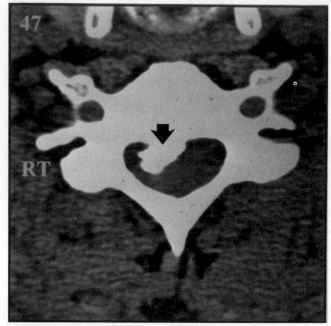

Figure 58.3 Classical OPLL, which was fully ossified (*large arrow*), originated at the mid C4 vertebral level on this transaxial non-contrast CT scan. Marked central and right-sided cord and nerve root compression resulted, with OPLL mass nearly touching the lamina dorsally.

Postoperatively, Myelo-CT studies help confirm whether decompression has been adequate or whether further surgery is warranted. Fujimura *et al.*[26] evaluated the amount of dorsal shift and expansion of the cervical cord following open-door laminoplasty performed in patients with OPLL. Postoperatively, OPLL patients demonstrated less dorsal shift of the cord but greater cord expansion, the degree of expansion positively correlating with outcome.

Documentation of Fusion Following Multilevel Anterior Cervical Surgery

Fusion criteria, documented on static radiographs and 2D CT studies performed immediately postoperatively and repeated at 3, 6, and 12 months postoperatively and included: (1) the presence of bony trabeculation and (2) presence or lack of bony lucency at the fibula strut allograft/vertebral body interface. Dynamic radiographs performed at similar intervals confirmed stability when less than 3.5mm of translation and less than 1mm of motion is demonstrated between the tips of adjacent spinous processes.

A potential additional criterion for fusion following multilevel ACF performed with fibula strut allograft, consisting of cephalad or caudad bony ingrowth from the vertebral end plate into the central canal, was also evaluated.[27] Eighteen patients with OPLL had average 2.9 level ACF performed with fresh frozen fibula strut allografts, accompanied by C2-T1 PWF. CT documentation of bony ingrowth was combined with other signs of fusion in 17 (94%) of 18 patients undergoing multilevel ACF/PWF. Bony ingrowth doubled from 3 to 6 months postoperatively, increasing rostrally from 1.5mm to 3.5mm, and caudally from 2.1mm to 4.6mm. Hounsfield Units, ranging from 500-900, confirmed the bony nature of this ingrow-

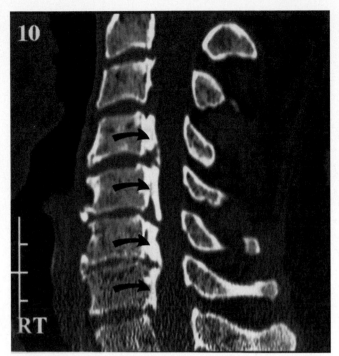

Figure 58.4 Continuous OPLL was readily demonstrated on this midline sagittal 2D CT reconstructed image extending from the C3-4 through the C7-T1 levels *(arrows)*. At all three interspaces, hypodense areas surrounded by ossification signaled OPLL's extension through the dura.

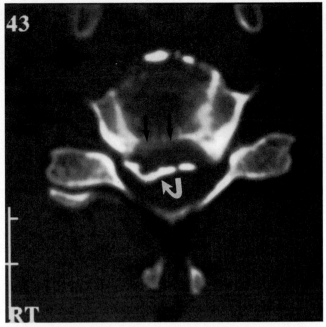

Figure 58.5 The "double layer" sign *(black arrows)* was documented on this transaxial non-contrast, bone window CT examination. Note the retrovertebral ossification which begins behind the vertebra, and then surrounds *(curved white arrow)* both the hypodense ligament and dura.

ing tissue. Although early bony ingrowth signaled progression toward fusion, its absence was not pathognomonic for a failure to fuse as observed in the eighteenth patient.

Computed Tomography Signs of Dural Penetrance

Anterior resection of OPLL rarely results in a CSF fistula if surgical resection is performed under an operating microscope. There is almost always a dural plane present. Preoperatively, CT signs of dural penetrance allow the surgeon to anticipate absence of dura and to plan how to manage the CSF fistula during and after surgery. This warrants not only direct dural repair where dural edges are available using bovine pericardial grafts, 7-0 Gortex sutures, and microdural staples, but it also includes the use of DuraGen, fibrin sealant, wound-peritoneal, and lumbo-peritoneal shunts.

Bone-window CT examinations proffer two signs of dural penetrance. First, the "double layer" sign is characterized by a hyperdense line of OPLL directly behind the vertebra, which continues to envelop a central hypodense mass representing hypertrophied PLL and penetrated dura (Figure 58.5).[28,29] The "double layer" sign has proven the most pathognomonic for absent dura at surgery, CSF fistulas being correlated with this sign 75% to 84% of the time. This "layer cake" image of the "double layer sign" reflects an "outside in" pattern of ossification. Hida et al.[29] used bone window CT examinations to determine whether a dural defect was present in 21 patients with cervical OPLL; CTs showed the double layer sign in 12 patients, 10 of whom exhibited dural defects at surgery.[29] When Epstein[28] studied the frequency of the dural penetrance resulting in CSF fistulas among 54 OPLL patients under-

going multilevel anterior corpectomies with fusion, only two had absent dura at surgery; one demonstrated the "double layer" CT sign. Now, out of a total of 85 patients undergoing multilevel ACF for OPLL, a total of three CSF fistulas has been observed, two others demonstrating the "single layer" sign characterized by a single solid ossified OPLL mass on CT, directly extending into the cervical canal.[28,30] Hida et al.[29] observed a lower 11% to 25% correlation of absent dura at surgery with this preoperative CT sign which typically occupied more than 50% of the spinal canal, the greatest focus of compression corresponding to the site of dural penetration.[29] When the "single layer sign" is accompanied by a lateral, irregular C-shaped configuration, it indicates that the dura has become imbricated in the growing OPLL mass and that a CSF fistula will more likely result from surgical extirpation (see Figure 58.4). For the "single layer sign," ossification appears to occur from the "inside-out," beginning centrally within the hypertrophied PLL ligament and extending to the periphery. At surgery, only one of nine patients showing the single layer sign developed a CSF leak during surgery.[29]

Diffuse Idiopathic Skeletal Hyperostosis (DISH)

DISH, an ossifying diathesis that involves extensive ossification of the anterolateral aspect of contiguous vertebral bodies, was readily demonstrated on preoperative CT examinations. DISH, typically observed in 15% to 30% of adults over age 65, and often asymptomatic, is far more prevalent than OPLL in North America.[9,31] OPLL is considered part of the diffuse ligamentous ossification seen in up to 50% of patients with DISH, but should only be resected either anteriorly or posteriorly if symptomatic.[32,33] As DISH often becomes massive before producing dysphagia, other etiologies of dysphagia must be sought before the surgical resection of DISH.[34] Furthermore, DISH excision may result in several months of dysphagia.[35]

OALL

OALL is defined by hypertrophy of the anterior longitudinal ligament, followed by progressive cartilaginous infiltration, and frank ossification. On T_1-weighted MR studies, the OALL mass appears hypointense, and fat, which is hyperintense, reflects active bone marrow production occurring within mature Haversian canals. On CT examinations, ventral OALL may become massive (Figure 58.6). However, massive OALL rarely produces dysphagia and should therefore only be resected once other etiologies for these symptoms have been ruled out. At surgery, the adequacy of OALL resection may be checked on routine intraoperative lateral radiographs or fluoroscopic images.

Conservative Treatment of OPLL

Conservative management of patients with OPLL may include the use of oral nonsteroidal or steroidal agents and epidural steroid injections. Immobilization in cervical orthoses is discouraged because these devices frequently exacerbate rather than relieve symptoms attributed to inadvertent hyperextension or hyperflexion. Multidisciplinary, comprehensive pain management centers may be used to manage older patients who are not considered candidates for surgical intervention based on significant comorbidities; cardiovascular disease, COPD, diabetes, and peripheral vascular disease. Nonsurgical management is also appropriate where severe long-term deficits are presumed to be fixed and irreversible, corresponding with MR documentation of myelomalacia (cell death, apoptosis), and cord atrophy.

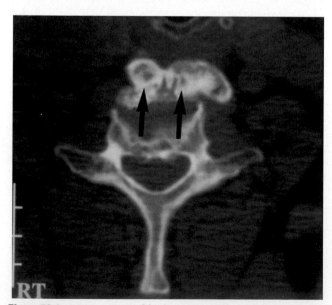

Figure 58.6 OALL was readily demonstrated on the transaxial bone window non-contrast CT study opposite the C5-6 level (*double arrows*).

Patients with OPLL, whether under or over age 65, with progressive myelopathy, MR evidence of cord edema, without significant medical risk factors, should be considered candidates for surgery. Operative intervention prior to the advent of minor cervical trauma is advantageous because myelopathic progression following these events is often permanent and irreversible.[22]

On the other hand, surgery for patients with OPLL over age 70 and with severe myelopathy and significant medical co-morbidities, is considered high risk. In Saunder's[36] series of 31 patients undergoing 4 level ACF, the three postoperative deaths corresponded with over age 70 and a history of cardiovascular or peripheral vascular disease. The causes of death included myocardial infarction, abdominal aortic aneurysm, and pulmonary embolism. Similarly, two of Epstein's[37] first 44 patients undergoing circumferential surgery for OPLL expired. The first patient, a 56-year-old with diabetes and two prior cardiac bypasses and bilateral femoral-popliteal bypass surgery, died within 48 hours of surgery from an acute myocardial infarction (MI). The second patient, over age 70, expired 3 weeks postoperatively from a myocardial infarction.

Role of Prophylactic Surgery for OPLL

Younger asymptomatic patients, under age 65, may be considered candidates for prophylactic decompression, if severe cervical OPLL is radiographically or physiologically documented. This population, with a longer life expectancy, is at greater risk for intercurrent trauma and resultant irretrievable myelopathy.[22,23] T_2-weighted MR studies demonstrating high cord signals, reflecting cord edema or myelomalacia, may signal the need for surgery. Similarly, abnormal SSEP responses may indicate subclinical dorsal cord compromise and the need to consider operative intervention. Surgery, performed prior to the onset or progression of a neurologic deficit correlated with better outcomes in 87% of the patients in Saunder's[36] series.

Anesthetic Protocol for OPLL Patients Undergoing Circumferential Cervical Surgery

Patients undergoing multilevel anterior corpectomy with fusion, posterior stabilization, and halo application for complex OPLL, are managed with a strict anesthetic protocol.[38,39] Avoiding emergent reintubation or tracheostomy following these procedures helps prevent acute graft and plate disruption, increased neurologic deficit, hypoxia, and even death. The strict anesthetic protocol begins with awake fiberoptic intubation and positioning under continuous intraoperative SSEP monitoring.[38] Eliminating cervical motion limits the potential for inadvertent hyperextension or hyperflexion cord injury. For the first postoperative night, patients are routinely kept intubated. This eliminates acute respiratory distress and the need for emergent reintubation in the immediate perioperative period. The first postoperative day, or thereafter, patients are electively fiberoptically extubated by an anesthesiologist. Parameters evaluated prior to extubation include: (1) direct fiberoptic evaluation of the trachea and vocal cords for swelling, (2) indirect assessment of swelling performed by letting down the endotracheal cuff checking for an air leak and the ability to verbalize, and (3) reviewing the patient's attendant medical risk factors. Where patients could not be extubated from postoperative days 1 to 7, elective tracheostomies were scheduled.

Fifty-eight patients undergoing multilevel circumferential surgery for OPLL with halo vests applied were managed with this strict protocol.[38] Patients had average three-level ACF with average 6.5 level PWF. Operations typically lasted 10 hours and required 2.6 units of blood in transfusion. Fiberoptic extubation was successfully accomplished the first postoperative day in 40 patients, and 15 patients were extubated between postoperative days 2 to 7. Three patients required elective tracheostomy performed on postoperative day 7. Using this protocol, only one patient required emergent reintubation 20 minutes after having been extubated on postoperative day 3. In her case, three risk factors were identified: a prior anterior surgical procedure (C4-7 ACF) 3 years earlier, a history of asthma, and the requirement for a second operation lasting over 10 hours (14-hour surgery). No patient in the series required an emergency tracheostomy.

Major risk factors positively correlated with delayed extubation or tracheostomy included in descending order: (1) surgical time over 10 hours (12 patients); (2) obesity greater than 220 lb (12 patients); (3) transfusions of over 4 units of blood (10 patients); (4) secondary anterior cervical surgery (9 patients); (5) anterior surgery, including the C2 level (7 patients); (6) four level ACF (5 patients); and (7) asthma (5 patients). Minor risk factors included advanced age (greater than age 65), severe preoperative neurologic deficits (Nurick Grade IV-V moderate/severe myelopathy), and intraoperative CSF fistula. Other factors observed in the literature known to contribute to airway complications included angioedema, recurrent laryngeal nerve palsy, dysphagia with or without esophageal perforation, and new cord injuries.[40]

Somatosensory Evoked Potential (SSEP) and Motor Evoked Potential (MEP) Monitoring

Performing continuous intraoperative SSEP monitoring during cervical procedures, including OPLL surgery, limits postoperative morbidity.[35,41,42] Monitoring technique included first obtaining baseline posterior tibial and ulnar SSEPs. Awake fiberoptic nasotracheal intubation is performed with the patient awake, under continuous SSEP monitoring. Similarly, positioning is also completed with the patient awake. This may include taping of the chin for anterior procedures or turning the patient prone for a posterior approach. Keeping the patient awake and avoiding induction while positioning allows potentials to be more readily compared with prepositioning baseline data. Loss or decrement of potentials may occur because of undue flexion or extension of the neck, or traction, rotation, or compression at the level of the shoulder, elbow, or wrist. To avoid SSEP "drop out," inhalation anesthetics (i.e., Isoflurane) are usually kept at concentrations below 0.4%, or a balanced narcotic technique is used.

A 50% decline in the amplitude and a 10% decrease in latency are defined as significant.[41] Such changes, observed 50 seconds for the first recording, and reproduced 100 seconds later, warrant immediate medical and surgical resuscitative measures. Medical measures include: the induction of hypertension, the warming of irrigating fluids, decreasing the concentration of inhalation anesthetic, and increasing oxygen concentration. Surgical resuscitative measures include: releasing distraction, removal of an over-sized graft, and cessation of manipulation. Epstein et al.[41] demonstrated that no instances of quadriplegia or death were encountered in 100 prospectively SSEP-monitored cases. These data compared favorably with the retrospective analysis of 218 unmonitored patients operated on by Epstein and four associates where eight patients became quadriplegic and one died.

In 1996, May et al.[43] successfully monitored SSEPs in 182 cervical procedures, yet 10 patients exhibited new postoperative neurologic deficits. Major risk factors that correlated with these new deficits included: (1) multisegmental surgery, (2) severe preoperative neurologic deficits, and (3) the use of instrumentation. Of interest, half of the patients with complete SSEP loss during surgery exhibited new postoperative neurologic deficits, and those with incomplete loss of SSEPs or with intraoperative recovery of potentials, did not. In both series, false positives were probably true positives, and the initiation of resuscitative maneuvers likely averted permanent neurologic injury in some of these individuals.

Intraoperative motor evoked potentials also provide continuous information regarding the status of the anterior cervical spinal cord. Gokaslan et al.[44] transcutaneously placed epidural electrodes to monitor anterior cervical cord function during 16 anterior cervical decompression and fusion procedures. They encountered no complications associated with electrode placement, demonstrated adequate baseline MEPs, and successfully monitored all patients. MEP preservation during surgery positively correlated with outcomes.

Surgery for OPLL

Much controversy surrounds whether anterior or posterior surgical approaches are superior for managing cervical OPLL. Anterior surgery offers direct OPLL removal, typically using multilevel corpectomies with fusion (ACF), and posterior procedures allow for indirect dorsal decompression of multilevel pathology using laminectomy with posterior fusion procedures or laminoplasty.

Dorsal Surgery

Older high-risk patients (greater than age 65) with significant multilevel OPLL, but an adequately preserved cervical lordotic curvature or hyperlordosis, may be managed with varied dorsal surgical decompressive approaches: laminectomy alone, laminectomy with dorsal fusion, or laminoplasty.[20,33,45-49] Posterior approaches effectively decompress the cervical cord in the presence of spondylosis, stenosis, and OPLL in the presence of an adequate cervical lordosis, as dorsal removal of shingled laminae and accompanying hypertrophied yellow ligament allows the cord to migrate away from ventrally situated pathology (Figure 58.7A,B). However, dorsal decompression is not appropriate in the presence of kyphosis, as removal of the posterior elements still leaves the cord tethered over ventral intrusions (Figure 58.7C).

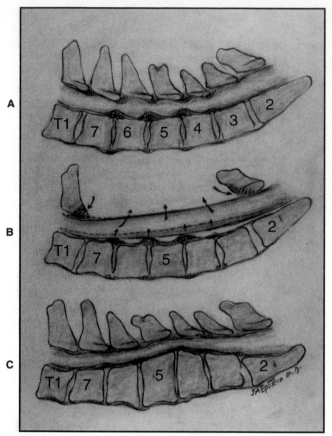

Figure 58.7 Dorsal decompression for cervical spondylosis, stenosis, and OPLL is only effective where the cervical lordotic curvature has been preserved. **(A)** Diffuse, multilevel cervical spinal stenosis is illustrated here along with adequate preservation of the cervical lordotic curvature. Observe the multilevel ventral spondylosis accompanied by dorsolateral compression from inward shingling of the lamina and hypertrophy of the yellow ligament. **(B)** Dorsal decompression, whether it consists of laminectomy or laminoplasty, offers dorsal migration of the cord away from ventrally situated osteophytes in the presence of an adequately preserved cervical lordotic curvature. **(C)** In the presence of severe kyphosis, dorsal decompression would fail to alleviate cord compression because the cord would remain tethered over the ventral pathology.

Laminectomy

Laminectomy alone may sufficiently decompress the cervical spinal canal in patients with OPLL if the cervical spine is stable (Figure 58.8). Laminectomy must be combined with medial facetectomies and foraminotomies restricted to less than 25% of the medial facet joint to preserve stability because greater than 25% facet removal correlated with greater pathologic motion.[50] When evaluating the long-term results of laminectomy in 44 patients with OPLL, Kato et al.[47] found a neurologic recovery rate of 44.2% one year postoperatively, a rate that remained nearly unchanged at 42.9% 5 years later. Nevertheless, outcomes worsened between 5 and 10 years postoperatively. Negative prognostic factors included older age at the time of the original surgery, more severe preoperative neurologic deficits, a history of new trauma, and the presence of ossification of the yellow ligament. Although

OPLL progression was observed in 70% of patients, this only contributed to deterioration in one instance. Furthermore, progression of kyphosis in 47% of patients did not appear to significantly contribute to deterioration.

Laminectomy with Posterior Fusion

Cervical laminectomy coupled with a posterior fusion is another alternative for the management of OPLL where the lordotic curvature is preserved. In some patients, prophylactic stabilization may be performed to avoid the evolution of instability, although in others, instability may already be present. Iatrogenic instability secondary to a failed laminectomy may also contribute to the need for simultaneous fusion.[50] Preoperative documentation of chronic olisthy, partial swan neck deformity, or hyperlordosis with excessive mobility constitute other reasons for considering posterior fusion.

Fusion Techniques

Fusion alternatives include facet-wiring techniques, insertion of lateral mass plates, or dorsal pedicle screw fixation.* Laminectomy with posterior facet wiring and fusion resulted in adequate fusion in five OPLL patients in Epstein's[45] series. Additionally, following failed anterior corpectomy and fusion procedures resulting in pseudarthrosis or anterior graft extrusion, secondary posterior spinous process wiring and fusion resulted in high fusion rates without significant complications in OPLL patients.[53] Alternatively, Hamanishi and Tanaka[33] observed no significant difference in outcomes when comparing laminectomy performed in 35 patients without instability to laminectomy with fusion performed in 34 unstable patients. Using the Short Form 36 (SF-36), Kumar et al.[48] evaluated patient-based outcomes in 25 patients undergoing laminectomy with lateral mass plating for unstable spondylotic myelopathy. None exhibited new postoperative instability or increased kyphosis, 80% showed good outcomes, 76% improved on myelopathy scores, and none developed delayed deterioration. Applying lateral mass plates in 43 patients, including 14 with post-laminectomy instability, Wellman et al.[49] encountered no significant complications out of 281 screws placed (average seven screws per patient). However, dorsal decompression with or without fusion did not suffice in a subset of Abumi and Kaneda's[51] patients with significant OPLL; following the application of pedicle screws for dorsal fixation after 26 laminectomies or laminoplasties, 15 patients additionally required anterior procedures. In Abumi's[52] et al. update 2 years later, postoperative radiographic studies demonstrated that 10/190 (5.3%) screws perforated the cortex of the pedicles but did not result in neurovascular complications.

Laminoplasty

Some surgeons consider the laminoplasty to be an optimal approach to multilevel OPLL. Irrespective of age, it simultaneously offers dorsal decompression while augmenting stability without the need for a formal fusion.[18,20,54,55]

---

*References 33,45,48,49,51,52.

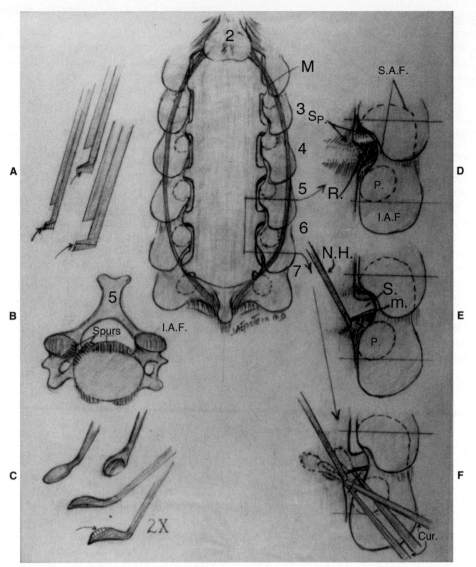

Figure 58.8 Cervical laminectomy may be performed in older patients with significant ventral OPLL where the lordotic curvature has been well-preserved. Illustrated here is how to perform a multilevel cervical laminectomy with medial facetectomy and foraminotomy. Additionally, partial excision of ventral OPLL or osteophytes with down-biting curettes is another option. **(A)** Angled and filed-down Kerrison rongeurs with thinned-down footplate are used in these cases, minimizing compression of the underlying neural elements during dissection. **(B)** Ventral OPLL and/or spurs may be decompressed indirectly with dorsal decompression alone where the cervical lordotic curvature has been well-preserved. Additionally, some degree of lateral and foraminal spur resection may be completed where needed with down-biting curettes. **(C)** The typical down-biting curettes with filed-down tips, which may be used for lateral and foraminal decompression of OPLL/spurs. **(C)** A laminectomy from C2-7 is illustrated here with careful preservation of the lateral two thirds of the individual facet joints at each vertebral level to preserve stability. In **(D)**, a medial facetectomy with foraminotomy is more specifically illustrated, the location of the spinal cord (*Sp*) and nerve root (*R*) extending laterally and foraminally in an upward direction being clearly delineated. Note the locale of the pedicle (*P*) with respect to the inferior aspect of the nerve root, and the necessity to remove only the medial aspect of the inferior and superior articular facet (*SAF*) for adequate decompression. **(E)** Using a small nerve hook (*NH*), the nerve root and its adhesions should be lysed to allow for mobilization of the nerve root over the underlying spur/OPLL. Careful dissection of both the sensory (*s*) and motor (*m*) portions of the root is critical to avoid new neural deficits. **(F)** With the down-biting curettes, dissection of spurs or OPLL underlying the exiting nerve root may be accomplished.

When Baisden et al.[56] compared the results of cervical decompression in a goat model using the laminoplasty versus the laminectomy, radiographic and biomechanical results confirmed that laminoplasty was superior in maintaining cervical alignment and avoiding postoperative spinal deformity.

Pros and Cons of Dorsal Approaches to OPLL

Dorsal Decompression of Multilevel OPLL

In Japan, varied expansive laminoplasty techniques are used to address multilevel OPLL; the greater the number of levels involved, the more likely they are to use the laminoplasty. However, improvement largely relies on whether there is a sufficient lordotic cervical curvature to allow for dorsal migration of the cord away from ventrally situated OPLL. Sodeyama et al.[55] compared the preoperative with postoperative Myelo-CT studies in 65 patients undergoing laminoplasty for OPLL; a mean dorsal cord shift of greater than 3mm correlated with good clinical outcomes (range 0-6.6mm). For lesions located at the rostral or caudal extremes of the canal, decompression had to be extended one level above or below this pathology to maximize dorsal cord shift. Morimoto et al.[18] demonstrated a 42% increase in the average postoperative AP canal diameter 3 years following laminoplasty. Additionally, a 96% bone fusion rate, with 83% preserved range of motion was also shown. Patients undergoing laminoplasty for OPLL improved from a preoperative JOA score of 9 to a postoperative score of 14.1.

Congenital Stenosis May Contraindicate a Dorsal Approach

Congenital cervical stenosis also helped determine whether laminoplasty would be effective in decompressing OPLL. Ishida et al.[57] performed laminoplasty for cervical myeloradiculopathy (63 patients) where the canal diameter was reduced to 14mm, but for those with OPLL, a canal diameter of 17mm (31 patients) was required for the cord to be adequately decompressed. For cases where OPLL was very extensive, laminoplasty was not appropriate.

Better Clinical Outcomes with Ventral Procedures

Clinical outcomes for patients with severe OPLL reflect the limitation of dorsal decompression. Clinical outcomes, as measured by Kawano et al.,[58] were better where anterior (48 patients) rather than dorsal (27 patients) surgical techniques were used to address OPLL. The overall mean improvement on the neurosurgical cervical spine scale score (NCSS) was 78% for those undergoing ventral compared with only 46.1% for those having posterior decompressions. Additionally, long-term follow-up scores were better for those having anterior rather than dorsal surgery. Anterior scores continued to rise and stabilize to 12.9 and 13.0, and those having laminoplasty showed a progressive decline from 10.4 to 9.7. Epstein[5,6,37,59,60] also observed better outcomes following anterior rather than posterior surgery for OPLL.

Increased OPLL Progression Following Dorsal Decompression

A major concern remains whether dorsal decompression of OPLL increases the rate of OPLL progression. Takatsu et al.[61] radiologically compared OPLL progression rates following 25 laminoplasties and 16 laminectomies versus 56 patients managed without surgery. No significant difference was observed in OPLL progression rates following either laminoplasty or laminectomy, but both procedures resulted in more rapid OPLL progression compared to those treated conservatively.

Long-Term Recovery Rates Following Dorsal Decompression of OPLL

Where OPLL extends up to the C2 level or down to the T1 level, these levels should be included in the original decompression. Otherwise, further OPLL expansion will warrant secondary surgery with its attendant greater morbidity. Using the JOA score, Kato et al.[47] discovered long recovery rates of 44.2% after 1 year, and 42.9% after 5 years in 44 patients undergoing laminectomy. However, long-term deterioration occurred 5 to 10 years later, JOA scores declining to 32.8%. Major negative prognostic factors included advanced age at the time of the original surgery, more severe preoperative myelopathy, and a history of trauma.

Ventral Surgical Procedures for the Management of OPLL

Many would agree that direct resection of ventral pathology, be it attributed to CSM and/or OPLL, results in improved postoperative neurologic outcomes. When Fessler et al.[62] studied neurologic outcomes for 93 patients undergoing anterior cervical surgery for spondylotic myelopathy, postoperative Nurick Scores improved in 86% of patients. Specifically, patients improved an average of 1.24 Nurick Grades. When compared with historical controls, poor outcomes following posterior surgery or no surgery were found. Those having laminectomy improved only 0.07 Nurick Grades and without surgery, patients deteriorated and showed an average of 0.23 Nurick Grades.

1-2 Level Ventral Cervical Procedures

Anterior cervical surgical procedures for OPLL and/or spondylostenosis offer direct ventral resection of the pathology (Figure 58.9). Few OPLL patients show symptoms with OPLL confined to a single interspace, more typically demonstrating multilevel disease with accompanying retrovertebral extension.

Non-Plated One- to Two-Level ADF. One-level ADF may be performed with a high incidence of successful fusion, while non-plated two-level ADF are associated with higher failure rates.[63,64] Epstein[64] demonstrated fusion rates of 99% for patients undergoing non-plated one-level ADF (78 patients) but only a 90% frequency of success followed non-plated two-level ADF (84 patients). Emery et al.[40] observed a 16% pseudarthrosis rate among 108 patients having predominantly one- to two-level, non-plated ADF.

Plating One- or Two-Level ADF. Plating one- and two-level ADF stabilized the anterior construct, facilitated fusion, and reduced the graft extrusion, pseudarthrosis, and kyphosis rates.[53,65] Bose[54,63] showed a 97.9% fusion rate with plates, and Connolly *et al.*[54,63] observed a 100% fusion rate among 42 plated average two level ADF.

One-Level Corpectomy/Fusion for OPLL. OPLL is rarely confined to two contiguous disc spaces; rather there is typically significant retrovertebral extension between adjacent interspaces. Therefore, two-level OPLL usually warrants performing a two-level discectomy with removal of the intervening vertebral body (one-level ACF). With this exposure, OPLL extending beyond the cephalad and caudad vertebral end plates may be removed by using angled 1- to 2-mm bayoneted curettes or small rotating Kerrison punches, while the posterior longitudinal ligament is excised.

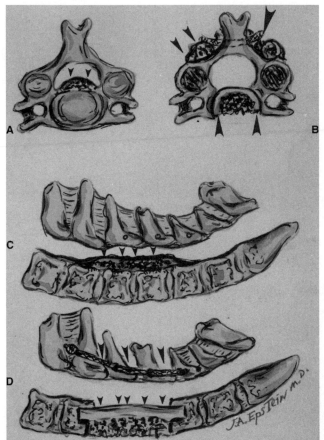

Figure 58.9 A non-plated C4-7 anterior corpectomy and fusion performed using a reversed iliac crest autograft is illustrated here, accompanied by a posterior wiring and fusion procedure. **(A)** OPLL is demonstrated filling the ventral aspect of the cervical spinal canal. **(B)** An anterior corpectomy and fusion graft has been applied ventrally and dorsal fusion has been performed using Songer cable wiring of a fibula strut allograft accompanied by en-lay application of iliac crest autograft. **(C)** This sagittal illustration demonstrates multilevel OPLL extending from the C4-7 levels contributing to marked cord compression. **(D)** Following anterior corpectomy and fusion from C4-7 of ventral OPLL with application of a reversed iliac crest strut graft, a posterior wiring and fusion procedure has also been performed to provide a posterior tension band.

The 10% or greater failure rates observed for non-plated two-level ADF prompted the application of plates to all one-level ACF constructs.[53,64] Reoperation rates to address graft extrusion, plate extrusion, or pseudarthrosis following 55 plated one-level ACF varied according to the type of plate applied. Plates included three Orion plates using a fixed plate/fixed screw design (Sofamor Danek, Memphis, TN), 12 Atlantis plates, using a fixed plate variable screw design (Sofamor Danek, Memphis, TN), and 40 ABC dynamic plates (Aesculap, Tuttlingen, Germany).[66] The ABC dynamic plates allow for up to 10mm of cephalad and caudad migration of the plates over screw heads that lock into longitudinal grooves in the plates. Results following application of both fixed-plate systems were suboptimal. One Orion plate extruded 6 weeks postoperatively, and two Orion plates resulted in pseudarthrosis. For the 12 Atlantis plates applied, four failed; one patient with pseudarthrosis required a secondary PWF 6 months later, and three developed delayed mid graft fractures 1 and 2 years later, warranting posterior wiring and fusion. Out of the total of 40 ABC plates applied, complications arose in four extremely obese patients. One patient developed an acute inferior graft and plate fracture within 2 weeks of surgery, warranting a C5-T1 ACF with PWF C2-T1. Two patients developed pseudarthrosis 6 months after a C2-4 ACF performed with a fibula strut graft, the other after a C5-7 ACF; both fused within 4 months after subsequent PWF. A fourth patient developed a delayed mid vertebral strut fracture 1 year postoperatively and required secondary PWF.[66] The overall failure rates were 7/15 (47%) for fixed compared with 4/40 (10%) for dynamic plates applied when performing one-level anterior corpectomy with fusion. The average cephalad migration of the ABC Aesculap plate was 6.6mm (range 3-10mm), and the average caudad migration, 5.7 (range 3-8mm). The lower failure rate for dynamic plates that demonstrated several mm of rostral and caudal migration indicated that the dynamic design contributed to reduced stress shielding and increased compression, both of which contributed to fusion and stability. Nevertheless, delayed iliac crest autograft strut fractures continued to be observed in subsequent larger series of one-level dynamic-plated ACF.[67,68] Furthermore, when 3- and 6-month postoperative x-ray and 2D-CT studies were separately interpreted by two radiologists following one-level ACF, the rates of fusion documented varied.[69] Three months postoperatively, 83% of the x-ray and only 50% of the 2D-CT studies confirmed fusion. Even 6 months postoperatively, 98% of x-ray studies and only 70% of 2D-CT studies revealed fusion.

Multilevel Ventral Corpectomy and Fusion

Better short- and long-term outcomes are associated with multilevel ventral corpectomy and fusion procedures performed to directly resect spondylosis, stenosis, and/or OPLL. Nevertheless, major complications are associated with these procedures.* In 76 patients with OPLL undergoing either non-plated ADF (average 3.5 levels) or ACF (average 3.0 levels), Epstein[76] found a 13% incidence of pseudarthrosis/instability within the first 6 postoperative months. Three of Saunder's[36] 31 non-plated patients

---

*References 30,37,60,70,72-75.

undergoing four-level ACF also failed acutely. In Macdonald et al.[77] series of 36 patients undergoing two- to four-level ACF, 15 performed with plates, the combined perioperative mortality, and major morbidity rate was 22%, even though 97% ultimately fused. Performing two-level multilevel ACF with fixed anterior plates, Vaccaro et al.[74] observed a 9% incidence of graft extrusion, the failure rate rising to 50% for three-level plated ACF. On the other hand, Eleraky et al.[78] found a fusion rate of 98.8%, a 3.2% neurologic complication rate, and 86.5% improvement rate after having plated one-level ACF (87 patients) and two- to three-level ACF (98 patients).

Results Using Fixed Versus Dynamic Plates

Complication rates were lower when dynamic rather than fixed plates were used to perform multilevel ACF/PWF. When Epstein[37] performed 22 multilevel (two- to four-level) ACF without ventral plates, but added PWF, three graft extrusions resulted. Adding fixed plates to another 22 of these multilevel constructs resulted in two immediate failures; inferior graft/plate extrusions.[60] When Atlantis plates (Sofamor Danek, Memphis, TN) were applied in 16 similar patients, three extruded 1 month (2 patients) and 4 months postoperatively; all included caudal graft, plate,

and screw extrusions.[30] After having performed 25 multilevel ACF/PWF with dynamic plates, only one patient developed a "partial" pseudarthrosis of the anterior graft demonstrated on sequential CT studies, warranting a second PWF (Figure 58.10).[79] The average dynamic plate migration for these multilevel ACF/PWF constructs was 6.1mm (range 4 to 10mm) cephalad, and 5.8mm (range 4 to 9mm) caudad. Dynamic plating similarly appeared to limit stress shielding, promoted graft settling, and fostered fusion in multilevel constructs.[80,81] Application of the Medical Outcomes Trust Short-Form 36 questionnaire (SF-36) preoperatively, and then 6 weeks, 3 months, 6 months, 1 year, and 2 years following circumferential cervical surgery in a subset of 47 out of 76 plated patients (36 fixed plates, 40 dynamic plates) who have undergone circumferential cervical surgery revealed that the majority of postoperative improvement occurred between 6 months and 1 year following surgery, with minimal additional improvement occurring within the second postoperative year.[82]

Dorsal Fusion Techniques

Posterior fusions may be completed using posterior wiring and fusion techniques, lateral mass screw/plating systems, or pedicle screw/rod instrumentation. The biomechanical

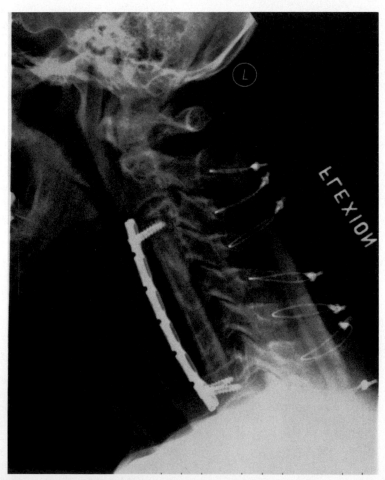

Figure 58.10 Presently, multilevel anterior corpectomy and fusion procedures are performed using fibula strut allografts with dynamic ABC Aesculap plates. Accompanying posterior wiring and fusions are completed by wiring split fibula strut allografts to the base of individual spinous processes with braided titanium cables, iliac crest, and autograft being placed over the decorticated lamina and facet joints and supplemented with ICM and allograft bone chips.

advantages of a posterior construct, or posterior "tension band" has been well documented. In a sagittal plane biomechanical study, Kirkpatrick et al.[73] demonstrated that posterior fusion reduced the range of motion by 62%, compared with 24% of strut grafting alone, and 43% following anterior strut graft and the application of an anterior plate. Of note, when performing posterior wiring and fusion following multilevel ACF, the inclusion of autogenous iliac crest graft is critical to achieving successful fusion.[83]

Complications of Multilevel ACF/PWF

Cord and Root Injuries

Complications of anterior cervical surgery include a 2% to 10% incidence of quadriplegia and up to a 17% incidence of root injury (typically C5 root).[40] The latter root injuries are often not the direct result of manipulation but result from rapid cord migration, a so-called untethering effect.[36] To address this "migration" Saunders recommended limiting the anterior trough to 15mm. Nevertheless, many North American patients with OPLL are large individuals, with interpedicular distances in the 18 to 20mm range. Here, troughs of only 15mm would leave significant amounts of OPLL unresected.

Ventral Floating Method: An Option for Anterior Opll Resection

Yamamura et al.[84] offered the anterior floating method as a technique for ventral OPLL resection where it occupies more than 60% of the spinal canal. This technique included marked lateral and cephalad/caudad resection and thinning of the vertebral bodies using air drills, and attempted to avoid the CSF fistulas typically produced by classic ventral OPLL resection techniques. Fusion was then performed using autogenous bone and a halo device. As this technique freed the ossified dura from its constraints, ventral migration of the remaining dura/OPLL mass would allow for adequate spinal cord and nerve root decompression. Long-term recovery rates of 71% using the JOA scale were observed using this procedure. However, as this procedure does not offer direct resection of OPLL mass, further progression of OPLL accompanied by retethering of the "floating OPLL" mass remains a major concern. Furthermore, technical risks including vertebral artery and root injury are associated with the extreme lateral resection technique.

REFERENCES

1. Epstein NE: Ossification of the posterior longitudinal ligament in evolution in 12 patients. *Spine* 19(6):673-681, 1994.
2. Miyasaka, H: Consideration on pathophysiology of OPLL. *Clin Orthop (Tokyo)* 10:1091-1096, 1975.
3. Epstein NE: Diagnosis and surgical management of ossification of the posterior longitudinal ligament. *Contemp Neurosurg* 22:1-6, 1992.
4. Epstein NE: Ossification of the posterior longitudinal ligament: diagnosis and surgical management. *Neurosurg Q* 2(3):223-241, 1992.
5. Epstein NE: The surgical management of ossification of the posterior longitudinal ligament in 51 patients. *J Spinal Disord Tech* 6(5):432-454, 1993.
6. Epstein NE: The surgical management of ossification of the posterior longitudinal ligament in 43 North Americans. *Spine* 19(6):664-672, 1994.
7. Koga H, Hayashi K, Taketomi E, et al: Restriction fragment length polymorphism of genes of the alpha 2(XI) collagen, bone morphogenetic protein-2, alkaline phosphatase, and tumor necrosis factor-alpha among patients with ossification of the posterior longitudinal ligament and controls from the Japanese population. *Spine* 21(4):469-473, 1996.
8. Koga H, Sakou T, Taketomi E, et al: Genetic mapping of ossification of the posterior longitudinal ligament of the spine. *Am J Hum Genet* 62(6):1460-1467, 1998.
9. Resnick D, Guerra J, Robinson CA: Association of diffuse idiopathic skeletal hyperostosis (DISH) and calcification and ossification of the posterior longitudinal ligament. *AJR* 131:1049-1053, 1978.
10. Terayama K: Genetic studies on ossification of the posterior longitudinal ligament of the spine. *Spine* 14(11):1184-1191, 1989.
11. Matsunaga S, Yamaguchi M, Hayashi K, Sakou T: Genetic analysis of ossification of the posterior longitudinal ligament. *Spine* 24(10):937-938, 1999.
12. Sakou T, Taketomie E, Matsunaga S, et al: Genetic study of ossification of the posterior longitudinal ligament in the cervical spine with human leukocyte antigen haplotype. *Spine* 16(11):1249-1252, 1991.
13. Ikegawa S, Kurokawa T, Hizuka N, et al: Increase of serum growth hormone-binding protein in patients with ossification of the posterior longitudinal ligament of the spine. *Spine* 18(13):1757-1760, 1993.
14. Yonemori I, Imamura T, Ishidou Y, et al: Bone morphogenetic protein receptors and activin receptors are highly expressed in ossified ligament tissues of patients with ossification of the posterior longitudinal ligament. *Am J Pathol* 150(4):1335-1347, 1997.
15. Motegi H, Yamazaki M, Goto S, et al: Proliferating cell nuclear antigen in hypertrophied spinal ligaments. Immunohistochemical localization of proliferating cell nuclear antigen in hypertrophied posterior longitudinal ligament of the cervical spine. *Spine* 23(3):305-310, 1998.
16. Epstein NE, Grande DA, Breitbart AS: In-vitro characteristics of cultured posterior longitudinal ligament tissue. *Spine* 27(1):56-58, 2002.
17. Breitbart AS, Grande DA, Kessler R, et al: Tissue engineered bone repair of calvarial defects using cultured periosteal cells. *Plastic Reconstr Surgery* 101:567-574, 1998.
18. Morimoto T, Matsuyama T, Hirabayashi H, et al: Expansive laminoplasty for multilevel cervical OPLL. *J Spinal Disord Tech* 10(4):296-298, 1997.
19. Okada K, Shirasaki N, Hayashi H, et al: Treatment of cervical spondylotic myelopathy by enlargement of the spinal canal anteriorly, followed by arthrodesis. *J Bone Joint Surg Am* 73(3):352-364, 1991.
20. Yonenobu K, Hosono N, Iwawaki M, et al: Laminoplasty versus subtotal corpectomy: a comparative study of results

in multisegmental cervical spondylotic myelopathy. *Spine* 17(11):1281-1284, 1992.

21. Yonenobu K, Hosono N, Iwasaki M, *et al:* Neurologic complications of surgery for cervical compression myelopathy. *Spine* 16(11):1277-1282, 1991.

22. Katoh S, Ikata T, Hirai N, *et al:* Influence of minor trauma to the neck on the neurological outcome in patients with ossification of the posterior longitudinal ligament of the cervical spine. *Paraplegia* 33(6):330-333, 1995.

23. Fujimura Y, Nakamura M, Toyama Y: Influence of minor trauma on surgical results in patients with cervical OPLL. *J Spinal Disord Tech* 11(1):16-20, 1998.

24. Koyanagi I, Iwasaki Y, Hida K, *et al:* Magnetic resonance imaging findings in ossification of the posterior longitudinal ligament of the cervical spine. *J Neurosurg* 88(2):247-254, 1998.

25. Baba H, Furusawa N, Imura S, *et al:* Late radiographic findings after anterior cervical fusion for spondylotic myeloradiculopathy. *Spine* 18(15):2167-2173, 1993.

26. Fujimura Y, Nishi Y, Nakamura M: Dorsal shift and expansion of the spinal cord after expansive open-door laminoplasty. *J Spinal Disord Tech* 10(4):282-287, 1997.

27. Epstein NE: Computed tomography (CT) validating bony ingrowth into fibula strut allograft: a criterion for fusion. *Spine J* 2:129-133, 2002.

28. Epstein NE: Identification of ossification of the posterior longitudinal ligament extending through the dura on preoperative CT examination of the cervical spine. *Spine* 26:182-186, 2001.

29. Hida K, Iwasaki Y, Kohanagi I, Abe H: Bone window computed tomography for detection of dural defect associated with cervical ossified posterior longitudinal ligament. *Neurol Med Chir (Tokyo)* Japan 37(2):173-175, 1997.

30. Epstein NE: Anterior approaches to cervical spondylosis and OPLL: review of operative techniques and assessment of 65 multilevel circumferential procedures. *Surg Neurol* 55:313-324, 2001.

31. Kissel P, Youmans JR: Posttraumatic anterior cervical osteophyte and dysphagia: surgical report and literature review. *J Spinal Disord Tech* 5(1):104-107, 1992.

32. Epstein NE: Simultaneous cervical diffuse idiopathic skeletal hyperostosis and ossification of the posterior longitudinal ligament resulting in dysphagia or myelopathy in two geriatric North Americans. *Surg Neurol* 53(5):427-431, 2000.

33. Hamanishi C, Tanaka S: Bilateral multilevel laminectomy with or without posterolateral fusion for cervical spondylotic myelopathy: relationship to type of onset and time until operation. *J Neurosurg* 85(3):447-451, 1996.

34. Oga M, Mashima T, Iwakuma T, Sugioka Y: Dysphagia complications in ankylosing spinal hyperostosis and ossification of the posterior longitudinal ligament. Roentgenographic findings of the developmental press of cervical osteophytes causing dysphagia. *Spine* 18(3):391-394, 1993.

35. McCafferty RR, Harrison MJ, Tamas LB, Larkings MV: Ossification of the anterior longitudinal ligament and Forrestier's disease: an analysis of seven cases. *J Neurosurg* 85(3):524-525, 1996.

36. Saunders RL, Pikus HJ, Ball P: Four-level cervical corpectomy. *Spine* 23(33):2455-2461, 1998.

37. Epstein NE: Circumferential surgery for the management of cervical ossification of the posterior longitudinal ligament. *J Spinal Disord Tech* 11(3):200-207, 1998.

38. Epstein NE: Can airway complications following multilevel anterior cervical surgery be avoided? *J Neurosurg* 94:185-188, 2001.

39. Emery SE, Smith MD, Bohlman HH: Upper-airway obstruction after multilevel cervical corpectomy for myelopathy. *J Bone Joint Surg Am* 73(4):544-551, 1991.

40. Emery SE, Bohlman HH, Bolesta MJ, Jones PK: Anterior cervical decompression and arthrodesis for the treatment of cervical spondylotic myelopathy. Two- to seventeen-year follow-up. *J Bone Joint Surg Am* 80(7):941-951, 1998.

41. Epstein NE: Evaluation of intraoperative somatosensory evoked potential monitoring during 100 cervical operations. *Spine* 18(6):737-747, 1993.

42. Epstein NE: Somatosensory evoked potential monitoring (SSEPs) in 173 cervical operations. *Neuro-Orthop (Springer-Verlag)* 20:2-21, 1996.

43. May DM, Jones SJ, Crockard HA: Somatosensory evoked potential monitoring in cervical surgery: identification of pre- and intraoperative risk factors associated with neurological deterioration. *J Neurosurg* 85(4):566-573, 1996.

44. Gokaslan ZL, Samudrala S, Deletis V, *et al:* Intraoperative monitoring of spinal cord function using motor evoked potentials via transcutaneous epidural electrode during anterior cervical spinal surgery. *J Spinal Disord Tech* 10(4):299-303, 1997.

45. Epstein NE: Laminectomy with posterior wiring and fusion for cervical OPLL, spondylosis, OYL, stenosis, and instability: a study of 5 patients. *J Spinal Disord Tech* 12:461-466, 1999.

46. Epstein NE: Posterior approaches in the management of spondylosis and ossification of the posterior longitudinal ligament. *Surg Neurol* 58:226-232, 2002.

47. Kato Y, Iwasaki M, Fuji T, *et al:* Long-term follow-up results of laminectomy for cervical myelopathy caused by ossification of the posterior longitudinal ligament. *J Neurosurg* 89(2):217-223, 1998.

48. Kumar VG, Rea GL, Mervis LJ, McGregor JM: Cervical spondylotic myelopathy: functional and radiographic long-term outcome after laminectomy and posterior fusion. *Neurosurgery* 44(4):771-777, 1999.

49. Wellman BJ, Follett KA, Traynelis VC: Complications of posterior articular mass plate fixation of the subaxial cervical spine in 43 consecutive patients. *Spine* 23(2):193-200, 1998.

50. Nowinski GP, Visarius H, Nolte LP, Herkowitz HN: A biomechanical comparison of cervical laminoplasty and cervical laminectomy with progressive facetectomy. *Spine* 18(14):1995-2004, 1993.

51. Abumi K, Kaneda K: Pedicle screw fixation for nontraumatic lesions of the cervical spine. *Spine* 22(16):1853-1863, 1997.

52. Abumi K, Kaneda K, Shono Y, Fujiya M: One-stage posterior decompression and reconstruction of the cervical spine by using pedicle screw fixation systems. *J Neurosurg* 90(suppl 1):19-26, 1999.

53. Epstein NE: Reoperation rates for acute graft extrusion and pseudarthrosis following one level anterior corpectomy and fusion with and without plate instrumentation: etiology and corrective management. *Surg Neurol* 56:73-81, 2001.

54. Bose B: Anterior cervical fusion using Caspar plating: analysis of results and review of the literature. *Surg Neurol* 49(1):25-31, 1998.

55. Sodeyama T, Goto S, Mochizuki M, *et al:* Effect of decompression enlargement laminoplasty for posterior shifting of the spinal cord. *Spine* 24(15):1527-1531, 1999.

56. Baisden J, Voo LM, Cusick JF, *et al:* Evaluation of cervical laminectomy and laminoplasty: a longitudinal study in the goat model. *Spine* 24(13):1283-1288, 1999.

57. Ishida Y, Ohmori K, Suzuki K, Inoue H: Analysis of dural configuration for evaluation of posterior decompression in cervical myelopathy. *Neurosurgery* 44(1):91-95, 1999.

58. Kawano H, Handa Y, Ishii H, *et al:* Surgical treatment for ossification of the posterior longitudinal ligament of the cervical spine. *J Spinal Disord Tech* 8(2):145-150, 1995.

59. Epstein NE: Advanced cervical spondylosis with ossification into the posterior longitudinal ligament and resultant neurologic sequelae. *J Spinal Disord Tech* 9(6):477-484, 1996.

60. Epstein NE: The value of anterior cervical plating in preventing vertebral fracture and graft extrusion following multilevel anterior cervical corpectomy with posterior wiring/fusion: indications, results, and complications. *J Spinal Disord Tech* 13:9-15, 2000.

61. Takatau T, Ishida Y, Suzuki K, Inoue H: Radiological study of cervical ossification of the posterior longitudinal ligament. *J Spinal Disord Tech* 12(3):271-273, 1999.

62. Fessler RG, Steck JC, Giovanini MA: Anterior cervical corpectomy for cervical spondylotic myelopathy. *Neurosurgery* 43(2):257-265, 1998.

63. Connolly PJ, Esses SI, Kostuik JP: Anterior cervical fusion: outcome analysis of patients fused with and without anterior cervical plates. *J Spinal Disord Tech* 9(3):202-206, 1996.

64. Epstein NE: Anterior cervical diskectomy and fusion without plate instrumentation in 178 patients. *J Spinal Disord Tech* 13:1-8, 2000.

65. Epstein NE: The management of 1 level anterior cervical corpectomy with fusion employing Atlantis hybrid plates: preliminary experience. *J Spinal Disord Tech* 13(4):324-328, 2000.

66. Epstein NE: The efficacy of anterior dynamic plates in complex cervical surgery. *J Spinal Disord Tech* 15(3): 221-227, 2002.

67. Epstein NE: Delayed iliac crest autograft fractures following plated single level anterior corpectomy with fusion. *J Spinal Disord Tech* 15(5):420-424, 2002.

68. Epstein NE: Anterior cervical dynamic ABC plating with single level corpectomy and fusion in 42 patients. *Spinal Cord* 41:153-158, 2003.

69. Epstein NE, Silvergleide RS: Documenting fusion following anterior cervical surgery: a comparison of roentgenogram versus two-dimensional computed tomographic findings. *J Spinal Disord Tech* 16(3):243-247, 2003.

70. Epstein NE: Vertebral body fractures following extensive anterior cervical surgical procedures for ossification of the posterior longitudinal ligament. *Neuro-Orthop (Springer-Verlag)* 21:1-11, 1997.

71. Epstein NE: Complications following surgical procedures of ossification of the posterior longitudinal ligament in the cervical spine warranting additional surgical correction. *Neuro-Orthop* 22:85-97, 1998.

72. Epstein NE: Circumferential surgery for spondylostenosis with kyphosis in two patients with athetoid cerebral palsy. *Surg Neurol* 52:339-344, 1999.

73. Kirkpatrick JS, Levy JA, Carillo J, Moeini SR: Reconstruction after multilevel corpectomy in the cervical spine: a sagittal plane biomechanical study. *Spine* 24(12):1186-1190, 1999.

74. Vaccaro AR, Falatyn SP, Scuderi GJ, *et al:* Early failure of long segment anterior cervical plate fixation. *J Spinal Disord Tech* 11(5):410-415, 1998.

75. Meding JB, Stambough JL: Critical analysis of strut grafts in anterior spinal fusions. *J Spinal Disord Tech* 6(2): 166-174, 1993.

76. Epstein NE: Evaluation and treatment of clinical instability associated with pseudarthrosis after anterior cervical surgery for ossification of the posterior longitudinal ligament. *Surg Neurol* 49(3):246-252, 1998.

77. Macdonald RL, Fehlings MG, Tator Ch, *et al:* Multilevel anterior cervical corpectomy and fibular allograft fusion for cervical myelopathy. *J Neurosurg* 86(6): 990-997, 1997.

78. Eleraky MA, Llanos C, Sonntag VK: Cervical corpectomy: a report of 185 cases and a review of the literature. *J Neurosurg* 90(suppl 1):35-41, 1999.

79. Epstein NE: A comparative analysis of plate/graft failure with correction following circumferential cervical spinal surgery. *Spinal Surg (Japan)* 16(1):1-8, 2002.

80. Epstein NE: From Postsurgical Imaging: Marked superior and inferior migration of a dynamic plate after multilevel anterior corpectomy and fusion with posterior wiring. *Spine J* 1:226-228, 2001.

81. Epstein NE: Fixed versus dynamic plate complications following multilevel anterior cervical corpectomy and fusion with posterior stabilization. *Spinal Cord* 41:379-384, 2003.

82. Epstein NE: Circumferential cervical surgery for ossification of the posterior longitudinal ligament: a multianalytic outcome study. *Spine* (in press), 2003.

83. Epstein NE: An analysis of combined Inductive-Conductive Matrix (ICM) and autologous bone graft in 61 posterior cervical fusions. *Spinal Surg* 17(1):1-6, 2003.

84. Yamamura I, Kurosa Y, Matuoka T, Shindo S: Anterior floating method for cervical myelopathy caused by ossification of the posterior longitudinal ligament. *Clinical Orthop Rel Res* 359:27-34, 1999.

CHAPTER 59

Scheuermann's Disease

Branko Prpa, Keith H. Bridwell, and Isador H. Lieberman

Scheuermann's Kyphosis

In 1920 Holger Werfel Scheuermann, a Danish surgeon, described a rigid kyphosis of the thoracic or thoracolumbar spine occurring in adolescents.[36] The disease, now known as *Scheuermann's disease,* manifests itself at puberty and involves ventral wedge formation of one or more vertebral bodies, leading to a rigid kyphotic deformity of the affected segments.[9,43] Scheuermann's disease typically involves the midthoracic spine with the apex at the T7 and T8 vertebrae.[34] Sorenson[40] defined the radiographic diagnosis of Scheuermann's kyphosis on the basis of anterior wedging of 5 degrees or more of at least three adjacent vertebral bodies. Scheuermann's disease typically involves the thoracic spine, but can also occur solely in the thoracolumbar spine in 25% of patients.

Incidence

Scheuermann's disease affects between 1% and 8% of the general population.[38,40] In a review of 1384 cadaveric specimens, Scoles *et al.*[38] reported a prevalence of 7.4%. Scheuermann's disease affects the growing, maturing spine and is usually identified in adolescents between 11 and 17 years of age. In Sorenson's review, 58% of those affected were male and 42% were female. There are, however, widely divergent reports regarding the relative gender prevalence. Bradford[5] reported a female-to-male ratio of 2:1, while Murray, Weinstein, and Spratt reported a 2:1 prevalence in males.[27] Researchers have not found a clear genetic predisposition for Scheuermann's disease, although a familial occurrence has been described.[9]

Pathogenesis

The etiology of Scheuermann's kyphosis remains unknown.[1,3,5] Many theories have been proposed to explain the progressive wedge shaping of the involved vertebrae. Scheuermann[36] considered the condition a form of avascular necrosis of the ring apophysis that leads to a growth arrest, resulting in wedging of the ventral portion of the vertebral bodies. However, Bick and Copel[4] later showed that the ring apophysis does not contribute to vertebral growth. Furthermore, avascular necrosis has never been identified in affected vertebral segments of patients with the disease.[1,5,26] Schmorl[37] postulated that herniations of disc material through the vertebral end plates (which now bear his name) lead to a loss of disc height and ventral wedging of the vertebral body. Subsequent studies dis-

proved these early theories but have not yet established a cause.

Osteoporosis may be an etiologic factor in the development of Scheuermann's kyphosis. Bradford *et al.*[6] prospectively studied 12 patients with an extensive osteoporosis work-up and iliac crest biopsy. The authors identified increased levels of serum alkaline phosphatase and urinary hydroxyproline, in conjunction with reduced bone mineral density. However, when compared to age-matched controls, no specific relationship could be identified. Bradford *et al.*[6] postulated that Scheuermann's disease may be related to a generalized skeletal disease that presents during the adolescent growth spurt. Gilanz *et al.*[14] subsequently reported on 20 adolescent patients 12 to 18 years of age with Scheuermann's kyphosis and could demonstrate no evidence of osteoporosis (as assessed by quantitative computed tomography).

Mechanical factors have also been postulated in the development of Scheuermann's kyphosis.[3,6] Strenuous physical activity has been associated with compression of the vertebrae of patients with this disease.[3] Ogden *et al.*[28] believe that the term *Scheuermann's disease* is a misnomer; they state that the changes noted radiographically are altered remodeling responses to abnormal biomechanical stresses and are not secondary to an underlying disease process. They theorized that the kyphosis occurs first and the ventral vertebral body is then subjected to increased forces that suppress ventral growth and perpetuate the deformity. The reported success of brace treatment lends support to the mechanical theory.[45] Lambrinudi[20] and others have suggested that the upright posture and tightness of the anterior longitudinal ligament of the spine contribute to the deformity. Most investigators believe that the growth plate becomes disorganized first and the emerging kyphosis follows. The kyphosis and growth plate changes may ultimately potentiate each other. The kyphosis likely results in increased pressure on the vertebral end plates ventrally, allowing for uneven growth of the vertebral bodies with wedging (as per Wolff's law).

Clinical Features

The onset of Scheuermann's disease usually appears around puberty, commonly as kyphosis of the thoracic (type I Scheuermann's) or thoracolumbar spine (type II Scheuermann's). These two entities differ both in location and by their clinical presentation. The deformity is often attributed to poor posture. This results in a delay in both diagnosis and treatment. Pain is often present; standing, sitting, and heavy physical activity may aggravate the pain (i.e., mechanical pain), which may or may not subside with cessation of growth. Adults who have untreated Scheuermann's disease may have severe back pain, especially when the deformity is advanced.

Patients will generally present with an angular thoracic or thoracolumbar kyphosis accompanied by a compensatory hyperlordosis of the lumbar spine. Their compensatory lordosis may lead to an increase in pelvic tilt.[43] Frequently, the cervical lordosis is increased with forward projection of the head. The kyphosis is fixed and remains apparent on hyperextension of the spine. In rare instances, advanced thoracic kyphosis can lead to thoracic spinal cord compression and paraparesis.[7] Pain, when present, is usually at the site of the thoracic deformity. Sorenson described pain as the major symptom in 50% of patients with advanced disease.[39]

In addition to the kyphosis of the thoracic spine, affected individuals demonstrate varying degrees of structural scoliosis.[6,26,34] Blumenthal et al.[3] noted 85% of lumbar scoliosis among 50 patients with type I Scheuermann's disease. Spondylolysis and spondylolisthesis are also common in the lumbar spine.[6,9] Ogilvie and Sherman[29] observed a 50% incidence of asymptomatic spondylolysis among 18 patients with type I disease. They postulated that the excessive hyperlordosis places stress on the pars of the L4 and L5 vertebrae, resulting in the spondylolysis.

Radiographic Features

Routine radiographic studies obtained for evaluation of the patient with Scheuermann's kyphosis should include anteroposterior and lateral radiographs of the entire spine via long films (scoliosis views) and a hyperextension lateral image of the thoracic spine. The lateral radiograph should be obtained with the patient standing, with knees and hips fully extended and arms out and away from the spine. The patient should be looking forward. The lateral radiograph should document the following typical changes of Scheuermann's kyphosis:

1. Schmorl's nodes
2. Kyphosis of the involved spinal segment
3. Ventral vertebral body wedging
4. End plate irregularity

Both the vertebral wedging and kyphosis should be measured by the Cobb method. When evaluating serial radiographs to document progression, care should be taken to ensure that the same end vertebral bodies are measured each time. The normal range of thoracic kyphosis is 20 to 45 degrees on a standing lateral radiograph[2,46] as measured by the Cobb method. Normal kyphosis increases with age and is slightly greater in women than in men.[12,13] Ventral wedge compression of one or more vertebral segments in association with kyphosis is the hallmark radiographic feature in Scheuermann's disease.[36] Wedging of at least 5 degrees of three or more vertebrae is diagnostic of Scheuermann's disease. The kyphosis in Scheuermann's disease is usually incompletely reducible with postural and positional changes. The vertebra with the greatest ventral deformity is located at the apex of the kyphotic curve. The kyphosis may approach 100 degrees in advanced cases with a compensatory hyperlordosis of both the cervical and lumbar spine.[43]

Early in the progression of the disease, the end plates may appear irregular.[34,37,43] The changes have been described as moth-eaten and relate to growth retardation rather than to a destructive process.[34] As the disease progresses, the growth plates will appear sclerotic, but despite interspace narrowing, the change is not associated with interbody fusion. The absence of fusion helps distinguish Scheuermann's from other kyphotic deformities of the spine.[3,5,34]

Natural History

The natural history of Scheuermann's disease remains very controversial. The condition tends to be symptomatic during the teenage years. However, in the late teenage years, it often produces less pain. In a long-term follow-up study, Sorenson noted pain in the thoracic region in 50% of patients during adolescence, with the number of symptomatic patients decreasing to 25% by the time of skeletal maturity.[40] Later, other authors offered a contrasting view, stating that adults with Scheuermann's kyphosis have a higher incidence of disabling back pain than do the normal population.[5,9] Murray et al.[27] performed a study in 67 patients with Scheuermann's kyphosis diagnosed by Sorenson's criteria (i.e., physical examination, trunk strength, radiography, a detailed questionnaire, and pulmonary function testing). The patients had an average kyphotic deformity of 71 degrees, and average follow-up was 32 years. An age-matched comparison group was used as a control. Normal or above normal averages for pulmonary function were found in patients in whom the kyphosis was less than 100 degrees. Patients in whom the kyphosis was greater than 100 degrees and the apex of the curve was in the first to eighth thoracic segments had restrictive lung disease. The authors concluded that patients may have functional limitations but these did not result in severe limitations due to pain or cause major interference with their lives. Lowe and Kasten state that adults with greater than 75 degrees of kyphosis can have severe thoracic pain secondary to spondylosis that can limit their activity.[24]

In summary, patients experience wide variations in the natural history of Scheuermann's kyphosis. There appears to be a subset of patients with refractory symptoms that justify the risk associated with aggressive treatments such as bracing and surgical management.

Treatment

The management of patients with symptomatic Scheuermann's kyphosis ranges from observation to combined ventral and dorsal reconstructive surgery. Treatment is based on the severity of the deformity, the presence of pain, and the age of the patient. The recommended treatment should be tailored to the individual on the basis of deformity progression, the severity of the curve, and symptomatology.

Anti-inflammatory Medications

Nonsteroidal anti-inflammatory drugs (NSAIDs) may be useful short-term adjuncts to nonoperative care of the adolescent. They may also be considered for longer-term care in the adult with spondylosis and back pain.

Exercise

Exercise has never been shown to improve or halt progression of fixed Scheuermann's kyphosis. However, a thoracic extension program, coupled with an aerobic exercise program, will improve conditioning and may alleviate pain. In the adult with spondylosis, flexion exercises may be added to improve trunk stability and help manage low back pain.

Brace Treatment

The few available brace treatment studies are retrospective, have different inclusion criteria, and do not have control groups. The initial report of Bradford *et al.*[8] regarding Milwaukee brace treatment of Scheuermann's kyphosis in 75 patients demonstrated a 40% decrease in mean thoracic kyphosis and a 35% decrease in mean lumbar lordosis after an average of 34 months of brace wear. Gutowski and Renshaw[15] reported on the use of Boston lumbar and modified Milwaukee orthoses for Scheuermann's kyphosis and abnormal juvenile round back, with an average 26-month follow-up. Of the 75 patients in their group, 31% rejected the brace within 4 months. Compliant patients had an improvement of 27% in the Boston group and 35% in the Milwaukee group. Whether the corrections were maintained over time is not known. Bracing can be expected to provide up to a 50% correction of the deformity, with some gradual loss of correction over time. Sachs *et al.*[35] followed 120 patients for more than 5 years after discontinuation of the brace and demonstrated that 69% still had improvement of 3 degrees or more.

The classic prerequisites for brace treatment of Scheuermann's kyphosis include a progressive curve beyond 45 degrees. Patients with a kyphosis of up to 65 degrees may be successfully treated. Curves greater than 74 degrees have been associated with higher failure rates.[35] Patients must have some flexibility and some remaining growth. The brace is typically worn for 23 hours a day for 1 to 2 years.

Surgical Treatment

The indications for surgical intervention remain unclear, since the natural history of Scheuermann's kyphosis remains controversial regarding pain, trunk deformity, disability, and self-esteem. The ultimate decision for surgical correction should be individualized. It may relate to the patient's symptoms, self-perception, and sense of self-esteem. The surgeon's training and level of skill in performing a safe, predictable correction also affect the decision-making process.

Surgical indications have evolved over the past 2 decades. The operative indications for Scheuermann's kyphosis are similar to those of patients with other deformity types: (1) progression of deformity, (2) neurologic compromise, (3) worsening pain, and (4) cosmesis.[35,39,42] Some authors also list unacceptable trunk appearance as an indication.[24] An adolescent with kyphosis greater than 75 degrees despite a trial of bracing may be a surgical candidate. An adult may become a candidate when severe refractory pain develops secondary to a curve of at least 60 degrees. Bradford and Garcia[9] have also described neurologic compromise in a patient with a thoracic disc herniation in conjunction with Scheuermann's disease, thus obligating surgical intervention.

The goal of surgical intervention is a solid arthrodesis throughout the length of the kyphosis; a ventral-only, ventral-dorsal, and dorsal-only approach can accomplish this. Kostuik[18] described a ventral-only approach with interbody fusion and ventral instrumentation with a Harrington distraction system augmented by postoperative bracing. He reported the results in 36 patients with a mean preoperative reduction from 75.5 to 60 degrees. Subsequently, ventral fusion has not gained significant acceptance for the correction of Scheuermann's kyphosis.

The correction of deformity by a dorsal instrumentation approach was originally reported by Bradford *et al.*[10] who noted excellent initial correction of deformity but loss of correction and pseudoarthrosis in kyphotic curves exceeding 70 degrees. They recommended a combined ventral-dorsal spine arthrodesis. Otsuka *et al.*,[30] using heavier Harrington compression rods in 10 patients, reported correction from a mean of 71 to 39 degrees at 26-month follow-up. They performed dorsal-only surgery if the kyphosis decreased to 50 degrees or less on a hyperextension lateral radiograph. The loss of correction after dorsal-only surgery has been attributed to the fusion being performed on the tension side of the spine, the failure of implants, the lack of ventral support, and inadequate correction of a severe deformity with a short construct.[23]

Strum *et al*[42] performed surgical instrumentation and fusion on 39 patients with Scheuermann's disease. They found single dorsal internal fixation and fusion was effective in correcting kyphosis (mean correction from 71.5 to 37.7 degrees) and arresting the progression in 30 of 39 patients at 72-month follow-up. The authors argued that a long dorsal fusion is the surgical treatment of choice, obviating the need for ventral approaches.

The ventral-dorsal approach is reserved for rigid curves (75 degrees or greater) that do not correct to less than 50 degrees on hyperextension lateral radiographs. Recently, the combined procedure has been performed at one operative sitting; however, some authors still advocate staged procedures. The ventral portion can be performed open or endoscopically.[16,22,25,32] The approach is typically performed on the right side to avoid the great vessels. A ventral release and bone graft is performed at all the levels that are wedged or have narrowed disc space. Transthoracic endoscopic techniques, compared with thoracotomy, provide a less invasive method of accessing the ventral spinal column, with benefits of an excellent exposure and minimal soft tissue disruption. With the simultaneous technique, staged or subsequent procedures can be eliminated and a circumferential structural release, as well as control of the mobilized spine, can be achieved. This simultaneous technique can be extended for use in correction of a variety of thoracic spinal pathologies.[22]

The precise determination of the vertebrae to include within the instrumented, corrected segment is important. Despite the early recognition that fusing too short results in persistent or recurrent deformity at follow-up,[8] this complication persists in even the most recent series.[24] Selection of fusion levels is integral in decision making, yet no well-established criteria that have been validated with long-term follow-up are available. In the standing patient with kyphosis, the greater the deformity is, the greater the compression moment across the thoracic spine.[47] When using operative techniques with claw constructs at the rostral (usually T2-3 and T4-5) and caudal (usually at L2-3) ends of the deformity, the remaining levels must be instrumented with the hooks placed in compression toward the apex. Using compression across the apex of the kyphosis lessens the actual bending of the rod and requires less force to be dissipated at either end of the construct.

Recently, the trend in the surgical treatment of Scheuermann's kyphosis has been toward instrumentation systems involving pedicle screw constructs. Pedicle fixation offers increased biomechanical integrity. However, the insertion of screws safely and reliably can be a technical challenge. Caution must be exercised. The choice of instrumentation system, whether hook or screw, should be left to the surgeon.

The problem of junctional kyphosis at the rostral or caudal end of the fusion mass has received significant attention in the recent literature.[21,33] Factors that may predispose the patient to junctional kyphosis include the following:

1. Osteoporosis may be an associated factor for junctional kyphosis at the middle or upper thoracic spine in adults.[21]
2. Instrumentation may be too short because of failure to accurately determine the end vertebra.[24] Many authors have reported that the instrumentation and fusion must extend over the entire length of the kyphosis to avoid loss of correction[41] and junctional kyphosis.[17] Instrumentation should not terminate at the middle or low thoracic level.[21]
3. Excessive intraoperative dissection of the soft tissues and ligaments of the most rostral and caudal vertebral levels may weaken the construct; wiring of the spinous processes may diminish the incidence of this complication.[19]
4. Some authors have reported that excessive correction of kyphosis may lead to junctional kyphosis.[24]
5. Finally, operative techniques using pure cantilever correction of a thoracic kyphosis frequently lead to junctional kyphosis.[11,21]

Junctional kyphosis has been reported with Cotrel-Dubousset instrumentation. It is likely related to sagittal balance and selection of fusion levels.[24,30] Lowe and Kasten[24] found that these patients tend to be in negative sagittal balance. This may be exaggerated by surgery, thus predisposing to junctional kyphosis. The most recent recommendations include fusion levels, the end vertebra of the kyphosis rostrally, and the extent of the fusion to the first lordotic disc beyond the transitional zone distally.[24,30] To adequately correct a typical Scheuermann kyphosis, dorsal corrective instrumentation from the T3 to the L2 level are necessary. Recommendations have also been made to limit the correction to 50% or less of the original deformity, in an attempt to prevent proximal junctional kyphosis.[24] Overcorrection should be avoided. The use of contemporary multisegmental rod, hook, and pedicle screw systems has increased the ability of the surgeon to obtain and maintain correction. Long-term follow-up of these newer techniques is needed to assess their efficacy. More in-depth research is needed to analyze the effect of living one's entire life with a 65-degree kyphosis as compared to having it corrected to 35 degrees and possibly subjecting patients to future problems with junctional kyphosis.

Most surgeons who treat patients with Scheuermann's kyphosis favor surgery only in the rare patient with advanced kyphosis refractory to external bracing.[17,35] The dorsal approach is advocated, unless ventral compressive pathology exists. A long dorsal stabilization and internal fixation construct with segmental fixation and the use of autologous fusion provides excellent results.[10,30-32] Cases 1 to 4 are provided to illustrate the aforementioned points.

Case 1. A male, 16 years and 9 months of age, with a 92-degree Scheuermann's kyphosis is shown in Figure 59-1A. It corrects to 48 degrees on a supine hyperextension lateral (Figure 59-1B). He is treated with ventral release/discectomy/morselized bone grafting, followed by dorsal instrumentation and fusion. The construct consists of six pedicle hooks/transverse process claws above apex. Multiple hooks and multiple pedicle screws were placed below the apex. His result at 3½ years following surgery is shown in Figure 59-1C. Clinical appearance before and after surgery is pictured in Figure 59-1D.

Case 2. A female, 12 years and 9 months of age, presented with a 90-degree Scheuermann's kyphosis (Figure 59-2A). On the hyperextension lateral, she corrects to roughly 70 degrees (Figure 59-2B). She was treated with multilevel ventral release/discectomy/morselized bone grafting with some cages ventrally. Following this, a dorsal fusion and instrumentation with mostly pedicle screws was performed. The 2-year postoperative result with correction to 56 degrees of kyphosis is shown in Figure 59-2C. Her clinical appearance preoperative is pictured in Figure 59-2D and at 2 years postoperative in Figure 59-2E.

Case 3. A female, 26 years and 6 months of age, initially presented with a 75-degree Scheuermann's kyphosis (Figure 59-3A). Her initial treating surgeons attempted a dorsal-only construct (Figure 59-3B). This construct failed, and her implants were removed. She subsequently progressed to a 95-degree kyphosis (Figure 59-3C). This deformity only corrected to 85 degrees with a supine hyperextension maneuver. She was then treated with a multilevel ventral release, followed by multiple Smith-Peterson osteotomies at essentially all levels and pedicle screw fixation at virtually all levels as well. She corrected to 44 degrees (Figure 59-3D). Her radiographic (Figure 59-3D) and clinical result following revision (Figure 59-3E) and at 1 year, 3 months postoperative (Figure 59-3F) are shown. She is converted from positive to negative sagittal balance.

Case 4.* A male, 19 years of age, presented with a 90-degree painful, progressive, and rigid Scheuermann's kyphosis (Figure 59-4A). His main concern was cosmesis. To avoid a front-back-front approach and a thoracotomy scar, a simultaneous anterior endoscopic release with interbody bone grafting and posterior segmental pedicle screw/hook instrumentation with bone grafting was recommended. In the operating room the patient was positioned prone for the two-team approach (Figure 49-4B). Correction was obtained by virtue of the multilevel releases with 4 to 5 degrees obtained at each level (Figure 59-4C-E). Final correction and sagittal balance was achieved and maintained at 45 degrees (Figure 49-4F). This case illustrates the utility and advantages of the simultaneous approach as an alternative to consider in rigid hyperkyphotic deformities.

---

*Case submitted by I. H. Lieberman, MD.

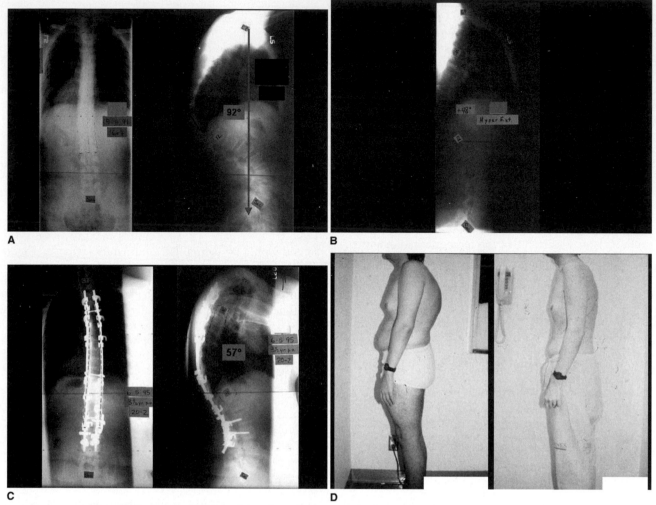

Figure 59-1 Case 1. **(A)** Upright AP/lateral x-rays preop. **(B)** Supine hyperextension lateral. **(C)** Upright AP and lateral x-rays, 3 years postop. **(D)** Preop *(left)* and postop *(right)*.

Other Kyphotic Disorders of the Growing Spine

Two other disorders associated with kyphosis occur in the juvenile spine. Round back deformity is a posture-related kyphosis that is reducible with extension.[8] It is the most common type of thoracic kyphosis identified in patients. Its etiology is unknown but is believed to be related to poor posture during spine maturation.[26] Balderston reported that it is more common in adolescent females and likely represents a compensatory slouch to developing breasts. Postural round back is differentiated from Scheuermann's disease by kyphosis that corrects with hyperextension, absence of ventral vertebral deformities, lack of interbody fusion, and absence of compensatory pelvic tilt and hamstring shortening.[5,8] The treatment of postural round back is observation. Occasional exercise and bracing are useful as an adjunct in patients with persistent pain.[26]

Congenital kyphosis of the spine is rare and results from the congenital absence or malformation of one or more vertebral segments.[26] It is characterized by two distinct forms: (1) congenital absence of one or more vertebra or (2) failure of segmentation of two or more vertebrae.[43] Failure of formation may lead to neurologic compromise. However, failure of segmentation does not, and it is the failure of segmentation that often looks very much like Scheuermann's kyphosis clinically and radiographically. Winter described 130 patients with congenital kyphosis of the spine.[48] Female to male ratio was 2:1. Eighty-six patients had failure of formation of one or more segments. The treatment of patients with congenital kyphosis revolves around preventing neurologic deterioration and arresting the progressive kyphosis. Bracing is ineffective in young patients. Dorsal instrumentation and fusion is recommended in patients less than 5 years of age with kyphosis less than 55 degrees.[26,33] Older patients with advanced kyphosis and neurologic involvement are typically managed with a ventral decompression and release, followed by a dorsal instrumentation and fusion.

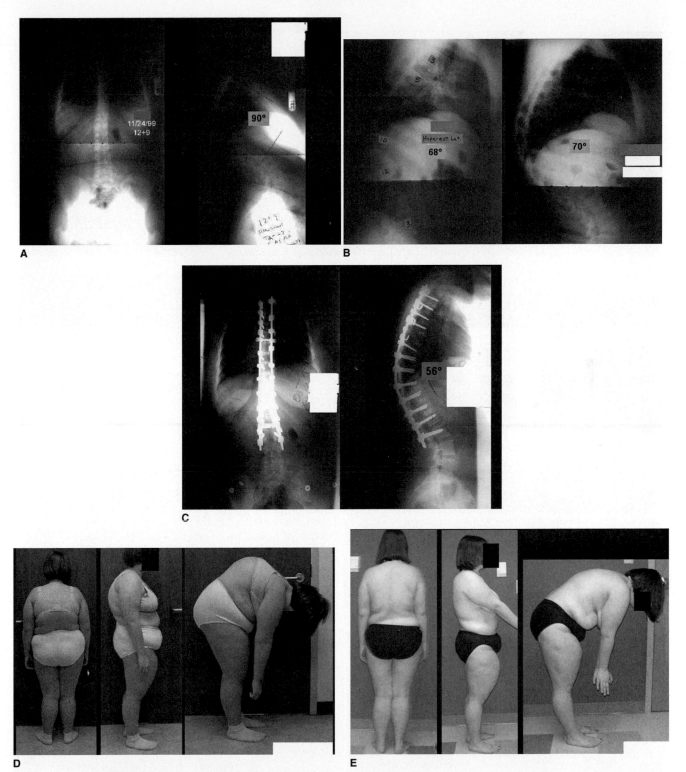

Figure 59-2 Case 2. (**A**) Upright AP/lateral x-rays preop. (**B**) Supine hyperextension lateral. (**C**) Upright AP/lateral x-rays, 2 years postop. (**D**) Preop. (**E**) Postop.

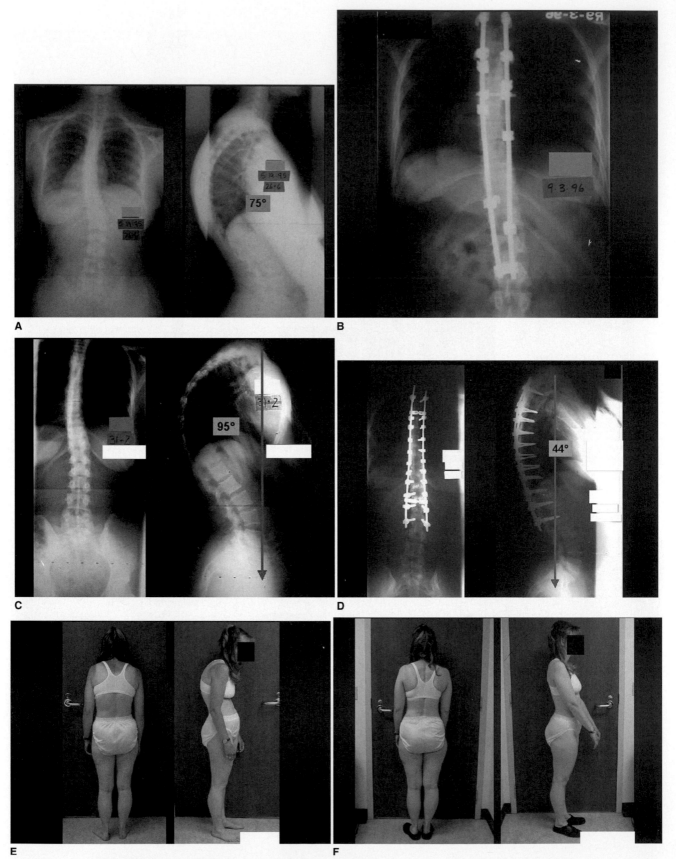

Figure 59-3 Case 3. **(A)** Initial presentation: upright AP/lateral x-rays. **(B)** PSF/PSSI. **(C)** Failed PSF/PSSI: upright AP/lateral x-rays. **(D)** Upright AP/lateral x-rays after revision reconstruction. **(E)** Preop revision reconstruction. **(F)** Postop revision reconstruction.

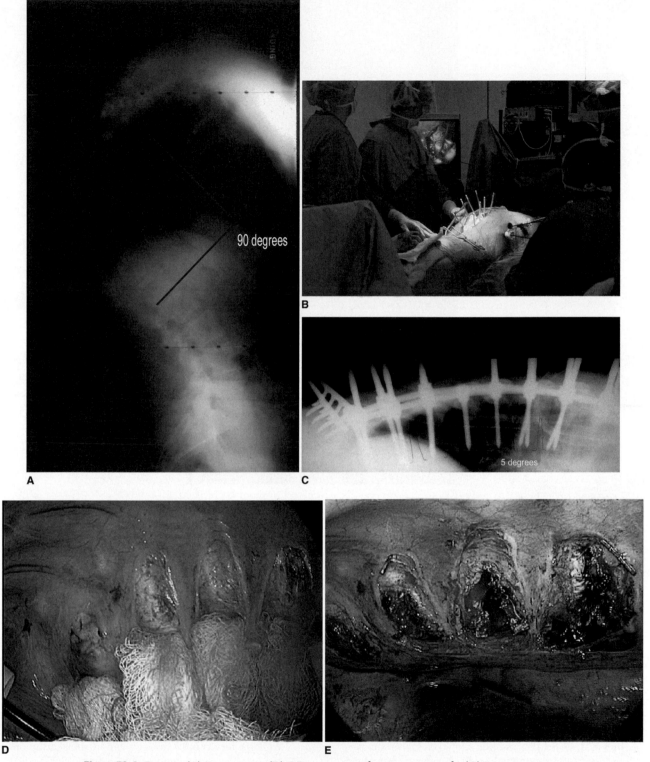

Figure 59-4 Case 4. **(A)** Preop x-ray. **(B)** OR set-up, simultaneous approach. **(C)** Intraop x-ray. **(D)** Precorrection video capture. **(E)** Postcorrection video capture.

Continued

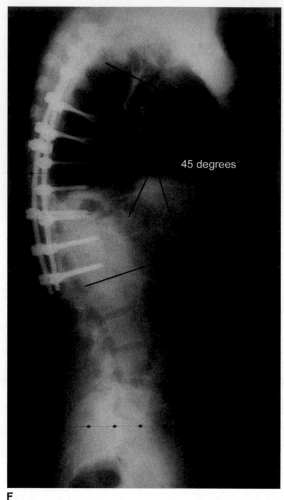

45 degrees

F

Figure 59-4 *cont'd* (F) Postop x-ray.

REFERENCES

1. Aufdermaur M: Juvenile kyphosis (Scheuermann's disease): radiography, histology, and pathogenesis, *Clin Orthop* 154:166-174, 1984.
2. Bernhardt M, Bridwell KH: Segmental analysis of the sagittal plane alignment of the normal thoracic and lumbar spines and the thoracolumbar junction, *Spine* 14:717-721, 1989.
3. Blumenthal SL, Roach J, Herring JA: Lumbar Scheuermann's: a clinical series and classification, *Spine* 12:929-932, 1987.
4. Bick EM, Copel JW: The ring apophysis of the human vertebra. Contribution to human osteogeny, *J Bone Joint Surg Am* 33:783, 1951.
5. Bradford DS: Juvenile kyphosis. In *Moe's Textbook of Scoliosis and Other Spinal Deformities*, ed 2. Philadelphia, WB Saunders, 1987, pp 347-368.
6. Bradford DS, Brown DM, Moe JH, Winter RB: Scheuermann's kyphosis: a form of osteoporosis? *Clin Orthop* 118:10, 1976.
7. Bradford DS, Garcia A: Neurological complications in Scheuermann's disease: a case report and review of the literature, *J Bone Joint Surg* 51A:567, 1989.
8. Bradford DS, Moe JH, Montalvo FJ: Scheuermann's kyphosis and roundback deformity: results of Milwaukee brace treatment, *J Bone Joint Surg Am* 51:567, 1969.
9. Bradford DS, Moe JH, Winter RB: Scheuermann's juvenile kyphosis and postural round back deformity. In Rothman RH, Simeone FA (eds): *The Spine*, vol 1. Philadelphia, WB Saunders, 1975, pp 361-379.
10. Bradford DS, Moe JH, Winter RB: Scheuermann's kyphosis: results of surgical treatment by posterior spine arthrodesis in 22 patients, *J Bone Joint Surg Am* 57:437, 1975.
11. Coscia MF, Bradford DS, Ogilvie JW: Scheuermann's kyphosis: results in 19 cases treated by spinal arthrodesis and L-rod instrumentation, *Orthop Trans* 12:255, 1988.
12. Fon GT, Pitt MJ, Thies AC: Thoracic kyphosis: range in normal subjects, *AJR* 134:979, 1980.
13. Gelb DE, Lenke LG, Bridwell KH, *et al*: An analysis of sagittal spinal alignment in 100 asymptomatic middle and older volunteers, *Spine* 20:1351-1358, 1995.
14. Gilanz V, Gibbens DT, Carlson M, King J: Vertebral bone density in Scheuermann's disease, *J Bone Joint Surg Am* 71:894, 1989.
15. Gutowski WT, Renshaw TS: Orthotic results in adolescent kyphosis, *Spine* 13:485, 1988.

16. Heniford BT, Matthews BD, Lieberman IH: Laparoscopic lumbar interbody spinal fusion, *Surg Clin North Am* 80(5):1487-1500, 2000.

17. Herndon WA, Emans JB, Micheli LJ: Combined anterior and posterior fusion for Scheuermann's kyphosis, *Spine* 6:125, 1980.

18. Kostuik JP: Anterior Kostuik-Harrington distraction systems, *Orthopedics* 11:1379, 1988.

19. La Grone MO: Loss of lumbar lordosis: a complication of spinal fusion for scoliosis, *Orthop Clin North Am* 19: 383-393, 1988.

20. Lambrinudi C: Adolescent and senile kyphosis, *Br Med J* 2:800, 1934.

21. Lettice J, Ogilvie J, Transfeldt E: Proximal junctional kyphos following Coutrel-Dubousset instrumentation in adult scoliosis, *Orthop Trans* 16:162, 1992.

22. Lieberman IH, Salo PT, Orr RD, Kraetschmer B: Prone position endoscopic transthoracic release with simultaneous posterior instrumentation for spinal deformity: a description of the technique, *Spine* 25: 2251-2257, 2000.

23. Lowe TG: Scheuermann's disease, *J Bone Joint Surg Am* 72:940, 1990.

24. Lowe TG, Kasten MD: An analysis of sagittal curves and balance after Coutrel-Dubousset instrumentation for kyphosis secondary to Scheuermann's disease, *Spine* 19:1680, 1994.

25. McLain RF, Lieberman IH: Endoscopic approaches to metastatic thoracic disease, *Spine* 25:1855-1858, 2000.

26. Moe JH, Winter RB et al: Juvenile kyphosis. In *Scoliosis and Other Spinal Deformities*, Philadelphia, WB Saunders, 1978, pp 331-343.

27. Murray PM, Weinstein SL, Spratt KF: The natural history and long-term follow-up of Scheuermann's kyphosis, *J Bone Joint Surg Am* 75:236, 1993.

28. Ogden JA, Ganey TM, Sasse J: Development and maturation of the axial skeleton. In Weinstein SL (ed): *The Pediatric Spine: Principles and Practice*, vol 1. New York, Raven Press, 1994.

29. Ogilvie JW, Sherman J: Spondylolysis in Scheuermann's disease, *Spine* 12:251, 1983.

30. Otsuka NY, Hall JE, Mah JY: Posterior fusion of Scheuermann's kyphosis, *Clin Orthop* 51:134, 1990.

31. Papagelopoulos PJ, Klassen RA, Peterson HA, Dekutoski MB: Surgical treatment of Scheuermann's disease with segmental compression and instrumentation, *Clin Orth Rel Res* 386:139-149, 2001.

32. Regan JJ, Yuan H, McCullen G: Minimally invasive approaches to the spine. In Springfield DS (ed): *Instructional Course Lectures,* vol 46. Rosemont, IL, American Academy of Orthopedic Surgeons, 1997, pp 127-141.

33. Reinhardt P, Bassett GS: Short segmental kyphosis following fusion for Scheuermann's disease, *J Spinal Disord* 3:162-168, 1990.

34. Rothman RH, Simeone FA: Scheuermann's juvenile kyphosis. In *The Spine*, ed 3, vol 1. Philadelphia, WB Saunders, 1980, pp 2380-2388.

35. Sachs B, Bradford DS, Winter R, Lonstein J: Scheuermann's kyphosis: follow-up of Milwaukee brace treatment, *J Bone Joint Surg Am* 69:50, 1987.

36. Scheuermann H: Kyphosis dorsalis juvenilis. *Ugeskr Laeger* 82:385-393, 1920.

37. Schmorl G: Die Pathogenese der juvenilen kyphose. *Fortschr Rontgenstr* 41:359, 1930.

38. Scoles PV, Latimer BM, Digiovanni BF, Vargo E: Vertebral alterations in Scheuermann's kyphosis, *Spine* 16:509, 1991.

39. Sorenson KH: *Scheuermann's juvenile kyphosis,* Copenhagen, Munksgaard, 1964.

40. Sorenson KH: *Scheuermann's juvenile kyphosis: clinical appearances, radiography, aetiology, and prognosis,* Copenhagen, Munksgaard, 1964.

41. Speck GR, Chopin DC: The surgical treatment of Scheuermann's kyphosis, *J Bone Joint Surg* 68B:189-193, 1982.

42. Strum PF, Dobson JC, Armstrong GWD: The surgical management of Scheuermann's, *J Bone Joint Surg Am* 18:685, 1993.

43. Tachdjian MO, editor: Scheuermann's juvenile kyphosis. In *Pediatric Orthopedics*, ed 2, vol 3. Philadelphia, WB Saunders, 1990, pp 2380-2390.

44. Tribus CB: Scheuermann's kyphosis in adolescents and adults: diagnosis and management, *J Am Acad Orthop Surg* 6:36, 1998.

45. Vendantam R, Lenke LG, Keeney JA, Bridwell KH: Comparison of standing sagittal spinal alignment in asymptomatic adolescent adults, *Spine* 23:211-215, 1998.

46. Wenger DR, Carollo JJ, Wilkerson JA Jr:. Biomechanics of scoliosis correction by segmental spinal instrumentation, *Spine* 7:260-264, 1982.

47. Winter RB, Moe JH, Wang JF: Congenital kyphosis: its natural history and treatment as observed in a study of one hundred thirty patients, *J Bone Joint Surg Am* 55A:189-193, 1973.

CHAPTER 60

Craniocervical Junction Deformities

Daniel K. Resnick

Abnormalities of the craniovertebral junction (CVJ) are caused by congenital disorders, degenerative disease, tumors, and trauma. Because of the complex anatomic configuration of this region, a number of craniometric and morphometric indices are used to define the limits of normal anatomy. Optimal treatment of abnormalities in this region should be designed to decompress the involved neural elements and provide structural support for the head. Depending on the anatomic configuration of the abnormality, decompression of the neural elements can be achieved with or without operative intervention. The ability to decompress the neural elements preoperatively greatly simplifies the surgical management of patients with abnormalities of the CVJ. The anatomic landmarks and indices used to define the normal and abnormal anatomy of the CVJ with regard to traumatic, degenerative, and congenital lesions are presented in this chapter. Also, the use of manual manipulation and craniocervical traction in the preoperative management of patients with abnormalities of the CVJ is discussed.

Clinical and Radiographic Anatomy of the Craniovertebral Junction

The CVJ consists of the cranial base, the atlas, and the axis. These structures, along with their associated ligaments, provide structural support for the head and protect the brainstem and upper cervical spinal cord. Simultaneously, these structures allow for significant movement in the sagittal (flexion or extension), coronal (lateral bending), and axial (rotation) planes. The anatomy of the CVJ reflects a compromise between structural strength and permissive flexibility. A thorough discussion of the embryology and anatomy of the CVJ has been presented elsewhere in this text, and therefore the following discussion is limited to an overview of the anatomic landmarks and indices used to define abnormal relationships.

The normal relationships among the occiput, atlas, and axis have been studied and are well-described. The use of computed tomography (CT) with sagittal reconstruction and multiaxial magnetic resonance imaging (MRI) has greatly enhanced the understanding and definition of abnormal anatomic relationships at the CVJ. In the case of

trauma, where previously normal anatomic relationships have been altered, a number of anatomic indices and reference points have been described. In patients with congenital disorders marked by ligamentous laxity, such as Down syndrome and Morquio's syndrome, abnormalities of normal anatomic relationships may or may not be relevant. Patients with diseases that result in cranial settling or basilar impression (e.g., osteogenesis imperfecta, rheumatoid arthritis) present with different sets of anatomic abnormalities described by separate sets of indices.

Trauma

Injury to the CVJ may be manifested by fracture or ligamentous injury related to the occiput, atlas, or axis. Radiographic criteria exist for definition of these injuries and for assessment of clinical stability. Occipital condyle fractures can be divided into three types. Type 1 injuries consist of a fracture of the occipital condyle with minimal or no displacement of fragments into the foramen magnum. This type of fracture is thought to result from axial loading. Type 2 condylar fractures occur as extensions of basilar skull fractures resulting from direct blows to the skull. Type 3 fractures are avulsion fractures of the condyle that are manifested by inferomedial displacement of fracture fragments toward the dens (traction by the alar ligaments). This type of fracture represents an avulsion of the alar ligament from the occipital condyle and is potentially unstable. The first two types of occipital condyle fractures are considered stable because the alar and tectorial membranes are intact.[2]

Normal plain radiographic relationships between the occiput and the atlas are defined by the Powers ratio, the basion-axial interval, and the measurement of the translational movement of the occiput on the atlas (only when chronic instability is in question).[16,30,46] The techniques used to determine these values are illustrated in Figure 60.1. Both Traynelis et al.[23] and Menezes and Piper[43] have classified atlanto-occipital dislocation (AOD) based on the relative position of the occiput. Type 1 dislocations, ventral dislocations of the occiput, are the most common type. Type 2 dislocations are the result of longitudinal dislocation of the occiput with separation of the occiput and the atlas, and type 3 injuries are characterized by dorsal dislocation of the occiput on the atlas. Radiographic findings associated with AOD are retropharyngeal hematoma, "bare" occipital condyles, and the presence of a prepontine epidural or subarachnoid hematoma on CT.[23,32] Multiplanar imaging with MRI and reconstructed CT may be very helpful in confirming the diagnosis in questionable cases. Because of the elastic recoil in the ligamentous structures of the neck, the deformity may reduce spontaneously. Standard radiographic imaging at this point may lead to a false-negative examination. A high index of suspicion, especially in the case of patients with severe neurologic injury without significant radiologic signs of trauma, should lead to a more comprehensive imaging work-up (Figure 60.2).

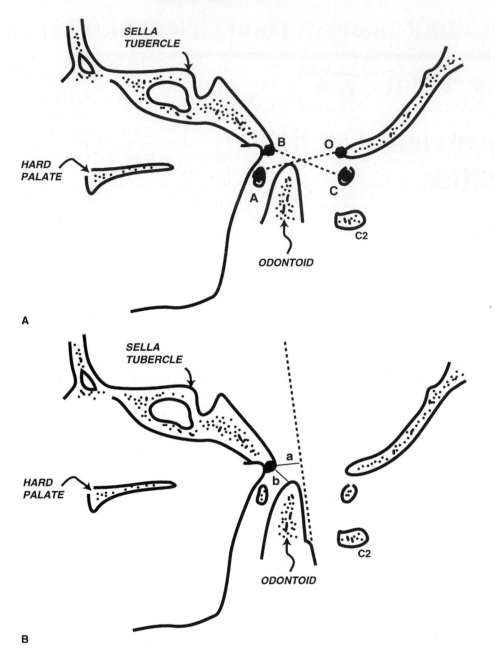

Figure 60.1 Atlanto-occipital (AO) joint evaluation. Evaluation of the relationships between the occiput and atlas is performed using one of several methods. **(A)** Calculation of the Powers ratio is determined by measuring the distance between the basion *(B)* and the midpoint of the dorsal arch of C1 *(C)*, and the distance between the opisthion *(O)* and the ventral arch of C1 *(A)*. The ratio BC/OA is said to be normal if the value is less than 0.9. Values between 0.9 and 1 are considered borderline, and values greater than 1 are diagnostic of anterior dislocation of the occiput on the atlas. Obviously, dorsal and longitudinal dislocations do not necessarily result in Powers ratios greater than 1. **(B)** The basion axial interval (BAI)/basion dental interval (BDI) method of evaluating the AO joint may be more accurate and is certainly applicable to a wider variety of abnormalities at this joint. The distance between the basion and the rostral extension of the dorsal cortical line of the axis defines the BAI. The basion should be no more than 12mm ventral to the caudal cortical line of the axis and can be as much as 4mm dorsal to it. Similarly, the distance between the basion and the superior cortex of the dens is less than 11.8mm in 95% of normal subjects.

Patients who survive the initial injury and who have preserved neurologic function below the level of injury should be immediately immobilized. Halo vest immobilization has been shown to be safe and effective for the prevention of delayed neurologic deterioration while the patient is stabilized and prepared for definitive treatment.[17] Early reduction followed by rigid fixation of the occiput to the upper cervical spine is recommended in order to avoid delayed neurologic deterioration. All attempts at reduction of AOD (especially dorsal [type 3])

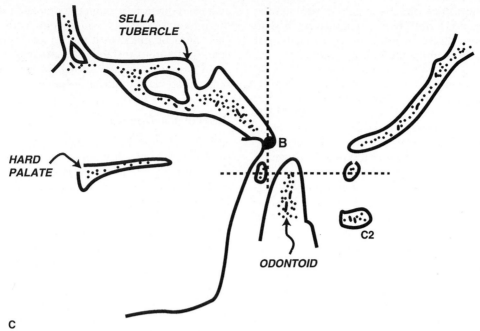

C

Figure 60.1 *cont'd* (C) In cases of suspected chronic instability of the AO joint, translational movement of the occiput on the axis can be measured. The position of the basion is determined in relation to a horizontal line connecting the ventral and dorsal rings of C1 in both flexion and extension. The total translational movement at the AO joint should not exceed 1mm (see text for references). (*Copyright University of New Mexico, Division of Neurosurgery, with permission.*)

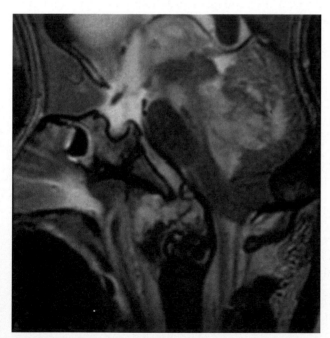

Figure 60.2 This MRI clearly demonstrates the degree of ligamentous disruption associated with atlantoaxial dislocation. This child, a victim of a high-speed motor vehicle accident, was unresponsive upon presentation to the emergency room. Initial cervical radiographs were interpreted as normal (although abnormalities are evident on retrospective review). A head CT demonstrated the premedullary hemorrhage, and an MRI was obtained. Note the distraction between the occiput and C1. This was not present on the initial plain films and is likely related to the use of a rigid cervical collar for immobilization of this highly unstable fracture.

should be performed under fluoroscopic guidance and with gentle manual manipulation. If the patient has residual neurologic function, then performance of the reduction with the patient sedated but awake allows for real-time monitoring of neurologic function. Somatosensory-evoked responses, when present, may provide some margin of safety in the anesthetized patient. Once the deformity is reduced, gentle compression is maintained with fixation of the halo ring to the operating table. *In situ* fixation is then performed. Patients with complete injuries or with concomitant severe head injuries should be immediately immobilized. Operative fixation may be performed on an elective basis if at all, depending upon the severity of the injury.[40]

Fractures of the atlas are commonly referred to as Jefferson fractures in reference to Geoffrey Jefferson[18] who reviewed 46 cases of C1 burst fractures in 1920. These types of fractures result from an axial load translated to the C1 via the wedge-shaped occipital condyles. These fractures are often detected with an open-mouth odontoid radiograph that demonstrates spreading of the lateral masses of C1 beyond the lateral borders of the C2 lateral masses. A critical determination in the treatment of patients with Jefferson fractures involves the integrity of the transverse ligament of the atlas. In a cadaver study, Spence *et al.*[41] found that the transverse ligament was likely intact if lateral mass spread (i.e., total of both sides) was less than 5.7mm and typically failed if the degree of spread totaled 6.9mm or more. The elastic recoil of the spinal ligaments may result in a false-negative study however, and in most cases, axial imaging through the craniovertebral junction is recommended. Failure of the transverse ligament can be directly visualized through the use of fine-cut axial CT or MRI.[11,12] The use of MRI in evaluating transverse ligament integrity has revealed that the ligament may be incompetent, despite lateral translation of less than 6.9mm.[12] Others have also noted that an abnormal (greater than 3mm) atlantodental interval (ADI) implies incompetence of the transverse ligament.[23,28] A study by Dickman et al.,[12] which evaluated the use of MRI in the assessment of transverse ligament competence, revealed that an abnormal ADI reliably predicted failure of the transverse ligament in the absence of a C1 ring fracture. In the case of a fracture through the transverse tubercle, 26% of patients with incompetent transverse ligaments had a normal ADI. Therefore, it appears prudent to study the CVJ with axial imaging techniques. Failure of the transverse ligament implies instability and, in the absence of a fracture through the transverse tubercle, the need for operative stabilization.[12,40] Atlas fractures without evidence of transverse ligament disruption are effectively managed by external immobilization.

Fractures of the odontoid process of the axis have been classified by Anderson and D'Alonzo[1] according to the site of the fracture. Rare type 1 fractures occur obliquely through the odontoid process, type 2 fractures occur through the base of the odontoid, and type 3 fractures occur through the body of the axis. A number of different management options exist for patients with odontoid fractures, depending on the degree of subluxation of the cranial fragment and the status of the transverse ligament. Ventral subluxations of 4 to 6mm have been associated with high rates of nonunion, as have dorsal subluxations of lesser degree. In these cases, surgical intervention is often recommended.[3,13] Reduction of the odontoid fragment and restoration of normal alignment are often achieved through the use of gentle traction and flexion (with dorsal subluxation) or extension (with ventral subluxation) under fluoroscopic guidance. Once the fragment is reduced, rigid external immobilization or internal fixation is used to secure the alignment. A complete radiographic work-up, including MRI, is advised in the management of odontoid fractures in order to define associated ligamentous injury.[12,33] As discussed earlier, failure of the transverse ligament implies significant instability of the atlantoaxial complex.

Fractures of the pars interarticularis of C2 are termed *hangman's fractures* because of their similarity to fractures suffered as a result of judicial hanging.[38] Effendi et al.[14] have classified these fractures into three types. Type 1 fractures are minimally displaced (less than 2mm) and minimally angulated. The disc space below the fracture is normal. Type 2 fractures are characterized by disruption of the C2-3 disc and displacement of the body of the axis. The body of the axis (dens) may be displaced and/or angulated ventrally or dorsally. Type 3 fractures are rare. In addition to displacement and angulation as seen in type 2 fractures, type 3 fractures are associated with locked facets between C2 and C3. The body of the axis is usually angulated and displaced ventrally in type 3 fractures.[14] If significant subluxation of C2 on C3 exists (greater than 3mm), operative intervention may be indicated for reduction and fixation.[14,15,27] In the case of a hangman's fracture without significant ligamentous injury, immobilization is an effective treatment option. A halo ring can be used to achieve reduction through traction and extension and then for immobilization in conjunction with a thoracic vest. Care must be taken with the use of traction when significant ligamentous instability exists (type 2 or 3) in order to avoid iatrogenic separation of C2 and C3 or inadvertent recapitulation of a judicial hanging.

Degenerative Disease

Abnormalities of bone metabolism, degeneration of synovial joints, or abnormal stresses placed on the CVJ may result in basilar impression. Paget's disease and osteogenesis imperfecta (discussed later) result in deformation of the skull base and migration of the foramen magnum and dens rostrally. Rheumatoid destruction of the synovial atlanto-occipital and lateral atlantoaxial joints causes a similar effect. A case of abnormal posture caused by torticollis, resulting in basilar impression, has also been reported.[22,37] Regardless of the cause, the principles of diagnosis and treatment remain the same.

The most common degenerative disorder that results in abnormalities of the CVJ is rheumatoid arthritis. This disease is estimated to affect 0.8% of the Caucasian adult population of the United States, or approximately 2.2 million people. The cervical spine is the second most commonly involved region of the body (following the hands and feet).[8] Changes observed in the cervical spine, and particularly at the CVJ, are progressive in nature. At the CVJ, changes consist of initial translational subluxation of C1 on C2, followed by vertical translation of C1 on C2.[8,26] As the lateral mass joints are eroded by inflammatory synovitis, ascension of the odontoid peg through the foramen magnum may occur, causing compression of the neural elements. Interestingly, defects in posterior column function appear to be the earliest signs of spinal cord dysfunction, indicating that the dorsal aspect of the spinal cord is especially sensitive to chronic injury by movement of the head.[36]

Assessment of transverse atlantoaxial subluxation in patients with rheumatoid disease uses the same criteria as for trauma (i.e., the ADI). As in trauma, an ADI greater than 3mm is considered abnormal.[28] Oda et al.[26] studied the progression of transverse atlantoaxial subluxation in a group of 49 patients with rheumatoid arthritis. They found a predictable progression from reducible ventral subluxation to irreducible subluxation to vertical subluxation of C1 on C2. Vertical subluxation is measured by measuring the vertical distance between the center of the pedicles of the axis to a line connecting the ventral and dorsal arch of the atlas (Figure 60.3). Vertical subluxation is said to exist if this distance is less than 13mm.[26,34]

Basilar impression refers to the ascension of medial structures into the posterior cranial fossa and is usually defined by an abnormal position of the dens with respect to the foramen magnum. Numerous anatomic indices are used for the diagnosis of basilar impression, including McRae's line, Chamberlain's line, Fishgold's digastric line, and Fishgold's bimastoid line.[6,19,20,22] The positions of these lines and the anticipated position of the dens are illustrated in Figures 60.4 and 60.5. Ascension of the dens causes compression of the ventral aspect of the brain stem and upper cervical spinal cord,

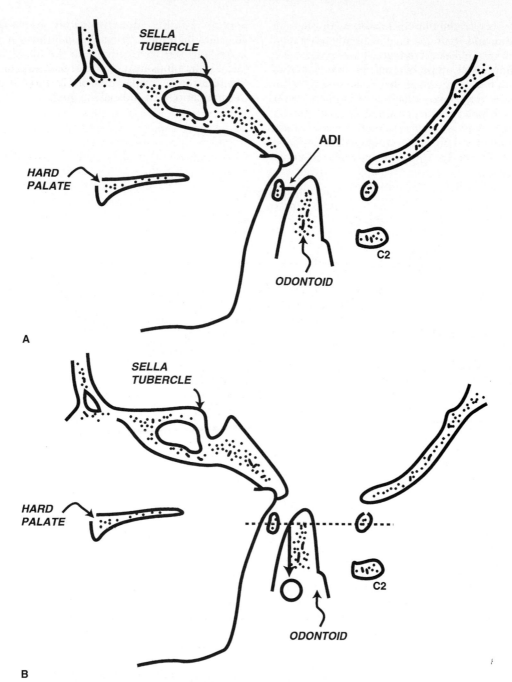

Figure 60.3 Horizontal and vertical translation of C1 on C2. **(A)** Horizontal translation of C1 on C2 can be assessed by measuring the ADI, the distance between the anterior dens and the posterior cortex of the ventral arch of C1. This interval should be 3mm or less in adults and 4.5mm or less in children. **(B)** Vertical translation of C1 and C2 can be assessed by measuring the perpendicular distance between the pedicle of C2 and a line connecting the midpoints of the anterior and posterior arches of C1. Vertical subluxation exists if this distance is less than 13mm (see text for references). *(Copyright University of New Mexico, Division of Neurosurgery, with permission.)*

which results in variable symptomatology including but not limited to myelopathy and lower cranial nerve deficits. The major goals of treatment for basilar impression are decompression of the neural elements and reestablishment of adequate support for the head. Decompression of the neural elements can be achieved directly through resection of the odontoid process and associated soft tissue pannus or indirectly through closed reduction of the deformity by using traction. The ability to achieve reduction of a deformity through axial traction and gentle manipulation may obviate the need for a ventral decompression procedure.

The determination that ventral lesions associated with basilar impression are irreducible can be made only after adequate attempts at reduction have been made through the use of traction and gentle manual manipulation. Long-standing lesions are unlikely to be reducible through manual manipulation. Therefore, a trial of craniocervical traction is warranted. Placement of a halo ring provides firm fixation for traction, allows the use of multiple points of skull fixation (which may be important in a patient with a weakened skull), and allows for fixation to the thoracic body jacket once the deformity is reduced. Traction is instituted with light weights (approximately 5lb); however,

heavier weights may ultimately be required. Most clinicians limit attempts at closed reduction of CVJ abnormalities to 5 to 7 days because the likelihood of further benefit after this time period is low and the incidence of complications related to prolonged immobilization increases.[22] The use of specially designed beds helps to reduce the incidence of these complications. Obviously, frequent neurologic and radiographic examinations are required in order to detect and prevent overdistraction. In most patients with degenerative conditions leading to

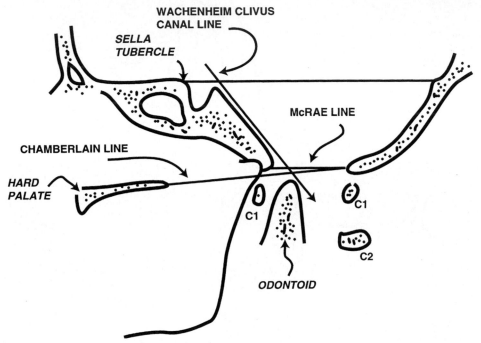

Figure 60.4 Landmarks and indices for basilar invagination: lateral view. There are a number of craniometric lines that aid in the diagnosis of basilar invagination. McRae's line joins the basion and opisthion. The length of this line should exceed 19mm, and the tip of the dens should be below this line. Chamberlain's line joins the dorsal aspect of the hard palate to the opisthion, and the tip of the dens should be at least 3.6mm below this line. Wachenheim's clivus canal line is a line drawn along the clivus into the cervical canal. The tip of the dens should be ventral and tangential to this line (see text for references). (*Copyright University of New Mexico, Division of Neurosurgery, with permission.*)

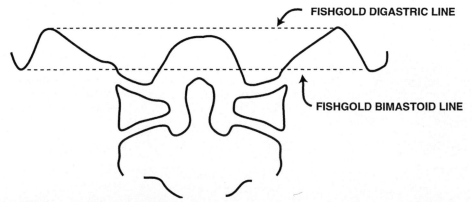

Figure 60.5 Landmarks and indices for basilar invagination: AP view. Fishgold's digastric line joins the digastric fossa bilaterally and corresponds to McRae's line on lateral radiographs; the tip of the dens should be below this line. Fishgold's bimastoid line connects the tips of the mastoid processes bilaterally. The tip of the dens can be up to 10mm above this line (see text for references). (*Copyright University of New Mexico, Division of Neurosurgery, with permission.*)

abnormalities of the CVJ, dorsal fixation is required after reduction or resection of a ventral mass.

Congenital Disorders

CVJ abnormalities are common in a number of inherited conditions, and the incidence of such abnormalities in certain disorders is well-known. For instance, the incidence of atlantoaxial subluxation is about 30% in Down syndrome and approaches 50% in Morquio's disease.[9] Other disorders are associated with CVJ abnormalities, such as Klippel-Feil deformity (Figure 60.6), Lesch-Nyhan syndrome, and osteogenesis imperfecta.[4,31,39,45] However, the incidence of such abnormalities is not firmly established.

The cause of CVJ abnormalities in these patients varies. In patients with C1-2 subluxation, the condition is likely related to ligamentous laxity, a common consequence of connective tissue disorders (e.g., Morquio's disease, Lesch-Nyhan syndrome) and a component of Down syndrome (Figure 60.7). Aberrant ossification of the dens may

also be accounted for by abnormal ligamentous laxity due to disturbances in the blood supply to the developing bone as a result of inordinate mobility.[9,42] In patients with osteogenesis imperfecta, abnormal collagen deposition results in the formation of brittle bone subject to multiple "microfractures." The cumulative effect of these microfractures is ascension of the dens and medial skull base, resulting in basilar invagination.

Treatment of these congenital lesions varies depending on the patient's symptoms and the syndrome involved. For example, repeated studies have demonstrated a tendency for children with Down syndrome to have increased atlantodental intervals and atlanto-occipital hypermobility.[5,7] Furthermore, the ligamentous laxity associated with Down syndrome can result in a devastating injury from trivial trauma.[25] Despite these findings, large cohort studies have not demonstrated increased rates of neurologic injury in children with Down syndrome and abnormal atlantodental intervals when compared with their peers. Nor have these studies demonstrated a protective effect of

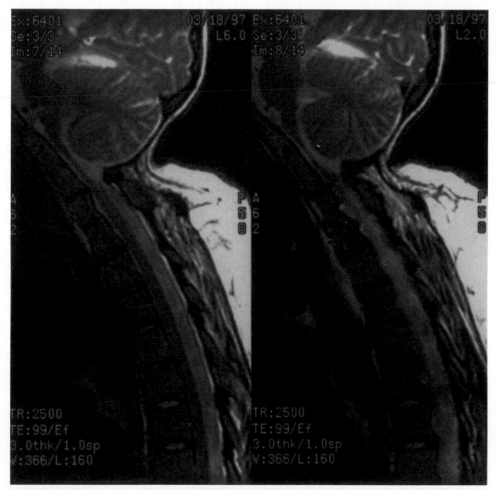

Figure 60.6 CVJ abnormalities in a patient with Klippel-Feil deformity. This patient complained of neck pain and headaches accompanied by speech and swallowing dysfunction and urinary incontinence. MRI of the CVJ demonstrated fusion of the clivus to the axis and marked narrowing of the foramen magnum with distortion of the brain stem. Because there was no ventral mass and because her bony deformity is fixed, she was offered dorsal decompression. Dorsal fixation was also recommended because of the belief that ventral fusion between the clivus and C2 would not provide sufficient support to resist further deformation. The patient has thus far declined surgical intervention.

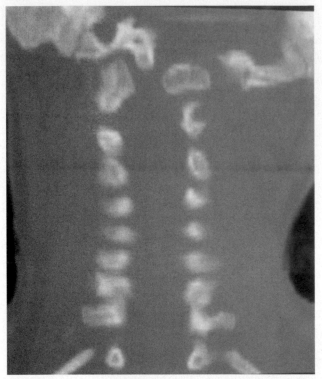

Figure 60.7 This coronal CT was obtained after an incidental abnormality was noted on a CT of the temporal bones (obtained for persistent ear infections). This child has Dubowitz syndrome, a hereditary condition associated with craniofacial abnormalities and ligamentous laxity. The scan shows lateral subluxation of the occiput on C1.

restricted activity.[7,24] Therefore, the usual indices of CVJ instability may not be applicable to the population of children with Down syndrome. Reduction and stabilization of the CVJ in these patients is probably not indicated unless the patient has clear signs of brain stem or upper cervical spinal cord compression.

In contrast, patients with Morquio's syndrome and other skeletal dysplasias are often found to have an os odontoideum in conjunction with ligamentous laxity (Figure 60.8).[35] The presence of an os odontoideum in this situation can be taken as evidence for instability, as the cartilaginous odontoid deforms with flexion or extension. Radiographically demonstrable C1-2 instability, as evidenced by changes in the ADI, is a late finding in these children, and when it occurs, myelopathy is nearly always present. Therefore, these patients benefit from prophylactic fusion before the onset of myelopathy. Although the ideal age for the operation has not been determined, Ransford et al.[35] suggest that surgery be performed at 4 years of age unless myelopathic signs begin to develop earlier. Interestingly, dorsal occipitoatlantoaxial fusion may result in complete ossification of the dens, lending support for the role of ligamentous laxity in the formation of an os odontoideum.[42]

The treatment of patients with congenital disorders of the CVJ varies depending on the syndrome, the symptomatology, and the relevant anatomy. The decision to surgically intervene in a patient with demonstrable atlantoaxial instability is highly dependent on the natural history of the dis-order (e.g., Down syndrome vs. Morquio's syndrome) and on the particular anatomy of the lesion. The use of traction for reduction of unstable lesions is recommended when there is a suspicion that a lesion may be reducible. Again, placement of a halo ring allows for the application of corrective forces, followed by fixation once reduction has been completed. In cases where radiographic information (see Figure 60.6) indicates the irreducibility of a lesion or that attempts at reduction have failed, surgery is indicated to decompress the neural elements and to stabilize the CVJ.

Tuite et al.[44] reviewed their experience with 27 pediatric patients who underwent transoral decompression procedures. The indications for surgery were irreducible atlantoaxial subluxation, basilar invagination, or tumor. The children suffered from a variety of congenital disorders, including Down syndrome, Morquio's syndrome, Klippel-Feil deformity, osteogenesis imperfecta, and spondyloepiphyseal dysplasia. They found that patients with conditions related to ligamentous laxity and patients with preoperative symptoms related to neural compression were at higher risk for significant morbidity with transoral procedures. Significant problems with speech and swallowing also occurred and were associated with lesions located above the foramen magnum.[44] The complications reported by this experienced group of physicians serve as indicators of the technical complexity of these procedures and the physiologic vulnerability of these patients.

Tumors

Tumors of the CVJ produce signs and symptoms of neural element compression (e.g., myelopathy, radiculopathy, cranial nerve deficits) and mechanical instability (e.g., pain, progressive deformity). The treatment of patients with these tumors is dependent on the patient's symptoms and age, the tumor type, and the anatomic configuration of the tumor. Piper and Menezes[29] reviewed a series of tumors affecting the axis and found that patients were generally affected later in life and presented with myelopathy, radiculopathy, or occipitocervical pain. Although the most commonly encountered tumor was a chordoma, other primary tumors were found, including osteoblastoma, eosinophilic granuloma, plasmacytoma, chondrosarcoma, and Ewing's sarcoma. Metastatic paraganglioma and breast carcinoma were also encountered.[29] Tuite et al.[44] reported six cases of chordoma involving the clivus resected through a transoral approach in children. These children presented with a variety of cranial nerve deficits, most commonly diplopia.

Treatment of these patients involves decompression of the neural structures and stabilization of the CVJ. The route of approach to a tumor depends on the tumor's location and mechanism of compression. Piper and Menezes[29] divide the axis into four zones (Figure 60.9) and tailor the surgical approach to the zone of involvement. A transoral approach (with or without division of the palate or mandible) is used for zone 1 tumors (ventral midline) involving the axis, atlas, and lower clivus. A lateral extrapharyngeal approach is used for tumors extending more laterally toward the lateral mass or more caudally (zone 2). A dorsolateral approach is used for tumors located dorsal to the ventrolateral mass, which may extend

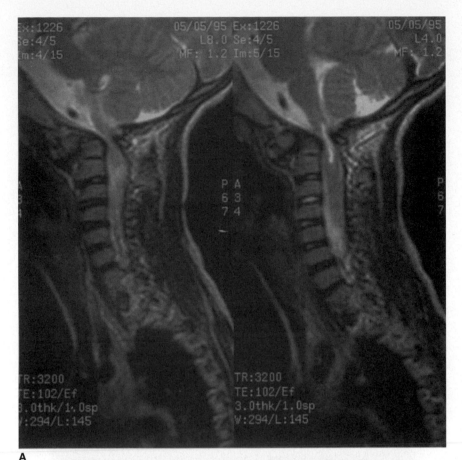

A

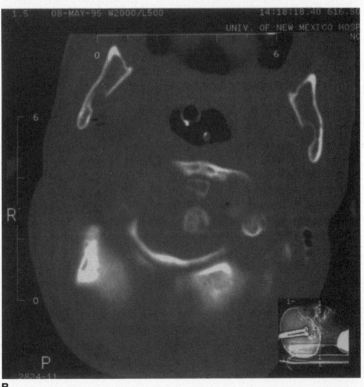

B

Figure 60.8 CVJ abnormalities in a patient with skeletal dysplasia. A young boy presented with progressive quadriparesis and spasticity. MRI (**A**), CT (**B**), and two-dimensional (**C**) and three-dimensional (**D**) reconstructions were performed to evaluate the CVJ abnormality. The lesion, an os odontoideum, with ventral and vertical subluxation of C1 on C2, proved to be irreducible. Therefore, a transoral resection of the ventral arch of C1 (*os*) and residual odontoid process was performed followed by dorsal decompression and fusion between the occiput and C3. The patient's neurologic status stabilized but did not improve. Note the dramatic signal change seen at the cervicomedullary junction in the preoperative MRI (**A**).

Continued

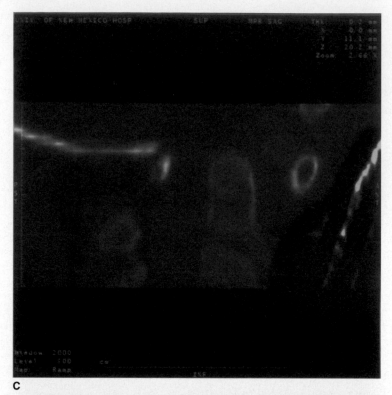

C

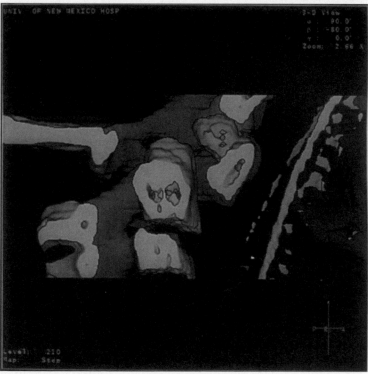

D

Figure 60.8 *cont'd*

into the dorsal fossa and/or occipital condyle (zone 3). Finally, dorsally located tumors (zone 4) are resected via a standard midline dorsal approach.[29]

The issue of immediate stabilization after resection of ventrally located tumors is controversial. Most clinicians agree that resection of the odontoid process renders the spine unstable.[10] However, Menezes[21] has reported that a substantial minority of patients (29 of 166) may not require dorsal stabilization after odontoid resection. Disagreement over the timing of dorsal stabilization also exists. Menezes maintains patients in a halo for 1 week after surgery to allow for wound healing ventrally and for assessment of instability. However, Crockard and Stevens[9] recommend that dorsal fixation be performed at the time of the ventral resection because most patients require dorsal stabilization not only for acute stabilization but also for chronic instability. An increased incidence of infection due to immediate dorsal surgery after "clean contaminated" ventral decompression through the oral cavity has not been reported.[44]

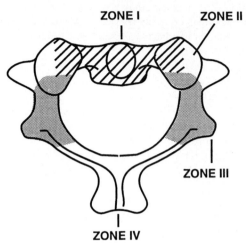

Figure 60.9 Anatomic zones for tumor resection at the CVJ. Menezes has divided the axis into zones that dictate the appropriate surgical approach for tumor resection. Zones I to IV are illustrated here. (See text for discussion and references.) *(Copyright University of New Mexico, Division of Neurosurgery, with permission.)*

Deformation Reduction

Perhaps the most important decision made in the treatment of patients with CVJ abnormalities concerns the method of deformity reduction. Depending on the anatomic configuration present in a given patient, immobilization, closed reduction followed by immobilization and/or fixation, or open reduction (by a ventral or dorsal route) may be necessary. Closed reduction is achieved through the use of axial traction, often employing a halo ring as the skull fixator and, in some cases, manual manipulation of the CVJ. For example, a patient with traumatic spondylolisthesis of C2 can be appropriately managed with mild axial traction in extension followed by capital flexion in order to reduce a ventrally displaced C2 body (Figure 60.10). Traction is always initiated with light weights (4lb) in order to avoid overdistraction in patients with ligamentous injury[14,33]; however, progression to heavier weights (up to 8 to 10lb) may be necessary in some cases.[14,23] A ventral mass, such as in a patient with C1-2 subluxation and pannus, can be effectively reduced (and thus decompressed) using axial traction, again in slight extension, obviating the need for ventral surgery.

In some patients, notably those with long-standing degenerative disorders or tumors, preoperative closed reduction is not possible. These patients require direct decompression of the neural elements via an appropriate surgical route (ventral for ventral pathology, lateral for lateral pathology, and dorsal for dorsal pathology), followed by reduction of deformity and possible fixation. Reduction of deformity is achieved in this instance by direct

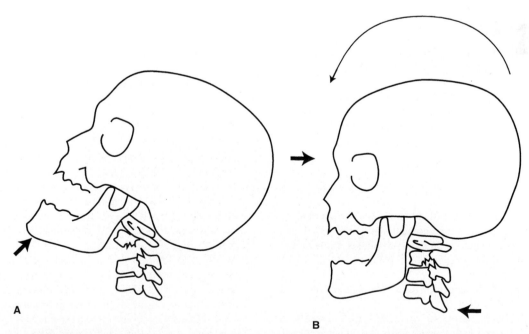

Figure 60.10 Cervical extension and capital flexion for reduction of traumatic spondylolisthesis of the axis. **(A)** A hangman's-type fracture results from forceful capital extension, with or without longitudinal distraction. **(B)** This type of fracture can be reduced with gentle manual manipulation through extension of the neck and capital flexion. Fixation with a halo orthosis is necessary to properly immobilize the fracture once reduction has been achieved. *(Copyright University of New Mexico, Division of Neurosurgery, with permission.)*

manipulation of the involved structures and is maintained by appropriate shaping of implants and postoperative immobilization.

Summary

Abnormalities of the CVJ can be caused by congenital disorders, degenerative changes, trauma, or tumors. The goal of treatment is decompression of neural elements and stabilization of the spine. Extensive morphometric and craniometric studies have been performed that allow for precise definitions of normal and abnormal anatomy. As experience with new imaging technologies increases, some of the older concepts regarding the anatomy and physiology of the CVJ are being revised. Craniocervical traction is a useful adjunct in the treatment of degenerative and many congenital disorders. It can be used for the treatment of some traumatic lesions of the CVJ. A thorough understanding of the anatomy of a given lesion is necessary prior to the institution of traction or the consideration of surgical intervention. Traction may obviate the need for ventral decompression in some cases and, when combined with rigid external fixation, may be the only treatment required for some traumatic and inflammatory conditions. When neural compression is found to be irreducible, surgical decompression is performed. The approach used for decompression is chosen based on the nature of the lesion and its location relative to the spinal cord and brain stem. Internal fixation is used when the primary disease process or the surgical remedy has rendered the spine unstable. Finally, it must be remembered that the anatomic complexity of this region, as well as the physiologic vulnerability of many patients, creates the potential for significant morbidity.

REFERENCES

1. Anderson LD, D'Alonzo RT: Fractures of the odontoid process of the axis, *J Bone Joint Surg Am* 56A:1663-1674, 1974.
2. Anderson PA, Montesano PX: Morphology and treatment of occipital condyle fractures, *Spine* 13:731-736, 1988.
3. Apuzzo MLJ, Heiden JS, Weiss MH *et al:* Acute fractures of the odontoid process: an analysis of 45 cases, *J Neurosurg* 48:85-91, 1978.
4. Baba H, Maezawa Y, Furusawa N, *et al:* The cervical spine in the Klippel-Feil syndrome: a report of 57 cases, *Int Orthop* 19:204-208, 1995.
5. Casey ATH, Crockard HA, Bland JM, *et al:* Predictors of outcome in the quadriparetic nonambulatory myelopathic patient with rheumatoid arthritis: a prospective study of 55 surgically treated Ranawat class IIIb patients, *J Neurosurg* 85:574-581, 1996.
6. Chamberlain WE: Basilar impression (platybasia), *Yale J Biol Med* 11:487, 1939.
7. Cremers MJ, Bol E, de Roos F, van Gijn J: Risk of sports activities in children with Down's syndrome and atlantoaxial instability, *Lancet* 342:511-514, 1993.
8. Crockard HA: Surgical management of cervical rheumatoid problems, *Spine* 20:2584-2590, 1995.
9. Crockard HA, Stevens JM: Craniovertebral junction anomalies in inherited disorders: part of the syndrome or caused by the disorder? *Eur J Pediatr* 154:504-512, 1995.
10. Dickman CA, Crawford NR, Brantley AGU, Sonntag VKH: Biomechanical effects of transoral odontoidectomy, *Neurosurgery* 36:1146-1153, 1995.
11. Dickman CA, Greene KA, Sonntag VKH: Injuries involving the transverse atlantal ligament: classification and treatment guidelines based upon experience with 39 injuries, *Neurosurgery* 38:44-50, 1996.
12. Dickman CA, Mamourian A, Sonntag VKH, *et al:* Magnetic resonance imaging of the transverse atlantal ligament for the evaluation of atlantoaxial instability, *J Neurosurg* 75:221-227, 1991.
13. Dunn ME, Seljeskog EL: Experience in the management of odontoid process injuries: an analysis of 128 cases, *Neurosurgery* 18:306-310, 1986.
14. Effendi B, Roy D, Cornish B, *et al:* Fractures of the ring of the axis: a classification based on the analysis of 131 cases, *J Bone Joint Surg Br* 63B:319-327, 1981.
15. Hadley MN, Dickman CA, Browner CM, *et al:* Acute axis fractures: a review of 229 cases, *J Neurosurg* 71:642-647, 1989.
16. Harris JH, Carson GC, Wagner LK: Radiological diagnosis of traumatic occipitocervical dissociation: 1. Normal occipitovertebral relationships on lateral radiographs of supine subjects, *AJR Am J Roentgenol* 162:881-886, 1994.
17. Heary RF, Hunt CD, Krieger AJ, *et al:* Acute stabilization of the cervical spine by halo vest application facilitates evaluation and treatment of multiple trauma patients, *J Trauma* 33:445-451, 1992.
18. Jefferson G: Fracture of the atlas vertebra: report of four cases and a review of those previously recorded, *Br J Surg* 7:407-422, 1920.
19. McGregor M: The significance of certain measurements of the skull in the diagnosis of basilar impression, *Br J Radiol* 21:171, 1948
20. McRae DL: Bony abnormalities in the region of the foramen magnum: correlation of anatomic and neurologic findings, *Acta Radiol* 40:335, 1953.
21. Menezes AH: Surgical approaches to the craniocervical junction. In Frymoyer JW (ed): *The adult spine: principles and practice*, New York, Raven Press, 1991.
22. Menezes AH: Congenital and acquired abnormalities of the craniovertebral junction. In Youmans JR (ed): *Neurological Surgery*, ed 4, Philadelphia, WB Saunders, 1995.
23. Menezes AH, Piper JG: Anatomy and radiographic pathology of injury to the occipitoatlantal complex. In Rea GL, Miller CA (eds): *Spinal trauma: current evaluation and management*, Park Ridge, IL, American Association of Neurological Surgeons, 1993.
24. Morton RE, Khan MA, Murray-Leslie C, Elliott S: Atlantoaxial instability in Down's syndrome: a five-year follow-up study, *Arch Dis Child* 72:115-118, 1995.
25. Nucci P, de Pellegrin M, Brancato R: Atlantoaxial dislocation related to instilling eyedrops in a patient with Down's syndrome, *Am J Ophthalmol* 122:908-910, 1996.
26. Oda T, Fujiwara K, Yonenobu K, *et al:* Natural course of cervical spine lesions in rheumatoid arthritis, *Spine* 20:1128-1135, 1995.
27. Papadopoulos SM: Biomechanics of occipito-atlanto-axial trauma. In Rea GL, Miller CA, editors: *Spinal trauma:*

current evaluation and management, Park Ridge, IL, American Association of Neurological Surgeons, 1993.

28. Penning L: Normal movements of the cervical spine, *AJR Am J Roentgenol* 130:317-326, 1978.

29. Piper JG, Menezes AH: Management strategies for tumors of the axis vertebra, *J Neurosurg* 84:543-551, 1996.

30. Powers B, Miller MD, Kramer RS, *et al:* Traumatic anterior atlanto-occipital dislocation, *Neurosurgery* 4:12-17, 1979.

31. Pozo JL, Crockard HA, Ransford AO: Basilar impression in osteogenesis imperfecta: a report of three cases in one family, *J Bone Joint Surg Br* 66B:233, 1984.

32. Przybylski GJ, Clyde BL, Fitz CR: Craniocervical junction subarachnoid hemorrhage associated with atlanto-occipital dislocation. *Spine* 21:1761-1768, 1996.

33. Przybylski GJ, Welch WC: Longitudinal atlantoaxial dislocation with type III odontoid fracture: case report and review of the literature, *J Neurosurg* 84:666-670, 1996.

34. Ranawat CS, O'Leary P, Pellicci P, *et al:* Cervical spine fusion in rheumatoid arthritis, *J Bone Joint Surg Am* 61A:1003-1010, 1979.

35. Ransford AO, Crockard HA, Stevens JM, *et al:* Occipito-atlanto-axial fusion in Morquio-Brailsford syndrome, *J Bone Joint Surg Br* 78B:307-313, 1996.

36. Rogers MA, Crockard HA, Moskovich R: Nystagmus and joint position sensation: their importance in posterior occipitocervical fusion in rheumatoid arthritis, *Spine* 19:16-20, 1994.

37. Ryken T, Menezes AH: Nonrheumatoid cranial settling, *Spine* 18:2525-2527, 1992.

38. Schneider RC, Livingston KE, Cave AJE, *et al:* "Hangman's fracture" of the cervical spine, *J Neurosurg* 22:141-154, 1965.

39. Shewell PC, Thompson AG: Atlantoaxial instability in Lesch-Nyhan syndrome, *Spine* 21:757-762, 1996.

40. Sonntag VKH, Dickman CA: Treatment of upper cervical spine injuries. In Rea GL, Miller CA (eds): *Spinal Trauma: Current Evaluation and Management,* Park Ridge, IL, American Association of Neurological Surgeons, 1993.

41. Spence KF Jr, Decker S, Sell KW: Bursting atlantal fracture associated with rupture of the transverse ligament, *J Bone Joint Surg Am* 52A:543-549, 1970.

42. Stevens JM, Kendall BE, Crockard HA, Ransford AO: The odontoid process in Morquio-Brailsford's disease: the effects of occipitocervical fusion, *J Bone Joint Surg Br* 73B:851-858, 1991.

43. Traynelis VC, Marano GD, Dunker RO, *et al:* Traumatic atlanto-occipital dislocation: case report, *J Neurosurg* 65:863-870, 1986.

44. Tuite GF, Veres R, Crockard HA, Sell D: Pediatric transoral surgery: indications, complications, and long-term outcome, *J Neurosurg* 84:573-583, 1996.

45. Wald SL, McLaurin RL: Anomalies of the craniocervical junction. In McLaurin RL, Venes JL, Schut L, Epstein F (eds): *Pediatric neurosurgery,* ed 2. Philadelphia, WB Saunders, 1989.

46. Wiesel SW, Rothman RH: Occipitoatlantal hypermobility, *Spine* 4:187-191, 1979.

CHAPTER 61

Subaxial Cervical Deformities

Paul M. Arnold and Dennis J. Maiman

Cervical kyphotic deformities are commonly observed and are often symptomatic, with patients presenting with complaints of neck pain, myelopathy, radiculopathy, or neck deformity with loss of mobility. The most common etiology of kyphosis is degenerative, but post-traumatic and postlaminectomy kyphosis are also frequently observed.

Cervical spine deformity may result from a variety of etiologies, including trauma; degenerative disease; congenital anomaly; infection; tumor; and iatrogenic causes, such as surgery and irradiation. Cervical deformities may also occur in patients with systemic arthritides, such as ankylosing spondylitis and rheumatoid arthritis. Likewise, patients with primary neurologic disorders such as athetoid cerebral palsy, spasmodic torticollis, and other movement disorders, as well as patients with neuromuscular disorders, are predisposed to develop cervical deformity caused by degeneration. Patients with bone disorders such as osteogenesis imperfecta and spondyloepiphyseal dysplasia may also develop deformity involving the cervical region.

Subaxial cervical deformities most commonly occur in the sagittal plane, primarily as kyphosis, although hyperlordosis or a mixed "swan-neck" deformity can also be observed. Deformity in the coronal plane, manifesting as a scoliosis or angulation, is uncommon in the cervical region when compared with the thoracic and lumbar regions.[25] Most cervical coronal deformities are the result of congenital vertebral anomalies.

Congenital vertebral lesions can be categorized as defects of segmentation and defects of formation. By far, the most common congenital defects of the subaxial cervical vertebrae are the defects of segmentation associated with the Klippel-Feil syndrome. Anomalies of vertebral formation are uncommon in this region of the spine. In the rare cases of hemivertebra of the cervical region, an angular coronal plane deformity may occur, with a risk of neurologic involvement, especially in the skeletally immature person. Trauma or postsurgical changes theoretically could produce a deformity with a coronal component. In practice, however, this is rare. Compensatory curves, which are occasionally observed in response to upper thoracic deformities, must be distinguished from a primary deformity affecting the cervical spine. Deformities in the coronal plane in adults are usually not severe and are infrequently associated with significant pain or neurologic symptoms. As a result, surgical treatment is rarely contemplated.

Significance of Cervical Kyphosis

A considerable variation in the degree of cervical lordosis can be observed in the average patient population. Degenerative changes associated with aging typically produce a straightening of the spine, but the limits of normality are not established.[10] After examining a group of asymptomatic patients, Gore et al.[11] concluded that the normal cervical spine has a lordotic curve measuring approximately 15 to 20 degrees from C1 to T1. Generally, cervical kyphosis is defined as a ventral or kyphotic angulation of 5 degrees or more. The incidence of straightening or kyphosis increases with age because the cervical discs contribute to the normal lordotic curve, and the loss of disc height associated with degenerative changes produces a straightening of the spine. In some patients, increases in thoracic kyphosis associated with aging may produce a compensatory increase in cervical lordosis.

After performing cadaver studies, Breig[4] first called attention to the motion and degree of elongation of the spinal cord that occur during flexion and extension movements of the cervical spine. According to his measurements, there may be as much as a 45 to 75mm change in length of the spinal cord as a result of flexion and extension movements. Furthermore, there is relative motion of the cord in relation to the underlying vertebrae. Flexion movements produce tensile forces within the cord and elongation, whereas extension causes shortening or compression of the cord. Flexion also produces a decrease in the anteroposterior dimension of the spinal cord, but because of straightening of the dura and ligamenta flava, the available canal diameter is actually increased. Extension produces the reverse changes. Changes in the normal configuration of the spinal canal caused by osteophyte formation, disc changes, or facet hypertrophy have the potential of compressing or stretching the cord. Instability that results from ligamentous laxity, particularly when associated with a short, angular kyphotic segment, has an increased likelihood of inducing trauma to the spinal cord or adjacent nerve roots. Frequently, examination of the spinal cord in the axial projection demonstrates flattening that is most marked at the kyphotic segment. The potential for neurologic deficit arising from kyphosis without actual compression is small but certainly not nonexistent.

The degree to which these dynamic changes are clinically manifest is difficult to determine. Current imaging studies are performed with the patient recumbent and with the cervical spine in a neutral or slightly extended position, and the images produced are static. Although flexion-extension magnetic resonance imaging (MRI) has been advocated, especially to evaluate craniocervical junction instability, it has yet to receive widespread clinical use.

The significance of cervical kyphosis in the production of chronic muscle fatigue and dorsal neck pain is unclear. Whereas many patients demonstrate reversal of normal cervical lordosis on plain radiographs, a very small number actually have refractory neck pain as a result of the deformity per se. Nonetheless, an occasional patient appears to have pain on this basis and requires careful evaluation and consideration for deformity correction and fusion (Figure 61.1).

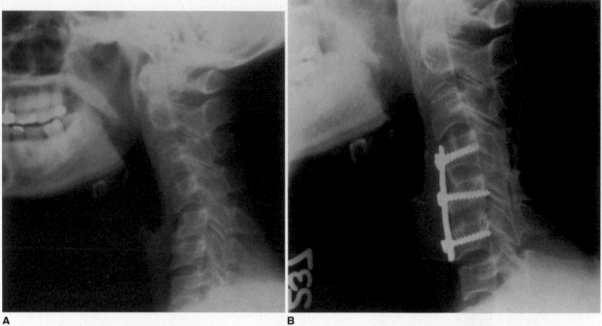

A   B

Figure 61.1 **(A)** Lateral cervical radiograph of a 53-year-old woman presenting with refractory posterior neck pain 6 months after a fall in which she had hyperflexion of her neck. Note the angulation and persistent fanning of the spinous processes at C4-5. **(B)** Postoperative radiograph demonstrating anterior interbody fusion augmented with plate fixation. The disc at C5-6 was markedly degenerative with osteophytes narrowing the canal and was therefore included in the fusion. The patient had immediate relief of her pain, and this has been maintained over 2 years of follow-up.

Postlaminectomy Kyphosis

Kyphosis is a well-recognized complication of laminectomy of the cervical spine.* The detachment of the dorsal paraspinous muscles, removal of the dorsal osseoligamentous complex, and occasional disruption of the facet complexes have all been recognized as potential causes of the development of a kyphotic deformity after laminectomy.[21]

The reported incidence of kyphosis after cervical laminectomy has been quite variable, although there is no doubt that it is considerably more common in the pediatric group. Reports of postlaminectomy kyphosis in series of pediatric patients range from 33% to 100%. Many of these patients, however, have other factors that predispose them to spinal deformity, such as bony tumors, neurofibromatosis, or irradiation. A recent series, which excluded these confounding factors, noted an incidence of kyphotic deformity of 53% in children.[3] Although the data are mixed, it appears that a younger age and a greater number of segments treated with laminectomy are associated with higher rates of deformity. Injury or resection of the facet joints also increases the probability of kyphosis. Laminectomy of C1 has a relatively low tendency to result in spinal deformity. Although it has not been conclusively demonstrated that the performance of laminoplasty as recommended by Raimondi *et al.*[19] will reduce the likelihood of postlaminectomy kyphosis in children, many neurosurgeons

who routinely perform cervical procedures on children perform laminoplasty, and some report evidence suggestive of benefit.[1] Prophylactic fusion should also be considered for patients undergoing laminectomy who are at high risk for developing kyphosis.[27] Dorsal fusions are much more effective at preventing kyphosis than at correcting kyphosis.

The incidence of postlaminectomy kyphosis in adults is relatively uncommon in the absence of an additional predisposing factor such as facet joint damage, prior ligamentous instability, ventral column compromise, neurologic deficit, or irradiation.[28,30] Adult cases will, nonetheless, be seen in any busy practice specializing in spinal problems (Figure 61.2). Recognition of the significance of this finding in terms of the probability of progression, the potential for symptoms, and the appropriate therapeutic options is essential for optimal management. Patients with the greatest risk of postlaminectomy kyphosis are those who have preoperative instability as well as those with straightening of the cervical spine.

In adults, when postlaminectomy kyphosis is mild, it is usually well tolerated, especially when there is associated stiffening of the spine from degenerative changes leading to loss of disc height and development of buttressing osteophytes. Progressive deformity, especially in a previously straight or lordotic spine, probably warrants close observation or consideration of treatment. Some surgeons routinely manage all cervical laminectomy patients in a hard cervical collar for several weeks postoperatively in an attempt to minimize the development of a postoperative deformity.

---

*References 3,5-7,14,15,17,23,27.

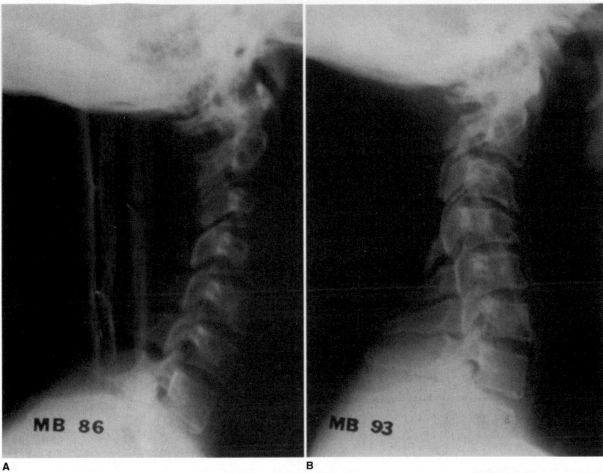

Figure 61.2 **(A)** Postoperative lateral cervical radiograph obtained after a C1-4 cervical laminectomy in a 20-year-old woman with longstanding shunted hydrocephalus. Surgery was performed to address progressing myelopathy that appeared to be related to dural fibrosis and stenosis causing spinal cord compression in the upper cervical spine. The patient improved after surgery. **(B)** Lateral cervical radiograph 7 years later, demonstrating the interval development of postlaminectomy kyphosis in this skeletally mature patient. At the time of this follow-up the patient was exhibiting recurrent symptoms of myelopathy and dorsal neck pain.

Surgical Correction of Cervical Kyphosis
Preoperative Assessment

Patients who present with kyphotic deformity of the cervical region generally have complaints of pain, neurologic symptoms, or both. Less frequently, they cite problems relating to the deformity itself, such as difficulty raising their head, looking forward, or opening their mouth. This latter group of patients encompasses patients with the more severe deformities.

The preoperative evaluation of all such patients should include a careful neurologic assessment to look for subtle signs of myelopathy or radicular involvement. Neuroradiologic imaging with MRI or myelography and postmyelographic computed tomography is important for evaluating spinal cord compression and the dimensions of the spinal canal. Assessment of the bony and ligamentous anatomy is also possible with these studies. Three-dimensional reconstructive CT has also been useful in assessing kyphosis, as bony detail, amount of deformity, and spinal canal encroachment can be visualized on one image (Figure 61.3). Plain cervical spine radiographs with flexion-extension views provide information about the levels involved in the deformity, its severity, and whether it appears fixed or rigid. The degree of spinal instability can also be assessed. Standing long-cassette films are helpful for evaluating overall sagittal spinal balance in patients with severe deformity. Concomitant thoracic kyphosis or fixed flexion contracture of the hip must be evaluated before consideration is given to lordosing a cervical kyphosis.

Most patients whose deformities do not reduce with neck extension should be given a trial of traction before surgery to determine the reducibility of the kyphosis. An exception to this is patients with minor deformity (which can often be reduced intraoperatively) or those with an obviously fixed kyphosis (e.g., ankylosing spondylitis). Traction is applied either with tongs or with a halo ring. Cervical halters are generally unsatisfactory because for most deformities, traction needs to be sustained to be effective. The amount of weight to apply is a matter of clinical judgment. The authors generally begin with 5 to 10 lb and increase the weight in a stepwise fashion, with regular assessment of neurologic function and patient tolerance and radiographic visualization of the degree of

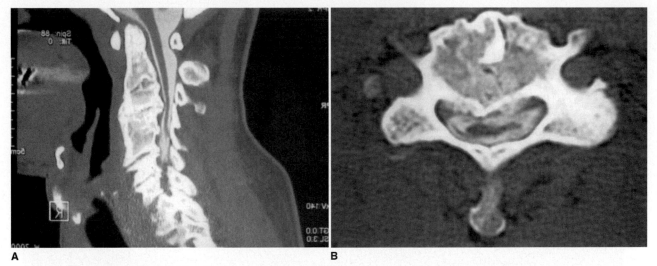

A　　　　　　　　　　　　　　**B**

Figure 61.3 **(A-B)** Three-dimensional reconstruction CT shows degenerative kyphosis with multilevel stenosis. This 62-year-old male had cervical myelopathy and required a combined ventral/dorsal procedure. His neck pain and paresthesias resolved, and his weakness and myelopathy improved.

reduction. Weights of more than 5 lb per level are usually not required. Close neurologic observation is imperative during traction because patients may demonstrate neurologic worsening that necessitates immediate discontinuation of traction. The optimal duration of traction is unclear; we usually apply traction for 48 hours or less before scheduled surgery.

If surgery is contemplated primarily for the treatment of pain believed to be the result of the deformity, other confounding conditions should be ruled out. In selected patients, psychologic screening may also be worthwhile for obtaining objective data regarding the likelihood of surgical success.

Surgical Techniques

The choice of operative technique for cervical deformity must be predicated on the type and severity of the deformity to be treated, the etiology of the deformity, neurologic symptomatology, posterior column integrity, the rigidity of the spine, and the experience of the surgeon. The indications for a ventral approach, a dorsal approach, or a combined ventral and dorsal approach are not absolute.

Ventral Surgery

A ventral approach is preferred for cases in which there is insufficient anterior column height or insufficient ability to bear an axial load, such as with collapse of a ventral bone graft or compression fracture, with ventral pathology such as tumor or associated spondylotic bars producing myelopathy, or with a deformity that is rigid or incompletely reducible. In addition, ventral surgery may be safer for the treatment of postlaminectomy kyphosis because surgery can be performed through an unoperated field (Figure 61.4). The ventral approach has other advantages, including the ability to ventrally decompress the spinal

cord and to use ventral interbody strut grafts that are loaded in compression, thereby enhancing fusion.[29]

In these cases, a ventral release, with or without ventral decompression of the spinal canal, is performed. If appropriate, the kyphotic deformity is then reversed, with reestablishment of some lordotic curve. Reversal of kyphosis should not be attempted in the face of significant radiologic evidence of spinal cord impingement unless surgical decompression is first performed (Figure 61.5). As noted above, extension of the cervical spine decreases the anteroposterior dimension of the spinal canal while increasing the thickness of the spinal cord. With a severe, rigid angular kyphotic deformity, dorsal decompression by means of laminectomy and foraminotomy should be considered before ventral osteotomy.

The surgical techniques for ventral decompression and fusion of deformity are quite similar to those used in the treatment of trauma or degenerative disease. Fiberoptic nasotracheal intubation is preferred to allow dental occlusion and maximal proximal exposure that is unimpeded by the mandible. The patient is positioned supine in traction with as much extension as is possible, as determined preoperatively. This may be facilitated by a roll placed dorsally in the cervical region. In cases in which spinal cord compression is observed, methylprednisolone as a 30 mg/kg IV bolus over 15 minutes followed by 5.4 mg/kg/hr IV continuous infusion can be given, although this is a controversial issue. If the patient awakens neurologically intact, the infusion is stopped. Otherwise infusion is continued for 23 hours. Prophylactic antibiotics are administered. When bicortical ventral fixation plates are used, C-arm fluoroscopy is routine. Plain radiography or fluoroscopy is also invaluable for assessing the degree of reduction and for graft placement. An intraoperative x-ray is performed at this time to assess spinal alignment. Significant deformity reduction is often evident after the placement of tong traction and general anesthesia. If autologous bone graft is to be used, the donor site and

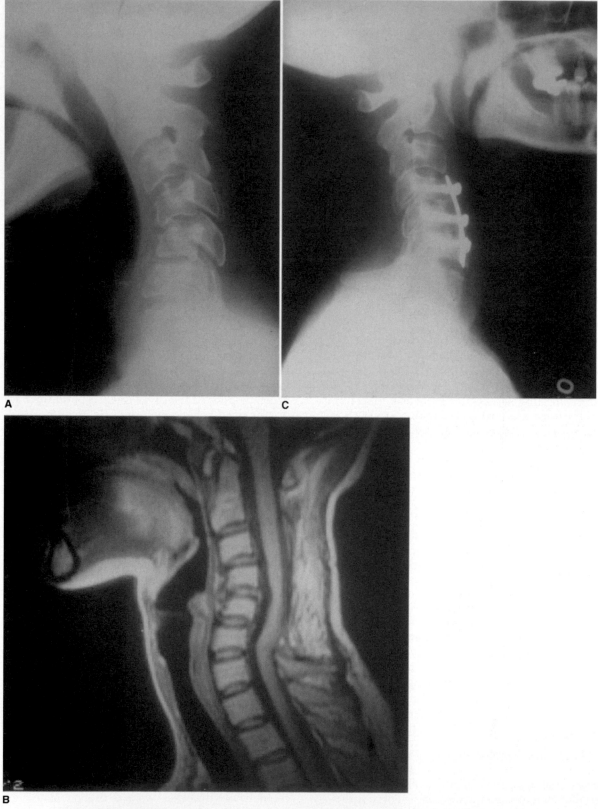

Figure 61.4 **(A-B)** Standing lateral cervical radiograph and sagittal T_1-weighted MRI image of a 38-year-old woman with severe dorsal neck pain and subtle signs of myelopathy. The patient had undergone cervical laminectomy several years previously. Note the development of a postlaminectomy "swan-neck" deformity in an adult. **(C)** Anterior interbody fusion and plating was performed to restore lordosis with resolution of the patient's pain and neurologic symptoms. On this film, performed 6 months postoperatively, there is slight kyphosis at C3-4 that may progress and will bear watching.

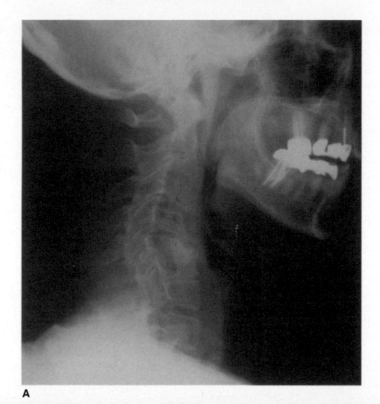

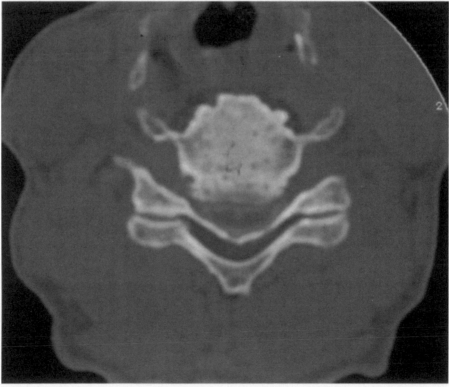

Figure 61.5 **(A)** Lateral cervical radiograph of a 71-year-old woman presenting with myelopathy. A kyphosis is observed from C4-6. **(B)** Computed tomographic myelogram at C5-6 demonstrating tight "circumferential" stenosis with shingling of the laminae. Because of the combination of dorsal and ventral cord compression, a posterior laminectomy was performed from C4-6 before repositioning the patient supine and carrying out C5 and C6 corpectomy, strut grafting, and anterior Caspar plate fixation from C4-7. The involved area progressed to solid fusion after immobilization in a rigid collar. Partial improvement of the myelopathy was observed.

cervical region are prepared simultaneously. The incision is centered at the middle of the deformity to be treated. A transverse incision placed in a skin crease is preferred for short (one to three) segment fusions or in people with short, thick necks. An incision along the ventral margin of the sternocleidomastoid muscle is used for longer fusions. Exposure of the ventral aspect of the spine is accomplished as described by Cloward[8] and Smith and Robinson.[20]

Dissection of the medial attachments of the longus colli muscles and placement of self-retaining retractors is followed by incision of the annulus fibrosus at the affected disc levels. The Caspar vertebral body distractor (Aesculap, San Francisco, CA) that uses screw posts placed into the vertebral bodies is a useful aid for reducing the kyphosis and placing ventral strut grafts (Figure 61.6). Excess intervertebral traction, however, may be injurious to the compromised spinal cord and thus should be used judiciously. The distraction posts are placed parallel to the vertebral end plates. After osteotomy or ventral release of annular attachments, the posts are used to affect reduction by positioning them in a parallel configuration. This maneuver realigns the spine and allows application of the retractor. The retractor then maintains the reduction and allows further distraction force to be applied. After a bone graft is inserted, the retractor is removed and a plate is applied. This technique should not be used if there is evidence of dorsal compression by laminae, ligaments, or other pathology.

The decompression is tailored according to the results of preoperative imaging. In some cases, multilevel discectomy with multiple interbody bone grafts is preferred. This is useful for kyphotic deformities extending over several motion segments. Plate fixation can then be segmental to provide greater rigidity. Alternatively, when there is a bony encroachment on the canal, trough corpectomy with strut grafting is performed. A strut graft spanning two disc spaces with an additional ventral interbody graft at the level above or below can also be used when required (Figure 61.7). This type of mixed construct provides the maximum number of sites for screw placement and allows for greater fixation and optimal reestablishment of lordosis. If two or more vertebral bodies are replaced, consideration should be given to adding posterior fixation.

Locking and nonlocking plates and slotted plates are used. For multisegment constructs, the latter system often provides more flexibility and is easier to apply. The variability in screw angulation allowed by the Caspar plate is helpful when plates are extended to C2 or C3. For one or two levels in the midcervical or lower cervical region, the Synthes (Paoli, PA) system may be easier to use. Fluoroscopy can be an aid to kyphosis reduction and plate application regardless of which system is employed. Fluoroscopic control is highly desirable when screws are placed into the dorsal vertebral body cortex. Steinmetz et al.[26] recently reported a series of 14 patients treated ventrally for postsurgical kyphosis. They employed intraoperative neck extension, as well as a dynamic, ventrally placed implant with multiple fixation points, to restore lordosis. The corrected 11 of 12 patients with this method (average 20 degrees correction) with minimal complications.

In most cases, postoperative immobilization is achieved with a rigid cervical collar that is worn for 6 weeks to

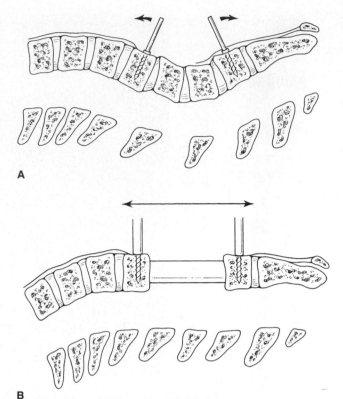

Figure 61.6 Use of the Caspar vertebral body distraction retractor to help maintain correction of kyphosis. (**A**) Initially, the distraction posts are inserted parallel to the end plates of the vertebral bodies. (**B**) When the deformity is corrected and the retractor is applied on the posts, it will maintain a more normal alignment as the site is prepared for strut grafting. Although the posts may be used as "handles" to aid in performing a reduction, this must be done with caution, or fracture of the vertebral body can result.

3 months. A halo vest or Minerva jacket may be used in cases in which fixation is suboptimal or when fusion is expected to be delayed. Patients with severe osteoporosis, high-grade instability noted preoperatively, or failed prior attempts at fusion perhaps should be included in this group. Herman and Sonntag[13] also noted the occasional need for halo immobilization in some high-risk patients after this type of procedure.

Complications. The potential complications associated with the ventral approaches are well known and include vocal cord palsy, hoarseness or dysphagia, injury to visceral structures (such as the esophagus or trachea), graft displacement, screw loosening or fracture, wound complications (such as infection), hematoma (which may be sufficient to cause respiratory embarrassment), and dehiscence.[12] The incidence of a number of complications can be reduced by periodically releasing or removing the retraction during the operation. Also, for procedures involving the lower cervical spine, a left-sided approach may reduce the likelihood of vocal cord paralysis in the event that there is a nonrecurrent right inferior laryngeal nerve.

Overdistraction of the cervical spine and placement of a strut graft that is too long for the corpectomy defect is a

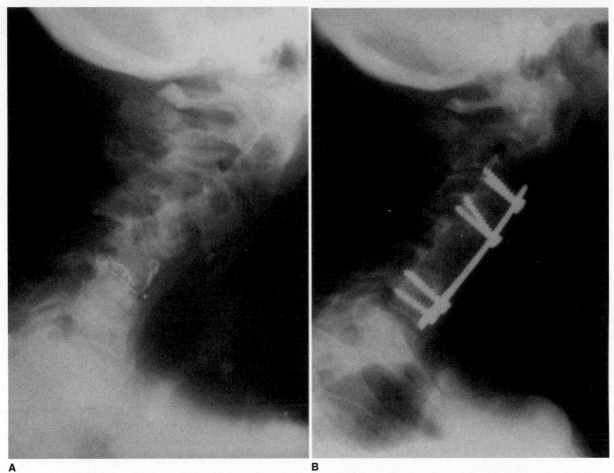

A   B

Figure 61.7 (**A**) Lateral cervical radiograph of a 70-year-old man with a painful, rigid cervical kyphosis resulting from multiple failed previous attempts at interbody fusion. Complaints included occipitocervical pain and an inability to maintain the head in an upright position. (**B**) Lateral radiograph obtained 18 months postoperatively demonstrating solid fusion with partial correction of the kyphotic deformity by means of corpectomy and osteotomy with strut grafting from C4-7, interbody grafting at C3-4, and ventral plating. Postoperatively, the patient was immobilized in a halo orthosis for 12 weeks.

common technical error. This situation preloads the construct, making telescoping, graft collapse, or displacement more likely. When a ventral plate is used, there must be no encroachment of the plate on the adjacent disc spaces, and screws must be placed appropriately. Meticulous sizing of the bone graft and any ventral plate is critical for avoiding complications and for long-term success.

Dorsal Fixation and Fusion Techniques

Dorsal fusion for cervical kyphotic deformity is primarily indicated as a prophylactic measure after laminectomy or when the deformity is the result of dorsal ligamentous insufficiency associated with the preservation of axial integrity of the anterior column, such as is seen acutely after ligamentous trauma (Figure 61.8). In these cases, the kyphosis usually will significantly or completely reduce with neck extension. Dorsal fusion is accomplished via standard techniques including interspinous wiring or lateral mass wire or plate fixation. Abumi *et al.*[2] recently reported a series of patients with cervical kyphosis who underwent placement of cervical pedicle screws to maintain correction. Dorsal surgical approaches for rigid or incompletely reducible kyphotic deformities have limited application and are biomechanically less sound. Nevertheless, certain circumstances may warrant their use as the sole operative treatment, especially if fusion *in situ* is being performed. More often, dorsal fusions are performed in conjunction with a dorsal decompression and ventral procedures when treating severe deformity associated with spinal cord compression.[14,18]

Postlaminectomy kyphosis is corrected less well by dorsal fixation and fusion than by ventral techniques. If this approach is to be used, lateral mass plates or interfacet wiring, combined with iliac strips or rib grafts are employed. Lateral mass plates have become the preferred fixation method because they provide greater rigidity than does wire fixation.[9] Complications associated with screw placement are uncommon if meticulous care is used to select screw entry points and the screws are angled appropriately rostrally and laterally to avoid the nerve root and vertebral artery. However, it must be cautioned that a

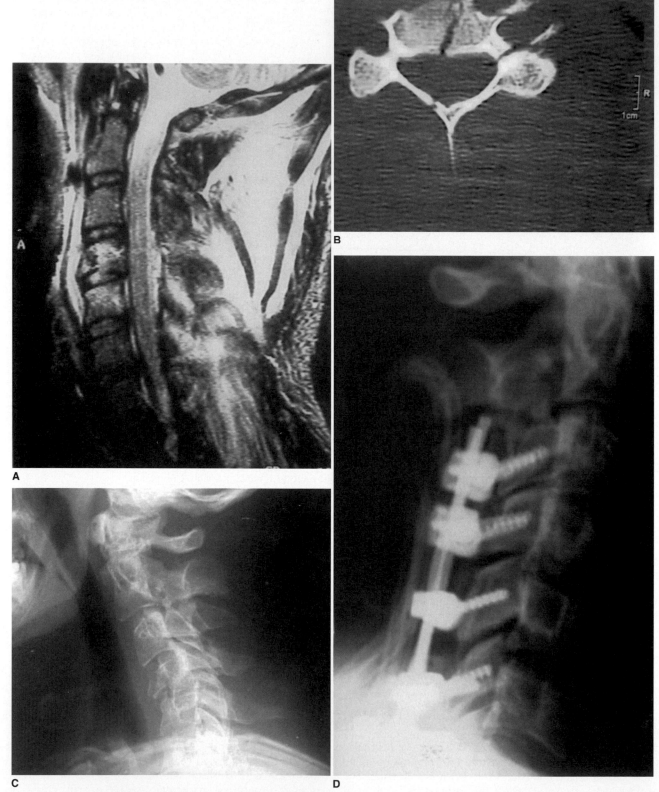

Figure 61.8 **(A-B)** A 22-year-old male involved in MVA. He was neurologically normal but had C4 and C5 fractures with normal alignment. The patient required anticoagulation and was placed in a halo. **(C)** Three weeks later he began experiencing neck pain, and a plain radiograph revealed kyphosis. **(D)** His anticoagulation was reversed and a posterior cervical fusion was performed.

deformity or prior surgery may obscure the anatomic land-marks so that great care is required for satisfactory screw placement. Frameless stereotaxy may be used in patients with previous surgery where standard landmarks may be lost. Bicortical purchase does not appear to be necessary for successful fixation in most cases. Fehlings and col-leagues[9] have obtained successful fusion results by using lateral mass plates without additional bone graft. This study, however, was heavily weighted with posttraumatic cases, so that careful consideration should be given to the use of autologous bone graft in deformity cases.

Combined Ventral and Dorsal Decompression and Fusion

Combined procedures involving both a ventral and a dor-sal approach are occasionally indicated, especially for the correction of rigid deformities (Figure 61.9). Other indi-cations include cases with both ventral and dorsal com-pression with radiculopathy secondary to foramental stenosis as a prominent feature, cases in which severe slip-page is associated with incompetent posterior ligamentous structures, and in trauma when there is compromise of the ventral and dorsal columns (Figure 61.10).

Patients with ankylosing spondylitis may present with a severe, rigid cervical kyphosis that limits the patient's abil-ity to look forward and that in some severe cases may limit jaw opening secondary to contact with the chest. Correction of this type of deformity will require osteotomy with resection of a portion of the dorsal elements. Different methods have been described for this proce-dure,[16,22,24] the most notable being the one advocated by Simmons,[24] in which a dorsal decompression is performed under local anesthesia at the C7-T1 level, with the patient in the seated position. The spine is fractured by forcibly extending the neck, which is held in traction by a halo ring. Usually the fracture in these patients occurs at the junc-tion between the vertebral end plate and the disc. Simmons advocates that the procedure be performed with the patient awake to provide for patient feedback during kyphosis reduction. Other surgeons have performed the procedure by using a general anesthetic and have moni-tored evoked potentials.

Summary

Deformity of the cervical spine is generally observed in the context of degenerative disease with its concurrent lig-amentous laxity, loss of disc height, and bony remodeling. Another relatively common circumstance is postlaminec-tomy kyphosis that tends to affect younger patients. Deformity resulting from congenital anomalies is uncom-mon in the lower cervical region. Surgical procedures may be indicated to treat neurologic symptoms (myelopathy) rather than the deformity itself. Ventral procedures are preferred in most cases of spinal cord compression or when the deformity is rigid. In irreducible kyphosis in which movement occurs across the angulated segment, decompression—combined with strut grafting and fusion in situ—may allow stabilization or improvement of neuro-logic symptoms. Severe kyphotic deformity may occasion-ally require correction for postural reasons. There is a small group of patients with neck pain and cervical defor-mity who benefit from reduction and fusion, although the methods to clearly identify patients suitable for surgery are not standardized. Careful patient selection is required for this difficult group.

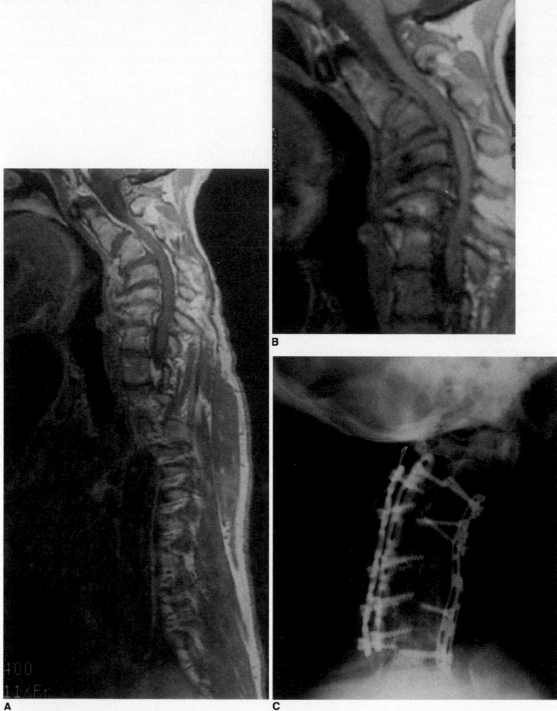

Figure 61.9 This 38-year-old right-handed man presented with progressive cervical myelopathy. The patient had a history of a cerebral palsy-like condition associated with mild spasticity, joint contractures, and thoracolumbar scoliosis. (**A**) Sagittal T_1-weighted MRI image demonstrating a kyphotic deformity of the cervical spine with associated thoracic lordoscoliosis. (**B**) Detailed sagittal MRI image of the cervical region demonstrating spinal cord impingement at multiple sites. Minimal preoperative reduction of this relatively rigid kyphosis was noted with cervical traction. (**C**) A ventral/dorsal decompression and fusion with internal fixation was performed from C2-7 by using titanium instrumentation. The kyphosis correction was a secondary goal of surgery and was partial. The patient, who required aids for ambulation preoperatively, now walks independently.

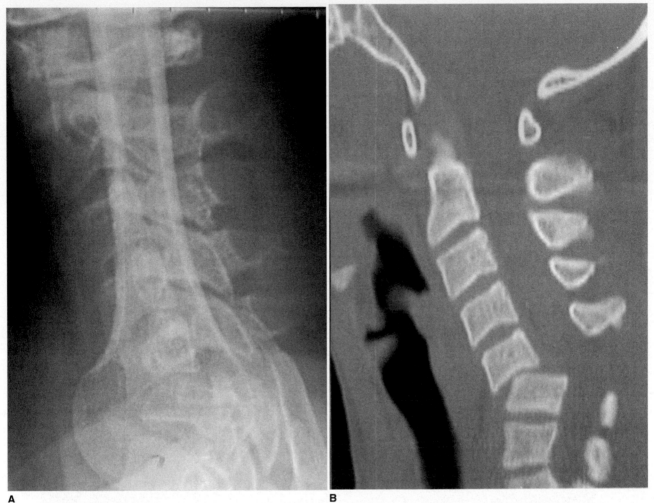

A   **B**

Figure 61.10 A 41-year-old female was involved in a MVA and complained of lower extremity painful dysesthesia. She was densely paraparetic with weakness in her distal upper extremities. Radiographic work-up included (**A**) plain x-rays, (**B**) CT scan, and (**C**) MRI. These studies revealed severe kyphosis at C5-6, with injury to the anterior and posterior columns. (**D**) She underwent a combined ventral/dorsal procedure. She is able to ambulate independently, and her dysesthetic pain has resolved.

Continued

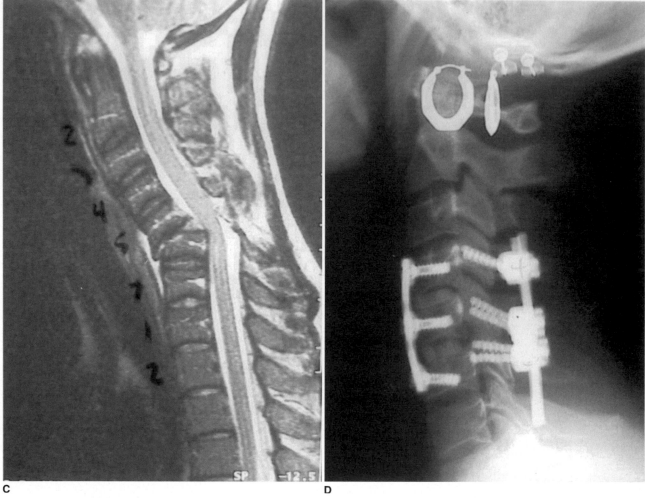

C   D

Figure 61.10 *cont'd*

REFERENCES

1. Abbott R, Feldstein N, Wisoff JH, *et al*: Osteoplastic laminotomy in children. *Pediatr Neurosurg* 18:153-156, 1992.

2. Abumi K, Shono Y, Taneichi H: Correction of cervical kyphosis using pedicle screw fixation systems. *Spine* 24:2389-2396, 1999.

3. Bell DF, Walker JL, O'Connor G, *et al*: Spinal deformity after multiple-level laminectomy in children. *Spine* 19: 406-411, 1994.

4. Breig A: *Biomechanics of the Central Nervous System.* Stockholm, Almquist and Wiskell, 1960.

5. Butler JC, Whitecloud TS: Postlaminectomy kyphosis: causes and surgical management. *Orthop Clin North Am* 23:505-511, 1992.

6. Callahan RA, Johnson RM, Margolis RN, Keggi KJ, Albright JA, Southwick WO: Cervical facet fusion for the control of instability following laminectomy. *J Bone Joint Surg* 59:991-1002, 1977.

7. Cattell HS, Clark GL Jr: Cervical kyphosis and instability following multiple laminectomies in children. *J Bone Joint Surg* 49:713-720, 1967.

8. Cloward RB: The anterior approach for removal of ruptured cervical discs. *J Neurosurg* 15:602-617, 1958.

9. Fehlings MG, Cooper PR, Errico TJ: Posterior plates in the management of cervical instability: long-term results in 44 patients. *J Neurosurg* 81:341-349, 1994.

10. Gay RE: The curve of the cervical spine: variations and significance. *J Manip Physiol Ther* 16:591-594, 1993.

11. Gore DR, Sepic SB, Gardner GM: Roentgenographic findings of the cervical spine in asymptomatic people. *Spine* 11:521-524, 1986.

12. Heller JG, Silcox DH III, Sutterlin CE: Complications of posterior plating. *Spine* 20:2442-2448, 1995.

13. Herman JM, Sonntag VKH: Cervical corpectomy and plate fixation for postlaminectomy kyphosis. *J Neurosurg* 80: 963-970, 1994.

14. Kaptain GJ, Simmons N, Replogle RE, Pobereskin L: Incidence and outcome of kyphotic deformity following laminectomy for cervical spondylotic myelopathy. *J Neurosurg (Spine 2)* 93:199-204, 2000.

15. Katsumi Y, Honma T, Nakamura T: Analysis of cervical instability resulting from laminectomy for removal of spinal tumor. *Spine* 14:1172-1176, 1989.

16. Lin SY, Wu HJ, Chien SH: Correction osteotomy of flexion deformity of cervical spine in ankylosing spondylitis, case report. *Kaohsiung J Med Sci* 6:454-460, 1990.

17. Mikawa Y, Shikata J, Yamamuro T: Spinal deformity and instability after multilevel cervical laminectomy. *Spine* 12:6-11, 1987.

18. Miyazaki K, Tada K, Matsuda Y, Okumo M, Yasuda T, Murakami H: Posterior extensive simultaneous multi-segment decompression with posterolateral fusion for cervical instability and kyphotic and/or S-shaped deformities. *Spine* 14:1159-1170, 1989.

19. Raimondi AJ, Gutierrez FA, Di Rocco C: Laminotomy and total reconstruction of the posterior spinal arch for spinal canal surgery in childhood. *J Neurosurg* 45:555-560, 1976.

20. Robinson RA, Smith GW: Anterolateral cervical disc removal and interbody fusion for cervical disc syndrome. *Bull Johns Hopkins Hosp* 96:223-224, 1955.

21. Saito T, Yammamuro T, Shikata J, *et al*: Analysis and prevention of spinal column deformity following cervical laminectomy. I. Pathogenetic analysis of postlaminectomy deformities. *Spine* 16:494-502, 1991.

22. Savini R, DiSilvestre M, Gargiulo G: Cervical osteotomy by the Simmons method in the treatment of cervical kyphosis due to ankylosing spondylitis, case report. *Ital J Orthop Traumatol* 14:377-383, 1988.

23. Sim FH: Swan neck deformity following extensive cervical laminectomy: a review of twenty-one cases. *J Bone Joint Surg* 56A:564-580, 1974.

24. Simmons EH: The surgical correction of flexion deformity of the cervical spine in ankylosing spondylitis. *Clin Orthop* 86:132-143, 1972.

25. Smith MD: Congenital scoliosis of the cervical or cervicothoracic spine. *Orthop Clin North Am* 25:301-310, 1994.

26. Steinmetz MP, Kager CD, Benzel EC: Ventral correction of postsurgical cervical kyphosis. *J Neurosurg (Spine 2)* 97:1-7, 2003.

27. Yasuoka S, Peterson HA, Laws ER Jr, MacCarty CS: Pathogenesis and prophylaxis of postlaminectomy deformity of the spine after multiple level laminectomy: difference between children and adults. *Neurosurgery* 9:145-52, 1981.

28. Zdeblick TA, Abitbol JJ, Kunz DN, *et al*: Cervical stability after sequential capsule resection. *Spine* 18:2005-2008, 1993.

29. Zdeblick TA, Bohlman HH: Cervical kyphosis and myelopathy. *J Bone Joint Surg* 71A:170-182, 1989.

30. Zdeblick TA, Zou, D, Warden KE, *et al*: Cervical stability after foraminotomy. A biomechanical in vitro analysis. *J Bone Joint Surg* 74A:22-27, 1992.

CHAPTER 62

Cervical Facet Dislocations: A Ventral Surgical Strategy for Decompression, Reduction, and Stabilization

Simcha J. Weller, Sait Naderi,
and Edward C. Benzel

Much controversy surrounds the management of subaxial cervical subluxations resulting from facet fracture-dislocation.* An initial attempt at closed reduction using skeletal traction is not without risk.† The most serious complication of cervical traction and closed reduction is the retropulsion of disc fragments into the spinal canal and resultant spinal cord compression (Figure 62.1). Several reports of neurologic deterioration after closed reduction in the setting of concurrent disc herniation have been described.[5,16,17,28,37] In addition, late instability is relatively common in patients treated with closed reduction alone, because of the concomitant presence of significant ligamentous disruption associated with these injuries.

The surgical technique for the open reduction of unstable cervical dislocations varies from surgeon to surgeon. Most reports have described dorsal reduction techniques.‡ However, the ventral surgical approach for reduction has its advocates. Several small series have been published describing the technique of ventral reduction of locked facets.§ Because of the popularization of dorsal fixation techniques (e.g., lateral mass plating and spinous process wiring), ventral reduction has not been widely used in clinical practice. However, an increasing concern has been raised regarding the danger associated with the dorsal reduction of a cervical spine dislocation in the presence of a ventral disc herniation.[5,6,17,28,37] Furthermore, because of the common coexistence of significant dorsal bony and soft tissue disruption, a three-vertebral segment (two-motion segment) dorsal fixation is commonly required to stabilize a two-vertebral segment (one-motion segment) instability. In addition, in dorsal reduction of locked facets it is commonly necessary to remove a significant portion of the involved facet(s), thus

often mandating a three-vertebral segment dorsal fixation procedure. Conversely, ventral reduction may be followed by arthrodesis of only a single-motion segment, thus sparing additional motion segments from arthrodesis.

Surgical Technique

Discectomy

The standard ventromedial approach is used through a transverse skin incision. After radiographic confirmation of the operative level, a discectomy is performed. A special consideration in the case of facet dislocation is the ventral translation (ventrolisthesis) of the rostral vertebral body on its caudal counterpart. This is often associated with some degree of kyphotic angulation and a resultant obscuration of the disc space, necessitating removal of the ventral aspect of the caudal end plate of the rostral vertebral body with a high-speed air drill (Figure 62.2). Care must be taken not to remove so much of the vertebral body as to preclude ventral screw-plate fixation. After exposure of the disc space, a standard discectomy is performed. The posterior longitudinal ligament is always removed, thus exposing the dura mater and ensuring adequate decompression.

Reduction

After completion of the discectomy, deformity reduction is attempted. Often, simple distraction is successful, because a potentially significant obstruction to reduction (the disc and annulus fibrosus) has been removed. However, if this maneuver fails, one of two intraoperative maneuvers may be used to facilitate reduction through the ventral approach: (1) the interbody spreader technique or (2) the vertebral body post technique. Failure to use either technique appropriately may result in failure of reduction.

Interbody Spreader Technique

A Cloward interbody spreader, or an equivalent device, is inserted into the disc interspace at a 30- to 40-degree angle (Figure 62.3A). Failure to place this device at an angle results in achieving only distraction force application (as simple distraction with tongs achieves). This does not result in the application of a bending moment, which is required for reduction with this technique.

While gradually applying distraction with the disc interspace spreader (applied in the midvertebral body region) (Figure 62.3B), the spreader is rotated rostrally. This applies a bending moment to the dislocated vertebral body while the facet dislocation is reduced by distraction. If the locked facets are disengaged, the vertebrae should realign. Distraction is then relaxed in the aligned position and the spreader removed (Figure 62.3C).

For bilateral facet dislocations, the intervertebral spreader should be placed in the midvertebral body region. For unilateral dislocations, the spreader should be placed on the side of the dislocation to facilitate the application of a torque about the long axis of the spine via the spreader. Placement of the intervertebral spreader too far ventrally may result in fracture of the end plate.

*References 2,3,8,13,18,20,24,25,30,33,36.
†References 1,11,19,22,34,35,39.
‡References 6,7,12,16,17,29,31,32.
§References 5,10,15,21,26,38.

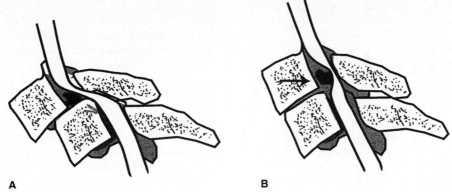

A   **B**

Figure 62.1 A typical bilateral facet dislocation with disc extrusion. Note that the spinal cord is compressed predominantly by the dislocated caudal vertebral body and rostral lamina before reduction (**A**). After reduction, the large fragment of extruded disc has been retropulsed into the spinal canal *(arrow)*, resulting in spinal cord compression (**B**). *(From University of New Mexico, Division of Neurosurgery, with permission.)*

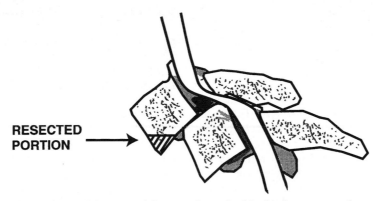

RESECTED
PORTION

Figure 62.2 The ventrocaudal aspect of the rostral vertebral body obscures visualization of the disc interspace, necessitating partial resection. *(From University of New Mexico, Division of Neurosurgery, with permission.)*

Vertebral Body Post Technique

If the aforementioned technique fails, the vertebral body post technique may be attempted. This technique uses a vertebral body distractor post. It is important to remember that parallel distraction via the vertebral body posts is equivalent to simple traction, in that these techniques do not apply a bending moment.

The vertebral body post technique usually involves placing the posts at an angle with respect to each other (Figure 62.4A). This allows for the application of a bending moment that unlocks the facets before the application of distraction forces (Figure 62.4B). Distraction should then allow for complete disengagement of the locked facets. Manual reduction via the placement of the dorsally directed pressure on the rostral vertebral body encourages reduction if the facets have been adequately disengaged (Figure 62.4C). Relaxation of the distraction forces then allows reengagement of the facets in a normal position. The placement of dorsally directed pressure on the rostral vertebral body, as described previously, may also be applied with the interbody spreader technique.

As an aside, unilateral facet dislocation reduction through a ventral approach may be achieved in a similar manner, with the application of torque about the long axis of the spine, thus facilitating the reduction of the rotatory component of the deformity (Figure 62.5). This tends to reduce the rotational component of the dislocation.

Special Considerations

When contemplating a ventral approach to the dislocated and unstable cervical spine, at least four factors must be considered: (1) the advantage of first performing a ventral discectomy before an attempt at reduction, (2) the feasibility of achieving a reduction by using a ventral approach, (3) the potential need for an accompanying dorsal procedure (failure of ventral reduction), and (4) the ability to obtain a stable construct through an isolated ventral approach. It is emphasized that each must be thoroughly addressed preoperatively.

Ventral Decompression Before Reduction

The incidence of extruded cervical disc herniation associated with cervical spine injury has been reported to be 0.7% to 42%.[5,16,17,27,37] Reduction of the dislocation with the potential for retropulsion of disc material into the reduced and realigned spinal canal may result in significant spinal cord encroachment.

Several authors have recommended a ventral decompression before reduction when they suspect the potential for reduction-induced spinal cord encroachment.[5,16,17,23,37] This relatively uncommon event may occur with either open or closed reduction strategies and is avoided by the removal of the potentially offending disc before reduction (see Figure 62.1). Although magnetic resonance imaging (MRI) is useful in predicting this event, it probably is not universally accurate. In fact, MRI may demonstrate the absence of intracanalicular disc fragments. Nevertheless, disc material could be retropulsed through a disrupted annulus into the spinal canal during reduction.[16]

Reduction Feasibility

Previous reports have addressed the ventral reduction of cervical spine dislocations.* The only relatively large series of ventral reduction of locked facets was by de Oliviera,[15] who reported ventral reduction in 15 cases. He reported no failure with this interbody spreader technique. An understanding of the case-specific anatomy and fundamental biomechanical principles allows ventral reduction to be much more successful than was generally thought. The key

*References 5,10,15,21,26,39.

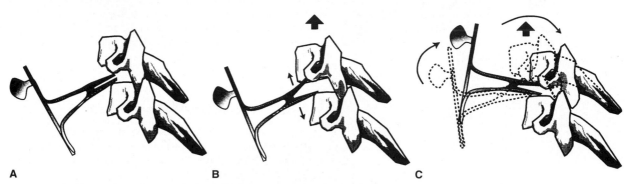

A   **B**   **C**

Figure 62.3 The interbody spreader technique for reduction of locked facets. After completion of discectomy, the spreader is placed into the disc interspace at a 30- to 40-degree angle. Note that the blades of the spreader should be placed deep enough to provide an adequate bending moment **(A)**. The application of traction *(large arrow)* and the simultaneous opening of the appropriately placed spreader *(small arrows)* create a bending moment and distraction of the disc interspace **(B)**. The application of a dorsally directed force by the spreader on the ventrocaudal aspect of the rostral vertebral body results in the realignment of the disengaged vertebrae **(C)**. *(From University of New Mexico, Division of Neurosurgery, with permission.)*

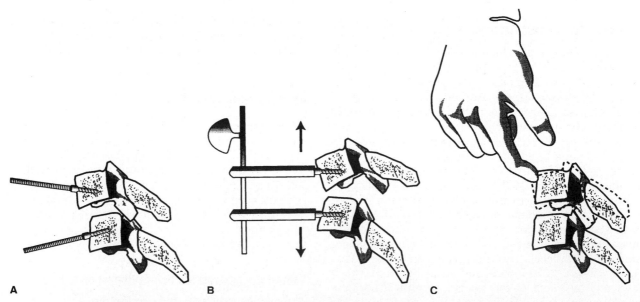

A   **B**   **C**

Figure 62.4 The vertebral body distractor post technique. **(A)** Placement of the posts at an angle with respect to each other allows for the application of a bending moment that helps disengage the dislocated facet joints. **(B)** The application of distraction forces *(arrows)* results in the realignment. Relaxation of the distraction can lead to reengagement of the facets in their normal position. This can be aided by the application of a dorsally directed force on the rostral vertebra **(C)**. *(From University of New Mexico, Division of Neurosurgery, with permission.)*

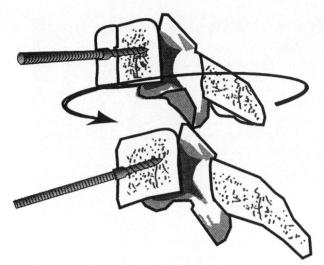

Figure 62.5 Appropriately placed posts and the application of torque about the long axis of the spine *(arrow)* can reduce the rotational component of a deformity. *(From University of New Mexico, Division of Neurosurgery, with permission.)*

is facet joint disengagement before an attempt at reduction. This requires the application of a bending moment to the unstable motion segment, followed by distraction, reduction, and finally, relaxation of the distraction.

Failure of Ventral Reduction

The failure of attempts at ventral deformity reduction is a reality. Therefore it behooves the spine surgeon to appropriately counsel the patient and family preoperatively regarding the possible need for a combined ventral and dorsal (and possibly, an additional ventral) approach. Although the latter may seem to be an excessive amount of surgical intervention, it provides the greatest chance for preservation and improvement of neurologic function. Significant comminution of the facets appears to be a risk factor for failure of ventral reduction. Therefore, in patients with this risk factor, consideration should be given to a dorsal reduction and arthrodesis if a disc herniation is not present.

Stability Acquisition via a Ventral Approach

Some authors have addressed the concern for stability acquisition in the circumferentially unstable spine (severe three-column injury)[14] via an isolated ventral approach.[9]

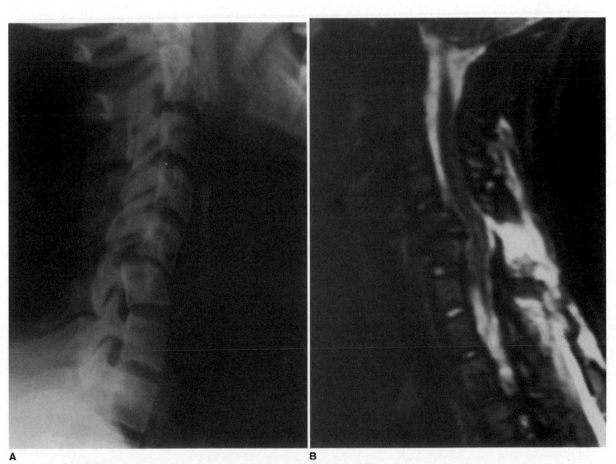

A   B

Figure 62.6 Lateral cervical radiograph of a neurologically intact 18-year-old woman who was involved in a diving accident, demonstrating a bilateral C5-6 facet dislocation (unilateral jumped facet, contralateral perched facet). Note the significant focal kyphosis with resultant obstruction of ventral access to the disc space (**A**). Preoperative T_2-weighted sagittal magnetic resonance image demonstrating a traumatic disc herniation at the level of the dislocation (**B**).

Continued

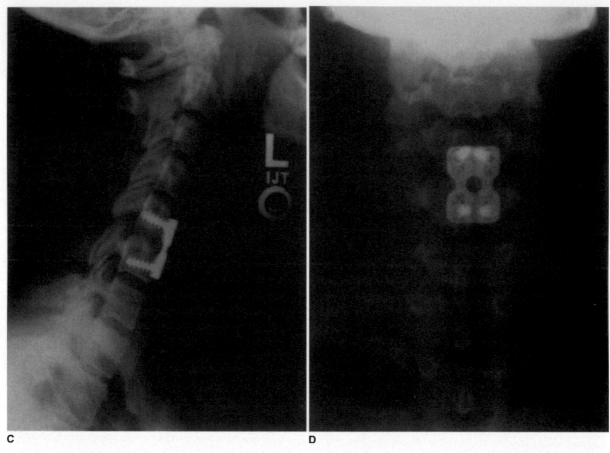

Figure 62.6 *cont'd* Postoperative lateral (**C**) and anteroposterior (**D**) radiographs after ventral decompression, reduction, and stabilization.

Most of these concerns have been directed at dislocations involving two or more motion segments (one or more vertebral body fractures) or after the use of dynamic fixation systems (nonfixed moment arms). However, with one-motion segment circumferential instability, the short bending moment applied by the implant (short implant) by way of the spine allows for greater stability acquisition potential.

Summary

A ventral approach to cervical dislocation and instability may be appropriate in more cases than previously thought. The ventral approach facilitates (1) ventral decompression before reduction (thus minimizing the chance for iatrogenic neurologic injury), (2) single-motion segment fixation (in contrast to two-motion segment fixation using a dorsal approach), and (3) stability acquisition through the application of effective ventral fixation techniques (Figure 62.6).

REFERENCES

1. Alexander EJ, Davis CT, Forsyth HF: Reduction and fusion of fracture dislocation of the cervical spine. *J Neurosurg* 27:588-591, 1967.

2. Argenson C, Lovet J, Sanouiller JL, de Peretti F: Traumatic rotatory displacement of the lower cervical spine. *Spine* 13:767-773, 1988.

3. Benzel E, Kesterson L: Posterior cervical interspinous compression wiring and fusion for mid to low cervical spinal injuries. *J Neurosurg* 70:893-899, 1989.

4. Benzel EC, Larson SJ: Functional recovery after decompressive spine operation for cervical spine fractures. *Neurosurgery* 20:742-746, 1987.

5. Berrington NR, van Staden JF, Willers JG, van der Westhuizen J: Cervical intervertebral disc prolapse associated with traumatic facet dislocations. *Surg Neurol* 40:395-399, 1993.

6. Beyer C, Cabanela M, Berquist T: Unilateral facet dislocations and fracture dislocations of the cervical spine. *J Bone Joint Surg* 73B:977-981, 1991.

7. Bohlman HH: Acute fractures and dislocations of the cervical spine. *J Bone Joint Surg* 61A:1119-1142, 1979.

8. Braakman R, Vinken PJ: Old luxations of the lower cervical spine. *J Bone Joint Surg* 50B:52-60, 1968.

9. Caspar W, Barbier DD, Klara PM: Anterior cervical fusion and Caspar plate stabilization for cervical trauma. *Neurosurgery* 25:491-502, 1989.

10. Cloward RB: Treatment of acute fractures and fracture-dislocations of the cervical spine by vertebra-body fusion. A report of eleven cases. *J Neurosurg* 18:201-209, 1961.

11. Cloward RB: Reduction of traumatic dislocation of the cervical spine with locked facets. Technical note. *J Neurosurg* 38:527-531, 1973.

12. Cooper PR, Cohen A, Rosiello A, Koslow M: Posterior stabilization of cervical spine fractures and subluxations using plates and screws. *Neurosurgery* 23:300-306, 1988.

13. Cotler HB, Miller LS, DeLucia FA *et al:* Closed reduction of cervical spine dislocations. *Clin Orthop* 214:185-199, 1987.

14. Denis F: Spinal instability as defined by the three-column spine concept in acute spinal trauma. *Clin Orthop* 189: 65-70, 1984.

15. de Oliviera JC: Anterior reduction of interlocking facets in the lower cervical spine. *Spine* 4:195-202, 1979.

16. Doran SE, Papadopulos SM, Ducker TB, Lillehei KO: Magnetic resonance imaging documentation of coexistent traumatic locked facets of the cervical spine and disc herniation. *J Neurosurg* 79:341-345, 1993.

17. Eismont FJ, Arena MJ, Green BA: Extrusion of an intervertebral disc associated with traumatic subluxation or dislocation of cervical facets. *J Bone Joint Surg* 73A: 1555-1560, 1991.

18. Evans DK: Reduction of cervical dislocations. *J Bone Joint Surg* 43B:552-555, 1961.

19. Hadley MN, Fitzpatrick BC, Sonntag VKH, Browner CM: Facet fracture dislocation injuries of the cervical spine. *Neurosurgery* 30:661-666, 1992.

20. Kleyn PJ: Dislocations of the cervical spine: closed reduction under anaesthesia. *Paraplegia* 22:271-228, 1984.

21. Kostuik JP, Connolly PJ: Anterior cervical plate fixation. In Garfin SR, Northrup BF (eds): *Surgery for the Spinal Cord Injuries.* Lippincott-Raven, New York, 1993, pp 163-173.

22. Maiman DJ, Banolat G, Larson SJ: Management of bilateral locked facets of the cervical spine. *Neurosurgery* 11:471-476, 1982.

23. Olerud C, Jonsson H Jr: Compression of the cervical spine cord after reduction of fracture dislocations. *Acta Orthop Scand* 62:599-601, 1991.

24. Osti OL, Fraser RD, Griffiths ER: Reduction and stabilization of cervical dislocation. *J Bone Joint Surg* 71B:275-282, 1989.

25. Perin N, Cooper PR: Posterior stabilization of the cervical spine using plates and screws. In Garfin SR, Bruce F, Northrup BF (eds): *Surgery for Spinal Cord Injuries.* Lippincott-Raven, New York, 1993, pp 113-122.

26. Rengachary SS, Duke DA: Stabilization of the cervical spine with the locking plate system. In Hitchon PW, Traynelis VC, Rengachary SS (eds): *Techniques in spinal fusion and stabilization.* Thieme Medical Publishers, Inc., New York, 1995, pp 176-190.

27. Rizzolo SJ, Piazza MR, Cotler JM *et al:* Intervertebral disc injury complicating cervical spine trauma. *Spine* 16 (Suppl 6):187-189, 1991.

28. Robertson PA, Ryan MD: Neurological deterioration after reduction of cervical subluxation: Mechanical compression by disc tissue. *J Bone Joint Surg* 74B:224-227, 1992.

29. Rorabeck C, Rock M, Hawkins R, Bourne R: Unilateral facet dislocation of the cervical spine. An analysis of the result of treatment in 26 patients. *Spine* 12:23-27, 1987.

30. Sabiston CP, Wing PC, Schweigel JF, Van Petegheim PK, Yu W: Closed reduction of dislocations of the lower cervical spine. *J Trauma* 28:832-835, 1988.

31. Schwarz N: Die verhakte Rotationssubluxation der Halswirbelsäule. *Unfallchirurg* 95:367-374, 1992.

32. Shapiro SA: Management of unilateral locked facet of the cervical spine. *Neurosurgery* 33:832-837, 1993.

33. Shrosbree RD: Neurological sequelae of reduction of fracture dislocations of the cervical spine. *Paraplegia* 17:212-221, 1979.

34. Sonntag VKH: Management of bilateral locked facets of the cervical spine. *Neurosurgery* 8:150-152, 1981.

35. Star AM, Jones AA, Cotler JM *et al:* Immediate closed reduction of cervical spine dislocations using traction. *Spine* 15:1068-1072, 1990.

36. Stauffer ES, Kelly EG: Fracture-dislocations of the cervical spine. *J Bone Joint Surg* 59A:45-48, 1977.

37. Tribus CB: Cervical disk herniation in association with traumatic facet dislocation. *Tech Orthop* 9:5-7, 1994.

38. Verbiest H: Anterior operative approach in cases of spinal cord compression by old irreducible displacement or fresh fracture of cervical spine. *J Neurosurg* 19:389-400, 1962.

39. Wolf A, Levi L, Mirvis S *et al:* Operative management of bilateral facet dislocation. *J Neurosurg* 75:883-890, 1991.

CHAPTER 63

Kyphotic Cervical Deformity Correction

Michael P. Steinmetz, Christopher Kager, Alexander R. Vaccaro, and Edward C. Benzel

The development of cervical spine deformity (e.g., kyphosis) may be secondary to advanced degenerative disease, trauma, neoplastic disease, or postsurgical causes.[15] Cervical spine deformity may also occur in patients with systemic arthritides, such as ankylosing spondylitis and rheumatoid arthritis. The most common cause is iatrogenic (postsurgical)[2] (Figure 63.1).

Subaxial cervical deformities most commonly occur in the sagittal plane, primarily as a kyphotic deformity. Coronal plane deformity, such as scoliosis, is uncommon in the cervical spine. If a coronal deformity is observed, it is most often the result of congenital vertebral anomalies.

The postoperative development of cervical kyphosis may follow both ventral and dorsal cervical approaches. Following ventral spine surgery, kyphosis may develop as a result of pseudoarthrosis[8,12] or failure to restore the anatomic cervical lordosis during surgery. Following dorsal surgery, kyphosis may develop and progress secondary to disruption of the natural stabilizing structures (tension band). The incidence of kyphosis in this situation may be as high as 21%.[16]

Whatever the cause, the development of cervical deformity should be avoided and corrected when appropriate. Cervical kyphosis is biomechanically unfavorable for the cervical musculature. Axial loads tend to cause further kyphosis via the application of the axial load through a moment arm-induced bending moment.[4] This is often associated with pain that is mechanical in nature.[17] Further and often excessive, degeneration of the cervical discs may occur, also contributing to cervical pain. In advanced cases, the patient's gaze, swallowing, and respiration may be adversely affected. In the spine's attempt to compensate for a severe cervical kyphosis, hyperlordosis of the lumbar spine may occasionally occur; this may potentially accelerate lumbar degenerative disease.

Clinical Presentation

Most patients complain of mechanical neck pain as a component of their symptoms. This pain is typically worse with exertion and is relieved by rest. As mentioned previously, the deformity places the adjacent cervical discs at risk for advanced degeneration. Therefore patients may present with radiculopathy. Patients may also be myelopathic or have a worsening myelopathy. As the kyphosis progresses, the stress on the ventral spinal cord increases. This may adversely affect the spinal cord vasculature and lead to even further myelopathic symptoms.[5,19]

Clinical Evaluation

The deformity should be evaluated by both static and dynamic (flexion/extension) radiographs of the cervical spine. The thoracic spine should also be evaluated if there is deformity at the cervicothoracic junction. In this manner, the deformity may be measured (sagittal angle) and any other abnormalities may be noted (e.g., subluxation, pseudoarthrosis). This strategy also assesses the flexibility of the cervical spine and determines the presence of ankylosed joints. If normal movement of the cervical spine on dynamic radiographs is present, and if a normal lordosis is achieved in extension, a dorsal surgical reconstruction procedure may adequately address the pathologic condition. Standing long-cassette radiographs are useful in the assessment of the overall sagittal balance. Thoracic hyperkyphosis or lumbar hyperlordosis must be taken into consideration when the treatment strategy is being designed.

All patients should be evaluated with preoperative magnetic resonance imaging or computed tomographic myelography. If a significant ventral compressive pathologic condition (disc, osteophyte) is present, a ventral decompressive procedure must be performed before the correction of the deformity.

Deformity Correction Strategies

The cervical spine may be exposed to coronal plane, rotational, or axial (subsidence) deformation stresses, but the most common deformity by far is in the sagittal plane (i.e., kyphosis). A common cause is iatrogenic.[2] This deformity may also accompany the pathologic entity of cervical spondylotic myelopathy.[4]

Sagittal plane deformity in the cervical spine may be addressed ventrally,[6,9,14,25] dorsally,[1,7] or both.[1,13,20,22] In general, if there is imaging evidence of ventral compression, a ventral procedure should be considered. If the deformity is fixed (joint ankylosis), a dorsal osteotomy may be used to correct the deformity. If the deformity is fixed but there is no ankylosis, a ventral decompression with fusion may be used to correct the kyphosis. Last, if the deformity is nonfixed (flexible), it may be corrected posturally or with traction then fused in the desired position dorsally.

Traction

Traction is often used as an initial tool in the evaluation of the surgical approach to cervical kyphosis. With traction, the deformity is corrected via the traction applied. Then dorsal fixation may be used to hold the correction and prevent further kyphotic progression. Typically, the patient is taken to the operating room with the traction applied, and the patient is fused in the corrected position. In the authors' experience, if the traction is to be useful in reducing a kyphotic deformity, the duration of traction required is generally 3 to 5 days. If no reduction is observed after 5 days, success with further traction is unlikely. Muscle relaxants may also be used to aid in the reduction process.

Ventral Strategies

The ventral approach to the cervical spine is a familiar approach with minimal morbidity. It allows decompression

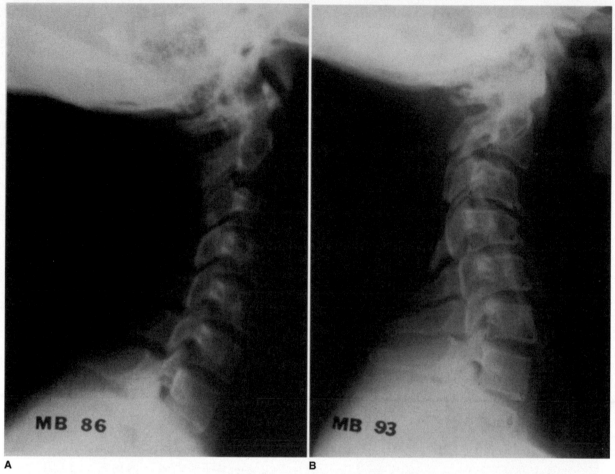

Figure 63.1 (**A**) Preoperative lateral cervical radiograph of a patient with progressive myelopathy. (**B**) Lateral cervical radiograph of the same patient 7 years after C1-4 laminectomy. The patient had mechanical neck pain and progressive myelopathy.

of ventral pathologic conditions, as well as reconstruction (deformity correction) with strut grafting and instrumentation. This strategy provides optimal ventral decompression of the spinal cord and permits the attainment of a lordotic cervical posture. In addition, it provides a superior surgical leverage for deformity correction than dorsal surgery.

A ventral strategy uses both posture and biomechanical principles to correct cervical deformity. Placing the head on a doughnut and/or towel to initially place the neck in a neutral position or in slight extension allows adequate exposure for the approach but does not compromise the spinal cord through extension over ventral conditions. After the decompression has been performed, removing the towels and/or doughnut extends the cervical spine (Figure 63.3).

Distraction posts should be placed in a convergent manner (Figure 63.4A). Distraction against posts placed in this manner provides cervical extension and furthers lordosis (Figure 63.4B).

The authors believe that long-segment corpectomies (e.g., C4, C5, and C6 corpectomies) should be avoided. Leaving an intermediate vertebral body (C5 in the aforementioned example) allows adequate decompression (Figure 63.5) and provides additional intermediate fixation points for deformity correction and increased security of fixation (Figure 63.6). An adequate or safe intermediate

point of fixation is present if a cerebrospinal fluid signal dorsal to such a vertebral body exists on a T_2-weighted magnetic resonance image (Figure 63.7).

There are many advantages for using multiple points of fixation with the ventral construct. When the intermediate screws are tightened, the spine is brought to the contoured construct (see Figure 63.6). This strategy not only achieves lordosis, but also provides three- or four-point bending forces to maintain the sagittal alignment following surgery. It also minimizes the chance of terminal screw-bone interface degradation.

When using this ventral strategy, the surgeon should consider using a dynamic ventral implant. These implants permit controlled deformation in the axial plane (axial subsidence), yet prevent deformation in the sagittal plane (kyphosis).[4] The controlled subsidence allows the bone graft(s) to absorb most of the axial forces, which, according to Wolff's law, should encourage bone healing.[4] The construct also off-loads stresses at the screw-bone interface. This further contributes to a diminished incidence of structural failure.

Steinmetz et al.[24] have shown that the aforementioned strategy is effective in the management of cervical kyphosis. Lordosis was achieved in all but one patient in their series. The average preoperative sagittal angle was 15 degrees of kyphosis. They were able to obtain 20 degrees of lordosis, which lead to an average postoperative sagittal angle of 5 degrees of lordosis. This angle was maintained during the follow-up period, with an average change in the sagittal angle of 2 degrees.

Dorsal Strategies

A dorsal strategy used alone for the correction of cervical deformity is not common. If the kyphosis is flexible

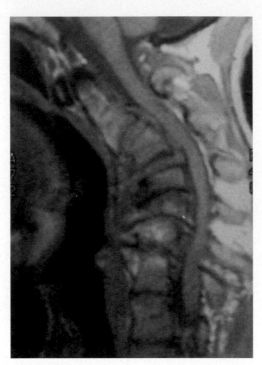

Figure 63.2 Lateral T_1-weighted cervical magnetic resonance image. The study demonstrates cervical kyphosis and ventral spinal cord compression at multiple sites.

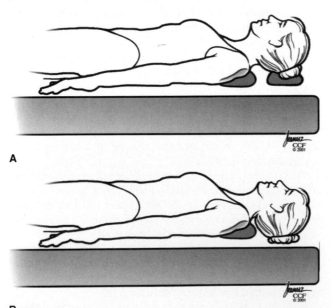

Figure 63.3 (**A**) Before decompression, the head is placed on a doughnut to keep it neutral or in slight extension. (**B**) After decompression has been performed, the doughnut is removed, and the neck is placed in extension.

(i.e., reducible with traction) and decompression is not required, a dorsal approach may be warranted. If decompression is required, it should be performed ventrally, and consideration should be given to a combined ventral and dorsal procedure.

Traction should be used to reduce the deformity, and the traction should be continued in the operating room. The patient's head is placed into a Mayfield-type head holder to maintain the reduction. A lateral preoperative cervical radiograph should be taken to ensure adequate deformity correction. A standard dorsal subperiosteal approach to the cervical spine is used. Interspinous wiring, lateral mass fixation, and pedicle screw fixation may be used to maintain the deformity correction (Figure 63.8). If laminectomy is performed, interspinous wiring may not be used because the spinous processes are removed.

Abumi et al.[1] have used cervical pedicle screws for the dorsal correction of cervical deformity. Kotani et al.[18] have shown that the cervical pedicle screw system is equivalent to combined ventral plate and dorsal wiring. Reports have shown that the lateral mass may not be an optimal stabilizing anchor for internal fixation in some patients.[3,11,13] Ventral release and fusion may be required for optimal deformity correction when lateral mass plate fixation is used.[1] Cervical pedicle screws may be biomechanically

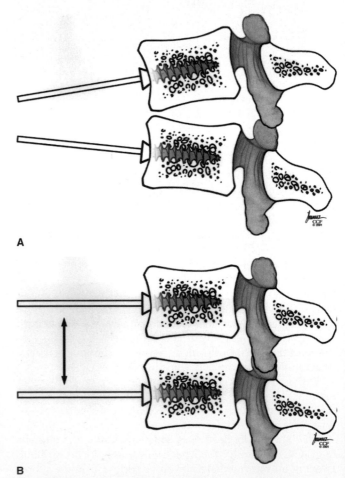

Figure 63.4 (**A**) The distraction posts are placed in a convergent manner. (**B**) Distraction against the posts (*arrow*) provides cervical extension and further lordosis.

superior as the stand-alone fixation construct. Abumi et al.,[1] using only cervical pedicle screws, were able to correct kyphosis from 28.4 to 5.1 degrees of kyphosis, with all patients achieving a solid arthrodesis. It should be emphasized that lordosis was not achieved with the dorsal-alone procedure, the kyphosis was only reduced.

Combined Ventral and Dorsal Approach

When the deformity is fixed and the dorsal elements are ankylosed, a combined ventral and dorsal approach may be required (Figure 63.9). In addition, if the deformity is at the cervicothoracic junction or crosses it, consideration should be given to a combined approach. In general, this approach permits ventral lengthening and dorsal shortening. It permits ventral decompression and release, with or without instrumentation, combined with dorsal instrumentation (Figure 63.10). The addition of the dorsal construct uses a long moment arm strategy to aid in deformity prevention.[4]

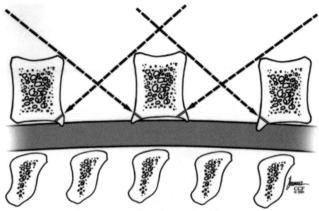

Figure 63.5 Leaving an intermediate body (one in which there is a cerebrospinal fluid signal dorsal to the body on a lateral T$_2$-weighted magnetic resonance image) permits complete spinal cord decompression, yet also provides a point for intermediate construct fixation. The arrows indicate the surgeon's field of view, demonstrating that adequate decompression may be performed while leaving an intermediate vertebral body.

When a combined approach is being planned, the goals of the operation should be clearly defined. This will aid the surgeon in choosing the order of the procedure. If ventral compression exists and the dorsal procedure is solely for supplemental instrumentation, the ventral decompression (discectomy or corpectomy) and grafting should be performed in the usual fashion first. Often, a ventral implant is also used. The patient may then be placed in a prone position and the dorsal procedure performed. Unless there is concomitant dorsal compression, laminectomy is often not performed, and a dorsal implant is placed (most often lateral mass plates). Interspinous wiring may also be used, but lateral mass fixation has been shown to provide greater rigidity than wire fixation alone.[11]

In cases involving conditions such as ankylosing spondylitis, a more extensive (e.g., 540-degree) procedure may be warranted. A dorsal osteotomy may be performed first. Simmons[23] has advocated performing this under local anesthesia in the seated position at the C7-T1 level. After the osteotomy has been performed, the patient may then be placed in the supine position and a ventral corpectomy performed to allow decompression and release for the correction of the deformity. Iliac crest bone grafting and ventral instrumentation may then be performed. Because of the large moment arm above and below the level of the fusion, dorsal instrumentation should also be used, thus aiding in the prevention of further deformity. Obviously, the order in which the stages of the operation are performed depends on the individual patient's situation.

If the deformity is to be corrected dorsally (e.g., using pedicle screws), the ventral decompression and release should be performed first without grafting or instrumentation. After the decompression, the patient is placed in a prone position to expose the dorsal cervical spine. An assistant may then adjust the head holder to achieve maximal lordosis. Because ventral decompression has been performed before the reduction, reduction should be safe. The dorsal construct (lateral mass fixation, pedicle screw construct) may then be placed to secure the deformity correction. Iliac crest may then be harvested to provide morselized bone for the dorsal fusion. The patient is again positioned supine, a ventral strut graft is placed, and a ventral implant secured. Using a combined ventral and dorsal approach with cervical pedicle screw instrumentation,

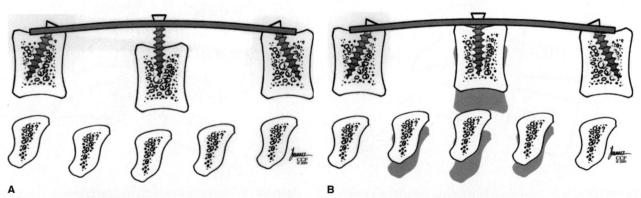

A   **B**

Figure 63.6 (A) After the construct has been secured at its rostral and caudal ends, the intermediate screws are placed. (B) When the intermediate screw is tightened, the spine is brought to the contoured implant. This allows the attainment of further lordosis.

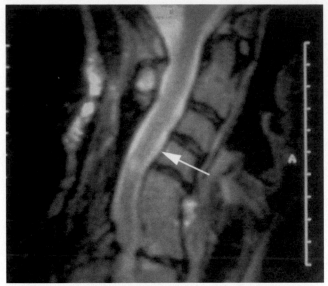

Figure 63.7 Lateral T$_2$-weighted magnetic resonance image. There is a cerebrospinal fluid signal dorsal to the C4 vertebral body *(arrow)*. This body will not be resected during the decompression. It will be left in place and used as an intermediate point of fixation.

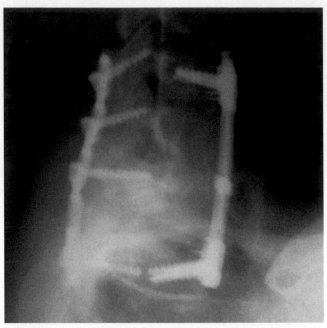

Figure 63.9 Lateral postoperative radiograph following a combined ventral and dorsal cervical deformity procedure. Instrumentation has been placed both ventrally and dorsally.

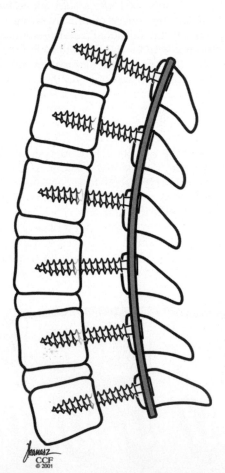

Figure 63.8 Lateral mass plate fixation has been performed to maintain the deformity correction, following a dorsal alone strategy.

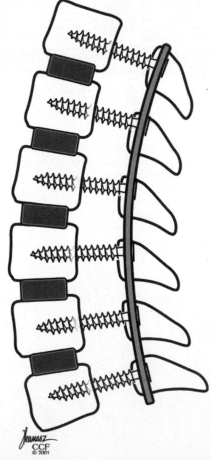

Figure 63.10 Ventral release with interbody strut grafting has been performed. Supplemental dorsal instrumentation has been added to maintain the correction and prevent deformity progression.

Abumi *et al.*[1] were able to improve an average preoperative kyphosis of 30.8 to 0.5 degrees at the final follow-up.

Osteotomy

Ankylosing spondylitis may produce an extreme fixed flexion deformity at the cervicothoracic junction. This extreme deformity may place the chin close to the chest, which may interfere with eating and respiration. Some have advocated treating this deformity by extension osteotomy at the cervicothoracic junction.[23,25] Essentially, the procedure, as initially described, is performed with the patient under local anesthesia, awake, and in a sitting position. After osteotomy, the deformity is corrected externally either by an articulated plaster jacket incorporating the head and neck[25] or by manual extension (intraoperatively). Stability is maintained by a halo jacket.[23]

McMaster[21] reported 15 patients with ankylosing spondylitis and flexion deformity who were treated by dorsal extension osteotomy and external fixation by halo (12 patients) or by internal fixation (3 patients). In brief, in these procedures, the cervicothoracic spine is exposed dorsally from C6 to T1. A wide laminectomy is performed at C7, with partial laminectomies of C6 and T1. The spinous process of C6 is also removed. The ankylosed C7-T1 facet joints are removed bilaterally to expose the C8 nerve roots beyond their intervertebral foramina (Figure 63.11). A portion of the C6 and T1 pedicles is removed to avoid impingement of the C8 nerve roots during the deformity

correction. Under electrophysiologic monitoring, the head is extended to correct the deformity (Figure 63.12). The correction is maintained in a halo vest or with internal fixation. The average correction obtained was 54 degrees. There were three neurologic complications. Four patients had subluxation of C7 on T1.

Recently, Duff *et al.*[10] reported one patient in whom a fixed flexion deformity was corrected using a single-stage two-level midcervical osteotomy. Internal fixation was used in this patient's case. Using the reported technique, the authors were able to achieve a correction of approximately 90 degrees of lordosis.

Today, many surgeons perform a ventral and dorsal approach in one surgery. Safety and control of deformity correction are the stated advantages of this combined approach.

Complications

Ventral Approach

The complications of the ventral approach are well known and are familiar to all spine surgeons. They include vocal cord palsy, dysphagia, tracheal or esophageal injury, graft failure (displacement), hardware failure (fracture), and wound complications (infection, hematoma). The incidence of these complications is probably greater in patients who have undergone deformity correction procedures, because most of these patients have had prior ventral cervical surgery, and the operation involves multiple spinal segments.

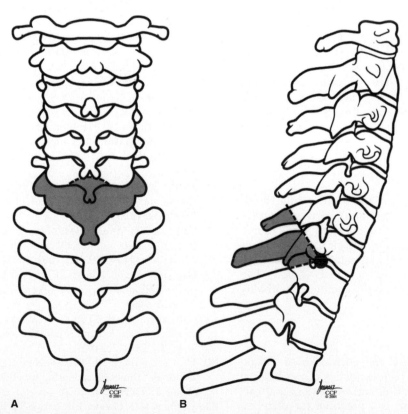

A   B

Figure 63.11 (**A**) Dorsal view of the bone removed (*shaded portion*) to perform the wedge osteotomy. (**B**) Lateral view of bone removed (*shaded portion*) to perform the wedge osteotomy.

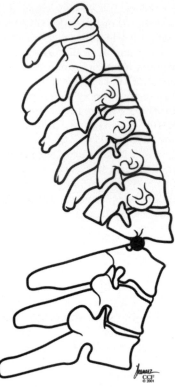

Figure 63.12 Dorsal wedge osteotomy has been performed. The spine is extended along the dorsal vertebral body and posterior longitudinal ligament.

Using biomechanically sound principles (e.g., using a dynamic implant when performing a ventral kyphosis correction) may lessen the hardware complications. A dynamic implant off-loads stresses at the screw-bone interface, which may be excessive in a large deformity correction case.[4] This lowering of stresses should contribute to a decreased incidence of hardware failure. In addition, using multiple points of intermediate fixation not only facilitates deformity correction, but also provides three- or four-point bending forces that help maintain sagittal alignment.

Dorsal Approach

Complications from the dorsal approach include hardware failure or fracture, nonunion, vertebral artery injury, and wound complications (infection, hematoma). The morbidity from the dorsal approach is greater compared with a ventral approach, and patients have considerably greater pain in the postoperative period. The combined approach obviously has the combined morbidity of both procedures.

Osteotomy

Dorsal wedge osteotomy for the correction of flexion deformity has a potentially high incidence of morbidity.[21] Complications include infection and respiratory and cardiovascular problems. There is a potential for vertebral artery injury during the osteotomy or neurologic injury during deformity correction. The resultant neurologic injury may range from minor nerve-root irritation to spinal cord compression and quadriplegia. After deformity correction, there is risk of subluxation of C7 on T1, with resultant bony nonunion.

Summary

Deformity of the cervical spine may follow prior surgery or may be a part of the aging process. It may lead to mechanical neck pain and progressive neurologic deficit. If the deformity is symptomatic, it should be corrected. Emphasis should also be placed on deformity prevention, such as restoring lordosis after a ventral decompressive procedure or using dorsal fusion and/or instrumentation after an extensive dorsal decompression. The authors believe a ventral approach is optimal in most cases. It permits decompression and provides a better surgical leverage for deformity correction than dorsal surgery does, while providing solid fixation points if intermediate fixation points are used. In cases in which the patient has a fixed deformity (ankylosing spondylitis), a combined approach may be used. Correction of cervical deformity is rewarding—most patients experience relief from their mechanical symptoms and an improvement in neurologic function.

REFERENCES

1. Abumi K, Shono Y, Taneichi H: Correction of cervical kyphosis using pedicle screw fixation systems. *Spine* 24:2389-2396, 1999.
2. Albert TJ, Vacarro A: Postlaminectomy kyphosis. *Spine* 23:2738-2745, 1998.
3. Anderson PA, Henley MB, Grady MS *et al:* Posterior cervical arthrodesis with AO reconstruction plates and bone graft. *Spine* 16:S72-S79, 1991.
4. Benzel EC: *Biomechanics of spine stabilization.* American Association of Neurological Surgeons, Rolling Meadows, IL, 2001.
5. Breig A, El-Nadi AF: Biomechanics of the cervical spinal cord: Relief of contact pressure on and overstretching of the spinal cord. *Acta Radiol Diagn* 4:602-624, 1964.
6. Buttler JC, Whitecloud TS III: Postlaminectomy kyphosis: Causes and surgical management. *Clin Orthop North Am* 23:505-511, 1992.
7. Callahan RA, Johnson RM, Margolis RN: Cervical facet fusion for control of instability following laminectomy. *J Bone Joint Surg* 59A:991-1002, 1977.
8. Caspar W, Pitzen T: Anterior cervical fusion and trapezoidal plate stabilization for re-do surgery. *Surg Neurol* 52: 345-352, 1999.
9. Cattrell HS, Clark GJ Jr: Cervical kyphosis and instability following multiple laminectomies in children. *J Bone Joint Surg* 49A:713-720, 1967.
10. Duff SE, Grundy PL, Gill SS: New approach to cervical flexion deformity in ankylosing spondylitis. *J Neurosurg (Spine 2)* 93:283-286, 2000.
11. Fehlings MG, Cooper PR, Errico TJ: Posterior plates in the management of cervical instability: Long-term results in 44 patients. *J Neurosurg* 81:341-349, 1994.

12. Geisler FH, Caspar W, Pitzen T, *et al:* Reoperation in patients after anterior cervical plate stabilization in degenerative disease. *Spine* 23:911-920, 1998.

13. Heller JG, Silcox DH III, Sutterlin CE III: Complications of posterior cervical plating. *Spine* 20:2442-2448, 1995.

14. Herman JM, Sonntag VK: Cervical corpectomy and plate fixation for post-laminectomy kyphosis. *J Neurosurg* 80: 963-970, 1994.

15. Johnston FG, Crockard HA: One stage internal fixation and anterior fusion in complex cervical spinal disorders. *J Neurosurg* 82:234-238, 1995.

16. Kaptain GJ, Simmons N, Replogle RE, *et al:* Incidence and outcome of kyphotic deformity following laminectomy for cervical spondylotic myelopathy. *J Neurosurg (Spine 2)* 93:199-204, 2000.

17. Katsuura A, Hukuda S, Imanaka T, *et al:* Anterior cervical plate used in degenerative disease can maintain cervical lordosis. *J Spine Disord* 9:470-476, 1996.

18. Kotani Y, Cunningham BW, Abumi K, McAfee PC: Biomechanical analysis of cervical stabilization systems: An assessment of transpedicular screw fixation in the cervical spine. *Spine* 19:2529-2539, 1994.

19. Masini M, Maranhao V: Experimental determination of the effect of progressive sharp-angle spinal deformity on the spinal cord. *Euro Spine J* 6:89-92, 1997.

20. McAfee PC, Bohlman HH, Ducker TB: One stage anterior cervical decompression and posterior stabilization. A study of one hundred patients with a minimum of two years of follow-up. *J Bone Joint Surg* 77A:1791-1800, 1995.

21. McMaster MJ: Osteotomy of the cervical spine in ankylosing spondylitis. *J Bone Joint Surg* 79B:197-203, 1997.

22. Savini R, Parisini P, Cervellati S: The surgical treatment of late instability of flexion-rotation injuries in the lower cervical spine. *Spine* 12:178-182, 1987.

23. Simmons EH: The surgical correction of flexion deformity of the cervical spine in ankylosing spondylitis. *Clin Orthop* 86:132-143, 1972.

24. Steinmetz MP, Kager C, Benzel EC: Ventral correction of postsurgical cervical kyphosis. *J Neurosurg (Spine 2)* 98:1-7, 2003.

25. Urist MR: Osteotomy of the cervical spine: Report of a case of ankylosing spondylitis. *J Bone Joint Surg* 40A:833-843, 1958.

26. Zdeblick TA, Bohlman HH: Cervical kyphosis and myelopathy: Treatment by anterior corpectomy and strut-grafting. *J Bone Joint Surg* 71A:170-182, 1989.

CHAPTER 64

Thoracic and Lumbar Deformities

Mark H. Bilsky, Oheneba Boachie-Adjei, Christopher B. Shields, and Nevan G. Baldwin

Techniques for the treatment of thoracic and lumbar spine deformities continue to evolve. The deformities addressed in this chapter are scoliosis, kyphosis, and spondylolisthesis. The segmental instrumentation systems currently used to correct these deformities lead to complications that are different from those observed historically with other nonsegmental instrumentation systems. With the use of segmental instrumentation systems, surgeons developed unique strategies and improved techniques to avoid these complications.

The following are necessary for thoracic and lumbar deformity correction: familiarity with their clinical presentation and symptomatology; a detailed differential diagnosis of the types of deformities; a precise radiographic assessment; and a thorough knowledge of the goals of treatment, whether treatment is nonoperative or surgical. This chapter addresses these issues as they affect the overall success of treatment.

Scoliosis

Scoliosis is a three-dimensional deformity that affects the spine in the coronal, sagittal, and axial planes. The primary goal of corrective surgery is to produce a balanced spine in all three planes. To achieve this goal, the surgeon must understand the cause of the curve and recognize the various implications of curve patterns. Scoliosis may begin before skeletal maturity (i.e., idiopathic or neurogenic) or it may arise after skeletal maturity as a result of degenerative changes or trauma.[152]

Idiopathic Scoliosis

Adolescent idiopathic scoliosis is the most common type of scoliosis, with a prevalence of 2% to 4% for curves of 10 degrees or greater.[34] For lateral curves greater than 20 degrees, the female/male ratio is 5.4:1.[79] Most children with curvature of the spine are referred to scoliosis clinics through school screening programs.[34,104] Adolescents with a suspected 10-degree curve on physical examination should have 36-inch standing posteroanterior (PA) and lateral radiographs taken. These should be repeated at 6-month intervals, and for those with curves greater than 20 degrees, follow-up should be at 4-month intervals. Curves greater than 20 degrees that demonstrate progression of greater than 5 degrees in any 4- to 6-month interval should be treated with an external orthosis, if the patient has at least a full year of growth remaining. Skeletally immature patients with 30- to 40-degree curves on first examination should be braced immediately. Skeletally immature patients with curves that are greater than 40 degrees despite adequate bracing may be candidates for surgical correction. Scoliosis patients who also have a significant thoracic lordosis that results in a clinically significant decreased anteroposterior (AP) chest diameter may also be candidates for corrective surgery because of the risk of pulmonary compromise.[50] Treatment parameters are based on criteria for adolescent scoliosis, including the degree of curvature, chronologic age, and the Risser sign (percentage of ossification of the iliac crest).

Neuromuscular Scoliosis

Rarely, scoliosis may be caused by a number of central nervous system disorders such as syringomyelia, diastematomyelia, tethered cord, or an intramedullary spinal cord tumor. Although neurogenic scoliosis accounts for less than 1% of cases seen in a general-screening scoliosis clinic, it is often the reason for referral to a neurosurgeon. Neurogenic scoliosis may be characterized by the following: (1) a rapid rate of curve progression unrelated to a growth spurt; (2) young age at presentation (younger than 11 years)[99]; (3) severe pain associated with the curve (particularly nocturnal); and (4) an abnormal neurologic examination, or dermatologic manifestations (i.e., skin dimpling) of an underlying disease (e.g., lipomyelomeningocele). Atypical curve patterns, such as a left convex thoracic or cervicothoracic curve, are highly suggestive of an underlying neurogenic cause. In patients who meet these criteria, a specific cause for the scoliosis may be identified with a cervical, thoracic, and lumbar screening magnetic resonance imaging (MRI) in up to 50% of patients.[2,59] This MRI is the best screening modality presently available to identify a neurogenic cause of scoliosis. In severe cases, the cause may be obscured because the curvature may take the spinal cord lesion out of the plane of the magnetic coil. If an MRI fails to image a specific defect in a patient in whom there is a high suspicion of an underlying neurogenic cause for the scoliosis, a complete myelogram should be performed, followed by a computed tomography (CT) scan.

In certain cases of neurogenic scoliosis, a significant improvement of the curve may be observed after treatment of the underlying disorder. However, in some instances, the curve may have developed significant structural characteristics that continue to progress despite successful neurosurgical intervention. Subsequent spinal instrumentation and fusion may be required. Conversely, failure to recognize a neurogenic cause before surgical correction may result in a significant neurologic deficit at the time of surgery. A high index of suspicion and a thorough workup and correction of the underlying neurogenic process is essential before operative correction of the scoliosis.

Adult Degenerative Scoliosis

Adult scoliosis is defined as scoliosis that occurs in patients older than 20 years of age.[141,152,153] Weinstein and

Ponseti,[155] in a 40-year follow-up of patients who had untreated idiopathic scoliosis from childhood, showed that thoracic curves 50 degrees or greater were likely to progress by 1 to 2 degrees/year in adulthood, as were lumbar curves and the lumbar portion of double major curves (Figure 64.1). Degenerative spine disease may result in the de novo creation of scoliosis in patients older than 65 years. Asymmetric degeneration of discs, osteoporosis, and compression fractures of vertebral bodies have all been implicated as the cause of adult degenerative scoliosis.[72]

Indications for operation in adult scoliosis include pain, progressive deformity, cardiopulmonary symptoms, and decompensation. Pain is the most common complaint in adult scoliosis.[92,160] There are several causes of the pain associated with the curve. Pain localized to the convexity of the curve is often the result of muscle spasm. Pain on the concave side of the curve may be localized to the back and nerve root. This may be the result of disc rupture or facet hypertrophy narrowing the lateral recess, resulting in the compression of the adjacent nerve root. Other potential causes for back pain include spinal stenosis, spinal tumors, sacroiliitis, arthritic hip disease, renal stones, and abdominal aortic aneurysms. A thorough investigation should be undertaken before attributing the pain to scoliosis. Surgery may be considered in patients with progressive scoliosis or decompensation confirmed by sequential imaging studies. In addition, patients with thoracic scoliotic curves greater than 80 degrees may be candidates for surgery, to prevent further pulmonary compromise or the development of cor pulmonale. Cosmesis is commonly the major complaint of these patients but is only a relative indication for corrective surgery, particularly in adults.

A number of factors must be considered before the correction of scoliosis. The scoliotic deformity is often coupled with thoracic hypokyphosis or relative lordosis. The primary goal of surgery is to correct the coronal, sagittal, and rotational balance of the patient. Scoliosis was initially defined as a lateral deviation in the normally straight vertical axis of the spine, and early attempts at surgical correction considered only the coronal plane deformity. Since the mid-1980s, the three-dimensional nature of the condition has been appreciated, and greater attention is now being paid to correcting and maintaining the normal sagittal contours, as well as correcting the rotational imbalance.

Dorsal Scoliosis Deformity Correction

Dorsal Spinal Instrumentation

Initially, surgical correction of scoliosis consisted of bone grafts, with postoperative placement in a Risser cast. This

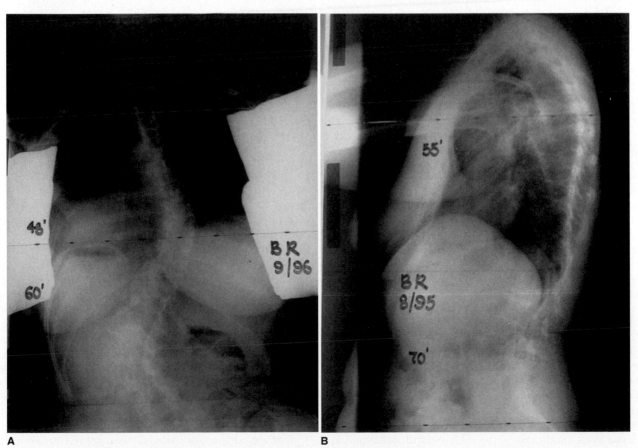

A   **B**

Figure 64.1 A 56-year-old woman with a history of untreated idiopathic scoliosis who developed progressive lumbar scoliosis, lower back pain, and limited function. Patient was treated with a one-stage anterior and posterior spinal fusion with segmental instrumentation. Anteroposterior (AP) (**A**) and lateral (**B**) radiographs showing 48-degree right thoracic 60-degree left lumbar scoliosis.

Continued

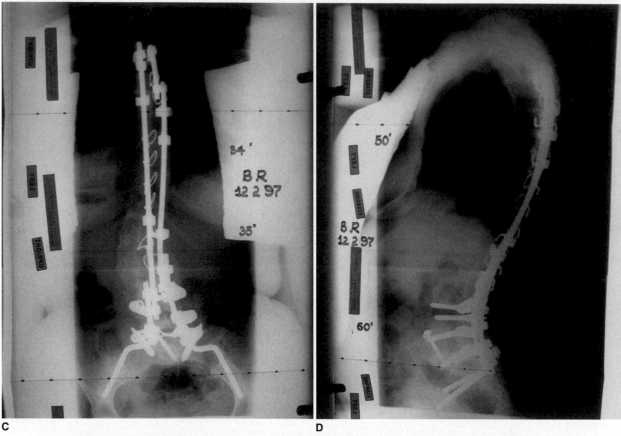

C   D

Figure 64.1 *cont'd* (**C**) Postoperative AP radiograph showing the segmental instrumentation
multi-hook, screw system (Isola) with Galveston fixation. Note ventral interbody fusion.
(**D**) Postoperative lateral radiograph showing the restoration of sagittal alignment with 50
degrees of thoracic kyphosis and 60 degrees of lordosis. Patient is 4 years postoperative and has
achieved solid arthrodesis and return to functional activities. (*Copyright Memorial Sloan-Kettering
Cancer Center.*)

procedure often failed to provide rigid fixation and
resulted in an unacceptably high pseudarthrosis rate. The
development of the Harrington distraction system proved
to be a major advance. It provided rigid internal fixation,
as well as significant correction of the coronal plane deformities, while the fusion ossified.[67-69] Thus the pseudarthrosis rate was reduced from approximately 50% with the
previous method to less than 5% with Harrington instrumentation.[68,115] Postoperative external orthosis was still
required to maintain adequate correction, but early
ambulation was possible with the addition of the internal
instrumentation.

Long instrumentation constructs often mandated that
the fusion be extended to the lower lumbar spine. This
resulted in an occasional junctional thoracolumbar kyphosis or loss of lumbar lordosis. Because Harrington instrumentation provided only distraction corrective forces to
the scoliotic spine, the result often was a thoracic or lumbar flat back syndrome.[27,89,114] This clinical syndrome is
characterized by low back pain, forward inclination of the
trunk, and the inability to stand erect. Furthermore, pure
distraction instrumentation did not provide an improvement of the thoracic sagittal contour and often increased
the degree of thoracic kyphosis.

The development of segmental instrumentation systems, and the use of these systems with autogenous fusion,
increased the surgeon's ability to achieve three-dimensional balance with improved correction in both the coronal and the sagittal planes. Luque rods, combined with
sublaminar wiring, achieved a marginally better overall
correction than did Harrington distraction rods and provided more stable fixation. However, the associated neurologic injuries from the placement and removal of the
wires were approximately four times greater than those
observed with Harrington instrumentation, with some
series experiencing up to a 10% incidence of associated
injuries.[73,145,157] The Wisconsin wiring technique, used in
conjunction with Luque rods, requires the use of the spinous processes for segmental fixation, obviating the need
for the passage of sublaminar wires.[39,80] Both of these systems require postoperative external orthosis to maintain
correction.

The introduction of Cotrel-Dubousset (C-D) instrumentation represented a significant advance in the surgeon's
ability to correct the three-dimensional deformity of scoliosis. When C-D instrumentation is used with cross-fixation,
an extremely rigid, stable construct can be achieved. This
may obviate the need for postoperative bracing. Whereas

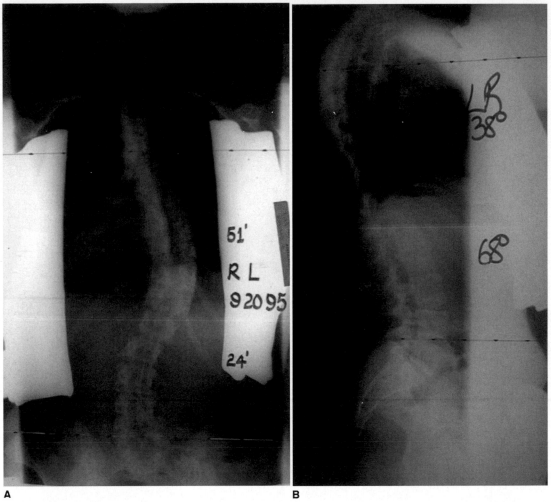

Figure 64.2 A 35-year-old female with progressive right thoracic scoliosis who was treated with posterior spinal fusion with segmental instrumentation. Preoperative anteroposterior (AP) (**A**) and lateral (**B**) radiographs showing severity of scoliosis.

Continued

Harrington instrumentation relies on distraction to provide transverse and axial forces to effect correction, C-D instrumentation adds a 90-degree derotation moment to the convex curve, which translates the coronal plane thoracic scoliosis into the desired kyphosis. This derotation force also translates the lumbar scoliotic curve into a relative lordosis. Therefore C-D instrumentation specifically addressed the rotational and sagittal deformity components of scoliosis for the first time.[30] Although the C-D system represents a leap in spinal deformity correction, a major problem with the original C-D instrumentation is its high profile. The surface area available for bone graft is also reduced, which presents a problem for patients with little soft tissue coverage.

From the concepts developed in the C-D system, a plethora of conceptually similar systems has been developed. These low-profile systems provide similar degrees of correction and fusion rates as were observed using the C-D instrumentation. Over the last 5 years, the use of sublaminar and pedicle hooks has been augmented or replaced with pedicle screw fixation. For added strength, sublaminar wires can also be used (Figure 64.2). The low-profile systems have resulted in a lower incidence of soft tissue complications and need for hardware removal.

Selection of Fusion Levels

Evaluation of curve patterns and spinal flexibility is essential for planning the correction of idiopathic scoliosis. Preoperative radiographs should include 36-inch PA and lateral films that image the spine from C7 to the sacrum. Lateral bending radiographs are necessary, not only to assess the degree of curve flexibility, but also to identify the primary structural curve. With this information, the surgeon may predict the extent of correction achievable at the time of surgery. Supine maximal traction radiographs may indicate the extent of axial correction that may be achieved. These supine maximal traction radiographs are more useful in identifying the flexibility of double major structural scoliotic curves than are lateral bending radiographs. The flexibility of an associated kyphotic deformity can be assessed by hyperextension films. Therefore a complete preoperative radiographic analysis is necessary for planning the correction of a rigid, complex deformity. Extensive preoperative imaging studies under stress are also necessary to enable the surgeon to select hook sites and to determine patterns that will lead to a balanced, corrected spine with minimal chance of decompensation.

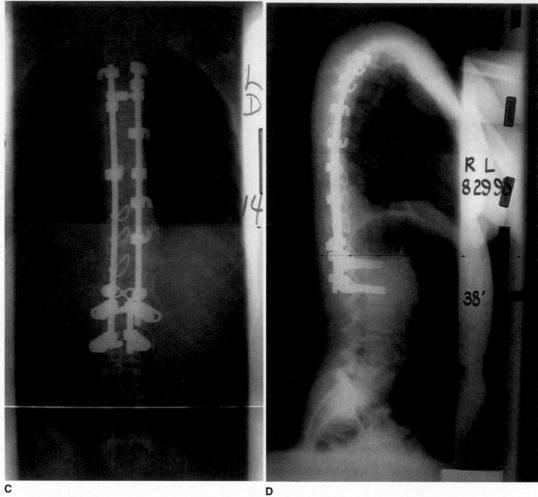

C   D

Figure 64.2 *cont'd* Postoperative AP (**C**) and lateral (**D**) radiographs showing excellent balance and coronal and sagittal plane alignments. (*Copyright Memorial Sloan-Kettering Cancer Center.*)

The correction of scoliosis requires a system of choosing fusion levels that ensure that fundamental principles of deformity correction are applied. Curve patterns were originally described by King *et al.*[87] for idiopathic thoracic scoliosis treated with Harrington instrumentation. Glassman[56] uses a slight modification of the King classification, in which he also considers the degree of compensatory curve flexibility (Table 64.1). Glassman's modification of the King classification is more applicable to segmental instrumentation correction. Types I, II, and V curves have both primary and compensatory curves, whereas Types III and IV curves consist of primary curves only. The compensatory curves may remain flexible or become rigid and fixed over time.

In Glassman's classification scheme, Types I and II are divided into two subgroups, A and B, based on the flexibility of the compensatory curve. Type A compensatory curves are flexible. Type B curves represent double major curves in which the normally flexible compensatory curve has become structurally rigid. In general, Type A curves require correction and fusion of only the primary curve. In Type B curves, both the primary and compensatory curves require correction and fixation.

The endpoints of the fusion are chosen as the Cobb end vertebrae, the most level disc space at the rostral and caudal ends of the curvature. Harrington's stable zone is defined as the vertebrae contained within the area created by two lines constructed perpendicular to the lumbosacral facets.[67] Both rostral and caudal endpoints should be within the stable zone on traction films to produce a spine that is well balanced over the pelvis. A further refinement of Harrington's stable zone is the central sacral line, which is defined by the highest vertebra bisected by a line drawn perpendicular to the horizontal line that connects the top of the iliac crests.[39] The caudal end vertebra is extended to ensure that the last disc space is horizontal on bending films.[56]

Preservation of motion segments in the caudal lumbar spine is critical to prevent the late development of accelerated degenerative changes and low back pain. Cochran *et al.*[25] found that 39% of patients fused to L3 subsequently developed low back pain and that extending the fusion level to L4 or L5 increased the percentage of patients with pain to 62% and 82%, respectively. In this series, the Harrington instrumentation was used with noncontoured rods. However, these results are probably applicable to all types of segmental spinal instrumentation. Ventral spinal

TABLE 64.1

Modified King Classification of Curves

Curve Type	Primary Curve	Compensatory Curve
IA	Left lumbar	Right thoracic curve: corrects more than 50% and to <40 degrees on traction or bending
IB	Left lumbar	Right thoracic curve: rigid
IIA	Right thoracic	Left lumbar curve: corrects more than 50% and to <30 degrees on traction or bending
IIB	Right thoracic	Left lumbar curve: rigid
III	Right thoracic	None
IV	Long right thoracolumbar curve (includes L4)	None
VA	Right thoracic	High left thoracic curve: corrects more than 50% and to <40 degrees on traction and bending
VB	Right thoracic	High left thoracic curve: rigid

(From Glassman SD: Hook pattern selection in the treatment of spinal deformity. In Holt RT [ed]: *Spine: State-of-the-Art Reviews,* vol 6, no 2. Hanley & Belfus, Philadelphia, 1992, p 331, with permission.)

instrumentation and fusion may be used to preclude the use of instrumentation to the lowest levels of the lumbar spine, thus saving important distal lumbar motion segments. Use of a ventral approach may allow for fusion to a level above the caudal Cobb end vertebrae with good results.

The fusion should never end at the apex of either the primary or the compensatory curve in either the sagittal or the coronal planes, because this may result in subsequent loss of curve correction (decompensation). The apical vertebra in the coronal plane deformity is recognized as the vertebra translated the farthest from the midline, and it is the vertebra that is maximally rotated. This apex is the site of maximal vertebral body deformity and curve rigidity, thus making it the most difficult area in which to achieve correction.

A marked decrease of thoracic kyphosis often occurs in conjunction with coronal plane translation. Correction of this kyphosis must also be considered. Thoracolumbar junctional kyphosis is also commonly observed with scoliotic deformity. The fusion should not end at the apex of this junctional kyphosis, although it appears that good correction of the coronal plane curvature can be achieved at this level. Ending the fusion at this level may lead to late decompensation with progressive kyphosis. To achieve a balanced spinal column, the surgeon must meticulously evaluate these features of scoliosis in all three dimensions when considering hook placement.

Operative Technique for Correction of a Type III Curve

For operative correction of a type III curve, the patient is placed prone on a Wilson or four-poster frame and a midline incision is made without regard to the scoliotic deformity. The lumbodorsal fascia is then opened over the spinous processes, and the muscle and ligamentous attachments are dissected off the lamina and transverse processes, using the cautery and subperiosteal dissection. Intraoperative radiograms are taken to confirm the levels to be included in the subsequent instrumentation. The interspinous ligaments are cut with a 10-Fr blade and resected with a Leksell rongeur between each spinous process. Facetectomies are then performed with a small osteotome, and each facet is decorticated with a curette

and packed with Gelfoam. The hook pattern, which was established preoperatively, is then placed.

A prototypical hook pattern is best illustrated when used to correct a Type III thoracic scoliosis (Figure 64.3). First, two upgoing hooks on the dorsal side of the curve apex are applied in distraction on the concave side of the curve. Next, a 90-degree rod derotation maneuver toward the convexity, combined with simultaneous distraction of the hooks, is performed. A second rod is then placed on the convex side in compression. The hook pattern on the convex side consists of a superior claw (a combination of upgoing and downgoing hooks at the rostral end vertebra), an upgoing apical pedicle hook, and an upgoing sublaminar hook at the caudal end vertebra. Sequential compression is applied to this rod, followed by cross-fixation at each end of the construct. Multiple corrective forces are applied with this procedure, including derotation and distraction, which result in coronal scoliosis correction, sagittal kyphosis restoration, and rib hump deformity reduction (Figure 64.4). Modification of these basic patterns is often necessary to address the structural rigidity of the compensatory curve.

After curve correction with instrumentation, a bone graft is harvested from the iliac crest. The dorsal elements are then meticulously decorticated with a small osteotome, and the bone graft is placed over the laminae, transverse processes, and facets, with particular attention to the facets.

Complications of Derotation Maneuver

Use of segmental instrumentation with the 90-degree derotation maneuver has been associated with a significantly higher rate of coronal decompensation than that obtained with Harrington instrumentation, particularly in the correction of Type IIB curves.[98,111,127,147] This greater decompensation may result from torque forces being delivered to the uninstrumented lumbar or thoracic spine. Essentially, derotation of the thoracic deformity results in a rotational moment that increases the rotation of both the rostral and the caudal structural compensatory curves. The correction of the primary structural curve does not address the compensatory curve's structural rigidity. Often, this leads to decompensation of the compensatory curve. This

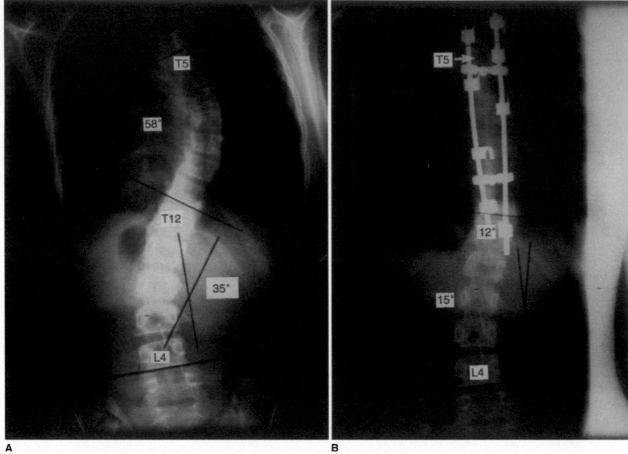

Figure 64.3 Type III idiopathic scoliosis correction with a Type III hook pattern.
(A) A 12-year-old had a preoperative primary thoracic curve measuring 58 degrees and a compensatory lumbar curve measuring 35 degrees. **(B)** Both the lumbar and thoracic curves corrected to 15 degrees, leaving the patient well balanced in the coronal plane.

causes a rapid increase in the magnitude of the compensatory curve (usually lumbar) and a significant deviation from the midline (i.e., listing). An understanding of this problem is essential to obtain a balanced correction. Avoidance of this problem may be achieved by decreasing the derotational force, increasing the intermediary hook's distraction force, and leaving the end hooks disengaged. In addition, a less than maximal curve correction may need to be accepted to avoid decompensation and to balance the degree of curve correction to match that of the compensatory residual curve. If the compensatory curve is deemed structural, it may need to be included in the primary fusion. If the structural compensatory curve is 40 degrees or less, an alternative may be to simply correct the primary curve to the same degree as the existing compensatory curve. This will lead to a balanced spine in the coronal plane. This, in turn, will prevent late decompensation.

Complication Avoidance and Treatment in Scoliosis Patients

Restoration of normal spinal alignment in scoliosis is not without risks. Not only does straightening the spine have a

risk of neurologic injury, but there are also a whole host of complications with respect to the fusion, instrumentation, and surgical approach.

Neurologic Injury and Monitoring

Although rarely encountered, a neurologic injury is by far the most serious injury that can occur while correcting a scoliotic spine. Manipulation of the spinal column in the presence of a syringomyelia or diastematomyelia may lead to postoperative neurologic deficits. The possibility of these neurogenic origins of scoliosis must be considered and addressed before correction of the curvature. In addition, children with ventriculoperitoneal shunts should be assessed for patency of the system and the presence of an adequate catheter length in the abdomen, because coronal plane correction can distract the abdominal catheter. This may result in acute shunt obstruction. In addition, patients who have more rigid curves with a severe degree of angulation (greater than 60 degrees) may be vulnerable to an increased risk of neurologic injury. This risk is related to an intrinsic shortening of the spinal column and the tremendous forces that must be applied to obtain correct

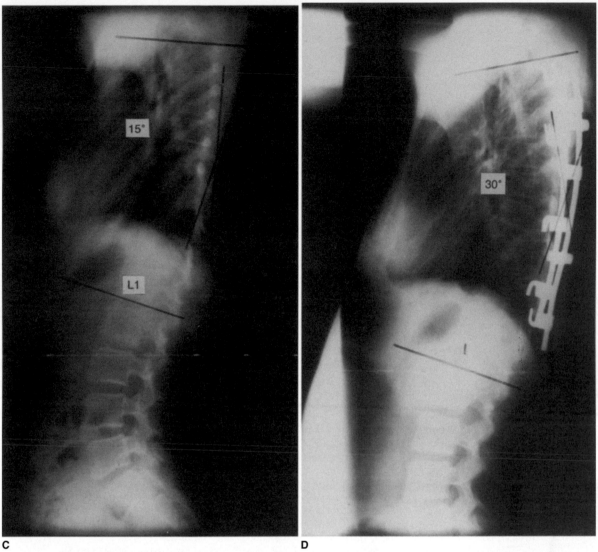

Figure 64.3 *cont'd* (**C**) Preoperative radiographs also revealed a thoracic hypokyphosis. (**D**) Thoracic hypokyphosis significantly improved postoperatively.

alignment. Patients with significant rigidity of the curvature should undergo ventral releases. This increases the flexibility of the spine, thereby decreasing the chance of neurologic injury.

To minimize the risk of neurologic complications, surgeons often recommend intraoperative monitoring with somatosensory-evoked potentials (SSEPs), motor-evoked potentials (MEPs), or both.[6] The Stagnara wake-up test is the gold standard and is performed intraoperatively to confirm the integrity of spinal cord function, even though spinal cord monitoring is used. SSEPs record ipsilateral dorsal column function predominantly, but they also record minor contributions from the spinothalamic and spinocerebellar tracts. Motor tracts are not directly monitored by SSEPs, but recent evidence suggests that significant neurologic injury is global and not selective to the anterior columns.[130] Several intraoperative factors may decrease the amplitude or prolong the latency of the SSEPs, leading to false-positive responses. These factors include equipment failure, electrode movement, hypotension, depth of anesthesia, use of halogenated anesthetic agents (e.g., isoflurane), hypoxia, core body hypothermia, and use of cold irrigating saline.[101] Correction of any of the factors thought to be abnormal should be carried out initially to see if the SSEPs return to baseline.

MEPs are sensitive and specific for predicting postoperative weakness because they specifically monitor descending motor tracts.[122] Three methods are available for motor tract assessment, including electrical and magnetic stimulation of the motor cortex and direct spinal cord stimulation. Transcranial magnetic stimulation (TCMS) is used most commonly. It is sensitive to anesthetic agents, such as isoflurane, enflurane, and propofol, which suppress the TCMS amplitude,[101] but neuromuscular blockade can be used.[63] Patients with a history of seizures are at increased risk, but there is no increased risk of seizures in the general population.[63] TCMS can rarely give accurate recording in patients with preexisting motor deficits.

The Stagnara wake-up test is routinely used in patients who undergo correction of spinal deformity, because false-negative and false-positive results are occasionally experienced with electrophysiologic testing. Despite its apparent

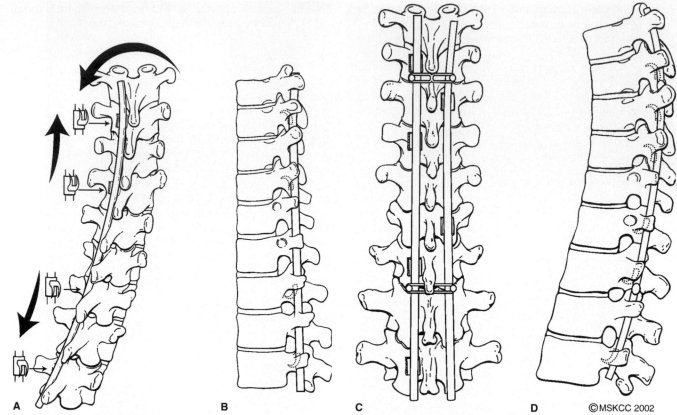

©MSKCC 2002

Figure 64.4 Derotation technique in Type III curve. (**A** and **B**) Distraction and derotation instrumentation (two upgoing hooks on the cephalic segment of the curve and two downgoing hooks on the caudal segment of the curve) is placed on the concave side of the curve at the preoperatively identified levels. (**A**) demonstrates rod and hook placement in the coronal plane, whereas (**B**) demonstrates placement in the sagittal plane. Gradual distraction *(small arrows in [A])* with a counterclockwise derotation moment *(large arrow in [A])* is applied to the spine intermittently, thereby correcting the coronal scoliotic deformity and decreasing the clockwise rotatory deformity of the spine (**C**), while restoring the normal kyphosis of the spine in the sagittal plane (**D**). A second rod is then placed on the convex side (**C**) of the curve in compression, thus providing for more corrective forces. Finally, crosslinks are applied (**C** and **D**) to biomechanically enhance the strength of the construct. Final spinal alignment in the coronal (**C**) and sagittal (**D**) planes is demonstrated. *(Copyright Memorial Sloan-Kettering Cancer Center.)*

crudeness, the Stagnara test remains the most specific criterion for intraoperative testing of neurologic function. This test is performed by decreasing the level of the anesthesia and reversing the muscle-relaxant activity. The operative field should be flooded with irrigation fluid to prevent the development of an air embolism, and the anesthesiologist should be alert to prevent the inadvertent dislodgment of the endotracheal tube. Patients are asked first to squeeze their hands and, second, to move their feet. The patients are encouraged to demonstrate adequate voluntary upper extremity motion before demonstrating lower extremity motion to ensure that there has been an adequate reversal of anesthetic agents and muscle relaxants. The wake-up test has several drawbacks including lack of sensory information, failure to provide real-time feedback, and inadvertent extubation.[123]

If a patient displays a significant reproducible SSEP change (amplitude decrease and latency prolongation of greater than 50%) or MEPs or cannot move his or her feet

during the Stagnara wake-up test, the surgical team should not proceed with the operation, but should observe the patient for 10 to 15 minutes. If hand movement is intact and the legs are paretic, the instrumentation should be relaxed. If neurologic function does not improve, the hardware should be removed. Myelography, postmyelographic CT, and MRI are all useful to determine the cause of the paresis if no intraoperative corrective measures result in improvement.

Blood Loss

A significant intraoperative blood loss should be anticipated; consequently, blood replacement should be planned for preoperatively. Despite the general blood supply being relatively safe, autologous and donor-directed blood donation and iron supplementation should be encouraged at least 4 weeks before elective operation. Intraoperative autologous transfusion, such as cell saver, can also be used. Intraoperative blood loss is decreased by meticulous control of muscle, epidural, and bone bleeding. Because bone decortication may cause a large blood loss, it is delayed until the end of the procedure, just before bone graft placement. Gelfoam soaked in thrombin is used to control bone bleeding; however, the extensive use of bone wax over the fusion site is not recommended because it may inhibit bone formation and it increases the incidence of pseudarthrosis.

Infection

Wound infection is a rare complication after correction of adolescent idiopathic scoliosis. It occurs more commonly in the surgical treatment of adult scoliosis and in post-myelomeningocele scoliosis. The guidelines outlined in this section apply to all spinal deformities for which instrumentation is used.

The prevention of wound infection should begin preoperatively, particularly in patients with myelomeningoceles, who frequently harbor chronic urinary tract infections (UTIs). Urine cultures and sensitivity should be performed preoperatively, and UTIs must be treated before the placement of spinal instrumentation because of the risk of bacteremic seeding of the metal construct.

Other risk factors associated with postoperative wound infection include prolonged surgery, previous spine surgery, the use of instrumentation, and poor soft tissue surgical technique.[75] Prophylactic antibiotics have been shown to decrease the infection rate.[8,150] Cefazolin (1 g/dose in adults and 12.5 mg/kg/dose in children) is administered as an intravenous drip 30 minutes before the surgical incision is made and is repeated every 6 hours during the procedure. Postoperatively, the antibiotic therapy is continued for 48 hours, at 6- to 8-hour intervals. Vancomycin (1 g every 12 hours for adults and 10 mg/kg every 6 hours for children) is substituted for the cefazolin for patients who are allergic to penicillin or who are in a hospital with a known methicillin-resistant *Staphylococcus aureus* colonization. It is important to maintain a therapeutic antibiotic level throughout the operation.[8]

Infections may present as an erythematous, hot, and tender wound, and possibly, as a fistulous tract draining purulent material within the first postoperative week. However, because some infections may be quite indolent, particularly gram-negative organisms and *Staphylococcus epidermidis*, a high index of suspicion is needed. Fever, leukocytosis, and an elevated sedimentation rate are indicators of infection. C-reactive protein may be a more sensitive indicator of the presence of an acute infection.[44,117,142] All acute bacterial spinal infections should be treated with multiple débridements. Delay of aggressive therapy may lead to development of a chronic infection, which will require hardware removal. Intravenous broad-spectrum antibiotics should be started at the first sign of infection and are then tailored to the organism after it has been cultured intraoperatively. Surgical treatment of an infected wound should include the following: (1) pulsatile lavage, (2) débridement of nonviable tissue, (3) use of antibiotic beads to increase the local concentration of the antibiotic, and (4) suction drainage between débridements. Three to four serial débridements are often needed. Following these recommendations will lead to a successful result 94% of the time, without removal of the hardware (unpublished personal data).

Pseudarthrosis

Pseudarthrosis is uncommon in corrective deformity surgery, but it may occur. Foremost in preventing this complication is meticulous technique, including proper exposure, decortication of bone and facets, preparation of the fusion bed, and use of autogenous bone grafts. The placement of two hooks at the same spinal level (with scoliosis surgery) must be avoided, because this may decrease the amount of bone available for adequate bone grafting at that level. A cancellous bone graft should be placed in the facet space to facilitate fusion. Decortication of spinous processes and the transverse processes should also be performed. Fusion is the critical part of these corrective procedures. Its success determines the success of the entire procedure. The instrumentation is only an adjunct for obtaining the initial spine correction and stabilization.

Ventral Scoliosis Deformity Correction

Ventral Fusion and Instrumentation

Some scoliosis problems can be adequately treated by ventral spinal fusion. In scoliosis, ventral fusion and instrumentation is particularly applicable for primary thoracolumbar and lumbar curves.

Potential advantages of anterior approaches include the ability to save spinal levels and thus motion segments. In addition, there are numerous other indications for anterior spinal instrumentation and fusion, including congenitally deformed vertebrae, extreme skeletal immaturity (younger than 10 years of age), and a rigid deformity.

Ventral fusion, when combined with a dorsal spinal fusion, may also be used to increase the chance of successful arthrodesis, especially when treating adult deformities, in which achieving a solid dorsal fusion is more difficult. An important indication for a ventral procedure with or without fusion is decompensation that results from the crankshaft phenomenon.[135] This phenomenon was initially observed by Dubousset et al.,[40] who noted 1-degree curve progression in all 40 patients who had a Risser score of less than one (idiopathic infantile and juvenile scoliosis) after dorsal fusion alone for the correction of their scoliosis. The only skeletally immature patient who did not experience decompensation of the primary curve underwent a ventral fusion as well. The crankshaft phenomenon results from continued growth of the ventral spine in the presence of dorsal growth arrest resulting from the dorsal instrumentation and arthrodesis. This spinal decompensation occurs in all three planes, but predominantly as a delayed axial rotation. Therefore ventral epiphysiodesis is recommended in patients younger than 10 years to create ventral growth arrest, thus preventing the crankshaft phenomenon.

Combined ventral and dorsal instrumentation and fusion procedures are often indicated. They allow for circumferential correction of the deformity and application of instrumentation with a minimal increase in morbidity. Studies have demonstrated that patients may tolerate these procedures better when they are performed sequentially in a single operation.[75,81,136] Combined ventral and dorsal approaches are particularly valuable to preserve lumbar motion segments by returning the spine to the stable zone while correcting the scoliosis. Other indications for combined procedures include the following: (1) myelomeningocele, when good dorsal bone stock is not available for fusion; (2) patients with a high likelihood of developing pseudarthrosis, such as smokers and those with neuromuscular scoliosis, osteoporosis, and rigid scoliotic deformities of greater than 75 to 80 degrees; and (3) pseudoarthrosis after a previous dorsal spine fusion. Ventral spinal procedures allow for direct visualization of the spinal deformity and the application of appropriate ventral corrective forces.

Ventral Instrumentation

The first ventral instrumentation, described in 1969 by Dwyer et al.,[41] consisted of inserting a staple and screw through the vertebral body, through which a flexible titanium wire was placed. Tightening the cable created a bending moment in the frontal plane, but did not improve the lumbar lordosis.[64] The lack of rigidity with this system led to a high pseudarthrosis rate.[85,164,165] In 1976, Zielke and Pellin[164] introduced a 3.2-mm threaded rod that provided a more rigid construct, with a subsequent decrease in the pseudarthrosis rate. This system provided good correction in the frontal plane and some correction of axial rotation, but resulted in lumbar kyphosis.[77,91,164] More recently, rigid rod systems have been introduced that allow for improvement in lumbar lordosis via derotation and in situ bending of the solid rod into lordosis. Like the C-D prototype system's dorsal correction of scoliosis, these rigid rod systems and, to a lesser extent, the Zielke system, can add a 90-degree derotation to sequentially applied compression forces.[48,151] This translates the lumbar or thoracolumbar scoliosis into the coronal midline and preserves a greater degree of the normal thoracolumbar and lumbar lordosis. These newer rigid rod systems include Isola, Texas Scottish Rite Hospital (TSRH), and Synergy. There is a hope that use of these more rigid rod systems will result in an even higher fusion rate than that obtained with the Zielke system (up to a 20% pseudarthrosis rate). These systems have a tendency to better preserve or restore normal thoracolumbar or lumbar sagittal plane alignments.

Technique for Insertion of Solid Rod Systems

Patients are positioned in the lateral decubitus position with the convex side of the scoliotic curve facing the surgeon. The technique for exposure of the spinal column is the same for both instrumented and noninstrumented ventral thoracic and lumbar procedures. Exposure of the thoracolumbar and lumbar curves is made with a transthoracic, retroperitoneal approach through a low thoracotomy incision, which requires resection of the tenth rib and detachment of the diaphragm. Alternatively, many surgeons are using thoracoscopic techniques for exposure and instrumentation. Regardless of whether an open or thoracoscopic technique is used, care must be taken to identify the major vessels and the ureters. Having exposed the

spine, the surgeon must first turn his or her attention to dissecting the soft tissue from the relatively avascular disc spaces before proceeding. An intraoperative radiograph or fluoroscopy is taken to confirm that the correct levels to be instrumented have been identified. The segmental vessels of each vertebral body to be instrumented are ligated on the ventral surface of the vertebral bodies to prevent interruption of collateral flow to the spinal cord. The discs are removed with sharp Cobb elevators, curettes, and large pituitary rongeurs. Particular attention should be paid to the complete removal of each disc and annulus in the dorsoventral corner of the disc space. This allows for greater flexibility in facilitating the derotation maneuver. The cartilaginous end plates are decorticated with an osteotome just before bone graft insertion. Bleeding after exposure of the dura and decortication of the vertebral bodies can be controlled with thrombin-soaked Gelfoam.

After discectomy and decortication, an awl is used to create a hole in each vertebral body, through which a screw is inserted. The screws are placed into each vertebral body as close to the spinal canal as possible. The screws should be aligned with each other. If the Zielke instrumentation is being used, the apical screw should be placed the most dorsally, with each successive screw placed slightly more ventrally, to facilitate the creation of a lordosis; however, this pattern of screw alignment is not necessary with the more rigid systems. A small block of bone obtained from a resected rib is placed within each disc space. With solid rod systems, a rod that is ³⁄₁₆ inch in diameter is cut to the appropriate length and contoured to create the desired end lordosis. The rod is attached to the screws just tight enough to allow for rotation of the system (function glide tight). The rod is then rotated 90 degrees to translate the lumbar scoliosis into the desired lordosis, using the wrench on the hexagonal end of the rod (Figure 64.5). The apical bolt is tightened, the end plates are decorticated, and bone grafts are placed, followed by sequential compression and bolt tightening from both ends toward the apex. Compression is continued until the disc spaces are parallel to each other (confirmed by a radiogram). The sagittal and coronal alignments must be checked to confirm correction of the curve in those planes as well (Figure 64.6).

Complications

Potential complications from the ventral approach include injury to the thoracic or abdominal aorta, vena cava, common iliac artery and vein, iliolumbar vein, kidney, ureter, thoracic duct, and spleen. Injury to the hypogastric sympathetic nerve plexus may result in retrograde ejaculation of sperm. A thorough knowledge of vertebral anatomy and experience with this approach minimizes the occurrence of these complications.

Segmental arteries should be ligated near the ventral midline of the vertebral body.[97] Sacrifice of the segmental arteries dorsally near the intervertebral foramen, particularly in the critical vascular zone of the spinal cord between the fourth thoracic vertebra and the thoracolumbar junction, leads to an increased risk of paraplegia.[37,38] Except in an extremely rare case, ligation of segmental arteries near the ventral midline of the vertebral body has

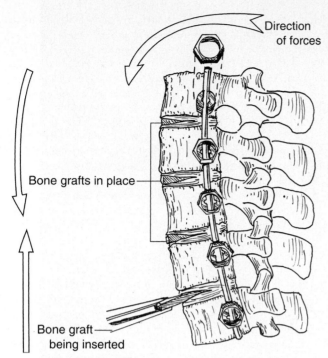

Direction of forces

Bone grafts in place

Bone graft being inserted

Figure 64.5 Example of a solid rod modification of the Zielke procedure for a primary Type I lumbar curve. After appropriate screw and rod placement on the ventral convex side of the curve following meticulous multilevel discectomies, a clockwise derotation moment is applied to the spine along with gradual compression (as noted by *arrows*). This shortens the anterior spinal column, thus rotating the spine back to the midsacral axis in the coronal plane. The disc spaces are packed with autogenous bone graft struts to maintain lordosis.

not been associated with spinal cord ischemia. Delayed vascular complications may arise from the instrumentation abutting the aorta of the iliac artery. The continuous pulsations of these arteries against the instrumentation may cause erosion of the vessel and result in hemorrhage. This is particularly true in the area of the thoracic spine. Although this complication has been reported specifically with the Dunn device when used ventrally for fracture reconstruction, this possibility should concern the surgeon when using any ventral instrumentation system. Surgeons should also avoid placing screws close to arteries. Limiting the application of ventral instrumentation systems to the right side of the spine and caudal to T11 greatly minimizes the possibility of this complication.

Failures with ventral instrumentation are often associated with pseudarthrosis. Instrumentation failure can result from rod or screw breakage or from uncoupling of the rod and screw. These complications are not uncommon with the Zielke instrumentation. The merits of the more rigid rod systems are not yet proven.

Late complications of ventral spinal scoliosis surgery include trunk decompensation, loss of lumbar lordosis, curve progression over uninstrumented segments, and low back pain. Trunk decompensation may occur from overcorrection of the lumbar or thoracolumbar curve that results in a shift in the curve from the midline. Compensatory curves may not compensate for this over-

correction. The rigid rod systems have a tendency to overcorrect curves because of the strong force they generate during curve correction. Careful monitoring of curve correction using intraoperative radiographs may prevent this from occurring.

Loss of lumbar lordosis, the result of placing the screws too ventral to the axis of rotation, can be prevented by placing the apical screw as dorsal as possible. In addition, the placement of bone blocks into the disc spaces before applying corrective forces helps prevent the development of kyphosis. Rigid ventral rod systems appear to prevent the development of kyphosis. Finally, curve decompensation may occur from improper selection of proximal and distal fusion levels. The development of low back pain occurs with greater frequency when the fusion is extended caudal to L3. This is probably the result of a loss of lumbar lordosis over the fused segments of the spine, with a resultant increase in lordosis below the fusion. This transfer of an increased load to the caudal motion segments may accelerate the development of disc and facet degeneration at the L4-5 and L5-S1 levels. As with dorsal spinal instrumentation, preserving motion segments in the caudal lumbar spine may prevent the development of low back pain.

Sagittal Plane Deformities: Thoracic Kyphosis and Flat Back Syndrome

Kyphosis is an excessive sagittal angular deformity that is beyond the established normal range. The normal range of the thoracic spine curvature is 25 to 40 degrees, with a transitional zone of approximately 40 to 55 degrees.[14] A kyphosis greater than 60 degrees in the thoracic spine is considered abnormal. However, at the thoracolumbar junction, the normal kyphosis is 0 degrees and the lumbar spine is normally lordotic. A posttraumatic deformity of greater than 30 degrees at the thoracolumbar junction[55] and a kyphosis of greater than 5 degrees in the lumbar spine are considered abnormal.[90]

There are several causes of kyphosis. Scheuermann's kyphosis is a prototypical cause of kyphosis and is considered to be of developmental origin. Some causes of kyphosis are posttraumatic fractures, osteomalacia, osteoporosis, and destruction of a vertebral body by tumor infiltration.

Nonoperative treatment of kyphosis can be successful in certain circumstances. The application of a Milwaukee brace for Scheuermann's kyphosis can result in complete correction of the deformity if it is applied during the adolescent growth spurt. Some patients with rigid Scheuermann's kyphosis require operative correction. Active intervention should be undertaken in postmenopausal women with thoracic osteoporotic compression fractures because of the high risk of developing significant kyphosis.[26] A clam shell or Jewett-type brace and antiinflammatory agents are indicated for the treatment of pain. Treatment also includes an active physical therapy program and daily calcium-replacement therapy to prevent and/or reverse the incidence of compression fractures and progressive kyphosis. More recently, kyphoplasty and vertebroplasty have been used to alleviate the painful deformities related to osteoporotic compression fractures. Short-term results have shown excellent pain control,

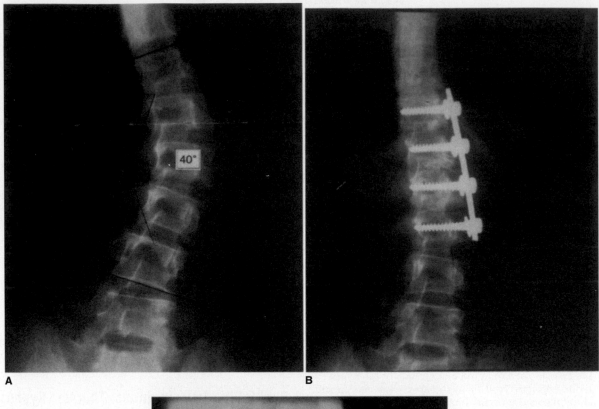

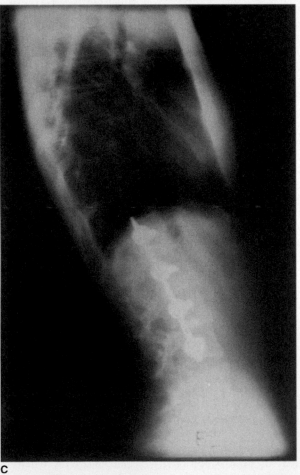

Figure 64.6 Type I unbalanced idiopathic scoliosis curve corrected with the vertebral body screw solid rod system. Type I idiopathic scoliosis corrected via a transdiaphragmatic retroperitoneal thoracolumbar approach with the vertebral body screw and solid rod instrumentation system. The curve was corrected from 40 degrees with a 2-cm right list (**A**) to 12 degrees with no list (**B**). Lumbar lordosis and motion segments preserved (**C**).

but long-term results are not known. This procedure is well covered in this text and is not covered in this chapter.[4,52,66,100,102,143]

This discussion is limited to posttraumatic deformities that should serve as a model for correction of other kyphotic deformities. Posttraumatic kyphosis usually results from a multicolumn fracture of the vertebral body, which causes a loss of support of the spinal segments and subsequent deformity. Posttraumatic kyphosis usually occurs at the thoracolumbar junction (T11, T12, L1 vertebrae), where the rigid thoracic spine makes the transition to the mobile lumbar spine. Depending on the mechanism and vector forces involved in the injury (i.e., flexion versus compression, axial loading versus rotation), a wide variety of injuries can occur, including burst fractures, fracture dislocations, and ligamentous injuries. An unstable injury may ensue, with the development of a posttraumatic kyphotic deformity. The resultant abnormal sagittal alignment shifts the spinal axis of rotation more ventrally, creating a moment arm that causes further kyphosis and a progressive delayed deformity.

Presentation

The most common presenting symptom of a delayed posttraumatic kyphosis is pain, either at the apex of the deformity or in the low back.[58,108,109,150] Pain at the apex is mechanical in nature and is made worse with movement or upright posture, but is improved by recumbency. Low back pain is the result of the compensatory hyperlordosis creating increased facet loading with resultant premature degeneration of the facet joints.

The progression of neurologic symptoms and signs may be the result of chronic compression or increased deformation of the spinal cord over the fixed kyphotic segment. Stenosis may also result from the spinal instability, producing myelopathy or radiculopathy. In addition, vascular insufficiency of the spinal cord, arachnoiditis, and the development of syringomyelia may contribute to increased neurologic symptoms. Other symptoms include progressive cosmetic deformity from instability resulting from a pseudarthrosis or nonunion of the fractured vertebral body.

Radiographic Assessment

Radiographic analysis begins with standard 36-inch PA and lateral plain radiographs. The classic deformity observed with posttraumatic deformity is a segmental kyphosis. The degree of kyphosis is measured according to the Cobb method. This measurement is taken from the angle of the caudal end plate of the vertebra above the defect and the intact caudal end plate of the involved vertebra. The sagittal index may be used as a predictor of progressive segmental kyphosis.[45] The sagittal index takes into account the normal contour at each motion segment for the thoracic (+5 degrees), thoracolumbar (0 degrees), and lumbar (10 degrees) spinal levels. The sagittal index is determined by subtracting the normal contour from the measured kyphotic deformity (i.e., degrees of measured kyphotic deformity less the degrees of normal contour equals the sagittal index). A sagittal index greater than 15 degrees is predictive of segmental instability with a potential for progression of the kyphosis. In addition, sequential radiographs may demonstrate global instability. Flexion and extension radiographs are contraindicated in the acute stage after injury because they may cause a progressive neurologic injury, but they may be useful in the evaluation of patients with longstanding kyphoses.

Other imaging studies are important to answer specific questions regarding mechanical instability or neurologic decompensation. CT scans and plain tomograms may identify a pseudarthrosis of the ventral and middle columns at the apex of the kyphosis. Myelography can supplement CT scans for determining the extent of spinal cord or nerve root compression. MRI may be used to determine the extent of neural compression, but it is also helpful because it directly images the soft tissues. MRI may also show ligamentous disruption, disc herniation, spinal cord edema or contusion, and syrinx formation.

Treatment: Ventral Principles

The treatment of these conditions must be tailored to each patient. Factors such as the nature of the injury, the age of the patient, underlying medical problems, available instrumentation, and the surgeon's skill and experience are important when planning treatment.

In the immediate posttraumatic period (within approximately 4 weeks of the injury), adequate spinal mobility often exists to allow for correction of the kyphotic deformity if only dorsal spinal fusion is used. Patients with ventral two-column injuries or with an isolated posterior column injury, who are neurologically normal without spinal cord or cauda equina compression, or who are paraplegic, may be treated with dorsal fusion alone, if there are sufficient intact vertebral bodies to maintain spinal stability (adequate axial load-bearing ability).[7] Prone lateral radiographs may help determine the flexibility of the spine, thereby assisting with the prediction of the extent of intraoperative reduction of the kyphosis that can be achieved with dorsal fusion alone. Reduction of a large kyphotic deformity (e.g., 30 degrees at the thoracolumbar junction) is important if a dorsal fusion is to be used alone, because restoration of the sagittal alignment reduces the tension placed on the fusion mass (by reducing the biomechanical disadvantage created by the pathologic bending moment), thus reducing the chance of the patient developing either a progressive kyphotic deformity and/or a pseudarthrosis.[128] Two methods commonly used to achieve reduction of the kyphotic deformity are the crossed-rod bending technique and the short-rod technique.

Surgical Technique for Dorsal Reduction of Acute Posttraumatic Kyphosis

Spinal reduction is often achieved by simply placing the patient on the spine frame. Additional correction is achieved with the use of dorsal instrumentation. After the skin incision is made, dissection of the soft tissue should progress from the caudal and rostral ends toward the level of the fracture to minimize neurologic injury, because the laminae may be fractured and the dorsal spinal ligaments may be completely disrupted. Laminar fractures are often associated with dural tears.[21] Great care should be taken

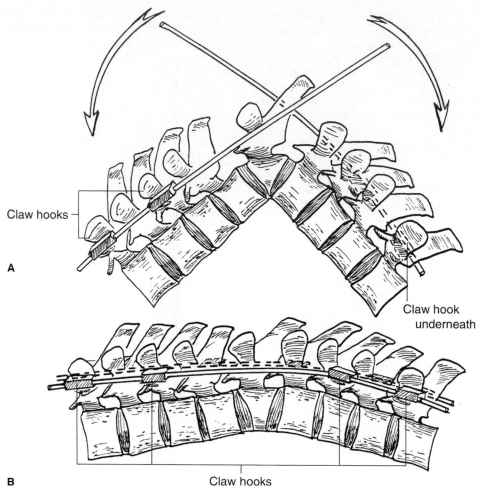

Figure 64.7 Crossed-rod bending technique for a reduction of kyphosis. **(A)** A claw-hook configuration is attached to each side of the spine with one claw-hook configuration cephalad and one claw-hook configuration caudal to the kyphotic deformity. After multiple dorsal osteotomies, downward force *(arrows)* is placed on the end of each rod. **(B)** This results in a reduction of the kyphosis. The free end of each rod is attached by an additional claw-hook configuration at opposite ends of the construct, completing it.

during the opening dissection to identify the abnormal anatomy and avoid further neurologic injury. Disrupted ligamentum flavum and bony fragments driven into the canal should be removed to provide for adequate decompression. When exploration is completed and the dura mater is repaired, attention is turned to spinal reduction. Laminectomy or multiple wedge osteotomies may be required for delayed injuries to improve correction of the deformity.

Crossed-Rod Technique

The crossed-rod technique consists of using a claw configuration at the rostral end of the rod that is attached to one side of the spine rostral to the deformity. A second rod and claw construct is attached to the opposite side of the spine, caudal to the deformity. The rods are crossed in the sagittal plane and are parallel to each other in the coronal plane on either side of the spine. The kyphosis is reduced by placing approximately equal downward forces on both the left and right rods. Then the free end of each rod is placed into a hook construct rostral or caudal to the apex of the

deformity. This maneuver brings the rods into a parallel orientation in both the sagittal and coronal planes (Figure 64.7). Finally, a cross-member is placed at each end of the construct, thus cross-fixing the two rods. This stabilizes the construct, thus creating greater biomechanical stability.

Placement of a Temporary Rod

A temporary compressive system is placed on one side of the spine, rostral and caudal to the kyphosis to allow for the application of gradual compression forces once the hooks and rods are inserted and tightened (Figure 64.8). The fracture is reduced with compression by the application of tension to the posterior column of the spine. Once proper reduction has been achieved by the temporary rod, a full-length compression construct is placed on the opposite side of the spine. An ideal construct consists of a set of hooks rostral to the kyphosis, placed over the rostral edge of the laminae, and a second set of hooks caudal to the kyphosis, placed at the caudal edge of the selected lamina. It is generally advisable to have at least two or three hooks in compression, both above and below the kyphosis, to

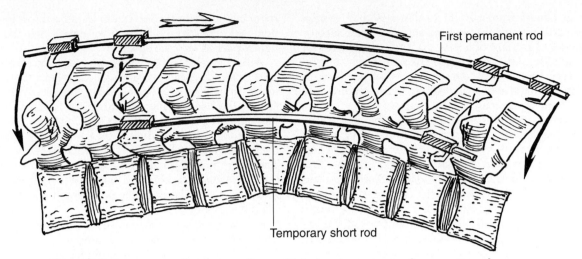

Figure 64.8 Temporary rod technique after multiple dorsal osteotomies for correction of a delayed deformity. Fracture reduction is achieved by applying gradual compression to a temporary, short-rod construct. A full-length construct is then placed on the opposite side of the spine in compression. The temporary rod is then replaced by a long-rod construct, completing the reduction. *Arrows* indicate the direction of the forces.

provide strong sublaminar fixation. After the permanent metal construct is inserted, the temporary rod is removed and another full-length compression construct is inserted in place. Finally, two horizontal crosslinks (one at each end) are inserted, connecting the rods and thereby stabilizing the construct.

Maintaining the deformity reduction obtained with instrumentation requires meticulous bone grafting techniques. Bone grafting requires that the surgeon adhere to the following principles: (1) attention should be paid to the removal of all soft tissue, (2) adequate facetectomies must be performed, (3) the cartilage of the facet joints are curetted, and (4) the facet joints are packed with a soft cancellous autograft. Adherence to these principles should result in a significant reduction of the deformity and achievement of a solid arthrodesis.

Ventral Techniques

Ventral decompression and fusion, which may improve the deformity correction and neurologic outcome, may be necessary for patients with posttraumatic kyphotic deformities. Patients who have an incomplete or progressive neurologic injury; a rigid, fixed kyphosis; or a significant loss of ventral and/or dorsal support may benefit from a ventral procedure. Incomplete or progressive neurologic deficits may result from bone fragments retropulsed into the anterior spinal canal (e.g., burst fractures) or from the kyphotic deformity producing chronic compression of the spinal cord. These two conditions may benefit from ventral spinal cord decompression.* This decompressive procedure is particularly important if a partial neurologic deficit exists, because significant neurologic recovery may occur. Ventral spinal approaches provide direct visualization for decompression of the spinal canal. In addition, correction of the deformity via a dorsal approach alone may distract the spinal cord over the kyphotic deformity, making the neurologic injury worse.

Therefore it is contraindicated to reduce fixed kyphotic deformities with dorsal distraction instrumentation before a ventral decompressive procedure.

Patients with rigid, fixed kyphotic deformities may also benefit from ventral decompression and fusion to achieve a better correction. Ventral spinal osteotomies are often necessary to improve spinal flexibility. The surgeon can achieve a better spinal reduction with fixed deformities than could be achieved by a dorsal procedure alone. In addition, ventral strut grafts have a biomechanical advantage over dorsal fusions because they provide maximal support (by augmenting axial load-bearing ability), thereby preventing progressive deformity. The ventral strut graft is under compression, which promotes vertebral body fixation, arthrodesis, and bone formation.[13,82]

Loss of significant ventral and/or dorsal support requires a ventral decompression and fusion. Fractures that result in a loss of ventral vertebral body bone stock are associated with a high failure rate with dorsal fusions alone.[128] Laminectomy is a common contributor to posttraumatic kyphosis.[10,31,156] In addition, the lack of dorsal elements may not provide sufficient surface area to achieve a solid posterior arthrodesis.

Ventral decompression and fusion should be augmented with either ventral instrumentation or dorsal fusion and instrumentation. Instrumentation decreases the rate of pseudarthrosis and graft extrusion. Commonly used ventral fixation devices include the Kaneda device[84] and Z-plate.[163] These devices should be used with caution at the thoracolumbar junction, because of the risk of vascular injury, as well as in patients with a significant posterior column injury.

Combined Techniques

Ventral and dorsal procedures may be performed in a single operation or in a staged manner. A combined procedure may be used, with the surgeon performing the ventral procedure first. Patients with a rigid deformity and a severe kyphosis (greater than 80 degrees in the thoracic

---

*References 11,13,23,32,35,93.

spine) may benefit from a 10- to 14-day period of traction (e.g., halo gravity traction) between staged ventral decompression and placement of a strut graft followed by dorsal instrumentation and fusion. Halo traction should not be used before the ventral decompressive procedure in patients harboring a neurologic deficit, because a progressive neurologic injury may develop (Figure 64.9).

The anterior column is approached via a thoracotomy or thoracolumbar approach. The correct spinal level is confirmed by intraoperative radiographs. The discs above and below the vertebrectomy site are removed initially. This helps the surgeon identify the dura mater before he or she performs the vertebrectomy. Osteotomes and Leksell rongeurs may be used to remove the fractured vertebral body. Extreme care should be exercised to prevent soft tissue and/or neural injury. As the dura is approached, small downbiting curettes may be used to remove bone fragments from the spinal canal. The vertebral body should be removed thoroughly, extending from pedicle to pedicle, to decompress the spinal canal adequately. The end plates of the vertebrae above and below the fractured vertebral body should be preserved to provide a solid base for strut grafting. The drill is used to decorticate the end plates in various spots to promote arthrodesis, but the cortical bone of the end plate is essentially left intact. Epidural venous hemorrhage can be brisk, particularly when bone fragments are removed. This bleeding can be controlled by gentle packing with Gelfoam or Oxycel at the site of hemorrhage.

Once the two ventral columns have been resected, a stout autogenous tricortical bone graft taken from the iliac crest is tapped into the vertebrectomy site, so that it abuts the rostral and caudal end plates tightly. The operating room table is then reduced from the flexed to a level position. A Kocher clamp is used to ensure that the graft is tightly packed into the space.

After the ventral decompression and placement of the strut graft, the patient is carefully placed in a Wilson frame in the prone position, with careful attention to avoid extension of the back. A long dorsal spinal fusion with instrumentation is performed next, beginning three levels above and ending two levels below the apex of the kyphosis in the lumbar spine (three levels below in the thoracic spine). This instrumentation may be placed in a compression pattern. Dorsolateral bone fusion is then performed after thorough decortication of the posterior elements, as previously described.

An external orthosis (e.g., clam shell or high Knight brace) should be applied postoperatively and maintained for 3 to 6 months, when some evidence of ventral and dorsal fusion should be observed.

Although there are several causes of postreduction neurologic decompensation, the major causes are deformity reduction over a fixed spinal canal mass and vascular insufficiency. The degree of reduction of the deformity must be tempered by the risk of neurologic injury. Resolution of symptoms created by the kyphosis is related more to the arthrodesis attained than by perfect curve correction. The surgeon must strike a balance between improved curve correction and the risk of increased neurologic injury.

Neurologic Injury

Anterior decompression is used before reduction of the deformity to reduce the risk of neurologic injury. As noted

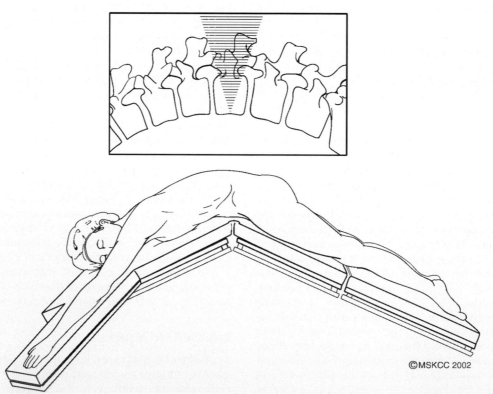

©MSKCC 2002

Figure 64.9 Intraoperative position with operating table flexed at the level of the deformity. (*Copyright Memorial Sloan-Kettering Cancer Center.*)

previously, the ventral decompression for burst fractures should be thorough, with the surgeon ensuring that all fragments are removed from the spinal canal. Meticulous technique must be used to ensure that no excessive pressure is placed on the neural elements during decompression or instrumentation. Intraoperative monitoring with SSEPs and the Stagnara wake-up test may be used to monitor spinal cord function in the same manner as described for scoliosis.

For a high-grade kyphosis, halo traction is used between the ventral decompression and strut grafting and the dorsal procedure. This provides for a gradual reduction of the deformity and for the opportunity to monitor an awake patient for signs of neurologic deterioration. Neurologic decompensation during halo traction necessitates immediate removal of the correcting forces. Radiographic imaging is necessary to determine the cause of the neurologic deterioration (i.e., increased kyphosis or spinal cord contusion that results from overdistraction).

Late neurologic decompensation may result from loss of correction and progression of the kyphosis with tethering of the spinal elements. Other causes for delayed neurologic deterioration include syringomyelia and arachnoiditis, which can be diagnosed with MRI or a myelogram.

Vascular Injury

Vascular causes of neurologic decompensation include blood loss (resulting in hypotension) and the sacrifice of major segmental arteries to the spinal cord. As with scoliosis, the normotensive anesthesia and ligation of segmental arteries near the anterior midbody of the vertebra help decrease the risk of this complication.

Graft Complications

Pseudarthrosis may present with instrumentation breakage or loss of correction, or both.[11,13,93] Repeat surgery for a pseudarthrosis with a resultant loss of correction may be necessary. Reduction of the deformity with a solid arthrodesis is necessary to balance the spine in the sagittal plane to prevent recurrent kyphosis.

Complications associated with ventral strut grafts used to reconstruct kyphotic deformities include pseudarthrosis, extrusion, fracture, and telescoping into the vertebral bodies. As has been previously noted, instrumentation improves the rate of arthrodesis with ventral strut grafts.[84,88,89,140]

Graft extrusion generally occurs ventrally and results in loss of correction and progression of the kyphosis. Dorsal graft extrusion can result in spinal cord compression with devastating neurologic consequences. These complications may result from poor graft quality, improper placement of the graft, or loss of end plate integrity. Keying the graft into the vertebral body is a method commonly used to prevent graft extrusion. This is done by creating troughs in the rostral and caudal vertebral bodies, into which the graft should fit tightly. This may increase the risk of the solid graft settling or telescoping into the soft cancellous bone of the vertebral body with a subsequent loss of correction. If this technique is used, a portion of the bone graft should maintain contact with the cortical end plate. A T-shaped graft is ideal for this purpose. The surgeon may choose to not key the graft into the vertebral body, but instead to decorticate the end plates in multiple areas and then tap the graft into place so that it abuts both rostral and caudal vertebral body end plates tightly. Dorsal instrumentation placed in compression, combined with spinal fusion, is then used to help lock the anterior strut graft into place. In addition, a shelf of bone can be maintained on the dorsal aspect of the vertebral body to protect against dorsal graft extrusion into the spinal canal.

Graft fracture is related to the intrinsic strength of the bone. A rib graft may be used, but it is weak and has a propensity to fracture when used as a strut in the thoracic or lumbar spine. A tricortical iliac crest bone graft provides rigid support but may not be long enough to reconstruct lengthy ventral defects created by the vertebrectomy. An allograft fibular strut or femoral ring graft provides extremely rigid axial support. However, an allograft takes approximately 2 years to become fully incorporated. Over this extended period, the graft may weaken, making it prone to fracture. Augmentation of the fibular strut graft with cancellous bone has been performed in an attempt to increase the rate of arthrodesis.

Flat Back Syndrome

The most common cause of flat back syndrome is iatrogenic secondary to failed spinal fusion with loss of lumbar lordosis. Other causes include posttraumatic, neuromuscular, or degenerative conditions or infection.[*]

Clinically, patients complain of difficulty with ambulation and severe back pain. They often assume a flexed knee-hip position in an attempt to compensate for the spinal deformity. Surgery is aimed a restoring the patient to an upright posture, achieving a horizontal visual field, and improving diaphragmatic respiration.

Initial surgical attempts using dorsal osteotomies to correct sagittal plane deformities resulted in complications related to lengthening of the anterior column, particularly stretching and disruption of the vascular structures and bowel.[94,138] To avoid these complications, Thomasen[144] described a corrective osteotomy that included removal of the L2 neural arch, lamina, and cancellous bone of the L2 vertebral body. This technique resulted in a 30- to 50-degree correction at a single level and avoided anterior column lengthening.[†] This eggshell procedure or transpedicular vertebrectomy with resultant anterior column shortening prevents the complications seen with posterior osteotomy techniques.

Eggshell Technique

Before surgery, radiographic evaluations, including MRI and CT myelogram, are used to evaluate the need for neural decompression. The amount of correction is estimated using standing full-length lateral spine radiographs. The osteotomy level is generally performed at L2 or L3 to provide adequate points of fixation, generally three levels above and below the osteotomy site.

---

*References 55,60-62,86,95,120,126.
†References 16,18,20,22,24,25,27,29,36,53,54.

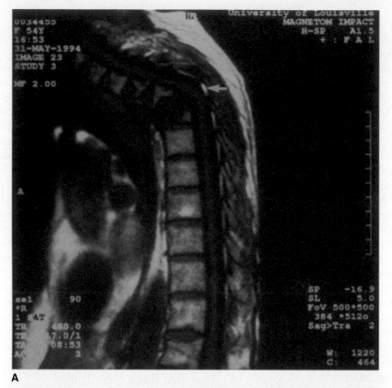

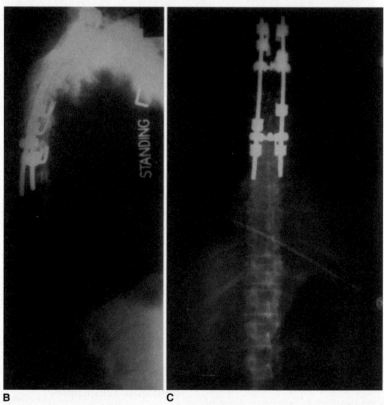

Figure 64.10 Posttraumatic kyphosis. A 54-year-old woman who was involved in a motor vehicle accident sustained an occult spinal fracture involving T4 and T5. Three months after her injury, the patient complained of severe back pain; she was noted to have a 90-degree kyphotic deformity of the upper thoracic spine and exhibited mild long-tract signs. (**A**) Magnetic resonance imaging showed collapse of the T4 and T5 vertebral bodies with tethering of the spinal cord anteriorly over the kyphosis *(arrow)*. A thoracotomy with T4 vertebrectomy with rib graft, as well as discectomies of T3-4, T4-5, and T5-6, was performed. After the patient was placed in halo traction for 10 days, the deformity decreased to 45 degrees. This was followed by a dorsal osteotomy, instrumental reduction, and a dorsal fusion. (**B**) Two years postoperatively, the patient showed a 20-degree kyphosis with resolution of her back pain. She was neurologically normal. (**C**) Anteroposterior radiographic view of instrumentation pattern.

The patient is positioned prone on a four-poster frame with the table flexed according to the deformity (Figure 64.10). Pedicle screw instrumentation is placed. For an L3 osteotomy, the L3 lamina, facet joints, transverse processes, and bilateral pedicles are resected. In addition, the overhanging L2 and L4 lamina are removed. The central dura and L2 and L3 nerve roots are completely mobilized.

Before dorsal wedge decancellation, temporary fixation is applied to one side of the spine to prevent collapse. The dura is carefully mobilized from the posterior aspect of the vertebral body. The amount of cancellous bone resected is predetermined based on preoperative radiographs and the degree of correction required. Correction is achieved by gradual extension of the operating table and closure of the osteotomy site, with the surgeon approximating the adjacent neural arches. Intraoperative radiographs are taken to confirm correction. The dura and nerve roots are directly observed during osteotomy closure. Pedicle resection provides a large area for the nerve roots to traverse. Both local bone and iliac crest are used for graft. Pedicle screws are secured with contoured rods. Postoperatively, patients are placed in a thoracolumbar sacral orthosis brace.

Complications

Neural compression is the most significant complication from this procedure. Monitoring SSEPs or MEPs may be important to prevent deficits. A Stagnara wake-up test is essential to assess neurologic function following deformity reduction, particularly to assess nerve root function.

Spondylolisthesis

Spondylolisthesis is a translational deformity of the spine in the sagittal plane in the lumbar spine that occurs in 6% of the population.[39] The deformity is usually stable and asymptomatic; however, it may become unstable with a progressive listhesis, causing low back pain and radiculopathy. An etiologic classification of spondylolisthesis has been developed[1,158,159] (Table 64.2).

General Conditions

Symptoms

The most common symptom of spondylolisthesis in both adolescents and adults is low back pain.[5] This pain is usually dull and aching and is aggravated by activity and improved by rest. Most commonly, an isthmic spondylolisthesis becomes symptomatic during the adolescent growth spurt,[3,70,133] whereas in degenerative spondylolisthesis, symptoms occur most often with increasing age. Adolescent patients with an L5-S1 isthmic spondylolisthesis rarely develop neurologic symptoms. Occasionally, however, radiculopathy results from a fibrocartilaginous bar that develops in the area of the lytic defect in the pars interarticularis, causing L5 nerve root compression. More rarely, a cauda equina syndrome develops in a high-grade spondylolisthesis. Because there is a relatively intact neural arch (spina bifida may be present) in the dysplastic (congenital) type of spondylolisthesis, cauda equina syndrome can occur with a lower-grade condition. Hamstring muscle tightness (Phalen-Dickson sign) may occur in all grades of spondylolisthesis.[125] This is thought to arise from a mild radiculopathy or cauda equina

TABLE 64.2

Classification of Spondylolisthesis

Type	Defect	Level	Associated Factors
Dysplastic	Congenital abnormalities of the facets and laminar arches	L5-S1	
Isthmic	Of the pars interarticularis (i.e., lytic-fatigue fracture; elongated but intact; acute fracture)	L5-S1	Spina bifida occulta; bipedal posture; heredity (Inuit)[109]; repetitive hyperextension exercises (weight lifting, gymnastics, football)[37,61,106]
Degenerative	Intersegmental instability secondary to facet-degenerating joint disease	L4-L5; L3-L4	Sacralization of L5
Traumatic	Facet and/or laminar arch fractures	L5-S1	Trauma
Pathologic	Destruction of the pars interarticularis, pedicle, and/or facets by generalized or localized bone disease	Any level	Tumor; osteoporosis; arthrogryposis
Postsurgical	Iatrogenic disruption of the intraspinous ligaments, disc, facet, and/or pars interarticularis	Previously decompressed level	Preexisting spondylolisthesis[66]

(Modified from Amundson G, Edwards CC, Garfin SR: Spondylolisthesis. In Rothman RH, Simeone FA [eds]: *The spine*, ed 3, vol 11. Philadelphia, WB Saunders, 1992, p 913, with permission.)

syndrome[3,33,125] or from the adjustment of the body to an altered center of gravity. Patients develop hip and knee flexion that results in a gait disturbance characterized as a *waddle*. In high-grade spondylolisthesis, the development of a lumbosacral kyphosis and other changes in spinal alignment result in flattened, heart-shaped buttocks and a shortened trunk. Paraspinal muscle spasm induced by the spondylolisthesis may result in a scoliotic curve that is structural and rigid.

In general, patients with degenerative spondylolisthesis develop neurologic symptoms in the fifth or sixth decades more often than those with isthmic spondylolisthesis. These neurologic symptoms are often related to anatomic changes associated with the degenerative spondylolisthesis, including herniated nucleus pulposus, degenerative disc disease, and facet arthropathy. In addition, as segmental spinal instability develops with a progressive slippage, foraminal impingement occurs.

Imaging

Spondylolisthesis is a common finding on plain radiographs, thus making it difficult to ascertain whether this deformity is the cause of the patient's low back pain. If the spondylolisthesis is thought to be asymptomatic, another pathologic condition may need to be identified. Sagittal translation (on plain lateral radiographs) may be graded according to Meyerding classifications as grades I through IV.[113] Radiographic evidence of instability can be identified by segmental vertebral body movement on lateral flexion and extension films. The best radiographic indicator of progressive ventral listhesis is a high slip angle.[132] Other features associated with spinal instability include a dome-shaped sacrum and a wedge-shaped L5 vertebral body.

MRI, myelograms, and postmyelographic CT scans are valuable diagnostic procedures in patients with neurologic symptoms. These studies specifically assess the severity of nerve root compression. MRI scans are particularly valuable for identifying evidence of degenerative disc disease associated with levels rostral to the spondylolisthesis. Bone scans[106,154] and single positron emission computed tomography scans[56,107] are valuable adjuncts for making a diagnosis of acute spondylolysis. Because the spondylolisthesis is asymptomatic in most cases, these imaging studies may also reveal abnormalities not associated with the spondylolisthesis that could be responsible for the patient's symptoms. In children and adolescents, this may include tethered cord, diastematomyelia, osteomyelitis, and tumor (osteoid osteoma, aneurysmal bone cyst, osteoblastoma, and eosinophilic granuloma).

Treatment Considerations

In most cases, nonoperative treatment methods are effective. These include nonsteroidal antiinflammatory medications, short-term bed rest, use of an external orthosis, a comprehensive exercise program, and physical therapy.[139] Most patients improve with this conservative treatment over 6 to 8 weeks.

Adolescent patients who are candidates for surgery include those (1) whose symptoms do not improve after a full course of nonoperative therapy and who continue to have persistent back pain and/or radiculopathy; (2) who have a progressive ventral listhesis documented by sequential radiographs, particularly when the slip is greater than 50%; and (3) who show radiographic signs of instability (i.e., movement on flexion and extension films, or a high slip angle).

A variety of surgical techniques has been applied to adolescents with isthmic spondylolisthesis. Patients with symptomatic spondylolysis may be treated with intersegmental wiring of the facet joints with localized bone fusion of the pars interarticularis defect.[15,43,148] This procedure is most effective in young patients with a spondylolysis and minimal ventral listhesis.

Dorsal *in situ* fusion is the preferred treatment for adolescent patients or young adults with spondylolisthesis.[65,110,119,129] A dorsolateral intertransverse process fusion provides the best fusion rates and clinical outcomes.[96,159] Dorsal interlaminar fusion is associated with a high pseudoarthrosis rate, because the pars interarticularis defect creates a disassociation of the vertebral body from the posterior spinal elements. Patients with low-grade spondylolisthesis at L5-S1 require dorsolateral fusion only at this spinal motion segment. The fusion should be extended to L4 for higher-grade slips. Extension of the fusion to L4 places the bone graft dorsal to the weight-bearing axis. This decreases the chance of bone resorption (which can occur along the lines of stress), which results in a pseudarthrosis and progressive spondylolisthesis. Pedicular instrumentation fixation with dorsolateral fusion has been used in adolescent patients with high-grade slips. Instrumentation provides resistance to the shear forces and decreases the segmental motion that occurs while the bone graft heals. Pedicle screws may also decrease the chance of further slip, which may occur as the immature fusion remodels and lengthens before obtaining a successful arthrodesis.

In situ fusion performed without decompression generally results in the resolution of minor radicular deficits and gait abnormalities,[83] but this may take up to 6 months. Decompressive laminectomy should be considered in adolescent patients with severe radiculopathy or evidence of neurogenic claudication. It is important during decompressive laminectomy to resect the fibrocartilage bar that impinges on the spinal canal and results in compression of the L5 nerve root. Decompression without fusion is contraindicated in children and adolescents because of the propensity of the spondylolisthesis to worsen in the skeletally immature patient.

Although dorsal *in situ* fusion is usually advocated for most spondylolisthetic deformities in adolescent patients, a number of other procedures have been described that reduce high-grade slips.* Reduction of the deformity provides a mechanical axis for fusion by restoring lumbar lordosis and decreasing the shear forces acting against the formation of a fusion mass. Deformity reduction may provide a better cosmetic appearance, improved gait, and increased fusion rates for patients with a pseudarthrosis after a previous fusion. However, the surgical and neurologic morbidity associated with these procedures is considerably higher than that encountered with *in situ* fusion. Reduction of the deformity stretches the con-

---

*References 12,14,19,51,118,131.

tracted L5 nerve root over the sacrum[124] and may result in a neurapraxic injury and foot drop. The most catastrophic complication of surgical reduction of the spondylolytic deformity is the development of a cauda equina syndrome. These deficits are often transient, but may be permanent.

Surgery is indicated in degenerative spondylolisthesis when nonoperative therapy has failed. The major indications for decompressive laminectomy include radiculopathy, neurogenic claudication, and/or back pain related to segmental spinal instability. The radiculopathy in an L4-5 degenerative spondylolisthesis commonly involves both the L4 and L5 nerve roots as opposed to a disc herniation, which generally affects only the L5 nerve root. The L4 nerve root is compressed between the hypertrophied L4-5 facet joint and the L5 vertebral body, and the L5 nerve root is compressed in the lateral recess. When this happens, both nerve roots must be decompressed.

Degenerative spondylolisthesis is associated with a dorsal shift of the axis of rotation from the nucleus pulposus to the facets. The facets become incompetent because of this increased load sharing. Radical resection of the already incompetent facet joint (greater than one third of the medial facet) and/or pars interarticularis may result in delayed segmental instability with increased back pain and radiculopathy. This complication necessitates reoperation and instrumented fusion.

Spinal arthrodesis after decompressive laminectomy for degenerative spondylolisthesis is recommended by a number of authors.* One prospective study clearly demonstrated improved long-term outcomes with simultaneous fusion with degenerative spondylolisthesis. Some authors advocate decompression alone; however, their follow-up periods may not have been long enough for proper outcome evaluations.[28,74,116] In general, decompressive laminectomy is not recommended without spinal arthrodesis, because there is a high probability of further slippage. This is a result of the removal of stabilizing structures necessary for decompression (i.e., dorsal spinal ligaments, facet capsules, ligamentum flavum, the disc at each level). Even with a limited decompression, some patients demonstrate a progression of the spondylolisthesis. Patients with a more radical procedure to ensure adequate decompression of the neural dorsal elements demonstrate progression of the spondylolisthesis.[74,103] When the surgeon performs a wide decompression of the neural elements with a dorsal spinal fusion, the risk of a progressive slip is decreased. Segmental spinal instability, which may result in incapacitating back pain and neurologic deficits, is also eliminated by creating a solid arthrodesis.[116] Rigid rod–pedicle screw fixation with posterolateral bone grafts provides better fusion rates than dorsolateral fusion alone.[17,105,163] Rigid rod or plate systems with dorsolateral bone grafts are recommended in all primary decompressions for spondylolisthesis and in all salvage procedures following postsurgical iatrogenic spondylolisthesis (Figure 64.11).

Dorsolateral Fusion and Pedicle Screw Fixation

The patient is placed prone in extension on an appropriate frame with the table flexed. A midline incision is made and

---

*References 17,46,72,103,112,162.

muscles are dissected off the spinous processes and laminae in a subperiosteal fashion using large Cobb elevators. An intraoperative cross-table lateral radiograph should always be taken to confirm that the surgeon is at the correct level. Care should be taken in the initial dissection and during subsequent lateral exposure of the spine to maintain the integrity of the facet capsule and the interspinous ligament of the most rostral level to be fused, because these structures contribute to spinal stability. For example, when a surgeon is performing a dorsolateral fusion for an L5-S1 spondylolisthesis, the facet capsule and interspinous ligament between L4-5 should be left intact, if possible. The decompressive procedure is then performed, after which the lateral exposure is accomplished. Meticulous removal of the soft tissues over the facets, pars interarticularis, transverse processes, and ala of the sacrum, using Cobb elevators, curved curettes, and osteotomes, must be performed. The facet cartilage should be removed with a small Leksell rongeur. Distortions of the normal anatomy that result from the spondylolisthesis may obscure identification of the transverse processes, particularly at the L5-S1 level. The ventral listhesis of the L5 vertebral body results in a more ventral location of the L5 transverse process relative to the ala sacralis. The L4 transverse process, which is in a more relatively dorsal location, may be easily mistaken for the L5 transverse process, especially with the higher-grade slips. Initial identification of the ala sacralis and the L4 transverse process, followed by dissection along the prerenal fascia, facilitates identification of the more deeply located L5 transverse process. It is imperative that this ventrally displaced transverse process be adequately exposed for incorporation into the posterolateral fusion. Decortication of the transverse processes and pars interarticularis is then accomplished, followed by the placement of strips of cancellous bone harvested from the posterior iliac crest. The bone grafts can be harvested through the midline incision by lateral dissection over the paraspinous fascia to avoid a second cutaneous incision and possible sectioning of the cluneal nerves.

Pedicular instrumentation may be used as an adjunct to dorsolateral fusion (see Figure 64.11). Anatomic changes with spondylolisthesis may greatly increase the difficulty of placing the screws. In isthmic spondylolisthesis at L5-S1, screw placement into the vertebral body of L5 is difficult because of the ventral translation and slip angle. It is often difficult to secure the rod to the screws, because the L5 and S1 screws lie in such close proximity to each other. With higher-grade slips, it may be necessary to extend the fusion to L4, placing pedicle screws in L4 and S1 without inclusion of L5. A cross-member is added to increase the stability of the construct. Finally, careful attention should be paid to maintaining the normal lumbar lordosis.

Anatomic Aspects of Pedicle Screw Fixation

A basic knowledge of lumbosacral spinal anatomy is essential for proper screw placement. The pedicles gradually decrease in diameter as they progress rostrally from the sacrum, making it difficult to place screws in the pedicles at L1-2. The coronal orientation is inclined at S1 approximately 30 degrees but decreases at each higher level

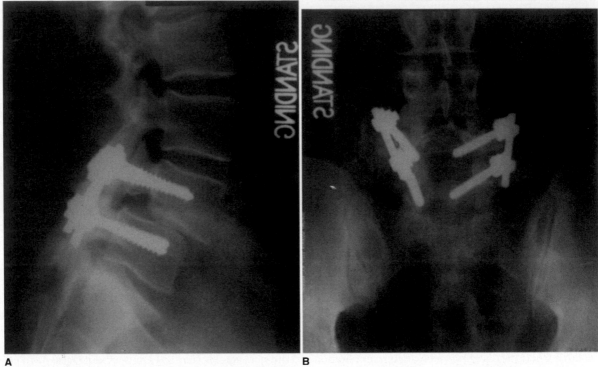

Figure 64.11 Pedicular screw instrumentation for a grade II spondylolisthesis. A 31-year-old patient with a 3-year history of low back pain and severe L4 and L5 radiculopathy presented with a grade II spondylolisthesis. The patient underwent an L4-5 decompression with pedicle screw instrumentation and posterolateral autologous iliac bone graft. One year postoperatively, the patient was asymptomatic and returned to light duty. Lateral (**A**) and anteroposterior (**B**) radiographic views.

approximately 5 degrees, to a near vertical orientation around L1 or L2. The transverse processes abut the pedicle and serve as a guide to pedicle entry. The orientation of the pedicle and the transverse process at each level varies slightly, so their relative orientation with an AP radiograph should always be checked.

The pedicle entry point is created using a rongeur at the junction of the pedicle and the transverse process. A small window into the pedicle is defined by a cancellous triangle. At this point, the pedicle orientation may be determined by a probe if a laminotomy has been performed. A sharp awl is used next to enlarge the entry point. A pedicular probe is then inserted to lengthen the hole before screw placement. Extreme caution should be taken not to plunge the probe into the spinal canal.

Thorough appreciation of the three-dimensional orientation of the pedicle is critical during pedicle probe placement. Precision may be increased by the use of radiographs, fluoroscopy, and electromyographic pedicle stimulation during placement of the screws. Sclerotic pedicles should first be enlarged with a tapping screw. There is some latitude for screw placement in the coronal, sagittal, and transverse planes within any given pedicle. Making use of this latitude enables the surgeon to place the screw heads in line, thus simplifying the placement of the rods. Intraoperative lateral radiographs or fluoroscopy may be used to confirm proper placement of the screws. A bone graft, harvested from the iliac crest, is then placed over the decorticated transverse processes, facets, and

pars interarticularis. The rods are then contoured with the proper amount of lordosis and attached to the pedicle screws.

Complications of Pedicle Screw Insertion

Attention to proper sagittal orientation is essential, because failure to restore or maintain lordosis leads to flat back syndrome. Ultimately, failure to maintain normal lumbar-sacral lordosis results in spinal imbalance with an increase of low back pain, unbalanced posture, and degeneration of adjacent spinal levels. Prevention of flat back syndrome may be accomplished by the proper positioning of the patient on the operating table and by *in situ* rod bending and placement to maintain lordosis.

Screws that breach the cortex of the pedicle and enter the spinal canal may result in a nerve root injury or a cerebrospinal fluid leak. Nerve root injury can best be avoided by careful placement of the pedicle screws. Nerve root injury most commonly occurs with breach of the caudomedial wall of the pedicle and impingement on the nerve as it travels around the pedicle to the intervertebral foramen or through the medial wall of the pedicle into the dural tube. Careful examination of preoperative CT scans, as well as plain AP and lateral radiographs, helps the surgeon determine the screw diameter appropriate for each pedicle. AP radiographs help determine the variability of the pedicle anatomy as it relates to the transverse process at each level to be instrumented. The intraoperative lateral radiographs help determine the angle at which the screw should be placed in the sagittal plane. If a laminotomy has been performed, the pedicle should be directly palpated with a probe to define the pedicle anatomy and to immediately identify a breach of the pedicle cortex during screw insertion. Pedicle screws that breach the cortex may not damage the nerve but may cause an irritation that results in postoperative radiculopathy. Although intraoperative radiographs should always be taken after pedicle screw placement to assess their proper position, these radiographs are reliable for identifying a breach of the pedicle only 85% of the time. Electrical pedicle screw stimulation may be used to record compound muscle action potentials from appropriate muscles in the leg.[59,121] Experience with this technique indicates that a stimulation threshold of greater than 15 mA is associated with a 98% confidence that the screw is entirely within the pedicle. If the stimulation threshold is between 10 and 15 mA, the pedicle should be explored for a possible breach of the cortex. If the stimulation threshold is less than 10 mA, the pedicle screw is usually in contact with a nerve root. The pedicle screw that is in contact with a nerve root should be replaced. Using the aforementioned criteria, researchers found that 9% of patients who radiographically were believed to have well-placed screws within the pedicle instead had low stimulation thresholds that required replacement or revision of the screws.[58]

Ventral perforations of the vertebral body may result in vascular injuries to the common iliac vessels. The most common cause of this complication is plunging too deep with the probe used to make the hole for the pedicle screw. Good control of this instrument is essential to prevent this complication from occurring. The surgeon's nondominant hand should be used to firmly grasp the shaft of this instrument while resting it against the patient's back. Vascular injury may be immediate from direct penetration of the vessel by the screw or the probe, or it may be delayed from repeated pulsations of major blood vessels against the metal threads of the screw. A screw length must be chosen that does not breach the ventral vertebral body cortex.

REFERENCES

1. Amundson G, Edwards CC, Garfin SR: Spondylolisthesis. In Rothman RH, Simeone FA (eds): *The spine,* ed 3, vol 11. WB Saunders, Philadelphia, 1992, p 913.
2. Arai S, Ohtsuka Y, Moriya H, *et al:* Scoliosis associated with syringomyelia. *Spine* 18:1591, 1993.
3. Barash HL, Galante JO, Lambert CL, Ray RD: Spondylolisthesis and tight hamstrings. *J Bone Joint Surg* 52A:1319, 1970.
4. Belkoff SM, Jasper LE, Stevens SS: An ex vivo evaluation of an inflatable bone tamp used to reduce fractures within vertebral bodies under load. *Spine* 27(15):1640, 2002.
5. Bellah RD, Summerville DA, Treves ST, Micheli LJ: Low-back pain in adolescent athletes: Detection of stress injury to the pars interarticularis with SPECT. *Radiology* 180:509, 1991.
6. Ben-David B: Spinal cord monitoring. *Orthop Clin North Am* 19:427, 1988.
7. Benson DR: Unstable thoracolumbar fractures with emphasis on the burst fracture. *Clin Orthop* 230:14, 1988.
8. Bergamini TM, Polk HC Jr: Pharmacodynamics of antibiotic penetration of tissue and surgical prophylaxis. *Surg Gynecol Obstet* 168:283, 1989.
9. Boachie-Adjei O, Girardi FP: Surgical treatment of rigid sagittal plane deformity. In Devlin VJ (ed): *Spine: State of-the-Art Reviews,* vol 12, no 1. Hanley & Belfus, Philadelphia, 1998, p 65.
10. Bohlman H: Late progressive paralysis and pain following fractures of the thoracolumbar spine. *J Bone Joint Surg* 58A:728, 1976.
11. Bohm H, Harms J, Donk R, Zielke K: Correction and stabilization of angular kyphosis. *Clin Orthop* 258:56, 1990.
12. Boos N, Marchesi D, Zuber K, Aebi M: Treatment of severe spondylolisthesis by reduction and pedicular fixation. A 6-year follow-up study. *Spine* 18:1655, 1993.
13. Bradford DS, Ganjavian S, Antonious D, *et al:* Anterior strut-grafting for the treatment of kyphosis. Review of experience with forty-eight patients. *J Bone Joint Surg* 64A:680, 1982.
14. Bradford DS, Gotfried Y: Staged salvage reconstruction of grade-IV and V spondylolisthesis. *J Bone Joint Surg* 69A:191, 1987.
15. Bradford DS, Iza J: Repair of the defect in spondylolysis or minimal degrees of spondylolisthesis by segmental wire fixation and bone grafting. *Spine* 10:673, 1985.
16. Bradford DS, Tribus CB: Current concepts and management of patients with fixed decompensated spinal deformity. *Clin Orthop* 306:64, 1994.
17. Bridwell KH, Sedgewick TA, O'Brien MF, *et al:* The role of fusion and instrumentation in the treatment of degenerative spondylolisthesis with spinal stenosis. *J Spinal Disord* 6:461, 1993.
18. Briggs H, Keats S, Schlesinger PT: Wedge osteotomy of spine with bilateral, intervertebral foraminotomy: Correction of flexion deformity in five cases of ankylosing arthritis of spine. *J Bone Joint Surg* 29:1075, 1947.
19. Burkus JK, Lonstein JE, Winter RB, Denis F: Long-term evaluation of adolescents treated operatively for spondylolisthesis. A comparison of in situ arthrodesis only with in situ arthrodesis and reduction followed by immobilization in a cast. *J Bone Joint Surg* 74A:693, 1992.
20. Camargo FP, Cordeiro EN, Napoli MM: Corrective osteotomy of spine in ankylosing spondylitis: Experience with 66 cases. *Clin Orthop* 208:157, 1986.
21. Cammisa FP Jr, Eismont FJ, Green BA: Dural laceration occurring with burst fractures and associated laminar fractures. *J Bone Joint Surg* 71A:1044, 1989.
22. Camp JF, Caudle R, Ashmun RD, Roach J: Immediate complications of Cotrel-Dubousset instrumentation to the sacro-pelvis: A clinical and biomechanical study. *Spine* 15:932, 1990.
23. Chang KW: Oligosegmental correction of post-traumatic thoracolumbar angular kyphosis. *Spine* 18:1909, 1993.
24. Cloward RB: Posterior lumbar interbody fusion updated. *Clin Orthop* 193:16, 1985.
25. Cochran T, Irstam L, Nachemson A: Long-term anatomic and functional changes in patients with adolescent idiopathic scoliosis treated by Harrington rod fusion. *Spine* 8:576, 1983.

26. Cortet B, Roches E, Logier R, *et al:* Evaluation of spinal curvatures after a recent osteoporotic vertebral fracture. *Joint Bone Spine* 69(2):201, 2002.

27. Cummine JL, Lonstein JE, Moe JH, *et al:* Reconstructive surgery in the adult for failed scoliosis fusion. *J Bone Joint Surg* 61A:1151, 1979.

28. Dall BE, Rowe DE: Degenerative spondylolisthesis. Its surgical management. *Spine* 10:668, 1985.

29. Dawson CW: Posterior osteotomy for ankylosis arthritis of the spine. *J Bone Joint Surg* 38A:1393, 1956.

30. Denis F: Cotrel-Dubousset instrumentation in the treatment of idiopathic scoliosis. *Orthop Clin North Am* 19:291, 1988.

31. Denis F, Armstrong GWD, Searls L, Motta L: Acute thoracolumbar back fractures in the absence of neurologic deficit. A comparison between operative and nonoperative treatment. *Clin Orthop* 189:142, 1984.

32. DeWald RL: Burst fractures of the thoracic and lumbar spine. *Clin Orthop* 189:150, 1984.

33. Deyerle WM: Lumbar-nerve-root irritation in children. *Clin Orthop* 21:125, 1961.

34. Dickson RA, Stamper P, Sharp AM, Harker P: School screening for scoliosis: Cohort study of clinical course. *Br Med J* 281:265, 1980.

35. Dimar JR, Wilde PH, Glassman SD, *et al:* Thoracolumbar burst fractures treated with combined anterior and posterior surgery. *Am J Orthop* 25:159, 1996.

36. Doherty JH: Complications of fusion in lumbar scoliosis: Proceedings of the Scoliosis Research Society. *J Bone Joint Surg* 55A:438, 1973.

37. Dommisse GF: The blood supply of the spinal cord. A critical vascular zone in spinal surgery. *J Bone Joint Surg* 56B:225, 1974.

38. Dommisse GF, Enslin TB: Hodgson's circumferential osteotomy in the correction of spinal deformity. *J Bone Joint Surg* 52B:778, 1970.

39. Drummond D, Guadagni J, Keene JS, *et al:* Interspinous process segmental spinal instrumentation. *J Pediatr Orthop* 4:397, 1984.

40. Dubousset J, Herring JA, Shufflebarger HL: The crankshaft phenomenon. *J Pediatr Orthop* 9:541, 1989.

41. Dwyer AF, Newton NC, Sherwood AA: An anterior approach to scoliosis: A preliminary report. *Clin Orthop* 62:192, 1969.

42. Edmonds HL, Paloheimo MP, Backman MH, *et al:* Transcranial magnetic motor evoked potentials (tcMMEP) for functional monitoring of motor pathways during scoliosis surgery. *Spine* 14:683, 1989.

43. Eingorn D, Pizzutillo PD: Pars interarticularis fusion in multiple levels of lumbar spondylolysis. A case report. *Spine* 10:250, 1985.

44. Ellitsgaard N, Andersson AP, Jensen KV, Jorgensen M: Changes in C-reactive protein and erythrocyte sedimentation rate after hip fractures. *Int Orthop* 15:311, 1991.

45. Farcy JP, Weidenbaum M, Glassman SD: Sagittal index in management of thoracolumbar burst fractures. *Spine* 15:958, 1990.

46. Feffer HL, Wiesel SW, Cuckler JM, Rothman RH: Degenerative spondylolisthesis. To fuse or not to fuse. *Spine* 10:287, 1985.

47. Ferguson RJ, McMaster JH, Stanitski CL: Low back pain in college football linemen. *J Sports Med* 2:63, 1975.

48. Fiore SM: Anterior spinal instrumentation. In Holt RT (ed): *Spine: State-of-the-Art Reviews,* vol 6, no 2. Philadelphia, Hanley & Belfus, 1992, p 311.

49. Fredrickson BE, Baker D, McHolick WJ, *et al:* The natural history of spondylolysis and spondylolisthesis. *J Bone Joint Surg* 66A:699, 1984.

50. Gagnon S, Jodoin A, Martin R: Pulmonary function test study and after spinal fusion in young idiopathic scoliosis. *Spine* 14:486, 1989.

51. Gaines RW, Nichols WK: Treatment of spondyloptosis by two stage L5 vertebrectomy and reduction of L4 onto S1. *Spine* 10:680, 1985.

52. Garfin SR, Yuan HA, Reiley MA: New technologies in spine: Kyphoplasty and vertebroplasty for the treatment of painful osteoporotic compression fractures. *Spine* 26(14):1511, 2001.

53. Gelb DE, Lenke LG, Bridwell KH, *et al:* An analysis of sagittal spinal alignment in 100 asymptomatic middle and older age volunteers. *Spine* 20:1351, 1995.

54. Gerscovich EO, Greenspan A, Montesano PX: Treatment of kyphotic deformity in ankylosing spondylitis. *Orthopedics* 17:335, 1994.

55. Gertzbein SD, Harris MB: Wedge osteotomy for the correction of post-traumatic kyphosis. A new technique and a report of three cases. *Spine* 17:374, 1992.

56. Glassman SD: Hook pattern selection in the treatment of spinal deformity. In Holt RT (ed): *Spine: State of the Art Reviews,* vol 6, no 2. Philadelphia, Hanley & Belfus, 1992, p 331.

57. Glassman SD, Dimar JR, Puno RM, *et al:* A prospective analysis of intraoperative EMG monitoring of pedicle screw placement with CT scan confirmation. *Spine* 20:1375, 1995.

58. Glassman SD, Farcy JPC: Late deformities. In Floman Y, Farcy JPC, Argenson C (Eds): *Thoracolumbar Spine Fractures.* New York, Lippincott-Raven, 1993, p 449.

59. Glassman SD, Nazar GB, Dimar JR *et al:* Neurogenic scoliosis in children. *J Ky Med Assoc* 92:19, 1994.

60. Graziano GP, Hensinger RN: Treatment of congenital lumbar lordosis in adults with a one-stage single-level anterior closing-wedge osteotomy. A report of two cases. *J Bone Joint Surg* 77A:1095, 1995.

61. Grubb SA, Lipscomb HJ: Diagnostic findings in painful adult scoliosis. *Spine* 17:518, 1992.

62. Grubb SA, Lipscomb HJ, Coonrad RW: Degenerative adult-onset scoliosis. *Spine* 13:241, 1998.

63. Gugino LD, Aglio LS, Segal ME, *et al:* Use of transcranial magnetic stimulation for monitoring spinal cord motor pathways. *Semin Spinal Surg* 9:315, 1997.

64. Hall JE, Gray J, Allen B: Current concepts: Dwyer instrumentation in anterior fusion of the spine. *J Bone Joint Surg* 59B:117, 1977.

65. Hanley EN Jr, Levy JA: Surgical treatment of isthmic lumbosacral spondylolisthesis. Analysis of variables influencing results. *Spine* 14:48, 1989.

66. Hardouin P, Fayada P, Leclet H, Chopin D: Kyphoplasty. *Joint Bone Spine* 69(3):256, 2002.

67. Harrington PR: Treatment of scoliosis. Correction and internal fixation by spine instrumentation. *J Bone Joint Surg* 44A:591, 1962.

68. Harrington PR: Technical details in relation to the successful use of instrumentation in scoliosis. *Orthop Clin North Am* 3:49, 1972.

69. Harrington PR: The history and development of Harrington instrumentation. *Clin Orthop* 93:110, 1973.

70. Haughton PR, Tullos HS: Spondylolisthesis in children. Observations and surgical treatment. *Clin Orthop* 79:75, 1971.

71. Healey JH, Lane JM: Structural scoliosis in osteoporotic women. *Clin Orthop* 195:216, 1985.

72. Herkowitz HN, Kurz LT: Degenerative lumbar spondylolisthesis with spinal stenosis. A prospective study comparing decompression with decompression and intertransverse process arthrodesis. *J Bone Joint Surg* 73A:802, 1991.

73. Herndon WA, Sullivan YA, Yngve DA, *et al:* Segmental spinal instrumentation with sublaminar wires. A critical appraisal. *J Bone Joint Surg* 69A:851, 1987.

74. Herron LD, Trippi AC: L4-5 degenerative spondylolisthesis. The results of treatment by decompressive laminectomy without fusion. *Spine* 14:534, 1989.

75. Holt RT, Johnson JR, Eldridge JC, Peress RE: An analysis of 107 cases of single stage anterior and posterior spine surgery. *Orthop Trans* 14:798, 1990.

76. Holt RT, Senter BS: Postoperative spinal infection. In Holt RT (ed): *Spine: State-of-the-Art Reviews,* vol 6, no 2. Hanley & Belfus, Philadelphia, 1992, p 389.

77. Horton WC, Holt RT, Johnson JR, Leatherman KD: Zielke instrumentation in idiopathic scoliosis: Late effects and minimizing complications. *Spine* 13:1145, 1988.

78. Jackson DW, Wiltse LL, Cirincione RJ: Spondylolysis in the female gymnast. *Clin Orthop* 117:68, 1976.

79. James JI: Idiopathic scoliosis. The prognosis, diagnosis, and operative indications related to curve patterns and the age at onset. *J Bone Joint Surg* 36B:36, 1954.

80. Jeng CL, Sponseller PD, Tolo VT: Outcome of Wisconsin instrumentation in idiopathic scoliosis. Minimum 5-year follow-up. *Spine* 18:1584, 1993.

81. Johnson JR, Holt RT: Combined use of anterior and posterior surgery for adult scoliosis. *Orthop Clin North Am* 19:361, 1988.

82. Johnson JTH, Robinson RA: Anterior strut grafts for severe kyphosis. Results of 3 cases with a preceding progressive paraplegia. *Clin Orthop* 56:25, 1968.

83. Johnson LP, Nasca RJ, Dunham WK: Surgical management of isthmic spondylolisthesis. *Spine* 13:93, 1988.

84. Kaneda K, Abumi K, Fujiya M: Burst fractures with neurologic deficits of the thoracic-lumbar spine. Results of anterior decompression and stabilization with anterior instrumentation. *Spine* 9:788, 1984.

85. Kaneda K, Fujiya N, Satoh S: Results with Zielke instrumentation for idiopathic thoracolumbar and lumbar scoliosis. *Clin Orthop* 205:195, 1986.

86. Kao-Wha C: Oligosegmental correction of post-traumatic thoracolumbar angular kyphosis. *Spine* 18:1909, 1993.

87. King HA, Moe JH, Bradford DS, Winter RB: The selection of fusion levels in thoracic idiopathic scoliosis. *J Bone Joint Surg* 65A:1302, 1983.

88. Kostuik JP: Anterior spinal cord decompression for lesions of the thoracic and lumbar spine, techniques, new methods of internal fixation results. *Spine* 8:512, 1983.

89. Kostuik JP: Anterior fixation for fractures of the thoracic and lumbar spine with or without neurologic involvement. *Clin Orthop* 189:103, 1984.

90. Kostuik JP: Anterior Kostuik-Harrington distraction systems for the treatment of kyphotic deformities. *Spine* 15:169, 1990.

91. Kostuik JP, Carl A, Ferron S: Anterior Zielke instrumentation for spinal deformity in adults. *J Bone Joint Surg* 71A:898, 1989.

92. Kostuik JP, Israel J, Hall JE: Scoliosis surgery in adults. *Clin Orthop* 93:225, 1973.

93. Kostuik JP, Matsusaki H: Anterior stabilization, instrumentation, and decompression for post-traumatic kyphosis. *Spine* 14:379, 1989.

94. La Chapelle EH: Osteotomy of the lumbar spine for correction of kyphosis in a cast of ankylosing spondylarthritis. *J Bone Joint Surg* 28:851, 1945.

95. Laroche M, Delisle MB, Aziza R *et al:* Is camptocormia a primary muscular disease? *Spine* 20:1011, 1995.

96. Laurent LE, Osterman K: Operative treatment of spondylolisthesis in young patients. *Clin Orthop* 117:85, 1976.

97. Lebwohl NH, Calancie B: Perioperative neurologic deficit: Surgical practices and intraoperative monitoring. In Holt RT (ed): *Spine: State of the Art Reviews,* vol 6, no 2. Philadelphia, Hanley & Belfus, 1992, p 403.

98. Lenke LG, Bridwell KH, Baldus C, *et al:* Cotrel-Dubousset instrumentation for adolescent idiopathic scoliosis. *J Bone Joint Surg* 74A:1056, 1992.

99. Lewonowski K, King JD, Nelson MD: Routine use of magnetic resonance imaging in idiopathic scoliosis patients less than eleven years of age. *Spine* 17(Suppl 6):S109, 1992.

100. Lin JT, Lane JM: Nonmedical management of osteoporosis. *Curr Opin Rheumatol* 14(4):441, 2002.

101. Linden RD, Johnson JR, Shields CB, *et al:* Intraoperative spinal cord monitoring with motor evoked potentials elicited by transcranial magnetic stimulation. In Bridwell KH, Dewald RL (eds): *The Textbook of Spinal Surgery,* ed 2. Philadelphia, Lippincott-Raven, 1997.

102. Linville DA 2nd: Vertebroplasty and kyphoplasty. *South Med J* 95(6):583, 2002.

103. Lombardi JS, Wiltse LL, Reynolds J, *et al:* Treatment of degenerative spondylolisthesis. *Spine* 10:821, 1985.

104. Lonstein JE, Winter RB: Adolescent idiopathic scoliosis. Nonoperative treatment. *Orthop Clin North Am* 19:239, 1988.

105. Lorenz M, Zindrick M, Schwaegler P, *et al:* A comparison of single-level fusions with and without hardware. *Spine* 16(Suppl 8):S455, 1991.

106. Lowe J, Schachner E, Hirschberg E, *et al:* Significance of bone scintigraphy in symptomatic spondylolysis. *Spine* 9:653, 1984.

107. Lusins JO, Elting JJ, Cicoria AD, Goldsmith SJ: SPECT evaluation of lumbar spondylolysis and spondylolisthesis. *Spine* 19:608, 1994.

108. Malcolm BW: Spinal deformity secondary to spinal injury. *Orthop Clin North Am* 10:943, 1979.

109. Malcolm BW, Bradford DS, Winter RB, Chou SN: Post-traumatic kyphosis. A review of forty-eight surgically treated patients. *J Bone Joint Surg* 63A:891, 1981.

110. Markwalder T-M, Battaglia M: Failed back-surgery syndrome. Part I: Analysis of the clinical presentation and results of testing procedures for instability of the lumbar spine in 171 patients. *Acta Neurochir Wien* 123:46, 1993.

111. Mason DE, Carango P: Spinal decompensation in Cotrel-Dubousset instrumentation. *Spine* 16 (Suppl 8):S394, 1991.

112. McGuire RA, Amundson GM: The use of primary internal fixation in spondylolisthesis. *Spine* 18:1662, 1993.

113. Meyerding HW: Spondylolisthesis. *Surg Gynecol Obstet* 54:371, 1932.

114. Moe JH, Denis F: The iatrogenic loss of lumbar lordosis. *Orthop Trans* 1:131, 1972.

115. Moe JH, Valuska JW: Evaluation of treatment of scoliosis by Harrington instrumentation. *J Bone Joint Surg* 48A:1656, 1966.

116. Montgomery DM, Fischgrund JS: Passive reduction of spondylolisthesis on the operating room table: A prospective study. *J Spinal Disord* 7:167, 1994.

117. Mustard RA Jr, Bohnen JM, Haseeb S, Kasina R: C-(S65) reactive protein levels predict postoperative septic complications. *Arch Surg* 122:69, 1987.

118. O'Brien JP, Mehdian H, Jaffray D: Reduction of severe lumbosacral spondylolisthesis. A report of 22 cases with a ten-year follow-up period. *Clin Orthop* 300:64, 1994.

119. Osterman K, Schlenzka D, Poussa M, et al: Isthmic spondylolisthesis in symptomatic and asymptomatic subjects, epidemiology, and natural history with special reference to disk abnormality and mode of treatment. *Clin Orthop* 297:65, 1993.

120. Otain K, Satomi K, Fujimura Y, et al: Spinal osteotomy to correct kyphosis in spinal tuberculosis. *Int Orthop* 3:229, 1979.

121. Owen JH, Kostuik JR, Gornet M, et al: The use of mechanically elicited electromyograms to protect nerve roots during surgery for spinal degeneration. *Spine* 19:1704, 1994.

122. Owen JH, Laschinger J, Bridwell K, et al: Sensitivity and specificity of somatosensory and neurogenic-motor evoked potentials in animals and humans. *Spine* 13:1111, 1988.

123. Padberg AM, Bridwell KH: Disorders of the pediatric and adolescent spine: Spinal cord monitoring current state of the art. *Orthop Clin North Am* 30(3):407, 1999.

124. Petraco DM, Spivak JM, Cappadona JG et al: An anatomic evaluation of L5 nerve stretch in spondylolisthesis reduction. *Spine* 21:1133, 1996.

125. Phalen GS, Dickson JA: Spondylolisthesis and tight hamstrings. *J Bone Joint Surg* 43A:505, 1961.

126. Pritchett JW, Bortel DT: Degenerative symptomatic lumbar scoliosis. *Spine* 18:100, 1993.

127. Richards SB, Birch JG, Herring JA, et al: Frontal plane and sagittal plane balance following Cotrel-Dubousset instrumentation for idiopathic scoliosis. *Spine* 14:733, 1989.

128. Roberson JR, Whitesides TE Jr: Surgical reconstruction of late post-traumatic thoracolumbar kyphosis. *Spine* 10:307, 1985.

129. Saraste H: Spondylolysis and spondylolisthesis. *Acta Orthop Scand Suppl* 251:84, 1993.

130. Schwartz DM, Sestokas AK, Turner LA, et al: Neurophysiological identification of iatrogenic neuronal injury during complex spinal surgery. *Semin Spine Surg* 10:242, 1998.

131. Schwend RM, Waters PM, Hey LA, et al: Treatment of severe spondylolisthesis in children by reduction and L4-S4 posterior segmental hyperextension fixation. *J Pediatr Orthop* 12:703, 1992.

132. Seitsalo S, Osterman K, Hyvarinen H, et al: Progression of spondylolisthesis in children and adolescents. A long-term follow-up of 272 patients. *Spine* 16:417, 1991.

133. Seitsalo S, Osterman K, Poussa M, Laurent LE: Spondylolisthesis in children under 12 years of age: Long-term results of 56 patients treated conservatively or operatively. *J Pediatr Orthop* 8:516, 1988.

134. Semon RL, Spengler D: Significance of lumbar spondylolysis in college football players. *Spine* 6:172, 1981.

135. Shufflebarger HL, Clark CE: Prevention of the crankshaft phenomenon. *Spine* 16(Suppl 8):S409, 1991.

136. Shufflebarger HL, Grimm JO, Bui V, Thomson JD: Anterior and posterior spinal fusion. Staged versus same-day surgery. *Spine* 6:930, 1991.

137. Simper LB: Spondylolysis in Eskimo skeletons. *Acta Orthop Scand* 57:78, 1986.

138. Smith-Peterson MN, Larson CB, Aufranc OE: Osteotomy of the spine for correction of flexion deformity in rheumatoid arthritis. *J Bone Joint Surg* 271, 1945.

139. Steiner ME, Micheli LJ: Treatment of symptomatic spondylolysis and spondylolisthesis with the modified Boston brace. *Spine* 10:937, 1985.

140. Streitz W, Brown JC, Bonnett CA: Anterior fibular strut grafting in the treatment of kyphosis. *Clin Orthop* 128:140, 1977.

141. Swank S, Lonstein JE, Moe JH, et al: Surgical treatment of adult scoliosis. A review of two hundred and twenty-two cases. *J Bone Joint Surg* 63A:268, 1981.

142. Thelander U, Larsson S: Quantitation of C-reactive protein levels and erythrocyte sedimentation rate after spinal surgery. *Spine* 17:400, 1992.

143. Theodorou DJ, Theodorou SJ, Duncan TD, et al: Percutaneous balloon kyphoplasty for the correction of spinal deformity in painful vertebral body compression fractures. *Clin Imaging* 26(1):1, 2002.

144. Thomasen E: Vertebral osteotomy for correction of kyphosis in ankylosing spondylitis. *Clin Orthop* 194:142, 1985.

145. Thompson GH, Wilber RG, Shaffer JW, et al: Segmental spinal instrumentation in idiopathic scoliosis. A preliminary report. *Spine* 10:623, 1985.

146. Thompson JD, Renshaw TS: Analysis of lumbar lordosis in posterior spine fusions for idiopathic scoliosis. *J Spinal Disord* 2:93, 1989.

147. Thompson JP, Transfeldt EE, Bradford DS, et al: Decompensation after Cotrel-Dubousset instrumentation of idiopathic scoliosis. *Spine* 15:927, 1991.

148. Tonino A, Van der Werf G: Direct repair of lumbar spondylolysis. 10-year follow-up of 12 previously reported cases. *Acta Orthop Scand* 65:91, 1994.

149. Transfeldt EE, Lonstein JE: Wound infections in elective reconstructive spinal surgery. *Orthop Trans* 9:128, 1985.

150. Transfeldt EE, White D, Bradford DS, Roche B: Delayed anterior decompression in patients with spinal cord and cauda equina injuries of the thoracolumbar spine. *Spine* 15:957, 1990.

151. Turi M, Johnston CE II, Richards BS: Anterior correction of idiopathic scoliosis using TSRH instrumentation. *Spine* 18:417, 1993.

152. Van Dam BE: Nonoperative treatment of adult scoliosis. *Orthop Clin North Am* 19:347, 1988.

153. Van Dam BE, Bradford DS, Lonstein JE, *et al:* Adult idiopathic scoliosis treated by posterior-spinal fusion and Harrington instrumentation. *Spine* 12:32, 1987.

154. Van den Oever M, Merrick MV, Scott JH: Bone scintigraphy in symptomatic spondylolysis. *J Bone Joint Surg* 69B:453, 1987.

155. Weinstein SL, Ponseti IV: Curve progression in idiopathic scoliosis. *J Bone Joint Surg* 65A:447, 1983.

156. Whitesides TE Jr: Traumatic kyphosis of the thoracolumbar spine. *Clin Orthop* 128:79, 1977.

157. Wilber RG, Thompson GH, Shaffer JW, *et al:* Postoperative neurological deficits in segmental spinal instrumentation. A study using spinal cord monitoring. *J Bone Joint Surg* 66A:1178, 1984.

158. Wiltse LL: Etiology of spondylolisthesis. *Clin Orthop* 10:48, 1957.

159. Wiltse LL, Newman PH, Macnab I: Classification of spondylolysis and spondylolisthesis. *Clin Orthop* 117:23, 1976.

160. Winter RB, Lonstein JE, Denis F: Pain patterns in adult scoliosis. *Orthop Clin North Am* 19:339, 1988.

161. York DH, Chabot RJ, Gaines RW: Response variability of somatosensory evoked potentials during scoliosis surgery. *Spine* 12:864, 1987.

162. Zdeblick TA: A prospective randomized study of lumbar fusion. Preliminary results. *Spine* 18:983, 1993.

163. Zdeblick TA: Z-plate anterior thoracolumbar instrumentation. In Errico TJ (ed): *Spine: State of the Art Reviews,* vol 8, no 2. Philadelphia, Hanley & Belfus, 1994, p 433.

164. Zielke K, Pellin B: Neue instrumente und implantate zur erganzung des Harrington-systems. *Z Orthop* 114:534, 1976.

165. Zielke K, Stunkat R, Beaujean F: Ventrale derotations: Spondylodese. Vorlaufigen ergebnisbericht über 26 operierte falle. *Arch Orthop Unfallchir* 85:257, 1976.

CHAPTER 65

Pediatric Spinal Deformities

Christopher I. Shaffrey, Gregory C. Wiggins,* and Mark F. Abel

In the pediatric age group, spinal deformity results from congenital anomalies, neuromuscular disorders, neurofibromatosis, connective tissue disorders, skeletal dysplasia (including dwarfing syndromes) as well as developmental (idiopathic) causes.[15,125] Idiopathic scoliosis, the most common deformity, is a diagnosis made after excluding generalized syndromes and congenital or inflammatory causes. In a university hospital pediatric spine practice, operative cases include patients with idiopathic scoliosis (about 25%) and neuromuscular and syndrome-related spinal deformities (about 30%), the remainder being patients with congenital deformities, neoplasms, trauma, or inflammatory conditions.

Each category of spinal deformity has a characteristic behavior that is dictated by the pathophysiology of the underlying condition. Scoliosis associated with cerebral palsy differs from idiopathic scoliosis that develops in an adolescent. This chapter describes the principles of treating pediatric spinal deformities, emphasizing congenital and idiopathic scoliosis. The discussion focuses on the evaluation, treatment, and potential complications of thoracic and lumbar deformities. Cervical, craniocervical, and dysraphic anomalies (sacral dysgenesis and meningomyelocele) are covered in other chapters. The terminology of spinal deformities, adopted by the Scoliosis Research Society, is used throughout this chapter (Appendix 65.1). Box 65.1 lists some categories of spinal deformities.

General Features

Scoliosis, kyphosis, and lordosis refer to deviations from normal spinal alignment. In the frontal plane, the spine is normally straight. In the sagittal plane, the thoracic region is kyphotic (range, 20 to 40 degrees), the lumbar region is lordotic, and the transition over the thoracolumbar region is relatively straight (Figure 65.1).[11] Scoliosis, curvature in the coronal plane, is also associated with transverse rotation, as well as with pathologic lordosis or kyphosis (Figure 65.2).[11,34-36,40,44] Therefore the descriptive terms *lordoscoliosis* and *kyphoscoliosis* are frequently used to characterize the three-dimensional character of the deformity. When more than one pathologic curvature exists along the length of the spine, the primary (or major) curve is designated on the basis of its size and rigidity. The secondary (or minor) curve(s), even if compensatory, may be rigid or have a "structural" component. Surgical planning must take into account the magnitude and flexibility of all the curves in all three planes.[8,16,45,69,112]

A radiographic classification of scoliosis, based on the location of the apical vertebra, designates cervical curves as having an apex between C1 and C6; cervicothoracic curves, an apex between C7 and T1; thoracic curves, an apex between T2 and T11; thoracolumbar curves, an apex between T12 and L1; lumbar curves, an apex between L2 and L4; and lumbosacral curves, an apex between L5 and S1.[13] The direction of the apex, whether right or left, is given, as is the diagnostic category, if known. Serial radiographs with measurements of scoliosis, kyphosis, and rotation are used to evaluate progression and the effect of treatment (Figure 65.3).[82,95,99,105] Myelography has largely been replaced by magnetic resonance imaging (MRI) to evaluate the spinal cord and conus medullarus.[14,111] Furthermore, the location of the kidneys and the disc interspace signal can be assessed with MRI. Software programs that examine computed tomography (CT) data and render three-dimensional images of the spine in any plane may have a place, along with radiographic tomography, for analyzing complex deformities. These imaging techniques define the shape of the involved and adjacent vertebrae, the anatomy of the individual segments, the spinal canal size, and the location of the neural elements. Treatments, which include bracing and surgery, are indicated for progressive deformity or for deformities that are destined to progress. However, the type of treatment is ultimately determined by the diagnosis and severity of the condition.*

Growth of the Spine

Pediatric spine deformities are usually not noticeable at birth. However, they all progress in proportion to spinal growth.[39,82,84] Therefore, anticipating and controlling the growth potential of the vertebral elements composing the deformity is the key to successful management. Diligent follow-up with concomitant radiographic analysis is critical to document progression and the need for intervention. Growth data have been studied extensively in relation to idiopathic scoliosis.[39] Two periods of rapid growth occur in children: (1) between birth and 3 years and (2) during the adolescent years. The timing and duration of the adolescent growth spurt can be determined by monitoring the growth velocity (Figure 65.4). According to Demiglio, in the adolescent growth spurt the thoracic spine grows 1.2 cm per year, whereas the lumbar spine grows 0.6 cm per year.[39] From these data one can calculate the effect of fusing spinal segments during puberty. However, the scoliotic spine does not grow linearly. Apical vertebral growth yields further rotation, displacement, and tilting of the vertebrae. As pointed out by Winter, a short, straight spine is preferable to a spine with severe scoliosis that compromises cardiopulmonary or neurologic function.[15]

Prediction of the spinal growth surrounding the time of puberty is based on physical and radiographic

---

*The views expressed in this material are those of the authors and do not reflect the official policy or position of the U.S. Government, the Department of Defense, or the Department of the Air Force.

---

*References 15,21,22,25,48,49,51,85,97,125,129,134,139.

Scoliosis: Idiopathic, neuromuscular, congenital
Kyphosis: Congenital, Scheuermann's
Spondylolysis, spondylolisthesis
Inflammatory conditions: Neoplasms and infection
Post-traumatic deformities

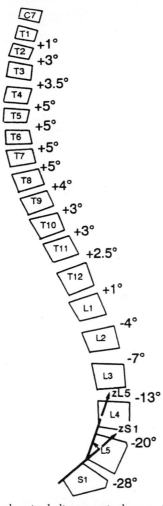

Figure 65.1 Spinal sagittal alignment is shown with the local angulation between vertebrae. Kyphosis is denoted by a positive value and lordosis by a negative value. Summation of the local angulation gives the regional kyphosis for the thoracic and lumbar spine; 40 degrees between T1 and T12 and 40 degrees between L1 and L5. (*From Bernhardt M, Bridwell KH: Segmental analysis of the sagittal plane alignment of the normal thoracic and lumbar spines and thoracolumbar junction. Spine 14:717-721, 1989, with permission.*)

examinations.[81,82] In girls, the development of pubic hair and breast buds marks the onset of the growth spurt. This corresponds to Tanner stage 2 and precedes the menarche. Skeletal age at this stage is approximately 11.5 years and can be determined radiographically from hand and wrist films.[52] The growth spurt ends at a skeletal age of 14 years, or approximately 1.5 years post menarche in girls. For boys, the onset of the growth spurts corresponds

closer to Tanner stage 3, when the pubic hair becomes curly. The skeletal age at onset is approximately 13 years and growth commonly continues until 18 years of age.

The Risser sign, another radiographic method for estimating the state of maturity, is based on the appearance and fusion of the iliac apophysis (Figure 65.5).[81,108] This apophysis begins to ossify ventrally and progresses in a dorsal direction until the entire iliac wing is capped. Finally, the apophysis fuses to the body of the ilium. The Risser stages range from 0 to 5, with stage 0 being the stage before ossification of the iliac apophysis. Stages 1 through 4 correspond to the sequential ossification of each quarter of the iliac crest, beginning with stage 1, in which ossification is present within the first 25% of the crest, and ending with stage 4, in which ossification covers 75% to 100% of the crest. The final stage (stage 5) is reached when the apophysis is closed and fused to the ilium, marking the end of growth. The appearance of the iliac ossification center signifies that puberty is under way in both boys and girls. In general, spinal growth is complete when Risser stage 4 is reached.

The estimation of the growth remaining is an integral part of planning all aspects of treatment for pediatric spinal deformities. Maintaining a growth rate chart is the ideal means of monitoring growth, but this is applicable only to the patient who presents early. Otherwise, the surgeon should consider physical findings such as the Tanner stage, in conjunction with historical information regarding the onset of menarche or the appearance of axillary hair in boys.[39,81]

Idiopathic Scoliosis: Early Onset and Adolescent Onset

Epidemiology and Classification

Idiopathic scoliosis has a familial tendency and a bimodal frequency distribution.[143] There is an early-onset variety with the majority of cases occurring in infancy, and a second major peak during adolescence. Accordingly, the Scoliosis Research Society adopted a scoliosis classification that is based on the age of onset: infantile scoliosis, 0 to 3 years; juvenile scoliosis, 3 to 9 years; and adolescent scoliosis, older than 9 years.[50] By far the most common variety is adolescent idiopathic scoliosis (AIS). However, in all age groups the incidence of scoliosis among relatives far exceeds its prevalence in the general population, and for first-degree relatives of affected adolescent girls, the incidence was 12%.[143] The infantile variety has a higher incidence in boys, whereas there is a higher prevalence of juvenile and adolescent scoliosis among girls.[64,71,143]

The cause of idiopathic scoliosis is not known, and therefore, the diagnosis is not made until all other causes of scoliosis have been excluded.[53,68,81] In idiopathic scoliosis, deformity is the primary reason for referral, because patients generally do not have symptoms. Occasionally, low-grade, activity-related backache can result from lumbar curves or curves in excess of 40 degrees. Atypical cases that do not fit the usual epidemiologic and clinical profile demand further evaluation to establish a diagnosis.[127,143]

The prevalence of AIS varies depending on the magnitude of the curve used for the diagnostic criterion.[20,123]

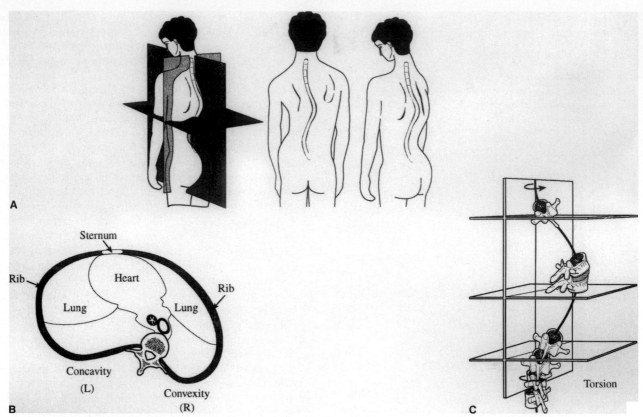

Figure 65.2 **(A)** Idiopathic scoliosis is a three-dimensional deformity, typically associated with thoracic hypokyphosis or lordosis. **(B)** Over time, the thoracic cage deforms so that the right dorsal rib angle becomes more prominent, and the left breast projects forward. **(C)** The end vertebrae of the scoliosis are most tilted, whereas the apical vertebrae are most rotated and laterally translated. Typically, a left lumbar curve is present in which the vertebrae are rotated in the opposite direction.

A curve of 10 degrees, as measured by the Cobb method, has been accepted as the lower limit to be considered diagnostic for idiopathic scoliosis. Using this diagnostic criterion, 2% to 3% of the adolescent population (10 to 16 years) has scoliosis. As the curve magnitude criterion increases, prevalence decreases. Curves in excess of 20 degrees have a prevalence of 0.3% to 0.5%, whereas the prevalence of curves in excess of 40 degrees is 0.1%. Treatment generally is not considered until curves exceed 20 degrees.

Early-onset idiopathic scoliosis, with a curve developing before the age of 8 years, is much less common but is associated with graver physiologic consequences.[144] Since curve progression is related to growth potential, the younger the patient is when the curve develops, the larger is the deformity at maturity. Curves developing before the age of 5 years have the potential of exceeding 100 degrees in magnitude, producing detrimental effects on the developing cardiopulmonary system.[41,64] Consequently, treatment approaches are recommended on the basis of patient age and magnitude of deformity.[46,110]

Adolescent Idiopathic Scoliosis
Clinical Features

Typically, AIS occurs in girls. The incidence in boys is approximately one-tenth that in girls.[40,143] The typical curve pattern is a right thoracic curve with an accompanying fractional left lumbar curve.[50,69] However, there are a variety of curve patterns. In order of frequency they include the following curves: right thoracic, left lumbar; right thoracolumbar; double thoracic; and left thoracic, right thoracolumbar.[125] The symptoms are minimal, and the patients present because of the deformity. Body asymmetry is noted, such as a trunk shift, unlevel shoulders, rib prominence, breast asymmetry, or waist asymmetry.[81] School screening has traditionally been a means of identifying these curves; however, there is no evidence that this has changed clinical outcomes.[21]

The natural history of AIS has been studied extensively by Weinstein, who followed the same group of patients for over 40 years,[123-127] and by Collis and Ponseti.[30] Before these studies, the prognosis for untreated curves was believed to be dismal because patients with all varieties of scoliosis were grouped together.[98,102] Factors that relate to progression of idiopathic curves include physiologic age, gender, curve magnitude, and curve type.[25,123] Progression is more likely in the younger patient, in girls, in patients with larger curves, and in patients with double curves. For example, a girl with a curve between 20 and 29 degrees and at a Risser stage of 0 to 1 has a 68% chance of curve progression, whereas if the Risser stage were 2 to 4, the risk is 23%.[25] During the adolescent years, curves typically progress an average of 1 degree per month and curves in

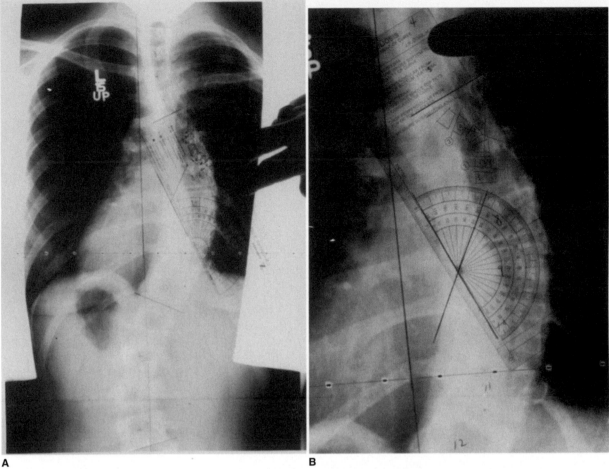

Figure 65.3 **(A)** The Cobb angle for scoliosis measurement is formed by the intersection of perpendicular lines drawn to the end plates of the most tilted vertebrae. **(B)** In this case, the Cobb angle measures 52 degrees. The same method is used for kyphosis measurement.

excess of 50 degrees have a high risk of progression even after skeletal maturity.[7,126] It is of note, however, that the relationship of symptoms to curve magnitude is not so straightforward, and many patients with severe curves have few symptoms. Lumbar curves are more likely to cause back pain. Finally, there is a significant inverse relationship between the pulmonary vital capacity and magnitude of thoracic scoliosis. Thoracic curves greater than 70 degrees are associated with a vital capacity less than that predicted for size.[1,28,127]

The physical examination should exclude other causes of scoliosis.[82,90] One should examine for skin lesions, subtle neurologic signs, body disproportions, and ligamentous laxity. The relationship of the head and trunk to the pelvis, level of the shoulders, leg length, and lateral body profile must be recorded (Figure 65.6). A major treatment objective is to center the head and trunk over the pelvis and to restore symmetry. The scoliometer or inclinometer is used to quantify the rib prominence and paralumbar prominence. A scoliometer reading greater than 5 degrees is associated with a scoliosis of at least 10 degrees. If a curve is noted, manipulation and bending can be done to assess flexibility. Finally, the physical maturity should be assessed and a Tanner rating assigned in order to determine the years of growth remaining. Maturation level is further cor-

roborated by historical information (about menarche) and radiographic analysis.

Atypical presentations demanding further evaluation with MRI include left thoracic curves, curves progressing more rapidly than expected, and curves associated with neurologic findings (Figure 65.7).[111] The neurologic findings may be subtle, such as asymmetric reflexes or absent abdominal (umbilical) reflexes.[90] Furthermore, the presence of pain, especially at night, suggests a diagnosis other than idiopathic scoliosis (Figure 65.8).

Radiographic Assessment

Standing radiographs should be obtained using a 36-inch film (long cassette) to include the cervicothoracic junction down to the middle of the pelvis.[82] Films are obtained in the posteroanterior (PA) direction to reduce radiation of the breasts. For the initial examination, frontal and sagittal (lateral) radiographs should be obtained to assess the deformity in both planes. However, subsequent films need only be in the frontal plane to limit radiation exposure unless a significant coexistent sagittal plane deformity is present. The Risser sign, the vertebral ring apophysis, and the triradiate cartilage of the acetabulum should be evaluated to help determine the amount of remaining spinal

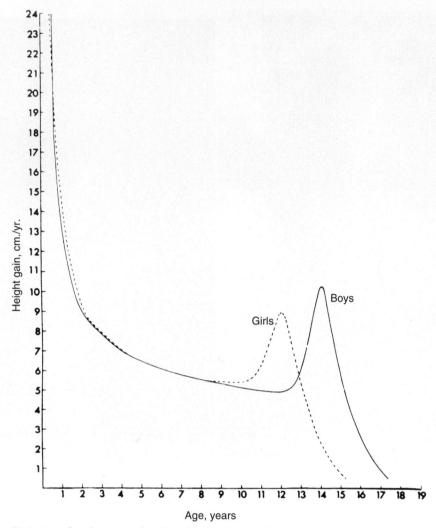

Figure 65.4 Growth velocity can be plotted by measuring height gain per year. The greatest velocity and propensity for scoliosis progression occur during the adolescent growth spurt. (*From Demiglio A: In* Moe's Textbook of Scoliosis and Other Spinal Deformities. *Philadelphia, WB Saunders, 1978, with permission.*)

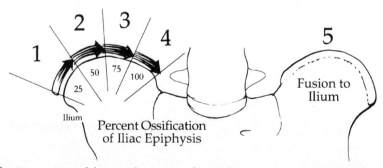

Figure 65.5 The Risser stage of iliac ossification can be used to estimate remaining maturity and growth.

growth. Once surgical treatment has been chosen, levels for instrumentation are determined by using right and left supine, side-bending films or traction films to assess the flexibility of the spine.

King *et al.*[69] developed the first important classification system for AIS on the basis of a review of frontal radiographs from 149 cases of idiopathic scoliosis. A cen-

ter sacral line was drawn on the standing PA radiographs through the center of the sacrum and perpendicular to the iliac crests. The vertebrae bisected most closely by this line were designated the *stable* vertebrae (Figure 65.9). The classification, which includes five curve patterns, is based on the number, flexibility, and deviation of the curves from the midline (Figure 65.10). Curve types

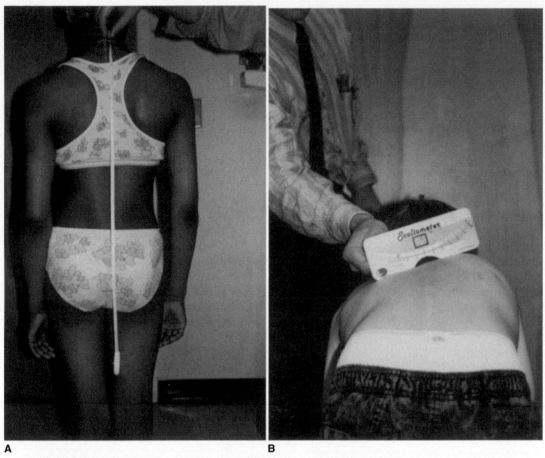

A   **B**

Figure 65.6 Body asymmetry produced by scoliosis is assessed by noting (**A**) the balance of the head and trunk over the pelvis by plumb line measurements, the level of the shoulders and iliac crests, and the definition of the waist and (**B**) the rib rotation by scoliometer (inclinometer) measurement.

I and II are double right thoracic and left lumbar curves in which the apical vertebrae of both curves are off the center sacral line. In a type I curve, the lumbar curve is dominant, meaning that it is of larger magnitude and less flexible on side bending than is the thoracic curve. In type II curves, the lumbar curve is of small magnitude than the thoracic curve and is usually more flexible. Type III and IV curves are single major thoracic or thoracolumbar curves in association with a fractional lumbar curve. Type III curves have the apex around T8 and end at L3 or higher. Type IV curves are longer so that L4 tilts into the curve. The type V curve is a double thoracic curve in which T1 tilts into the upper thoracic curve. Vertebral levels included in the fusion will depend on the deformity pattern, severity, and flexibility of the curves.

Ideally, a classification system is used to assess a clinical entity, enable surgeons to recommend treatments, and allow comparison of different treatment methods.[32] The King classification system has been used extensively. However, since it was based only on the PA radiograph, this system did not consider scoliosis as a three-dimensional deformity. Intraobserver and interobserver reliability is only poor to fair.[32,75] Lenke et al.[77] recently developed a classification system to address these issues and attempt to:

- Be comprehensive
- Consider sagittal alignment
- Define treatment standards
- Be based on objective criteria
- Have good interobserver and intraobserver reliability
- Be easily understood (Figure 65.11)

The classification system was based on standing long-cassette coronal, lateral, right and left side-bending radiographs. The curves are classified according to curve type (1 to 6) and curve flexibility combined with a lumbar spine modifier (A, B, or C) and a sagittal thoracic modifier (−, N, or +).[77] A structural proximal thoracic curve has a minimum residual coronal curve on side-bending radiographs of at least 25 degrees (with or without a positive first thoracic tilt) and/or kyphosis (from the second to the fifth thoracic level) of at least +20 degrees. A structural main thoracic curve has a minimum residual coronal curve of at least 25 degrees and/or thoracolumbar kyphosis (from the tenth thoracic to the second lumbar level) of at least +20 degrees. A structural thoracolumbar/lumbar curve also has a minimum residual coronal curve of at least 25 degrees and/or thoracolumbar kyphosis (from the tenth thoracic to the second lumbar level) of at least +20 degrees even though sagittal malalignment may be due to a rotational deformity instead of a true kyphosis. A minor curve is structural if these criteria are present.

The structural curve types are main thoracic (type 1), double thoracic (type 2), double major (type 3), triple

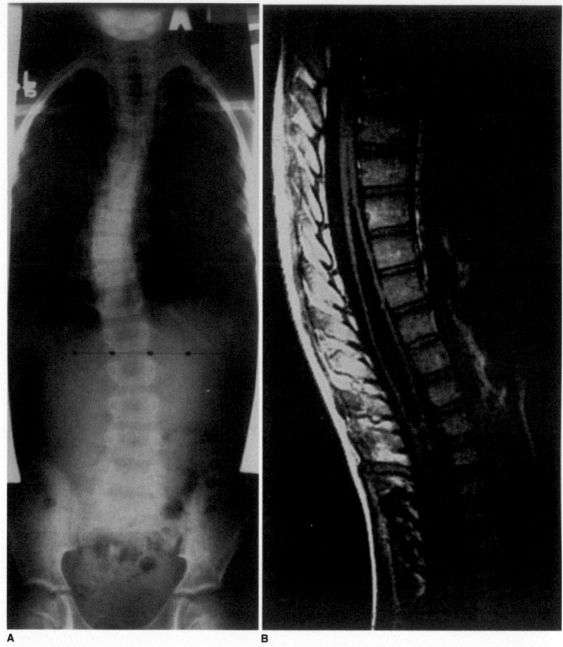

Figure 65.7 **(A)** A 10-year-old boy with a left thoracic curve has a normal neurologic examination. **(B)** Because of the atypical features (male gender and left thoracic curve) an MRI scan was obtained, uncovering a large syrinx.

major (type 4), thoracolumbar/lumbar (type 5), and thoracolumbar/lumbar main thoracic (type 6). The left and right side-bending radiographs determine which curves are structural and nonstructural. The lumbar spine modifier is determined on the basis of the relationship of the center sacral vertical line (CSVL) to the lumbar curve on the coronal radiograph. The lumbar modifiers quantify the amount of lumbar curve as A (minimal), B (moderate), and C (large). The CSVL either (A) runs through the lumbar vertebra to the stable vertebrae, (B) runs between the medial border of the lumbar concave pedicle and the concave lateral margin of the apical vertebrae, or (C) falls completely medial to the entire concave lateral aspect of the apical ver-

tebrae. The sagittal thoracic modifier describes overall thoracic kyphosis: hypokyphosis (−), a curve less than +10 degrees; normal (N), a curve +10 to +40 degrees; or hyperkyphosis (+), a curve more than +40 degrees.

The intraobserver reliability has been shown to be greater than that of the King classification.[77] The authors have proposed that only the structural curves need to be fused. In a roundtable discussion format, seven cases were presented to 28 scoliosis surgeons. There was 84% agreement on classification of the curve type, 86% agreement on lumbar modifier, and 90% agreement on thoracic modifier.[76] However, when asked to pick the proximal and distal level for fusion, the operative approaches used and levels

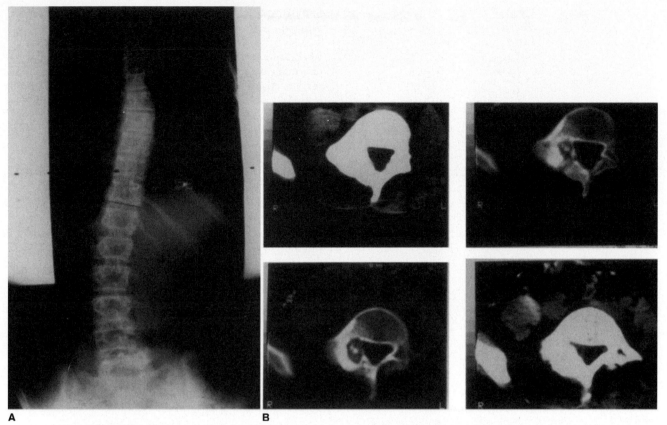

Figure 65.8 (**A**) A 13-year-old girl presented with upper back pain and a right thoracic scoliosis. (**B**) Because of the atypical history of pain, a bone scan and CT scan were obtained, revealing an osteoid osteoma in the T8 pedicle.

picked varied widely. There was an average of five different proximal and four different distal fusion levels chosen for each case.[76] This new classification system seems to address some of the shortcomings of the King classification system. Only time and more investigation will determine if using the new classification will help standardize the assessment and standardize the treatment of AIS.

Bracing for AIS

Brace treatment of AIS is recommended to minimize progression in a growing patient for curves greater than 25 degrees and less than 40 degrees.[85] Indications are listed in Box 65.2. For example, a girl in Risser stage 0 to 1 with a curve between 20 and 29 degrees has a 70% chance of progression and should be placed in a brace at presentation.[25] If a patient is followed at an earlier stage, bracing is initiated if progression (an increase of 5 degrees or more) beyond 20 degrees is documented. Adolescents with curves in excess of 45 degrees are treated surgically, because even after skeletal maturity, curves of this magnitude have a high probability of progressing.[7,126,127] However, bracing may be attempted for curves of this magnitude in juveniles, with the intent of slowing progression prior to a planned surgical procedure. The bracing is not used as a definitive treatment but rather as an attempt to obtain additional spinal growth prior to fusion. In all cases, bracing should be abandoned if the attempt to control progression of deformity fails.

If strict indications for bracing are followed, approximately 11% to 55% of braced patients progress 5 degrees or more and 3% to 25% of patients require surgery.[85] Lonstein and Winter reviewed brace treatment in 1020 patients and found 22% required surgery. In patients with a curve between 20 and 29 degrees, 51% progressed if the Risser sign was 0 to 1 but only 15% did so if the Risser sign was greater than 2. Similarly, if the curve was 30 to 39 degrees, 53% of patients with a Risser sign of 0 to 1 progressed, whereas only 25% of patients with a Risser sign greater than 2 progressed. Nevertheless, these rates of progression were less than those observed in a similar group that did not receive treatment. This series confirmed again that the more immature the patient, and the greater the curve, the more likely the progression.

A variety of braces are available, but the most extensive studies have involved the Milwaukee brace (cervicothoracolumbosacral orthosis) and the underarm brace (thoracolumbosacral orthosis) exemplified by the Boston brace.[48,85] If the apex of the curve is at T8 or lower, an underarm orthosis should suffice. A Milwaukee-type brace is needed to control curves with an apex above T8. Several studies have demonstrated that bracing for 16 to 24 hours per day throughout growth halts curve progression but does not correct the existing curve.[51] The presence of thoracic lordosis may contraindicate bracing unless it can be successfully accomplished without further compromising pulmonary function.

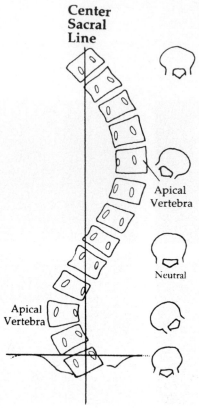

Figure 65.9 The center sacral line is the perpendicular to a horizontal line across the iliac crest, passing vertically through the sacral spinous processes. Vertebrae bisected by the center sacral line are designated as the stable vertebrae.

Early-Onset Scoliosis (Age Younger than 8 Years)
Clinical Features

Idiopathic scoliosis most commonly develops during late childhood (juvenile type) or adolescence and can create serious cosmetic and functional problems. However, pulmonary compromise is an additional concern in the rare cases of scoliosis developing before 5 years of age.[33,64] According to the study of Nilsonne and Lundgren, severe curves (greater than 100 degrees) resulted in death from cardiac or pulmonary causes in 60% of cases.[102] The significant morbidity and mortality associated with scoliosis developing before 5 years of age underscores the importance of identifying these patients early before significant symptoms develop.[64] Because idiopathic infantile scoliosis is so rare, meticulous examination of these patients and radiography are mandatory to exclude congenital or neurologic causes of the scoliosis. Routine brain stem and spinal cord MRI is reasonable for excluding central nervous system abnormalities, such as syringomyelia in patients younger than 8 years presenting with a spinal deformity of greater than 20 degrees.[111]

In comparison with adolescent and juvenile idiopathic scoliosis, the curves in infantile scoliosis are commonly (in 50% to 75% of patients) left thoracic curves, with boys more commonly affected than are girls.[64] Increased risk of curve progression is associated with double curves, large curves, and in patients with significant rotational deformity. Mehta found that risk of progression was related to the rib vertebral angle difference (RVAD).[95] This angle is formed by a line along the rib head and a perpendicular with the base of the apical vertebra (Figure 65.12). If the difference between the angles on the concave and convex side exceed 20 degrees, progression appears to be likely.[26,95]

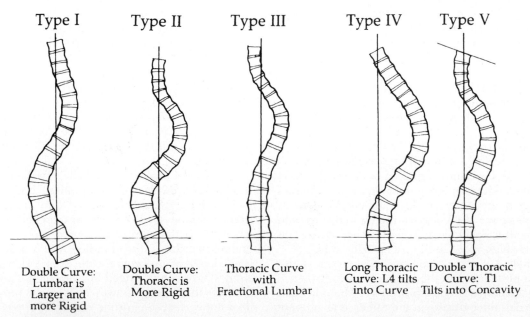

Figure 65.10 King classification for idiopathic scoliosis (*From King HA, Moe JH, Bradford DS, et al: The selection of fusion levels in thoracic idiopathic scoliosis.* J Bone Joint Surg Am 65:1302-1313, 1983, with permission.)

Curve Type

Structural criteria
(minor curves)

Proximal thoracic:
- Side bending Cobb ≥25°
- T2–T5 kyphosis ≥+20°

Main thoracic:
- Side bending Cobb ≥25°
- T10–L2 kyphosis ≥+20°

Thoracolumbar/lumbar:
- Side bending Cobb ≥25°
- T10–L2 kyphosis ≥+20°

*Major = largest Cobb measurement, always structural
Minor = all other curves with structural criteria applied

Location of apex
(SRS definition)

Curve	Apex
Thoracic	T2–T11/12 disc
Thoracolumbar	T12–L1
Lumbar	L1/2 disc–L4

Modifiers

Lumbar spine modifier	CSLV to lumbar apex
A	CSVL between pedicles
B	CSVL touches apical body(ies)
C	CSLV completely medial

Thoracic sagittal profile T5–T12	
– (hypo)	<10°
N (normal)	10°–40°
+ (hyper)	>40°

Curve type (1–6) + lumbar spine modifier (A, B, or C) + thoracic sagittal modifier (–, N, or +)

Figure 65.11 Lenke classification of adolescent idiopathic scoliosis. Synopsis of all necessary criteria for curve classification. *CSVL*, Center sacral vertical line; *SRS*, scoliosis Research Society. (*From Lenke LG, Betz RR, Harms J, et al: Adolescent idiopathic scoliosis: a new classification to determine extent of spinal arthrodesis. J Bone Joint Surg Am 83-A:1169-1181, 2001, with permission.*)

Indications for bracing in idiopathic scoliosis

Curves are 25-40 degrees and growth is remaining
Curves are progressing (increasing 5 degrees or more) above 20 degrees
Thoracolumbosacral orthosis: If curve apex is at T8 or below
Modified Milwaukee (cervicothoracolumbosacral) orthosis: If apex is above T8

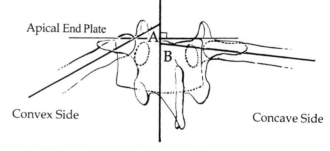

Rib-Vertebral Angles

Figure 65.12 Dorsal view of apical vertebrae from a left thoracic, infantile curve. The rib-vertebra angles are formed between a perpendicular to the vertebral end plates and a line along the corresponding rib head. If the rib-vertebra angle difference (B – A) is greater than 20 degrees, curve progression is more likely. (*Data from Mehta MH: The rib-vertebra angle in the early diagnosis between resolving and progressive infantile scoliosis. J Bone Joint Surg Br 54:230-243, 1972.*)

Treatment

Observation is a reasonable course of action until the curve reaches 30 degrees, because bracing and casting are difficult in small children.[64,93] Curves less than 35 degrees with RVAD of less than 20 degrees have a good response to bracing, whereas curves greater than 45 degrees with RVAD greater than 20 degrees have a poor prognosis for avoiding further progression and surgery.[66] If the early-onset curve fails to be halted by several attempts at casting or bracing, surgery should be considered once the curves exceed 55 to 60 degrees. Spinal instrumentation without fusion is the preferred technique for patients aged younger than 9 years. This technique involves the insertion of distraction rods along the subfascial space, with hooks placed on the end vertebrae.[41] Only the hook sites

are stripped of periosteum. Serial distraction is carried out every 6 to 9 months with the ratcheted distraction rod. The patient is protected in a brace at all times, and once adolescence is reached, a formal instrumentation and fusion is carried out. Complications with this technique are common and include hook dislodgment, rod breakage, skin breakdown, and early fusion without bone graft. Yet despite the frequent complications, subfascial instrumentation for early-onset or juvenile scoliosis is a reasonable alternative to the inevitable cardiopulmonary problems associated with curve progression. Some surgeons perform ventral discectomy over the apical segments as the initial procedure, followed by dorsal subcutaneous rod insertions.[122] This makes sense in the more severe curves and in the presence of thoracic lordosis.

Crankshaft Phenomenon

The crankshaft phenomenon has been used to explain curve progression in preadolescent patients after dorsal instrumentation and fusion.[45,46,110] Sanders et al. analyzed 43 patients with idiopathic scoliosis after dorsal instrumentation and fusion.[110] The mean age of the patients was 12.4 years at the time of fusion. Eleven patients demonstrated the crankshaft phenomenon. Of these 11 patients, 10 had open triradiate cartilages and 7 had progression of the RVAD of 10 degrees or more. The authors recommended ventral discectomy to accompany dorsal instrumentation and fusion in patients aged younger than 10 years, in older premenarchal patients who have a Risser sign of 0, or in patients in whom the triradiate cartilages are open.

In conclusion, the large amount of spinal growth remaining increases the complexity of deformity treatment in juvenile and preadolescent patients. If the curve is progressing and measures 55 to 60 degrees, fusion is preferred to allowing the curve progression. Frequently, a ventral and dorsal fusion with instrumentation is required to prevent crankshafting. Winter has pointed out that although fusion guarantees shortening of the trunk in these patients (approximately 0.1 cm per segment per year of growth), untreated scoliosis produces further curvature rather than longitudinal growth.[15,122]

Surgical Approaches to the Spine

The dorsal approach to the spine is used most commonly. The patient is positioned on a four-post scoliosis frame that allows the abdomen to hang freely, thus reducing venous pressure and bleeding (Figure 65.13). The entire back and iliac crests are prepared within the surgical field. The tissue dissection is the same along the entire length of the dorsal spine, but the orientation and configuration of the vertebrae vary and must be studied. Exposure of the spine is carried out to the tips of the transverse processes. If a hook-and-rod system is employed, hook sites are prepared after exposure. It is important to perform facetectomies and graft at all levels instrumented included any intervening uninstrumented levels before placing the rods in position, otherwise access to the facets will be blocked.

Ventral approaches differ considerably at different levels. It is wise to solicit the assistance of a thoracic or general surgeon if such procedures are not performed routinely by the spine surgeon. The ventral approach to the lumbar spine, from L2 to L5, is retroperitoneal on the convex side of the deformity. The bifurcation of the common iliac vessels, at the L4-5 disc, makes access below this level more difficult. Exposure of the L5-S1 disc space often requires a transabdominal approach. The thoracolumbar junction is approached through the bed of the tenth or eleventh rib (Figure 65.14). The diaphragm is detached and repaired after completion of the procedure. Above the diaphragm, a transpleural approach is generally employed. However, retropleural access is possible in young patients with thick parietal pleura.

Theoretically, with a retropleural approach, one can avoid using a tube thoracostomy. The thoracic spine below T4 is approached through the rib above the level of greatest concern. Approach to the cervicothoracic junction presents a challenge if a vertebrectomy is planned. Options include ventrolateral thoracotomy through the fourth rib and scapular elevation. The right side is preferred, with ligation of the azygous vein. A ventral cervical approach can be combined with a high thoracotomy or median sternotomy to expose several vertebrae at the cervicothoracic junction. The presence of the aortic arch, brachycephalic vessels, sympathetic chain, recurrent laryngeal nerve, thoracic duct, esophagus, and trachea make any wide exposure to this region a challenge.

Open ventral approaches have been the mainstay of anterior spinal surgery. Postoperative pain and pulmonary problems have led to the development of alternatives to an open ventral approach. Although thoracoscopy was first used in the 1920s, this technique was not utilized until the past 20 years.[63] Video-assisted thorascopic surgery (VATS) has widely been accepted for nonspinal surgery since the early 1980s.[37,67] The advantages of VATS include decreased morbidity, improved cosmesis, and improved shoulder girdle and chest wall muscle function.[58,73] The application of this technology to pediatric spinal deformity is relatively recent. This technology does have a significant learning curve.[101] Several studies have demonstrated that anterior release and discectomy performed either by VATS or by standard thoracotomy produce similar results on the mobility of the spine.[100,121] This is an evolving technology including new forms of segmental spinal instrumentation that can be placed thoracoscopically that has promise to minimize operative trauma while still obtaining successful anterior release, deformity correction, instrumentation, and fusion.

Instrumentation for Spinal Deformity
Surgical Treatment

Typically, surgical treatment of AIS is accomplished with dorsal instrumentation and fusion. However, if the curve exceeds 75 degrees and does not correct to 50 degrees on side-bending radiographs, a ventral approach might be considered for improving correction and for enhancing fusion by performing discectomies and releasing the anterior longitudinal ligament. Ventral approaches are also used to arrest the growth of the vertebrae in immature patients in whom progression, because of crankshafting, may be a problem (Figure 65.15). Finally, ventral instrumentation is now being considered for lumbar curves or thoracolumbar curves in order to spare lumbar motion segments (Figures 65.16 and 65.17).

Dorsal Instrumentation

Dorsal spinal instrumentation for the correction of deformity has evolved rapidly since the introduction of distrac-

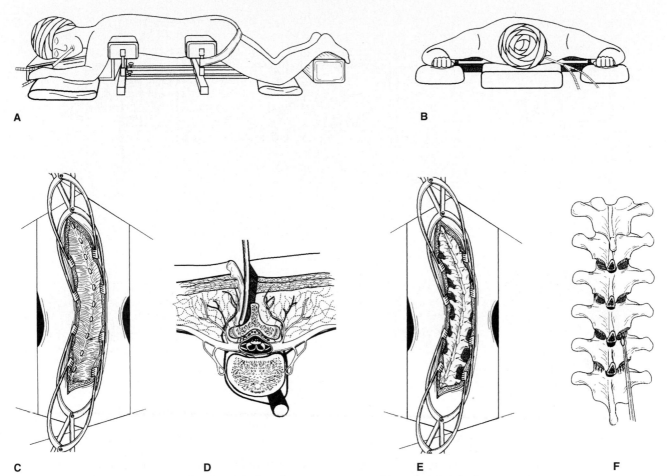

Figure 65.13 The dorsal approach to the spine is commonly employed. **(A)** The patient is positioned on a frame that allows the abdomen to hang freely and the hips to be slightly flexed. **(B)** Pressure on the eyes and axilla should be avoided. **(C)** A midline incision is made down to the spinous processes. **(D)** Elevators are used to strip subperiosteally to the tips of the transverse processes. **(E)** When the facets are exposed, hook sites are prepared, and remaining facets are grafted before rod placement.

tion rods and hooks by Harrington in 1960.[57] In this evolution the primary emphasis has been on more secure fixation and three-dimensional correction.[17,18,45,106] Surgical instrumentation systems are available from several manufacturers, and the application principles and designs share many similarities.[80,106] All employ segmental anchors linked to longitudinal elements (rods) (Figure 65.18).

There are several segmental anchor options including hooks, wires, or pedicle screws. Hooks vary in width, blade angle, and blade depth to accommodate the changes in canal dimension throughout the length of the spine. A bifid hook may be employed to gain purchase on the thoracic pedicles, whereas in other areas of the spine, the hook blade lies flat. The hook bodies may be opened or closed. The open hook design allows the rod to be placed after hooks are positioned on the strategic vertebrae. The linkage between the open hook and the rod includes sleeves, caps, bars, or eye bolts, depending on the manufacturer.

Rod diameters and strength can be varied to accommodate differences in body habitus. Rods with a diameter of ¼ inch (6.5 mm) are used in most cases. However, for small adolescents or children, ³⁄₁₆-inch rods (5.0 mm) are available. Strength varies inversely with rod diameter, but

strength can also be influenced by the manufacturing technique and metal type. As a compromise, 5.5-mm rods are available that are manufactured to provide a strength that approximates that of the 6.5-mm rods.

Rigid constructs produce more "stress shielding" of the bone, whereas smaller rods and hook designs have lower profiles and less stress shielding at the cost of reduced strength. It is emphasized that the minimum strength needed to avoid bracing, maintain correction, and minimize stress shielding has not been defined. Stainless steel has traditionally been used for rod construction, but rods made from titanium, which is stronger, lighter, and has less tissue reaction have become readily available. Titanium has the advantage of fewer artifacts on MRI so that its use in conjunction with spinal canal decompression may be preferred.

Varying amounts of rotational, tilting (coronal and sagittal), axial, and translational forces are exerted by the various segmental anchors (Figure 65.19). Therefore, the anchor can be tailored to the specific deformity and to the corrective force required. In addition, the rods are crossfixed to enhance stability of the construct and to couple the forces of the dual hook-rod constructs. The hook-rod linkage can produce coronal and sagittal plane tilting and

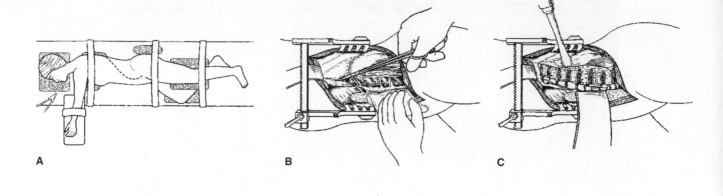

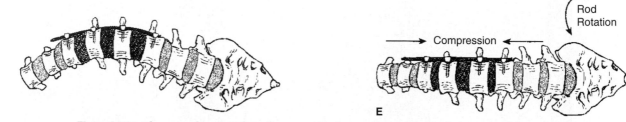

Figure 65.14 The ventral approach to the upper lumbar or thoracolumbar spine is used for discectomy or instrumentation. **(A)** A lateral decubitus position is used with the convexity up. The T11 rib is generally excised, and the retroperitoneal space is entered through its bed. **(B)** The kidney is brought ventrally, and the diaphragm is opened to expose the vertebrae. **(C)** Segmented vessels are ligated, and the psoas muscle is elevated and retracted dorsally. **(D)** A thorough discectomy is performed between the segments to be instrumented. Vertebral body screws are placed perpendicular to the vertebrae along the midlateral line, beginning with the end vertebrae. The rod is positioned within the screw head and held. **(E)** Ventral rotation of the rod converts scoliosis into lordosis and translates the apex toward the midline. The rod is then fixed within the screws, and bone graft is added between the vertebrae. Compression provides further scoliosis correction and locks the graft into place.

axial compression or distraction. Because the lamina is dorsal to the center of the vertebrae, hook compression produces lordosing forces, and conversely, hook distraction produces kyphosing forces. Hook claws (lamina-lamina, lamina-transverse process, or lamina-pedicle) provide secure fixation at the termini of the construct. Wires provide strong translational forces and are anchored through the spinous process or under the lamina.[90] The lamina is stronger and closer to the vertebral body center (instantaneous axis of rotation) than is the spinous process, so greater translational force can be exerted with sublaminar wires.[3,8,42] However, the risk of neurologic injury increases with insertion and retrieval of sublaminar wires, compared with spinous process wires.[128]

Pedicle screws can produce sagittal plane tilting, rotation, axial compression or distraction, and translation of instrumented vertebrae (see Figure 65.19). Unlike the use of pedicle hooks, some controversy surrounds the use of pedicle screws in the thoracic spine. Early reports of screw breakage, pull-out, and neurologic injury have been followed by numerous reports describing improved deformity correction compared with hooks with a comparable complication rate. At first, pedicle screws were used to anchor the caudal end of the construct in the lumbar pedicles.[9,56] As the unique complexity of pediatric thoracic pedicle anatomy has been better understood,

thoracic pedicle screws have been increasingly used to treat scoliosis (Figure 65.20)[103] Despite theoretical concerns about the risks of placement of pedicle screws in the rotated spine, several studies have shown that for properly trained spinal surgeons, thoracic pedicle screws for pediatric deformity are safe.[9,19,103,117] Biomechanically, thoracic pedicle screws have been shown to have higher pull-out strength than hooks.[78] Clinically, thoracic pedicle screws permit greater curve correction than hooks, restore thoracic kyphosis in hypokyphotic spines, and potentially decrease the number of fused levels.[79,115,116,118,119]

Deacon and Dickson are credited with the concept that scoliosis is pathologic lordosis associated with vertebral rotation; thus the term *lordoscoliosis* correctly describes the majority of thoracic curves.[35,36,40] With the three-dimensional pathoanatomy in mind, Dubousset and Cotrel introduced the technique of concave rod insertion, followed by rod rotation back to midline in order to convert the lordoscoliosis to pure thoracic kyphosis (Figure 65.21).[45] Strategic vertebrae, including the end vertebra and the rigid intermediate vertebra, were instrumented with hooks. Although conceptually correct, subsequent studies have shown that "derotation" of the vertebrae is limited.[17] Although some rotation may occur, most of the thoracic correction is achieved by distraction and apical translation.

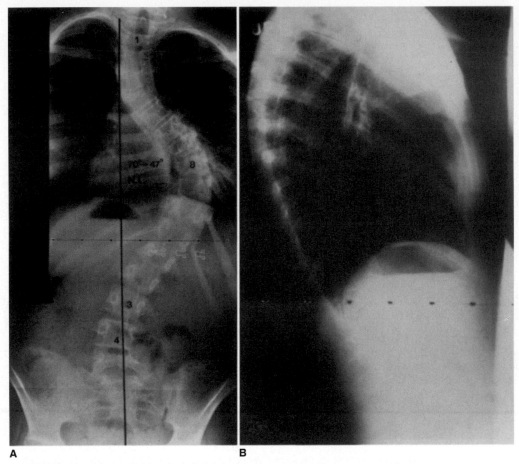

Figure 65.15 (**A**) Twelve-year-old female, Tanner stage 2, Risser stage 0, with King type V idiopathic curve pattern. The upper thoracic curve measures 45 degrees with the right shoulder down and the lower thoracic curve, 70 degrees. The stable vertebra is L3 and the neutral vertebra is T12. (**B**) Sagittal contours are relatively normal. *Continued*

Other researchers, such as the designers of the Isola instrumentation, have substituted wires as anchors for the intermediate vertebrae about the apex.[8] These developers reasoned that wires exert strong translational forces for more effective correction of the rigid apical segment. Furthermore, when wires are used to supplement hooks, hook displacement, which commonly occurs on the intermediate vertebrae, is minimized. A typical construct for AIS includes hooks at the termini, wires attached to apical vertebrae for translation, and cross-fixation to enhance stability of the construct (see Figure 65.15). Apical translation can also be achieved by using two rods on the concave side. The smaller, inner rod is attached to the intermediate vertebrae, and the outer, concave rod to the end vertebrae (Figure 65.22). A threaded connector is used to pull the inner rod to the outer rod, thus translating the apex to the midline. The Luque technique, designed for long neuromuscular curves, employs sublaminar wires and rods only (Figure 65.23). With the rod attached to the end of the spine, cantilever and translational forces are exerted to achieve correction (Figure 65.24).

In the development of spinal systems, three principles have evolved for selection of the levels to instrument and fuse: (1) Instrumentation should begin and end in the stable zone; (2) instrumentation at a junctional zone between

kyphosis and lordosis should be avoided; and, (3) the concave rod should be inserted first, if the major curve is lordotic, and distractive forces should be applied. Conversely, the convex rod is inserted first and hooks are compressed if correction of a kyphotic primary curve is desired. Some surgeons have published recommendations for the hook configuration and insertion sequences in order to correct the variety of idiopathic curve types.[8,45,112] In all cases, attempts are made to correct frontal and sagittal alignment but not at the expense of a well-balanced spine. A more successful clinical outcome results from a procedure that has a plumb line passing from the center of the C7 vertebrae through the center of the sacrum at the completion of the procedure than results from a greater degree of coronal correction but with coronal imbalance. Meticulous facetectomy, decortication, and autologous bone grafting are essential to achieve lasting correction of spinal deformities. Hardware loosening, loss of correction, pain, and rod breakage are potential problems if fusion is not achieved.

Ventral Instrumentation

At approximately the same time that Harrington developed dorsal instrumentation for scoliosis correction in the

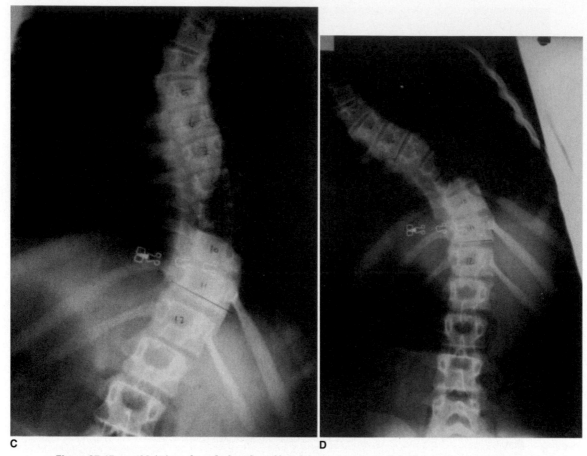

C   D

Figure 65.15 *cont'd* (C) Right side-bending film shows correction of the lower thoracic curve to 47 degrees. (D) Left side–bending film shows complete correction of the fractional lumbar curve whereas the upper thoracic curve reduces to 35 degrees. The L1-2 space opens to the right on this film.

United States, Dwyer, in Australia, developed the first ventral system.[47] Dwyer reasoned that better correction could be achieved by instrumenting the vertebral bodies after a ventral release and discectomy. Dwyer's ventral approach and the instrumentation (vertebral body screw and staple-and-cable construct) were the prototypes for other systems.[27,47] Newer systems for ventral instrumentation of scoliotic deformities use a rod and vertebral body screws. The rigidity of the rods minimizes the kyphosing tendency that was commonly observed with Dwyer's cables. These newer ventral instrumentation systems are ideally suited for a lumbar or a thoracolumbar scoliosis with a minimal or flexible thoracic curve. For this curve pattern, fusion to L4 is necessary, using the current dorsal constructs. However, powerful corrective forces can be exerted when ventral instrumentation is coupled with thorough discectomies. In most cases, one lumbar motion segment is spared with the ventral construct (see Figure 65.25).

The ventral procedure is performed via a retroperitoneal thoracolumbar approach to the curve convexity (see Figure 65.14).[47] The vertebral discs to be spanned by the instrumentation must be exposed sufficiently to allow complete removal back to the posterior longitudinal ligament. Therefore, the psoas muscle is mobilized and segmental vessels are ligated to achieve the exposure. After

discectomy, the vertebral end plates are removed to expose bleeding surfaces for fusion. Gelfoam is used temporarily after discectomy to control bleeding while the implants are inserted. The vertebral body screws vary in diameter from 5.5 to 7.0mm. Pull-out strength increases in proportion to major screw diameter and thread depth. The screws are inserted in the midlateral point of the vertebral body until a thread penetrates the far cortex to maximize holding power. Screw length can be measured before insertion, and the direction can be judged by looking across the disc space. With proper exposure, a finger can be placed on the far side of the vertebral body to avoid prominence of the tip. The end screws are placed first, followed by the intermediate screws for ease of alignment. The rod is held within the screw head and rotated to convert the scoliosis into lordosis. After rotation, the disc spaces are visibly opened ventrally. The space should be filled with bone graft. Rib graft harvested at the time of the surgical approach is the ideal bone source. Once the ventral disc spaces have been propped open, the morcellized rib is used to fill the remainder of the space. Vertebral compression and definitive tightening of the screws to the rod are then carried out to stabilize the construct. The rods vary from 4.8 to 6.5mm in diameter and are strong enough that postoperative bracing or casting may not be needed.

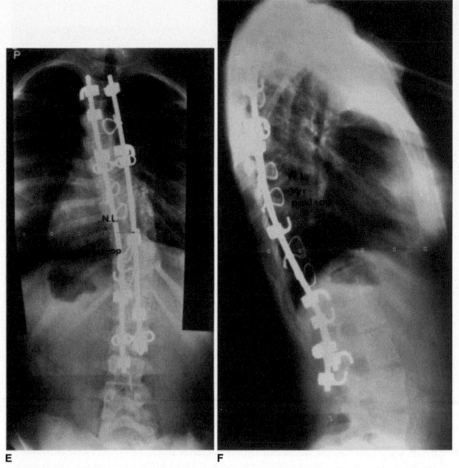

E   **F**

Figure 65.15 *cont'd* (E) Surgical correction involved ventral discectomies from T7 to T11 followed by dorsal instrumentation and fusion from T2 to L2 (using ¾₆-inch rods). Distraction was used across the concavities, apical translation with sublaminar wires and compression over the convexities. **(F)** Final correction shows balanced residual curves of 30 degrees and normal sagittal contours.

At the present time, ventral instrumentation and fusion is a commonly used option for both Lenke type 1 and Lenke type 5 curve patterns. It may also be used as an adjunct in combination with posterior transpedicular instrumentation for the treatment of more severe Lenke type 6 thoracolumbar curves to save fusion levels.

Pelvic Fixation

Fixation to the pelvis is indicated when the scoliosis extends to L5 and includes a fixed spinopelvic deformity.[141] Hook-rod constructs to achieve pelvic fixation were subject to failure because the sacral laminae were poorly developed and hook purchase on the alae was inadequate.[23,57] Currently, four techniques have evolved for instrumentation to the pelvis (Figure 65.25). The Luque-Galveston technique, developed by Allen and Ferguson, consists of contoured Luque rods placed between the cortical tables of the ilium.[4,5] Replacing the intrailiac portion of this technique with a screw and innovative rod connectors has simplified this procedure. Typically, this technique is used for neuromuscular scoliosis with significant pelvic obliquity (frontal plane) (see Figure 65.23). Because these

techniques compromise the sacroiliac joints and affect the ability to ambulate, spinopelvic fixation is rarely used for treatment of AIS. Jackson developed a technique for correction of lumbosacral kyphosis by using fixation within the cortical walls of the sacrum and S1 pedicle screws to anchor the rods to the sacrum.[114] The Dunn technique is another method for increasing sacral fixation. This is frequently utilized in patients with spinal deformity secondary to myelodysplasia and no neurological function below the L4 level. With this technique, contoured rods are passed through the S1 foramen, coming to rest on the anterior sacrum, between the internal iliac vessels.[91] This technique is especially effective in myelodysplasia because these patients frequently have osteopenic bone that precludes pedicular fixation for correction of the lumbosacral kyphosis.

Thoracoplasty

Despite the attention given to the frontal plane deformity, patients with scoliosis are often most concerned with the resultant breast and rib asymmetry. Chest wall deformities result from the transverse plane malrotation and rib

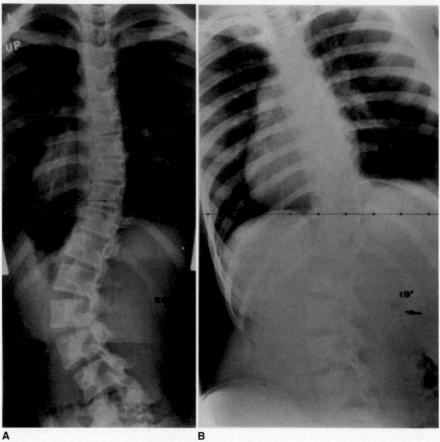

Figure 65.16 (**A**) Thirteen-year-old female with 50 degrees left lumbar idiopathic scoliosis. Vertebral ring apophyses are visible, signifying further spinal growth potential. (**B**) Left side-bending film shows the curve is flexible, correcting to 19 degrees.

dysplasia associated with scoliosis. Typically, a right dorsal rib prominence is observed with ventral projections of the left chest (see Figure 65.2). Obviously, these chest wall and rib changes are more significant in early-onset scoliosis.

Currently, thoracoplasty is an option for removing the prominent rib sections on the convex side of the thoracic scoliosis. The procedure was performed along with dorsal fusion for treatment of idiopathic scoliosis decades ago.[62] Steel reported his experience with 398 cases of thoracoplasty performed in conjunction with dorsal spinal fusion.[113] His technique is the one used most commonly. Despite his enthusiastic report, the procedure is performed more commonly after surgery, when a severe rib prominence results from the crankshaft phenomenon.[16,59] The hesitancy of surgeons in performing the procedure stems from the reported deterioration in pulmonary function observed in some patients postoperatively.[87] Owen et al.[104] found a significant reduction in pulmonary functions in a group of patients undergoing thoracoplasty together with Harrington rod insertion compared with a group that had dorsal instrumentation alone. Therefore, baseline pulmonary function should be checked before thoracoplasty, and the procedure should not be performed if the forced vital capacity is less than 60% of the predicted value. Adults, likewise, are more prone to significant pulmonary compromise after thoracoplasty. Thoracic transpedicular instrumentation has greater ability

to correct chest wall deformity that traditional hook-rod techniques. With this improved correction, the routine use of thoracoplasty is becoming less common.

The surgical approach may be performed via a midline incision or via an incision over the rib prominence. If the surgical incision is centered over the convex rib prominence, it must be long enough to reach all the ribs in the curve. An alternative approach, if done in conjunction with a dorsal spinal fusion, is to use the midline incision with flap elevation laterally to the dorsal axillary line for rib exposure. If a ventral fusion (Box 65.3) is being performed, the thoracoplasty can be performed via the thoracotomy exposure. On the average, seven ribs are excised from the dorsal axillary line to the junction with the transverse process. The excised ribs are used for bone graft if the procedure is done along with spinal fusion. Rib exposure is done by subperiosteal dissection so that the pleura is not violated. However, if the pleura is inadvertently opened, treatment requires suturing the defect and inserting a thoracostomy tube if necessary. Some surgeons advocate prophylactic thoracostomy tube insertion after thoracoplasty.

Thoracoplasty is performed primarily to address the cosmetic deformity produced by the convex rib prominence.[87] Therefore, the indications are somewhat subjective. Measurements of the chest wall deformity are generally performed with the inclinometer (scoliometer),

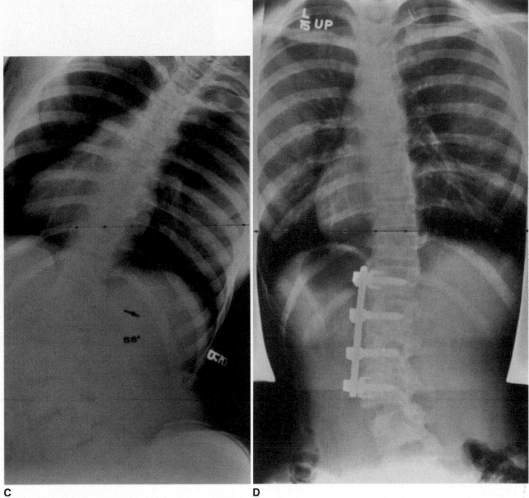

Figure 65.16 *cont'd* (C) L3-4 opens to the left on the right side-bending film. (D) Treatment consisted of ventral instrumentation from T12 to L3 using vertebral body screws and ¼-inch rods. Residual scoliosis measures 25 degrees; however, three lumbar discs were preserved.

Continued

and measurements in excess of 15 degrees are considered significant enough to warrant the procedure. In the young patient with good pulmonary function, the procedure will effectively reduce the hump back deformity, thus improving the patient's body image. These positive effects are worthwhile in carefully selected cases, provided the risks are considered and explained.

Expansion Thoracoplasty

Congenital scoliosis can also be treated with expansion thoracoplasty via lengthening of the concave hemithorax with rib distraction by means of a prosthetic rib distracter—with apparent growth of the concave side of the curve and the unilateral unsegmented bar. Campbell *et al.*[24] reported on 21 patients with congenital scoliosis and fused ribs were treated with expansion thoracoplasty by means of a vertical, expandable, titanium prosthetic rib. After expansion thoracoplasty, both the concave and the convex side of the thoracic spine and unilateral unsegmented bars appeared to grow in these patients. Although the follow-up period was

only an average of 3.3 years, the results were promising and could potentially provide a better alternative to either growth type rods or early arthrodesis.

Conclusions

The major goals of instrumentation for spinal deformities are to obtain and to maintain correction until the fusion is solid. Steps leading to a firm arthrodesis include facet excision, decortication, and onlay grafting from autologous sources if possible. Implants ultimately fail if a fusion is not achieved. Generally, dorsal instrumentation and fusion suffice for adequate correction of the coronal and sagittal plane deformities in AIS. The patient should be warned that some rotational deformity (prominence of one breast or rib prominence) might persist. If the rib prominence is severe, thoracoplasty (medial rib resection) can be performed.[87,113] A ventral release and ventral discectomy should be performed for severe curvature (greater than 75 degrees with minimal correction on bending) and in immature patients susceptible to the crankshaft phenomenon.[42,110]

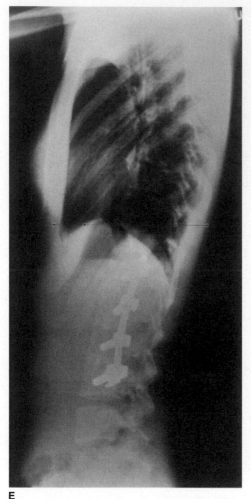

E

Figure 65.16 *cont'd* (**E**) Sagittal contours were normalized postoperatively.

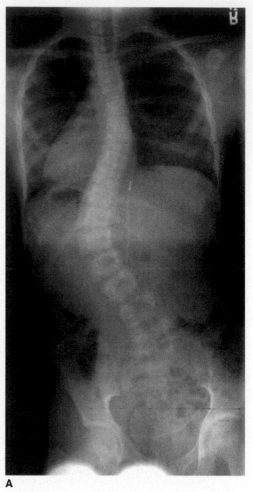

A

Figure 65.17 Sixteen-year-old female with a King type I idiopathic curve.

Congenital Spinal Deformities: Scoliosis, Kyphosis, and Lordosis
Epidemiology and Clinical Features

Congenital spinal anomalies are estimated to occur with an incidence of 0.5 to 1 per 1000 births and usually arise as sporadic cases, with a 1% chance of transmission.[129,132,137,142] However, when the spinal anomaly is a component of a multisystem anomaly, the risk of transmission rises to 5% to 10%.[142] A wide variety of associated anomalies can accompany congenital spinal deformities.[60,72,92,137,138] Renal abnormalities occur in 20% to 30% of cases. Cardiac abnormalities, which are often observed in association with chest deformities (pectus carinatum or excavatum), occur in 10% of cases.[43,60,92,137] Intraspinal anomalies, such as stenosis, diastematomyelia, and tethering of the spinal cord, occur in 5% to 35% of congenital spinal deformities. They may be signaled by the presence of dorsal midline skin lesions (such as hairy patches or deep dimples), asymmetric foot deformities (cavus or flat feet), muscle weakness, or spasticity.[14,92] Sight and hearing can also be congenitally impaired.[60] All of these systems must be thoroughly examined when a congenital spinal

deformity is discovered. Renal ultrasonography, cardiac consultation, and MRI of the entire brain stem and spinal cord are essential to the complete evaluation. The uncovered organ system defect may be more significant for the patient's well-being than is the spinal deformity. Some common syndromes that have congenital scoliosis as a feature are discussed in Chapter 4.

Radiographic and Other Imaging Evaluations

Imaging techniques are performed to determine the type and location of the vertebral anomaly, the presence of compensatory curves, the flexibility of the curves, the size of the spinal canal, and the status of the underlying nervous system elements.

Radiographs of the entire spine, including frontal and sagittal views, should be performed with the patient standing to assess trunk balance and the stable zone. Serial radiographic measurements, performed over the same vertebral levels and demonstrating a 5-degree increase, have classically been the criteria for establishing progression. Side-bending and traction views are used to assess the flexibility of the scoliotic deformity before surgical correction.[94,129] Polycycloidal tomography can be used to better characterize the size, shape, and position of the vertebral

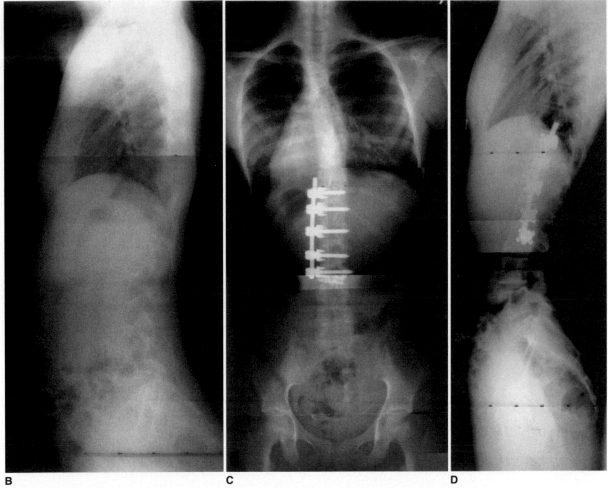

B   C   D

Figure 65.17 *cont'd* (**A**) PA and (**B**) lateral radiographs reveal a 61 degrees lumbar curve and compensatory flexible thoracic curve. (**C**) Treatment consisted of ventral release and instrumentation from T11 to L3 with near-complete correction of the lumbar curve. Three lumbar discs were preserved. (**D**) She maintained normal lumbar lordosis postoperatively.

anomaly. Computer software has been developed that renders *three-dimensional* images from CT scan data to assess spinal canal size and shape (Figure 65.26).[45] The location of a hemivertebra in the transverse plane, the length of an unsegmented bar, the status of the adjacent disc space, and the presence or absence of dorsal elements can be determined with these techniques. MRI of the entire brain stem and spinal cord has replaced myelography as a mandatory component of evaluating congenital spinal deformities for the presence of intraspinal anomalies and spinal cord impingement and for determining the relationship of neural elements to the deformity.[14,92]

Classification and Prognosis

The predominant congenital deformity usually exists as a scoliosis, kyphosis, or lordosis. However, just as with idiopathic scoliosis, most are multiplane deformities. Description of the congenital deformity should include the area of the spine involved, the type of vertebral anomaly, and the configuration of the deformity, because these factors have implications for evaluation and treatment.[94,129,137] For example, a thoracic lordoscoliosis can jeopardize the pulmonary vital capacity and may require a

combined ventral and dorsal approach, whereas a thoracic kyphoscoliosis may be treated successfully with dorsal surgery alone.[74,137] Similarly, deformities in the lumbosacral region tend to produce more trunk decompensation than do deformities higher in the spine (Figure 65.27). Thoracic and thoracolumbar kyphosis is reported to be associated with neurologic impairment at presentation in 10% to 20% of cases.[92,140] Cervical, cervicothoracic, and high thoracic anomalies produce shoulder asymmetry, head tilting, and facial flattening.

A classification system for congenital spinal deformities based on the embryologic development of the spine was refined by Winter *et al.*[137] This system allows 80% of deformities to be classified; however, for the remaining 20%, classification is obscured by the multiplicity of defects. Spinal anomalies are classified as failures of segmentation, failures of formation, and mixed anomalies (Figure 65.28). This classification provides a prognostic guide for treatment. In general, 75% of congenital scoliotic deformities progress, with the rate varying with the type.

Defects of segmentation can be unilateral or bilateral. A block vertebra is a bilateral segmentation defect that causes the spine to shorten, but it has little propensity for scoliosis progression. However, unilateral unsegmented

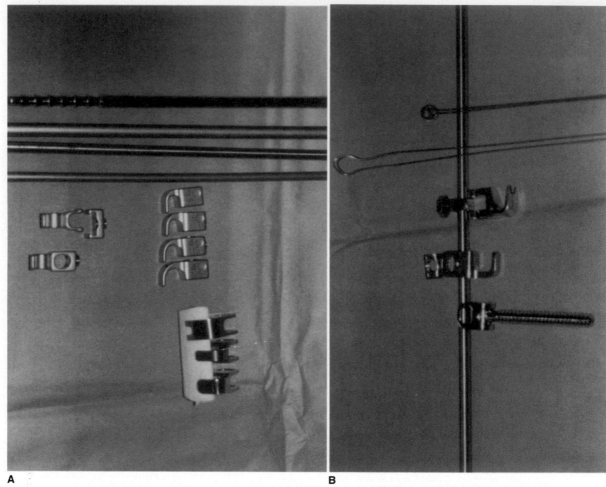

A   **B**

Figure 65.18 Spinal implants include longitudinal elements (rods) and segmental anchors (hooks, wires, and screws). **(A)** Rod sizes vary from ³⁄₁₆ inch (5.0 mm) to ¼ inch (6.25 mm). The ratcheted Harrington distraction rod is rarely used. Variations in hook designs include bifid pedicle hooks, flat laminar hooks, different body-shoe distances, and open or closed bodies. **(B)** Anchoring of vertebrae to the rod may be achieved by pedicle screws, hooks, and wires (sublaminar and spinous process).

bars have a high frequency of progressing because growth potential exists on only one side of the spine. An unsegmented bar opposite a hemivertebra has the poorest prognosis for rapid progression and should be surgically treated at an early stage to prevent severe deformity (Figure 65.29). In McMaster's series, these deformities progressed at a rate of least 6 degrees per year, and all exceeded 50 degrees by 4 years of age.[94,137] Early in the course, a segmentation defect can appear as a narrow disc space that progressively narrows with growth until fusion occurs (Figure 65.30). If growth in other parts of the spinal segment continues, scoliosis or kyphosis will develop.

Defects of formation is the other large class of congenital spinal deformities. In these cases, there is an absence or maldevelopment of a part of the spine that may produce sagittal or coronal plane deformity. Bifid or absent dorsal elements, hemivertebra, and wedge vertebrae are examples of defects of formation. When spina bifida is associated with defects of the neural elements (meningomyelocele), the spasticity and partial paralysis play a major role in the natu-

ral history of the spinal deformity. Dorsal element deficiency can be present without spinal cord dysraphism. Recognizing deficiencies of the dorsal element is important before the dorsal surgical exposures.

Hemivertebra, another type of formation failure, may involve mild wedging to complete absence of one side of the vertebra. There are four types of hemivertebra: (1) *fully segmented*, with growth plates present both rostrally and caudally: (2) *semisegmented*, with only one end plate open; (3) *unsegmented*, with fusions or slit end plates; and (4) *incarcerated*, with an ovoid, small hemivertebra tucked into the side of the spine and associated with minimal or no deformity (see Figure 65.28). Hemivertebra can occur in isolation or in association with other spinal anomalies at different levels and on different sides of the spinal column (see Figures 65.23 and 65.24). The prognosis varies and is based on the type, location, and number of hemivertebrae. In general, 25% of hemivertebrae progress rapidly, 25% do not progress, and 50% progress slowly.[94,134] The presence of open vertebral growth plates dictates the tendency to progress, so that

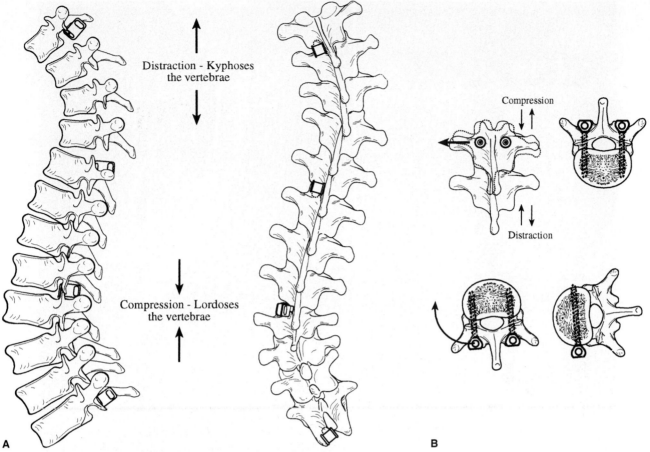

Figure 65.19 Implant-derived forces. **(A)** Distraction across the concavity corrects scoliosis and produces kyphosis. Similarly, compression across the convexity reduces scoliosis and produces lordosis. **(B)** Hooks and pedicle screws can be employed for sagittal or coronal tilting of the vertebrae as the axial force (distraction or compression) is applied. In addition, rotational forces can be exerted with pedicle and vertebral body screws.

the fully segmented hemivertebra, with a functional plate rostrally and caudally, has the greatest propensity to progress. Incarcerated and unsegmented hemivertebrae have little tendency for progression. Treatment is recommended for severe deformity or with curves greater than 30 to 40 degrees when curve progression has been documented to be 10 degrees or more.

Congenital lordosis is most commonly due to dorsal segmentation defects, whereas kyphotic deformities can result from both segmentation defects and failure of formation. A mild scoliosis frequently coexists with congenital lordosis and kyphosis. If the segmentation defect involves the dorsal and lateral side of the spinal column (dorsolateral bar), growth results in lordosis and scoliosis. Ventral bars result in progressive kyphosis and scoliosis if located to one side of the midsagittal plane. Similarly, a partial vertebra located dorsolaterally will result in a kyphoscoliosis. Kyphosis resulting from defects of formation manifests as sharper, more angulated deformities that are more likely to evolve into paraplegia, especially if dorsal elements are deficient or if the deformity is in the thoracic spine (see Figures 65.26).[134,140] Kyphosis stemming from failure of formation (hemivertebra) progresses an average of 7 degrees

per year.[140] Kyphosis resulting from segmentation failure is more rounded, but progressive deformity can still develop. Winter estimates that 95% of congenital kyphoses progress.[129,132]

Treatment

Ideally, surgical arthrodesis is performed early to prevent deformity progression, and correction becomes the goal when patients present later with a severe deformity. Obviously, prevention is preferable because procedures necessary to achieve correction are usually more complex. The surgical options include (1) dorsal fusion, (2) ventral fusion, (3) combined ventral and dorsal fusion, (4) hemivertebra excision, (5) spinal osteotomy and fusion, and (6) expansion thoracoplasty. Box 65.4 lists some intraoperative considerations. Surgical planning considerations are given in Box 65.5.

Dorsal spinal fusion is the "gold standard" for both congenital scoliosis and kyphosis. Using this approach in 290 cases, Winter arrested curve progression in 86% of cases.[138] To be successful, the dorsal arthrodesis must include the entire curve, from stable vertebra to stable vertebra. Dorsal fusion should always involve bilateral

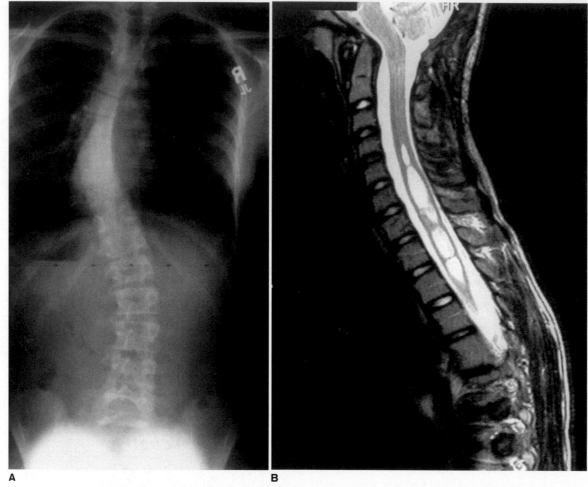

Figure 65.20 (**A**) Twelve-year-old female with King type II idiopathic curve pattern. Since she had a neurologic deficit, an MRI was performed (**B**) revealing a complex cervicothoracic syrinx. After the syrinx was treated, she underwent T4-12 instrumented fusion with pedicle screws.

facet excision, decortication of lamina and transverse processes, and onlay grafting, preferably from autogenous sources. Postoperative casting is used for 3 months to obtain correction, followed by bracing for an additional 6 to 9 months while the fusion matures. One year of postoperative casting and bracing is particularly important when dorsal fusion is under tension, for example, when it is used to treat kyphosis.

The crankshaft phenomenon or bending of the dorsal fusion mass may occur in some very young patients, younger than 5 years of age, with congenital scoliosis (see Figure 65.29).[135] Twelve of 32 patients aged younger than 5 years in Winter's series showed progression after dorsal spinal arthrodesis for congenital scoliosis. On the basis of these and similar experiences, ventral discectomy and fusions are performed with greater frequency in conjunction with dorsal fusion for congenital scoliosis in very young patients less than 5 years of age. A "wait and see" approach can be adopted after a dorsal fusion in a young patient with a mild kyphotic or scoliotic deformity. However, careful measurements of all the radiographs over the same levels must be performed at every visit to avoid the insidious progression that can occur as the fusion mass bends. When thoracic lordosis is part of the defor-

mity, ventral discectomy and fusion is recommended to avoid progressive thoracic encroachment.

Congenital Kyphosis

In mild cases of congenital kyphosis, spontaneous correction after dorsal fusion alone can occur in young patients (younger than 5 years of age) with kyphosis less than 50 degrees.[135] When the focal kyphosis exceeds 50 degrees, correction requires ventral release followed by dorsal fusion. If the ventral release is not performed, the pseudarthrosis rate may be as high as 54% compared with 13% when combining ventral and dorsal fusion.[140] The ventral approach is performed to release the ventral tether or to decompress the spinal canal. Winter *et al.*[140] recommended routine re-exploration of the dorsal bone graft 6 months after a dorsal approach if ventral fusion was not performed. However, instrumentation was not used in this series.[140]

Congenital Thoracic Lordosis

Congenital thoracic lordosis is a rare but particularly dangerous deformity that compromises pulmonary function as deformity progresses.[136] This is a rare indication for iso-

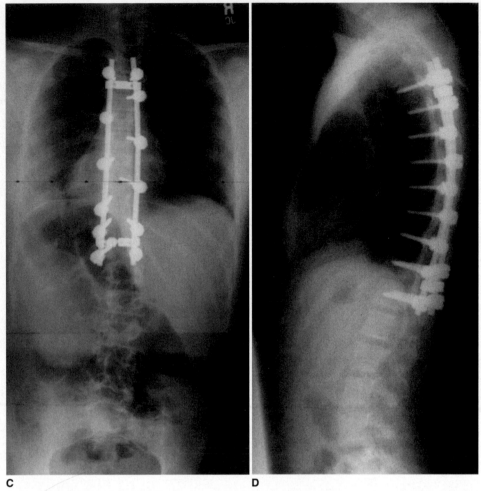

C   D

Figure 65.20 *cont'd* Postoperative **(C)** AP and **(D)** lateral images show near-complete correction of structural curve with normal sagittal plane balance.

lated ventral fusion. For severe deformities, correction can only be achieved by staged ventral wedge osteotomies, followed by dorsal instrumentation and fusion.[131,132,136] Complications, including death, are particularly high after surgical treatment of severe thoracic lordosis.

Convex Ventral and Dorsal Hemiepiphyseodesis

In 1955, Roaf[109] described the technique of ventral and dorsal convex hemiepiphyseodesis in humans on a large scale. When congenital scoliosis is due to one or two ipsilateral, fully segmented hemivertebrae, ventral convex discectomy and ventral convex fusion are carried out to arrest convex growth and thus potentiate correction by preferential concave growth.[6,12] Winter* stated that the procedure provided the best results in patients aged younger than 5 years with curves less than 40 degrees (Figure 65.31). The technique is not recommended for kyphotic deformities and has limited application in patients aged older than 5 years. Of 13 patients treated by this technique, Winter et al. found curve improvement (a true epiphyseodesis effect) in 5 patients, fusion with curve stabilization in 7 patients, and failure with

progression in 1 patient (because of inadequate size of fused area).[133]

Excision of Hemivertebrae

Combined ventral and dorsal approaches are used for excision of hemivertebrae.[13,70,74] Although excisions have been performed at the thoracic and lumbar levels, ideally this procedure is reserved for an L5 hemivertebra at the lumbosacral junction with trunk decompensation (see Figure 65.27). The retroperitoneal and dorsal approaches can be performed at a single setting, with minimal risk of neurologic injury. Excision of hemivertebrae at other levels is usually reserved for severe kyphotic deformities, with or without neurologic defects. In these cases, the excision is performed to decompress the spinal cord that is tented over the apex of the kyphosis (see Figure 65.26).

After ventral exposure, vertebrectomy for decompression is begun at a level above the apex by hollowing out the center of the vertebral body. This process of hollowing the center is carried out caudally to a level below the apical hemivertebra. When the vertebral body centers have been removed, curettes are used to work carefully, proceeding dorsally until the dorsal cortex is reached. Bleeding is

---

*References 6,12,130,132,133.

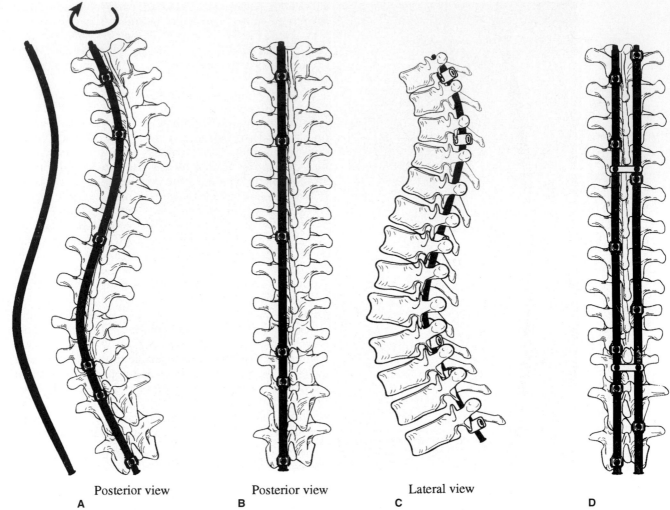

Posterior view   Posterior view   Lateral view

A   B   C   D

Figure 65.21 Scoliosis correction by rod rotation. **(A)** Hooks are placed on the end, intermediate, and apical vertebrae to produce segmental forces. The rod is contoured to fit the scoliosis, placed within the hooks, and rotated to the left. **(B)** This converts the right lordoscoliosis into thoracic kyphosis and the left lumbar scoliosis into lumbar lordosis. Some apical translation occurs with rotation. The downgoing L3 laminar hook and upgoing L4 laminar hook produce a claw for enhanced stability. **(C)** The right hooks are inserted to apply compression across the thoracic convexity and lumbar distraction across the concavity. **(D)** The two rods are linked with two cross-connectors to produce a rigid construct with 10 points of fixation to the spine.

controlled with bone wax, Gelfoam, and packing techniques. The hard, dorsal cortex is distinctly different from the cancellous bone of the body. When the dorsal cortex is reached, it is carefully windowed above the apex. Again, by working caudally from the window, the cortex and posterior longitudinal ligament are removed over the extent of the kyphotic apex. An adequate decompression should expose dura mater and epidural fat.

Failure to remove the posterior longitudinal ligament may prevent the spinal cord from moving ventrally into the cavity created by the decompression. If scoliosis accompanies kyphosis, the decompression must include the pedicles on the concave side.

When the ventral spinal cord decompression has been achieved, the strut grafts are placed across the apex of the deformity. The vertebral bodies rostral and caudal to the apex are gently distracted, and the struts (obtained from

rib, iliac crest, or fibula) are inserted into hollowed-out slots on the end plates. The distraction force should only be enough to securely lock the ventral struts into position. Distraction is then released, and the compression force locks the struts into position. Because of the inordinate risk of neurologic injury with distraction for congenital kyphosis, intraoperative spinal cord monitoring ideally should be used if distraction is anticipated or planned. Dorsal arthrodesis is usually performed as a second stage, approximately 2 weeks later, using compression constructs combined with concave distraction if concomitant scoliosis exists.

Use of Bracing, Cast, and Instrumentation

Congenital spinal deformities are rigid, and correction, by whatever means, is achieved through the mobile segments

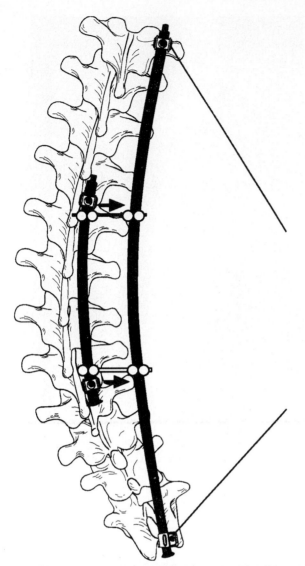

Figure 65.22 Two-rod translation. If the curve is rigid, a short rod across the apex can be translated to a longer rod attached to the end vertebrae. Threaded cross-fixation devices are designed to produce transverse traction and apical translation to the midline.

should be performed. Tethered cords and diastematomyelia must be corrected before instrumentation is attempted. Furthermore, instrumentation appropriate to the patient's size must be chosen. Intraoperative spinal cord monitoring is preferred when instrumentation is to be employed.

The endpoints of instrumentation are chosen so that the head is centered over the pelvis in both the frontal and sagittal planes. Bending and traction radiographs help predict correction and determine the endpoints of instrumentation. The compensatory curve need not be included in the fusion, unless it is anticipated that the structural component of the compensatory curve is sufficient to cause trunk decompensation. Highly flexible compensatory curves need not be included but must be followed carefully to ensure that progression does not occur postoperatively. If progression is documented and growth remains, bracing until maturity is recommended.

Dorsal instrumentation is reversed for the thoracic and lumbar deformities in adolescents or when significant instability is created by combined ventral and dorsal osteotomies. Deformities at the cervicothoracic junction are extremely difficult to treat with dorsal instrumentation systems because the space available in the spinal canal is limited. Therefore, for cervical and upper thoracic anomalies, halo casts are used. Halo traction can be used between reconstructive stages and later attached to a thoracic cast (Figure 65.32). In some cases, ventral instrumentation can be achieved by adapting cervical plates.

Pitfalls of Treatment

The primary treatment goal for congenital spinal anomalies is to prevent deformity by early fusion. Some anomalies such as unilateral bars invariably progress and should be fused at presentation, whereas others should be followed until progression is documented. Measuring all the films at each follow-up, using the same levels for comparison, and considering both the frontal and the sagittal deformities, are necessary to document the insidious progression that can occur. The current films should also be compared with the initial films to not miss a slowly progressive deformity. Early fusion of progressive deformities allows the greatest trunk height to be achieved.[122,134,137] Furthermore, failure to recognize progression may lead to a more severe deformity and necessitate riskier surgery. Rapid growth during the first 2 years of life and during puberty mandates more frequent monitoring during these periods.

Spinal cord compression can develop in association with congenital spinal anomalies and is invariably due to ventral compression associated with kyphosis (see Figure 65.26). Therefore, decompression should always be approached ventrally. Often, laminectomy leads to further instability and should be avoided.[140] Of all pediatric spinal deformities, iatrogenic spinal cord injury occurs with the greatest frequency in association with treatment of congenital spinal deformities. Distraction forces are particularly risky, especially with kyphosis, a tether, or diastematomyelia. Implants inserted into the spinal canal may exacerbate congenital stenosis. All of these potential complications underscore the importance of thoroughly

above and below the anomaly. Children tolerate casts well, and often, satisfactory correction can be maintained without instrumentation and the attendant risk of spinal cord injury. Underarm casts are used for thoracolumbar anomalies. If the curve apex is above T8, the cast must extend above the shoulders to obtain sufficient corrective force. If the curve is below L3, inclusion of the thigh(s) should be considered to reduce bending stress on the bone graft. The casts are best applied using a Risser table, to exert corrective forces while the plaster is rolled. Incorporation and remodeling of the fusion mass require approximately 1 year.

Instrumentation may be employed to improve or maintain correction of congenital spinal deformities; however, the risk of neurologic impairment after surgery is highest in this group.[54,131,132] The risks result from the small spinal canal size, the severity of deformities, and the frequent presence of intraspinal anomalies, such as diastematomyelia or tether.[54] Therefore, before a hook or wire is inserted in the spinal canal, MRI of the entire spinal cord

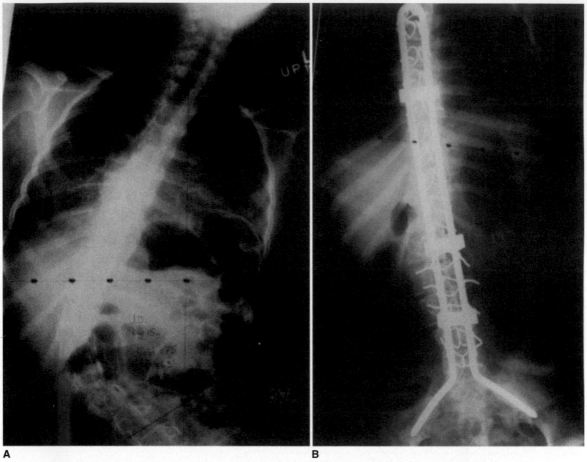

A   B

Figure 65.23 (**A**) Fifteen-year old female, Tanner stage 2, with cerebral palsy has a 75 degrees neuromuscular scoliosis with pelvic obliquity and severe left trunk shift. (**B**) Correction was achieved with dorsal instrumentation and fusion to the pelvis using the Luque-Galveston technique, a unit rod, and 16-gauge sublaminar wires. Trunk and pelvic alignment have been restored.

assessing the spinal column and cord with the appropriate imaging studies and monitoring with evoked potentials intraoperatively.

Summary

Of all pediatric spinal deformities, congenital spinal deformities are the most challenging because they occur in small children and are frequently associated with other organ system defects. Progression of the primary curve or of the compensatory curve can occur insidiously as these young patients grow. Therefore, diligent follow-up is required, and the three-dimensional aspects of the deformity must be appreciated. If progression is documented, surgical treatment is performed. The technique and approach vary with the type of deformity and the estimate of the growth potential of the anomalous segment. The goals of treatment are to halt progression of the deformity and to achieve trunk and head balance over the pelvis. The surgeon should not hesitate to engage the assistance of other specialists in the preoperative assessment and surgical approach to these complex deformities. Finally, periodic postoperative evaluation until skeletal maturity is mandatory to be sure that progression of the primary or compensatory curve does not occur.

Neuromuscular Spinal Deformity and Pelvic Obliquity

Spinal deformity commonly develops in association with neuromuscular conditions. Conditions associated with spasticity, such as cerebral palsy, have particularly rigid curves that often include the pelvis (see Figure 65.23). Other neuromuscular conditions associated with weakness or hypotonia, such as muscular dystrophy, have collapsing kyphoscoliosis. Friedreich's ataxia and Charcot-Marie-Tooth disease have deformities that fall between these extremes. In general, constructs to correct neuromuscular scoliosis include more vertebrae, with anchors on every level to provide the stability necessary to overcome the deforming forces and to allow early mobilization without a brace. In neuromuscular scoliosis associated with pelvic obliquity, fixation should be extended to the pelvis to align the trunk over a level pelvis so that balanced seating can be achieved.[83] The goals of spinal deformity correction are listed in Box 65.6.

Complications of Spinal Instrumentation and Fusion

Since the 1970s, spine surgery techniques and options have expanded dramatically. Ventral approaches to the spine

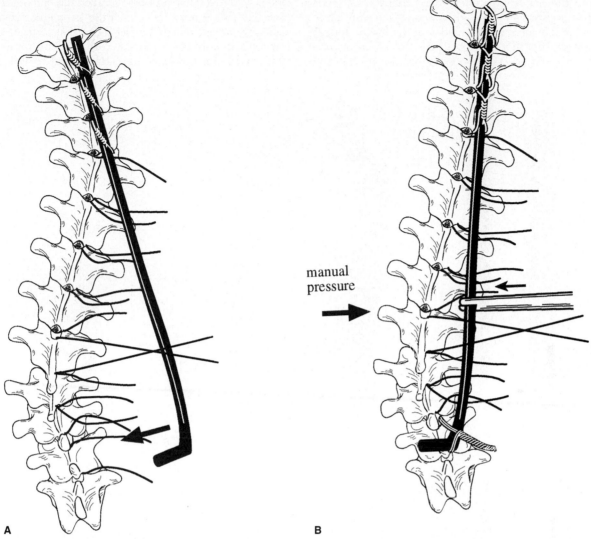

manual
pressure

A

B

Figure 65.24 Cantilever correction. (**A**) The right rod is anchored to the end of the spine via sublaminar wires, and cantilever force is applied to bring the upper segment to the midline. (**B**) The intermediate vertebrae are then translated to the rod via sublaminar wires that are sequentially and gradually tightened.

have become routine, and there has been a burgeoning of instrumentation for correction of deformity. Although the use of segmental instrumentation in place of casts to correct spinal deformity has been a vast improvement, the attendant risks of the surgery have increased. Furthermore, more follow-up is needed to determine whether newer constructs will reduce the incidence of lumbar arthritis caudal to the constructs (Figure 65.33).[29,31] Finally, spinal deformity can be associated with other organ system compromise. Therefore, a comprehensive preoperative evaluation is mandatory. Even if the patient is a healthy adolescent with idiopathic scoliosis, the magnitude of the surgery results in disturbances of organ systems that must be recognized and managed carefully to avoid complications. Some of the potential problems are listed in Box 65.7.

Trunk Decompensation

The goal of scoliosis surgery has always been to halt progression by bone fusion and to obtain correction of

deformity. An improved understanding of the three-dimensional nature of the deformity has occurred in parallel with the development of new techniques and instrumentation to correct all aspects of the scoliosis, including frontal and sagittal spine contours and trunk balance. Furthermore, the surgeon should seek to obtain correction with fusion of as few segments as possible, especially preserving lumbar vertebrae. Therefore, choosing levels for instrumentation and fusion becomes a critical component of the surgical planning process. Mistakes in choosing levels can result in persistent deformity or trunk decompensation (Figure 65.34). It must be remembered that surgery for idiopathic scoliosis is most often performed in growing patients, and therefore, despite instrumentation and grafting, growth still occurs both within and, to a greater extent, outside the instrumented area. Consequently, both improper levels of instrumentation and further spinal growth contribute to the problems of trunk decompensation and deformity progression after surgery (Box 65.8).[16,59,69,88]

Before the era of instrumentation, Hibbs *et al.*[61] performed scoliosis surgery through a window in a cast. All the
vertebrae of the curve were included in the fusion, and the
patients were kept in a cast for a period of a year or more
until fusion occurred. Moe[96] popularized the concept that

the neutrally rotated vertebrae marked the end of the curve
and that fusion must include all the intervening segments.
Harrington[57] introduced dorsal distraction instrumentation
for scoliosis correction and stated that the instrumentation
must end within the stable zone. Harrington, as well as Moe,

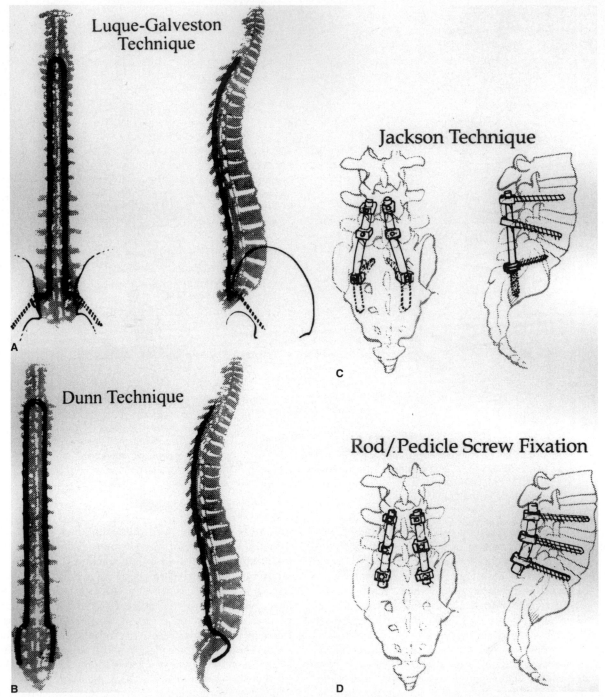

Figure 65.25 Spinopelvic fixation. **(A)** The Luque-Galveston technique is used for correction of
pelvic obliquity by passing the lower ends of the rods between the inner and outer cortical
tables of the ilium. **(B)** The Dunn technique is used for correction of lumbar kyphosis as seen in
myelodysplasia. The lower portion of the rods are passed anteriorly through the S1 foramen to
lie on the front of the sacrum. **(C)** The Jackson technique is used for correction of lumbosacral
or lower lumbar kyphosis as seen in spondylolisthesis. The lower portions of the rods are passed
into channels created in the body of the sacrum, whereas the upper rod is affixed to pedicle
screws. **(D)** S1, S2, and the lumbar pedicle screws can also be fixed to rods to achieve
lumbosacral arthrodesis.

understood that in some cases, the lesser curves (fractional curves and compensatory curves) did not need to be included in the fusion.[96] For example, in King type II curves, instrumentation of the thoracic curve alone led to some spontaneous improvement in the compensatory lumbar curve, thus maintaining trunk balance. King *et al.*[69] reviewed the cases of Moe to test the effectiveness of these concepts. One hundred forty-nine cases were studied with frontal plane radiographs and grouped into five categories as previously outlined (see Figure 65.10). For all curve types, instrumentation to the stable vertebra resulted in optimal frontal plane balance. For type I curves, both thoracic and lumbar components needed to be included, because the lumbar curve was the more structural. For type II curves, selective thoracic fusion to the lower thoracic stable vertebrae

resulted in some spontaneous correction of the lumbar curve, reasonable compensation, and preservation of lumbar motion segments. Thoracolumbar (type IV) and thoracic (type III) curves were both fused to the stable vertebrae. For double thoracic (type V) curves, both curves required instrumentation in order to produce level shoulders. Although this review provided a practical classification system and guidelines for treatment, it has several deficiencies. The cases were all treated with Harrington distraction instrumentation, rather than with the newer segmental systems. Furthermore, spinal flexibility, as demonstrated by bending radiographs did not play an obvious role in the selection of the levels to instrument. Harrington's technique provided primarily coronal plane correction by distraction, whereas the newer techniques allow greater apical translation and rotation, thus inducing greater correction. Greater correction may imply that fewer segments are fused in some cases, but it may also impart torsional forces in unfused segments, resulting in persistent or new deformity.[16] Trunk decompensation occurs when correction of the upper spine exceeds the capacity of the lower uninstrumented segment of the spine to correct spontaneously. In this situation, the lower spinal segments remain structurally deformed, leaving an oblique take-off from the sacrum. The problem produces cosmetic deformity and theoretically predisposes to arthritis by asymmetric loading of the vertebral segments.

The most predictable trunk balance is achieved by instrumentation to the stable vertebra. However, for double

---

BOX 65.3

Indications for ventral fusion

Release for severe deformity (focal kyphosis greater than 50 degrees; rigid scoliosis greater than 75 degrees)
Spinal cord decompression
Prevention of crankshaft phenomenon
Instrumentation of lumbar or thoracolumbar idiopathic scoliosis

---

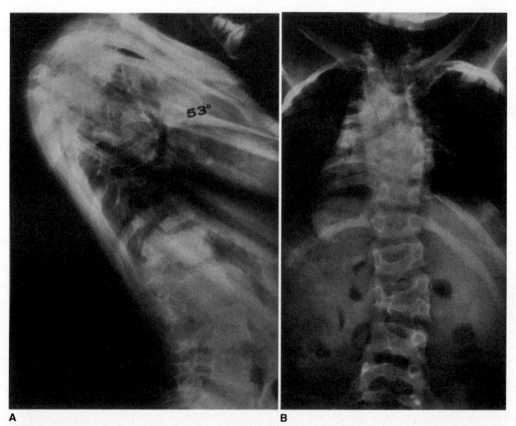

A   **B**

Figure 65.26 **(A)** Eight-year-old male presented with severe cervicothoracic kyphosis measuring 53 degrees secondary to a congenital left hemivertebra at T2. Clonus and hyperreflexia were noted. **(B)** Frontal radiograph shows multiple vertebral anomalies; however, head and trunk alignment are satisfactory.

Continued

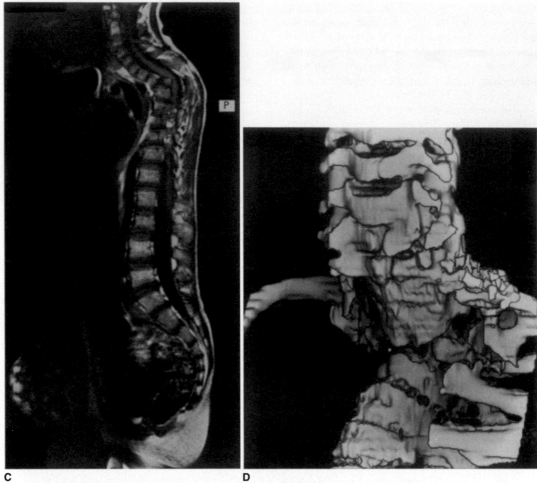

Figure 65.26 *cont'd* **(C)** MRI scan reveals spinal cord impingement and narrowing of the canal.
(D) Three-dimensional CT images demonstrate the left posterior location of the hemivertebra,
behind the conjoined T1-T2 rib head. Decompression and hemivertebrectomy was achieved by
a high left thoracotomy and T3 rib resection. The scapula was elevated for this approach, and
the T3 rib was used as a strut graft.

major curves (King type I and type II curves), L4 may be
the lower stable vertebra. Therefore, surgeons are faced
with a dilemma, because the weight of evidence suggests
that early lumbar arthritis often develops when fusions are
carried to L4 and below. An alternative for King type II
curves is selective fusion of the thoracic component, stopping at the neutral and stable lower *thoracic* vertebrae, usually T11 or T12. For selective fusions, the caudal curve must
be flexible, and the apex of the rostral curve must not be
translated past the midline. Distraction and transverse traction should be used and rotation should be avoided for
selective instrumentation of King type II curves because the
counter-rotation created in the lumbar spine when rotational maneuvers are used may limit the improvement in
the lumbar curves.[16-18] Furthermore, partial instrumentation of the caudal curve must be avoided. For flexible King
type III and type IV curves, stopping at the neutral vertebrae may produce acceptable results if the neutral vertebrae are brought into the stable zone with side bending, and
the underlying disc space opens toward the apex. For large
structural lumbar curves (King type I and type II curves),
the lumbar component must be included to achieve correc-

tion adequately. Regrettably, this implies that the fusion
usually needs to go to L4 (Figure 65.35). The alternative for
isolated lumbar and thoracolumbar curves is ventral instrumentation to L3 (see Figure 65.16).

The authors have attempted to reconcile differences
between the King and Lenke classification systems in
determining fusion levels. Both systems will be used
for the description of fusion levels that are typically used
for each curve pattern. The use of ventral and transpedicular instrumentation systems may potentially save fusion
levels compared with what is classically described. In the
Lenke classification, the extent of arthrodesis and instrumentation of the main thoracic curve, the major curve in
types 1 through 4, is influenced by an increased kyphosis
in the proximal thoracic and thoracolumbar/lumbar
regions. In types 5 and 6, the thoracolumbar/lumbar
curve is the major curve, and the main thoracic curve is
nonstructural in type 5 and structural in type 6. For
Lenke type 6 (King type 1) curves, both thoracic and lumbar components should be included in the construct,
because the lumbar curve is more structural. For Lenke
type 1 and the rare Lenke type 3 A or B curves (King type

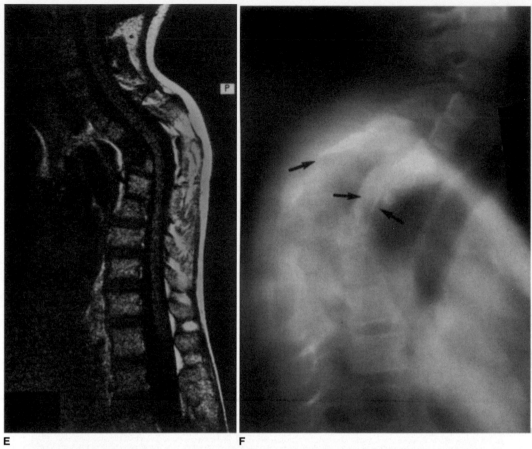

E

F

Figure 65.26 *cont'd* (**E**) Postoperative MRI shows the canal has been widened and the cord decompressed. (**F**) Tomogram demonstrates the ventral strut graft and a dorsal laminar defect that was addressed by posterior autogenous grafting 2 weeks later. The patient was confined in a halo cast for 3 months followed by a cervicothoracic orthosis for 3 months. Neurologic symptoms resolved after the decompression.   *Continued*

II curves), a selective thoracic fusion to the lower thoracic stable vertebrae results in some spontaneous correction of the lumbar curve, reasonable compensation, and preservation of lumbar motion segments. Lenke type 5 thoracolumbar (King type IV) and Lenke type 1 thoracic (King type III) curves were both fused to the stable vertebrae, in the lumbar and thoracic spine respectively. For Lenke type 2 double thoracic (King type V) curves, both curves required instrumentation in order to produce level shoulders.

Postoperative Fluid Management

Fluid administration in the range of 3 to 12L is common during long procedures for instrumentation and fusion. In general, crystalloid accounts for two thirds of the fluid administered, and colloid, including blood products, for the other one third. Patients commonly have a net positive fluid balance of 3 to 6L at the conclusion of the procedure. The use of hypotensive anesthetic techniques compounds the problem of massive fluid shifts, with pooling in the extravascular spaces. Fortunately, the patients are generally young and healthy so that these fluid shifts do not present major problems (provided that an accurate record of intake and output is kept). The use of a Foley catheter

and intravenous administration during the first 3 days after surgery allows for a more accurate accounting of fluid balance.

Antidiuretic hormone (ADH) is a polypeptide hormone released from the posterior lobe of the pituitary when baroreceptors in the aortic arch, carotid artery, and atrium signal a low blood pressure. ADH, in turn, changes the permeability of the distal renal tubules so that free water is retained and urine osmolality is increased. Release is also stimulated by central neural mechanisms, by emotional and physical stress such as surgery, and by certain anesthetic agents. A combination of these factors leads to the syndrome of inappropriate ADH secretion after scoliosis surgery.[10,89] The response is inappropriate because serum osmolality shortly after surgery is normal, whereas ADH serum levels are peaking. Consequently, the syndrome of inappropriate ADH results in low urine output for the first several postoperative days and a gradual reduction of serum osmolality as reflected by hyponatremia, and in dilutional anemia. Although serum ADH levels return to normal by postoperative day 1, the serum sodium level and the hematocrit continue to drop until day 3 postoperatively.

The effects of ADH are exacerbated by use of hypotonic parenteral solutions. Furthermore, pulmonary

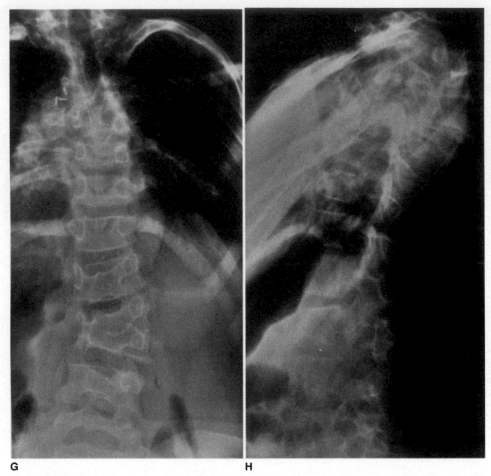

Figure 65.26 *cont'd* (**G**) Frontal alignment 1 year postoperatively. (**H**) Lateral alignment 1 year postoperatively.

edema can result from the injudicious use of fluid boluses in the early postoperative period to treat the low urine output. Proper management begins with a careful accounting of fluid balance from the time of surgery. If persistent blood loss (drain output), hypotension, and tachycardia suggest true intravascular depletion, administration of blood or colloid may be the prudent course. In many cases, however, fluid retention is driven by the ADH release, not by intravascular depletion. The proper management is to use isotonic fluids, administered postoperatively at rates sufficient to compensate for insensible losses and daily catabolic activity (maintenance rates). The postoperative diuresis generally begins on the second postoperative day and continues for several days. It is accompanied by a return of serum osmolality and sodium concentration to normal levels.

Infections

Postoperative infections are inevitable in this modern era of spinal instrumentation because of the large amount of metal implanted, including rods, cross-fixators, and multiple hooks. The routine use of perioperative antibiotics has kept the incidence of infection for idiopathic cases to approximately 1 per 100 cases, whereas for neuromuscular cases the rate rises to approximately 5%.[83,120] Patients with

meningomyelocele have infection rates of approximately 10%. Factors that predispose to infection include development of a hematoma, poor skin (meningomyelocele), concurrent infections such as urinary tract infection, and poor nutrition. All of these factors can be controlled to a certain extent.

Persistent fever with a temperature higher than 101.5°F after the fifth day postoperatively should heighten suspicions of an acute wound infection. Evaluation includes a comprehensive culture of tissues including blood, urine, pulmonary fluids, and wound aspirates. A purulent aspirate or a persistent large hematoma should be treated aggressively by irrigation in the operating room. Prompt irrigation should be followed by administration of parenteral antibiotics until culture results have been obtained. If an established infection is found, loose bone graft should be removed. Most surgeons close over a drain. Other options include closing over a close suction-irrigation system or leaving the wound open for packing with healing by secondary intention. The latter method is generally reserved for failure of the other options. Similarly, the duration of antibiotic administration and the route of administration will vary. Commonly, parenteral use of antibiotics for at least 3 weeks, followed by oral administration for 3 weeks, is prescribed. The sedimentation rate is a useful marker to follow; however, it may not

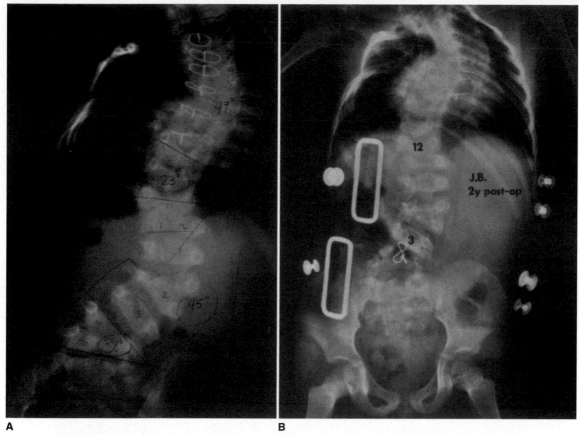

A   B

Figure 65.27 (**A**) Two-year-old male with Goldenhar's syndrome (oculoauriculovertebral dysplasia) has multiple organ system anomalies including vertebral, cardiac, and renal anomalies and Sprengel's deformity. The L5 hemivertebra was addressed to reduce the right trunk shift. (**B**) Frontal radiograph 1 year post hemivertebrectomy shows some improvement. A Milwaukee brace is currently employed to maintain the trunk alignment.

normalize for several weeks after treatment of the acute inflammation. Therefore, undertreatment is unlikely using this parameter as a guide.

Delayed infections are now well recognized after spinal surgery.[107] Affected patients present with back pain and signs of inflammation or drainage months to years after spinal surgery. The most common organisms are *Staphylococcus epidermidis*, *Propionibacterium acnes*, and other skin flora. These organisms of low virulence are believed to contaminate the wound at the time of surgery, and infection remains subclinical for an extended period.[107] Treatment of these infections should follow the same guidelines as for acute infections. Aggressive irrigation and debridement followed by wound drainage is the first treatment. Healing by secondary intention may be necessary for failure of the initial attempts. Rarely will the hardware have to be removed to control spinal infections. In fact, every attempt to salvage the instrumentation should be made. Pseudarthrosis is common after infections and, if symptomatic, it should be treated by autogenous grafting once the infection has been treated. Postoperative antibiotics should be used for several weeks after the grafting to reduce the chance of a recurrence.

Hemostasis

Bleeding is an obvious consequence of spinal surgery, but the routine use of hypotensive anesthesia and the use of frames to suspend the abdomen are techniques to reduce bleeding. Nevertheless, bleeding from the decorticated bony surfaces usually continues postoperatively. Hence, the placement of closed wound drains is a popular measure to reduce hematoma formation. The authors place the drains superficial to the paraspinal muscle fascia after first carrying out a meticulous, fluid-tight muscle repair. Generally, drainage tapers off after 36 hours, and the drains are pulled. Persistent bleeding may reflect uncorrected coagulopathy. Use of vitamin K supplements or administration of blood products such as platelets and fresh frozen plasma may be necessary in some cases. If blood loss is expected to exceed 1000 ml, intraoperative cell savers should be considered.

Nutritional Management

Patients with neuromuscular scoliosis, particularly those with cerebral palsy, are at risk of having nutritional deficiencies. Many of these patients cannot eat or swallow efficiently, and the surgery often involves a long fusion with

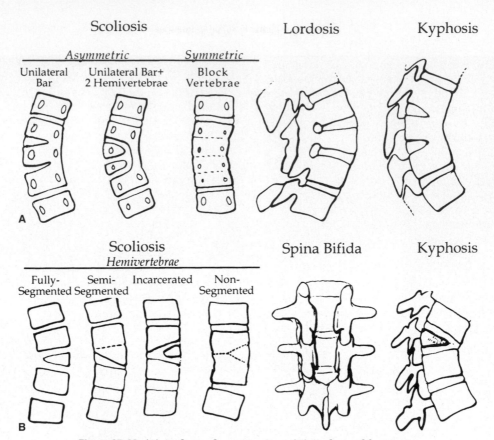

Scoliosis Lordosis Kyphosis

Asymmetric *Symmetric*

Unilateral Bar   Unilateral Bar + 2 Hemivertebrae   Block Vertebrae

A

Scoliosis Spina Bifida Kyphosis

Hemivertebrae

Fully-Segmented   Semi-Segmented   Incarcerated   Non-Segmented

B

Figure 65.28 (**A**) Defects of segmentation. (**B**) Defects of formation.

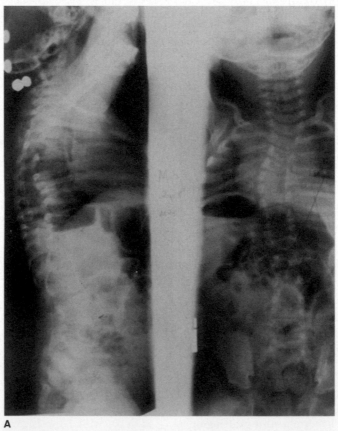

A

Figure 65.29 (**A**) Progressive lordoscoliosis developed in a 2-year-old male with multiple pterygium syndrome. The vertebral deformities included a concave thoracic bar from T5 to T8, block vertebrae from T8 to T12, and laminar synostosis from L2 to L5.

extensive exposure. Use of a feeding tube does not guarantee adequate nutrition. Several studies have demonstrated the association of malnutrition with poor wound healing and an impaired immune response.[65] Jevsevar and Karlin[65] reviewed the infection rates of 44 cerebral palsy patients and found the group with serum albumin less than 3.5mg percent, or a total lymphocyte count less than 1.5g/L, to have a significantly greater number of postoperative infections. On the basis of these studies, all patients with neuromuscular scoliosis should have their nutritional status determined. The amount of time required to feed these patients should be considered because many have difficulty swallowing, and they are susceptible to aspiration pneumonia. If the laboratory studies suggest significant protein malnutrition, or feeding and swallowing difficulties are suspected, supplemental feeding via a gastrostomy is a prudent measure before the surgery. Furthermore, the inevitable postoperative ileus may preclude feeding for 2 to 5 days postoperatively. Therefore, a central line, placed at surgery, is used to give parenteral nutrition until oral feeding is fully instituted.

Pseudarthrosis and Metal Failure

The use of spinal instrumentation has enhanced the spine surgeon's ability to achieve correction. However, halting progression and maintaining correction is ultimately dependent on achieving a bony fusion. Factors that impact the ability to obtain fusion include the source of the bone graft, surgical technique, magnitude of the deformity, and healing potential of the patient.

Autogenous bone graft produces the best fusion and is the preferred source, if available. However, in patients with severely osteopenic bone, such as those with cerebral palsy and muscular dystrophy, or in small children, adequate autograft may not be available, and allogenic bone will have to be used. Cancellous graft is preferred for placement within the denuded facets, on the decorticate laminae, and on transverse processes. If structural stability is needed, such as after a vertebrectomy, then a cortical graft, either from fibula, rib, or tricortical iliac crest, is used. Fusions occur best when the bone is under compression, such as at the concavity of the scoliosis, and they heal poorly when under excessive tension, such as that associated with a large kyphotic deformity.

Attention to surgical detail should enhance fusion rates. Thorough facetectomies should be carried out, and the graft should be placed within the joints before the rods are placed. When rods are in place, access to the facets is limited. Hook claws or pedicle screws should be considered in areas in which bending loads are high, such as at the end of the construct. For severe deformities and in certain patient populations, ventral discectomy and fusion is recommended. The indications for ventral discectomy and

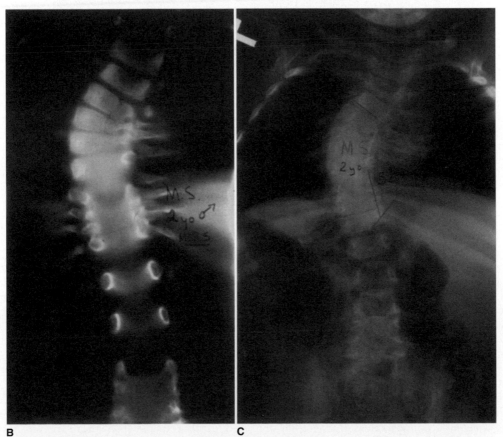

B   C

Figure 65.29 *cont'd* **(B)** Tomograms show the segmentation defect in the thoracic spine with open disc spaces on the convex side of the deformity. **(C)** When the thoracic curve reached 52 degrees, a dorsal fusion was carried out from T4 to T8. Progression continued because of further ventral growth and thus left thoracotomy spand discectomy were carried out from T5 to T8.   *Continued*

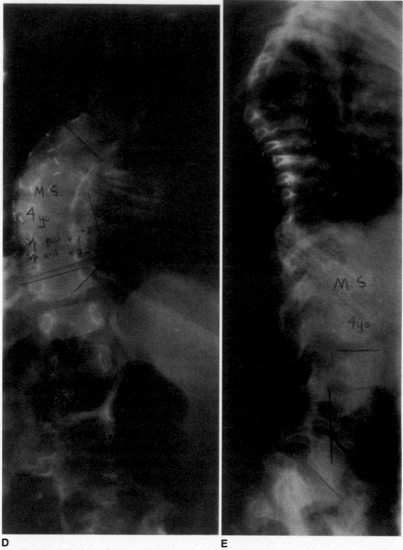

D   E

Figure 65.29 *cont'd* (**D**) Nineteen months after the initial procedures and 7 months after the anterior discectomy, the scoliosis measures 58 degrees. (**E**) Lateral radiographs show the thoracic lordosis and lumbar dorsal synostoses. In the presence of thoracic lordosis, a combined ventral and dorsal arthrodesis should have been done initially. These vertebral anomalies result in severe trunk shortening. However, the goal is prevention of cardiopulmonary complications.

fusion include a long kyphosis greater than 70 degrees or a congenital kyphosis greater than 50 degrees. Certain patient groups, including those with Marfan's syndrome and neurofibromatosis, heal poorly. Thus, as a routine, ventral fusion is recommended to enhance fusion. As conventional wisdom has dictated, there is a race with time between the fatigue life of the implants and the formation of a solid bony fusion.

One or more of the following symptoms and signs usually indicates the presence of a pseudarthrosis: pain, progressive deformity, or implant failure (rod breakage or hook pull-out). Imaging studies such as tomography or bone scans can be used to confirm the diagnosis and the location of the pseudarthrosis.[120] If the signs of pseudarthrosis are present, exploration and grafting of the defect are recommended. The defect is usually found in an area of tension. Treatment entails removal of all fibrous tissue, copious bone grafting, and instrumentation designed to produce compression across the site. Cultures are obtained routinely because of the high association between infections and pseudarthroses.

Neurologic Complications

Before the use of instrumentation for spinal deformity correction, surgically induced neurologic injury was rare. Neurologic complications are the inevitable consequence of more invasive techniques. The exact incidence can only be estimated because there is no national registry. However, the Scoliosis Research Society surveyed its members in 1993 and reported a 0.6% incidence of neurologic injury associated with scoliosis correction and a 1.4% incidence associated with all categories of spinal deformity. The vast majority of cases involved nerve root

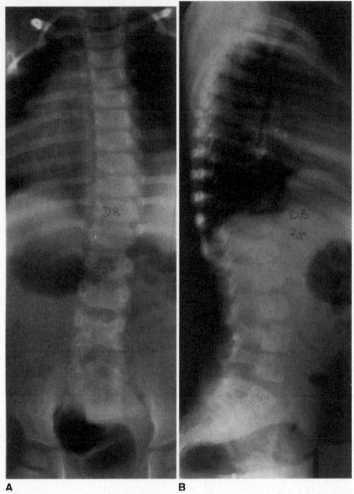

Figure 65.30 (**A**) At the age of 2 years, a 10 degrees left lumbar and 12 degrees right thoracolumbar curve was observed. The lumbar spine is shortened because of a segmentation defect. (**B**) The L3-4 disc space is narrow on the lateral radiograph.

Continued

damage, and most patients recovered. However, cases of complete or partial spinal cord injury were reported. Therefore, an understanding of the risk factors and avoidance techniques is crucial to minimizing this complication.

Neurologic injury results from direct trauma, such as with hooks, screws, wires, or bony impingement of the spinal cord and from indirect injury from excessive distraction or ischemia. A combination of both direct and indirect mechanisms may also be responsible in some cases. Spinal cord injury from hook or screw impingement may result in partial paralysis, such as Brown-Séquard syndrome. The anterior cord syndrome occurs with anterior spinal artery damage after a ventral approach. Recovery from neurologic deficits is most likely if correction of the offending lesion is possible and is instituted early. Therefore, methods to monitor spinal cord function intraoperatively are important in deformity correction.

In 1973, Vauzelle and Stagnara introduced the wake-up test to confirm spinal cord conduction after instrumentation.[55] To perform the test, anesthesia is lightened until the patients can follow commands to move their feet.

When both feet have been observed to move, the anesthetic is deepened, and the procedure is completed. Complications with this technique include extubation and air embolus. Furthermore, incomplete, subtle neurologic deficits can be missed, and this technique is not applicable to most neuromuscular cases.

Direct monitoring of spinal cord function is the other method for intraoperative confirmation of spinal cord conduction.[128] Presently, posterior column function is monitored by recording somatosensory-evoked potentials. Stimulating electrodes are placed over peripheral nerves in the lower extremities and recording is carried out via scalp, neck, or spinous process electrodes. A positive result is considered to be an acute change of 50% in amplitude or 15% in latency. However, this method is not foolproof. False results (both false-positive and false-negative) can occur if the core temperature drops or if the level of halogenated anesthetic agents become too high.[2] Clearly, factors involving the surgeon and technician impact the utility of evoked-potential monitoring. Furthermore, some motor function could be lost without a change in the

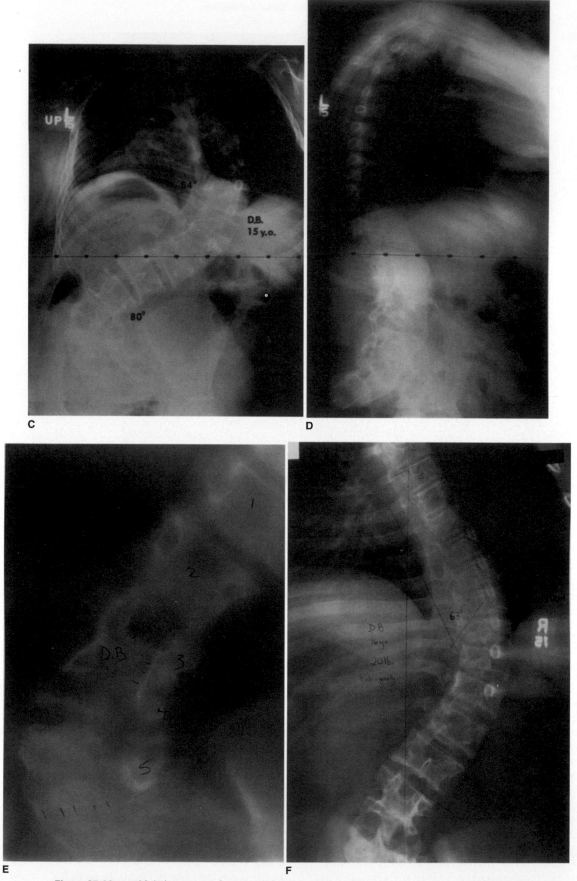

Figure 65.30 *cont'd* (**C**) Presented again at the age of 15 with a severe 84 degrees right thoracic and 80 degrees left lumbar curve. (**D**) Lateral radiograph shows increased thoracic kyphosis and lumbar lordosis. (**E**) Tomogram defines a right lumbar synostosis and an open L1-2 disc space. (**F**) Traction film, obtained while the patient was undergoing gradual preoperative halo traction, shows the right thoracic curve corrected to 63 degrees.

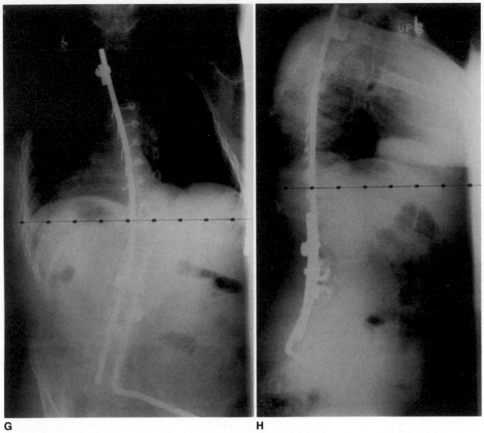

G **H**

Figure 65.30 *cont'd* (**G**) Reconstruction was carried out via dorsal instrumentation and fusion from T2 to the sacrum using spinous process wires on the intermediate vertebrae and hooks on the end vertebrae. After surgery, 3 months were spent in a spinopelvic orthosis that incorporated a thigh. (**H**) Reduction of thoracic kyphosis and lumbar lordosis is evident in the sagittal plane.

65.5

BOX

Considerations for surgical planning of scoliosis correction

Magnitude of scoliosis
Flexibility of scoliosis
Relative heights of shoulders
Deformity in sagittal plane
Stability of vertebrae
Neutrally rotated vertebrae
Skeletal age
Status of the cord (need for MRI)
Status of pulmonary and other organ systems
Availability of blood
Radiographic imaging capabilities

65.4

BOX

Intraoperative considerations for scoliosis correction

Positioning to relieve pressure and free abdomen
Inserting vascular access monitoring lines: arterial, peripheral, and central lines
Inserting Foley catheter
Monitoring spinal cord evoked potentials
Using cell saver

BOX 65.6

Goals of spinal deformity correction

Normal coronal and sagittal alignment
Shoulders level and head centered over pelvis
Preservation of as many motion segments as possible
Fusion and arrest of progression

BOX 65.8

Causes of spinal decompensation

Instrumentation cephalic of stable vertebra
Partial instrumentation into the lower structural curve
Progressive scoliosis below instrumentation
Excessive correction or translation of upper curve

Data from Bridwell,[16] Bridwell et al.,[18] and Mason and Carango.[88]

BOX 65.7

Complications of spinal instrumentation and fusion

Arthritis: Distal fusion, spondylolysis
Metal failure: Hook dislodgment, rod breakage
Pseudarthrosis
Neurologic: Peripheral nerve; cord injury (complete or
    incomplete)
Gastrointestinal: Ileus, superior mesenteric artery syndrome
Urologic: Retention, infection
Electrolytes: Syndrome of inappropriate antidiuretic
    hormone (ADH) secretion, hypokalemia
Hematologic: Bleeding, disease transmission
Infection: Early, late

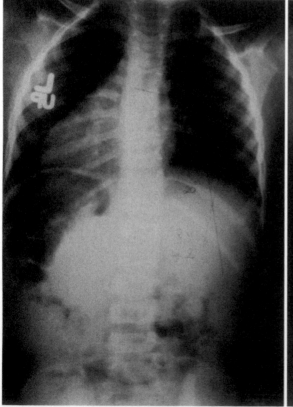
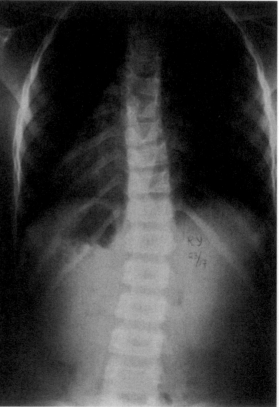

A   **B**

Figure 65.31 (**A**) Two-year-old female with left thoracic 20 degrees scoliosis resulting from hemivertebrae. (**B**) Eighteen months later, the curve measured 28 degrees and a compensatory 17 degrees right thoracolumbar curve had developed.

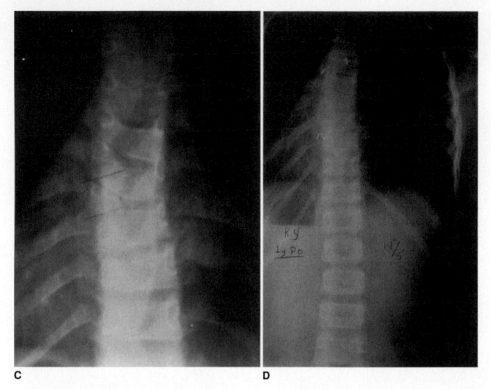

C   D

Figure 65.31 *cont'd* (**C**) Tomograms show fully segmented contiguous hemivertebrae. Treatment consisted of convex hemiepiphyseodesis from T6 to T10 via an anterior and posterior approach. (**D**) One year postoperatively, reduction of deformity resulted from concave growth, and the right thoracic curve measured 14 degrees and the left thoracolumbar curve, 5 degrees.

sensory potentials. Concomitant monitoring of anterior column function (motor-evoked potentials) is another alternative but is technically challenging.

If a neurologic complication is suspected, on the basis of an abnormal wake-up test, immediate correction of hypotension and release of distraction should be undertaken.[55] If the wake-up test continues to be abnormal, one should consider removal of the instrumentation. Similarly, if evoked potentials remain abnormal after correction of physiologic parameters, distraction should be relieved and implants should be removed in an attempt to restore cord function. Often, with an acute change in the evoked potentials, reversal of the previous step (removal of a hook or reduction of distraction) will restore the potentials. The ability to monitor continuously is a major advantage of evoked-potential monitoring (compared with the wake-up test).

Patient factors associated with increased neurologic complications include kyphosis (congenital or otherwise), congenital deformity, neurofibromatosis, sublaminar wires, rigid curves, and combined ventral-dorsal approaches.[86] Kyphotic deformities place the spinal cord on stretch. Therefore, compression or shortening of the spinal column should be employed for correction.[140] Congenital deformities have a high incidence of occult intraspinal anomalies that could lead to spinal cord injury if these problems are not addressed before scoliosis is corrected.[92] The tight angular curves associated with neurofibromatosis put the spinal cord at risk in patients. In addition, neurofibromas may occupy space within the spinal canal, producing a relative stenosis. Both insertion and removal of sublaminar wires is associated with a higher incidence of neurologic complications, in comparison with hook and rod systems.[128] However, this is a useful technique for correction in neuromuscular deformities and rigid curves. Spinous process wires are a suitable alternative for lesser deformities and do not carry the risk of cord injury. Finally, severe deformities that require a combined ventral and dorsal approach are more likely to result in neurologic deficits. Spinal cord ischemia may play a role in the pathophysiology. Therefore, if possible, the goal should be to spare the segmental vessels. The segmental vessels can be clamped during observation of the evoked potentials (preferably motor-evoked potentials) before ligation.

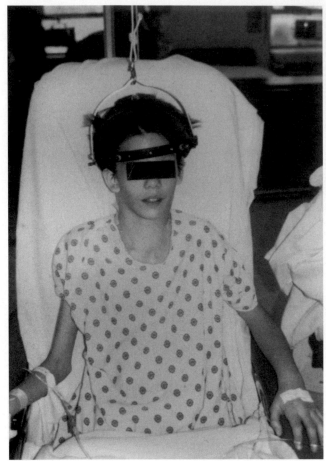

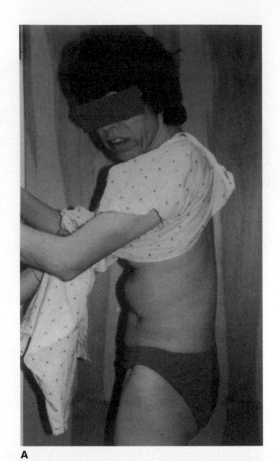

A

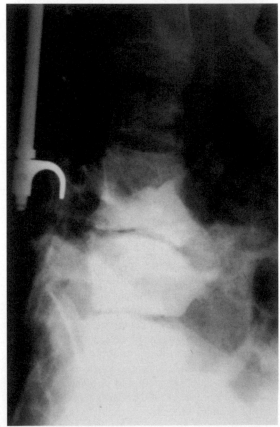

B

Figure 65.32 Halo traction can be used to obtain gradual correction of spinal deformity. Up to 20 lb may be used and suspended via a frame and pulleys over the bed or over chairs. Traction in the awake, alert patient reduces risk of neurologic injury.

Figure 65.33 **(A)** Thirty-six-year-old female with lower back pain, 22 years after a Harrington distraction rod insertion from T4 to L4. Flattening of the lumbar spine is clinically apparent. **(B)** Radiograph shows severe degenerative changes including disc space narrowing and diffuse osteophyte formation.

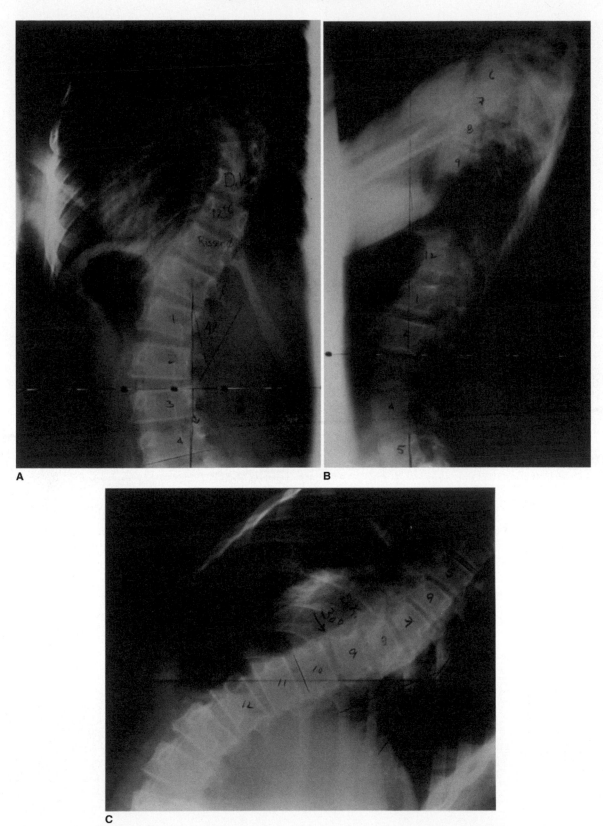

Figure 65.34 (**A**) A King type II curve pattern is noted with 56 degrees right thoracic and 42 degrees left lumbar curves in a 12-year-old girl with idiopathic scoliosis. Note that T11 is neutral and T12 is the lower thoracic stable vertebra. Only 11 ribs are present. (**B**) Mild hypokyphosis is noted on the lateral radiograph. (**C**) Right side-bending film shows correction to 30 degrees of the thoracic curve. *Continued*

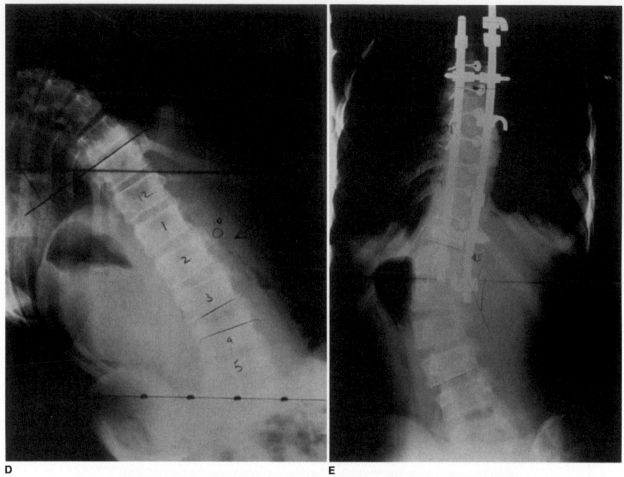

D

E

Figure 65.34 *cont'd* (**D**) Left side-bending film shows complete correction of the lumbar curve. (**E**) Dorsal instrumentation from T3 to T12 was carried out with apical translation using spinous process wires. Postoperatively, decompensation to the left results because correction of the thoracic curve exceeded the capacity of the lower curve to correct. Bracing postoperatively did improve trunk balance.

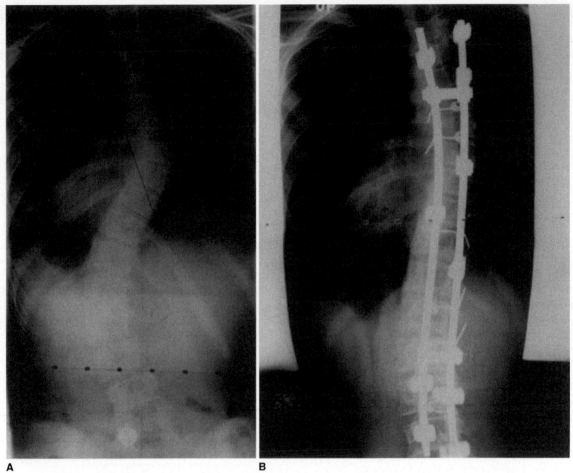

Figure 65.35 **(A)** Thirteen-year-old female, Tanner stage 3, with 48 degrees right thoracic and 51 degrees left lumbar curves. Bending films showed the lumbar curve to be more flexible (King type II curve pattern). **(B)** Instrumentation and fusion was carried out from T4 to L4, the lower stable vertebra. The lumbar curve was included because of the large size. Richards ¼-inch rods were used, supplemented with spinous process wires to promote apical translation.

REFERENCES

1. Aaro S, Ohlund C: Scoliosis and pulmonary function. *Spine* 9:220-222, 1984.
2. Abel MF, Mubarak SJ, Wenger DR, *et al:* Brainstem evoked potentials for scoliosis surgery: a reliable method allowing use of halogenated anesthetic agents. *J Pediatr Orthop* 10:208-213, 1990.
3. Allen BL, Jr., Ferguson RL: The Galveston technique for L rod instrumentation of the scoliotic spine. *Spine* 7:276-284, 1982.
4. Allen BL, Jr., Ferguson RL: The Galveston technique of pelvic fixation with L-rod instrumentation of the spine. *Spine* 9:388-394, 1984.
5. Allen BL, Jr., Ferguson RL: L-rod instrumentation for scoliosis in cerebral palsy. *J Pediatr Orthop* 2:87-96, 1982.
6. Andrew T, Piggott H: Growth arrest for progressive scoliosis. Combined anterior and posterior fusion of the convexity. *J Bone Joint Surg Br* 67:193-197, 1985.
7. Ascani E, Bartolozzi P, Logroscino CA, *et al:* Natural history of untreated idiopathic scoliosis after skeletal maturity. *Spine* 11:784-789, 1986.
8. Asher MA: Isola Instrumentation. In Weinstein SL (ed): *Pediatric Spine: Principles and Practice.* Philadelphia: Lippincott-Raven, 1994.
9. Barr SJ, Schuette AM, Emans JB: Lumbar pedicle screws versus hooks. Results in double major curves in adolescent idiopathic scoliosis. *Spine* 22:1369-1379, 1997.
10. Bell GR, Gurd AR, Orlowski JP, *et al:* The syndrome of inappropriate antidiuretic-hormone secretion following spinal fusion. *J Bone Joint Surg Am* 68:720-724, 1986.
11. Bernhardt M, Bridwell KH: Segmental analysis of the sagittal plane alignment of the normal thoracic and lumbar spines and thoracolumbar junction. *Spine* 14:717-721, 1989.
12. Bradford DS: Partial epiphyseal arrest and supplemental fixation for progressive correction of congenital spinal deformity. *J Bone Joint Surg Am* 64:610-614, 1982.
13. Bradford DS, Boachie-Adjei O: One-stage anterior and posterior hemivertebral resection and arthrodesis for congenital scoliosis. *J Bone Joint Surg Am* 72:536-540, 1990.
14. Bradford DS, Heithoff KB, Cohen M: Intraspinal abnormalities and congenital spine deformities: a

radiographic and MRI study. *J Pediatr Orthop* 11:36-41, 1991.

15. Bradford DS, Lonstein JE, Moe JH, *et al: Moe's Textbook of Scoliosis and Other Spinal Deformities.* Philadelphia, WB Saunders, 1989.

16. Bridwell KH: Adolescent idiopathic scoliosis: surgical treatment. In Weinstein SL (ed): *The Pediatric Spine: Principles and Practice.* Philadelphia, Lippincott-Raven, 1994.

17. Bridwell KH, Betz R, Capelli AM, *et al:* Sagittal plane analysis in idiopathic scoliosis patients treated with Cotrel-Dubousset instrumentation. *Spine* 15:921-926, 1990.

18. Bridwell KH, McAllister JW, Betz RR, *et al:* Coronal decompensation produced by Cotrel-Dubousset "derotation" maneuver for idiopathic right thoracic scoliosis. *Spine* 16:769-777, 1991.

19. Brown CA, Lenke LG, Bridwell KH, *et al:* Complications of pediatric thoracolumbar and lumbar pedicle screws. *Spine* 23:1566-1571, 1998.

20. Bunnell WP: The natural history of idiopathic scoliosis. *Clin Orthop* 229:20-25, 1988.

21. Bunnell WP, MacEwen GD: Non-operative treatment of scoliosis in cerebral palsy: preliminary report on the use of a plastic jacket. *Dev Med Child Neurol* 19:45-49, 1977.

22. Bunnell WP, MacEwen GD, Jayakumar S: The use of plastic jackets in the non-operative treatment of idiopathic scoliosis. Preliminary report. *J Bone Joint Surg Am* 62: 31-38, 1980.

23. Camp JF, Caudle R, Ashmun RD, *et al:* Immediate complications of Cotrel-Dubousset instrumentation to the sacro-pelvis. A clinical and biomechanical study. *Spine* 15:932-941, 1990.

24. Campbell RM, Jr., Hell-Vocke AK: Growth of the thoracic spine in congenital scoliosis after expansion thoracoplasty. *J Bone Joint Surg Am* 85-A:409-420, 2003.

25. Carr WA, Moe JH, Winter RB, *et al:* Treatment of idiopathic scoliosis in the Milwaukee brace. *J Bone Joint Surg Am* 62:599-612, 1980.

26. Ceballos T, Ferrer-Torrelles M, Castillo F, *et al:* Prognosis in infantile idiopathic scoliosis. *J Bone Joint Surg Am* 62:863-875, 1980.

27. Chan DP: Zielke instrumentation. *Instr Course Lect* 32:208-209, 1983.

28. Chapman EM, Dill DB, Graybill A: The decrease in functional capacity of the lungs and heart resulting from deformity of the chest: pulmonocardiac failure. *Medicine* 18:167-202, 1939.

29. Cochran T, Irstam L, Nachemson A: Long-term anatomic and functional changes in patients with adolescent idiopathic scoliosis treated by Harrington rod fusion. *Spine* 8:576-584, 1983.

30. Collis DK, Ponseti IV: Long-term follow-up of patients with idiopathic scoliosis not treated surgically. *J Bone Joint Surg Am* 51:425-445, 1969.

31. Connolly PJ, Von Schroeder HP, Johnson GE, *et al:* Adolescent idiopathic scoliosis. Long-term effect of instrumentation extending to the lumbar spine. *J Bone Joint Surg Am* 77:1210-1216, 1995.

32. Cummings RJ, Loveless EA, Campbell J, *et al:* Interobserver reliability and intraobserver reproducibility of the system of King et al. for the classification of

adolescent idiopathic scoliosis. *J Bone Joint Surg Am* 80:1107-1111, 1998.

33. Davies G, Reid L: Effect of scoliosis on growth of alveoli and pulmonary arteries and on right ventricle. *Arch Dis Child* 46:623-632, 1971.

34. Deacon P, Archer IA, Dickson RA: The anatomy of spinal deformity: a biomechanical analysis. *Orthopedics* 10: 897-903, 1987.

35. Deacon P, Dickson RA: Vertebral shape in the median sagittal plane in idiopathic thoracic scoliosis. A study of true lateral radiographs in 150 patients. *Orthopedics* 10:893-895, 1987.

36. Deacon P, Flood BM, Dickson RA: Idiopathic scoliosis in three dimensions. A radiographic and morphometric analysis. *J Bone Joint Surg Br* 66:509-512, 1984.

37. DeCamp MM, Jr., Jaklitsch MT, Mentzer SJ, *et al:* The safety and versatility of video-thoracoscopy: a prospective analysis of 895 consecutive cases. *J Am Coll Surg* 181:113-120, 1995.

38. Demiglio A: In *Moe's Textbook of Scoliosis and Other Spinal Deformities.* Philadelphia, WB Saunders, 1978.

39. Demiglio A, Bonnel F: Growth of the spine. In Raimondi AJ, Choux M, Dirocco C (eds): *The Pediatric Spine.* New York, Springer-Verlag, 1989, pp 39-83.

40. Dickson RA: The aetiology of spinal deformities. *Lancet* 1:1151-1155, 1988.

41. Dickson RA: Early-onset idiopathic scoliosis. In Weinstein SL (ed): *The Pediatric Spine: Principles and Practice.* Philadelphia, Lippincott-Raven, 1994, pp 421-430.

42. Dickson RA, Archer IA: Surgical treatment of late-onset idiopathic thoracic scoliosis. The Leeds procedure. *J Bone Joint Surg Br* 69:709-714, 1987.

43. Drvaric DM, Ruderman RJ, Conrad RW, *et al:* Congenital scoliosis and urinary tract abnormalities: are intravenous pyelograms necessary? *J Pediatr Orthop* 7:441-443, 1987.

44. Dubousset J: Three-dimensional analysis of the scoliotic deformity. In Weinstein SL (ed): *The Pediatric Spine: Principles and Practice.* Philadelphia, Lippincott-Raven, 1994.

45. Dubousset J, Cotrel Y: Application technique of Cotrel-Dubousset instrumentation for scoliosis deformities. *Clin Orthop* 264:103-110, 1991.

46. Dubousset J, Herring JA, Shufflebarger H: The crankshaft phenomenon. *J Pediatr Orthop* 9:541-550, 1989.

47. Dwyer AF: Experience of anterior correction of scoliosis. *Clin Orthop* 93:191-214, 1973.

48. Emans JB, Kaelin A, Bancel P, *et al:* The Boston bracing system for idiopathic scoliosis. Follow-up results in 295 patients. *Spine* 11:792-801, 1986.

49. Federico DJ, Renshaw TS: Results of treatment of idiopathic scoliosis with the Charleston bending orthosis. *Spine* 15:886-887, 1990.

50. Goldstein LA, Waugh TR: Classification and terminology of scoliosis. *Clin Orthop* 93:10-22, 1973.

51. Green NE: Part-time bracing of adolescent idiopathic scoliosis. *J Bone Joint Surg Am* 68:738-742, 1986.

52. Greulich WW, Pyle SI: *Radiographic Atlas of Skeletal Development of the Hand and Wrist.* Stanford, Stanford University Press, 1950.

53. Hadley-Miller N, Mims B, Milewicz DM: The potential role of the elastic fiber system in adolescent

idiopathic scoliosis. *J Bone Joint Surg Am* 76:1193-1206, 1994.

54. Hall JE, Herndon WA, Levine CR: Surgical treatment of congenital scoliosis with or without Harrington instrumentation. *J Bone Joint Surg Am* 63:608-619, 1981.

55. Hall JE, Levine CR, Sudhir KG: Intraoperative awakening to monitor spinal cord function during Harrington instrumentation and spine fusion. Description of procedure and report of three cases. *J Bone Joint Surg Am* 60:533-536, 1978.

56. Hamill CL, Lenke LG, Bridwell KH, *et al:* The use of pedicle screw fixation to improve correction in the lumbar spine of patients with idiopathic scoliosis. Is it warranted? *Spine* 21:1241-1249, 1996.

57. Harrington PR: Technical details in relation to the successful use of instrumentation in scoliosis. *Orthop Clin North Am* 3:49-67, 1972.

58. Hazelrigg SR, Landreneau RJ, Boley TM, *et al:* The effect of muscle-sparing versus standard posterolateral thoracotomy on pulmonary function, muscle strength, and postoperative pain. *J Thorac Cardiovasc Surg* 101:394-400; discussion 400-391, 1991.

59. Hefti FL, McMaster MJ: The effect of the adolescent growth spurt on early posterior spinal fusion in infantile and juvenile idiopathic scoliosis. *J Bone Joint Surg* Br 65:247-254, 1983.

60. Hensinger RN, Lang JE, MacEwen GD: Klippel-Feil syndrome; a constellation of associated anomalies. *J Bone Joint Surg Am* 56:1246-1253, 1974.

61. Hibbs RA, Risser JC, Ferguson AB: Scoliosis treated by the fusion operation: an end-result study of three hundred and sixty cases. *J Bone Joint Surg* 13:91-104, 1931.

62. Hoke M: A study of a case of lateral curvature of the spine: a report on an operation for the deformity. *Am J Orthop Surg* 1:168-208, 1903.

63. Jacobeaus J: The cauterization of adhesion in pneumo-thorax treatment of tuberculosis. *Surg Gynecol Obstet* 32:493-500, 1921.

64. James JIP, Lloyd-Roberts GC, Pilcher MF: Infantile structural scoliosis. *J Bone Joint Surg Br* 41:719-735, 1959.

65. Jevsevar DS, Karlin LI: The relationship between preoperative nutritional status and complications after an operation for scoliosis in patients who have cerebral palsy. *J Bone Joint Surg Am* 75:880-884, 1993.

66. Kahanovitz N, Levine DB, Lardone J: The part-time Milwaukee brace treatment of juvenile idiopathic scoliosis. Long-term follow-up. *Clin Orthop* 167:145-151, 1982.

67. Kaiser LR: Video-assisted thoracic surgery. Current state of the art. *Ann Surg* 220:720-734, 1994.

68. Kindsfater K, Lowe T, Lawellin D, *et al:* Levels of platelet calmodulin for the prediction of progression and severity of adolescent idiopathic scoliosis. *J Bone Joint Surg Am* 76:1186-1192, 1994.

69. King HA, Moe JH, Bradford DS, *et al:* The selection of fusion levels in thoracic idiopathic scoliosis. *J Bone Joint Surg Am* 65:1302-1313, 1983.

70. King JD, Lowery GL: Results of lumbar hemivertebral excision for congenital scoliosis. *Spine* 16:778-782, 1991.

71. Koop SE: Infantile and juvenile idiopathic scoliosis. *Orthop Clin North Am* 19:331-337, 1988.

72. Kuhns JG, Hormell RS: Management of congenital scoliosis. *Arch Surg* 65:250-263, 1952.

73. Landreneau RJ, Hazelrigg SR, Mack MJ, *et al:* Postoperative pain-related morbidity: video-assisted thoracic surgery versus thoracotomy. *Ann Thorac Surg* 56:1285-1289, 1993.

74. Leatherman KD, Dickson RA: Two-stage corrective surgery for congenital deformities of the spine. *J Bone Joint Surg Br* 61-B:324-328, 1979.

75. Lenke LG, Betz RR, Bridwell KH, *et al:* Intraobserver and interobserver reliability of the classification of thoracic adolescent idiopathic scoliosis. *J Bone Joint Surg Am* 80:1097-1106, 1998.

76. Lenke LG, Betz RR, Haher TR, *et al:* Multisurgeon assessment of surgical decision-making in adolescent idiopathic scoliosis: curve classification, operative approach, and fusion levels. *Spine* 26:2347-2353, 2001.

77. Lenke LG, Betz RR, Harms J, *et al:* Adolescent idiopathic scoliosis: a new classification to determine extent of spinal arthrodesis. *J Bone Joint Surg Am* 83-A:1169-1181, 2001.

78. Liljenqvist U, Hackenberg L, Link T, *et al:* Pullout strength of pedicle screws versus pedicle and laminar hooks in the thoracic spine. *Acta Orthop Belg* 67:157-163, 2001.

79. Liljenqvist UR, Halm HF, Link TM: Pedicle screw instrumentation of the thoracic spine in idiopathic scoliosis. *Spine* 22:2239-2245, 1997.

80. Logue E, Sarwark JF: Idiopathic scoliosis: new instrumentation for surgical management. *J Am Acad Orthop Surg* 2:67-77, 1994

81. Lonstein JE: Embryology and spine growth, in Bradford DS, Lonstein JE, Moe JH, et al (eds): *Moe's Textbook of Scoliosis and Other Spinal Deformities.* Philadelphia, WB Saunders, 1987, pp 25-40.

82. Lonstein JE: Patient evaluation, in Bradford DS, Lonstein JE, Moe JH (eds): *Moe's Textbook of Scoliosis and Other Spinal Deformities.* Philadelphia, WB Saunders, 1987.

83. Lonstein JE, Akbarnia A: Operative treatment of spinal deformities in patients with cerebral palsy or mental retardation. An analysis of one hundred and seven cases. *J Bone Joint Surg Am* 65:43-55, 1983.

84. Lonstein JE, Carlson JM: The prediction of curve progression in untreated idiopathic scoliosis during growth. *J Bone Joint Surg Am* 66:1061-1071, 1984.

85. Lonstein JE, Winter RB: The Milwaukee brace for the treatment of adolescent idiopathic scoliosis. A review of one thousand and twenty patients. *J Bone Joint Surg Am* 76:1207-1221, 1994.

86. Lonstein JE, Winter RB, Moe JH, *et al:* Neurologic deficits secondary to spinal deformity. A review of the literature and report of 43 cases. *Spine* 5:331-355, 1980.

87. Manning CW, Prime FJ, Zorab PA: Partial costectomy as a cosmetic operation in scoliosis. *J Bone Joint Surg Br* 55:521-527, 1973.

88. Mason DE, Carango P: Spinal decompensation in Cotrel-Dubousset instrumentation. *Spine* 16:S394-403, 1991.

89. Mason RJ, Betz RR, Orlowski JP, *et al:* The syndrome of inappropriate antidiuretic hormone secretion and its effect on blood indices following spinal fusion. *Spine* 14:722-726, 1989.

90. McCarthy RE: Evaluation of the patient with deformity. In Weinstein SL (ed): *The Pediatric Spine: Principles and Practice.* Philadelphia, Lippincott-Raven, 1994, pp 185-224.

91. McCarthy RE, Dunn H, McCullough FL: Luque fixation to the sacral ala using the Dunn-McCarthy modification. *Spine* 14:281-283, 1989.

92. McMaster MJ: Occult intraspinal anomalies and congenital scoliosis. *J Bone Joint Surg Am* 66:588-601, 1984.

93. McMaster MJ, Macnicol MF: The management of progressive infantile idiopathic scoliosis. *J Bone Joint Surg Br* 61:36-42, 1979.

94. McMaster MJ, Ohtsuka K: The natural history of congenital scoliosis. A study of two hundred and fifty-one patients. *J Bone Joint Surg Am* 64:1128-1147, 1982.

95. Mehta MH: The rib-vertebra angle in the early diagnosis between resolving and progressive infantile scoliosis. *J Bone Joint Surg Br* 54:230-243, 1972.

96. Moe JH: Methods of correction and surgical techniques in scoliosis. *Orthop Clin North Am* 3:17-48, 1972.

97. Moe JH, Kharrat K, Winter RB, et al: Harrington instrumentation without fusion plus external orthotic support for the treatment of difficult curvature problems in young children. *Clin Orthop* 185:35-45, 1984.

98. Nachemson A: A long-term follow-up study of non-treated scoliosis. *Acta Orthop Scand* 39:466-476, 1968.

99. Nash CL, Jr., Moe JH: A study of vertebral rotation. *J Bone Joint Surg Am* 51:223-229, 1969.

100. Newton PO, Cardelia MJ, Farnsworth CL, et al: A biomechanical comparison of open and thorascopic anterior spinal release in a goat model. *Spine* 23:530-535, 1998.

101. Newton PO, Shea KG, Granlund KF: Defining the pediatric spinal thoracoscopy learning curve: sixty-five consecutive cases. *Spine* 25:1028-1035, 2000.

102. Nilsonne U, Lundgren KD: Long-term prognosis in idiopathic scoliosis. *Acta Orthop Scand* 39:456-465, 1968.

103. O'Brien MF, Lenke LG, Mardjetko S, et al: Pedicle morphology in thoracic adolescent idiopathic scoliosis: is pedicle fixation an anatomically viable technique? *Spine* 25:2285-2293, 2000.

104. Owen R, Turner A, Bamforth JS, et al: Costectomy as the first stage of surgery for scoliosis. *J Bone Joint Surg Br* 68:91-95, 1986.

105. Perdriolle R, Vidal J: Thoracic idiopathic scoliosis curve evolution and prognosis. *Spine* 10:785-791, 1985.

106. Phillips WA, Hensinger RN: Wisconsin and other instrumentation for posterior spinal fusion. *Clin Orthop* 229:44-51, 1988.

107. Richards BS: Delayed infections following posterior spinal instrumentation for the treatment of idiopathic scoliosis. *J Bone Joint Surg Am* 77:524-529, 1995.

108. Risser JC, Norquist DM, Cockrell BR, Jr., et al: The effect of posterior spine fusion on the growing spine. *Clin Orthop* 46:127-139, 1966.

109. Roaf R: Wedge resection for scoliosis. *J Bone Joint Surg Br* 37:97-101, 1955.

110. Sanders JO, Herring JA, Browne RH: Posterior arthrodesis and instrumentation in the immature (Risser-grade-0) spine in idiopathic scoliosis. *J Bone Joint Surg Am* 77:39-45, 1995.

111. Schwend RM, Hennrikus W, Hall JE, et al: Childhood scoliosis: clinical indications for magnetic resonance imaging. *J Bone Joint Surg Am* 77:46-53, 1995.

112. Shufflebarger HL: Theory and mechanisms of posterior derotation spinal systems. In Weinstein SL (ed): *The Pediatric Spine: Principles and Practice*. Philadelphia, Lippincott-Raven, 1994.

113. Steel HH: Rib resection and spine fusion in correction of convex deformity in scoliosis. *J Bone Joint Surg Am* 65:920-925, 1983.

114. Stefee A, Edwards CC, Yuan HA, et al: *Spinal Instrumentation Techniques*. Rosemont, IL, Scoliosis Research Society, 1994.

115. Suk SI, Kim WJ, Kim JH, et al: Restoration of thoracic kyphosis in the hypokyphotic spine: a comparison between multiple-hook and segmental pedicle screw fixation in adolescent idiopathic scoliosis. *J Spinal Disord* 12:489-495, 1999.

116. Suk SI, Kim WJ, Lee CS, et al: Indications of proximal thoracic curve fusion in thoracic adolescent idiopathic scoliosis: recognition and treatment of double thoracic curve pattern in adolescent idiopathic scoliosis treated with segmental instrumentation. *Spine* 25:2342-2349, 2000.

117. Suk SI, Kim WJ, Lee SM, et al: Thoracic pedicle screw fixation in spinal deformities: are they really safe? *Spine* 26:2049-2057, 2001.

118. Suk SI, Lee CK, Kim WJ, et al: Segmental pedicle screw fixation in the treatment of thoracic idiopathic scoliosis. *Spine* 20:1399-1405, 1995.

119. Suk SI, Lee CK, Min HJ, et al: Comparison of Cotrel-Dubousset pedicle screws and hooks in the treatment of idiopathic scoliosis. *Int Orthop* 18:341-346, 1994.

120. Trendwell SJ: Complications of Spinal Surgery. In Weinstein SL (ed): *The Pediatric Spine: Principles and Practice*. Philadelphia, Lippincott-Raven, 1994, pp 1761-1786.

121. Wall EJ, Byulsi-Austrow DI, Shelton FS, et al: Endoscopic discectomy increases thoracic spine flexibility as effectively as open discectomy: A mechanical study in a porcine model. *Spine* 23:9-16, 1998.

122. Warner WC: Juvenile idiopathic scoliosis. In Weinstein SL (ed): *The Pediatric Spine: Principles and Practice*. Philadelphia, Lippincott-Raven, 1994.

123. Weinstein SL: Adolescent idiopathic scoliosis: prevalence and natural history. In Weinstein SL (ed): *The Pediatric Spine: Principles and Practice*. Philadelphia, Lippincott-Raven, 1994.

124. Weinstein SL: Idiopathic scoliosis. Natural history. *Spine* 11:780-783, 1986.

125. Weinstein SL: *The Pediatric Spine: Principles and Practice*. Philadelphia: Lippincott-Raven, 1994.

126. Weinstein SL, Ponseti IV: Curve progression in idiopathic scoliosis. *J Bone Joint Surg Am* 65:447-455, 1983.

127. Weinstein SL, Zavala DC, Ponseti IV: Idiopathic scoliosis: long-term follow-up and prognosis in untreated patients. *J Bone Joint Surg Am* 63:702-712, 1981.

128. Wilber RG, Thompson GH, Shaffer JW, et al: Postoperative neurological deficits in segmental spinal instrumentation. A study using spinal cord monitoring. *J Bone Joint Surg Am* 66:1178-1187, 1984.

129. Winter RB: *Congenital Deformities of the Spine*. New York, Thieme, 1983.

130. Winter RB: Convex anterior and posterior hemiarthrodesis and hemiepiphyseodesis in young children with progressive congenital scoliosis. *J Pediatr Orthop* 1:361-366, 1981.

131. Winter RB, Leonard AS: Surgical correction of congenital thoracic lordosis. *J Pediatr Orthop* 10:805-808, 1990.

132. Winter RB, Lonstein JE, Boachie-Adjei O: Congenital spinal deformity. *Instr Course Lect* 45:117-127, 1996.

133. Winter RB, Lonstein JE, Denis F, *et al:* Convex growth arrest for progressive congenital scoliosis due to hemivertebrae. *J Pediatr Orthop* 8:633-638, 1988.

134. Winter RB, Lonstein JE, Drogt J, *et al:* The effectiveness of bracing in the nonoperative treatment of idiopathic scoliosis. *Spine* 11:790-791, 1986.

135. Winter RB, Moe JH: The results of spinal arthrodesis for congenital spinal deformity in patients younger than five years old. *J Bone Joint Surg Am* 64:419-432, 1982.

136. Winter RB, Moe JH, Bradford DS: Congenital thoracic lordosis. *J Bone Joint Surg Am* 60:806-810, 1978.

137. Winter RB, Moe JH, Eilers VE: Congenital scoliosis: a study of 234 patients treated and untreated. Part 2 Treatment. *J Bone Joint Surg Am* 50:1-15, 1968.

138. Winter RB, Moe JH, Lonstein JE: Posterior spinal arthrodesis for congenital scoliosis. An analysis of the cases of two hundred and ninety patients, five to nineteen years old. *J Bone Joint Surg Am* 66:1188-1197, 1984.

139. Winter RB, Moe JH, MacEwen GD, *et al:* The Milwaukee brace in the non-operative treatment of congenital scoliosis. *Spine* 1:85-96, 1976.

140. Winter RB, Moe JH, Wang JF: Congenital kyphosis. Its natural history and treatment as observed in a study of one hundred and thirty patients. *J Bone Joint Surg Am* 55:223-256, 1973.

141. Winter RB, Pinto WC: Pelvic obliquity. Its causes and its treatment. *Spine* 11:225-234, 1986.

142. Wynne-Davies R: Congenital vertebral anomalies: aetiology and relationship to spina bifida cystica. *J Med Genet* 12:280-288, 1975.

143. Wynne-Davies R: Familial (idiopathic) scoliosis. A family survey. *J Bone Joint Surg Br* 50:24-30, 1968.

144. Wynne-Davies R: Infantile idiopathic scoliosis. Causative factors, particularly in the first six months of life. *J Bone Joint Surg Br* 57:138-141, 1975.

APPENDIX 65.1

Spinal Deformity Terminology

Adolescent scoliosis: Spinal curvature presenting at or about the onset of puberty and before maturity.

Apical vertebra: The most rotated vertebra in a curve; the most deviated vertebra from the vertical axis of the patient.

Body alignment, balance, compensation: 1. The alignment of the midpoint of the occiput over the sacrum in the same vertical plane as the shoulders over the hips. 2. (*roentgenology*) When the sum of the angular deviations of the spine in one direction is equal to that in the opposite direction, curves are compensated.

Cervical curve: Spinal curvature that has its apex from C1 to C6.

Cervicothoracic curve: Spinal curvature that has its apex at C7 or T1.

Compensation: Accurate alignment of the midline of the skull over the midline of the sacrum.

Compensatory curve: A curve that can be structural, above or below a major curve that tends to maintain normal body alignment.

Congenital scoliosis: Scoliosis resulting from congenitally anomalous vertebral development.

Curve measurement: 1. *Cobb method:* Select the upper and lower end vertebrae. Erect perpendiculars to their transverse axes. These perpendiculars intersect to form the angle of the curve. If the vertebral end plates are poorly visualized, a line through the bottom or top of the pedicles may be used. 2. *Ferguson method:* Draw two lines from the center of the superior and inferior end vertebral bodies to the center of the apical vertebral body. These lines intersect to form the angle of the curve.

Double structural curve (double major scoliosis): A scoliosis with two structural curves. Two structural curves in the same spine, one balancing the other.

Double thoracic curve (scoliosis): A scoliosis with a structural upper thoracic curve, a larger, more deforming lower thoracic curve, and a relatively nonstructural lumbar curve.

End vertebra: The most rostral vertebra of a curve whose superior surface tilts maximally toward the concavity of the curve surface or the most caudal vertebra of a curve whose inferior surface tilts maximally toward the concavity of the curve.

Fractional curve: A compensatory curve that is incomplete because it returns to the erect position. Its only horizontal vertebra is rostral or caudal.

Full curve: A curve in which the only horizontal vertebra is at the apex.

Functional curve (nonstructural curve): A curve that has no structural component and that corrects or overcorrects on recumbent side-bending radiographic views.

Idiopathic scoliosis: A structural spinal curvature for which no cause is established.

Iliac epiphysis (iliac apophysis): The epiphysis along the wing of the ilium.

Iliac epiphysis sign (iliac apophysis sign): In the anteroposterior (AP) radiographic view of the spine, when the excursion of ossification in the iliac epiphysis (apophysis) reaches its ultimate medial migration; vertebral growth may be complete.

Inclinometer: An instrument used to measure the angle of thoracic inclination or rib hump.

Infantile scoliosis: Spinal curvature that develops during the first 3 years of life.

Juvenile scoliosis: Spinal curvature that develops between the skeletal age of 3 years and the onset of puberty.

Kyphos: A change in the alignment of a segment of the spine in the sagittal plane that increases the posterior convex angulation.

Kyphoscoliosis: Lateral curvature of the spine associated with either increased posterior, or decreased anterior, angulation in the sagittal plane in excess of the accepted normal angulation for that region. In the thoracic region, 20 degrees to 40 degrees of kyphosis is considered normal.

Lordoscoliosis: Lateral curvature of the spine associated with an increase in anterior curvature or a decrease in posterior angulation. In a thoracic spine in which posterior angulation is normally present, less than 20 degrees would constitute lordoscoliosis.

Lumbar curve: Spinal curvature that has its apex from L1 to L4.

Lumbosacral curve: Spinal curvature that has its apex at L5 or lower.

Major curve: Term used to designate the larger (largest) curve(s), usually structural.

Minor curve: Term used to refer to the smaller (smallest) curve(s).

Neutral vertebra: Vertebra with no transverse plane rotation so that on the frontal plane AP radiograph, the spinous process is located midway between the pedicles. It is often found at the transition zone between two curves and often is the most tilted vertebra.

Pelvic obliquity: Deviation of the pelvis from the horizontal in the frontal plane. Fixed pelvic obliquities can be attributable to contractures either above or below the pelvis.

Primary curve: The first or earliest of several curves to appear, if identifiable.

Rib hump: The prominence of the ribs on the convexity of a spinal curvature, usually due to vertebral rotation. It is best exhibited on forward bending.

Skeletal age (bone age): The age obtained by comparing an AP radiographic view of the left hand and wrist with the standards of the Greulich and Pyle Atlas.[53]

Stable vertebra: The vertebra most closely bisected by the center sacral line on the frontal view. The line is drawn by making a perpendicular to a line across the top of the sacrum or iliac crest, which passes through the sacral spinous processes. It denotes the vertebra that is situated over the center of the sacrum.

Structural curve: A segment of the spine with a fixed lateral curvature. Radiographically, it is identified in supine lateral side-bending views by the failure to correct. There may be multiple structural curves.

Thoracic curve: Scoliosis in which the apex of the curvature is between T2 and T11.

Thoracolumbar curve: Spinal curvature that has its apex at T12 or L1.

Transitional vertebra: Vertebra that is neutral in relation to rotation, usually at the end of a curve.

Vertebral end plates: The superior and inferior plates of cortical bone of the vertebral body adjacent to the intervertebral disc.

Vertebral growth plate: The cartilaginous surface covering the top and bottom of a vertebral body that is responsible for the linear growth of the vertebra.

Vertebral ring apophyses: The most reliable index of vertebral immaturity, seen best in lateral radiographs or in the lumbar region in side-bending AP views.

CHAPTER 66

Deformity Correction

James S. Harrop, Michael P. Steinmetz,
and Edward C. Benzel

Subaxial Cervical Spine

The vertebral or spinal column provides humans with the ability to maintain an upright posture, protects the neural and visceral organs (i.e., heart, lungs, abdominal contents), and aids with mobility. The cervical spine provides a transition from the rigid thoracic spine to the cranium and provides the ability to alter position in order to improve swallowing function and optimize hearing and sight. Numerous forces, both internal and external, may affect the structure and position of the cervical spine such that it becomes deformed or is altered from its normal anatomic alignment.

Spinal deformities are more often encountered in the thoracic and lumbar spine. However, the cervical spine may also develop structural deformities secondary to congenital disorders, neuromuscular diseases,[80] trauma,[81] neoplastic disease,[5] or previous spine surgery.[44] These deformities may also occur in patients with systemic arthritides, such as ankylosing spondylitis and rheumatoid arthritis. This chapter reviews the normal subaxial cervical anatomy, alignment, biomechanical properties, etiologies of deformities, and treatment strategies. Traumatic and posttraumatic kyphosis are not discussed since they are covered extensively elsewhere in this text.

Anatomy

The cervical spine consists of seven vertebrae (C1-7) (Figure 66.1).[28] C1 and C2 are anatomic and functionally unique, which allows for the transition and attachment of the cervical spine to the cranium. These vertebrae (C1-2) are not considered when discussing the subaxial cervical spine (C3-7).

Vertebral Body and Disc

The size of the subaxial cervical vertebral bodies (C3-7) generally increases from rostral to caudal (see Figure 66.1). The exception is the C6 body, which is slightly decreased in size compared to C5.[8,60,107] This increase in vertebral body's width, depth, and total end plate cross-sectional area allows greater loads to be supported and forces to be dispersed.[75] The majority of these physiologic loads are carried through the dorsal cervical vertebral body in a flexion posture while in extension the loads are carried through the dorsal elements (articular columns).[107]

The intervertebral disc connects the vertebral end plates and is composed of the cartilaginous end plate,

annulus fibrosus, and nucleus pulposus. The disc heights are not symmetric, with the ventral height being greater than the dorsal height (see Figure 66.1). This contributes to the lordotic curvature of the cervical spine.[19,60]

The pedicles are horizontal columns of bone that connect the vertebral body to the dorsal elements (Figure 66.2). The cervical pedicles have an elliptical shape, with the height being greater than the width.[75,103] The cortical bone surface of the cervical pedicles is similar on the rostral and caudal portion, but the lateral wall thickness is significantly less than the medial wall thickness.[76] These pedicles insert into the vertebral body with transverse angle ranges from −8 to 11 degrees from the horizontal, and the sagittal angles ranging from 40 to 29 degrees.[75]

Articulations

There are four articular surfaces between adjacent vertebral segments in the subaxial cervical spine, one set located on the vertebral body and another set involving the dorsal elements. The articulations located on the rostral, lateral dorsal aspect of the vertebral body are termed the uncovertebral or Luschka joints. These "joints" articulate with the caudal, dorsal, lateral aspect of the rostral vertebral body (Figure 66.3).[8] The heights of the uncinate process gradually increase as one descends the spine at each segment from C3-7, while the length and width remained relatively constant.[103] These joints are actually believed to be degenerative clefts and not true joints since they are not present at birth and develop during adolescence.[10,33]

The dorsal elements of the cervical spine allow a large degree of mobility due to a pair of segmental articulations in the form of facet joints (see Figure 66.3). These are apophyseal joints and are composed of a loose but strong capsule and synovial lining. The cervical facet joints are oriented at approximately 45 degrees in the coronal plane and 80 to 90 degrees in the sagittal plane.[8,78] This facet orientation permits a large degree of sagittal plane motion, flexion, and extension, but limits or restricts translation and lateral movements or bending.[8,83]

Ligaments (ALL, PLL, Capsular, Flavum)

The anterior longitudinal ligament (ALL) and the posterior longitudinal ligament (PLL) are the two major ligaments in the cervical spine and are attached directly to the vertebral body. The ALL is a fibrous band that attaches to the edges of the vertebral bodies (C2 to sacrum) and that is diminished in width at the disc spaces. It provides significant support and resists cervical extension.[106] The PLL also is continuous from C2 to the sacrum but differs from the ALL in that it narrows over the vertebral bodies and then widens at the disc interspace where it is interwoven with the annulus fibrosis. This ligament resists flexion and has half the strength of the ALL.[106]

Numerous other ligaments also support the dorsal cervical spine. These include the ligamentum flavum, the capsular, and the interspinous ligaments. The ligamentum flavum extends from the undersurface of the lamina to the adjacent rostral lamina. This ligament has the highest amount of elastin in the human body. It also has a baseline amount

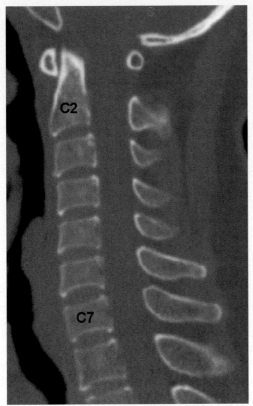

Figure 66.1 This is a sagittal CT reformatted image of the cervical spine. The rest of the cervical spine vertebral bodies, C3 through C7, increase in size ventrally to caudally with the exception of C6, which is slightly decreased. Also note that the disc spaces are increased ventrally compared with dorsally, particularly at C5-6, increasing the overall lordosis of the cervical spine.

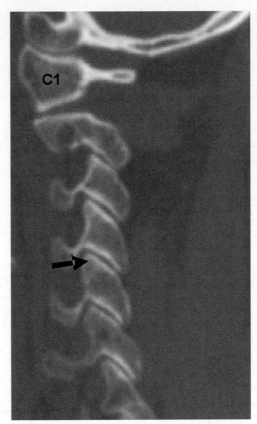

Figure 66.3 Lateral portion of sagittal CT reformat images of cervical spine from occiput to thoracic junction. Note the facet joints (*arrow*) articulate with approximately a 45-degree angulation. This provides for a great degree of mobility in flexion and extension.

of strain in the neutral position such that with extension the ligament does not relax and buckle in to the spinal canal. The capsular ligaments attach circumferentially around the facet joints and are the strongest ligaments in the cervical spine. The interspinous ligament is a relatively weak ligament that spans between adjacent spinous processes.

Normal Cervical Alignment

The cervical spine permits head rotation, flexion, and extension to maintain the line of sight, while also placing the cranium over the pelvis and supporting a balanced upright posture. Hardacker et al. demonstrated that a plumb line dropped from the tip of the odontoid process would fall ventral to the seventh cervical vertebra, hence sagittal balance[9] (Figure 66.4).

It is difficult to define spine deformity based on clinical observation alone. Gross deformities may be determined through observation of the tragus' relationship to the spinous process of C7 in the sagittal plane. However, these physical examination findings have been found to be inaccurate in most circumstances. In general, surface contour has not been shown to correlate with vertebral body location and position.[43,85] Therefore, radiographs are essential to attempt to objectively understand and document spinal alignment.

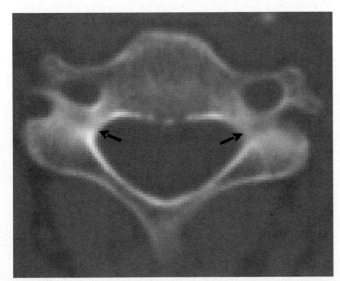

Figure 66.2 Axial CT scan of the cervical spine. The cervical pedicles (*arrows*) are horizontal columns of bones that connect the vertebral bodies to the dorsal elements.

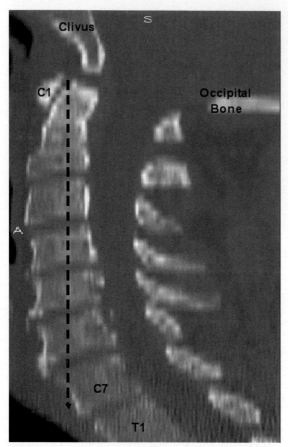

Figure 66.4 This is a plumb line drop from the tip of the odontoid process, falls ventral to the seventh cervical vertebra typically between 0-2 cm.

Presently, there is no accepted standard measurement algorithm for sagittal or coronal cervical spinal curvature. The most commonly used method is the Cobb angle technique that places parallel lines from the caudal and rostral aspects of the vertebral bodies and then measures the intersection angle of these perpendicular lines[16] (Figure 66.5A). Inaccuracy of the Cobb method has been reported since it is based on the noncuboidal shape of the vertebral bodies, where the vertebral body end plate to dorsal cortical angle is greater than 90 degrees.[30] Harrison used tangential lines to the dorsal vertebral bodies (Figure 66.5B) and calculated the "normal" cervical (C2-7) lordosis to be 26 degrees (C2 and C7).[30] Based on these results and engineering principles, he concluded that the tangential technique is more accurate at assessing the cervical angle than the Cobb method, which from C1-7, overestimated, and from C2-7, underestimated the lordosis.[30]

Cervical Alignment—Neutral

The length of the cervical spinal canal measured in the sagittal plane during flexion (kyphotic posture) is greater than during extension (lordotic posture).[79] Therefore, the normal cervical lordosis allows the neural elements to traverse the spinal canal through a shorter course without ventral compression. The lordotic curvature might also protect against neural injury since axial loads are dispersed dorsally onto the facet joints and large articular pillars, rather than the vertebral body (as seen in kyphosis).

A number of disease processes affect the spine, in particular the thoracic and lumbar spine's sagittal balance, which in turn affects the entire spine's sagittal balance. The flexibility of the cervical spine allows it the ability to compensate for misalignment of the thoracic and lumbar spine. Therefore, an increased lordotic cervical posture has been observed when there was a concurrent exaggerated thoracic kyphosis.[29,38,39,59] This compensation permits the maintenance of the overall sagittal balance (i.e., head over the pelvis).

Hardacker *et al.* measured the cervical curvature of 100 volunteers and recorded the mean total cervical lordosis alignment (foramen magnum to C7 inferior end plate) as 40 degrees with a standard deviation of 9.7 degrees where the majority of the lordotic curve was at the C1-2 junction and only 6 degrees was present from C4-7.[29] Despite no patient having an overall cervical kyphotic posture, 39% had a segmental kyphotic angle greater than 5 degrees, typically at C4-5 and C5-6, based on individual segmental angles analysis.[29] Gore *et al.*[26] also measured mean lordotic angles in the cervical spine of osteoarthritis patients from perpendicular lines of the C2 and C7 bodies and observed a 16- to 22-degree lordosis for men and a 15- to 25-degree lordosis in women. Others have measured the C2-7 lordotic curvature to be approximately 14 degrees.[72,111] While numerous studies have shown a wide range for cervical lordosis, slight head extension (0 to 13.9 degrees) has been shown to not affect the cervical spine alignment.[31]

Overall, there is not an accepted range defined as "normal" for cervical posture. While definitive angles have not been calculated, studies have shown that due to aging and degenerative changes the cervical spine has an increase in the lordotic angle.[26,29,40] This lordotic angle increased with aging,[29] from approximately 15 degrees in the third decade to 22 to 25 degrees in the seventh decade.[26]

Cervical Alignment—Dynamic Movement

The cervical spine, also, allows a great degree of flexibility, and dynamic images (flexion and extension radiographs) permit an assessment of the intersegmental motion related to this flexibility. Flexion and extension radiographs of normal individuals have shown that the greatest motion occurs at C4-5 and C5-6 and the least at C2-3.[40,45,58,79] Lin *et al.*[58] further demonstrated that the spine moved from a lordotic position in extension to a nearly parallel position with flexion, such that all intervertebral differences in angular displacement were less than 7 degrees and translation was less than 0.6mm. The total range of motion (ROM) from C2-7 was reported from 50 degrees to greater than 90 degrees with a normal gaussian distribution and a mean of 67 degrees.[58] This ROM is affected by the stiffing of the spine, which occurs throughout the normal aging process.[100]

Degenerative Changes

Cervical spondylotic myelopathy is a pathological process that affects the aging spine. Gore et al. showed that 90% of asymptomatic males, age 60 to 65 years, had degenerative changes on cervical roentgenographic studies.[26] As a

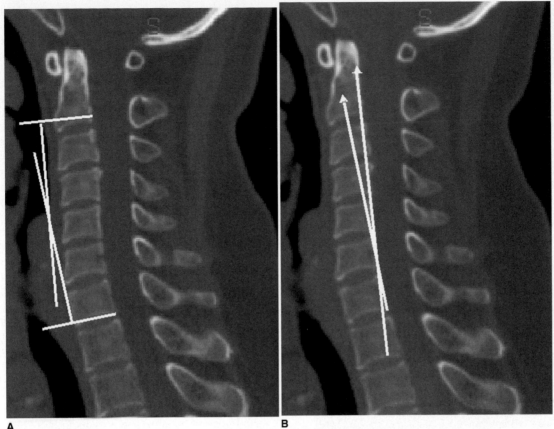

A   B

Figure 66.5 (**A**) Cobb lines are drawn from the inferior end plate of the superior body and from the inferior end plate of the caudal vertebral body. Perpendicular lines are drawn and the angle of intersecting lines is measured. (**B**) Harrison's tangential lines to the dorsal vertebral bodies typically performed at C2 and C7.

result of aging, the vertebral discs dehydrate and the vertebral column loses height (Figure 66.6). This loss of height results in a decreased tension of the ligamentum flavum. The loss of tension on the ligament causes it to shorten and results in buckling of the ligament into the spinal canal, with possible spinal cord compression. Also, degenerative and osteophytic changes take place in the facet joints, along with vertebral disc space junction. The result is a stiffening or rigidity of the cervical spine and a decreased ROM. Holmes illustrated this by showing that the spine segments with the greatest motion migrates from C5-6 to C4-5 with aging.[40]

The overall alignment of the cervical spine should not assume a kyphotic posture due to the normal aging process (see Figure 66.6). Gore showed that, despite the decrease in the intervertebral distance, the overall lordotic curve (C2-7) increased with aging in 200 asymptomatic adults.[26]

Cervical Spine Biomechanical Principles

The position, posture, and motion of the cervical spine are complex processes that direct and manipulate forces on and around the spine. These forces allow the cervical spine to maintain an upright and lordotic posture. Due to the significant mobility of the cervical spine, the displacement of loads can be variable through different anatomic structures depending on the position of the spine during loading. For example, applied axial loads, with the spine in extension, are dispersed through the facet and dorsal articular column, while in flexion the vertebral body supports the majority of the load.

The point or position in the vertebral body that all other points rotate about when a movement occurs is termed the instantaneous axis of rotation (IAR). This is not a static point, but rather is dynamic and changes with position, posture, and direction of movements. Also, each segment has a unique IAR for every movement; it is influenced by spine alignment, anatomy, muscle, and loads exerted. White and Panjabi[40] theorized that in the sagittal plane for flexion and extension, the IAR is located in the ventral portion of the vertebral body. Therefore, each vertebral body has its own IAR for each directional movement. The summation of all the IAR movements dictates spinal column orientation and motion (Figure 66.7).

These forces that act upon the spinal column have both a direction and a magnitude and are, therefore, referred to as force vectors. The perpendicular distance between a force vector and the IAR is defined as the lever or moment arm. The combination of the force vector and the lever arm results in a bending moment about the IAR. Therefore, the IAR can be thought of as a fulcrum, such that with flexion all points ventral to it come together and all points dorsal spread apart[8] (see Figure 66.7).

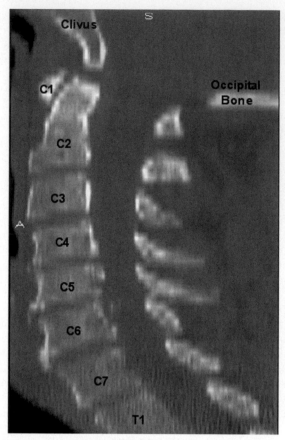

Figure 66.6 CT reformatted sagittal images of degenerative cervical spine. Note the osteophyte formations and loss of disc height.

The muscle and ligament complexes of the cervical spine have a significant effect on the support, motion, and stability of the cervical spine. The effectiveness of each ligament is not only related to the strength of that ligament but also the moment arm through which the ligament acts[8,77] (Figure 66.8). A weaker ligament with a longer level arm might provide more support and strength to the spine than a very strong ligament located on the spinal column, with a short lever arm.

Multiple studies have illustrated the importance of intact and functioning cervical musculature to support and maintain the cervical lordosis. Nolan and Sherk performed a biomechanical analysis of the extensor musculature of the cervical spine and demonstrated that the semispinalis muscle acted as a dynamic stabilizer and the removal of its attachments resulted in the loss of cervical lordosis.[70] Iizuka et al.[41] reattached the semispinalis cervicis muscle after laminoplasty and found that attachment of the extensor musculature on serial MRIs correlated with a maintained cervical lordosis in the postoperative period.

The majority of the cervical spine's ligamentous and muscle complexes support and attach to the dorsal aspect of the spine. These structures, along with the laminae, provide a lever arm, which allows the cervical spine to maintain a lordotic curve. Panjabi showed that without muscular support, the osteoligamentous cervical spine would buckle and fail at only one fifth the weight of the human head.[73,74] These cervical spine specimens (Co-T1) failed with increasing loads of only 11N,[73] while in vivo load testing has shown load ranges from 53N to 1175N.[32,67] This data has to be taken in the context that in vitro models comparing segmental vertebral body motions do not correlate well with in vivo data.[74]

The human body's center of gravity is located approximately 4cm ventral to the sacrum. Therefore, in the sagittal plane, this center of gravity is ventral to the vertebral body. In the standing individual, a plumb line dropped from the tip of the odontoid process, falls slightly ventral (0 to 2cm) to the ventral surface of the C7 vertebral body (see Figure 66.4). The cervical IAR is also located ventral to the vertebral bodies. Therefore, there is a constant

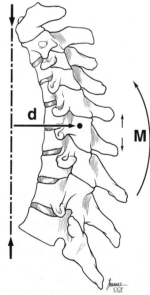

Figure 66.7 The instantaneous axis of rotation (IAR), point in figures, is defined as the position of vertebral body that all other points rotate about when movement occurs. The perpendicular distance (d) between the force vector and instantaneous axis of rotation is defined as lever or moment arm (M). The combination of both the force vector and lever arm results in bending moment about the IAR. (Courtesy of Cleveland Clinic Foundation, 2003.)

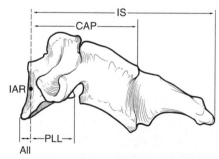

Figure 66.8 The lever arm of the ligaments to the IAR (instantaneous axis of rotation) greatly influences the stability of the spine. The weaker interspinous ligaments work at the greatest distance from the IAR and therefore provide significant resistance to gravitational influences. Although the dorsal elements have weaker ligaments in general, they have much longer lever arms on which they act, and therefore providing a substantial posterior tension band. *ALL,* Anterior longitudinal ligament; *CAP,* capsular ligaments; *IS,* interspinous ligaments; *PLL,* posterior longitudinal ligament.

attraction or force drawing or pulling the spine towards the center of gravity. Newton's first law indicates an object at rest tends to stay at rest while an object in motion tends to stay in motion with the same speed and in the same direction unless acted upon by an unbalanced force. Therefore, as long as the spine has the ability to resist against these gravitational forces through a strong tension band in the form of the dorsal musculoligamentous complex the spine will maintain a lordotic curvature. Otherwise, the cervical spine will gravitate to its lowest energy state or a kyphotic posture, which implies that the cervical spine, without resisting forces, would prefer to be located over at the center of gravity or zero energy state.

The strong muscles and ligaments of the cervical spine are able to maintain this lordotic posture against the gravitation forces due to their increased distance or greater lever arm relative to the IAR (see Figure 66.8). This increased distance creates a mechanical advantage that the muscles and ligaments use to maintain a lordotic curvature. If the muscles and ligaments are weakened either due to congenital diseases, or iatrogenic causes (postsurgical) such a dorsal "anchor" will have a less substantial effect. Then, despite the mechanical advantage provided by the increased lever arm, the cervical spine will migrate further ventrally and the result will be a loss of the lordotic curvature. The ventral migration towards the IAR causes the lever arm that the compromised dorsal muscles and ligaments are acting through to be shorter (Figure 66.9). The shorter lever arm and the weakened dorsal tension band, ligaments, and muscles, fail to provide ample support. This in turn results in further progression of the kyphotic defor-mity. This cycle of impaired muscles and shorter lever arm continues until a significant deformity with possible neurologic findings results. The aforementioned may be illustrated in a patient with Marfan's syndrome. In this disorder, the affected individuals have an increased laxity of their ligamentous structures and therefore are at an increased risk for abnormal cervical alignment. Hobbs et al.[39] confirmed this by showing that 36% of patients with this disorder had absence of the normal cervical lordosis.

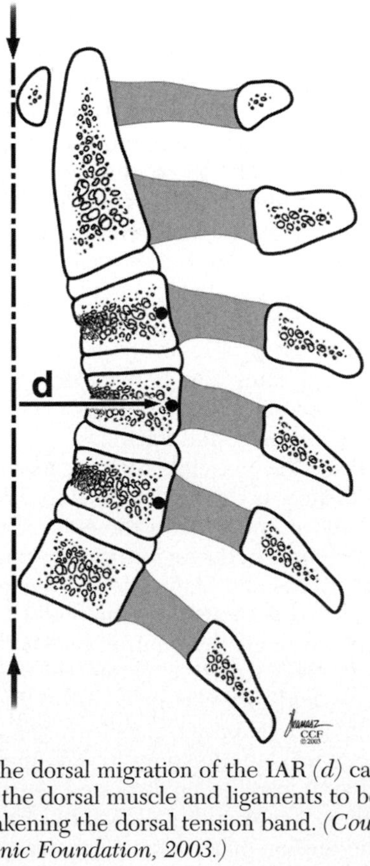

Etiologies and Treatment Approaches

Subaxial cervical deformities can develop in any plane or direction, but most commonly occur in the sagittal plane, primarily as a kyphotic deformity, and rarely as coronal plane abnormalities (i.e., scoliosis). Cervical and cervicothoracic scoliosis are extremely rare disorders and only sparse reports of their occurrences are available in the literature. However, there are multiple causes for kyphotic deformities, resulting either through congenital or acquired disorders. Congenital diseases create structural spinal disorders due to abnormalities of the bones either focally in the vertebral bodies (Klippel-Feil, hemiverte-bra);[94,95,108] systemic disorders (dystrophic dystonia, Larsen's syndrome);[27,54,65,86,87] or the muscle and ligamentous structures (Marfan's syndrome, Prader-Willi syndrome).[39,102] Acquired kyphotic cervical spine disorders may be secondary to spinal tumors (neurofibromatosis),[69] occupational exposures,[50] iatrogenic causes (postlaminectomy, pseudoarthrosis),[2,21] and traumatic injuries.

Cervical and Cervicothoracic Scoliosis

Smith defined cervical and cervicothoracic scoliosis as a structural curvature of the cervical or cervicothoracic region resulting from an osseous abnormality, such as a block vertebrae or unilateral bar, that is visible on either anterodorsal or lateral radiographs (Figure 66.10).[94,95] Other etiologies include a failure of segmentation, block vertebrae, a failure of formation, hemivertebrae, or a combination of these anomalies.[94,95] Cervical scoliosis is occasionally associated with unilateral congenital nerve defects in the upper extremity.[108] This disorder typically occurs in children and they present early due to cosmetic concerns of malpositioning of the head. Cervical spine alignment abnormalities do not have the ability to form a rostral compensatory curve since the head is the rostral terminus of the spine.

Treatment options vary depending on the degree of curvature, the anatomical abnormalities, and the age and medical condition of the patient. Bracing is the least invasive technique, but is unfortunately not an optimal treatment strategy since most deformities are due to segmental, formation, and developmental disorders. They, therefore, are usually associated with a large curve. In the few patients with a kyphotic angle less than 30 degrees that passively correct past the neutral plane, bracing is the best treatment option.[94,95] These patients must be able to wear their brace for extended periods and be followed clinically with serial imaging and clinical examinations for signs of curve progression.

Figure 66.9 The dorsal migration of the IAR (*d*) causes the lever arms of the dorsal muscle and ligaments to be shorter, therefore weakening the dorsal tension band. (*Courtesy Cleveland Clinic Foundation, 2003.*)

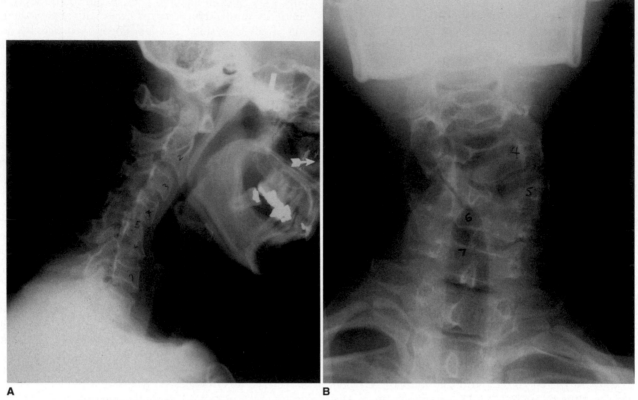

A   B

Figure 66.10 Adult patient presenting with radiculopathy who is noted to have a congenital hemivertebra and kyphotic deformity (**A**) and resultant scoliosis as seen on her anteroposterior radiograph (**B**).

Unfortunately, most patients present with severe curves (i.e., greater than 40 degrees), rigidity, severe torticollis, and lateral tilting that does not respond to bracing.[94,95] Smith *et al.*[94,95] advocated operative treatment strategy for these patients via a dorsal fusion of the structural portion of the curve. Surgical dissection must be meticulous since the incidence of bone abnormalities and absent lamina has been reported to be as high as 30%.[95] Fortunately, these curves are usually flexible due to the young age of the patient population and can be manipulated intraoperatively. Smith,[95] using this dorsal arthrodesis technique, had a solid fusion in 20 of 21 patients, with an average follow-up of 17 years. If the curves are stiff and rigid, the use of traction preoperatively increases the mobility of the spine. Winter[109] had two cases of cervical scoliosis with associated arm paralysis and advocated early surgical intervention for progressive spinal deformity. Deburge[18] reported one patient with a cervical scoliosis secondary to a hemivertebra and Klippel-Feil syndrome that was treated with a staged ventral and dorsal procedure.

Postsurgical Kyphosis

The postoperative development of a cervical kyphotic deformity may follow either a ventral or dorsal cervical spine operation. Following ventral surgery, kyphosis may develop secondary to pseudoarthrosis or inadequate restoration of the anatomic cervical lordosis.[2,14,25] However, to a greater degree, kyphosis occurs iatrogenically due to the destruction of the dorsal tension band after cervical laminectomy (Figure 66.11).[2,21]

Historically, dorsal operations for cervical decompression have been felt to result in cervical instability and the formation of kyphotic or swan-neck deformities due to the excessive resection of the facet joints and loss of integrity of the muscle and ligamentous complex (dorsal tension band). Several *in vitro* studies have confirmed these suspicions, demonstrating that the cervical spine loses its stability if the facet joint is resected bilaterally after laminectomy.[14,83,84,111] Zdeblick *et al.*[111] further defined this process through progressively greater facetectomies, and showed that greater than 50% of facet joint resection resulted in the cervical spine being unable to maintain strain, torsional stiffness, and flexion.

The biomechanical principle that fosters the creation of a kyphotic deformity is the loss of the dorsal tension band. As illustrated above, the IAR for the cervical bodies lies in the ventral vertebral body region in the neutral position (see Figure 66.7). Pal and Sherk[72] tested the load transmission in cadaver and demonstrated that 36% of axial forces were displaced through the ventral vertebral body while the majority or 64% was transmitted through the dorsal columns (facets and articular processes). The loss of the dorsal muscle and ligament tensile force and support (i.e., after a cervical laminectomy) results in the weight of the head and axial loads to be displaced ventrally onto the vertebral bodies. These additional ventral forces cause an increase in the tension on the dorsal ligaments and muscles

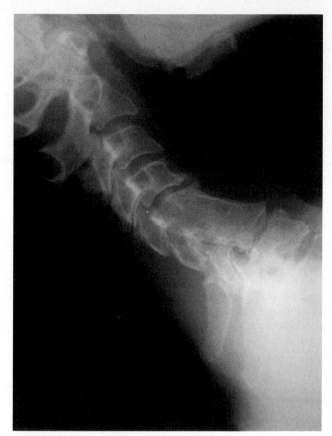

Figure 66.11 Lateral radiograph in a patient presenting with a postlaminectomy kyphosis and previous anterior fusion. Note the absence of the posterior spinous process and lamina and a resulting severe kyphotic deformity.

that are maintaining cervical alignment. If the muscles and ligaments are weakened or the bony structures are excessively resected (i.e., greater than 50% of the facet joint), then the ventral forces might overcome the weakened dorsal tensile forces, resulting in migration of the curve to a straight or kyphotic posture. As this occurs, further loads create a kyphotic bending moment, which leads to further kyphosis. Thus, a vicious cycle is created, and the resultant curve progression may lead to compression of the spinal cord and neurologic deficit. As the kyphosis progresses further, the increased stress on the ventral spinal cord may adversely affect the spinal cord vasculature and lead to even further myelopathic symptoms.[11,61] Also, this kyphotic posture or angle places a large degree of strain on the dorsal muscles, which has been shown to correlate with neck pain,[6,49] including mechanical pain.[48] Eventually, the dorsal cervical musculature fatigues, permitting greater kyphosis, and even greater mechanical pain.

Children are the most vulnerable to develop structural deformities after laminectomy.[4,7,15] These patients typically have laminectomies for the management of intradural tumors. Cervical laminectomy combined with the underlying disease state and compromised neurologic status adds to the stress on the spine, and markedly increases the incidence of postsurgical kyphosis. Bell[7] reviewed 132 children who underwent cervical laminectomies and reported a 15% incidence of hyperlordosis and a 38% incidence of kyphotic deformities. Aronson[4] noted instability in 95%

of the patients that had a laminectomy with concurrent suboccipital craniectomy.

The incidence of postlaminectomy kyphosis in the adult population has not been defined, but may be as high as 21%.[12,46] However, it is known that the patient population with a kyphotic spinal alignment prior to laminectomy is at the greatest risk of developing a progressive kyphotic deformity.[66,91] Mikawa *et al.*[66] examined 64 patients for an extended period of time (i.e., 26 years) and analyzed their cervical alignment after laminectomy. In this population, 36% had a change in their alignment, but only 14% were classified as developing a kyphotic deformity. Of note, no patient experienced neurologic sequelae as a result of the changes in their cervical alignment.

Ankylosing Spondylitis

Ankylosing spondylitis, also referred to as Marie-Strumpell disease, is a seronegative spondyloarthropathy that primarily affects the spine, hips, and sacroiliac joints. The cervical spine is commonly affected and has radiographic manifestations of the disease in over 48% of patients.[57] This disorder is a continuum from soft tissue disease to the destruction and fusion of the joints.[24] These patients' spines gradually ossify, and over time, the ligamentous insertion sites on the bone, including the discs, fuse into a rigid circumferential kyphotic position (Figure 66.12).[35,64]

The cervical spine kyphotic deformities limit horizontal gaze. The result of extreme cervical deformity is a chin on chest deformity with the inability for the patient to perform daily activities due to poor line of sight, difficulty opening their mouths, and mastication difficulties. Prior to treating cervical or gaze abnormalities, full 36-inch radiographs of the entire spine should be performed. This permits assessment of the overall sagittal balance, including lumbar or thoracic kyphosis. Also, horizontal gaze abnormalities can be a result of hip-flexion contractures, which must also be evaluated and ruled out as the underlying pathology.[56]

Smith-Peterson *et al.*[96] first describe the osteotomy technique to restore sagittal balance. The ankylosis of the vertebral bodies in these patients makes the spine essentially a rigid column and concurrently creates a kyphotic deformity. These patients are very vulnerable to fractures due to the long rigid moment arm, confined with poor bone quality.[17,99] It is this principle of a long ossified lever arm that facilitates restoration of horizontal gaze and correction of the kyphotic deformity through a dorsal osteotomy.

Once the patient is determined to be an appropriate surgical candidate, the location of the site for deformity correction must be determined. The majority of authors advocate treating this deformity by extension osteotomy at the cervicothoracic junction.[89,92,104] This level is chosen since it is caudal to the majority of the eloquent cervical spinal cord, the exiting C8 nerve roots are very mobile and resistant to traction or manipulation, and the vertebral arteries have not yet entered the foramen transversarium.[92,93] The procedure, as initially described, is performed under local anesthesia with the patient awake and sitting. Removing all of the C7, the caudal portion of C6, and the rostral portion of the T1 laminae, along with the

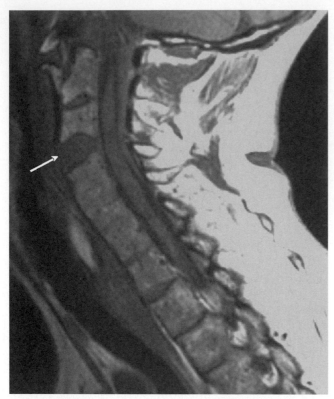

Figure 66.12 Cervical spine ankylosing spondylitis. Note the circumferential autofusion of the spine. Prior to fracture, the patient had a severe kyphotic or chin on chest deformity. As a result of the fall and hyperextension injury *(arrow)*, the spine was fractured at the superior apex of the autofused spine. The result was a normalization of the patient's overall sagittal alignment.

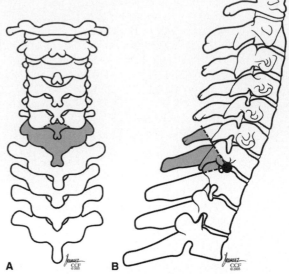

Figure 66.13 (**A**) Dorsal view of the bone removed *(shaded portion)* to perform the wedge osteotomy. (**B**) Lateral view of bone removed *(shaded portion)* to perform the wedge osteotomy. *(Courtesy Cleveland Clinic Foundation, 2003.)*

C7-T1 facet joints is required to perform the wedge osteotomy (Figure 66.13). The deformity is then corrected externally either by an articulated plaster jacket incorporating the head and neck[104] or by manual extension (intraoperatively).[92,93] Stability is maintained with an *in situ* fusion along with a halo-jacket,[92] or with internal fixation with instrumentation.[63,99]

Urist was the first to perform a dorsal cervicothoracic reduction osteotomy,[104] which Simmons modified and popularized (the dorsal laminectomy technique) (see Figure 66.13). McMaster *et al.*[63] reported 15 patients with ankylosing spondylitis and flexion deformity that were treated by dorsal extension osteotomy and external fixation by halo (12 patients) or by internal fixation (3 patients). Their surgical technique consisted of additionally resecting a portion of the C6 and T1 pedicles to avoid impingement of the C8 nerve roots during the deformity correction. Under electrophysiological monitoring, the head is extended that permits an average deformity correction of 54 degrees. Others have also shown that the application of dorsal instrumentation, such as lateral mass plates and intraspinous wiring, is well tolerated and has allowed immobilization in a cervical collar without the use of a halo apparatus.[20,90,99] Duff *et al.*[20] reported one patient in whom a fixed flexion deformity was corrected, (approximately 90 degrees of lordosis), utilizing a single-stage two-level midcervical osteotomy.

Some surgeons use both a ventral and dorsal approach for correction of rigid ankylosed cervical deformities. Safety and control of deformity correction are the stated advantages of this combined approach.[90] After the osteotomy has been performed, the patient may then be placed in the supine position and a ventral corpectomy performed to allow decompression and release for the correction of the deformity. Iliac crest bone grafting and ventral instrumentation may then be performed. Due to the large moment arm above and below the level of the fusion, dorsal instrumentation should also be used, thus aiding in the prevention of further deformity.

Congenital—Larsen's Syndrome

In 1950, Larsen *et al.*[54] described a clinical syndrome in six patients consisting of: ventral dislocation of the knee, dislocation of the elbows and hips, equinovarus deformity of the feet, and typical facies (i.e., increased intracanthral distance, prominent forehead, depressed nasal bridge). Since this initial series, others have noted that spinal skeletal abnormalities are also associated with this syndrome and in particular the progression of cervical kyphotic deformities.[42,55,65,97]

These kyphotic deformities can be very impressive and cause neurologic injury due to spinal cord compression at the apex of the curve. The kyphosis typically develops due to marked hypoplasia of one to two vertebral bodies with concurrent dorsal element anomalies.[42,65] Due to the severe degree of kyphosis, these cervical deformities are diagnosed at a young age. Johnson *et al.*,[42] noting the severe neurologic compromise associated with these deformities, emphasized the need to make the diagnosis of cervical kyphosis when Larsen's syndrome is suspected.

An early operative treatment of this cervical kyphosis has been advocated due to the often associated severe neurologic morbidity and mortality at a young age (less than 2 years).[42,65,68] Ventral cervical fusions play a limited role in these pediatric patients since they limit future ventral axial growth, while permitting further dorsal growth. The end result is lengthening the dorsal column, while the ventral column is fixed, which creates further propagation of the kyphotic deformity. However, with extreme deformities, a ventral fusion and strut graft optimizes the deformity correction. Francis et al.[23] performed this technique in one child with a severe kyphosis (168 degrees) with neurologic deficits, and observed a complete neurologic recovery.

Therefore, a dorsal arthrodesis is typically used for the treatment of this patient population.[42,65] A dorsal arthrodesis provides a tension band, but also allows the ventral column to continue with axial growth, thus increasing the cervical lordosis.[88] Johnson[42] showed that in two of the four patients he treated with a dorsal arthrodesis, spinal alignment corrected into a lordotic posture on follow-up. These patients must be followed serially, since the continued growth can cause hyperlordosis and dorsal compression from the fusion mass.[42]

Congenital—Diastrophic Dysplasia

Diastrophic dysplasia is a rare autosomal recessive disease manifested as short-limbed, short stature, multiple joint contractures, early degeneration of joints, and spinal deformities.[47,82,86,87,105] The spinal anomalies can be manifested as cervical kyphosis, scoliosis, and exaggerated lumbar lordosis. The cervical spine in these patients typically assumes a kyphotic alignment due to midcervical vertebral body hypoplasia. However, unlike other systemic bone disorders that affect the cervical spine these patients' cervical kyphotic deformities have been reported to spontaneously resolve.[9,82,86,87]

Remes et al.[86] reported on the natural history of this disorder; that is, resolution of the cervical kyphosis and vertebral body hypoplasia. In the 25 patients that had radiographs taken prior to the age of 2 the incidence of a kyphotic deformity was 96%. With advanced age, the incidence of kyphosis reduced to only 29 of 120 patients (24%).[86] Therefore, in approximately 75% of these patients, kyphosis resolved after the age of 2 years. The remodeling of the vertebral bodies in the pediatric population allows further ventral support, and along with the strengthening of the dorsal musculature and ligamentous complex, allows these patients to obtain a lordotic cervical curvature.[86,101]

Patients with kyphotic deformities less than 60 degrees or resolving curves without neurologic symptoms can be followed clinically and with serial radiographs. A kyphotic deformity angle greater than 60 degrees and round or triangular dorsally displaced vertebral bodies at the apex were signs of a poor prognosis. Curves greater than 60 degrees are at a biomechanical disadvantage and remodeling and repair of the ventral spine is not sufficient to restore alignment. These patients, along with patients with progressive curves or those patients with neurologic symptoms due to the kyphotic deformity, should be treated surgically. If left untreated, these severe kyphotic deformities can cause medullary compression, resulting in respiratory depression and possibly death.[47,82] When surgical treat-ment is required, a combined ventral and dorsal procedure has been reported as a favored technique.[9,37,53,86]

Surgical Techniques

Sagittal plane deformity in the cervical spine may be surgically treated through a ventral,[14,25,36,110] dorsal,[1,13] or combined approach.[1,34,51,62] In general, if there is imaging evidence of ventral compression of the cervical spinal cord, a ventral procedure should be performed combined with a dorsal approach. If there is no radiographic or clinical evidence of spinal cord compression and the deformity is flexible (nonfixed), the deformity may be corrected posturally or with traction, then fused in the desired position dorsally. If the kyphotic deformity is fixed or rigid, a ventral decompression with fusion following deformity correction may be used to address the kyphosis. If the deformity is fixed and there is evidence of ankylosis of the facet joints, a ventral decompression and bone grafting, combined with a dorsal osteotomy and fusion should be considered, often with combined ventral and dorsal instrumentation. Lastly, ankylosing spondylitis patients with ankylosis of the vertebral bodies and long ossified vertebral columns can be treated with a dorsal osteotomy reduction and fusion.

The reduction of the deformity through positioning, traction, or intraoperative manipulation allows the spine to be positioned optimally for fusion. The use of instrumentation or external immobilization will provide interim rigidity and support. However, the ultimate goal of surgical intervention is a solid arthrodesis and maintaining the deformity correction.

Traction

Traction is often useful as an initial tool in the evaluation of the surgical approaches to cervical kyphosis, after obtaining dynamic cervical radiographs and assessing the flexibility of the cervical spinal deformity. Traction over an extended period (multiple days) affords the spine the opportunity to gradually respond to external forces that are directed and controlled by the surgeon. Traction can be used to maintain a position; yet it may also be used to correct the deformity as well. The patient can then be taken to the operating room and a dorsal fixation performed to maintain the adjusted cervical alignment and prevent further kyphotic progression. The duration of traction required to reduce kyphotic deformities typically takes 3 to 5 days. If there is only a limited or no reduction of the deformity after 3 days, further traction is unlikely to be beneficial. Muscle relaxants and a gradual increase of the weight may also be used to aid in the reduction process.

Postlaminectomy kyphotic deformities typically develop over an extended period of time and are more difficult to manage due to the rigid nature of the deformity. During the time interval that the kyphosis develops, the spine ages and becomes stiffer due to the loss of disc height, along with the development of osteophytes and other degenerative changes. These changes make traction more difficult in these spondylotic patients. Sims et al.[91] were not able to reduce kyphotic deformities in 8 of 17 postlaminectomy patients and only had complete reduction in 3 patients.

Although reducing kyphotic deformities with traction may be difficult in these patients, any improvement or increased flexibility is advantageous intraoperatively.

Ventral Approach

The ventral approach to the cervical spine provides direct access to the ventral column and provides the greatest ability to correct kyphotic deformities while simultaneously decompressing the neural elements. The use of an isolated ventral technique for deformity correction obligates the determination of the dorsal element mobility preoperatively. This surgical approach provides optimal ventral decompression of the spinal cord and permits the attainment of a lordotic cervical posture via a variety of strategies. This ventral decompression of the apex of the kyphotic deformity can result in an improved neurologic outcome (Figure 66.14).[36]

The ventral deformity correction technique involves multiple components (or stages), including positioning the patient in an extended position on the operating table, local distraction and extension via segmental distraction techniques (i.e., the use of Caspar distractors initially placed in a convergent fashion), further extension after neural decompression, the use of lordotic-shaped bone grafts, and the use of multiple instrumentation fixation points and bending moments. The distraction of the vertebral bodies for the bone graft increases the tension of the dorsal longitudinal ligament and reduces buckling of

this ligament. This elimination of dorsal ligamentous buckling increases the area in the spinal canal for the spinal cord. This distraction also allows the neural foramen to widen due to the increased distance between the pedicles.

The ventral approach and correction of the cervical deformity uses both posture and biomechanical principles. The initial positioning on the operating table by placing the head and neck in a neutral position or in slight extension not only increases the exposure but helps reduce the kyphotic deformity (Figure 66.15). It is important to test the limits of patient tolerance to neck extension prior to placing the patient under general anesthesia in order to not compromise the spinal cord. This may occur as the spinal cord is draped over ventral kyphotic pathology (osteophytes) as the neck is extended. The physician should access the cervical alignment from the intraoperative images obtained during the localization portion of the procedure; this should also permit an estimation of the correction desired.

Local traction through the use of distraction devices (i.e., the Caspar technique) may further aid with kyphotic deformity correction. The distraction posts should be placed in a convergent manner (Figure 66.16A), since the distraction posts have a mechanical advantage due to an increased lever arm. When the posts are distracted the long lever arms cause the vertebral end plates to become parallel, resulting in an increase in the cervical extension and, lordosis (Figure 66.16B). After the decompression has been completed, the neck and head may be further extended and positioned in a more lordotic alignment. This may be accomplished by having the anesthesiologist remove the previously placed doughnut from under the patient's head, thus further extending the spine (see Figure 66.15).

Resection of the kyphotic apex and reconstruction of the cervical spine into a lordotic posture is the ultimate goal of the procedure. There are multiple strategies to achieve this goal. One technique is to leave an intermediate vertebral body (C5 in the preceding example) in the area of decompression. This allows adequate decompression, since the dorsal intermediate vertebral body can be resected from both a rostral and caudal direction

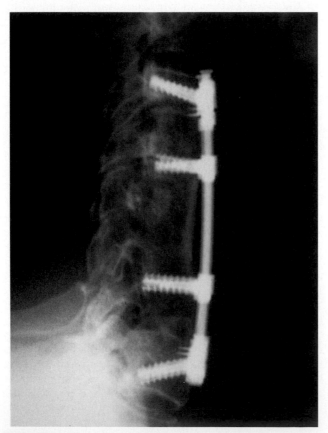

Figure 66.14 Ventral approach to a kyphotic deformity in patient illustrated in Figure 66.11. Note the reduction of the kyphotic deformity and a more natural lordotic curvature.

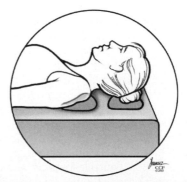

Figure 66.15 Diagram when positioning on the operating table where the patient is continued in the neutral to slightly extended position with both a shoulder roll and donut. After surgical decompression, the headrest may be removed along with further extension and reduction of the kyphotic deformity. (*Courtesy Cleveland Clinic Foundation, 2003.*)

(Figure 66.17). Perhaps most importantly, the retention of the intermediate vertebral body provides an additional intermediate point of fixation for further deformity correction (see discussion that follows), while increasing the security of the instrumentation (see Figure 66.17).

There are numerous biomechanical and clinical advantages associated with the use of multiple points of fixation ventrally. When the intermediate screws are tightened, the spine is brought to the contoured construct (see Figure 66.17). This strategy not only achieves lordosis, but also provides three or four point bending force application, which serves to maintain the sagittal alignment and to prevent rotational and translational forces. Hence, this strategy minimizes the chance of terminal screw-bone interface degradation. The intermittent vertebral bodies provide additional bone surface to induce fusion, thereby requiring a shorter bone graft. A long iliac bone graft or fibular graft is typically straight and therefore the end result of the reconstruction will be straighter, rather than the natural lordotic curvature.

The lordotic curve can be further enhanced by the contour of the bone graft. Constructing or designing the ventral portion of the graft to be longer than the dorsal portion positions the end plates in a convergent manner and results in a more lordotic posture. Also, if an autologous tricortical iliac crest graft is to be used, the cortical bone should be placed ventrally. The crestal portion of the graft should provide greater subsidence prevention ability

than cancellous bone. This as well promotes the restoration of a lordotic curvature.

A dynamic ventral implant should be considered when using this ventral strategy. These implants permit controlled deformation in the axial plane (axial subsidence), yet prevent deformation in the sagittal plane (kyphosis) (see Figure 66.14).[8] The controlled subsidence allows the bone graft(s) to absorb most of the axial forces, which should encourage bone healing via Wolff's Law.[8] The implant design also off-loads stresses at the screw-bone interface. This further contributes to a diminished incidence of structural failure. Steinmetz et al.[98] utilizing this technique, were able to maintain their 20-degree lordotic correction (−5 degrees preoperatively to 15 degrees postoperatively) with less than a 2-degree kyphosis with a 13-month average follow-up.

Dorsal Approach

The use of a single staged dorsal strategy for the correction of cervical deformity is not common in the adult population. If there is a ventral vector compressing and distorting the neural elements then a ventral procedure should be performed and then only if necessary followed by a subsequent dorsal procedure. However, if the kyphotic deformity is flexible and ventral decompression is not required, a dorsal approach may be warranted (Figure 66.18). Additionally, the technique of cervical traction followed by dorsal fixation is effective only if the spinal canal compression is dorsal and there is no significant ventral compression.[66,91]

Cervical traction may be used to maximally reduce the kyphotic deformity. If used, this traction should be maintained in the operating room or once in the operating room, the traction can be switched to a Mayfield headrest. A lateral preoperative cervical radiograph should be

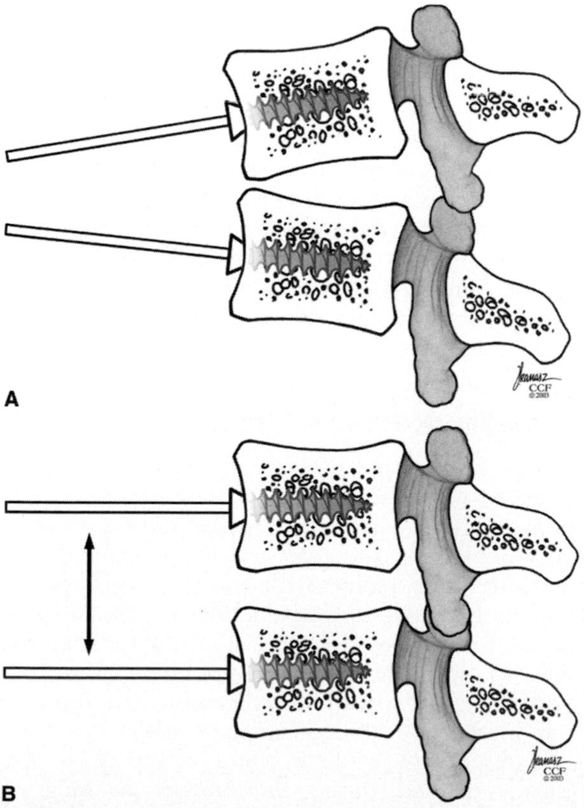

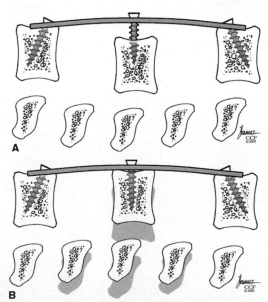

Figure 66.16 **(A)** The distraction posts are placed in a convergent manner. **(B)** Distraction against the posts provides cervical extension and further lordosis. *(Courtesy Cleveland Clinic Foundation, 2003.)*

Figure 66.17 **(A)** After the construct has been secured at its rostral and caudal ends, the intermediate screws are placed. **(B)** When this intermediate screw is tightened, the spine is brought to the contoured implant. This allows the attainment of further lordosis. *(Courtesy Cleveland Clinic Foundation, 2003.)*

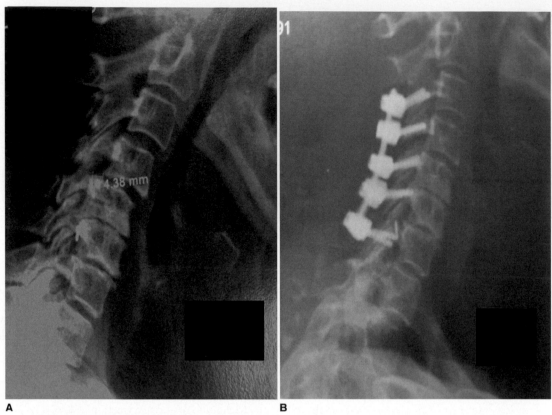

Figure 66.18 Kyphotic deformity with 4mm of subluxation at C4-5 (**A**), which increases to 7mm with flexion and reduces on extension. Posterior reduction with laminectomy due to cervical stenosis and myelopathy with a posterior instrumented fusion (**B**).

obtained to ensure adequate cervical alignment. A standard dorsal subperiosteal approach to the cervical spine is then performed.

Once the spine in exposed, there are numerous techniques to optimize fusion and maintain the deformity correction. External immobilization, interspinous wiring, lateral mass fixation, and pedicle screw fixation may all be used to maintain the deformity correction. While lateral mass fixation is the most commonly used method, some reports have shown that the lateral masses may not be the optimal stabilizing anchor for some patients.[3,22,34] When placing lateral mass fixation, the rostral lateral quadrant is devoid of vascular and nervous structures, making it the safest target for placing lateral mass screws.[71] Interspinous wiring may not be used if laminectomy is performed, due to removal of the spinous processes.

Abumi *et al.*[1] utilized cervical pedicle screws fixation for the dorsal correction of cervical deformities. Kotani *et al.*[52] has shown that the cervical pedicle screws are equivalent to combined ventral plate and dorsal wiring and cervical pedicle screws may be superior biomechanically as a stand-alone fixation construct. Abumi *et al.*,[1] utilizing only cervical pedicle screws were able to correct flexible cervical kyphotic deformities from 28.4 to 5.1 degrees of kyphosis, with all patients achieving a solid arthrodesis. These patient's cervical kyphotic deformities were only reduced and then fused into a neutral position. It should,

however, be emphasized that lordosis was not achieved with this dorsal procedure alone. Also, the technique of cervical pedicle screw fixation can result in severe neurologic and vascular consequences due to the proximity of the vertebral artery, nerve roots, and cervical spinal cord. Despite no clinical sequelae in their patients, this cervical pedicle screw technique had a 6.3% pedicle perforation and malposition rate.[1]

Combined Ventral and Dorsal Approaches

Combined ventral and dorsal approaches allow ventral lengthening and concurrent dorsal shortening to maximize cervical deformity correction. This technique permits ventral decompression and release, with or without ventral instrumentation, along with dorsal decompression, release, and possible instrumentation (Figure 66.19). The addition of the dorsal construct uses a long moment arm strategy to aid in deformity prevention.[8] Ventral release and fusion may be required for the optimal deformity correction when using lateral mass plate fixation.[1]

The ultimate goals of the operative procedure should be clearly defined, during the strategy planning stage. There are multiple combined approach strategies to approach a cervical deformity. The surgeon can use a ventral-dorsal, dorsal-ventral, ventral-dorsal-ventral, or a dorsal-ventral-dorsal technique. The particular anatomic

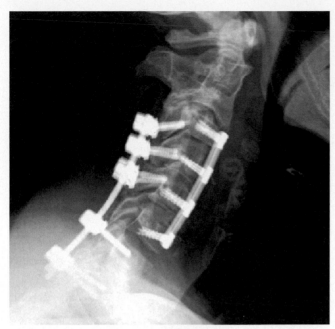

Figure 66.19 Postoperative radiographs after an anteroposterior decompression and fusion with both a lengthening of the anterior column and shortening of the posterior column that allows for a reduction deformity and the development of a lordotic posture.

constraint of each patient and surgical goals permit the surgeon to choose the sequence of operative approaches.

When ventral compression exists, and the dorsal procedure is solely for supplemental instrumentation for stability, the ventral decompression (discectomy or corpectomy) and grafting should be performed first. Oftentimes a ventral-dorsal technique with a ventral and dorsal implant is used. A laminectomy is not necessary unless there is concomitant dorsal compression. The lateral masses are exposed, decorticated and then a dorsal implant is placed, most often lateral mass plates or rods. Interspinous wiring may also be used, but lateral mass fixation has been shown to provide greater rigidity than wire fixation alone.[22]

If an inadequate deformity correction is accomplished through an anterior technique, then the dorsal elements have to be released further. The ventral-dorsal-ventral technique can be used, since it allows further dorsal deformity correction after the dorsal release. Once this is achieved, additional ventral correction strategies can be employed followed by instrumentation if appropriate. Unfortunately, instrumentation cannot be placed after the initial ventral decompression since this would lock the vertebral bodies in position and limit further dorsal correction.

Another ventral-dorsal-ventral strategy can be accomplished by using cervical pedicle screws. The ventral decompression and release should be performed first without grafting or instrumentation. After decompression, the patient is placed in the prone position to expose the dorsal cervical spine. An assistant may then adjust the head holder to achieve maximal lordosis. Since ventral decompression has been performed before this reduction, further dorsal reduction should be safe. The dorsal con-

struct (lateral mass fixation or pedicle screw construct) may then be placed to secure the deformity correction. Iliac crest may then be harvested to provide morselized bone for the dorsal fusion and a ventral strut graft. The patient is again placed in the supine position, the ventral strut graft is placed, and a ventral implant is secured. Abumi *et al.*,[1] utilizing a combined ventral/dorsal approach with cervical pedicle screw instrumentation, were able to improve an average preoperative kyphosis of 30.8 to 0.5 degrees of kyphosis at the final follow-up.

Patients with kyphotic deformities and ankylosed or fused posterior elements may benefit from a dorsal-ventral or a dorsal-ventral-dorsal procedure. The dorsal technique permits the release of the posterior fusion and removal of previous instrumentation. No attempt to reduce the deformity should be performed after the dorsal release if there is any ventral compression. Once the dorsal elements are released the patient can be turned supine and the ventral procedure performed. This ventral operation permits release of the ventral bodies and deformity correction. Any ventral compression can be removed and once the deformity is corrected an implant can be placed for stability. Depending on the quality of the patient's bone and the surgeon's satisfaction with the implant and bone graft stabilization the decision of dorsal stability can be addressed. If the graft does not appear to be stable then a dorsal-ventral-dorsal procedure can be performed with supplement instrumentation on the dorsal elements.

Summary

Cervical spine deformities result from a variety of causes. They may result in and present with mechanical neck pain and/or progressive neurologic deficit. If the patient is symptomatic or quality of life is threatened as a result of the deformity, surgical correction should be considered. Emphasis should also be placed on further deformity prevention, such as restoring lordosis after a ventral decompression procedure or using dorsal fusion and/or instrumentation after an extensive dorsal decompression. The ventral approach is optimal in most cases of kyphotic cervical deformities since it permits decompression and permits a "better surgical leverage" than dorsal surgery for deformity correction. The ventral approach also provides numerous solid fixation points and the number may be increased if intermediate points of fixation are employed. In cases where a fixed deformity exists, a combined approach may be warranted. Overall, the correction of cervical deformities is rewarding, since the majority of patients obtain relief of their mechanical symptoms and enjoy an improvement of neurologic function.

REFERENCES

1. Abumi K, Shono Y, Taneichi H, *et al*: Correction of cervical kyphosis using pedicle screw fixation systems. *Spine* 24(22):2389-2396, 1999.
2. Albert TJ, Vacarro A: Postlaminectomy kyphosis. *Spine* 23(24):2738-2745, 1998.

3. Anderson PA, Henley MB, Grady MS: Dorsal cervical arthrodesis with AO reconstruction plates and bone graft. *Spine* 16:S72-79, 1991.

4. Aronson DD, Kahn RJ, Canady A: Cervical spine instability following suboccipital decompression and cervical laminectomies for Arnold-Chiari syndrome (abstract). Presented at the 56th annual meeting of the American Academy of Orthopaedic Surgeons, Las Vegas, 1989.

5. Asazuma T, Yamagishi M, Nemoto K, *et al:* Spinal fusion using a vascularized fibular bone graft for a patient with cervical kyphosis due to neurofibromatosis. *J Spinal Disord* 10(6):537-540, 1997.

6. Batzdorf U, Batzdorff A: Analysis of cervical spine curvature in patients with cervical spondylosis. *Neurosurgery* 22(5):827-36, 1988.

7. Bell DF, Walker JL, O'Connor G, Tibshirani R: Spinal deformity after multiple-level cervical laminectomy in children. *Spine* 4:406-11, 1994.

8. Benzel EC: *Biomechanics of Spine Stabilization*. Chicago, IL, American Association of Neurological Surgeons, 2001.

9. Bethem D, Winter RB, Lutter L: Disorders of the spine in diastrophic dwarfism. *J Bone Joint Surg Am* 62A: 529-536, 1980.

10. Bland JH, Boushey DR: Anatomy and physiology of the cervical spine. *Semin Arthritis Rheum* 20:1-20, 1990.

11. Breig A, El-Nadi AF: Biomechanics of the cervical spinal cord: Relief of contact pressure on and overstretching of the spinal cord. *Acta Radiol Diagn* 4:602-624, 1964.

12. Butler JC, Whitecloud TS 3rd: Postlaminectomy kyphosis. Causes and surgical management. *Orthop Clin of North Am* 23(3):505-511, 1992.

13. Callahan RA, Johnson RM, Margolis RN: Cervical facet fusion for control of instability following laminectomy. *J Bone Joint Surg Am* 59A:991-1002, 1977.

14. Caspar W, Pitzen T: Ventral cervical fusion and trapezoidal plate stabilization for re-do surgery. *Surg Neurol* 52: 345-352, 1999.

15. Cattell HS, Clark GL Jr: Cervical kyphosis and instability following multiple laminectomies in children. *J Bone Joint Surg Am* 49(4):713-720, 1967.

16. Cobb JR: Chapter outlines for the study of scoliosis. In Edwards JW (ed): *Outlines for the Study of Scoliosis: Instructional Course Lecture,* vol 5. Ann Arbor, MI, American Academy of Orthopedic Surgeons, 1948, pp 261-275.

17. Cooper C, Carbone L, Michet CJ, *et al:* Fracture risks in patients with ankylosing spondylitis: A population-based study. *J Rheumatol* 21:1877-1882, 1994.

18. Deburge A, Briard J: Cervical hemivertebrae excision. A report of a case. *J Bone Joint Surg Am* 63A:1335-1339, 1981.

19. Depalma AF, Rothman RH: *The Intervertebral Disc*. Philadelphia, WB Saunders, 1970, pp 5-46.

20. Duff SE, Grundy PL, Gill SS: New approach to cervical flexion deformity in ankylosing spondylitis. *J Neurosurg (Spine 2)* 93:283-286, 2000.

21. Fager CA: Laminectomy and kyphotic deformity. *J Neurosurg* 95(1 Suppl):157-158, 2001

22. Fehlings MG, Cooper PR, Errico TJ: Dorsal plates in the management of cervical instability: Long-term results in 44 patients. *J Neurosurg* 81:341-349, 1994.

23. Francis WR Jr, Noble DP: Treatment of cervical kyphosis in children. *Spine* 13(8):883-887, 1988.

24. Freeman GE: Correction of severe deformity of the cervical spine in ankylosing spondylitis with the halo device. *J Bone Joint Surg* 43A:547-552, 1961.

25. Geisler FH, Caspar W, Pitzen T: Reoperation in patients after ventral cervical plate stabilization in degenerative disease. *Spine* 23:911-920, 1998.

26. Gore DR, Sepic SB, Gardner GM: Roentgenographic findings of the cervical spine in asymptomatic people. *Spine* 11:521-4, 1986.

27. Goto S, Kobayashi Y, Saisu T, Moriya H. Cervical myelopathy caused by destructive kyphotic spine in Cushing's disease. *J Bone Miner Metab* 17(4):301-307, 1999.

28. Gray H: *Anatomy, Descriptive and Surgical*. Pick TP, Howden R (eds). American ed, revised from 15 ed English. New York, Bounty Books, 1977.

29. Hardacker JW, Shuford RF, Capicotto PN, Pryor PW: Radiographic standing cervical segmental alignment in adult volunteers without neck symptoms. *Spine* 22(13):1472-1480; discussion 1480, 1997.

30. Harrison DE, Harrison DD, Cailliet R, *et al:* Cobb method or Harrison dorsal tangent method: which to choose for lateral cervical radiographic analysis. *Spine* 5(16):2072-2078, 2000.

31. Harrison DE, Harrison DD, Janik TJ, *et al:* Slight head extension: does it change the sagittal cervical curve? *Eur Spine J* 10(2):149-153, 2001.

32. Hattori S, Oda H, Kawai S, *et al:* Cervical intradiscal pressure in movements and traction of the cervical spine. *Z Orthop* 119:568-569, 1998.

33. Hayashi K Yabuki T: Origin of the uncus and of Luschka's joint in the cervical spine. *J Bone Joint Surg Am* 67(5):788-791, 1985.

34. Heller JG, Silcox III DH, Sutterlin CE III: Complications of dorsal cervical plating. *Spine* 20:2442-2448, 1995.

35. Herbert JJ: Vertebral osteotomy for kyphosis, especially in Marie-Strumpell arthritis: A report of fifty cases. *J Bone Joint Surg Am* 41(2):291-302, 1959.

36. Herman JM, Sonntag VK: Cervical corpectomy and plate fixation for postlaminectomy kyphosis. *J Neurosurg* 80(6):963-970, 1994.

37. Herring JA: The spinal disorders in diastrophic dwarfism. *J Bone Joint Surg Am* 60(2):177-182, 1978.

38. Hilibrand AS, Tannenbaum DA, Graziano GP, *et al:* The sagittal alignment of the cervical spine in adolescent idiopathic scoliosis. *J Pediatr Orthop* 15(5):627-632, 1995.

39. Hobbs WR, Sponseller PD, Weiss AP, Pyeritz RE: The cervical spine in Marfan syndrome. *Spine* 22(9):983-989, 1997.

40. Holmes A, Wang C, Han ZH, Dang GT: The range and nature of flexion-extension motion in the cervical spine. *Spine* 19(22):2505-2510, 1994.

41. Iizuka H, Shimizu T, Tateno K, *et al:* Extensor musculature of the cervical spine after laminoplasty: morphologic evaluation by coronal view of the magnetic resonance image. *Spine* 26(20):2220-2226, 2001.

42. Johnston CE 2nd, Schoenecker PL: Cervical kyphosis in patients who have Larsen syndrome. Comment on: *J Bone Joint Surg Am* 1996 Apr;78(4):538-45. *J Bone Joint Surg Am* 79(10):1590-1591, 1997.

43. Johnson GM: The correlation between surface measurement of head and neck posture and the anatomic position of the upper cervical vertebrae. *Spine* 23(8): 921-927, 1998.

44. Johnston FG, Crockard HA: One stage internal fixation and anterior fusion in complex cervical spinal disorders. *J Neurosurg* 82:234-238, 1995.

45. Johnson RM, Hart DL, Simmon EF, *et al:* Cervical orthosis: a study comparing their effectiveness in restricting cervical motion in normal subjects. *J Bone Joint Surg Am* 59A:332-339, 1977.

46. Kaptain GJ, Simmons NE, Replogle RE, Pobereskin L: Incidence and outcome of kyphotic deformity following laminectomy for cervical spondylotic myelopathy. *J Neurosurg* 93(2 Suppl):199-204, 2000.

47. Kash IJ, Sane SM, Samaha FJ, Briner J: Cervical cord compression in diastrophic dwarfism. *J Pediatr* 84: 862-864, 1974.

48. Katsuura A, Hukuda S, Imanaka T, *et al:* Anterior cervical plate used in degenerative disease can maintain cervical lordosis. *J Spinal Disord* 9:470-476, 1996.

49. Kawakami M, Tamaki T, Yoshida M, *et al:* Axial symptoms and cervical alignments after cervical ventral spinal fusion for patients with cervical myelopathy. *J Spinal Disord* 12(1):50-56, 1999.

50. Kelkar P, O'Callaghan B, Lovblad KO: Asymptomatic grotesque deformities of the cervical spine. An occupational hazard in railway porters. *Spine* 23(6): 737-740, 1998.

51. Kokubun S, Ozawa H, Sakurai M, Ishii Y: One-stage ventral and dorsal correction of severe kyphosis of the cervical spine in neurofibromatosis. A case report. *Spine* 18(15):2332-2335, 1993.

52. Kotani Y, Cunningham BW, Abumi K, McAfee PC: Biomechanical analysis of cervical stabilization systems: An assessment of transpedicular screw fixation in the cervical spine. *Spine* 19:2529-2539, 1994.

53. Krecak J, Starshak RJ: Cervical kyphosis in diastrophic dwarfism: CT and MR findings. *Pediatr Radiol* 17(4): 321-322, 1987.

54. Larsen LJ, Schottstaedt ER, Bost FC. Multiple congenital dislocations associated with characteristic facial abnormalitiy. *J Pediatr* 37:574-581, 1950.

55. Latta RJ, Graham CB, Aase J, *et al:* A skeletal dysplasia with multiple joint dislocations and unusual facies. *J Pediatr* 78:291-298, 1971.

56. Law WA. Osteotomy of the spine. *J Bone Joint Surg* 41A:291-302, 1962.

57. Lee HS, Kim TH. Yun HR, *et al:* Radiologic changes of cervical spine in ankylosing spondylitis. *Clin Rheumatol* 20(4):262-266, 2001.

58. Lin RM, Tsai KH, Chu LP, Chang PQ: Characteristics of sagittal vertebral alignment in flexion determined by dynamic radiographs of the cervical spine. *Spine* 26(3):256-261, 2001.

59. Loder RT: The sagittal profile of the cervical and lumbosacral spine in Scheuermann thoracic kyphosis. *J Spinal Disord* 4(3):226-231, 2001.

60. Lu J, Ebraheim NA, Yang H, Rollins J, Yeasting RA: Anatomic bases for ventral spinal surgery: surgical anatomy of the cervical vertebral body and disc space. *Surg Radiol Anat* 21(4):235-239, 1999.

61. Masini M, Maranhao V: Experimental determination of the effect of progressive sharp-angle spinal deformity on the spinal cord. *Eur Spine J* 6:89-92, 1997.

62. McAfee PC, Bohlman HH, Ducker TB: One stage ventral cervical decompression and dorsal stabilization. A study of one hundred patients with a minimum of two years of follow-up. *J Bone Joint Surg Am* 77:1791-1800, 1995.

63. McMaster MJ: Osteotomy of the cervical spine in ankylosing spondylitis. *J Bone Joint Surg Br* 79B:197-203, 1997.

64. Mehdian H, Jaffray D, Eisenstein S: Correction of severe cervical kyphosis in ankylosing spondylitis by traction. *Spine* 17(2):237-240, 1992.

65. Micheli LJ, Hall JE, Watts HG. Spinal instability in Larsen's syndrome: report of three cases. *J Bone Joint Surg Am* 58(4):562-565, 1976.

66. Mikawa Y, Shikata J, Yamamuro T: Spinal deformity and instability after multilevel cervical laminectomy. *Spine* 12:6-11, 1987.

67. Moroney SP, Schultz AB, Miller JA: Analysis and measurement of neck loads. *J Orthop Res* 6:713-20, 1988.

68. Muzumdar AS, Lowry RB, Robinson CE: Quadriplegia in Larsen's syndrome. *Birth Defects Orig Art Ser* 13:202-211, 1977.

69. Nemoto K, Asazuma T, Amako M, *et al*. Vascularized fibula graft for spinal fusion in severe cervical kyphosis due to neurofibromatosis *J Reconstr Microsurg* 13(8): 559-562, 1997.

70. Nolan JP, Sherk HH: Biomechanical analysis of the extensor musculature of the cervical spine. *Spine* 13:9-11, 1988.

71. Pait GT, McAllister PV, Kaufman HH: Quadrant anatomy of the articular pillars (lateral cervical mass) of the cervical spine. *J Neurosurg* 82:1011-1014,1995.

72. Pal GP, Sherk HH: The vertical stability of the cervical spine. *Spine* 13(5):447-449, 1988.

73. Panjabi MM, Cholewicki J, Nibu K, *et al:* Critical loads of the human cervical spine: an in vitro experimental study. *Clin Biomech (Bristol, Avon)* 13:11-17, 1998.

74. Panjabi MM, Miura T, Cripton PA, *et al:* Development of a system for in vitro neck muscle force replication in whole cervical spine experiments. *Spine* 26(20):2214-2219, 2001.

75. Panjabi MM, Duranceau J, Goel V, *et al:* Cervical human vertebrae quantitative three-dimensional anatomy of the middle and lower regions. *Spine* 16(8):861-869, 1991.

76. Panjabi MM, Shin EK, Chen NC, Wang JL: Internal morphology of human cervical pedicles. *Spine* 25(10):1197-1205,2000.

77. Panjabi MM, Greenstein G, Duranceau J, *et al:* Three-dimensional quantitative morphology of lumbar spinal ligaments. *J Spinal Disord* 4:54-72, 1991.

78. Panjabi MM, Oxland T, Takata K, *et al:* Articular facets of the human spine. *Spine* 18(10):1298-1310, 1993.

79. Penning L: Normal movements of the cervical spine. *AJR Am J Roentgenol* 130:317-326, 1978.

80. Piccirilli CB, Chadduck WM: Cervical kyphotic myelopathy in a child with Morquio syndrome. *Childs Nerv Syst* 12(2):114-116, 1996.

81. Polly DW, Klemme WR, Shawen S: Management options for the treatment of posttraumatic thoracic kyphosis. *Semin Spine Surg* 12:110-116, 2000.

82. Poussa M, Merikanto J, Ryoppy S, *et al:* The spine in diastrophic dysplasia. *Spine* 16:881-887, 1991.

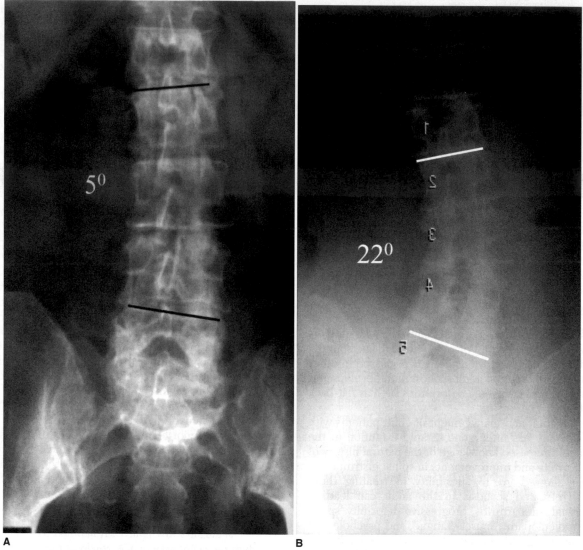

A   **B**

Figure 67.1 Supine (**A**) and standing (**B**) AP lumbar radiographs demonstrating the increase of the lumbar scoliosis from 5 to 22 degrees with change in position.

similar findings in 1986. They reviewed 187 random cases of untreated idiopathic scoliosis evaluated from 15 to 47 years (average 33 years) after the end of growth. All curves increased an average of 0.4 degrees per year after skeletal maturity. The thoracic curves progressed more than lumbar, lumbar more than thoracolumbar, and thoracolumbar more than double major curves.

Despite agreement concerning curve progression, there remains controversy regarding the incidence of back pain, cardiorespiratory complications, and mortality related to adult spinal deformity. In contrast to adolescents who are usually asymptomatic, adults with deformity tend to present with back pain. It can arise from muscle fatigue, trunk imbalance, facet arthropathy, or degenerative disc disease. Low back pain, however, is ubiquitous among the adult population. Therefore, determining if back pain is related to the deformity becomes more difficult. In spite of complaints of back symptoms ranging from 40% to 90% of patients with idiopathic curves, long-term follow-up studies find that

the incidence of back pain is no greater than the general population.* A recent study by Weinstein and associates[200] followed 117 patients with late onset idiopathic scoliosis, and 62 matched control patients for 50 years. They reported that 61% of patients with late onset idiopathic scoliosis complained of chronic back pain whereas only 35% of their matched controls had chronic back pain. On closer investigation, whereas back pain was more prevalent, it was minor and did not result in a significant difference in activities. They concluded that untreated idiopathic adolescent scoliosis causes little physical impairment other than back pain and cosmetic concerns.

Several authors have tried to correlate the degree of curve and the incidence of back pain. Independently, studies by Collis and Ponseti[48] in 1969 and Edgar and Mehta[62] in 1988 failed to find a correlation between back symp-

---

*References 6,13,34,49,61,65,95,102,142.

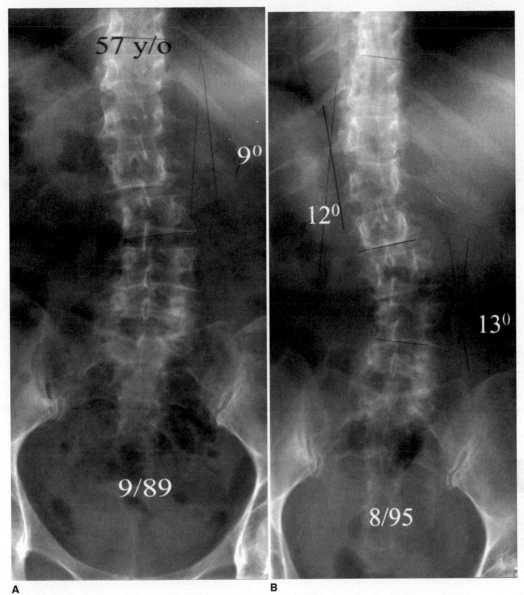

A **B**

Figure 67.2 **(A-D)** A series of AP lumbar spine radiographs from age 57 through 70, which demonstrates a progression of lumbar scoliosis from 9 to 33 degrees after skeletal maturity.

Continued

toms and the degree or type of curve. However, two other papers found a correlation between curve severity and back pain.[70,102] In 1981, Kostuik and Bentivoglio[102] noted that as the degree of curvature increased, the severity of pain increased, especially for curves more than 45 degrees. In addition, patients without back pain tended to have smaller curves. Back pain, in this population, was related to curve magnitude, facet sclerosis, and radiologic changes at the apex of the curve. It was not related to the age of the patient.

Surgeons have also tried to compare surgically treated patients with control subjects. Connolly and associates[49] reviewed 83 patients treated with Harrington instrumentation and 60 control patients. Seventy-six percent of the treated patients and 50% of the control patients complained of chronic low back pain. As expected a higher incidence of degenerative changes was noted with fusions

into the lower spine, and sagittal imbalance (flat-back) was associated with a poor result. Twenty-two percent of patients underwent additional procedures, and 17% felt the goals of surgery had not been accomplished.

In addition to back pain, adult patients with significant scoliosis are more likely to experience symptoms of spinal stenosis and radiculopathy from rotatory subluxation. Fortunately, paresis or paraplegia from untreated scoliosis in the absence of true kyphosis has not been reported.

Pulmonary function may also be compromised as adolescents with scoliosis advance into adulthood. Decreased vital capacity may occur in patients with severe thoracic curves, especially in the presence of thoracic lordosis, which effectively decreases the anterior-posterior chest diameter.[189] Ascani and associates[7] documented that 35% of their patients with untreated severe thoracic scoliosis complained of cardiopulmonary

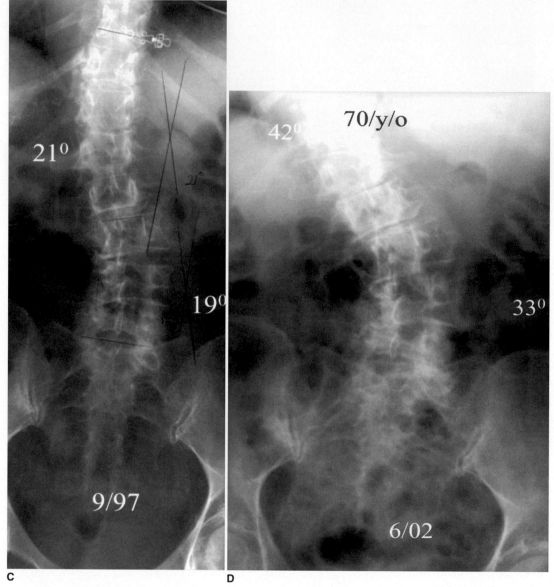

21⁰

19⁰

9/97

C

42⁰   70/y/o

33⁰

6/02

D

Figure 67.2 *cont'd*

symptoms. In a recent report with 50-year follow-up, Weinstein and associates[200] found that 22% of patients complained of shortness of breath during everyday activities compared with 15% of 53 controls. An increased risk of shortness of breath was also associated with the combination of a Cobb angle greater than 80 degrees and a thoracic apex. It is therefore possible to imagine that a progressive thoracic deformity could cause deterioration of lung function and cor pulmonale. However, Pehrsson and associates[151] reported a 20-year follow-up in untreated scoliosis showing no difference in pulmonary function other than what was predicted by declining age. Evidence is lacking to suggest progression of pulmonary disease in an adult with previous normal pulmonary function after skeletal maturity without pre-existing pulmonary disease or history of smoking.

Older studies looking at mortality of untreated scoliosis had significantly higher rates of mortality as compared with more recent studies. Nilsonne and Lundgren[146] in

1968 reviewed 102 patients with idiopathic scoliosis who had been followed for 50 years. They reported a mortality rate twice that of the general population with right heart failure (cor pulmonale) accounting for 60% of the deaths. Another study in 1968 by Nachemson[143] reported long-term follow-up of patients with untreated scoliosis. Of the 117 patients, 20 were dead with 16 related to cardiopulmonary disease. In 1986, Ascani and associates[7] reported a 17% mortality rate in an unselected group of 187 patients with untreated scoliosis who were followed from 15 to 47 years after skeletal maturity. This was twice that of the general population. All of the patients had severe thoracic scoliosis and died of cardiopulmonary complications. In contrast, in a recent 50-year follow-up of 117 patients with untreated scoliosis and 62 matched volunteers, there was no difference in probability of survival.[200]

Several investigators have documented social disturbances. Appearance and health have become increasingly important for social acceptance. Not being able to perform up to expectations, whether it is real or perceived, because of a deformity can create a significant social burden. In 1968, Nilsonne and Lundgren[146] found that almost half of their patients, mainly those with severe deformities, were not working. Ascani and co-workers[7] also reported a low marriage rate in women. The same year Nachemson[143] found that 30% of patients were on disability and none of the full-time employed patients were employed in heavy manual labor. Patients with a pre-existing curve may migrate toward less physically demanding occupations or may be more likely to miss work if they have a physically demanding job.[87,136]

Psychological factors have not been well documented in adults, but patients with adolescent idiopathic scoliosis show a greater frequency of suicidal ideation and feelings of poor body development.[75,150] Ascani and associates[7] reported real psychological disturbances in 19% of their patients. These patients were more commonly women or had thoracic curves (greater than 40 degrees). Despite these reports, Collis and Ponseti,[48] in their 1969 study, found few psychiatric disturbances related to scoliosis. In their study, 90% of patients were married and lived productive lives. Nineteen percent admitted psychological reactions to their deformity, but none required psychiatric counseling.

Patient Presentation

Spinal deformity in an adult has a significant impact on that patient's perception of his or her health. Schwab and colleagues[165] in 2003 surveyed 22 patients with adult scoliosis using the Medical Outcomes Survey Short-Form 36 (SF-36). This is considered to be a generic measure of health values that are not age, treatment, or disease specific. Therefore, it is a universal measure of health assessment. The average age was 63 years. The patients with adult scoliosis averaged much lower scores than norms for both the general U.S. population and the U.S. population for ages 55 to 64. In fact, these patients had lower scores compared with norms of patients with co-morbid conditions such as back pain and hypertension. These data demonstrate the significant effect adult scoliosis has on a patient's perception of health.

Adolescents with idiopathic scoliosis rarely have complaints other than cosmesis. Adults with deformity, however, present with a variety of complaints. They include pain, curve progression, neurological symptoms including radiculopathy and neurogenic claudication, cardiopulmonary compromise, cosmesis, or problems from previous surgeries. The incidence of pain associated with adult scoliosis is controversial. Reports range from 40% to 90%.[48,62,95,102,142] Back pain is more commonly seen in lumbar curves and in thoracolumbar and lumbar curves larger than 45 degrees with apical rotation and coronal imbalance.[102,195] The patients' complaints are similar to those of patients with lumbar degenerative disease without deformity. The pain typically starts on the convexity, possibly because of muscle fatigue. As time progresses, pain can develop on the concavity. This can be secondary to asymmetric loading and facet arthropathy. With time, radicular pain can develop secondary to narrowing of the neuro-

foramina caused by lateral listhesis, facet arthropathy, or bulging of degenerative discs.

In addition to pain, some patients present with curve progression. As discussed earlier, adolescent curves can progress, even after skeletal maturity. In a 1969 study, Vanderpool and colleagues[195] documented a six-fold increase in the incidence of scoliosis in patients older than 50 who had osteoporosis as compared with a control group. Some patients will develop a *de novo* deformity in adulthood. Robin and co-workers[159] documented that 10% of their subjects developed scoliosis *de novo* during a 7- to 13-year follow-up period. However, they found no direct relationship between the presence or progression of scoliosis and osteoporosis. Although the precise etiology of *de novo* adult scoliosis is uncertain, many of these patients seem to develop the scoliosis in the setting of degenerative disc pathology. Asymmetric disc degeneration has been suggested as one etiology; occasionally tumors or infection, causing asymmetric vertebral destruction, may underlie a new scoliotic curve.

Cardiopulmonary compromise in patients with severe thoracic scoliosis (more than 60 degrees) with an effective thoracic lordosis is well recognized. However, adults without previous pulmonary compromise or history of smoking rarely present with new cardiopulmonary symptoms as the main reason for evaluation. Increasingly, because of cosmetic complaints, adults are seeking surgical evaluation for deformity. Considering the significant risks, surgery in adults based entirely on improving appearance is controversial.

Surgical intervention in adolescent scoliosis has increased as the instrumentation has allowed for better correction of the coronal plane deformity. Harrington rods revolutionized the treatment of adolescent scoliosis in the 1960s, but consequences of the shortcoming of this system have gradually been recognized. With the development of segmental instrumentation and then pedicle screw fixation, more patients (both adolescent and adult) have undergone surgical correction of deformities with improvement in the coronal and sagittal alignment of the spine. Not all deformity correction surgery is successful, and a variety of complications are associated with the procedure, especially for surgery in adult patients. There is a growing population of patients who have undergone previous surgery and either have curve progression, pseudarthrosis, pain, or poor coronal or sagittal balance in whom further problems such as flat-back syndrome arise.

Patient Evaluation

The assessment of a patient with spinal deformity has many components used in evaluating any patient with back pain or lower extremity neurologic complaints. More focus is needed on the history of the curvature, whether symptoms are long-standing or recent, and which activities improve or worsen pain. Frequently, evaluating an adult with deformity is more difficult than an adolescent. Adult deformity patients tend to have more pain and often have other conditions that complicate the assessment such as hip or knee arthritis. It is difficult to interpret if the pain is secondary to the deformity itself, caused by neurological compromise or the effect of deconditioning. The criteria for operative treatment are undergoing evolution. Many aspects of the timing of surgery, the optimal surgical approach, and number of levels of the spine that need to be treated are not yet clearly defined. In addition, surgical treatment of adult spinal deformities carries a significantly higher rate of complications and longer recovery periods than those for adolescent patients.

A complete history and physical examination followed by the appropriate radiographic studies is essential. The history should focus on the pain (location, radiation, aggravating and alleviating factors, and temporal course). It is important to rule out other causes of back discomfort such as osteoporotic fracture, infection, or tumor. In addition, a relevant family history of deformity is obtained. The importance of social and family history and occupational history cannot be overemphasized. Depression, substance abuse, and nicotine use can result in poor outcomes.

The physical examination should be complete. It is important to examine the patient's skin for signs of intraspinal pathology, such as café au lait spots, nevi, or hairy patches. The cosmetic appearance of the deformity can be documented by observing the rib hump, asymmetry of the trunk, and the spinal balance in both the frontal and lateral planes. Additionally, the rigidity of the deformity can be evaluated subjectively in the clinic. Performing a thorough neurologic examination is important; however, cardiopulmonary and general psychiatric evaluations are important if surgical intervention is considered.

Imaging Studies

No evaluation of spinal deformity is complete without a thorough radiologic evaluation. If available, previous studies (including old chest radiographs and scout films for other studies) should be reviewed to document curve progression. Full-length (14 × 36 inch), standing posterior-anterior (PA) and lateral radiographs are the most important radiographs to assess spinal deformity. They will allow evaluation of each curve (structural and compensatory) magnitude, axial rotation, lateral translation, and global balance (coronal and sagittal). When surgery is considered, dynamic views (side bending to the left and right) assessing curve flexibility are obtained.

Supine lateral bending films, with the patient giving maximal effort, help to evaluate flexibility of the coronal deformity and plan fixation levels (Figure 67.3). Flexion and extension views help to determine the rigidity or flexibility of sagittal plane deformities and to assess for coexistent spinal instability. Traction views may be helpful in determining the flexibility of deformities over 60 degrees.[154,196] Other techniques have been advocated in order to determine curve flexibility during preoperative planning to select proximal and distal fixation levels. Some have advocated the use of a fulcrum bending view. In this view, the patient is in the lateral decubitus position with the apex of the primary curve over a large bolster. Bridwell and associates[197] have advocated the use of a "push-prone radiograph" in which the pelvis of the prone patient is stabilized, while the surgeon applies lateral pressure to the major curve. They concluded that this technique allows better estimation of the effects that correction of the primary curve has on the curves above and below the level of fusion.

If a patient has symptoms of radiculopathy, neurogenic claudication, or any neurologic abnormality, intraspinal imaging is mandatory. Magnetic resonance imaging (MRI) is now the preferred imaging technique. MRI is able to evaluate spinal cord pathology and nerve root compression. Occasionally, in patients with previous metallic implants (due to artifacts), or very large curves, myelography and post myelography computerized tomography (CT) become necessary. The widespread use of titanium alloy implants, which cause less MRI artifact, and advances in imaging techniques may obviate the need for myelography in the future.

Other Studies

Discography as a means of evaluating the source of pain remains controversial.[47,92] A recent position paper by the North American Spine Society supported the use of discography in the "assessment of discs before fusion to determine if the discs within the proposed fusion segment are symptomatic and to determine if discs adjacent to this segment are normal."[80] The information obtained from the procedure is highly variable and is related to the patient's ability to reliably localize the pain and the practitioner performing the study. The false-positive rate and difficulty of a patient to separate spinal from non-spinal sources of pain has been questioned.[41,42] Carragee and associates[40] demonstrated that high-intensity zones in discs did not correlate with positive discography. The same group[39] also reported that patients with abnormal psychological profiles had significantly higher rates of positive disc injections than either asymptomatic volunteers or symptomatic subjects with normal psychological screening. Despite this, several studies using discography to localize pain seemed to show the usefulness of discography in the preoperative assessment.[56,99-102] However, patients with discogram-positive low back pain who do not undergo an operation may improve without an operation.[176] In a 2002 study by Madan and associates,[130] discography did not improve surgical outcomes after circumferential fusion for lumbar discogenic back pain. Certainly the value of discography in predicting the results of surgical fusion can be disputed. Discography is most commonly used for longer fusion in adults to assess the L4-5 and L5-S1 levels. If no significant degeneration exists and the levels are painless on discography, stopping a fusion short of the sacrum or pelvis can be considered.

Pulmonary function testing is performed on patients with thoracic curves greater than 70 degrees, in patients who complain of pulmonary symptoms, or in those with history of pulmonary disease such as chronic smokers. This information is especially helpful if a thoracoplasty is considered to be part of the operative therapy. Lenke and colleagues[125] demonstrated that adults who undergo thoracoplasty experience a 27% decline in pulmonary function by 3 months that did not improve after 2 years. This is in contrast to adolescents who experience a decline in pulmonary function but usually regain the function by the 2-year follow-up.

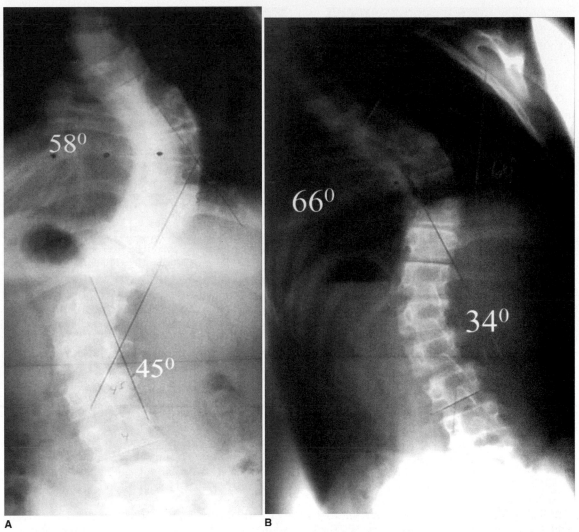

Figure 67.3 Standing PA (**A**) left side–bending (**B**) and right side–bending (**C**) radiographs demonstrating moderate correction of the lumbar curve from 45 to 34 degrees and no significant change in the thoracic curve from 58 to 54 degrees.

Continued

Treatment

Non-Operative Treatment

The initial treatment of adults with deformity is the same as the treatment of patients with mechanical back pain without deformity. The pain can be treated with non-steroidal anti-inflammatory drugs and non-narcotic analgesics. Chronic narcotics should be discouraged because of a risk of dependency and tolerance. Additionally, high levels of narcotics can complicate the postoperative pain management leading to respiratory depression or inadequate analgesia caused by narcotic tolerance. Although bracing has not been shown to prevent curve progression, the stabilizing effect may be beneficial in pain relief.[144,145,190] Epidural steroid injections, nerve root blocks, and facet injections may also be of value in the conservative management of a patient with adult spinal deformity.

Physical therapy or water aquatic therapy should be instituted to promote spinal motion, maintenance of muscle tone, and aerobic activities. Many of the adults with spinal deformity are significantly deconditioned. The activity is designed to counteract a sedentary lifestyle. If obesity is a problem, the patient is encouraged to lose weight. Patients are also encouraged to stop smoking, which is known to contribute to respiratory dysfunction in addition to the inhibitory effects nicotine has on bone fusion. If they do require operative intervention, any conditioning they can do preoperatively will aid them during postoperative recovery. Therefore, all patients should undergo a reasonable non-operative course of treatment before considering surgical intervention.

Operative Treatment

Indications

The operative indications for adults with spinal deformity are not as clearly defined as for adolescents with spinal deformity. There are two major groups of patients. One

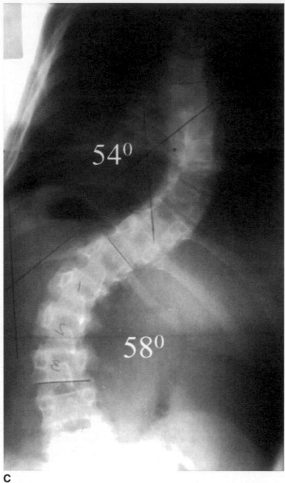

54⁰

58⁰

C

Figure 67.3 *cont'd* (**C**) Radiographs demonstrating moderate correction of the lumbar curve from 45 to 34 degrees and no significant change in the thoracic curve from 58 to 54 degrees.

Progressive pain related to deformity
Deformity progression:
   Thoracic curve greater than 50-60 degrees
   Lumbar curve greater than 45 degrees
Neurologic deficit:
   Radiculopathy
   Neurogenic claudication
Salvage/reconstructive surgery

ment with recumbency are the best candidates for surgical correction of the deformity.

Curve progression is another indication for surgical intervention. Younger patients (<40) with thoracic curves greater than 50 to 60 degrees or lumbar curves greater than 45 degrees have a high risk of progression. At a younger age, these curves are more likely to be flexible and amenable to a single stage anterior or posterior procedure. As these patients age, the curve becomes rigid requiring more extensive surgery.

Coronal or sagittal imbalance is another indication for surgical intervention. Truncal imbalance of greater than 4 cm is more common in the older population and impacts ability to perform activities of daily living. This imbalance can lead to deformity progression and referred muscular pain in an attempt to balance the spine. Severe sagittal imbalance is particularly disabling and can limit standing or ambulating to very brief periods.

Neurologic deficits are rare in younger patients. If present, they mandate MRI evaluation looking for syringomyelia, congenital anomalies of the spinal column or cord, spinal cord tumors, cord compression, or infection. Neurologic complaints are more common in the older patient population and associated with extensive degenerative changes causing spinal or foraminal stenosis. With the degenerative changes come symptoms of neurogenic claudication.

With the advent of Harrington distraction instrumentation, the deformity of AIS was corrected in the coronal plane and maintained until arthrodesis was obtained. However, the spinal distraction used for this technique led to a loss of lumbar lordosis and the development of flat-back syndrome in thoracolumbar and lumbar curves. A large population of patients now undergo surgical correction for deformity as an adolescent with distraction instrumentation. They can present with flat-back syndrome, adjacent degenerative changes, or adjacent level kyphosis.

group consists of the patients with adolescent idiopathic scoliosis (AIS) who present in young adulthood, whereas the other group consists of older patients (usually >50) with either progression deformity or new onset of deformity. The younger patients tend to have outcomes similar to AIS with relatively low morbidity. However, the older patients have more chronic disease (diabetes, cardiac disease, pulmonary disease), greater frequency of spinal degenerative disease, and poorer bone quality; thus they have a substantial risk for complications with large reconstructive procedures. Indications for surgery include unrelenting pain, deformity progression, neurologic deficit, and salvage reconstruction following previous surgery (including flat-back syndrome) (Box 67.1).

Pain is a very common complaint and is the main complaint in many adult patients with scoliosis. As discussed earlier, determining the source of pain remains challenging. As patients age, they develop more spinal degenerative disease and also present more often with pain. As with any surgery, finding the source of pain and focusing the surgery to address that pathology will more predictably lead to a successful outcome. Patients who have significant pain with standing or ambulation but substantial improve-

General Considerations

Surgical treatment of spinal deformities in adults is often challenging. The deformities are often rigid and unbalanced in either the coronal or sagittal planes. The bone is frequently osteopenic, affecting fixation points and the choice of fixation devices. Associated neurologic complaints such as radiculopathy and neurogenic claudication are frequent. Often the patients have had prior decompressive surgical procedures without instrumentation or fusion that has resulted in further progression of the deformity, worsening pain, or further neurologic compromise.

The goals of surgical intervention include pain relief, prevent progression of deformity, solid fusion, rigid internal fixation, and finishing with a balanced spine (Box 67.2).

Segmental instrumentation has replaced Harrington distraction rods as the fixation of choice in spinal deformities. Whereas the Harrington rods limited correction to the coronal plane and potentially had detrimental effects on sagittal balance, segmental instrumentation allows the surgeon to simultaneously address the coronal and sagittal balance. With the greater flexibility of the instrumentation, patients who in the past would not have been candidates for surgical intervention are now undergoing deformity correction. Patients with previous fusion are at an increased risk for degeneration in adjacent motion segments.[66,108,109,121] The risk may increase in proportion to the extent of the prior fusion into the lumbar region.[2] These patients may require extension of the fusion. In 1992 Paonessa and Engler[148] reviewed 103 idiopathic scoliosis patients fused with Harrington rods to L3 or lower and a control group of 29 patients fused to L2 or above. They found a higher rate of secondary surgeries for complications or late disc disease below the fusion, a higher back pain score, and more difficulties with normal daily activities in the study group. This was especially true in the patients older than 30 who were fused to L3 or distally. In 1995, Connolly and associates[49] reviewed 83 patients who had Harrington instrumentation for idiopathic scoliosis into the lumbar spine at an average 12-year follow-up. They found a higher incidence of low back pain for fusions performed at or below L2.

Overall, it is important to remember that the amount of correction of the deformity is not as important as leaving the patient with a balanced spine in both the coronal and sagittal plane. Correction of a thoracic rib prominence is less important in an adult. Although used in adolescents to correct the rib prominence, thoracoplasty is rarely used in older adults because of increased complications and worsening of pulmonary function. Overcorrection of a primary curve should be avoided because any secondary curve in an adult is more likely to be less flexible than an adolescent and may result in spinal imbalance.

Osteoporosis is a significant problem in adult deformity patients and may dictate the type of fixation used. Segmental fixation provides improved purchase in weakened osteoporotic bone by spreading the forces of correction over multiple fixation points. There are three types of fixation used: sublaminar wires, laminar/pedicle/transverse process hooks, and pedicle screws. Since sublaminar wires or cables have been associated with an increased risk of neurologic injury,* they should be used with caution except in specific instances where the patient has a preexisting deficit. Lumbar pedicle screws are superior to hooks and provide better three-dimensional control.[8] Pedicle screw pullout has been correlated with bone mineral density.[83] Undertapping or not tapping the pedicle is another technique to improve screw purchase and diminish the risk of pullout. Two recent studies demonstrated that pedicle screws have the greatest pullout strength of the three systems, even in the thoracic spine.[88,128] Other techniques such as adding a laminar hook at the same level[84] or triangulating the pedicle screws with cross links[160] can increase the pullout strength. In addition, long fusions to the sacrum should be avoided if possible.

Undoubtedly the most important item to consider preoperatively is the expected outcome. Patients must have a realistic outcome or they will be dissatisfied with the procedure despite a technical success. In general, studies report 30% to 50% deformity correction with 60% to 95% reduction in pain severity.* Satisfaction with the procedure is generally high. Simmons and associates[173] reviewed 40 patients with painful adult idiopathic scoliosis and found a 90% success rate. Hu and associates[91] retrospectively evaluated the outcomes of 84 patients over the age of 40 who underwent major spinal reconstructive surgery. They found that 81% of patients were satisfied with the surgery with significant improvements in many areas of functional status. Dickson and colleagues[59] compared a group of 81 patients treated for adult scoliosis with 30 patients who declined surgery. They were followed for an average of 5 years. The treated patients reported a significantly greater decrease in pain and fatigue and significantly more improvement in self-image and in the ability to perform physical, functional, and positional tasks than did the untreated patients. Albert and colleagues[5] in 1995 studied 55 adult deformity patients before and, on average, 2 years after surgery with the SF-36. Using this validated medical outcome instrument, they demonstrated statistically significant improvements in postoperative scores for physical function, social function, bodily pain, and perceived health change. They found no significant differences in self-reported health function parameters related to age (> 40 vs. < 40), end vertebral level of fusion, or presence of complications after surgery.

Thoracic Curves

For many deformities, there are several surgical options. Anterior-only, posterior-only, combined (anterior and posterior), and vertebral resection (for severe curves) have all been advocated for different types of deformities. Thoracic curvatures less than 70 degrees that are mobile can be treated with a single stage posterior approach or anterior approach. Radical facetectomies, convex rib resections, and concave rib head resections allow additional mobility for a posterior-only surgery. Thoracic curve greater than 70 degrees or with rigid components often respond better with

*References 6,53,61,62,101,148.
*References 34,48,77,78,105,155,168,183,185.

BOX 67.2

Goals of surgery

Pain relief
Prevent progression
Solid arthrodesis
Rigid internal fixation
Global spine balance (coronal and sagittal)

a combined anterior release followed by a posterior instrumentation procedure (Figure 67.4). In the setting of a severe (>90 degrees) and rigid deformity, spinal column resection (vertebrectomy) may allow for deformity correction while protecting from neurologic injury.[16,24,182]

Fixed kyphosis

Another special group of patients are those with fixed thoracic kyphosis or kyphoscoliosis. If left untreated, they can result in symptoms of compressive myelopathy. Most of the techniques used were developed for resection of hemivertebra causing kyphosis.[11,21,35,116,170] Most of these reports were in children with hemivertebra with relatively flexible remaining spinal segments. Leatherman[118,119] reported vertebral body resection using a staged anterior and posterior approach with approximately 47% deformity correction. Chewning and Heinig[46] described an "entire osteotomy" technique using an anterior and posterior or posterior-alone approach, but they did not report outcomes.

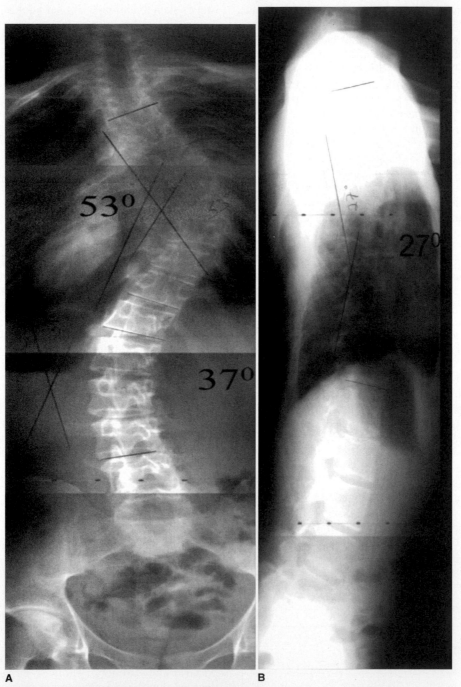

Figure 67.4 A 23-year-old female with pulmonary dysfunction. PA **(A)** and lateral **(B)** radiographs demonstrate thoracic and lumbar scoliosis with 27 degrees of thoracic lordosis. The patient underwent multilevel anterior release followed by T3-L2 posterior instrumented arthrodesis. Postoperative PA **(C)** and lateral **(D)** radiographs demonstrate global coronal and sagittal balance with recreation of 12 degrees of thoracic kyphosis.

The concept of correcting deformities completely from behind is not new. Gertzbein and Harris[72] introduced "wedge osteotomy for post-traumatic kyphosis." Lehmer and associates[122] performed posterior transvertebral osteotomies to correct kyphosis in 38 patients with post laminectomy or post fracture kyphosis. They were able to obtain and maintain correction in 93% of patients with an average of 35 degrees of correction. However, 19.5% of patients developed new neurologic deficits and in 7.3% they were permanent. Despite the risks, 76% of patients stated they would repeat the surgery and 90%

recommended it to another person. Kawahara and associates[97] treated seven patients with sagittal kyphosis mostly after fracture. They performed a closing wedge osteotomy for the first 30 to 35 degrees of correction and then moved the hinge posteriorly to create an opening osteotomy to obtain more correction. They were able to correct the average kyphosis from 67 to 18 degrees. Another series by Shimode and associates[169] treated seven patients age 8 to 31 with rigid kyphosis or kyphoscoliosis by posterior wedge osteotomy. They obtained 54% correction with improvement of the global

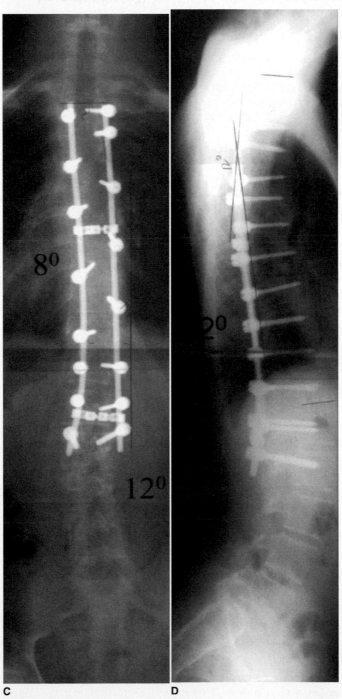

Figure 67.4 *cont'd*

sagittal alignment from 21mm of anterior balance to 3mm. More importantly, they did not experience any permanent neurologic deficits. The important lessons from these series are to obtain adequate fixation points, completely expose the target vertebrae, and control the shortening of the spine through the use of precontoured or temporary rods (Figure 67.5). Finally, the role of intraoperative monitoring should not be understated in attempting to avoid postoperative neurologic deficits.

Thoracolumbar and Lumbar Curves—Anterior

Thoracolumbar and lumbar curves without kyphosis in younger patients can be treated with anterior instrumentation (Figure 67.6).[206] In the presence of kyphosis, an anterior-only approach is contraindicated because it leads to further kyphosis that might result in sagittal plane imbalance. Any osteoporosis is also a contraindication because of a high risk for failure of the bone-vertebral body interface. The ideal curve is a mobile deformity with preserved lumbar lordosis. The advantages of this technique include superior correction, fewer motion segments fused, and a lower incidence of nonunion.[76,78,81,104,147] Anterior interbody fusion is also advocated for long fusions to the sacrum to prevent pseudarthrosis.[103-105]

Preoperative planning is critical when this approach is selected. A fixed secondary lumbosacral curve that is not included in the fusion can lead to a fixed coronal imbalance. Additionally, it is difficult and not advised to place anterior instrumentation below L4. The iliolumbar veins hinder extension of instrumentation to L5 or the sacrum. They need to be identified and ligated to allow the common iliac vein to be mobilized. Instrumentation should not contact the aorta or iliac arteries because of concerns about vessel erosion with the risk of exsanguination. Approaching the L4-5 and L5-S1 interspaces from an anterolateral approach can be technically very difficult and is also a limit to the anterior approach for deformity correction.

Thoracolumbar and Lumbar Curves—Posterior

Patients with thoracolumbar or lumbar curves may also present with symptoms of neural compression resulting from lumbar stenosis. A posterior approach is preferred when there are symptoms related to spinal stenosis or radiculopathy. This allows direct decompression of the neural elements. Surgical adjuncts to this approach include ventral releases for rigid curves and rib excision for improved cosmesis in the presence of a rib hump. When correcting a curve from posteriorly, it is important to not end the construct at the thoracolumbar junction. Older patients may develop a progressive junctional kyphosis. In addition, the instrumentation should not stop in the mid-thoracic spine because a junction kyphosis may occur.[20,23] In certain patients, it may be beneficial to extend the fusion posteriorly up to T2, T3, or T4 to avoid postoperative junctional kyphosis.

Another group of patients are those with symptomatic lumbar stenosis in the setting of a lumbar scoliosis. These patients are best approached posteriorly to perform the decompression, followed by instrumented fusion. It may be possible to decompress a single level without violating the facet joints and not perform a fusion. However, if multiple levels need to be decompressed, or it is necessary to sacrifice the facet to obtain decompression, a fusion should be incorporated as part of the procedure. In 1992, Simmons and Simmons[174] retrospectively reviewed 40 patients average age 61.5 years who underwent decompression and pedicle screw instrumented fusion for lumbar stenosis with lumbar scoliosis. The follow-up averaged 44 months. They obtained an average of 19 degrees of correction (from 37 to 18 degrees). Eighty-three percent of the patients complained of significant pain preoperatively, whereas 93% stated they had no or minimal pain postoperatively. Marchesi and Aebi[131] reported a series of 27 patients with an average age of 60 who underwent posterior instrumented fusion for adult degenerative scoliosis. They obtained greater than 50% curve correction with 86% of patients stating their walking distance had increased. There was a 4% pseudarthrosis rate. In 1994, Grubb and colleagues[78] reported 28 patients with

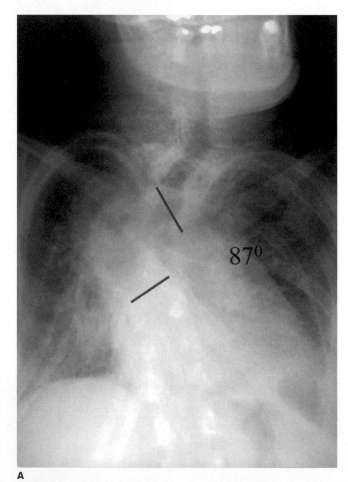

A

Figure 67.5 A 68-year-old patient with PA (**A**) radiograph and sagittal reconstruction of a CT scan (**B**) demonstrating an 87-degree thoracic kyphoscoliosis. The kyphosis is so severe that a conventional axial MRI (**C**) scan actually views two vertebrae in cross-section. The patient underwent posterior-only exposure, vertebral column resection, and reconstruction from T1 to L2. Postoperative PA (**C**) and lateral (**D**) radiographs demonstrate correction of the coronal deformity with significant improvement in the thoracic kyphosis.

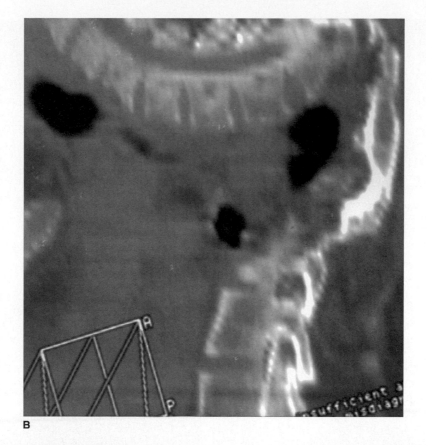

B

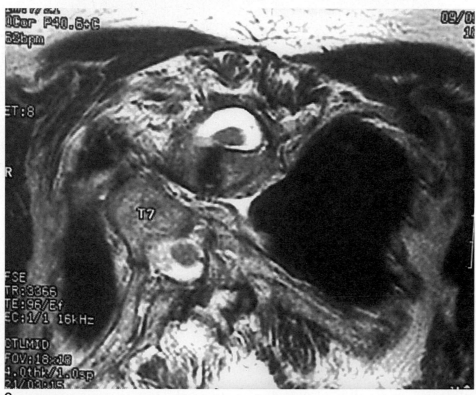

C

Figure 67.5 *cont'd*

Continued

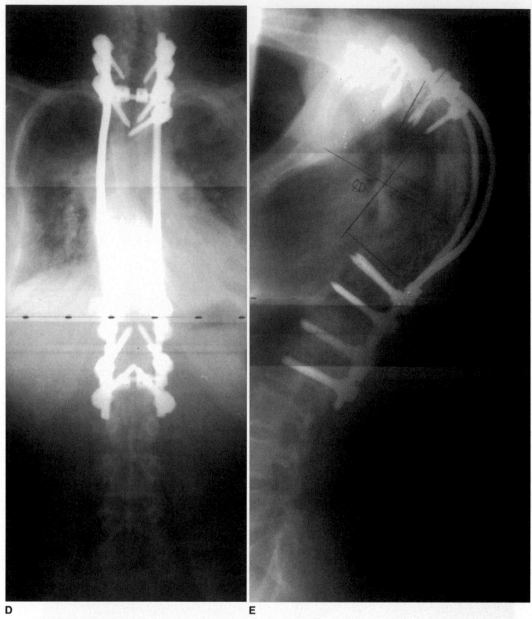

D   **E**

Figure 67.5 *cont'd*

idiopathic scoliosis and 25 patients with degenerative sco-liosis treated with posterior instrumented fusion. After a minimum 2-year follow-up, the idiopathic patients had an 80% reduction in pain whereas the degenerative patients had a 70% pain reduction. Both groups reported improved function such as standing and walking. However, there was a 17.5% pseudarthrosis rate, all in patients fused to the sacrum by posterior instrumentation only.

Patients may also present with a balanced double curve. The most common group of patients with double curves will present with balanced curves that are less than 30 degrees. These patients do not need surgical interven-tion. Patients with balanced thoracic and lumbar curves less than 60 degrees can be satisfactorily treated with pos-terior instrumented fusion. The need for a combined approach increases as the curves become more rigid or the patient has a sagittal or coronal imbalance.

Combined Procedures

Some problems can occur with posterior fusion and instru-mentation alone. They include minimal correction of the curve, pseudarthrosis, and persistent decompensation of the spine. In 1973 Kostuik and associates[105] reported 57 adult deformity patients with 48% correction after poste-rior spinal fusion using Harrington instrumentation. They observed a 14% loss of correction over time and 7% pseudarthrosis rate. This is a similar rate as observed by other authors. Byrd and associates[34] reported better cor-rection and decreased pseudarthrosis rate with a two-staged approach versus posterior fusion alone.

Patients with severe rigid structural deformities may present as a consequence of an untreated idiopathic curve usually with a significant kyphosis (Figure 67.7). As the curve rigidity increases, the need for a combined

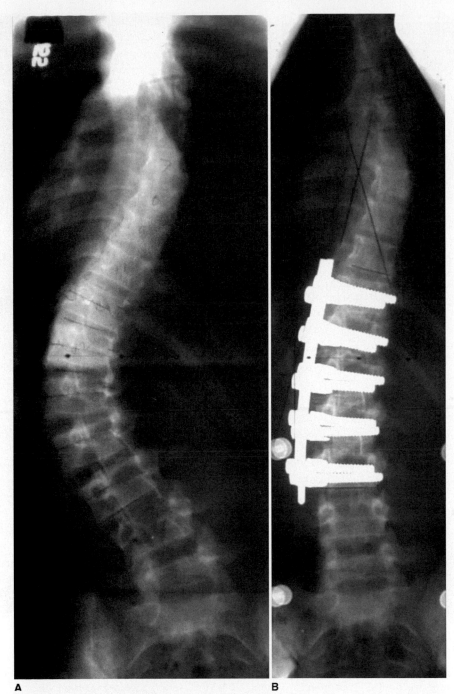

A   **B**

Figure 67.6 PA (**A**) radiograph of a 24-year-old female with progressive thoracic and lumbar scoliosis. Her thoracolumbar curve is structural. She underwent an anterior approach with structural allograft at the lumbar levels and allograft at the thoracic levels from T11-L3. Postoperative PA (**B**) radiograph demonstrates good correction of the thoracolumbar curve. The thoracic curve will need to be followed for evidence of progression.

procedure increases. Rigid curves more often require a combined approach to correct and stabilize the deformity. The absolute indications for combined surgery versus posterior fusion and instrumentation remain unclear at best. Combined surgery does allow better correction, and the reestablishment of the lumbar lordosis; it also increases the likelihood of a solid arthrodesis.[23] In lumbar curves that exceed 50 degrees, a combined approach is favored (Figure 67.8). The first stage is an aggressive

anterior release with placement of structural allograft supplemented with autograft or alternative bone graft material in the lumbar disc spaces followed by instrumented posterior fusion. An anterior paramedian approach has been recently advocated to perform anterior release and structural grafting to enhance coronal and sagittal deformity correction. This procedure is currently under investigation. Its long-term success is not known.

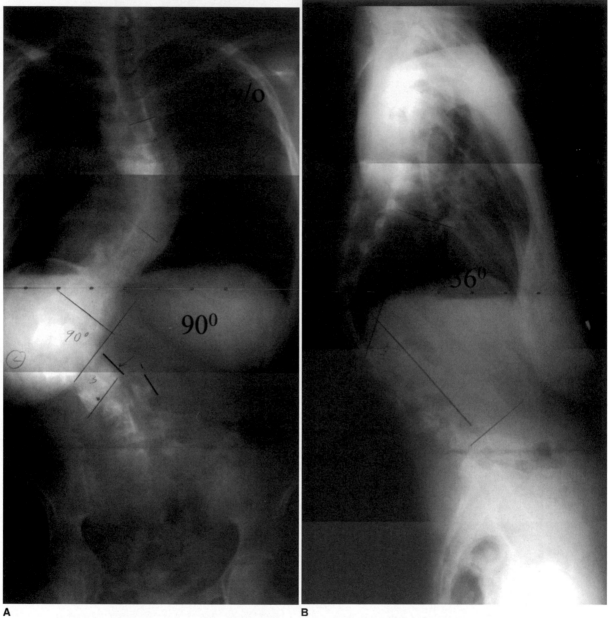

A   **B**

Figure 67.7 A 27-year-old female with PA (**A**) and lateral (**B**) radiographs demonstrating severe thoracolumbar kyphoscoliosis with 36 degrees of kyphosis and a 54-degree structural thoracic curve in addition to a lateral listhesis at L3-4. The patient underwent anterior release and placement of structural allograft from L2-3 through L4-5 followed by posterior instrumented arthrodesis T3-L5.

In 1980, Kostuik[100] reported 85 patients with severe rigid deformities measuring greater than 90 degrees. The majority were thoracic or thoracolumbar idiopathic curves. All patients underwent posterior release and anterior osteotomies followed by a posterior instrumented fusion in a delayed fashion. The idiopathic curves averaged 48% correction, and the authors cited the combined approach as the main reason for a lower incidence of pseudarthrosis as compared with posterior-instrumented fusions. In 2003, Shapiro and colleagues[168] reported 16 patients with adult idiopathic scoliosis, low back pain, and spinal stenosis. They underwent anterior discectomies with allograft fusion and then posterior decompression

and instrumented posterolateral fusion. The mean age was 66 years with a minimum of 2 years follow-up. The curve correction averaged 50.4%. Complications occurred in 75% of the patients with 10 major complications in 10 patients (8 required re-operation). Despite the high risk of complications, 94% of patients were satisfied with their treatment. The Oswestry disability back pain improved from 44.3 to an average of 26.7, and 69% of patients stated they had significant pain relief.

In severe cases, vertebral column resection either with a combined approach or completely posterior approach is another alternative.[16,24,182] Bradford and colleagues[16,23,24] advocate a combined approach for severe

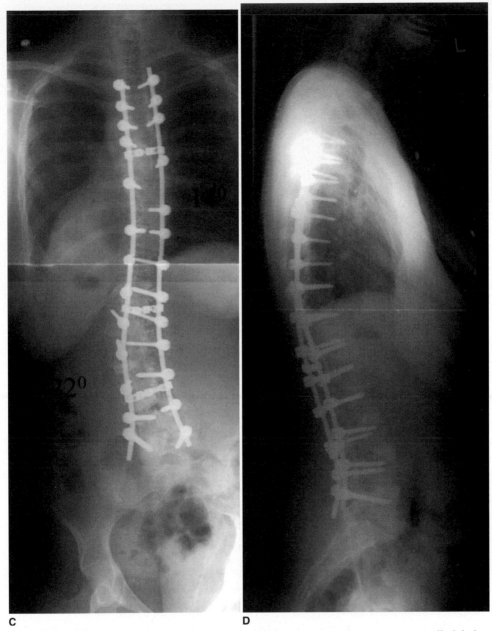

C   D

Figure 67.7 *cont'd* Postoperative PA (**C**) and lateral (**D**) radiographs demonstrate overall global sagittal and coronal balance in addition to correction of the lumbar lateral listhesis.

spinal deformities with spinal imbalance. They perform an anterior exposure over the convexity of the deformity (and the vertebral bodies are decancellated back to the posterior longitudinal ligament), remove the pedicles, perform complete discectomies, and then replace the cancellous bone while closing the periosteal flap. In the second procedure, the posterior spine is exposed, remaining pedicles removed, and instrumented arthrodesis performed. Bradford and associates[16,24] reported their retrospective series of 24 patients with an average age of 27. They were followed 2 to 10 years. The scoliosis was improved 52% and the coronal and sagittal decompensation by 82 and 87%, respectively. They had complications in 58% of their patients but stated that there were no major complications and the complications were transient.

Fusion to the Sacrum

Arthrodesis to the sacrum in patients with adult scoliosis should be avoided if possible, because the complication rates are higher, especially pseudarthrosis at the lumbosacral junction.[78] However, there are some circumstances that would indicate extending the fusion to the sacrum. It is necessary to fuse to the sacrum if a patient has an unbalanced lumbosacral curve: where balance is not achieved on bending films, tilting of the L5 vertebral body of greater than 10 degrees, severe disc degeneration at the L5-S1 level, prior or proposed laminectomy of L5, or spondylolisthesis at the L5 levels is present.

A combined approach is favored when fusing to the sacrum to maximize the fusion rate, maintain or reestablish lumbar lordosis, and prevent hardware failure. Posterior

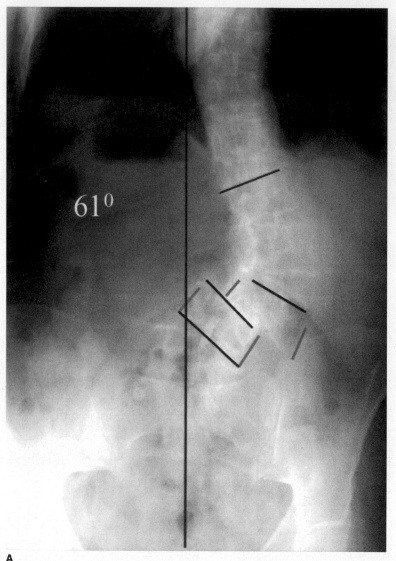

A

Figure 67.8 PA (**A**) and lateral (**B**) radiographs of a 56-year-old patient with progressive degenerative lumbar scoliosis with a lateral listhesis at L3-4 and loss of lumbar lordosis. The patient underwent a combined approach with placement of structural allograft at L2-3 and L3-4 followed by posterior instrumented arthrodesis from T10-S1. Postoperative PA (**C**) and lateral (**D**) radiographs demonstrate reduction of the lateral listhesis, improvement of the lumbar scoliosis to 21 degrees, and creation of lumbar lordosis.

instrumentation and fusion alone carries a 15% to 20% rate of pseudarthrosis even with newer stiffer instrumentation.[78,89] The preferred method is a structural allograft filled with autogenous bone. Femoral ring allograft has been shown to provide maintenance of lordosis and to achieve solid anterior fusion better than autograft.[32,33] Structural allograft provides a large surface area for structural support and a large area for autogenous bone graft or alternative bone graft to be placed in the middle for the allograft. Allograft also comes in a variety of sizes with varying lordotic angles and can also be shaped to provide optimal correction of the coronal plane deformity while maintaining lumbar lordosis. Since 66% of the total lumbar lordosis occurs at L4-5 and L5-S1, it is important to maintain this lordosis and prevent flat-back syndrome.[94]

Alternatives to structural allograft including anterior cage constructs have gained popularity but add additional

costs. The use of growth factors such as rhBMP-2, OP-1, and GDF-5 may revolutionize the way a fusion is obtained. Multiple animal studies demonstrate superior results with these substances over autogenous bone graft in achieving a solid arthrodesis.* Recent studies using recombinant bone morphogenic protein in threaded titanium cages have indicated good clinical results.[30,31] Although promising, the cost of alternative bone graft material may prohibit routine use. The difficult patient with diminished bone stock or with the use of nicotine may be a good candidate for alternative fusion material.[171,172]

Long fusions to the sacrum run a higher risk of pseudarthrosis. Posterior pedicle screw fixation alone is frequently inadequate and leads to an unacceptable

---

*References 17,18,50,51,129,140,158,161-164.

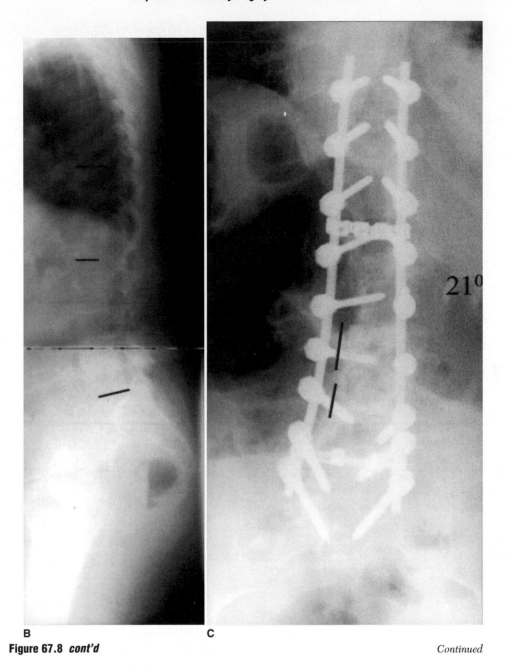

B   **C**

Figure 67.8 *cont'd*   *Continued*

pseudarthrosis rate.[78] There are many instrument techniques available to span the lumbosacral junction or spinopelvic junction. They include: medially directed bicortical sacral promontory screws, laterally directed sacral alar screws, sacral screws with intrasacral rods (Jackson Technique), Luque-Galveston intrailiac rods, and iliac screws.[15,38,73,93,149] Although easier to insert than the Luque-Galveston rods, iliac screws can be prominent but are very effective in and frequently require a delayed operation for removal.[23,63] Adding a structural interbody fusion significantly diminishes the rate of pseudarthrosis.[101] Kostuik[104,107] showed good and fair postoperative results in 93% of patients, as long as a solid fusion was obtained and lumbar lordosis was restored.

Complications

Complication avoidance is especially important in adult deformity patients. The results of operative correction of adult deformity have improved significantly as the techniques of anesthesia, blood salvage, and instrumentation systems have improved. The incidence of complications depends on the approach, level of deformity, age of patient, and experience of the surgeon. Age is a major determinant of complications. McDonnell and colleagues[132] retrospectively reviewed 447 patients undergoing a variety of anterior thoracic or lumbar spine procedures for a variety of indications. For patients 3 to 23 years old, they documented 9% major and 20% minor complications. For the age group 21 to 40 years, they

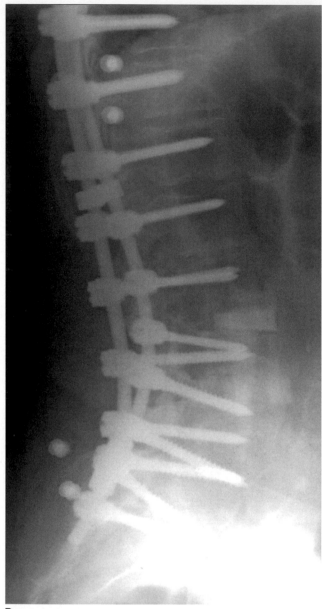

D

Figure 67.8 *cont'd*

found 6% major and 21% minor complications. In the age group 41 to 60, the complication rate was 14% major and 27% minor. The oldest patients, aged 61 to 85 years, had 32% major and 40% minor complications. The authors clearly documented for these procedures that the complication rate dramatically increased especially in the oldest patient group.

Although major complications can occur, neurologic injury occurs in less than 1% to 5% of cases. Significant risk factors for major intraoperative neurologic deficits include hyperkyphosis and combined surgery.[27] Neurologic deficits do not have to present immediately after the surgical procedure has finished. Delayed paraplegia is a devastating complication that can occur several hours after spinal reconstruction surgery. Postoperative hypovolemia and mechanical tension on spinal vessels along the concavity of the curve have been implicated as

the cause of spinal cord ischemia, which leads to delayed postoperative paraplegia.[186] Therefore, it is imperative to maintain adequate volume and blood pressure in the patients during the postoperative period.

Postoperative visual loss is another devastating complication. There have been several case reports.[3,60,120,138] One review estimated that the risk after major spinal surgery was 0.05% and 1%.[204] In 2000, Cheng and associates[45] surveyed neurosurgeons and identified 24 patients with visual loss. They stated that many patients had risk factors of hypotension, low hematocrit, and coexisting disease. In 1997, Myers and associates[141] surveyed the members of the Scoliosis Research Society and reviewed the cases reported in the literature. They reviewed 37 patients with postoperative blindness. Ninety-two percent had undergone posterior instrumented fusion. Although most had a significant episode of intraoperative hypotension, there was no difference in hematocrit of blood pressure values compared with a matched control group. Blindness was caused by ischemic optic neuropathy, retinal artery occlusion, and cortical blindness. Eleven patients had bilateral blindness, and 15 were completely blind in at least one eye. Unlike delayed postoperative paraplegia that may resolve after adequate volume support, the visual losses were permanent in most patients.

Surgical procedures should be designed to obtain stability that allows for early ambulation with minimal or no external support. Adult patients tend to tolerate external orthosis poorly. Since many of these deformities are rigid, combined surgery may be the preferred method. Same day combined procedures are preferable to staged procedures if they can be performed within a reasonable period (e.g., 12 hours). If staged procedures are performed too closely together, the patient can become malnourished. In a study by Dick and associates,[58] 7 of 11 staged procedure patients and 10 of 13 combined procedure patients developed postoperative malnutrition. The only infections occurred in the staged patients. The combined group had 30% less hospital costs and a shorter hospital stay. Not surprisingly, all patients reported that they would prefer to have both operations performed on the same day as opposed to staged operations. Lenke and associates[126] prospectively demonstrated that it takes 6 to 12 weeks to return to baseline nutritional status and that as the number of fusion levels increase, the time to return to nutritional baseline increases. Therefore, if a surgical procedure needs to be staged, the patient should receive hyperalimentation between the stages to reduce the risk of malnutrition-related complications.[90]

Electrolyte abnormalities can occur after spinal surgery. Callewart and colleagues[36] reported a prospective study that evaluated 101 operations in 96 patients. Forty-four percent of patients developed postoperative hyponatremia. They documented a 6.9% rate of SIADH. Patients undergoing revision surgery had a two to four times greater risk than patients having the primary procedure. They also noted an increased risk of developing SIADH as the blood loss increased.

Infection rates depend on the approach and the age of the patient. Infection rates in scoliosis surgery are between 1% and 2%, whereas adults have a higher infection rate at 3% to 5%. Infection after anterior surgery alone is around

1%.[202] Despite a low rate of infection, a deep infection can have significant sequelae and may require multiple operations to eradicate the infection. Pseudarthrosis is another serious complication that may require revision surgery. Weis *et al.*[202] reported a 38% pseudarthrosis rate at 37 months follow-up that increased to 64% if the sacrum was included in the fusion. Others have documented that posterior instrumentation and fusion alone to the sacrum carries a 15% to 20% rate of pseudarthrosis even with newer stiffer instrumentation.[78,89]

Revision Surgery

Many patients achieve acceptable results with surgical intervention. However, there are a number of patients who may benefit from revision or salvage procedures. Painful pseudarthrosis, adjacent level degeneration, residual deformity, progressive deformity, and flat-back syndrome are some of the indications for revision surgery. The surgical goals are the same as the index procedure: obtain a solid fusion, provide rigid internal fixation, and finish with adequate spinal balance in both coronal and sagittal planes (Figure 67.9). In other words, the procedure should end with the head over the pelvis in both the coronal and sagittal planes. Although the goals are the same, revision surgery is more complicated because of previous dissection, fixation sites already used, and potentially rigid residual deformity.

The presence of a pseudarthrosis on postoperative imaging does not necessarily mean that the pseudarthrosis is symptomatic. The management of the pseudarthrosis depends on the level, presence of deformity, implanted hardware, and ultimately the presence of pain or disability. A painful pseudarthrosis in the setting of a progressive deformity and hardware loosening is the clearest indication for revision surgery. However, most patients will not have such a clear indication for revision surgery.

Choosing the type of surgery for revision depends on several factors: number of pseudarthroses, level of pseudarthrosis, presence of deformity, and presence of neurologic compression. A single level anterior interbody arthrodesis, with or without instrumentation, is the best revision for a single level pseudarthrosis after a posterior instrumented fusion. If there are several levels of pseudarthrosis, the whole posterior instrumentation should be removed, copious autogenous bone graft applied, and re-instrumentation placed under compression. Additionally, a second anterior arthrodesis over the levels of pseudarthrosis should be considered.

Longer fusions may develop adjacent level disc degeneration. Some of these patients will develop symptomatic stenosis. If the stenosis is not associated with deformity, limited decompression (sparing the midline posterior elements) may be sufficient. If the patient also has junctional kyphosis, coronal deformity, or an insufficiency fracture, the fusion should be extended with instrumentation (Figures 67.10 and 67.11).

Progressive deformity can be seen in adult patients above or below a previous fusion performed during childhood. This occasionally occurs because the initial fusion

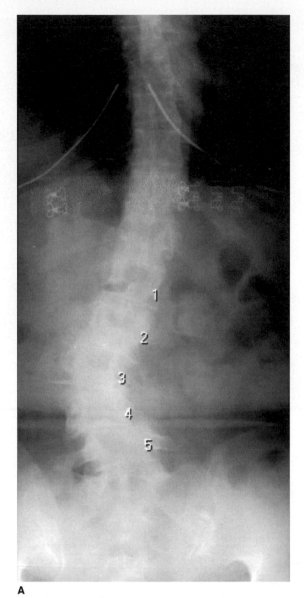

A

Figure 67.9 PA (**A**) and lateral (**B**) radiographs of a 55-year-old female with post-laminectomy lumbar scoliosis and kyphosis. She underwent a combined procedure with placement of structural allografts from L2-3 through L4-5 and posterior instrumented arthrodesis from T11-L5. Postoperative PA (**C**) and lateral (**D**) radiographs demonstrate good correction of the scoliosis with correction of the lumbar kyphosis and recreation of physiologic lumbar lordosis.

Continued

did not incorporate sufficient levels.[23] If the patient has good bone quality, the junctional deformity can be treated by posterior extension of the fusion along with instrumentation. However, if the patient is osteopenic, has a rigid deformity, or has an unbalanced spine, a combined approach is recommended.

Iatrogenic Flat-Back

Iatrogenic loss of lordosis is now frequently recognized as a complication following thoracolumbar instrumentation,

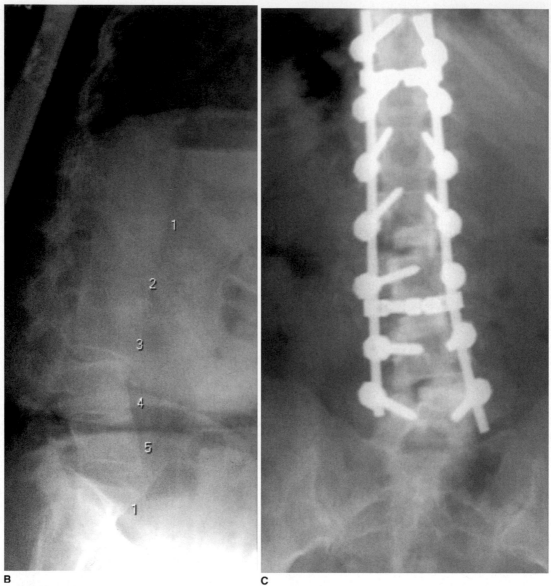

B

C

Figure 67.9 *cont'd*

especially with distraction instrumentation spanning the lumbar spine.* When lumbar lordosis is diminished enough to create an imbalance with the center of gravity of the head anterior to the sacrum, it is described as positive sagittal balance. Historically, loss of lumbar lordosis resulted from the use of distraction instrumentation across the lumbar spine used for the treatment of scoliosis. Over time, this loss of lumbar lordosis and loss of the ability of other spinal segments to compensate resulted in progressive positive sagittal balance. The symptom complex that develops as the body's compensatory mechanisms fail has been described as *flat-back syndrome*. More recently, the term *flat-back syndrome* has been used to describe symptoms resulting from iatrogenic loss of lumbar lordosis with forward inclination of the trunk, inability to stand upright, and back pain.

---

*References 1,104,106,111,112,137.

Etiology

There is a spectrum of etiologies that can lead to flat-back syndrome. Several factors have been identified as contributing to the syndrome, including distraction instrumentation into the lower lumbar spine or sacrum, pseudarthrosis resulting in loss of sagittal plane correction, fixed thoracic hyperkyphosis, hip flexion contractures, and preexisting thoracolumbar kyphosis.[112]

The use of distraction instrumentation into the lower lumbar spine or sacrum is the single biggest risk factor for developing flat-back syndrome. Distraction instrumentation allowed greater correction to be obtained and maintained in the frontal plane while causing sagittal imbalance. The magnitude of loss of lordosis increases the farther distally the instrumentation is placed. Aaro and Ohlen[1] studied 96 patients with Harrington distraction instrumentation. Patients instrumented to T12 had a lumbar lordosis of −38 degrees while patients instrumented to L5 had a lumbar lordosis of

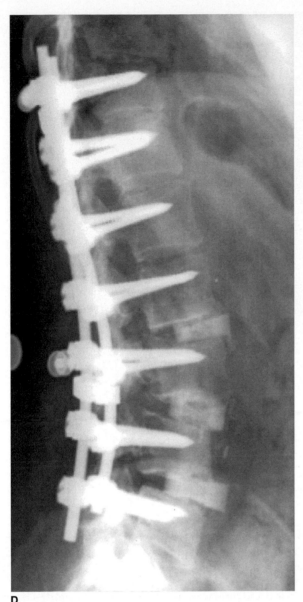

D
Figure 67.9 *cont'd*

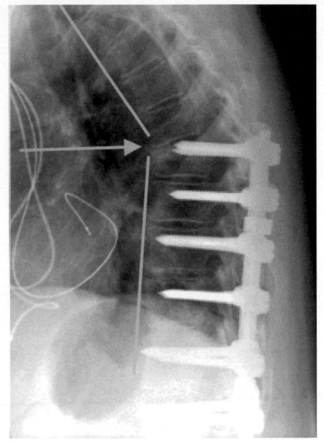

Figure 67.10 Lateral radiograph demonstrating postoperative junctional kyphosis in a patient who had the fusion stopped at the apex of the thoracic kyphosis.

only −16 degrees. In 1990, Swank and associates[184] reviewed 43 patients with radiographs before and after Harrington instrumentation into the lumbar spine for scoliosis. Lordosis decreased progressively in lower levels of fusion. The increase in lordosis below the fusion did not compensate for the overall loss of lordosis in the fused spine.

The incidence of flat-back syndrome varies by study and to a greater extent by the distal level of the distraction instrumentation. Swank and associates[183] in 1981 reported on 222 adult patients who underwent operations for scoliosis. With an average of 3.9 years of follow-up, they noted a 5% incidence of symptomatic loss of lumbar lordosis. In 1983, Kostuik and Hall[104] reviewed 45 adult patients with fusion to the sacrum for scoliosis. Of the patients, 22 (49%) were noted to have loss of lumbar lordosis. Thirteen (29%) underwent corrective osteotomies with improvement in their pain. In another study, van Dam and associates[191] reviewed 91 adult patients who underwent Harrington instrumentation for scoliosis. The average fol-

low-up was 3.5 years. None was fused to the sacrum. Some flattening of the lumbar spine was found (10 degrees or more in 43% of patients instrumented to L4 or L5). However, only 2 of 35 patients developed symptoms with one who underwent a corrective osteotomy.

Pseudarthrosis may also contribute to postoperative loss of lumbar lordosis. Lagrone and associates[112] noted that 20% of their patients undergoing corrective osteotomies for flat-back syndrome had a pseudarthrosis with progressive loss of sagittal plane balance. Preexisting thoracolumbar kyphosis is another contributing factor to the development of flat-back syndrome.[111] Usually the thoracolumbar junction is straight. Frequently in lumbar or thoracolumbar scoliosis, the thoracolumbar junction is kyphotic while the lumbar spine compensates by hyperlordosis. If instrumented with distraction instrumentation, the lumbar spine may not be able to compensate.

The principal cause of loss of lumbar lordosis with modern spinal instrumentation systems using transpedicular instrumentation is patient positioning that reduces lumbar lordosis. Positions that have been demonstrated to reduce lumbar lordosis include both "knee-chest" and kneeling positions. Lumbar lordosis has been demonstrated convincingly to be reduce the flexion of the hips that normally occurs with either the "knee-chest" or kneeling positions such as those used with an Andrews-type table (Orthopaedic Systems, Inc., Hayward, CA).[9,153] Conversely, lumbar lordosis is accentuated by positioning the patients

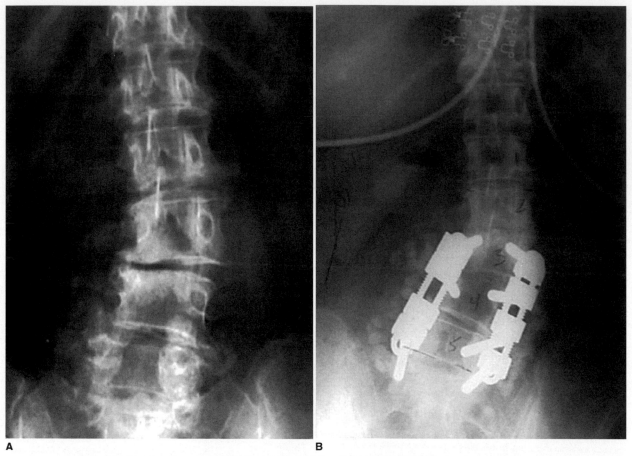

A   B

Figure 67.11 AP radiograph (**A**) of a 65-year-old female who developed progressive lumbar scoliosis after lumbar laminectomy. She underwent a local L3-5 instrumented fusion and developed junctional scoliosis (**B**) and kyphosis (**C**).

with the hips fully extended, such as on a Jackson Table (Orthopaedic Systems, Inc., Hayward, CA).[179]

Segmental distraction with transpedicular instrumentation for "foraminal enlargement" or during device or bone graft placement for posterior interbody lumbar fusion or transforaminal interbody lumbar fusion can also induce focal kyphosis. Although the loss of lumbar lordosis may not be as dramatic as was classically seen with Harrington instrumentation, the compensatory mechanisms are less in older patients and flat-back syndrome can still develop.

Clinical Presentation

Flat-back syndrome is characterized by loss of the normal lumbar lordosis resulting in a typical clinical syndrome characterized by (1) forward inclination of the trunk, (2) inability to stand erect without knee flexion, and (3) pain.[57] The patients require first extension of the hips and then knee flexion and cervical extension to maintain horizontal gaze. Because of the strain of trying to achieve the erect posture, pain and fatigue may be noted in the cervical, thoracic, and lumbar spine.

Normal Sagittal Alignment

Any discussion of deformity regarding sagittal alignment would not be complete without a discussion of "normal"

sagittal balance. At birth, the human spine has a kyphotic curvature that encompasses the entire spine. As the child begins to ambulate and develop an upright posture, the spinal column develops a compensatory lordosis in the cervical and lumbar spine. The two lordotic curves balance the thoracic kyphosis, resulting in lining the head up over the pelvis.

Propst-Proctor and Bleck[156] reviewed lateral radiographs of 104 children and found lumbar lordosis from top of L1 to bottom of L5 averaged −40 degrees in normal children and −48.5 degrees in those with scoliosis. In adults, the same measurements by Stagnara and associates[178] demonstrated an average lordosis of −42 degrees with a range from −18 to −69 degrees. When the same patients were measured from the top of L1 to the top of the sacrum, the range changed to between 33 and 79 degrees. In asymptomatic patients over the age of 40, Gelb and associates[71] found the T12-S1 lordosis to average −64 degrees ± 10 degrees. This just confirms a wide range of "normal" lumbar lordosis.

The absolute value of the lumbar lordosis or the thoracic kyphosis is of little significance. What is important clinically is the overall sagittal balance of the spine.[111] The head should be over the sacrum in both the frontal and sagittal planes. The global sagittal balance can be determined by obtaining a full-length lateral radiograph of the spine with the knees fully extended. A plumb line is

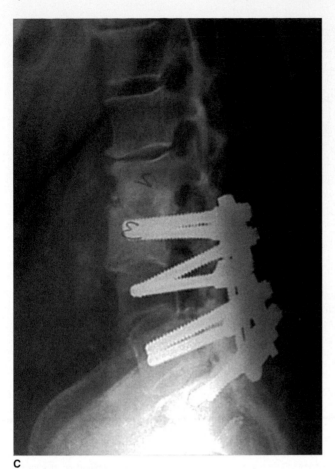

C

Figure 67.11 *cont'd*

dropped from the dens (or the middle of C7 if the dens is not visualized). Neutral sagittal balance exists when a plumb line, dropped from the body of C7, intersects the rostral-dorsal corner of the S1 vertebral body. If the plumb line falls behind the lumbosacral disc, it is termed *negative balance*. If the plumb line falls in front of the lumbosacral disc, this is positive sagittal balance. The "C7-S1 distance" is the distance from this plumb line to the anterior aspect of the sacrum. If the plumb line falls within 2cm of the anterior aspect of the sacrum, this is considered normal in patients without scoliosis or with idiopathic scoliosis without surgery.[135] Gelb and associates[71] evaluated 100 asymptomatic volunteers without history of spinal deformity who were over the age of 40. They found the C7-S1 distance to fall 3.2cm ± 3.2cm behind the sacrum.

Prevention

The surgical treatment of flat-back deformity is an extensive operation that can have perioperative complications in upwards of 60% of patients.[112] Most patients are improved over their preoperative status, but few are completely relieved of their symptoms. In their review of surgical correction of flat-back syndrome, Lagrone and associates[112] noted that 47% of patients complained of leaning forward and 36% continued to have back pain. This was over an average of 6 years follow-up. Therefore prevention is the best way to treat this deformity.

Proper patient positioning and avoidance of distraction instrumentation, especially to the lower lumbar spine and sacrum, are the primary methods to avoid postoperative loss of lumbar lordosis. The use of segmental instrumentation, particularly multisegmental pedicle screw instrumentation systems, has allowed greater maintenance of lumbar lordosis. Bridwell and associates[26] studied 160 patients treated with segmental instrumentation. They found that this segmental instrumentation to the mid and distal lumbar spine could preserve and, at times, enhance lumbar lordosis. In 1992, Lenke and associates[124] reported their experience in 95 patients treated with segmental instrumentation with an average follow-up of 35 months. They concluded that the segmental instrumentation helped to preserve segmental lumbar lordosis. In the following year the same group determined that segmental instrumentation allowed maintenance of the sagittal alignment while diminishing the number of lumbar levels that were included in the fusion.[123] By including less distal levels in the fusion, they are able to maintain more distal levels to allow compensation for any fusion level loss of sagittal balance.

There is an increasing incidence of loss of lumbar lordosis as the fusion extends distally to the sacrum.[104,112] If fusion to the sacrum is determined to be necessary, distraction instrumentation should be avoided. Alternative forms of instrumentation include the Galveston technique of inserting L-rods into the pelvis and pedicle screw fixation. Deciding on the proximal end of the fusion is also important. If the fusion is stopped at or just below the apex of the thoracic or thoracolumbar kyphosis, the patient will be at risk of "falling off" proximal to the fusion.[111] This would tend to increase the kyphosis and increase the problem of loss of sagittal balance. By extending the proximal fusion above the apex of the kyphosis, this complication can be avoided.

Surgical Planning

The goal of surgery is to restore the sagittal balance such that the plumb line intersects the posterosuperior corner of the S1 vertebra (i.e., to end up with the head centered over the sacrum). This allows the patient to stand without knee flexion and hip hyperextension, thereby diminishing the overall pain.

The decision regarding where to place the osteotomy depends on the site of the deformity. Patients with flattening of the lumbar spine without thoracolumbar kyphosis can be treated by osteotomies below the level of the conus medullaris. This provides adequate lordosis without jeopardizing the spinal cord. If there is co-existing thoracolumbar kyphosis, this also needs to be addressed. If it is flexible and corrects on hyperextension radiographs, osteotomies can be performed in the lumbar spine and the fusion can be extended proximally into the thoracic spine. If it is not flexible, either an osteotomy can be performed at the apex of the kyphosis (usually thoracolumbar junction), or an osteotomy or larger magnitude or multiple levels of osteotomies can be performed.

There have been several types of osteotomies described to correct sagittal imbalance. Extension (Smith-Petersen), polysegmental, and closing wedge osteotomies have all

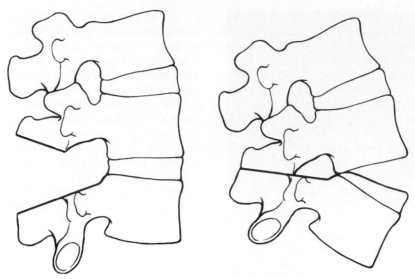

Figure 67.12 Line drawing of extension (Smith-Petersen) osteotomy. Note that the correction is obtained through rupture of the anterior longitudinal ligament, thus lengthening the anterior spine. *(From Wiggins GC, Ondra SL, Shaffrey CI: Management of iatrogenic flat-back syndrome. Neurosurg Focus 15:Article 8, 2003.)*

been described to treat fixed sagittal deformities. Many of these osteotomies were initially described to treat deformity as a result of ankylosing spondylitis and have been adapted to treat flat-back syndrome.*

Extension (Smith-Petersen) Osteotomy

In 1945, Smith-Petersen and associates[177] were first to describe a posterior osteotomy for the correction of fixed sagittal deformity in patients with rheumatoid arthritis. The osteotomy involves removing the posterior elements, undercutting the adjacent spinous processes, and then closing the osteotomy, thus creating an opening of the spine (extension) anteriorly through the disc space (Figure 67.12). The posterior aspect of the disc space is the axis of rotation. The extension osteotomy creates hyperextension by closing the posterior elements and opening the anterior elements. In 1946 La Chapelle[110] described a modification of the technique by adding an anterior release. The anterior release was performed as a second operation and included packing of bone obtained from the tibia into the disc space.

Various series report the use of extension osteotomies, mainly in the treatment of ankylosing spondylitis.* Although extension osteotomy can correct the deformity, the technique does carry significant morbidity and mortality. By lengthening the anterior column, there is risk of injury to anterior vascular structures and neural elements. Law[113] in 1959 reported his experience in 100 patients, of which 80 were available for review. Eight patients (10%) died of complications related to the procedure. Neurologic complications have been reported in up to

30% of patients.[113,133] Forceful hyperextension of the spine may cause rupture of the aorta or inferior vena cava, which are frequently calcified in patients with ankylosing spondylitis.[127,199] As the anterior spine is lengthened, the superior mesenteric artery can stretch over the third part of the duodenum and lead to acute dilatation of the stomach and paralytic ileus in the early postoperative period.[134,175] This results in an increased incidence of emesis and aspiration.

Pseudarthrosis is another reported complication. The osteotomy creates a gap through the disc space. In a standing position, 80% to 90% of axial compressive forces pass through the anterior lumbar column and only 10% to 20% pass through the posterior column.[10] This makes the extension osteotomy biomechanically unstable. In 1947 Briggs and associates[29] added a spinous process plate to aid in the postoperative stability of the spin. In 1985, McMaster[133] reported the addition of Harrington compression hooks to secure the osteotomy. In 1995, Weale and associates[198] describe the addition of transpedicular screws and cable in 37 patients. They noted a loss of correction of 15 degrees in the patients without fixation and 4.8 degrees in the patients with internal fixation. Some authors suggest a simultaneous or staged anterior fusion to help reduce the pseudarthrosis rate.[106,110-112]

The extension osteotomy can obtain a significant degree of correction at one level. The reported average correction in most series is around 32 degrees.* The general rule is one degree of correction for every 1mm of bone resected posteriorly.[25] Unfortunately the correction is lost over time. McMaster[133] reported a 5-degree loss of correction over 3 years even with patients in a plaster jacket postoperatively. Lagrone and associates[112] also report a 5-degree loss of correction over 6 years despite

---

*References 4,16,22,37,43,44,64,69,70,74,82,86,98,110,117,127,133,134, 175,177,181,192,205.
*References 4,29,64,68,74,86,106,110,113-115,127,133,134,175,177.

*References 68,74,106,112,133,198.

the addition of Harrington compression rods. With the addition of a pedicle screw and cable system, Weale and associates[198] also had a mean loss of 4.8 degrees. This is despite revision in several of their patients because of loss of correction within 4 weeks of operation.

Overall, extension osteotomy can correct the sagittal plane deformity. The procedure inherently lengthens the anterior spine and places vascular and neural structures at risk. In addition, the spine is relatively unstable after this procedure, resulting in pseudarthrosis and loss of correction.

Polysegmental Osteotomies

Extension osteotomies produce correction by creating a sharp lordotic angle and elongation of the anterior column that may result in significant complications. In 1949, Wilson and Turkell[205] reported on the use of multiple osteotomies to correct the sagittal balance in a patient with ankylosing spondylitis. This was achieved through polysegmental posterior lumbar osteotomies (Figure 67.13). This technique involves removing the facet joints at several levels and then compressing the posterior elements to create a lordosis. The correction is obtained through the deformation of the disc spaces without rupture of the anterior longitudinal ligament.

Several authors advocate polysegmental lumbar osteotomies to create a harmonious lumbar lordosis.* Wilson and Turkell[205] first reported the use of osteotomies alone. Simmons[175] added the use of internal fixation (Harrington compression rod) to thoracic posterior wedge osteotomies and an anterior strut. In the lumbar spine, this device failed.[22,82,157] In 1990 Hehne and associates[85] reported their experience in 177 patients with ankylosing spondylitis treated with polysegmental lumbar

---

*References 44,82,85,157,193,205.

osteotomies using transpedicular screw and threaded rods. Average correction was 44 degrees, about 9.5 degrees per segment. Complications include 2.3% mortality, 2.3% non-reversible neurologic deficit, and 18% reversible complications. Despite the use of postoperative body casts, there was an average loss of 20% of the correction with implant breakage in 4 patients.

Using a similar method, Chen[44] in 1998 reported his experience with 16 patients. The average correction was 25.8 degrees, or 5 degrees per segment. The average loss of correction was 0.9 degrees per segment with early rod breakage in 25% of patients. In 1988, van Royen and associates[193] reported their experience with 21 patients. They had average curve improvement of 25.6 degrees, 9.5 degrees per segment, and mean loss of 10.7 degrees over the whole fusion. Forty-three percent of their patients had a postoperative complication. Insufficient correction or loss of correction led to implant failure and loss of correction.

Closing Wedge Osteotomy

A closing wedge osteotomy is the next technique described to correct the deformity without lengthening the anterior spine. In 1963, Scudese and Calabro[166] were the first to describe a monosegmental intravertebral closing wedge posterior osteotomy of the lumbar spine. Then Thomasen[188] reported on 11 patients with ankylosing spondylitis treated with posterior closing wedge osteotomies. He used spinous process plates in 4 and spinous process wiring in 2 patients. A closing wedge osteotomy (Figure 67.14) involves the complete removal of a wedge of bone with the base at the spinous processes and the apex at the anterior margin of the vertebral body. Care is taken to adequately undercut the dorsal elements the level above and below the primary osteotomy level to ensure that the neural elements are not constricted. A version of the closing wedge osteotomy

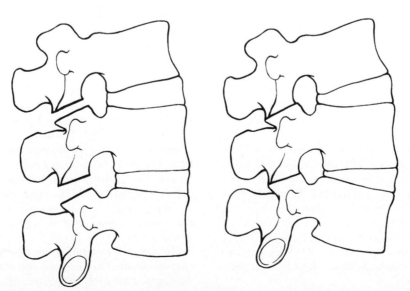

Figure 67.13 Line drawing of polysegmental osteotomy. The correction is obtained through disc deformation without rupture and compression of the osteotomy with instrumentation. (*From Wiggins GC, Ondra SL, Shaffrey CI: Management of iatrogenic flat-back syndrome.* Neurosurg Focus 15:Article 8, 2003.)

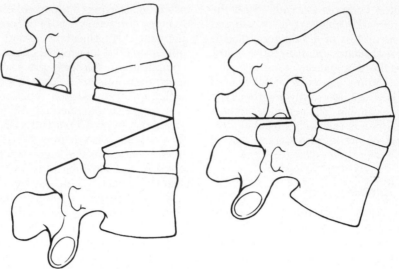

Figure 67.14 Line drawing of closing wedge osteotomy. The axis of rotation is the anterior margin of the vertebral body. This osteotomy places two large cancellous surfaces together to obtain fusion. Note that two nerve roots will now exit through one larger neuroforamen. *(From Wiggins GC, Ondra SL, Shaffrey CI: Management of iatrogenic flat-back syndrome. Neurosurg Focus 15:Article 8, 2003.)*

described as the pedicle subtraction osteotomy has gained popularity in correcting significant sagittal plane and coronal plane deformities. This aggressive osteotomy removes the posterior elements, including the pedicle and transverse process. With this technique, removal of up to 6cm of bone is possible with resultant sagittal plane correction of up to 60 degrees. By performing an asymmetric removal of the posterior elements, correction of both sagittal and coronal plane deformities can be performed (Figures 67.15 and 67.16).

This procedure is technically demanding, and substantial blood loss typically occurs from the epidural venous plexus or from the cancellous bone surfaces. With the removal of the pedicle bilaterally, two nerve roots exit through the reconstructed neural foramina at the level of the osteotomy. Care must be taken during the closure of the osteotomy that impingement of the thecal sac or nerve roots does not occur.

Since the original description, there have been many reports of using these techniques for fixed sagittal plane deformities of different etiologies ranging from ankylosing spondylitis to trauma to flat-back deformity.* A recent report by Bridwell and associates[28] reviewed 27 patients with fixed sagittal imbalance treated with pedicle subtraction closing wedge osteotomy. The etiologies were varied (14 idiopathic scoliosis, 8 degenerative scoliosis, 3 post traumatic, and 2 ankylosing spondylitis). Average correction was 33.5 degrees immediately postoperatively and 34.5 degrees with a minimum of 2 years follow-up. Sagittal plumb line improved from 17.74 to 1.99cm immediately postoperatively and to 4.23cm on final follow-up. Twenty-four complications occurred in these 27 patients.

There are several advantages of pedicle subtraction closing wedge osteotomy. Correction is obtained through all

three columns of the spine. This allows for correction in both the sagittal and coronal plane. By resecting more bone on the convexity of the deformity, coronal deformities can also be corrected at the same level.[28] In addition, the spine is not lengthened, thereby avoiding the vascular and abdominal complications associated with extension osteotomies. The bone surface for fusion is large and placed under compression by the mechanics of the osteotomy. The instrumentation is therefore used to maintain the alignment as opposed to create the desired alignment.

Comparison of Techniques

In 1999, van Royen and De Gast[192] performed a meta-analysis of the literature to compare opening wedge, polysegmental, and closing wedge osteotomies in the treatment of ankylosing spondylitis. They included 41 articles with 856 patients reported between 1945 and 1998. Only 16 studies on 523 patients met the inclusion criteria. Perioperative mortality was highest in opening wedge osteotomies (5.8%) and least in closing wedge osteotomies (1.3%). Neuropraxia was reported in 11.3% of polysegmental osteotomies and 7.8% of closing wedge osteotomies. As the polysegmental osteotomies are closed, the neuroforamen is narrowed and can create new radiculopathy. In addition, paralysis was seen in 3.1% of opening wedge osteotomies and 2% of polysegmental osteotomies, and it did not occur in closing wedge osteotomies.

In 330 of the patients the degree of surgical correction was reported. The average correction was a similar 35 to 40 degrees for each technique. However, there was significantly more loss of correction in both opening wedge osteotomy (3.9%) and polysegmental osteotomy (6.0%) than closing wedge osteotomy (2.7%). Reported patients results were similar, with good outcomes ranging from

---

*References 12,28,37,43,54,67,72,79,96-98,117,122,139,187,188,194.

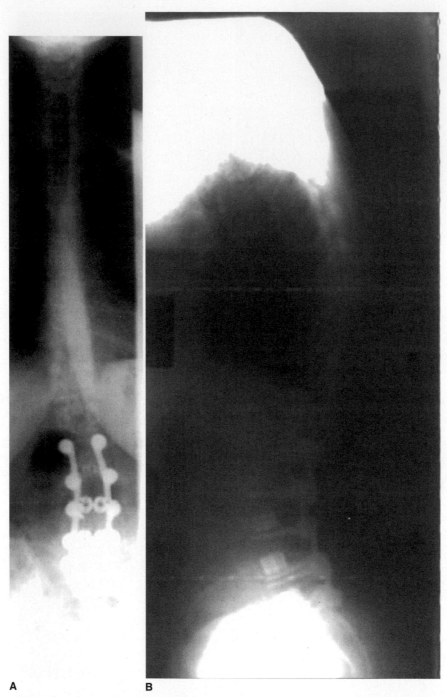

A   **B**

Figure 67.15 This is a 40-year-old patient who underwent a laminectomy, posterior lumbar interbody fusion, and then an instrumented fusion. AP (**A**) and lateral (**B**) radiographs demonstrate positive sagittal balance with a mild lumbar scoliosis. She had severe back pain and an inability to stand more than 10 minutes. The patient underwent pedicle subtraction osteotomy at L2 with extension of her fusion. Postoperative AP (**C**), lateral (**D**), and lumbar lateral (**E**) radiographs demonstrate correction of the lumbar scoliosis and restoration of sagittal balance. Sagittal reconstruction (**F**) of a computed tomography scan demonstrates the closure of the osteotomy and sagittal correction. (*From Wiggins GC, Ondra SL, Shaffrey CI: Management of iatrogenic flat-back syndrome.* Neurosurg Focus 15:Article 8, 2003.)

Continued

69% to 78%. The authors concluded that there was insufficient evidence to conclude that one surgical technique is preferable over the other. However, there was a trend toward less serious complication for closing wedge osteotomy with greater maintenance of correction.

Booth and associates[19] reviewed a consecutive series of flat-back deformity in 28 patients. They had a minimum of 2 years follow-up with an average of 3.6 years. Three patients had extension osteotomies alone, three patients had closing wedge osteotomies alone, and the

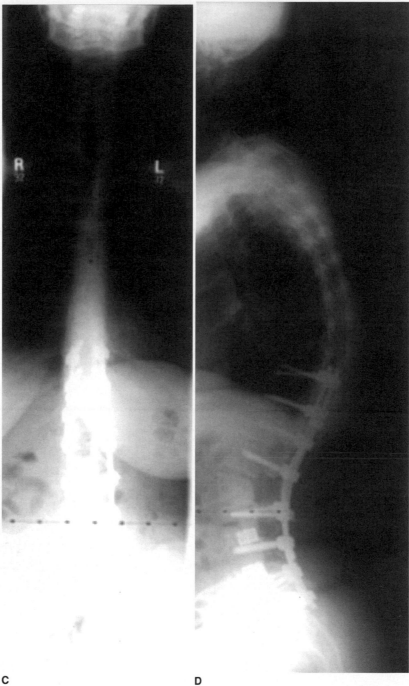

C   D

Figure 67.15 *cont'd*

remainder underwent a variety of anterior and posterior procedures. All patients were instrumented with hook-rod-screw systems. There were seven patients with 11 complications. There were no deaths, and no patient suffered a neurologic deficit. All the complications occurred in patients who underwent anterior and posterior procedures. All patients completed outcome questionnaires. Seventy-nine percent reported a decrease in pain as a result of the procedure. Fifty percent reported increased function. Although the numbers are small, this study demonstrates good outcomes for patients who underwent surgical correction of flat-back syndrome.

Summary

Adult scoliosis occurs in a challenging and rewarding patient population. The patients have more co-morbidities and risks than adolescents with spinal deformity. In addition, complete correction is not the goal. Finishing with a pain-free, well-balanced spine in both the coronal and sagittal planes with the head centered over the pelvis is the goal. Advances in surgical technique and especially rigid segmental internal fixation have increased our ability to internally stabilize the spine. With this increase in surgical instrumentation, we have to guard against iatrogenic complications such as flat-back syndrome.

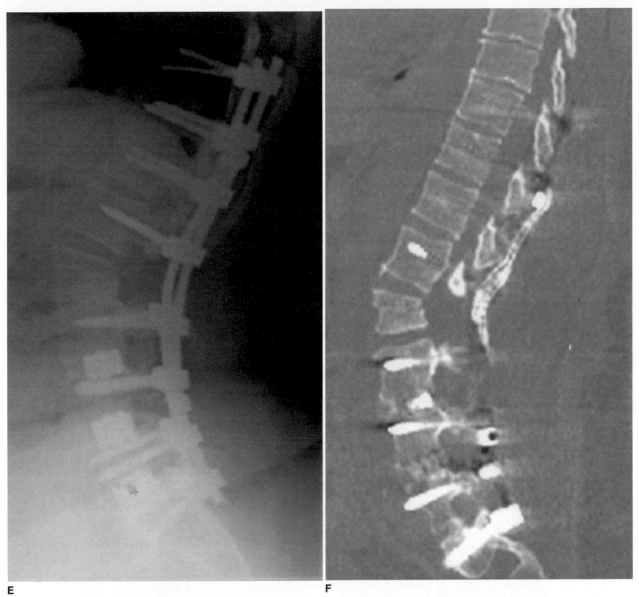

E

F

Figure 67.15 *cont'd*

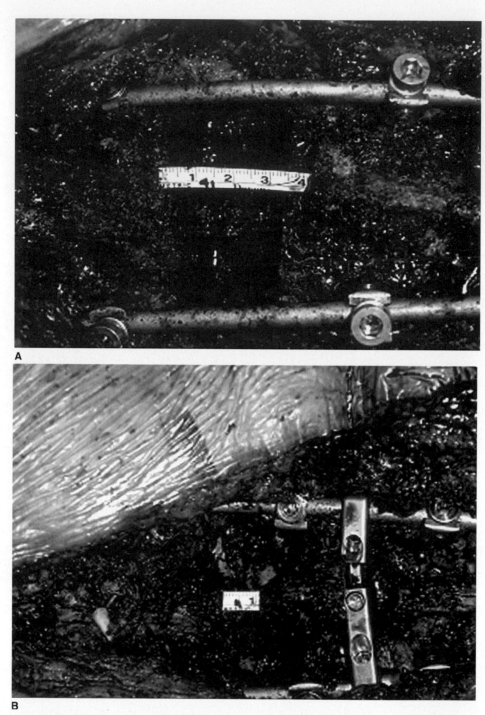

Figure 67.16 Pre-closure (**A**) and post-closure (**B**) intraoperative photographs from the patient in Figure 67.4 demonstrate the amount of closure obtained at the osteotomy. *(From Wiggins GC, Ondra SL, Shaffrey CI: Management of iatrogenic flat-back syndrome. Neurosurg Focus 15:Article 8, 2003.)*

REFERENCES

1. Aaro S, Ohlen G: The effect of Harrington instrumentation on the sagittal configuration and mobility of the spine in scoliosis. *Spine* 8:570-575, 1983.

2. Abitbol JJ, Dowling TJ, Benz RJ, *et al:* Adult scoliosis. In Herkowitz HN, Garfin SR, Balderston RA, *et al* (eds): *Rothman-Simeone, The Spine,* vol 1, ed 4. Philadelphia, WB Saunders, 1999, pp 809-834.

3. Abraham M, Sakhuja N, Sinha S, *et al:* Unilateral visual loss after cervical spine surgery. *J Neurosurg Anesthesiol* 15:319-322, 2003.

4. Adams JC: Techniques, dangers, and safeguards in osteotomy of the spine. *J Bone Joint Surg Br* 34:226-232, 1952.

5. Albert TJ, Purtill J, Mesa J, *et al:* Health outcome assessment before and after adult deformity surgery. A prospective study. *Spine* 20:2002-2004; discussion 2005, 1995.

6. Allen BL, Jr., Ferguson RL: The Galveston technique for L rod instrumentation of the scoliotic spine. *Spine* 7:276-284, 1982.

7. Ascani E, Bartolozzi P, Logroscino CA, *et al:* Natural history of untreated idiopathic scoliosis after skeletal maturity. *Spine* 11:784-789, 1986.

8. Barr SJ, Schuette AM, Emans JB: Lumbar pedicle screws versus hooks. Results in double major curves in adolescent idiopathic scoliosis. *Spine* 22:1369-1379, 1997.

9. Benfanti PL, Geissele AE: The effect of intraoperative hip position on maintenance of lumbar lordosis: a radiographic study of anesthetized patients and unanesthetized volunteers on the Wilson frame. *Spine* 22:2299-2303, 1997.

10. Bergmark A: Stability of the lumbar spine. A study in mechanical engineering. *Acta Orthop Scand Suppl* 230: 1-54, 1989.

11. Bergoin M, Bollini G, Taibi L, *et al:* Excision of hemivertebrae in children with congenital scoliosis. *Ital J Orthop Traumatol* 12:179-184, 1986.

12. Berven SH, Deviren V, Smith JA, *et al:* Management of fixed sagittal plane deformity: results of the transpedicular wedge resection osteotomy. *Spine* 26:2036-2043, 2001.

13. Bjure J, Nachemson A: Non-treated scoliosis. *Clin Orthop* 93:44-52, 1973.

14. Blount WP, Mellencamp D: The effect of pregnancy on idiopathic scoliosis. *J Bone Joint Surg Am* 62:1083-1087, 1980.

15. Boachie-Adjei O, Bradford D: The Cotrel-Dubousset system—results in spinal reconstruction. Early experience in 47 patients. *Spine* 16:1155-1160, 1991.

16. Boachie-Adjei O, Bradford DS: Vertebral column resection and arthrodesis for complex spinal deformities. *J Spinal Disord* 4:193-202, 1991.

17. Boden SD, Schimandle JH, Hutton WC: 1995 Volvo Award in basic sciences. The use of an osteoinductive growth factor for lumbar spinal fusion. Part II: Study of dose, carrier, and species. *Spine* 20:2633-2644, 1995.

18. Boden SD, Schimandle JH, Hutton WC, *et al:* 1995 Volvo Award in basic sciences. The use of an osteoinductive growth factor for lumbar spinal fusion. Part I: Biology of spinal fusion. *Spine* 20:2626-2632, 1995.

19. Booth KC, Bridwell KH, Lenke LG, *et al:* Complications and predictive factors for the successful treatment of flatback deformity (fixed sagittal imbalance). *Spine* 24:1712-1720, 1999.

20. Bradford DS: Adult scoliosis. Current concepts of treatment. *Clin Orthop* Apr:70-87, 1988.

21. Bradford DS, Boachie-Adjei O: One-stage anterior and posterior hemivertebral resection and arthrodesis for congenital scoliosis. *J Bone Joint Surg Am* 72:536-540, 1990.

22. Bradford DS, Schumacher WL, Lonstein JE, *et al:* Ankylosing spondylitis: experience in surgical management of 21 patients. *Spine* 12:238-243, 1987.

23. Bradford DS, Tay BK, Hu SS: Adult scoliosis: surgical indications, operative management, complications, and outcomes. *Spine* 24:2617-2629, 1999.

24. Bradford DS, Tribus CB: Vertebral column resection for the treatment of rigid coronal decompensation. *Spine* 22:1590-1599, 1997.

25. Bridwell KH: Osteotomies for fixed deformities in the thoracic and lumbar spine. In Bridwell KH, DeWald RL (eds): *The Textbook of Spinal Surgery,* ed 2. Philadelphia: Lippincott-Raven, 1997, pp 821-835.

26. Bridwell KH, Betz R, Capelli AM, *et al:* Sagittal plane analysis in idiopathic scoliosis patients treated with Cotrel-Dubousset instrumentation. *Spine* 15:644-649, 1990.

27. Bridwell KH, Lenke LG, Baldus C, *et al:* Major intraoperative neurologic deficits in pediatric and adult spinal deformity patients. Incidence and etiology at one institution. *Spine* 23:324-331, 1998.

28. Bridwell KH, Lewis SJ, Lenke LG, *et al:* Pedicle subtraction osteotomy for the treatment of fixed sagittal imbalance. *J Bone Joint Surg Am* 85-A:454-463, 2003.

29. Briggs H, Keats S, Schlesinger PT: Wedge osteotomy of the spine with bilateral intervertebral foraminotomy: correction of flexion deformity in five cases of ankylosing arthritis of the spine. *J Bone Joint Surg* 29:1075-1082, 1947.

30. Burkus JK, Dorchak JD, Sanders DL: Radiographic assessment of interbody fusion using recombinant human bone morphogenetic protein type 2. *Spine* 28:372-377, 2003.

31. Burkus JK, Gornet MF, Dickman CA, *et al:* Anterior lumbar interbody fusion using rhBMP-2 with tapered interbody cages. *J Spinal Disord Tech* 15:337-349, 2002.

32. Buttermann GR, Glazer PA, Hu SS, *et al:* Anterior and posterior allografts in symptomatic thoracolumbar deformity. *J Spinal Disord* 14:54-66, 2001.

33. Buttermann GR, Glazer PA, Hu SS, *et al:* Revision of failed lumbar fusions. A comparison of anterior autograft and allograft. *Spine* 22:2748-2755, 1997.

34. Byrd JA 3rd, Scoles PV, Winter RB, *et al:* Adult idiopathic scoliosis treated by anterior and posterior spinal fusion. *J Bone Joint Surg Am* 69:843-850, 1987.

35. Callahan BC, Georgopoulos G, Eilert RE: Hemivertebral excision for congenital scoliosis. *J Pediatr Orthop* 17: 96-99, 1997.

36. Callewart CC, Minchew JT, Kanim LE, *et al:* Hyponatremia and syndrome of inappropriate antidiuretic hormone secretion in adult spinal surgery. *Spine* 19: 1674-1679, 1994.

37. Camargo FP, Cordeiro EN, Napoli MM: Corrective osteotomy of the spine in ankylosing spondylitis. Experience with 66 cases. *Clin Orthop* Jul:157-167, 1986.

38. Camp JF, Caudle R, Ashmun RD, *et al:* Immediate complications of Cotrel-Dubousset instrumentation to the sacro-pelvis. A clinical and biomechanical study. *Spine* 15:932-941, 1990.

39. Carragee EJ, Chen Y, Tanner CM, *et al:* Provocative discography in patients after limited lumbar discectomy: A controlled, randomized study of pain response in symptomatic and asymptomatic subjects. *Spine* 25: 3065-3071, 2000.

40. Carragee EJ, Paragioudakis SJ, Khurana S: 2000 Volvo Award winner in clinical studies: Lumbar high-intensity zone and discography in subjects without low back problems. *Spine* 25:2987-2992, 2000.

41. Carragee EJ, Tanner CM, Khurana S, *et al:* The rates of false-positive lumbar discography in select patients without low back symptoms. *Spine* 25:1373-1380; discussion 1381, 2000.

42. Carragee EJ, Tanner CM, Yang B, *et al:* False-positive findings on lumbar discography. Reliability of subjective concordance assessment during provocative disc injection. *Spine* 24:2542-2547, 1999.

43. Chen IH, Chien JT, Yu TC: Transpedicular wedge osteotomy for correction of thoracolumbar kyphosis in ankylosing spondylitis: experience with 78 patients. *Spine* 26:E354-360, 2001.

44. Chen PQ: Correction of kyphotic deformity in ankylosing spondylitis using multiple spinal osteotomy and Zielke's VDS instruments. *Taiwan Yi Xue Hui Za Zhi* 87:692-699, 1988.

45. Cheng MA, Sigurdson W, Tempelhoff R, Lauryssen C: Visual loss after spine surgery: a survey. *Neurosurgery* 46:625-630; discussion 630-621, 2000.

46. Chewning SJ, Heinig CF: Osteotomy. In Weinstein SL (ed): *The Pediatric Spine: Principles and Practice,* vol 2. New York: Raven Press, 1994, pp 1443-1458.

47. Collins CD, Stack JP, O'Connell DJ, *et al:* The role of discography in lumbar disc disease: a comparative study of magnetic resonance imaging and discography. *Clin Radiol* 42:252-257, 1990.

48. Collis DK, Ponseti IV: Long-term follow-up of patients with idiopathic scoliosis not treated surgically. *J Bone Joint Surg Am* 51:425-445, 1969.

49. Connolly PJ, Von Schroeder HP, Johnson GE, *et al:* Adolescent idiopathic scoliosis. Long-term effect of instrumentation extending to the lumbar spine. *J Bone Joint Surg Am* 77:1210-1216, 1995.

50. Cook SD, Dalton JE, Tan EH, *et al:* In vivo evaluation of anterior cervical fusions with hydroxyapatite graft material. *Spine* 19:1856-1866, 1994.

51. Cook SD, Rueger DC: Osteogenic protein-1: biology and applications. *Clin Orthop* Mar:29-38, 1996.

52. Cotrel Y, Dubousset J, Guillaumat M: New universal instrumentation in spinal surgery. *Clin Orthop* 227:10-23, 1988.

53. Cummine JL, Lonstein JE, Moe JH, *et al:* Reconstructive surgery in the adult for failed scoliosis fusion. *J Bone Joint Surg Am* 61:1151-1161, 1979.

54. Danisa OA, Turner D, Richardson WJ: Surgical correction of lumbar kyphotic deformity: posterior reduction "eggshell" osteotomy. *J Neurosurg* 92:50-56, 2000.

55. Denis F: Cotrel-Dubousset instrumentation in the treatment of idiopathic scoliosis. *Orthop Clin North Am* 19:291-311, 1988.

56. Derby R, Howard MW, Grant JM, *et al:* The ability of pressure-controlled discography to predict surgical and nonsurgical outcomes. *Spine* 24:364-371; discussion 371-362, 1999.

57. DeWald RL: Revision surgery for spinal deformity. *Instr Course Lect* 41:235-250, 1992.

58. Dick J, Boachie-Adjei O, Wilson M: One-stage versus two-stage anterior and posterior spinal reconstruction in adults. Comparison of outcomes including nutritional status, complications rates, hospital costs, and other factors. *Spine* 17:S310-316, 1992.

59. Dickson JH, Mirkovic S, Noble PC, *et al:* Results of operative treatment of idiopathic scoliosis in adults. *J Bone Joint Surg Am* 77:513-523, 1995.

60. Dilger JA, Tetzlaff JE, Bell GR, *et al:* Ischaemic optic neuropathy after spinal fusion. *Can J Anaesth* 45:63-66, 1998.

61. Dwyer AF: Experience of anterior correction of scoliosis. *Clin Orthop* 93:191-214, 1973.

62. Edgar MA, Mehta MH: Long-term follow-up of fused and unfused idiopathic scoliosis. *J Bone Joint Surg Br* 70: 712-716, 1988.

63. Emami A, Deviren V, Berven S, *et al:* Outcome and complications of long fusions to the sacrum in adult spine deformity: luque-galveston, combined iliac and sacral screws, and sacral fixation. *Spine* 27:776-786, 2002.

64. Emneus H: Wedge osteotomy of spine in ankylosing spondylitis. *Acta Orthop Scand* 39:321-326, 1968.

65. Epstein JA, Epstein BS, Jones MD: Symptomatic lumbar scoliosis with degenerative changes in the elderly. *Spine* 4:542-547, 1979.

66. Etebar S, Cahill DW: Risk factors for adjacent-segment failure following lumbar fixation with rigid instrumentation for degenerative instability. *J Neurosurg* 90:163-169, 1999.

67. Farcy JP, Schwab F: Posterior osteotomies with pedicle substraction for flat back and associated syndromes. Technique and results of a prospective study. *Bull Hosp Jt Dis* 59:11-16, 2000.

68. Farcy JP, Schwab FJ: Management of flatback and related kyphotic decompensation syndromes. *Spine* 22:2452-2457, 1997.

69. Fazl M, Bilbao JM, Hudson AR: Laceration of the aorta complicating spinal fracture in ankylosing spondylitis. *Neurosurgery* 8:732-734, 1981.

70. Fowles JV, Drummond DS, L'Ecuyer S, *et al:* Untreated scoliosis in the adult. *Clin Orthop* Jul-Aug:212-217, 1978.

71. Gelb DE, Lenke LG, Bridwell KH, *et al:* An analysis of sagittal spinal alignment in 100 asymptomatic middle and older aged volunteers. *Spine* 20:1351-1358, 1995.

72. Gertzbein SD, Harris MB: Wedge osteotomy for the correction of post-traumatic kyphosis. A new technique and a report of three cases. *Spine* 17:374-379, 1992.

73. Glazer PA, Colliou O, Lotz JC, *et al:* Biomechanical analysis of lumbosacral fixation. *Spine* 21:1211-1222, 1996.

74. Goel MK: Vertebral osteotomy for correction of fixed flexion deformity of the spine. *J Bone Joint Surg Am* 50:287-294, 1968.

75. Goldberg MS, Mayo NE, Poitras B, *et al:* The Ste-Justine Adolescent Idiopathic Scoliosis Cohort Study. Part II: Perception of health, self and body image, and participation in physical activities. *Spine* 19:1562-1572, 1994.

76. Goldstein JM, Nash CL, Jr., Wilham MR: Selection of lumbar fusion levels in adult idiopathic scoliosis patients. *Spine* 16:1150-1154, 1991.

77. Grubb SA, Lipscomb HJ, Coonrad RW: Degenerative adult onset scoliosis. *Spine* 13:241-245, 1988.

78. Grubb SA, Lipscomb HJ, Suh PB: Results of surgical treatment of painful adult scoliosis. Spine 19:1619-1627, 1994.

79. Guven O, Bezer M, Gokkus K, *et al:* Transpedicular decancellation osteotomy in the treatment of peridural fibrosis. *Arch Orthop Trauma Surg* 121:517-520, 2001.

80. Guyer RD, Ohnmeiss DD: Lumbar discography. *Spine J* 3:11S-27S, 2003.

81. Hall JE: Dwyer instrumentation in anterior fusion of the spine. *J Bone Joint Surg Am* 63:1188-1190, 1981.

82. Halm H, Metz-Stavenhagen P, Zielke K: Results of surgical correction of kyphotic deformities of the spine in ankylosing spondylitis on the basis of the modified arthritis impact measurement scales. *Spine* 20:1612-1619, 1995.

83. Halvorson TL, Kelley LA, Thomas KA, *et al:* Effects of bone mineral density on pedicle screw fixation. *Spine* 19:2415-2420, 1994.

84. Hasegawa K, Takahashi HE, Uchiyama S, *et al:* An experimental study of a combination method using a pedicle screw and laminar hook for the osteoporotic spine. *Spine* 22:958-962; discussion 963, 1997.

85. Hehne HJ, Zielke K, Bohm H: Polysegmental lumbar osteotomies and transpedicled fixation for correction of long-curved kyphotic deformities in ankylosing spondylitis. Report on 177 cases. *Clin Orthop* Sep:49-55, 1990.

86. Herbert JJ: Vertebral osteotomy for kyphosis, especially in Marie-Strumpell arthritis. *J Bone Joint Surg Am* 41:291-302, 1959.

87. Herndon WA, Sullivan JA, Yngve DA, *et al:* Segmental spinal instrumentation with sublaminar wires. A critical appraisal. *J Bone Joint Surg Am* 69:851-859, 1987.

88. Hitchon PW, Brenton MD, Black AG, *et al:* In vitro biomechanical comparison of pedicle screws, sublaminar hooks, and sublaminar cables. *J Neurosurg* 99:104-109, 2003.

89. Horton WC, Holt RT, Muldowny DS: Controversy. Fusion of L5-S1 in adult scoliosis. *Spine* 21:2520-2522, 1996.

90. Hu SS, Fontaine F, Kelly B, *et al:* Nutritional depletion in staged spinal reconstructive surgery. The effect of total parenteral nutrition. *Spine* 23:1401-1405, 1998.

91. Hu SS, Holly EA, Lele C, *et al:* Patient outcomes after spinal reconstructive surgery in patients > or = 40 years of age. *J Spinal Disord* 9:460-469, 1996.

92. Ito M, Incorvaia KM, Yu SF, *et al:* Predictive signs of discogenic lumbar pain on magnetic resonance imaging with discography correlation. *Spine* 23:1252-1258; discussion 1259-1260, 1998.

93. Jackson RP, McManus AC: The iliac buttress. A computed tomography study of sacral anatomy. *Spine* 18:1318-1328, 1993.

94. Jackson RP, McManus AC: Radiographic analysis of sagittal plane alignment and balance in standing volunteers and patients with low back pain matched for age, sex, and size. A prospective controlled clinical study. *Spine* 19:1611-1618, 1994.

95. Jackson RP, Simmons EH, Stripinis D: Incidence and severity of back pain in adult idiopathic scoliosis. *Spine* 8:749-756, 1983.

96. Jaffray D, Becker V, Eisenstein S: Closing wedge osteotomy with transpedicular fixation in ankylosing spondylitis. *Clin Orthop* Jun:122-126, 1992.

97. Kawahara N, Tomita K, Baba H, *et al:* Closing-opening wedge osteotomy to correct angular kyphotic deformity by a single posterior approach. *i* 26:391-402, 2001.

98. Kim KT, Suk KS, Cho YJ, *et al:* Clinical outcome results of pedicle subtraction osteotomy in ankylosing spondylitis with kyphotic deformity. *Spine* 27:612-618, 2002.

99. Kostuik JP: Anterior Kostuik-Harrington distraction systems for the treatment of kyphotic deformities. *Spine* 15:169-180, 1990.

100. Kostuik JP: Recent advances in the treatment of painful adult scoliosis. *Clin Orthop* Mar-Apr:238-252, 1980.

101. Kostuik JP: Treatment of scoliosis in the adult thoracolumbar spine with special reference to fusion to the sacrum. *Orthop Clin North Am* 19:371-381, 1988.

102. Kostuik JP, Bentivoglio J: The incidence of low-back pain in adult scoliosis. *Spine* 6:268-273, 1981.

103. Kostuik JP, Carl A, Ferron S: Anterior Zielke instrumentation for spinal deformity in adults. *J Bone Joint Surg Am* 71:898-912, 1989.

104. Kostuik JP, Hall BB: Spinal fusions to the sacrum in adults with scoliosis. *Spine* 8:489-500, 1983.

105. Kostuik JP, Israel J, Hall JE: Scoliosis surgery in adults. *Clin Orthop* 93:225-234, 1973.

106. Kostuik JP, Maurais GR, Richardson WJ, *et al:* Combined single stage anterior and posterior osteotomy for correction of iatrogenic lumbar kyphosis. *Spine* 13:257-266, 1988.

107. Kostuik JP, Musha Y: Extension to the sacrum of previous adolescent scoliosis fusions in adult life. *Clin Orthop* Jul:53-60, 1999.

108. Kumar MN, Baklanov A, Chopin D: Correlation between sagittal plane changes and adjacent segment degeneration following lumbar spine fusion. *Eur Spine J* 10:314-319, 2001.

109. Kumar MN, Jacquot F, Hall H: Long-term follow-up of functional outcomes and radiographic changes at adjacent levels following lumbar spine fusion for degenerative disc disease. *Eur Spine J* 10:309-313, 2001.

110. La Chapelle EH: Osteotomy of the lumbar spine for correction of kyphosis in a case of ankylosing spondylarthritis. *J Bone Joint Surg* 28:851-858, 1946.

111. La Grone MO: Loss of lumbar lordosis. A complication of spinal fusion for scoliosis. *Orthop Clin North Am* 19:383-393, 1988.

112. Lagrone MO, Bradford DS, Moe JH, *et al:* Treatment of symptomatic flatback after spinal fusion. *J Bone Joint Surg Am* 70:569-580, 1988.

113. Law WA: Lumbar spinal osteotomy. *J Bone Joint Surg Br* 41:270-278, 1959.

114. Law WA: Osteotomy of the spine. *Clin Orthop* 66:70-76, 1969.

115. Law WA: Surgical treatment of rhematic diseases. *J Bone Joint Surg Br* 34:215-225, 1952.

116. Lazar RD, Hall JE: Simultaneous anterior and posterior hemivertebra excision. *Clin Orthop* Jul:76-84, 1999.

117. Lazennec JY, Saillant G, Saidi K, *et al:* Surgery of the deformities in ankylosing spondylitis: our experience of lumbar osteotomies in 31 patients. *Eur Spine J* 6:222-232, 1997.

118. Leatherman KD: The management of rigid spinal curves. *Clin Orthop* 93:215-224, 1973.

119. Leatherman KD, Dickson RA: Two-stage corrective surgery for congenital deformities of the spine. *J Bone Joint Surg Br* 61-B:324-328, 1979.

120. Lee AG: Ischemic optic neuropathy following lumbar spine surgery. Case report. *J Neurosurg* 83:348-349, 1995.

121. Lee CK: Accelerated degeneration of the segment adjacent to a lumbar fusion. *Spine* 13:375-377, 1988.

122. Lehmer SM, Keppler L, Biscup RS, *et al:* Posterior transvertebral osteotomy for adult thoracolumbar kyphosis. *Spine* 19:2060-2067, 1994.

123. Lenke LG, Bridwell KH, Baldus C, *et al:* Ability of Cotrel-Dubousset instrumentation to preserve distal lumbar motion segments in adolescent idiopathic scoliosis. *J Spinal Disord* 6:339-350, 1993.

124. Lenke LG, Bridwell KH, Baldus C, *et al:* Cotret-Dubousset instrumentation for adolescent idiopathic scoliosis. *J Bone Joint Surg Am* 38:1056-1067, 1992.

125. Lenke LG, Bridwell KH, Blanke K, *et al:* Analysis of pulmonary function and chest cage dimension changes after thoracoplasty in idiopathic scoliosis. *Spine* 20:1343-1350, 1995.

126. Lenke LG, Bridwell KH, Blanke K, *et al:* Prospective analysis of nutritional status normalization after spinal reconstructive surgery. *Spine* 20:1359-1367, 1995.

127. Lichtblau PO, Wilson PD: Possible mechanism of aortic rupture in orthopaedic correction of rheumatoid spondylitis. *J Bone Joint Surg Am* 38:123-127, 1956.

128. Liljenqvist U, Hackenberg L, Link T, *et al:* Pullout strength of pedicle screws versus pedicle and laminar hooks in the thoracic spine. *Acta Orthop Belg* 67:157-163, 2001.

129. Lovell TP, Dawson EG, Nilsson OS, *et al:* Augmentation of spinal fusion with bone morphogenetic protein in dogs. *Clin Orthop:*266-274, 1989.

130. Madan S, Gundanna M, Harley JM, *et al:* Does provocative discography screening of discogenic back pain improve surgical outcome? *J Spinal Disord Tech* 15:245-251, 2002.

131. Marchesi DG, Aebi M: Pedicle fixation devices in the treatment of adult lumbar scoliosis. *Spine* 17:S304-309, 1992.

132. McDonnell MF, Glassman SD, Dimar JR 2nd, *et al:* Perioperative complications of anterior procedures on the spine. *J Bone Joint Surg Am* 78:839-847, 1996.

133. McMaster MJ: A technique for lumbar spinal osteotomy in ankylosing spondylitis. *J Bone Joint Surg Br* 67:204-210, 1985.

134. McMaster MJ, Coventry MB: Spinal osteotomy in ankylosing spondylitis. Technique, complications, and long-term results. *Mayo Clin Proc* 48:476-486, 1973.

135. Moe JH: The iatrogenic loss of lumbar lordosis. *Orthop Trans* 1:131, 1977.

136. Moe JH, Purcell GA, Bradford DS: Zielke instrumentation (VDS) for the correction of spinal curvature. Analysis of results in 66 patients. *Clin Orthop* Nov:133-153, 1983.

137. Moskowitz A, Moe JH, Winter RB, *et al:* Long-term follow-up of scoliosis fusion. *J Bone Joint Surg Am* 62:364-376, 1980.

138. Murphy MA: Bilateral posterior ischemic optic neuropathy after lumbar spine surgery. *Ophthalmology* 110:1454-1457, 2003.

139. Murrey DB, Brigham CD, Kiebzak GM, *et al:* Transpedicular decompression and pedicle subtraction osteotomy (eggshell procedure): a retrospective review of 59 patients. *Spine* 27:2338-2345, 2002.

140. Muschler GF, Hyodo A, Manning T, *et al:* Evaluation of human bone morphogenetic protein 2 in a canine spinal fusion model. *Clin Orthop:*229-240, 1994.

141. Myers MA, Hamilton SR, Bogosian AJ, *et al:* Visual loss as a complication of spine surgery. A review of 37 cases. *Spine* 22:1325-1329, 1997.

142. Nachemson A: Adult scoliosis and back pain. *Spine* 4:513-517, 1979.

143. Nachemson A: A long-term follow-up study of non-treated scoliosis. *Acta Orthop Scand* 39:466-476, 1968.

144. Nachemson A: Physiotherapy for low back pain patients. A critical look. *Scand J Rehabil Med* 1:85-90, 1969.

145. Nachemson AL, Bjure JC, Grimby LG, *et al:* Physical fitness in young women with idiopathic scoliosis before and after an exercise program. *Arch Phys Med Rehabil* 51:95-98 passim, 1970.

146. Nilsonne U, Lundgren KD: Long-term prognosis in idiopathic scoliosis. *Acta Orthop Scand* 39:456-465, 1968.

147. Nuber GW, Schafer MF: Surgical management of adult scoliosis. *Clin Orthop* Jul:228-237, 1986.

148. Paonessa KJ, Engler GL: Back pain and disability after Harrington rod fusion to the lumbar spine for scoliosis. *Spine* 17:S249-253, 1992.

149. Pashman RS, Hu SS, Schendel MJ, *et al:* Sacral screw loads in lumbosacral fixation for spinal deformity. *Spine* 18:2465-2470, 1993.

150. Payne WK 3rd, Ogilvie JW, Resnick MD, *et al:* Does scoliosis have a psychological impact and does gender make a difference? *Spine* 22:1380-1384, 1997.

151. Pehrsson K, Bake B, Larsson S, *et al:* Lung function in adult idiopathic scoliosis: a 20-year follow-up. *Thorax* 46:474-478, 1991.

152. Perennou D, Marcelli C, Herisson C, *et al:* Adult lumbar scoliosis. Epidemiologic aspects in a low-back pain population. *Spine* 19:123-128, 1994.

153. Peterson MD, Nelson LM, McManus AC, *et al:* The effect of operative position on lumbar lordosis. A radiographic study of patients under anesthesia in the prone and 90-90 positions. *Spine* 20:1419-1424, 1995.

154. Polly DW, Jr., Sturm PF: Traction versus supine side bending. Which technique best determines curve flexibility? *Spine* 23:804-808, 1998.

155. Ponder RC, Dickson JH, Harrington PR, *et al:* Results of Harrington instrumentation and fusion in the adult idiopathic scoliosis patient. *J Bone Joint Surg Am* 57:797-801, 1975.

156. Propst-Proctor SL, Bleck EE: Radiographic determination of lordosis and kyphosis in normal and scoliotic children. *J Pediatr Orthop* 3:344-346, 1983.

157. Puschel J, Zielke K: [Corrective surgery for kyphosis in bekhterev's disease -indication, technique, results (author's transl)]. *Z Orthop Ihre Grenzgeb* 120:338-342, 1982.

158. Riew KD, Wright NM, Cheng S, *et al:* Induction of bone formation using a recombinant adenoviral vector carrying the human BMP-2 gene in a rabbit spinal fusion model. *Calcif Tissue Int* 63:357-360, 1998.

159. Robin GC, Span Y, Steinberg R, *et al:* Scoliosis in the elderly: a follow-up study. *Spine* 7:355-359, 1982.

160. Ruland CM, McAfee PC, Warden KE, *et al:* Triangulation of pedicular instrumentation. A biomechanical analysis. *Spine* 16:S270-276, 1991.

161. Sandhu HS, Kanim LE, Kabo JM, *et al:* Evaluation of rhBMP-2 with an OPLA carrier in a canine posterolateral (transverse process) spinal fusion model. *Spine* 20: 2669-2682, 1995.

162. Sandhu HS, Kanim LE, Kabo JM, *et al:* Effective doses of recombinant human bone morphogenetic protein-2 in experimental spinal fusion. *Spine* 21:2115-2122, 1996.

163. Sandhu HS, Kanim LE, Toth JM, *et al:* Experimental spinal fusion with recombinant human bone morphogenetic protein-2 without decortication of osseous elements. *Spine* 22:1171-1180, 1997.

164. Sandhu HS, Toth JM, Diwan AD, *et al:* Histologic evaluation of the efficacy of rhBMP-2 compared with autograft bone in sheep spinal anterior interbody fusion. *Spine* 27:567-575, 2002.

165. Schwab F, Dubey A, Pagala M, *et al:* Adult scoliosis: a health assessment analysis by SF-36. *Spine* 28:602-606, 2003.

166. Scudese VA, Calabro JJ: Vertebral wedge osteotomy. Correction of rhematoid (ankylosing) spondylitis. *JAMA* 186:627-631, 1963.

167. Shands AR, Jr., Eisberg HB: The incidence of scoliosis in the state of Delaware; a study of 50,000 minifilms of the chest made during a survey for tuberculosis. *J Bone Joint Surg Am* 37-A:1243-1249, 1955.

168. Shapiro GS, Taira G, Boachie-Adjei O: Results of surgical treatment of adult idiopathic scoliosis with low back pain and spinal stenosis: a study of long-term clinical radiographic outcomes. *Spine* 28:358-363, 2003.

169. Shimode M, Kojima T, Sowa K: Spinal wedge osteotomy by a single posterior approach for correction of severe and rigid kyphosis or kyphoscoliosis. *Spine* 27:2260-2267, 2002.

170. Shono Y, Abumi K, Kaneda K: One-stage posterior hemivertebra resection and correction using segmental posterior instrumentation. *Spine* 26:752-757, 2001.

171. Silcox DH 3rd, Boden SD, Schimandle JH, *et al:* Reversing the inhibitory effect of nicotine on spinal fusion using an osteoinductive protein extract. *Spine* 23:291-296; discussion 297, 1998.

172. Silcox DH 3rd, Daftari T, Boden SD, *et al:* The effect of nicotine on spinal fusion. *Spine* 20:1549-1553, 1995.

173. Simmons ED, Jr., Kowalski JM, Simmons EH: The results of surgical treatment for adult scoliosis. *Spine* 18:718-724, 1993.

174. Simmons ED Jr., Simmons EH: Spinal stenosis with scoliosis. *Spine* 17:S117-120, 1992.

175. Simmons EH: Kyphotic deformity of the spine in ankylosing spondylitis. *Clin Orthop* Oct:65-77, 1977.

176. Smith SE, Darden BV, Rhyne AL, *et al:* Outcome of unoperated discogram-positive low back pain. *Spine* 20:1997-2000; discussion 2000-1991, 1995.

177. Smith-Petersen MN, Larson CB, Aufranc OE: Osteotomy of the spine for correction of flexion deformity in rheumatoid arthritis. *J Bone Joint Surg* 27:1-11, 1945.

178. Stagnara P, De Mauroy JC, Dran G, *et al:* Reciprocal angulation of vertebral bodies in a sagittal plane: approach to references for the evaluation of kyphosis and lordosis. *Spine* 7:335-342, 1982.

179. Stephens GC, Yoo JU, Wilbur G: Comparison of lumbar sagittal alignment produced by different operative positions. *Spine* 21:1802-1807, 1996.

180. Strayer III LM: The incidence of scoliosis in the postpartum female on Cape Cod. *J Bone Joint Surg Am* 55:436, 1973.

181. Styblo K, Bossers GT, Slot GH: Osteotomy for kyphosis in ankylosing spondylitis. *Acta Orthop Scand* 56:294-297, 1985.

182. Suk SI, Kim JH, Kim WJ, *et al:* Posterior vertebral column resection for severe spinal deformities. *Spine* 27:2374-2382, 2002.

183. Swank S, Lonstein JE, Moe JH, *et al:* Surgical treatment of adult scoliosis. A review of two hundred and twenty-two cases. *J Bone Joint Surg Am* 63:268-287, 1981.

184. Swank SM, Mauri TM, Brown JC: The lumbar lordosis below Harrington instrumentation for scoliosis. *Spine* 15:181-186, 1990.

185. Takahashi S, Delecrin J, Passuti N: Surgical treatment of idiopathic scoliosis in adults: an age-related analysis of outcome. *Spine* 27:1742-1748, 2002.

186. Taylor BA, Webb PJ, Hetreed M, *et al:* Delayed postoperative paraplegia with hypotension in adult revision scoliosis surgery. *Spine* 19:470-474, 1994.

187. Thiranont N, Netrawichien P: Transpedicular decancellation closed wedge vertebral osteotomy for treatment of fixed flexion deformity of spine in ankylosing spondylitis. *Spine* 18:2517-2522, 1993.

188. Thomasen E: Vertebral osteotomy for correction of kyphosis in ankylosing spondylitis. *Clin Orthop* Apr:142-152, 1985.

189. Upadhyay SS, Mullaji AB, Luk KD, *et al:* Relation of spinal and thoracic cage deformities and their flexibilities with altered pulmonary functions in adolescent idiopathic scoliosis. *Spine* 20:2415-2420, 1995.

190. van Dam BE: Nonoperative treatment of adult scoliosis. *Orthop Clin North Am* 19:347-351, 1988.

191. van Dam BE, Bradford DS, Lonstein JE, *et al:* Adult idiopathic scoliosis treated by posterior spinal fusion and Harrington instrumentation. *Spine* 12:32-36, 1987.

192. Van Royen BJ, De Gast A: Lumbar osteotomy for correction of thoracolumbar kyphotic deformity in ankylosing spondylitis. A structured review of three methods of treatment. *Ann Rheum Dis* 58:399-406, 1999.

193. van Royen BJ, de Kleuver M, Slot GH: Polysegmental lumbar posterior wedge osteotomies for correction of kyphosis in ankylosing spondylitis. *Eur Spine J* 7:104-110, 1998.

194. van Royen BJ, Slot GH: Closing-wedge posterior osteotomy for ankylosing spondylitis. Partial corporectomy and transpedicular fixation in 22 cases. *J Bone Joint Surg Br* 77:117-121, 1995.

195. Vanderpool DW, James JI, Wynne-Davies R: Scoliosis in the elderly. *J Bone Joint Surg Am* 51:446-455, 1969.

196. Vaughan JJ, Winter RB, Lonstein JE: Comparison of the use of supine bending and traction radiographs in the selection of the fusion area in adolescent idiopathic scoliosis. *Spine* 21:2469-2473, 1996.

197. Vedantam R, Lenke LG, Bridwell KH, *et al:* Comparison of push-prone and lateral-bending radiographs for predicting postoperative coronal alignment in thoracolumbar and lumbar scoliotic curves. *Spine* 25: 76-81, 2000.

198. Weale AE, Marsh CH, Yeoman PM: Secure fixation of lumbar osteotomy. Surgical experience with 50 patients. *Clin Orthop* Dec:216-222, 1995.

199. Weatherley C, Jaffray D, Terry A: Vascular complications associated with osteotomy in ankylosing spondylitis: a report of two cases. *Spine* 13:43-46, 1988.

200. Weinstein SL, Dolan LA, Spratt KF, *et al:* Health and function of patients with untreated idiopathic scoliosis: a 50-year natural history study. *JAMA* 289:559-567, 2003.

201. Weinstein SL, Ponseti IV: Curve progression in idiopathic scoliosis. *J Bone Joint Surg Am* 65:447-455, 1983.

202. Weis JC, Betz RR, Clements DH 3rd, *et al:* Prevalence of perioperative complications after anterior spinal fusion for patients with idiopathic scoliosis. *J Spinal Disord* 10: 371-375, 1997.

203. Wiggins GC, Ondra SL, Shaffrey CI: Management of iatrogenic flat-back syndrome. *Neurosurg Focus* 15:Article 8, 2003.

204. Williams EL: Postoperative blindness. *Anesthesiol Clin North Am* 20:605-622, viii, 2002.

205. Wilson MJ, Turkell JH: Multiple spinal wedge osteotomy. Its use in a case of Marie-Strumpell spondylitis. *Am J Surg* 77:777-782, 1949.

206. Zielke K, Stunkat R, Beaujean F: [Ventrale derotations-spondylodesis (author's transl)]. *Arch Orthop Unfallchir* 85:257-277, 1976.

CHAPTER 68

Ankylosing Spondylitis

Darren Bergey, Robert S. Pashman, and J. Patrick Johnson

Introduction

Ankylosing spondylitis is a seronegative spondyloarthropathy that primarily affects the axial skeleton, including ligaments and articulations of the pelvis and spinal column. It is estimated to occur in 0.02% of the population. Although once believed to affect men predominantly, recent evidence suggests women are affected equally but experience milder symptoms. The HLA-B27 antigen is positive in 80% to 90% of patients with ankylosing spondylitis as compared with 8% of the general population of American Caucasians.[28] This strongly suggests that HLA-B27 antigen is important in the pathogenesis of ankylosing spondylitis. Its precise role remains unclear; however, it is generally understood that an inflammatory response is incited by environmental or infectious agents, and hosts are rendered susceptible by HLA-B27 or related antigens.[37]

Similar to rheumatoid arthritis, the pathophysiology of ankylosing spondylitis remains unclear. The basic pathologic process is an inflammatory focus, predominantly lymphocytic, that targets both articular joints as well as the insertion of ligaments, tendons, and capsules to bone (entheses). Reactive bone formation at these entheses, termed *enthesopathy*, ultimately results in progressive ankylosis of the axial skeleton, typically involving the sacroiliac, apophyseal, and costovertebral joints. The course of the disease includes progressive enchondral ossification of cartilage, resulting in the characteristic joint stiffness and ankylosis. Symptoms usually begin in at the sacroiliac joints and progress proximally in the spine.

The "Romanus lesion" is an erosion of the anterior and lateral border of the vertebral end plate at the site of vascular attachment of the annulus fibrosus. This lesion represents a focal area of spondylitis, ultimately resulting in syndesmophyte formation and ossification of the annulus fibrosus. These osseous changes result in the classic "bamboo spine" appearance radiographically, which is the hallmark of ankylosing spondylitis.

Clinical Presentation

Ankylosing spondylitis typically presents in healthy adults during the second or third decade of life. Sacroiliitis or low back pain is typically the initial manifestation of the disease. Pain may be unilateral or bilateral and may include radicular symptoms extending into the buttocks or thigh. This radicular pain seldom extends below the knee. Symptoms are usually worse in the morning and improve with activity. This clinical feature distinguishes ankylosing spondylitis from mechanical low back pain, which generally worsens with activity and improves with rest. Night pain relieved by activity is not an uncommon feature of ankylosing spondylitis.[28]

In patients with an uncontrolled inflammatory phase of the disease, the lumbar, thoracic, and cervical spine become progressively ankylosed and kyphotic. This usually progresses in a caudal to cranial direction. According to Simkin and colleagues, kyphosis is produced when the patient assumes a "flexed posture in an attempt to unload the facets, thereby reducing joint pressure and alleviating pain."[51] Compensatory flexion contractures of the hips and knees may develop as the patient attempts to maintain an erect posture. Following the inflammatory phase, the patient is typically stiff and kyphotic but relatively pain free. Significant spinal deformity and functional disability may be the end result. Carette and associates[13] studied 150 war veterans for a mean of 38 years and found that, despite severe limitations in spinal motion, 50% of the patients functioned well. Those with more severe deformities, however, may be unable to stand upright, lose horizontal gaze, and develop the so-called chin-on-chest deformity.

Spinal fracture and spondylodiscitis are clinical manifestations of ankylosing spondylitis that are of specific interest to spine surgeons. Ossification of the disc space occurs centripetally through the annulus fibrosus, and only rarely is the center of the disc involved. This incomplete ossification combined with stress concentration from loss of polysegmental spinal motion and secondary osteopenia predispose patients to spinal fracture and nonunion (spondylodiscitis).[26] Spondylodiscitis presents as focal pain with coexisting erosive sclerotic changes in adjacent vertebral bodies. It is uncertain whether this is a primary inflammatory process or the result of trauma. Radiographically, the appearance of spondylodiscitis, pseudarthrosis, and discitis are very similar.

Neurologic decline in the patient with ankylosing spondylitis is uncommon, exclusive of fractures. However, neurologic injury can be a significant complication of spinal fracture, and the diagnosis should not be missed. Severe spinal deformities, together with spondylodiscitis and acute fracture, provide the most common indication for spine surgery in the patient with ankylosing spondylitis.

Surgical Management

General Principles

Because ankylosing spondylitis may lead to severe flexion deformities of the spine, the goal in treatment of these patients is early recognition and adequate medical therapy in an attempt to control the disease progress and prevent associated deformities. However, patients may still become grossly deformed and functionally disabled. Spinal osteotomy may be indicated to correct the deformity and achieve upright posture.

Two considerations determine the technique and location of the osteotomy: the region of the spinal deformity that maximally influences sagittal alignment and a surgical procedure that minimizes the surgical risk. It is important to reemphasize that the overall spinal balance as well as the hips must be evaluated to delineate the primary site of deformity. In some patients, more than one of these sites may contribute to the deformity. The lumbar spine is the most common site of deformity, followed by the thoracic and cervical regions. Accurate measurement of the deformity is required for surgical planning, and Simmons[52] advocates the chin-brow to vertical angle as the most effective and reproducible measurement of deformity (Figure 68.1).

Deformities isolated to the lumbar spine are corrected by a lumbar osteotomy procedure. The osteotomy is preferred below the level of the conus medullaris and is usually performed at L3 to avoid acute angular correction at the cord level.[52] Most lumbar-thoracic kyphotic deformities can also be addressed through a single lumbar osteotomy. The correction should be planned so that the plumb line from C7 falls within the body of S1. Even in cases in which the thoracic kyphosis is greater than normal, a compensatory lumbar osteotomy may correct sagittal plane malalignment and allow the patient to have forward gaze with the hips and knees fully extended. In cases of severe thoracic kyphosis, where the lumbar and cervical lordosis have been at least partially maintained, thoracic osteotomy by a combined anterior and posterior

approach may be indicated. When the primary deformity is at the cervical-thoracic junction, resulting in a "chin-on-chest" deformity, an extension osteotomy of the cervical spine is indicated. The C7-T1 junction is the preferred location because it places the osteotomy below the entrance of the vertebral arteries into the transverse processes at C6 and uses the relatively large spinal canal-to-cord area ratio to safely obtain correction.

The influence of severe hip flexion contractures, with or without associated hip joint disease, is critical in the preoperative assessment. Soft tissue releases about the hips, or more commonly, total hip joint arthroplasty, may be sufficient in itself to allow the patient to stand reasonably upright and see straight ahead, irrespective of the spinal deformity.[5] These should be performed prior to any surgical correction of spinal deformity.

Preoperatively, patients should be screened for cardiac and pulmonary abnormalities that can be associated with extraarticular manifestations of ankylosing spondylitis. Although pulmonary function abnormalities secondary to decreased thoracic expansion have not carried anesthetic risk for most patients,[20] 10% will have cardiac

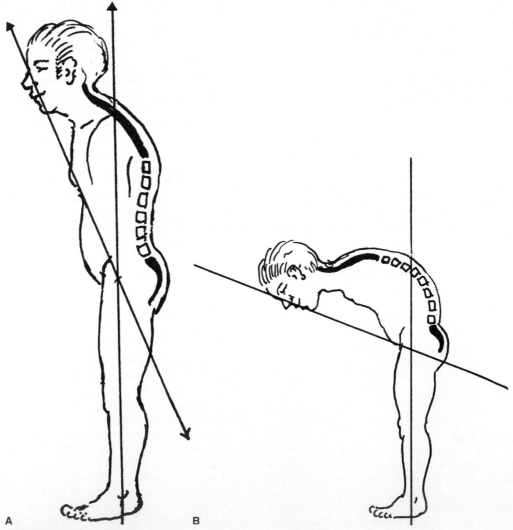

Figure 68.1 Measurement of sagittal plane deformity with chin-brow to vertical angle. (**A**) Lesser deformity. (**B**) Greater deformity.

pathology, generally either aortic stenosis or conduction abnormalities.

Although local anesthesia has been reported in the treatment of these spinal deformities,[32,57] general anesthesia is preferred. Intubation is facilitated by the use of fiberoptic guidance in cases where cervicothoracic kyphosis complicates easy passage of the endotracheal tube. After the patient has been anesthetized and intubated, the operating table must be modified according to the patient's spinal deformity. The table is flexed into a position where the apex of the table is under the primary spinal deformity. Bolsters are used to free the abdomen and protect bony prominences and peripheral nerves in the extremities.

Lumbar Osteotomy

Smith-Petersen and colleagues[55] first proposed lumbar osteotomy for the correction of spinal deformity caused by ankylosing spondylitis in 1945. They performed a V-shaped wedge resection osteotomy at the L3-4 level. The spinous processes were removed at the appropriate angle as were the L3-4 lamina. The osteotomy was extended laterally to include the bilateral facet joints. The lamina and pedicles were undercut to prevent impingement of the dura or nerve roots on closure of the osteotomy site. This osteotomy wedge was then closed and the deformity corrected via forceful manipulation through hyperextension. This maneuver caused fracture of the anterior and middle columns, allowing the osteotomy to close. Osteotomes may be used to complete the fracture if the manual maneuver is unsuccessful. Local bone grafts were placed across the osteotomy sites, and the patient was immobilized in a postoperative cast for 2 months followed by a back brace for 1 year. Six patients were reported, and detailed results are not described.

Simmons[52] used the Smith-Petersen osteotomy and popularized the use of local anesthetic for both lumbar and cervical osteotomies, arguing that two thirds of the 8% to 10% mortality and 30% neurologic complications documented in previous studies were related to the use of general anesthesia. In his series of 90 patients, he was able to show that correction can be reliably achieved through this posterior osteotomy without a secondary ventral approach, paralleling the experience of other authors.[25,26,37,54,63] His

series reported a 40- to 104-degree correction with an average of 56 degrees (Figure 68.2). The chin-brow to vertical angle improved from an average of 60 degrees preoperatively to 5 degrees postoperatively.

The most common complication associated with this procedure is neurologic compression. In Simmons series, 7 (8%) patients developed nerve root or cauda equine symptoms postoperatively.[52] Such complications can be minimized by adequate decompression and undercutting of the lamina prior to closure of the osteotomy site and rigid stabilization. If these complications occur, prompt reexploration and decompression should be performed.

This osteotomy advocated by Smith-Peterson and Simmons uses the middle column as the fulcrum for closure of the posterior osteotomy and has the inherent risk of placing the spinal cord on stretch. Thomasen reported a spinal column shortening osteotomy via a posterior approach that utilized a decancellization procedure[56] (Figure 68.3). The decancellization procedure, also known as an "eggshell osteotomy" or "pedicle subtraction osteotomy," is performed by removing a wedge of the posterior elements of L3 as well as bilateral pedicles. This is followed by resection of the posterior vertebral cortex as well as the cancellous bone of the vertebral body. The ventral cortex of the

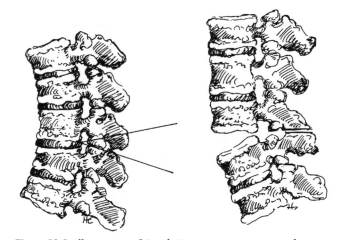

Figure 68.2 Illustration of Smith-Petersen osteotomy technique.

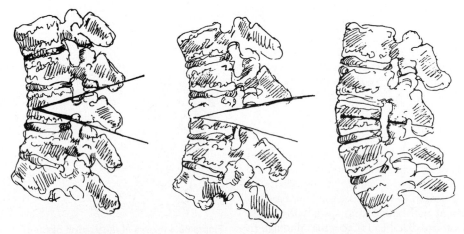

Figure 68.3 Illustration of pedicle subtraction osteotomy (PSO) technique.

vertebral body is left intact and is the fulcrum for closure, effectively shortening the spinal canal and achieving angular correction. Moreover, removal of the pedicle creates a "super-foramen," which transmits the nerve roots from the adjacent segments and decreases the chance for root compression. Generous undercutting/decompression of the supra- and sub-adjacent laminar edges are performed to ensure adequate space for the redundant dura that may be produced during closure of the osteotomy. Segmental spinal fixation that utilizes multiple pedicle screws and/or hook constructs is used to allow for immediate patient mobilization. The table is carefully extended, closing the osteotomy. If necessary, closure can be augmented by pressure on the patient's shoulders or legs and by compression between the pedicle screws once the rods are placed. A wake-up test is routinely performed to assess neurologic function. Finally, a local bone graft is applied and augmented with iliac crest autograft or banked bone, as needed. Thomasen reported 12 to 50 degrees of correction in 11 patients, with 5 of the 11 having a correction of less than 35 degrees.[56] He concluded that this small degree of correction was all that was required to obtain an erect posture. This technique is the procedure of choice at this time.

Thoracic Osteotomy

Thoracic osteotomies are rarely required in patients with ankylosing spondylitis. As stated previously, if the thoracic kyphosis is mild or moderate and associated with a flat or kyphotic lumbar spine, the deformity can be addressed with a lumbar spine osteotomy. The rare patient will have severe thoracic kyphosis with minimal loss of lumbar or cervical lordosis. This is the patient in whom a thoracic osteotomy may be indicated.

Smith-Petersen pointed out in 1945 that single-stage posterior thoracic osteotomy correction is compromised by stiffness of the costovertebral joints. The authors favor a two-stage procedure that consists of a first-stage transthoracic approach creating osteotomies through the ossified thoracic disc spaces. Ventral interbody fusion is performed with autogenous cancellous bone graft. This is followed at the same sitting or 1 week later by posterior, multiple-level Smith-Peterson osteotomies with segmental instrumentation. Dural adhesions to the lamina that formed during the inflammatory phase of the disease can be encountered during dorsal osteotomy and likewise may make passage of sublaminar wires used in the Luque technique more difficult. The authors therefore prefer to stabilize the osteotomy with hook-rod compression instrumentation or thoracic pedicle screws. The approach is similar to that used for severe juvenile kyphosis.[7,9]

Cervical Osteotomy

Cervical osteotomy may occasionally be indicated when the primary deformity is isolated at the cervical-thoracic junction. In 1953, Mason and associates[40] reported successful correction of flexion deformity of the cervical-thoracic spine in a patient with ankylosing spondylitis. They performed the osteotomy distal to C7 to avoid damage to the vertebral arteries. In 1958, Urist[59] reported a success-

ful osteotomy at the cervical-thoracic junction in a patient awake under local anesthesia.

Simmons[53] has reported experience in 95 patients, consisting of a wide laminectomy from C6 to T1 with osteotomy at the C7-T1space. The entire posterior arch of C7 is resected, as is the inferior half of C6 and the upper half of T1. The lamina are undercut, and complete foraminotomies are performed to prevent impingement of the C8 nerve root. The amount of bone to be resected is based on the preoperative chin-brow to vertical angle. This angle is transferred to the lateral radiograph, with the apex of the angle at the posterior edge of the C7-T1 disc space. Following bony decompression, Simmons extended the neck and "cracked" the anterior column (Figure 68.4). An osteotome may be used to perform an anterior osteotomy in a more controlled fashion. Simmons performed the procedure under local anesthesia with halo control and then fixed the halo to a body cast that was worn for 4 months. There were no mortalities, and C8 weakness was the primary morbidity, occurring in 18 patients, with 5 being permanent deficits.

The most popular technique for cervical osteotomy is that described by Urist and Simmons.[53,59] We prefer general anesthetic with controlled halo correction, followed by either an intraoperative wake-up test or spinal cord monitoring. Lateral mass screws are used in the cervical spine, with thoracic pedicle screws placed in the upper thoracic spine for internal fixation. Halo and vest supplementation may or may not be used.

Complications

Postoperative ileus is common in these patients. Nasogastric drainage is essential. Although aortic rupture has been reported,[39,50,60] the case in question occurred after closed forceful osteoclasis of severe kyphosis in a patient who had previously been treated with radiation therapy for ankylosing spondylitis. The authors believe that the fear and likelihood of this complication has been greatly overstated.

It has been stated in review of several series[43-57] that mortality has varied from 8% to 10%, and neurologic complications have occurred in up to 30% of patients. However, these quotes may be misleading. In our analysis of the 14 largest series consisting of 5 or more cases reported,* a total of 427 cases, we find a 4% incidence of neurologic complications and a 5% mortality rate. However, and perhaps even more

---

*References 17-21,36-39,43,53,54,56,57.

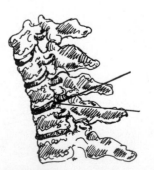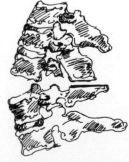

Figure 68.4 Cervical illustration of Smith-Petersen osteotomy technique.

importantly, it appears that in 8 of these reports, consisting of 74 patients, there were no neurologic deficits. In 9 of these series with a total of 85 patients,[17-21,39,54,56] no deaths were reported. In the single largest study, 177 patients reported by Hehne and associates,[24] there was 2.3% mortality and 2.3% irreversible root lesions. Based on the authors' review of the published data and their own experience, it appears that neurologic complications and mortality can be greatly lessened if not prevented altogether by careful attention to four critical factors: (1) avoiding compression of neurologic tissue, (2) monitoring neurologic function during the osteotomy (by wake-up test), (3) using internal fixation, and (4) avoiding translational displacement at the osteotomy site.

Fractures

Osteoporosis and stress concentration secondary to long, stiff lever arms enhance the susceptibility of the ankylosing spondylitis patients to acute spinal fracture. Hunter and Dubo[30] and Hyman et al.[31] noted that 75% of fractures occur in the cervical or cervicothoracic junction, 14% in the thoracic spine, and 5% in the lumbar spine.

Cervical fractures commonly involve both anterior and posterior columns, and this fact probably explains the increased rates of mortality and neurologic complication seen in patients with ankylosing spondylitis as compared with fractures in normal spines.[6,9,44] A review by Trent and colleagues[58] summarizing the world literature points out that thoracolumbar fractures in patients with ankylosing spondylitis commonly occur between T9 and L2 and are associated with a 25% incidence of neurologic deficit at initial presentation, with subsequent poor prognosis for recovery. All authors stress the importance of a high index of suspicion in any ankylosing spondylitis patient with acute onset of new focal pain or deformity. Occult fractures must be suspected, and tomography is often required to fully evaluate the symptomatic areas.

Treatment of the ankylosing spondylitis patient with an acute fracture begins with positioning and transport in the prefracture alignment. Extending the neck in the case of cervical fracture or positioning the patient supine in the case of thoracic or lumbar fractures can have serious neurologic consequences.[58] Both operative[6,8,34,57] and nonoperative management of these fractures have been described in the literature with similar good outcomes for solid union. Clearly, surgery is indicated in cases of progressive neurologic deficit. With current advancements in spinal fixation techniques, we believe that aggressive surgical management leads to earlier mobilization and may avoid the secondary complications of prolonged bed rest.

Spondylodiscitis

Histopathologic features of both inflammatory enthesis and post-traumatic nonunion[2-5] are noted in the entity termed *spondylodiscitis*. The true etiology remains controversial. Unlike acute fractures, spondylodiscitis is viewed as a stable lesion because of its lack of involvement of both anterior and posterior columns. The stability of this type of lesion accounts for its low incidence of associated neuro-

logic deficit. In contrast to acute fractures, spondylodiscitis more commonly occurs in the thoracic and lumbar spine. Nonoperative treatment has been associated with spontaneous healing of these defects.* Hehne and associates have reported a 97% fusion rate at 2 years in the operative treatment of spondylodiscitis by pedicle screw fixation in 28 patients.[24] Ho and colleagues, reporting the experience at the University of Hong Kong, observed excellent results with anterior spinal fusion in 16 patients.[27]

Our current practice for the treatment of both acute fractures and spondylodiscitis in patients with ankylosing spondylitis and no neurologic deficit is early operative treatment with posterior segmental fixation. Patients with neurologic deficit in whom a compressive lesion can be identified may also benefit from anterior decompression. These recommendations are based on an approach that parallels the treatment of fractures in normal spines. Early fixation decreases the chance of progressive deformity as well as the untoward effects of prolonged recumbence and secondary pulmonary and vascular complications in the non-operated patient.[22,45]

ACKNOWLEDGMENTS

The authors acknowledge Helen Cambron, RN, FNP-C, for her illustrative contribution to this chapter.

*References 3-23,29,33,47,49,61,64.

REFERENCES

1. Adams JC: Technique, dangers and safeguards in osteotomy of the spine. *J Bone Joint Surg* 34B:226-232, 1952.
2. Agarwal AK, Reidbord HE, Kraus DR, Eisenbeis CH Jr: Variable histopathology of discovertebral lesion (spondylodiscitis) of ankylosing spondylitis. *Clin Exp Rheumatol* 8:67-69,1990.
3. Baggenstoss AH, Bickel WH, Ward LE: Rheumatoid granulomatous nodules as destructive lesions of vertebrae. *J Bone Joint Surg* 34A:601-609, 1952.
4. Ball J: The Heberden oration, 1970. Enthesopathy of rheumatoid and ankylosing spondylitis. *Ann Rheum Dis* 30:213-223,1971.
5. Bisia RS, Ranawat CS, Inglis AE: Total hip replacement in patients with ankylosing spondylitis with involvement of the hip. *J Bone Joint Surg* 58A:233-238, 1976.
6. Bohlman HH: Acute fractures and dislocations of the cervical spine: an analysis of three hundred hospitalized patients and review of the literature. *J Bone Joint Surg* 61A:1119-1142, 1979.
7. Bohm H, Harms J, Donk R, Zieike K: Correction and stabilization of angular kyphosis. *Clin Orthop* 258:56-61, 1990.
8. Bradford DS, Schumacher WL, Lonstein JE, Winter RB: Ankylosing spondylitis: Experience in surgical management of 21 patients. *Spine* 12:238-243, 1987.
9. Bradford DS. In Kane WJ (ed): *Kyphosis: Current Orthopaedic Management*. New York, Churchill-Livingstone, 1981.
10. Briggs H, Keats S, Schlesinger PT: Wedge osteotomy of the spine with bilateral intervertebral foraminotomy. *J Bone Joint Surg* 29:1075-1082, 1947.

C H A P T E R 6 9

Intramedullary Spinal Cord Lesions

Paul C. McCormick and John A. Anson

Surgery, once used for the diagnosis of intramedullary spinal cord tumors alone, now represents the most effective treatment of benign well-circumscribed tumors (which constitute the majority of intramedullary neoplasms).* Long-term tumor control or cure, with preservation of neurologic function, can be achieved in most patients with microsurgical removal alone.[4,5] The benign nature of most intramedullary neoplasms, advances in microsurgical techniques, early clinical diagnosis with magnetic resonance imaging (MRI), and the ineffectual or inconsistent treatment response of most intramedullary tumors to radiation therapy largely account for the expanded role of surgery in the management of these lesions.[8,14] Therefore, optimization of surgical treatment is the key to successful management of patients with intramedullary mass. This includes early diagnosis and aggressive primary treatment, the avoidance of technical and judgmental errors and their associated complications, and a strict adherence to contemporary microsurgical technique.

Patient Evaluation

The main benefit of surgery for an intramedullary tumor is prophylactic. Preservation, rather than restoration, of neurologic function is the most likely outcome after successful surgical treatment. In fact, significant improvement of a severe or long-standing preoperative neurologic deficit rarely occurs after a technically successful surgical excision. Surgical morbidity is also greater in patients with more significant preoperative deficits. This creates a therapeutic irony in which the risk of surgery is actually less in patients with minimal or no objective neurologic deficit. Thus, early clinical diagnosis and, if possible, definitive initial treatment are critical to successful clinical management of most intramedullary tumors.

Because of the slow growth rate of benign tumors and the availability of MRI, most patients with intramedullary tumors are diagnosed before the onset of significant neurologic deficit. Gadolinium-enhanced MRI is the procedure of choice for imaging and preoperative evaluation of an

intramedullary tumor. Spinal cord enlargement and tumor enhancement are the characteristic findings (Figure 69.1). Polar cysts are often present. Ependymomas are usually symmetrically located and exhibit uniform tumor enhancement, whereas astrocytomas are associated with a more variable appearance with respect to tumor margins and enhancement patterns (Figure 69.2). Prediction of these tumor types on MRI appearance is often inaccurate, predominantly because of the variability of presentation on MRI scans, and is therefore avoided because it may unfairly influence the surgical objective. Hemangioblastomas usually appear as an intensely enhancing eccentric mass or nodule. There is often diffuse spinal cord enlargement that may extend a considerable distance from the tumor (Figure 69.3). The cause of this tumor enlargement is most likely vasogenic edema.[12]

Patient Selection

Whereas early diagnosis is routinely achieved with gadolinium-enhanced MRI, the sensitivity of MRI has far exceeded its specificity. Acute inflammatory conditions or demyelinating conditions such as multiple sclerosis or transverse myelitis are exquisitely imaged with MRI. These are not surgical lesions, and biopsy for diagnosis usually reveals only a nonspecific inflammatory response. This rarely provides a specific diagnosis, prognosis, or treatment options. In most cases, patients with these conditions can be distinguished on the basis of clinical presentation and MRI appearance. These patients usually have symptoms of either acute or subacute onset of significant neurologic deficit. MRI typically shows patchy or focal gadolinium enhancement that may be confined to the white matter (Figure 69.4). Spinal cord enlargement is subtle or, more likely, absent. In contrast, patients with benign intramedullary tumors usually experience a significant spinal cord enlargement with minimal, if any, objective neurologic deficit. Thus, a patient who shows symptoms of an acute or subacute onset of a significant neurologic deficit in the absence of obvious spinal cord enlargement usually harbors a nonsurgical inflammatory lesion.

Obviously, there are exceptions. Malignant or hemorrhagic tumors may have a rapidly progressive or acute presentation in the absence of significant spinal cord enlargement. Conversely, chronic inflammatory or demyelinating conditions may have a more insidious or chronic progressive course that may mimic an intramedullary neoplasm. Surgical exploration for diagnostic biopsy may be required in some cases.

Surgical Objectives

The most important factor influencing the surgical objective is the nature of the tumor-spinal cord juncture. This juncture can be assessed accurately only through an adequate myelotomy, which extends over the entire rostrocaudal

---

*References 3,5,6,8,11,13,15.

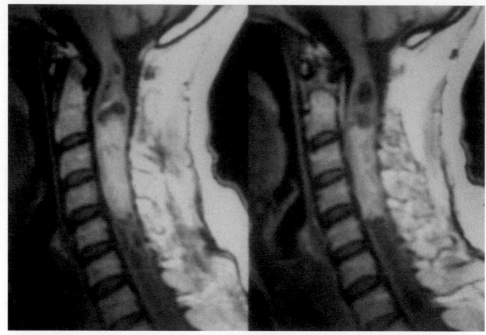

Figure 69.1 Gadolinium-enhanced sagittal MRI shows upper cervical intramedullary enhancing mass. Significant spinal cord enlargement is present over several spinal cord segments, although the solid tumor extends only from C2 to C5. A small rostral and a large caudal polar cyst account for the remainder of the spinal cord enlargement. At surgery, a benign ependymoma was totally removed.

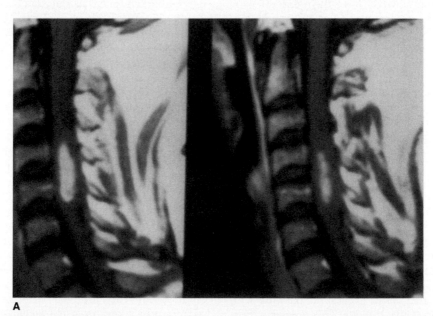

A

Figure 69.2 Gadolinium-enhanced (**A**) sagittal and (**B**) axial MRI scans show a focal, uniformly enhancing intramedullary mass. Irregular tumor margins are apparent on the axial view. At surgery, a focal benign astrocytoma with infiltrating margins was radically, but subtotally, resected.

extent of the tumor. Benign tumors, such as ependymomas and hemangioblastomas, although unencapsulated, are noninfiltrative lesions that typically exhibit a distinct tumor-spinal cord interface. Gross total removal is the treatment of choice in these cases. Astrocytomas are more variable. Unlike the consistently benign histology, circumscribed nature, and natural history of ependymoma and hemangioblastoma, astrocytomas are much more variable with

respect to histology, physical characteristics, and natural history. Although some benign astrocytomas are well circumscribed and allow gross total resection, most exhibit variable infiltration into the surrounding spinal cord. This is often reflected in a gradual transition zone between the tumor and spinal cord. There is rarely a definitive dissection plane. Thus, whereas gross total resection may be achieved in some cases, the extent of removal is uncertain and poorly

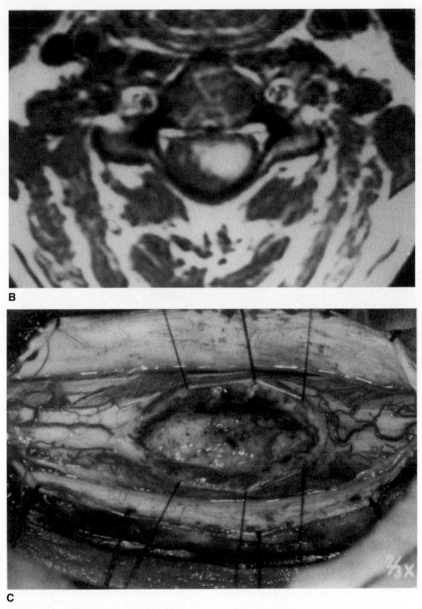

Figure 69.2 *cont'd* **(C)** Intraoperative photograph after tumor resection demonstrates indistinct infiltrating tissue margins.

defined in most cases. Furthermore, more peripheral dissection beyond what is clearly tumor tissue risks loss of neurologic function from the resection of infiltrated, yet functionally viable, spinal cord parenchyma. The surgical objective for spinal cord astrocytomas remains unclear. Specifically, a correlation between the extent of resection and tumor control has not been definitively established.[9,10] Because preservation of neurologic function, rather than complete tumor resection, is the more prudent treatment objective in these cases, tumor removal is limited to tissue that is clearly distinguishable from the surrounding spinal cord. Therefore, the extent of tumor removal varies. Diffusely infiltrative tumors without a definite mass are biopsied, whereas gross total resection may be possible in well-circumscribed examples. Variable degrees of resection will account for the remainder of astrocytomas.

The management of less common intramedullary mass lesions is also dictated by the nature of the tumor-spinal cord juncture. Metastatic spinal cord tumors, for example, usually appear as a well-circumscribed focal mass amenable to gross total resection. Post-resection radiation therapy, as is the case with intracranial metastasis, however, may reduce the risk of local tumor recurrence. Intramedullary lipomas are inclusion tumors that result from disordered embryogenesis (most likely from a defective cleavage of germ cell layers). These are not true neoplasms. They enlarge slowly through continued fat deposition in metabolically normal cells. Gross total resection is not possible because these lesions insinuate into functional spinal cord tissue at their margins. Conservative internal decompression results in long-term clinical stabilization, in most cases.

Cavernous angiomas are congenital vascular malformations that may appear as an intramedullary mass lesion. Most of these lesions are well circumscribed and can be completely excised.[3]

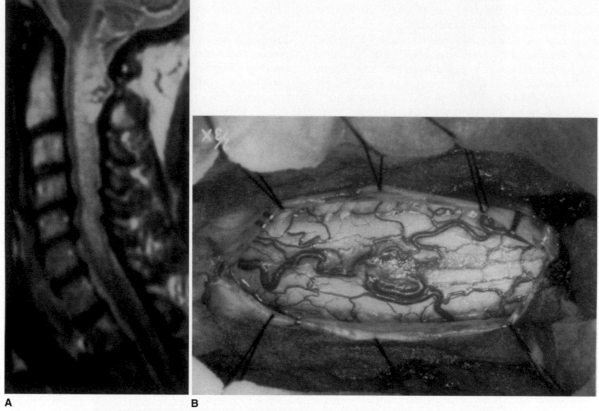

Figure 69.3 (**A**) Sagittal MRI demonstrates a focal dorsal mass at the C2 level. Note diffuse spinal cord enlargement. (**B**) Intraoperative photograph demonstrates orange pia-based hemangioblastoma with associated epipial draining veins.

Intraoperative biopsy is performed primarily to corroborate the gross surgical findings and, more often, the tumor-spinal cord juncture. Determining the surgical objective solely on the basis of biopsy obtained through a small myelotomy should be avoided for two reasons. First, interpretation of tiny biopsy fragments is often inaccurate or nondiagnostic and may consist of only peritumoral gliosis that may be erroneously interpreted as an infiltrating astrocytoma. Second, it is difficult, if not impossible, to assess accurately the nature of the tumor-spinal cord juncture through a tiny myelotomy.

Biopsy results may be particularly helpful in some instances. Identification of a histologically malignant tumor, for example, independently signals an end to the procedure because aggressive surgery is of no benefit for malignant intramedullary neoplasms.[2] In other cases in which the tumor-spinal cord juncture may not be apparent, the confident histologic identification of an ependymoma reassures the surgeon that a plane must exist and that surgical removal should continue.

Surgical Technique

After intubation and administration of perioperative steroids and antibiotics, the patient is turned to the prone position. A Mayfield skull clamp is used for cervical and upper thoracic lesions. Neck flexion and head elevation (i.e., military prone position) reduce the spinal curvature at these levels. Sensory and motor evoked potential monitoring may be used throughout the procedure. The acquired data, however, rarely influence the surgical technique or the surgical objective.[1]

A midline incision and subperiosteal bony dissection is accomplished. A standard laminectomy is performed. This should extend to at least one segment above and one segment below the solid tumor component. The facet joints are preserved, if possible. Delayed instability rarely occurs after laminectomy for intramedullary tumor removal in adults. Although laminoplasty may be a reasonable option, it is not required.

Strict hemostasis must be secured before opening the dura to prevent ongoing contamination into the dependent microsurgical field. Wide, moist, cottonoid "wall-offs" cover the exposed muscles. Surgicel is generously spread over the lateral gutters to prevent contamination of the operative field with blood. The dura mater is opened in the midline and tented laterally to the muscles with sutures (Figure 69.5A).

The arachnoid is opened separately, and the spinal cord is inspected for any surface abnormality. Most glial tumors appear with only localized spinal cord enlargement. The spinal cord may be rotated. Occasionally, the overlying spinal cord may be thinned or even transparent secondary to a large or eccentrically located tumor or polar cyst. Ultrasonography is useful for tumor localization and assurance of adequate bony exposure.

Rarely, an exophytic component of a benign glial tumor may extend into the subarachnoid space through a nerve root entry zone. Malignant neoplasms may replace surface spinal cord tissue or fungate through the pia into the subarachnoid space. Most hemangioblastomas arise from the dorsal half of the spinal cord with a visible pial attachment (see Figure 69.3B).[7] The size of the pial attachment may bear no relationship to the underlying embedded portion of the tumor.

Exposure of most intramedullary glial neoplasms is through a dorsal midline myelotomy. Eccentrically located tumors that abut the pia may be exposed via an off-midline myelotomy that extends longitudinally from both ends of the visible tumor.

The dorsal midline septum is identified as the midpoint between corresponding dorsal root entry zones. Bipolar cautery marks the dorsal midline over the extent of the intended myelotomy. The myelotomy is begun with a microknife in an avascular pial segment at the point of maximum spinal cord enlargement. The pia is a white, glistening fibrocartilaginous membrane that is tightly applied to the outer glial limiting membrane of the spinal cord. The pia is sharply incised over the entire extent of the tumor. Midline crossing epipial vessels are sequentially cauterized and divided. The myelotomy is deepened by gentle spreading with blunt microforceps and dissectors. Fibrous gliosis at the polar margins of the tumor may require sharp dissection with a microknife. The myelotomy continues until the entire rostrocaudal extent of the

dorsal tumor surface has been identified (Figure 69.5B). Although the myelotomy must extend a few millimeters beyond the solid portion of the tumor, it is not necessary to completely expose polar cysts. Sizes 6-0 pial sutures are placed and hung on mosquito clamps to maintain gentle traction (Figure 69.5C). Evaluation of the tumor-spinal cord interface and frozen section biopsy examination (to a lesser extent) determine the appropriate treatment objective. Ependymomas are usually characterized by a glistening reddish or brownish-red surface that may be slightly lobulated (see Figure 69.5C). Blood vessels often course over the tumor surface. These tumors are clearly distinguishable from the surrounding spinal cord on the basis of color and texture. Although unencapsulated, these tumors do not infiltrate and can be easily distinguished and separated from the surrounding spinal cord. Astrocytomas are more heterogeneous with respect to physical characteristics and abut the spinal cord. Intratumoral cysts are quite common, but tumor color and consistency are variable. In adults, most astrocytomas appear as a definable intramedullary mass with a gradual and indistinct transition between the tumor mass and surrounding spinal cord (see Figure 69.2C). This reflects the infiltrative nature of these neoplasms.

The technique of tumor removal depends upon its juncture with the spinal cord and its size. Development of the tumor-spinal cord juncture is preferred for circumscribed tumors with a well-defined plane. The dorsal tumor surface is exposed with pial sutures and gentle,

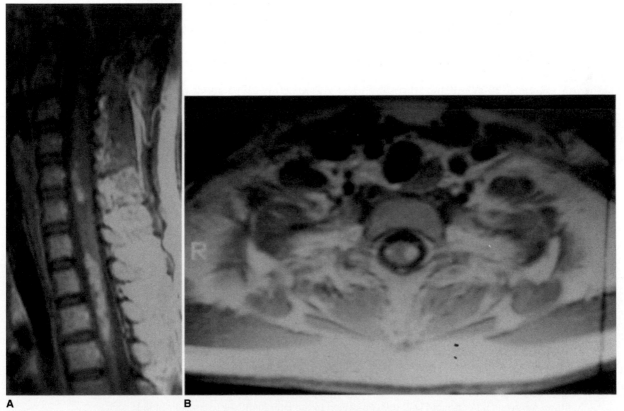

A   **B**

Figure 69.4 Gadolinium-enhanced (**A**) sagittal and (**B**) axial MRI scans in patient with acute onset of significant neurologic deficit demonstrate patchy white matter enhancement without spinal cord enlargement. The clinical presentation and radiographic appearance are consistent with transverse myelitis. Surgery is not indicated in this patient.

blunt lateral displacement of the overlying dorsal hemi-cords with dissectors. Fibrous and vascular attachments that tether the spinal cord to the tumor surface are systematically cauterized and divided. The development of the lateral and polar tumor margins is facilitated by forceps traction on the tumor and gentle pial suture and manual dissector countertraction on the spinal cord (Figure 69.5D). Larger tumors require internal decompression with an ultrasonic aspirator or laser to allow better visualization and mobilization of the lateral and ventral tumor margins. Infiltrating tumors are removed using an "inside-out" technique. Internal decompression is continued peripherally until the clear distinction of the tumor and spinal cord is no longer obvious (see Figure 69.2C).

The technique of hemangioblastoma removal differs because of its vascularity and pial attachment. Internal decompression is not an option (because of the vascularity). Instead, the pial attachment should be circumferentially incised. Systematic cautery on the tumor surface shrinks the tumor bulk to allow adequate mobilization and dissection from the surrounding spinal cord. Small polar longitudinal myelotomies may improve visualization of large tumors embedded in the spinal cord, with only a small exposed pial surface attachment. After completion of tumor resection, the pial sutures are removed. No attempt is made to suture the dorsal hemicords. The subarachnoid space is copiously irrigated with warm saline. Meticulous multilayer closure is then performed to prevent cerebrospinal fluid (CSF)

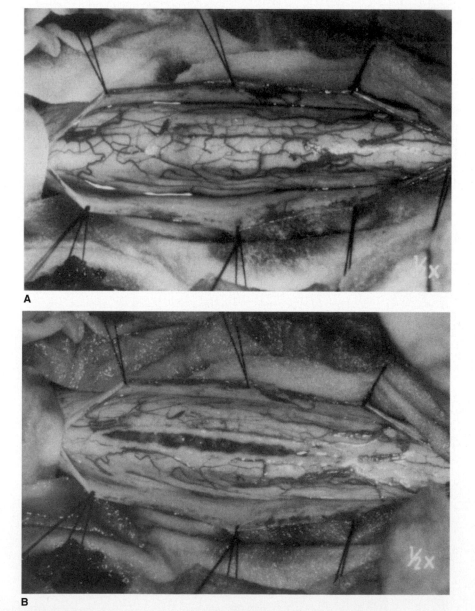

Figure 69.5 (**A**) Initial exposure of spinal cord. The dura mater is tented to the muscles with suture. Surgicel and cottonoid wall-offs are placed in the lateral gutters to prevent blood drainage into the dependent operative field. The spinal cord is swollen without visible surface abnormality. (**B**) A midline myelotomy has been performed. The tumor is encountered at a depth of about 2mm. The myelotomy extends over the entire rostrocaudal extent of the tumor mass.

leakage. This is particularly important in patients who have undergone previous surgery and radiation therapy. There is a high risk of CSF fistula in these patients. An autologous thoracodorsal fascia dural patch graft may be used after biopsy of infiltrative or malignant tumors.

Postoperative Management

Postoperative management is standard. Early mobilization is encouraged to prevent the complications of recumbency, such as deep venous thrombosis and pneumonia. Paretic patients are particularly vulnerable to thromboembolic complications. Subcutaneous heparin (5000 units bid) is begun on the second postoperative day in these patients. Orthostatic hypotension may occasionally occur after removal of upper thoracic and cervical intramedullary neoplasms. This is usually a self-limiting problem that can be managed with liberal use of fluids and more gradual mobilization. A posterior fossa syndrome occasionally occurs after removal of a high cervical intramedullary neoplasm. This is effectively managed with steroids, although a spinal tap may be required to rule out meningitis. CSF fistulas are aggressively managed. An early return to the operating room for wound revision is recommended to prevent this complication in selected cases.

Despite confident gross total resection, benign intramedullary tumors present a continued risk of

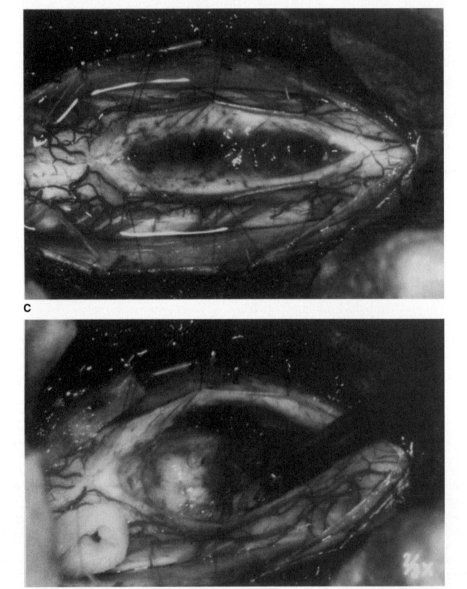

C

D

Figure 69.5 *cont'd* (C) Photograph after exposure of the dorsal tumor surface demonstrates glistening appearance of an intramedullary ependymoma that is clearly separate from the surrounding spinal cord. Exposure is maintained with pial traction. Sutures are hung over the edge of the wound by mosquito clamps. (**D**) Development of the lateral and ventral tumor margins is performed with forceps traction on the tumor against gentle countertraction on the surrounding cord tissue.
Continued

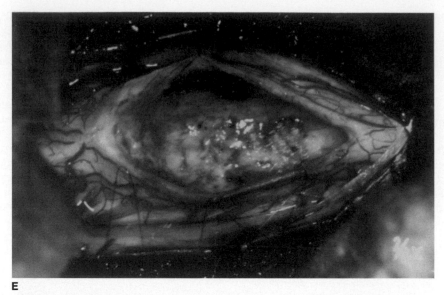

E

Figure 69.5 *cont'd* (**E**) Intraoperative photograph after gross total resection of an intramedullary ependymoma shows clean tumor margins without evidence of residual tumor.

recurrence. Long-term clinical and radiographic follow-up is warranted in these patients. An early postoperative MRI (6 to 8 weeks after surgery) establishes the completeness of resection and serves as a baseline against which further studies can be compared. Serial gadolinium-enhanced MRI scans are obtained yearly because radiographic evidence of tumor recurrence usually precedes clinical symptoms. Surgical reexploration, if clinically appropriate, can then be performed with minimal surgical morbidity. Exposure of the spinal cord at reoperation can be technically difficult. There is often tethering of the spinal cord to the dural suture line at the previous myelotomy site. If the dura was not closed at the previous surgery, then the spinal cord may be densely adherent to the thick epidural scar. In either case, normal dura should be exposed above and below the tethered segment, even if additional bone removal is required. The dura mater or scar is opened as an ellipse around the tether. Meticulous sharp dissection is carried centrally to free the dorsal surface of the spinal cord.

Nearly all patients experience dorsal column dysfunction postoperatively. This probably results from the dorsal midline myelotomy. Patients often complain of numbness or paresthesias with minimal objective discriminative or proprioceptive deficits. These subjective complaints usually improve with time but do not resolve totally. Postoperative neurologic function usually correlates with the preoperative neurologic deficit. The new onset of significant objective neurologic deficits rarely occurs in patients with minimal or no preoperative deficits. Conversely, worsening of an existing preoperative deficit often occurs postoperatively.

Summary

Surgery represents the only established effective treatment modality for benign intramedullary neoplasms. Optimization of surgical outcome, therefore, is the most important treatment consideration. Aggressive initial management, appropriate judgment and technique, and adherence to strict microsurgical techniques are the most effective methods of avoiding complications and ensuring an optimal treatment outcome.

REFERENCES

1. Adams DC, Emerson RG, Heyer EJ, *et al:* Intraoperative evoked potential monitoring with controlled neuromuscular blockade. *Anesth Analg* 77:913-918, 1993.
2. Cohen AR, Wisoff JH, Allen JC, *et al:* Malignant astrocytomas of the spinal cord. *J Neurosurg* 70:50-54, 1989.
3. McCormick PC: Spinal ependymoma. *Neurosurg Q* 3: 178-191, 1993.
4. McCormick PC: Anatomic principles of the intradural spinal surgery. *Clin Neurosurg* 41:204-223, 1994.
5. McCormick PC, Stein BM: Intramedullary tumors in adults. *Neurosurg Clin North Am* 1:609-630, 1990.
6. McCormick PC, Stein BM: Spinal cord tumors in adults. In Youmans JR (ed): *Neurological Surgery,* ed 4. Philadelphia, WB Saunders, 1996, pp 3102-3122.
7. McCormick PC, Michelson WJ, Post KD, *et al:* Cavernous malformations of the spinal cord. *Neurosurgery* 23:459-463, 1988.
8. McCormick PC, Torres R, Post KD, *et al:* Intramedullary ependymoma of the spinal cord. *J Neurosurg* 72:523-533, 1990.
9. Rossitch E, Zeidman S, Burger PC, *et al:* Clinical and pathological analysis of spinal and astrocytomas in children. *Neurosurgery* 27:193-196, 1990.
10. Sandler HM, Papadopoulos SM, Thuntan AF, *et al:* Spinal cord astrocytoma: results of therapy. *Neurosurgery* 30: 490-493, 1992.
11. Sloof JL, Kernohan JW, MacCarthy CS: *Primary Intramedullary Tumors of the Spinal Cord and Filum Terminale.* Philadelphia, WB Saunders, 1964.

12. Solomon RA, Stein BM: Unusual spinal cord enlargement related to intramedullary hemangioblastoma. *J Neurosurg* 68:550-553, 1988.

13. Stein BM, McCormick PC: Intramedullary neoplasms and vascular malformations. *Clin Neurosurg* 39:361-387, 1992.

14. Whitaker SJ, Bessell EM, Ashley SE, *et al:* Post-operative radiotherapy in the management of spinal cord ependymoma. *J Neurosurg* 74:720-728, 1991.

15. Wood EH, Berne AS, Taveras JM: The value of radiation therapy in the management of intrinsic tumors of the spinal cord. *Radiology* 63:11-24, 1954.

CHAPTER 70

Intradural Extramedullary Spinal Lesions

Barry D. Birch, Paul C. McCormick, and Daniel K. Resnick

Before the advent of microsurgical techniques, surgery of many spinal cord neoplasms consisted primarily of open biopsy and radiation therapy.[43,48,49] Recent technologic advances in neurosurgery and diagnostic imaging have expanded the role for operative treatment of spinal tumors. Although Horsely performed the first successful excision of a spinal tumor in 1887, and Elsberg and Frazier advocated resection of spinal tumors in the early part of the twentieth century, consistently acceptable morbidity and mortality were not realized until recently.[3,9,17,26] Magnetic resonance imaging (MRI) has facilitated preoperative localization and surgical planning. The use of intraoperative neurologic monitoring and ultrasound has led to reduced operative morbidity. Advances in microsurgical techniques and the development of ultrasonic aspiration and laser technology have established microsurgical removal as the most effective treatment for benign intradural extramedullary tumors.

Incidence and Pathology

Tumors of the spine are anatomically classified by their relationship to the dura mater and spinal cord parenchyma. Intradural tumors can be intramedullary or extramedullary and account for roughly three fourths of all spinal tumors.[9,19,20,43] Intradural neoplasms make up approximately 10% of primary central nervous system tumors in adults,[22,43] and about two-thirds are extramedullary, histologically benign, and well circumscribed. Meningioma, schwannoma, and filum terminale ependymoma are the most common histopathologic lesions in this location. Meningiomas and nerve sheath neoplasms account for 80% of extramedullary spinal cord tumors, and filum terminale ependymomas make up 15% of these lesions. The remaining 5% includes paragangliomas, drop metastases, and granulomas, all of which are rare.

Meningiomas

Meningiomas arise from arachnoid cap cells embedded in the dura mater near the nerve root sleeve, reflecting their predominant lateral location and meningeal attachment. Other possible cells of origin include fibroblasts associated with the dura or pia mater, which may account for the occa-

sional ventral or dorsal location of these tumors. Meningiomas occur in all age groups, but most arise in persons between the fifth and seventh decades of life. Women account for 75% to 85%, and about 80% are thoracic.[23,31,44] The upper cervical spine and foramen magnum are also common sites (Figure 70.1).[46] Here, meningiomas often occupy a ventral or ventrolateral position and may adhere to the vertebral artery near its intradural entry and initial intracranial course. Low cervical and lumbar meningiomas are infrequent. Most spinal meningiomas are entirely intradural; however, about 10% can be both intradural and extradural or entirely extradural.[31] Meningiomas are generally solitary, but multiplicity can be observed in patients with neurofibromatosis. The overall incidence of multiplicity in the spine is 1% to 2%.[33]

Gross characteristics range from smooth and fibrous to the more frequent variegated, fleshy, friable appearance. Microscopic calcification may occur. The dural attachment is often broader than expected, but en plaque examples are unusual. Bony involvement does not occur in the spine because of the well-defined epidural space.

Nerve Sheath Tumors: Schwannoma and Neurofibroma

Nerve sheath tumors are categorized as either schwannomas or neurofibromas. Although evidence from tissue culture, electron microscopy, and immunohistochemistry supports a common Schwann cell origin of neurofibromas and schwannomas, the morphologic heterogeneity of neurofibromas suggests participation of additional cell types such as perineural cells and fibroblasts. Neurofibromas and schwannomas merit separate consideration because of distinct demographic, histologic, and biologic characteristics. A schwannoma appears grossly as a smooth, globoid mass that does not produce enlargement of the nerve but is suspended eccentrically from it by a discrete attachment. The histologic appearance consists of elongated bipolar cells with fusiform, darkly staining nuclei arranged in compact interlacing fascicles that tend to palisade (Antoni A pattern). A loosely arranged pattern of stellate cells (Antoni B pattern) is less common.[22] The histologic appearance of a neurofibroma consists of an abundance of fibrous tissue and the conspicuous presence of nerve fibers within the tumor stroma.[39] Grossly the tumor produces fusiform enlargement of the involved nerve, which makes it impossible to distinguish between them. Multiple neurofibromas establish the diagnosis of neurofibromatosis, but this syndrome should be considered even in patients with solitary involvement.

Nerve sheath tumors account for about 25% of intradural spinal cord tumors in adults.[24,31] Most are solitary schwannomas occurring throughout the spinal canal. The fourth through sixth decades of life represent the peak incidence of occurrence, and men and women are equally affected. Most nerve sheath tumors arise from a dorsal nerve root. Ventral root tumors are more commonly neurofibromas. Most nerve sheath tumors are entirely intradural, but in 10% to 15% of cases they extend through the dural root sleeve as a dumbbell-shaped tumor with both intradural and extradural components (Figure 70.2).[31] About 10% of nerve sheath tumors are epidural or paraspinal in location. Intramedullary

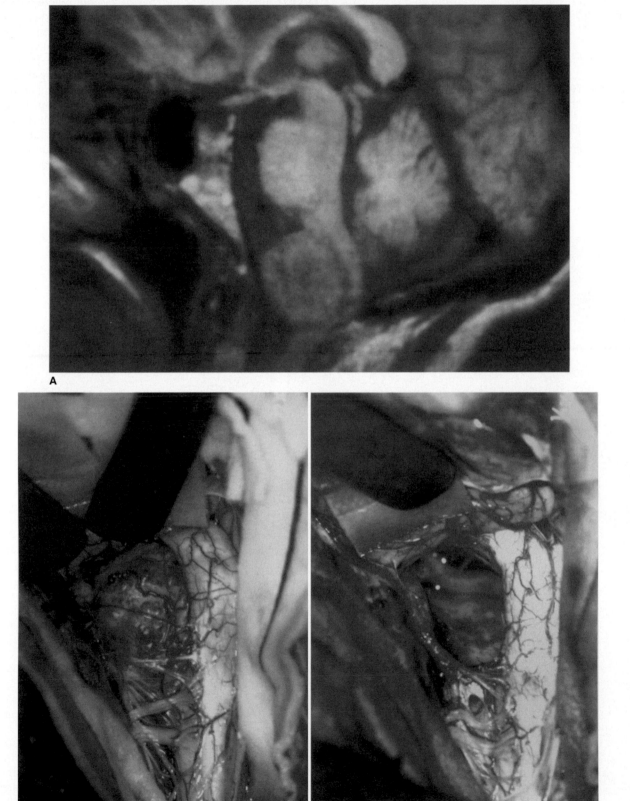

Figure 70.1 Foramen magnum meningioma. (**A**) T1-weighted MRI demonstrates ventral location with dorsal displacement of the spinal cord. (**B**) Dorsolateral approach prior to resection. (**C**) Appearance after gross total resection.

accounts for 1% and are believed to arise from the perivascular nerve sheaths that accompany penetrating spinal cord vessels. Centripetal growth of a nerve sheath tumor can also result in subpial extension, and this occurs most often with plexiform neurofibromas. In these cases, both intramedullary and extramedullary tumor components are apparent. Brachial or lumbar plexus neurofibromas can extend centrally into the intradural space along multiple nerve roots. Conversely, retrograde intraspinal extension of a paraspinal schwannoma usually remains epidural.

About 2.5% of intradural spinal nerve sheath tumors are malignant,[42] and at least one-half of these occur in patients with neurofibromatosis. Malignant nerve sheath tumors carry a poor prognosis, and survival is generally less than 1 year. These tumors must be distinguished from the rare cellular schwannoma, which has aggressive histologic features but is associated with a favorable prognosis.

Filum Terminale Ependymoma

Although filum ependymomas have been classified as intramedullary lesions by virtue of the neuroectodermal derivation of the filum terminale, it is appropriate to consider them with extramedullary tumors from an anatomic and surgical perspective.[26,43] About 40% of spinal canal ependymomas arise within the filum terminale (Figure 70.3),[43] most occurring in its proximal intradural portion. Astrocytomas, oligodendrogliomas, and paragangliomas can also originate in the filum but are rare. Filum terminale ependymomas occur throughout life but are most common in the third to fifth decades. Men are slightly more commonly affected. Filum ependymomas and cauda equina nerve sheath tumors occur with about equal frequency in men and women.[12,32]

Lesions are typically red, sausage-shaped growths with moderate vascularity. Although unencapsulated, they are

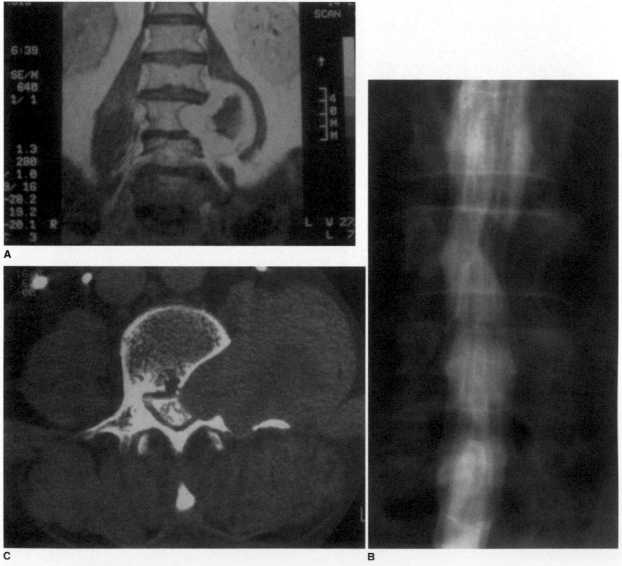

Figure 70.2 Dumbbell-shaped schwannoma. **(A)** Coronal lumbar MRI after intravenous gadolinium, demonstrating extension through the neural foramen into the paraspinal region. **(B)** AP myelogram shows intradural component of the tumor. **(C)** Axial CT myelogram image demonstrates relationship to the dura mater and bony erosion.

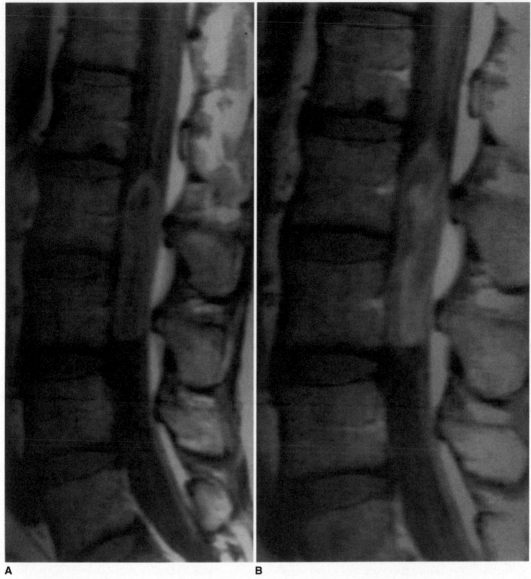

A

B

Figure 70.3 Filum terminale ependymoma. Sagittal T_1-weighted MRI (**A**) before and (**B**) after intravenous gadolinium. Origin from the filum terminale is apparent on both images.

usually well circumscribed and may be covered by arachnoid. Myxopapillary ependymoma is the most common histologic type encountered. The microscopic appearance consists of a papillary arrangement of cuboidal or columnar tumor cells surrounding a vascularized core of hyalinized and hypocellular connective tissue.[22] Nearly all are histologically benign.[45] These tumors, however, tend to be more aggressive in younger age groups.[5]

Miscellaneous Pathology

Extramedullary masses can be neoplastic or non-neoplastic. Paragangliomas are rare tumors of neural crest origin arising from the filum terminale or cauda equina.[38] They are benign and usually nonfunctioning tumors that histologically resemble extra-adrenal paraganglia. They appear grossly as well-circumscribed vascular tumors and may be clinically and radiographically indistinguishable from filum terminale ependymomas. Identification of dense-core neu-

rosecretory granules on electron microscopy establishes the diagnosis, and complete removal can be accomplished in most cases. Cavernous malformations, hemangioblastomas, and ganglioneuromas may involve an intradural nerve root and appear as an extramedullary mass. These lesions can be observed clinically as nerve sheath tumors with early radicular symptoms. Ganglioneuromas may be manifested as dumbbell-shaped tumors in pediatric patients.

Dermoids, epidermoids, lipomas, teratomas, and neurenteric cysts are inclusion lesions resulting from disordered embryogenesis.[1,36] They can occur throughout the spinal canal but are more common in the thoracolumbar and lumbar spine. Intramedullary locations have also been reported. Associated anomalies such as cutaneous lesions, sinus tracts, occult ventral or dorsal rachischisis, and split cord malformations may be present.[18,36] Inclusion tumors and cysts are generally seen as masses, but recurrent meningitis, tethered cord syndrome, or congenital deformities may be the predominant clinical finding.

Non-neoplastic lesions may also appear as extramedullary masses, arachnoid cysts being a well-known example. These cysts are most common in the thoracic spine and are usually dorsal to the spinal cord.[30] Intraspinal aneurysms are extremely rare. Herniated intervertebral disks have occasionally been reported to rupture through the dura and appear as an intradural extramedullary mass.[27]

Inflammatory pathologies such as sarcoidosis, tuberculoma, and subdural empyema are rarely seen as intradural mass lesions.[14,21,27] Although spinal carcinomatous meningitis frequently complicates systemic cancer, secondary metastatic mass lesions of the intradural extramedullary compartment are rare. Malignant intracranial neoplasms that oppose the subarachnoid space or ventricles are the most likely intracranial tumors to demonstrate cerebrospinal fluid (CSF) drop metastasis into the spinal subarachnoid space.[3] Systemic cancer accesses the subarachnoid space either through direct dural root sleeve penetration or, more commonly, hematogenously via the choroid plexus.[34,37]

Clinical Features

Extramedullary spinal cord lesions cause a variety of clinical signs and symptoms, and no particular clinical syndrome is pathognomonic. In general, pain followed by progressive neurologic deficit is the clinical course most often encountered. The classic syndrome historically ascribed to intradural extramedullary tumors consists of progression through segmental, hemicord, and transverse cord dysfunction.[8,15] This presentation, however, is rarely observed in current clinical practice and is not specific to extramedullary lesions. Generally, the clinical features of most extramedullary tumors reflect a slow-growing intraspinal mass. Specific manifestations are variable and determined mainly by tumor location. Upper cervical and foramen magnum tumors are often ventral and are frequently accompanied by suboccipital pain, distal arm weakness, and hand intrinsic muscle weakness and atrophy causing clumsiness.[46] The etiology of this well-known syndrome is uncertain, but it most likely results from venous insufficiency. Increased intracranial pressure and hydrocephalus can occur rarely with an extramedullary tumor at any level but are more common with upper cervical lesions.[13] The mechanism is probably related to elevation of the CSF protein and resulting impaired CSF flow and absorption. Segmental motor weakness and long tract signs are the hallmarks of low-cervical and mid-cervical tumors. Early signs and symptoms are typically asymmetric, which reflects the predominantly lateral location of most intradural tumors. Brown-Sequard's syndrome, characterized by ipsilateral corticospinal spinal tract and posterior column and contralateral spinothalamic tract dysfunction, is common.

Thoracic tumors frequently produce long-tract signs, and corticospinal tracts are particularly vulnerable. Initial signs of stiffness and early muscle fatigue eventually give way to spasticity. Weakness usually begins distally, particularly with dorsiflexion of the ankle and large toe. Sensory gait ataxia may result from bilateral posterior column compression with dorsal midline tumors. Bowel and bladder functions are not significantly impaired until late in the clinical course. Filum ependymomas are characterized most frequently by back pain and subsequent asymmetric radiation to both legs. Increased pain on recumbency, an important clinical feature of extramedullary tumors, is most often associated with large cauda equina lesions. Subarachnoid hemorrhage has also been reported as a typical feature of an extramedullary tumor.[7]

Imaging Evaluation

The mainstay of imaging diagnosis for all spinal cord tumors is magnetic resonance imaging (MRI). It provides spatial and contrast resolution of neural structures that is unattainable by any other imaging modality. Plain radiographs are of little use in the modern diagnosis of spinal cord tumors because they do not image soft tissue adequately. However, the effects of intraspinal tumors on the vertebral elements are sometimes evident. Nerve sheath tumors can cause enlargement of the intervertebral foramina. This finding may be important in patients imaged for other reasons. Myelography alone has a very limited role in the workup of spinal cord tumors and is seldom performed without subsequent computed tomography (CT). Intradural extramedullary tumors typically produce rounded filling defects of the dye column on a plain myelogram. CT and CT myelography (myelo-CT) greatly enhance anatomic details compared to plain radiographs and myelography. CT provides excellent visualization of osseous structures, but soft tissue detail is inferior to that provided by MRI. For extramedullary tumors, myelo-CT allows excellent visualization of tumors arising in the region of the neural foramen, and accompanying bony changes are well demonstrated. MRI with and without intravenous contrast is the optimal initial radiographic examination for patients suspected of having an intradural extramedullary spinal lesion.

Lesion signal abnormalities, CSF capping, and spinal cord or cauda equina displacement identify most extramedullary masses in a technically adequate MRI study.[2] The diagnosis of lipoma, neurenteric cysts (dermoid or epidermoid), arachnoid cysts, or vascular pathology can be established on the basis of imaging characteristics alone. Gadolinium-enhanced images markedly increase the sensitivity of MRI, particularly for small tumors.

Most extramedullary tumors are isointense or slightly hypointense with respect to the spinal cord on T_1-weighted images. Nerve sheath tumors are more likely to be hyperintense to the spinal cord than meningiomas on T_2-weighted images. Cauda equina tumors usually demonstrate increased signal intensity with respect to CSF on both T1 and T2 pulse sequences. However, small cauda equina tumors are easily overlooked on noncontrast scans.[2,11]

Virtually all extramedullary spinal tumors demonstrate some degree of contrast enhancement. Meningiomas typically exhibit intense uniform enhancement, although nonenhancing calcifications or intratumoral cysts may be seen. Enhancement of the adjacent dura, a "dural tail," strongly supports the diagnosis of meningioma (Figure 70.4). Although most nerve sheath tumors and filum ependymomas also demonstrate uniform contrast uptake, heterogeneous enhancement from intratumoral cysts, hemorrhage, or necrosis is frequent (Figure 70.5).

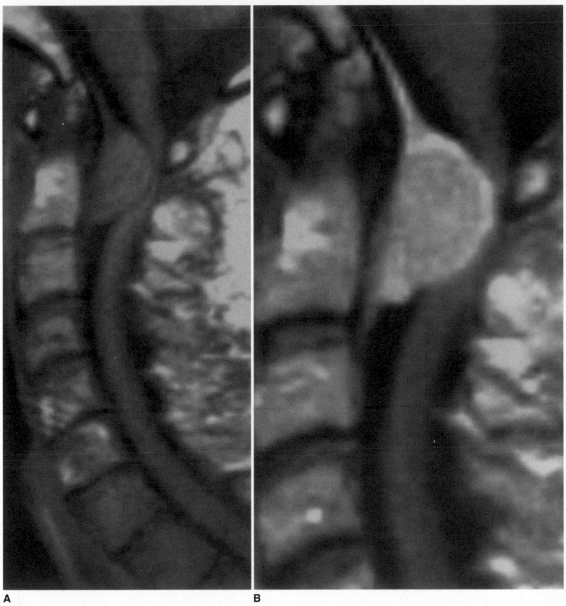

Figure 70.4 High cervical meningioma. Sagittal T_1-weighted MRI (**A**) before and (**B**) after intravenous gadolinium. Enhancing dural tails are evident.

Currently, myelography and myelo-CT are not often used for the evaluation of intradural pathology. Nevertheless, the spatial resolution of myelo-CT remains superior to that of MRI. For tumors that are closely applied to the surface of the spinal cord and when the MRI is equivocal with respect to an intramedullary or extramedullary location, myelo-CT can provide better resolution. The intradural or extradural distribution of a paraspinal or dumbbell-shaped tumor is also better visualized with myelo-CT than with MRI (see Figure 70.2C).

Management

After clinical and imaging evaluation reveal a lesion that is believed to be a spinal cord tumor, tissue diagnosis is necessary. The surgical objective for most intradural extramedullary spinal cord lesions is gross total removal,

and surgical planning must proceed accordingly. Immediately preoperatively, patients are given high-dose glucocorticoids and intravenous antibiotics. Most tumors are accessible with the patient in the prone position. For cervical lesions, stabilization of the head and neck in pins is necessary. Adequate exposure is crucial and is dictated by the location and extent of the lesion. Intraoperative monitoring with somatosensory evoked potentials (SSEP) and motor evoked potentials (MEP) should be considered. Intraoperative ultrasound is often useful in localizing and delineating the extent of the pathology. Competent dural closure is essential. Steroids are tapered postoperatively, and early mobilization and rehabilitation are encouraged.

Surgical Considerations

The optimal treatment of intradural extramedullary tumors is surgical excision. For nerve sheath lesions this

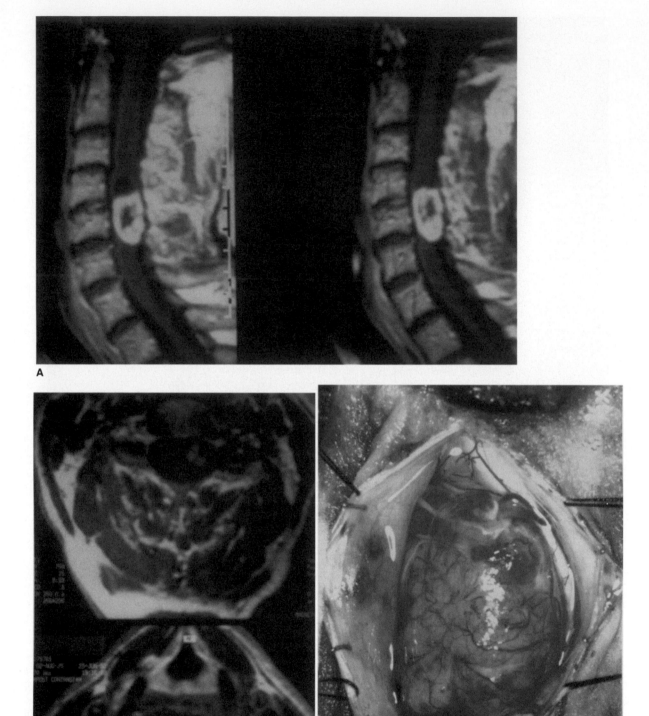

A

B   C

Figure 70.5 Cystic schwannoma. (**A**) Sagittal and (**B**) axial T_1-weighted MRI after intravenous gadolinium; a small apical syrinx and heterogeneous enhancement are demonstrated. (**C**) Intraoperative photograph showing encapsulated tumor with a densely adherent arachnoid layer.

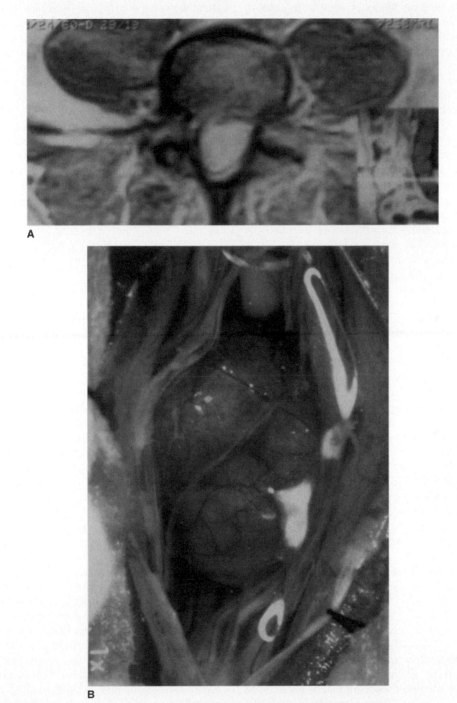

Figure 70.6 Cauda equina schwannoma. (**A**) Axial T$_1$-weighted MRI after intravenous gadolinium; a homogeneously enhancing lesion is apparent. (**B**) Dorsolateral location is evident with displacement of the cauda equina ventrolaterally.

can be accomplished in nearly all cases through standard laminectomy.[26] Recurrences are rare when gross total removal has been achieved. Most nerve sheath tumors are dorsal or dorsolateral to the spinal cord and are easily seen after opening the dura mater (Figure 70.6). Ventral tumors may require dentate ligament section to achieve adequate visualization, and lumbar tumors may be covered by the cauda equina or conus medullaris. The nerve roots must be separated to provide adequate visualization.

Laminectomy provides adequate exposure for spinal meningiomas in most cases. Unilateral laminectomy and facetectomy can be used for eccentrically located or ventral tumors. Large ventral tumors can also be approached satisfactorily through standard dorsal exposures because they have already provided the necessary spinal cord retraction. Suture retraction on a divided dentate ligament or on noncritical dorsal nerve roots provides additional ventral exposure. Depression of the paraspinal muscle mass with table-mounted retractors further facilitates ventral access. Alternatively, a costotransversectomy or lateral extracavitary approach can be used for ventral thoracic tumors. The extreme lateral approach is used when there is a significant ventral tumor component above the foramen magnum.[41] Resection of ventrally located cervical nerve sheath tumors through a ventral corpectomy approach has also recently been reported.[35] Similarly, a thoracoscopic approach to ventral thoracic tumors has also been decribed.[6] Both of these techniques have been described via case reports, however, and the reader is cautioned that intradural tumor resection from a ventral approach is technically challenging.

The role of surgery in treating filum terminale ependymomas depends on the size of the tumor and its relationship to the surrounding roots of the cauda equina. Gross total en bloc resection should be attempted whenever possible. This can usually be accomplished for small and moderate-sized tumors that remain well circumscribed within the fibrous coverings of the filum terminale and are easily separated from the cauda equina nerve roots. A portion of uninvolved filum terminale is generally present between the tumor and spinal cord. Amputation of the afferent and efferent filum segments is required for tumor removal. Internal decompression is not used for small and moderate-sized tumors because it can increase the risk of CSF dissemination. Recurrences after successful en bloc resection are rare.

Adjuvant Therapy

The effects of postoperative radiation therapy on spinal meningiomas and nerve sheath tumors have not been extensively studied. Radiation treatment can be considered for subtotally resected lesions that are recurrent and histologically and clinically aggressive. It is probably best to wait until reoperation is complete before instituting therapy. Biologically aggressive filum ependymomas, which are more common in the younger population, demonstrate early tumor recurrence and can be treated with radiation therapy. If significant tumor burden is present after initial surgery, however, as in the case of known CSF dissemination, postoperative radiation therapy is given as a primary adjunct. Postoperative radiation therapy is delayed in situ-

ations where piecemeal total or near total removal has been accomplished. In these cases, tumor recurrences can be treated with repeat surgery and followed by radiation therapy. While the response of spinal cord ependymomas to radiation therapy is unpredictable, there is some evidence that long-term control can be achieved with radiation therapy in some patients.[47] This response cannot be predicted individually. Because prior radiation therapy markedly increases the morbidity of future surgical prospects, it is generally delayed in situations where further surgery may be contemplated. The role of stereotactic radiosurgery in the management of inoperable or recurrent tumors is currently being evaluated as well.[29]

Recently, a phase III study was conducted looking at the use of etoposide as salvage chemotherapy in patients with recurrent spinal cord ependymomas. Ten patients were treated and five achieved stable disease status. However, most of these patients had intramedullary tumors, so these results may not be relevant to the more benign tumors of the cauda equina.[4]

Operative Technique

Meningioma

A variety of strategies can be used for removal of spinal meningiomas. Dorsal and dorsolateral lesions are delivered away from the spinal cord with traction on the open dural margins, and circumscribing excision of the dural origin completes the removal. For lateral and ventral tumors, the arachnoid over the exposed portion of the tumor is incised and reflected so that the dissection can proceed directly on the tumor surface (Figure 70.7). The rostral and caudal tumor poles should be identified. Small cotton pledgets can be placed in the spinal lateral canal gutters on either side of the tumor to minimize blood spillage into the subarachnoid space. The exposed tumor surface is then cauterized to diminish tumor vascularity and to shrink tumor mass. Large tumors are bisected and debulked through a central trough. The tumor segment apposing the spinal cord is then delivered into the resection cavity with gentle traction and surface dissection. The remaining dura-based tumor is amputated from the dural attachment, and the attachment is then extensively coagulated. Alternatively, the dural base can be excised and replaced with a thoracodorsal fascia patch graft. All blood and debris are irrigated from the subarachnoid space with warm saline, and arachnoid adhesions holding the cord in a deformed position are divided. These maneuvers can diminish the risk of postoperative complications such as spinal cord tethering, arachnoiditis, delayed syrinx formation, and hydrocephalus, which occasionally complicate extramedullary tumor removal. Rarely, a spinal meningioma extends through a dural nerve root sleeve and appears as a dumbbell-shaped tumor. The techniques for removal are similar to those described here for nerve sheath tumors.

Nerve Sheath Tumors

Surgical exposure of nerve sheath tumors depends on the specific anatomy of the lesion. Tumors that are small and strictly intradural can be approached via dorsal laminectomy. Ventrally located tumors may require facetectomy, transthoracic, or far lateral approaches. Once exposure is achieved, a plane of dissection directly on the tumor surface must be identified.

There is usually an arachnoid membrane tightly applied to the tumor surface (see Figure 70.5C). This is the fenestrated arachnoid layer that separately ensheaths each dorsal and ventral nerve root within the subarachnoid space.[25] This layer is sharply incised and reflected off the tumor

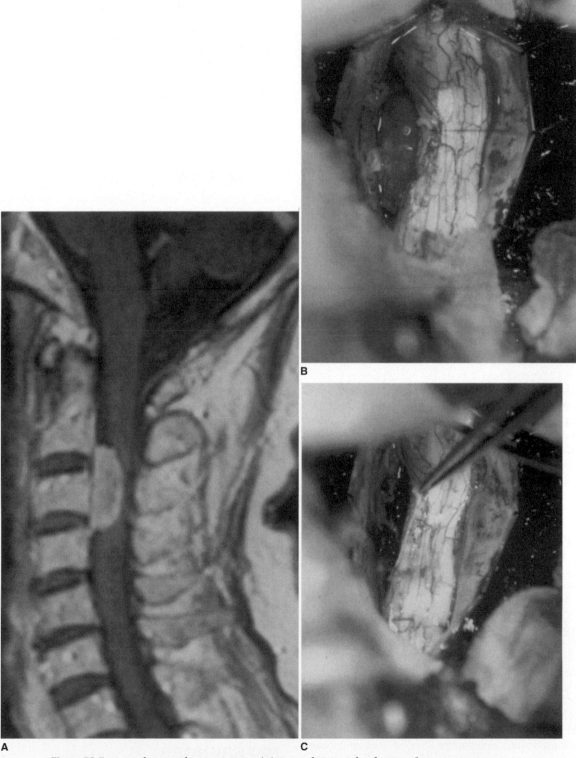

Figure 70.7 Ventral cervical meningioma. (**A**) Sagittal T_1-weighted MRI after intravenous gadolinium. (**B**) Exposure after arachnoid dissection and section of the dentate ligaments. (**C**) Appearance after gross total resection.

surface. The tumor capsule is cauterized to diminish vascularity and shrink tumor volume. Tumor removal requires identification and division of the proximal and distal nerve root tumor attachments, which may not be immediately apparent with large tumors. Internal decompression with a laser or ultrasonic aspirator is used in such cases. Sacrifice of the nerve root of origin is usually required for tumor removal. Occasionally, some fascicles of the nerve root can be preserved, especially for smaller tumors. It is usually possible, however, to preserve the corresponding intradural nerve root because the fenestrated arachnoid sheaths allow anatomic separation of the dorsal and ventral nerve roots to a point just distal to the dorsal root ganglion. In a typical case involving dorsal root tumor origin, for example, it is possible to preserve the ventral root which is tightly applied to the ventral tumor surface. Extension of a dumbbell-shaped tumor through the root sleeve, however, usually necessitates resection of the entire spinal nerve.[25] This rarely causes significant nerve deficit, even at the cervical and lumbar enlargements. The function of the involved root has probably already been compensated for by adjacent roots. A very proximal tumor origin may be partially embedded in the epipial tissue or may elevate the pia to occupy a subpial location. The tumor-cord junction may be difficult to develop in these cases and requires resection of a segment of pia to effect complete removal.

Filum Ependymoma

The exposure for resection of filum ependymomas is standard dorsal laminectomy over the involved levels. Removal consists of developing a clean arachnoid plane around the lesion and separating it from the involved nerve roots. Large filum terminale ependymomas, however, can present significant problems for surgical resection. These tumors have been present for many years and involve a risk of CSF tumor dissemination. Unencapsulated, pliable neoplasms can insinuate among the roots and within the arachnoid sheaths of the cauda equina, compartmentalized by innumerable arachnoid septae. Filum ependymomas can also spread as contiguous tumor sheaths along the arachnoid septae that act as scaffolding for surface growth. CSF dissemination may occur because of the subarachnoid location. Tumor removal in these cases is necessarily piecemeal and is almost always subtotal. Dense tumor attachments to the roots of the cauda equina present significant risks of postoperative deficits because of the manipulation required for removal.

Outcome

The results of surgery for intradural extramedullary spinal cord tumors are usually excellent. Neurologic morbidity is typically less than 15%, and mortality is extremely uncommon.[10,26] Complications are generally related to wound healing and CSF leakage. As most patients have not received radiation therapy, conservative treatment with lumbar drainage is sufficient management for CSF leakage in most cases. Neurologic complications, such as new deficits or exacerbation of existing ones, are uncommon but are most often associated with manipulation of the cauda equina. Motor and sensory deficits typically improve after surgery, but return of bladder function is variable. Improvement in preoperative deficits is typical and may be dramatic early in the postoperative period. Recovery is related to the duration and severity of the existing deficit and the age of the patient.

Meningioma

Recurrence of spinal meningiomas after total resection is about 1% at 5 years and 6% at 14 years. Subtotally resected lesions have average recurrence rates of approximately 15%.[23,44] Dural resection versus coagulation apparently does not significantly affect recurrence.[44] Meningiomas with extradural spread or en plaque lesions are more difficult to remove and tend to recur more frequently. These lesions are also associated with greater degrees of postoperative morbidity. These factors must be balanced when planning the extent of resection.

Nerve Sheath Tumors

Total removal of neurofibromas and schwannomas not associated with neurofibromatosis is generally curative.[26,40] However, tumors with extensive paraspinal involvement that are subtotally resected have a definite propensity to recur. Deficits resulting from sacrifice of the involved nerve roots are usually minor and well tolerated. Patients with multiple lesions from neurofibromatosis should usually be observed. Resection is reserved for progressive and symptomatic focal lesions.

Filum Ependymoma

Neurologic deterioration after removal of filum ependymomas is more frequent than that associated with nerve sheath tumors and meningiomas.[2,28,45] Lesions involving the conus medullaris or intimately adherent to many roots of the cauda equina carry the highest risk of postoperative morbidity. Recurrence after gross total resection is rare, and subtotally removed lesions recur in approximately 20% of cases. Survival after total removal is almost 100%.[26,45] Incompletely resected lesions treated with postoperative radiation therapy are associated with 5- and 10-year survival rates of 69% and 62%, respectively.[16,47] Subtotally removed lesions should be frequently followed by MRI.

Summary

Treatment of intradural extramedullary spinal cord lesions remains a gratifying area of neurosurgery. Advances in imaging sensitivity and refinement of microsurgical skills have allowed removal alone to be viewed as definitive treatment in most cases. Early diagnosis and aggressive definitive treatment, when possible, optimize the management of most of these neoplasms.

REFERENCES

1. Agnoli AL, Laun A, Schonmayr R: Enterogenous intraspinal cysts. *J Neurosurg* 61:834-840, 1984.

2. In Amour TE, *et al* (eds): *MRI of the Spine*. New York, Lippincott-Raven, 1994, 299-434.

3. Calvo FA, Hornedo J, De La Terra A: Intracranial tumors with risk of dissemination in neuroaxis. *Int J Radiat Oncol Biol Phys* 9:1297-1301, 1983.

4. Chamberlain MC: Salvage chemotherapy for recurrent spinal cord ependymoma. *Cancer* 95:997-1002, 2002.

5. Davis C, Barnard RO: Malignant behavior of myxopapillary ependymoma. *J Neurosurg* 62:925-929, 1985.

6. Dickman CA, Apfelbaum RI: Thoracoscopic microsurgical resection of thoracic schwannoma: a case report. *J Neurosurg* 88:898-902, 1998.

7. Divitiis ED, Maiuri F, Corriero G: Subarachnoid hemorrhage due to a spinal neurinoma. *Surg Neurol* 24:187-190, 1985.

8. Elsberg CA: *Tumors of the Spinal Cord and the Symptoms of Irritation and Compression of the Spinal Cord and Nerve Roots: Pathology, Symptomatology, Diagnosis, and Treatment*. New York, PB Heuber, 1925.

9. Elsberg CA: *Surgical Disease of the Spinal Cord, Membranes, and Nerve Roots*. New York, PB Heuber, 1941.

10. Epstein FJ, Farmer JP: Pediatric spinal cord tumor surgery. *Neurosurg Clin North Am* 1:569-590, 1990.

11. Epstein NE, Bhuchar S, Gavin R: Failure to diagnose conus ependymomas by magnetic resonance imaging. *Spine* 14:134-137, 1989.

12. Fearnside MR, Adams CBT: Tumours of the cauda equina. *J Neurol Neurosurg Psychiatry* 41:24-31, 1978.

13. Feldman E, Bromfield E, Navia B: Hydrocephalic dementia and spinal cord tumor. *Arch Neurol* 43:714-718, 1986.

14. Fraser RAR, Ratzan K, Wolpert SM: Spinal subdural empyema. *Arch Neurol* 28:235-238, 1973.

15. Frazier CH: *Surgery of the Spine and Spinal Cord*. New York, Appleton, 1919.

16. Garrett PG, Simpson WJK: Ependymomas: results of radiation treatment. *Int J Radiat Oncol Biol Phys* 9: 1121-1124, 1983.

17. Gowers W, Horsley V: A case of tumor of the spinal cord. Removal. Recovery. *Med Chir Trans* 71:377-428, 1888.

18. Gregorios JB, Gree B, Page L: Spinal cord tumors presenting with neural tube defects. *Neurosurgery* 19: 962-966, 1986.

19. Guidetti B, Fortuna A: Differential diagnosis of intramedullary and extramedullary tumours. In Vinken PJ, Bruyn GW (eds): *Handbook of Clinical Neurology*. Amsterdam, Elsevier, 1975, pp 51-75.

20. Guidetti B, Mercuri S, Vagnozzi R: Long-term results of the surgical treatment of 129 intramedullary spinal gliomas. *J Neurosurg* 54:323-330, 1981.

21. Holtzman RNN, Hughes JEO, Sachdev RK: Intramedullary cysticercosis. *Surg Neurol* 26:187-191, 1986.

22. Kernohan JW, Sayre GP: *Tumors of the Central Nervous System*. Fascicle 35. Washington, DC, Armed Forces, Institute of Pathology, 1952.

23. Levy WJ, Bay J, Dohn DF: Spinal cord meningioma. *J Neurosurg* 57:804-812, 1982.

24. Levy WJ, Latchaw J, Hahn JF: Spinal neurofibromas: a report of 66 cases and a comparison with meningiomas. *Neurosurgery* 18:331-334, 1986.

25. McCormick PC: Anatomic principles of intradural surgery. *Clin Neurosurg* 41:204-223, 1994.

26. McCormick PC, Post KD, Stein BM: Intradural extramedullary tumors in adults. *Neurosurg Clin North Am* 1:591-608, 1990.

27. McCormick PC, Stein BM: Miscellaneous intradural pathology. *Neurosurg Clin North Am* 1:687-700, 1990.

28. McCormick PC, Torres R, Post KD: Intramedullary ependymoma of the spinal cord. *J Neurosurg* 72:523-533, 1990.

29. Murphy MJ, Adler JR, Jr., Bodduluri M, *et al:* Image guided surgery for the spine and pancreas. *Comput Aided Surg* 5:278-288, 2000.

30. Nabors MW, Pait TG, Byrd EB: Updated assessment and current classification of spinal meningeal cysts. *J Neurosurg* 68:366-377, 1988.

31. Nittner K: Spinal meningiomas, neurinomas and neurofibromas, and hourglass tumours. In Vinken PH, Bruyn GW (eds): *Handbook of Clinical Neurology*. New York, Elsevier, 1976, pp 177-322.

32. Norstrom CW, Kernohan JW, Love G: One hundred primary caudal tumors. *JAMA* 178:1071-1077, 1961.

33. Okazaki H: *Fundamentals of Neuropathology*. New York, Igaku-Shoin, 1983.

34. Olson ME, Chernick NL, Posner JB: Infiltration of the leptomeninges by systemic cancer. *Arch Neurol* 30:122-137, 1974.

35. O'Toole JE, McCormick PC: Midline ventral intradural schwannoma of the cervical spinal cord resected via anterior corpectomy with reconstruction: technical case report and review of the literature. *Neurosurgery* 52(6):1482-1485, 2003.

36. Pang D: Split cord malformation. Part II: clinical syndrome. *Neurosurgery* 31:481-500, 1992.

37. Perrin RG, Livingston KE, Asrabi B: Intradural extramedullary metastasis. *J Neurosurg* 56:835-837, 1982.

38. Reyes MG, Torres H: Intrathecal paraganglioma of the cauda equina. *Neurosurgery* 15:578-582, 1984.

39. Russel DS, Rubinstein LJ: *Pathology of Tumors of the Central Nervous System*. Baltimore, Williams & Wilkins, 1989, pp 192-214.

40. Schwade JG, Wara WM, Sheline GE: Management of primary spinal cord tumors. *Int J Radiat Oncol Biol Phys* 4:389-393, 1978.

41. Sen CN, Sekhar LN: An extreme lateral approach to intradural lesions of the cervical spine and foramen magnum. *Neurosurgery* 27:197-204, 1990.

42. Seppala MT, Haltia MJJ: Spinal malignant nerve sheath tumor or cellular schwannoma? A striking difference in prognosis. *J Neurosurg* 79:528-532, 1993.

43. Sloof JL, Kernohan JW, MacCarthy CS: *Primary Intramedullary Tumors of the Spinal Cord and Filum Terminale*. Philadelphia, WB Saunders, 1964.

44. Solero CL, Fornari M, Giombini S: Spinal meningiomas: review of 174 operated cases. *Neurosurgery* 25:153-160, 1989.

45. Sonneland PRW, Scheithauer BW, Onofrio BM: Myxopapillary ependymoma: a clinicopathologic and immunocytochemical study of 77 cases. *Cancer* 56:883-893, 1985.

46. Stein BM, Leeds NE, Taveras JM: Meningiomas of the foramen magnum. *J Neurosurg* 20:740-751, 1963.

47. Whitaker SJ, Bessel EM, Ashley SE: Post-operative radiotherapy in the management of spinal cord ependymoma. *J Neurosurg* 74:720-728, 1991.

48. Woltman HW, Kernohan JW, Adson AW, *et al:* Intramedullary tumors of the spinal cord and gliomas of intradural portion of filum terminale: fate of patients who have these tumors. *Arch Neurol Psychiatry* 65:378-393, 1951.

49. Wood EHB, Taveras JM: The value of radiation therapy in the management of intrinsic tumors of the spinal cord. *Radiology* 63:11-24, 1954.

CHAPTER 71

Spinal Intradural Vascular Malformations

Jonathan A. White, Thomas A. Kopitnik, and H. Hunt Batjer

Spinal vascular malformations are indeed a family of lesions. They involve abnormalities of the arteries or veins surrounding the spinal column, spinal cord, and nerve roots. They are relatively rare[18,30,81] and may appear as a hemorrhage, myelopathy, radiculopathy, or back pain.[2,3,25,51] These lesions can be divided into two broad categories: lesions that are intradural and lesions whose abnormal arterial connections are extradural. Extradural lesions are the most common and account for approximately 80% of spinal vascular malformations and are considered in another chapter. This chapter discusses the intradural lesions and includes: glomus arteriovenous malformations, juvenile arteriovenous malformations, and intradural direct arteriovenous fistulas. Cavernous malformations of the spinal cord and intradural spinal aneurysms will also be discussed. In addition to discussing the symptoms, diagnosis, treatment, natural history, and outcomes of these lesions, an attempt will be made to contrast the demographics and symptoms of these lesions with the extradural lesions.

History and Nomenclature

The early classification of spinal arteriovenous malformations (AVMs) occurred prior to the advent of spinal angiography. Patients with signs and symptoms of myelopathy were taken to surgery and the lesions were characterized based on their pathologic appearance.[10,12,19,33,38]

With the advent of spinal angiography in the 1960s, a more refined nomenclature developed based on the pattern of arterial input and venous drainage.[22,23,24] This resulted in the creation of the terms *type I, type II*, and *type III AVMs* still in common use today.[30,31,68]

Type I lesions are dural arteriovenous fistula whose single or occasionally multiple arteriovenous connection lay within the dura of the nerve root sheath and result in a dilated, arterialized coronal venous plexus.[29,45] Prior to angiography, this dilated vein was erroneously felt to be the site of pathology rather than the arteriovenous connection that is the true source of pathology. Surgical treatment consisted of stripping the veins, often with poor results.[48] With the recognition of the fistulous component of this lesion, surgical therapy has been directed at ligation of the abnormal arteriovenous connection and has led to significantly better outcomes. Since the type I lesions have their abnormal arteriovenous connections within the leaves of the dura, they are

considered in more detail in the chapter on extradural vascular lesions.

Type II lesions, or glomus AVMs, are analogous to intracranial AVMs and consist of a tightly packed nidus of vessels over a short segment of the spinal cord. These lesions tend to present at an earlier age than the type I lesions and tend to occur at the cervicothoracic junction rather than at the thoracolumbar junction.[18,67] Like type I lesions they may be amenable to surgical excision. Type III lesions, or juvenile AVMs, arise in single or multiple adjacent somites and therefore are frequently both extradural and intradural and may involve soft tissue and bone, in addition to the spinal cord and dura.[44,58] In the cord they form a diffuse nidus with normal spinal cord existing between loops of abnormal vessels. The embryologic term *metameric* was historically used in connection with these lesions because it connotes involvement of tissue derived from the entire somite.[36] Surgical cure of these metameric or type III lesions (juvenile AVMs) is difficult and often requires a multidisciplinary approach.

Shortly after the introduction of the type I-III concept an additional type IV lesion was proposed by Heros *et al.*[34] This lesion is a direct connection between an intradural artery and vein in the subarachnoid space without a definable nidus. The lesions are frequently ventral and involve the anterior spinal artery. Surgical cure is possible when the lesions are small. Embolization may be a helpful adjuvant and may be palliative for the larger lesions.

The understanding and classification of spinal vascular malformations continues to evolve. Recently, a type V spinal AVM has been proposed based on the observation that some type III AVMs are outside the spinal cord and dura and are therefore not truly metameric.[60] Their epidural location drastically changes the potential for treatment. Spetzler *et al.*,[79] in addition to their other nomenclature contributions, have proposed that juvenile AVMs of the conus medullaris be considered a separate category of spinal AVM because complex juvenile lesions at the level of the conus may have a more favorable prognosis with surgical resection.

With the advent of MRI, cavernous malformations of the spinal cord have been identified with increasing frequency.* Like their intracranial counterparts, they are sinusoidal venous channels that appear with stair-step neurologic decline from repeat hemorrhage. Some controversy exists over the indication for surgical resection of these lesions. Intradural spinal aneurysms are also being diagnosed with increasing frequency and may be traumatic, flow related from AVM feeding vessels, or rarely congenital such as an aneurysm of a posterior inferior cerebellar artery that has a spinal origin. These lesions appear with subarachnoid hemorrhage and may require direct surgical repair or endovascular vessel sacrifice.

Embryology and Vascular Anatomy

The fetal spinal vascular network develops in four stages.[86] The first, or "primitive segmental stage," occurs between weeks 2 and 3 of gestation. During this stage, 31 pairs of

---

*References 1,6,10,11,13,14,17,18,21,32,37,39,41,42,50-52, 55-57,63,65,69,77,78,87,88,93.

segmental vessels originate from paired dorsal aortas and grow toward the neural tube along the developing nerve roots. The segmental vessels divide into ventral and dorsal branches and form capillary networks on the ventrolateral surface of the neural tube. These networks ultimately develop into paired primitive ventral arterial tracts, the precursors of the anterior spinal artery. The anterior spinal artery develops when these paired ventral arterial tracts fuse during the third stage of development.

The second, or "initial," stage occurs between weeks 3 and 6 of development and is significant for development of dorsal arterial anastomoses, separate and distinct from the ventral spinal vascular system. At this stage, longitudinal venous channels also develop on both the ventral and dorsal spinal cord surfaces. These venous channels eventually expand and give rise to an interconnected capillary network. It is within this second stage that maldevelopment theoretically leads to the genesis of vascular malformations that persist after birth and into adulthood.

The transitional stage is the third embryologic stage of spinal vascular development and occurs between the sixth week and fourth month of fetal growth. The major development in this stage is the formation of the adult pattern of vascular supply. The primitive ventral longitudinal arterial tracts fuse and the number of segmental arteries supplying the spinal cord is reduced.[83] By 10 weeks' gestational age, adult patterns of superficial spinal cord vessels are present. The last stage, called the "terminal stage," occurs after 4 months of development and is the phase of maturation and increased tortuosity of the major spinal cord vessels.

The most likely stage of embryologic development at which spinal vascular malformations can arise is the second stage (3 to 6 weeks). Maldevelopment in this stage leads to persistence of thin-walled tortuous vessels that exhibit primitive capillary interconnections, arteriovenous shunts, and poorly developed elastic and medial layers that closely resemble intracranial angiomas.[19] The concept that intradural vascular malformations are congenital and are the result of fetal vascular maldevelopment is supported by the fact that 20% of patients with intradural AVMs have other associated congenital vascular anomalies (see Table 71.1). Furthermore, these malformations are present in younger patients and are distributed throughout the entire spinal axis. This favors a common dysembryogenic basis of intradural spinal and other vascular malformations.

In the adult the anterior spinal artery arises from the fusion of a contribution from each of the vertebral arteries. It supplies the ventral two-thirds of the spinal cord, including the lateral corticospinal tracts. It narrows as it descends but is reinforced by blood vessels at some segmental levels of the spinal column. At each segmental level a dorsal ramus of the intercostal artery enters the intervertebral foramen and gives rise to three branches: a dural branch, a radicular branch, and a medullary branch. The radicular and dural branches go to the nerve root and dura, respectively, and the medullary branch augments the flow to the anterior spinal artery. As mentioned, in fetal life during the third stage of vascular development most of the medullary branches involute leaving the distal portion of the cord relatively ischemic. In the upper lumbar region at one segmental level the medullary artery does not involute and augments the supply of blood to the cord. This retained medullary vessel arises somewhere between T8 and L4, most often on the left, and is known as the *arteria radicularis magna*, or *artery of Adamkiewicz*. This still leaves a zone relatively vulnerable to ischemia in the upper thoracic region. The paired posterior spinal arteries run the length of the spine and supply the posterior third of the cord.

Venous drainage of the cord follows the arterial supply. Radial veins coalesce from the cord and anastomose to become the coronal venous plexus, a plexus of veins on the cord surface. At segmental levels medullary veins leave the coronal plexus and exit the intervertebral foramen to join the epidural venous plexus. This epidural plexus communicates with the venous sinuses of the cranial dura and drain into ascending lumbar veins and the azygous venous system.

Glomus Arteriovenous Malformations

Glomus, or type II, spinal AVMs are high-flow malformations in which a tightly packed malformation nidus is located within a short segment of the pia or the spinal cord parenchyma. They may occur anywhere along the longitudinal axis of the spinal cord, although some reports indicate a higher incidence of glomus AVMs in the cervicothoracic junction.[18,67] The feeding arteries of glomus AVMs usually arise from distinct medullary arteries and also supply the spinal cord.[28] The malformations are frequently found in the ventral aspect of the spinal cord and derive their blood supply from medullary branches of the anterior spinal artery. Venous drainage is through the coronal venous plexus, and, unlike dural (type I) AVMs, the venous drainage usually occurs in both a rostral and a caudal direction (Figure 71.1).[75] With dural lesions, caudal venous drainage is extremely rare.

The clinical symptoms of glomus-type intramedullary AVMs is usually apoplectic in nature because of sudden hemorrhage from the malformation. These AVMs usually become symptomatic before adulthood and frequently appear with subarachnoid hemorrhage (SAH). Neurologic symptoms often involve the upper extremities, if the nidus

---

TABLE 71.1
Congenital Vascular Anomalies Associated with Intradural Spinal Arteriovenous Malformations

Congenital Anomaly	Reference
Brain arteriovenous malformation	Brion *et al.*[12]; Bruni *et al.*[13]; Di Chiro and Wener[22]; Hebold[38]; Jellinger *et al.*[43]
Cerebral aneurysm	Aminoff and Logue[2]; Djindjian[25]; Djindjian *et al.*[26]; Hebold[38]
Vascular agenesis	Hebold[38]
Rendu-Osler-Weber syndrome	Doppman *et al.*[31]; Hebold[38]
Klippel-Trénaunay-Weber syndrome	Cogen and Stein[15]; Hebold[38]; Heros *et al.*[40]
Soft-tissue hemangiomas	Djindjian *et al.*[27]
Hemangioblastomas	Hall *et al.*[35]

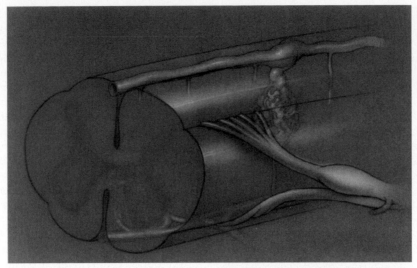

Figure 71.1 Spinal cord glomus arteriovenous malformation with arterial feeding from the anterior spinal artery and bidirectional venous drainage.

is in or near the cervical portion of the spinal cord. By comparison, upper extremity involvement is exceedingly rare in the more commonly observed dural (type I) AVMs. There is no gender predilection for intradural AVMs, whereas at least 85% of spinal dural AVMs occur in males. SAH or intramedullary hemorrhage occurs in 50% of patients with intradural vascular malformations and is attributed to the frequently associated presence of arterial or venous aneurysms.[18,27,76] Of 54 patients with confirmed intradural spinal AVMs who were studied at the National Institute of Health, 30 patients (52%) had experienced SAH and 24 patients (44%) had aneurysms associated with either the draining or feeding vasculature.[76] SAH occurs as the initial symptom most commonly in glomus-type malformations, whereas weakness is most common in any other spinal vascular malformation.

At the time of diagnosis, most patients with intradural AVMs have some motor and sensory deficit. Spastic paraparesis and pain and temperature sensory deficits are the most frequent neurologic findings during onset.[76] A bruit heard over the affected dermatome may also be present. With intradural AVMs specific neurologic symptoms reflect the location of the nidus along the longitudinal axis of the spinal cord. Strenuous activity or postural changes rarely exacerbate the symptoms of intradural glomus-type AVMs, although this is a common finding with dural type I lesions or juvenile (type III) spinal malformations.

The differential diagnosis encompasses numerous conditions that may mimic the symptoms of an intradural AVM. Because of the relatively rare incidence of intradural spinal vascular malformations, other diagnoses are more tenable. They include: degenerative diseases, neoplasms, infections, trauma, demyelinating or neurodegenerative diseases, and developmental and acquired conditions. The apoplectic nature of spinal SAH, which occurs in at least one-half of patients with intradural glomus AVMs, is the single distinguishing event that strongly implicates an intradural vascular malformation as the etiology.

Adequate and appropriate radiologic investigation is paramount for confirming the diagnosis of an intradural

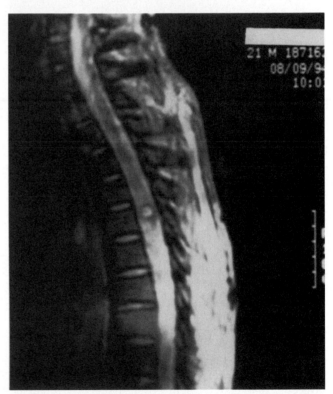

Figure 71.2 Sagittal MRI scan of glomus arteriovenous malformation.

vascular malformation. Plain spine radiographs may be useful to rule out other pathology and have been found by some to be abnormal in patients with high-flow intradural AVMs. Rosenblum *et al.*[76] found that 15% of patients with intradural AVMs had widened interpeduncular distances on plain spine radiographs. No increase in spinal canal dimension was observed with type I dural lesions.

Although total spine myelography was the radiologic test of choice for many years, most patients now undergo MRI as a screening test instead of myelography (Figure 71.2). Although the sensitivity of myelography and

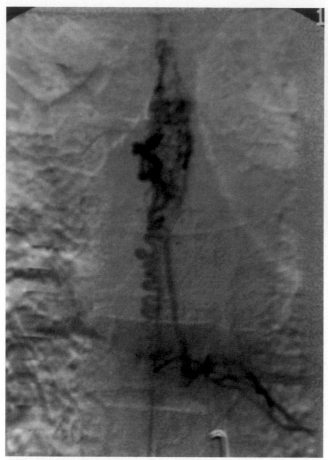

Figure 71.3 Anteroposterior spinal arteriogram of juvenile spinal arteriovenous malformation.

Favorable features for surgical resection of a glomus AVM include the radiographic appearance of a compact nidus located in an accessible portion of the spinal cord and an informed patient who understands the risks and the potential benefits of the procedure.[64] The operative procedure requires precise localization of the nidus and adequate exposure to minimize spinal cord manipulation. Use of the operative microscope and microsurgical technique is mandatory to minimize trauma to the spinal cord. Dissection is initially directed at the feeding vessels entering at the periphery of the lesion. The plane of dissection is deepened until the arterial supply has been eliminated and only venous drainage remains. The venous drainage is divided and the nidus delivered out of the spinal cord. The presence of an intramedullary clot is helpful for defining the periphery of the nidus, although SAH hampers visualization. Surgery is best not attempted in the period immediately after an acute spinal SAH and should be delayed.

The embolization of type II spinal AVMs through endovascular techniques can be a useful adjunct to surgical resection. Preoperative embolization may reduce the blood flow and the number of vessels supplying the malformation and thus decreases the technical difficulty of surgical resection. The risk of embolization of glomus AVMs is the inadvertent occlusion of radiculomedullary afferent vessels supplying vital regions of the adjacent spinal cord parenchyma and potential worsening of the patient's neurologic status.[5] Embolization has been advocated as a sole treatment for these lesions in some cases[9] and has been shown to favorably alter the hemodynamics of the lesions.[84] The high tendency toward revascularization and need for frequent repeat procedures is a significant limitation of this strategy. Newer embolic agents such as onyx may reduce the revascularization rate.[59]

Juvenile Arteriovenous Malformations

Juvenile, or type III, spinal AVMs are extremely rare, formidable lesions that constitute approximately 7% of all spinal AVMs.[15,54] These AVMs can be distinguished from glomus, or type II, malformations by several characteristics. Juvenile spinal AVMs are exceedingly rare, large, high-flow intramedullary AVMs. They usually have multiple feeding vessels over several spinal segments and often extend into and involve the epidural space, vertebrae, paravertebral musculature, and soft tissues (see Figure 71.3).[44,58] Juvenile malformations may have integumentary representation with cutaneous extension of AVM within the somites corresponding to the spinal level of involvement.[47] They are frequently located in the cervical or upper thoracic region and involve several spinal segments. The entire transverse area of the spinal cord is usually involved with malformation, and functional neural tissue is present within the interstices of the lesion (Figure 71.4).

Subarachnoid, or intramedullary hemorrhage, is an uncommon occurrence in juvenile type III spinal AVMs.[76] The typical symptom is one of progressive neurologic deterioration that occurs during early adulthood or adolescence. Postural changes, Valsalva's maneuver, and pregnancy have been reported to exacerbate the clinical

computed tomography (CT) for detecting a spinal AVM is high, the anatomic information is nonspecific.[66] Selective spinal angiography with high-resolution digital imaging remains the diagnostic test of choice to provide the most precise anatomic information (Figure 71.3).

The indications for surgical resection of glomus, or type II, spinal AVMs are difficult to generalize because of the rarity of these lesions, the variability of symptoms, and the poorly understood natural history of these malformations. Several authors have reported excellent results with surgical resection of glomus AVMs, although extrapolation of these results, obtained by highly specialized microvascular surgeons, to a general neurosurgical practice would be grossly misleading.[61] Rosenblum[76] reported a series of 43 patients who underwent surgery to resect intradural spinal malformations. In 22 patients (51%) the neurologic status was unchanged, 14 patients (33%) improved, and 6 patients (14%) were neurologically worse after surgery. In this series, residual malformation was detected in one-third of the patients who underwent postoperative angiography.[76] This is extremely important if the natural history of intramedullary spinal AVMs parallels that of cranial AVMs, because partial resection offers no benefit but poses a tremendous risk. A more recent series reported 6 of 15 (40%) patients improved, 8 of 15 (53%) patients were stable, and 1 (7%) patient became worse after resection of a type II lesion.[16]

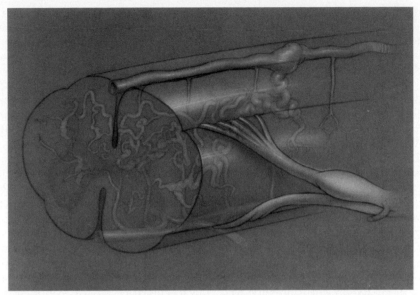

Figure 71.4 Spinal cord juvenile AVM with multiple arterial feeders and functional neural tissue within the interstices of the lesion.

symptoms.[2,26,49,63,80] There may be an overlying bruit if significant soft-tissue involvement is present.[15]

Due to the extensive involvement of the spinal cord, type III spinal AVMs can only rarely be removed with acceptable morbidity.[22,23,53,54] Touho et al.[85] and Spetzler et al.[80] have reported cases of successful removal of juvenile spinal AVMs in patients who had a definable nidus within the spinal cord. Malis[53,54] described his experience in the treatment of spinal AVMs. He reported a series of 43 patients in which 3 patients underwent attempted surgical resection of type III malformations. In this series 1 patient died, 1 had no improvement of severe neurologic deficits, and 1 patient was left paraplegic after attempted surgical resection.[53,54] Ommaya et al.[68] and others[25] have reported some success with arterial embolization as the sole treatment regimen. Hall et al.[35] reported delayed recanalization of spinal AVMs that had previously undergone complete angiographic embolization as the only treatment. Similarly, Bao and Ling[7] reported that 17 of 22 (75%) patients with a type III lesion, treated with embolization, required repeat embolization because of recanalization or clinical recurrence. Cyanoacrylate, a more permanent liquid embolic agent may provide higher cure rates but is difficult to control.[7]

Intradural Arteriovenous Fistulas

True intradural or perimedullary AV fistulas are very rare, with only a few cases reported over the past decade.[4,40,71,82] Heros et al.[40] suggested classifying true intradural fistulas separately from previously described spinal AV malformations and proposed referring to them as type IV spinal AVMs. Others have subsequently reported similar cases that could be classified as type IV spinal AVMs.[2,82] These lesions are direct AV fistulas that involve the normal arterial supply of the spinal cord and drain into the coronal venous plexus that often becomes dilated and aneurysmal. Of those cases

reported in the United States, 10 of 14 patients had AV fistulas involving the anterior spinal artery, whereas 4 patients of the cases reported by Tomlinson et al.[2,40,82] had posterior spinal artery supply of the fistula.

Three types of intradural extramedullary fistulas have been described based on radiographic appearance and intraoperative observations. The first type may be a simple connection between an elongated but normal-caliber, anterior spinal artery and the coronal venous plexus as described by Aminoff et al.[4] The second type consists of a dilated anterior spinal artery with a fistulous connection to a dilated aneurysmal venous system, similar to the case reported by Heros et al.[40] The third type consists of a large fistula from multiple arterial pedicles with rapid blood flow and a massively dilated system of draining veins.[34,72,90]

The etiology of intradural direct AV fistulas remains unclear, although a congenital etiology is a likely possibility. In the patients reported by Aminoff et al.[4,40] and Heros et al.,[4,40] the symptoms and history were inconsistent with fistulas of an acquired nature. Wakai et al.[90] have also reported a similar case in a 9-year-old child in whom an unusual intradural AV fistula was treated. This patient suffered two distinct SAHs separated by approximately 1 year. The patient underwent three negative cerebral arteriograms before an MRI scan was obtained that demonstrated a spinal intradural AV fistula. The typical symptoms are usually related to progressive neurologic deterioration rather than hemorrhage, although SAH can occur and may be a repetitive occurrence if the fistula remains undiagnosed and untreated. In patients with these rare lesions, symptoms of progressive myelopathy may be due to compressive mass effect from venous aneurysms, arterial vascular steal phenomenon, venous hypertension, or subacute intraparenchymal hemorrhage.

The diagnosis is usually confirmed with selective spinal angiography. Treatment is contingent on the precise localization and anatomic delineation of the fistula. Surgical interruption of the AV fistula is the definitive treatment when feasible. Because of the frequent involvement of the anterior spinal artery and the commonly ventral location of the fistulas, complex ventral spinal approaches are often necessary to adequately expose the fistula for resection.[40,92] When the arterial feeders are separated from the venous outflow, complete removal of the dilated venous structures is hazardous and usually unnecessary.

If the fistula is of giant proportions and the risks of surgical intervention are deemed too great, endovascular occlusion techniques may be considered. Hall *et al.*[35] reported six patients who were followed after complete embolization of spinal AVMs. Three patients underwent endovascular treatment of type I spinal AV fistulas, whereas three patients underwent embolization of glomus malformations as the sole treatment modality. All but one patient developed recanalization of the malformation and four of the six patients had symptomatic recurrence.[35] Definitive treatment of spinal intradural direct AV fistulas by endovascular techniques is feasible, but the long-term efficacy remains to be demonstrated. Furthermore, endovascular occlusion of feeding arteries in too proximal a location may result in delayed recruitment of collateral arterial channels, whereas extremely distal occlusion may compromise already tenuous venous outflow and precipitate neurologic deterioration.[34,71] Endovascular treatment as the sole modality is perhaps most useful with giant AV fistulas and least appropriate for small fistulas of the first type.

Cavernous Angiomas

Spinal cavernous malformations are rare and represent 5% to 12% of all spinal vascular malformations.[42] Most spinal cavernous malformations arise within the vertebral bodies, although many reports of intradural and intramedullary cavernous malformations exist.* Cavernous angiomas occur throughout the nervous system. They are vascular malformations, pathologically composed of closely opposed, blood-filled spaces lined by a single layer of epithelium. The vessel walls of the malformation vary from thin capillary-sized vessels to thick, hyalinized vessels densely packed with collagen. Typically, there are no elastic fibers and no smooth muscle within the walls,[63] and the vessels of the cavernous malformations are arranged in a sinusoidal network without intervening neural tissue. The neural parenchyma surrounding these malformations is often gliotic and hemosiderin laden.[57,77] According to McCormick and Nofzinger,[57] spinal cavernous malformations are pathologically indistinguishable from cerebral cavernous malformations.

The clinical symptoms of patients with intradural spinal cavernous malformations is usually progressive paraparesis and sensory loss, along with pain. Symptoms may exist or progress over many years and in the pre-MRI era, diagnosis was difficult, and cavernous angioma was often confused with multiple sclerosis.[56,70] Symptoms appear most commonly during the fourth decade, although as many as 10% may occur in children.[20] Females account for 70% of patients diagnosed with spinal cavernous malformations.[14,63] These lesions may occur anywhere along the neuroaxis and occur with equal frequency in the cervical and thoracic

cord. The average size at diagnosis is 17mm and is similar to cranial cavernous malformations; no correlation between size and the incidence of hemorrhage has been shown.[74] Familial cavernous malformations account for 50% of all cases of central nervous system cavernous angiomas, and in these cases, genetic transmission is believed to be autosomal dominant.[37,73] Spontaneous development of new cavernomas has been documented in rare patients followed for existing lesions,[78] and patients with cavernous malformations of the spine have an increased risk of multiple neuroaxis cavernous malformations.[89]

Cavernous malformations produce symptoms through repetitive hemorrhages. Typically, hemorrhage is associated with small amounts of bleeding into the surrounding neural parenchyma. In rare cases of intradural extramedullary cavernomas, SAH has been reported.[1,13,39,69,87] In a literature review by Canavero *et al.*,[14,74] the risk of hemorrhage was estimated to be 1.6% per person-year of exposure. This is roughly two times the estimated annual risk of hemorrhage with cranial cavernous malformations. Pregnancy appears to statistically increase the risk of hemorrhage, as does a cervical location of the cavernoma.[14,88]

Before the availability of MRI, cavernous malformations of the spinal cord were difficult to visualize radiographically. Myelography is uniformly unreliable and may only reveal subtle widening of the spinal cord. CT may also demonstrate pathologic spinal cord widening or the presence of acute hemorrhage, calcifications, or a syrinx cavity. Angiography is uniformly negative and carries unnecessary risk because the diagnosis can be confirmed with MRI. MRI is the diagnostic procedure of choice for intradural cavernous malformations and is virtually 100% reliable. The appearance of spinal cavernous malformations on MRI scans is similar to that of cerebral lesions. There is typically mixed signal intensity on both T_1- and T_2-weighted images that variably enhance with gadolinium (Figure 71.5). Regions of acute hemorrhage, edema, or hemosiderin deposition may be observed immediately surrounding these lesions. Hemosiderin deposition produces a ring-like region of decreased signal intensity on both T_1- and T_2-weighted images.[32]

Optimal treatment of a spinal cavernous malformation remains unclear. In the review of 57 patients by Canavero *et al.*,[14] the single most important factor relating to outcome was neurologic status at onset of symptoms. When neurologic status was poor, patients typically did poorly with surgical treatment. In their review, the age of the patient, site of the lesion, duration of the condition, and extent of removal had no significant impact on outcome. Because neurologic improvement is common after a bleeding episode, the reported improvement with surgical resection may be coincidental.

The goal of microsurgical removal of cavernous malformations is to prevent further hemorrhage and subsequent neurologic deterioration. Intraoperative ultrasonography is useful for precise intraoperative localization and for limiting the length of the myelotomy.[52] After exposure of the involved spinal cord, slight staining of the dorsal surface is often observed. A myelotomy is made over the region of staining, and microsurgical technique under high magnification is used to dissect the gliotic plane surrounding the lesion. Bleeding on the periphery of the malformation is usually due to low-flow, low-pressure vessels that are easily controlled

---

*References 1,6,10,11,13,14,17,18,21,32,37,39,41,42,50-52, 55-57,63,65,69,77,78,87,88,93.

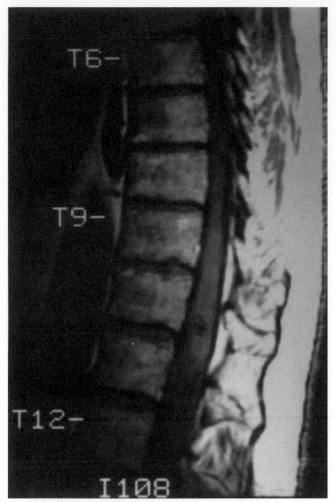

Figure 71.5 T$_1$-weighted sagittal MRI scan of thoracic cavernous malformation.

with bipolar electrocoagulation. The resected lesions resemble small "berries" of vascular tissue similar to cerebral cavernous malformations. Preoperative treatment of patients with high-dose steroids and the use of intraoperative somatosensory evoked potentials may be useful to minimize the inherent morbidity of intramedullary spinal cord surgery.

Although some surgeons have reported good results with radiosurgery for occult vascular malformations of the brain, others have reported poor results and have pathologically confirmed post-treatment radiation necrosis when brain stem lesions have been treated with stereotactic radiosurgery.[46,91] Because of the lack of evidence of therapeutic benefit and the risk of radionecrosis, microsurgical resection, if clinically warranted, appears to be the only therapeutic treatment option. There is no apparent indication for radiosurgery in the treatment of spinal cavernous malformations.

REFERENCES

1. Acciarri N, Padovani R, Pozzati E, *et al:* Spinal cavernous angioma: a rare cause of subarachnoid hemorrhage. *Surg Neurol* 37:453, 1992.

2. Aminoff MJ, Logue V: Clinical features of spinal vascular malformations. *Brain* 97:197, 1974.

3. Aminoff MJ, Logue V: The prognosis of patients with spinal vascular malformations. *Brain* 97:211, 1974.

4. Aminoff MJ, Gutin PH, Norman D: Unusual type of spinal arteriovenous malformation. *Neurosurgery* 22:589, 1988.

5. Anson JA, Spetzler RF: Interventional neuroradiology for spinal pathology. *Clin Neurosurg* 39:388, 1992.

6. Anson JA, Spetzler RF: Surgical resection of intramedullary spinal cord cavernous malformations. *J Neurosurg* 78:446, 1993.

7. Bao Y, Ling F: Classification and therapeutic modalities of spinal vascular malformations in 80 patients. *Neurosurgery* 40(1):75-81, 1997.

8. Barrow DL, Awad IA (eds): *Spinal Vascular Malformations.* Illinois, AANS, 1999.

9. Biondi A, Merland JJ, Reizine D, *et al:* Embolization with particles in thoracic intramedullary arteriovenous malformations: long-term angiographic and clinical results. *Radiology* 177(3):651-658, 1990.

10. Bergstrand A, Hook O, Lidvall H: Vascular malformations of the spinal cord. *Acta Neurol Scand* 40:169, 1964.

11. Bicknell JM, Carlow TJ, Kornfeld M: Familial cavernous angiomas. *Arch Neurol* 35:746, 1978.

12. Brion S, Netzky MG, Zimmermann HM: Vascular malformations of the spinal cord. *Arch Neurol Psychiatry* 68:339, 1952.

13. Bruni P, Massari A, Greco R, *et al:* Subarachnoid hemorrhage from cavernous angioma of the cauda equina: case report. *Surg Neurol* 41:226, 1994.

14. Canavero S, Pagni CA, Duca S, *et al:* Spinal intramedullary cavernous angiomas: a literature metaanalysis. *Surg Neurol* 41:381, 1994.

15. Cogen P, Stein BM: Spinal cord arteriovenous malformations with significant intramedullary components. *J Neurosurg* 59:471, 1983.

16. Connolly ES, Jr., Zubay GP, McCormick PC, *et al:* The posterior approach to a series of glomus (type II) intramedullary spinal cord arteriovenous malformations. *Neurosurgery* 42(4):774-786, 1998.

17. Cosgrove GR, Bertrand G, Fontaine S, *et al:* Cavernous angiomas of the spinal cord. *J Neurosurg* 68:31, 1988.

18. Criscuolo GR, Long DM: Vascular anomalies of the spinal cord. In Frymoyer, Dueker, Hadler, *et al* (eds): *The Adult Spine: Principles and Practice.* Philadelphia, JB Lippincott, 1991, p 679.

19. Cushing H, Bailey P: *Tumors Arising from the Blood Vessels of the Brain: Angiomatous Malformations and Hemangioblastomas.* Springfield, IL, Charles C. Thomas, 1928.

20. Deutsch H, Shrivistava R, Epstein F, *et al:* Pediatric intramedullary spinal cavernous malformation. *Spine* 26(18):E427-E431, 2001.

21. DiChiro G: Combined retino-cerebellar angiomatosis and deep cervical angiomas: case report. *J Neurosurg* 14:685, 1957.

22. DiChiro G, Wener L: Angiography of the spinal cord: a review of contemporary techniques and applications. *Neurosurgery* 39:1, 1973.

23. DiChiro G, Doppman JL, Ommaya AK: Selective arteriography of arteriovenous aneurysms of the spinal cord. *Radiology* 88:1065, 1967.

24. DiChiro G, Doppman JL, Ommaya AK: Radiology of spinal arteriovenous malformations. *Prog Neurol Surg* 4:329, 1971.

25. Djindjian R: Embolization of angiomas of the spinal cord. *Surg Neurol* 4:411, 1975.

26. Djindjian M, Djindjian R, Rey A, *et al:* Intradural extramedullary spinal arteriovenous malformations fed by the anterior spinal artery. *Surg Neurol* 8:85, 1977.

27. Djindjian R, Hurth M, Houdart R: Angiomas medullaires, dysplasies vasculaires segmentaires ou generalisees et chacomatoses. *Rev Neurol* 124:121, 1971.

28. Doppman JL: The nidus concept of spinal cord arteriovenou malformations: a surgical recommendation based upon angiographic observations. *Br J Radiol* 44:758, 1971.

29. Doppman JL, DiChiro G, Dwyer AJ, *et al: Selective Arteriography of the Spinal Cord.* St. Louis, Warren H. Green, 1969.

30. Doppman JL, DiChiro G, Dwyer AJ, *et al:* Magnetic resonance imaging of spinal arteriovenous malformations. *J Neurosurg* 66:830, 1987.

31. Doppman JL, DiChiro G, Oldfield EH: Origin of spinal arteriovenous malformation and normal cord vasculature from a common segmental artery: angiographic and therapeutic considerations. *Radiology* 154:687, 1985.

32. Fontaine S, Melanson D, Cosgrove R, *et al:* Cavernous hemangiomas of the spinal cord: MR imaging. *Radiology* 166:839, 1988.

33. Gaupp J: Casustische Beitrage zur pathologischen Anatomie des Rηckenmarks und seiner Haute. *Beitr pathol Anat* 2:510, 1987.

34. Gueguen B, Merland JJ, Riche MC, *et al:* Vascular malformations of the spinal cord: intrathecal perimedullary arteriovenous fistulas fed by medullary arteries. *Neurology* 37:969, 1987.

35. Hall WA, Oldfield EH, Doppman JL: Recanalization of spinal arteriovenous malformations following embolization. *J Neurosurg* 70:714, 1989.

36. Hamilton MG, Anson JA, Spetzler RF: Arteriovenous and other vascular malformations of the spine. In Menezes AH, Sonntag VKH (eds): *Principles of Spinal Surgery.* New York, McGraw-Hill, 1996.

37. Hayman LA, Evans RA, Ferrell RE: Familiar cavernous angiomas: natural history and genetic study over a 5-year period. *Am J Med Genet* 11:147, 1982.

38. Hebold O: Aneurysmen der kleinsten Rηckenmarkgefasse. *Arch Psychiatr Nervenkr* 16:813, 1885.

39. Heimberger K, Schnaberth G, Koos W, *et al:* Spinal cavernous hemangioma (intradural-extramedullary) underlying repeated subarachnoid hemorrhage. *J Neurol* 226:289, 1982.

40. Heros RC, Debrun GM, Ojemann RG, *et al:* Direct spinal arteriovenous fistula: a new type of spinal AVM. *J Neurosurg* 64:134, 1986.

41. Houdart R, Djindjian R, Hurth M: Les angiomes de la monlle. Itude clinique. Mϑcanism de α atteinte medullairs. Possibilities therapeutiques. A propos de 32 cas. *Rev Neurol* 118:97-110, 1968.

42. Jellinger K: Pathology of spinal vascular malformations and vascular tumors. In Pia HW, Djindjian R (eds): *Spinal Angiomas: Advances in Diagnosis and Therapy.* Berlin, Springer-Verlag, 1978, 18.

43. Jellinger K, Minauf M, Garzuly F, *et al:* Angiodysgenetische nekrotisierende myelopathie. *Arch Psychiat Nervenkr* 21:377, 1968.

44. Kaplan P, Hollenberg RD, Fraser FC: Spinal arteriovenous malformation with hereditary cutaneous hemangiomas. *Am J Dis Child* 130:1329, 1976.

45. Kendall BE, Logue V: Spinal epidural angiomatous malformations draining into intrathecal veins. *Neuroradiology* 13:181, 1977.

46. Kondziolka D, Lunsford D, Coffey RJ, *et al:* Stereotactic radiosurgery of angiographically occult vascular malformations: indications and preliminary experience. *Neurosurgery* 27:892, 1990.

47. Krayenbuhl H, Benini A, Bollinger A, *et al:* Ein Fall von Klippel-Trenaunay-Weber Syndrom mit arteriovenoser Fistel in Bereich der Brustwirbel S≡ule. *Neurochirurgia* 13:228, 1970.

48. Krayenbuhl H, Yasargil MG, McClintock HG: Treatment of spinal cord vascular malformations by surgical excision. *J Neurosurg* 30:427-431, 1969.

49. Kulkarni MV, Burks DD, Price AC, *et al:* Diagnosis of spinal arteriovenous malformation in a pregnant patient by MR imaging. *J Comput Assist Tomogr* 9:171, 1985.

50. Lindboe CF, Nordal JH: Multiple neurilemmomas of the cauda equina, cavernous hemangioma of the spinal cord, and degeneration of the lateral corticospinal tracts in a man with a clinical diagnosis of multiple sclerosis. *Clin Neuropathol* 4:260, 1985.

51. Logue V: Angiomas of the spinal cord: review of the pathogenesis, clinical features and the results of surgery. *J Neurol Neurosurg Psychiatry* 42:1, 1979.

52. Lunardi P, Acqui M, Ferrante L, *et al:* The role of intraoperative ultrasound imaging in the surgical removal of intramedullary cavernous angiomas. *Neurosurgery* 34:520, 1994.

53. Malis, LI: Microsurgery for spinal and arteriovenous malformations. *Clin Neurosurg* 26:543, 1979.

54. Malis LI: Arteriovenous malformations of the spinal cord. In Youmans JR (ed): *Neurological Surgery*, 2nd ed., vol 3. Philadelphia, WB Saunders, 1982, p 1850.

55. McCormick PC: Spinal vascular malformations. *Semin Neurol* 13:349, 1993.

56. McCormick PC, Michelsen WS, Post KD, *et al:* Cavernous malformations of the spinal cord. *Neurosurgery* 2:459, 1988.

57. McCormick WF, Nofzinger JD: "Cryptic" vascular malformations of the central nervous system. *J Neurosurg* 24:865, 1966.

58. Merry GS, Appleton DB: Spinal arterial malformation in a child with hereditary hemorrhagic telangiectasia. *J Neurosurg* 44:613, 1976.

59. Molyneux AJ, Coley SC: Embolization of spinal cord arteriovenous malformation with an ethylene vinyl alcohol copolymer dissolved in dimethyl sulfoxide (onyx liquid embolic system): report of two cases. *J Neurosurg* 93 (Suppl 2):304-308, 2000.

60. Morgan H, Morrill K: Vascular lesions of the spine. In Batjer HH, Loftus CM (eds): *Textbook of Neurological Surgery.* Philadelphia, Lippincott-Williams & Wilkins, 2003, pp 1847-1857.

61. Morgan MK: Outcome from treatment for spinal arteriovenous malformation. *Neurosurg Clin N Am* 10(1):113-119, 1999.

62. Newman MJD: Spinal angioma with symptoms in pregnancy. *J Neurol Neurosurg Psychiatry* 21:38, 1958.

63. Ogilvy CS, Louis DN, Ojemann RG: Intramedullary cavernous angiomas of the spinal cord: clinical presentation, pathological features, and surgical management. *Neurosurgery* 31:219, 1992.

64. Ohata K, Takami T, El-Naggar A, *et al:* Posterior approach for cervical intramedullary arteriovenous malformation with diffuse-type nidus: report of three cases. *J Neurosurg* 91(Suppl 1):105-111, 1999.

65. Ojemann Rg, Crowell RM, Ogilvy CS: Management of cranial and spinal cavernous angiomas. *Clin Neurosurg* 40:98, 1993.

66. Oldfield EH, Doppman JL: Spinal arteriovenous malformations. *Clin Neurosurg* 34:161, 1986.

67. Ommaya AK: Spinal arteriovenous malformations. In Williams RH, Rengachary SS (eds): *Neurosurgery*, vol 2. New York, McGraw-Hill, 1985, p 1495.

68. Ommaya AK, DiChiro G, Doppman J: Ligation of arterial supply in the treatment of spinal cord arteriovenous malformations. *J Neurosurg* 30:69, 1969.

69. Pagni CA, Canavero S, Forni M: Report of a cavernoma of the cauda equina and review of the literature. *Surg Neurol* 33:124, 1990.

70. Pia HW: Diagnosis and treatment of spinal angiomas. *Acta Neurochir* 28:1, 1973.

71. Riche MC, Melke JP, Merland JJ: Embolization of spinal cord vascular malformations via the anterior spinal artery. *Am J Neuroradiol* 4:378, 1983.

72. Riche MC, Scialfa G, Gueguen B, *et al:* Giant extramedullary arteriovenous fistula supplied by the anterior spinal artery: treatment by detachable balloons. *Am J Neuroradiol* 4:391, 1983.

73. Rigamonti D, Hadley MN, Drayer BP, *et al:* Cerebral cavernous malformations: incidence and familiar occurrence. *N Engl J Med* 319:343, 1988.

74. Robinson JR, Awad IA, Little JR: Natural history of the cavernous angioma. *J Neurosurg* 75:709, 1991.

75. Rosenblum BR, Oldfield EH, Doppman JL: Pathogenesis of spinal arteriovenous malformations. *Surg Forum* 37:489, 1987.

76. Rosemblum BR, Oldfield EH, Doppman JL, *et al:* Spinal arteriovenous malformations: a comparison of dural arteriovenous fistulas and intradural AVMs in 81 patients. *J Neurosurg* 67:795, 1987.

77. Russell DS, Rubinstein LJ: *Pathology of Tumors of the Nervous System*. 5th Ed. London, E. Arnold, 1989.

78. Scott RM, Barnes P, Kupsky W, *et al:* Cavernous angiomas of the central nervous system in children. *J Neurosurg* 76:38, 1992.

79. Spetzler RF, Detwiler PW, Riina HA, *et al:* Modified classification of spinal cord vascular lesions. *J Neurosurg* 96(Suppl 2):145-156, 2002.

80. Spetzler RF, Zabramski JM, Flom RA: Management of juvenile spinal AVMs by embolization and operative excision. *J Neurosurg* 70:629, 1989.

81. Symon L, Kuyama H, Kendall B: Dural arteriovenous malformations of the spine: clinical features and surgical results in 55 cases. *J Neurosurg* 60:238, 1984.

82. Tomlinson FH, Rufenacht DA, Sundt TM, *et al:* Arteriovenous fistulas of the brain and the spinal cord. *J Neurosurg* 7:16, 1993.

83. Torr JB: The embryological development of the anterior spinal artery in man. *J Anat* 91:587, 1957.

84. Touho H, Karasawa J, Ohnishi H, *et al:* Hemodynamic evaluation of spinal arteriovenous malformations before and after embolization: preliminary report. *Neurol Med Chir (Tokyo)* 35(7):445-449, 1995.

85. Touho H, Karasawa J, Shishido H, *et al:* Successful excision of a juvenile-type spinal arteriovenous malformation following intraoperative embolization. *J Neurosurg* 75:647, 1991.

86. Turnbull IM: Bloody supply of the spinal cord. In Vinken PJ, Bruyn GW (eds): *Handbook of Clinical Neurology*, vol 12. Amsterdam, North Holland, 1972, p 478.

87. Veda S, Saito A, Inomori S, *et al:* Cavernous angioma of the cauda equina producing subarachnoid hemorrhage: case report. *J Neurosurg* 66:134, 1987.

88. Villani RM, Arienta C, Caroli M: Cavernous angioma of the cenral nervous system. *J Neurosurg Sci* 33:229, 1989.

89. Vishteh AG, Zabramski JM, Spetzler RF: Patients with spinal cord cavernous malformations are at an increased risk for multiple neuroaxis cavernous malformations. *Neurosurgery* 45(1):30-32, 1999.

90. Wakai S, Inoh S, Iwanaga H, *et al:* Successful surgical obliteration of a huge intradural arteriovenous fistula of the spinal cord in a child. *Childs Nerv Syst* 8:347, 1992.

91. Weil S, Tew JM, Seiner L: Comparison of radiosurgery and microsurgery for treatment of cavernous malformation of the brain stem. *J Neurosurg* 72:336A, 1990.

92. Williams FC, Zabramsic JM, Spetzler RF, *et al:* Anterolateral transthoracic transvertebral resection of an intramedullary spinal arteriovenous malformation. *J Neurosurg* 71:1004, 1991.

93. Wyburn-Mason R: *The Vascular Abnormalities and Tumors of the Spinal Cord and the Membranes*. London, Henry Kimpton, 1943.

CHAPTER 72

Spinal Dural Vascular Malformations

Peter A. Rasmussen, H. Hunt Batjer, and Robert F. Spetzler

The most common type of spinal arteriovenous malformation (AVM) is the dural, or type I, AVM. First described by Gaupp[16] in 1888 as "hemorrhoids of the pia mater," spinal dural AVMs have recently become better recognized and understood with the advent of modern superselective neuroangiography. As a distinct subtype of spinal AVMs, these lesions, known as spinal dural arteriovenous fistulas (AVFs) require specific treatments that differ from those for intradural or intraparenchymal vascular malformations. At present, these AVMs are best treated surgically, although endovascular techniques may play an increasing role in the future.

Spinal Vascular Anatomy

A comprehensive knowledge of the vascular anatomy of the spinal cord is necessary to understand the pathologic and clinical aspects of spinal dural AVFs and their differentiation from other spinal AVMs. The spinal cord receives its blood supply from three separate longitudinal vessels—one anterior spinal artery and two posterior spinal arteries (Figure 72.1).

The anterior spinal artery is formed by the convergence of branches from each of the distal intradural vertebral arteries and descends in the anterior median sulcus. Additional contributions are received from radiculomedullary arteries branching from the vertebral, ascending cervical, intercostal, and lumbar arteries. These arteries make a characteristic hairpin turn as they join with the anterior spinal artery. The largest of these is the artery of Adamkiewicz, or arteria radicularis magna. Usually arising from a lower intercostal artery on the left side, this vessel supplies the anterior two-thirds of the thoracic spinal cord and conus medullaris. Another large radicular artery from the C5 or C6 level often predominates in the cervical region and is known as the artery of cervical enlargement. As they enter the dura mater at the level of the nerve root sleeve, the radiculomedullary arteries give off small branches that supply the dura. These are the vessels that form the enlarged arterial feeders to spinal dural AVFs.

The posterior spinal arteries course along the dorsolateral aspect of the spinal cord behind the dorsal nerve roots. They also receive supply from radiculomedullary arteries. The two posterior spinal arteries supply the posterior one-third of the spinal cord, including the posterior columns and portions of the lateral columns of the spinal cord. They

join with the distal anterior spinal artery at the end of the conus medullaris to form the cruciate anastomosis.

The venous drainage of the spinal cord is via small radial veins that run from the center to the periphery of the cord and into the coronal venous plexus that ascends and descends along its posterior surface. These surface veins converge to form medullary veins that exit at the root sleeve. It is the coronal veins along the dorsal spinal cord surface that become dilated and tortuous in patients with spinal dural AVFs, often forming a convoluted vascular mass along the posterior aspect of the cord.

Classification

Although this chapter addresses only spinal dural AVFs, the classification system for spinal AVMs should be understood to appreciate the differences between these lesions and other types of AVMs. To recognize and properly categorize spinal AVFs is important for treatment decisions, particularly between dural and intramedullary lesions. Historically, spinal dural AVMs were first referred to as *angioma racemosum venosum* by Wyburn-Mason[41] in his 1943 monograph. This was later shortened to just *angioma racemosum* by Bergstrand[8] and Krayenbuhl.[22] Malis[24] later referred to them as *long dorsal AVMs*. Currently, *dural AV fistula* or *type I spinal AVM* are the most appropriate terms.[3,20]

Type II spinal AVMs, also known as *glomus AVMs*, represent intramedullary AVMs with a true compact nidus.[24,41] Type III spinal AVMs are also known as *juvenile AVMs* and are much less common. They are larger, more extensive lesions that often involve both intramedullary, extramedullary, and extradural spaces over more than one spinal level.[24,38] Last, type IV AVMs are intradural extramedullary AV fistulas that were first described by Djindjian[10] and later classified as type IV lesions by Heros.[19] Unlike type I dural AV fistulas that arise from dural branches, these lesions are fed from the anterior spinal artery or, less commonly, from the posterior spinal artery. They flow directly into an enlarged venous outflow tract, lie outside the spinal cord and its pia mater, and vary in size and flow.[6]

Pathophysiology

It is important to understand that the clinical signs and symptoms develop because of venous hypertension of the spinal cord. The fact that the patient has a small AVM of the dura is inconsequential. What is of utmost importance, however, is that the venous outflow of this AVM is into the coronal venous plexus of the spinal cord. This leads to venous congestion of the plexus, stagnation of arterial flow through the spinal cord, decreased perfusion pressure, ischemia, and edema formation.

It is easiest to think of spinal dural AV fistulas as consisting of two relevant compartments: a vascular malformation (AVM) nidus located in the spinal dura and the medullary vein and coronal venous plexus draining the AVM. Usually, a single radiculomedullary artery enters the dural root dorsolaterally at the dural root sleeve. This artery supplies an arteriovenous malformation that is typically embedded

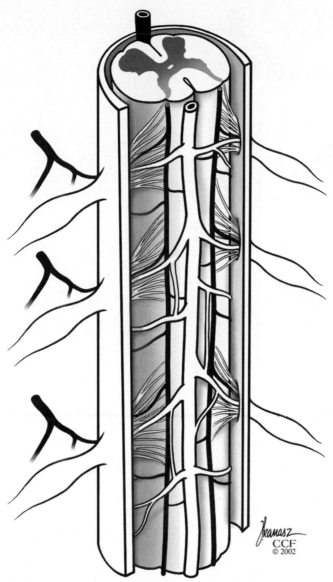

Figure 72.1 Normal vascular anatomy of the spinal cord. The radiculomedullary artery enters the dura at the root sleeve, supplying the anterior and posterior spinal arteries.

within the dura mater around the proximal nerve root sleeve and/or adjacent spinal dura (Figure 72.2). The venous outflow of the AVM is then via retrograde flow through a medullary vein that has anastomosis with the coronal venous plexus. It is this medullary vein and coronal venous plexus that is obvious on the superselective spinal angiogram. This medullary vein and coronal venous plexus are normal but dilated from the flow through the AVM lying in the dural wall.

The radiculomedullary arterial feeder tends to be separate from the branch that normally penetrates the dura to supply the anterior or posterior spinal arteries. Occasionally, however, a single vessel supplies both the malformation and the anterior spinal artery.

Although most spinal dural AVFs have a single arterial feeder, some may have two arterial feeders that enter at separate levels.[5,24] The additional feeders appear to travel within the dura mater to the fistula nidus located in the wall of the dura, where they converge and communicate with the

intradural efferent medullary vein. No valves are present within the radial veins or coronal plexus and, therefore, the increased pressure is transmitted to the spinal cord parenchyma. It is critical to recognize the additional feeding branches when these are present, because failure to obliterate all inflow channels can lead to recurrence of the AVF.[32]

On angiography, the nidus appears as a small area of fine vessels near the neuroforamen. From there, outflow of the fistula passes intradurally through the medullary vein and then into the dorsal venous plexus along the spinal cord surface. This plexus becomes dilated and tortuous because of the arterialized venous pressure and may extend over the full length of the cervical, thoracic, and lumbar spine.

Clinical Characteristics

Most patients with type I dural AVFs are between ages 40 and 70, with few showing symptoms before age 30.

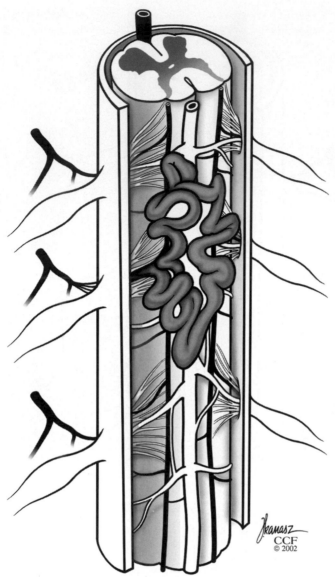

Figure 72.2 Spinal dural AVF. The nidus is located in the dura mater at the root sleeve, at which it is usually supplied by a single arterial feeder and at which it drains into an enlarged intradural (medullary) vein running to the dorsal venous plexus.

Over 80% of patients are male, and no familial tendency has been identified.[36,40] This differs from types II and III spinal AVMs, which typically appear in patients under age 40 and have less male predominance. This age discrepancy suggests that type I lesions may be acquired rather than congenital.

The typical pattern of symptoms and clinical course was first described by Aminoff and Logue,[1,2] and this description has been supported by other more recent reports.[28,32,36,40] The most common symptom associated with dural AVFs is pain, which may be local, radicular, or nonspecific. Most patients also experience leg weakness and sensory changes by the time of diagnosis.[36,40] Spastic paraparesis, along with loss of pain and temperature sensation, is the most common neurologic pattern. Most patients have a distinct sensory level corresponding to the level of the vascular nidus. Disturbances of bladder, bowel, and sexual function are less common initially but become more frequent over time.

Most patients experience a gradual onset of symptoms and a slowly progressive clinical deterioration.[1,2] Only 10% to 15% of patients experience an acute onset of symptoms, in contrast to patients with types II and III AVMs that lead to an acute onset of symptoms in more than 50% of patients. The progressive neurologic deterioration occurring with these lesions was first documented by Aminoff and Logue.[2] At 6 months after onset of symptoms, only 56% of patients had unrestricted activity, and 19% were severely disabled. At 3 years after onset, only 9% had no restrictions, and 50% were severely disabled.

Because of the infrequency and gradual course of spinal dural AVFs, symptoms are often present long before the diagnosis of spinal dural AVF is made. In Symon's[40] series of 55 patients, only 33% were diagnosed within 1 year of symptom onset, and 66% were not diagnosed for more than 3 years. In fact, given the large amount of edema found on T2 MRI, many patients will have undergone spinal cord biopsy in search of a tumor prior to proper diagnosis. On rare occasions, onset of symptoms can be acute, caused by thrombosis within the draining medullary veins. This produces a catastrophic, acute necrotizing myelitis that is often referred to as Foix-Alajouanine syndrome.[15] Subarachnoid hemorrhage (SAH) is extremely uncommon with spinal dural AVMs.[36,40] In contrast, other types of spinal AVMs, particularly type II lesions, have a significant incidence of SAH.

Exercise and certain postures can exacerbate symptoms in patients with dural AVMs.[1,36,40] Because almost all dural AVMs have rostrally directed venous outflow, the greater venous hydrostatic pressure in the upright position may explain why symptoms worsen with standing.[34] Types II and III AVMs, which have both rostral and caudal venous drainage, do not produce symptoms that change with position. Worsening symptoms have also been associated with physical activity, probably because of increased draining venous pressure during systemic hypertension.[18]

The key to making a timely diagnosis of spinal dura AVF lies with a physician aware of this condition and who has a high clinical suspicion for the presence of this lesion.

Radiologic Evaluation

Since the first diagnosis of spinal AVM was made by myelography in 1927,[34] most patients have undergone myelography as part of their radiologic evaluation. Although the typical findings of tortuous channels outlined by intrathecal contrast are almost pathognomonic for spinal AVM, in recent years myelography has largely been replaced by magnetic resonance imaging (MRI) as the initial study.[30] Irregular, serpentine flow void signals suggest vessels can often be seen along the posterior surface of the cord (Figure 72.3). MRI can also differentiate type I from type II and type III lesions, and it is the test of choice for visualizing spinal cord cavernous malformations. Moreover, T2-weighted MRI images often suggest extensive edema of the cord.[13,25]

The definitive radiologic study for spinal dural AVFs is selective spinal angiography. Aortography may demonstrate the general location of the AVM; however, this large volume contrast injection may limit the extent of the superselective injections available because of contrast load reasons. Generally, bilateral selective injections of radiculomedullary branches are performed in both AP and lateral views to demonstrate the precise location, extension, hemodynamic characteristics, and venous drainage of the lesion. Multiple levels above and below the nidus must be studied to identify any additional feeding vessels. It is also essential to visualize the anterior spinal artery above and below the AVM to determine whether it has a supply in common with the AVM. Although this is a rare configuration with dural AVFs, it is a critical factor in planning treatment. Most dural AVFs are located along the dorsal aspect of the spinal cord, although 15% of patients may have dilated veins anterior to the cord, and almost all of these lesions are found in the midthoracic to lower thoracic or thoracolumbar region.[24,36,40] This distribution differs from that of other types of spinal AVMs, which occur throughout the length of the spinal cord. If there is high clinical and radiographic suspicion of the presence of a spinal dural AVF, selective angiography is not complete until all possible vessels that may contribute to the spinal vascula-

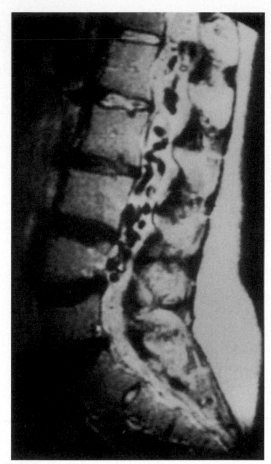

Figure 72.3 MRI scan showing the typical serpiginous flow void within the canal, suggesting the presence of a type I dural AVF.

ture have been imaged. This includes vertebral, external carotid, and sacral arteries. Occasionally, before this can be accomplished, the maximum volume of contrast that the patient's kidneys can safely tolerate is reached. Therefore, scheduling the spinal angiogram over 2 days time will allow for this possibility and completing the examination.

Characteristically, the radiculomedullary feeding vessel is observed to disperse into a cluster of small abnormal vessels within or adjacent to the dura within the neural foramen (Figures 72.4 and 72.5). The transition from artery to vein, representing the AV fistula itself, is usually observed at the medial margin of this cluster. When additional feeders are present, they usually run within the dura to the level of the fistula. Flow is then seen progressively throughout the dilated dorsal venous plexus that typically extends for three to five spinal segments, but occasionally, dilated veins will be seen extending over the full length of the cervical, thoracic, and lumbar regions. The blood flow is slow through the intradural veins, and 16 to 20 seconds are often required for contrast to clear.[32] Associated arterial or venous aneurysms are extremely uncommon with dural AVFs, in contrast to intramedullary lesions.

Venous drainage from dural AVFs is typically in a rostral direction,[36] unlike that from intramedullary AVFs, which drain both rostrally and caudally. It has been

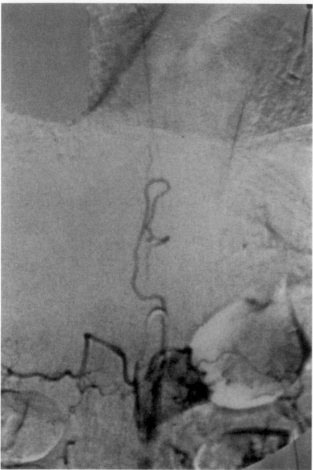

Figure 72.4 Spinal angiogram showing the characteristic appearance of a spinal dural AVM. The feeding vessel goes into the cluster of small vessels at the nidus in the root sleeve dura, which then drains into the dilated dorsal coronal venous plexus.

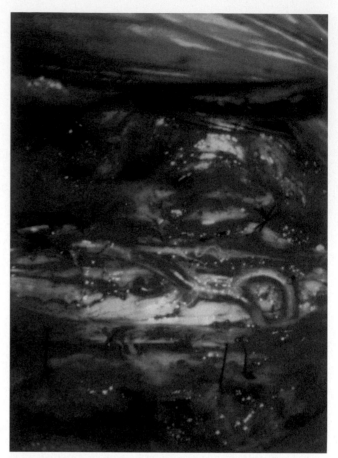

Figure 72.5 Intraoperative photograph of a spinal dural AVF. The intradural vein is seen entering from the dura and communicating with the enlarged dorsal venous plexus.

suggested that this rostral drainage of dural AVFs, along with their occurrence in the lower spine, is additional evidence for an acquired etiology of dural AVFs.[36] The pattern of venous drainage through anatomically normal, but dilated, venous channels, despite increased hydrostatic pressure, supports theories that a diminished, rather than an increased, venous outflow may be associated with the formation of dural AVFs. Congenital malformations would be expected to occur along the entire spinal axis, as seen with intramedullary AVMs.

Complete neuroradiologic evaluation of these lesions allows for planning accurate surgical and possible endovascular treatment.

Endovascular Treatment

Embolization of spinal dural AVFs has been reported, most commonly with cyanoacrylate "glue" or with polyvinyl alcohol (PVA) particles.[17,26-28,30] Because the spinal arteries do not participate in the dural fistula, these lesions are potentially well suited for endovascular treatment, with minimal risk to the normal spinal cord.

The goal of endovascular treatment is the same as that for surgery, namely, to interrupt the fistula itself, including the distal feeding vessel and most importantly the proximal efferent intradural arterialized vein.[4] Because most patients improve after obliteration of the fistula, thus making excision of the venous plexus unnecessary, several authors[9,27,29] have recommended embolization as the initial treatment of choice.

The most important factor that determines the feasibility of embolizing a dural AVF is the normal supply to the spinal cord. An anterior spinal artery supplied by the same arterial feeder as the AVF is a relative contraindication to embolization.[7,26] Inability to selectively catheterize the radiculomedullary artery because of its size or configuration is another contraindication. The second most important factor that determines the feasibility of embolization is the durability of the embolic agents. Previous reports concerning the use of PVA suggest a high rate of recurrence within only a few months of treatment.[16,26] Experience with the use of PVA would indicate that this material is not a permanent embolic agent. Cyanoacrylate glues such as n-butyl cyanoacrylate (NBCA) are likely to be more permanent.

In addition to treatment failure, the complications of endovascular treatment include direct clinical or neurologic deterioration. Neurologic deterioration after embolization is usually due to inadvertent occlusion of feeding arteries to the normal spinal cord because of an unrecognized connection, improper placement or dislodgment of the catheter, improper particle size, or failure to discontinue embolization when the fistula is occluded.[7,26,35] With dural AVFs, the greatest risk of deterioration is from occlusion of the venous drainage at a site considerably distal from the fistula.[11] This would occlude normal venous drainage of the spinal cord. Distal occlusion can aggravate venous hypertension, impede normal blood flow through the spinal cord, and potentially cause enlargement or rupture of the AVF.

Several large series of patients, in which surgical and endovascular treatments were compared, showed comparable clinical results with the two approaches.[26,27,30] Failures included a number of patients in whom the dural AVF could not be successfully obliterated initially, patients in whom interruption of the fistula had failed at a later stage, and one patient who became paraplegic after the cyanoacrylate embolus migrated into the distal veins.[23,26,27,30]

Late recanalization after initial obliteration with PVA particles is a well-recognized phenomenon.[12,17,28,30] Of 17 patients with these lesions reported from the Mayo clinic, 14 underwent embolization with PVA particles or microfibrillary collagen.[28] Although initial obliteration of the AVM was accomplished in all but one patient, delayed follow-up angiography demonstrated recanalization in 13 of the 15 patients studied, with the average time for recanalization being only 5 months. Similar results have been reported from the National Institutes of Health in 2 of 3 patients[17] and by Djindjian,[12] who found recanalization in 10 of 12 patients. PVA is not an adequate embolization material for the sole treatment of these lesions and should be used only for preoperative embolization of lesions that will then be treated surgically. Recanalization is less common after embolization with cyanoacrylate glue.[23] However, the distal extent of embolization with glue is more difficult to regulate because of its polymerization characteristics, making complications from normal venous obstruction more likely. In addition, microcatheters have been glued in place with the use of cyanoacrylates. Because of the greater risk of complications with glue and the high rate of recanalization with particulate embolization, direct surgical treatment is generally considered preferable in suitable patients.

It is likely, however, that as newer embolic agents with better material properties become available that the role of endovascular treatment of these lesions will be more prominent.

Surgical Treatment

Although Krause[21] performed the first surgical exposure of a spinal AVM in 1910, the first successful surgical treatment of a spinal dural AVF, at the T9 sensory level, was reported by Elsberg[14] in 1916 in a patient with paraparesis. He ligated and excised a large "vein" that traversed the dura adjacent to the T8 nerve root, and the patient made a complete neurologic recovery. A number of subsequent reports, however, described poor results,[8,31,39] and it was not until the advent of modern neuroangiography, which

allowed preoperative evaluation of these lesions, that therapy improved.[22,37]

For many years the standard surgical treatment for dural AVFs included stripping the enlarged venous plexus from the dorsal spinal cord.[24,37,42] It has subsequently become clear, however, that this extensive resection is unnecessary and, also, potentially dangerous. Obliteration of the AV fistula alone is sufficient to eliminate the AVM in the dural sleeve. Surgery is much safer without resection of the dorsal veins, because manipulation of the spinal cord is minimized, risk to normal vessels is diminished, and the operation is shortened. In addition to complicating the surgery, resection of the dorsal vessels may injure the spinal cord by interrupting its normal venous drainage because the radial veins have no anastomotic system within the spinal cord parenchyma.[32]

The authors' approach to type I spinal AVFs is to obliterate the dural fistula surgically by interrupting the arterialized medullary vein without resection of the enlarged dorsal veins. The surgical technique is as follows: Patients are positioned on a Wilson frame, Jackson table, or on chest rolls, and the appropriate level is verified by radiology. A standard approach to the dorsal spinal elements is performed. A laminectomy is performed using a high-speed air drill. Alternatively, a one-piece laminectomy may be performed as in a laminoplasty.

Once the laminectomy is completed, the operating microscope is used. The dural surface is carefully examined for evidence of the nidus, although it is often located too far laterally to be seen easily. After meticulous hemostasis is achieved, the dura is opened longitudinally, with care being taken to leave the underlying arachnoid intact. The dura mater is retracted laterally using 4-0 sutures. The arachnoid is then opened separately under the microscope. After dividing the small arachnoid adhesions to the spinal cord, it is held up to the dural edges with small hemoclips. The intradural arterialized vein is located, the preoperative angiogram serving as a guide. The vessel is carefully dissected free from surrounding tissues and the arachnoid. This should be done with sharp dissection with microscissors. It is best to avoid blunt dissection, which can tear small vessels from the radial spinal cord veins and cause bleeding and impaired venous drainage. After the intradural arterialized vein is freed, it is coagulated with bipolar cautery and divided. Alternatively, a temporary aneurysm clip can be applied to the vessel, and observation of the coronal venous plexus for a color change to a more purplish hue may provide the surgeon with reassurance prior to definitive occlusion. Often, there is a lengthy intradural segment that is quite long and that may be resected. At this point, the inner dural surface should be carefully inspected and coagulated. Care should be taken to identify and interrupt any other feeding vessels running in or under the dura from adjacent levels. When the nidus and efferent vein have been obliterated, the large dorsal veins should have decreased turgor and flow. The surgeon should allow several minutes for direct inspection because the venous plexus can remain arterialized for 5 to 10 minutes as a result of the sluggish venous outflow. Microvascular Doppler imaging can be of assistance if insonation is performed before and after venous interruption. If the veins do not become blue and soft after 5 to 10 minutes, additional feeders should be

TABLE 72.1

Reported Results of Surgical Series of Fistula Obliteration for Spinal Dural AVFs

Reference	Year	No. of Patients with Surgery	No. of Patients Improved	No. of Patients Stabilized	No. of Patients Worsened
Ommaya et al.[33]	1969	9	5	4	0
Oldfield et al.[32]	1983	5	4	1	0
Symon et al.[40]	1984	46	32	?	?
Rosenblum et al.[36]	1987	27	19	7	0
Mourier et al.[30]	1989	20	10	9	1
Anson and Spetzler[4]	1994	24	17	6	1
Totals		131	87	27	2

sought and interrupted. There is no need to resect or strip the dorsal venous plexus from the dorsal surface of the spinal cord. Attempting this only causes bleeding and interferes with normal venous drainage of the spinal cord and may lead to venous infarction.

Once the dural fistula has been completely obliterated, the arachnoid is let down from its dural clips but not sutured. The dura is closed with a running suture (4-0 to 6-0) in a watertight fashion. The lamina segment may be replaced, usually being reattached with 2-0 sutures or craniotomy plates. It is brought laterally to abut the bone on one side to improve refusion. Instrumentation and fusion are rarely indicated. The wound is then closed in the usual fashion. A drain is not routinely placed.

All patients undergo postoperative spinal angiography, usually the day after surgery. If residual flow through the AVF is present, reoperation is performed.

With this basic approach, good surgical results were achieved in 24 patients with spinal dural AVFs.[5] Of the 24 patients, 17 improved, 6 remained unchanged, and 1 slightly worsened.

Similarly, good results after obliteration of the dural AV fistula alone have been reported by others (see Table 72.1). One of the largest series was reported by Symon et al.,[40] who operated on 50 of 55 patients with dural AVFs. Through a limited laminectomy, this group identified the communication between the AVM and the dorsal venous plexus. If the nidus was accessible on the dura it was coagulated or excised. If the nidus was separated from the coronal plexus by several levels, it was left undisturbed, and the intradural arterialized vein was interrupted. Improvement after surgery was related mainly to preoperative disability, with 65% of patients with severe preoperative disabilities and 80% of moderately disabled patients showing improvement. The authors[40] stressed that attempts to resect the coronal venous plexus are unnecessary and potentially damaging. Although previously considered a factor, spinal cord compression by these enlarged veins is improbable. Furthermore, because obliteration of the fistula causes collapse of the veins, resection to "decompress" the spinal cord is not a reasonable indication.

Rosenblum et al.[36] reported surgical results in 27 patients with spinal dural AVMs and 54 patients with intradural AVMs. After surgical obliteration of the AV fistula, 72% of patients improved and 28% stabilized, in comparison with surgical results in 43 patients treated

for intramedullary AVMs, in which 33% improved, 51% remained unchanged, and 14% worsened. Outcome after surgery did not correlate with the presence or degree of preoperative sensory loss or with the rate of neurologic deterioration. There was a direct correlation, however, between preoperative and postoperative motor function.

Similarly, good results were described by Oldfield et al.[32] in five patients treated by coagulating and excising the cluster of abnormal vessels at the nidus and by dividing the intradural arterialized vein. In all patients, neurologic function improved progressively within days of surgery.

Summary

Although spinal dural AVFs are rare lesions, it is important to recognize and treat them appropriately. If left untreated, they almost invariably cause progressive neurologic deterioration, with paraparesis, sensory symptoms, and urinary disturbances, as well as pain. Unlike intradural spinal AVMs, these lesions usually appear in men older than age 40, have a gradual onset of symptoms that is often affected by activity, and usually localize to the lower half of the spinal column. Spinal cord dysfunction is produced by venous hypertension and not by compression or vascular steal as once thought.

After initial diagnosis by MRI or myelography, selective spinal angiography is critical for precise characterization of the number and nature of the arterial feeders, as well as of the intradural draining vein. Although endovascular treatment can be of short-term effectiveness, at present it carries greater risk and has a poorer outcome than does surgery. Surgical treatment should be aimed at complete obliteration of the dural nidus and intradural efferent draining vein, without resection of the enlarged dorsal venous plexus. With appropriate surgical treatment, the outcome in patients who are not already severely disabled is excellent, and risk is minimal.

REFERENCES

1. Aminoff MJ, Logue V: Clinical features of spinal vascular malformation. *Brain* 97:197-210, 1974.
2. Aminoff MJ, Logue V: The prognosis of patients with spinal vascular malformations. *Brain* 97:211-218, 1974.

3. Anson JA, Spetzler RF: Classification of spinal arteriovenous malformations and implications for treatment. *BNI Quarterly* 8:2-8, 1992.

4. Anson JA, Spetzler RF: Interventional neuroradiology for spinal pathology. *Clin Neurosurg* 39:388-417, 1992.

5. Anson JA, Spetzler RF: Spinal dural arteriovenous malformations. In Barrow W, Awad I (eds): *Dural Arteriovenous Malformations*. Park Ridge, IL, American Association of Neurologic Surgeons, 1993, pp 175-191.

6. Barrow DL, Colohan AR, Dawson R: Intradural perimedullary arteriovenous fistulas (type IV spinal cord arteriovenous malformations). *J Neurosurg* 81:221-229, 1994.

7. Berenstein A, Kricheff, II: Catheter and material selection for transarterial embolization: technical considerations. Part II: Materials. *Radiology* 132:631-639, 1979.

8. Bergstrand A, Hook O, Lidvall H: Vascular malformations of the spinal cord. *Acta Neurol Scand* 40:169-183, 1964.

9. Choi IS, Berenstein A: Surgical neuroangiography of the spine and spinal cord. *Radiol Clin Am* 26:1131-1141, 1988.

10. Djindjian M, Djindjian R, Rey A, *et al:* Intradural extramedullary spinal arteriovenous malformations fed by the anterior spinal artery. *Surg Neurol* 8:85-93, 1977.

11. Djindjian R: Embolization of angiomas of the spinal cord. *Surg Neurol* 4:411-420, 1975.

12. Djindjian R, Merland JJ, Djindjian M, *et al:* Embolization in the treatment of medullary arteriovenous malformations in 38 cases (In French). *Neuroradiology* 16:428-429, 1978.

13. Doppman JL, DiChiro G, Dwyer AJ, *et al:* Magnetic resonance imaging of spinal arteriovenous malformations. *J Neurosurg* 66:830-834, 1987.

14. Elsberg CA: *Diagnosis and Treatment of Surgical Diseases of the Spinal Cord and Its Membranes*. Philadelphia, WB Saunders, 1916, pp 194-204.

15. Foix CH, Alajouanine TH: La myélite nécrotique subaigue. *Rev Neurol (Paris)* 46:1-42, 1926.

16. Gaupp J: Hämorrhoiden der pia mater spinalis im gebietedes lendenmarks. *Beitr Pathol* 2:516-518, 1888.

17. Hall WA, Oldfield EH, Doppman JL: Recanalization of spinal arteriovenous malformations following embolization. *J Neurosurg* 70:714-720, 1989.

18. Hassler W, Thron A, Grote EH: Hemodynamics of spinal dural arteriovenous fistulas: an intraoperative study. *J Neurosurg* 70:360-370, 1989.

19. Heros RC, Debrun GM, Ojemann RG, *et al:* Direct spinal arteriovenous fistula: a new type of spinal AVM. Case report. *J Neurosurg* 64:134-139, 1986.

20. Kendall BE, Logue V: Spinal epidural angiomatous malformations draining into intrathecal veins. *Neuroradiology* 13:181-189, 1977.

21. Krause F: *Chirurgie des Gehirns und Ruckenmarks nach eigenen Erfahrungen, II: band*. Berlin, Urban and Schwarzenberg, 1911, pp 775-776.

22. Krayenbuhl H, Yasargil MG, McClintock HG: Treatment of spinal cord vascular malformations by surgical excision. *J Neurosurg* 30:427-435, 1969.

23. Lundqvist C, Berthelsen B, Sullivan M, *et al:* Spinal arteriovenous malformations: neurological aspects and results of embolization. *Acta Neurol Scand* 82:51-58, 1990.

24. Malis LI: Arteriovenous malformations of the spinal cord. In Youmans JR (ed): *Neurological Surgery: A Comprehensive Reference Guide to the Diagnosis and Management of Neurosurgical Problems,* ed 2. Philadelphia, WB Saunders, 1982, pp 1850-1874.

25. Masaryk TJ, Ross JS, Modic MT, *et al:* Radiculomeningeal vascular malformations of the spine: MR imaging. *Radiology* 164:845-849, 1987.

26. Merland JJ, Reizine D: Embolization techniques in the spinal cord. In Dondelinger RF, Rossi P, Kurdziel JC, *et al.* (eds): *Interventional Radiology*. New York, Thieme, 1990, pp 433-442.

27. Merland JJ, Reizine D: Treatment of arteriovenous spinal-cord malformations. *Semin Interv Radiol* 4:281-290, 1987.

28. Morgan MK, Marsh WR: Management of spinal dural arteriovenous malformations. *J Neurosurg* 70:832-836, 1989.

29. Mourier KL, Gelbert F, Reizine D, *et al:* Phase contrast magnetic resonance of the spinal cord: preliminary results in spinal cord arteriovenous malformations. *Acta Neurochir (Wien)* 123:57-63, 1993.

30. Mourier KL, Gelbert F, Rey A, *et al:* Spinal dural arteriovenous malformations with perimedullary drainage: indications and results of surgery in 30 cases. *Acta Neurochir (Wien)* 100:136-141, 1989.

31. Newman MJD: Racemose angioma of the spinal cord. *QJ Med* 28:97-108, 1959.

32. Oldfield EH, Di Chiro G, Quindlen EA, *et al:* Successful treatment of a group of spinal cord arteriovenous malformations by interruption of dural fistula. *J Neurosurg* 59:1019-1030, 1983.

33. Ommaya AK, Di Chiro G, Doppman J: Ligation of arterial supply in the treatment of spinal cord arteriovenous malformations. *J Neurosurg* 30:679-692, 1969.

34. Perthes G: Ueber das rankenangiom der weichen haute des gehirns und ruckenmarks. *Deutsche Ztschr Chir* 203: 93-103, 1927.

35. Riché MC, Melki JP, Merland JJ: Embolization of spinal cord vascular malformations via the anterior spinal artery. *Am J Neuroradiol* 4:378-381, 1983.

36. Rosenblum B, Oldfield EH, Doppman JL, *et al:* Spinal arteriovenous malformations: a comparison of dural arteriovenous fistulas and intradural AVMs in 81 patients. *J Neurosurg* 67:795-802, 1987.

37. Shephard RH: Some new concepts in intradural spinal angioma. *Riv Patol Nerv Ment* 86:276-283, 1965.

38. Spetzler RF, Zabramski JM, Flom RA: Management of juvenile spinal AVMs by embolization and operative excision: case report. *J Neurosurg* 70:628-632, 1989.

39. Svien HJ, Baker HL Jr.: Roentgenographic and surgical aspects of vascular anomalies of the spinal cord. *Surg Gynecol Obstet* 112:729-735, 1961.

40. Symon L, Kuyama H, Kendall B: Dural arteriovenous malformations of the spine: clinical features and surgical results in 55 cases. *J Neurosurg* 60:238-247, 1984.

41. Wyburn-Mason R: *The Vascular Abnormalities and Tumors of the Spinal Cord and Its Membranes*. London, Henry Kimpton, 1943.

42. Yasargil MG, DeLong WB, Guarnaschelli JJ: Complete microsurgical excision of cervical extramedullary and intramedullary vascular malformations. *Surg Neurol* 4: 211-214, 1975.

CHAPTER 73

Cauda Equina Syndrome

Michael G. Fehlings, Seth M. Zeidman, and Y. Raja Rampersaud

Cauda equina syndrome (CES) is a complex of symptoms and signs including low back pain, unilateral or bilateral radiculopathy, lower extremity motor weakness, sensory disturbance including saddle anesthesia, and loss of visceral function (i.e., bladder and bowel incompetence ranging from frequency to bladder and anal sphincter paralysis, and erectile dysfunction) that results from either acute or chronic cauda equina compression (Box 73.1). This syndrome is characterized by a variable clinical presentation that is dependent on the anatomic location (lumbar, sacral, or coccygeal/focal central or complete compression), rapidity, and duration of compression of the cauda equina. Motor weakness involving the lumbar, sacral, and coccygeal roots in isolation or in combination is often present. There is often hypesthesia or anesthesia in the dermatomal distribution of L3 to Coc1, inclusive. Radicular signs and symptoms may be either unilateral or bilateral. Bowel or bladder dysfunction is common and represents the hallmark signs and symptoms of CES. The knee and ankle jerk may be absent. There are typically no upper motor neuron findings, and the Babinski sign is absent. CES, particularly if unrecognized and untreated, often results in paraplegia, severe paraparesis, permanent bladder and bowel incontinence, or sexual dysfunction.

Pathophysiology

Spinal nerve root compression commonly occurs in conditions such as acute herniated disc, spinal stenosis, trauma (e.g., burst fractures), metastatic or primary tumors of the spine, or spinal infections (e.g., epidural abscess) (Box 73.2). Acute CES most commonly presents secondary to lumbosacral intervertebral disc prolapse (Figure 73.1). However, the pathophysiology of the symptoms and signs related to spinal nerve root compression remains poorly defined.

Several experimental studies have assessed the pathophysiologic mechanism of CES. Delamarter et al.[9,10] developed an animal model of CES, subjecting 30 beagle dogs to L6-7 laminectomy and cauda equina compression. Neurologic recovery was assessed in animals undergoing 75% constriction of the cauda equina followed by immediate, early, or delayed decompression. The first group was constricted and immediately decompressed. The remaining groups were constricted for 1 hour, 6 hours, 24 hours, and 1 week, respectively, before being decompressed. Evoked potentials were measured before and after surgery, before and after decompression, and 6 weeks after decompression. Six weeks after decompression, all dogs were killed, and the neural elements were analyzed histologically. After compression, all 30 dogs

had significant lower extremity weakness, tail paralysis, and urinary incontinence. All dogs recovered significant motor function by 6 weeks after decompression. The dogs with immediate decompression typically recovered neurologic function within 2 to 5 days. The dogs receiving 1- and 6-hour compression recovered within 5 to 7 days. Dogs receiving 24 hours of compression remained paraparetic for 5 to 7 days, with bladder dysfunction persisting for 7 to 10 days and tail dysfunction for up to 4 weeks. The dogs with compression for 1 week were paraparetic and incontinent during the duration of cauda equina compression. They recovered the ability to walk by 1 week and regained bladder and tail control by the time of euthanasia. Immediately after compression, all five groups demonstrated at least 50% deterioration of the posterior tibial evoked potential amplitudes.[10] Delamarter[10] demonstrated axoplasmic flow blockade and wallerian degeneration of the motor nerve roots distal to the constriction and of the sensory roots proximal to the site of constriction, as well as posterior column degeneration. Severe arterial narrowing occurred at the level of the constriction with venous congestion of the roots and dorsal root ganglia of the seventh lumbar and first sacral nerves.[9] Evoked potentials were the most sensitive predictor of neural compression, revealing neurologic abnormalities before the appearance of neurologic signs and symptoms.[9] Cystometrograms were not sensitive until severe compression was achieved. Bladder dysfunction was correlated with axoplasmic flow blockade and early sensory changes during neurovenous congestion.

Olmarker et al.[43-47] developed an experimental model of acute, graded compression of the cauda equina in pigs that accurately mimics the neural and vascular anatomy of the human cauda equina. There were structural and vascular differences between spinal nerve roots and peripheral nerves that could contribute to differences in compression susceptibility between these two parts of the nervous system. Pressure transmission from the balloon to the nerve roots permitted determination of occlusion pressures for the arterioles, capillaries, and venules of the cauda equina.[47] Arteriolar blood flow ceased when the applied pressure approached mean arterial blood pressure. Capillary blood flow was dependent on flow in connected venules, and the blood flow in some venules ceased at 5 to 10mmHg despite venous occlusion pressures ranging from 5 to 60mmHg. Compression up to 200mmHg for 2 hours did not induce a no-reflow phenomenon upon compression release. However, transient hyperemia was noted at all pressure-time relations studied, indicating nutritional deficit in the compressed segment during compression. Signs of edema were observed in nerve roots exposed to compression for 2 hours at either 50 or 200mmHg. The nutritional supply to the cauda equina was impaired at low pressure levels (less than 10mmHg).[44,45] Thus diffusion from adjacent tissues with a better nutritional supply, including the cerebrospinal fluid, could not compensate completely for compression-induced effects on the transport of nutrients. However, a certain nutritional supply to the compressed segment was present even at 200mmHg compression. A rapid compression rate resulted in more pronounced effects on the nutritional supply than did a slow compression rate. Nutritional impairment was observed both within and outside the compressed nerve segment. An increase in vascular permeability was induced

Clinical features of cauda equina syndrome

Low back pain
Unilateral or bilateral radiculopathy
Motor weakness of the lower extremities
Sensory disturbance including saddle anesthesia
Loss of visceral function (i.e., bladder and bowel
   incontinence)

Causes of cauda equina syndrome

Disc herniation
Trauma
Spinal stenosis
Tumors: primary and secondary
Infection
Arteriovenous malformation
Hemorrhage (subarachnoid, subdural, epidural)
Ankylosing spondylitis
Iatrogenic causes
   Continuous spinal anesthesia
   Postsurgery
   Post-intradiscal therapy
   Post-chiropractic manipulation

by compression at 50mmHg for 2 minutes.[46] The magnitude of this permeability increase was dependent on both the magnitude and the duration of compression. The permeability increase was more pronounced for the rapid compression onset rate than for the slow compression onset rate at all pressure-time relations studied. Reduction of muscle action-potential amplitude in tail muscles, after stimulation cranial to the compression zone, was induced by compression at 100 and 200mmHg for 2 hours.[44,46]

Pedowitz et al.[49] and Rydevik et al.[51,52] presented an experimental model of compression-induced functional changes of the porcine cauda equina that permits electrophysiologic investigation of the neurophysiologic changes induced by nerve root deformation. In several studies, they compared the effects of various pressures and durations of acute compression on spinal nerve root conduction in the pig cauda equina. Changes in both afferent (compound nerve action potentials) and efferent (compound motor action potentials) conduction were induced at an acute pressure threshold of 50 to 75mmHg. Higher compression pressures produced a differential recovery in afferent and efferent conduction.[51,52] Efferent conduction and afferent conduction were monitored during compression for 2 or 4 hours with compression pressures of 0 (sham treatment), 50, 100, or 200mmHg. Recovery was monitored for 1.5 hours. No significant deficits in spinal nerve root conduction were observed with 0 or 50mmHg compression, whereas significant deficits were induced by 100 and 200mmHg compression. Variance analysis demonstrated significant effects of compression pressure and duration on conduction, with a significant difference

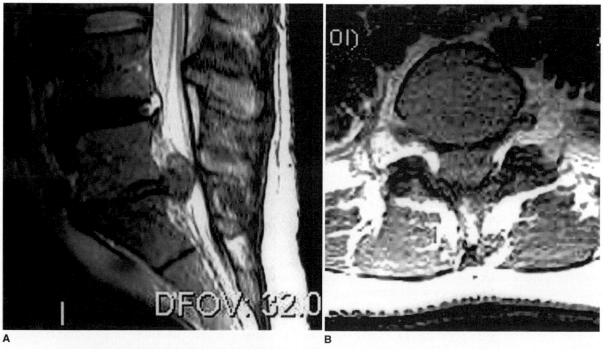

A   B

Figure 73.1 Thirty-year-old woman with acute cauda equina syndrome secondary to a large herniated disc at the L5-S1 level. The patient's initial symptoms included urinary retention (postvoid residual = 200ml), saddle anesthesia, and S1 motor-sensory radiculopathy. **(A)** T_2-weighted midsagittal magnetic resonance image (MRI). **(B)** Axial MRI demonstrating complete occlusion of the spinal canal at L5-S1.

Continued

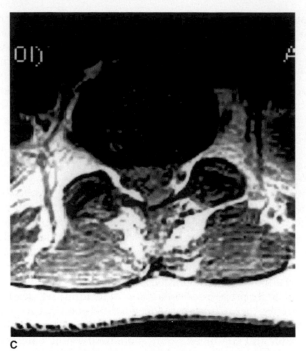

Figure 73.1 *cont'd* (C) Axial MRI caudal to area of maximal compression **(B)** demonstrating displacement of the S1 roots and compression of the central sacral roots. Patient underwent urgent surgical (less than 24 hours of bladder symptoms) decompression with complete recovery of bladder function, sensation, and radiculopathy.

between efferent and afferent conduction at the end of the recovery period, suggesting a synergistic interaction between biomechanical and microvascular mechanisms in the production of nerve root conduction deficits.[49]

Compression of the spinal nerve roots often occurs at multiple levels simultaneously; however, the basic pathophysiology of multilevel compression is poorly defined. Using a thermal diffusion technique, Takahashi *et al.*[62] quantitated intraneural blood flow in the uncompressed segment between two compressive balloons in the porcine cauda equina. At 10mmHg compression, there was a 64% reduction of total blood flow in the uncompressed segment compared with precompression values. Total ischemia occurred at pressures 10 to 20mmHg less than the mean arterial blood pressure. After two-level compression at 200mmHg for 10 minutes, there was a gradual recovery of the intraneural blood flow toward the baseline. Recovery was less rapid and less complete after 2 hours of compression. Double-level compression of the cauda equina induced blood flow impairment, not only at the sites of compression but also in the intermediate nerve segments located between two compression sites, even at very low pressures.

Cauda Equina Syndrome Secondary to Disc Herniation
Epidemiology

CES secondary to a large central disc herniation is a relatively uncommon entity, but its clinical importance far exceeds its rarity (see Figure 73.1).

The incidence of CES has been estimated to range from 1.2% to 6%. In 1970, Raaf[50] reported an incidence of 2% in 624 patients with protruded discs. In 1972, Spangfort[60] reported a 1.2% incidence in 2504 cases, and his review of the literature found a total incidence of approximately 2.4%. In 1986, Kostuik *et al.*[30] reported a 2.2% incidence of CES in patients admitted for lumbar laminectomy. In 1990, Gleave and MacFarlane[18] reported cauda equina paralysis secondary to lumbar disc prolapse in 3.2% of cases; this probably overestimated the true incidence because they did not consider nonoperatively treated patients.

Clinical Syndrome

CES can mimic the typical presentation of a lumbar intervertebral disc herniation with low back pain and unilateral radiculopathy. However, back and perianal pain often predominates, and radicular symptoms may be minimal. Severe back pain, often out of proportion with the radicular pain, should alert the physician to a possible CES lesion and mandates periodic evaluation to exclude a progressive neurologic deficit. Accurate diagnosis may be delayed if the lesion is incomplete or evolving. CES often presents with abnormal radicular signs and normal or upper motor neuron lesion activity, but it can present as a lower motor neuron lesion.

Clinical presentation varies depending on the level and location of the disc herniation. For example, a large central disc herniation can compress several or all of the traversing cauda equina roots. A disc at L2-3 with complete compression may present with motor-sensory disturbance from L3 (+L2) to S5. An L5-S1 disc may cause CES without motor or sensory loss in the lower extremities. This scenario happens when the herniation is focally central and compresses the lower centrally located sacral nerve roots, serving bowel and bladder function, but leaves the S1 roots unaffected. If slowly progressive, large central disc herniations can also mimic the presentation of an intraspinal tumor.

When compromised, the centrally placed sacral fibers to the lower abdominal/pelvic viscera produce the symptoms characterizing cauda equina compression. Initial leg pain may be followed by foot numbness and difficulty with ambulation. Sensory deficits are common and often involve the lower sacral roots. Perianal numbness, saddle dysesthesia or anesthesia, and a loss of the anal reflex or diminished rectal tone characterize the syndrome. Difficulty with urination, including either frequency or retention with overflow incontinence, can develop relatively early in the clinical course. The onset of bladder and rectal paralysis with saddle anesthesia should be viewed with a high index of suspicion in any patient with backache and sciatica. In men, a recent history of impotence can often be elicited. This should be clarified as to whether the impotence is pain mediated or neurologically (unable to obtain an erection) mediated.

Some reports contend that bilateral sciatica is a necessary component of CES, but a number of large series refute this notion. In a review of 31 patients by Kostuik *et al.*[30] in 1986, sciatica was bilateral in 14 patients and unilateral in 17. Severe saddle anesthesia was indicative of a poor prognosis for recovery, particularly for return of bladder and bowel function.[30] However, any correlation of factors such as severity of somatic signs and symptoms, symptom duration before surgical decompression, and the size and location of disc protrusion with recovery of bowel and bladder function was unclear.

Clinical Course

Tay and Chacha[63] reported eight cases observed over a 5-year period that fell into three clinical groups. The first group of patients noted sudden onset of symptoms without previous back problems. The second group noted recurrent episodes of backache and sciatica, with the most recent episode resulting in cauda equina involvement. The final group of patients had slowly evolving backache and sciatica that progressed to cauda equina paralysis. Disc prolapse occurred between the L5 and S1 vertebrae in 50% of the patients, most of whom had no limitation in straight-leg raising. Urgent myelography and disc removal within 2 weeks of symptom onset resulted in substantial recovery of motor and bladder function within 5 months of surgery. Sensory and sexual function recovery was incomplete for as long as 4 years postoperatively.[63]

Choudhury and Taylor[5] reported on 42 patients with lumbar disc disease and herniation who presented with CES. Simple disc herniation accounted for the syndrome in only five cases. Associated structural lesions were noted in the remaining 37 cases, and operative manipulation and trauma during disc removal through an interlaminar approach was reported in two patients.[5]

Lafuente et al.[33] noted sacral sparing and preservation of sphincter control in 8 of 14 cases of cauda equina compression from central lumbar disc herniation and postulated that the triangular shape of the lumbar spinal canal may be one factor for this constellation of findings, because the increase in linear strain on the stretched roots of the cauda equina is least in the more centrally placed lower sacral roots. Kostuik et al.[30] identified two distinct modes of presentation. The first was an acute mode (in 10 patients) in which there was an abrupt onset of severe symptoms and signs and a slightly poorer prognosis after decompression, especially for the return of bladder function. The second mode of presentation (in 21 patients) had a more protracted onset, characterized by prior symptoms for varying time intervals before the gradual onset of CES. All patients reported preoperative urinary retention. Bladder function was the most seriously affected function preoperatively and remained so postoperatively. The prognosis for return of motor function was good. Of 30 operated patients, 27 regained normal motor function.[30]

Diagnostic Imaging

Diagnosis and treatment are often delayed because of lack of recognition of the condition and failure to appreciate the surgical imperative for its treatment. Once cauda equina compression is recognized or suspected, magnetic resonance imaging (MRI) is the investigation of choice. If an MRI is contraindicated, of poor quality because of motion artifact (patients with CES are often in severe pain), or unavailable, computed tomography (CT)–myelography is

recommended. CT alone can be misleading in cases of complete canal occlusion (Figure 73.2).

Surgical Therapy

Urgent surgical intervention should be commenced after diagnosis. Choudhury and Taylor[5] advocated wide laminectomy with excision of the overhanging facet joints and adequate visualization of the lumbar nerve roots. This yielded good or excellent results in 95% of patients and fair results in the remainder. No postoperative spinal instability or significant morbidity was reported.[5]

A routine microdiscectomy interlaminar approach necessitates retraction on already severely compromised nerve roots. Furthermore, because of the extent of compression, these roots often have no available canal space, thus retraction not only increases traction but also may cause direct compression (against the disc or the overlying lamina). For the same reason, the use of large punches with a thick footplate is also not recommended (compresses underlying roots against the herniated disc) (Figure 73.3). Consequently, the authors advocate a wide bilateral decompression (laminectomy and medial ⅓ facetectomy). To avoid iatrogenic compression of the cauda equina, the surgeon can perform the laminectomy using a high-speed burr to thin out the lamina and then curettes and small punches lateral to the area of maximal compression to release the medial portion of the lamina (see Figure 73.3). Once the lamina is released, it can be safely lifted away from the cauda equina. The decompression should be adequate enough to allow access lateral to the thecal sac and traversing roots at the level of the affected disc space and/or the sequestered fragment. The surgeon should carefully perform retrieval of the herniated fragment to avoid creating a further mass effect and therefore increased traction on the less mobile central sacral roots. This can be accomplished by performing a lateral annulotomy and discectomy and then pushing the central fragment back into the disc space with a reverse-angle curette. If the fragment is sequestered, it should be manipulated in a lateral direction using a nerve hook or angled curette and then retrieved. Before closure, the surgeon should confirm adequate decompression.

Timing of Surgical Intervention

With respect to CES resulting from lumbar disc herniation, controversy persists regarding the definition, cause, diagnosis, and timing of surgical intervention. Conventional wisdom has been that early detection of CES is essential to maximize the probability of neurologic recovery after decompressive laminectomy and discectomy.[16] Some have gone so far as to advocate the necessity for decompression within 6 hours of presentation.[11] However, data supporting immediate intervention are far from clear.

Kostuik et al.[30] reported 31 patients with CES secondary to a central disc lesion. The average time to surgical decompression after initial presentation ranged from 1.1 days for the group with more acute lesions to 3.3 days for the second group. There was no correlation between these times and return of function. The authors recommended early surgery but noted that decompression did not have to be immediate.[30]

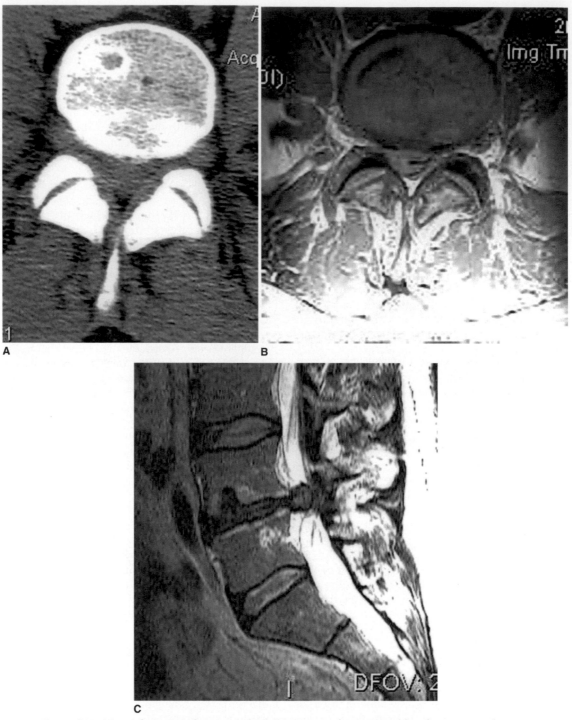

Figure 73.2 (**A**) Axial computed tomography (CT) at L4-5 of a 43-year-old male patient with right L5 radiculopathy and abnormal perineal sensation. Axial (**B**) and sagittal (**C**) magnetic resonance image (MRI) of the same patient. As can be seen, the contrasting effect of epidural fat or cerebrospinal fluid in CT can be lost because of massive disc herniations causing near or complete occlusion of the spinal canal. This patient's CT was interpreted as equivocal for an L4-5 disc herniation. Consequently, MRI and CT-myelography are the imaging modalities of choice for the evaluation of CES.

Shapiro[56] studied 14 patients with acute CES from herniated lumbar discs who all presented with bilateral sciatica and leg weakness; 93% had bladder or bowel dysfunction. All patients were emergently studied with CT, myelography, or MRI. Nine patients had large or massive

herniations, and five had smaller herniations superimposed on preexisting stenoses. The time to surgery ranged from less than 24 hours to more than 30 days. Postoperatively, six patients (43%) were normal, four patients (28.5%) had chronic pain and numbness, and four patients (28.5%)

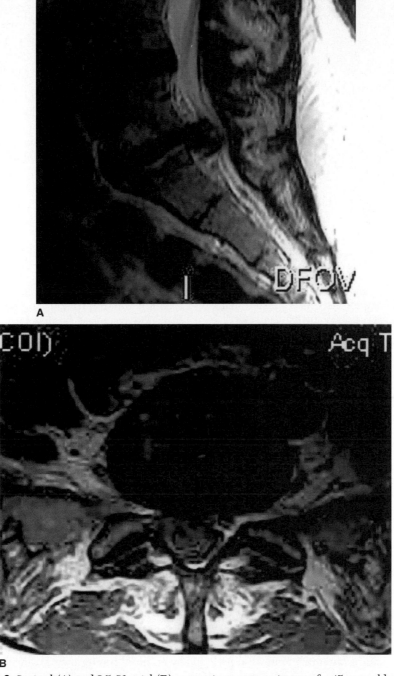

Figure 73.3 Sagittal (**A**) and L5-S1 axial (**B**) magnetic resonance image of a 45-year-old woman with CES demonstrating severe compression of the cauda equina.

Continued

had persistent incontinence and weakness. Of the 10 patients without postoperative incontinence, 7 underwent surgery within 48 hours of onset. Of the four patients with persistent incontinence, all underwent surgery 48 hours or more after presentation.[56]

The onset of bladder paralysis is an important indicator for urgent surgery. Dinning and Schaeffer[13] reported a significant difference in the outcome of patients operated on within 24 hours of bladder paralysis compared with those operated on after this period. Thus it would appear that urgent decompression is superior to delayed surgery with regard to the recovery of neurologic function, but the necessity to perform immediate surgery (within 6 hours of presentation) is less clear. Hussain *et al.*[27] recently reported on 20 patients with CES from herniated lumbar disc. Nine patients underwent emergent decompression (less than 5 hours from time of presentation to the surgical unit), and the remainder had their surgery the next day but within 24 hours. At a mean of 16 months follow-up, there was no difference in urologic or quality-of-life outcome between the emergent and delayed groups.[27]

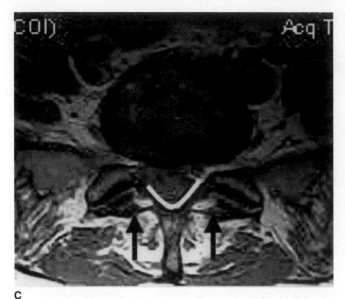

C

Figure 73.3 *cont'd* (C) The cauda equina *(outlined in white)* is draped over the disc and compressed between the disc and lamina. Removal of the lamina (medial to the *black arrows*) by sublaminar placement of standard spinal punches (see text) would obviously cause further compression of the roots. Wide bilateral laminectomy is required to gain safe access to the disc. Following appropriate decompression of cauda equina, care also has to be taken when retrieving large disc fragments to avoid excessive traction or mass effect on the tented traversing nerve roots.

Cauda Equina Syndrome Resulting From Intradural Disc Rupture

There is a strong association between the presence of intradural disc rupture and the development of CES. Dinning and Schaeffer[13] reported that intradural sequestration of disc fragments occurs in 7.5% of cases, although in most other series the rate is less than 1%. Spangfort[60] detected no differences in age or sex distribution. Lower lumbar discs were the most commonly affected levels; however, there was a significantly larger number of high lumbar herniations leading to this problem than to other disc syndromes. Myelography typically demonstrates complete block, and at surgery, intradural fragments of sequestrated disc material can be found (Figure 73.4). Intradural exploration or transdural sequestrectomy avoids traction on already compromised nerve roots and is often safer than extradural sequestrectomy.

Cauda Equina Syndrome Secondary to Trauma

Patients with sacral fracture or dislocation and CES have been reported. Schnaid *et al.*[54] reported CES complicating acute lumbosacral fracture or dislocation 3 weeks postinjury. Isolated transverse sacral fractures are rare, but extensive neurologic deficits may accompany these injuries. Extradural hemorrhage can accompany these fractures and produce a serious neurologic deficit requiring urgent sacral laminectomy.[15]

Hilibrand *et al.*[26] reported CES associated with acute spondylolytic spondylolisthesis after major trauma. The deformity progressed from grade III to grade V (spondyloptosis), and the patient developed CES. The patient was managed with posterior reduction and arthrodesis followed by an anterior arthrodesis, and the neurologic deficits resolved. Although minor or repetitive trauma is often associated with spondylolysis, high-energy trauma may produce a more severe form of spondylolysis with spondylolisthesis. These deformities are more unstable, with instability similar to that of a fracture-dislocation, and they have a greater propensity to progress than does the usual form of spondylolytic spondylolisthesis.[26]

Dorsal dural lacerations associated with lumbar burst fractures can occur and are produced by dural impaction within a fractured lamina. Neural elements can be extruded outside the dura mater and be trapped in a lamina fracture. Preoperative appreciation of this diagnosis is imperative and is based on clinical presentation, fracture pattern, and radiographic findings. Denis and Burkus[12] recommended extraction of entrapped neural elements from the fractured lamina by laminoplasty of the dorsal neural arch. Neurologically impaired patients with lumbar burst fractures and radiographic evidence of dorsal displacement of the neural elements in the lamina fracture should undergo dorsal exploration of the spinal canal, extraction of cauda equina neural elements, and repair of the dural laceration before any spinal reduction maneuver is attempted.[12]

Intradural lumbar arachnoid diverticula are rare but can cause mild compression of the cauda equina and produce debilitating symptoms. A chronic posttraumatic lumbar intradural arachnoid cyst causing CES has been reported.[69]

Cauda Equina Syndrome Secondary to Primary or Secondary Neoplasms

Primary extradural or intradural tumors may rarely present with acute CES.[11] For example, myxopapillary ependymomas of the conus or filum may present acutely with subarachnoid hemorrhage and cauda equina dysfunction.[1,36]

Metastatic tumors to the lumbosacral spine can create CES by one of two means: (1) cauda equina compression by epidural tumor and (2) vertebral instability resulting in canal compromise and subsequent cauda equina compression (Figure 73.5). The most common clinical manifestation is pain with or without concomitant nerve root signs. Regardless of the cause, the major goal of treatment is prompt decompression of the neural elements with stabilization or, at a minimum, avoidance of destabilization of the spine.

Indications for surgical intervention in patients with CES secondary to metastatic tumors include unknown tumor with rapid compression, previous irradiation precluding further radiotherapy, radioresistant tumor, neurologic deterioration during radiotherapy, and pathologic fracture/instability producing neural compression.

Spiegelmann *et al.*[61] reported a patient with acute myelogenous leukemia with CES as the presenting symptom. Woo *et al.*[66] reported 97 Chinese patients with multiple

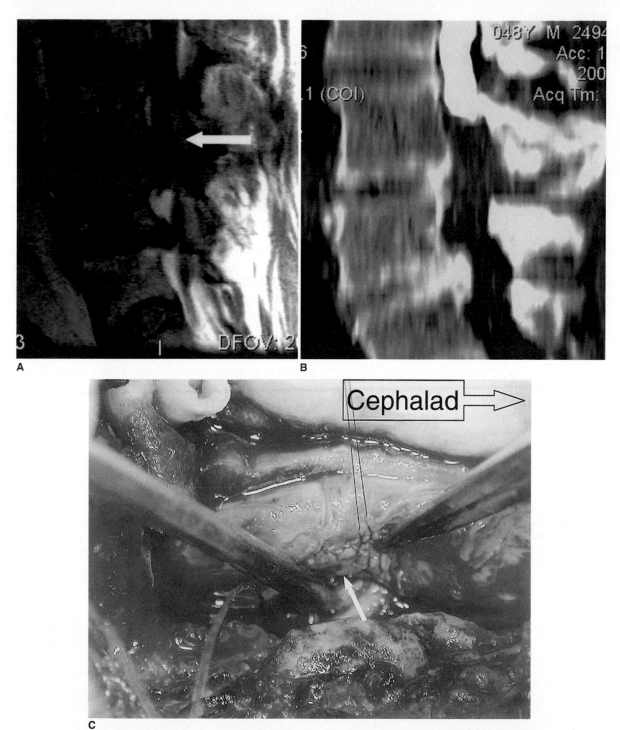

Figure 73.4 Patient is a 48-year-old man who presented with a 2-week history of severe low back pain and 24-hour history of progressive frank CES with complete loss of erectile, bladder, and bowel function, as well as right bilateral L4-S1 leg weakness. He had a right L3-4 microdiscectomy 2 years previously. **(A)** T1 sagittal magnetic resonance image (MRI) demonstrating intradural disc herniation *(arrow)*. Because of uncontrollable pain, the patient was unable to lie flat for the rest of the MRI and underwent a computed tomography (CT)–myelogram in the lateral decubitus position. **(B)** Sagittal reformatted CT demonstrating complete myelographic block at the rostral aspect of the L3 vertebral body. Patient underwent urgent (less than 12 hours from presentation to emergency) surgical decompression. **(C)** Intraoperative picture demonstrating wide decompression, release of previous epidural scar, and small defect (5mm) in the dura. The defect was enlarged, and a massive intradural sequestered disc fragment *(white arrow)*. *Continued*

myeloma, of whom 23.7% had cauda equina or spinal cord compression. Predictive features for spinal cord compression include paraprotein type, hemoglobin level, and extent of bone lesion at initial hematologic diagnosis. They concluded that vertebral cortex involvement

predisposes the patient to spinal cord compression.[66] Rarely, patients with gynecologic tumors may present with acute CES.[11]

Cauda Equina Syndrome Secondary to Ankylosing Spondylitis

CES may occur as a neurologic complication of longstanding ankylosing spondylitis. The syndrome is uncommon, and its pathophysiology is poorly defined. There are several case reports of slowly progressive CES in patients with longstanding ankylosing spondylitis, with loss of lower spinal motor and sensory root function. The pathogenesis of CES in ankylosing spondylitis may be demyelination, postirradiation ischemia, or compression from spinal arachnoiditis, or it may arise in association with massive dural ectasia.[29,40,59]

Symmetric neurologic deficits typically progress slowly and occur late in the evolution of spondylitis, long after the onset of the condition and well after the rheumatologic symptoms have abated. The initial symptom is typically disturbance of sphincter control with subsequent changes in ankle reflexes and cutaneous sensation, particularly in the sacral dermatomes. Variable lower nerve root involvement has been reported. Typical findings include cutaneous sensory impairment of the lower limbs and perineum with sphincter disturbances. Motor impairment occurs less commonly, and associated pain is inconsistent. Eventually, patients experience cutaneous sensory loss in the fifth lumbar and sacral dermatomes and develop a

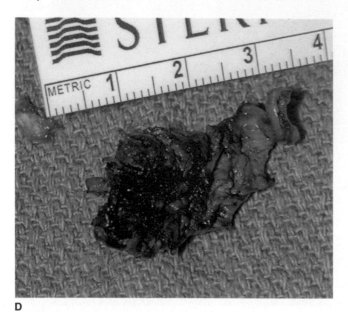

D

Figure 73.4 *cont'd* (**D**) was removed. At 2 years follow-up, the patient has some residual right L5 weakness; a functional bladder with normal postvoid residuals; good, but not normal, bowel function; and incomplete erectile dysfunction that has responded to medical management.

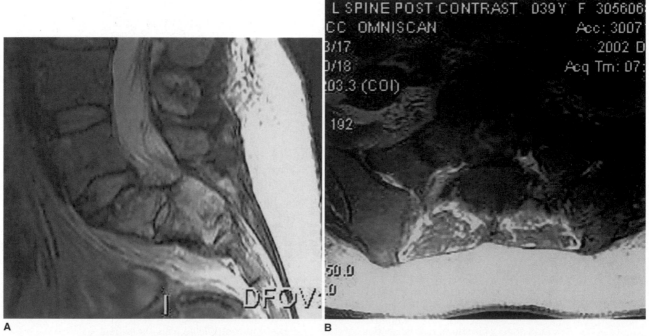

A   **B**

Figure 73.5 Sagittal (**A**) and L5-S1 axial (**B**) magnetic resonance image (MRI) of a 39-year-old woman with low back pain and urinary incontinence. She had no leg symptoms. MRI demonstrated multiple spinal metastases of unknown origin with complete compression of the sacral cauda equina by tumor extending posterior from the body of S2. Patient underwent urgent surgical decompression and postoperative palliative radiation. She had rapid resolution of her pain, but at 6-month follow-up, she still required in-and-out catheterization. Her tumor is an adenocarcinoma, but extensive investigations have not identified the origin.

lower motor neuron urinary sphincter disturbance with loss of rectal sphincter tone and with incontinence or severe constipation. Some patients have mild to moderate weakness in the lumbosacral myotomes or pain in the rectum or lower limbs.[3]

A cauda equina–like syndrome with neuropathic bladder is a rare but well-described complication of longstanding ankylosing spondylitis. Diverticula from the subarachnoid space may erode into the lumbosacral vertebrae. These spinal diverticula can be demonstrated by CT.[21] Electromyographic (EMG) abnormalities are typically consistent with multiple lumbosacral radiculopathies.[3]

The clinical diagnosis of CES can be adequately confirmed with plain radiology, electromyography, and CT. CT and MRI represent noninvasive means of establishing the diagnosis of CES in patients with ankylosing spondylitis.[59] MRI of the CES in patients with ankylosing spondylitis aids in the diagnosis and may provide valuable insight into the pathophysiology of this condition.[65] The features observed on MRI are pathognomonic, allowing accurate noninvasive diagnosis of the disorder.[42]

CT-myelography of the lumbosacral spine typically shows dilation of the spinal canal and lumbar sac with multiple posterior arachnoid diverticula eroding the laminae and spinous processes. Young et al.[67] found no compressive lesions with myelography, and foraminal encroachment was not seen. The pathogenesis of these erosions may be related to arachnoiditis in the early phase of the spondylitis.[20] Recognition of this syndrome, coupled with CT of the lower spinal canal, allows the clinician to avoid myelography, a procedure that is often difficult to perform in these patients because of associated spine abnormalities.

Early investigators concluded that surgery for CES secondary to ankylosing spondylitis was neither beneficial nor indicated and that it should be avoided.[3,59] However, surgery may be indicated in some patients, particularly when there is nerve root compression by the arachnoid cysts and when the patient is treated before irreversible damage to the cauda equina has occurred.[57]

Cauda Equina Syndrome Secondary to Arteriovenous Malformation or Hemorrhage

Spinal subdural hematoma is a rare cause of cauda equina compression that can occur in patients with a bleeding diathesis. Johnson et al.[28] reported a case of subacute lumbar subdural hematoma that was demonstrated by MRI. Laus et al.[34] reported three cases of CES resulting from epidural hematoma secondary to Coumadin-induced coagulopathy. They recommended anticoagulant correction with appropriate medications and hemoderivatives, with surgical treatment for the severe cases. Schmidt et al.[53] presented a patient with acute CES from a ruptured aneurysm in the sacral canal. The lesion was associated with pathologic enlargement of the lateral sacral arteries bilaterally, which occurred to provide cross-pelvic collateral flow in response to the diversion of the right internal iliac artery for renal transplantation. The patient showed signs and symptoms of spontaneous spinal epidural hemorrhage. In addition to angiography and partial embolization

of the vascular supply, contrast-enhanced, high-resolution CT was essential in the diagnosis and treatment of this aneurysm.[53]

CES caused by massive spontaneous subarachnoid hemorrhage from an intradural angioblastic meningioma of the filum terminale has been reported.[32] Kulali et al.[32] reviewed six cases of spontaneous spinal subarachnoid hematoma caused by subarachnoid hemorrhage from a spinal tumor with acute compression of the adjoining nervous structures. Likewise, Malbrain et al.[36] reported a patient with acute CES resulting from intratumoral and spinal subarachnoid hemorrhage from a filum terminale ependymoma after therapy with oral anticoagulants. Only 13 cases of spinal subarachnoid hemorrhage caused by cauda equina ependymoma have been reported.

Iatrogenic Cauda Equina Syndrome

Postsurgical Cauda Equina Syndrome

Postoperative CES may develop as a result of intraoperative injury or after a normal baseline postoperative neurologic examination. CES developing postoperatively is often reversible if recognized and corrected expeditiously. Delay in diagnosis or treatment can result in a permanent neurologic deficit. Postoperative CES may develop because of hematoma formation, malpositioned or excessively large autologous fat graft, epidural abscess, or failure to relieve spinal stenosis.

Laus et al.[35] analyzed the complications resulting from the surgical treatment of lumbar stenosis and reported 4 cases of CES in 96 patients undergoing multiple bilateral laminectomies. Maurice-Williams and Marsh[38] reported four cases of cauda equina lesions after dorsal surgery for severe dysplastic spondylolisthesis, three cases after in situ fusion and one case after decompressive laminectomy. The mechanism of nerve root injury was postulated to be mechanical, occurring during decortication before bone grafting.[38]

Schoenecker et al.[55] identified 12 patients who developed CES after in situ bilateral posterolateral arthrodesis for grades III or IV lumbosacral spondylolisthesis. No mention of direct cauda equina injury was noted in the operative reports. Five of the 12 patients eventually recovered completely. The remaining seven patients had a permanent residual neurologic deficit, manifested by complete or partial inability to control the bowel and bladder. Schoenecker et al.[55] postulated that preoperative sacral nerve root dysfunction in a patient with lumbosacral spondylolisthesis is an indication for cauda equina decompression concomitant with the arthrodesis. They recommended immediate decompression, including resection of the posterosuperior rim of the dome of the sacrum and the adjacent intervertebral disc for acute CES after in situ arthrodesis for spondylolisthesis.

McLaren and Bailey[39] reported six cases of acute CES after lumbar discectomy in a series of 2842 lumbar discectomies. Five patients had coexisting bony spinal stenosis at the level of the disc protrusion that was not decompressed at the time of surgery. Inadequate decompression played a role in the postoperative neurologic deterioration. Bowel and bladder recovery was good when the cauda equina was decompressed early, sensory recovery was universally good, and motor recovery was poor if a severe deficit developed before decompression. McLaren and Bailey[39] advised urgent decompression of postoperative CES if cauda equina compression is radiographically confirmed. Bowen and Ferrer[4] reported a case of CES that resulted from displacement of a hook plate into the canal at L5, eroding the dura and pressing on the nerve roots. Removal of the hook and fusion of L5 and S1 relieved the symptoms.

The overall incidence of neurologic deficit after lumbar spine surgery is approximately 0.2%. The key principles in its management are vigilance in diagnosis and expeditiousness in decompression. The authors use electrophysiologic monitoring, including somatosensory evoked potentials, as an intraoperative adjunct when decompressing lesions involving the cauda equina. During resection of large tumors involving nerve roots or during surgery for congenital malformations such as tethered cord, intraoperative stimulation of nerve roots and recording of EMG activity from selected muscles including the tibialis anterior, gastrocnemius, and perianal sphincter are performed.[25,31]

Cauda Equina Syndrome After Intradiscal Therapy

Automated percutaneous lumbar discectomy for contained herniated lumbar discs has a low associated morbidity. Epstein[14] reported cauda equina injury after a left-sided L5-S1 automated percutaneous discectomy. Despite delayed surgery, which included excision of a sequestrated L5-S1 disc and intradural exploration, S1 radiculopathy, sacral numbness, and overflow incontinence persisted. Onik et al.[48] reported CES secondary to a Nucleotome probe placed in the thecal sac, reviewed the landmarks for the thecal sac, and emphasized the preventable nature of this complication.

Hedtmann et al.[23] reported two patients who developed CES after intradiscal collagenase therapy secondary to large extruded disc fragments. Smith et al.[58] similarly reported three cases of acute disc herniation causing cauda equina compression syndrome after chemonucleolysis. All three patients had myelographic blocks and, despite emergency decompression procedures, were left with residual neurologic deficits.

Postchiropractic Cauda Equina Syndrome

CES has been implicated as a potential complication of spinal manipulation. Multiple cases of CES have been reported to result from chiropractic lumbar spinal manipulation.[8,17,37] Haldeman and Rubinstein[22] identified 10 reported cases of CES in patients who underwent manipulation between 1911 and 1989 and presented three new cases in which cauda equina symptoms occurred after lumbar manipulation. Kostuik et al.[30] reported three patients who developed CES after chiropractic manipulation of the spine.

Cauda Equina Syndrome Secondary to Continuous Spinal Anesthesia

CES may occur after continuous spinal anesthesia.[19] In the described cases, there was evidence of a focal sensory block

and, to obtain adequate analgesia, the patients were given a dose of local anesthetic that was greater than the dose usually administered with a single-injection technique. The combination of maldistribution and a relatively high dose of local anesthetic was postulated to result in neurotoxic injury. The increased incidence of CES associated with the use of microcatheters and continuous spinal anesthesia prompted the U.S. Food and Drug Administration to issue a safety alert.[19]

Cauda Equina Syndrome Caused by Infection

CES can present in association with lumbar spinal infections that result in an epidural abscess or pathologic fracture (Figure 73.6). CES typically results from direct compression of the cauda equina, but may also occur secondary to subarachnoid vascular injury or thrombosis.[7] Management consists of early detection, antibiotic and surgical decompression, and débridement with or without spinal stabilization.

Arend et al.[2] described a patient who developed toxic shock syndrome, meningitis, and CES several days after lumbar laminectomy. Enterotoxin-producing *Staphylococcus aureus* was cultured from the surgical wound and the cerebrospinal fluid. The patient recovered from toxic shock syndrome but remained partially paralyzed. CES was postulated to result from the neurotoxic effects of the intrathecally produced *S. aureus* exotoxins.[2]

Crawfurd et al.[6] presented five patients who were human immunodeficiency virus (HIV) positive who had symptoms initially thought to be indicative of lumbar disc lesions. Signs of nerve root or cauda equina compression were noted in all five patients, but lumbar imaging studies demonstrated no evidence of compressive lesions. Therefore physicians must exercise caution in diagnosing nerve root compression in HIV-positive patients. Likewise,

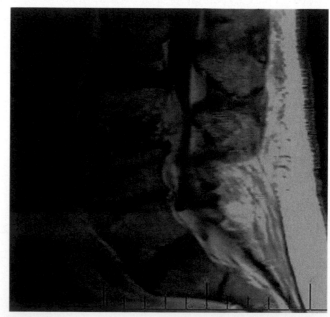

Figure 73.6 Gadolinium-enhanced T$_1$-weighted magnetic resonance imaging scan of a 70-year-old diabetic woman with cauda equina compression from an epidural abscess.

Zeman and Donaghy[68] reported a case of CES in the context of acute infection with HIV and emphasized the importance of considering the possibility of primary HIV infection in a wide range of self-limiting neurologic disorders.

Diagnostic Pitfalls

Tullberg and Isacson[64] reported 19 patients with normal lumbar myelograms and symptoms consistent with CES. Two patients had thoracic lesions, one with a tumor and the other with a herniated disc, that were discovered on a second myelogram. One patient was considered to have hysterical paresis. In three other patients, the symptoms were attributed to diseases not related to the spine. Thirteen patients recovered spontaneously. The authors concluded that the prognosis for patients with signs of compression of the cauda equina is favorable, provided the myelography results are normal and surgical exploration is not indicated. However, if severe unexplained symptoms persist, and the CT-myelogram is normal, the authors recommend myelography of the thoracic spine.[64]

A high level of suspicion should be maintained. If lumbosacral compression is not demonstrated, then imaging to rule out a proximal lesion should be pursued.

Prognosis for Recovery of Bladder Dysfunction

CES must be considered for prompt surgical intervention, because spontaneous neurologic recovery is uncommon. If incontinence is present, prompt surgery can possibly lessen the likelihood of future urinary dysfunction and maintain whatever function is still preserved. Similarly, severe paresis or paraplegia merits the consideration for prompt and generous decompression. Patients with CES should undergo emergent radiologic evaluation and urgent surgical intervention if indicated.

Gleave and MacFarlane[18] reviewed 932 patients who underwent surgery for prolapsed lumbar intervertebral disc and identified a group of 33 patients with acute urinary retention. No identifiable factor predisposed this group of patients to CES. The mean duration of bladder paralysis before operation was 3.6 days. Ultimately, 79% of patients claimed full recovery of bladder function, but only 22% were left without sensory deficits in the limbs or perineum. There was no correlation between recovery and the duration of bladder paralysis before surgery, except in three patients in whom there was no sciatica and in whom the correct diagnosis was delayed for many days. Retention developing less than 48 hours after acute prolapse was associated with a worse prognosis.

Hellstrom et al.[24] urodynamically evaluated bladder function after surgery in 17 patients with CES caused by lumbar intervertebral disc herniation. At the 3-year follow-up, 10 patients (59%) reported normal bladder function, whereas seven patients (41%) noted obstruction or incontinence. Urodynamic function was normal in four patients (24%), three patients (18%) had no detrusor contraction, two patients (12%) used the detrusor but strained during voiding, and three patients (18%) had an unstable detrusor; the remaining five patients (29%) had either an increased bladder capacity or a decreased maximal flow rate. Neurologic findings were normal in two patients (12%). Bladder function is often substantially disturbed in patients with asymptomatic CES, and therefore urodynamic testing is warranted in all patients with CES. Urgent surgical intervention may improve long-term bladder function. Regeneration of the autonomic nervous supply to the bladder and genitals often requires several months or even years.

Nielsen et al.[41] reported that among 1972 patients operated for lumbar disc herniation in a 7-year period (from 1971 to 1978), CES was diagnosed in 26 patients. Twenty-two patients had follow-up visits 4 to 72 months postoperatively (average, 37 months). At follow-up, half of the patients had a history of normal micturition, and only six patients had a serious complaint of micturition. One third of the patients were free from lumbar or sciatic pain, whereas two thirds complained of distressing pain and neurologic symptoms. The urodynamic investigation revealed complete bladder emptying in all but one patient. In half of the patients, normal detrusor contraction was demonstrated, whereas one third of the patients voided by straining only. Preoperative micturition symptoms exceeded 2 days in almost all patients voiding by straining. This finding indicates a connection of early diagnosis and treatment with the degree of detrusor damage.

Summary

CES is a complex of low back pain, saddle anesthesia, bowel and bladder dysfunction or incontinence that is often associated with radiculopathy, and lower extremity motor weakness that occasionally progresses to paraplegia.

Patients with CES should undergo rapid radiologic evaluation and surgical intervention. It is prudent to adhere to a few simple principles during evaluation of patients with acute back pain or lumbosacral trauma (Box 73.3). It is important to maintain a high index of suspicion for the diagnosis of CES and its implications both diagnostically and prognostically. It is essential that these patients are specifically asked about urinary incontinence and retention and that their bladder and bowel functions are monitored vigilantly. If the clinician is suspicious, he or she should obtain a postvoid residual urine volume. In addition, trauma patients often receive an indwelling catheter at the time of their admission to the emergency department. This catheter should be removed and checked for postvoid residual urine volume as quickly as

---

73.3

BOX

Recommendations for evaluating patients with acute back pain or lumbosacral trauma

Maintain a high index of suspicion
Perform a rectal examination
Perform appropriate imaging studies
Perform early operation

possible. A rectal examination and evaluation of perianal sensation is mandatory when assessing any patient with acute onset of severe back pain or significant lumbosacral trauma. Imaging studies to determine the nature of the lesion (e.g., disc herniation, fracture, hematoma, tumor) must be performed expeditiously. If one imaging study (e.g., MRI) is inadequate, a complementary study (e.g., CT-myelography) should be obtained. If surgical management is indicated, meticulous surgical technique is critical to avoid additional nerve root traction or compression.

REFERENCES

1. Admiraal P, Hazenberg GJ, Algra PR, et al: Spinal subarachnoid hemorrhage due to a filum terminale ependymoma. *Clin Neurol Neurosurg* 94:61-72, 1992.
2. Arend SM, Steenmeyer AV, Mosmans PC, et al: Postoperative cauda syndrome caused by *Staphylococcus aureus*. *Infection* 21:248-250, 1993.
3. Bartleson JD, Cohen MD, Harrington TM, et al: Cauda equina syndrome secondary to long-standing ankylosing spondylitis. *Am Neurol* 14:662-669, 1983.
4. Bowen JR, Ferrer J: Spinal stenosis caused by a Harrington hook in neuromuscular disease. A case report. *Clin Orthop* 80:179-181, 1983.
5. Choudhury AR, Taylor JC: Cauda equina syndrome in lumbar disc disease. *Acta Orthop Scand* 51:493-499, 1980.
6. Crawfurd EJ, Baird PR, Clark AL: Cauda equina and lumbar nerve root compression in patients with AIDS. *J Bone Joint Surg* 69B:36-37, 1987.
7. Currier BL, Eismont FJ: Infections of the spine. In Rothman RH, Simeone FA (eds): *The Spine*, ed 3. Philadelphia, WB Saunders, 1992.
8. Dan NG, Saccasan PA: Serious complications of lumbar spinal manipulation. *Med J Aust* 2:672-673, 1983.
9. Delamarter RB, Bohlman HH, Dodge LD, Biro C: Experimental lumbar spinal stenosis. Analysis of the cortical evoked potentials, microvasculature, and histopathology. *J Bone Joint Surg* 72A:110-120, 1990.
10. Delamarter RB, Sherman JE, Carr JB: Cauda equina syndrome: Neurologic recovery following immediate, early, or late decompression. *Spine* 16:1022-1029, 1991.
11. den Boon J, Avezaat CJ, van der Gaast A et al: Conus-cauda syndrome as a presenting symptom of endodermal sinus tumor. *Gynecol Oncol* 57:121-125, 1995.
12. Denis F, Burkus JK: Diagnosis and treatment of cauda equina entrapment in the vertical lamina fracture of lumbar burst fractures. *Spine* 16:S433-439, 1991.
13. Dinning TA, Schaeffer HR: Discogenic compression of the cauda equina: A surgical emergency. *Aust NZ J Surg* 63:927-934, 1993.
14. Epstein NE: Surgically confirmed cauda equina and nerve root injury following percutaneous discectomy at an outside institution: A case report. *J Spinal Disord* 3:380-382, 1990.
15. Fisher RG: Sacral fracture with compression of cauda equina: Surgical treatment. *J Trauma* 28:1678, 1988.
16. Floman Y, Wiesel SW, Rothman RH: Cauda equina syndrome presenting as a herniated lumbar disk. *Clin Orthop* 147:234, 1980.
17. Gallinaro P, Cartesegna M: Three cases of lumbar disc rupture and one of cauda equina associated with spinal manipulation (chiropraxis). *Lancet* 1(8321):411, 1983 [letter].
18. Gleave JR, MacFarlane R: Prognosis for recovery of bladder function following lumbar central disc prolapse. *Br J Neurosurg* 4:205-209, 1990.
19. Griffith RW: Complications of continuous spinal anesthesia. *CRNA* 3:164-169, 1992.
20. Grosman H, Gray R, St Louis EL: CT of long-standing ankylosing spondylitis with cauda equina syndrome. *Am J Neuroradiol* 4:1077-1080, 1983.
21. Haddad FS, Sachdev JS, Bellapravalu M: Neuropathic bladder in ankylosing spondylitis with spinal diverticula. *Urology* 35:313-316, 1990.
22. Haldeman S, Rubinstein SM: Cauda equina syndrome in patients undergoing manipulation of the lumbar spine. *Spine* 17:1469-1473, 1992.
23. Hedtmann A, Steffen R, Kramer J: Prospective comparative study of intradiscal high-dose and low-dose collagenase versus chymopapain. *Spine* 12:388-392, 1987.
24. Hellstrom P, Kortelainen P, Kontturi M: Late urodynamic findings after surgery for cauda equina syndrome caused by a prolapsed lumbar intervertebral disk. *J Urol* 135:308-312, 1986.
25. Herdmann J, Dvorak J, Vohanka S: Neurophysiological evaluation of disorders and procedures affecting the spinal cord and the cauda equina. *Curr Opin Neurol Neurosurg* 5:544-548, 1992.
26. Hilibrand AS, Urquhart AG, Graziano GP, Hensinger RN: Acute spondylolytic spondylolisthesis: Risk of progression and neurological complications. *J Bone Joint Surg* 77A:190-196, 1995.
27. Hussain SA, Gullan RW, Chitnavis BP: Cauda equina syndrome: Outcome and implications for management. *Br J Neurosurg* 17(2):164-167, 2003.
28. Johnson PJ, Hahn F, McConnell J, et al: The importance of MRI findings for the diagnosis of nontraumatic lumbar subacute subdural haematomas. *Acta Neurochir (Wien)* 113:186-188, 1991.
29. Koenigsberg RA, Klahr J, Zital L, et al: Magnetic resonance imaging of the cauda equina syndrome in ankylosing spondylitis. *J Neuroimaging* 5:46-48, 1995.
30. Kostuik JP, Harrington I, Alexander D, et al: Cauda equina syndrome and lumbar disc herniation. *J Bone Joint Surg* 68A:386-391, 1986.
31. Kothbauer K, Schmid UD, Seiler RW, Eisner W: Intraoperative motor and sensory monitoring of the cauda equina. *Neurosurgery* 34:702-707, 1994.
32. Kulali A, von Wild K, Hobik HP: Subarachnoid haemorrhage with acute cauda symptom due to spinal tumour. *Neurochirurgia (Stuttg)* 32:87-90, 1989.
33. Lafuente DJ, Andrew J, Joy A: Sacral sparing with cauda equina compression from central lumbar intervertebral disc prolapse. *J Neurol Neurosurg Psychiatr* 48:579-581, 1985.
34. Laus M, Alfonso C, Giunti A: Lumbosciatic pain and coagulopathies. *Chir Organi Mov* 76:229-236, 1991.
35. Laus M, Pignatti G, Alfonso C et al: Complications in the surgical treatment of lumbar stenosis. *Chir Organi Mov* 77:65-71, 1992.

36. Malbrain ML, Kamper AM, Lambrecht GL *et al:* Filum terminale ependymoma revealed by acute cauda equina compression syndrome following intratumoral and spinal subarachnoid hemorrhage in a patient on oral anticoagulants. *Acta Neurol Belg* 94:35-43, 1994.

37. Malmivaara A, Pohjola R: Cauda equina syndrome caused by chiropraxis on a patient previously free of lumbar spine symptoms. *Lancet* 2:986-987, 1982 [letter].

38. Maurice-Williams RS, Marsh HT: Priapism as a feature of claudication of the cauda equina. *Surg Neurol* 23:626-628, 1985.

39. McLaren AC, Bailey SI: Cauda equina syndrome: A complication of lumbar discectomy. *Clin Orthop* 204: 143-149, 1986.

40. Mitchell MJ, Sartoris DJ, Moody D, Resnick D: Cauda equina syndrome complicating ankylosing spondylitis. *Radiology* 175:521-525, 1990.

41. Nielsen B, de Nully M, Schmidt K, Hansen RI: A urodynamic study of cauda equina syndrome due to lumbar disc herniation. *Urol Int* 35:167-170, 1980.

42. Normand JP, Dufour M, Lang JY *et al:* Radiographic features of cauda equina syndrome complicating ankylosing spondylitis. *Can Assoc Radiol J* 45:58-61, 1994.

43. Olmarker K, Holm S, Rosenqvist AL, Rydevik B: Experimental nerve root compression: A model of acute, graded compression of the porcine cauda equina and an analysis of neural and vascular anatomy. *Spine* 16:61-69, 1991.

44. Olmarker K, Holm S, Rydevik B: Importance of compression onset rate for the degree of impairment of impulse propagation in experimental compression injury of the porcine cauda equina. *Spine* 15:416-419, 1990.

45. Olmarker K, Rydevik B, Hansson T, Holm S: Compression-induced changes of the nutritional supply to the porcine cauda equina. *J Spinal Disord* 3:25-29, 1990.

46. Olmarker K, Rydevik B, Holm S: Edema formation in spinal nerve roots induced by experimental, graded compression. An experimental study on the pig cauda equina with special reference to differences in effects between rapid and slow onset of compression. *Spine* 14:569-573, 1989.

47. Olmarker K, Rydevik B, Holm S, Bagge U: Effects of experimental graded compression on blood flow in spinal nerve roots: A vital microscopic study on the porcine cauda equina. *J Orthop Res* 7:817-823, 1989.

48. Onik G, Maroon JC, Jackson R: Cauda equina syndrome secondary to an improperly placed nucleotome probe. *Neurosurgery* 30:412-414, 1992.

49. Pedowitz RA, Garfin SR, Massie JB *et al:* Effects of magnitude and duration of compression on spinal nerve root conduction. *Spine* 17:194-199, 1992.

50. Raaf J: Removal of protruded lumbar intervertebral discs. *J Neurosurg* 32:604-611, 1970.

51. Rydevik B: Neurophysiology of cauda equina compression. *Acta Orthop Scand Suppl* 251:52-55, 1993.

52. Rydevik BL, Pedowitz RA, Hargens AR *et al:* Effects of acute, graded compression on spinal nerve root function and structure. An experimental study of the pig cauda equina. *Spine* 16:487-493, 1991.

53. Schmidt RH, Grady MS, Cohen W, *et al:* Acute cauda equina syndrome from a ruptured aneurysm in the sacral canal. Case report. *J Neurosurg* 77:945-948, 1992.

54. Schnaid E, Eisenstein SM, Drummond WJ: Delayed post-traumatic cauda equina compression syndrome. *J Trauma* 25:1099-1101, 1985.

55. Schoenecker PL, Cole HO, Herring JA, *et al:* Cauda equina syndrome after in situ arthrodesis for severe spondylolisthesis at the lumbosacral junction. *J Bone Joint Surg* 72A:369-377, 1990 [comments].

56. Shapiro S: Cauda equina syndrome secondary to lumbar disc herniation. *Neurosurgery* 32:743-746, 1993 [comments].

57. Shaw PJ, Allcutt DA, Bates D, Crawford PJ: Cauda equina syndrome associated with multiple lumbar arachnoid cysts in ankylosing spondylitis: Improvement following surgical therapy. *J Neurol Neurosurg Psychiatr* 53: 1076-1079, 1990.

58. Smith S, Leibrock LG, Gelber BR, Pierson EW: Acute herniated nucleus pulposus with cauda equina compression syndrome following chemonucleolysis: Report of three cases. *J Neurosurg* 66:614-617, 1987.

59. Soeur M, Monseu G, Baleriaux WD *et al:* Cauda equina syndrome in ankylosing spondylitis: Anatomical, diagnostic, and therapeutic considerations. *Acta Neurochir (Wien)* 55:303-315, 1981.

60. Spangfort EV: The lumbar disc herniation: A computer-aided analysis of 2,504 operations. *Acta Orthop Scand Suppl* 142:1-95, 1972.

61. Spiegelmann R, Ram Z, Findler G *et al:* Spinal cord involvement as the presenting symptom of acute monocytic leukemia. *Surg Neurol* 29:145-148, 1988.

62. Takahashi K, Olmarker K, Holm S *et al:* Double-level cauda equina compression: An experimental study with continuous monitoring of intraneural blood flow in the porcine cauda equina. *J Orthop Res* 11:104-109, 1993.

63. Tay EC, Chacha PB: Midline prolapse of a lumbar intervertebral disc with compression of the cauda equina. *J Bone Joint Surg* 61B:43-46, 1979.

64. Tullberg T, Isacson J: Cauda equina syndrome with normal lumbar myelography. *Acta Orthop Scand* 60: 265-267, 1989.

65. Tullous MW, Skerhut HE, Story JL *et al:* Cauda equina syndrome of long-standing ankylosing spondylitis. Case report and review of the literature. *J Neurosurg* 73: 441-477, 1990.

66. Woo E, Yu YL, Ng M *et al:* Spinal cord compression in multiple myeloma: Who gets it? *Aust NZ J Med* 16: 671-675, 1986.

67. Young A, Dixon A, Getty J *et al:* Cauda equina syndrome complicating ankylosing spondylitis: Use of electromyography and computerised tomography in diagnosis. *Ann Rheum Dis* 40:317-322, 1981.

68. Zeman A, Donaghy M: Acute infection with human immunodeficiency virus presenting with neurogenic urinary retention. *Genitourin Med* 67:345-347, 1991.

69. Zuccarello M, Powers G, Tobler WD *et al:* Chronic posttraumatic lumbar intradural arachnoid cyst with cauda equina compression: Case report. *Neurosurgery* 20: 636-638, 1987.

CHAPTER 74

Primary Bony Spinal Lesions

Patrick W. Hitchon, Mark H. Bilsky, and Michael J. Ebersold

Primary tumors of the spine are extremely uncommon. In a review of 6221 bone tumors at the Mayo Clinic, Dahlin[16] found that less than 10% of all primary tumors involved the spine. In a recent, even more extensive review at the Mayo Clinic, Unni *et al.* (unpublished data, personal communication, 2000) reviewed 8091 skeletal bone tumors in patients who underwent surgery. Of these 8091 skeletal tumors distributed throughout the skeleton, 2334 were benign and 5757 were malignant. A further analysis of this group revealed that 510 tumors involving the spine were malignant and only 145 were benign. A more detailed grouping of the benign tumors is presented in Table 74.1. Not all patients with benign or malignant tumors undergo surgery. Therefore these numbers are somewhat misleading because they are underestimates.

The presenting symptoms of night pain, pain at rest, or progressive neurologic deficit should prompt the clinician to entertain the diagnosis of benign or malignant disease of the spine. The primary complaint of most patients with primary tumors of the spine is pain. In a recent review, more than 84% of the patients complained of pain, either localized to the back (60.2%) or radicular (24%). There was no apparent difference between the pain symptoms in patients with benign disease involving the spine and those with malignant disease involving the spine.[57] Fifty-five percent of the patients with malignant spine tumors and 35% of the patients with benign tumors demonstrated objective evidence of neurologic deficits. It is suspected that with the advent and increased availability of magnetic resonance imaging (MRI), the number of patients presenting with neurologic deficits will decrease.

Although a rapidly progressive neurologic deficit is more suggestive of a malignant tumor or a pathologic fracture, it is not uncommon for patients with benign tumors involving the spine to experience rather rapid progressive neurologic deterioration. Nevertheless, because of the slow growth of these benign tumors of the spine, there is often a prolonged interval between the onset of symptoms and the diagnosis.

The data presented in Table 74.1, contrasted with those in Table 74.2, demonstrate the relative frequency or infrequency of these primary tumors involving the spine. Chordoma is listed among the malignant tumors involving the spine, although tumor growth in some patients with chordoma is extremely slow. Conversely, giant cell tumor is considered a benign tumor, although this particular lesion, in some cases, can be aggressive in nature, and early tumor recurrence is common, even after aggressive but subtotal tumor removal.

Often, plain radiographs demonstrate the site of the lesion and, in many cases, can be diagnostic. Computed tomography (CT) and MRI are often extremely valuable for defining the extent and precise location of the lesion. The need for myelography to diagnose and define benign tumors of the spine has been nearly eliminated by these two imaging advances. However, angiography can often be of significant benefit in determining or confirming the nature of the lesion. In addition, angiography may be used for accurate definition of the vascular extent of the lesion and for preoperative embolization, when appropriate. Often, preoperative embolization can decrease the operative blood loss and therefore the postoperative morbidity. Aneurysmal bone cysts, giant cell tumors, and hemangiomas, in particular, should be considered for preoperative embolization.

Some of the primary tumors of the spine have very characteristic imaging findings. The clinician should be aware of the classical radiographic findings associated with these tumors, because this knowledge is not only helpful for identifying the cause of the symptoms, but may also be of value by limiting additional testing. Several of the common spinal lesions have unique features and are presented in the pages that follow.

Management

Surgery

A major advance in the treatment of primary spine tumors is the concept of marginal or wide "en bloc" vertebral body resection (i.e., en bloc spondylectomy). For primary tumors at extraspinal sites, the long-term local tumor control, survival, and cure are dependent on en bloc tumor resection to achieve a marginal, wide, or radical resection.* Although intralesional resection of spine tumors results in good neurologic outcomes, local recurrence rates remain high. For this reason, there has been resurgent interest in treating primary spinal tumors with en bloc resection. En bloc spine resections are characterized as marginal, wide, or radical, based on the surgical margin obtained. As applied to the spine, a marginal resection dissects through the pseudocapsule of the tumor, and wide resection provides a cuff of normal tissue (more than 2mm of healthy bone, reactive periosteum, or pleura). Radical resection is not applicable to the spine, because it requires resection of the entire spinal compartment from coccyx to skull. Marginal en bloc resection or intralesional resection with an adjuvant (e.g., phenol, liquid nitrogen, methylmethacrylate) may be curative for aneurysmal bone cysts, giant cell tumors, osteoid osteomas, and osteoblastomas. Evidence is mounting that wide en bloc resections for primary tumors such as chondrosarcoma, chordoma, osteogenic sarcoma, and Ewing's sarcoma[6,8,26,45a,54a] may effect a longer disease-free interval and a potential cure, as is seen for primary tumors arising at extraspinal sites.[8]

En bloc resection of primary spine tumors to achieve a marginal or wide resection is dependent on the pattern of tumor at presentation. According to the Weinstein,

---

*References 11,13,18,20,21a,27a,32a.

TABLE 74.1

Skeletal Distribution of Benign Tumors*

Tumor Type	Number of patients with	
	Tumors Involving the Spine	Benign Skeletal Tumors
Osteochondroma	19	748
Chondroma	5	290
Chondroblastoma	1	119
Chondromyxoid fibroma	1	45
Osteoid osteoma	30	332
Osteoblastoma	29	87
Giant cell tumor	32	574
Fibous histiocytoma	0	9
Hemangioma	28	109
Lipoma	0	7
Neurilemmoma	0	14
Total	145	2334

From Unni KK et al: Unpublished data, personal communication, 2000.
*Only those patients undergoing surgery and therefore having tissue available for pathologic review are included in this table.

TABLE 74.2

Skeletal Distribution of Malignant Tumors*

Tumor Type	Number of patients with	
	Tumors Involving the Spine	Malignant Skeletal Tumors
Myeloma	232	803
Lymphoma	82	694
Chondrosarcoma	54	892
Secondary chondrosarcoma	7	121
Dedifferentiated Chondrosarcoma	1	120
Mesenchymal chondrosarcoma	4	25
Osteosarcoma	37	1649
Periosteal osteosarcoma	0	69
Ewing's tumor	16	514
Malignant giant cell tumor	2	35
Adamantinoma	0	36
Malignant fibrous histiocytoma	2	83
Deshmoid fibroma	0	12
Fibrosarcoma	9	255
Chordoma	51	356
Hemanangioendothelioma	13	80
Hemangiopericytoma	1	13
Total	511	5757

From Unni KK et al: Unpublished data, personal communication, 2000.
*Only those patients undergoing surgery and therefore having tissue available for pathologic review are included in this table.

Boriani, Biagini (WBB) classification,[9] the vertebra is divided into 12 radiating zones (numbered 1 through 12, clockwise) and into 5 layers (A to E, from paravertebral to dural involvement). In addition, the longitudinal extent of the tumor is noted. Tumors involving the posterior elements or those contained within the vertebral body can potentially be resected in an en bloc fashion. Vertebral body tumors with unilateral pedicle involvement or small paraspinal masses may also be considered for en bloc resection. Tumors with extensive epidural tumor are not considered for en bloc resection, because the risk of neurologic injury is extremely high. In addition, resecting the dura as a margin may increase the risk of intradural seeding.[2]

Radiation

Primary tumors may benefit from neoadjuvant or postoperative adjuvant radiation or chemotherapy. In general, the more benign tumors (e.g., osteoid osteoma, osteoblastoma, osteochondroma) have a poor response rate to these therapeutic modalities, and gross resection of the tumor will affect a cure. A significant concern in patients radiated for the more benign tumors is the development of postradiation sarcomas. In a review of 59 operated spinal sarcomas at Memorial Sloan-Kettering Cancer Center (MSKCC), seven patients had postradiation sarcomas at a median interval of 14 years from the time of radiation.[2] Other tumors such as osteogenic sarcoma and Ewing's sarcoma may benefit from neoadjuvant chemotherapy followed by resection. Chondrosarcoma and chordoma are extremely radiotherapy and still chemotherapy resistant, but positive surgical margins are irradiated.

A great challenge in radiotherapy to the spine is that the dose the spinal cord can tolerate is significantly lower than the dose required to achieve local tumor control. Several strategies have evolved in an attempt to deliver tumoricidal doses of radiation while avoiding radiation-induced myelopathy. These advances include brachytherapy; proton beam therapy; and newer modalities of three-dimensional conformal radiation therapy (3D-CRT), such as intensity-modulated radiation therapy (IMRT). All three techniques provide a higher tumoral dose of radiation with reduced damage to surrounding tissues and potentially smaller fields compared with conventional external beam techniques.

Intraoperative radiation therapy (IORT) involves the delivery of a custom-designed electron beam or high-dose-rate brachytherapy that precisely demarcates the tumor volume. Lead shields and gold foil are used to shield the spinal cord. In a retrospective review by Seichi et al.,[48a] 37 patients underwent IORT with electron beams following surgical resection to a total dose of 2000cGy, a dose estimated by the authors to be biologically equivalent to 4500cGy of conventional fractionated external beam radiation therapy. Twenty-two patients also received fractionated external beam radiotherapy to a median dose of 3400cGy. One patient in whom the spinal cord was not shielded developed symptomatic radiation myelopathy. Local control was achieved in all patients at a median follow-up of 11 months. Unfortunately, this technique is somewhat labor-intensive, and dosimetry considerations are difficult to predict around the spinal cord. Although brachytherapy offers high-dose focal radiation, the spinal cord must be shielded,[12] which limits its usefulness in patients with epidural tumor. Brachytherapy will probably be largely replaced with 3D-CRT, as has already occurred with its use in treating brain tumors.

Proton beam therapy has an inherent geometric advantage over therapy with photons and electrons because of the finite range of penetration in tissues (Bragg-peak effect). Photon beams can be designed such that there is a uniform dose to the target volume (i.e., tumor) and minimal dose delivery to the critical surrounding tissues (e.g., spinal cord, bowel, esophagus). Proton beam treatment plans are often supplemented with additional photon beam therapy to improve tumoral coverage. A major drawback for proton beam therapy is the limited availability of treatment centers in the United States to accommodate the demands for treating primary tumors, particularly chordomas and chondrosarcomas. Currently, only two centers offer proton beam therapy–Massachusetts General Hospital (Boston, MA) and Loma Linda University Medical Center (Loma Linda, CA).

Similar to proton beam therapy, 3D-CRT is a method of irradiating a tumor volume with an array of photon beams that are individually shaped to conform to a 3D rendering of the target. Treatment planning considers dose inhomogeneities caused by the differing electron densities of various tissues and calculates the resulting dose distribution using sophisticated algorithms. Intensity modulated radiation therapy (IMRT) represents an advanced form of 3D-CRT in which multileaf collimators are used to dynamically change the field shape during treatment, thus permitting the delivery of an inhomogenous dose that conforms more tightly to the target region. Because of the precise dosimetry demands of IMRT, accurate delivery requires reproducible patient setup and positioning. Various body frames have been developed at MSKCC to provide quick and reliable patient setup to deliver fractionated treatments. Preliminary data suggest that IMRT may improve the clinical outcome of inoperable tumors and those tumors requiring a boost after surgical resection. The wider availability of IMRT or similar photon applications (e.g., CyberKnife) compared with the availability of proton beam therapy may improve spine surgeons' ability to offer high-dose fractionated therapy for primary spine tumors.

Hemangioma

Hemangioma is one of the common benign lesions involving the spinal axis. It is often discovered incidentally during evaluation of patients with back or neck pain. The relatively low incidence, noted in Table 74.1, confirms that most patients with hemangioma are not treated surgically. Several studies have demonstrated that this entity may affect as much as 10% to 12% of the population.* Spine surgeons become involved with the treatment of hemangioma when the lesion causes spinal cord or nerve root compression. In general, decompres-

---

*References 3,11,22,33,43,44.

sive surgery should be reserved for this specific group, because such surgery is usually not required for the management of pain that is not associated with neurologic involvement. In a recent review at the Mayo Clinic, it was demonstrated that, in fact, it is rare for incidental hemangiomas associated with pain alone to progress to spinal cord compression. Only 2 of 59 patients with previously diagnosed asymptomatic or painful lesions later developed spinal cord compression. Patients with asymptomatic lesions do not require further evaluation unless pain or neurologic deficits develop. Patients with painful lesions should be followed closely, with a combination of radiographic studies and periodic neurologic evaluations.

In the past, subtotal tumor removal with postoperative irradiation was often considered the treatment of choice in symptomatic tumors. The development of modern spine surgery techniques and the advancements made possible by a skilled surgical team and modern instrumentation have now made total removal of these lesions a viable option in many cases. Preoperative embolization has also significantly decreased intraoperative and postoperative morbidity.

Imaging

Plain radiography, tomography, and CT can often clearly demonstrate the typical coarsened trabeculae within the involved vertebrae, with a characteristic honeycombed appearance. Gadolinium enhancement and MRI evidence of a soft tissue component are often observed (Figure 74.1).

Histology

Most of the trabeculae are atrophic because of the abnormal blood vessels, although some become thickened and sclerotic. Microscopically, there are two main types of trabeculae. These are characterized by cavernous or capillary vessels. In some cases, adipose tissue may be found within the lesion.[22] Malignant degeneration is not known to occur.[21] Spinal cord compression may arise from the expansile nature of the vertebral body, an associated soft tissue component of the tumor that rests within the spinal canal, a compression fracture of the weakened vertebral body, or rarely, an epidural hemorrhage.

Management

The management scheme should depend on the size, extent, and location of the lesion; the patient's general age and health; and the patient's clinical course and neurologic findings. Surgical decompression is recommended if there is progressive neurologic decline. It is important for the spine surgeon to be familiar with the variety of available surgical approaches so that the most appropriate technique can be used to remove the tumor. Many patients for whom laminectomy and postoperative radiation therapy would have been recommended can now be treated using a lateral or ventral surgical approach to the lesion. Laminectomy followed by radiation therapy of lesions involving the vertebral body yielded a 93% rate of neurologic recovery, without recurrent symptoms, in a 52-month

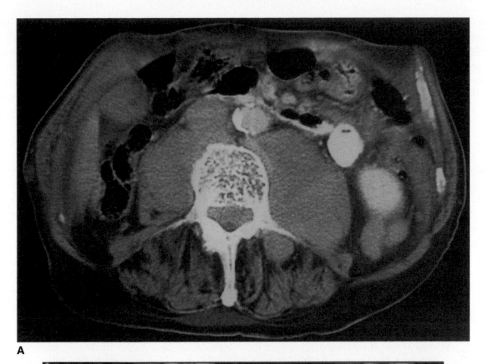

A

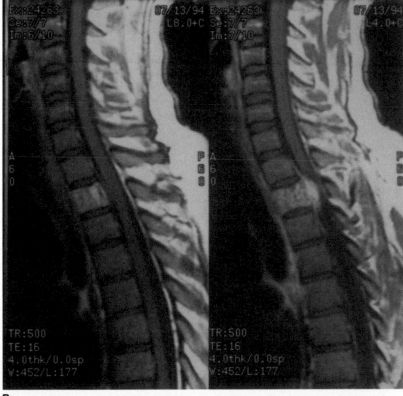

B

Figure 74.1 (**A**) Computed tomographic scan of vertebral body demonstrating the typical trabeculated appearance of a hemangioma of the lumbar spine. (**B**) T_1-weighted sagittal magnetic resonance image of the thoracic spine demonstrates an indeterminate mass, later pathologically proven to be a hemangioma involving the body and right pedicle of T2. This hemangioma displaced the thecal sac and produced mild to moderate deformity of the adjacent thoracic spinal cord. In asymptomatic patients, this appearance is often an incidental finding.

follow-up period.[40] Laminectomy without radiation therapy for subtotal tumor resections resulted in tumor control rates of 70% to 80%.[1,17,32,36,40] It appears that postoperative irradiation reduces the risk of tumor recurrence in patients after subtotal tumor removal. Nevertheless, because of the potential morbidity and relative lack of efficacy associated with radiation therapy, total lesion removal often should be attempted.

Aneurysmal Bone Cysts

Aneurysmal bone cysts are benign, proliferative nonneoplastic lesions that may occur in any part of the skeleton. Although this is not a tumor per se, its classical appearance and presentation should be familiar to clinicians dealing with spine lesions. Approximately 20% of lesions occur in the spine, with a predilection for the lumbar spine. Lesions are often not confined to a single vertebra; instead they bridge two or more levels in approximately 40% of cases.[28,55] Although primary aneurysmal bone cysts are of unknown cause, a secondary form of aneurysmal bone cyst has been described that arises within eosinophilic granulomas, simple bone cysts, osteosarcomas, chondroblastomas, or giant cell tumors.[55]

Aneurysmal bone cysts of the spine typically present in young patients in their second decade, with a slight predominance in women.[27] In one series, 60% of lesions arose in the neural arch and 40% arose in the body.[43] Pain that occurs especially at night and that is localized to the site of the mass is the most common presenting complaint.[38] The presence or absence of a neurologic deficit depends on the site of the tumor and on the degree of compression of adjacent neural elements. Symptoms and signs may vary, from cord compression with myelopathic findings to radicular features of single root involvement. The clinical course is commonly progressive over several months because of the slow growth of these lesions, although rapid growth can also occur.

Imaging

Anatomic delineation of aneurysmal bone cysts is often best achieved with plain radiography and CT, which accurately define the degree of bone destruction and full extent of the lesion (Figure 74.2*A,B*). MRI can be helpful for defining a spinal cord compressive component, and it readily demonstrates the full epidural extent of the mass. The rather classical appearance of the involved vertebra is that of a multiloculated, expansile, highly vascular mass with eggshell-like cortical bone and blood product fluid levels. Collapse of involved bodies and involvement of adjacent ribs may also be observed.

Selective spinal angiography has both diagnostic and, potentially, therapeutic value.[38] In addition to defining the relationship of the arterial supply of the lesion to the arterial supply of the cord, angiography also defines the involvement of the vertebral arteries with cervical lesions. The anatomic location of the artery of Adamkiewicz in lower thoracic or upper lumbar lesions can be defined clearly with spinal angiography. Finally, preoperative embolization is a useful adjunct that may decrease the intraoperative blood loss (Figure 74.2*C*).

Histology

Microscopically, aneurysmal bone cysts are characterized by spaces separated by septa that contain fibroblasts and giant cells. Reactive new bone is usually present. Although mitotic activity is brisk, there is no cytologic atypia. The lesions are lytic and expansile, and they extend to the cortex and occasionally violate the periosteum. Hemorrhage is common. The lesions contain sinusoidal vessels with hypervascular stroma, and multinucleated giant cells, monocytes, and macrophages are common.

Management

Complete surgical resection is the treatment of choice with aneurysmal bone cysts of the spine, especially in patients who have a neurologic deficit. The approach (ventral, dorsal, or dorsolateral) depends on the exact location and extent of the lesion. An eggshell-thin cyst of subperiosteal new bone that is continuous with adjacent cortex is observed at surgery. This delineates the extent of the lesion, and its removal often results in intense bleeding. The core of the tumor consists of soft, fleshy, vascular tissue, as well as a cystic trabeculation of the interior of the mass containing unclotted blood. The mass may invade adjacent soft tissue or surround the thecal sac. Although there may be some concern about using a cell saver when removing tumors from any location in the body, there appears to be no contraindication to this procedure when removing aneurysmal bone cysts. Subtotal surgical excision is followed by a high incidence of recurrence, which is usually rapid (within 1 year, and often within 4 months).[26]

There seems to be little justification for needle biopsy. The results are likely to be negative, and the procedure is potentially dangerous owing to risk of epidural hematoma. Rarely, spontaneous disappearance of aneurysmal bone cysts has been reported to occur. Despite the inherent technical difficulties of excision that are related to location and extent of the lesion, the prognosis is excellent with complete excision. Therefore this should be the goal of surgical intervention.

Giant Cell Tumor

Giant cell tumors of the spine are locally aggressive benign primary bone tumors that constitute 4.2% of bone tumors in Dahlin's series.[16] Approximately 6.5% of all giant cell tumors occur in the spine,[47] with half occurring in the sacrum, followed by the thoracic and cervical spines in frequency.[25] The mean age of involvement is approximately 30 years, with a range of 13 to 62 years.[26,58] In most reviews, the incidence in women appears to outnumber that in men by a ratio of 2:1.[26,48] Most patients present with pain localized to the site of the lesion and, occasionally, with a neurologic deficit, depending on the location. Malignant transformation occurs in approximately 10% of cases. Some giant cell tumors are biologically aggressive lesions.

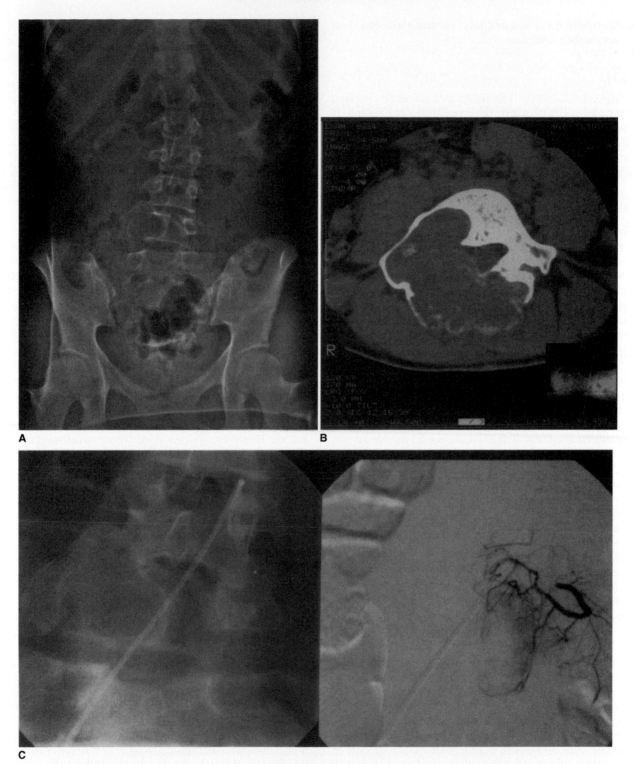

Figure 74.2 Aneurysmal bone cyst. (**A**) Plain radiograph of lumbar spine demonstrating the typical appearance of a lytic, eccentric, expansile lesion of the vertebral body and dorsal elements of L5, as observed with an aneurysmal bone cyst. (**B**) Computed tomographic scan of lumbar spine demonstrating the lytic lesion of the dorsal elements and the vertebral body, with the tumor having an osseous shell consisting of a thin rim of cortical bone surrounding the mass. (**C**) Plain and subtracted angiographic views display the typical segmental vascular supply of an aneurysmal bone cyst with vascular staining.

In patients with these tumors, local recurrence is common after incomplete resection.

Imaging

The diagnosis of giant cell tumors may be made from plain radiographs and CT scans (Figure 74.3). The lesion is characterized as a destructive, expansile mass within the sacrum or other vertebrae. MRI reveals a heterogeneous, cystic, compartmentalized mass that may contain blood degradation products.

Histology

Grossly, the giant cell tumor is soft and fleshy and has a characteristic tan-brown color. Areas of necrosis and yellow discoloration may be found. Microscopically, these tumors show a combination of mononuclear cells and giant cells. The mononuclear cells are round to oval, and the nuclei are similar to those of the giant cells. Areas of necrosis and cystic change may be observed.

Management

In a review of 24 patients with giant cell tumor of the spine, pain was the presenting symptom in all cases, and half of the patients also had a neurologic deficit.[48] All patients were treated with surgical curettage or en bloc resection, depending on the location and extent of the tumor. Ten patients had recurrences, and seven of these were treated with irradiation. The most acceptable treatment approach seems to be an attempted wide resection. Preoperative tumor embolization may be beneficial.

Radiation therapy may be considered with subtotal surgical excision. Giant cell tumors can recur relatively early after even the most radical surgical excision. In such cases, it may be reasonable to consider radiation therapy if it is believed that further excisional attempts will also be unsuccessful. Because of the risk of sarcomatous changes, radiation therapy should be reserved for patients with recurrent or residual disease after attempted resection.[50] In the spine, wide resection may cause destabilization and may necessitate instrumentation of the spine and fusion.[23] However, total excision is curative if it is achieved.[49]

Because of their location, sacral lesions pose specific problems. Complete eradication of the tumor usually necessitates sacrifice of bowel and bladder control. For this reason, some authors propose irradiation as the primary form of treatment. However, sacrectomy with attempted wide excision is warranted with acceptance of inevitable neurologic sequelae, if it is believed that such surgery can result in total tumor removal and cure.

Osteoid Osteoma

Osteoid osteoma is a relatively common benign neoplasm that occurs in the spine and accounts for 21% of surgically managed benign lesions. Typically, it has a central nidus of interlacing osteoid and woven bone within a loose vascular stroma, surrounded by an osteosclerotic rim. These lesions are sharply demarcated from surrounding bone (Figure 74.4). The nidus is rarely greater than 1.5cm in diameter, and lesions larger than this are categorized as osteoblastomas. The distinction between the two lesions is often unclear, and they may represent a continuum.

Most patients are young, with half of all cases occurring in the second decade, with a marked predominance of males. Typically, the neural arch elements are affected, most commonly in the lumbar spine. In a series of 33 patients, the patients invariably presented with pain, which increased with exercise and was classically relieved with aspirin.[41] Associated features included the presence of radicular symptoms referable to the underlying root and antalgic scoliosis. A neurologic deficit was present in only two patients (both with cervical lesions). Osteoid osteoma is the most common cause of painful scoliosis in adolescents. This deformity can be corrected with resection of the osteoid osteoma alone if surgery is within 15 months of onset of symptoms or before the development of a structural curve.[41] Fifteen months appears to be the critical cut-off point after which spontaneous correction does not occur after surgery.

Imaging

Osteoid osteomas are best imaged by CT, which reveals the lucent nidus with surrounding sclerotic changes. Technetium bone scans show an intense focal increase in activity on intermediate and delayed films at the site of the lesion. However, lesions may be missed on plain radiographs and MRI scans.

Management

The definitive treatment for osteoid osteomas is complete surgical excision. The diagnosis is often missed initially, in the absence of a neurologic deficit, leading to a prolonged duration of symptoms.

Osteoblastoma

Osteoblastomas are uncommon lesions, constituting approximately 0.36% of all primary bone tumors that are treated with surgery. Thirty-three percent of these lesions occur in the spine. Osteoblastomas represent a histologic continuum of osteoid osteoma, the difference being the size of the lesions. Osteoblastomas are lesions that are greater than 1.5cm in diameter. Patients are usually in their second or third decade at presentation,[55] and there is a male/female predominance of 2:1.[7] Osteoblastomas are distributed throughout the spine, and in the series by Boriani et al.,[7] 16 of 30 lesions occurred in the lumbar spine, 8 in the thoracic spine, and 6 in the cervical spine. Two thirds of these lesions are confined to the dorsal elements. As observed with other benign spinal neoplasms, pain is the most common presenting complaint, and it may be associated with scoliosis and neurologic deficit. Unlike osteoid osteomas, osteoblastomas can progressively enlarge. The radiologic work-up of these lesions should include plain radiography and CT. These scans may show a well-defined, lobulated, lytic, expansile mass that usually involves the neural arch structures. Fifty percent of lesions

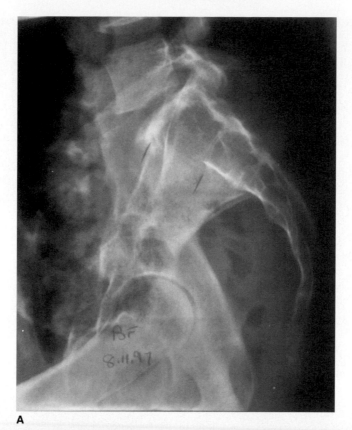

A

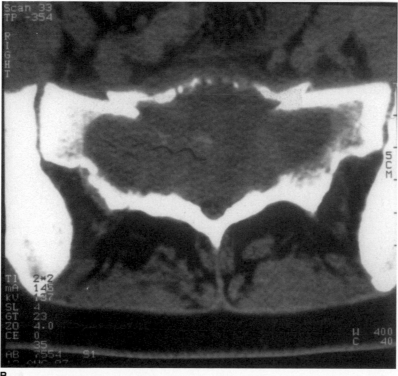

B

Figure 74.3 Giant cell tumor in a 17-year-old girl with several years of low back pain and a 1-year history of leg weakness and urinary retention and constipation. The lateral plane film (**A**) demonstrates a lytic lesion of S1, with erosion of the anterior cortex. The computed tomographic scan (**B**) demonstrates the expansile intramedullary tumor with extension into the spinal canal. *Continued*

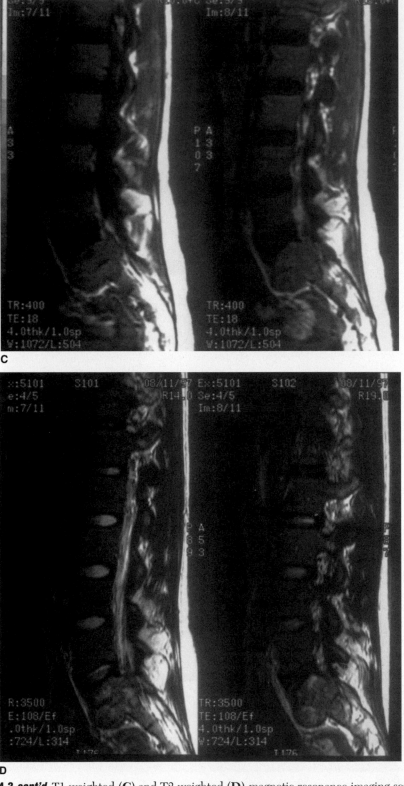

Figure 74.3 *cont'd* T1-weighted (**C**) and T2-weighted (**D**) magnetic resonance imaging scans reveal the bony tumor arising from S1 with extension anteriorly and posteriorly.

are radiolucent with a sclerotic rim. As with osteoid osteomas, MRI is often less informative than CT for defining these lesions. Unlike osteoid osteomas, bone scans often are not necessary for diagnosis but may be helpful with smaller lesions. Osteoblastomas should be treated surgi-

cally with total resection. Approximately 10% of lesions recur after surgery.

It is important to remember that both osteoid osteoma and osteoblastoma should be considered in any young patient with back or neck pain, painful scoliosis, or

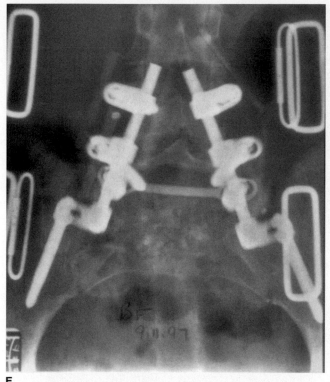

E

Figure 74.3 *cont'd* One month following posterior decompression and stabilization, radiographs (**E**) show satisfactory alignment with hardware in place. The patient later underwent anterior resections 5 and 26 months following the first operation. She is doing well, without recurrence or radiation.

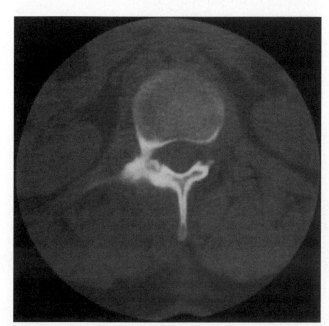

Figure 74.4 Osteoid osteoma. Computed tomographic scan of the lumbar spine demonstrates the distinctive osteoblastic lesion or nidus with the associated surrounding zone of sclerosing bone in a typical osteoid osteoma. In this patient, it involves the facet joint.

radicular pain. These lesions often become symptomatic before they are visible on plain radiographs.

Management

Although osteoid osteoma and osteoblastoma form a histologic continuum, and the duration of symptoms is prolonged in many cases because of diagnostic difficulties, a number of differences exist. Osteoid osteomas are small lesions that are not progressive and that have even been described to exhibit spontaneous regression. Patients with these lesions are treated most commonly because of persistent pain. Conversely, osteoblastomas demonstrate progressive enlargement, with the potential for malignant transformation. Thus they are managed both for pain and for progressive enlargement and destructiveness of the lesion. There is a much higher recurrence rate with osteoblastomas.

Both osteoid osteomas and osteoblastomas may cause scoliosis and neurologic deficit, the latter being more common with osteoblastoma. With larger, aggressive lesions, radiation therapy and embolization may be considered as adjuncts to surgical resection, but the potential risks of radiation therapy must be considered, including the risk of sarcomatous transformation.

Osteochondromas

Osteochondromas constitute 9.2% of all primary bone tumors that are treated surgically, but they rarely occur in the spine (2.5% of all osteochondromas). They consist of cartilage-covered cortical bone with underlying medullary bone, both types of bone being contiguous with their counterparts in the parent bone. The cartilaginous cap undergoes ossification to form the osteochondroma.

Histologically, the cartilaginous cap and underlying bone are identical to normal bone. The tumors can be solitary or multiple, and most present in the third decade. There is a male/female predominance of 2:1. The lesions affect the transverse or spinous processes, and half of all lesions occur in the cervical spine. Lesions are best diagnosed by plain radiography and CT. Patients usually have localized pain; neurologic deficit is uncommon. Rarely, osteochondromas may also be a manifestation of hereditary multiple osteochondromas. Only 1% of solitary lesions undergo malignant transformation. Surgical excision is the treatment of choice.

Other Benign Primary Spine Tumors

The other benign tumors that affect the spine are uncommon, as evidenced from Table 74.1. However, the indications for surgical intervention for these rare lesions and the goals of treatment are similar to those for the more common spine lesions already discussed.

Plasma Cell Tumors

Plasma cell tumors of the spine (multiple myeloma and solitary plasmacytoma) are the most common type of malignant

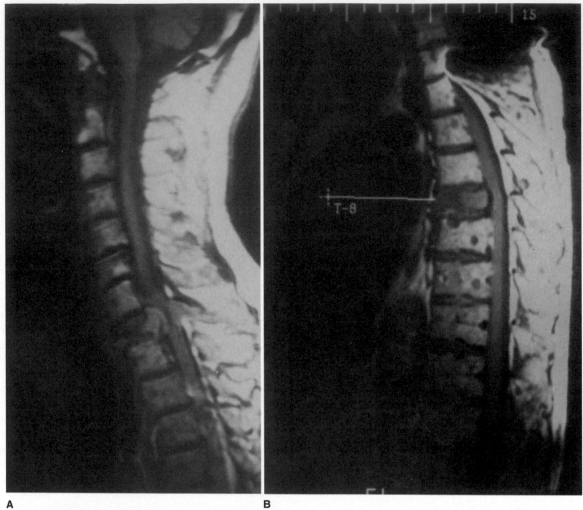

A   B

Figure 74.5 A 63-year-old man presenting with paraparesis and Brown-Séquard's syndrome. (**A**) Pathologic fracture involving T1 with retropulsion of bone and circumferential spinal cord compression by a solitary plasmacytoma (sagittal T_1-weighted magnetic resonance image [MRI]). A bone scan and skeletal survey were negative for other lesions. (**B**) A progressive increase in pain and paraparesis developed 18 months later. Sagittal T_1-weighted MRI shows a pathologic fracture at T8 with spinal cord compression. Multiple other lytic lesions of bone, secondary to multiple myeloma, are also noted. Bone marrow aspirate revealed plasma cell infiltrates, and bone scan showed increased uptake in the left clavicle.

primary tumors involving the spine (see Table 74.2). Multiple myeloma is the most common plasma cell tumor, characterized by multiple bony lesions, infiltration of the bone marrow by plasma cells, and a marked reduction of normal immunoglobulins.[31,36,43,47] Conversely, solitary plasmacytoma constitutes only 3% of plasma cell tumors. Patients with this condition are characterized by one or, at most, two bony lesions. The bone marrow is negative for plasma cell infiltrates, and serum-protein electrophoresis results are normal. A small monoclonal spike that disappears with treatment may reflect local lesions only.

Plasma cell tumors of the spine usually present with pain and, in advanced cases, with myelopathy. The duration of symptoms before diagnosis may vary; however, in general, symptoms worsen considerably in the 6 to 12 months before presentation. The incidence of multiple myeloma is the same in both males and females, whereas with solitary plasmacytoma, a twofold to threefold higher incidence is

encountered in males. The vertebral column is affected in approximately 45% of patients with plasma cell neoplasms. The diagnosis of solitary plasmacytoma is established histologically by either a needle biopsy or an open procedure. Multiple myeloma is usually diagnosed definitively by a bone marrow biopsy, the presence of multiple bony lesions on bone survey, and an abnormal monoclonal immunoglobulin spike on serum or urine electrophoresis. Most patients with multiple myeloma present with Bence Jones proteinuria, reflecting the spillover of monoclonal immunoglobulin fragments into the urine.

Management

The treatment of choice for solitary plasmacytoma in the absence of instability or rapid paralysis is radiation therapy. However, approximately 50% of all solitary plasmacytoma cases progress to multiple myeloma within 5 years, most commonly within 2 years (Figure 74.5). When the diagnosis of multiple myeloma is established, chemotherapy is indicated, although prognosis at that time is poor, with a median survival thereafter of 2 years and a 5-year survival of 18%.[43,58] The dose of radiation to the spine for plasmacytoma varies from 35 to 50Gy, although some oncologists favor larger doses. Chemotherapy is generally withheld until progression to multiple myeloma is documented.[43] It is recommended that patients with a diagnosis of solitary plasmacytoma be followed closely for the development of indexes characteristic of multiple myeloma. Whether chemotherapy should be instituted after the diagnosis of solitary plasmacytoma of bone remains unclear.[30]

Chordoma

Chordoma constitutes approximately 5% of malignant tumors involving the spine (see Table 74.2). The tumor originates from primitive remnants of the notochord. Fifty percent of all chordomas are sacrococcygeal, 40% are sphenoccipital, and the remaining 10% involve the mobile intermediate regions of the spine.[2,47,54,58] These tumors, considered to be of low-grade malignancy, are extremely difficult to resect because of their proximity to the spinal cord and cauda equina. In addition, in 5% to 10% of cases, they tend to metastasize within 1 to 10 years of the diagnosis. Fifty percent of all chordomas occur in the fifth to seventh decades of life, with a mean age of onset of approximately 50 years.[2,47,54] Men are twice as likely to be afflicted with this tumor as women.

Chordomas arise from the vertebral body, with ensuing ventral and dorsal extension. Pain is the presenting symptom in 75% of cases, with sphincter disturbance in 20% and radicular motor or sensory deficits in 10% of patients. These tumors can affect two adjacent vertebral bodies, while sparing the intervertebral disc.

Histology

Histologically, chordomas consist of two cell types: a small, compact stellate cell that is considered to be the precursor of the more prevalent and larger physaliphorous cell containing mucinous vacuoles.[2,54] These tumors have a characteristic lobular appearance on MRI. They can often be diagnosed by radiologic studies, including plain radiography. On plain radiographs, calcification can be observed in 40% of cases, and it is twice as likely to be observed by CT. Chordomas are generally avascular and are not associated with excessive intraoperative blood loss.

Management

The optimal treatment of chordomas is wide en bloc resection. The location of these lesions (close to neural structures) renders cure extremely unlikely. Ventral approaches with corpectomy and stabilization may contribute to improved outcome. With involvement of the sacrococcygeal spine, resection can be accomplished by either ventral, dorsal (Figure 74.6), or combined approaches.[27,35,37,54] These approaches are geared for the widest possible resection of tumor, with sparing of as many nerves as possible.[46]

Generally sparing the S3 nerve root on either side may be sufficient for bladder and fecal continence.

Although no prospective randomized studies have been conducted, radiation therapy is recommended.[10,30,46] A retrospective study involving 21 patients with spinal chordomas favored a combination of surgery and irradiation over surgery alone.[29] There is no evidence that doses higher than 40 to 55Gy are more likely to be associated with better results.[10] Neither is there evidence in support of treatment with more than a single fraction per day. The disease-free survival time for five patients with lumbosacral tumors treated with surgery and irradiation was 6.6 years compared with 4.1 years for seven patients treated with surgery alone ($p = .08$).[30] The actuarial 5-year disease-free survival for patients with lumbosacral tumors treated with surgery and irradiation was 60% versus 28% in patients treated with surgery alone ($p = .09$). The often-quoted 5-year survival has ranged, depending on the source, from 50% to 77%, with a 10-year survival of 50%.[46,52] There is currently no evidence to support chemotherapy for treatment of chordoma.

Primary Spinal Ewing's Sarcoma

Ewing's sarcoma constitutes 6% of all primary malignant bone tumors[10]; however, primary spinal involvement occurs in only 3.5% of all patients with Ewing's sarcomas.[25,49] This tumor afflicts males more commonly than females (2:1 ratio), and 88% of cases present in the first two decades of life.[10,25] In terms of the level of involvement, frequency decreases in a caudal to rostral progression, with more than 50% of all cases occurring in the sacrum.[10,25,49] The most common presenting feature is pain, with or without radicular involvement, depending on the level. In general, two of three patients present with a neurologic deficit (Figure 74.7). The duration of symptoms can range from 1 to 30 months; most symptoms are 1 year or less in duration. A rectal mass may be encountered on examination, considering that there is sacral involvement in one of four patients with primary spinal Ewing's sarcoma. In half of the cases, a lytic process is observed on plain radiographs, whereas other cases show blastic or mixed features.[25,49] A paravertebral soft tissue mass may occur independently or concurrently with bony involvement. This may be best appreciated on CT or MRI scans (Figure 74.7C and D). Confirmation of diagnosis has been accomplished more commonly by laminectomy, particularly in the presence of neurologic deficit. With the advent of CT-guided biopsies, needle aspiration has been undertaken in some patients.

Histology

Histologically, Ewing's sarcoma consists of infiltrating sheets of small, round to oval cells with a scant amount of cytoplasm that tests positive for glycogen.[10] These tumors are fragile and vascular. Intraoperative bleeding can be extensive, particularly with spinal involvement. Grossly, these tumors are gelatinous in consistency and gray-white in color. The borders of these lesions are poorly outlined, with extension into the bony trabeculae, as well as into the paravertebral soft tissues.

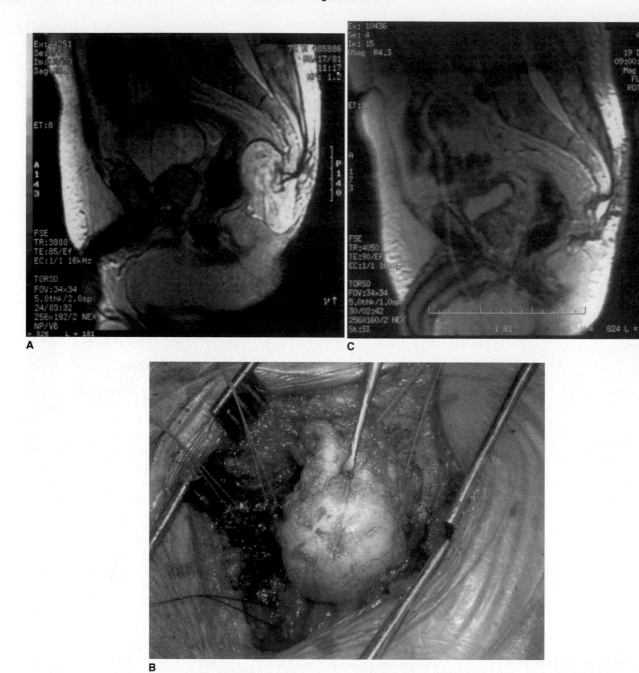

Figure 74.6 An 80-year-old man presenting with rectal bleeding resulting from rectal adenocarcinoma. During his work-up, a presacral mass was discovered. A T_2-weighted magnetic resonance image (MRI) in the sagittal plane demonstrated a soft tissue mass arising from the lower sacrum and coccyx (**A**). Through a posterior midline approach, the chordoma was removable with distal amputation of the sacrum and coccyx (**B**). An MRI 7 months postoperative shows the resection bed devoid of tumor (**C**).

Management

When surgical excision is attempted, preoperative embolization is recommended.[10,49] Optimal treatment after diagnosis is provided by a combination of radiation therapy and chemotherapy.[19,39] Local radiation therapy to the spine is usually given at a dose of 50 to 55Gy, with inclusion of an adequate margin as deemed appropriate by CT or MRI. Higher doses, when delivered to the spine, can be associated with postradiation myelopathy.[49] The accepted chemotherapy protocol developed by the Intergroup Ewing's Sarcoma Study (IESS) consists of cyclophosphamide, vincristine, actinomycin, and doxorubicin. This regimen, when administered in addition to local radiation therapy, has proven superior to a three-drug regimen with local irradiation or to a four-drug regimen with bilateral pulmonary radiotherapy.[39] The IESS protocol was tested in 342 patients and involved mostly appendicular, pelvic, and rib tumors. As expected, the

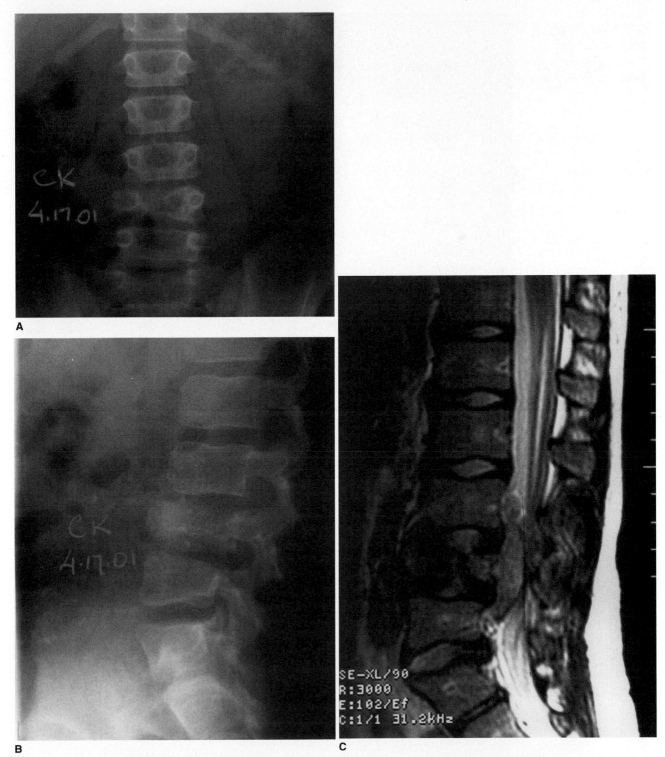

Figure 74.7 A 10-year-old boy presents with a 4-month history of low back pain and right leg weakness. Anteroposterior (**A**) and lateral (**B**) radiographs show a pathologic fracture of L4. T₂-weighted sagittal (**C**) and axial (**D**) images show the exophytic Ewing's sarcoma extending into the spinal canal and compressing the thecal sac. Because of tumor vascularity, the tumor was embolized preoperatively.

Continued

most favorable results were encountered with distal appendicular disease, and the worst were encountered with pelvic involvement. Younger patients (less than 10 years of age) were observed to have an associated 71% 5-year survival, compared with 46% in patients older than 15 years of age. A more intense chemotherapeutic and radiation therapy protocol (the IESS-II protocol) was developed for the treatment of pelvic and sacral Ewing's sarcoma.[19] With this regimen consisting of four-agent chemotherapy before and after high-dose local irradiation,

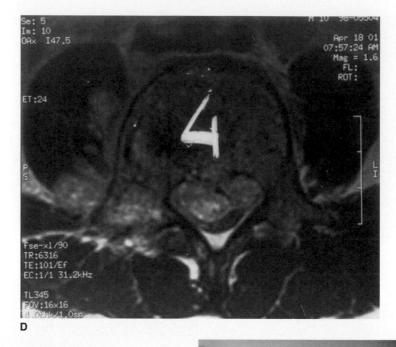

D

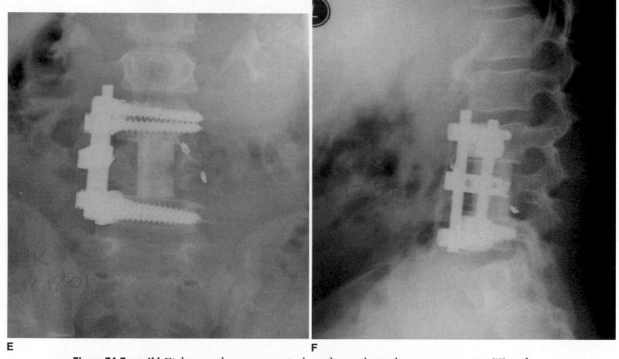

E   **F**

Figure 74.7 *cont'd* Eight months postoperatively, radiographs in the anteroposterior (**E**) and lateral (**F**) projections show the alignment to be satisfactory, with the hardware and femoral allograft in place. The endovascular coils are seen in both projections.

a survival pattern was achieved that is comparable with that achieved for disease in nonpelvic sites.

The role of surgery in the treatment of Ewing's sarcoma remains controversial. Indications for operation include high-grade epidural compression with symptomatic neurologic progression, stabilization, poor response to neoadjuvant chemotherapy or radiotherapy, and radiographic residual tumor post-neoadjuvant treatment.[49] When surgery is indicated for diagnosis or for neural decompression, an attempt at maximal resection should be undertaken.[49] These procedures routinely entail bony fusions with spinal implants to restore stability and prevent progressive deformity and neurologic deficit. Decompressive laminectomy may be associated with significant complications, including instability and progressive angulation.[24]

In an attempt to identify certain prognostic factors associated with Ewing's sarcoma, a retrospective study was conducted with 46 patients, 43 with osseous involvement and 3 with extraosseous involvement. An attempted resection was performed in 12 patients but not in the remaining 34 patients.[45] This analysis demonstrated that survival is improved in patients with local disease, tumors less than

500ml in volume, peripheral involvement only, and gross total resection, compared with patients who have metastatic involvement, tumor volume greater than 500ml, central involvement, and no resection. This analysis suggested that aggressive surgery with radiation therapy might be an important prognostic factor.

Ewing's sarcoma remains recalcitrant to surgical treatment. The best prognosis is provided by local irradiation and chemotherapy. A retrospective review of 36 patients who had primary involvement of the spine with Ewing's sarcoma yielded a 5-year survival of 33% with a mean survival of 2.9 years. Nine patients treated with the IESS regimen remained disease free at follow-up.[45]

Osteosarcoma

Osteosarcomas are primary malignant tumors of the bone. Spinal involvement is uncommon, present in only 37 of 1649 osteosarcomas (2.2%) (see Table 74.2). Osteosarcomas occur most commonly in the second decade of life, have a slight predilection for males,[16] and are the most common primary malignant bone tumor in the pediatric population. They usually arise in the vertebral body and occur throughout the spine. Pain is the most common presenting feature and may or may not be associated with a neurologic deficit, depending on the extent of spinal involvement with tumor.

Pathologically, osteosarcomas are firm and calcified and consist mostly of sarcomatous connective tissue that forms osteoid tissue or bone. They can be categorized further based on the dominant line of histologic differentiation into osteoblastic (55%), fibroblastic (23%), and chondroblastic (22%) types.[16]

Osteosarcomas usually arise de novo or may occur secondarily in previously irradiated bone, usually several years later (Figure 74.8). Postirradiation osteosarcomas occurred in 16 of 600 cases in Dahlin's series.[16] They may also occur as a secondary phenomenon in bone in older patients with Paget's disease, mostly those patients older than 60 years of age, or in osteochondromas. Two of 600 osteosarcomas in Dahlin's series arose from the latter lesion. Plain radiographs and CT scans of osteosarcomas may demonstrate osteolytic or osteoblastic changes. MRI is superior for showing tumor extent within the bone marrow and associated soft tissue and for delineating epidural tumor extension. Prognosis with this tumor is poor. Shives et al.[51] reviewed 27 cases of spinal osteosarcoma and reported a median survival of 10 months from diagnosis.

Management

Multimodality therapy to treat spinal osteogenic sarcoma was originally described by Sundaresan et al.[53] in 1988. Eleven patients underwent neoadjuvant chemotherapy followed by aggressive resection and postoperative irradiation. In this limited series, there were five long-term survivors.

A more recent series by Ozaki et al.[41a] reported on 22 patients who received neoadjuvant chemotherapy regimen according to the Cooperative Osteosarcoma Study Group (COSS) followed by resection. Four different chemotherapy protocols were used. All patients received preoperative high-dose methotrexate and doxorubicin in combination with a variety of other agents including cisplatin, ifosfamide, bleomycin, actinomycin D, and alpha-interferon. COSS 96 used both preoperative and postoperative chemotherapy. Twelve patients underwent tumor resection, including two wide, three marginal, and seven intralesional excisions. Eight patients were irradiated.

The median survival was 23 months. Patients with metastases ($p = .004$), large tumors (greater than 10cm) ($p = .010$), and sacral tumors ($p = .048$) had a worsened survival compared with those with no metastases, small tumors, and nonsacral tumors. This was a significant difference between the 17 patients who underwent intralesional excision or no surgery and the five patients who underwent marginal or wide excisions ($p = .033$). Postoperative irradiation extended overall survival in patients who underwent intralesional or no resection ($p = .059$).[41a] In this series, patients received conventional external photon beam irradiation (median tumoral dose 45Gy). No patient underwent either proton beam or IMRT irradiation.

Chondrosarcoma

Chondrosarcomas are primary malignant tumors arising from cartilaginous elements. They are rare tumors, constituting 892 of the 5751 malignant skeletal tumors (see Table 74.2). In this series, 54 tumors (6%) occurred in the spine. Like osteosarcomas, chondrosarcomas show a predilection for males; however, unlike osteosarcomas, they occur in middle-aged and older patients. Chondrosarcoma may arise de novo as a primary lesion or may occur as a secondary tumor from a preexisting solitary osteochondroma (1%) or from hereditary multiple exostosis (20%).[51]

Pain, the most common presenting symptom, may be indolent, leading to a delay in diagnosis. Pathologically, chondrosarcomas do not demonstrate neoplastic osteoid tissue or bone evolving from a sarcomatous matrix. Instead, they display nuclear pleomorphism, with numerous mitoses surrounded by a myxoid matrix. In addition to this conventional chondrosarcomatous appearance, variants may be subcategorized as predominantly myxoid, mesenchymal, or dedifferentiated.

Imaging

Plain radiographs and CT scans demonstrate osteolytic lesions with a calcified matrix. The amount of calcification correlates with the degree of differentiation. MRI is the study of choice for demonstrating the adjacent soft tissue and epidural extent of tumor spread. MRI also demonstrates the heterogeneity of the lesion (Figure 74.9). Of note, lesions that are more malignant tend to have larger amounts of soft tissue components, more irregular calcification, and more extensive bone destruction.

Management

Although chondrosarcomas are slowly growing lesions, they have a relatively poor overall prognosis. Survival correlates with degree of malignancy. Because of the spinal location, total resection is usually not possible.

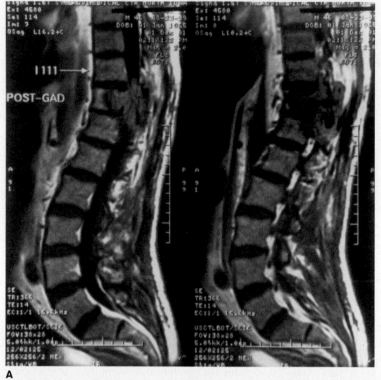

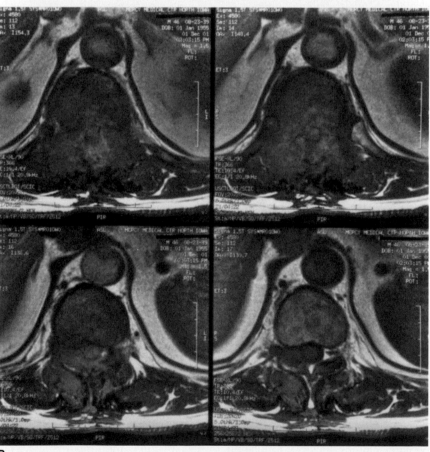

Figure 74.8 A 46-year-old man presented with rapidly progressive spinal pain and paraparesis of 3 months' duration. Past medical history indicated that 15 years earlier he had undergone surgery for a conus myxopapillary ependymoma. This had been followed by a full course of radiation therapy. His condition necessitated emergency decompression that revealed osteosarcoma. Sagittal T_1-weighted (**A**) and axial MRI without (**B**) and with (**C**) enhancement revealed a destructive bone tumor involving $T1_1$ and $T1_2$, with extension into the canal and neural foramina.

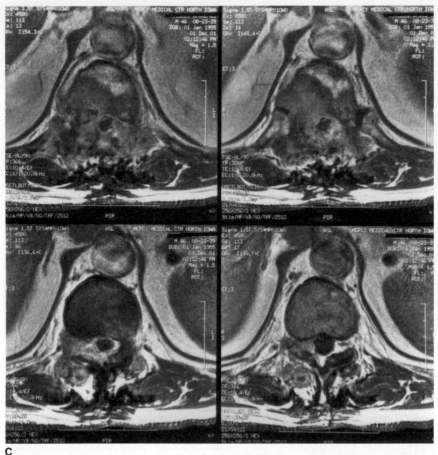

C

Figure 74.8 *cont'd*

Continued

This, combined with resistance of the tumor to chemotherapy and radiation therapy, establishes a tendency for local recurrence of tumor. However, small numbers of long-term survivors with low-grade lesions have been observed. Such patients can be managed with multiple local excisions. Complete excision is the goal of surgery, considering the propensity of the tumor for local recurrence.

In a series of predominantly low-grade chondrosarcomas, Boriani et al. showed improved local control with marginal or wide resections compared with intralesional resection. In this series, 17 of 18 patients undergoing intralesional resection had a local recurrence within 36 months. Two patients who had en bloc resections but contaminated margins (i.e., intralesional resections) recurred at 12 and 32 months. At a median follow-up of 81 months, only one patient undergoing marginal or wide resection had recurrence at 48 months. The patients in this series had predominantly posterior-element tumors and no epidural extension.

Despite the relative radioresistance of chondrosarcoma, we recommend high-dose 3D-CRT, using either proton beam or IMRT, following resection in patients with high-grade tumors following either intralesional resections or en bloc excisions with positive histologic margins.

Indications for Surgery

The goal of management of spine tumors is to establish a definitive diagnosis, decompress the neural elements, maintain or achieve spinal stability, and if possible, cure the patient.[23,48] In the case of benign tumors involving the spinal axis, cure can often be achieved if proper consideration is given to size, extent, and location of the tumor.

Not every patient with a primary tumor of the spine is a candidate for surgery. For example, hemangioma is often an incidental finding, and surgery is not appropriate unless there are specific clinical symptoms or signs. In general, progressive neurologic loss is a rather definite indication that surgery should at least be considered in the patient with a benign lesion. The patient's age, his or her general well-being, and the expected morbidity of the surgical procedure are all factors that must be considered.

If the patient is a reasonable surgical candidate, progressive neurologic loss is definitely a reason to consider surgery. In patients with malignant disease in whom diagnosis is already established, radiation therapy is often an appropriate alternative. The pros and cons of radiation therapy or open surgery must be considered. Pain is also a common indication for surgery in patients with benign tumors. This pain may be a result of recent spinal instability, of nerve root compression, or simply, of the ever-expanding mass that results in secondary soft tissue irritation and pain.

Progressive tumor enlargement can often result in a loss of stability of the spine, compression fractures, and secondary spinal deformity. A progressive spinal deformity often proves to be the specific concern that leads to consideration for surgery.

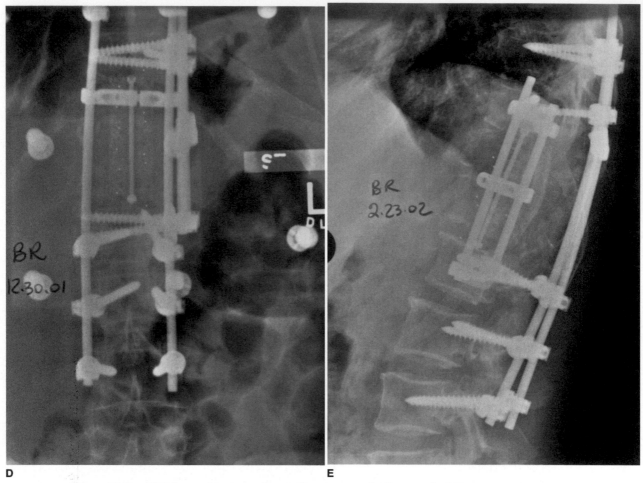

D　　　　　　　　　　　　　　　　　　　　**E**

Figure 74.8 *cont'd* The cord is circumferentially compressed. Three weeks following emergency decompression, the patient underwent T11-12 corpectomy, anterior stabilization, and posterior instrumentation from T8 to L3 (**D** and **E**). Motor performance improved, but pain control has remained the major problem.

Avoidance of Complications

Advances in radiologic imaging, especially MRI and CT, have resulted in better preoperative planning. Knowing the extent and precise location of the tumor certainly can result in an optimally planned surgical approach. Improvements in preoperative angiography and embolization have significantly decreased intraoperative blood loss with some of the more vascular benign and malignant tumors. With lesions such as the aneurysmal bone cyst, the use of the cell saver has resulted in a decreased requirement for administration of blood products. This, in turn, can significantly decrease the likelihood of intraoperative or postoperative complications from transfusion. With benign lesions especially, because there is often adequate time for preoperative planning, the practice of autodonation of blood can significantly decrease the risks of transfusion reaction.

Wound healing, especially in patients who have previously undergone extensive radiation therapy, can be a significant problem. The plastic surgeon can assist significantly in planning the surgical incision to maximize options for wound closure (see Chapter 88).

Often, incomplete lesion removal results in early recurrence. When appropriate, every attempt should be made to perform the procedure definitively during the first operation. To achieve the best outcomes with the least morbidity, the surgical team dealing with these lesions must be very comfortable with a variety of ventral and dorsal approaches to the spine, so that the best method can be selected for the lesion at hand.

When the tumor has been removed and the spinal cord and nerve roots decompressed, bone grafting, with or without instrumentation, should be considered. Many of the complications that result from spine surgery involve the destabilizing effects of surgery. If spinal instability has resulted from the tumor or the surgical treatment of the tumor, it is necessary to supplement the surgical procedure with a fusion of the unstable segments.

Over time, most spinal instrumentation constructs fatigue, loosen, and fail unless bony fusion ensues. In the case of malignant disease, the limited life expectancy of the patient may, in fact, make bony fusion unnecessary. On the other hand, when clinicians are dealing with benign disease, it is important that they recognize the limitations of instrumentation without fusion. The purpose of the instrumentation is to

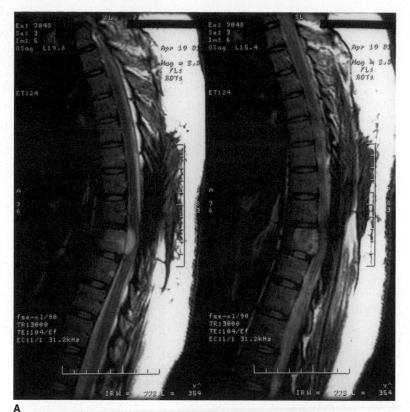

A

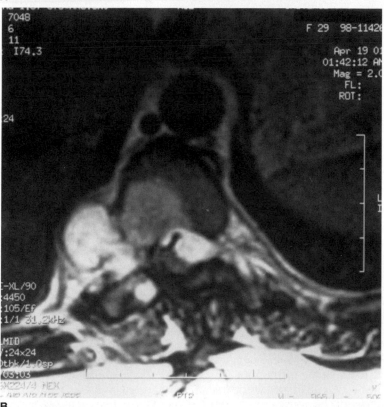

B

Figure 74.9 A 29-year-old woman presented with pain and paraparesis necessitating emergency decompression 5 months earlier. The pathologic condition was low-grade chondrosarcoma. Sagittal **(A)** and axial **(B)** magnetic resonance imaging (MRI) scans show a tumor arising from the body of T10 extending into the canal compressing the cord primarily on the patient's left side. There is also tumor extension into the paravertebral space on the right side. Through a right thoracotomy approach, the patient underwent a T10 corpectomy with tumor resection and anterior stabilization. Because of recurrence and paraparesis, posterior decompression with instrumentation was necessary 5 months later.

Continued

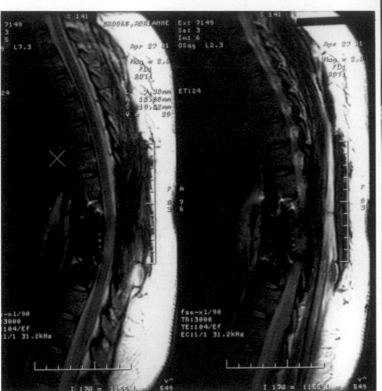

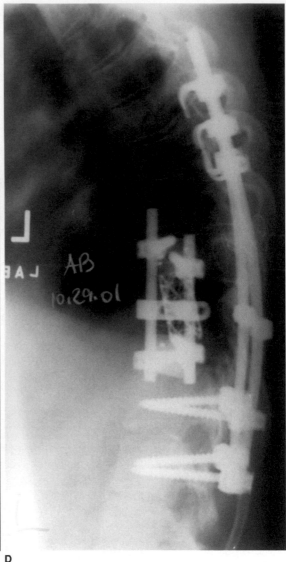

C   D

Figure 74.9 *cont'd* Postoperative sagittal MRI (**C**) shows the decompression and the hardware artifact. Plain lateral radiograph (**D**) shows the anterior titanium mesh graft and the anterior and posterior screw and hook fixation. The patient received postoperative radiation and has subsequently required further surgery for recurrence.

maintain stability and proper spinal alignment while the bony fusion is occurring. A fusion is much more likely to occur if movement at the fusion site is minimized. This can often be accomplished without instrumentation.

One of the disadvantages of using metal implants is the interference with CT and MRI. Some of the new alloys produce fewer imaging artifacts, and these alternatives, although more expensive, should be considered in some cases. Titanium implants have major advantages over stainless steel in MRI tumor recurrence. Titanium implants should be standard for spine tumor reconstruction. Other materials such as carbon fiber (e.g., OCELOT Stackable Cage System, DePuy Spine, Johnson & Johnson, Raynham, MA) were developed to readily show tumor recurrence, as well as osteointegration of bone graft, on imaging.[5]

Although the goal of surgical treatment of benign tumors involving the spine is usually total removal of the pathologic process, there are situations in which the massive size of the lesion, the benign nature of the lesion, and the overall age and status of the patient need to be considered in the decision-making process. Overaggressive surgery should be avoided. The unnecessary removal of additional bone can further compromise future stability and may necessitate more elaborate stabilization procedures than might otherwise be required.

The only legitimate method of acquiring a cure in patients with both benign and malignant tumors involving the spine is total removal of the lesion. Although total removal is often impossible to accomplish with malignant tumors, it should certainly be the goal with many benign lesions. Clearly, with a malignant diffuse process, extremely radical resections may be unwarranted.

Management of Complications

The best way to deal with complications of spine surgery is to minimize their occurrence. Some of the more common complications include inadequate wound healing (possibly related to previous radiation therapy or infection), cerebrospinal fluid leaks, deep infections, and inadequate stabilization efforts (see Chapter 88).

Cerebrospinal fluid leaks should be treated aggressively, because a persistent leak significantly increases the likelihood of infection. Although it is occasionally possible to stop a leak by simply reinforcing the skin closure with additional sutures, methods that are more elaborate are sometimes necessary. Spinal drainage via a catheter placed somewhat remote to the wound site may decrease the pressure head and allow for proper wound healing. However, if the site of the dural injury is known, it is often more appropriate to reopen that section of the wound and repair the site of the dural leak. In other cases, unhealthy, nonviable tissue overlying the dura mater may require débridement so that more viable tissue can be approximated. For patients who have received previous radiation therapy or undergone multiple surgical procedures, the assistance of a plastic surgeon may be valuable.

A deep wound infection often complicates stabilization efforts. Clearing an infection may be almost impossible if there is instrumentation at the site of infection. Nevertheless, occasionally, severe spinal instability makes it necessary to leave the instrumentation in place until the infection can be brought under control. This allows time for the bony fusion to mature. The instrumentation can then be removed and the antibiotics continued. In some cases, the implant can be salvaged.

The need for adequate and appropriate nutritional supplementation, physical therapy, and emotional support cannot be overstated. Because of the significant costs of hospitalization and of improper antibiotic use or inadequate or inappropriate nutrition, other health care professionals must help meet these needs, when appropriate, to assist the surgical team.

Summary

Primary tumors that involve the spinal axis, although rare, are often best managed by surgery. It may be the only method to effect a cure in some patients. A failure to recognize primary spinal lesions may result in the inappropriate use of other tests to rule out metastatic disease. It is important for clinicians to recognize that they should be prepared to achieve a total removal of this lesion, if the potential gain justifies the morbidity. A subtotal removal may require early reoperation. Certainly, the best time to accomplish total tumor removal is at the first surgical procedure. Proper preoperative planning and, when appropriate, preoperative embolization often results in satisfactory patient outcomes.

REFERENCES

1. Bergstrand A, Hook O, Lidvall H: Vertebral hemangiomas compressing the spinal cord. *Acta Neurol Scand* 39:59, 1963.
2. Bilsky MH, Boland PJ, Panageas KS, et al: Intralesional resection of primary and metastatic sarcoma involving the spine: Outcome analysis of 59 patients. *Neurosurgery* 49:1277, 2001.
3. Bjornsson J, Wold LE, Ebersold MJ, Laws ER: Chordoma of the mobile spine: A clinicopathologic analysis of 40 patients. *Cancer* 71:735, 1993.
4. Blankstein A, Spiegelmann R, Shacked I, et al: Hemangioma of the thoracic spine involving multiple adjacent levels: Case report. *Paraplegia* 26:186, 1988.
5. Boriani S, Biagini R, Bandiera S, et al: Reconstruction of the anterior column of the thoracic and lumbar spine with a carbon fiber stackable cage system. *Orthopedics* 25:37-42, 2002.
6. Boriani S, Biagini R, De Iure F, et al: En bloc resections of bone tumors of the thoracolumbar spine. A preliminary report on 29 patients. *Spine* 21(16):1927-1931, 1996.
7. Boriani S, Capanna R, Donati D, et al: Osteoblastoma of the spine. *Clin Orthop* 278:37, 1992.
8. Boriani S, De Iure F, Bandiera S, et al: Chondrosarcoma of the mobile spine: report on 22 cases. *Spine* 25(7):804-812, 2000.
9. Boriani S, Weinstein JN, Biagini R: Primary bone tumors of the spine. Terminology and surgical staging. *Spine* 22: 1036-1044, 1997.
10. Bradway JK, Pritchard DJ: Ewing's tumor of the spine. In: Sundaresan N, Schmidek HH, Schiller AL, Rosenthal DI (eds): *Tumors of the Spine: Diagnosis and Clinical Management*. Philadelphia, WB Saunders, 1990, p 235.
11. Brady MS, Gaynor JJ, Brenan MF: Radiation-associated sarcoma of bone and soft tissue. *Arch Surg* 127:1379-1385, 1992.
12. Byrne TN: Spinal cord compression from epidural metastases. *N Engl J Med* 327:614-619, 1992.
13. Conlon KC, Casper ES, Brennan MF: Primary gastrointestinal sarcomas: analysis of prognostic variables. *Ann Surg Oncol* 2:26-31, 1995.
14. Cummings BJ, Hodson DI, Bush RS: Chordoma: The results of megavoltage radiation therapy. *Int J Radiat Oncol Biol Phys* 9:633, 1983.
15. Dagi TF, Schmidek HH: Vascular tumors of the spine. In: Sundaresan N, Schmidek HH, Schiller AL, Rosenthal DI (eds): *Tumors of the Spine: Diagnosis and Clinical Management*. Philadelphia, WB Saunders, 1990, p 181.
16. Dahlin DC: *Bone Tumors: General Aspects and Data on 6,221 Cases*. Charles C Thomas, Springfield, IL, 1978.
17. Dahlin DC, Coventry MB: Osteogenic sarcoma, a study of 600 cases. *J Bone Joint Surg* 49A:101, 1967.
18. Dirix LY, Vermeulen P, De Wever I, Van Oosterom AT: Soft tissue sarcoma in adults. *Curr Opin Oncol* 9:348-359, 1997.
19. Djindjian M: Vertebral hemangiomas with neurologic symptoms: Summary. *Neurochirurgie* 35:264, 1989.
20. Enneking WF: A system of staging musculoskeletal neoplasms. *Clin Orthop* 204:9-24, 1986.
21. Evans RG, Nesbit ME, Gehan EA et al: Multimodal therapy for the management of localized Ewing's sarcoma of pelvic and sacral bones: A report from the second intergroup study. *J Clin Oncol* 9:1173, 1991.

21a. Farhood AI, Hajdu SI, Shiu MH, Strong EW. Soft tissue sarcomas of the head and neck in adults. *Am J Surg* 160: 365-369, 1990.

22. Faria SL, Schlupp WR, Chiminazzo H Jr: Radiotherapy in the treatment of vertebral hemangiomas. *Int J Radiat Oncol Biol Phys* 11:387, 1985.

23. Fox MW, Onofrio BW: The natural history and management of symptomatic and asymptomatic vertebral hemangiomas. *J Neurosurg* 78:36, 1993.

24. Gokaslan ZL, Romsdahl MM, Kroll SS, *et al:* Total sacrectomy and Galveston L-rod reconstruction for malignant neoplasms. *J Neurosurg* 87:781, 1997.

25. Grubb MR, Currier BL, Pritchard DJ, Ebersold MJ: Primary Ewing's sarcoma of the spine. *Spine* 19:309, 1994.

26. Hart RA, Boriani S, Biagini R, Currier B, Weinstein JN: A system for surgical staging and management of spine tumors. A clinical outcome study of giant cell tumors of the spine. *Spine* 22:1773, 1997.

27. Hay MC, Paterson D, Taylor TKF: Aneurysmal bone cysts of the spine. *J Bone Joint Surg* 60B:406, 1978.

27a. Heslin MJ, Lewis JJ, Nadler E, *et al:* Prognostic factors associated with long-term survival for retroperitoneal sarcoma: implications for management. *J Clin Oncol* 15: 2832-2839, 1997.

28. Huth JF, Dawson EG, Eilber ER: Abdominal sacral resection for malignant tumors of the sacrum. *Am J Surg* 48:157, 1984.

29. Karparov M, Kitov D: Aneurysmal bone cysts of the spine. *Acta Neurochir (Wien)* 39:101, 1977.

30. Keisch ME, Garcia DM, Shibuya RG: Retrospective long-term follow-up analysis in 21 patients with chordomas of various sites treated at a single institution. *J Neurosurg* 75:374, 1991.

31. Kempin S, Sundaresan N: Disorders of the spine related to plasma cell dyscrasias. In: Sundaresan N, Schmidek HH, Schiller AL, Rosenthal DI (eds): *Tumors of the Spine: Diagnosis and Clinical Management.* Philadelphia, WB Saunders, 1990, p 214.

32. Kostuik JP, Errico TJ, Gleason TF, *et al:* Spinal stabilization of vertebral column tumors. *Spine* 13:250, 1988.

32a. Kraus DH, Dubner S, Harrison LB, *et al:* Prognostic factors for recurrence and survival in head and neck tissue sarcomas. *Cancer* 74: 697-702, 1994.

33. Krueger EG, Sobel GL, Weinstein C: Vertebral hemangioma with compression of spinal cord. *J Neurosurg* 18:331, 1961.

34. Lang EF Jr, Peserico L: Neurologic and surgical aspects of vertebral hemangiomas. *Surg Clin North Am* 40:817, 1960.

35. Localio SA, Eng D, Ranson JH: Abdominosacral approach for retrorectal tumors. *Ann Surg* 191:555, 1980.

36. Loftus CM, Michelsen CB, Rapoport F, Antunes JL: Management of plasmacytomas of the spine. *Neurosurgery* 13:30, 1983.

37. McAllister VL, Kendall BE, Bull JW: Symptomatic vertebral haemangiomas. *Brain* 98:71, 1975.

38. McCarty CS, Waugh JM, Mayo CW, Coventry MB: The surgical treatment of presacral tumor: A combined problem. *Mayo Clin Proc* 27:73, 1952.

39. Mohan V, Ardra MM, Gupta RP *et al:* Aneurysmal bone cysts of the dorsal spine. *Arch Orthop Trauma Surg* 108:390, 1989.

40. Nesbit ME, Gehan EA, Burget EO: Multimodal therapy for the management of primary, nonmetastatic Ewing's sarcoma of bone: A long-term follow-up of the first intergroup study. *J Clin Oncol* 8:1664, 1990.

41. Nguyen JP, Djindjian M, Pavlovitch JM, *et al:* [Vertebral hemangioma with neurologic signs. Therapeutic results. Survey of the French Society of Neurosurgery.] *Neurochirurgie* 35:299, 1989 (French).

41a. Ozaki T, Flege S, Liljenqvist U, *et al:* Osteosarcoma of the spine: experience of the Cooperative Osteosarcoma Study Group. *Cancer* 94:1069-1077, 2002.

42. Pettine KA, Klassen RA: Osteoid osteoma and osteoblastoma of the spine. *J Bone Joint Surg* 68A:354, 1986.

43. Poor MM, Hitchon PW, Riggs CE Jr: Solitary spinal plasmacytomas: Management and outcome. *J Spinal Disord* 4:295, 1988.

44. Reizine D, Laredo JD, Riche MC *et al:* Vertebral hemangiomas. In: Jeanmart L (ed): *Radiology of the spine: Tumors.* Springer-Verlag, Berlin, 1986, p 73.

45. Rosenblum BR, Camins MB: Bony lesions of the cervical spine. In Camins MB, O'Leary P (eds): *Disorders of the cervical spine.* Baltimore, Williams & Wilkins, 1992, p 519.

45a. Russo P, Brady MS, Conlon K, *et al:* Adult urological sarcoma. *J Urol* 147:1032-1036, 1992.

46. Sailer SL, Harmon DC, Mankin HJ, *et al:* Ewing's sarcoma: Surgical resection as a prognostic factor. *Int J Radiat Oncol Biol Phys* 15:43, 1988.

47. Samson IR, Springfield DS, Suit HD, Mankin HJ: Operative treatment of sacrococcygeal chordoma: A review of twenty-one cases. *J Bone Joint Surg* 75A:1476, 1993.

48. Sanjay BKS, Sim FH, Unni KK, *et al:* Giant cell tumors of the spine. *J Bone Joint Surg* 75B:148, 1993.

48a. Seichi A, Kondoh T, Hozumi T, Karasawa K: Intraoperative radiation therapy for metastatic spinal tumors. *Spine* 24:470-473, 1999.

49. Sharafuddin MJA, Haddad FS, Hitchon PW, *et al:* Treatment options in primary Ewing's sarcoma of the spine: Report of seven cases and review of the literature. *Neurosurgery* 30:610, 1992.

50. Shikata J, Yamamuro T, Shimizu K *et al:* Surgical treatment of giant cell tumors of the spine. *Clin Orthop* 278:29, 1992.

51. Shives TC, Dahlin DC, Sim FH *et al:* Osteosarcoma of the spine. *J Bone Joint Surg* 68A:660, 1986.

52. Shives TC, McLeod RA, Unni KK *et al:* Chondrosarcoma of the spine. *J Bone Joint Surg* 71A:1158, 1989.

53. Sundaresan N, Rosen G, Huvos AG, Krol G: Combined treatment of osteosarcoma of the spine. *Neurosurgery* 23:714-719, 1988.

54. Sundaresan N, Rosenthal DI, Schiller AL, Krol G: Chordomas. In: Sundaresan N, Schmidek HH, Schiller AL, Rosenthal DI (eds): *Tumors of the Spine: Diagnosis and Clinical Management.* Philadelphia, WB Saunders, 1990, p 292.

54a. Talac R, Yaszewski MJ, Currier BL, *et al.* Relationship between surgical margins and local recurrence in sarcomas of the spine. *Clin Orthop* Apr:127–132, 2002.

55. Turcotte RE, Sim FH, Unni KK: Giant cell tumors of the sacrum. *Clin Orthop* 291:215, 1993.

56. Vandertop WP, Pruijs JEH, Snoeck IN, *et al:* Aneurysmal bone cyst of the thoracic spine: Radical excision with use of the Cavitron. *J Bone Joint Surg* 76A:608, 1994.

57. Weinstein JN: Surgical approach to spine tumors. *Orthopedics* 12:897, 1989.

58. Weinstein JN, McLain RF: Primary tumors of the spine. *Spine* 12:843, 1987.

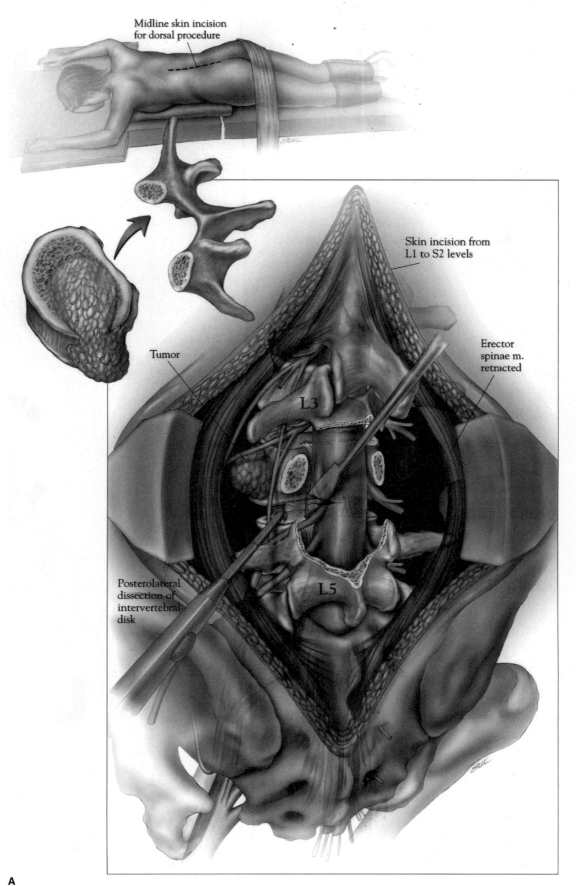

Midline skin incision
for dorsal procedure

Skin incision from
L1 to S2 levels

Erector
spinae m.
retracted

Tumor

L3

Posterolateral
dissection of
intervertebral
disk

L5

A

Figure 75.1 **(A)** Illustration of the anatomy as visualized from the posterior approach. During this
part of the procedure, the surgeon removes the posterior vertebral elements en bloc, exposing the
dura mater and involved nerve roots. A partial discectomy is also performed during this part of
the operation. Inset: Illustration of patient positioning for the posterior-approach stage of the
procedure, showing skin incisions involved. *Continued*

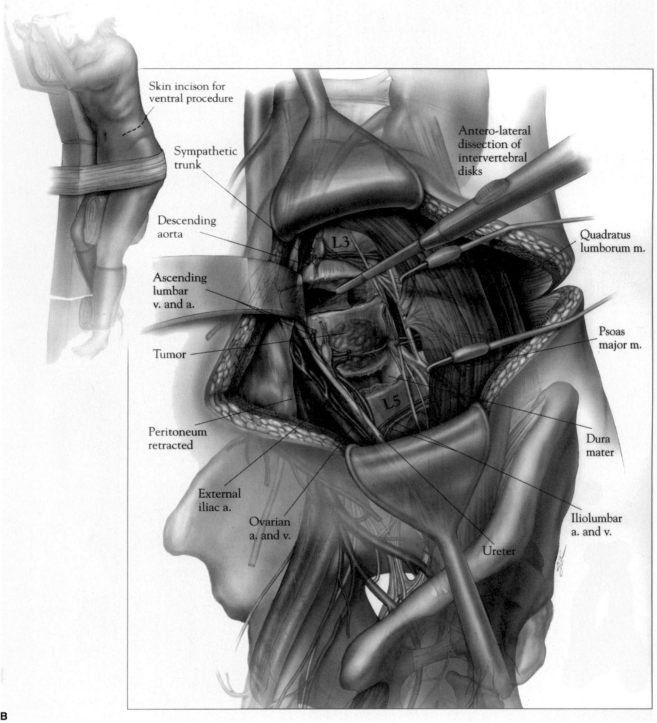

B

Figure 75.1 *cont'd* (B) Illustration of anatomy as visualized from the anterolateral approach. During this part of the procedure, the surgeon completes the discectomy and divides the ligamentous attachments of the vertebral body to allow for the en bloc removal of the anterior part of the involved vertebra. *Inset*: Illustration of patient positioning for the anterolateral-approach part of the procedure, showing the skin incision involved. *a*, artery; *v*, vein.

Partial mobilization of the sacrum facilitates identification of the sacrospinous and sacrotuberous ligaments, which are then transected. The rectum is dissected from the distal sacrococcygeal attachments. The previously placed silastic sheath, visualized at this point, serves as a guide in this dissection. Sacral nerve roots are divided as they exit the sacrum, protecting the sciatic nerves from injury. The entire sacrum, along with the neoplasm, is then removed en bloc (see Figure 75.2, *lower left*).

A vertebral spacer, such as autograft, fresh and/or frozen allograft, alumina ceramic vertebral prosthesis (Kyocera, Kyoto, Japan), apatite-wollastonite glass-ceramic prosthesis (Lederle, Tokyo, Japan), or titanium mesh cylinder (MOSS Miami, DePuy Motech, Warsaw, IN), is inserted properly to the anchor holes within the remaining healthy vertebrae. After checking the appropriate position of the vertebral spacer radiographically, the surgeon adjusts the posterior instrumentation to slightly compress the inserted vertebral spacer. Finally, Marlex mesh (CR Bard Inc., Billerica, MA) is placed to cover the entire ventral and dorsal reconstructed areas to reduce bleeding.

5. Postoperative management. Draining by suction is the preferred treatment for patients 2 to 3 days after surgery, and the patient is allowed to begin walking 1 week after surgery. The patient wears a thoracolumbar orthosis for 2 to 3 months until the bony union or incorporation of the artificial vertebral prosthesis is attained.

Lower lumbar spondylectomy is depicted in Figure 75.1.

Total Sacrectomy and Reconstruction for Malignant Neoplasms

Primary sacral neoplasms involving S1 and S2 are amenable to complete en bloc resections for possible cure. Tumors selected for the surgery ideally have a low propensity for metastasis and yet are symptomatic and unresponsive to noninterventional therapy (e.g., giant-cell tumors and low-grade malignant tumors such as chondrosarcomas and chordomas).

Subtotal resection of the sacrum caudal to the midportion of the S1 vertebral body does not destabilize the pelvis. However, total sacrectomy requires establishment of a bilateral union between the lumbar spine and the ilium, as well as reconstruction of the pelvic ring.[5,16] Preservation of the lumbar roots allows ambulation; however, urinary bladder, rectosigmoid colon, and sexual function are markedly altered, although manageable with rehabilitation. The indications for sacrectomy suggested by Gokaslan et al.[14] are as follows:

1. Intractable pain
2. Impairment of sacral nerve functions
3. Localized progressive disease
4. The absence of effective noninterventional treatments

Two patients with localized primary giant cell tumors have been treated by Gokaslan.[14] This is a complex operation.

The Galveston L-rod technique used in this study[2] is recommended by Gokaslan[14] as the optimal reconstructive method after total sacrectomy. Each Galveston rod forms a one-piece bridge between the lumbar spine and ilium, and the transiliac rod completes the pelvic ring. Augmented by both autologous and allogeneic bone grafts, this instrumentation system prevents both caudal migration and axial rotation of the spinal column, while simultaneously preventing the open-book phenomenon with the use of a threaded transiliac rod placed more anteriorly on the

ilium. This system provides stability around the horizontal axis of the spinal column while preventing rotation around this axis.[14]

Surgical Technique

Surgery was performed in two stages, with an interval of 21 (Case 1) and 17 (Case 2) days between stages.

Stage I. The goal of this stage is to mobilize and dissect visceral and vascular structures from the ventral portion of L5 and the sacrum. A midline celiotomy is performed through an abdominal incision made to expose this region, and the rectosigmoid colon is dissected from the presacral fascia to the coccygeal region. The internal iliac arteries and veins and the lateral and median sacral vessels are divided at their origin to allow ample exposure of the first and second anterior sacral nerve roots (Figure 75.2, *upper left*). The common iliac vessels, distal vena cava, and aorta are mobilized after division of small posterior vessels arising from these structures. Lateral dissection of the ala of the sacrum allows identification of the lumbar trunk (L4-5) of the lumbosacral plexus. The sacroiliac joint is identified lateral to these nerve roots, and bilateral partial ventral sacroiliac osteotomy is performed (see Figure 75.2, *upper right*). The lumbosacral disc is exposed and removed along with the anterior aspect of the annulus fibrosis. The ventral sacral periosteum is electrocoagulated, and the S1-3 ventral nerve roots are divided at their foramina, if they are not obscured by the tumor.

A flexible, thin silastic sheath is placed dorsal to the vascular structures and the rectum, isolating them from the lumbar vertebrae and sacrum. This inhibits formation of adhesions between these structures and aids in the performance of the second stage of the operation. After Stage I, a significant ileus lasting approximately 8 days occurs because of interruption of the autonomic presacral nerves.

Stage II. Stage II is begun by reopening the celiotomy incision. A unilateral myocutaneous pedicle flap fed by the inferior epigastric vessels is mobilized to the pelvic inlet, dorsal to the rectosigmoid colon but ventral to the previously placed silastic sheath (see Figure 75.2, *center left*). The abdominal incision is closed, and the patient is placed in the prone jackknife position for sacral resection through the dorsal midline approach.

The dorsal incision extends from L2 to beyond the coccyx, leaving skin, subcutaneous tissue, and muscle in place over the sacrum to facilitate en bloc resection. The posterior iliac crests, greater sciatic foramina, and sciatic nerves are exposed bilaterally, as are the L3-5 spinous processes, facet joints, and transverse processes. An L5 laminectomy exposes the thecal sac and cauda equina below this level. Sacral nerve roots are then divided, and the thecal sac is closed with a double layer of sutures. The remaining posterior L5-S1 intervertebral disc is excised, and the posterosuperior iliac spines are removed, facilitating bilateral osteotome cuts lateral to the ala of the sacrum and parallel to the sacroiliac joints, thus completing the osteotomy cuts made in these planes during the Stage I procedure (see Figure 75.2, *center right*).

the vena cava. A straight, vertical midline incision is made over the spinous processes and is extended three vertebrae above and below the involved segment(s). The paraspinal muscles are dissected from the spinous processes and the laminae and then are retracted laterally. If the patient underwent posterior biopsy, the tracts are dissected carefully in a manner similar to that used in the limb-salvaging procedure. After a careful dissection of the area around the facet joints, a large retractor (termed the *articulated spinal retractor*) is applied. (The articulated spinal retractor has a uniaxial joint in each limb and was designed for this surgery.) By spreading the retractor and detaching the muscles around the facet joints, the surgeon then obtains a wider exposure. The surgical field must be wide enough on both sides to allow dissection under the surface of the transverse processes. In the thoracic spine, the ribs on the affected level are transected 3 to 4cm lateral to the costotransverse joint, and the pleura is separated bluntly from the vertebra. For the surgeon to expose the superior articular process of the uppermost vertebra, the spinous and the inferior articular processes of the neighboring vertebra are osteotomized and removed with dissection of the attached soft tissues, including the ligamentum flavum.

2. Introduction of the T-saw guide. To make an exit for the T-saw guide through the nerve root canal, the surgeon dissects and removes the soft tissue attached to the inferior aspect of the pars interarticularis, using utmost care not to damage the corresponding nerve root. A C-curved, malleable T-saw guide then is introduced through the intervertebral foramen in a cephalocaudal direction. In this procedure, the tip of the T-saw guide should be introduced along the medial cortex of the lamina and the pedicle so that the spinal cord and the nerve root are not injured. After the T-saw guide is passed, its tip at the exit of the nerve root canal can be found beneath the inferior border of the pars interarticularis. In the next step, a flexible, multifilament 0.54mm diameter thread-wire saw is passed through the hole in the T-saw guide and is clamped with a T-salo clamp at each end. The T-saw guide is removed, and tension on the thread-wire saw is maintained. When two or three vertebrae are resected, the thread-wire saw is inserted into a thin polyethylene tube (T-saw catheter), and the saw and tube are passed under the lamina. This procedure also is applied to the contralateral side.

3. Cutting the pedicles and resection of the dorsal element. While tension is maintained, the thread-wire saw is placed beneath the superior articular and transverse processes with a specially designed T-saw manipulator. With this procedure, the thread-wire saw placed around the lamina is wrapped around the pedicle. With a reciprocating motion of the thread-wire saw, the pedicles are cut, and then the whole dorsal element of the spine (the spinous process, the superior and inferior articular processes, the transverse process, and the pedicle) is removed in one piece. The cut surface of the pedicle is sealed with bone wax to reduce bleeding and to minimize

contamination by tumor cells. To maintain stability after segmental resection of the anterior column, the surgeon performs a temporary posterior instrumentation.

Step 2: en bloc corpectomy (resection of the ventral column of the vertebra)

1. Blunt dissection around the vertebral body. At the beginning of the second step, the segmental arteries must be identified bilaterally. The spinal branch of the segmental artery, which runs along the nerve root, is ligated and divided. This procedure exposes the segmental artery, which appears just lateral to the cut edge of the pedicle. In the thoracic spine, the nerve root is cut on the side from which the affected vertebra is removed. The blunt dissection is performed anteriorly on both sides through the plane between the pleura (or the iliopsoas muscle) and the vertebral body. Usually, the lateral aspect of the body is dissected easily with a curved vertebral spatula. Then the segmental artery should be dissected from the vertebral body. By continuing dissection of both lateral sides of the vertebral body ventrally, the aorta is carefully dissected dorsally from the ventral aspect of the vertebral body with a spatula and the surgeon's fingers. When the surgeon's fingertips meet with each other anterior to the vertebral body, a series of spatulas, starting from the smallest size, is inserted sequentially to extend the dissection. A pair of the largest spatulas is kept in the dissection site to prevent the surrounding tissues and organs from iatrogenesis and to make the surgical field wide enough for manipulating the ventral column.

2. Passage of the thread-wire saw. Thread-wire saws are inserted at the proximal and distal cutting levels of the vertebral bodies where grooves are made along the desired cutting line using a V-notched osteotome after the disc levels have been confirmed using needles.

3. Dissection of the spinal cord and removal of the vertebra. Using a cord spatula, the surgeon mobilizes the spinal cord from the surrounding venous plexus and the ligamentous tissue. The teeth-cord protector, which has teeth on both edges to prevent the thread-wire saw from slipping, then is applied. The thread-wire saw cuts the ventral column of the vertebra and the anterior and posterior longitudinal ligaments. After cutting the anterior column, the surgeon again checks the mobility of the vertebra to ensure a complete corpectomy. The freed ventral column is rotated around the spinal cord and removed carefully to avoid injury to the spinal cord. With this procedure, a complete ventral and dorsal decompression of the spinal cord (circumspinal decompression) and total en bloc resection of the vertebral tumor are achieved.

4. Ventral reconstruction and dorsal instrumentation. Bleeding, which occurs mainly from the venous plexus within the spinal canal, should be arrested completely. An anchor hole on the cut end of the remaining vertebra is made on each side to seat the graft.

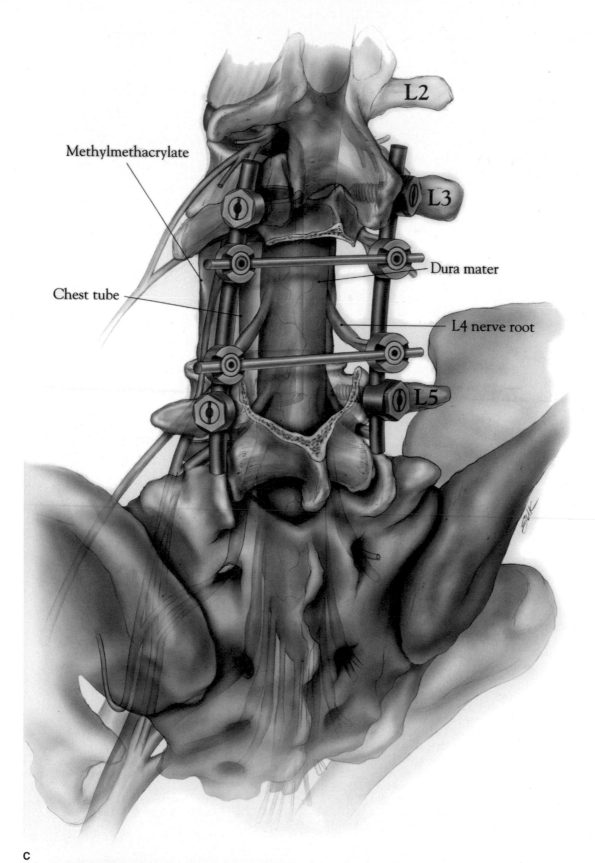

Methylmethacrylate

Chest tube

L2

L3

Dura mater

L4 nerve root

L5

C

Figure 75.1 *cont'd* (C) Illustration (posterior view) showing the posterior instrumentation, in which pedicle screws were used, and the anterior reconstruction of the L4 vertebral body with part of a chest tube and methylmethacrylate.   *Continued*

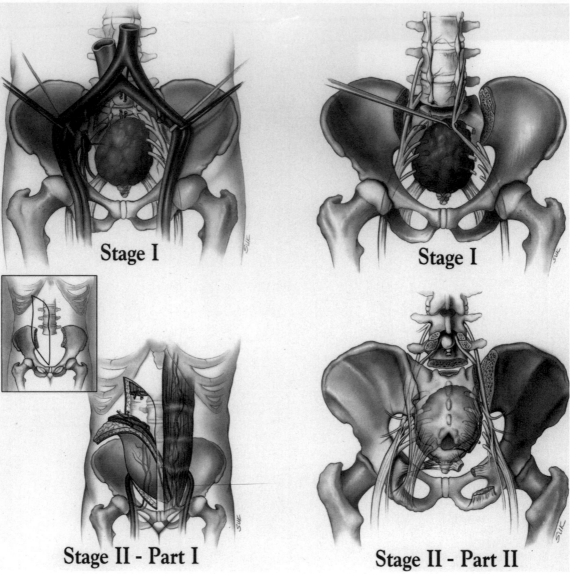

Figure 75.2 Illustrations depicting the operative fields during Stages I and II of total sacrectomy. *Upper left*: Stage I. Ventral view of lumbosacral region after median celiotomy. Inferior vena cava and aorta (and their main branches) are mobilized, allowing a clear view of the L5-S1 disc space and permitting retraction of these vessels for lumbar trunk (L4-5 nerve roots) identification. Median and lateral sacral vessels and internal hypogastric vessels are ligated. The S1 foramina and nerve roots are also visualized bilaterally; the tumor usually obscures the lower sacral nerve roots (S2-5). Visualized sacral roots are then transected ventrally while the lumbar trunk is preserved. *Upper right*: Stage I. Ventral view of lumbosacral region with the vessels removed. Nerve roots at S1-3 are transected ventrally. Using a diamond burr, the surgeon performs partial (ventral) sacroiliac osteotomy lateral to the lumbar trunk. *Center left*: Stage II, Part I. Ventral view of abdominal wall while the patient is supine. A vascularized musculus rectus abdominis with an island of skin and subcutaneous adipose tissue is harvested from the location outlined in the *inset*. Taking care to preserve the inferior epigastric vessels, the surgeon places this flap in the abdominal cavity and closes the incision. *Center right*: Stage II, Part II. Dorsal view of the lumbosacral region while the patient is in the jackknife position after completion of L5 laminectomy and bilateral L5-S1 foraminotomy. The completed L5-S1 discectomy and dorsal sacroiliac osteotomy are also shown. The thecal sac is ligated distal to the takeoff of the L5 nerve roots bilaterally.

Reconstruction of the Sacrum

Two vertical L-shaped rods are positioned bilaterally in a manner allowing fixation to the L3-5 pedicles on each side, according to the Galveston technique. Two to three cross-connecting rods are used to secure the vertical rods to each other. Distally, the vertical rods are directed laterally into the ilium between the two cortices. A transverse threaded rod (transiliac bar) is placed to fix opposing iliac bones to each other and thereby prevent axial rotation of

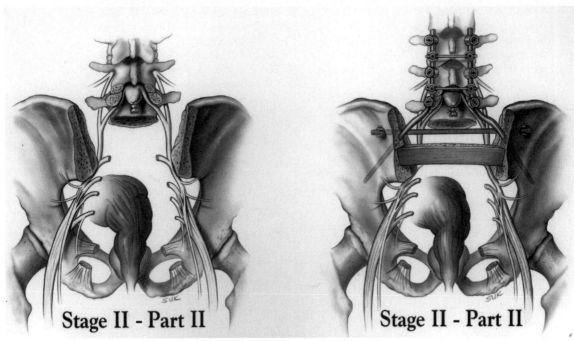

Figure 75.2 *cont'd* *Lower left*: Stage II, Part II. Dorsal view of lumboiliac region after en bloc removal of sacrum. The cut ends of nerve roots S1-4 are shown bilaterally, as are the bilaterally preserved lumbar trunk and remaining sciatic nerve. Sacrotuberous and sacrospinous ligament cut ends are also depicted. The dorsal rectal wall is viewed ventrally. *Lower right*: Stage II, Part II. Dorsal view of the lumbosacral region after en bloc removal of sacrum. The cut ends of nerve roots S1-4 are shown bilaterally, as are the bilaterally preserved lumbar trunk and remaining sciatic nerve. Sacrotuberous and sacrospinous ligament cut ends are also depicted. The dorsal rectal wall is viewed ventrally. *Lower right*: Stage II, Part II. Dorsal view of the lumbosacral region after reconstruction. Pedicle screws are seen bilaterally at L3-5 along with rods that are attached to the screws and bent (L-shaped) and embedded between the cortices of the remaining ilia as reported in the Galveston technique. A threaded rod (transiliac bar) is placed ventral to the Galveston rods but dorsal to the lumbar trunk, and the ends outside the iliac cortical surface are secured with C-shaped clamps. The tibial allograft is seen bridging the defect between the remaining ilia.

the lumboiliac union (see Figure 75.2, *lower right*). Both autologous (from posterior iliac crests) and allogeneic bone grafts are placed to promote fusion of the transverse processes and lamina from L3 distally to the medioposterior aspect of the transected ilium bilaterally. A tibial allograft strut is used to close the space between the two ilia, and a bone fusion promoter (e.g., Grafton) and bone chips (allograft) are added across the graft area to facilitate fusion of the entire defect (see Figure 75.2).

The previously mobilized rectus abdominis myocutaneous pedicle flap is advanced through the pelvis, positioned over the reconstructed area, and secured to gluteus muscles and skin after closed drains are placed.

Summary

TES and total sacrectomy are technically demanding procedures with significant associated morbidity and mortality. The patients who are candidates for these procedures should be carefully chosen using a multidisciplinary approach. In properly selected cases, en bloc resection of these neoplasms should be the goal of surgical treatment, because it provides improved overall disease-free survival rates and functional outcome, as well as pain control.

REFERENCES

1. Adachi B: *Das arteriensystem der japaner*. Maruzen Publishing, Kyoto, Tokyo, 1928.
2. Allen BL Jr, Ferguson RL: The Galveston technique for L rod instrumentation of the scoliotic spine. *Spine* 7:276, 1982.
3. Askin GN, Webb JK: The management of spinal neoplasia. In Torrens MJ, Dickinson RA (eds): *Operative Spinal Surgery*. Churchill Livingstone, Edinburgh, 1991.
4. Barwick KW, Huvos AG, Smith J: Primary osteogenic sarcoma of the vertebral column: Clinicopathologic correlation of ten patients. *Cancer* 46:595, 1980.
5. Blatter G, Ward EGH, Ruflin G, *et al:* The problem of stabilization after sacrectomy. *Arch Orthop Trauma Surg* 114:40, 1994.
6. Boriani S, Biagini R, De Iure F, *et al:* Vertebrectomia lombare per neoplasia ossea: Tecnica chirurgica. *Chir Organi Mov* 79:163, 1994.
7. Boriani S, Chevalley F, Weinstein J, *et al:* Chordoma of the spine above the sacrum: Treatment and outcome in 21 cases. *Spine* 21:1569, 1996.
8. Bradford DS, Bueff HU: Miscellaneous problems: Benign and malignant tumors of the spine. In Lonstein JE, Bradford DS, Winter RB, Ogilvie JW (eds): *Moe's Textbook*

of Scoliosis and Other Spinal Deformities, ed 3. WB Saunders, Philadelphia, 1995.

9. Bridwell KH, Ogilvie JW: Primary tumors of the spine (benign and malignant). In Bridwell KH, DeWald RH (eds): *The textbook of spinal surgery*, vol 2. JB Lippincott, Philadelphia, 1991.

10. De Santis E, Gasparini G, Pallotta F, Lisai P: Cordoma: Rassegna di 11 casi. *Arch Tutti Chir Organi Mov* 38:323, 1990.

11. Dreghorn CR, Newman RJ, Hardy GJ, Dickman RA: Primary tumors of the axial skeleton: Experience of the Leeds Regional Bone Tumor Registry. *Spine* 15:137, 1990.

12. Enneking WF, Spanier SS, Goodmann MA: A system for the surgical staging of musculoskeletal sarcoma. *Clin Orthop* 153:106, 1980.

13. Fujita T, Ueda Y, Kawahara N, *et al:* Local spread of metastatic vertebral tumors. A histologic study. *Spine* 22:1905, 1997.

14. Gokaslan Z, Romsdahl M, Kroll S, *et al:* Total sacrectomy and Galveston L-rod reconstruction for malignant neoplasms. *J Neurosurg* 87:787, 1997.

15. Grubb MR, Currier BC, Pritchard DJ, Ebersold MJ: Primary Ewing's sarcoma of the spine. *Spine* 19:309, 1994.

16. Gunterberg B, Romanus B, Stener B: Pelvic strength after major amputation of the sacrum. An experimental study. *Acta Orthop Scand* 47:635, 1976.

17. Hermann G, Sacher M, Lanzieri CF, *et al:* Chondrosarcoma of the spine: An unusual radiographic presentation. *Skeletal Radiol* 14:178, 1985.

18. Kawahara N, Tomita K, Baba H, *et al:* Cadaveric vascular anatomy for total en bloc spondylectomy in malignant vertebral tumors. *Spine* 21:1401, 1996.

19. Keish ME, Garcia DM, Shibuya RB: Retrospective long term follow-up analysis in 21 patients with chordomas of various sites treated at a single institution. *J Neurosurg* 75:374, 1991.

20. Loftus CM, Michelsen CB, Rapoport F, Antunes JL: Management of plasmacytomas of the spine. *Neurosurgery* 13:30, 1983.

21. Lubicky JP, Patel NS, De Wald RL: Two-staged spondylectomy for a giant-cell tumor of L4. *Spine* 8:112, 1983.

22. Lybert MLM, Meerwalddt JH: Chordoma: Report on treatment results in eighteen cases. *Acta Radiol Oncol* 25:41, 1986.

23. Magerl F, Coscia MF: Total posterior vertebrectomy of the thoracic or lumbar spine. *Clin Orthop* 232:62, 1988.

24. Marmor E, Rhines L, Weinberg J, Gokaslan Z: Total en bloc lumbar spondylectomy. *J Neurosurg* 95(2 Suppl):264, 2001.

25. McLain RF, Weinstein JN: Solitary plasmacytomas of the spine: A review of 84 cases. *J Spinal Disord* 2:69, 1989.

26. Parke WW, Whalen JL, Van Demark RE, Kambin P: The infra-aortic arteries of the spine: Their variability and clinical significance. *Spine* 19:1, 1994.

27. Poor MM, Hitchon PW, Riggs CE Jr: Solitary spinal plasmacytomas. Management and outcome. *J Spinal Disord* 1:295, 1988.

28. Rich TA, Schiller A, Suit HD, Mankin HJ: Clinical and pathological review of 48 cases of chordoma. *Cancer* 56:182, 1985.

29. Roy-Camille R, Saillant G, Bisserie M, *et al:* Resection vertebrale totale dans la chirurgie tumorale au niveau du rachis dorsal par voie posterieure pure. *Rev Chir Orthop* 67:421, 1981.

30. Savini R, Gherlinzoni F, Morandi M, *et al:* Surgical treatment of giant-cell tumor of the spine: The experience at the Instituto Orthopedico Rizzoli. *J Bone Joint Surg* 65A:1283, 1983.

31. Shapiro S: Myelopathy secondary to leiomyosarcoma of the spine: Case report. *Spine* 17:249, 1992.

32. Stener B: Total spondylectomy in chondrosarcoma arising from the seventh thoracic vertebra. *J Bone Joint Surg* 53B:288, 1971.

33. Stener B: Complete removal of vertebrae for extirpation of tumors. *Clin Orthop* 245:72, 1989.

34. Stener B: Technique of complete spondylectomy in the thoracic and lumbar spine. In Sundaresan N, Schmidek HH, Schiller AL, Rosenthal DI (eds): *Tumors of the Spine: Diagnosis and Clinical Management*. Philadelphia, WB Saunders, 1990.

35. Sundaresan N, Rosen G, Huvos AG, Krol G: Combined treatment of osteosarcoma of the spine. *Neurosurgery* 23:714, 1988.

36. Sundaresan N, Rosental DI, Schiller AL, Krol G: Chordomas. In Sundaresan N, Schmidek HH, Schiller AL, Rosenthal DI (eds): *Tumors of the Spine: Diagnosis and Clinical Management*. Philadelphia, WB Saunders, 1990.

37. Tomita K, Kawahara N, Baba H, *et al:* Total en bloc spondylectomy for solitary spinal metastasis. *Int Orthop* 18:291, 1994.

38. Tomita K, Kawahara N, Baba H, *et al:* Total en bloc spondylectomy: A new surgical technique for primary malignant vertebral tumors. *Spine* 22:324, 1997.

39. Tomita K, Kawahara N, Mizuno K, *et al:* Total en bloc spondylectomy for primary malignant vertebral tumors. In: Rao RS, Deo MG, Sanghvi LD, Mittra I (eds): *Proceedings of the XVI International Cancer Congress, New Delhi, India, October 30-November 5, 1994*. Monduzzi Editore, Bologna, 1994.

40. Tomita K, Kawahara N, Takahashi K, *et al:* Total en bloc spondylectomy for malignant vertebral tumors. *Orthop Trans* 18:1166, 1994.

41. Tomita K, Kawahara N, Toribatake Y, *et al: Oncological radical surgery for primary vertebral tumours: Total en bloc spondylectomy*. Presented at the 62nd Annual Meeting of the American Academy of Orthopaedic Surgeons, Orlando, Florida, February 16, 1995.

42. Tsuchiya H, Yasutake H, Yokogawa A, *et al:* Effect of chemotherapy combined with caffeine for osteosarcoma. *J Cancer Res Clin Oncol* 118:567, 1992.

43. Weinstein JN: Differential diagnosis and surgical treatment of primary benign and malignant neoplasms. In Frymoyer JW, Ducker TB, Halder NM, *et al* (eds): *The Adult Spine: Principles and Practice*, vol 1. New York, Raven Press, 1991.

44. Weinstein JN, McLain RF: Primary tumors of the spine. *Spine* 12:843, 1987.

45. Winter RB, Denis F, Lonstein JL, Caramelia J: Techniques of surgery: Anatomy of thoracic intercostals and lumbar arteries. In Lonstein JL, Bradford DS, Winter RB, Ogilvie JW (eds): *Moe's Textbook of Scoliosis and Other Spinal Deformities*, ed 3. Philadelphia, WB Saunders, 1994.

CHAPTER 76

Metastatic Spine Tumors

Mark H. Bilsky and Todd W. Vitaz

The development of better neo-adjuvant strategies for the treatment of primary solid tumor malignancies has led to significant improvements in loco-regional control. Therefore, patients with these tumors are surviving longer and thus more patients are developing metastatic disease. As a result, the incidence of spine metastases has increased in recent years. Between 5% and 10% of patients will develop symptomatic spine metastases at some point during their disease course.[10,215] The vast majority of these include disease of the vertebral body, with or without epidural compression; however, in rare instances tumors may also spread intradurally. Breast, prostate, and lung cancers are the most common primary tumors that spread to the spine; however, hematologic malignancies, such as myeloma and Hodgkin's disease, are also frequently seen (Table 76.1).[77]

The early diagnosis and treatment of metastatic spine tumors is essential to reducing pain, preserving or improving neurologic function, and improving quality of life. Radiation therapy (RT), surgery, and chemotherapy continue to be important treatment options for these patients. While these modalities are all essential for treating metastatic spine tumors, no prospective trial has established the role of any modality as first-line therapy. The decision-making process for each patient must be individualized based on the patient's symptoms and disease presentation as well as the institutional experience and individual preferences of the treating physician.

At Memorial Sloan-Kettering Cancer Center (MSKCC), treatment decisions are based on a conceptual framework that evaluates biomechanical, neurologic, and oncologic considerations in the context of a patient's medical co-morbidities and the extent of disease. Biomechanical issues include the presence of mechanical pain, pattern of bone involvement, and the presence of coronal (scoliosis) and sagittal (kyphosis) plane deformities. Neurologic issues include the presence and degree of radiculopathy, myelopathy, and radiographic epidural spinal cord compression. Oncologic issues reflect the radiation and/or chemosensitivity of a given tumor type. The evaluation of patients based on these concepts has provided a more objective rationale to make treatment decisions. This chapter reviews the physiology, presentation, imaging considerations, and treatment options that must be considered to determine the optimal treatment paradigm for each individual patient.

Pathophysiology of Epidural Spine Metastasis

Tumor cells predominantly metastasize to heavily vascularized skeletal structures (red bone marrow) such as vertebral bodies, ribs, or proximal long bones.[152] The predilection to metastasize to a specific area of the spine is based on the volume and number of vertebral bodies; thus 70% of metastases are found in the thoracic spine, 20% in the lumbar spine, and 10% in the cervical spine.

Blood Supply

The high propensity for metastatic vertebral body involvement is related to physiologic properties of blood flow. Batson's plexus has been implicated in the wide dissemination of prostate cancer to the spine and accounts for the high percentage of vertebral body disease, as opposed to posterior element involvement.[152] This system is a high volume, low pressure, valveless network of veins that communicates with the pelvic plexus and intercostal veins. Arterial spread has also been implicated as a potential cause and intracardiac injection of tumor cells in animals results in patterns of metastatic tumor similar to those observed in clinical scenarios.[7,155,182] Such tumor embolization may explain the predilection for bone metastases to occur at the terminal end of major feeding arteries that supply the bone,[194,214] and may be the route for dissemination to the dorsal spinal elements (i.e., laminae and pedicles) (Figure 76.1).

Seed and Soil Theory

Certain tumors such as lung, prostate, and breast have a strong predilection for metastasizing to bone. In 1889, Paget proposed the "seed and soil" theory of distant metastases.[120,166] A great deal of research has been conducted recently to elucidate the mechanisms of distant spread and the creation of osteolytic and osteoblastic metastases. Tumor dissemination is a multistep process that involves specific tumor and host tissue interactions termed the *metastatic cascade* (Figure 76.2). Angiogenesis not only allows for growth of the tumor at the primary site but it also gives these cells access to the systemic circulation. Cell adhesion molecules, such as laminins, integrins, and E-cadherin, allow tumor cells to attach to other tumor cells and to extracellular structures such as the basement membranes of blood vessels.[*] Next, proteolytic enzymes, such as matrix metalloproteinases and type IV collagenase, are released, which cause destruction of the basement membrane, allowing the malignant cells to gain access into the intravascular space and then exit this space at some distant site.[†] Once situated at these distant sites, the cells must be able to continue to replicate and induce further angiogenesis in order to form a metastatic deposit. This process is mediated by numerous growth factors, as well as the uncoupling of other cellular processes such as cell-cell suppression, angiogenesis, and bone turnover.[‡] In fact, only

---

[*]References 10,13,87,93,130,138,155,159,160,185,190,201,214.
[†]References 11,31,62,63,72,90.
[‡]References 4,13,31,62,63,87,90,93,130,138,155,159,160,173,185,190, 201,214.

1% of tumor cells that reach the intravascular space survive, with even fewer being able to establish a foothold at a distant site and grow into a micrometastatic deposit.[118]

The osteolysis that is associated with many bone metastases is not simply a mechanism of tumor replacing or destroying bone, but a complex process centered on the activation of osteoclasts causing dysregulated bone remodeling.[104] This has been well elucidated in a breast cancer model where parathyroid hormone-related peptide (PTH-rP) released by tumor cells was found to stimulate osteoclastic bone resorption.[152] In addition, the local release of TGF-B also increases the activity of PTH-rP, and other cytokines, most notably interleukin-6 (IL-6), enhance PTH-rp activity via up-regulation of osteoclast progenitor cells.[45,170,222,230] Conversely, osteoblastic metastases, which are most commonly seen with prostate cancer, arise as a result of stimulation of osteoblasts via a numerous regulatory proteins such as TGF-B, fibroblast growth factors, prostate specific antigen, and bone morphogenic protein.[§]

Contiguous Spread

The spine may also be involved by the growth of surrounding lesions, such as chest wall, mediastinal and paraspinal masses, with extension into the spinal canal through the neuroforamen. This pattern is most commonly seen in neuroblastoma, sarcoma, and superior sulcus lung (Pancoast's) tumors. Tumors may grow through the neuroforamen to involve the epidural space causing spinal cord compression, without involvement of the surrounding bony structures. Because of the absence of bone involvement, these patients do not present with typical prodromal pain complaints unless they have pain attributed to the paraspinal or rib lesions. However, these patients have a much higher incidence of neurologic deficit from spinal cord or lower cervical nerve root compression at the time of diagnosis. In addition, metabolic imaging studies, such as radionucleotide bone scans, may be falsely negative because of the limited bone disease; thus underscoring the necessity of magnetic resonance imaging (MRI) for the evaluation of back pain in cancer patients (Figure 76.3).

Presentation

Pain is the most common presenting symptom in patients with metastatic tumors to the spine. This often precedes the

TABLE 76.1	
Review of Primary Cancers with Spinal Metastases seen at M.D. Anderson Cancer Center, 1984-1994*	
Primary Site	**% of all Spine Metastases (n = 11,884)**
Breast	30.2
Lung	20.3
Blood	10.2
Prostate	9.6
Urinary tract	4.0
Skin	3.1
Unknown primary	2.9
Colon	1.6
Other	18.1

*Adapted from Gokaslan ZL, York JE, Walsh GL, *et al:* Transthoracic vertebrectomy for metastatic spinal tumors. *J Neurosurg* 89:599-609, 1998.

§References 1,29,30,32,41,42,53,85,86,95,115,126,136,137,157,175-177, 202,203.

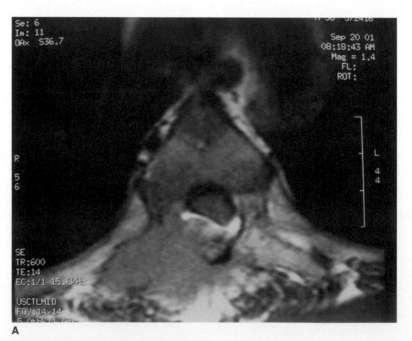

A

Figure 76.1 (A-B) Axial T$_2$-weighted MR images from a patient with metastatic hepatocellular carcinoma involving the right pedicle and dorsal elements with epidural disease resulting in spinal cord compression and deformation.

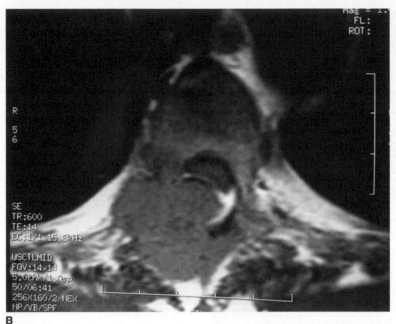

B

Figure 76.1 *cont'd*

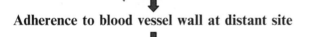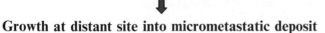

Growth at primary site

⬇

Angiogenesis

⬇

Loss of cell-cell adhesion

⬇

Migration across basement membrane and
entrance into intravascular space

⬇

Adherence to blood vessel wall at distant site

⬇

Migration across basement membrane and
entrance into extracellular space

⬇

Growth at distant site into micrometastatic deposit

⬇

Angiogenesis

⬇

Growth into Macrometastatic Lesion

Figure 76.2 Metastatic cascade.

development of other neurologic symptoms by weeks or months. Back pain in a cancer patient should be assumed to be from metastatic disease until proven otherwise. Two distinct types of back pain are encountered in these patients: (1) biologic (i.e., tumor-related) and (2) mechanical.[19]

Biologic pain predominantly affects patients during the night or early in the morning and generally improves as the day progresses. A variety of causes have been proposed as a mechanism for this type of pain, including the local release of cytokines, periosteal irritation, stimulation of intraosseous nerves, and increased pressure or mass effect from tumor tissue in the bone.[77] Biologic pain generally responds to the administration of low-dose steroids (e.g., Dexamethasone 12mg per day). Definitive treatment of the underlying tumor with radiation or surgery often relieves this pain. Recurrence of biologic pain following treatment may be a harbinger of locally recurrent tumor.

Mechanical pain results from a structural abnormality of the spine, such as a lytic bone destruction of the vertebral body or facet joints resulting in instability. The diagnosis of instability in patients with spine metastasis is based almost solely on clinical symptoms as opposed to radiographic findings.[165] Radiographic criteria of instability have been developed for trauma but these are not necessarily applicable to pathologic fractures. With the exception of the atlanto-axial spine, the authors have not found dynamic radiographic findings to be helpful in determining which patients require surgical intervention or in predicting response to other treatment modalities.[19] Mechanical pain is typically worsened with movement and maneuvers that increase the axial load of the spine, such as sitting or standing. Patients with thoracic or thoracolumbar compression fractures may also develop an unstable kyphosis, in which the pain is worsened when the patient lies flat (secondary to extension or straightening of the kyphosis). Mechanical pain does not typically respond to steroids, but may be relieved with narcotics or an external orthosis, pending definitive therapy. Patients with intractable mechanical pain are often considered strong candidates for operation. One should avoid the use of an external orthosis in these patients unless their medical condition precludes surgery. Cancer patients do not tolerate such devices because of their limited physiologic reserves.

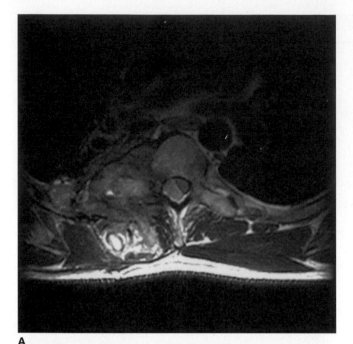

A

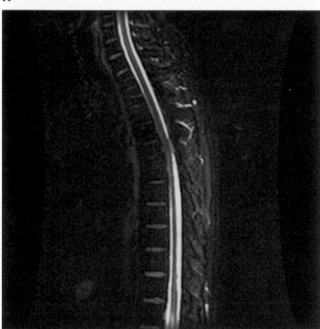

B

Figure 76.3 **(A)** Axial MRI from a 37-year-old patient with Ewing's sarcoma with a T5 paraspinal mass with extension through the neuroforamen resulting in high-grade spinal cord compression without significant involvement of the vertebral body or posterior elements. **(B)** Sagittal STIR image showing lack of signal change.

Neurologic signs and symptoms often begin with nerve root symptoms (radiculopathy), which are often overlooked by the patient and primary care provider until signs of spinal cord compression develop. Radiculopathy in the cervical or lumbar spine causes pain or weakness in the classic dermatomal distributions. However, thoracic radiculopathy occurs as a band-like pain at a segmental level. In the lumbar spine, patients may present with a mechanical radiculopathy resulting from a mildly unstable

compression fracture with extensive tumor in the neuroforamen. In recumbency or sitting, these patients have no radiculopathy, but severe, unremitting leg pain develops with increased axial loading when standing. Recognition of this entity is important as these patients generally respond only to operative management. Mechanical radiculopathy must be differentiated from hip or long-bone fractures by radiographic and clinical examinations.

Myelopathy begins as hyperreflexia, a Babinski reflex, and clonus, but progresses to weakness, proprioceptive sensory loss, and loss of pain and temperature below the level of the spinal cord compression. Proprioception can be very disabling, preventing ambulation even in patients with normal motor power. Isolated loss of bowel and bladder function in the absence of motor or sensory symptoms most often results from compression at the conus medullaris (tip of the spinal cord at approximately L1) or from tumor compressing the lower nerve roots in the sacrum or pelvis. In lesions above the conus medullaris, autonomic dysfunction is frequently a late finding.[79]

A comprehensive neurologic examination should be performed on all patients with suspected spine metastases. This is essential because patients will often have numerous lesions and it is important to determine which one is causing the symptoms. In addition, it is also important to adequately rule out other causes for these symptoms such as brain metastasis, leptomeningeal tumor, peripheral neuropathy, or paraneoplastic disease. Any patient with facial weakness or other cranial neuropathies requires cranial imaging prior to surgical intervention for metastatic spine disease. In addition, focal extremity weakness with normal or decreased reflexes may be caused by plexus or peripheral nerve compression from other metastases or as a result of toxicity from chemotherapeutic agents. As well, many of these patients will have been treated with long courses of corticosteroids and have developed a steroid-induced myopathy. Classically this involves the girdle muscles of the hips and shoulders. Patients will describe difficulty raising from the seated position.[23] Finally, in order to serially follow a patient's improvement or deterioration during the course of treatment, the patient's neurologic status must be adequately documented at the time of presentation.

The last step of the pretreatment evaluation should include objective scoring measures such as a pain assessment, quantitative neurologic score, and general performance score. Visual analog pain scales are most commonly used for pain assessment and objective neurologic scales, such as the Frankel grading system and ASIA score, can also be used (Table 76.2).[70,94] Performance status reflects ambulation, medical co-morbidities, and extent of disease. A patient may have normal motor strength but be unable to ambulate due to loss of proprioception, severe mechanical pain, lower extremity fracture, poor nutritional status, or poor pulmonary function. The ECOG (Eastern Cooperative Oncology Group) performance status is also commonly used in cancer patients as a functional assessment (Table 76.3).[55]

Evaluating Metabolic and Physiologic Issues

Cancer patients tend to be older than patients undergoing surgery for elective spine disorders, and have a high

TABLE 76.2

Impairment Scales

Grade	Description of Deficit below the Level of the Lesion
ASIA Scale	
A	Complete: No motor or sensory function
B	Incomplete: Sensory but no motor function
C	Incomplete: Some motor function is preserved but a majority of the muscle groups have a grade <3
D	Incomplete: Some motor function preserved but a majority of the muscle groups have a grade >3
E	Normal sensory and motor function
Frankel Scale	
A	Complete loss of motor and sensory function
B	Complete loss of motor, some preservation of sensory function
C	Sensory function useless, some motor function preserved but not enough to be functional
D	Sensory function useful, weak but useful motor function
E	Neurologically intact

TABLE 76.3

ECOG Performance Status

Grade	Description
0	Fully active, able to carry on all pre-disease performance without restriction
1	Restricted in physically strenuous activity but ambulatory and able to perform light work
2	Ambulatory and capable of all self-care but unable to perform work activities (bedridden <50% of the time)
3	Capable of only limited self-care (bedridden >50% of the time)
4	Completely disabled, not capable of any self-care (bedridden 100% of the time)

incidence of medical co-morbidities such as pulmonary, renal, and cardiovascular disorders. This may affect treatment decisions. In addition, there are several other physiologic derangements that are common among cancer patients. Hypercalcemia occurs in 10% to 20% of all cancer patients with the highest incidence in patients with lung and breast tumors.[149] The pathophysiologic abnormalities that lead to this condition are believed to be secondary to the multifactorial effects of increased bone turnover and increased calcium reabsorption in the proximal renal tubules. However, immobilization and dehydration have also been shown to be contributing factors especially in patients with end stage disease.[102,149,166] Hypercalcemia is commonly treated with IV fluid rehy-

dration and bisphosphonate administration and if left untreated, it can result in cardiac or kidney dysfunction, and even death in extreme cases.[102]

Coagulation abnormalities are also frequently observed in this patient population. This can result from metastatic tumor spread to the liver, toxic side effects of chemotherapeutic agents or thrombocytopenia as a result of bone marrow suppression, extensive RT, or antiplatelet antibodies. In addition, many patients who develop spinal cord compression from spinal metastases are actively receiving chemotherapy for the treatment of disease at other sites. A major concern is that many of these agents (e.g., doxorubicin) affect blood counts 2 to 3 weeks after their administration and if not monitored can result in life-threatening pancytopenia. Often, the oncologist will be able to accurately predict when blood counts will drop, based on the type of chemotherapeutic agent. Fortunately, the administration of filgrastim (Amgen Inc., Thousand Oaks, CA), a granulocyte stimulating colony factor, can rapidly reverse neutropenia within 24 to 48 hours. Operations should be delayed until the absolute neutrophil count is greater than 1.0 (white blood cell count ✕ percentage of neutrophils).

Imaging

Advances in imaging have facilitated earlier diagnosis of spine metastases due to the improved sensitivity of imaging studies, as well as the ability to adequately rule out other disorders with these same radiographic tests. MRI has revolutionized the assessment of metastatic spine tumors, but many imaging modalities continue to play a role in the work-up of these patients. The ideal imaging study should be 100% sensitive and specific in identifying tumors, while also providing precise anatomic detail plus being able to identify distant metastases. No single imaging modality accomplishes all of these goals. Therefore, it is important to understand the advantages and disadvantages of the available imaging modalities.

Plain radiographs are relatively poor screening tests for metastases. Visualization of a radiolucent defect on plain radiographs requires at least 50% destruction of the vertebral body. However, metastatic tumors often infiltrate the bone marrow of the vertebral body without destroying the cortical bone. Nevertheless, compression and burst fractures are readily identified. Sagittal (kyphosis) and coronal (scoliosis) plane deformities are often observed. Dynamic flexion and extension films may be used to detect instability, although they are rarely necessary and may put the patient at risk for progressive spinal cord injury. Postoperatively, plain films are the best imaging modality for assessing spinal alignment and structural integrity of the instrumentation.

The advantage of a 99mTc-MDP bone scan is its ability to screen the entire skeleton with a single image.[5] Patients with spinal tumors often have other associated bone lesions that may be responsible for symptoms. However, bone scans rely on an osteoblastic reaction or bone deposition to detect spinal metastases so that rapidly progressive, destructive tumors may not be detected.[5,78] In addition, this technique is relatively insensitive for multiple myeloma and tumors confined to the bone marrow.[78]

TABLE 76.4

MSKCC Epidural Spinal Cord Compression Grading Scale

Grade°	Description
0	No subarachnoid space compression
1	Subarachnoid space partially obliterated without spinal cord compression
2	Subarachnoid space partially obliterated with spinal cord compression
3	Subarachnoid space completely obliterated with cord compression

°Determined at level of worst compression.

Fractures, degenerative disease, and benign disorders of the spine (Schmorl's nodes, hemangioma) all also result in increased tracer uptake, but contiguous spread of a lesion through the neuroforamen may be negative. In a review by Avrahami, 21 out of 40 patients (52%) with tumor diagnosed with MRI and symptoms referable to spine metastasis had negative computed tomography (CT) and bone scans.[9] Frank *et al.*[69] reviewed a series of 95 patients in which 28% had negative bone scans with MRI demonstrating tumor.

Until MRI became widely available, myelography and postmyelogram CT were the best diagnostic imaging modalities for assessing acute spinal cord compression. Currently, the risks associated with myelography, including acute neurologic decompensation in patients with high-grade blocks, have limited its role.[147,219] CT continues to be useful for assessing the degree of bone destruction, as well as determining when bone rather than tumor is causing spinal cord compression. However, these techniques continue to be essential for evaluating patients with spinal instrumentation and the presence of recurrence or disease progression.[82,162]

MRI is the most sensitive and specific modality for imaging spinal metastases. Sagittal screening images of the entire spine reveal bone, epidural, and paraspinal tumor.[183] The extent and degree of spinal cord compression can be readily appreciated, especially on T_2-weighted images (Table 76.4). Hybrid scans of the brachial or lumbosacral plexus may reveal tumor in patients with extremity weakness that is not entirely related to spinal cord or root involvement. Contrast (Gd-DPTA) is not typically given unless there is a concern for leptomeningeal metastases.[145]

Common imaging sequences used to evaluate spinal metastases are T_1- and T_2-weighted. Tumor on a T_1-weighted image is hypointense relative to the normal marrow signal. However, if contrast is given, tumor may possibly be overlooked because it may appear isointense to normal bone. The ports from prior spinal radiation can be discerned on T_1-weighted images as a hyperintense signal change. This may assist in making acute therapeutic decisions when radiation port films are not available (Figure 76.4). Tumor is hyperintense relative to marrow on standard T_2-weighted imaging and produces a myelogram effect, with cerebrospinal fluid appearing hyperintense. Unfortunately, the recently developed timesaving fast spin echo T-2 techniques may decrease tumor conspicuity. This

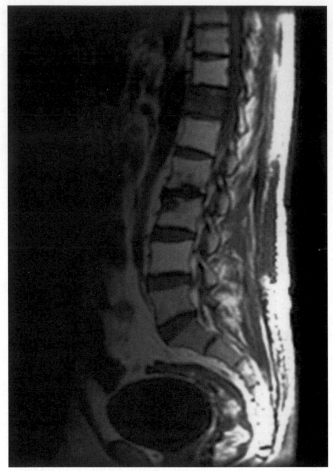

Figure 76.4 Sagittal T_1-weighted MRI from a patient with metastatic hepatocellular carcinoma illustrating T12 vertebral body lesion and previous radiation ports (hyperintense marrow signal) extending from T11-L4.

decreased conspicuity can be compensated for by using short tau inversion recovery (STIR) techniques. STIR images show enhanced contrast between the lipid marrow (hypointense) and tumor (hyperintense) and may be the most sensitive screening modality for tumor, but give less anatomic detail than standard T-1 or fast spin echo T-2 images (Figure 76.5).[54,99,143,208] Because of the high rate of multiple noncontiguous lesions, the screening of the entire spine, with sagittal sequences followed by axial imaging through any areas of abnormality, is often prudent.

Metastatic dissemination to bone usually occurs with multiple synchronous lesions. Isolated metastases to the vertebral body are rare and should be differentiated from primary bone tumors. The most common tumors to present as a solitary vertebral body lesion are thyroid, renal, and plasmacytoma. With rare exception, patients presenting with a solitary metastasis eventually develop widespread tumors.[46,141,167]

Tumors may be difficult to differentiate from osteomyelitis, osteoporotic compression fractures, and treatment effect. However, discitis and osteomyelitis are more likely to cause changes in the end plates and disc spaces, whereas tumors rarely, if ever, involve the disc space (Figures 76.6 and 76.7). Osteoporotic compression

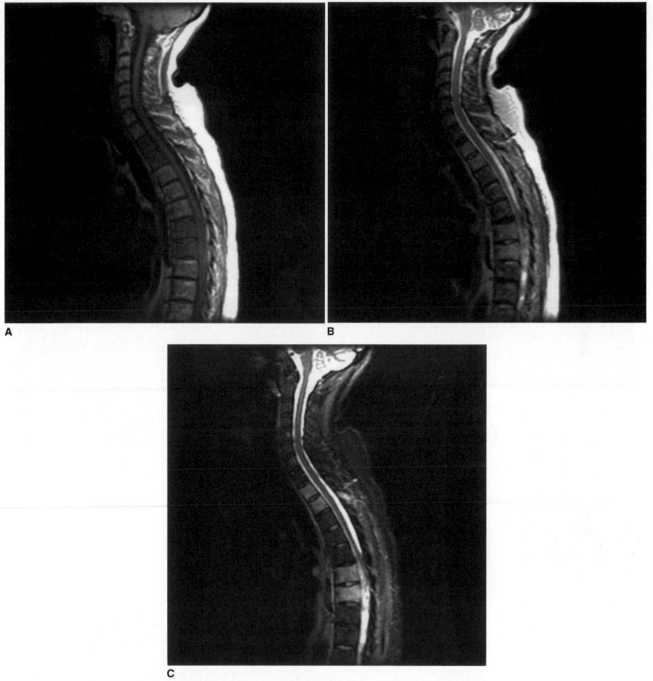

Figure 76.5 (**A**) Sagittal T$_1$-weighted, (**B**) T$_2$-weighted, and (**C**) STIR images from a patient with lymphoma. (Same patient as Figure 76.11.)

fractures are extremely common in the cancer population and have been differentiated from pathologic fractures with 94% accuracy based on T1-weighted imaging characteristics.[146] Osteoporotic fractures are more commonly thoracic, lack signal change, have band-like abnormality and do not involve the pedicle or have contour abnormality (Figure 76.8). Pathologic fractures showed homogeneously decreased signal, and a convex vertebral contour involving the pedicles and lumbar location (Figure 76.9).

In addition, 2-[F-18] flouro-2-deoxy-D-glucose (FDG-PET) can also be used for differentiating osteoporotic from pathologic compression fracture, as well as

for determining the viability of previously treated bone tumors.[44] Osteoporotic compression fractures greater than 3 days from the onset of symptoms are generally hypometabolic with a standardized uptake value (SUV) of less than three and most tumors have an SUV greater than three. FDG-PET has been useful in directing the biopsy to a specific hypermetabolic site in the vertebral body, increasing the chance of successfully making a diagnosis. Other radionuclide scans may be helpful for screening specific tumor types including 131I scans for papillary thyroid cancer, MIBG scans for neuroblastoma, and somatostatin scans for neuroendocrine tumor.

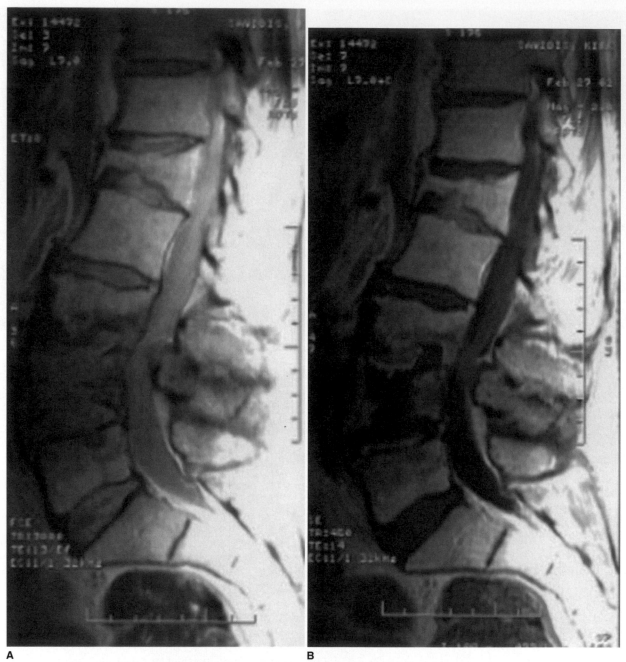

Figure 76.6 Sagittal T_1-weighted MR image without (**A**) and with (**B**) contrast from a patient with osteomyelitis involving L3 and L4. Note the significant bone destruction as well as involvement of the intervening disc space. An incidental L1 osteoporotic compression fracture is also seen. (Same patient as Figure 76.10.)

Estimating Tumor Burden in Other Regions

At MSKCC, tumor staging is usually performed in conjunction with the primary oncologists who have a better appreciation of the patient's disease in terms of overall aggressiveness and degree of progression. Typically, this is done with radiographic studies including chest radiographs and CT of the chest, abdomen, and pelvis. MRI of the head, bone scans, PET scans or serum markers, such as prostate specific antigen (PSA) or carcinoembryonic antigen (CEA), may also be helpful in selected cases.

The presence of distant metastases to extraspinal sites and active disease at the primary site are not contraindications to spine surgery, but recognizing the extent of disease is important for decision making. In patients with diffusely metastatic or rapidly progressive tumor, options such as RT may be more appropriate. However, the appropriateness of surgical interventions is often based more on the patient's overall medical condition as opposed to tumor burden. Even in cases with limited life expectancy (3 to 6 months), decompression and stabilization may help preserve neurologic function, and thus quality of life, as

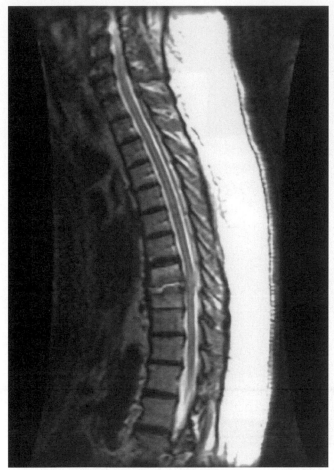

Figure 76.7 Sagittal T$_2$-weighted MRI from a patient with metastatic breast cancer who presented with severe mechanical back pain in the absence of myelopathy or constitutional symptoms. A lesion is seen at the T8-9 disc space with signal change and end plate edema. Biopsy of this lesion confirmed an infectious cause.

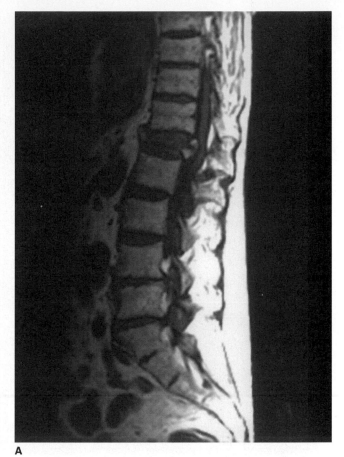

A

Figure 76.8 MR images from a 77-year-old female with an osteoporotic compression fracture who presented with severe mechanical back pain and myelopathy (**A**) sagittal T$_1$-weighted.
Continued

well as palliate pain symptoms with an acceptable level of morbidity.

Treatment

There are three primary treatment modalities available for the treatment of spinal metastases: (1) chemotherapy, (2) radiation therapy (RT), and (3) surgery.

Chemotherapy

Chemotherapy not only includes antitumor medications, but also drugs that can prevent or ameliorate the effects of tumor, such as steroids or bisphosphonates. The role of antitumor chemotherapy in the treatment of metastatic spine tumors is relatively limited, except for chemosensitive tumors, such as neuroblastoma, Ewing's sarcoma (PNET), osteogenic sarcoma, germ cell tumors, and lymphoma.[81] At MSKCC, chemotherapy is often considered the primary treatment for patients with these tumors even in the presence of epidural compression.

Steroids typically have two indications for the treatment of patients with metastatic spine tumors. The first is for the control of biologic pain, which usually only requires low doses that are often associated with a rapid and dramatic improvement in the patient's pain control. The second indication is for the control of vasogenic edema to help reduce or stabilize neurologic dysfunction in the preoperative and immediate postoperative periods. The optimal dose used to treat patients with acute spinal cord compression is controversial.* Complications from steroids are more common with higher dose regimens and include hyperglycemia, gastrointestinal hemorrhage, intestinal perforation, and avascular necrosis of the hip. Steroids are not required to prevent acute RT complications, as they do for brain RT, and thus may not need to be given in fully ambulatory patients undergoing RT for malignant spinal cord compression.[127] In situations in which patients present with a spinal mass, without a history of cancer, one must resist the temptation to deliver steroids prior to biopsy. The oncolytic effects of these drugs on certain tumors, such as lymphoma and thymoma, can be rapid, thus affecting biopsy results. Rapid neurologic deterioration is an obvious exception to this strategy (Figure 76.10).[172]

---

*References 26,80,89,108,122,191.

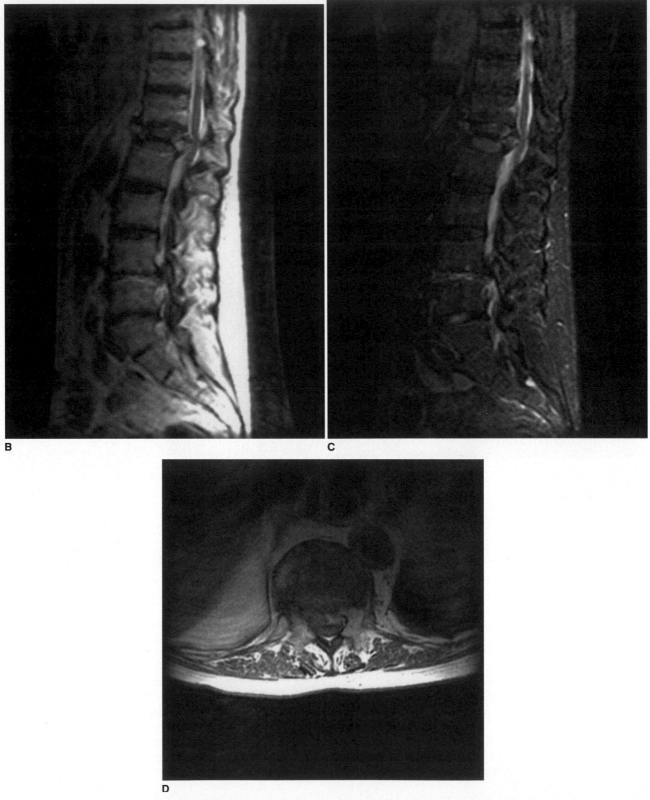

Figure 76.8 *cont'd* **(B)** T$_2$-weighted, **(C)** STIR, and **(D)** axial T$_1$-weighted sequences. The patient underwent decompression and fusion and as expected there was no evidence of tumor in the specimen.

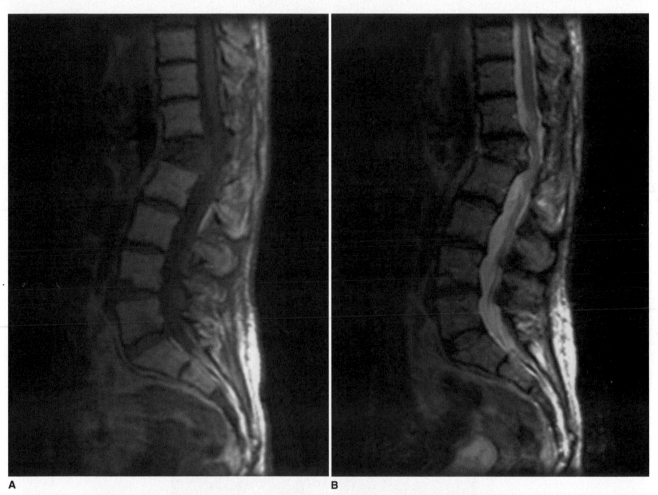

A   B

Figure 76.9 Images from a 66-year-old female with metastatic breast cancer and myelopathy and back pain. Imaging revealed a L1 compression deformity with signal changes consistent with metastatic tumor (**A**) sagittal T_1-weighted, (**B**) T_2-weighted.   *Continued*

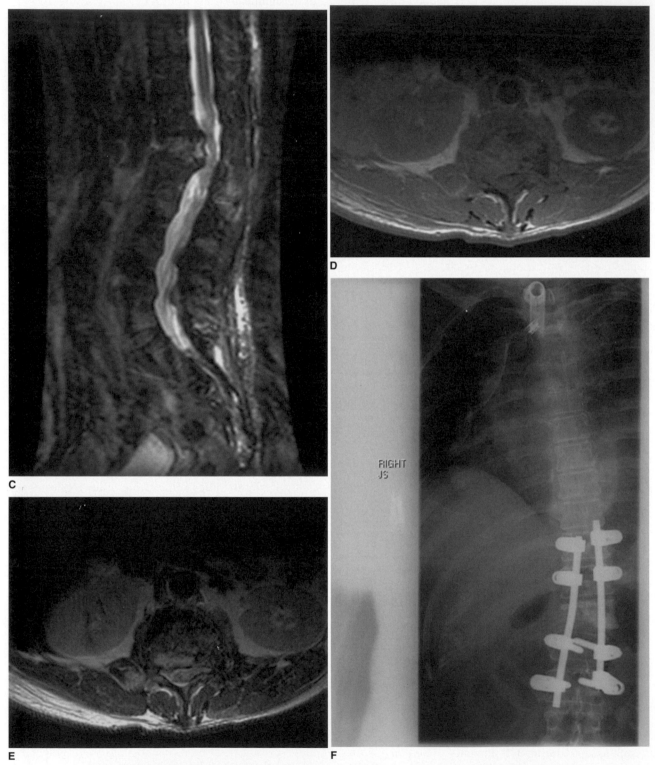

Figure 76.9 *cont'd* (**C**) STIR, (**D**) axial T$_1$-weighted, and (**E**) T$_2$-weighted sequences. The patient underwent decompression and fusion with evidence of tumor at the time of operation; (**F**) AP view.

In the past several years substantial research has shown that tumor cells can secrete substances such as PTH-rP, cytokines, and interleukins that affect the balance between osteoblastic bone formation and osteoclastic bone turnover.[206,224,227] These substances lead to osteoclast activation and increased bone turnover. Therefore, it has been hypothesized that the inhibition of these pathways limits the progression of such metastasis.[150,151,225,226] Bisphosphonates are a class of drugs that are rapidly becoming an integral part of treatment regimens for cancer patients because of their ability to inhibit osteoclast reabsorption of bone matrix and thus decrease bone turnover.[21,67,120,224]

Randomized clinical trials evaluating the use of these medications have shown significant decreases in the rate of skeletal-related complications, such as compression fractures, hypercalcemia, and the need for radiation to bone metastases in patients with breast cancer and multiple myeloma.* In addition, other studies in patients with breast cancer have shown that use of these compounds prior to the development of bone metastasis may decrease the rate of future bone metastasis and skeletal-related complications when compared to the group receiving placebo, as well as decreasing tumor-related pain.† These findings have been confirmed by laboratory experiments that have shown that these agents decrease the adherence of tumor cells to bone structures.[20,124,210] However, studies evaluating the efficacy of these compounds for other types of malignancies, such as prostate cancer, have shown mixed results.[116,187] Unfortunately, none of these compounds have ever been shown to improve survival.[119,120,125,174]

Three generations of bisphosphonates are currently available. Etidronate and clodronate belong to the first generation, pamidronate and alendronate are second-generation compounds, and zoledronate is the third-generation compound.[125] Most bisphosphonates are available as intravenous and oral preparations. Gastrointestinal side effects predominate, especially esophagitis and diarrhea. However, administration with a full glass of water may limit many of these complaints. Other problems such as fever, fatigue, or headache have also been described.[16,125]

Radiation Therapy

Based on several comparative studies that demonstrated no difference in outcome between patients undergoing external photon beam RT versus laminectomy without dorsal segmental fixation (often in combination with RT), RT replaced laminectomy as first-line therapy for patients with spinal metastasis with epidural compression in the 1970s.‡ However, approximately 75% of patients in these studies were nonambulatory at the time of presentation.[65] Patients undergoing RT alone showed a 79% rate of maintaining ambulation and a 42% rate of return to ambulation in paraparetic patients with a 21% risk of neurologic decompensation during RT. Patients undergoing either laminectomy alone or with postoperative RT had a 48% to 67% rate of maintaining ambulation with a 33% rate of

recovering ambulatory status in paraparetic patients with 17% to 52% showing neurologic deterioration following surgery. However, the posttreatment morbidity was shown to be significantly less from RT than from surgery.

A key study showing the benefit of RT was a retrospective review of 235 patients by Gilbert, in which analysis was based on the radiation sensitivity of the tumor and preoperative functional status.[74] The overall rate of postoperative ambulation in the laminectomy and RT versus RT alone was 46% and 49%, respectively. Patients with radiosensitive tumors (breast, myeloma, lymphoma) had better functional neurologic outcome compared to less radiosensitive tumors (lung, colon, renal cell), regardless of the treatment. Those patients ambulatory at the outset of treatment also had better outcomes compared to those paraparetic (nonambulatory) or paraplegic.

More recent radiation studies have confirmed the utility of this modality for the treatment for spinal metastases.[128] Maranzano[128] conducted a prospective trial over a 6-year period in which 275 patients were treated with RT for metastatic spinal cord compression, with a median follow-up of 49 months. Patients who were end stage or who had strong surgical indications were excluded from analysis. In addition, 25 patients who died during their course of RT because of nonrelated issues were also excluded. Twenty patients (7%) underwent surgery as initial treatment, either for histologic diagnosis, vertebral body collapse with bone impingement in the spinal canal, prior RT, or spinal instability. All patients were treated to a total dose of 3000cGy using two different fractionation schedules. Patients were divided into radiosensitive (e.g., breast, prostate, lymphoproliferative) and radioinsensitive tumors (e.g., lung, renal, colon). The overall rate of maintaining or improving to ambulatory status was 76% and the rate of improving sphincter control was 44%. Patients who were functionally normal or had minor abnormalities had a 94% rate of maintaining ambulation following treatment, regardless of the radiosensitivity of the lesion. Sixty percent of nonambulatory patients returned to ambulation post-RT and this was found to be heavily dependent on the radiosensitivity of the tumor. The improved rates of maintaining ambulation, compared to older studies, may be reflective of excluding deaths and maintaining stringent surgical criteria for initial therapy.

The standard RT treatment for palliation of spinal metastases is 10 daily fractions of 300cGy (total dose of 3000cGy). Either a single dorsal field or opposed fields are used to encompass the involved segment, with a margin of one or two levels above and below the involved region.[18] Spinal cord or cauda equina tolerance to RT is the limiting factor preventing the use of doses greater than 3000cGy. Higher doses of RT place the patient at an increased risk for pathologic radiation myelopathy and functional spinal cord transection.[18] However, the limited life expectancy of these patients may make it possible to re-irradiate the spine with limited additional risk.[184]

Newer Radiation Techniques

Recent advances in radiation oncology have permitted newer treatment approaches for many spine lesions. These include intraoperative RT (IORT), three-dimensional

---

*References 14-16,34,46,49,92,104,119,120,125,141,167,204,205,211.
†References 36,57,59,60,66,68,76,105,119,175,205,212.
‡References 24,35,37,52,71,74,83,107,109,121,131,158,188, 213,218,219,221,228.

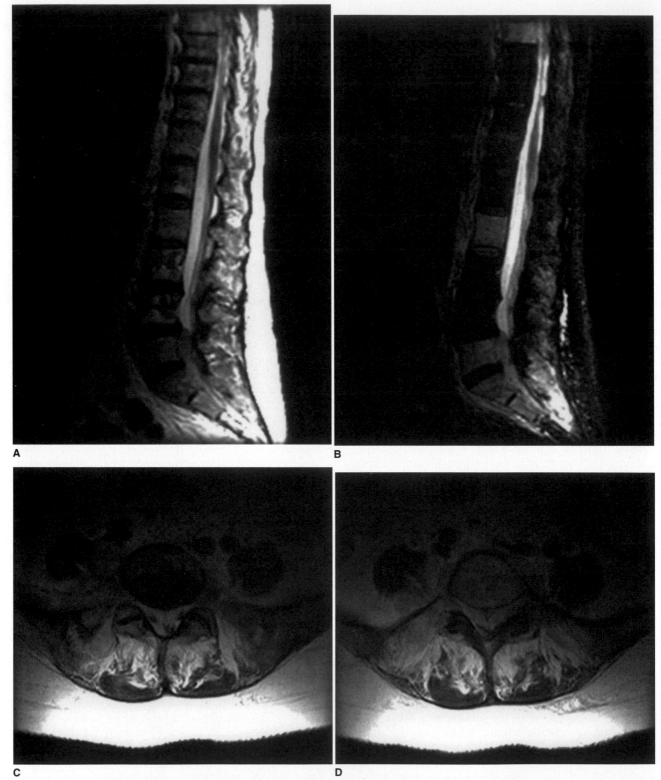

Figure 76.10 **(A)** Sagittal T_2-weighted and **(B)** STIR sequences from a 63-year-old woman without prior history of cancer who presented with diffuse nocturnal back pain followed by rapidly progressive bowel and bladder dysfunction. T_2-weighted axial images through the L5 and S1 levels **(C-D)** showed significant epidural tumor with encasement and dorsal displacement of the nerve roots. Steroids were initially withheld and the patient was taken emergently to the operating room where open biopsy was consistent with lymphoma. The patient's neurologic function improved immediately following decompression and initiation of steroids. (Same patient as Figure 76.6.)

conformal RT (3D-CRT), and intensity-modulated RT (IMRT). All three technologies improve the therapeutic ratio by providing a highly conformal dose of radiation to the tumor while sparing the surrounding structures. IORT involves the delivery of a custom-designed electron beam or high-dose rate brachytherapy photon beam to tumor volume while lead shields and gold foil are used to shield the spinal cord.[84,186]

Three D-CRT uses a method of irradiating a tumor volume with an array of x-ray beams similar to stereotactic radiosurgery for the treatment of intracranial lesions. The radiation beams are individually shaped to conform to a 3-dimensional rendering of the target sparing surrounding structures. Treatment planning considers dose inhomogeneities caused by the differing electron densities of various tissues, such as bone and muscle, and calculates the resulting dose distribution using sophisticated algorithms.

IMRT represents an advanced form of 3D-CRT in which multileaf collimators are used to dynamically change the field shape during treatment, thus permitting the delivery of an inhomogeneous dose that conforms more tightly to the target region. Advances in the development of noninvasive stereotactic body frames have enabled reliable localization of the paraspinal lesions with an error of less than 2mm. At MSKCC, patient immobilization for CT-guided radiotherapy relies on a stereotactic body frame (SBF) that uses several pressure points to guarantee a reliable "rigid" immobilization of the appendicular and axial skeleton during the course of the entire treatment process. The frame has a removable ventral and fixed dorsal CT-localization fiducial plate that establishes an independent coordinate system to accurately localize patient anatomy.

Such approaches may permit the delivery of a higher dose of radiation to a target tissue, while maintaining the dose delivered to the spinal cord within an acceptable tolerance level (Figure 76.11). This may improve the clinical outcome for patients with inoperable lesions, as well as in those requiring a radiation boost following surgical resection. To date, 12 of the initial 6 patients with paraspinal tumors have been treated at MSKCC with this technology. Four received previous radiation ranging from 3000cGy to 4000cGy. IMRT doses varied pending on the pathology of the lesion but ranged from 1600cGy in 8 fractions to 6660cGy in 37 fractions. The follow-up of these patients is too short to determine any conclusions about the long-term control rates using this new technology, but there was no acute toxicity.

Surgery

The role of surgery in the treatment of spinal metastases is still being defined, but the goal of this intervention is palliative, focusing on the reduction of pain, preservation of neurologic function, and restoration of mobility. Results using laminectomy as initial therapy, either alone or with adjuvant radiation, yielded relatively poor outcomes. Laminectomy alone does not provide exposure to resect lateral and ventral epidural or vertebral body tumors and therefore has higher associated failure rates. Additionally, the resection of the dorsal elements, without the employment of spinal instrumentation, often leads to progressive kyphosis and increased mechanical pain and neurologic deficits.

The development of newer surgical techniques and approaches has improved surgical outcomes because of the resulting ability to perform more extensive tumor

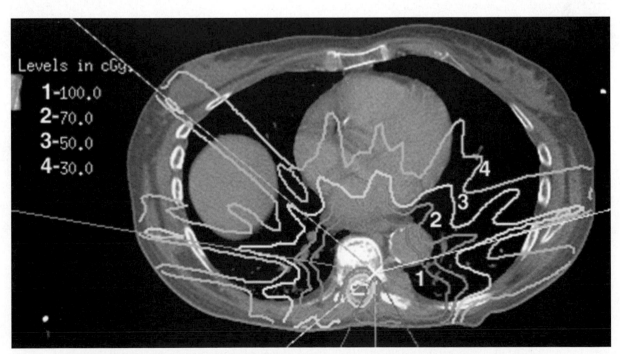

Figure 76.11 Treatment planning showing isodose curves for a patient with recurrent malignant fibrous histiocytoma undergoing IMRT. The 100% isodose curve is a 2mm margin from the spinal cord. (Same patient as Figure 76.5.)

resection and spinal cord decompression and reconstruction procedures. These include ventral transcavitary, and dorsolateral transpedicular approaches.* The decision to use a particular surgical approach is dependent on the location of the bone, epidural and paraspinal tumor, type of reconstruction required, patient comorbidities, extent of disease, and surgeon familiarity. Regardless of the approach, the goal is epidural decompression with the greatest possible cytoreduction.

Results using these techniques have improved surgical outcomes compared to patients treated with laminectomy. Resection of the tumor with spinal fixation permits for immediate neural decompression and spinal column stabilization, which is frequently associated with rapid diminution in the patient's pain. Multiple series reporting pain outcomes have shown a 76% to 100% improvement when either anterior or posterolateral approaches are used.† Functional and neurologic improvements have been observed in 50% to 76% of patients. Patients treated prior to the development of neurologic symptoms (ASIA E, ECOG 0) maintained function in greater than 95% of cases.‡ The percentage of ambulatory patients has risen significantly since the advent of MRI and is greater than 80% in most modern studies.[79]

As with RT, preoperative neurologic and functional status and favorable tumor histology are factors that impact outcome. Kelkamp and Samii reviewed 101 patients who underwent surgery for metastatic spinal tumor prior to receiving adjuvant therapy (RT or chemotherapy).[110] The types of procedures included dorsolateral (79%), ventral transcavitary (12%), and anterior and dorsal approaches (9%). Of the patients who were ambulatory preoperatively, 96% maintained ambulation. Only 22% of nonambulatory patients regained ambulation for the same duration. These findings compare similarly to those of the Maranzano study where patients were preferentially treated with RT.[110,128] Patients with favorable tumor histology (e.g., breast, kidney, thyroid, prostate) had significantly better neurologic outcome and survival than those with unfavorable histologies (lung, gastrointestinal tract, and unknown primary). As has been observed in other studies, local recurrence rates are significant.[197] In this study, 58% recurred after 6 months, 69% at 1 year, and 96% after 4 years. Factors predictive of low recurrence rates included preoperative ambulatory status, favorable tumor histology, tumor in the cervical spine, low number of affected vertebral bodies, complete resection, and elective surgery. At MSKCC, the authors aggressively approach many patients with tumor recurrence including reoperation and IMRT.

A review of multiple surgical series shows complication rates ranging from 10% to 52%.§ Complications include DVT, myocardial infarction, and pneumonia. Surgical complications include failed fixation requiring revision and postoperative hematoma. Wound dehiscence and infection are complications predominantly observed with dorsolateral approaches in up to 15% of cases. Mortality rates are as high as 13% and are frequently related to the medical or oncologic condition of the patients.

Treatment Decision Making

At MSKCC, radiation therapy is first-line for most patients who present with metastatic spine tumors. Surgery is reserved for a variety of indications based on the three previously mentioned issues: oncologic, biomechanical, and neurologic. Patients with radioresistant tumors (e.g., sarcoma, renal cell carcinoma), spinal instability, and/or a pathologic fracture with bone in the spinal canal are considered for surgery prior to RT (Table 76.5 and Box 76.1).[18] Patients with significant mechanical or radicular pain complaints may only marginally improve with RT alone. In addition, patients with circumferential epidural tumor that is moderately to highly radioresistant are more likely to worsen during RT when compared to other patterns of epidural tumor and are considered for surgery as initial treatment. A frequently reported indication for surgery is the absence of a diagnosis. This, however, can frequently be established with CT-guided needle biopsy or thoracoscopic biopsy.

Following prior RT that has reached spinal cord tolerance, patients are considered for surgery based on progression of neurologic symptoms, radiographic progression of tumor, and spinal instability. Contraindications to surgery include a limited life expectancy, significant medical comorbidities and extensive disease. Additionally paraplegic patients are rarely operated on because of the significantly low rate of recovery, particularly after 24 hours.

TABLE 76.5

Radiosensitivity of Various Metastatic Spine Tumors

Sensitivity	Tumor Histology
Low	Sarcoma
	Renal cell
	Lung
	Colon
Intermediate	Breast
	Prostate
High	Lymphoma
	Myeloma

BOX 76.1

Surgical indications

Primary surgery
Radioresistant tumor
Spinal instability
Pathologic fracture with bone in the canal
Circumferential or high-grade epidural tumor compression for moderately to highly radioresistant tumor
Occult primary tumor

Surgery following radiation/chemotherapy
Progressive neurologic symptoms
Radiographic tumor progression with high-grade compression
Spinal instability

*References 3,12,25,27,38,79,110,113,168,169,195,196,197,200,215.
†References 3,12,25,27,38,79,110,111,168,169,195-197,200,215.
‡References 3,12,17,25,27,38,79,110,111,168,169,195-197,200,215.
§References 3,12,25,38,79,110,111,168,169,195-197,215.

Operative Considerations and Techniques

The approach to tumor resection and spinal reconstruction is dependent on the location of epidural, vertebral body, and paraspinal tumor involvement. The spinal level also is important in decision making and thus, atlanto-axial, subaxial, thoracic, and lumbar tumors are considered separately.

Atlanto-axial Tumor

Atlanto-axial tumors often present with severe neck pain that is frequently associated with a rotational component. Occasionally these tumors present with occipital neuralgia from C2 nerve root involvement or cranial neuropathies from base of skull involvement. Epidural tumor and myelopathy are rare at presentation. Despite the severity of mechanical neck pain, the majority of patients can be treated nonoperatively with RT or chemotherapy (Figure 76.12).[19,171,199] Patients undergoing nonoperative management are maintained in a hard-collar until 6 weeks after the completion of therapy. Operations, as initial therapy, are reserved for patients with significant fracture subluxations, defined as an odontoid fracture with greater than

5mm subluxation or greater than 3.5mm subluxation and greater than 11-degree angulation. Other indications for operation include prior RT to overlapping ports (e.g., head and neck cancers) and unknown primary tumors.

Using this algorithm, 33 patients were treated over a 6-year period. Twenty-five initially received RT and/or chemotherapy with 23 of the 25 (92%) obtaining significant pain relief.[19] Five patients subsequently underwent operation, but only one for a new fracture subluxation that occurred 1 month following the completion of RT. Two patients had subluxations greater than 5mm at presentation, but refused operation. Two had neoadjuvant chemotherapy, with a planned resection.

Thirteen patients underwent operations, 8 as initial therapy and 5 following prior therapy. All operations involved dorsal fixation with or without a dorsal decompression. Ventral decompression was not necessary in any patient because spinal cord decompression was obtained with fracture reduction and instrumentation.[171,199] A wake-up test and intraoperative radiographs should be obtained following reduction and hardware placement. C1 to C2 or C3 fusion is performed in patients following fracture reduction with either a dorsal wiring technique or using the Apofix device (Medtronic, Sofamor Danek, Memphis,

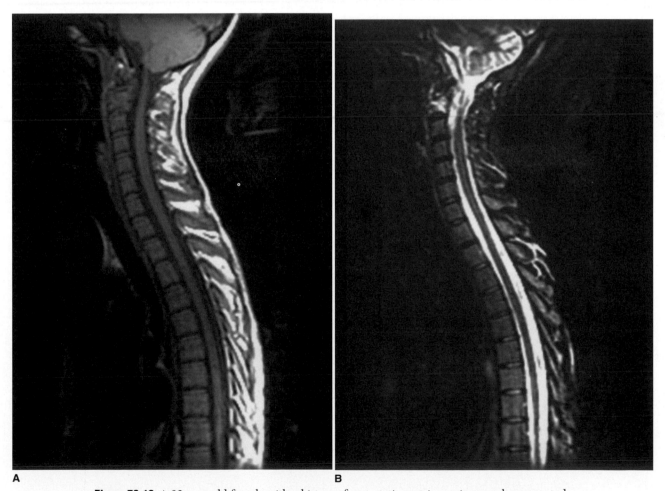

A   B

Figure 76.12 A 32-year-old female with a history of metastatic gastric carcinoma who presented with a 2-week history of severe neck pain worsened with rotation, **(A)** sagittal T_1-weighted, **(B)** T_2-weighted.

Continued

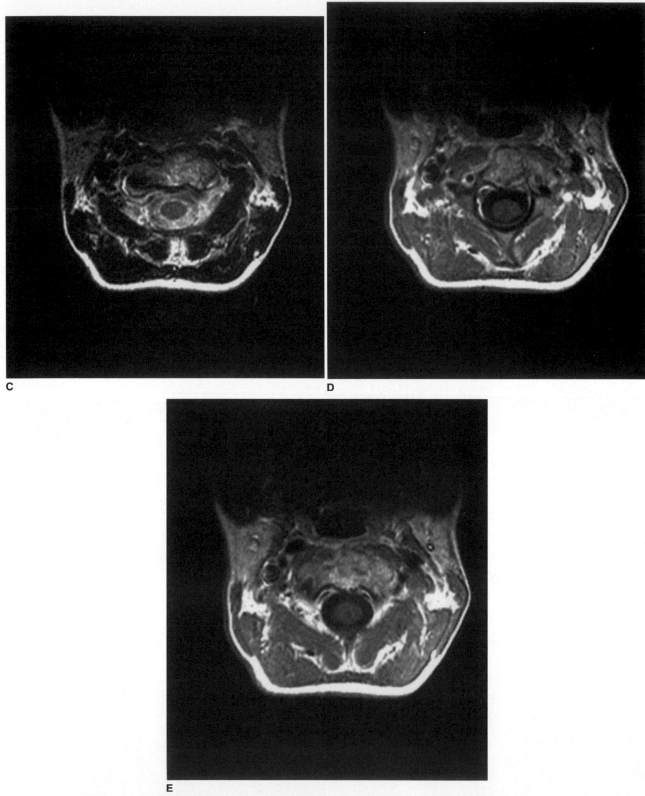

Figure 76.12 *cont'd* (**C**) Axial T_2-weighted, (**D**) T_1-preweighted and (**E**) T_1-weighted postcontrast sequences showing tumor involving the C2 vertebral body. The patient was treated with radiation with complete resolution of her pain.

TN). Transarticular screws have become very popular in traumatic atlanto-axial fractures, but have little role in pathologic fractures, because of the preponderance of lytic destruction of the ventral spinal elements. Occipitocervical fixation is reserved for patients in whom the fracture cannot be reduced, necessitating a C1 laminectomy for decompression. Other indications for occipitocervical fixation included a breach of the dorsal C1 or C2 arch or destruction of the occipital condyles. Occipitocervical fixation can be achieved with the lateral mass plates or more recently with screw-rod combinations. Systems, such as Summit (Johnson & Johnson, Depuy-Acromed, Boston MA) allow the cranial screws to be placed in the midline keel of the suboccipital region and distribute the force laterally providing excellent skull fixation. At a median follow-up of 9 months in our series, there were no fixation failures or symptomatic tumor recurrence. All operated patients had significant and durable pain relief.[19]

Subaxial Cervical Spine Tumors

RT remains the primary treatment for metastatic tumors in the cervical spine; however, tumors in the subaxial cervical spine often present with marked instability pain and epidural compression requiring operation. In contrast to the atlanto-axial spine, mechanical instability pain resulting from a compression or burst fracture is generally an indication for surgery. Further, lytic destruction of the vertebral body and concomitant posterior element tumor virtually always results in instability pain.

Preoperative assessments of the vertebral artery and vocal cord function are essential to good surgical outcomes. The patency of the vertebral artery can often be assessed preoperatively using magnetic resonance angiograms. If one plans to aggressively resect tumor from the vertebral artery, a preoperative angiogram and a balloon occlusion test may be used to definitively establish whether the contralateral vertebral artery can maintain adequate flow.

Another important preoperative consideration is vocal cord function. Recurrent laryngeal nerve palsy may occur secondary to tumor infiltration, even though the patient may not report a history of or exhibit hoarseness. The authors routinely employ a preoperative assessment with a fiberoptic laryngoscopy. If a paralyzed vocal cord is identified, the surgical approach should be on the same side. Fortunately, a unilateral, paralyzed vocal cord can be managed postoperatively with a relatively simple procedure involving medialization of the vocal cord with a Teflon (polytetrafluoroethylene) injection.[112]

Subaxial spine tumors arising from the vertebral body should be addressed with a ventral approach and vertebral body resection.* The ventral Smith-Robinson approach[179] provides excellent exposure from C3 to C7 and usually T1 can be reached. High cervical approaches (e.g., C3 corpectomy) may require the specialized services of the head and neck team to avoid trauma to the superior laryngeal and hypoglossal nerves, especially in previously radiated patients or those with large paraspinal masses. Placement of a nasogastric tube following induction helps identify location of the esophagus during the dissection.

Tumor resection is initiated by resecting the mass ventral to the spine until the disc spaces are identified. The disc spaces are generally preserved and can help with identification of the posterior longitudinal ligament (PLL). The tumor can then be intralesional resected to the level of the PLL. Resection of the PLL provides a normal plane on the ventral dura mater. Once this is identified, the nerve roots can be identified laterally and the lateral paraspinal mass dissected. Tumor can be dissected from the vertebral arteries using tenotomy scissors. Rarely, tumor infiltrates the vertebral artery wall, necessitating sacrifice.

A number of materials can be used for ventral strut grafts including PMMA and Steinman pins or filled into a chest tube, cages, or structural autograft or allograft. For metastatic cancer reconstruction, we have most often used fibula allograft and a ventral cervical plate, as these provide better deformity reduction and fixation than pins and cement.[33,51,139] Cutting flanges into the rostral and caudal aspect of a titanium mesh cage can also provide excellent structural support without the need to place a cervical plate (Figure 76.13).

Dorsal instrumentation is generally used if more than one vertebral body and/or dorsal element tumor are resected.[100,140,168,209] Lateral mass plates or screw-rod systems both provide excellent fixation. Dorsal element tumor resection often requires facetectomies in addition to laminectomy, which places additional strain on the hardware. For this reason, the instrumentation is extended for several additional levels adjacent to the decompression in order to achieve more points of bone fixation. Sublaminar wires are sometimes used to augment screw fixation. If a vertebral artery has been sacrificed or injured, screws should be avoided on the contralateral side to prevent damage to the patent vertebral artery. In these circumstances, sublaminar wires or hooks provide acceptable alternatives in selected cases.

Thoracic and Lumbar Spine Tumors

Thoracic and lumbar spine tumors can be treated via ventral, dorsolateral, or combined approaches. The choice of the approach is dependent on the location of bone and paraspinal tumor, pattern and degree of epidural compression, and instrumentation requirements. At MSKCC, ventral transcavitary approaches are used for isolated one- or two-level vertebral body tumors with unilateral epidural extension. The ventral approaches have been well described in this text and will not be covered in detail here. Standard thoracotomy and retroperitoneal approaches are used for thoracic and lumbar tumors, respectively. Thoracolumbar tumors are generally approached through a T10 thoracotomy, but the diaphragm is not cut along its entire length. In cancer patients, a modification of the standard thoracolumbar approach is to detach only the insertions of the diaphragm at the level of the spine. This technique provides excellent exposure and more rapid closure.

The ventral approach to the cervicothoracic junction (C7-T3) depends on the location of the tumor. A hemi-clamshell thoracotomy ("trap door" approach) is useful for vertebral body tumors with ventral mediastinal extension. This approach requires a dissection along the ventral border of the sternocleidomastoid muscle, extending down

*References 8,96,100,129,135,189.

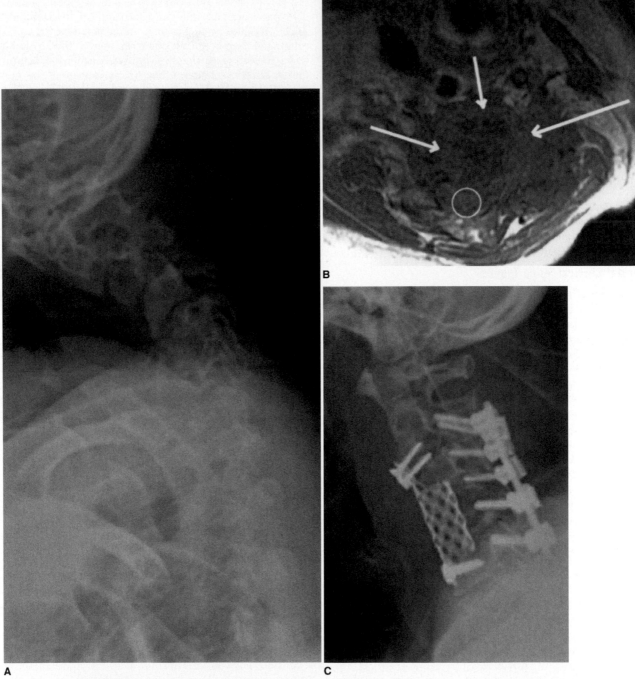

Figure 76.13 Images from a 45-year-old patient with metastatic epithelioid sarcoma to C5-6 presents with compression fracture and marked kyphosis. **(A)** Lateral cervical radiographs showing deformity **(B)** T_1-weighted image shows destruction of vertebral body *(arrows)*, facet joints and marked spinal cord compression *(circle)*. **(C)** Postoperative radiographs shows anterior reconstruction using a titanium cage with the flanges cut and secured to the vertebral body. This was augmented with posterior fixation using a screw-rod system.

the sternum and across the fourth interspace.[156] It is more easily accomplished from the right to avoid operating over the aortic arch, but carries a higher risk of recurrent laryngeal stretch injury. More recently for limited resections extending to T2, we have used an ventral sternocleidomastoid incision and manubrial osteotomy.[44] A dorsolat-

eral thoracotomy provides exposure for spine tumors with a lateral paraspinal component, extension to the lower trunk of the brachial plexus and dorsal mediastinal structures. This technique requires elevation of the scapula to provide lateral exposure and is most often used for resection of superior sulcus tumors.

The technique for tumor resection in the thoracic and lumbar spine is similar to that for the cervical spine. The disc spaces serve as normal anatomical landmarks, especially in the presence of a large paraspinal mass. The pleura are reflected and the rib heads are resected from the affected levels and two adjacent segments. The disc spaces are exenterated and intralesional resection is accomplished to identify the PLL. The PLL should be resected to obtain a margin on the ventral dura mater. The pedicle on the side of the approach should also be removed to aid in resection of epidural tumor and to identify normal lateral dura. Following resection, anterior strut grafts can be placed. Most commonly PMMA is used either with Steinman pins or using the chest tube technique.[144] Autologous rib graft may be available, but generally does not provide adequate ventral support. Femoral allograft or cages packed with autologous rib graft are a good alternative to PMMA and pins. These should be supplemented with a ventral plate, screw rod system, and/or dorsal fixation.

Dorsolateral Transpedicle Approach (PTA)

At MSKCC, dorsolateral transpedicle approaches (PTAs) for thoracic and lumbar tumor decompression have largely replaced the ventral, transcavitary approaches.[*] Many patients have patterns of tumor involving the vertebral body that are not readily amenable to a ventral approach, requiring both ventral and dorsal approaches to achieve adequate decompression and fixation. Indications include patients with three-column tumor involvement, multilevel vertebral body or epidural tumor, vertebral body tumor with bilateral or circumferential epidural spinal cord compression, or major spinal deformity. Additionally, some patients are poor candidates for ventral approaches because of poor pulmonary function, previous surgery or RT, or unresectable ventral masses.[17] Advantages of the PTA include starting the dissection of the tumor from a normal dural plane, readily resecting circumferential epidural tumor and achieving ventral and dorsal fixation from a single approach. The disadvantage is no direct visualization of the ventral dura mater, but this is overcome with sharp dissection of the PLL from the ventral dura.

The PTA is initiated with a long dorsal midline incision, followed by dissection of the muscles off of the lamina and facets to the tips of the transverse processes. Following muscle dissection, bone removal is performed using a high-speed drill with a matchstick side-cutting burr, such as the M-8 burr (Medtronic Midas Rex, TX). The lamina, pars interarticularis, and facets at the level(s) of the tumor and one-half level above and below are removed. The pedicles are drilled flush with the vertebral body. The presence of ventral epidural tumor extending from the dorsal vertebral body precludes the use of Kerrison rongeurs and the drill is used to dissect to the level of the dura mater or ligamentum flavum. Epidural tumor is resected dorsal and lateral to the dura using tenotomy scissors starting from a normal dural plane. Care must be taken to identify the thoracic nerve roots, which are double ligated with vascular clips. In the lumbar spine, the

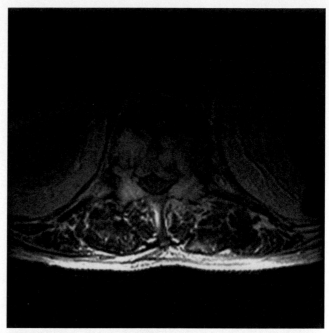

Figure 76.14 Axial T_1-weighted MRI of a lesion involving the ventral vertebral body and pedicles. The PLL (*dark line ventral to spinal cord*) is resistant to tumor spread but is displaced dorsally by the tumor creating the V sign.

nerve roots are preserved. Lumbar nerve roots are identified at their takeoff from the thecal sac and can be dissected to the lumbosacral plexus using tenotomy scissors. A minority of patients may develop dysesthetic pain or lose nerve root function from aggressive tumor resection and devascularization of the root.

The removal of dorsolateral bone opens a wide corridor lateral to the thecal sac providing access to the ventral vertebral body. Intralesional vertebral body resection is performed using curettes and pituitary rongeurs. Following removal of tumor and infiltrated bone in this region, attention is then turned towards the epidural disease on the ventral aspect of the thecal sac. The PLL typically provides a barrier to tumor invasion and remains preserved in most instances. The intact PLL is identified by the V sign on preoperative imaging (Figure 76.14). The plane between the PLL and thecal sac can usually be developed and resected sharply. Curettes should not be used to remove the PLL as this may cause excessive traction on the spinal dura.

Anterior reconstruction is then initiated with the placement of Steinman pins. A right angle clamp is used to create a starting point in the adjacent vertebral bodies. The Steinman pins are then driven into this bone using a needle driver. Next, methylmethacrylate impregnated with tobramycin is injected around the pins and compressed against the end plates.

Dorsal instrumentation is performed according to the surgeon's preference. Pedicle screws have largely replaced sublaminar hooks in our practice. Cervicothoracic junction dorsolateral instrumentation is difficult because of the additional stresses placed on the hardware by the transition from fixed thoracic, kyphotic spine to the mobile, lordotic cervical spine. The most reliable fixation in this region has been with 5mm sublaminar hooks in the cervical spine connected to thoracic hooks or pedicle screws with a one-quarter inch titanium rod. More recently, the authors have begun using a hybrid pedicle screw–lateral mass plate system. However, the jury is still out on which technique has better long-term results (Figure 76.15).

Case Presentations

Case 1

A 54-year-old male with a known history of neuroendocrine carcinoma who presented with back pain and early myelopathy with sensory loss and four out of five muscle power that improved to five out of five (ASIA D, ECOG 2) following high-dose dexamethasone. The patient had received previous radiation to this lesion approximately 9 months earlier and was thus taken for dorsolateral spinal decompression and instrumentation following preoperative embolization (Figure 76.16). He returned to an ASIA E, ECOG 0 and was independently ambulatory.

Case 2

A 67-year-old male with known history of prostate cancer who presented with mechanical back pain, thoracic radiculopathy, and loss of proprioception prohibiting ambulation; ASIA D, ECOG 3. Because of the circumferential pattern of epidural tumor in a moderately resistant tumor (i.e., hormone-refractory prostate cancer) and mechanical back pain, operation was recommended. The patient refused secondary to personal matters and was treated with radiation and high-dose steroids. The patient

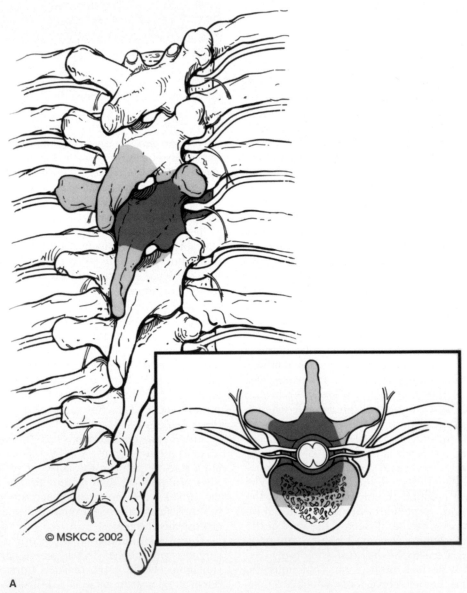

A

Figure 76.15 (A) Illustration depicting the bone and tumor removal in a PTA. The dorsal elements including lamina, facet joints, pedicles, and involved segment are resected with a high-speed drill. The vertebral body, adjacent disc spaces, and PLL are removed.

showed progressive neurologic symptoms during RT, and died at 6 weeks following treatment of sepsis, related to paralysis (Figure 76.17).

Case 3

A 34-year-old male without known history of cancer who presented with severe incapacitating mechanical back pain and radiculopathy, which rendered the patient bedridden (ASIA C, ECOG 4). Work-up revealed multiple bone lesions and serum and urine protein electrophoresis were consistent with multiple myeloma. Even though we primarily treat this radiosensitive tumor with upfront RT, we elected to proceed with dorsolateral decompression and instrumentation because of the patient's severe mechanical pain, which we felt would not improve with radiation alone. Immediately following surgery the patient began

radiation for his other lesions and his spine was radiated 6 weeks later. The patient is now fully ambulatory with minimal narcotic requirements (Figure 76.18).

Complication Avoidance: Intraoperative Strategies

Neurologic Injury

The most serious intraoperative complication in the treatment of spine metastasis is neurologic injury. In older surgical series this occurred in as many as 20% of patients. However, with newer surgical approaches and techniques this is much less common. The risks of neurologic injury can be minimized by several intraoperative maneuvers. First, the surgeon must be extremely careful

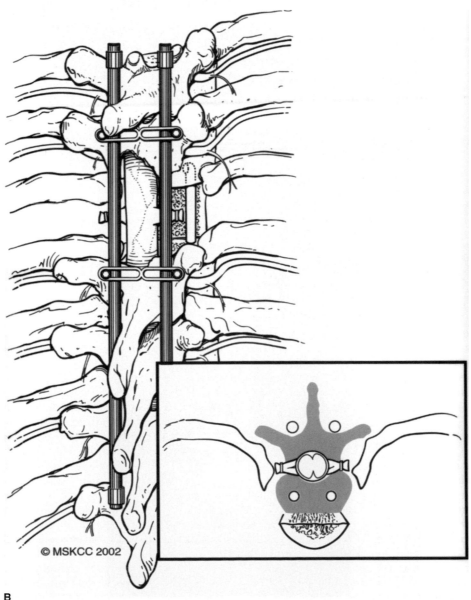

Figure 76.15 *cont'd* (B) Illustration depicting reconstruction with PMMA and Steinman pins in the vertebral body defect, augmented with dorsal segmental fixation.

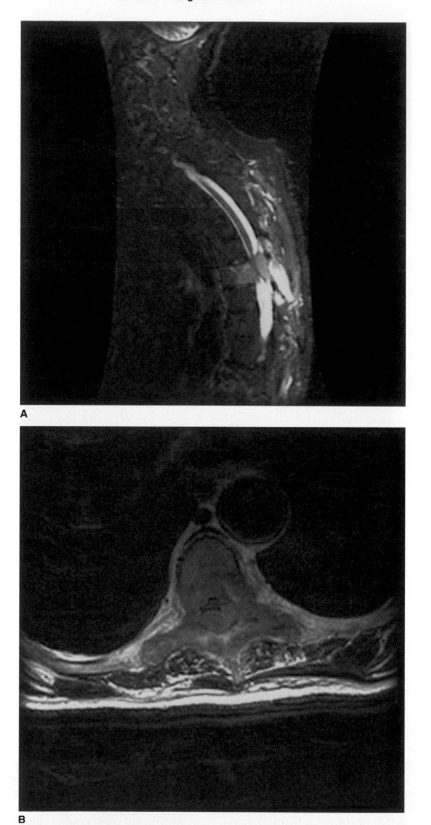

A

B

Figure 76.17 Images from Case 3 *(see text)*: **(A)** sagittal STIR, **(B-C)** axial T$_2$-weighted images.

has occurred. If waterlight dural closure is not possible, options include the use of bovine pericardial patch grafts, DuraGen (Integra Neurosciences, New Jersey), and/or fibrin glue. Controlled lumbar drainage (10ml/hr) is often used for 2 to 3 days postoperatively to help seal the leak.

Intraoperative Hemorrhage

One of the most frequent intraoperative complications is excessive blood loss. This can occur because of either arterial, venous, or capillary bleeding from the tumor, bone, or surrounding muscle. While preoperative embolization is

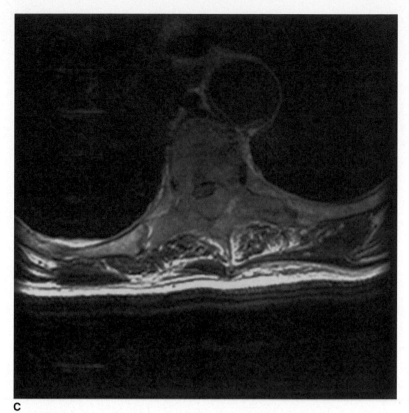

Figure 76.17 *cont'd*

helpful for selected cases where tumors are known to have large arterial feeders it has no role in prevention of venous or capillary bleeding, which can be just as vigorous. Adequate packing cannot typically be performed early on during the procedure because of the proximity of the spinal cord. Therefore, tumor resection should be done expeditiously once all of the bone work is finished. Finally, in lesions that are expected to be very vascular we often place the instrumentation prior to tumor resection. This facilitates a more rapid placement of the rods at the conclusion of the procedure and reduces the length of time for oozing of the tumor cavity.

Embolization is performed for hypervascular tumors (e.g., renal cell, papillary thyroid carcinoma, leiomyosarcoma) 1 or 2 days prior to operation as this has been shown to dramatically reduce intraoperative blood loss. In the authors' series of 25 patients operated via a dorsolateral approach with circumferential instrumentation, embolization successfully reduced operative blood loss for hypervascular tumors (i.e., renal, thyroid, angiosarcoma) to the same level as those not requiring embolization (1900 and 1620mls, respectively).[17,161,198]

In addition to embolization, the authors have found several other steps helpful for controlling intraoperative bleeding. A new commercially available thrombin/collagen particle mixture termed *FloSeal* (Baxter Healthcare Corporation, California) has proven useful. Studies have shown this product to work two to three times faster than other agents.[163] FloSeal is provided in a gel form with a syringe applicator that can be easily applied or packed into any space. In addition, dilute hydrogen peroxide is also effective for controlling venous oozing especially from the

deep bone resection cavities. To prevent postoperative seromas one or two deep subfascial drains may be placed and left in place until output is less than 30ml per day.

During these procedures, close monitoring of the ongoing blood loss is essential as it is not unusual to lose over 3 or 4L throughout the case. For vascular lesions, blood transfusions are usually initiated before excessive blood loss has occurred in order to prevent significant anemia or hypotension. In addition, for every 6 units of packed red blood cells 6 units of platelets and 4 units of fresh frozen plasma perhaps should be administered to prevent dilutional/transfusion thrombocytopenia and coagulopathy. Postoperatively these parameters are frequently monitored and corrected as required for the first 3 to 4 days.

Postoperative Mechanical Pain and Hardware Failure

Instrumentation with either pedicle screws or sublaminar hooks is performed following surgical decompression in a majority of patients undergoing surgical intervention for metastatic spine disease. Many of these patients have preexisting mechanical instability as a result of tumor-related bone destruction, iatrogenic instability as a result of intraoperative bone removal, or are at risk for delayed instability secondary to tumor progression. The addition of instrumentation prevents the delayed development of mechanical back pain and often adds only 30 to 60 minutes to the case. Many of these patients require longer fusion segments, as opposed to patients with degenerative disease because of tumor involvement in surrounding bone. Autogenic bone graft is not typically used because of the short life expectancy of these patients and concomitant

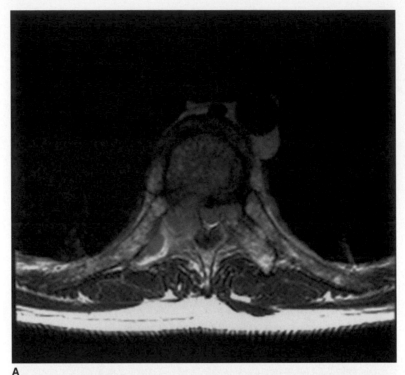

A

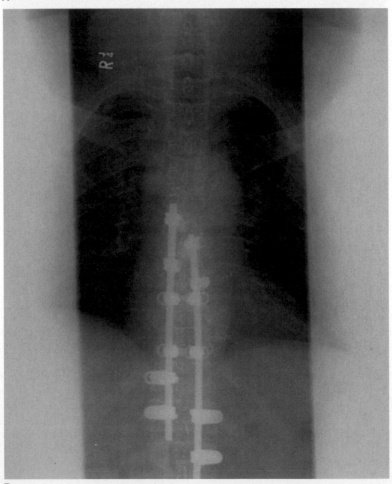

B

Figure 76.18 Images from Case 4 *(see text)*: **(A)** axial T$_2$-weighted MRI, **(B)** AP, radiograph.

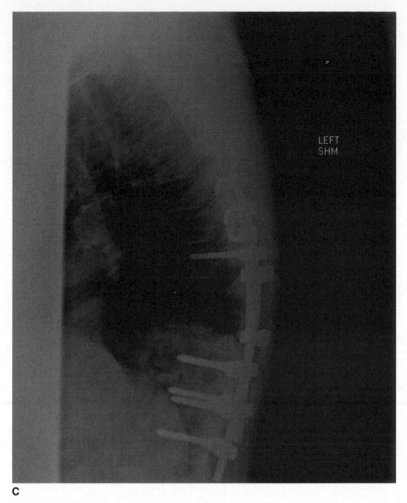

C

Figure 76.18 *cont'd* (C) Lateral postoperative radiograph.

use of postoperative radiation in some patients. The routine use of external orthosis is not supported as these can compromise pulmonary function and wound healing in patients with minimal reserves.

Complication Avoidance: Postoperative Strategies

Patients undergoing surgery for the treatment of spinal metastasis typically have poor functional reserve and are often malnourished secondary to the nitrogen wasting effects of their cancer and the numerous prior treatments and surgeries. Therefore, these patients are at an extremely high risk for adverse postoperative complications.

Pulmonary Management

Pulmonary function is often diminished in these patients, many of whom have extremely poor pulmonary reserve. This may be secondary to prior thoracotomy with pulmonary resection, pulmonary metastasis, pleural effusions, history of smoking, poor muscular tone, and interstitial pulmonary fibrosis secondary to chemotherapy. At MSKCC, all patients obtain a preoperative chest radiograph, and any patients with prior thoracotomy, any previously men-

tioned risk factor, or a history of dyspnea, are evaluated with preoperative pulmonary function tests. Postoperatively, all patients are placed on a Flexicair mattresses (Hill-Rom, Batesville, Indiana). This achieves two goals: (1) patients are rotated in a semi-upright position, which maximizes pulmonary function, and (2) pressure on the wound is minimized by rotation of the bed, thus constantly changing the pressure points of the skin against the mattress. In addition, close monitoring of volume status should be performed as many of these patients require large volume transfusions of blood products and thus pulmonary edema can occur.

Acute Renal Insufficiency

Although this complication occurs rarely following spine surgery, its development may push a patient with marginal reserve over the edge and lead to progressive deterioration of functional status or death. Patients who have undergone preoperative embolization or prior nephrectomy for renal cell carcinoma are at the highest risk. Other risk factors include diabetes mellitus, hypertension, and chronic renal insufficiency. Adequate hydration, frequent monitoring of serum BUN and creatinine levels, and prevention of intraoperative or postoperative hypotension best prevents acute renal insufficiency. Once this condition develops it can be managed by careful rehydration and renal dose dopamine. It often necessitates consultation with a nephrologist.

Deep Venous Thrombosis

Another complication in this population is the development of deep venous thrombosis (DVT) and the associated risk of pulmonary embolus. The cause of DVTs in this population is thought to be multifactorial and not simply a result of immobility. Many solid tumors release cytokines and other tissue factors that have procoagulant effects. Perioperative prophylaxis with pneumatic compression boots and subcutaneous heparin is helpful, but not fool proof in decreasing the rate of postoperative DVT. Patients are mobilized as soon as possible postoperatively. When DVTs are present preoperatively, they are managed with inferior vena cava filter placement. Postoperatively, they are treated with either inferior vena cava filters and/or anticoagulation.

Postoperative Pain Management

The adequate control of cancer-related and postoperative pain can also be very challenging in this population, and when not managed appropriately, it can lead to immobilization. A significant number of these patients may have chronic pain syndromes and require large doses of narcotics typically in the form of delayed-release oral or transdermal preparations. This makes postoperative pain control difficult because of tolerance to these agents. At MSKCC, all patients receive narcotics (morphine, fentanyl, or hydromorphone) via PCA postoperatively for several days with frequent dosing modifications until adequate pain control is established and are then switched to equianalgesic doses of oral or transdermal medications.

Wound Healing Complications

One of the most frustrating complications seen in our patient population is the development of wound dehiscences and infections following dorsal surgical approaches. Not only do wound infections/dehiscences place the patient at risk for other morbidities, but in many circumstances, require them to undergo repeated procedures for the treatment of this complication.

While ventral approaches provide direct access to the ventral spinal cord and are associated with a significantly lower rate of wound complications, they are more difficult for patients with metastatic cancer to tolerate. Many of these patients have had previous procedures through the abdomen and chest; in addition these patients as a group also have poor functional, nutritional, and physiologic reserve.

The downside of such dorsal approaches is that these patients have a much higher rate of wound dehiscence and infection because of prior radiation, corticosteroids, and malnourishment.* Numerous studies have shown the deleterious effects that radiation has on wound healing including inhibition of fibroblast outgrowth, reduced collagen

formation, and decreased wound tensile strength.[50,73,91,106] Even when radiation has been performed at a remote time course, the negative affects that this has on the microvasculature results in hyalinization of vessels and diminished blood flow in the radiation field greatly impacting on wound healing.[73,91,101] Patients are at greatest risk when radiation precedes surgery by less than 6 weeks and in these patients we now perform prophylactic rotational flaps.[50,73] In addition, the authors now try to rapidly wean steroids postoperatively in any patient who has undergone decompression and is neurologically normal.

Finally, many of these patients must undergo numerous surgical procedures that lead to further fibrosis and decreased vascularity in the surrounding soft tissue. These factors all lead to decreases in the bulk and quality of soft tissue available for covering such complicated wounds. The authors have found the use of rotational flaps very advantageous for the treatment of such wound healing complications. These flaps permit for laterally situated muscle that exists outside the RT port to be brought into the defect and help to fill dead space. These flaps have been shown in both clinical and animal studies to improve wound healing and control bacterial contamination.* While several other treatment strategies, such as suction irrigation systems, serial débridements with antibiotic-impregnated beads, and vacuum packs, exist for the treatment of complicated spine wounds all of these fail to correct the soft tissue problems and fill the dead space that results.[75,117,192,217,229] The advantage of using rotational flaps over the other methods is that soft tissue is brought in over the instrumentation and patients can be débrided and irrigated once followed by advancement flaps at a second sitting. This facilitates earlier definitive wound closure and thus mobilization and restoration of normal postoperative course in these patients allowing earlier hospital discharge while at the same time having high rates of instrument salvage. At MSKCC, we have treated 13 patients who developed deep wound dehiscence and/or infection with this strategy. Intravenous antibiotics were continued for 6 to 8 weeks depending on the bacteria and the response to treatment. This strategy has allowed for great success in managing these difficult wounds with no failures and only two complications (wound seromas). In addition, in the past year, three superficial wounds that did not extend through the paraspinal muscle fascia were treated with the use of vacuum packs, with success.[226]

*References 6,28,61,77,91,133,135,153,180,181,220.

REFERENCES

1. Achbarou A, Kaiser S, Tremblay G, et al: Urokinase overproduction results in increased skeletal metastasis by prostate cancer cells in vivo. *Cancer Res* 54:2372-2377, 1994.
2. Adami S, Salvagno G, Guarrera G, et al: Dichloromethylene diphosphonate in patients with prostatic carcinoma metastatic to the skeleton. *J Urol* 134:1152-1154, 1985.
3. Akeyson E, McCutcheon IE: Single-stage posterior vertebrectomy and replacement combined with posterior instrumentation for spinal metastasis. *J Neurosurg* 85: 211-20, 1996.

*References 40,47,56,97,117,132,142,148,217.

4. Albelda SM, Buck CA: Integrins and other cell adhesion molecules. *FASEB J* 4:2868-2880, 1990.

5. Algra RR, Heimans JJ, Valk J, et al: Do metastases in vertebrae begin in the body or pedicles? Imaging study in 45 patients. *AJR Am J Roentgenol* 158:1275-1279, 1992.

6. Anthony JP, Mathes SJ, Alpert BS: The muscle flap in the treatment of chronic lower extremity osteomyelitis. *Plast Reconstr Surg* 88:311-315, 1991.

7. Arguello F, Baggs RB, Frantz CN: A murine model of experimental metastases to bone and bone marrow. *Cancer Res* 48:6876-81, 1988.

8. Atanasiu J, Badatcgeff F, Pidhorz L: Metastatic lesions of the cervical spine. *Spine* 1993;18:1279-128.

9. Avrahami E, Tadmor R, Kaplinsky N: The role of T2-weighted gradient echo in MRI demonstration of spinal multiple myeloma. *Spine* 18:1812-1815, 1993.

10. Barron KD, Hirano A, Araki S: Experiences with metastatic neoplasms involving the spinal cord. *Neurology* 9:91-106, 1959.

11. Basset P, Bellocq JP, Wolf C, et al: A novel metalloproteinase gene specifically expressed in stromal cells of breast carcinomas. *Nature* 348:699-704, 1990.

12. Bauer HCF, Wedin R: Survival after surgery for spinal and extremity metastases: prognostication of 241 patients. *Acta Orthop Scand* 66(2):143-146, 1995.

13. Behrens J, Mareel MM, Van Roy FM, Birchmeier W: Dissecting tumor cell invasion: epithelial cells acquire invasive properties after the loss of uvomorulin-mediated cell-cell adhesion. *J Cell Biol* 108:2435-2447, 1989.

14. Berenson JR, Lichtenstein A, Porter L, et al: Efficacy of pamidronate in reducing skeletal events in patients with advanced multiple myeloma. Myeloma aredia study group. *N Engl J Med* 334:488-493, 1996.

15. Berenson JR, Lichtenstein A, Porter L, et al: Long-term pamidronate treatment of advanced multiple myeloma patients reduces skeletal events. Myeloma aredia study group. *J Clin Oncol* 16:593-602, 1998.

16. Berenson JR, Rosen LS, Howell A, et al: Zoledronic acid reduces skeletal-related events in patients with osteolytic metastases: a double-blind, randomized dose-response study. *Am Cancer Soc* 91(7):1191-1200, 2001.

17. Bilsky M, Boland P, Lis E, et al: Single-stage posterolateral transpedicle approach for spondylectomy, epidural decompression and circumferential fusion of spinal metastases. *Spine* 25:2240-2250, 2000.

18. Bilsky M, Lis E, Raizer J, et al: The diagnosis and treatment of metastatic spinal tumor. *Oncologist* 4:459-69, 1999.

19. Bilsky MH, Shannon FJ, Sheppard S, et al: Diagnosis and management of a metastatic tumor in the atlantoaxial spine. *Spine* 27(10):1062-1069, 2002.

20. Boissier S, Magnetto S, Frappart L, et al: Bisphosphonates inhibit prostate and breast carcinoma cell adhesion to unmineralized and mineralized bone extracellular matrices. *Cancer Res* 1997;57:3890-3894.

21. Boonekamp PM, van der Wee-Pals LJA, van Wijk-van Lennep MML: Two modes of action of bisphosphonates on osteoclastic resorption of mineralized matrix. *Bone Mineral* 1:27-39, 1986.

22. Boriani S, Biagini R, De Iure F, et al: Resection surgery in the treatment of vertebral tumors. *Chir Organi Mov* 83 (1-2):53-64, 1998.

23. Bowyer SL, LaMothe MP, Hollister JR: Steroid myopathy: incidence and detection in a population with asthma. *J Allergy Clin Immunol* 76:234, 1985.

24. Brice J, McKissock W: Surgical treatment of malignant extradural spinal tumours. *Br Med J* 1:1341-1344, 1965.

25. Bridwell KH, Jenny AB, Saul T, et al: Posterior segmental spinal instrumentation (PSSI) with posterolateral decompression and debulking for metastatic thoracic and lumbar spine disease: limitations and technique. *Spine* 13:1383-1394, 1988.

26. Byrne TN: Spinal cord compression from epidural metastases. *N Engl J Med* 327:614-619, 1992.

27. Cahill DW, Kumar R: Palliative subtotal vertebrectomy with anterior and posterior reconstruction via a single posterior approach. *J Neurosurg* 90(1 suppl):42-47, 1999.

28. Calderon W, Chang N, Mathes SJ: Comparison of the effect of bacterial inoculation in musculocutaneous and fasciocutaneous flaps. *Plast Reconstr Surg* 77:785-782, 1986.

29. Canalis E, Centrella M, McCarthy T: Effects of basic fibroblast growth factor on bone formation in vitro. *J Clin Invest* 81:1572-1577, 1988.

30. Canalis E, Lorenzo J, Burgess WH, Maciag T: Effects of endothelial cell growth factor on bone remodeling in vitro. *J Clin Invest* 79:59-58, 1987.

31. Carr I, Orr FW: Current reviews: invasion and metastasis. *Can Med Assoc J* 128:1164-1167, 1983.

32. Charhon SA, Chapuy MC, Delving EE, et al: Histomorphometric analysis of sclerotic bone metastases from prostatic carcinoma with special references to osteomalacia. *Cancer* 51:918-924, 1983.

33. Clarke CR, Keggi KJ, Panjabi MM: Methylmethacrylate stabilization of the cervical spine. *J Bone Joint Surg Am* 66:40-46, 1984.

34. Clemens MR, Fessele K, Heim ME: Multiple myeloma: effect of daily dichloromethylene bisphosphonate on skeletal complications. *Ann Hematol* 66:141-146, 1993.

35. Cobb CA, Leavens ME, Eckles N: Indications for nonoperative treatment of spinal cord compression due to breast cancer. *J Neurosurg* 47:653-658, 1977.

36. Coleman RE, Woll PJ, Miles M, Scrivener W, Rubens RD: Treatment of bone metastases from breast cancer with (3-amino-1-hydroxy-propylidene)-1, 1-bisphosphonate (APD). *Br J Cancer* 58:621-625, 1988.

37. Constans JP, DeDivitiis E, Donzelli R, et al: Spinal metastases with neurological manifestations: review of 600 cases. *J Neurosurg* 59:111-118, 1983.

38. Cooper P, Errico T, et al: A systematic approach to spinal reconstruction after anterior decompression for neoplastic disease of the thoracic and lumbar spine. *Neurosurgery* 32:1-8, 1993.

39. Cresswell SM, English PJ, Hall RR, et al: Pain relief and quality-of-life assessment following intravenous and oral clodronate in hormone-escaped metastatic prostate cancer. *Br J Urol* 76:360-365, 1995.

40. Cruse PJ, Foord R: A five-year prospective study of 23,649 surgical wounds. *Arch Surg* 107:206-210, 1973.

41. Dallas SL, Miyazono K, Skerry TM, Mundy GR, Bonewald LF: Dual role for the latent transforming growth factor-beta binding protein in storage of latent TGF-beta in the extracellular matrix and as a structural matrix protein. *J Cell Biol* 1995;131:539-549, 1995.

42. Dallas SL, Park-Snyder S, Miyazono K, *et al:* Characterization and autoregulation of latent TGFb complexes in osteoblast-like cell lines: production of a latent complex lacking the latent TGFb-binding protein (LTBP). *J Biol Chem* 1994;269:6815-6822, 1994.

43. Darling GE, McBroom R, Perrin R: Modified anterior approach to the cervicothoracic junction. *Spine* 20(13):1519-1521, 1995.

44. Dehodashti F, Siegal BA, Griffeth LK, *et al:* Benign versus malignant intraosseous lesions: discrimination by means of PET with 2-[F-18] fluoro-2-deoxy-D-glucose. *Radiology* 2000(1): 243-247, 1996.

45. de la Mata J, Uy HL, Guise TA, *et al:* Interleukin-6 enhances hypercalcemia and bone resorption mediated by parathyroid hormone-related protein in vivo. *J Clin Invest* 95:2846-2852, 1995.

46. Delmas PD: The use of clodronate in multiple myeloma. *Bone* 12(Suppl 1):S31-S34, 1994.

47. Dickhaut SC, DeLee JC, Page CP: Nutritional status: Importance in predicting wound-healing after amputation. *J Bone Joint Surg Am* 66:71-75, 1984.

48. Dickman CA, Rosenthal D, Karahalios DG, *et al:* Thoracic vertebrectomy and reconstruction using a microsurgical thoracoscopic approach. *Neurosurgery* 38(2):279-293, 1996.

49. Diel IJ, Solomayer EF, Costa SD, *et al:* Reduction in new metastases in breast cancer with adjuvant clodronate treatment. *N Engl J Med* 339:357-363, 1998.

50. Disa JJ, Smith AW, Bilsky MK: Management of radiated reoperative wounds of the cervicothoracic spine: the role of the trapezius turnover flap. *Ann Plast Surg* 47:394-397, 2001.

51. Dunn EJ: The role of methylmethacrylate in the stabilization and replacement of tumors of the cervical spine: a project of the Cervical Spine Research Society. *Spine* 2:15-24, 1977.

52. Dunn, RC Jr., Kelly WA, Wohns RNW, *et al:* Spinal epidural neoplasia: a 15-year review of the results of surgical therapy. *J Neurosurg* 52:47-51, 1980.

53. Dunstan CR, Garrett IR, Adams R, *et al:* Systemic fibroblast growth factor (FGF-1) prevents bone loss, increases new bone formation, and restores trabecular microarchitecture in ovariectomized rats. *J Bone Miner Res* 10(suppl 1):279, 1995.

54. Dwyer AJ, Frank JA, Sank VJ, *et al:* Short T1 inversion-recovery pulse sequence: analysis and initial experience in cancer imaging. *Radiology* 1988;168: 827-836, 1988.

55. *Eastern Cooperative Oncology Group Performance Status Scale.* Eastern Cooperative Oncology Group. Revised March 25, 1998.

56. Ehrlich HP, Hunt TK: Effects of cortisone and vitamin A on wound healing. *Ann Surg* 167:324-328, 1968.

57. Elomaa I, Blomqvist C, Grohn P et al: Long-term controlled trial of bisphosphonate in patients with osteolytic bone metastases. *Lancet* 1:146-149, 1983.

58. Elomaa I, Kylmala T, Tammela T, *et al:* Effect of oral clodronate on bone pain—a controlled study in patients with metastatic prostate cancer. *Int Urol Nephrol* 24: 159-166, 1992.

59. Ernst DS, Brasher P, Hagen N, *et al:* A randomized, controlled trial of intravenous clodronate in metastatic bone disease and pain. *J Pain Symptom Manage* 13: 319-26, 1997.

60. Ernst DS, MacDonald N, Paterson AHG, *et al:* A double-blind crossover trial of intravenous clodronate in metastatic bone pain. *J Pain Symptom Manage* 7:4-11, 1992.

61. Eshima I, Mathes SJ, Paty P: Comparison of the intracellular bacterial killing activity of leukocytes in musculocutaneous and random-pattern flaps. *Plast Reconstr Surg* 86:541-545, 1990.

62. Fidler IJ, Poste G: The cellular heterogeneity of malignant neoplasms: implications for adjuvant chemotherapy. *Semin Oncol* 12:207-221, 1985.

63. Fidler IJ: Tumor heterogeneity and the biology of cancer invasion and metastasis. *Cancer Res* 38:2651-2660, 1978.

64. Fidler MW: Radical resection of vertebral body tumours. A surgical technique used in ten cases. *J Bone Joint Surg Br* 76(5):765-772, 1994.

65. Findlay GFG: Adverse effects of the management of malignant spinal cord compression. *J Neurol Neurosurg Psychiatry* 47:761-768, 1984.

66. Flanagan AM, Chambers TJ: Inhibition of bone resorption by bisphosphonates: Interactions between bisphosphonates, osteoclasts, and bone. *Calcif Tissue Int* 49:407-415, 1991.

67. Fleisch H: Bisphosphonates—history and experimental basis. *Bone* 8(Suppl 1):523-528, 1987.

68. Fleisch H: Bisphosphonates: a new class of drugs in diseases of bone and calcium metabolism. *Recent Results Cancer Res* 116:1-28, 1989.

69. Frank JA, Ling A, Patronas NJ, *et al:* Detection of malignant bone tumors: MR Imaging vs Scintigraphy. *AJR Am J Roentgenol* 1990;155:1043-1048.

70. Frankel HL, Hancock DO, Hyslop G, *et al:* The value of postdural reduction in the initial management of closed injuries in the spine with paraplegia and tetraplegia. I. Comprehensive management and research. *Paraplegia* 7:179-192, 1969.

71. Friedman M, Kim TH, Panahon AM: Spinal cord compression in malignant lymphoma: treatment and results. *Cancer* 37:1485-1491, 1976.

72. Garbisa S, Pozzatti R, Muschel RJ, *et al:* Secretion of type IV collagenolytic protease and metastatic phenotype: induction by transfection with c-Ha-ras but not c-Ha-ras plus AD2-Ela. *Cancer Res* 47:1523-1528, 1987.

73. Ghogawala Z, Mansfield FL, Borges LF: Spinal radiation before surgical decompression adversely affects outcomes of surgery for symptomatic metastatic spinal cord compression. *Spine* 26:818-824, 2001.

74. Gilbert R W, Kim J H, Posner JB: Epidural spinal cord compression from metastatic tumor: diagnosis and treatment. *Ann Neurol* 3:40-51, 1978.

75. Glassman SD, Dimar JR, Puno RM, Johnson JR: Salvage of instrumented lumbar fusions complicated by surgical wound infection. *Spine* 21:2163-2169, 1996.

76. Glover D, Lipton A, Keller A, *et al:* Intravenous pamidronate disodium treatment of bone metastases in patients with breast cancer: a dose-seeking study. *Cancer* 74:2949-2955, 1994.

77. Gokaslan ZL, York JE, Walsh GL, *et al:* Transthoracic vertebrectomy for metastatic spinal tumors. *J Neurosurg* 89:599-609, 1998.

78. Gosfield E, Alavi A, Kneeland B: Comparison of radionuclide bone scans and magnetic resonance imaging in detecting spinal metastases. *J Nucl Med* 34(12): 2191-2198, 1993.

79. Graham GP, Dent CM, Burgess N, *et al:* Urinary retention in prostatic carcinoma: obstructive or neurogenic? *Br J Hosp Med* 49(10):733-734, 1993.

80. Greenberg HS, Kim JH, Posner JB: Epidural spinal cord compression from metastatic tumor: results with a new treatment protocol. *Ann Neurol* 8(4):362-366, 1980.

81. Grubb MR, Currier BL, Pritchard DJ, *et al:* Primary Ewing's sarcoma of the spine. *Spine* 19(3):309-313, 1994.

82. Gundry CR, Fritts HM: Magnetic resonance imaging of the musculoskeletal system: the spine. *Clin Orthop* 346:262-278, 1998.

83. Hall A, Mackay N: The results of laminectomy for compression of the cord or cauda equina by extradural malignant tumour. *J Bone Joint Surg Br* 55:497-505, 1973.

84. Hamilton AJ, Lulu B, Stea B, *et al:* The use of gold foil wrapping for radiation protection of the spinal cord for recurrent tumor therapy. *Int J Rad Oncol Biol Phys* 32(2):507-511, 1995.

85. Harris SE, Bonewald LF, Harris MA, *et al:* Effects of transforming growth factor beta on bone nodule formation and expression of bone morphogenic protein 2, osteocalcin, osteopontin, alkaline phosphatase, and type 1 collagen mRNA in long-term cultures of fetal rat calvarial osteoblasts. *J Bone Miner Res* 9:855-863, 1994.

86. Harris SE, Boyce B, Feng JQ, *et al:* Antisense bone morphogenetic protein 3 (BMP 3) constructions decrease new bone formation in prostate cancer model. *J Bone Miner Res* 7(suppl 1)abstr:92, 1992.

87. Hashimoto M, Niwa O, Nitta Y, *et al:* Unstable expression of E-cadherin adhesion molecules in metastatic ovarian tumor cells. *Jpn J Cancer Res* 80:459-463, 1989.

88. Heary R, Vaccaro A, Benevenia J, Cotler JM: "En bloc" vertebrectomy in the mobile lumbar spine. *Surg Neurol* 50:(6):548-556, 1998.

89. Heimdal K, Hirschberg H, Slettebo H, *et al:* High incidence of serious side effects of high-dose dexamethasone treatment in patients with epidural spinal cord compression. *J Neurosurg* 12:141-144, 1992.

90. Heppner G: Tumor heterogeneity. *Cancer Res* 214: 2259-2265, 1984.

91. Hochberg J, Ardenghy M, Yuen J, *et al:* Muscle and musculocutaneous flap coverage of exposed spinal fusion devices. *Plast Reconstr Surg* 102(2):385-389, 1998.

92. Hortobagyi GN, Theriault RL, Porter L, *et al:* Efficacy of pamidronate in reducing skeletal complications in patients with breast cancer and lytic bone metastases. *Protocol* 19 Aredia Breast Cancer study group. *N Engl J Med* 335: 1785-1791, 1996.

93. Hynes RO: Integrins: versatility, modulation, and signaling in cell adhesion. *Cell* 69:11-25, 1992.

94. International standards for neurological and functional classifications of spinal cord injury. Chicago, American Spinal Injury Association 1982 (revised 1996).

95. Izbicka E, Dunstan C, Esparza J, *et al:* Human amniotic tumor which induces new bone formation in vivo produces a growth regulatory activity in vitro for osteoblasts identified as an extended form of basic fibroblast growth factor (bFGF). *Cancer Res* 56:633-636, 1996.

96. Jenis GL, Dunn EJ, An HS: Metastatic disease of the cervical spine. A review. *Clin Orthop* 359:89-103, 1999.

97. Jensen JE, Jensen TI, Smith TK, *et al:* Nutrition in orthopedic surgery. *J Bone Joint Surg Br* 64:1263-1272, 1982.

98. Johnston F, Uttley D, Marsh HT, *et al:* Synchronous vertebral decompression and posterior stabilization in the treatment of spinal malignancy. *Neurosurgery* 25:872-876, 1989.

99. Jones KM, Schwartz RB, Mantello MT, *et al:* Fast spin-echo MR in the detection of vertebral metastases: comparison of three sequences. *AJNR Am J Neuroradiol* 15(3):401-407, 1994.

100. Jonsson B, Jonsson Jr H, Karlstrom G, *et al:* Surgery of cervical spine metastases: a retrospective study. *Eur Spine J* 3:76-83, 1994.

101. Joseph DL, Shumrick DL: Risks of head and neck surgery in previously irradiated patients. *Arch Otolaryngol* 97: 306-314, 1973.

102. Kanis JA, Percival RC, Yates A, Urwin GH, Hamdy NA: Effects of diphosphonates in hypercalcemia due to neoplasia. *Lancet* 1:615-616, 1986.

103. Kanis JA, McCloskey EV: Bone turnover and biochemical markers in malignancy. *Cancer Suppl* 80(8):1538-1546, 1997.

104. Kanis JA, McCloskey EV, Powles T, *et al:* A high incidence of vertebral fracture in women with breast cancer. *Br J Cancer* 79(7-8):1179-1181, 1999.

105. Kanis JA, Powles T, Paterson AH, *et al:* Clodronate decreases the frequency of skeletal metastases in women with breast cancer. *Bone* 19:663-667, 1996.

106. Ketcham AS, Hoye RC, Chretien PB, Brace KC: Irradiation twenty-four hours preoperatively. *Am J Surg* 118:691-697, 1969.

107. Khan F, Glicksman A, Chu F, *et al:* Treatment by radiotherapy of spinal cord compression due to extradural metastases. *Radiology* 89:495-500, 1967.

108. Kim RY, Spencer SA, Meredith RF, *et al:* Extradural spinal cord compression: analysis of factors determining functional prognosis. Prospective study. *Radiology* 176:279-282, 1990.

109. Kleinman WB, Kiernan HA, Michelsen WJ: Metastatic cancer of the spinal column. *Clin Orthop* 136:166-172, 1978.

110. Klekamp J, Samii H: Surgical results for spinal metastases. *Acta Neurochir (Wien)* 140:957-967, 1998.

111. Kostuik JP: Anterior spinal cord decompression for lesions of the thoracic and lumbar spine, techniques, new methods of internal fixation results. *Spine* 8(5):512-531, 1983.

112. Kraus DH, Ali MK, Ginsberg RJ, *et al:* Vocal cord medialization for unilateral paralysis associated with intrathoracic malignancies. *J Thorac Cardiovasc Surg* 11(2):334-339, 1996.

113. Kylmala T, Tammela T, Risteli L, *et al:* Evaluation of the effects of oral clodronate on skeletal metastases with type 1 collagen metabolites. A controlled trial of the Finnish Prostate Cancer Group. *Eur J Cancer* 291:821-825, 1993.

114. Kylmala T, Tammela TLJ, Lindholm, *et al:* The effect of combined intravenous and oral clodronate treatment on bone pain in patients with metastatic prostate cancer. *Ann Chirurg Gynecol* 83:316-319, 1994.

115. Langenstroer P, Tang R, Shapiro E, *et al:* Endothelin-1 in the human prostate: tissue levels, source of production and isometric tension studies. *J Urol* 150:495-499, 1993.

116. Lee MV, Fong EM, Singer FR, Guenette RS: Bisphosphonate treatment inhibits the growth of prostate cancer cells. *Cancer Res* 61:2602-2608, 2001.

117. Levi AD, Dickman CA, Sonntag VK: Management of postoperative infections after spinal instrumentation. *J Neurosurg* 86:975-980, 1997.

118. Liotta LA, Kohn E: Cancer invasion and metastases. *JAMA* 263:1123-1126, 1990.

119. Lipton A, Theriault RL, Hortobagyi GN, *et al:* Pamidronate prevents skeletal complications and is effective palliative treatment in women with breast carcinoma and osteolytic bone metastases: Long term follow-up of two randomized, placebo-controlled trials. *Am Cancer Soc* 88(5):1082-1090, 2000.

120. Lipton A: Bisphosphonates and breast carcinoma. *Cancer* 80(8):1668-1673, 1997.

121. Livingston KE, Perrin RG: The neurosurgical management of spinal metastases causing cord and cauda equina compression. *J Neurosurg* 49:839-843, 1978.

122. Loblaw AD, Laperriere NJ: emergency treatment of malignant extradural spinal cord compression: an evidence-based guideline. *J Clin Onc* 16(4):1613-1624, 1998.

123. Magerl F, Coscia M: Total posterior vertebrectomy of the thoracic and lumbar spine. *Clin Orthop* 232:62-69, 1988.

124. Magnetto S, Boissier S, Delmas P, Clezardin P: Additive antitumor activities of toxoids in combination with the bisphosphonate ibandronate against invasion and adhesion of human breast carcinoma cells to bone. *Int J Cancer* 83:263-269, 1999.

125. Major PP, Lipton A, Berenson J, Hortobagyi G: Oral bisphosphonates: a review of clinical use in patients with bone metastases. *Am Cancer Soc* 88(1):6-14, 2000.

126. Mansson PE, Adams P, Kan M, McKeehan WL: HBGF1 gene expression in normal rat prostate and two transplantable rat prostate tumors. *Cancer Res* 49:2485-2494, 1989.

127. Maranzano E, Latini P, Beneventi S, *et al:* Radiotherapy without steroids in selected metastatic spinal cord compression patients. *Am J Clin Oncol* 19(2):179-83, 1996.

128. Maranzano E, Latini P: Effectiveness of radiation therapy without surgery in metastatic spinal cord compression: final results from a prospective trial. *Int J Rad Onc Biol Phys* 32(4):959-967, 1995.

129. Marchesi DG, Boos N, Aebi M: Surgical treatment of tumors of the cervical spine and first two thoracic vertebrae. *J Spinal Disord* 6(6):489-496, 1993.

130. Mareel MM, Behrens J, Birchmeier W, *et al:* Down-regulation of E-cadherin expression in Madin-Darby canine kidney (MDCK) cells inside tumors of nude mice. *Int J Cancer* 47:922-928, 1991.

131. Marshall LF, Langfitt TW: Combined therapy for metastatic extradural tumors of the spine. *Cancer* 40:2067-2070, 1977.

132. Massie JB, Heller JG, Abitbol JJ, *et al:* Postoperative posterior spinal wound infections. *Clin Orthop* 284:99-108, 1992.

133. Mathes SJ, Alpert BS, Chang N: Use of the muscle flap in chronic osteomyelitis: experimental and clinical correlation. *Plast Reconstr Surg* 69:815-821, 1982.

134. Mathes SJ, Teng L, Hunt TK: Coverage of the infected wound. *Am J Surg* 198:420-427, 1983.

135. Matsui H, Tatezaki S, Tsuji H: Ceramic vertebral body replacement for metastatic spine tumors. *J Spinal Disord* 7(3):248-254, 1994.

136. Matuo Y, Nishi N, Matsui S, *et al:* Heparin binding affinity of rat prostate growth factor in normal and cancerous prostate; partial purification and characterization of rat prostate growth factor in the Dunning tumor. *Cancer Res* 47:188-192, 1987.

137. Mayahara H, Ito T, Nagai H, *et al:* In vivo stimulation of endosteal bone formation by basic fibroblast growth factor in rats. *Growth Factors* 9:73-80, 1993.

138. Mbalaviele G, Dunstan CR, Sasaki A, *et al:* E-cadherin expression in human breast cancer cells suppresses the development of osteolytic bone metastases in experimental metastases model. *Cancer Res* 56:4063-4070, 1996.

139. McAfee P, Bohlman H, Ducker T, Eismont F: Failure of stabilization of the spine with methylmethacrylate. A retrospective analysis of twenty-four cases. *J Bone Joint Surg* 65-A:1145-1157, 1986.

140. McAfee PC, Bohlman HH: One-stage anterior cervical decompression and posterior stabilization with arthrodesis. A study of twenty-four patients who had a traumatic or neoplastic lesion. *J Bone Joint Surg* 71-A:78-88, 1989.

141. McCloskey EV, Spector TD, Eyres KS, *et al:* The assessment of vertebral deformity: a method for use in population studies and clinical trials. *Osteoporos Int* 3:138-147, 1993.

142. McPhee IB, Williams RP, Swanson CE: Factors influencing wound healing after surgery for metastatic disease of the spine. *Spine* 3:726-732, 193, 1998.

143. Mehta RC, Marks MP, Hinks RS, *et al:* MR evaluation of vertebral metastases: T1-weighted, short-inversion-time inversion recovery, fast spin-echo, and inversion-recovery fast spin-echo sequences. *AJNR Am J Neuroradiol* 16(2):281-288, 1995.

144. Miller DJ, Lang FF, Walsh FL, *et al:* Coaxial double-lumen methylmethacrylate reconstruction in the anterior cervical and upper thoracic spine after tumor resection. *J Neurosurg* 92(2):181-190, 2000.

145. Moulopoulos LA, Kumar AJ, Leeds N: A second look at unenhanced spinal magnetic resonance imaging of malignant leptomeningeal disease. *Clinical Imag* 21(4):252-259, 1997.

146. Moulopoulos LA, Yoshimitsu K, Johnston DA, *et al:* MR prediction of benign and malignant vertebral compression fractures. *J Magn Reson Imag* 6(4):667-674, 1996.

147. Mullan J, Evans JP: Neoplastic disease of the spinal extradural space: a review of 50 cases. *Arch Surg* 1957;74:900-909.

148. Mullen JL, Buzby GP, Matthews DC, Smale BF, Rosato EF: Reduction of operative morbidity and mortality by combined preoperative and postoperative nutritional support. *Ann Surg* 192:604-613, 1980.

149. Mundy G: Hypercalcemia of malignancy revisited. *J Clin Invest* 82:1-6, 1988.
150. Mundy GR, Yoneda T: Bisphosphonates as anticancer drug. *N Engl J Med* 339:357-363, 1998.
151. Mundy GR, Yoneda T: Facilitation and suppression of bone metastasis. *Clin Orthop* 312:34-44, 1995.
152. Mundy GR: Mechanisms of bone metastasis. *Cancer Suppl* 80(8):1546-1556, 1997.
153. Murphy RC, Robson MC, Heggers JP, Kadowski M: The effect of microbial contamination on musculocutaneous and random flaps. *J Surg Res* 41:75-80, 1986.
154. Muscle and musculocutaneous flap coverage of exposed spinal fusion devices. *Plastic Recon Surg* 102:385-389, 1998.
155. Nakai M, Mundy GR, Williams PJ, *et al:* A synthetic antagonist to laminin inhibits the formation of osteolytic metastases by human melanoma cells in nude mice. *Cancer Res* 52:5395-5399, 1992.
156. Nazzaro JM, Arbit E, Burt M: "Trap door" exposure to the cervicothoracic junction. Technical notes. *J Neurosurg* 80:338-341, 1994.
157. Nelson JB, Hedican SP, George D, *et al:* Identification of endothelin-1 in the pathophysiology of metastatic adenocarcinoma of the prostate. *Nat Med* 1:944-949, 1995.
158. Nicholls PJ, Jarecky TW: The value of posterior decompression by laminectomy for malignant tumors of the spine. *Clin Orthop* 201:210-212, 1985.
159. Nip J, Shibata H, Loskutoff DJ, *et al:* Human melanoma cells derived from lymphatic metastases use integrin alpha v beta 3 to adhere to lymph node vitronectin. *J Clin Invest* 90:1406-1413.
160. Oka H, Shiozaki H, Kobayashi K, *et al:* Expression of E-cadherin cells adhesion molecules in human breast cancer tissue and its relationship to metastasis. *Cancer Res* 53:1696-1701, 1993.
161. Olerud C, Jonsson H, Lofberg AM, *et al:* Embolization of spinal metastases reduces perioperative blood loss: 21 patients operated on for renal cell carcinoma. *Acta Orthop Scand* 64(1):9-12, 1993.
162. Ortiz O, Pait TG, McAllister P, *et al:* Postoperative magnetic resonance imaging with titanium implants of the thoracic and lumbar spine. *Neurosurgery* 38(4): 741-745, 1996.
163. Oz M., Cosgrove DM III, Badduke BR, *et al:* Controlled clinical trial of a novel hemostatic agent in cardiac surgery. The Fusion Matrix Study Group. *Ann Thorac Surg* 69(5):1376-1382, 2000.
164. Paget S: The distribution of secondary growths in cancer of the breast. *Lancet* 1:571-573, 1989.
165. Panjabi MM, White AA: Basic biomechanics of the spine. *Neurosurgery* 7:76-93, 1980.
166. Paterson A: The potential role of bisphosphonates as adjuvant therapy in the prevention of bone metastases. *Cancer* 88:3038-3046, 2000.
167. Paterson AHG, Powles TJ, Kanis JA, *et al:* Double-blind controlled trial of oral clodronate in patients with bone metastases from breast cancer. *J Clin Oncol* 11:59-65, 1993.
168. Perrin RG, McBroom RJ: Anterior versus posterior decompression for symptomatic spinal metastasis. *Can J Neur Sci* 14:75-80, 1987.
169. Perrin RG, McBroom RJ: Spinal fixation after anterior decompression for symptomatic spinal metastasis. *Neurosurgery* 22(2):324-327, 1998.
170. Pfeilschifter J, Mundy GR: Modulation of transforming growth factor beta activity in bone cultures by osteotropic hormones. *Proc Natl Acad Sci USA* 84:2024-2028, 1987.
171. Phillips E, Levine AM: Metastatic lesions of the upper cervical spine. *Spine* 14:1071-1077, 1989.
172. Posner JB, Howieson J, Cvitkovic E: "Disappearing" spinal cord compression: oncolytic effect of glucocorticoids (and other chemotherapeutic agents) on epidural metastases. *Ann Neurol* 2:409-413, 1977.
173. Poste G: Pathogenesis of metastatic disease: implications for current therapy and for the development of new therapeutic strategies. *Cancer Treat Rep* 70:183-199, 1986.
174. Powles TJ, Paterson AHG, Neventaus S, *et al:* Adjuvant clodronate reduces the incidence of bone metastases in patients with primary operable breast cancer. *Proc Am Soc Clin Oncol* 17:468, 1998.
175. Rabbani SA, Desjardins J, Bell AW, *et al:* Identification of a new osteoblast mitogen from a human prostate cancer cell line, PC-3. *J Bone Miner Res* 5:549, 1990.
176. Rabbani SA, Desjardins J, Bell AW, *et al:* An amino-terminal fragment of urokinase isolated from prostate cancer cell line (PC-3) is mitogenic for osteoblast-like cells. *Biochem Biophys Res Commun* 173:1058-1064, 1990a.
177. Rabbani SA, Mazar AP, Bernier SM, *et al:* Structural requirements for the growth factor activity of the amino-terminal domain of urokinase. *J Biol Chem* 267:14151-14156, 1992.
178. Ramasastry SS, Schlechter B, Cohen M: Reconstruction of posterior trunk defects. *Clin Plast Surg* 22:167-185, 1995.
179. Robinson R, Riley L: Techniques of exposure and fusion of the cervical spine. *Clin Orthop* 109:78-84.
180. Russell RC, Graham DR, Feller AM, *et al:* Experimental evaluation of the antibiotic carrying capacity of a muscle flap into a fibrotic cavity. *Plast Reconstr Surg* 81:162-166, 1988.
181. Saliban AH, Tesoro VR, Wood DL: Stages of transfer of a free microvascular latissimus dorsi myocutaneous flap using saphenous vein grafts. *Plast Reconstr Surg* 71: 543-547, 1983.
182. Sasaki A, Alcalde RE, Nishiyama A, *et al:* Angiogenesis inhibitor TNP-470 inhibits human breast cancer osteolytic bone metastases in nude mice through the reduction of bone resorption. *Cancer Res* 58(3):462, 1998.
183. Schiff D, O'Neill BP, Wang CH, *et al:* Neuroimaging and treatment implications of patients with multiple epidural spinal metastases. *Cancer* 83(8): 1593-1601, 1998.
184. Schiff D, Shaw EG, Cascino TL: Outcome after spinal reirradiation for malignant epidural spinal cord compression. *Ann Neurol* 37:583-589, 1995.
185. Seftor REB, Seftor EA, Gehlsen KR, *et al:* Role of the alpha v beta 3 integrin in human melanoma cell invasion. *Proc Natl Acad Sci USA* 89:1557-1561, 1992.
186. Seichi A, Kondoh T, Hozumi T, *et al:* Intraoperative radiation therapy for metastatic spinal tumors. *Spine* 24(5):470-473, 1999.
187. Smith JA: Palliation of painful bone metastases from prostate cancer using sodium etidronate: results of a

randomized, prospective, double-blind placebo-controlled study. *J Urol* 141:85-87, 1989.

188. Smith R: An evaluation of surgical treatment for spinal cord compression due to metastatic carcinoma. *J Neurol Neurosurg Psych* 28:152-158, 1965.

189. Solini A, Orsini G, Broggi S: Metal cementless prosthesis for vertebral body replacement of metastatic malignant disease of the cervical spine. *J Spinal Disord* 2(4):254-262, 1989.

190. Sommers CL, Thompson EW, Torri JA, *et al:* Cell adhesion molecule uvomorulin expression in human breast cancer cell lines: relationship to morphology and invasive capacities. *Cell Growth Differ* 2:365-372, 1991.

191. Sorensen S, Helweg-Larsen S, Mouridsen H, *et al:* Effect of high-dose dexamethasone in carcinomatous metastatic spinal cord compression treated with radiotherapy: a randomized trial. *Eur J Cancer* 1:22-27, 1994.

192. Sponseller PD, LaPorte DM, Hungerford MW, *et al:* Deep wound infections after neuromuscular scoliosis surgery: a multicenter study of risk factors and treatment outcomes. *Spine* 25:2461-2466, 2000.

193. Steffee A, Stikowski D, Topham LS, *et al:* Total vertebral body and pedicle arthroplasty. *Clin Orthop* 203:203-208, 1986.

194. Sugiyama A: Study of vertebral metastasis by MR imaging: significance of T2 weighted image (gradient field echo) and metastatic pattern. *Nippon Igaku Hoshasen Gakkai Zasshi* 54(8):767, 1994.

195. Sundaresan N, Choi IS, Hughes JE, *et al:* Treatment of spinal metastases from kidney cancer by presurgical embolization and resection. *J Neurosurg* 73:548-554, 1990.

196. Sundaresan N, DiGiacinto G, Krol G, Hughes JE: Spondylectomy for malignant tumors of the spine. *J Clin Oncol* 7:1485-1491, 1989.

197. Sundaresan N, DiGiacinto GV, Hughes JE, *et al:* Treatment of neoplastic spinal cord compression: results of a prospective study. *Neurosurgery* 29(5):645-650, 1991.

198. Sundaresan N, Galicich JH, Bains MS, *et al:* Vertebral body resection in the treatment of cancer involving the spine. *Cancer* 53:1393-1396, 1984.

199. Sundaresan N, Galicich JH, Lane JM, Greenberg HS: Treatment of odontoid fractures in cancer patients. *J Neurosurg* 54:187-192, 1981.

200. Sundaresan N, Steinberger AA, Moore F, *et al:* Indications and results of combined anterior-posterior approaches for spine tumor surgery. *J Neurosurg* 85:438-446, 1996.

201. Takeichi M: Cadherin cell adhesion receptors as a morphogenetic regulator. *Science* 251:1451-1455, 1991.

202. Takuwa Y, Masaki T, Yamashita K: The effects of the endothelin family peptides on cultured osteoblastic cells from rat calvariae. *Biochem Biophys Res Commun* 170:998-1005, 1990.

203. Takuwa Y, Ohue Y, Takuwa N, Yamashita K: Endothelin-1 activates phospholipase C and mobilizes Ca2+ from extra and intracellular pools in osteoblastic cells. *Am J Physiol* 257:E797-E803, 1989.

204. Terpos E, Plermos J, Tsionos K, *et al:* Effect of pamidronate administration on markers of bone turnover and disease activity in multiple myeloma. *Eur J Haematol* 65:331-336, 2000.

205. Theriault RL, Lipton A, Hortobagyi GN, *et al:* Pamidronate reduces skeletal morbidity in women with advanced breast cancer and lytic bone lesions: a randomized, placebo-controlled trial. *J Clin Oncol* 17(3):846-854, 1999.

206. Thomas RJ, Guise TA, Yin JJ, *et al:* Breast cancer cells interact with osteoblasts to support osteoclasts formation. *Endocrinology* 140:4451-4458, 1999.

207. Tomita K, Kawahara N, Baba H, *et al:* Total en bloc spondylectomy for solitary spinal metastasis. *Int Orthop* 18:291-298, 1994.

208. Traill Z, Richards MA, Moore NR: Magnetic resonance imaging of metastatic bone disease. *Clin Orthop* 312: 76-88, 1995.

209. Vaccaro AR, Falatyn SP, Scuderi GJ, *et al:* Early failure of long segment anterior cervical plate fixation. *J Spinal Disord* 11:410-415, 1998.

210. Van der Pluijm G, Vloedgraven H, van Beek E, *et al:* Bisphosphonates inhibit the adhesion of breast cancer cells to bone matrices in vitro. *J Clin Invest* 98:698-705, 1996.

211. Van Holten-Verzantvoort AT, Bijvoet OL, Cleton FJ, *et al:* Reduced morbidity from skeletal metastases in breast cancer patients during long-term bisphosphonates (APD) treatment. *Lancet* 11:983-985, 1987.

212. Van Holten-Verzantvoort AT, Zwinderman AH, Aaronson NK, *et al:* The effect of supportive pamidronate treatment on aspects of quality of life of patients with advanced breast cancer. *Eur J Cancer* 27:544-549, 1991.

213. Vieth R, Odom G: Extradural spinal metastases and their neurosurgical treatment. *J Neurosurg* 23:501-508, 1965.

214. Yoneda T: Arterial microvascularization and breast cancer colonization in bone. *Histol Histopathol* 12(4):1145, 1997.

215. Vleminchx K, Vakaet L, Mareel M, *et al:* Genetic manipulation of E-cadherin expression by epithelial tumor cells reveals an invasion suppressor role. *Cell* 66:107-119, 1991.

216. Walsh GL, Gokaslan ZL, McCutcheon IE, *et al:* Anterior approaches to the thoracic spine in patients with cancer: indications and results. *Ann Thorac Surg* 64:1611-1618, 1997.

217. Warnold I, Lundholm K: Clinical significance of preoperative nutritional status in 215 noncancer patients. *Ann Surg* 199:299-305, 1984.

218. Wendt JR, Gardner VO, White JI: Treatment of complex postoperative lumbosacral wounds in nonparalyzed patients. *Plast Reconstr Surg* 101:1248-1253, 1998.

219. White W, Patterson R, Bergland R: The role of surgery in the treatment of spinal cord compression by metastatic neoplasm. *Cancer* 27:558-561, 1971.

220. Wild WO, Porter RW: Metastatic epidural tumor of the spine. *Arch Surg* 87:825-830, 1962.

221. Wilhelmi BJ, Snyder N, Colquhoun T, *et al:* Bipedicle paraspinous muscle flaps for spinal wound closure: an anatomic and clinical study. *Plast Reconstr Surg* 106: 1305-1311, 2000.

222. Wright R: Malignant tumours of the spinal extradural space: results of surgical treatment. *Ann Surg* 157: 227-231, 1963.

223. Yin JJ, Chirgwin JM, Taylor SD, *et al:* Dominant negative blockade of the transforming growth factor B (TGFB) type II receptor decreases breast cancer-mediated osteolysis. *J Bone Miner Res* 11(suppl 1):180, 1996.

224. Yoneda T, Michigami T, Yi B: Actions of bisphosphonate on bone metastasis in animal models of breast carcinoma. *Cancer* 88(12):2979-2988, 2000.

225. Yoneda T: Cellular and molecular mechanisms of breast and prostate cancer metastasis to bone. *Eur J Cancer* 34:240-245, 1998.

226. Yoneda T: Mechanisms of preferential metastasis of breast cancer to bone. *Int J Oncol* 9:103-109, 1996.

227. Yonida, JJ, Selander K, Chirgwin JM, *et al:* TGFb signaling blockade inhibits PTH-rP secretion by breast cancer cells and bone metastasis development. *J Clin Invest* 103:197-206, 1999.

228. Young RF, Post EM, King GA: Treatment of spinal epidural metastases. *J Neurosurg* 53:741-748, 1980.

229. Yuan-Innes MJ, Temple CL, Lacey MS: Vacuum-assisted wound closure: a new approach to spinal wounds with exposed hardware. *Spine* 26:E30-E34, 2001.

230. Zakalik D, Diep D, Hooks MA, *et al:* Transforming growth factor beta increases stability of parathyroid hormone related protein messenger RNA. *J Bone Miner Res* 7(suppl 1)abstr:104, 1992.

CHAPTER 77

Metabolic Bone Disease

Daniel J. Mazanec, Ran Vijai P. Singh,
Sonia Suys, and Parley W. Madsen III

Metabolic bone diseases represent a diverse group of skeletal disorders characterized by reduced bone mass (osteoporosis), defective bone mineralization (osteomalacia), or disordered bone remodeling (Paget's disease). Although these conditions are frequently asymptomatic, clinical consequences of interest to the spine specialist include vertebral fragility fracture with or without instability or neural compression, bone pain, spinal stenosis, or even cauda equina syndrome. Furthermore, surgical therapy may be significantly affected by coexisting metabolic bone disease. For example, pagetic bone may bleed excessively. Pedicle screw fixation may be difficult in osteoporotic bone.

In addition to surgical considerations, medical evaluation and management of metabolic bone disease is crucial to a successful therapeutic outcome. For many patients, the presenting symptom of previously unrecognized asymptomatic osteoporosis is spinal pain from an atraumatic vertebral compression fracture. In addition to managing the acute fracture, it is the responsibility of the spine specialist to ensure that appropriate medical assessment and treatment of the underlying metabolic bone disease is carried out.

Osteoporosis

Definition and Classification

A recent NIH consensus conference defined osteoporosis as "a skeletal disorder characterized by compromised bone strength predisposing a person to increased risk of fracture."[4] Bone fragility is a consequence of decreased bone density or mass, a reduced capacity to repair microfractures, or architectural changes with reduced bone strength. Bone mineral density (BMD) accounts for about 70% of bone strength. Osteoporosis is considered *primary* when it occurs in association with menopause (type I) or normal aging (type II).[122] *Secondary* osteoporosis occurs as a consequence of a variety of genetic disorders, endocrine diseases, gastrointestinal diseases, nutritional deficiencies, medications, malignancies, hypogonadism, and alcoholism (Box 77.1). As many as 50% of men with osteoporosis and 11% to 31% of women have at least one secondary factor contributing to their osteoporosis.[43,44]

Peak bone mass (PBM) is reached by 30 to 35 years of age. After the age of 35 and before the onset of menopause, bone mass gradually decreases.[216] This process affects men and women equally at a rate of approximately 0.3% per year.[88] Accelerated loss of bone mass begins in women at menopause, continuing for 10 to 15 years at a rate of approximately 3% per year.[43,88] This is primarily a result of estrogen deficiency. After the age of 70, bone mass decreases at a slower rate (which is comparable in men and women). Late, postmenopausal bone loss occurs as a result of vitamin D deficiency and resistance, physiologic hyperparathyroidism, and local secretion of bone-resorbing cytokines.[43,235]

The risk of osteoporosis is determined not only by the rate of bone loss but also by the PBM achieved during the second and third decade of life. Peak bone mass is influenced by genetic factors that are believed to account for approximately 60% to 70% of the variation in bone density.[43] Since achievement of genetically determined maximum peak bone mass occurs primarily before the age of 20 years, osteoporosis later in life may be regarded as a pediatric disease with geriatric consequences.[232] Juvenile calcium intake is positively associated with bone mass in the fourth decade of life.[211] Physical activity is another factor that positively influences achievement of optimal bone mass.

Incidence, Epidemiology, and Risk Factors

Current estimates suggest that 10 million Americans have osteoporosis and 18 million additional individuals meet World Health Organization (WHO) criteria for reduced bone mass (osteopenia), a prevalence of 12% to 15%.[8] The clinical manifestation of osteoporosis is fracture. In 1995, medical costs for the treatment of osteoporotic fractures were estimated at $14.6 billion.[240] The probability that a 50-year-old white woman will have a hip fracture during her lifetime is 14%, more than twice the risk for a male. Twenty-five percent of women over 50 years will sustain a symptomatic vertebral fracture.[50] The risk for African-Americans is about half that of Caucasians.

Only about one third of osteoporotic vertebral fractures are symptomatic, but nearly all are associated with a significant increase in mortality and functional and psychological impairment.[182] In a recent prospective cohort study, the presence of a vertebral compression fracture was associated with a 23% increase in age-adjusted mortality.[132] Vertebral fractures are also associated with significant morbidity including abdominal symptoms and pulmonary compromise, with a reduction in vital capacity of nearly 10% for each fracture.[267] Osteoporotic hip fracture is associated with a mortality rate of 20% at 1 year. Furthermore, hip fracture is associated with a dramatic decline in quality of life with one third of survivors unable to live independently. Eighty percent of women over 75 years of age indicated they would prefer death to a hip fracture resulting in nursing home placement.[202]

BMD represents the major, but not the only, factor predicting risk of fracture. Bone mineral density measured by using dual-energy x-ray absorptiometry (DEXA) has been demonstrated to predict fracture risk.[26,269] For each standard deviation below mean young adult peak bone density, the relative risk of fracture is approximately 1.5 to 2.0.[191] Other risk factors for fragility fractures are related to increased incidence of falls and include impaired vision; use of opiates, benzodiazepines, antihypertensives, and antipsychotics; inactivity; and muscle weakness.[61] Other clinical risk factors for osteoporotic fracture include low body weight, advancing age, previous fracture, and a resting pulse greater than 80bpm.[128,253,295]

The primary risk factors for primary osteoporosis in women are related to estrogen deficiency: postmenopausal status; nulliparity; late menarche; early menopause (before age 45), either natural or surgical; and secondary amenorrhea related to exercise or eating disorders.[43,287] Other risk factors for low bone mass include increased age, white race, low weight and body mass index (BMI), and family history of osteoporosis.[60,192] Environmental factors including smoking, excessive alcohol intake, poor calcium intake, and lack of physical exercise may account for about 30% of the variation in bone density.

As already noted, secondary causes are identified in at least one half of men with osteoporosis and almost one third of women. Secondary causes typically fall into one of the following groups: endocrine, drugs, gastrointestinal, neoplastic, and rheumatic/inflammatory (Box 77.2).

In men with osteoporosis, the most common secondary causes include hypogonadism, glucocorticoid use, and alcoholism.[210,216] In women with bone loss, secondary causes are most often present in the pre- or perimenopausal age groups and include hypoestrogenemia,

---

BOX 77.1

Etiology of osteoporosis

Primary
Common
Type I: Postmenopausal osteoporosis
Type II: Senile osteoporosis

Rare
Idiopathic juvenile osteoporosis
Transient painful osteoporosis of the hip
Idiopathic osteoporosis

Secondary
Drugs
Glucocorticoids
Heparin
Anticonvulsants
Methotrexate
Oral tetracycline
Loop diuretics
Aluminum antacids
High doses of vitamin A

Endocrine disorder
Hypogonadism
Cushing syndrome
Hypoparathyroidism
Hypothyroidism
Growth hormone deficiency

Diet
Malabsorption syndrome
Dietary calcium or fluoride deficiency
Starvation
High-fiber and protein diet (increased renal calcium loss)
Scurvy
Excess alcohol (a low amount of alcohol is protective)

Disease
Osteogenesis imperfecta
Hypophosphatasia
Hemolytic anemia
Renal tubular acidosis
Rheumatoid arthritis
Immobilization
Liver disease
Multiple myeloma
Leukemia

BOX 77.2

Risk factors for osteoporosis

Genetic: family history
Racial: black < white or asian
Hormonal

Decreased levels of gonadal hormone
Premature menopause
Anorexia nervosa, sport, (natural or surgical) luteinizing hormone agonists
Late menarche
Tubal ligation
Partial hysterectomy
Vegetarian diet: high fecal excretion of estrogens
Increased hepatic conversion to inactive metabolites (cigarette smoking, anorexia, high protein diet)
Increased levels of parathyroid hormone, thyroid hormone, adrenal corticosteroids

Nutritional
Decreased calcium, phosphorus, vitamin D
Excess protein, alcohol, caffeine

Lifestyle
Sedentary, little exercise, smoking

Mechanical
Local and systemic factors governing bone function
Inactivity
Increased parathyroid hormone secondary to reduced calcium absorption
Increased dietary protein with consequentially increased renal loss of calcium
Lack of dietary calcium or fluoride
Inadequate exogenous vitamin D
Hormone deprivation at time of menopause: decreased estrogens

Drugs
Glucocorticoids, thyroxine, anticonvulsants, minor tranquilizers, heparin anticoagulants, lithium, loop diuretics, cytotoxic therapy, chronic use of phenothiazines, theophylline, or calcium-channel blockers

glucocorticoid therapy, thyroid hormone excess, and anticonvulsant therapy.[202]

Diagnosis

Although painful fracture represents the most obvious clinical marker for osteoporosis, most patients are asymptomatic. Since at least 30% of bone mass must be lost before osteopenia is visible on a standard radiograph, more-sensitive tests are required for earlier detection in the absence of fracture (Figure 77.2).[287] The primary role of plain radiographs is to identify the presence of fracture, although without comparison films the age of the fracture cannot usually be determined (Figure 77.1). Osteoporotic vertebral compression fractures are typically wedged ventrally. Patients with midthoracic or thoracolumbar fractures have a 98% chance of having generalized osteoporosis. In contrast, fractures above T6 are rarely osteoporotic and those above T4 are most often caused by metastatic disease or spondylitis.[16] Dorsal wedging of the vertebra should raise the suspicion of Paget's disease or malignancy.

Several more-sensitive measurements of bone mass—including forearm single photon absorptiometry (SPA), spinal and hip dual photon absorptiometry (DPA), quantitative ultrasound of the calcaneus (QUS), and dual energy x-ray absorptiometry (DEXA) of the hip and spine—have been demonstrated to predict osteoporotic fracture risk.[22,95,105,109,191] Because low bone mass is the strongest predictor of future fracture, the WHO has defined osteoporosis and osteopenia on the basis of bone mineral density (BMD) assessed by these techniques[14] (Table 77.1). A T score is defined as the number of standard deviations above or below the average BMD for healthy young white females. In contrast, the Z-score is defined as the number of standard deviations above or below the average BMD for age- and sex-matched controls. Osteoporosis is present when the T score is at least −2.5. Severe osteoporosis is defined as a T score at least −2.5 in the presence of one or more fragility fractures. A low Z score suggests relative bone loss as compared with the patient's peer group and suggests secondary causes of bone loss may be present.

Because of wide availability, high precision (1% to 2%), low radiation exposure (in comparison with quantitative CT), and comparatively low cost, DEXA has been widely adopted as the standard in bone mass measurement. DEXA uses two x-rays of differing energy to distinguish between bone and adjacent noncalcified tissues. Since the axial skeleton contains more metabolically active trabecular bone than appendicular sites, BMD is most often measured in the lumbar spine. However, in older patients, hypertrophic osteoarthritic spinal changes may spuriously elevate lumbar BMD measurements by DEXA. In such patients, measurement at the hip is more accurate. Measurement of BMD at a particular site predicts fracture risk at that site as well at other skeletal sites.[57,191] For each standard deviation of decrease in BMD of the hip, the risk of fracture increases 2.6 times.[178] Serial BMD measurements in the same patient should be performed on the same machine if possible because variability between BMD assessed by equipment of different manufacturers is considerable.[159]

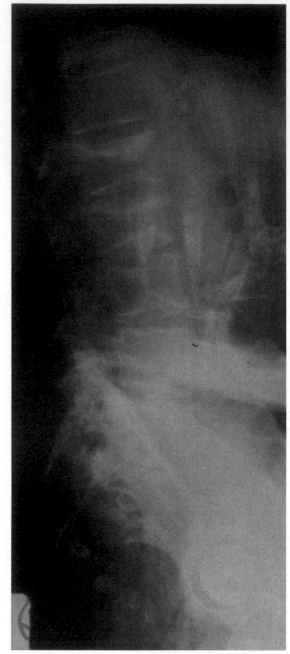

Figure 77.1 Lateral radiograph of the lumbosacral spine demonstrating diffuse osteopenia with multiple compression fractures (L2-4). Note the thin uninterrupted anterior and posterior cortical margins of the vertebral bodies.

Markers of bone turnover—formation or resorption—are of limited value in the diagnosis of osteoporosis.[74] Indices of bone formation include bone-specific alkaline phosphatase and osteocalcin. Markers for resorption include pyridinoline or deoxypyridinoline collagen cross-links linked to C-terminal (CTx) or N-terminal (Ntx) telopeptides. Since high bone turnover is a strong predictor of increased fracture risk and these biochemical markers respond within 2 to 3 months of initiation of therapy, they may be most useful in monitoring clinical response to treatment.[195,247]

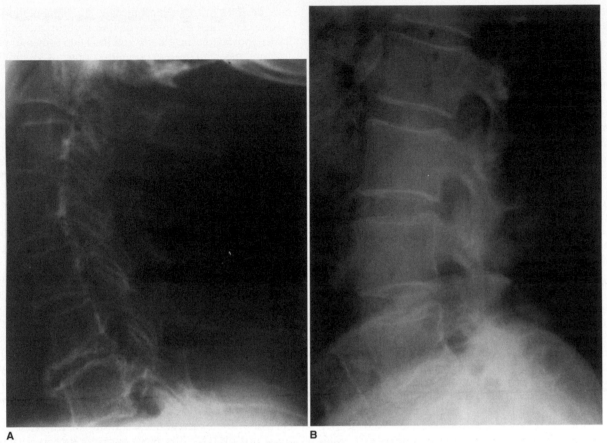

Figure 77.2 Lateral radiographs of the cervical (**A**) and lumbosacral (**B**) spine documenting diffuse osteopenia and degenerative changes that are more prominent on the cervical study. Note the increased radiodensity of the subchondral bone at the inferior and superior vertebral body margins. The vertical trabeculae are prominent.

TABLE 77.1

Osteoporosis and Osteopenia: WHO Criteria

Classification	Criteria
Normal	BMD up to ± 1 SD of the mean of the young adult reference range
Osteopenia	BMD between 1 and 2.5 SD below the mean of the young adult reference range
Osteoporosis	BMD greater than 2.5 SD below the mean of the young adult reference range
Severe osteoporosis	BMD greater than 2.5 SD below the mean of the young adult reference range in the presence of one or more insufficiency fractures

BMD, Bone material density; *SD,* standard deviation.

Osteoporosis is often unrecognized—and untreated—in high-risk patients or even in persons who have already sustained an osteoporotic fragility fracture.[278] From a preventive medicine standpoint, the issue of osteoporosis is frequently not addressed even in higher-risk populations. Fewer than 50% of perimenopausal and postmenopausal women report discussing osteoporosis with their primary care physician, and only 9% had had bone density measurement.[94] In a review of hip fracture patients recently treated at four different medical centers, only 12% to 24% of patients were subsequently referred for bone density testing.[110] The responsibility and opportunity for ensuring appropriate screening and treatment in vertebral fracture patients frequently rests with the treating spinal specialist.

The objective of screening is identification of individuals at increased risk of fracture. As noted earlier, bone density is the strongest predictor of future fracture. Current recommendations for populations who should have BMD measured include persons with a history of previous fragility fracture (hip, vertebrae, wrist), all women age 65 years and older, women over 60 who have risk factors as noted above, and persons who have diseases associated with bone loss—for example, rheumatoid arthritis.[206,217,218,293] Other suggested indications for BMD measurement include patients with mild asymptomatic hyperparathyroidism or radiographic osteopenia and patients initiating probable long-term corticosteroid therapy. Current evidence does not support routine screening of all perimenopausal women, as its value in directing preventive therapy against future fractures has not been established.[202]

In most patients with osteoporosis, laboratory studies are normal. However, patients should be screened for the common secondary causes. This is particularly important in men under 65 years of age, since more than 50% will be found to have a secondary cause. Any patient whose BMD reveals a Z score well below the mean should undergo careful screening as well. Initial general screening should include a complete blood count, erythrocyte sedimentation rate, serum calcium, phosphorus, alkaline phosphatase, creatinine, AST, TSH, and serum protein electrophoresis. In male patients, serum testosterone should be obtained. Other studies including 24-hour urinary calcium, PTH, and 25-hydroxyvitamin D levels, and serum immunoelectrophoresis, should be obtained selectively based on the results of preliminary testing and risk factor assessment.

Treatment

The primary objective of osteoporosis treatment is prevention of fractures. Ensuring acquisition of optimal bone mass during youth by ingesting adequate amounts of calcium, exercising regularly, and avoiding negative factors such as smoking and high caffeine, protein, and phosphorous intake represents an important but unproved strategy. In adults, adherence to similar behavioral and lifestyle guidelines may be effective in preventing bone loss. An NIH Consensus Conference has made age- and gender-specific recommendations for calcium intake[203] (Table 77.2). Calcium supplements alone have little impact on prevention of bone loss in perimenopausal women.[251] In older patients, however, there is considerable evidence that calcium with or without vitamin D retards bone loss and reduces fracture risk.[42,56,66,241] As intestinal calcium absorp-

tion declines with increasing age, supplementation with vitamin D, which enhances calcium absorption, is particularly important in the elderly and has been shown to reduce fracture risk.[165] The recommended dose of vitamin D is 400 IU before age 70 and 800 IU after age 70 years.

Regular weight-bearing exercise has been demonstrated to produce a modest increase in BMD of up to 3% in younger women.[90] Similarly, studies in older patients suggest endurance and resistance exercise increases bone mass.[63,271] Whether these exercise-induced increases in BMD reduce fracture risk remains unproved.

Until very recently, estrogen (hormone replacement therapy [HRT]) was the mainstay for prevention of bone loss in perimenopausal and postmenopausal women. Estrogen therapy begun in the immediate perimenopausal period diminishes the accelerated bone loss that typically occurs and ultimately reduces subsequent fracture risk.[87,163,296] In 1984, an NIH Consensus Conference on Osteoporosis recommend HRT for all postmenopausal women under the age of 60 years.[204] However, a recent placebo-controlled comparison of estrogen plus progesterone in more than 16,000 postmenopausal women found significant increases in risk of invasive breast cancer, cardiac events, venous thromboembolism, and stroke.[306] Although this study did demonstrate a reduction in hip fracture risk, the authors concluded that the results were not consistent with HRT as a viable intervention for primary prevention of a chronic disease. Largely as a result of this study, long-term use of HRT for prevention of osteoporosis is no longer recommended for most women.

Alternative approaches to HRT for osteoporosis prevention in postmenopausal women and other groups include raloxifene and oral bisphosphonates. Raloxifene is a selective estrogen receptor modulator (SERM) that has estrogen-like agonist effects on bone and lipids and estrogen-antagonist effects on the breast and uterus.[141] Raloxifene has been demonstrated to prevent bone loss in postmenopausal women.[68] In postmenopausal women with established osteoporosis, the drug significantly increased spinal and hip BMD and reduced vertebral fractures by 30% to 50%.[86,177] Reduction of hip fracture risk has not been demonstrated. Raloxifene is associated with an increased risk of venous thromboembolism and is contraindicated in persons with a history of deep venous thrombosis or pulmonary embolism. Hot flashes are noted in up to 50% of persons taking the drug.

Currently available oral bisphosphonates include alendronate and risedronate. Etidronate, pamidronate, and zoledronic acid are available but not approved for use in osteoporosis. These agents are potent inhibitors of osteoclastic bone resorption and effectively reduce bone turnover. Alendronate and risedronate are available in daily or weekly dosing forms and have been shown to be effective in prevention and treatment of postmenopausal osteoporosis. Both drugs have also been shown to effectively retard glucocorticoid-induced osteoporosis.[48,264] In postmenopausal patients with established osteoporosis, both alendronate and risedronate have been shown to reduce vertebral and nonvertebral fragility fractures by approximately 50%.[27,59,112,240] Etidronate is administered in a cyclic fashion and has been shown to reduce vertebral but not

TABLE 77.2	
Recommendations for Optimal Calcium Intake	
Age Group	**Optimal Intake of Calcium (mg/day)**
Infants	
Birth-6 months	400
6 mo-1 yr	800
Children	
1-5 yr	800
6-10 yr	800-1200
Adolescents/young adults	
11-24 yr	1200-1500
Men	
25-65 yr	1000
Over 65 yr	1500
Women	
25-50 yr	1000
Over 50 yr (postmenopausal)	
On estrogens	1000
Not on estrogens	1500
Over 65 yr	1500
Pregnant or nursing	1200-1500

Data from National Institutes of Health Consensus Development Conference.[203]

nonvertebral fracture rates.[54] Zoledronic acid is administered by intravenous infusion and offers potential for once-yearly effective therapy.[242] The most common adverse reaction to alendronate or risedronate is esophagitis.

Calcitonin is a physiologic antiresorptive hormone that decreases osteoclast formation, attachment, and bone resorption.[41] Calcitonin has been demonstrated to decrease serologic markers of bone turnover by 10% to 20%.[219] Calcitonin is administered subcutaneously or intranasally. The intranasal form has been demonstrated to reduce the risk of new vertebral fracture by 33% in postmenopausal women with established osteoporosis.[41] No effect on nonvertebral fractures has been demonstrated. Unlike other antiresorptive agents, some patients experience an analgesic effect from calcitonin that may be of benefit in patients with symptomatic vertebral compression fractures.[227] This effect may be mediated modulation of beta-endorphin levels.[100]

Teriparatide (recombinant human parathyroid hormone 1-34) has recently been approved for treatment of osteoporosis. Unlike the other available agents that are primarily antiresorptive, teriparatide is anabolic, increasing bone turnover and stimulating osteoblasts to a greater extent than osteoclasts.[67] Teriparatide is the 34 N-terminal fragment of PTH that in postmenopausal women with existing osteoporosis has been shown to increase bone mass by about 10% and reduce vertebral and nonvertebral fracture risk by more than 50%.[53,205] The drug is administered by daily subcutaneous self-injection. Recommended duration of treatment is 2 years, and observation studies suggest continued benefit for at least 18 months after discontinuation.[164] Side effects seen in clinical trials include mild hypercalcemia, leg cramps, nausea, and dizziness. The most serious concern is the risk of osteogenic sarcoma, because rat studies found a dose-dependent increase in tumors in teriparatide-treated animals.[294] The risk in humans is believed to be small. Currently, this agent should be reserved for patients at high risk for fracture or who are unresponsive to or intolerant of antiresorptive drugs.

Current consensus recommendations for who should be treated for osteoporosis include all persons with prior fragility fractures, women with BMD T scores of −2.0 and below and women with T scores of −1.5 and below who have additional risk factors for fracture.

Osteomalacia

Osteomalacia is a metabolic bone disorder characterized by deficient mineralization of newly formed matrix or osteoid. Overall, there is a decreased, normal, or increased amount of bone with decreased mechanical properties. The diminished deposition of mineral is caused by a decrease in the calcium phosphate product, which could be the result of either a low plasma calcium or a low plasma phosphate level. This is caused most commonly by abnormal vitamin D metabolism or altered phosphate reabsorption (Box 77.3).[16,193] Particularly in the elderly, osteoporosis and osteomalacia may coexist. It is difficult to determine the incidence of osteomalacia because most patients are asymptomatic.

Osteomalacia is a disease not only of the elderly. However, the infantile form of the disease (rickets) has been uncommon in the United States since the routine fortification of milk with vitamin D. Primary osteomalacia in adults is uncommon, and spinal problems are rarely the major complaint. In adults, most cases are secondary to kidney, gastrointestinal, or liver disease.[25]

Diagnosis

Patients with osteomalacia typically present with bone pain. This is associated with a proximal myopathy caused by calcium deficiency in some patients. In advanced cases, pain is accompanied by bony deformities. Early in the course of the disorder, muscular abnormalities cause abnormal loading of the vertebral bodies before they become pathologically involved. These patients experience pain when the spine is loaded by weight bearing or by action of the musculature. Typically, patients at rest do not experience pain.

The radiographic confirmation of osteomalacia is difficult because some findings, such as osteopenia, are nonspecific. Gross deformities of the bone skeleton are associated with this disorder. Areas of spongy bone show a decreased number of trabeculae, and the remaining trabeculae appear prominent. Pseudofractures or Looser's zones are lucent areas that are oriented at right angles to the cortex that incompletely span the diameter of the bone. These lines represent areas of inadequately mineralized osteoid.[225] A technetium-99m bone scan reveals increased uptake in the regions with fractures or in Looser's zones.

Laboratory findings in osteomalacia vary by etiology (Table 77.3). In vitamin D-deficient states, for example, alkaline phosphatase is elevated and serum calcium typically decreased.

In some cases, particularly when osteomalacia is suspected in patients with coexisting osteoporosis, a transiliac, tetracycline-labeled bone biopsy may be indicated. This is an invasive diagnostic tool and should, therefore, be used only if the result would alter treatment. Histology in osteoporosis reveals a decrease in bone mass, with a normal mineral-to-organic matrix ratio.[175] This is clearly distinguished from osteomalacia, in which the mineral-to-organic matrix ratio is, by definition, low and the total amount of bone may be reduced, normal, or increased.[16,25] Bone histology provides the only certain method of proving the diagnosis of osteomalacia.[29]

Treatment

The aim of treating established osteomalacia is to relieve symptoms, increase bone strength by promoting osteoid mineralization, and correct secondary hyperparathyroidism. Osteomalacia resulting from a low vitamin D intake or from limited sun exposure can be treated with adequate calcium and 2000 to 4000 IU of vitamin D daily (equivalent to 25 to 50μg vitamin D) for 6 to 12 weeks, at which time the dose can be reduced to 200 to 400 IU daily.[154] This regimen results in substantial mineral deposition within 1 week. Phosphate-related osteomalacia is less predictable and therefore is often not amenable to

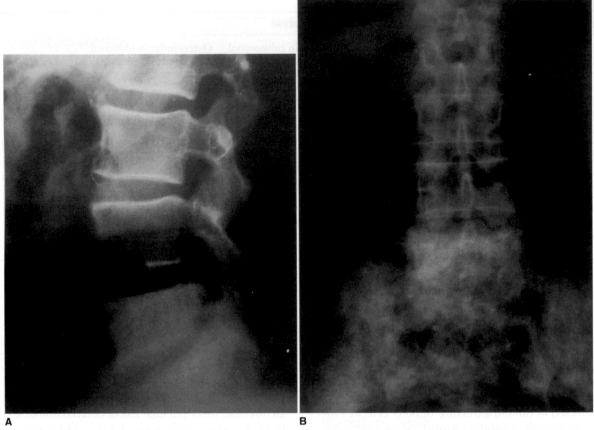

A   **B**

Figure 77.3 Lateral (**A**) and anteroposterior (**B**) radiographs of the lumbosacral spine in a patient with Paget's disease of the spine. There is increased anteroposterior width of the L5 vertebral body compared to the immediately superior body. The anteroposterior view shows increased density of the bone on the right side of the L5 vertebra, the sacrum, and the ilium. There is also coarsening of the trabeculae in the same distribution consistent with Paget's disease.

density with trabecular and cortical thickening has been described (Figure 77.3).[75] The skull may become flattened and mottled. Characteristically, the bones in Paget's disease demonstrate localized enlargement. The increase in bone size is deceptive, however, as pagetic bone does not have the compressive or tensile strength of normal bone and readily deforms with weight-bearing stress. The thick, massive pelvis is mottled and resembles a trefoil because the pressure of the femoral heads causes protrusion acetabuli.[134]

Radionuclide bone scanning is more sensitive than plain radiography for the detection of Paget's, revealing areas of increased uptake ("hot spots") in active disease sites.[161] During the inactive phase, increased uptake is often present at pseudofracture and compression sites.

Laboratory results in Paget's disease typically show an increase in serum alkaline phosphatase levels, reflecting increased bone formation. This corresponds with the extent and activity of the disease. Urinary hydroxyproline is a marker of resorption and is also elevated. In patients with monostotic involvement, these values may be normal. In such patients, serum bone-specific alkaline phosphatase may be a more-sensitive marker of increased bone formation and may be useful in monitoring disease activity.[7] Other studies including serum calcium and phosphorus are usually normal as long as formation and resorption remain balanced.[24,79,155,304]

Treatment

The primary indication for treatment of Paget's disease is pain, which most commonly is bony in origin or articular. Paget's disease may lead to anatomic malalignment of joints with accelerated degenerative joint disease. In such patients, treatment of Paget's will not alleviate pain of arthritic change. Traditionally, most patients with Paget's who are asymptomatic were not treated. However, the availability of newer, safer therapeutic agents has led to changes in indications for treatment. Patients with bone pain or joint pain should be treated. Asymptomatic patients at risk of complications of the disease such as hearing loss caused by basilar skull involvement, spinal nerve entrapment with spinal disease, and fracture caused by lytic findings in the lower-extremity long bones should be treated as well. Prior to elective surgery involving pagetic bone or operative procedures associated with prolonged immobilization, drug treatment is indicated, because suppression of disease activity reduces the risk of hypercalcemia and excessive blood loss. Patients with an early onset of the disease in areas in which disabling deformity or neurologic complications are anticipated should be considered for treatment.

Effective therapeutic agents decrease bone resorption by suppressing osteoclastic activity. Calcitonin is a polypeptide hormone that causes an acute decrease in osteoclastic activity, followed some time later by a reduction in the number of osteoclasts. This results in an early significant hypocalcemia and an initial positive calcium balance lasting 1 to 4 weeks. Pain relief is usually apparent within 2 weeks. Hydroxyproline exertion decreases within days,[28] and alkaline phosphatase levels decrease within a few weeks. Typically, these levels decrease by about 50% and remain decreased as long as treatment is continued. In about 20% of persons, alkaline phosphatase and hydroxyproline levels slowly return to pretreatment levels despite continuing therapy.[69] Calcitonin may stabilize hearing loss and has been reported to reverse paraparesis caused by Paget's disease.[189,281] Similarly, high-output cardiac failure and bony osteolytic lesions improve with calcitonin therapy.[274]

Side effects of calcitonin include nausea and vomiting as well as generalized flushing. Nasal calcitonin causes fewer adverse reactions. Some patients develop resistance to calcitonin that is related to development of calcitonin antibodies in patients treated with porcine or salmon calcitonin or to down-regulation of calcitonin receptors with secondary hyperparathyroidism.[273]

Bisphosphonates are synthetic analogs of inorganic pyrophosphate that bind the surface of hydroxyapatite and are localized at the site of active bone formation. They decrease bone resorption and formation by decreasing osteoclastic activity and number.[2,152,277] Currently available oral agents of this class include etidronate sodium, alendronate, and risedronate. All are poorly absorbed and must be taken without food. Pamidronate is poorly tolerated orally and therefore administered intravenously.[168] Etidronate, the first-generation agent of this class, is associated with a mineralization defect—osteomalacia—at higher doses.[3] This is not a problem with second-generation drugs. As with calcitonin, diphosphonates produce a 50% decrease in serum alkaline phosphatase and urinary hydroxyproline in most patients. Unlike calcitonin, however, these effects are sustained for months or years after therapy is discontinued.[69]

Diphosphonates improve bone pain, neurologic complications, and radiographic findings in patients with Paget's disease.[69]

Surgical Therapy

Surgery for Osteoporosis

The majority of osteoporotic spinal fractures are stable, with a small risk of associated neurologic injury, healing to complete resolution in 2 to 3 months.[139,290] Traditional "conservative" treatment consists of adequate analgesia and a short period of bed rest for pain control. Mobilization is encouraged as early as possible. Patients with minimal vertebral compression should avoid compression overload for 12 weeks. In more-severe vertebral compression, temporary bracing may be necessary, although it is usually poorly tolerated by elderly patients. Extension exercises are very valuable for increasing the strength of the back musculature and for improving balance but have little effect on long-term complications.[46] Loss of height in one vertebra or several adjacent verte-

brae of 40% to 50% or more of the normal vertebral height or angulation of more than 20 degrees is responsible for different spinal mechanics that may eventually result in painful degenerative changes.[133,146]

Recently, two new procedures have become available to treat acute osteoporotic compression fractures.[96] Vertebroplasty involves fluoroscopically guided percutaneous injection of polymethylmethacrylate cement into the collapsed vertebrae. The procedure immediately stabilizes the fracture with significant pain relief in up to 95% of patients.[18] In addition to decreased pain, improvement in patient function has been demonstrated.[313] Cement leakage outside of the vertebral body is common, occurring in 50% to 67% of patients, but clinical complications such as radiculopathy or cord compression are rare.[64,126,263] Other concerns include fat embolism, temperature increases resulting from cement polymerization, and the possibility of increased risk of vertebral fractures adjacent to the treated vertebra.[124] Further study is necessary to determine which patients should be considered for this procedure.

Kyphoplasty was introduced in 1998 for treatment of symptomatic compression fractures. The procedure involves fluoroscopically guided introduction of an inflatable bone tamp into the fractured vertebra. Inflation of the bone tamp is intended to create a cavity as well as reexpand the vertebral body. The cavity is then filled with PMMA. In contrast to vertebroplasty, the creation of a cavity permits injection of thicker cement under lower pressure, reducing the risk of leakage.[96] Experience with kyphoplasty to date suggests fracture pain relief is achieved in more than 90% of patients.[96,162] A potential advantage of this procedure over vertebroplasty is the potential to restore fractured vertebral height, minimizing long-term biomechanical consequences of one or more wedge fractures. Studies are currently under way to further assess this possibility. The appropriate duration of conservative treatment after vertebral fracture before considering kyphoplasty is not established but earlier intervention in patients with acute thoracolumbar junction fractures in an effort to preserve spinal sagittal alignment should be considered.[224]

In patients with acute neurologic symptoms or instability, early surgery may be indicated. After a fracture has healed, surgery may be required if (1) the patient has continuing intense pain, (2) the patient has significant symptomatic or increasing deformity, (3) degenerative changes are severe, or (4) late neurologic deficits occur.[180] There is some controversy over the ideal time for intervention. One group advocates initial bracing. At follow-up, if there is increased deformity or if there is considerable pain, delayed stabilization and fusion are performed.[31] Another group opts for early stabilization and fusion because a dorsal approach is possible, whereas with delayed surgery, a ventral approach is usually necessary.[146]

A variety of problems are associated with surgery for osteoporosis because the mechanical properties of the bone are greatly diminished. This is extremely important when internal fixation is used. Postoperative assessment of the fusion mass is less straightforward in osteoporosis, as development of a solid fusion may occur more slowly. Most osteoporotic patients are elderly, with coexisting significant comorbid medical disease that may represent at least a relative contraindication for operation. Surgery, however, should not be denied solely on the basis of age.[134]

The purpose of most operative procedures in osteoporosis is to obtain a solid fusion—that is, bony union across a vertebral space after surgical manipulation.[158] This involves grafting across a surgically prepared intervertebral space and limiting motion until the graft has incorporated and union has been accomplished. In most cases, some form of spinal instrumentation is used as the supporting and immobilizing construct for the graft site. Spinal fusion is indicated for the treatment of deformity, fractures, spondylolisthesis, or disc disease, which can be associated with osteoporosis.[134] A successful fusion depends on the quality of the fusion site and the bone graft, as well as on systemic and local factors.[158] In all spinal surgery, but especially surgery on osteoporotic spines, it is important to optimize all these components.

The fusion site is the primary source of viable cells for bone growth because very few cells in the autogenous graft survive. It is therefore of the utmost importance to handle and prepare the tissue bed carefully. Adequate blood supply is the source of nutrients and paracrine signals, a vehicle for endocrine stimuli, and a pathway for the recruitment of osteoprogenitor and inflammatory cells. Any avascular, nonviable or heavily traumatized tissue should be removed during preparation of the graft bed.[158] Some authors suggest that a limited postoperative hematoma may form an osteoconductive meshwork and that the platelets trapped in it release growth factors.[55] The early inflammatory response after grafting is a potent mediator of osteoinduction. Local bone is a reservoir of osteogenic cells and osteoinductive proteins and provides an osteoconductive surface. To maximize the exposed surface area of cancellous bone, the fusion site is decorticated with an osteotome or rongeur. The use of a power burr or cautery could potentially cause thermal necrosis.[158]

Bone graft accelerates the normal regenerative capacity of bone, and an ideal graft has osteogenic (cells), osteoinductive (matrix proteins, growth factors, paracrine stimuli), and osteoconductive (extracellular matrix) properties.[229] The most effective graft material, having all these characteristics, is autologous cancellous bone. Grafting with autologous cortical bone is less successful because it contains fewer cells that are located deep within the matrix. The lack of marrow cells in cortical bone decreases the osteogenic capabilities of this material. The osteoinductive and osteoconductive properties of cortical bone are lower because of the low surface area-to-weight ratio. This type of graft also forms a barrier to vascular ingrowth and remodeling, but its mechanical strength is high, and therefore it is used often in ventral vertebral fusion.[158] A vascularized autologous graft offers a clear advantage in a number of cases.[158,300] Ventral iliac crest, fibula, and rib grafts have been used in this manner. The improved vascularization of this graft greatly improves incorporation in irradiated areas and in ventral spinal fusions in which donor vessels are readily available. These grafts are seldom indicated in osteoporotic patients, because most of these patients are elderly, and the use of this graft increases the operative time considerably and carries its own morbidity.[158] Frozen or freeze-dried allografts are other alternatives, because these avoid the morbidity associated with

graft harvest. They have been used in areas in which an insufficient amount of donor material is available in settings that require a significant mechanical function of the graft. Freeze-drying causes a 50% reduction in the mechanical strength of the graft.[91]

Several systemic and local factors are known to play an important role in healing after all types of surgery (Box 77.4). An attempt should be made to optimize all of these factors, especially during the first 7 postoperative days, the critical period for fusion. Local electrical stimulation has been used in the treatment of bony nonunion, and it may be useful in spinal fusion.[21,208] Although electrical stimulation has not been evaluated in osteoporosis, it has been used because its potential benefits are believed to outweigh possible risks.[133] The effect of osteoporosis on spinal fusion is poorly understood, partly because it is difficult to separate BMD from other variables such as age and age-related physiologic and metabolic changes. The quality of the bone marrow and the number of cells, for instance, are greatly decreased in the elderly, regardless of BMD.[158]

A good fusion depends on limitation of movement at the graft site. A recent study documents decreased rates of pseudoarthrosis with the use of rigid internal fixation when dorsolateral fusions were performed.[308] Mechanical stability is, for the most part, controlled by the surgeon. A good internal fixation, limiting patient activity, and use of external immobilization devices reduce movement. In metabolic bone disease, the bone in the fusion graft may have been replaced by structurally inferior bone.[136]

Dorsolateral fusion is preferred for a dorsal fusion. It incorporates the dorsal elements, including the facet joints, the pars interarticularis, and the transverse processes. The indications for ventral fusion have expanded over the years and include, among others, degenerative disease and spondylolisthesis. Either a vertebrectomy with strut grafting or an interbody fusion can be performed.

Some complications of spinal fusion are worth mentioning, because careful surgical technique can greatly diminish their incidence. The consequences of hemorrhage can be quite grave, especially in the osteoporotic elderly patient who may have preexisting cardiovascular disease. When the patient is positioned prone, bleeding is considerable, because of venous obstruction. The use of a frame or the knee-chest position decreases bleeding because of reduced external pressure on the abdomen. Decortication should be done only after complete bony exposure, soft-tissue excision, and graft harvest to minimize the time of bleeding. Oozing from the bone should not be treated with bone wax because this retards osteogenesis.[99] The paraarticular vessels—that is, the dorsal muscular branches of the segmental lumbar arteries—are often disrupted during bony exposure. They have a fairly consistent anatomic location and should be cauterized when dissecting lateral to the facet joints.[173]

The occurrence of pseudoarthrosis depends on the number of levels fused, the actual levels fused, the type of fusion, and the surgical technique. Failure to achieve a fusion is reported to be between 0% and 56%.[35,302] The wide range of nonunion is caused, in part, by the difficult assessment of true pseudoarthrosis. No consistent definition is used in the literature, making comparison of study results difficult. Most authors use the absence of

77.4

BOX

Local and systemic factors affecting bone healing

Positive factors	Negative factors
Systemic factors	
Nutritional status	
Hormones	Drugs
Insulin	Corticosteroids
Testosterone	NSAIDs
Estrogen	Chemotherapeutic drugs
Growth hormone	Sepsis
Parathyroid hormone	Anemia
Calcitonin	Obesity
Anabolic steroids	Tobacco
Vitamins A and D	Hormone deficiency
	Vitamin intoxication
Local factors	
Increased surface area	
Mechanical stability	Radiation
Mechanical loading	Denervation
Presence of bone marrow	Tumor
Factors promoting angiogenesis	Local bone disease
Osteoporosis	Movement
Bone wax	
Sepsis	

NSAIDs, Nonsteroidal anti-inflammatory drugs.

movement on flexion-extension radiographs and the presence of bony trabeculae across the fusion site as their criteria. Clinical results have been quite satisfactory without bony union, and even a solid fusion has been accompanied by a clinically unsatisfactory result. The clinical outcome is a more accurate assessment of the result of a spinal fusion. If symptoms persist despite an adequate time for fusion to occur (6 to 12 months), reexploration of the fusion mass should be strongly considered. If, on the contrary, there is radiographic evidence of pseudoarthrosis, but the patient is clinically asymptomatic, the approach of the surgeon should be conservative. A number of factors other than metabolic abnormalities may be responsible for pseudoarthrosis.[233,268] Of the patients with pseudoarthrosis, 58% have a decreased BMD, and some authors have therefore suggested that there is an association between low BMD and failure of fusion. This analysis may not be correct, because the incidence of low BMD in successful fusion is not known and could have been even higher. Moreover, only 14.9% of patients with nonunion have abnormal laboratory findings.[268]

Dorsal midline lumbar fusions are often complicated by postfusion stenosis. The cross section of the spinal canal is diminished after fusion because of thickening of the laminae. Sometimes the fusion mass shows overgrowth at its rostral end. This mass dips down ventrally and causes spinal cord compression. This complication can be avoided by dorsolateral fusion.[157]

Several studies on the effect of fusion on spinal bone density have shown a temporary decrease in BMD.[166] In the vertebrae above the fusion, the BMD decreases by 15.7% in the first 3 to 12 months after surgery. This bone loss may be because of the use of immobilization, the surgical procedure, or the postoperative bracing. At the end of the first year, however, 60% of patients had a BMD 10% above baseline. Of the 40% of patients remaining, 12% had BMDs that had reached baseline, and 28% had BMDs below baseline. This is partly explained by Frost's concept of bone remodeling, that after any significant injury, bone turnover accelerates for 6 to 12 months.[92]

In osteoporosis, the amount of bone graft is often insufficient, because the bone consists of a thin cortex with interposed fatty material. When fibular autografts are used in older patients, thrombophlebitis and fractures are more frequent. For dorsal fusion, dorsal iliac crest graft and allograft may be morcellized and used as a paste. In ventral fusion, a tricortical graft is used, but even this may offer poor structural support. The strength of the graft can be enhanced with a suitable allograft, such as a femur or tibial segment, that can be packed with the autograft.

Instrumentation for Internal Fixation
Early Devices

Spinal instrumentation is used as a fixation method to hold the spine in position until the bony graft is incorporated and as a technique to correct deformity. In 1953, the Harrington rod was developed for the correction of postpolio scoliosis; it consists of threaded rods that can either distract or compress the spine with hooks.[97] With this original design, there were frequent problems with hook disengagement, rod failure, and recurrence of the deformity. The distraction rod was eventually modified by increasing the rod diameter and changing to a ratcheting hook mechanism, and the location of the hook sites was adjusted by

placing the rostral hooks three levels above the injury level and the caudal hooks two levels below.[230] With these modifications, the Harrington rod construct became the first clinically useful spinal instrumentation system. After additional modifications that improved the performance of the construct, the Harrington fixation system became the gold standard to which others' systems were compared.[174,246] Subsequent universal fixation systems have been marketed in the United States. Postoperatively, 6 months of external immobilization is recommended. The authors use a bivalved, plastic thoracolumbar orthosis.

Other systems have been developed since the introduction of the Harrington hook-and-rod system in an attempt to obviate some of the shortcomings inherent in the design of the initial fixation system and to increase internal stability, thereby rendering external fixation unnecessary. One is the Luque instrumentation system, which consists of smooth L-shaped rods, two of which can be placed to overlap, forming a rectangle. The rods can then be contoured to the spine and fixed segmentally with sublaminar wires. The attachment of a Harrington rod implant to the spine at laminae other than at the two distal hook sites results in increased construct stability, obviating the need for external bracing.[170]

Although segmental fixation results in both improved rotational and translational stability, the placement of sublaminar wires has been associated with significant risks to the integrity of the nervous tissue.[131,172,299] The passage of sublaminar wires can damage the spinal cord and nerve roots in the spinal canal, but the risk of injury can be decreased with the use of proper technique during the placement. The wires should not be passed laterally, the radius of curvature of the wire should be less than the laminar width, and the bend of the wire tip should not exceed 45 degrees.[104] Wires can be placed transforaminally if the laminae are not intact. Braided cables have replaced the solid wires and have reduced the potential for inadvertent injury to the spinal cord. When the cables are placed under the lamina, they avoid the inadvertent injury caused by displacement of a solid wire into the spinal canal before or during fixation to the rod.[174]

Luque fixation is not adequate for the fixation of fractures resulting from an axial injury mechanism, because there is no resistance to this deformity vector, but the fixation system is used for the treatment of scoliosis and of pathologic fractures without significant axial compromise.[174] The Luque system has been modified by Ferguson and Allen in the Galveston technique for pelvic fixation, and Asher et al.[10] reported modifications of this fixation technique that ultimately resulted in the Isola universal fixation system.

The technique of segmental wiring was incorporated by Drummond to stabilize Harrington distraction constructs and was named the *Wisconsin* wiring technique.[4,76] This resulted in rotational and translational stability in addition to that afforded by segmental sublaminar wiring, with the wires being placed at the base of the spinous processes and thereby reducing the chance of inadvertent compression of the spinal cord by avoiding the placement of wires in the spinal canal. Winter et al.[301] described the use of a Moe rod, which is a modified Harrington rod with a square end, to engage a similarly

modified caudal hook and segmental wiring. This construct was also reported to enhance the rotational stability of the construct as compared with a conventional Harrington construct. Edwards described the use of an "anatomic" hook that increased the surface area of the hook engaging the lamina and thereby decreased the risk of hook cutout. He also described the use of polypropylene sleeves to focus the reduction vector of the construct and to increase the construct resistance to rotational and translational deforming forces.[81] Alterations were made to the Harrington rod system by researchers at the Texas Scottish Rite Hospital, and an intermediate hook was developed for additional bone fixation. They also developed cross-fixators that markedly increased rotational stability, initially for the Luque rods, but these were also used to stabilize Harrington distraction rod constructs. These modifications ultimately resulted in the Texas Scottish Rite Hospital universal fixation system.[12]

Universal Hook-And-Rod Fixation

Cotrel-Dubousset generated a universal spine fixation system that used multiple hooks rather than the two distal hooks of the Harrington distraction system.[51] This system used "claws" that were paired hooks, one directed caudally and the other directed rostrally on the lamina of the same or adjacent vertebral levels. These additional hooks decreased the significant failure rate of the rostral hook in Harrington distraction constructs. The use of multiple hooks also allows the correction of focal deformities, which was not possible with the Harrington distraction constructs in which only distraction over the entire length of the instrumented spine was possible. The ability to correct deformities in multiple planes was especially useful for scoliosis. With biplanar deformities, this system allowed restoration of the sagittal curve, as well as correction of the coronal abnormalities. The ability to correct multiple deformities was also useful in treatment of traumatic spine injuries, tumors, and spondylolisthesis.[51,107] The additional hooks on the construct were advantageous for use in osteoporotic spines, because the load on individual hooks was reduced. This, in turn, reduced the chance of the hook fracturing the osteoporotic lamina. The universal spine fixation system was used with two devices for transverse traction to secure the rods to each other and to improve rotational stability of the constructs. In the majority of cases, postoperative bracing was not believed to be necessary. Pedicle screws could be added to the construct, if necessary, to decompress the spinal canal or in the absence of adequate dorsal elements or with degenerative curves, tumors, or spondylolisthesis.

Pedicle Fixation

Boucher is credited with the first use of the pedicle screw for spinal fixation and Roy-Camille with the development and first use of a plate-and-pedicle screw construct for fixation of the spine in 1963.[28,300] Although Harrington, in 1969, attempted to attach pedicle screws placed in L4 pedicles to a distraction rod using wires, the first practical pedicle

screw-rod construct was reported by Cotrel in 1985.[111,300] Pedicle screw systems were developed simultaneously in Ohio, Vermont, Gotenburg, and Dravos, and all systems used connectors to attach the screws solidly to the fixation construct.[72,149,283] The advantage of pedicle screw fixation is the ability to control the three spinal columns simultaneously through a dorsal approach and the necessity to immobilize only a limited number of segments.[1] The latter factor is of particular advantage in the lumbar spine.[300] Currently, a large number of fixation systems are available.[171,259,283] Whereas the Roy-Camille and Steffee instrumentation systems allow plate contouring to retain the sagittal plane of the curvature, the inability to apply compressive or distractive forces to the instrumented spinal segments is a significant limitation.[260,284] The use of pedicle screws with universal fixation systems is not so limited, and local compression and distraction with pedicle screws is possible. The use of cross-fixators to attach the construct rods rigidly to each other not only increases rotational stability but also increases screw

pullout strength.[261] Pedicle screw systems are used for treatment of existing spinal instability, such as postlaminectomy spondylolisthesis or symptomatic pseudoarthrosis; treatment of potential instability in spinal stenosis; surgical treatment of degenerative scoliosis, unstable fractures, and spinal osteotomies; and ventral strut grafting in tumors, infections, and trauma. Kostuik acknowledged that other surgeons had experienced difficulty with pedicle screw fixation of the osteoporotic spine but reported no difficulty except for sacral fixation (Figure 77.4).[144]

Ventral Devices

Despite the availability of various ventral instrumentation systems, their utility in the surgical treatment of osteoporosis has been limited. Dwyer and Zielke developed compressive devices implanted via a retroperitoneal approach. Both systems relied on transvertebral coronal plane screws connected by a flexible steel cable in the

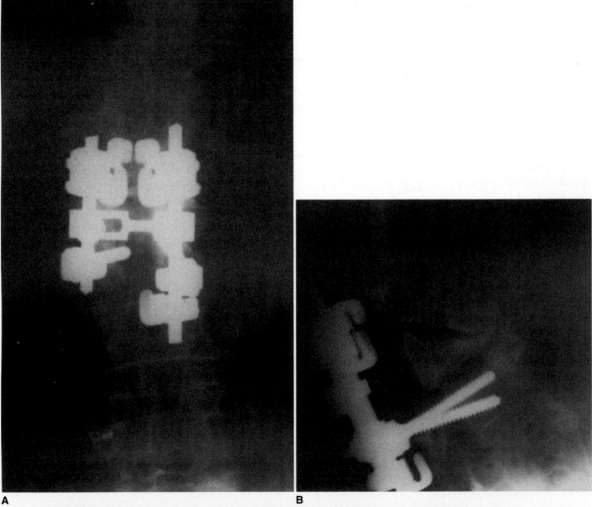

A   B

Figure 77.4 Anteroposterior (**A**) and lateral (**B**) plain films of an 84-year-old woman with a thoracolumbar compression fracture treated posteriorly with a dorsal, short segment universal construct. The films were taken 6 weeks after surgical treatment when the deformity recurred. The construct consisted of bilateral pedicle screws placed in the immediately inferior vertebral body. A laminar hook is placed on one side. A single-level claw was placed bilaterally on the immediately superior lamina that has failed.

Dwyer system and by a fully threaded compressive rod in the Zielke system. The Zielke fixation system allows rotational control and the use of an outrigger that greatly reduces the tendency for kyphosis. The Kostuik-Harrington construct is a modification of the Harrington distraction device for use ventrally. The Yuan I-plate, the Kaneda device, and several low-profile, multihole plate constructs have been used for short segment instrumentation.[82] Ventral devices allow a ventral strut to be placed in a kyphotic deformity, but the exposure requires approaching the great vessels of the abdomen and lower thoracic area. The Dunn device was withdrawn from the market after reports of injury to the great vessels.[32,79,125] Kaneda et al.[136] reported the successful treatment of patients with neurologic deficit secondary to osteoporotic collapse of vertebral bodies with a ventral decompression, grafting with ceramic implants, and fixation with the Kaneda device. Kostuik recommended the use of polymethylmethacrylate (PMMA) to secure screws placed in the vertebral body via a ventral approach but cautioned that PMMA be limited to the first sacral pedicle dorsally because of potential leakage of the cement into the spinal canal from undetected breaches in the pedicle cortex.[145]

The Surgical Management of Structurally Deficient Bone

Despite the severe spinal deformity caused by spinal compression fractures in osteoporosis, nerve root compression and spinal cord compression have been relatively rare.* Osteoporotic fractures with the following characteristics are more commonly associated with spinal cord compression: (1) patients older than 70 years (2) fractures in the upper thoracic spine with spinal cord compression in which a vascular factor may aggravate the mechanical compression, and (3) presence of angular deformities. Wedge compression fractures, by definition, involve only the ventral part of the vertebral body. Osteoporotic collapse affects the cancellous part of the vertebral body.[70] In these fractures, the dorsal cortical wall is preserved. Therefore, usually, neither wedge compression fracture nor osteoporotic collapse is accompanied by spinal cord compression. Neurologic abnormalities, when present, consist of varying degrees of lower extremity paresis or sensory loss, and in 6% to 7% of patients, bladder dysfunction with or without bowel dysfunction is present.[270] For spinal fractures with acute neurologic problems, the main mode of treatment is decompression.[234] Because the majority of symptomatic fractures involve failure of the middle column, they may be unstable,[70] and therefore a simple laminectomy is contraindicated because the mechanical integrity of the posterior column would be compromised, increasing the stability of the spine.[123]

In the lower thoracic and lumbar spine, the preferred treatment is a one-stage dorsal decompression and stabilization procedure.[83] The retropulsed aspect of the vertebral body is resected by curettage under intraoperative ultrasonic guidance, and bone graft is placed both ventrally and dorsolaterally. Fixation should be performed with a pedicle screw or hook via a universal fixation

system, or alternatively, Harrington rods and sublaminar wires that incorporate two or three levels above and two levels below the fracture should be used. Shorter dorsal constructs are associated with early failure of the fusion and fixation.[188] Ventral decompression and fixation are advocated by some surgeons, mainly in patients who are active and who have only moderate osteoporosis. Reinforcement of ventrally placed vertebral body fixation screws with PMMA has been reported to increase the stability of the construct.[146] There is controversy over which procedure provides the greatest chance of recovery: a ventral approach or dorsal stabilization.[184,270] A third approach combines dorsal stabilization and fusion with a vertebrectomy via a ventral approach. Some wedge fractures with significant compression deformity cause compression of the spinal cord at the upper and lower margins of the vertebral body.[270] These fractures are treated by spinal realignment with instrumentation and decompression (ventral or laminectomy) when necessary.

The indications for treatment of deformity arising from osteoporotic fractures are progressive severe deformity (usually with disabling pain), early neurologic problems (a rare occurrence), late neurologic problems (spinal stenosis), or chronic incapacitating pain unresponsive to bracing, exercises, or medication.[135] Scoliosis in elderly women is a marker for osteoporosis and compression fractures.[114] Kyphosis is positively correlated with a low BMD[292] and compression fractures. Treatment of scoliosis with Harrington rods produces good results in 70% of patients but has a rate of pseudoarthrosis formation of 11%.[144] Pedicle screws are reported to be much more reliable than laminar hooks when used with Cotrel-Dubousset instrumentation.[144] Coe et al.[45] tested various systems in a dorsally directed load-to-failure model and showed that the Harrington hook fixation has a significantly higher pullout resistance capability than other systems tested. (The order of increasing pullout resistance was [1] Cotrel-Dubousset, [2] Drummond spinous process wires, [3] Steffee VSP transpedicular screws, and [4] Harrington hook.) They also showed that the failure of Harrington instrumentation does not correlate with BMD, in contrast to the other systems. They concluded that Harrington laminar hooks were superior in metabolic bone disease associated with a decreased BMD.

It should be noted that the failure mode for screws in the clinical situation was rarely pullout but, more often, screw metal fatigue or screw loosening. The drawbacks of the Harrington fixation method are the need to incorporate two levels above and three levels below the diseased vertebral level and the inability to employ the technique after an extensive laminectomy. A two-stage procedure has been necessary to treat a kyphoscoliosis. The ventral approach consists of a multilevel discectomy filling the disc space with morcellized bone graft. The dorsal procedure involves universal instrumentation, especially in a thoracolumbar curve in which it is important to restore the lordosis. Screw fixation rather than the use of sublaminar hooks is recommended, although sublaminar cabling and multiple sublaminar hook techniques, combined with long rod length, have been advocated by others.[80] Kyphosis can be treated with Harrington instrumentation, with one of its modifications, or with some form of ventral fixation

---

*References 9,117,138,140,223,266.

device. Pedicle screw-plate fixation can be used solely or in combination with a ventral approach (Figure 77.5).

Progressive angular deformity or instability are the bases of increasing spinal stenosis or late neurologic deficits.[146,180] The preferred treatment for this is laminectomy. The addition of fusion is definitely advisable if more than two levels are to be decompressed or if there is a coexisting spondylolisthesis.[283] Progressive slip after a laminectomy for decompression is observed in as many as 62% of osteoporotic patients, and hence, the addition of fusion is advocated in all cases.[144,234] Fusion should preferably be combined with some form of internal fixation such as dorsal pedicle screw fixation or ventral stabilization to increase the fusion rate.[308] A tricortical graft is recommended as an interbody graft because a bicortical graft contains only two thin pieces of cortex and provides limited structural support.[146] The authors have successfully used allograft tibia or fibula struts packed with autograft as a vertebral body graft.

The indications for pedicle screw constructs have continued to increase over the years. Pedicle screws have been used for the treatment of fresh fractures, malunion, dislocations, tumor resection, arthrosis, and deformities.[254,257,258] This form of treatment, with certain modifications when used in the osteoporotic spine, has approached the characteristics of its use in normal bone.

In comparison with other systems, pedicle screw constructs have much lower failure rates, and the treatment supports the purpose of surgical intervention—that is, the reduction of vertebral displacement (thereby providing realignment and decompression of the spinal canal), exploration of the spinal canal, stabilization of the spinal column, and facilitation of patient care.[260]

Pedicle screw constructs are indicated for the treatment of focal deformity. If vertebral collapse and focal kyphosis are minimal, maximal deformity has already occurred at the time of injury, and chronic deterioration is not expected. In this situation, rehabilitation is the treatment of choice. If the deformity is stable but considerable, there may be mechanical, functional, neurologic, or cosmetic consequences. Treatment is conservative, but surgery is indicated if conservative treatment fails. If the pathology is located at the thoracolumbar junction, with displacement of the dorsal rostral corner of the vertebral body, spinal canal stenosis is likely. Surgery, with resection of the responsible fragment and pedicle screw fixation, is indicated.[260]

Instability is an indicator of the risk of displacement and depends on the relative contribution of disc, ligament, and bone injury. The diagnosis of disc or ligament injury is often difficult to make but can be inferred from the initial displacement of the fragments, from the thickness and the

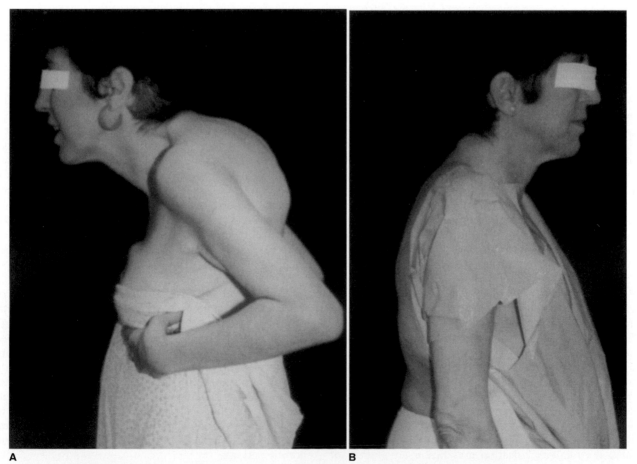

A   **B**

Figure 77.5 A 55-year-old woman with a severe kyphotic deformity of the thoracic spine secondary to multiple compression fractures of an osteoporotic spine. (**A**) Preoperative and (**B**) postoperative lateral photographs.   *Continued*

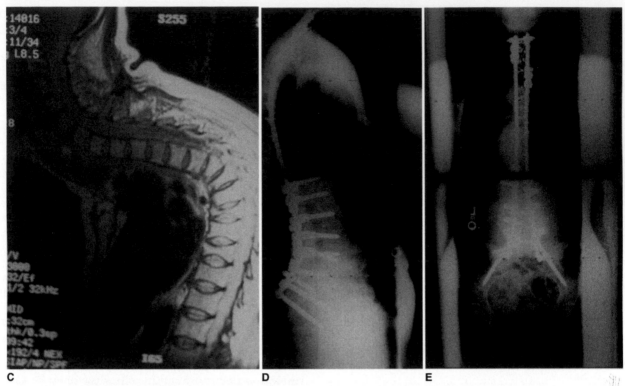

Figure 77.5 *cont'd* (**C**) Preoperative proton density sagittal magnetic resonance imaging scan of the cervical and thoracic spine. Postoperative lateral (**D**) and anteroposterior (**E**) radiographs of the instrumented spine. Note the bilateral iliac screws, lumbar pedicle screws, thoracic and lower cervical sublaminar cables, and cross-links. The patient was treated ventrally with multiple corpectomies and grafts prior to the placement of dorsal instrumentation and dorsolateral autograft. (Photographs courtesy of Dr. N. Lebwohl.)

regularity of the disc, from the presence of associated facet injury, and from the interspinous distance. Major bone injuries produce significant callus and heal spontaneously, whereas ligament or disc injuries never attain stability spontaneously. Significant bone lesions are nearly always associated with considerable ligament and disc injury. Small lesions with no displacement are treated conservatively. Moderate lesions are at risk of gradual displacement and should be treated with reduction and fixation if a significant bone, disc, or ligament injury is present. Severe lesions are likely to suffer sudden unexplained displacement and should be treated with internal fixation, including pedicle screws or hooks, with a universal spine fixation system.[260] Most lesions in osteoporosis are stable, but because of the change in mechanics after long-term deformity, late instability can become a problem.

Different treatment modalities are appropriate for different levels of fractures. Thoracic fractures have an inherent stability because of the presence of the thoracic cage. Conservative treatment with an external orthosis is usually sufficient for these fractures. If an operative procedure is necessary, a dorsal fixation with a Harrington system or dorsal universal fixation system, including pedicle screws, may be employed. At the thoracolumbar junction, simple reduction or internal fixation and fusion are indicated, depending on the severity of the injury. In this area, safeguarding mobility is important, but securing construct strength is a primary concern. Therefore, osteosynthesis

should be extended two levels above and below the diseased level. With a lesion at L2 to L4, pedicle screw constructs are indicated, with the fusion kept as short as possible and spanning only three vertebrae. Mobility is very important at this level. If significant vertebral body or disc collapse is present at this level, the patient may benefit from complementary ventral stabilization and fusion. Injuries of L5 are uncommon, but conservative treatment provides poor results, with a high incidence of secondary low back pain. Pedicle screw constructs fixing L4 to the sacrum, coupled with fusion, are the appropriate form of treatment.[260]

Fractures associated with vertebral displacement or the presence of a bony fragment within the spinal canal can lead to neurologic involvement. Immediate surgical intervention is usually not required, but increased perisurgical complications in the first 5 days after injury have been reported. In patients with a complete cord syndrome or in the case of neurologic deterioration in a patient with an incomplete spinal cord injury, emergency intervention may be necessary. Although one author advised surgical intervention, which consisted of reduction of the fracture, decompressive laminectomy, and pedicle screw construct fixation, others favor a ventral approach, even with osteoporotic patients.[134,146,260]

Before embarking on pedicle screw fixation, a detailed knowledge of the anatomic features of the pedicle and it surroundings is necessary to avoid potential problems and complications. The transverse diameter of the pedicle is 4.5mm at T5, and it gradually increases to 7 to 8mm at the thoracolumbar junction and to 18mm at L5.[260,310] In general, the sagittal diameter is slightly larger at all levels. The pedicle is angled less than 10 degrees ventromedially in the thoracic spine and about 30 degrees at L5, in the transverse plane.[260] In the sagittal plane, the pedicles are orientated 15 to 17 degrees ventrally in the thoracic spine; they are neutral in the lumbar spine and are directed 18 degrees caudally at L5. The ventrodorsal distance from the ventral vertebral cortex to the dorsal is used to avoid retraction on the spinal cord. A laminectomy, extended laterally to include the articular mass, the pedicle, and even the transverse process, allows access to the dorsal vertebral body without distorting the spinal cord.

Transpedicular fixation of the spine is accomplished with the patient in the prone position and through a midline incision made to expose the lamina, pars, facets, and transverse processes. Several different approaches have been described, but the authors prefer to remove the caudal lateral facet with a rongeur and to make a shallow pilot hole with a high-speed drill. A probe connected to evoked electromyographic monitoring may then be used to determine the optimal depth and track for screw placement.[34]

Pedicle screw fixation has been a highly useful technique in the hands of experienced surgeons, but there are reports of significant rates of penetration of the pedicle or vertebral body cortex. This complication has been reported to be reduced by using radiographic methods to determine the correct position, but Weinstein reported that even with a careful surgical technique and image intensifier control, penetration of the pedicular cortex occurred in 21% of cases.[65,103,288] A screw inserted to an inadequate depth was more likely to pull out.[149] Whitecloud[298] showed that because of the curvature of the ventral vertebral body and angulation of the screw, a lateral radiograph is inadequate for determining the exact penetration of the vertebral body.

Dural tears should be repaired immediately, and dural leaks that are noticed only later usually require exploration and closure of the fistula. Nerve roots can be injured by a drill, curette, or eccentrically placed screws (116%).[38,260] They can also be damaged by late screw cutout or as a result of spinal canal exploration during decompression surgery.[259]

The optimal position of pedicle screws along the axis incorporates the largest available diameter in the sagittal and transverse plane. Inadvertent penetration of the pedicular cortex has resulted in damage to some of the surrounding structures: to the medial side of the pedicle, the dural sac with the spinal cord, or the spinal nerve roots; caudally, to the nerve root as it exits the intervertebral foramen[46,262]; and laterally, to the rostral spinal nerve. Damage to nerve roots is most likely to occur by violation of the medial-caudal and extended at least 6mm into the spinal canal.[38] The lumbosacral plexus is found along the ventral ala of the sacrum, whereas the presacral plexus lies ventral to the L5-S1 disc space and sacral promontory.[103] The aorta and inferior vena cava lie ventral to the vertebral bodies and branch into the common iliac vessels at the L4-5 disc. They continue as the common, external, and internal iliac vessels along the ventral sacrum.

Originally, pedicle instrumentation consisted of plates with multiple holes for semirigid fixation. Currently, screws connect with certain fixation devices such as plates and rods in a rigid or nonrigid fashion.[260] The universal systems allow interval pedicle fixation to control lordotic, kyphotic, and rotational forces and use cross-fixators to increase the rigidity of the constructs and the pullout force of the screws.

Reduction of the bony deformity is obtained in different ways. The prone surgical position reduces most of the focal kyphosis. The application of the universal fixation and the pull of the screws further reduce the spinal deformity. Removal of a compressive fragment requires laminectomy. Below L2 a simple laminectomy is sufficient, because the dura mater can be retracted to gain access to the dorsal vertebral body. Above L2 an enlarged dorsal approach is used to avoid retraction on the spinal cord. A laminectomy, extended laterally to include the articular mass, the pedicle, and even the transverse process, allows access to the dorsal vertebral body without distorting the spinal cord.

If the nerve injury was caused by a screw, it usually resolves after removal of the offending screw.[259] Careful postoperative monitoring with early computed tomography scan or magnetic resonance imaging should lead to early decompression when needed. Titanium devices minimize imaging artifacts.[236]

Infection is more prevalent (at 2% to 6%) with this type of surgery[65,260] because of the extensive dissection and the length of the procedure. The number of surgical instruments employed is large, and the risk of glove perforation is also considerable. The use of intraoperative imaging creates more traffic in the operating room.

In very thin patients, the implant may be very prominent and may cause skin necrosis from postoperative orthosis pressure. Adjusting the brace and using extensive padding have obviated this complication. The implant is left in situ until the fusion is solid, and only exposure of the instrumentation warrants removal of the device.

Loss of stabilization is caused by poor fixation as a result of osteoporosis, improperly placed screws, improper instrumentation design, or improper implantation.[147,215] Postoperative immobilization with a body jacket until there is radiographic evidence of healing decreases the risk of screw cutout or implant failure. Within 1 year, 15% of implants must be removed, mainly as a result of pain or discomfort. The radiographic rate of implant failure at 6 months is 5% to 31%.[19,65,176,311] A faulty design or manufacture has been implicated in early system failure. Breakage at the connection between the plate and the screw has been reduced by allowing slight motion between the screw and the longitudinal connector in the semi-rigid systems and by redesigning the screws. Screw fracture (4%) is lower in screws that have a larger diameter or that are placed more deeply within the vertebral body.[310] Often, screw breakages occur when the fusion is already solid (5 to 24 months). Screw loosening (in some series, 20%) has become less of a problem since redesign of the screws.[19,147,261,284]

Biochemical Considerations

Several tests have been used in experimental settings to evaluate the resistance of failure of spinal instrumentation.[1] Panjabi[221] suggested three biochemical tests to evaluate spinal instrumentation. The strength of the spinal construct is determined from destructive tests, stability is measured by nondestructive tests with physiologic loads, and fatigue failure is assessed with load deformation tests. Destructive tests assess the ultimate strength of the fixation with a load large enough to cause failure, but spinal instrumentation seldom fails with this method. Nondestructive tests apply cyclic loading to determine the failure as a result of fatigue. Although this is a much more realistic mode of failure, the test was rather impractical. To mimic a clinically relevant situation, the system would have to be put through 1 to 4×10^6 cycles of loading. Load deformation testing measures the change in angle or length in response to a given load. It allows calculation of the tensile strength (stress that causes fatigue failure) and the endurance limit (stress below which the metal does not fail). This approaches the real-life situation, because the goal of spinal instrumentation is to stabilize the spine until the fusion matures. These variables are tested in the 6 degrees of freedom of the vertebra: movement in ventrodorsal, mediolateral, and rostrocaudal directions and rotation in the frontal, sagittal, and horizontal planes.

Failure results from failure of the metal components (e.g., screw or plate fatigue).[190] The quality of the different components depends on the design of the components and the properties of the metal. Failure also occurs at the metal-metal juncture, but the most common method of breakdown is at the bone-metal juncture.[45,215] Screws fail by pullout, cutout, or loosening. These events destabilize the construct and consequently make nonunion more likely. The rate of failure is grossly affected by bone quality and is much higher in osteoporotic bone.[1,121,282] Other important factors that determine the stability of fixation are the technique of implantation of the construct and the inherent properties of the device, especially the screws. Individual juncture stresses are decreased when the load is spread over a larger area.

In the osteoporotic spine, the primary stability of the implant is low, and consequently, failure is frequent, especially after mobilization begins. The maximum pullout force of pedicle screws in osteoporotic bone is about half that in the normal spine.[150,289,310] This pullout force decreases caudally to rostrally and is minimal at T4-5. It correlates highly with the BMD.[45,289] Several methods have been described for increasing the implant stability to normal or near normal. The use of these techniques is necessary when BMD drops to less than 0.7 g/cm^2 in the lumbar spine or to less than 0.85g/cm^2 in the thoracic spine.[289]

From axial pullout experiments, the most important factor in screw loosening is poor bone quality.[310] Because there are no means to improve this, other variables are manipulated to improve the holding power of the screws. Partially threaded screws have a better purchase if they are inserted less deeply so that the larger threaded portion of the screw is located within the pedicle. Fully threaded screws have a higher pullout force than partially threaded screws. A larger diameter screw also greatly reduces the risk of loosening. This is taken into consideration by determining the proper size of the screw on the basis of the pedicle anatomy before inserting the pedicle screw. All lumbar pedicles should be able to take at least 6.5mm screws, but in the series of Zindrick et al.,[312] multiple lumbar pedicles (L1-3) had a diameter less than 6.5mm and, in some cases, even less than 4.5mm. Although an attempt should be made to place the largest screw possible, a potential fracture of the pedicle must be avoided by not choosing an excessively large screw. The depth of insertion of the screws in the severely osteoporotic spine has little influence on their holding power unless the ventral cortex is penetrated, because deeper insertion engages only poor quality bone. Screw design contributes little to screw purchase.[149,310] Bone cement provides an anchoring effect because of its penetration into the intratrabecular spaces.[309] Methylmethacrylate doubled the load-to-failure with dorsally directed forces.[282,286,311] When PMMA is used, the size of the screw becomes less important. Although the use of cement greatly augments the stability of the construct, the risk of infection is slightly higher, and the cement can migrate into the spinal canal or foramen. The latter situation has caused damage to the cord or the nerve roots. Extrapedicular cement that has leaked retroperitoneally can cause problems with removal in revision surgery. If revision becomes necessary, the pedicle is useless for fixation, even with PMMA. PMMA is possibly toxic or carcinogenic, and the long-term effects on the soft tissues and the bone-cement junction are not well established. For this reason, other biodegradable materials are being tested. Wittenberg et al.[303] demonstrated that the reinforcement provided by polypropylene fumarate is similar to that of PMMA, but polypropylene fumarate is eventually resorbed and replaced by host bone. Further studies with this compound will be necessary before clinical use is initiated. Reinsertion of screws in salvage procedures performed for improperly placed screws or loosened screws in pseudoarthrosis relies on three factors to ensure adequate fixation: (1) PMMA used in salvage procedures after previous screw loosening has restored the pullout force to the original value; (2) insertion of PMMA under pressure can double the pullout force resistance capability[310]; and (3) in revision procedures, the outcome can also be improved by using larger screws with a more aggressive design (greater thread depth and increased pitch) or by using longer screws, engaging the ventral cortex.[188]

Cyclic loading tests reveal that holding power can be greatly increased by inserting the screws more deeply. Placing the screws all the way up to the ventral cortex instead of only 50% of the way results in a significant increase in the number of cycles and a 91% increase in medial-lateral cycles before failure occurs. Engaging the ventral cortex is followed by an additional increase in the number of cycles of 194% in the rostral-caudal direction.[310] After penetration of the ventral cortex, cycling in the medial-lateral direction results in pedicle fracture or bending of the crew, which implies that this configuration is so strong that the construct does not loosen.[310] These and other biomechanical studies have helped determine the optimal depth of penetration.[84,147,310] In the thoracic and lumbar spine, 60% of the fixation strength was located in the pedicles, 15% to 20% was in the cancellous bone of the vertebral body, and the remaining 20% to 25%

was derived from engagement of the ventral cortex. Considerable clinical data suggest that penetration of the ventral cortex is not routinely necessary, especially in view of the added risk to the ventral structures.[145,256,257,284] In the sacral region, 60% of the fixation strength arises from the ventral cortex. Therefore, routine engagement of the ventral cortex in osteoporotic sacral bone is a rational procedure.

Cross-fixation, triangulation, and the placement of screws at intermediate levels are other means to diminish the failure rate. Since the introduction of pedicle screw systems, most surgeons have recommended the use of screws at all vertebral levels.[167,259,284] Occasionally, Horowitch[120] left out a level in a long fusion. Recently, Krag[148] suggested using screws only in the top and bottom vertebrae, regardless of the length of the fusion. Dick et al.[71] demonstrated a significant increase in stability in all planes (axial, flexion, rotation) after the insertion of screws at the intermediate levels. The recommendation for screw placement in all vertebral levels in osteoporotic bone is rational because the load is divided over all the screws, and the chance of failure is thus decreased. Triangulation of the construct increases the stability of the fixation. Failure of spinal instrumentation at the bone-metal juncture is the result of a suboptimal attachment of the construct to the vertebra. If instrument failure occurs away from the bone-metal link, it implies that the connection between the bone and the device is optimal and that the fixation strength depends on the material properties of the vertebra. The limiting factor in this case is the quality of the underlying bone. With a single pedicle screw, the strength of the fixation relies on the volume of bone within the screw thread. With a triangular construct, the strength of the fixation depends not only on the bone within the trapezoid formed by the screws. These constructs, therefore, provide a significantly greater fixation than do conventional pedicle screw or sublaminar hook systems, even in osteoporotic spine.[261] Cross-fixation provides a considerable improvement in rotational stability.* Pintar and colleagues[226] noted that rotational stability is more pronounced with medially placed constructs (rod placed medially to the screw) compared with laterally placed constructs (rod placed laterally to the screw), regardless of the presence of a transverse connector. They also found that rotational instability increases with longer rods. For lateral rods, the transverse connectors offer an advantage, primarily for the longer rods (15 to 18cm). With medial placement of the rods (the most commonly used configuration), transverse connectors greatly increase the rotational stability for all rod lengths. Until the rod is more than 15cm long or more than three vertebral levels long, one transverse fixator is equivalent to two.

Over the years, several articles have reported the advantages of pedicle screw fixation over systems relying on sublaminar hooks or wires.[73,167,259] Plate screws are compatible with universal fixation systems and provide three-dimensional correction of deformities via control of all three columns of the spine. They allow strong fixation from a dorsal approach and incorporate only a small number of vertebrae in the fusion.[259,283] Rigid pedicle screw

systems have been advocated over semirigid systems (e.g., Roy-Camille plate system), because semirigid systems allow a toggling motion between the screw and the rod or plate, which increases the risk of a pseudoarthrosis.[13] Rigid pedicle screw systems permit less motion and therefore have a higher rate of fusion. However, because of their rigidity, these systems are associated with an increased incidence of device-related osteoporosis as a result of stress shielding.[166,186] Early design pedicle screws fractured in rigid constructs. This type of fixation, however, failed more frequently at the bone-metal juncture.[33,160] They were also responsible for the so-called transitional syndrome, which consisted of increased osteoarthritis at the levels adjacent to a stiff spinal construct. Therefore, although some surgeons have advocated the use of semirigid systems, our preference remains rigid universal fixation titanium constructs.

The ventral approach has been used less frequently in osteoporotic patients because of the perception that these procedures are associated with increased risk to a generally older population. In a limited number of patients who are quite active or fairly young, ventral instrumentation is indicated, mainly in the presence of major spinal canal involvement or neurologic injury after a vertebral body fracture from an axial load.[102,143] In this procedure, the disc and end-plates on either side of the fractured vertebra are removed, and distraction is applied (either manually or with the instrumentation) to restore the normal vertebral body height. A tricortical interbody autograft or a combination of autograft and allograft is used. Most surgeons recommend the use of some form of internal fixation, because the bone graft alone cannot control rotation adequately, the osteoporotic bone does not withstand the normal load in the upright position, and correction is lost. Ventral plates provide only fixation, whereas distractive constructs (Kostuik-Harrigton, Dunn, Zielke, and Kaneda devices) provide additional correction. Kostuik et al.[145] recommended dorsal fixation and fusion after ventral instrumentation and fusion in "markedly osteoporotic patients." Because of their location, the latter systems pose a potential risk of damage to the great vessels. Inadvertent injury to the ureters or the great vessels has been reported as a potential complication in cases in which the ventral spine has been previously exposed.[145] Vertebral implants provide significant stability in axial compression but do not provide torsional stability. Postoperatively, patients are placed in a thoracolumbar spinal orthosis for 6 months and are followed at monthly intervals for the first 3 months.

Surgery in Patients with Concomitant Osteoporosis

The most common indication for spinal surgery in older patients with osteoporosis has been degenerative disease. Dorsal fixation with a universal spinal system, including pedicle screws, or ventral decompression and fusion, are the treatments of choice.

Surgery in Patients with Paget's Disease

Spinal surgery is not the preferred treatment in patients with Paget's disease. However, some specific problems have been described that require intervention by a spine

---

*References 1,10,37,71,185,226.

surgeon. One third of patients with osteitis deformans have vertebral pathology. Of these, one third have symptomatic spinal stenosis and one half have back pain.[6,137] Spinal cord compression and nerve root lesions are more common in the thoracic spine, because the spinal canal of the lumbar spine is more spacious and because of the presence of the spinal cord in the thoracic spine.[113] Collapse of the vertebral body with intrusion of bone into the spinal canal has caused cord injury. Additional causes of neurologic deficit include spinal artery steal phenomenon, with blood being shunted away from the spinal cord to the pagetic vertebra and new bone forming, with narrowing of the spinal canal or the neuroforamen. The site of compression can be identified by plain radiograph, myelography, computed tomography, or magnetic resonance imaging (MRI). In some patients with bony overgrowth, deterioration can occur after lumbar puncture because of obstruction to the flow of contrast medium by a complete spinal subarachnoid block, but the ability to obtain a computed tomography or MRI scan has obviated this concern.

Sadar et al.[265] reported 86 patients in the medical literature up to 1972 who had neurologic dysfunction attributable only to Paget's disease of the vertebral column and added four more cases. Of these patients, 71% met the criteria for surgical intervention and underwent a decompressive laminectomy. Although 55 patients had "definite but variable degrees of improvement" of the preoperative neurologic deficit, 4 had only minimal improvement, 2 were unchanged, and 1 was worse. There were 7 operative deaths.

Usually the progression of compression can be halted or even reversed by medical treatment, causing a decrease in vascularity and possibly even a reduction in the actual size of the bone. A decompressive procedure is indicated if the neurologic deficit progression cannot be prevented by drug treatment and long tract signs or sphincter disturbances are present. Although improvements in surgical techniques and perioperative care have taken place since the review of the literature by Sadar et al.,[265] pagetic patients, with involvement of the spinal column, present a challenge for the spine surgeon. Decompression more completely ameliorates the symptoms associated with stenosis as compared with those resulting from a vascular abnormality.

Low back pain is a common presentation in Paget's disease because of the loss of lumbar lordosis, the simian posture, and the altered gait dynamics as a result of protrusion acetabuli and bowed extremities. Lumbar back pain is a consequence of unrelated osteoarthritis or disc disease. Treatment for osteoarthritis is the same as in the general population: anti-inflammatory drugs, strengthening exercises, and lumbar support. Spinal fusion is used only if more conservative therapy has failed and a correctible lesion is present. Spinal fusion is performed via a dorsal or ventral approach, as previously described.

Some specific problems have been encountered in surgery for Paget's disease. Bleeding is often considerable, because of the high vascularity of pagetic bone. Preoperative administration of calcitonin greatly diminishes disease activity and, therefore, reduces blood loss. During the sclerotic phase, drilling and removal of bone is difficult, whereas in the osteolytic stage, the bone is abnormally soft, and the holding power of internal fixation devices is decreased. Bone healing is delayed and nonunion is more frequent during the sclerotic phase. Long periods of immobilization are avoided, thereby decreasing disuse osteoporosis or hypercalcemia.

Osteosarcoma is a rare complication, but it has a poor prognosis, regardless of the treatment. Sadar et al.[265] warned that pagetic patients with sarcomatous changes present with rapidly decreasing neurologic function and with pain as the dominant symptom. In selected cases, a ventral vertebrectomy and fusion is indicated.[150,265]

Another rare complication of Paget's disease is basilar impression, first described by Rokitansky in 1844. Subsequently, secondary platybasia because of bony softening and molding in Paget's disease was described by others.[119,297,307] High cervical laminectomy and suboccipital decompression have resulted in dramatic recovery. In this procedure, laminectomy of the upper cervical vertebrae is performed, the bone over the cerebellar hemispheres is rongeured away, and an allograft duraplasty is performed.

Surgery in Patients with Osteomalacia

Surgery is seldom necessary in osteomalacia. In this condition, the main characteristic is weak, osteopenic bone. The surgeon therefore relies on the same surgical principles as in osteoporosis.

Summary

Spinal surgery is challenging in the osteoporotic patient but should not be denied a patient if the proper indications exist. Segmental fixation devices, better pre- and postoperative care, and judicious use of PMMA have made the success rate of spinal surgery acceptable in osteoporosis.

When surgery is indicated, universal fixation systems, combined with meticulous grafting technique, afford the highest success rate. A ventral decompression and fusion is advocated in a select group of patients, either in combination with dorsal surgery or, rarely, as the sole treatment. There are few indications for spinal surgery in Paget's disease and osteomalacia.

REFERENCES

1. Albert TJ, Jones TJ, Balderstone RA: Spinal instrumentation. In Rothman RH, Simeone FA (eds): The Spine, ed 3, vol II. Philadelphia, WB Saunders, 1992, p 1777.
2. Alden JC: Osteoporosis: a review. Clin Ther 11:3, 1989.
3. Alexandre CM, Chapuy MC, Vignon E, et al: Treatment of Paget's disease of bone with ethane-1-hydroxy 1,1, diphosphonate (EHDP) at a low dosage (5 mg/kg/day). Clin Orthop 174:193-205, 1983.
4. Allen BL, Ferguson RJ: The Galveston technique of pelvic fixation with L rod instrumentation of the spine. Spine 9:388, 1984.
5. Aloia JF, Cohn SH, Vaswani A, et al: Risk factors for postmenopausal osteoporosis. Am J Med 78:95, 1985.

6. Altman RD: Articular complications of Paget's disease of bone. *Semin Arthritis Rheum* 23:248, 1994.

7. Alvarez L, Guanbens N, Peris P, *et al*: Discriminative value biochemical markers of bone turnover in assessing the activity of Paget's disease. *J Bone Miner Res* 10:458-465, 1995.

8. America's bone health: the state of osteoporosis and low bone mass in our nation. Washington (DC): National Osteoporosis Foundation, 2002.

9. Arciero RA, Leung KYK, Pierce JH: Spontaneous unstable burst fracture of the thoracolumbar spine in osteoporosis. *Spine* 14:114, 1989.

10. Asher MA, Carson WL, Heinig CF, *et al*: A modular rod linkage system to provide rotational stability. *Spine* 13:272, 1988.

11. Asher MA, Strippgen WE, Heinig CF, Carson WL: Isola spinal implant system: principles, design, and applications. In An HS, Cotler JM (eds): *Spinal Instrumentation*. Baltimore, Williams & Wilkins, 1992, p 325.

12. Ashman RB: History and development of the TRSH system. In Ashman RB, Herring JA, Johnston JA, *et al* (eds): *TRSH Universal Spinal Instrumentation*. Dallas, Hundley & Associates, 1993, p 1.

13. Ashman RB, Birch JG, Bone LB, *et al*: Mechanical testing of spinal instrumentation. *Clin Orthop* 227:113, 1988.

14. Assessment of fracture risk and its application to screening for postmenopausal osteoporosis. Report of a WHO Study Group. *World Health Org Techn Rep Ser* 843:1-129, 1994.

15. Avioli LV: *The Osteoporotic Syndrome: Detection, Prevention and Treatment*. Orlando, Grune & Stratton, 1983.

16. Avioli LV, Lindsay R: The female osteoporotic syndrome(s). In Avioli LV, Krane SM (eds): *Metabolic Bone Disease and Related Disorders*. Philadelphia, WB Saunders, 1990, p 397.

17. Barker DJP: The epidemiology of Paget's disease. *Metab Bone Dis Rel Res* 4&5:531, 1981.

18. Barr JD, Barr MS, Lemley TJ, McCann RM: Percutaneous vertebroplasty for pain relief and spinal stabilization. *Spine* 25:923-928, 2000.

19. Barry HC: Incidence. In: *Paget's Disease of Bone*. England, E&S Livingston Ltd., 1969, p 17.

20. Basle MF, Russel WC, Gowsami KKA, *et al*: Paramyxovirus antigens in osteoclasts of Paget's bone tissue detected by monoclonal antibodies. *J Gen Virol* 66:2103, 1985.

21. Bassett CAL, Mitchell SN, Gaston SR: Pulsing electromagnetic field treatment in ununited fractures and failed arthrodeses. *JAMA* 247:263, 1982.

22. Bauer DC, Gluer CC, Cauley JA, *et al*: Broadband ultrasonic attenuation predicts fractures strongly and independently of densitometry in older women. *Arch Intern Med* 157:629-634, 1997.

23. Bergkvist L, Adami H, Persson I, *et al*: The risk of breast cancer after estrogen and estrogen-progestin replacement. *N Engl J Med* 321:293, 1989.

24. Bernstein J, Lane MJ: Metabolic bone disorders of the spine. In Rothman RH, Simeone FA (eds): *The Spine*, ed 3, vol II. Philadelphia, WB Saunders, 1992, p 1381.

25. Biyvoet OLM, van der Sluys Veer J, Jansen AP: Effects of calcitonin in patients with Paget's disease, thyrotoxicosis, or hypercalcemia. *Lancet* 1:876, 1968.

26. Black D, Cummings SR, Genant HK, *et al*: Axial and appendicular bone density predicts fractures in older women. *J Bone Miner Res* 7:633-638, 1997.

27. Black DM, Cummings SR, Karpf DB, *et al*: Randomized trial of effect of alendronate on risk of fracture in women with existing vertebral fractures: Fracture Intervention Trial Research Group. *Lancet* 348:1535-1541, 1996.

28. Boucher HH: A method of spinal fusion. *J Bone Joint Surg* 41B:248, 1959.

29. Boyce BF: Uses and limitations of bone biopsy in management of metabolic bone disease. *Baillieres Clin Endocrinol Metab* 2:31, 1988.

30. Boyce BF, Smith L, Fogelman I, *et al*: Focal osteomalacia due to low dose diphosphonate therapy in Paget's disease. *Lancet* 1:821, 1984.

31. Bracken MB, Webb SB, Wagner FC: Classification of acute spinal cord injury: implications for management. *Paraplegia* 15:319, 1978.

32. Brown L, Birdwell KH, Holt RH, Jennings J: Aortic erosions and lacerations associated with the Dunn anterior spinal instrumentation. Presented at the 20th Annual Meeting of the Scoliosis Research Society, San Diego, 1985.

33. Burton CV: The liabilities of fusion. In Cauthen JC (ed): *Lumbar Spine Surgery*. Baltimore, Williams & Wilkins, 1987.

34. Calanci B, Madsen PW, Lebwohl N: Stimulus-evoked EMG monitoring during transpedicular lumbosacral spine instrumentation. *Spine* 19:2780, 1994.

35. Cameron HU, Bridges A: Pseudoarthrosis in lumbar spine fusion. *Prog Clin Biol Res* 187:479, 1985.

36. Campodarve I, Ulrich U, Bell, *et al*: Urinary N-telopeptide of type I collagen monitors bone resorption and may predict change in bone mass of the spine in response to hormone replacement therapy. *Abstract* · *J Bone Miner Res*, suppl 10:S17, 1995.

37. Carson WL, Duffield RC, Arendt M, *et al*: Internal forces and moments in transpedicular spine instrumentation: the effect of pedicle screw angle and transfixation—the 4R-4Bar linkage concept. *Spine* 15:893, 1990.

38. Castro WHM, Halm H, Jerosch J, *et al*: Accuracy of pedicle screw placement in lumbar vertebrae. *Spine* 21:1320, 1996.

39. Cauley JA, Gutai JP, Sandler RB, *et al*: The relationship of endogenous estrogen to bone density and bone area in normal postmenopausal women. *Am J Epidemiol* 124:752, 1986.

40. Chalmers J: Osteomalacia. *J R Coll Surg Edinb* 13:255, 1968.

41. Chesnut CH, Silverman S, Andriano K, *et al*: A randomized trial of nasal spray salmon calcitonin in postmenopausal women with established osteoporosis: the prevent recurrence of osteoporotic fracture study. *Am J Med* 109:267-276, 2000.

42. Chevalley T, Rizzoli R, Nydegger V, *et al*: Effects of calcium supplements on femoral bone mineral density and vertebral fracture rate in vitamin-D-replete elderly patients. *Osteoporos Int* 4:245-252, 1994.

43. Clark BL: Diagnosis and management of postmenopausal osteoporosis. *JCOM* 9:397-408, 2002.

44. Clark J, Tamenbaum C, Posnett K, *et al*: Laboratory testing in healthy osteopenic women. *J Bone Miner Res* 12:S141, 1997.

45. Coe JD, Warden KE, Herzig MA, McAfee PC: Influence of bone mineral density on the fixation of thoracolumbar implants: A comparative study of transpedicular screws, laminar hooks and spinous process wires. *Spine* 15:902, 1990.

46. Cohen LD: Fractures of the osteoporotic spine. *Orthop Clin North Am* 21:143, 1990.

47. Cohen MS, Wall EJ, Brown RA, *et al*: Cauda equina anatomy II: Extrathecal nerve roots and dorsal root ganglia. *Spine* 15:1244, 1990.

48. Cohen S, Levy RM, Keller M, *et al*: Risedronate therapy prevents corticosteroid-induced bone loss: a twelve-month, multicenter, randomized, double blind, placebo-controlled, parallel group study. *Arthritis Rheum* 42:2309-2318, 1999.

49. Collins DH: Paget's disease of bone: incidence and subclinical forms. *Lancet* 2:51, 1956.

50. Cooper C, Atkinson EJ, O'Fallon WM, Melton LJ III: Incidence of clinically diagnosed vertebral fractures: a population-based study in Rochester, Minnesota, 1985-1989. *J Bone Miner Res* 7:221-227, 1992.

51. Cotrel Y, Dubousset J, Guillaumat M: A new universal instrumentation in spinal surgery. *Clin Orthop* 227:10, 1988.

52. Coventry MB, Topper EM: Pelvic instability: a consequence of removing iliac bone for grafting. *J Bone Joint Surg* 54A:83, 1972.

53. Crandall C: Parathyroid hormone for treatment of osteoporosis. *Arch Intern Med* 162:297-309, 2002.

54. Cranney A, Welch V, Adachi JD, *et al*: Etidronate for treating and preventing postmenopausal osteoporosis. *Cochrane Database Syst Rev* 2001; (4): CD003376 (latest version 25 March 2001).

55. Cruess RL: Healing of bone, tendon, and ligament. In Rockwood CA, Green DP (eds): *Fractures.* Philadelphia, Lippincott-Raven, 1984, 153.

56. Cumming RG, Cumings SR, Nevitt MC, *et al*: Calcium intake and fracture risk: results from the study of osteoporotic fractures. *Am J Epidemiol* 145:926-934, 1997.

57. Cummings SR, Black DM, Nevitt MC, *et al*: Bone density at various sites for prediction of hip fractures. *Lancet* 341:72-75, 1993.

58. Cummings SR, Black DM, Rubin SM: Lifetime risk of hip, Colles or vertebral fracture and coronary heart disease among white postmenopausal women. *Arch Intern Med* 149:2445, 1989.

59. Cummings SR, Black DM, Thompson DE, *et al*: Effect of alendronate on risk of fracture in women with low bone density but without vertebral fractures: results from the Fracture Intervention Trial. *JAMA* 280:2077-2082, 1998.

60. Cummings SR, Kelsey JL, Nevitt MC, O'Dowd KJ: Epidemiology of osteoporosis and osteoporotic fractures. *Epidemiol Rev* 7:178-208, 1985.

61. Cummings SR, Nevitt MC, Browner WS, *et al*: Risk factors for hip fracture in white women. *N Engl J Med* 332:767-773, 1995.

62. Dalen N, Feldreich AL: Osteopenia in alcoholism. *Clin Orthop* 99:210, 1974.

63. Dalsky GP, Stocke KS, Ehsani AA, *et al*. Weight-bearing exercise training and lumbar bone mineral content in postmenopausal women. *Ann Intern Med* 108:824-828, 1988.

64. Daramond H: Percutaneous vertebroplasty with polymethylmethacrylate: technique, indications, and results. *Radiol Clin North Am* 36:533-546, 1998.

65. Davne SH, Myers DL: Complications of lumbar spinal fusion with transpedicular instrumentation. *Spine* 17(suppl):S184, 1992.

66. Dawson-Hughes B, Harris SS, Krall EA, Dallal GE: Effect of calcium and vitamin D supplementation on bone density in men and women 65 years of age or older. *N Engl J Med* 337:670-676, 1997.

67. Deal C, Gideon J: Recombinant human PTH 1-34 (Forteo): an anabolic drug for osteoporosis. *Cleve Clin J Med* 70:585-601, 2003.

68. Delmas PD, Bjarnason NH, Mitlak BH, *et al*. Effects of raloxifene on bone mineral density, serum cholesterol concentrations, and uterine endometrium in postmenopausal women. *N Engl J Med* 337:1641-1647, 1997.

69. Delmas PD, Meunier PJ: The management of Paget's disease of bone. *N Engl J Med* 336:558-566, 1997.

70. Denis F: The three column spine and its significance in the classification of acute thoracolumbar spinal injuries. *Spine* 8:817, 1983.

71. Dick JC, Jones MP, Zdeblick TA, *et al*: A biomechanical comparison evaluating the use of intermediate screws and cross-linkage in lumbar pedicle fixation. *J Spinal Disord* 7:402, 1994.

72. Dick W: The fixateure interne as a versatile implant for spine surgery. *Spine* 12:882, 1987.

73. Dickman CA, Yahiro MA, Lu HTC, Melkerson MN: Surgical treatment alternatives for fixation of unstable fractures of the thoracic and lumbar spine. *Spine* 19(suppl):S2266, 1994.

74. Dominguez Cabrera C, Sosa Henriquez M, Traba ML, *et al*: Biochemical markers of bone formation in the study of postmenopausal osteoporosis. *Osteoporosis Int* 8: 147-151, 1998.

75. Douglas DL, Bickerstaff DR: Metabolic bone disease. Part 2. *Surgery* 78:1882, 1990.

76. Drummond DS: Harrington instrumentation with spinous process wiring for idiopathic scoliosis. *Orthop Clin North Am* 19:281, 1988.

77. Dubois-Dalcq M, Coblentz JM, Pleet AB: Subacute sclerosing panencephalitis: unusual nuclear inclusions and lengthy clinical course. *Arch Neurol* 31:355, 1974.

78. Dull TA, Henneman PH: Urinary hydroxyproline as an index of collagen turnover in bone. *N Engl J Med* 268:132, 1963.

79. Dunn HK: Anterior spine stabilization and decompression for thoracolumbar injuries. *Orthop Clin North Am* 17:113, 1986.

80. Edwards CC, Levine AM: Early rod-sleeve stabilization of the injured thoracic and lumbar spine. *Orthop Clin North Am* 17:121, 1986.

81. Eismont FJ: personal communication.

82. Eismont FJ, Garfin SR, Abitbol J: Thoracic and upper lumbar spine injuries. In Browner BD, Jupiter JB, Levine AM, Trafton PG (eds): *Skeletal Trauma,* vol. 1. Philadelphia, WB Saunders, 1992, p 179.

83. Eismont FJ, Green BA, Berkowitz BM, *et al*: The role of intraoperative ultrasonography in the treatment of thoracic and lumbar fractures. *Spine* 9:782, 1984.

84. Ekstrom L, Hanssoon T, Afonja A: The pullout strength of intrapedicular screws in relation to the vertebral bone mineral content. Presented at First World Conference on Biomechanics. La Jolla, California, August 1990.

85. Escalas F, DeWald RL: Combined traumatic arteriovenous fistula and ureteral injury: a complication of iliac bone grafting. *J Bone Joint Surg* 59A:270, 1977.

86. Ettinger B, Black DM, Mitlak BH, *et al*: Reduction of vertebral fracture risk in postmenopausal women with osteoporosis treated with raloxifene. Results from a 3-year randomized trial. *JAMA* 282: 637-645, 1999.

87. Ettinger B, Genant HK, Cann CE: Long-term estrogen replacement therapy prevents bone loss and fractures. *Ann Intern Med* 102:319, 1985.

88. Firooznia H, Golimbu C, Rafii M, Schwartz MS: Rate of spinal trabecular bone loss in normal perimenopausal women: CT measurement. *Radiology* 161:735, 1986.

89. Francis RM: The calcium controversy. In Smith R (ed): *Osteoporosis*. London, Royal College of Physicians of London, 1990, p 125.

90. Friedlander AL, Genant HK, Sadowsky S, *et al*: A two-year program of aerobics and weight-training enhances bone mineral density of young women. *J Bone Miner Res* 10:574-585, 1995.

91. Friedlander GE, Mankin HJ: Bone banking: current methods and suggested guidelines. *AAOS Instr Course Lect* 30:36, 1981.

92. Frost HM: Symposium on osteoporosis. *Orthop Clin North Am* 12:725, 1981.

93. Galibert P, Deramond H: La vertebroplasty acrylique percutanée comme traitement des angiomes vertébraux et des affections dolorigenes et fragilisantes du rachis. *Chirurgie* 116;362, 1990.

94. Gallagher TC, Geling O, Comite F: Missed opportunities for prevention of osteoporotic fracture. *Arch Intern Med* 162:450-456, 2002.

95. Gardsell P, Johnell O, Nilsson E: Predicting fractures in women by using forearm bone densitometry. *Calcif Tissue Int* 44:235-242, 1989.

96. Garfin SR, Yan HA, Reiley MA. Kyphoplasty and vertebroplasty for the treatment of painful osteoporotic compression fractures. *Spine* 26:1511-1515, 2001.

97. Garrington PR: The history and development of Harrington instrumentation. *Clin Orthop* 227:3, 1988.

98. Gaxier KL, Holbrook TL, Kelsey JL, Stauffer RN: The Frequency of Occurrence, Impact, and Cost of Musculoskeletal Conditions in the United States. The American Academy of Orthopaedic Surgeons, Chicago, 1984.

99. Geary JR, Frantz VK: New absorbable bone wax: experimental and clinical studies. *Ann Surg* 132:1128, 1947.

100. Gennari C, Agnusdei D, Camporeale A: Use of calcitonin in the treatment of bone pain associated with osteoporosis. *Calcif Tissue Int* 49(suppl 2):S9-S13, 1991.

101. Georgis T, Rydevik B, Weinstein JN, Garfin SR: Complications of pedicle screw fixation. In Garfin SR (ed): *Complications of Spine Surgery*. Baltimore, Williams & Wilkins, 1989, p 200.

102. Gertzbein SD, Court-Brown CM, Marks P, *et al*: The neurological outcome following surgery for spinal fractures. *Spine* 13:641, 1988.

103. Gertzbein SD, Robbins SE: Accuracy of pedicular screw placement in vivo. *Spine* 15:11, 1990.

104. Goll SR, Balderston RA, Stambough JL, *et al*: Depth of intraspinal wire penetration during passage of sublaminar wires. *Spine* 13:503, 1988.

105. Grampp S, Genant HK, Mathur A, *et al*: Comparisons of non-invasive bone mineral measurements in assessing age-related loss, fracture discrimination, and diagnostic classification. *J Bone Miner Res* 12:697-611, 1997.

106. Gruber HE, Ivey JL, Baylink DJ, *et al*: Long-term calcitonin therapy in postmenopausal osteoporosis. *Metabolism* 33:295, 1984.

107. Gurr KR, McAfee PC: Cotrel-Dubousset instrumentation in adults: a preliminary report. *Spine* 13:510, 1988.

108. Guyer PB, Chamberlain AT: Paget's disease of bone in two American cities. *BMJ* 280:985, 1980.

109. Hans D, Dargent-Molina P, Schott AM, *et al*: Ultrasonographic heel measurements to predict hip fracture in elderly women: the EPIDOS prospective study. *Lancet* 348: 511-514, 1996.

110. Harrington JT, Broy SB, Derosa AM, *et al*: Hip fracture patients are not treated for osteoporosis: A call to action. *Arthritis Rheum* 47:651-654, 2002.

111. Harrington PR, Tullos H: Reduction of severe spondylolisthesis in children. *South Med J* 62:1, 1969.

112. Harris ST, Watts NB, Genant HK, *et al*: Effects of risedronate treatment on vertebral and nonvertebral fractures in women with postmenopausal osteoporosis: a randomized controlled trial: Vertebral Efficacy with Risedronate Therapy (VERT) study group. *JAMA* 282:1344-1352, 1999.

113. Hartman JT, Dohn DF: Paget's disease of the spine with cord or nerve-root compression: report of six cases. *J Bone Joint Surg* 48A:1079, 1966.

114. Healey JH, Lane M: Structural scoliosis in osteoporotic women. *Clin Orthop* 195:216, 1985.

115. Heaney RP, Gallagher JC, Johnston CC, *et al*: Calcium nutrition and bone health in the elderly. *Am J Clin Nutr* 36(suppl):986, 1982.

116. Heath DA: The role of Mitramycin in the management of Paget's disease. *Metab Bone Dis Rel Res* 4&5:343, 1981.

117. Heggeness MJ: Spine fracture with neurological deficit in osteoporosis. *Osteoporos Int* 3:215, 1993.

118. Henneman PH, Dull TA, Avioli I, *et al*: Effect of aspirin and corticosteroids on Paget's disease of bone. *Trans Stud Coll Physicians Phila* 31:10, 1963.

119. Homen EA: Zur Kenntnis der rachitischen Deformationen der Schadelbasis und der basalen Schadelhyperostosen. *Dtsch Z Nervenheilk* 20:3, 1901.

120. Horowitch A, Peek RD, Thomas JC, *et al*: The Wiltse pedicle screw fixation system: early clinical results. *Spine* 14:461, 1989.

121. Huvos AG: Osteogenic sarcoma of bones and soft tissues in older persons: a cliniocopathological analysis of 117 persons older than 60 years. *Cancer* 57:1442, 1989.

122. Jackson JA, Kleerekoper M: Osteoporosis in men: diagnosis, pathophysiology, and prevention. *Medicine* 69:137, 1990.

123. James KS, Wenger KH, Schiegel JD, *et al*: Biomechanical evaluation of the stability of thoracolumbar burst fractures. *Spine* 19:1731, 1994.

124. Jarvik JG, Kallmes DF, Mizra SK. Vertebroplasty. Learning more, but not enough. *Spine* 28:1487-1489, 2003.

125. Jendrisak MD: Spontaneous abdominal aortic rupture from erosion by a lumbar spine fixation device: a case report. *Surgery* 99:631, 1986.

126. Jense ME, Evans AJ, Mathis JM, *et al*: Percutaneous polymethylmethacrylate vertebroplasty in the treatment of osteoporotic vertebral body compression fractures: technical aspects. *Am J Neuroradiol* 18:311-323, 1997.

127. Jensen GF, Christiansen C, Boesen J, *et al*: Epidemiology of postmenopausal spinal and long bone fractures. *Clin Orthop* 166:75, 1982.

128. Johnell O, Gullberg B, Kanis JA, *et al*: Risk factors for hip fractures in European women. *J Bone Miner Res* 10: 1802-1815, 1995.

129. Johnson BE, Lucasey B, Robinson RG, Lukert BP: Contributing diagnoses in osteoporosis. The value of a complete medical evaluation. *Arch Intern Med* 149: 1069-1072, 1989.

130. Johnston CC, Epstein S: Clinical, biochemical, epidemiologic and economic features of osteoporosis. *Orthop Clin North Am* 12:559, 1981.

131. Johnston CE II, Happel LT, Norris R, *et al*: Delayed paraplegia complicating sublaminar segmental spinal instrumentation. *J Bone Joint Surg* 65A:556, 1986.

132. Kado D, Browner W, Palermo L, *et al*: Vertebral fractures and mortality in older women. A prospective study. *Arch Intern Med* 159: 1215-1220, 1999.

133. Kahanovitz N: Osteoporosis and fusion. *AAOS Instr Course Lect* 41:231, 1992.

134. Kane WJ: Osteoporosis, osteomalacia and Paget's disease. In Frymoyer JW (ed): *The Adult Spine: Principles and Practice*. Philadelphia, Lippincott-Raven, 1991, p 637.

135. Kaneda A, Yamaaura I, Kamikozura M, *et al*: Paraplegia as a complication of corticosteroid therapy: a case report. *J Bone Joint Surg* 66A:783, 1984.

136. Kaneda K, Asano S, Hashimoto T, *et al*: The treatment of osteoporotic posttraumatic vertebral prosthesis. *Spine* 17(suppl):S295, 1992.

137. Kaplan FS: Paget's disease of bone: orthopedic complications. *Semin Arthritis Rheum* 23:250, 1994.

138. Kaplan PA, Orton DF, Asleson RJ: Osteoporosis with vertebral compression fractures, retropulsed fragments, and neurological compromise. *Radiology* 165:533, 1987.

139. Kaufer H: Fractures and dislocations of the spine. In Rockwood C, Green D (eds): *Fractures*. Philadelphia, Lippincott-Raven, 1975, p 817.

140. Kempinsky WH: Osteoporotic kyphosis with paraplegia. *Neurology* 8:181, 1958.

141. Khovidhunkit W, Shoback DM: Clinical effects of raloxifene hydrochloride in women. *Ann Intern Med* 130:431-439, 1999.

142. Kleerekoper M: Extensive personal experience: the clinical evaluation and management of osteoporosis. *J Clin Endocrinol Metab* 80:757, 1995.

143. Kostuik JP: Anterior fixation for burst fractures of the thoracic and lumbar spine with and without neurological involvement. *Spine* 13:286, 1988.

144. Kostuik JP: Compression fractures and surgery in the osteoporotic patient. In Frymoyer JW (ed): *The Adult Spine: Principles and Practice*, vol 1. Philadelphia, Lippincott-Raven, 1991, 661.

145. Kostuik JP, Errico TJ, Gleason TF: Techniques of internal fixation for degenerative conditions of the spine. *Clin Orthop* 203:219, 1986.

146. Kostuik JP, Huler RJ, Esses SI, Stauffer ES: Thoracolumbar spine fracture. In Frymoyer JW (ed): *The Adult Spine: Principles and Practice*, vol 2. Philadelphia, Lippincott-Raven, 1991, p 1269.

147. Krag MH: Biomechanics of transpedicle spinal fixation. In Weinstein JN, Wiesel SW (eds): *The Lumbar Spine*. Philadelphia, WB Saunders, 1990, p 916.

148. Krag MH: Biomechanics of thoracolumbar spinal fixation. *Spine* 16:84, 1991.

149. Krag MH, Beynnon BD, Pope MH, *et al*: An internal fixator for posterior application to short segments for the thoracic, lumbar, or lumbosacral spine: design and testing. *Clin Orthop* 203:75, 1986.

150. Krag MH, Van Val ME, Beynnon BD: Placement of transpedicular vertebral screws close to anterior vertebral cortex: description of methods. *Spine* 14:879, 1989.

151. Krag MH, Weaver DL, Beynnon BD, Haugh LD: Morphometry of the thoracic and lumbar spine related to transpedicular screw placement for surgical spinal fixation. *Spine* 13:27, 1988.

152. Krane SM: Etidronate disodium in the treatment of Paget's disease of the bone. *Ann Intern Med* 96:619, 1982.

153. Krane SM: Paget's disease of bone. In Wilson JD (ed): *Harrison's Principles of Internal Medicine*, ed 12, vol 2. New York, McGraw-Hill, 1991, p 1938.

154. Krane SM, Holick MF: Metabolic bone disease. In Wilson JD (ed): *Harrison's Principles of Internal Medicine*, ed 12, vol 2. New York, McGraw-Hill, 1991, p 1921.

155. Krane SM, Simon LS: Metabolic consequences of bone turnover in Paget's disease of bone. *Clin Orthop* 217:26, 1987.

156. Kurz LT, Garfin SR, Booth RE: Harvesting autogenous iliac bone grafts: a review of complications and techniques. *Spine* 14:1324, 1989.

157. Kurz LT, Samberg LC, Herkowitz HN: Iliac bone grafting: techniques of harvesting and complications. In Garfin SR (ed): *Complications of Spine Surgery*. Baltimore, Williams & Wilkins, 1989, p 323.

158. Lane JM, Muschler GF: Spinal fusion: principles of bone fusion. In Rothman RH, Simeone FA (eds): *The Spine*, ed 3, vol 2. Philadelphia, WB Saunders, 1992, p 1739.

159. Laskey MA, Crisp AJ, Cole TJ, Compston JE. Comparison of the effect of different reference data on Lunar DPX and Hologic QDR 1000 dual-energy X-ray absorptiometers. *Br J Radiol* 65:1124-1129, 1992.

160. Lee CK: Accelerated degeneration of the segment adjacent to a lumbar fusion. *Spine* 13:375, 1988.

161. Lentle BC, Russell AS, Heslip PG, Percy JS: The scintigraphic findings in Paget's disease of bone. *Clin Radiol* 27:129, 1976.

162. Lieberman IH, Dudeney S, Reinhardt MK, Bell G: Initial outcome and efficacy of "Kyphoplasty" in the treatment of painful osteoporotic vertebral compression fractures. *Spine* 26:1631-1638, 2001.

163. Lindsay R, Hart DM, Aitken JM, *et al*: Long-term prevention of postmenopausal osteoporosis by oestrogen: evidence for an increased bone mass after delayed onset of oestrogen treatment. *Lancet* 1: 1038-1041, 1976.

164. Lindsay R, Scheele WH, Clancy AD. Incident vertebral fractures during an 18 month observational period following discontinuation of LY 333334 (recombinant human parathyroid hormone (1-34) rh PTH (1-34) use in postmenopausal women with osteoporosis (abstract). *J Bone Miner Res* 16 (suppl 1) S175, 2001.

165. Lips P, Graafmans WC, Ooms ME, et al: Vitamin D supplementation and fracture incidence in elderly persons: a randomized placebo-controlled trial. *Ann Intern Med* 124:400-406, 1996.

166. Lipscomb HJ, Grubb SA, Talmage RV: Spinal bone density following spinal fusion. *Spine* 14:477, 1989.

167. Louis R: Fusion of the lumbar and sacral spine by internal fixation with screw plates. *Clin Orthop* 201:18, 1986.

168. Lufkin EG, Argueta R, Whitaker MD, et al: Pamidronate: a unrecognized problem in gastrointestinal tolerability. *Osteoporos Int* 4:320-322, 1994.

169. Lufkin EG, Ory SJ: Estrogen replacement therapy for the prevention of osteoporosis. *Am Fam Physician* 40:205, 1989.

170. Luque ER, Cardoso A: A treatment of scoliosis without arthrodesis or external support: preliminary report. *Orthop Trans* 1:37, 1977.

171. Luque ER, Rapp GF: A new semi-rigid method for interpedicular fixation of the spine. *Orthopedics* 11:1445, 1988.

172. MacEwen, Bunnell WP, Sriram K: Acute neurological complications in the treatment of scoliosis: a report of the Scoliosis Research Society. *J Bone Joint Surg* 57A:404, 1975.

173. MacNab I, Dall D: The blood supply of the lumbar spine and its application to the technique of intertransverse lumbar spinal fusion. *J Bone Joint Surg* 53B:628, 1971.

174. Madsen PW, Lee TT, Eismont FJ, Green BA: Diagnosis and management of thoracic spine fractures. In Youmans JR (ed): *Neurological Surgery*, ed 4, vol 4. Philadelphia, WB Saunders, 1995, p 2043.

175. Malluche HH, Faugere MC: Bone biopsies: Histology and histomorphometry of bone. In Avioli LV, Krane SM (eds): *Metabolic Bone Disease and Clinically Related Disorders*. Philadelphia, WB Saunders, 1990, p 283.

176. Marchesi DG, Thalgott JS, Aebi M: Application and results of the AO internal fixation system in nontraumatic indications. *Spine* 16(suppl):S162, 1991.

177. Maricic M, Adachi JD, Sarkar S, et al: Early effects of raloxifene on clinical vertebral fractures at 12 months in postmenopausal women with osteoporosis. *Arch Intern Med* 162:1140-1143, 2002.

178. Marshall D, Johnell O, Wedel H: Meta-analysis of how well measures of bone mineral density predict occurrence of osteoporotic fractures. *BMJ* 312:1254-1259, 1996.

179. Martin AD, Houston CS: Osteoporosis, calcium and physical activity. *Can Med Assoc J* 136:587, 1987.

180. Maruo S, Tatekawa F, Nakano K: Paraplegia caused by vertebral compressive fracture in senile osteoporosis. *Orthopedics* 125:320, 1987.

181. Maurice PF, Lynch TN, Bastomy CH, et al: Metabolic evidence of suppression of Paget's disease of bone by aspirin. *Trans Assoc Am Physicians* 75:20-28, 1962.

182. Mazanec DJ, Mompoint A, Podichetty VK, Potnis A: Vertebral compression fractures: manage aggressively to prevent sequelae. *Cleve Clin J Med* 70: 147-156, 2003.

183. Mazzuoli GF, Passeri M, Gennari C, et al: Effects of salmon calcitonin in postmenopausal osteoporosis: a controlled double-blind clinical study. *Calcif Tissue Int* 38:3, 1986.

184. McAfee PC, Bohlman HH, Yuan HA: Anterior decompression of traumatic thoracolumbar fractures with incomplete neurological deficit using a retroperitoneal approach. *J Bone Joint Surg* 67A:89, 1985.

185. McAfee PC, Ruland CM, Warden KE, et al: Triangulation of pedicular instrumentation: a biomechanical analysis. Presented at the Annual Meeting of the Scoliosis Research Society, Dallas, Texas, September, 1990.

186. McAfee PC, Sutterlin C, Gurr K, et al: Device-related osteoporosis with spinal instrumentation. *Spine* 14:919, 1989.

187. McLain RF, Fry MF, Mosley TA, Sharkey NA: Lumbar pedicle screw salvage: pullout testing of three different pedicle screw designs. *J Spinal Disord* 8:62, 1995.

188. McLain RF, Sparling E, Bensen DR: Early failure of short-segment pedicle instrumentation for thoracolumbar fractures. *J Bone Joint Surg* 75A:162, 1993.

189. Melick RA, Ebeling P, Hjorth RJ: Improvement in paraplegia in vertebral Paget's disease treated with calcitonin. *BMJ* 1:627-628, 1976.

190. Melick RA, Martin TJ: Paget's disease in identical twins. *Aust NZ J Med* 5:564, 1975.

191. Melton LJ, Atkinson EJ, O'Fallon WM, et al: Long-term fracture prediction by bone mineral assessed at different sites. *J Bone Miner Res* 10:1227-1233, 1993.

192. Melton LJ, Kan SH, Frye MA, et al: Epidemiology of vertebral fractures in women. *Am J Epidemiol* 192:1000, 1989.

193. Melton LJ, Riggs BL: Impaired bone strength and fracture patterns at different skeletal sites. In Unthoff HK, Stahl E (eds): *Current Concepts of Bone Fragility*. Berlin, Springer-Verlag, 1986, p 149.

194. Melton LJ, Riggs BL: Risk factors for injury after a fall. *Clin Geriatr Med* 1:525, 1985.

195. Miller PD, Baram DT, Bilezkian JP, et al: Practical clinical application of biochemical markers of bone turnover (consensus of an expert panel). *J Clin Densitom* 2:323-342, 1999.

196. Mills BG, Frautso A, Singer FR, et al: Multinucleated cells formed in vitro from Paget's bone marrow express viral antigens. *Bone* 15:443-448, 1994.

197. Mills BG, Singer SR: Nuclear inclusions in Paget's disease of bone. *Science* 194:201, 1976.

198. Mills BG, Singer SR, Weiner LP, et al: Evidence of both respiratory syncytial virus and measles virus antigens in the osteoclasts of patients with Paget's disease of bone. *Clin Orthop* 183:303, 1984.

199. Milne JS, Williamson J: A longitudinal study of kyphosis in older people. *Age Ageing* 12:225, 1983.

200. Montagu MFA: Paget's disease (osteitis deformans) and heredity. *Am J Human Genet* 1:94, 1949.

201. Munk-Jensen N, Pors Nielson S, Obel EB, Bonne Eriksen P: Reversal of postmenopausal vertebral bone loss by estrogen and progestogen: a double-blind placebo controlled study. *Br Med J (Clin Res)* 269:1150, 1988.

202. National Institutes of Health Consensus Development Panel. Osteoporosis prevention, diagnosis, and therapy. *JAMA* 285:785-795, 2001.

203. National Institutes of Health Consensus Development Conference: Prophylaxis and treatment of osteoporosis. *Am J Med* 90:107, 1991.

204. National Institutes of Health Consensus Development Conference: Statement on osteoporosis. *JAMA* 252:799, 1984.

205. Neer RM, Arnaud CD, Zanchetta JR, *et al*. Effect of parathyroid hormone (1-34) on fractures and bone mineral density in postmenopausal women with osteoporosis. *N Engl J Med* 344:1434-1441, 2001.

206. Nelson HD, Helfand M, Woolf SH, Allan JD. Screening for postmenopausal osteoporosis: a review of the evidence for the U.S. Preventive Services Task Force. *Ann Intern Med* 137:529-541, 2002.

207. Nerubay J, Marganit B, Bubis JJ, *et al*: Stimulation of bone formation by electrocurrent on spinal fusion. *Spine* 11:167, 1986.

208. Newman FW: Paget's disease. *J Bone Joint Surg* 28:798, 1946.

209. Newton-John HF, Morgan DB: The loss of bone with age, osteoporosis, and fractures. *Clin Orthop* 71:229, 1970.

210. Nguyen TV, Eisman JA, Kelly PJ, Sambrook PN. Risk factors for osteoporotic fractures in elderly men. *Am J Epidemiol* 144: 255-263, 1996.

211. Nieves JW, Golden AL, Siris E, *et al:* Teenage and current calcium intake are related to bone mineral density of the hip and forearm in women aged 30-39 years. *Am J Epidemiol* 141:342-351, 1995.

212. Nordin BEC, Horsman A, Crilly RG, *et al*: Treatment of spinal osteoporosis in postmenopausal women. *Br Med J* 280:451, 1980.

213. Obrant KJ, Beugner V, Johnel O, *et al*: Increasing age-adjusted risk of fragility fractures: a sign of increasing osteoporosis in successive generations. Editorial. *Calcif Tissue Int* 44:157, 1989.

214. O'Doherty DP, Bickerstaff DR, McCloskey EV, *et al*: Treatment of Paget's disease of bone with aminohydroxybutylidene bisphosphonate. *J Bone Miner Res* 5:483, 1980.

215. Okuyama K, Sato K, Abe E, *et al*: Stability of transpedicle screwing for the osteoporotic spine: an in vitro study of the mechanical stability. *Spine* 18:2240, 1993.

216. Orwoll ES. Osteoporosis in men. *Endocrinol Metab Clin North Am* 27:349-367, 1997.

217. Royal College of Physicians: *Osteoporosis: Clinical Guidelines for Prevention and Treatment*. London, Royal College of Physicians of London, 1999.

218. Osteoporosis: review of the evidence for prevention, diagnosis and treatment and cost-effectiveness analysis. National Osteoporosis Foundation. *Osteoporosis Int* 8 (suppl 4):S7-S80, 1998.

219. Overgaard K: Effect of intranasal salmon calcitonin therapy on bone mass and bone turnover in early postmenopausal women: a dose-response study. *Calcif Tissue Int* 55: 82-86, 1994.

220. Paget J: On a form of chronic inflammation of bones (osteitis deformans). *Med-Chir Trans* 60:37, 1877.

221. Panjabi MM: Biomechanical evaluation of spinal fixation devices. I. A conceptual framework. *Spine* 133: 1129, 1988.

222. Parfitt AM: Osteomalacia and related disorders. In Avioli LV, Krane SM (eds): *Metabolic Bone Disease and Clinically Related Disorders*. Philadelphia, WB Saunders, 1990, p 329.

223. Parfitt AM, Duncan H: Metabolic bone disease affecting the spine. In Rothman RH, Simeone FA (eds): *The Spine*. Philadelphia, WB Saunders, 1975, p 599.

224. Phillips FM: Minimally invasive treatments of osteoporotic vertebral compression fractures. *Spine* 28: S45-S53, 2003.

225. Pitt MJ: Rickets and osteomalacia. In Resnick D, Niwayama G (eds): *Diagnosis of Bone and Joint Disease*. Philadelphia, WB Saunders, 1981, p 1682.

226. Pintar AP, Maiman DJ, Yoganandan N, *et al*: Rotational stability of a spinal pedicle screw/rod system. *J Spinal Disord* 8:49, 1995.

227. Pontiroli AE, Pajetta E, Scaglia L, *et al*: Analgesic effect of intranasal and intramuscular salmon calcitonin in post-menopausal osteoporosis: a double-blind, double placebo study. *Aging Clin Exp Res* 6: 459-463, 1994.

228. Power ML, Heany RP, Kalkwarf HJ, *et al*: The role of calcium in health and disease. *Am J Obstet Gynecol* 181:1560-1569, 1999.

229. Prolo DJ, Rodrigo JJ: Contemporary bone graft physiology and surgery. *Clin Orthop* 200:322, 1985.

230. Purcell GA, Markolf KL, Dawson EG: Twelfth thoracic first lumbar vertebral mechanical stability of fractures after Harrington-rod instrumentation. *J Bone Joint Surg* 63A:71, 1981.

231. Pygott F: Paget's disease of bone: the radiological incidence. *Lancet* 1:1170, 1957.

232. Raisz LG. Physiology and pathophysiology of bone remodelling. *Clin Chem* 45:1353-1358, 1999.

233. Raney FL, Kolb FO: The effect of metabolic bone disease on spinal fusion. In White AH, Rothman RH, Ray CD (eds): *Lumbar Spine Surgery: Techniques and Complications*. St. Louis, CV Mosby, 1987.

234. Ray CD: Extensive lumbar decompression: Patient selection and result. In White AH, Rothman R, Ray CD (eds): *Lumbar Spine Surgery: Techniques and Complications*. St Louis, CV Mosby, 1987, p 165.

235. Ray NF, Chan JK, Thamer M, Melton LJ: Medical expenditures for the treatment of osteoporotic fractures in the United States in 1995: report from the National Osteoporosis Foundation. *J Bone Miner Res* 12:24-35, 1997.

236. Razak N, Madsen PW: Titanium TSRH instrumentation for thoracic and lumbar instability. Presented at American Association of Neurological Surgeons, Annual Meeting, Minneapolis, Minnesota, April 30, 1996.

237. Rebel A, Malkani D, Basel M, Bregeon C: Osteoclast ultrastructure in Paget's disease. *Calcif Tissue Res* 20:187, 1976.

238. Recker RR: Low bone mass may not be the only cause of skeletal fragility in osteoporosis. *Proc Soc Exp Biol Med* 191:272, 1989.

239. Reddy SV, Singer FR, Mallette L, Roodman GD: Detection of measles virus transcripts in peripheral blood mononuclear cells and marrow mononuclear cells from

patients with Paget's disease. Abstract. *J Bone Miner Res* 10(suppl):S154, 1995.

240. Reginster J, Minne HW, Sorensen OH, *et al*: Randomized trial of the effects of risedronate on vertebral fractures in women with established postmenopausal osteoporosis: Vertebral Efficacy with Risedronate Therapy (VERT) study group. *Osteoporosis Int* 11:83-91, 2000.

241. Reid IR, Ames RW, Evans MC, *et al*: Effect of calcium supplementation on bone loss in postmenopausal women. *N Engl J Med* 328:460-464, 1993.

242. Reid IR, Brown JP, Burckhardt P, *et al*: Intravenous zoledronic acid in postmenopausal women with low bone mineral density. *N Engl J Med* 346:653-661, 2002.

243. Resnick D, Niwayama G: Intervertebral disc herniation: cartilaginous Schmorl's nodes. *Radiology* 126:57, 1978.

244. Resnick D, Niwayama G: Osteoporosis. In Resnick D, Niwayama G (eds): *Diagnosis of Bone and Joint Disease*. Philadelphia, WB Saunders, 1981, 1638.

245. Resnick D, Niwayama G: Paget's disease. In Resnick D, Niwayama G (eds): *Diagnosis of Bone and Joint Disease*. Philadelphia, WB Saunders, 1981.

246. Riebel GD, Yoo JU, Frederickson BE, *et al*: Review of Harrington rod treatment of spinal trauma. *Spine* 18:479, 1993.

247. Riggs BL. Are biochemical markers for bone turnover clinically useful for monitoring therapy in individual osteoporotic patients? (editorial) *Bone* 6:551-552, 2000.

248. Riggs BL, Melton LJ: Involutional osteoporosis. *N Engl J Med* 314:1676, 1986.

249. Riggs BL, Melton LJ: *Osteoporosis: Etiology, Diagnosis and Management*. Philadelphia, Lippincott-Raven, 1988.

250. Riggs BL, Wahner HW, Melton LJ, *et al*: Rates of bone loss in appendicular and axial skeletons of women. *J Clin Invest* 77:1487, 1986.

251. Riis B, Thomsen K, Christiansen C. Does calcium supplementation prevent postmenopausal bone loss? A double-blind, controlled clinical study. *N Engl J Med* 316:173-177, 1987.

252. Roodman GD: Osteoclast function in Paget's disease and multiple myeloma. *Spine* 16(suppl):S91, 1991.

253. Ross PD: Prediction of fracture risk II. *Am J Med* 312:260-269, 1996.

254. Roy-Camille R: Tumeur du rachis. In: Troisièmes Journées de la Pitié. Paris, Masson, 1983, 151.

255. Roy-Camille R, Saillant F, Berteaux D, Salgado V: Osteosynthesis of the thoracolumbar spine fractures with metal plates screwed through the vertebral pedicles. *Reconstr Surg Traumatol* 15:2, 1976.

256. Roy-Camille R, Saillant G, Berteaux D, *et al*: Vertebral osteosynthesis using metal plates: its different uses. *Chirurg* 105:597, 1979.

257. Roy-Camille R, Saillant G, Coulson JP, Couchard P: Spondylolisthesis L4-L5 et L5-S1. In Roy-Camille R (ed): *Troisièmes Journées de la Pitié*. Paris, Masson, 1983, p 91.

258. Roy-Camille R, Saillant G, La Presle PH, *et al*: A secret in spinal surgery: the pedicle. Presented at the 51st meeting of the American Academy of Orthopedic Surgeons. Atlanta, February, 1984.

259. Roy-Camille R, Saillant G, Mazel C: Internal fixation of the lumbar spine with pedicle screw plating. *Clin Orthop* 203:7, 1986.

260. Roy-Camille R, Saillant G, Mazel C: Plating of thoracic thoracolumbar, and lumbar injuries with pedicle screw plates. *Orthop Clin North Am* 17:147, 1986.

261. Ruland CM, McAfee PC, Warden KE, Cunningham BW: Triangulation of pedicular instrumentation: a biomechanical analysis. *Spine* 16(suppl):S270, 1991.

262. Rydevik B, Lundborg G, Skalak R: Pathoanatomy and pathophysiology of nerve root compression. *Spine* 9:7, 1984.

263. Ryu KS, Park CK, Kim MC, Kang JK: Dose-dependent epidural leakage of polymethylmethacrylate after percutaneous vertebroplasty in patients with osteoporotic vertebral compression fractures. *J Neurosurg* 96(suppl1):56-61, 2002.

264. Saag KG, Emkey R, Schnitzer TJ, *et al*: Alendronate for the prevention and treatment of glucocorticoid-induced osteoporosis. Glucocorticoid-Induced Osteoporosis Intervention Study Group. *N Engl J Med* 339:292-299, 1998.

265. Sadar ES, Waldon RJ, Grossman HH: Neurological dysfunction in Paget's disease of the vertebral column. *J Neurosurg* 37:661, 1972.

266. Salomon C, Chopin D, Benoist M: Spinal cord compression: an exceptional complication of spinal osteoporosis. *Spine* 13:222, 1988.

267. Schlaich C, Minne HW, Bruckner T, *et al*: Reduced pulmonary function in patients with spinal osteoporotic fractures. *Osteoporosis Int* 8:261-267, 1998.

268. Schofferman J, Schofferman L, Zucherman J, *et al*: Metabolic bone disease in lumbar pseudoarthrosis. *Spine* 15:687, 1990.

269. Schott AM, Cormier C, Hans D, *et al*. How hip and whole-body bone mineral density predict hip fracture in elderly women: the EPIDOS prospective study. *Osteoporosis Int* 8:247-254, 1998.

270. Shikata J, Yamamuro T, Lida H, *et al*: Surgical treatment for paraplegia resulting from vertebral fractures in senile osteoporosis. *Spine* 15:485, 1990.

271. Simkin A, Ayalon J, Leichter I: Increased trabecular bone density due to bone-loading exercises on postmenopausal osteoporotic women. *Calcif Tiss Int* 40:59-63, 1987.

272. Simmons EH, Capicotto WN: Posterior transpedicular Zielke instrumentation of the lumbar spine. *Clin Orthop* 236:180, 1988.

273. Singer FR, Fredericks RS, Minkin C: Salmon calcitonin therapy for Paget's disease of bone: The problem of acquired clinical resistance. *Arthritis Rheum* 23: 1148-1154, 1980.

274. Singer FR, Krane SM: Paget's disease of bone. In Avioli LV, Krane SM (eds): *Metabolic Bone Disease and Clinically Related Disorders*. Philadelphia, WB Saunders, 1990, p 546.

275. Singer FR, Mills BG: The etiology of Paget's disease of bone. *Clin Orthop* 127:37, 1977.

276. Singer FR, Schiller AI, Pyle EB, Krane SM: Paget's disease of bone. In Avioli LV, Krane SM (eds): *Metabolic Bone Disease*. New York, Academic Press, 1977, p 558.

277. Siris RS: Extensive personal experience: Paget's disease of bone. *J Clin Endocrinol Metab* 80:335, 1995.

278. Siris ES, Miller PD, Barrett-Connor E, *et al*: Identification and fracture outcomes of undiagnosed low

bone mineral density in postmenopausal women: results from the national osteoporosis risk assessment. *JAMA* 286:2815-2822, 2001.

279. Siris RS, Ottman R, Flaster E, Kelsey JL: Familial aggregation of Paget's disease. *J Bone Miner Res* 6:495, 1991.

280. Siris RS, Weinstein R, Altman R, *et al*: Comparative study of alendronate versus etidronate for the treatment of Paget's disease of bone. *J Clin Endocrinol Metab* 81:961, 1996.

281. Solomon LR, Evans JM, Canty DP, Gill NW: Effects of calcitonin treatment on deafness due to Paget's disease of bone. *BMJ* 2:485-487, 1977.

282. Soshi S, Shiba R, Kondo H, Murota K: An experimental study on transpedicular screw fixation in relation to osteoporosis of the lumbar spine. *Spine* 16:1335, 1991.

283. Steffee AD, Sitkowski DJ: Posterior lumbar interbody fusion and plates. *Clin Orthop* 227:99, 1988.

284. Steffee AD, Biscup RS, Sitkowski DJ: Segmental spine plates with pedicle screw fixation: A new internal fixation device for disorders of the lumbar and thoracic spine. *Clin Orthop* 203:45, 1986.

285. Steffee AD, Sitkowski DJ: Reduction and stabilization of grade IV osteoporosis. *Clin Orthop* 227:82, 1988.

286. Steinmann JC, Herdowitz HN, El-Kommos H, Wesolowski P: Spinal pedicle fixation: Confirmation of an image-based technique for screw placement. *Spine* 18:1856, 1993.

287. Stephen AB, Wallace WA: The management of osteoporosis. *J Bone Joint Surg Br* 83-B:316-323, 2001.

288. Stevenson JC, Lees B, Devenport M, *et al*: Determinants of bone density in normal women: risk factors for future osteoporosis. *Br Med J (Clin Res)* 298:924, 1989.

289. Strempel AV, Kuhle J, Plitz W: Stabiltat von pedikelschrauben–Teil 2: Maximale Auszugskrafte unter Berucksichtigung der Knochendichte. *Z Orthop* 132:32, 1994.

290. Stulberg BN, Watson JT: Management of orthopaedic complication of metabolic bone disease. *Cleve Clin J Med* 56:696, 1989.

291. Thevenon A, Pollez B, Cantegrit F, *et al*: Relationship between kyphosis, scoliosis, and osteoporosis in the elderly population. *Spine* 12:744, 1987.

292. Thompson PW: Assessment of the skeleton. In Stevenson J (ed): *Osteoporosis*. Surrey, Reed Business Publishing Group, 1991, p 29.

293. U.S. Preventive Services Task Force: Screening for osteoporosis in postmenopausal women: recommendations and rationale. *Ann Intern Med* 137:526-528, 2002.

294. Vahle JL, Sato M, Long GG, *et al*: Skeletal changes in rats given daily subcutaneous injections of recombinant human parathyroid hormone (1-34) for 2 years and relevance to human data. *Toxicol Pathol* 30:312-321, 2002.

295. Wasnich RD, Davis JW, Ross PD: Spine fracture risk is predicted by non-spinal fractures. *Osteoporos Int* 41-5, 1994.

296. Weiss NS, Ure CL, Ballard JH, *et al*: Decreased risk of fracture of the hip and lower forearm with postmenopausal use of estrogen. *N Engl J Med* 303:1195-1198, 1980.

297. Whitecloud TS, Butler JC, Cohen JL, Candelora PD: Complications with the variable spinal plating system. *Spine* 14:472, 1989.

298. Whitecloud TS, Skalley TC, Cook SD, Morgan EL: Roentgenographic measurement of screw penetration. *Clin Orthop* 245:57, 1989.

299. Wilber RG, Thompson GH, Shaffer JW, *et al*: Postoperative neurologic deficits in spinal instrumentation: a study using spinal cord monitoring. *J Bone Joint Surg* 66A:1178, 1984.

300. Wiltse LL: History of pedicle screw fixation of the spine. *Spine: State of the Art Reviews* 6:1, 1992.

301. Winter RB, Lonstein JE, Vandenbrink, *et al*: Harrington rod with sublaminar wires in the treatment of adolescent idiopathic thoracic scoliosis: a study of sagittal plane correction. *Orthop Trans* 11:89, 1987.

302. Wisneki RJ, Rothman RH: Posterior intertransverse fusions: indications, pathomechanics, and results. In White AH, Rothman RH, Ray CD (eds): *Lumbar Spine Surgery: Techniques and Complications*. St Louis, CV Mosby, 1987.

303. Wittenberg RH, Lee K, Shea M, *et al*: Effect of screw diameter insertion technique and bone cement augmentation on pedicular screw fixation strength. *Clin Orthop* 296:278, 1993.

304. Woodard HQ: Longterm studies of the blood chemistries in Paget's disease of bone. *Cancer* 12:1226, 1959.

305. Wolfe SA, Kawamoto HK: Taking the iliac bone graft: a new technique. *J Bone Joint Surg* 58A:70, 1978.

306. Writing Group for the Women's Health Initiative Investigators. Risks and benefits of estrogen plus progestin in healthy postmenopausal women: principal results from the Women's Health Initiative randomized controlled trial. *JAMA* 288:321-333, 2002.

307. Wycis HT: Basilar impression (platybasia): a case secondary to advanced Paget's disease with severe neurological manifestations, successful surgical result. *J Neurosurg* 1:299, 1994.

308. Yamagata M, Kitahara H, Minami S, *et al*: Mechanical stability of the pedicle screw fixation systems for the lumbar spine. *Spine* 17:51, 1992.

309. Young RL, Goldzieher JW: Current status of postmenopausal estrogen therapy. *Drugs* 33:95, 1987.

310. Zdeblick TA: A prospective, randomized study of lumbar fusion: preliminary results. *Spine* 18:983, 1993.

311. Zindrick MR, Knight BW, Patwardhan, *et al*: The effect of polymethylmethacrylate augmentation upon pedicle screw fixation in the spine. Presented at the meeting of the International Society for the Study of the Lumbar Spine, Dallas, Texas, June 5, 1986.

312. Zindrick MR, Wiltse LL, Widell EH, *et al*: A biomechanical study of intrapeduncular screw fixation in the lumbar spine. *Clin Orthop* 203:99, 1986.

313. Zoarski GH, Snow P, Olan WJ, *et al*: Percutaneous vertebroplasty for osteoporotic compression fractures: Quantitative prospective evaluation of long-term outcome. *J Vasc Interv Radiol* 13:1390-1480, 2002.

314. Zuckerman J, Hsu K, White A, Wynne G: Early results of spinal fusion using variable spine plating systems. *Spine* 13:570, 1988.

CHAPTER 78

Foramen Magnum Lesions

Jean-Valéry C.E. Coumans, Cary D. Alberstone, and Russ P. Nockels

Tumors in the region of the foramen magnum have long challenged surgeons who confront not only the difficulties of diagnosis but also the technical obstacles of a hazardous tumor resection. In the past, determined efforts often ended in respiratory failure and death. In the 1954 series of Love et al.,[45] for example, 34 of 74 patients died postoperatively, most often as a result of respiratory failure. However, with the advent of magnetic resonance imaging (MRI) and microsurgical technique, surgical outcome has greatly improved as reflected by the results of larger, more recent series.[27,28,49,77]

A wide array of tumors, both malignant and benign, arise in the region of the foramen magnum. Collectively they comprise about 5% of all spinal tumors and 1% of intracranial tumors.[75] It is useful to divide all foramen magnum tumors into intra-axial, intradural extramedullary, and extradural masses. Each location is associated with a specific group of tumors and special topographic relationships that present unique surgical considerations.

More than 90% of foramen magnum tumors are intradural extramedullary tumors and most commonly occur ventrolaterally in relation to the spinal cord. The majority of these tumors are meningiomas and neurofibromas, the former being twice as common as the latter.[75] Intra-axial tumors, such as brain stem gliomas, and extradural tumors, such as chordomas, comprise less than 10% of foramen magnum tumors.[27]

The results of surgical management of these tumors have greatly improved over the years, because with the advent of advanced microsurgical techniques and a detailed knowledge of foramen magnum anatomy, these lesions are now amenable to safe surgical resection. Given the variable pathologic anatomy in the region of the foramen magnum and the availability of a variety of surgical options with varying advantages and disadvantages, the surgeon must carefully choose an appropriate surgical approach. The rational basis for this selection is outlined below, with emphasis on the problems presented by intradural extramedullary lesions.

This chapter reviews the clinical features, microsurgical anatomy, and three surgical approaches to tumors in the region of the foramen magnum. It is emphasized that early diagnosis, a thorough knowledge of microsurgical anatomy, and selection of the appropriate surgical approach all contribute to an optimal patient outcome.

History

A foramen magnum tumor was first described by Hallopeau in 1874[31] in a case report of a 50-year-old woman who presented with spastic upper extremity weakness that progressed to quadriparesis with brain stem signs. The patient eventually died of respiratory failure. Autopsy revealed a foramen magnum tumor, "the size of a small chestnut," that caused compression of the lateral funiculi of the spinal cord bilaterally.

Although early attempts at surgical removal of foramen magnum tumors were met with disastrous consequences,[1,25] Elsberg and Strauss[24] successfully removed a foramen magnum meningioma from a woman, aged 36 years, who presented with Brown-Séquard syndrome. Despite several intraoperative episodes of respiratory failure, the patient enjoyed full neurologic recovery postoperatively. The report of this case in 1929 was accompanied by the first systematic evaluation of foramen magnum tumors.

In their classic 1938 treatise, Cushing and Eisenhardt[18] divided foramen magnum tumors into craniospinal and spinocranial tumors on the basis of their predominant anatomic location and associated clinical symptomatology. Since this account by Cushing and Eisenhardt, several series of patients with foramen magnum tumors have been reported in the literature.*

In an effort to approach both ventral and ventrolateral lesions more safely than is possible dorsally, two other surgical approaches are now available to the surgeon. The transoral approach was originally described by Kanavel in 1919[36] in a report on the transoral removal of a bullet that was lodged between the atlas and the base of the skull. Although the technique has been described most commonly as an approach to extradural lesions,[5,17,21,29] intradural lesions have also been treated.[15,16,50,51] Like the transoral approach, the far lateral approach was originally described to manage vertebral and vertebrobasilar artery lesions rather than foramen magnum tumors,[33] but this approach has since been modified and adopted to deal with tumors in the region of the foramen magnum.[64,69]

Pathology and Epidemiology

Major features of the largest series of foramen magnum tumors are presented in Table 78.1. As mentioned earlier, tumors in the region of the foramen magnum are best categorized into intra-axial, intradural extramedullary, and extradural tumors.

Intra-axial tumors are predominantly brain stem gliomas but also include gangliogliomas, anaplastic astrocytomas, ependymomas, and cavernous hemangiomas. Caudal extension of medulloblastomas and hemangioblastomas into the foramen magnum occurs in children and adults, respectively.[55] Intradural extramedullary tumors consist mainly of meningiomas and nerve sheath tumors and a much smaller number of epidermoid tumors and paragangliogliomas.[26,55]

*References 13,22,27,28,45,49,65,70,72,77.

TABLE 78.1

Series of Extramedullary Foramen Magnum Tumors

Reference	Time Span	No. of Patients	Tumor Location	Tumor Type	Age Range	Mean Duration: Symptom Onset to Diagnosis
Symonds and Meadows[72] (1937)	? yr	5	2 VL, 1 V, 1 L, 1 DL	4 meningiomas, 1 neurofibroma	38-57 yr	3.5 yr
Smolik and Sachs[65] (1956)	4 yr	6	2 L, 1 DL, 1 VL	6 meningiomas	33-56 yr	2.5 yr
Stein et al.[70] (1963)	? yr	25	21 VL, 3 D, 1 L, 1 V	25 meningiomas	27-88 yr	<5 yr
Guidetti and Spallone[28] (1980)	26 yr	18	12 VL, 3 DL, 3 V	11 meningiomas, 7 neurofibromas	13-65 yr	3.5 yr
Meyer et al.[49] (1982)	58 yr	102	61 V, 21 D, 20 L	78 meningiomas, 23 neurofibromas, 1 teratoma	12-81 yr	2.25 yr
George et al.[27] (1993) 32 osseous	10 yr	230	56% L, 31% V, 13% D	106 meningiomas, 49 neurofibromas, 28 chordomas, tumors,[°] 15 others[†]	47 yr (mean)	2.25 yr
Total	24.5 yr	386	38% V, 14% VL, 31% L, 14.5% D, 2% DL	NA	25.69 yr	3.2 yr

D, Dorsal; *DL,* dorsolateral; *L,* lateral; *NA,* not applicable; *V,* ventral; *VL,* ventrolateral.
°Nineteen primary and 13 metastatic osseous tumors.
†Includes 4 melanomas, 3 hemangioblastomas, 3 dermoid or epidermoid cysts, 2 ependymomas, 1 cavernoma, 1 angiomyolipoma, and 1 cholesterin cyst.

Extradural neoplasms are primarily osteocartilaginous tumors, of which chordoma is, by far, the most common. Chondromas and chondrosarcomas may also arise in this region.[55] Occasionally, meningiomas extend extradurally. This type of meningioma is associated with more aggressive pathologic features and clinical course.

This distribution of tumors is reflected in the series of George et al.[27] They reviewed 230 cases of extramedullary intradural and extradural tumors of the foramen magnum (intra-axial tumors were excluded). Among these tumors, 177 were intradural, 55 were extradural, and 42 tumors were both intradural and extradural. The intradural tumors that comprised almost 80% of the cases reviewed included meningiomas (60%) and neurofibromas (30%). Fifty percent of extradural tumors were chordomas. The most frequently occurring tumors (in order of decreasing frequency) were meningioma (106 cases), neurofibroma (49 cases), and chordoma (28 cases).

The topography of foramen magnum tumors is of special interest to surgeons. George et al.[27] defined ventral tumors as those that are attached to the foramen magnum (dura, spinal root, or spinal cord) on both sides of the midline, lateral tumors as those between the midline and the dentate ligament, and dorsal tumors as those behind the dentate ligament. Using these strict criteria, George et al.[26,27] found that among the 106 meningiomas in their series, 56% occurred laterally, 31% ventrally, and

13% dorsally. Other authors have reported a similar distribution.[22,28,49,70,77]

The relative rarity of foramen magnum tumors belies their clinical importance. Compared with other central nervous system neoplasms, foramen magnum tumors occur infrequently: they account for only 5% of all spinal neoplasms and 1% of all intracranial neoplasms. Considering meningiomas alone, those occurring in the region of the foramen magnum account for only 1.2% to 3.2% of meningiomas.[22,70,77]

Among the large series, the age range of patients with foramen magnum tumors was 2 to 81 years, but the majority of these tumors occur around the fifth decade.° The average time between onset of symptoms and diagnosis was 2.5 years. The mean age was 47 years, with a female-to-male ratio of 1.5:1.[27] These figures are consistent among authors.[28,49,70,77] Female predominance of meningiomas in general is also a consistent finding.

Besides neoplasms, other entities can present as foramen magnum lesions. Calcium pyrophosphate deposition in the transverse ligament can form a tumor-like mass that compresses the cervicomedullary junction.[6] This condition is common in the elderly and rarely becomes symptomatic. It can be diagnosed by CT scan, which demonstrates calcification around the odontoid. Tuberculosis can also affect the cervicomedullary junction in isolation.[39] Although uncommon, this condition is likely to increase with the recent resurgence of tuberculosis associated with HIV. A recent series of 29 cases of craniocervical tuberculosis describes frequent destruction of the condyles, clivus,

°References 22,28,44,45,49,65,70,72,77.

and of the dens and anterior arch of the atlas. The majority of patients harbored space-occupying soft tissue masses in the epidural and paravertebral spaces, large enough to cause myelopathy in 12 out of 29 cases. Cervicomedullary compression can also occur in craniometaphyseal dysplasia,[19] a sclerosing bone disorder characterized by bony encroachment of neural foramina.

Clinical Presentation

Many authors have noted that there are no signs or symptoms that are pathognomonic for foramen magnum tumors.[22,35] As early as 1937, Symonds and Meadows observed that "the clinical picture which results from compression of the spinal cord at, or near, the level of the foramen magnum is not always easy of recognition."[72] Indeed, the clinical presentation of foramen magnum tumors is usually variable and includes such ubiquitous symptoms as neck pain and limb dysesthesias, which are also associated with several more common diseases. The rarity of foramen magnum tumors may therefore cause them to be overlooked by clinicians.[57] Even a series as recent as that of George et al.,[27] which reviews 230 cases of foramen magnum tumors from 1985 to 1995, reports a misdiagnosis rate as high as 13.5%.

The most common presenting symptoms of foramen magnum tumors, in order of decreasing frequency, are suboccipital or neck pain, dysesthesias of the extremities more frequent in the upper than in the lower extremities, gait disturbance, and weakness more frequent in the upper extremities than in the lower. Other common early symptoms include clumsiness of the hands, bladder disturbance, dysphagia, nausea and vomiting, headache, "drop attacks," and dizziness.[22,28,49,70]

Suboccipital or upper cervical pain, probably caused by irritation of the C2 nerve root, is the most common presenting complaint and may precede other symptoms by months or years. C2 distribution sensory loss frequently accompanies the pain, and together, these symptoms should suggest the diagnosis of foramen magnum tumor. In the series of Stein et al.,[70] Meyer et al.,[49] and Guidetti and Spallone,[28] suboccipital or upper cervical neck pain was the initial complaint in 65% to 80% of patients. By the time of admission, 100% of Guidetti and Spallone's patients complained of neck pain.

Limb dysesthesias are frequently present and may occur in the form of a burning[28,77] or cold[7,24] sensation; proprioceptive loss is also common.[62] Weakness typically accompanies the sensory changes and tends to involve the upper extremities more than the lower extremities, and the ipsilateral side more than the contralateral side.[22] An unusual feature of the weakness is its occasional association with wasting of the intrinsic hand muscles.[38,53] Taylor and Byrnes[74] have cogently argued, on the basis of their own experimental evidence, that foramen magnum lesions produce hand wasting by causing venous obstruction in the upper cervical cord, which leads to venous infarction in the lower cervical gray matter.

The initial neurologic examination of the patient with a foramen magnum tumor most commonly reveals weakness, sensory loss, hyperreflexia, Babinski sign, and spastic gait. Typically, the weakness first affects the ipsilateral arm and then evolves over time into a progressive spastic quadriparesis. Sensory loss may involve the modalities of pain and temperature, proprioception, or both. The burning and cold dysesthesias have been mentioned. Other less common, but still frequent, signs include nystagmus (classically, downbeat), accessory nerve palsy, and atrophy of the intrinsic muscles of the hand. Infrequent signs include atrophy of the arms and legs, papilledema, Horner's syndrome, and cranial neuropathies involving cranial nerves V, VII to X, and XII.[62]

As mentioned above, the nonspecific signs and symptoms produced by foramen magnum tumors must be distinguished from several more common conditions. Although modern neuroimaging has lessened this problem, the neurosurgical literature is replete with examples of patients with tumors in the region of the foramen magnum that were misdiagnosed on initial presentation. Even the most recent series of foramen magnum tumors found a 13.5% incidence of misdiagnosis.[27] The failure to establish the correct diagnosis most commonly occurs because a foramen magnum tumor has not been included in the differential diagnosis.[10] The clinical entities most commonly confused with foramen magnum tumors include cervical spondylosis, multiple sclerosis, syringomyelia, intramedullary tumors, carpal tunnel syndrome, normal pressure hydrocephalus, Chiari malformation, and amyotrophic lateral sclerosis.

Cervical spondylosis presents with upper extremity paresthesias and weakness in association with gait and bladder disturbance. Unlike foramen magnum tumors, however, cervical spondylosis infrequently produces pain in the C2 distribution and is not associated with cranial neuropathies.

Multiple sclerosis and syringomyelia may also mimic foramen magnum tumors with chronic symptoms of motor-sensory changes, and gait and bladder disturbances. However, the course of multiple sclerosis is typically marked by exacerbations and remissions, and its symptoms do not usually include neck pain. Furthermore, syringomyelia is not associated with neck pain or cranial nerve deficits.

Intramedullary tumors, although otherwise similar to foramen magnum tumors in their clinical presentation, usually do not produce pain in the C2 distributions.

Carpal tunnel syndrome shares extremity dysesthesia and weakness with foramen magnum tumors but is otherwise clinically distinguishable.

Normal pressure hydrocephalus may cause gait and bladder disturbance also seen with foramen magnum tumors. Neck pain, sensory changes, and cranial nerve involvement, however, are all absent.

Finally, Chiari malformations may present with symptoms that are clinically indistinguishable from foramen magnum tumors, requiring imaging examination to make the diagnosis.

Although foramen magnum tumors share multiple signs and symptoms in common with other more frequently occurring diseases, the presence of hypalgesia in the C2 region and 11th cranial nerve palsy are two of the most reliable, clinically helpful signs.

Surgical Anatomy

A thorough knowledge of foramen magnum anatomy is critical to safe surgical exposure in this region. For a more detailed review of the microsurgical anatomy, the reader is referred to the elegant anatomical studies of Oliveira et al.,[52] Rhoton et al.,[58] and Wen et al.[76]

Osseous Structures

The foramen magnum is formed by the occipital bone, which consists of three parts: basilar, lateral, and squamosal. The basilar part is formed by a fusion between the occipital bone and the clivus. The lateral parts consist of the occipital condyles, which articulate with the atlas. Behind and above the foramen is the occipital squama whose internal surface is marked by a prominent midline ridge, the internal occipital crest, which serves as the attachment for the falx cerebelli. The anterior margin of the foramen magnum is termed the basion and the opposite margin, the opisthion. The shape of the foramen magnum is variable. It is generally oval in shape, and the wider portion is located dorsally.[52] It measures on average 35 mm in length and 29 mm in width. The foramen magnum transmits the medulla oblongata, the meninges, the ascending portion of the spinal accessory nerve, and the vertebral, anterior, and posterior spinal arteries.

The occipital condyles are located lateral to the ventral half of the foramen magnum. The occipital condyles are oval and their inferior surface is convex. They are oriented in a posterolateral to anteromedial direction. They articulate with the superior facet of the atlas, which overlies its lateral mass. The anatomy of the occipital condyles, as it pertains to the transcondylar approach, has been reviewed.[23]

The hypoglossal canal is located within the occipital bone, ventral to the junction between the anterior and middle third of the occipital condyles.[76] The hypoglossal nerve is the only structure that travels through the hypoglossal canal. The jugular foramen is located lateral to the ventral half of the occipital condyles, at the junction of the petrous part of the temporal bone and the occipital bone. It is irregular in shape and has a smaller anterior part and a larger dorsal division. The anterior part transmits the inferior petrosal sinus and the glossopharyngeal nerve. The posterior part transmits the vagus and spinal accessory nerves, the internal jugular vein, the meningeal branches of the ascending pharyngeal and occipital arteries.[52]

Muscles

The muscles of the foramen magnum region can be divided into superficial and deep layers. The muscles of the superficial layer consist of the trapezius, the sternocleidomastoid, the splenius capitis, and the longissimus capitis muscles. The trapezius arises from the medial third of the superior nuchal line and extends medially to the ligamentum nuchae and laterally to the spine of the scapula and the lateral third of the clavicle. The sternocleidomastoid attaches to the lateral half of the superior nuchal line and the adjacent portion of the mastoid process, and to the sternum and medial clavicle. The splenius capitis attaches to the lateral part of the superior nuchal line and to the spinous processes of C7 to T4. Lateral to this muscle lays the longissimus capitis muscle. This muscle arises from the articular processes of the last four cervical vertebrae and the transverse processes of the first five thoracic vertebrae. It inserts in the posterior part of the mastoid process.

Deep to the splenius capitis is the semispinalis capitis muscle. This muscle arises from the tip of the transverse processes of the first six thoracic vertebra and inserts between the superior and inferior nuchal lines. The deepest layer is comprised of a group of four small suboccipital muscles: the rectus capitis posterior major and minor, and the obliquus capitis inferior and superior. The rectus capitis posterior major is attached to the spinous process of C2 and inserts into the lateral part of the inferior nuchal line. The rectus capitis posterior minor arises from the tubercle of C1 and insets into the medial part of the inferior nuchal line. The superior obliquus capitis extends from the transverse process of C2 to the occipital bone, between the superior and inferior nuchal lines, laterally. The inferior obliquus capitis extends from the spinous process of C2 to the transverse process of C1.

Neural Structures

Neural structures in the region of the foramen magnum include the caudal medulla, caudal vermis, cerebellar tonsils, fourth ventricle, rostral spinal cord, lower cranial nerves, and upper cervical nerves.

The medulla blends into the spinal cord just rostral to the emergence of the dorsal and ventral rootlets that form the first cervical nerve. It is the medulla, therefore, and not the spinal cord that occupies the foramen magnum.

The dentate ligaments attach medially to the pia mater of the spinal cord and laterally to the dura mater, midway between the dorsal and ventral roots. Whereas its medial attachment is continuous, laterally the dentate ligament forms triangular processes that attach to the dura mater at intervals. Division of the upper two triangular processes may facilitate exposure of ventral tumors.

Cranial Nerves

Any of the lower four cranial nerves may be affected by lesions arising in the foramen magnum. The hypoglossal nerve is formed by a series of rootlets that arise in the ventrolateral sulcus between the pyramid and the olive, along a line that is continuous with the ventral spinal roots. The hypoglossal rootlets course ventrolaterally through the subarachnoid space on their way to the hypoglossal canal, passing dorsally in relation to the vertebral artery. If the course of the vertebral artery is short and straight, there may be no contact between the artery and the hypoglossal nerve. A tortuous vertebral artery, on the other hand, may displace the nerve dorsally and medially against the medulla, stretching and damaging its fibers.[71] Infrequently, the artery passes through the rootlets of the nerve.[52]

The glossopharyngeal, vagus, and cranial portions of the accessory nerves all arise in series along the dorsolateral sulcus, between the olive and the tuber cinereum. They exit the skull together through the jugular foramen. The cranial part of the accessory nerve is joined by a spinal part that arises as a series of rootlets between the ventral and dorsal rootlets and ascends through the foramen magnum between the dentate ligament and the dorsal roots. The hypoglossal nerve, and less commonly, the glossopharyngeal, vagus, and accessory nerves may be displaced dorsomedially by a thickened and atheromatous vertebral artery.[71]

Spinal Nerve Roots

The C1 nerve root often lacks a dorsal rootlet. The accessory nerve frequently contributes a root to the C1 nerve root when the C1 dorsal root, as is commonly the case, is absent. Before exiting the dura mater, the C1 ventral root and the dorsal root, if present, attach to the dorsal caudal surface of the intradural segment of the vertebral artery. The ventral and dorsal roots then exit the dura around the vertebral artery and unite within or just beyond the dural exit.

Vascular Structures

The arteries in the region of the foramen magnum include the vertebral and posterior inferior cerebellar arteries, the anterior and posterior spinal arteries, and the meningeal branches of the vertebral and carotid arteries.

In most individuals, the left vertebral artery is dominant. After ascending through the C1 foramina, the vertebral arteries continue medially with the C1 nerve root along a groove on the rostral surface of the dorsal arch of the atlas, behind the lateral mass. Frequently, this groove forms a complete bony canal that surrounds the vertebral artery.[52] Between C6 and C2, the vertebral arteries are thus protected dorsally by the lateral masses. However, as the arteries course dorsal to the C1 lateral mass and enter the region of the foramen magnum, they lose their dorsal bony protection.

From the rostral surface of the dorsal arch of the atlas, the arteries enter the vertebral canal by passing ventral to the lateral border of the atlanto-occipital membrane. This segment of the vertebral artery is partially covered by the atlanto-occipital membrane, the rectus capitis posterior major, and the superior and inferior oblique muscles, and, importantly, is also surrounded by a venous plexus.

Before entering the dura mater, the vertebral artery gives rise to the posterior meningeal and posterior spinal arteries, branches to the deep cervical musculature, and, infrequently, the posterior inferior cerebellar artery. Lang found only a 4% incidence of an extradural origin of the posterior inferior cerebellar antery.[41]

After giving off these branches, the vertebral arteries enter the dura mater just caudal to the lateral edge of the foramen magnum behind the occipital condyles, accompanied by the first cervical nerve and the posterior spinal artery.[52]

The initial intradural segment of the vertebral artery passes rostral to the dorsal and ventral roots of the first cervical nerve and ventral to the posterior spinal artery, the dentate ligament, and the spinal portion of the accessory nerve. In its ascent along the lower lateral and upper ventral aspect of the medulla, the vertebral artery remains ventral to the lower cranial nerves.[75] Variations in this relationship do exist, however, and the vertebral artery may lie dorsal to some cranial nerve rootlets.[75] Connections between the

hypoglossal nerve, glossopharyngeal nerve, spinal accessory nerve, and the C2 cervical root provide the anatomic substrate for various "neck and tongue" syndromes.[54]

As the vertebral arteries ascend ventromedially along the lateral and then the ventral surface of the medulla, they run adjacent to the occipital condyles, the hypoglossal canals, and the jugular tubercles and then come to rest on the clivus. At or near the pontomedullary junction, the arteries join together to form the basilar artery. The precise point at which the arteries join will vary with the size and tortuosity of the vessels.[52]

The posterior inferior cerebellar artery usually originates from the intradural portion of the vertebral artery just above the foramen magnum, although it rarely arises extradurally at or below the foramen.[52] As mentioned, 4% of the posterior inferior cerebellar arteries examined by Lang arose extradurally.[40] In its course along the anterolateral and then the posterolateral medulla, this artery may pass rostrally, caudally, or between the hypoglossal rootlets or above, below, or between the rootlets of the glossopharyngeal, vagus, and accessory nerves.[43] Like the vertebral artery, the relationship between the posterior inferior cerebellar artery and the lower cranial nerves is an intimate one and frequently leads to deformation and stretching of the nerves.

After passing through or around the rootlets of the nerves, the posterior inferior cerebellar artery comes to lie dorsal to the glossopharyngeal, vagus, and accessory nerves and then takes a variable course to reach the dorsal medulla where it bifurcates into a medial and a lateral trunk.[43] The medial trunk supplies the vermis and the adjacent cerebellar hemisphere; the lateral trunk supplies the tonsil and hemispheres.

The anterior spinal artery is usually formed by the union of the paired anterior ventral spinal arteries. These arise from the vertebral artery, supply the paramedial ventral medulla, converge, and run caudally along the ventral median fissure of the spinal cord. In a common variant, the anterior spinal artery may arise from a single vertebral artery, supplemented by supply from vertebral radicular branches at C2 or C3.[40] The posterior spinal arteries have widely variable origins. They may arise from the posterior inferior cerebellar artery or from the intra- or extradural segment of the vertebral artery.[40]

The arteries that supply the dura mater in the region of the foramen magnum include the paired anterior and posterior meningeal branches of the vertebral artery, the ascending pharyngeal artery, the meningohypophyseal trunk of the intracavernous internal carotid artery, and the occipital artery. A variable number of radiculomuscular branches also arise from the extradural vertebral artery.[40] The size and flow of any of these vessels may markedly increase when supplying a dura-based tumor of the foramen magnum.

The venous sinuses most proximal to the foramen magnum include (1) the marginal venous sinus that is formed by the dura lining the rim of the foramen magnum; (2) the occipital venous sinus that is formed by the cerebellar falx; and (3) the basilar venous plexus that is the anastomosis connecting the cavernous sinus on each side, extending along the clivus from the dorsum sellae rostrally to the ventral rim of the foramen magnum caudally.

The veins in the region of the foramen magnum are located both extradurally and intradurally. Extradural veins comprise the epidural venous plexus, which is formed by veins in the epidural space, and vertebral venous plexus, which is formed by veins in the deep muscles surrounding the cervical vertebrae. Intradural veins drain the lower part of the cerebellum and brain stem and the upper part of the spinal cord. Dorsally these veins drain into the dural sinuses surrounding the foramen magnum and torcula. Ventrally and laterally they drain into the superior petrosal sinus.

Alteration of Anatomy by the Tumor

The most important consideration in the selection of a surgical approach is the topographic relationship between the tumor and the neurovascular structures. These structures include the rostral spinal nerve roots, the glossopharyngeal, vagus, accessory, and hypoglossal nerves, and the vertebral artery and its branches. Obviously, the direction of displacement of the neurovascular structures varies with the location and size of the tumor (Figure 78.1). Although there are variations, the following guidelines generally apply:

1. Dorsal midline tumors displace neurovascular structures ventrally.
2. Ventral midline tumors displace neurovascular structures dorsally.
3. Ventrolateral tumors displace the spinal cord and brain stem dorsomedially, the cranial and spinal nerves dorsally, and the vertebral artery and its branches ventrally.

Selection of a Surgical Approach

Although many surgical approaches to the region of the foramen magnum have been described, the following three are the most common: (1) the dorsal approach, (2) the far lateral approach, and (3) the transoral approach. The advantages and disadvantages of each of these approaches are outlined in Table 78.2.[75]

The first step in deciding between these approaches is to determine the topographic relationship of the tumor to the neurovascular structures.

The dorsal approach is the most familiar and least technically demanding of the three approaches. It is best suited for dorsal midline tumors that require neither retraction of the spinal cord or brain stem nor proximal vascular control of the vertebral artery to address ventral or lateral components of the lesion. The disadvantages of this approach include its poor visualization of the spinal cord-tumor juncture with tumors that are more ventrolateral and its lack of provision for proximal vascular control.

Although it involves more dissection and greater bone removal, the far lateral approach overcomes the disadvantages of the strict dorsal approach by allowing the dissection of the spinal cord-tumor juncture to be carried out under direct vision and by providing excellent control of the vertebral artery.[3,37,63,75] It may also be used to approach ventrally located tumors because it exposes the entire ventral aspect of the thecal sac. Compared with the transoral approach, the instrumentation is also simpler and the risk of infection is minimized. Also, in contrast to the transoral approach, destabilization of the craniocervical junction can be addressed with a fusion and instrumentation procedure. The latter is performed easily concomitantly.

TABLE 78.2		
Advantages and Disadvantages of Surgical Approaches to the Foramen Magnum		
Approach	**Advantages**	**Disadvantages**
Posterior	Most familiar	Poor visualization of cord-tumor interface
	Least demanding	
	Minimal risk of infection	Exposure limited by neurovascular structures
	Permits stabilization and fusion for craniocervical instability	Limited proximal control of vertebral artery
Far lateral	Minimal risk of infection	More complex exposure
	Direct visualization of cord-tumor interface	Associated with postoperative hydrocephalus
	Exposes anterior aspect of thecal sac	Time consuming
	Obviates need for cord retraction	
	Excellent proximal control of vertebral artery	
	Rarely produces craniocervical instability	
	Permits stabilization and fusion for craniocervical instability	
Transoral	Obviates need for cord retraction	Deep operative field
	No neurovascular obstacles in midline	Limited lateral exposure
	Exposes midline of anterior thecal sac	Cord-tumor interface not seen until end of operation
		High risk for CSF leak and meningitis
		Destabilizes craniocervical junction
		Stabilization or fusion of craniocervical junction requires separate incision
		No proximal control of vertebral artery

The transoral approach is best suited for midline ventral tumors, especially extradural ones. Its advantages include lack of neurovascular obstacles and avoidance of any retraction of the neuraxis. The drawbacks of the transoral approach, however, are many: laterally placed or broad-based tumors are inadequately exposed; vascular control is lacking; the spinal cord-tumor juncture is not observed until the end of the operation; and iatrogenic spinal destabilization, which invariably occurs, requires a separate stabilizing procedure. Furthermore, because the operative field is necessarily contaminated and because a watertight dural closure is difficult to achieve, there is a high incidence of postoperative cerebrospinal fluid (CSF) fistula and meningitis.

Surgery
Preoperative Considerations

The administration of corticosteroids may improve patient symptoms during the preoperative planning stage. Patients should be informed of the possible need for a tracheotomy and gastrostomy. Prophylactic antibiotics should be administered before operation. If the transoral approach is to be used, first obtaining nose and throat bacterial cultures may guide the choice of antibiotics.

Before induction of anesthesia, sequential compression stockings are applied as prophylaxis for deep venous thrombosis. An assessment is made of the patient's toler-

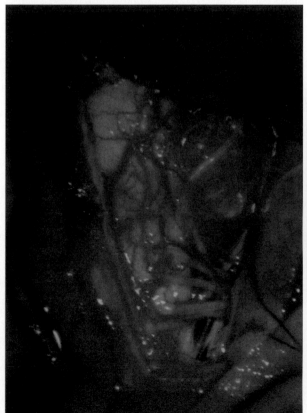

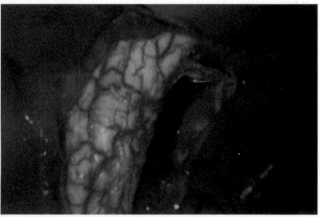

Figure 78.1 A 64-year-old woman presented with a progressive quadriparesis. (**A**) Sagittal T_1-weighted magnetic resonance imaging scan of the cervicomedullary junction shows a ventrally located, well-delineated isointense mass at the foramen magnum causing dorsal displacement of the medulla and upper cervical spinal cord. (**B**) Intraoperative photograph shows the tumor and its relation to the hypoglossal and accessory nerves.
(**C**) Intraoperative photograph after resection of the tumor. The patient experienced full neurologic recovery.

ance to neck flexion to avoid neurologic injury during positioning.

A lumbar drain is inserted before beginning any far lateral approach or any transoral operation in which the dura is likely to be violated. CSF can be drained at a rate of 10 to 20 ml/hr for the first two postoperative days. This may reduce the amount of suboccipital pain, some of which may be related to blood in the CSF. Furthermore, it reduces the need for a CSF shunting procedure after the far lateral approach. In cases of postoperative CSF leak that persists, despite several days of CSF drainage, a lumboperitoneal shunt may be placed.

Electrophysiological monitoring, including somatosensory evoked potentials and brain stem auditory evoked potentials, is employed in most cases. The vagus nerve can be monitored using an electromyographic endotracheal tube.[4] Electromyography can also be performed on the accessory and hypoglossal nerves. The pre- or perioperative placement of a ventriculostomy should be considered when hydrocephalus is present or seems likely to occur. Finally, the surgical approach should be selected on the basis of the location of the tumor and its relationship to the neural and osseous structures.

Dorsal Approach

The prone, three-quarter prone (park bench), or semi sitting position may be chosen. For tumors limited to the dorsal space, the prone position is the simplest and safest. For tumors that extend laterally, the three-quarter prone position may be better. Access to the ventral foramen magnum region is further facilitated by turning the head to the side of the lesion. Three-point rigid fixation of the head aids proper positioning.

Either a vertical midline, a vertical paramedian, or a hockey-stick incision is used. The former is adequate for true dorsal lesions; the latter two are best for more lateral lesions. Whatever incision is chosen, it must be long enough to accommodate a suboccipital craniectomy and a C1-2 laminectomy. The hockey-stick incision angles rostrolaterally above the inion and can accommodate a burr hole for ventricular puncture.

After an incision is made deep to the subcutaneous tissues, the underlying fascia is divided in a Y-shaped fashion. The upper limbs of the Y run along the superior nuchal line, leaving a fascial cuff attached to the bone to facilitate closure. The caudal limb of the incision extends downward in the midline to the spinous process of C2 or lower. After hemostasis is obtained, a subperiosteal dissection is carried out to expose the occipital squama and the spinous processes and laminae of C1 and C2.

Traditionally, two burr holes are next placed bilaterally in the occipital bone. After the dura mater is separated, bone cuts are made transversely and down to the foramen magnum rim with a high-speed drill. Alternatively, in younger patients without significant tension in the posterior fossa, the craniotomy can be started from the rim of the foramen magnum using the high-speed drill without burr holes. The craniotomy is carried rostrally to the caudal edge of the transverse sinus. Caudally, the dorsal rim of the foramen magnum is removed. Bilateral laminectomies are then made at the upper one or two cervical vertebrae

(depending on the caudal extent of the tumor). These should be carried out widely, although disruption of the facet joints should be avoided unless absolutely necessary.

The dura mater is opened in a Y-shaped configuration. The rostral limbs of the Y are placed just below the transverse sinus, and the caudal limb is carried downward in the midline to expose the full extent of the tumor. Should the occipital sinus bleed, it may be ligated with 4-0 nylon or coagulated with bipolar cautery. Dural tack up sutures are then placed to expose cerebellum, the arachnoid is incised in the midline, and the cisterna magna is opened. Full exposure of tumors that attach to the roof or the floor of the fourth ventricle may require resection of a cerebellar tonsil or splitting of the inferior vermis.

Dorsally located tumors are directly accessible with this approach and usually present little risk of vascular injury or cranial neuropathy. By contrast, ventrolateral lesions require care to avoid injury to the vertebral or posterior inferior cerebellar arteries, which may be attached to or encased by the tumor. Furthermore, ventrolateral lesions tend to displace the spinal cord dorsally, stretching one or more rootlets of the cranial nerves or rostral spinal roots over the tumor.

Tumor resection is carried out between the involved rootlets in a piecemeal fashion, with care taken to avoid injury to the radicular vessels that run along the rostral cervical nerve roots. Sectioning the dentate ligaments may improve exposure.

The tumor capsule is best opened sharply. The ultrasonic aspirator can be useful for debulking the intracapsular portion of the tumor. The tumor capsule itself is dissected free from surrounding neurovascular structures and is excised along with involved dura mater.

The need for the radical resection of meningioma-involved dura mater to prevent tumor recurrence is controversial.[42,67] Curettage of the inner surface of tumor-involved dura with a Penfield dissector or a small curette, followed by bipolar coagulation, may be sufficient to allay tumor recurrence when involved dura mater cannot be completely excised.

A watertight dural closure is necessary to prevent the development of a postoperative pseudomeningocele. To avoid neural compression or leakage, a dural graft may be constructed to ensure that the dura mater is not closed under tension.

Far Lateral Approach

The far lateral approach is best suited for tumors located ventrally or ventrolaterally.[3,37,63,75] This provides exposure of the ventral brain stem and makes excessive retraction of neural elements unnecessary. At least fifteen variations exist in the far lateral approach, as described in the literature. One should therefore tailor the amount and the order of the dissection and bone removal to the pathology. It is important to weigh the added morbidity of extensive dissection against its associated gain in visualization and surgical freedom of movement.[68] Immediately after anesthesia is induced and before surgery, a lumbar drain is inserted. The patient is then positioned in a modified park bench position. The lower arm is allowed to drop from the end of the table, where it is cradled in a sling. The head is flexed, rotated downward, and tilted away from the ipsilateral shoulder for maximal opening of the space between the atlas and the foramen magnum. The upper shoulder is pulled down toward the feet with tape to create a larger space for movement of the microscope. The entire body is secured with tape to allow full rotation of the table. Alternatively, this operation has been performed in the sitting position. This may provide the advantage of improved visualization caused by a reduction of venous distension and bleeding, but is associated with air embolism. This is especially true when working around the vertebral artery and hypoglossal nerve, which are surrounded by a rich venous plexus.

An inverted J-shaped incision is begun at the mastoid prominence, curved to the midline, and extended caudally to the C6 level (Figure 78.2A). The nuchal fascia is cut transversely, leaving a 1-cm cuff for reattachment. The paraspinal muscles are split and elevated from the spinous processes and lamina. The muscle flap is dissected from the suboccipital bone to the mastoid process, and the entire flap is retracted laterally and caudally with fishhooks that are attached to a table-mounted device, such as a Leyla bar. The midline aspect of the wound is retracted contralaterally with fishhooks from a second Leyla bar. The lateral mass of C1 and the vertebral artery from C1 to the dura mater are exposed. Bleeding from the venous plexus surrounding the vertebral artery is controlled with bipolar cauterization and packing with Surgicel. Care must be taken to avoid injury to the vertebral artery or to one of its extracranial branches. Occasionally, the posterior inferior cerebellar artery arises extracranially, and could be inadvertently coagulated and divided.[59] It has even been noted to originate between C1 and C2.[73] The same is true

of a hypoplastic vertebral artery.[76] The dorsal arch of C1 is then removed with a high-speed drill (Midas Rex; Midas Rex Institute, Inc., Forth Worth, TX), with a B1 bit and footplate. The ipsilateral lamina is cut at its far lateral extent, as well as on the contralateral side, slightly across the midline. The C1 arch is saved and replaced at closure.

A suboccipital craniotomy is performed with the same drill. The drilling begins at the foramen magnum and extends contralaterally across the midline and ipsilaterally as far laterally as possible. The ipsilateral rim of the foramen magnum is removed with a bone rongeur to the occipital condyle. The dorsal occipital condyle and the rostral lateral mass and facet of C1 are removed by using the drill with the B1 bit. The safest technique is to drill away the inner portion of the occipital condyle, leaving a thin shell of cortical bone to protect the surrounding structures. The shell is carefully removed with small curettes and rongeurs until the dorsolateral third of the condyle has been removed (see Figure 78.2B). Bleeding from the condylar veins can be controlled easily with bone wax. The extradural vertebral artery should be protected with a small dissector while the condyle is being drilled. The hypoglossal canal is located in the ventral medial third of the condyle and is not threatened by removal of the dorsolateral third. Occasionally, a total condylectomy is necessary to remove an extradural lesion with condylar involvement.[68]

The dura mater is opened over the midline of the upper cervical spinal cord. At its caudal extent above C2, the dural incision is curved to the ipsilateral side. Rostrally, the dural opening extends in a curvilinear fashion to the rostral lateral aspect of the craniotomy. This configuration allows the dural flap to be hinged laterally, where it is tented up with 4-0 sutures. Because the occipital condyle

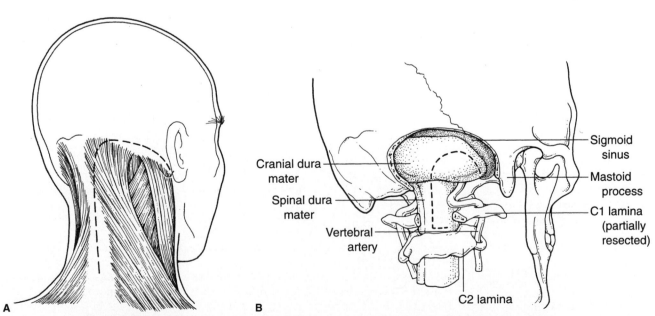

Figure 78.2 (A) Skin incision for the far lateral approach. The inverted J-shaped incision begins at the mastoid process, curves medially to the midline, and extends caudally to the C6 level. **(B)** Far lateral bone opening. A lateral suboccipital craniotomy is extended laterally to include the posterolateral one third of the occipital condyle and caudally to include the ipsilateral portion of the dorsal C1 arch.

is extensively removed, excellent visualization of the proximal intradural vertebral artery is achieved after the dura is opened. Minimal retraction of the cerebellar hemisphere improves the more distal exposure of the vertebral artery and the tumor (Figure 78.3).

After resection of the tumor, the dura mater is closed in a watertight fashion, and both the suboccipital bone flap and the C1 arch are replaced. The wound is closed in layers. If the headholder is first repositioned in a more neutral position, the nuchal fascia is easier to reapproximate.

As with any posterior fossa operation, communicating hydrocephalus can develop after the far lateral approach is performed. A postoperative computed tomography (CT) scan should be performed, even in asymptomatic patients. The extensive muscle dissection involved in the far lateral approach causes considerable pain during the first 2 to 3 days after surgery. Therefore, patients should be given sufficient analgesics.

The stability of the craniocervical junction is an important issue to address following the far lateral approach.[8,68] The surgeon must carefully balance the trade-off between improving visualization and causing instability. In a series of 25 patients with a far lateral approach, Bejjani et al.[8] performed an occipitocervical fusion in eight cases. The authors delineated three indications for fusing across the occipitocervical region: the presence of a painful head tilt, instability on flexion-extension radiographs or complete resection of the occipital condyle. As a general rule, patients with less than 70% removal of the condyle do not require fusion. This corresponds to resection up to the hypoglossal canal. Any further resection increases the likelihood of craniocervical instability.

Transoral Approach

The transoral approach has been widely used for the treatment of extradural lesions and bony abnormalities of the craniovertebral junction.[*] This approach also provides the most direct access to the intradural foramen magnum

---

[*]References 2,5,17,20,21,29,46,48,56,61.

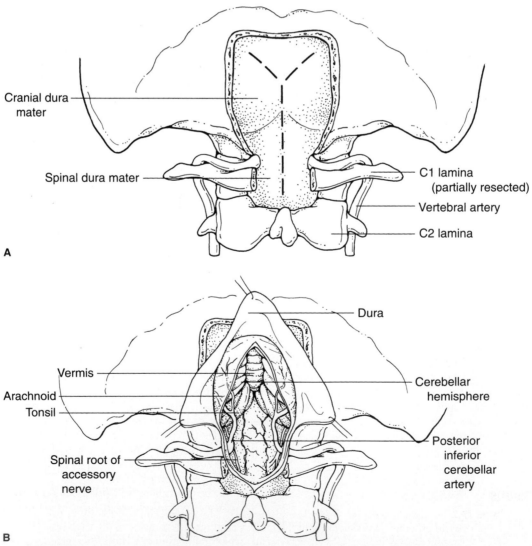

Figure 78.3 (**A**) Suboccipital bone opening and dural incision. The arch of C1 has been removed. (**B**) Exposure of cervicomedullary junction following suboccipital craniectomy.

lesions located at the ventral midline.* The lateral exposure achieved by this approach, however, is limited by the vertebral arteries, the hypoglossal nerves, and the jugular foramen structures. A further disadvantage of this approach is the inability to directly close the dura mater in a watertight fashion, leading to increased risk of CSF leak and postoperative meningitis.

Although a tracheotomy can be performed preoperatively when necessary, most surgeons use endotracheal intubation, keeping the tube depressed below the oral retractor. In all cases in which the dura mater may be penetrated or is going to be penetrated, a lumbar drain is inserted immediately after induction of anesthesia and before surgery.

The patient is positioned supine with the head in three-point fixation. An oral retraction system is then placed, with care taken to avoid injury to the teeth. Attention must also be given to tongue retraction, which can result in postoperative swelling and can lead to airway compromise. Periodic release of the tongue blade intraoperatively, in addition to pre- and postoperative steroid administration, may help prevent this complication. Direct application of steroid ointment to the tongue and oropharyngeal mucosa is very helpful in reducing swelling.

Improved exposure of the dorsal nasopharynx is obtained by suturing the uvula to a rubber catheter passed through the nose and applying gentle upward retraction. This elevates the uvula and soft palate out of the way for C1-2 exposure. If necessary for exposure of the caudal clivus, the soft palate and uvula can be divided to expose the pharyngeal wall. The latter is incised in the midline. The soft palate incision should be brought to one side of the uvula, leaving it intact to the opposite side (Figure 78.4A). Dissection is continued through the prevertebral musculature and prevertebral fascia, which are retracted laterally. Next, the anterior atlanto-occipital and longitudinal ligaments are detached from the clivus and the upper cervical vertebrae. The drill is then used to remove the lower third of the clivus, the ventral C1 arch, the odontoid peg, and part of the C2 body (see Figure 78.4B). Care is taken to avoid excessively lateral dissection that might injure the vertebral arteries, the hypoglossal nerves, or the jugular foramen structures. Once it is adequately exposed, the dura mater is opened in a cruciate fashion.

After excision of the tumor, the dura mater is closed. This may be accomplished by primary closure, including duraplasty, but this is difficult and is rarely watertight. The dural closure may be further sealed with fibrin glue. Where approved, bonding material (Tisseel; Immuno, Austria) can be applied over the incision. A fat graft may be used as an additional seal and to obliterate the retropharyngeal space. Finally, the longus colli muscle is reapproximated with single interrupted Vicryl sutures, and the pharyngeal and soft palate mucosa are closed with running chromic gut suture.

Surgical Results

The surgical results from more recent series are generally good. Most patients with extramedullary foramen mag-

num tumors not only tolerate surgery well but also enjoy good to excellent neurologic recovery. The best chance to achieve complete tumor resection and to effect a cure is at the time of the first surgery.

Meyer et al.[49] reviewed 102 patients with benign extramedullary foramen magnum tumors who underwent operation at the Mayo Clinic between 1924 and 1982. They found a 5% mortality rate and an additional 5% rate of tumor-related deaths (from recurrence) within 3 years of surgery. However, the long-term survival rate was 90%, with 75% of the patients returning to productive lives and 12% being only mildly impaired.

George et al.[27] found a 77% rate of complete tumor removal, a 16% rate of subtotal removal, and only a 7% rate of partial removal. Complete tumor removal was least frequently achieved with ventrally located tumors (69%, versus 81% for lateral tumors and 86% for dorsal tumors). Furthermore, gross total resection was more often attained among intradural tumors (83% versus 50% for extradural tumors). George et al.[27] also observed superior results with the far lateral approach, compared with the standard dorsal approach, for both ventral and lateral tumors: 86% gross total resection with the far lateral approach versus 71% with the straight posterior approach.

Samii et al.[60] obtained a complete resection of craniocervical junction meningiomas in 25 out of 40 patients. There was a marked disparity in the rate of complete removal between patients with encapsulated lesions compared to patients with en plaque or aggressive lesions. Incomplete tumor removal was found to be independently associated with encasement of the vertebral artery, an en plaque pattern, infiltrative growth and an intracranial origin.

Experience with the transoral approach to intradural extramedullary tumors is limited. It is absent in the reports of both Meyer et al.[49] and George et al.[27] Among seven ventrally located intradural lesions at the craniovertebral junction, including three meningiomas, two schwannomas, a neurenteric cyst, and a basilar-anterior inferior cerebellar artery junction aneurysm, Crockard et al. achieved a total removal of both schwannomas, a subtotal removal of two of the three meningiomas, a total removal of the neurenteric cyst, and a successful clipping of the aneurysm.[16,17,50] Major postoperative complications included spinal instability (two patients), CSF leakage (three patients), and velopharyngeal insufficiency (three patients).

Chono et al.[12] successfully removed a ventrally located foramen magnum meningioma with the transoral approach. The procedure was complicated by a CSF leak that required reoperation; a ventral occipitocervical fusion was performed. Bonkowski et al.[9] reported the successful removal of a ventrally located foramen magnum meningioma by the transoral approach that was uncomplicated by spinal instability or CSF leakage. The authors' avoidance of CSF leakage may in part be related to their innovative application of a bone baffle.

The best predictors of poor outcome are the presence of a large ventrally located tumor and poor preoperative neurologic status.* Tumor-related deaths most commonly result from respiratory failure.

___

*References 9,12,14,15,50,51.

*References 13,28,45,49,70,72.

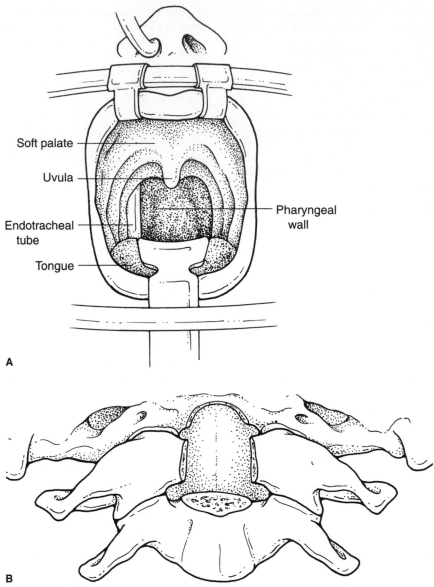

Figure 78.4 (**A**) The transoral incision begins in the midline of the hard palate and is carried down to one side of the uvula. (**B**) The lower third of the clivus, the ventral C1 arch, the odontoid peg, and part of the C2 body are removed using a high-speed drill with the diamond burr.

Complications

The intraoperative and postoperative complications of surgery in the region of the foramen magnum may be divided into categories, as formulated by Sen *et al.*[64] as follows: (1) neurologic, (2) CSF leakage, (3) vascular, (4) infections, and (5) systemic.

Neurologic Complications

Neurologic complications may be caused by intradural or extradural hematoma formation, cerebellar contusion, or injury to the cranial nerves. Postoperative hematoma is best prevented by meticulous hemostasis at the time of operation. Particular attention should be paid to obtaining

excellent surgical exposure to prevent undetected bleeding in areas of the wound that are not well visualized. Wide exposure also minimizes the need for excessive retraction. Routine postoperative computed tomography may be used to detect the development of any hematoma or hydrocephalus. Cerebellar contusion is best avoided by applying only gentle retraction at the time of exposure and by providing intermittent periods of relaxation.

The glossopharyngeal, vagus, accessory, and hypoglossal nerves are vulnerable to injury during surgery in the region of the foramen magnum, particularly because of their proximity to and frequent involvement with the lesion.[47,66] Gentle and meticulous surgical technique provides the best chance of protecting these structures that may be inadvertently sectioned or stretched. In a series of ventral foramen magnum meningiomas,[4] glossopharyngeal and vagus nerve dysfunction was the most common complication postoperatively.

Injury to the glossopharyngeal or vagus nerves causes dysfunction of the pharynx and larynx. Clinically, these patients can present with hoarseness, poor cough, stridor, dysphagia, or aspiration, with the symptoms ranging from the mildly annoying to those that are life-threatening.

Hoarseness and a poor cough may be further evaluated by indirect or fiberoptic laryngoscopy to determine the status of the vocal cord. The evaluation of dysphagia and aspiration is best made with a fluoroscopic barium swallow study that assesses the patient's ability to handle both thin and thick barium preparations and to protect the tracheobronchial tree from the swallowed material. Poor performance on this test suggests the need for a tracheotomy and nasogastric tube or a gastrostomy. In rare instances, intractable aspiration must be managed with laryngotracheal separation.

The accessory nerve is divided into cranial and spinal portions. The cranial portion carries fibers that join the vagus nerve to innervate the muscles of the pharynx and larynx. Recognition and management of damage to these fibers follows the guidelines outlined above.

The spinal portion of the accessory nerve innervates the sternocleidomastoid and trapezius muscles. Injury to these fibers presents clinically with inability to turn the head toward the side of the lesion (sternocleidomastoid muscle paralysis) and inability to shrug the ipsilateral shoulder (trapezius muscle paralysis). Inadvertent division of the accessory nerve should be repaired, if possible, primarily at the time of surgery. The marked decrease in range of motion of the shoulder that results from trapezius muscle paralysis may lead to adhesive capsulitis. Physiotherapy helps maintain the range of motion of the scapulohumeral joint to minimize this pathologic process.

Injury to the hypoglossal nerve results in paralysis of the ipsilateral intrinsic tongue muscles. Unilateral hypoglossal nerve injury causes the tongue to deviate toward the side of the lesion and is fairly well tolerated. Bilateral paralysis produces an immobile tongue, associated with profound difficulties in swallowing and speaking.

Concomitant lesions of the glossopharyngeal, vagus, and accessory nerves magnify the effects of a hypoglossal nerve lesion. Depending on the severity of injury, patients may require only minimal speech and swallowing therapy, or they may require a comprehensive speech and swallowing rehabilitation program with or without a tracheotomy and gastrostomy. In general, patients with preoperative cranial nerve deficits are at lower risk for postoperative aspiration pneumonia, since they have already adapted to a slowly progressive dysfunction of the lower cranial nerves.[60]

Velopharyngeal insufficiency is a unique complication of the transoral approach. Three of the seven patients of Crockard's series developed this problem postoperatively.[15] It probably results from removal of the bony support of the dorsal pharynx and should be distinguished from a cranial nerve palsy.[14] Because it appears related to bony removal, velopharyngeal insufficiency does not occur after transoral procedures for extradural lesions.[30,48]

Placement of "bone baffle" has been proposed to prevent this complication.[9]

CSF Leakage

CSF leakage is one of the more common complications of surgery in the region of the foramen magnum. Because of its association with an increased risk of CSF infection, every attempt should be made to ensure a watertight dural closure. Construction of a dural graft is often necessary to achieve this. Placement of a lumbar spinal fluid drain may also help prevent (or treat) postoperative CSF leakage. This is particularly useful during a transoral surgical approach, which is most likely to result in a postoperative CSF leak.

Once the problem is recognized, the initial management of a CSF leak is with a lumbar spinal fluid drain. If this measure fails to stop the leak, surgical reexploration and dural repair may be necessary. In addition to predisposing to meningitis, a CSF leak can produce a pseudomeningocele. This has been associated with postoperative neurologic deterioration.[11,32,34]

Vascular Injury

All the vessels in the region of the foramen magnum are at risk for iatrogenic injury, particularly the vertebral artery, which may be attached to, or encased by, the tumor. Good preoperative planning is the best defense against vascular injury at the time of surgery. Preoperative angiography may be useful if the magnetic resonance imaging scan suggests vertebral artery involvement. Proximal vertebral artery involvement requires extradural control. Dissection should be carried out along a plane that is parallel to the path of the artery. Blunt dissection should be avoided when separating the tumor from the artery to prevent irregular tears that are difficult to repair.

If sharp dissection is complicated by a major arterial laceration, the artery should be repaired primarily. Irregular tears produced by blunt dissection may require the application of a vein patch graft or the fashioning of a vein graft reconstruction. Sacrifice of a vertebral artery should be avoided and should never be done without ensuring an adequate contralateral collateral supply.

Infections

Prophylactic intraoperative antibiotics are used routinely and should be given before the skin is incised (the potential for infection starts with this step). Repeated dosing may be required to maintain adequate tissue concentration of the antibiotic. Proper tissue handling will help avert tissue devitalization and desiccation that may later form the nidus for infection. Copious irrigation is performed intermittently throughout the procedure, particularly before closure. Postoperative CSF leakage, which may lead to meningitis, should be prevented or promptly recognized and addressed.

Systemic Complications

The most common life-threatening systemic complications include lower extremity deep venous thrombosis,

69. Spetzler RF, Grahm TW: The far lateral approach to the inferior clivus and the upper cervical region: technical note. *Barrow Neurological Institute Quart* 6:35-38, 1990.

70. Stein BM, Leeds NE, Taveras JM, Pool JL: Meningiomas of the foramen magnum. *J Neurosurg* 10:1740-1751, 1963.

71. Sunderland S: Neurovascular relations and anomalies at the base of the brain. *J Neurol Neurosurg Psychiatry* 11:243-257, 1948.

72. Symonds CP, Meadows SP: Compression of the spinal cord in the neighborhood of the foramen magnum. *Brain* 60:52-84, 1937.

73. Tanaka A, Kimura M, Yoshinaga S, Tomonaga M: Extracranial aneurysm of the posterior inferior cerebellar artery: case report. *Neurosurgery* 33:742-745, 1993.

74. Taylor AR, Byrnes DP: Foramen magnum and high cervical cord compression. *Brain* 977:473-480, 1974.

75. Tuite GF, Crockard HA: The far lateral approach to the foramen magnum. In Torrens M, Dickson RA (eds): *Practice of Surgery*. New York, Churchill Livingstone (In press).

76. Wen HT, Rhoton AL, Katsuta T, Oliveira de E: Microsurgical anatomy of the transcondylar, supracondylar, and paracondylar extensions of the far-lateral approach. *J Neurosurg* 87:555-585, 1997.

77. Yasuoka S, Okazaki H, Daube JR, MacCarty CS: Foramen magnum tumors: *J Neurosurg* 49:828-838, 1978.

CHAPTER 79

Sacral Lesions

Donald A. Smith and David W. Cahill

Reviews of sacral lesions have repeatedly emphasized their rarity, their highly variable pathology, and the frequent delay in their diagnosis[9,20,22,26,29] Because many of these lesions are malignant and are far advanced at the time of presentation, their surgical management becomes complex, necessarily taking account of neurologic, colorectal, urologic, and orthopedic considerations. In the case of high sacral lesions, definitive resection may compromise lumbopelvic stability and require purposeful sacrifice of bladder, bowel, and sexual functions. The resultant creation of a very large tissue void, sometimes within a previously irradiated field, raises additional reconstructive issues if difficulties with wound healing and wound sepsis are to be averted. The conflict arising between the goals of functional preservation of the individual versus cure of the disease process in a region that traditionally has been regarded as a surgical boundary zone among several different subspecialists is not unlike the dilemma that confronts the skull base surgeon. This chapter outlines an approach to sacral lesions from an anatomic and pathologic perspective and reviews possibilities for resection and reconstruction and methods of avoiding complications.

Clinical Presentation and Investigations

Sacral tumors are relatively rare, comprising between 1% and 7% of all spinal tumors coming to clinical attention. Low back, pelvic, or gluteal pain, and sciatica are the earliest and almost universal symptoms. However, the nonspecific nature of these complaints and their high prevalence in the general population frequently delays rigorous investigation. Plain film examinations are not sensitive, and routine lumbar myelography, computed tomography (CT), and magnetic resonance imaging (MRI) studies often fail to visualize the sacrum below the S2 segment. Many patients are misdiagnosed with lumbar disc disease and may even undergo ill-advised surgery. All too commonly, the true diagnosis is disclosed late in the course of illness, when pain is unrelenting, after bowel and bladder control have been affected or when a large presacral mass is detected at rectal examination.

Radiographic studies directed specifically at the sacrum are the primary clinical investigative tool. Plain radiographs are relatively insensitive and abnormal in only 50% of cases of sacral tumors. Overlying bowel gas is a frequent source of obscuration, and destructive changes must be far advanced before they become evident on plain radiographs. Lateral films must include the entire sacrum and coccyx; anteroposterior films should display the sacrum en face. Because of the acute angulation of the sacrum with respect to the lumbar spine, and because of the curved surface of the sacrum itself, this is accomplished only by a transpelvic view, directing the central beam rostrally into the hollow of the sacrum. Lesions with sharply defined sclerotic rims imply a chronic process, with reactive changes in the bone connoting benignancy. Destructive and erosive processes without sharply marginated borders are suggestive of a malignant condition.

Imaging

CT and MRI are very sensitive techniques and are the current mainstays of neuroradiologic diagnosis. CT provides excellent definition of the cortical and cancellous anatomy of the sacrum and dorsal pelvic ring. Presacral and postsacral soft-tissue masses and any contained tumor calcifications are also well shown, and the abdomen can be staged for signs of further visceral dissemination. In order to assess optimally the full extent of tumor within the spinal canal it may be necessary to precede this study with the instillation of intrathecal contrast. This technique demonstrates lesions within the spinal canal down to the level of termination of the thecal sac at the S2 level.

Multiplanar imaging capabilities and the exquisite rendition of soft-tissue structures are the principal advantages of MRI. The midsagittal view is particularly helpful for defining the rostral limit of sacral involvement that is critical to surgical planning, whereas axial scans depict the tumor's relationship to the sacroiliac joints. Intra- and extradural involvement throughout the entire length of the sacral canal is readily assessed. CT and MRI provide complementary information.

Nucleide bone scans are mainly relevant as screening examinations during the phase of primary diagnosis or to rule out widespread bony metastasis during preoperative staging. In the former situation, a positive scan is entirely nonspecific and will serve only to prompt more definitive CT and MRI studies. Furthermore, a negative scan does not exclude disease, either for reasons of spatial resolution, obscuration by nucleide elimination in the bladder, or for lack of an osteoblastic response in the bony surround. Multiple myeloma and lymphoma are tumors that are typically undetected with routine bone scanning. The role of PET scanning in the overall work-up of sacral lesions is yet to be determined; at the moment it may be most useful as a measure of systemic burden in patients evaluated for potential metastatic spread. Prior to the availability of CT and MRI, conventional tomography, intravenous pyelography, and barium enemas were often a routine part of the diagnostic evaluation. Today these studies have relatively less to contribute to surgical planning. Angiography with potential tumor embolization is still a worthwhile consideration in vascular lesions such as giant cell tumors and aneurysmal bone cysts.

Biopsy

If a primary rectal malignancy with local involvement of the sacrum is suspected, endoscopy with biopsy of any suspicious endoluminal lesions is appropriate. In the case of masses extrinsic to the rectal mucosa, transrectal biopsy is discouraged, because this violation of previously uninvolved tissue planes could then commit the patient to an otherwise unneeded bowel resection. If a major sacral resection is planned, it is frequently advisable to obtain baseline urodynamic studies to objectively assess voiding functions preoperatively.

Often, the combination of anatomic localization and imaging characteristics, when taken in the context of a specific clinical setting, suggests a short list of possible pathologic diagnoses. Preoperative biopsy should be reserved for those patients in whom exact knowledge of the pathologic diagnosis would influence the decision to operate or would alter the scope of surgery. Although open biopsies and transrectal biopsies were common in the past; almost all biopsies are now performed percutaneously under CT guidance. The trajectory of the biopsy should be considered to allow for its easy inclusion within the boundaries of any subsequent surgical resection. Biopsy has particular relevance in hematopoietic malignancies that may be best treated with irradiation and combination chemotherapy. Lesions that are metastatic to the sacrum from remote sites are considered for operation only under special circumstances. This rarely occurs outside the context of a known primary tumor with widely disseminated disease, and so this is an uncommon indication for biopsy. In patients who are deemed unsuited for a major operative procedure because of medical infirmity, a biopsy is warranted to establish a diagnosis and indicate the most appropriate therapeutic alternatives.

Most primary malignancies of the sacrum are locally aggressive tumors, metastasizing only late in the course of disease or not at all. Nonetheless, chest radiography and CT of the chest and abdomen, as well as a bone scan, are probably prudent, because evidence of remote disease may well alter the decision for surgery and the method of treatment. Cancers of the rectum and pelvic organs with sacral involvement must be thoroughly staged before any consideration of surgery.

Osseoligamentous Anatomy

The relevant sacral anatomy has been presented in Chapter 20. Certain aspects of the bony and ligamentous anatomy are reviewed here as they pertain to lumbopelvic stability. The adult sacrum is composed of five fused vertebral segments. The ventral surface of the sacrum is concave in both sagittal and axial planes. The corrugated lateral aspects of the first two to three sacral segments articulate with the ilium on either side. These joint surfaces diverge rostrally to create a wedgelike configuration that locks the sacrum into the dorsal pelvic ring, like a keystone within an arch.

The sacrum is secured within this ring by very strong sacroiliac joints and supporting ventral and dorsal ligamentous groups. The ventral surface of the sacroiliac joint is spanned by ventral sacroiliac ligaments that blend with the periosteum. Obliquely directed iliolumbar ligaments that attach to the transverse processes of L5 and course caudally and laterally to insert on the ilium or merge with the ventral sacroiliac ligament provide additional reinforcement (Figure 79.1). The dorsal ligamentous complex is very strong and is composed of interosseous ligaments and a dorsal sacroiliac group. The interosseous ligaments connect the sacral tuberosities immediately rostral to the sacral articular surfaces to the overhanging bone of the iliac tuberosities. The posterior sacroiliac ligaments are anchored in the interval from the posterior superior to the posterior inferior iliac spines; their rostral portions attach at the two rostral sacral eminences, and their caudal portions blend with the sacrotuberous ligaments below.

In an upright posture, the center of gravity shifts ventral to the sacroiliac joint. This exerts an angular force on the sacrum to depress the sacral promontory and elevate the coccyx about a transverse axis of rotation centered in the S2 body. The forces that tend to rotate the coccyx dorsally and upward are strongly counteracted by the tension-banding effect of the sacrotuberous and sacrospinous ligaments (Figure 79.2). Both ligaments attach at the lower two sacral eminences and along the coccyx and span to the ischial tubercle and the ischial spine, respectively. The sacrospinous ligament also serves to demarcate the greater from the lesser sciatic foramen. The reciprocal tendency for the sacral promontory to rotate ventrally and downward is similarly counteracted by the "checkrein" effect of the iliolumbar and posterior sacroiliac ligaments.

Clinical Biomechanics

Integrity of the pelvic ring depends on ligamentous stabilization ventrally at the pubic symphysis and dorsally at each of the sacroiliac joints. The sacroiliac, sacrotuberous, and sacrospinous ligaments are responsible for dorsal stabilization. As long as the sacroiliac joint and its investing ligaments are not violated, sacropelvic stability is unaltered. It is for this reason that distal sacral resections (below S2) and simple sacral laminectomies are not significantly destabilizing. There are few biomechanical studies on the effects of higher sacral amputations that involve the sacroiliac joints. Gunterberg et al.[11] have conducted some preliminary studies in cadavers and indicate that the ability of the sacroiliac joints to resist axial loading is lost in proportion to the extent of sacroiliac joint disruption. Amputations through the level of the S1 foramina sacrifice approximately 50% of the joint surface and are associated with a 50% reduction in tolerance to axial loading. The amount of the sacroiliac joint that must be preserved to maintain clinical stability is unknown and could be expected to vary according to body habitus, activity, and quality of the underlying tissues. Stener's experimental and clinical experience appear to indicate that resection through even the midbody of the S1 vertebra, leaving about one-third of the sacroiliac joint intact, is still compatible with clinical stability.[25] Resections higher than this level or through the entirety of the sacroiliac joint require lumbopelvic stabilization.

Sacral Neuroanatomy

The thecal sac tapers abruptly upon entry into the sacral canal, terminating typically at the S2 level. From the distal sac emerge the lower sacral and coccygeal nerves, segre-

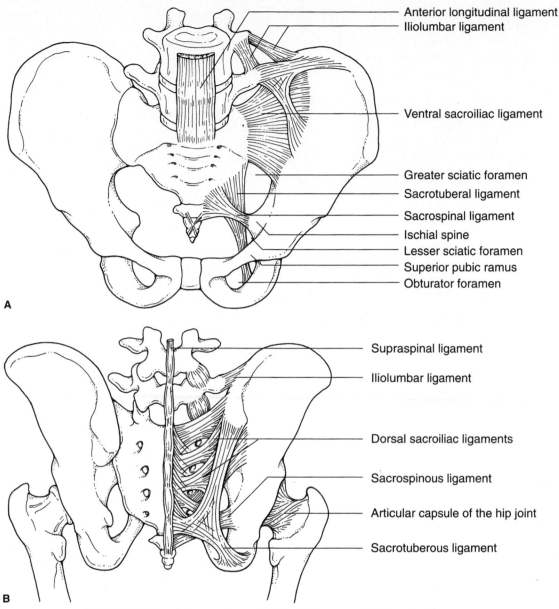

Figure 79.1 Ligamentous anatomy. (**A**) Ventral sacrum. (**B**) Dorsal sacrum.

gated as ventral and lateral roots, as well as the filum terminale. The upper four sacral roots exit the sacrum caudally and laterally through paired ventral and dorsal foramina. Inferiorly, the sacral canal terminates in the sacral hiatus from which the fifth sacral roots, the coccygeal roots, and the filum terminale emerge. Paired sacral plexi lie to either side of the bony sacrum on the ventral fascia of the piriformis muscles. Each plexus is formed from the confluence of a lumbosacral trunk derived from ventral L4 and L5 roots coursing caudally and laterally over the sacral alae with contributions from the ventral rami of S1 to S3 (Figure 79.3). The upper part of the plexus is often intersected by the superior gluteal artery, whereas its lower part is penetrated by the inferior gluteal artery. The largest and most important branch of the sacral plexus is the sciatic nerve, which forms at the level of the S3 foramina. It is accompanied in its exit from the greater sciatic notch by other sacral plexus branches including the superior and inferior gluteal nerves, and branches to the quadratus femoris, gemelli, and obturator internus muscles.

Medial and caudal to the sacral plexus, branches of the ventral rami of S2 to S4 join to form the pudendal nerve. The pudendal nerve is unique in exiting the greater sciatic foramen only to reenter the lesser sciatic foramen by passing around the sacrospinous ligament. It innervates the coccygeal and levator muscles of the pelvic floor as well as the external anal sphincter. The often ill-defined coccygeal plexus derives from the fourth and fifth sacral roots and the coccygeal roots. It subserves perianal sensation.

Both the sympathetic and parasympathetic nerves have an intimate relationship with the sacrum. The sympathetic chains course caudally into the pelvis, closely applied to the ventral surface of the sacrum. While at this level they lack white rami communicantes and there are small ganglionic enlargements just medial to the ventral foramina.

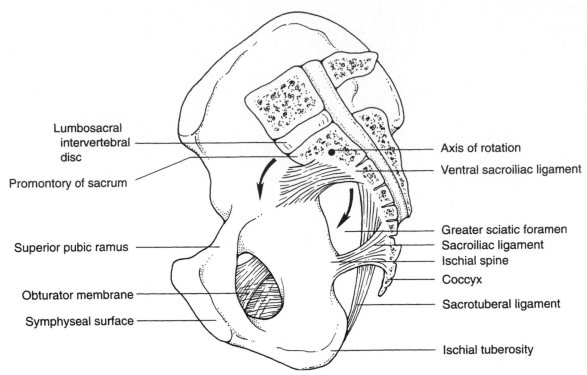

Figure 79.2 Rotational forces acting on the sacrum counteracted by ligamentous structures.

The two trunks unite in the midline over the coccyx to form the ganglion impar. The sympathetic trunks distribute gray rami communicantes to several of the sacral roots and contribute fine filamentous branches to the superior hypogastric plexus. The superior hypogastric plexus is the caudal continuation of the periaortic sympathetic plexus. It overlies the L5-S1 disc and the upper sacrum medial to the sympathetic trunks. Like the coccygeal plexus, it is somewhat ill defined.

At the S1-2 level, fibers of the superior hypogastric plexus diverge inferolaterally and cross the sympathetic trunks to form two laterally arrayed inferior hypogastric (pelvic) plexi that overlie the surface of the obturator internus muscles at the S2-4 levels. The parasympathetic contribution to the pelvic plexi is derived from small fibers that originate from the ventral S2-4 nerve roots that comprise the pelvic splanchnic nerves. From both the superior hypogastric and the pelvic plexi, small fibers are distributed distally to the various pelvic organs. The sympathetic system supports male fertility by promoting timely transport of spermatozoa from the testes to the seminal vesicles and coordinated antegrade ejaculation out of the urethra. The parasympathetic system is primarily responsible for the vascular reflexes that sustain erectile functions.

Classification of Sacral Lesions

A wide variety of neoplastic and nonneoplastic processes may present as sacral and presacral lesions (Box 79.1). Currently, there is no unified schema for their classification and staging. As with other pathologic entities, they may be categorized according to etiologic, biologic, or anatomic criteria. Some of these lesions such as cysts, meningoceles, and lipomas are non-neoplastic. Tumors are divisible into those that arise from neural tissues or their supporting elements, those that originate in bone, and those that are the result of hematogenous spread from a remote primary or from direct extension from local gynecologic or colorectal malignancy.

When formulating surgical objectives to deal with tumors of the sacrum, one must appraise the anatomic extent of the lesion and its likely biologic behavior. Anatomic considerations direct the surgeon to the lesion, whereas biologic considerations dictate the scope of the surgery. Of prime importance is whether the process is merely expansile but contained within its anatomic borders, or whether it has a fundamentally invasive or infiltrative character. Approximately one-half of sacral tumors are benign, encapsulated lesions and usually can be dealt with by lesional resection, even in a piecemeal fashion. Low-grade malignancies with infiltrative borders require a more aggressive approach with en bloc resection and a wide local excision with a circumferential margin of uninvolved tissue to effect cure. Certain higher-grade or disseminated malignancies are best treated not with surgical resection, but with irradiation or chemotherapy. In undertaking radical treatments of sacral lesions, the goal of achieving tumor control or cure must be balanced against the functional consequences of therapy and the anticipated longevity of the patient.

Neurogenic Lesions

Neurogenic lesions within the sacrum are relatively rare. Only 1% to 5% of spinal schwannomas arise at this level.[1]

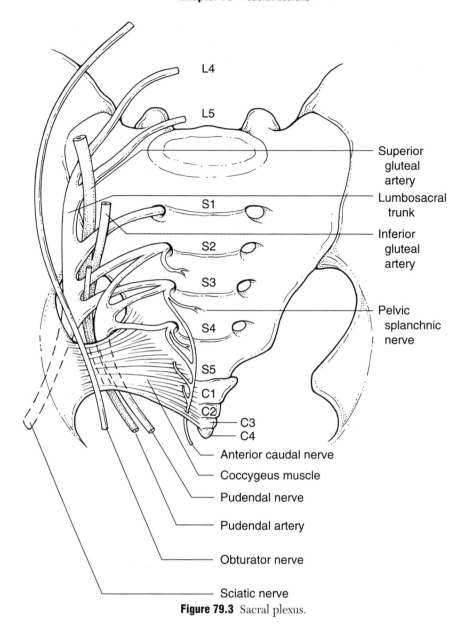

Figure 79.3 Sacral plexus.

Like neurogenic lesions elsewhere in the spine, they tend to originate in the spinal canal itself or in close relation to the nerve roots or their coverings. They may exist intradurally or extradurally. With continued growth they can expand to fill the sacral canal or grow out of the ventral or dorsal sacral foramina to variable degree. The majority of such lesions coming to surgical attention will be largely confined to the spinal canal and can be treated by lesional excision in the same fashion as similar lesions are treated elsewhere in the spine. In cases of long-delayed diagnosis, growth into the sacrum and presacral space can be quite massive, creating what has been termed a "giant" sacral tumor.[1] The sacrum itself becomes highly excavated in the course of this expansion, but the bony interface remains well marginated, containing a "pushing" rather than an infiltrative border. Giant sacral neurofibromas, schwannomas, and ependymomas occur with roughly equal rarity, whereas giant sacral meningiomas are exceedingly uncommon. Total lesional resection of these tumors with significant intrasacral and presacral extension can be a formidable undertaking, but it is potentially curative. Subtotal resection may result in clinical recurrence, but often this is quite delayed. Malignant neurogenic tumors such as malignant schwannoma or malignant ependymoma tend to disseminate within the neuraxis before local bony invasion becomes an issue.

Primary Osseous Tumors

Primary osseous tumors of the sacrum are histologically and biologically heterogeneous. Unlike neurogenic lesions, because they arise in the bone matrix itself, even benign osseous tumors lack a definitive tumor capsule. They can be categorized either as tumors of low biologic activity that respond well to intralesional curettage, or as

minimize the risk of creating a cerebrospinal fluid fistula. Sacral laminectomy is less well suited as a definitive exposure in lesions that originate outside the sacral canal or that have developed significant extension into the pelvis via the neural foramina or through sacral replacement.

Dorsal Sacrectomy

Dorsal sacrectomy, as described by MacCarty et al.[15] is an excellent procedure for dealing with lesions of the sacrum below the level of the sacroiliac joints. The capacity to address the presacral extension of tumor and the potential to perform a genuine oncologic procedure including en bloc resection of tumor with a circumferential margin of uninvolved tissues distinguishes this from simple sacral laminectomy. These advantages are particularly relevant to osseous lesions of the sacrum that are more often malignant and that are more likely to present with a presacral mass. This is generally suitable for tumors whose superior limit can be reached on digital rectal examination. It should not be employed in cases with primary rectal involvement.

Patients are placed in a prone position over padded bolsters to allow the abdomen to hang free to minimize compression of the vena cava. The anus may be temporarily purse-string closed. A midline incision is made that extends from the lumbosacral junction to the coccyx. The incision can be modified to an ellipse to incorporate any previous biopsy tract. The overlying soft tissues are reflected in routine fashion to expose the bony sacrum dorsally. If preoperative imaging studies indicate tumor eruption out of the sacral hiatus or dorsal foramina, then the soft-tissue dissection is altered to leave an island of sacrospinalis musculature and fat overlying the dorsal surface of the sacrum and a cuff of gluteal musculature attached laterally. In these circumstances, the sacral periosteum should not be incised or dissected. The anococcygeal ligament is divided at a distance from the sphincter, and finger dissection is used to mobilize the rectum and develop the presacral space. The sacrotuberous and sacrospinous ligaments are detached from the lateral edges of the lower sacrum. This uncovers the piriformis and coccygeal muscles that are divided to reveal the lower elements of the sacral plexi. For malignant lesions such as chordoma the transverse sacral osteotomy should extend one whole segment rostral to the level of radiographically involved bone. This determines the level at which the sacral nerves must be divided, and the procedure is facilitated through a limited sacral laminectomy immediately rostral to the level of the intended amputation. The sacral plexi and sciatic nerves are quite lateral at this point and are only rarely involved directly by tumors of the lower sacrum. The pudendal nerves exiting the greater sciatic foramen and reentering the lesser foramen should also be identified and protected except when they are too intimate with the tumor to be spared. The transverse sacral osteotomy is then completed through any remaining dorsal elements and all of the ventral sacrum using an osteotome. A protected finger inserted into the presacral space at the level of the intended sacral division helps provide additional tactile guidance for the osteotomy and for the subsequent release of any soft-tissue attachments. The specimen is freed circumferentially and can be removed from the field. Bleeding from the sacral stump is controlled with bone wax, and considerable care is taken to

secure hemostasis in the presacral soft tissue because a large dead space cavity will result from the resection. The median and lateral sacral arteries and their accompanying veins are usually the major sources of this bleeding. Large-bore, closed suction wound drains are used to collapse dead space and evacuate any postoperative bleeding. The wound is reapproximated in a layered, tensionless fashion according to individual preference. This may necessitate mobilization of soft-tissue flaps but can generally be achieved without resorting to more elaborate reconstructive measures.

Dorsal sacrectomy works well for smaller lesions of the mid and distal sacrum not yet requiring resection through the level of the sacroiliac joint. Although MacCarty et al.[15] described amputation as high as the first sacral segment, this is a less attractive method in our view, as the ability to accurately dissect tissue planes of the upper presacrum is unpredictable from this approach, thereby risking a major vascular injury, inadvertent entry into the rectum, or violation of the tumor capsule during attempts to osteotomize the ventral sacrum and sacroiliac joints from behind. These difficulties are best addressed by combining the techniques of dorsal sacrectomy with a ventral approach for lesions requiring amputation through the level of the sacroiliac joints.

Sacral Resection Using Combined Ventral and Dorsal Approaches

A sequential ventral and dorsal approach to facilitate high sacral amputation was described by Bowers in 1948.[6] Transabdominal exposure was used to gain control of the hypogastric vessels and enable a safer dorsal sacrectomy. The ventral approach allows mobilization of the rectum off of the tumor under direct vision rather than by blind finger dissection. Furthermore, should the rectum be involved by tumor either as a consequence of direct extension or because of seeding from an injudicious transrectal biopsy, it can be isolated for en bloc resection with the sacral specimen. This is impossible from the dorsal approach alone.

Localio et al.[14] popularized a synchronous abdominosacral approach for sacral lesions. They favored a lateral decubitus position with the left side uppermost, thereby enabling simultaneous ventral and dorsal exposure without need for patient repositioning. The abdominal approach begins through an obliquely oriented flank incision centered midway between the costal margin and the iliac crest. The retroperitoneum is dissected, and the descending colon and rectum are mobilized rightward. The internal iliac arteries and veins are controlled with vessel loops, and the entire perimeter of the tumor mass is defined ventrally. Tumor vessels, which usually emanate from the lateral and median sacral arteries, are interrupted directly. The sacrum is exposed through a separate dorsal incision, and with division of the anococcygeal ligament, the two wounds are communicated. As for dorsal sacrectomy, the lateral muscular attachments onto the sacrum and sacroiliac joint are released. With the hypogastric vessels temporarily occluded, the sacrotuberous and sacrospinous ligaments are detached and the posterior sacroiliac ligaments are divided rostrally up to the intended level of amputation. The sacrum and sacroiliac joint can then be osteotomized ventrally and dorsally under direct vision. Localio *et al.*[14] suggested that this technique of synchronous abdominosacral resection resulted in less blood loss than did sequential resection. They reported succinctly on five patients with chordoma operated via this approach, two of whom were alive and without evidence of disease at 7- and 8-year follow-ups. The present authors' primary objection to this exposure relates to the awkwardness of operating on a patient in the lateral position. Although it is indeed possible to expose the sacrum ventrally and dorsally simultaneously in the lateral position, it is more difficult to expose both of them well. The lateral position also complicates efforts at soft-tissue reconstruction and mechanical stabilization that are integral to the success of these procedures.

A sequential ventral and dorsal approach with pedicled rectus abdominis pull-through flap reconstruction is favored for high sacral resections. The technique of surgical resection is essentially similar to that described by Stener and Gunterberg.[25] The rectus abdominis pull-through flap was originally described for reconstruction and repair of perineal wounds.[24,31] Its routine use in the closure of the large surgical voids created by high sacrectomy has virtually eliminated problems with prolonged wound drainage and breakdown.[3,7,17] Although the surgery is necessarily interrupted by the need for patient repositioning, the superior visibility and the working ease made possible through the sequential approach more than justifies this inconvenience.

A low-residue diet and mechanical bowel preparation are begun preoperatively. Broad-spectrum antibiotic prophylaxis is utilized. Blood loss can be substantial, and adequate transfusion reserves and IVs for volume resuscitation should be secured in advance. The use of the cell saver has been eschewed because of the potential for tumor dissemination. The operation begins with abdominal exposure. Incisions for a transversely oriented myocutaneous flap based on the upper rectus abdominis muscles are outlined in the epigastrium; a midline lower abdominal entry is employed (Figure 79.4). Although the sacrum can be exposed ventrally by bilateral extraperitoneal dissection, the authors generally favor a transperitoneal route. After the bowel has been packed off, the dorsal parietal peritoneum is opened to one side, the ureters are identified, and the iliac vessels are dissected bilaterally. If the rectum is to be spared, it is mobilized off of the tumor capsule ventrally after incision of the retrorectal peritoneal reflection.

The tumor capsule is outlined circumferentially. Bleeding from the venous plexus in the loose areolar tissue surrounding the tumor can be profuse. The internal iliac arteries and veins are ligated along with any tumor vessels. In some cases, it may not be possible to attain absolute hemostasis until after the tumor is completely resected.

High sacral resections require mobilization of the iliac veins medially and laterally during the osteotomies. The surgeon is advised to preemptively ligate the iliolumbar veins entering their back wall, lest they be avulsed during these maneuvers and become a source of troublesome bleeding. The sacral foramina are visualized ventrally. These serve as the landmarks to guide the ventral sacral osteotomy. In high sacrectomies, the periosteum is incised transversely at the sacral promontory and is reflected downward to the level of the intended amputation. Inevitably, this measure divides the sympathetic trunks and, in high sacral resections, also sacrifices the hypogastric plexus. The lumbosacral nerve trunks coursing caudolaterally over the sacral alae and the sacroiliac joints are dissected free and protected. A transverse osteotomy is then begun through the ventral sacrum at the selected level (Figure 79.5). Usually this incorporates the ventral sacral foramina, in which case the sacral nerves exiting at that level are first dissected out and preserved. If the osteotomy must transect the midbody of S1 above the foramina, it will not be feasible to save any of the sacral nerves. Because the midportion of the osteotomy enters the sacral canal, this is best performed with a chisel to minimize the chance of premature entry into the thecal sac. A lateral radiograph with a radiographic marker in place is a useful cross-check against the preoperative imaging studies before definitive osteotomy. The bone cuts are extended inferolaterally into the sacroiliac joints, with care taken to protect the lumbosacral trunks and any remaining sacral roots. The apically convex course of the osteotomy parallels the path of the nerves to be spared. A chisel osteotome is favored for this, as saws and drills are more apt to entrain adjacent soft-tissues. The peritoneal investment and the periosteum are incised caudally as far as the greater sciatic notch, and the cortex is scored ventrally to create a stress riser that facilitates subsequent completion osteotomy from behind. Waxing the osteotomy cuts helps reduce bleeding and improves visibility.

In those cases in which the rectum is to be resected, the rectosigmoid junction is mobilized in preparation for division with a mechanical stapler. The stapled-closed stumps of bowel may then be invaginated and oversewn with serosal sutures to lessen the chances of wound soilage. The rostral and middle rectal vessels are isolated and divided, and the rectovesical or rectouterine peritoneal reflection is incised to allow access to the pelvic floor. Peritoneal adhesions between the tumor mass and the bladder or pelvic side walls should not be simply lysed, because this may indicate a need for pelvic exenteration if the surgery is to have a curative intent. Wide local excision including bladder, prostate, vagina, cervix, or endopelvic fascia and contained vessels may be required in such cases.[27,30] Access for deep pelvic dissection can be enhanced through division of the symphysis pubis and introduction of a rib spreader to open the pelvic ring ventrally.

At this point, a rectus abdominis myocutaneous flap based on the inferior epigastric vessels is prepared. The ventral abdominal wall skin island is sealed with iodine-impregnated plastic adhesive dressing and then stowed within the pelvis. It may be helpful for the purposes of hemostasis and for anatomic demarcation during the subsequent dorsal approach to insinuate large sheets of gelatin sponge into the plane of dissection between the sacrectomy specimen with any attached presacral mass and the iliac vessels, sacral plexi, and ureters remaining undisturbed. If required, a colostomy is performed, and the wound is closed according to preference.

The patient is then repositioned prone on a padded thoracoabdominal rest, allowing the abdomen to hang

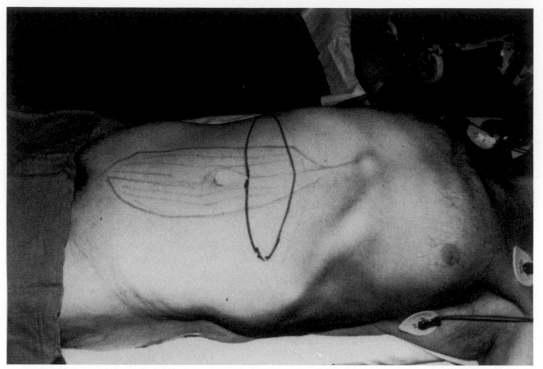

Figure 79.4 Outlines indicating where incisions will be made for the rectus abdominis flap and the abdominal entry.

free. Dorsally a midline incision extending from the L5-S1 interlaminar space to the level of the external anal sphincter is outlined. If the rectum is to be included with the specimen, the caudal limb of the incision continues as an ellipse encircling the anus. Alternatively, the perineal dissection may be performed during the abdominal exposure if the patient is operated in the lithotomy position with the buttocks elevated on a small cushion. Any skin compromised by tumor, previous biopsy, radiation change, or prior surgery should also be excised with the specimen. Dissection through the soft tissues is deepened in a conically widening fashion: at the summit is any involved skin and at the base is the biopsy tract and any tumor erupting out of the dorsal sacrum (Figure 79.6). This again reemphasizes the objective of an en bloc resection with a margin of healthy, uninvolved tissues.

Rostrally, the interspinous and interlaminar ligaments at L5-S1 are dissected out to enable isolation of the thecal sac in preparation for its ligation immediately below the level of exit of the last nerve roots to be preserved. If the S2 roots are to be spared, a limited rostral sacral laminectomy is needed to allow their visualization. Dorsally, the sacrospinalis muscles are sectioned transversely, and the dorsal sacroiliac ligament is released from the ilium. Laterally, the gluteal musculature is transected, leaving a cuff attached at its sacral origin. This uncovers the piriformis muscles that are, in turn, divided at their musculotendinous junction (Figure 79.7). The superior gluteal vessels and nerves are found at the upper border of the piriformis, and the inferior gluteal vessels, the sciatic, pudendal, and posterior femoral cutaneous nerves are found exiting the pelvis at its lower edge. These should be identified carefully and preserved whenever possible.

If rectal resection is not planned, the caudal border of the specimen is freed by division of the anococcygeal ligament just proximal to the anal sphincter. The sacrotuberous ligament is detached from the ischial tuberosity, and the coccygeal muscles are cut. The sacrospinous ligament is conveniently detached by an osteotomy cut across the base of the ischial spine. If the rectum is to be included with the specimen, the anus is dissected circumferentially with additional division of the levator musculature.

The soft-tissue dissection is now concluded, and the field is prepared for completion osteotomy. A finger is introduced through the anococcygeal interval and the greater sciatic notch on either side to redevelop the presacral space and palpate the previously outlined osteotomy cuts from within the pelvis (Figure 79.8). This helps guide the dorsal cuts to ensure an accurate intercept with the ventral osteotomies. The osteotomy along the ilium can exit into the sciatic notch either medial or lateral to the ischial spine. The sacrum is free and can be lifted out of the wound dorsally when the lower sacral roots coursing laterally toward the sacral plexi and pudendal nerves are sequentially divided (Figure 79.9). Bleeding can be profuse at this stage. Bone edges should be waxed expeditiously and bleeding from larger vessels promptly secured with ligatures or hemoclips.

Removal of the sacrum in this manner creates a large trapdoor opening into the pelvis. It is desirable to obliterate as much of this dead space as possible. Toward this end, the gluteal muscles can be reapproximated to bone or to one another, a measure that may also enhance their function postoperatively by reestablishing an origin for them. Large-bore, bulb-type closed suction drains are placed into the wound depth and tunneled out to a remote point of exit

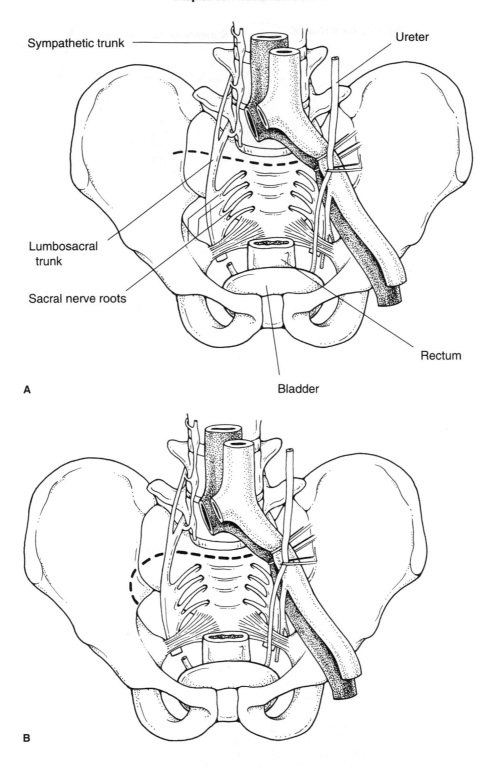

Figure 79.5 **(A)** Ventral transverse sacral osteotomy. **(B)** Extent of ventral osteotomy across the sacroiliac joint and exiting into the sciatic notch.

after copious antibiotic wash. The rectus abdominis myocutaneous flap, which had been previously positioned in the pelvis during the abdominal phase of the procedure, is now retrieved through the sacrectomy window. The flap is trimmed as needed to match the contours of the soft-tissue defect overlying the sacrum and sewn into place in a layered fashion (Figure 79.10). The authors have been far more satisfied with this reconstructive method than with the alternatives of primary closure or reconstruction with reversed latissimus dorsi flaps, gluteal flaps, or gracilis flaps. Microvascular free flap reconstruction is yet another option, but this further escalates the technical requirements of an already arduous procedure. The rectus abdominis pull-through flap is recommended especially in the frequent circumstances of previous surgery or irradiation, when the prospects for successful primary closure are remote. It largely averts problems with rectal prolapse into the wound during defecation and obviates the need for mesh closure of the dorsal peritoneal or fascial defect.

Total Sacrectomy

Tumors whose surgical extirpation requires total or near-total sacrectomy present an additional challenge because of the difficulties in reestablishing lumbopelvic stability. The precise extent of sacroiliac joint that must be preserved in a given individual to maintain clinical stability is

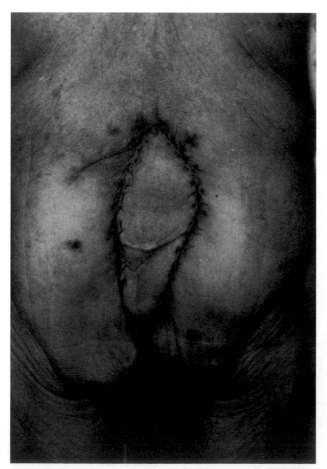

Figure 79.10 Sacrectomy defect closed with rectus abdominis pull-through flap.

unknown. Experience indicates that preservation of the upper half of the S1 segment is generally sufficient for this purpose.[11,25] Involvement of the upper S1 segment has been regarded by some surgeons as a contraindication to surgery on account of the extreme instability that would result from its resection. Certainly if less than 50% of the S1 segment remains intact, strong consideration should be given to supplemental stabilization.

Only a very limited number of cases of total sacrectomy have been reported in the literature. The methods of sacral resection and soft-tissue reconstruction in total sacrectomy are fundamentally similar to those just discussed. Rather than a transverse osteotomy through the upper sacrum, however, the lowermost disc space is divided, and the caudal end plate of L5 thoroughly denuded of soft tissue and cartilage. With the spine functionally disconnected from the sacrum, some method of lumbopelvic fixation is required.

Current posterior instrumentation requires significant adaptation to secure fixation to the posterior pelvic ring. The Galveston technique, which employs segmental fixation to at least the lower three lumbar segments coupled to L-shaped rods driven into each ilium, is applicable to this reconstructive problem.[2] However, the posterior pelvis has been "sprung" through removal of the sacral keystone, and any further axial loading will cause the iliac wings to splay further apart with the symphysis pubis acting as a hinge. These forces can be counteracted in part through application of a contoured, transverse reconstruction plate or a "sacral bar" that reestablishes continuity of the dorsal pelvic ring. Jackson and Gokaslan have recently reviewed their experience with neoplasms at the lumbosacral junction. They described their modification of the Galveston technique using pedicle screw fixation in the lumbar spine and threaded transiliac rods to reconstruct the posterior pelvic ring in those patients undergoing upper sacrectomy.[10,13]

Previous descriptions of total sacrectomy with instrumented lumbopelvic reconstructions by Shikata et al.[23] and Tomita et al.[33] incorporated a direct linkage of the lumbar fixation to transverse pelvic fixators. Shikata reported a technique for telescoping the lumbar spine downward into the sacrectomy defect and then transfixing the L5 body with a transverse sacral bar. Ideally the construct should incorporate a large bone graft locked into place between the two iliac bones by some type of a compression plate and should have sufficient immediate strength to function as a new foundation for the spine. Salehi et al.[21] have cleverly addressed this reconstructive problem by seating the inferior end plate of L5 atop a large titanium mesh cage, which itself is transfixed by a transiliac rod in conjunction with a Galveston-type posterior instrumentation.

The volume requirement for graft material to span the void between the iliac bones and the spine is enormous. Autologous bone is preferred and may be obtained from the iliac wings, greater trochanters, fibulae, and ribs, but will almost certainly require supplementation with allograft. Other bone substitutes and graft-promoters may have a role to play in the future. The reader is referred to Chapter 109 for a review of the current state of the art of complex lumbosacralpelvic reconstruction. Ambulation is begun cautiously, and use of a molded external orthosis with thigh extension may be advisable.

Postoperative Care, Rehabilitative Concerns, and Results

Patients undergoing major sacral resections are cared for in an intensive care unit postoperatively. Ongoing assessments are made of any continuing need for blood and blood product replacements. Major fluid shifts are anticipated, and strict vigilance is required if either under-replacement or over-replacement is to be avoided. Clotting parameters and electrolyte status must be carefully monitored in light of these replacements. Nursing the patient initially on an air bed is a justifiable precaution to guard against sacral decubiti and wound breakdown. Antibiotics are continued for 24 hours after removal of the last wound drain. Aggressive prophylaxis against deep vein thrombosis (DVT) with sequential compression devices on the lower extremities and fractionated heparin is advised in view of recumbency, dissection of the pelvic veins, and possible neurologic deficit. Every attempt is made to mobilize the patient as soon as the cardiopulmonary reserve and perceived dorsal pelvic ring stability allow. Indwelling bladder catheters are discontinued within the first several days postoperatively, but one must reckon with a high incidence of at least temporary voiding dysfunction during early convalescence. This is most appropriately dealt with by a program of scheduled intermittent catheterizations. Fecal incontinence, if persistent, can generally be accommodated with a constipating diet and prompted evacuation by digital stimulation, enema, or oral laxatives as for spinal cord injury patients. Clinical observations indicate that functional urinary and fecal continence is generally achievable if at least one S3 nerve root can be preserved.[32] The objective of providing the patient with a genuine oncologic procedure however should not be compromised by the attempt to preserve continence. In males, the extensive dissection of the sympathetic and parasympathetic plexi will expectedly diminish erectile function and the capacity for antegrade ejaculation. Patients should be counseled preoperatively about the potential consequences of sacral resection for anogenital and reproductive function. Currently, many surgical and nonsurgical options exist to help address both the physical and psychological ramifications of these surgeries.

Somatic sensory and motor deficits that result from sacral resection are generally well compensated. If the S1 roots, lumbosacral trunks, and sciatic nerves can all be preserved, the disability in the legs is very minor. With sacrifice of the S1 roots there is a noticeable decrement in plantar flexion power, although this is accommodated by hypertrophy of the lateral gastrocnemius muscles with time. Loss of the L5 roots or injury to the lumbosacral trunks adds to this the further difficulty of foot drop, which may in part be counteracted through the use of anti-flexion orthoses. The glutei, which are the main physiologic extensors of the hips, are often greatly impaired after upper sacral resection as a result of detachment from their origin, denervation, or diminished blood supply. Loss of gluteal function becomes especially evident upon attempts to rise from a seated posture or ascend stairs. In time, increased hamstring and adductor magnus function may help compensate this loss. Sensory loss is rarely of a magnitude to impact protective sensibilities adversely or cause a sensory ataxia. Perineal hypesthesia is of course anticipated; the legs are affected to the degree that the lumbosacral trunk, the posterior femoral cutaneous nerve, and the S1 root are compromised. Generally, this is a lesser problem than are the concomitant motor deficits.

The main sources of surgical mortality in upper sacral resection are intraoperative blood loss and postoperative wound sepsis. This has generally ranged from 0% to 15% in various reports.[14,29,30,34,38] Wound complications, including prolonged drainage, delayed breakdown, infections, seromas, cerebrospinal fluid leaks, and pelvic prolapse were common in the past and have probably been underreported. Sung et al.[29] and Touran et al.[34] have acknowledged wound complication rates of 11% and 25%, respectively. Surgical results, with respect to survival and cure of disease, are difficult to summarize owing to the long natural history of many of the treated conditions, and the vagaries of reporting, operative technique, and follow-up. Furthermore, the reported series are generally small and were accrued over many years. Nonetheless, the overall experience with benign tumors seems to be highly encouraging.[1,9,26,29] The experience with chordoma, as expected, is less favorable, with recurrences reported in at least one-third to one-half of patients followed for more than 2 years. The disease-free survival seems to be enhanced when the goal of wide local excision can be realized.[5] Sundaresan et al. had no local recurrences over a 7-year period in a subgroup of patients with sacral chordoma in whom this objective was achieved.[28] In higher-grade malignancies, such as primary and recurrent rectal carcinomas, the results are less encouraging. Using judicious case selection, preoperative irradiation, and surgical techniques emphasizing en bloc resection, Temple and Ketcham[30] have reported a mean survival of 3 years and an 18% cure rate with complete 5-year follow-up in this very difficult group of patients. The sporadic reports of sacral resection for other high-grade malignancies such as osteogenic sarcoma, malignant schwannoma, and neurofibrosarcoma have generally indicated poor outcomes.

Summary

The tremendous advances in neuroimaging since the early 1980s have greatly simplified the diagnosis of sacral tumors. The majority of tumors arising in the sacral canal or in the distal bony sacrum have been well handled by conventional techniques. Tumors with more proximal involvement necessitating total sacrectomy pose the greatest management challenges. At times, past results have been compromised by an insufficient appreciation of the need for en bloc resection of malignant lesions with an inviolate margin of normal tissue. Otherwise, patients may be condemned to early recurrence or remote dissemination. At other times, surgical efforts have been diminished by suboptimal wound closure. As with cranial base surgery, the best results are achieved by drawing upon the expertise of a multidisciplinary surgical team. The collaborative input of oncologic and plastic surgeons may be of major assistance to the spine surgeon who undertakes a high or total sacral resection. In our experience the imperative for a tensionless wound closure with obliteration of dead space by viable, nonirradiated tissues has been best satisfied by the rectus abdominis pull-through flap. The issue of how best to reconstruct the lumbopelvic junction after total or near total sacrectomy is not yet answered. Current methods of pelvic stabilization, sacral replacement, and lumbopelvic fixation are technically daunting solutions to this problem. Sacrectomy for malignant disease remains a highly morbid undertaking with a significant chance for local failure. It is obvious that physical methods of tumor extirpation are relatively crude and that biologic barriers will only be overcome when these mechanical techniques can be mated to therapies directed to the molecular genetics of the neoplastic process itself.

REFERENCES

1. Abernathy C, Onofrio B, Scheithauer B, et al: Surgical management of giant sacral schwannomas. J Neurosurg 65:286-295, 1986.
2. Allen BL Jr, Ferguson RL: The Galveston technique for L-rod instrumentation of the scoliotic spine. Spine 7: 276-284, 1982.
3. Alper M, Bilkay U, Kececi Y, et al: Transsacral usage of a pure island TRAM flap for a large sacral defect: a case report. Ann Plast Surg 44:417-421, 2000.
4. Bergh P, Gunterberg B, Meis-Kindblom JM, Kindblom LG: Prognostic factors and outcome of pelvic, sacral, and spinal chondrosarcomas: a center-based study of 69 cases. Cancer 91:1201-1212, 2001.
5. Bergh P, Kindblom LG, Gunterberg B, et al: Prognostic factors in chordoma of the sacrum and mobile spine: a study of 39 patients. Cancer 88:2122-2134, 2000.
6. Bowers RF: Giant cell tumor of the sacrum. A case report. Ann Surg 1:1164-1172, 1948.
7. Cahill DW: Surgical approaches to the lumbar spine and sacrum. In GL Rea (ed): Spine Tumors. Rolling Meadows, IL, American Association of Neurological Surgeons, 1994, pp 89-103.
8. Cummings BJ, Hodson DI, Bush RS: Chordomata: the results of megavoltage radiation therapy. Int J Radiat Oncol Biol Phys 99:635-642, 1983.
9. Feldenzer JA, McGauley JL, McGillicuddy JE: Sacral and presacral tumors: problems in diagnosis and management. Neurosurgery 25:884-891, 1989.
10. Gokaslan ZL, Romsdahl MM, Kroll SS, et al: Total sacrectomy and Galveston L-rod reconstruction for malignant neoplasms. Technical note. J Neurosurg 87: 781-787, 1997.
11. Gunterberg B, Romanus B, Stener B: Pelvic strength after major amputation of the sacrum. Acta Orthop Scan 47:635-642, 1976.
12 Ishii K, Chiba K, Watanabe M, et al: Local recurrence after S2-3 sacrectomy in sacral chordoma. Report of four cases. J Neurosurg 97(1 Suppl):98-101, 2002.
13. Jackson RJ, Gokaslan ZL: Spinal-pelvic fixation in patients with lumbosacral neoplasms. J Neurosurg 92(1 Suppl): 61-70, 2000.
14. Localio SA, Eng K, Ranson JH: Abdominosacral approach for retrorectal tumors. Ann Surg 191:555-560, 1980.
15. MacCarty CS, Waugh JM, Mayo CW, Coventry MD: The surgical treatment of presacral tumors: a combined problem. Proc Staff Meet Mayo Clin 27:73-84, 1952.
16. Marcove RC, Sheth DS, Brien EW, et al: Conservative surgery for giant cell tumors of the sacrum. The role of cryosurgery as a supplement to curettage and partial excision. Cancer 74:1253-1260, 1994.
17. Miles WK, Chang DW, Kroll SS, et al: Reconstruction of large sacral defects following total sacrectomy. Plast Reconstr Surg 105:2387-2394, 2000.
18. Ozaki T, Liljenqvist U, Halm H, et al: Giant cell tumor of the spine. Clin Orthop 401:194-201, 2002.
19. Papagelopoulos PJ, Choudhury SN, Frassica FJ, et al: Treatment of aneurysmal bone cysts of the pelvis and sacrum. J Bone Joint Surg Am 83-A:1674-1681, 2001.
20. Raque GH Jr, Vitaz TW, Shields CB: Treatment of neoplastic diseases of the sacrum. J Surg Oncol 76:301-307, 2001.
21. Salehi SA, McCafferty RR, Karahalios D, Ondra SL: Neural function preservation and early mobilization after resection of metastatic sacral tumors and lumbosacropelvic junction reconstruction. J Neurosurg 97(1 Suppl):88-93, 2002.
22. Sar C, Eralp L : Surgical treatment of primary tumors of the sacrum. Arch Orthop Trauma Surg 122:148-155, 2002.
23. Shikata J, Yamamuro T, Kotoura Y, et al: Total sacrectomy and reconstruction for primary tumors. J Bone Joint Surg Am 70A:122-125, 1988.
24. Skene AI, Gault DT, Woodhouse CRJ, et al: Perineal, vulval and vaginoperineal reconstruction using the rectus abdominis myocutaneous flap. Br J Surg 77:635-637, 1990.
25. Stener B, Gunterberg B: High amputation of the sacrum for extirpation of tumors. Spine 3:351-366, 1978.
26. Stewart RJ, Humphreys WG, Parks TG: The presentation and management of presacral tumors. Br J Surg 73: 153-155, 1986.
27. Sugarbaker PH: Partial sacrectomy for en bloc excision of rectal cancer with posterior fixation. Dis Col Rect 25: 708-711, 1987.
28. Sundaresan N, Huvos AG, Krol G, et al: Surgical treatment of spinal chordomas. Arch Surg 122:1479-1482, 1987.
29. Sung HW, Shu WP, Wang HM, et al: Surgical treatment of primary tumors of the sacrum. Clin Orthop 215:91-98, 1987.
30. Temple WJ, Ketcham AS: Sacral resection for control of pelvic tumors. Am J Surg 163:370-374, 1992.
31. Tobin GR, Day TG: Vaginal and pelvic reconstruction with distally based rectus abdominis myocutaneous flaps. Plast Reconstr Surg 81:62-69, 1988.
32. Todd LT Jr, Yaszemski MJ, Currier BL, et al: Bowel and bladder function after major sacral resection. Clin Orthop 397:36-39, 2002.
33. Tomita K, Tsuchiya H: Total sacrectomy and reconstruction for huge sacral tumors. Spine 15:1223-1227, 1990.
34. Touran T, Frost DB, O'Connell TX: Sacral resection. Arch Surg 125:911-913, 1990.
35. Turcotte RE, Sim FH, Unni KK: Giant cell tumor of the sacrum. Clin Orthop 291:215-221, 1993.
36. Venkateswaran L, Rodriguez-Galindo C, Merchant TE, et al: Primary Ewing tumor of the vertebrae: clinical

characteristics, prognostic factors and outcome. *Med Pediatr Oncol* 37:30-35, 2001.

37. Weber KL, Nelson H, Gunderson LL, Sim FH: Sacropelvic resection for recurrent anorectal cancer. a multidisciplinary approach. *Clin Orthop* 372:231-240, 2000.

38. Wuisman P, Lieshout O, Sugihara S, van Dijk M: Total sacrectomy and reconstruction: oncologic and functional outcome. *Clin Orthop* 381:192-203, 2000.

CHAPTER 80

Tarlov Cysts

Jean-Marc Voyadzis and Fraser C. Henderson

Tarlov or perineurial cysts are lesions of the nerve root most often found in the sacral region. They were first discovered serendipitously by Tarlov in 1938 during his autopsy studies of the filum terminale at the Montreal Neurological Institute.[37] Since his seminal report, more than 100 cases of symptomatic Tarlov cysts have been published in the literature.[*] The advent of computed tomography (CT) and magnetic resonance imaging (MRI) has enhanced our ability to recognize them as a cause of sacral neurologic dysfunction.

The treatment of symptomatic Tarlov cysts remains a matter of debate. Various therapeutic strategies from the minimally invasive to complete surgical excision of cyst and root have been attempted with variable results.[†] Furthermore, many surgeons are reluctant to operate on sacral root cysts based on anecdotal evidence of treatment failures.[3,32] In this chapter the pathologic, radiologic, and clinical characteristics of Tarlov cysts are presented and the curative approaches to these lesions and their associated complications discussed.

Histopathologic Composition

Tarlov distinguished these cysts from other extradural meningeal lesions on the basis of several important findings.[33,34,37] First, the cyst forms between the endoneurium and perineurium generally at, or beyond the junction of the dorsal ganglion and the posterior nerve root and, most commonly, at S2 or S3. Second, the lining of these lesions contains nerve fibers and/or ganglion cells, which may surround the entire cavity. Third, the cysts are not in contact with the cerebrospinal fluid (CSF) of the subarachnoid space. Tarlov noted these cysts were often multiple, were extended around the circumference of the nerve, and could enlarge to impinge upon neighboring nerve roots and cause significant bony erosion. These characteristics clearly distinguished them from meningeal diverticula. Meningeal diverticula are proximal to the dorsal root ganglion, freely communicate with the subarachnoid space, and possess a lining composed of arachnoid membrane and dura mater devoid of neural tissue.

In the authors' series of 10 consecutive patients harboring symptomatic Tarlov cysts,[38] most, but not all of the specimens studied demonstrated neural tissue within the cyst wall. Others contained ganglion cells and two cysts were completely devoid of neural tissue. The variable histologic presentation of these cysts could represent different stages of evolution. Furthermore, meningeal lesions of the thecal sac from the meningeal diverticulum to the Tarlov cyst may represent a morphologic continuum of disease with a common origin.[9] In one report, a cyst of the lumbar nerve roots is described for which histologic findings are suggestive of both meningeal diverticula and Tarlov cysts.[4] Another presented a patient with multiple coexisting lesions.[16]

Origin of Tarlov Cysts

The pathogenesis of Tarlov cysts remains unclear. Tarlov[34,35,37] proposed that ischemic degeneration, inflammation, or hemorrhage either infiltrating from the subarachnoid space or of traumatic origin could lead to cyst formation. A number of patients harboring symptomatic Tarlov cysts in the literature have a history of trauma to the sacral area.[*] Half of the cases the authors studied had evidence of old hemorrhage in the form of hemosiderin deposits and two cases had foci of dystrophic calcification within the cyst wall suggestive of previous trauma.[38] Other authors suggested that Tarlov cysts form as a result of arachnoidal proliferation[20] or an obstruction of perineural lymphatic flow.[7] A developmental origin of Tarlov cysts is supported by Nabors et al.,[14] although the cysts have not been described in children[7,28,39] and an association between Tarlov cysts and spinal dysraphism is not well established. Only two patients with symptomatic Tarlov cysts and spina bifida have been reported.[15,38]

Struly et al.[28,29] and Smith[26] proposed that Tarlov cysts form as a result of increased CSF hydrostatic pressure. The following findings led to their hypothesis: First, cysts containing neural tissue and located at the junction of the nerve root and the dorsal root ganglion were also identified at the cervical, thoracic, and lumbar levels.[10,25,26,28,29] Second, the microscopic communication between the cysts and the subarachnoid space established myelographically suggests that CSF could flow along the nerve root and produce a dilatation within, due to either higher hydrostatic pressure, or inherent, traumatic or iatrogenic weakness in the nerve root sheath.[28] Third, the frequency and size of nerve root cysts along the spinal cord can be correlated with the rostral-caudal hydrostatic pressure gradient.[10,26,28] Several reports on patients with Tarlov cysts have documented either a history of straining or coughing or an exacerbation of symptoms by these maneuvers.[†] Authors of one recent study found that lumbar CSF drainage significantly alleviated symptoms in three of their patients with symptomatic cysts.[1]

Clinical Presentation

Tarlov[36] was the first to establish the clinical significance of these lesions when he documented a case in which removal of the cyst relieved sciatica. Since then, more than

[*]References 2,6,8,11,13-15,22,23,29,31,33,34,38-40.
[†]References 5,6,13,21,24,33,38,39.

[*]References 2,8,11,15,22,23,33,36,38.
[†]References 8,13,14,23,28,31,35,38.

100 cases have been reported describing a causal relationship between these cysts and signs and symptoms of nerve root compression.* The symptoms occasionally produced by these lesions are variable. Patients may complain of progressive pain in the lower back, sacrum, lower extremities, coccyx, rectum, vagina, or penis. They can also experience other sensory disturbances such as hypoesthesias or paresthesias over the buttocks, perineal area, and lower extremities. Motor weakness, bladder and bowel incontinence, impotence, and dyspareunia have also been documented.[38] Two patients in our series had symptoms contralateral to the origin of the cyst demonstrating that the mass effect of Tarlov cysts is sufficient to cause contralateral findings.[38] Tarlov cysts were also implicated as the underlying cause of bilateral adnexal[19] and presacral masses[12]; however, the free communication between these cysts and the thecal sac documented in both reports suggests that these lesions were probably meningeal diverticula, not Tarlov cysts. Most Tarlov cysts are asymptomatic, and discovered incidentally during myelography, CT, or MRI usually when the patient is in the fourth or fifth decade of life. Women appear to develop symptomatic Tarlov cysts more often than men.[5,13,15,28]

Diagnosis

Following Tarlov's initial report, authors of several studies[22,31] demonstrated that the cysts did eventually fill with

---

*References 2,6,8,11,13-15,22,23,29,31,33,34,38-40.

radiopaque dye on myelography, proving that there is a communication between the subperineurial space of the cyst and the subarachnoid space; however, it is not free enough to allow immediate visualization with oil myelography. With time, hours, days or weeks, the pulsatile pressure of the CSF gradually forces the contrast material into the subperineurial space.[33] This phenomenon of delayed myelographic filling is used to distinguish between Tarlov cysts and meningeal diverticula. Tarlov cysts may be observed to fill more readily with metrizamide myelography, a water-soluble contrast material with a lower viscosity than its oil-based counterpart.[15] MRI is now the gold standard for detecting extradural spinal masses[21] (Figures 80.1 and 80.2) although CT without contrast is still considered an excellent study. [8,24,30,40] To truly distinguish Tarlov cysts from other extradural meningeal lesions, a lumbo-sacral myelogram followed by immediate and delayed (1 hour) CT of the sacrum is required (Figure 80.3).

Treatment and Complications

There has been a great deal of controversy regarding the means of treatment of symptomatic Tarlov cysts and the efficacy thereof. Authors of one report of four patients with symptomatic Tarlov cysts found that percutaneous fibrin glue therapy was effective in alleviating symptoms, although three patients developed postprocedural aseptic meningitis.[17] The effectiveness of percutaneous drainage of Tarlov cysts was assessed in another study.[18] Four of the five

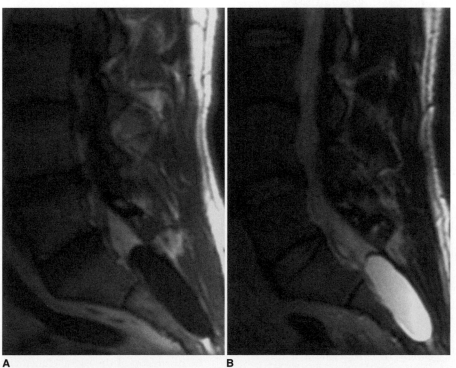

A   **B**

Figure 80.1 Imaging studies. **(A-B)** T_1- and T_2-weighted sagittal MRI of the sacrum demonstrating a 5 × 2 cm cystic lesion occupying the sacral canal at S2 with compression of both S2 nerve root sleeves and sacral erosion. (*From Voyadzis JM, Bhargava P, Henderson FC: Tarlov cysts: a study of 10 cases with review of the literature.* J Neurosurg 95:25-32, 2001.)

patients in that series suffered a recurrence of symptoms. In our experience, three patients preoperatively underwent percutaneous aspiration of their cysts; none improved.[38] In fact, one patient experienced marked worsening of her symptoms. This deterioration may have been the result of hemorrhage of the cyst wall, or nerve root injury.

Neurosurgical techniques include sacral laminectomy alone,[21,24] complete excision of cyst and root [14,33,39] or cyst fenestration and imbrication.[5,13] In a retrospective review of eight patients with symptomatic sacral cysts by Mummaneni et al.,[13] four of eight improved markedly

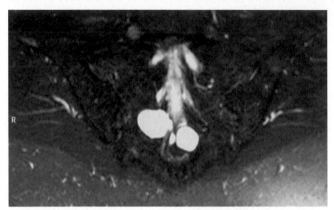

Figure 80.2 T_2-weighted coronal MRI of the sacrum demonstrating bilateral S3 Tarlov cysts.

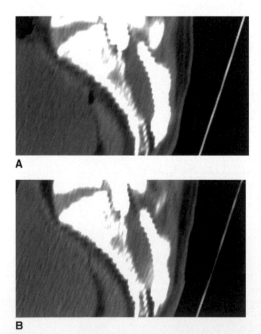

Figure 80.3 Imaging studies. (A) Immediate postmyelogram sagittal CT of the sacrum demonstrating the lesion with an intracystic density measurement of 20 Hounsfield units (HU). (B) Delayed (1 hour) postmyelogram CT demonstrating a significant increase in density within the cyst (75 to 137HU) consistent with delayed communication of the lesion with the thecal sac. (From Voyadzis JM, Bhargava P, Henderson FC: Tarlov cysts: a study of 10 cases with review of the literature. J Neurosurg 95:25-32, 2001.)

with regard to radicular pain following microsurgical cyst fenestration and imbrication with or without postoperative lumbar drainage with a mean follow-up of 19 months. Caspar et al.[5] recently reported excellent results from a series of 15 patients treated by cyst excision combined with duraplasty or cyst wall plication with a mean follow-up of 60 months. All patients underwent lumbar drainage and bed rest for 10 days postoperatively. It is unclear, however, whether all patients underwent a CT myelogram to distinguish Tarlov cysts from sacral meningoceles or diverticula. Both aforementioned studies reported no CSF leaks or new postoperative neurologic deficits. In our series of 10 cases, 7 patients reported significant improvement of pain and partial or complete resolution of neurologic deficits at an average follow-up of 17.6 months.[38] The authors found that patients with neurologic deficits that are anatomically related to Tarlov cysts greater than 1.5cm in diameter enjoyed substantial improvement following resection. Furthermore, there was a very strong correlation between the presence of radicular symptoms and excellent outcome. The recovery or improvement of bladder control after surgery in 3 of these patients with larger cysts was very gratifying. Those patients that did not experience substantial pain relief complained of nonradicular symptoms such as coccydynia, dyspareunia or proctalgia. There were no CSF leaks in our series postoperatively. One patient with a large cyst (2.5cm) developed overflow incontinence postoperatively. A second patient suffered from urinary incontinence and numbness in the left inner buttock that subsequently resolved. This was due to excessive traction on the sacral roots during resection.

Illustrative Case

History. A 46-year-old man presented with an 8-month history of increasing sacral, left buttock, and left posterior thigh and leg pain. His pain was a 6 out of 10 by visual analog scale (VAS), worsened by standing and walking, and relieved by sitting.

Examination. There was no tenderness to palpation or percussion of the lumbar and sacral spine. Strength and tone were normal. Deep tendon reflexes were 2+ and symmetric. Sensation to light touch, pinprick, proprioception, and vibration were intact. Sphincter tone was normal.

Radiologic Findings. MRI demonstrated a 5 × 2cm cystic mass occupying the sacral canal with bony erosion and compression of sacral nerve roots (see Figure 80.1). CT scan with immediate and delayed (1 hour) myelography demonstrated delayed contrast enhancement of the intraspinal cyst (see Figure 80.3).

Operation. Sacral laminectomy and dissection: the cyst originating from the right S2 nerve root was compressing both S2 nerve root sleeves and causing bony erosion of the sacral canal. The Tarlov cyst was then resected and the neck ligated (Figure 80.4).

Histologic Findings. A cyst wall of relatively uniform thickness composed of dense collagen bundles with sparse cellularity along with some loose areolar tissue was observed. No ganglion cells or nerve bundles were identified (Figure 80.5).

Postoperative Course. Postoperative hospital stay was uneventful. He noted substantial pain relief on the left posterior thigh and leg in the immediate postoperative period. He was discharged on postoperative day 3. At 22 months follow-up, he no longer had any pain: 0/10 by VAS.

Surgical Technique

An incision is made from L5 to S3, and the involved sacral laminae are entirely exposed. The laminectomy is performed with a Kerrison rongeur, care being taken to preserve the integrity of the Tarlov cyst, which frequently erodes the overlying bone. The terminal thecal sac is identified, and then dissected free from the overlying cyst or cysts. Each Tarlov cyst is dissected from surrounding structures to reveal its origin in the dorsal root ganglion of the respective sacral root (Figure 80.6A). The smaller cysts are easily dissected; the larger cysts appear initially to be fused to the surrounding structures. With patience, however, the cyst wall is dissected away from adjoining root sleeves and sacrum with which the diaphanous cyst closely approximates. A small neck is demonstrated in some cases; in others, a neck to the cyst is not identified. In a meningeal diverticulum, the small neck fills and drains directly from and into the thecal sac. Compressing a meningeal diverticulum results in collapse of the mass; a Valsalva maneuver immediately causes the sac to fill with spinal fluid. The Tarlov cyst on the other hand will burst if compressed and not refill. After the neck of the Tarlov cyst has been developed down to the ganglion, a clip is placed across the neck, and the cyst is cut distal to the clip. If the neck to the cyst is not identified, then the cyst wall is resected down to the ganglion (Figure 80.6B). Care is taken to avoid large neural elements that lie along the *ventral* aspect of the cyst wall. Several 6-0 Prolene stitches are placed to imbricate the remaining root sleeve (Figure 80.6C). A Valsalva maneuver is performed to ensure that there is no leakage of spinal fluid. Gelfoam and fibrin glue are placed over the cut neck or cyst origin along the root. The wound is closed in watertight layers. In our experience, 3 days of bedrest and acetazolamide without lumbar drainage have been sufficient to prevent pseudomeningocele and delayed leakage of spinal fluid.

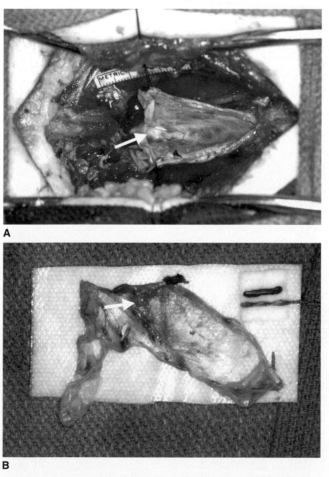

Figure 80.4 Intraoperative photographs. **(A)** *Left:* rostral; *Right:* caudal. The Tarlov cyst has been dissected and the neck *(arrow)* developed down to reveal its origin at the dorsal root ganglion. **(B)** The resected Tarlov cyst. *(From Voyadzis JM, Bhargava P, Henderson FC: Tarlov cysts: a study of 10 cases with review of the literature.* J Neurosurg 95:25-32, 2001.*)*

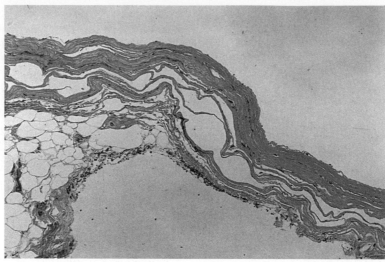

Figure 80.5 Dense collagenous bundles along with loose vascularized fibrofatty tissue *(lower left)* (H&E, ×120). *(From Voyadzis JM, Bhargava P, Henderson FC: Tarlov cysts: a study of 10 cases with review of the literature.* J Neurosurg 95:25-32, 2001.)

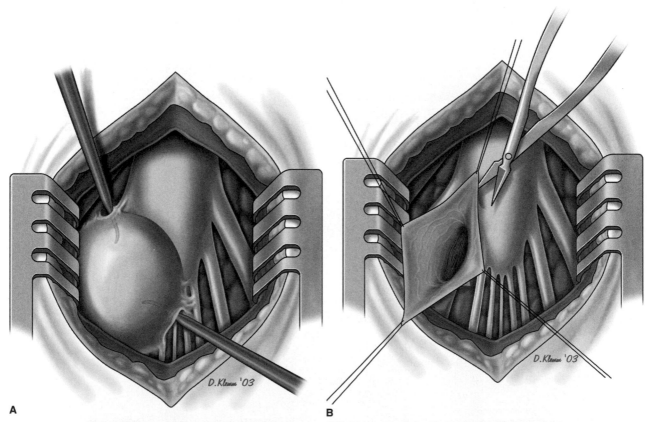

A   **B**

Figure 80.6 Drawings of a left sacral Tarlov cyst. (**A**) Exposure of the Tarlov cyst following sacral laminectomy. (**B**) Resection of the cyst wall containing wispy nerve fibers and preservation of underlying root fibers.

Summary

Tarlov cysts should be recognized as an important clinical entity in the differential diagnosis of sacral radiculopathy and sacral pain syndromes, particularly in women. The advent of CT and MRI has enhanced our ability to detect these lesions. Diagnosis is made by MRI followed by CT with immediate and delayed myelography. Elevated CSF pressure and trauma may play a role in their pathogenesis.

The management of symptomatic Tarlov cysts continues to be a matter of debate. Several retrospective reviews have demonstrated that symptomatic relief can be achieved with microsurgical excision and cyst imbrication with or without postoperative lumbar drainage in carefully

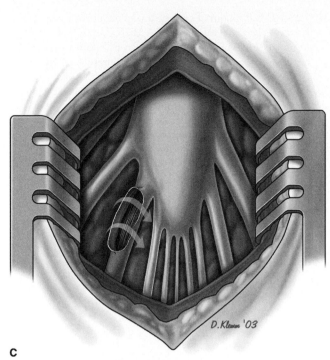

C

Figure 80.6 *cont'd* **(C)** Imbrication of remnant of the perineurial sleeve over root fibers.

selected cases. Patients with large cysts (>1.5cm), radicular symptoms, and urinary incontinence have enjoyed substantial relief from surgery.

REFERENCES

1. Bartels RH, van Overbeeke JJ: Lumbar cerebrospinal fluid drainage for symptomatic sacral nerve root cysts: an adjuvant diagnostic procedure and/or alternative treatment? Technical case report. *Neurosurgery* 40: 861-864, 1997.
2. Basauri L, Hudson H, Bardales A: Case reports and technical notes: diverticuli of the nerve root sheaths. *J Neurosurg* 31:680-682, 1969.
3. Benzel E: Microsurgical treatment of symptomatic sacral Tarlov cysts (comment). *Neurosurgery* 47:78, 2000 (comment).
4. Bucci MN, McGillicuddy JE: Spinal extradural meningeal cysts that contain nerve fibers: case report. *Neurosurg* 21:411-413, 1987.
5. Caspar W, Papavero L, Nabhan A, *et al:* Microsurgical excision of symptomatic sacral perineurial cysts: a study of 15 cases. *Surg Neurol* 59:101-106, 2003.
6. Davis DH, Wilkinson JT, Teaford AK, Smigiel MR: Sciatica produced by a sacral perineurial cyst. *Texas Medicine* 83: 55-56, 1987.
7. Dickenman RC, Chason JL: Cysts of dorsal root ganglia, report of 29 cysts and review of the literature. *Arch Pathol* 77:366-369, 1964.
8. Foreman SM, Centeno R, Kerber CW: Diagnosis of perineurial arachnoid cysts using computed tomography: technical and clinical considerations. *J Manipulative Physiol Ther US* 9(1):23-26, 1986.
9. Fortuna A, La Torre E, Ciapetta P: Arachnoid diverticula: a unitary approach to spinal cysts communicating with the subarachnoid space. *Acta Neurochir* 39:259-268, 1977.
10. Holt S, Yates PO: Cervical nerve roots "cysts." *Brain* 87:481-490, 1964.
11. Kageyama Y, Machida A, Okada M, *et al:* Sacral perineurial cyst with ossification of the arachnoid membrane. *Rev Rhum* 65(2):153-156, 1998.
12. Maleci A, Bianco F, Onnis G, Di Lorenzo N: Iatrogenic spinopelvic cerebro-spinal fluid fistula: case report. *J Neurosurg Sci Ital* 39:261-263, 1995.
13. Mummanemi PV, Pitts LH, McCormack BM, *et al:* Microsurgical treatment of symptomatic Tarlov cysts. *Neurosurgery* 47:74-78, 2000.
14. Nabors NW, Pait TG, Byrd EB, *et al:* Updated assessment and current classification of spinal meningeal cysts. *J Neurosurg* 68:366-377, 1988.
15. Nishiura I, Koyama T, Handa J: Intrasacral perineurial cyst. *Surg Neurol* 23:265-269, 1985.
16. North RB, Kidd DH, Wang H: Occult, bilateral anterior sacral and intrasacral meningeal and perineurial cysts: case report and review of the literature. *Neurosurgery* 27: 981-986, 1990.
17. Patel MR, Louie W, Rachlin J: Percutaneous fibrin glue therapy of meningeal cysts of the sacral spine. *AJR Am J Roentgenol* 168:367-370, 1997.
18. Paulsen RD, Call GA, Murtagh FR: Prevalence and percutaneous drainage of cysts of the sacral nerve root sheath (Tarlov cysts). *AJNR Am J Neuroradiol* 15:293-297, 1994.
19. Raza S, Klapholz H, Benacerraf BR: Tarlov cysts: a cause of bilateral adnexal masses on pelvic sonography. *J Ultrasound Med* 13:803-805, 1994.
20. Rexed BA, Wennstrom KG: Arachnoidal proliferation and cystic formation in the spinal nerve-root pouches of man. *J Neurosurg* 16:73-84, 1959.
21. Rodziewics GS, Kaufman B, Spetzler RF: Diagnosis of sacral perineurial cysts by nuclear magnetic resonance. *Surg Neurol* 22:50-52, 1984.
22. Schreiber F, Haddad B: Lumbar and sacral cysts causing pain. *J Neurosurg* 8:504-509, 1951.
23. Seaman WB, Furlow LT: The myelographic appearance of sacral cysts. *J Neurosurg* 13:88-94, 1956.
24. Siqueira EB, Schaffer L, Kranzler LI, Gan J: CT characteristics of sacral perineural cysts: report of two cases. *J Neurosurg* 61:596-598, 1984.
25. Smith DT: Multiple meningeal diverticula (perineurial cysts) of the cervical region disclosed by pantopaque myelography: report of a case. *J Neurosurg* 19:599-601, 1962.
26. Smith DT: Cystic formations associated with human spinal nerve roots. *J Neurosurg* 18:654-660, 1961.
27. Stella L, Gambardella A, Maiuri F: Giant sacral perineurial cyst. *Clin Neurol Neurosurg* 91:343-346, 1989.
28. Strully K: Meningeal diverticula of sacral nerve roots (perineurial cysts). *JAMA* 161:1147-1152, 1956.
29. Strully K, Heiser S: Lumbar and sacral cysts of meningeal origin. *Radiology* 62:544-549, 1954.
30. Tabas J, Deeb Z: Diagnosis of sacral perineurial cysts by computed tomography. *J Comput Tomogr* 10:255-259, 1986.
31. Taheri ZE, Riemenschneider P, Ecker A: Case reports and technical notes: Myelographic diagnosis of sacral perineurial cyst. *J Neurosurg* 9:93-95, 1952.

32. Tarlov E: Occult, bilateral anterior sacral and intrasacral meningeal and perineurial cysts: case report and review of the literature. *Neurosurgery* 27:986, 1990 (comment).

33. Tarlov IM: Spinal perineurial and meningeal cysts. *J Neurol Neurosurg Psychiatry* 33:833-843, 1970.

34. Tarlov IM: *Sacral Nerve-Root Cysts: Another Cause of the Sciatic or Cauda Equina Syndrome.* Springfield, IL, Charles C. Thomas, 1953, pp 56-116.

35. Tarlov IM: Cyst of the sacral nerve roots: clinical significance and pathogenesis. *Arch Neurol Psychiatry* 68:94-108, 1952.

36. Tarlov IM: Cysts (perineurial) of the sacral roots: another cause (removable) of sciatic pain. *JAMA* 138:740-744, 1948.

37. Tarlov IM: Perineurial cysts of the spinal nerve roots. *Arch Neurol Psychiatry* 40:1067-1074, 1938.

38. Voyadzis JM, Bhargava P, Henderson FC: Tarlov cysts: a study of 10 cases with review of the literature. *J Neurosurg* 95:25-32, 2001.

39. Wilkins RH: Intraspinal cysts. In Wilkins RH, Rengachary SS (eds): *Neurosurgery.* New York, McGraw-Hill, 1996, pp 2061-2070.

40. Willinsky RA, Fazl M: Computed tomography of a sacral perineural cyst. *J Comput Assist Tomogr* 9:599-601, 1985.

Index

Note: Page numbers followed by the letter b refer to boxes; those followed by the letter f refer to figures, those followed by the letter t refer to tables.

A

ABC™ Plating System, 27, 1432
ABCs. *See* Aneurysmal bone cysts
Abdominal aorta, branches of, 302f
Abscess
  epidural. *See* Epidural abscess
  retropharyngeal, spinal surgery and, 235
Abulcasis, 2
Accessory atlantoaxial, atlanto-occipital joint,
    265f
Accessory nerve, 270f
ACD. *See* Anterior cervical discectomy
ACDF. *See* Anterior cervical discectomy and
    fusion
Acquired immunodeficiency syndrome (AIDS),
    Cryptococcus and, 39
Actinomyces, 38
Actinomyces israelii, 2021
Actinomycosis
  causes of, 38
  management of, 38
  signs of, 38
  symptoms of, 38
Acupuncture, low back pain and, 1957
Acute transverse myelitis autoimmune
    (ATMA), 52
Acute transverse myelitis necrotizing (ATMN),
    52
ADI. *See* Atlantodens interval
Adolescent idiopathic scoliosis (AIS), 874
  bracing for, 831, 833b
  classification of, 825–826
  clinical features of, 826–827, 829f, 830f, 831f
  early-onset (age younger than 8 years)
    clinical features of, 832, 833f
    crankshaft phenomenon, 834
    surgical approach to, 834, 835f, 836f
    treatment of, 833–834
  epidemiology of, 825–826
  instrumentation for
    dorsal, 834–837, 844f, 845f, 846–847f,
      848f, 849f, 850f, 851f
    ventral, 836f, 837–839, 852f
  pelvic fixation for, 839, 850f, 852f
  radiographic assessment of, 827–831, 832f,
    833f
  surgical treatment of, 834, 837–839f,
    840–843f
  thoracoplasty and, 839–841, 853b
    expansion, 841
Adrenomyeloneuropathy (AMN), 53
Adson approach (dorsal transsacral approach),
    anterior sacral meningocele and,
    1162
Adult discitis, 37
Advanced trauma life support (ATLS), 1227
Aerobic activity, for back/neck pain, 1955, 1958
Agenesis, sacral, 79–80, 79f
AIDS. *See* Acquired immunodeficiency
    syndrome
Air embolism, spine surgery and, 234

AIS. *See* Adolescent idiopathic scoliosis
Alar ligament
  atlanto-occipital joint, 265f
  right, 278f
Albee, Fred, 11, 11f
ALIF. *See* Anterior lumbar interbody fusion
A-line™ Cervical Plating System, 27
Alkaline phosphate (ALP), metastatic disease
    and, 40
Allografts, 169–170
  bone graft harvesting and, 1253
  cons of, 194–195
  pros of, 194
ALP. *See* Alkaline phosphate
ALS. *See* Amyotrophic lateral sclerosis
AMN. *See* Adrenomyeloneuropathy
Amphotericin-B, 39
Amyotrophic lateral sclerosis (ALS), 53, 54
Androgens, spinal fusion and, 173
Anesthesia
  airway management and
    cervical spine injury and, 1831, 1831f
    extubation, 1831
    intubation difficulty, 1829, 1830f
    laryngeal mask airway, 1831
    preoperative evaluation, 1829
    rheumatoid arthritis and, 1831
  crisis
    air embolism, 2194, 2196
    prone cardiopulmonary arrest, 2194,
      2195f, 2196f
  fluid/blood therapy
    blood loss/replacement, 1833–1834
    induced hypotension, 1834
    pharmacologic aids, 1834
  monitoring
    general, 1825–1826
    neurophysiologic
      in awake patient, 1826
      motor evoked potentials, 1828
      nonparalytic anesthesia/intraoperative
        monitoring, 1827
      somatosensory spinal evoked potentials,
        1827–1828, 1828t
      wake-up test, 1826–1827
  pharmacology
    ideal agent, 1824
    induction, 1824
    inhalation agents, 1824–1825
    Ketamine, 1824
    muscle relaxants, 1825
    narcotics, 1825
    Propofol, 1824
  positioning
    peripheral nerve injury and, 1832
    postoperative visual loss, 1832, 1832f,
      1833f
    sitting, 1832–1833
    spinal cord infarction, 1833
  preoperative assessment of
    laboratory studies, 1823

Anesthesia *(Continued)*
    rheumatoid arthritis considerations and,
      1823
    scoliosis considerations and, 1823
    spinal cord injury considerations and,
      1823
  techniques
    general anesthesia, 1829
    regional analgesia, 1828–1829
    regional anesthesia, 1828
Aneurysmal bone cysts (ABCs), 42–43, 43f
  histology of, 996
  imaging of, 996, 997f
  management of, 996
Ankylosing spondylitis (AS), 45, 93–94, 404
  cauda equina syndrome and, 986–987
  clinical manifestations of, 704–705
  clinical presentation of, 931
  fractures and, 935
  management of, 45
  pathogenesis of, 703
  pathology of, 703, 704f, 705f
  patient population with, 45
  radiologic features of, 705
  signs of, 45
  spinal deformity and, 712, 714
    correction of, 714, 714f
    lumbar osteotomy
      cervical, 720
      complications of, 719–720
      historical aspects of, 716–718, 718f, 719f
      results of, 719–720
      surgical technique, 718–719, 720–722f
      types of, 716–718, 718f, 719f
    preoperative planning of, 714–716, 714f,
      715f, 716–717f
  spinal fractures and, 706–712, 706f,
    707–712f
    cervical, 707–711
    lumbar, 711–712, 712–713f
    thoracic, 711–712, 712–713f
    upper cervical, 711
  spondylodiscitis and, 723–724, 724–725f,
    935
  surgical conditions involving spine, 706
  surgical management of, 931–935
    cervical osteotomy, 934, 934f
    complication in, 934–935
    general principles in, 931–933, 932f
    lumbar osteotomy, 933–934, 933f
    thoracic osteotomy, 934
  symptoms of, 45
Annular degeneration. *See* Black disc disease
Annulus fibrosus, 279f
Anomalous nerve root, anatomy of, 132, 132f
Anterior arch, atlanto-occipital joint, 264
Anterior atlanto-occipital membrane, 278f
Anterior caudal nerve, 304f
Anterior cervical discectomy (ACD). *See*
    Anterior cervical discectomy and
    fusion